THIRD EDITION

DIAGNOSTIC PATHOLOGY
MOLECULAR ONCOLOGY

VASEF • AUERBACH

BOCKLAGE • CHABOT-RICHARDS • AGUILERA • KARNER • LOO • KLETECKA

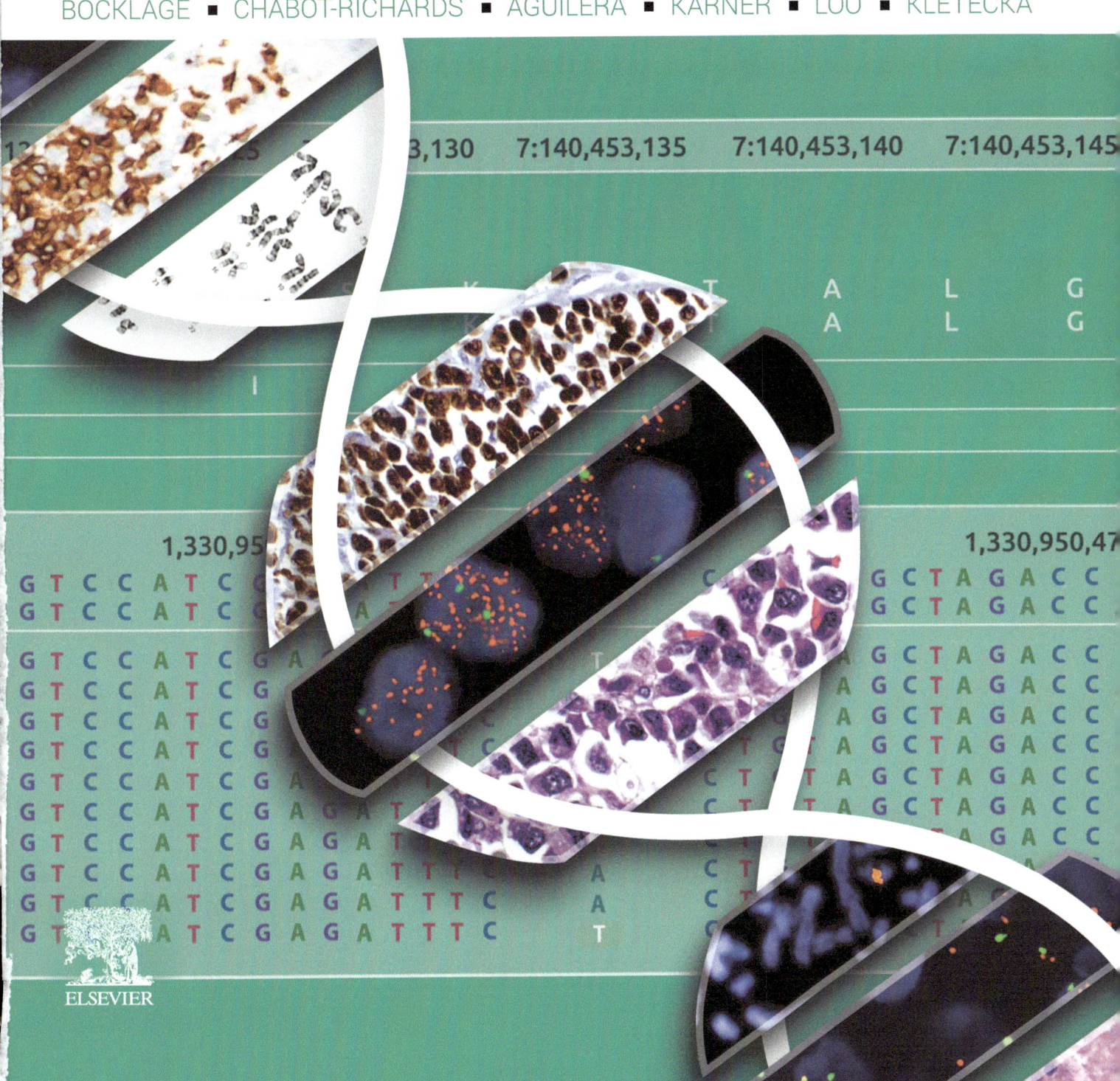

ELSEVIER

DIAGNOSTIC PATHOLOGY
MOLECULAR ONCOLOGY

THIRD EDITION

Mohammad A. Vasef, MD
Professor
Department of Pathology
Director of MGP Fellowship Program
Medical Director of Molecular Diagnostics
The University of New Mexico Health Sciences Center
TriCore Reference Laboratories
Albuquerque, New Mexico

Aaron Auerbach, MD, MPH
Director of Medical Education
Senior Hematopathologist
Joint Pathology Center
Silver Spring, Maryland

Thèrése Bocklage, MD
Professor and Director of Anatomic Pathology
Department of Pathology and Laboratory Medicine
Director, Biospecimen Procurement and
Translational Pathology Shared Resource Facility of
the Markey Cancer Center
University of Kentucky College of
Medicine and UK Healthcare
Lexington, Kentucky

Devon Chabot-Richards, MD
Associate Professor
Department of Pathology
The University of New Mexico Health Sciences Center
Medical Director of Molecular Oncology Laboratory
TriCore Reference Laboratories
Albuquerque, New Mexico

Nadine Aguilera, MD
Professor
Department of Pathology
Section Head of Hematopathology
University of Virginia Health System
Charlottesville, Virginia

Kristin Hunt Karner, MD
Associate Professor
Department of Pathology
University of Utah Health Sciences Center
Medical Director, Hematopathology
ARUP Laboratories
Salt Lake City, Utah

Eric Y. Loo, MD
Associate Professor
Department of Pathology & Laboratory Medicine
Dartmouth Health
Lebanon, New Hampshire

M. Carmen Frias Kletecka, MD
Medical Director, Molecular Diagnostics Laboratory
Pathology & Laboratory Medicine Service
West Los Angeles VA Medical Center
US Department of Veterans Affairs
Los Angeles, California

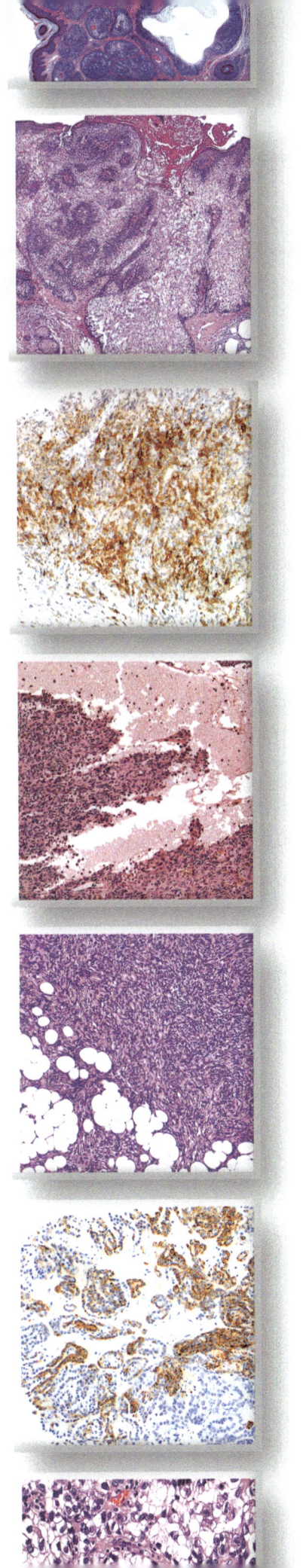

Elsevier
1600 John F. Kennedy Blvd.
Ste 1800
Philadelphia, PA 19103-2899

DIAGNOSTIC PATHOLOGY: MOLECULAR ONCOLOGY, THIRD EDITION

ISBN: 978-0-443-11220-1

Copyright © 2024 by Elsevier. All rights reserved.

No part of this publication may be reproduced or transmitted in any form or by any means, electronic or mechanical, including photocopying, recording, or any information storage and retrieval system, without permission in writing from the publisher. Details on how to seek permission, further information about the Publisher's permissions policies and our arrangements with organizations such as the Copyright Clearance Center and the Copyright Licensing Agency, can be found at our website: www.elsevier.com/permissions.

This book and the individual contributions contained in it are protected under copyright by the Publisher (other than as may be noted herein).

Notices

Practitioners and researchers must always rely on their own experience and knowledge in evaluating and using any information, methods, compounds or experiments described herein. Because of rapid advances in the medical sciences, in particular, independent verification of diagnoses and drug dosages should be made. To the fullest extent of the law, no responsibility is assumed by Elsevier, authors, editors or contributors for any injury and/or damage to persons or property as a matter of products liability, negligence or otherwise, or from any use or operation of any methods, products, instructions, or ideas contained in the material herein.

Previous edition copyrighted 2020.

Library of Congress Control Number: 2023946498

The identification of specific products or scientific instrumentation is considered an integral part of the scientific endeavor and does not constitute an endorsement or implied endorsement on the part of the author(s), DoD, or any component agency. The views expressed in this book are those of the author(s) and do not necessarily reflect the official policy of the Department of Defense or the U.S. Government.

Printed in the United States of America

Last digit is the print number: 9 8 7 6 5 4 3 2

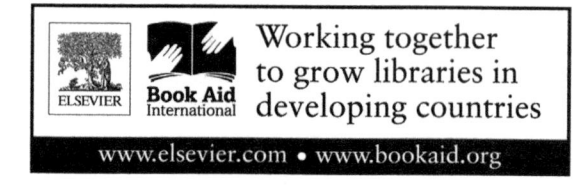

ELSEVIER | Book Aid International — Working together to grow libraries in developing countries
www.elsevier.com • www.bookaid.org

DEDICATIONS

To my mother, Shamsi, and my father, Rahim, for their inspiration.

To my dear wife, Fatemeh, and our wonderful children, Yashar and Idean.

To my sisters, Najeebeh and Soudabeh.

Special thanks to Aaron Auerbach for his amazing partnership and contributions,
to my colleagues in the Department of Pathology at the University of New Mexico Health
Sciences Center, and to the Molecular Diagnostics team at TriCore Reference Laboratories,
and in honor of Jim Gale and Tom Williams.

Thanks,

MAV

Much love to my shining stars, Suzanne, Zachary, and Ben,
for their support with all of my endeavors.

Mi familia, Ann Auerbach, Don Auerbach, Shayna Auerbach,
Jahna Auerbach, Laurie Freed, and Hal Freed, gracias por su apoyo.

As always, thank you to Mohammad Vasef as a great collaborator and pathologist.

Thank you to my Joint Pathology Center colleagues,
especially Joel Moncur, Tom Baker, Alejandro Luina Contreras, Justin Wells, and John Schmieg
for their support of my academic efforts.

Friendship is the spice of life, and thank you to Aaron Levine, Rebecca Levine,
Jake Levine, and Mara Levine for all the adventures.

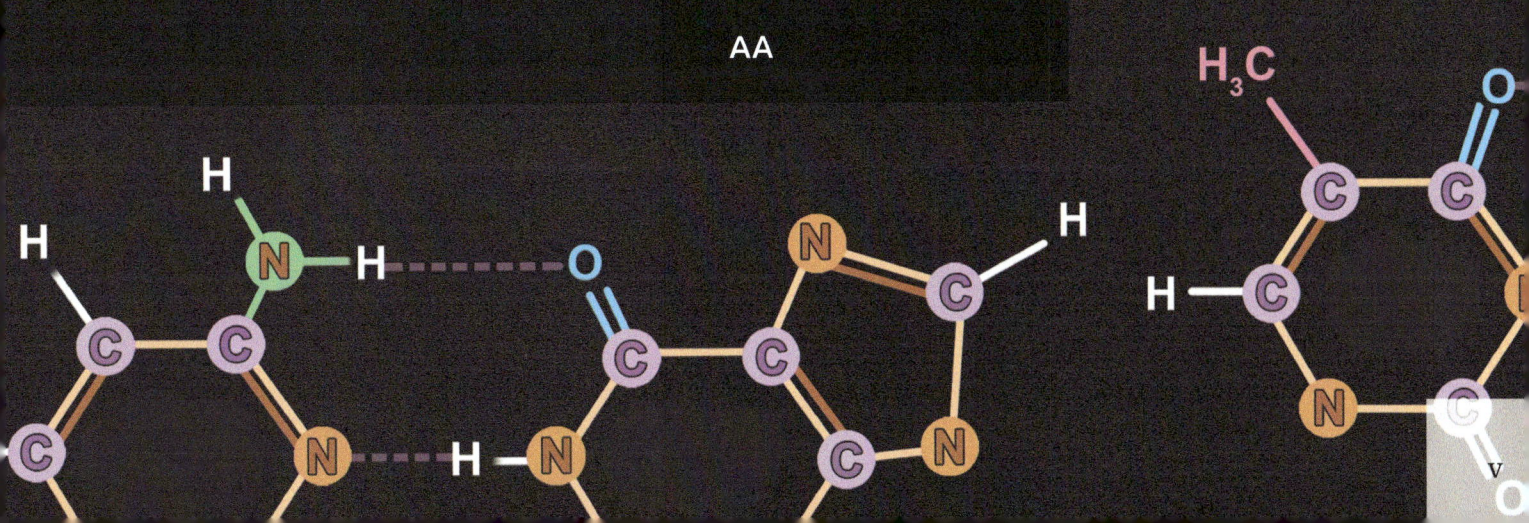

AA

CONTRIBUTING AUTHORS

Rania Bakkar, MD
Associate Professor
Department of Pathology
City of Hope National Cancer Center
Duarte, California

Marc Barry, MD
Associate Professor
Department of Pathology
University of Utah Health Sciences Center
Huntsman Cancer Institute
Salt Lake City, Utah

David Cassarino, MD, PhD
Consultant Dermatopathologist and Staff Pathologist
Southern California Permanente Medical Group
Los Angeles Medical Center
Los Angeles, California

Joanna L. Conant, MD
Assistant Professor
Department of Pathology and Laboratory Medicine
Robert Larner, M.D. College of Medicine
at the University of Vermont
University of Vermont Health Network
Burlington, Vermont

Edgar Fischer, MD, PhD
Professor
Department of Pathology
The University of New Mexico Health Sciences Center
Albuquerque, New Mexico

Michael M. Franklin, DO
Hematopathology Fellow
The University of New Mexico Health Sciences Center
Albuquerque, New Mexico

Rama Gullapalli, MD, PhD
Assistant Professor
Department of Pathology
Department of Chemical and Biological Engineering
The University of New Mexico Health Sciences Center
Albuquerque, New Mexico

David G. Hicks, MD
Professor and Director of IHC-ISH Laboratory and Breast
Subspecialty Service
University of Rochester Medical Center
Rochester, New York

Giovanni Insuasti-Beltran, MD
Associate Professor of Pathology
Medical Director, Molecular Oncology
and Flow Cytometry Laboratories
Director, Hematopathology Fellowship
Wake Forest University – Atrium
Health Wake Forest Baptist
Winston-Salem, North Carolina

Nancy Joste, MD
Professor
Department of Pathology
The University of New Mexico Health Sciences Center
Albuquerque, New Mexico

Lesley Lomo, MD
Associate Professor
Department of Pathology
University of Utah Health Sciences Center
Huntsman Cancer Institute
Salt Lake City, Utah

Amer Mahmoud, MD, FCAP
Hematopathology and Molecular Genetic Pathology
Pathology Associates of Albuquerque
Presbyterian Hospital
Clinical Assistant Professor
Department of Pathology
The University of New Mexico Health Sciences Center
Albuquerque, New Mexico

Elisabeth Rushing, MD
Medica Laboratories
Zurich, Switzerland
Cantonal Hospital of Lucerne
Lucerne, Switzerland

Von Samedi, MD, PhD
Professor of Pathology
Director, Head & Neck Pathology
Director, Residency Program
University of Colorado School of Medicine
Aurora, Colorado

John Schmieg, MD, PhD
Staff Hematopathologist
Staff Molecular Pathologist
The Joint Pathology Center
Silver Spring, Maryland

Khalil Sheibani, MD, FCAP
Pathologist
Department of Pathology
Orange County Global Medical Center
Santa Ana, California

Jeremy C. Wallentine, MD
Staff Pathologist
Intermountain Health and Utah Pathology Services, Inc.
Intermountain Medical Center
Salt Lake City, Utah

Guanghua Wang, MD
Director of Molecular Diagnostics Laboratories
Senior Staff Pathologist in Molecular Pathology
and GI/Hepatic Pathology
The Joint Pathology Center
Silver Spring, Maryland

Yongjie Zhou, MD, PhD
Office of Therapeutic Products
Center for Biologics Evaluation and Research
US Food and Drug Administration
Silver Spring, Maryland

ADDITIONAL CONTRIBUTORS

Daniel Babu, MD
Carlos Bueso-Ramos, MD, PhD
David R. Czuchlewski, MD
Kathryn Foucar, MD
Joshua Anspach Hanson, MD
Sibel Kantarci, PhD
Susan C. Lester, MD, PhD
David R. Lucas, MD
Anna P. Matynia, MD
L. Jeffrey Medeiros, MD
Roberto N. Miranda, MD
Kaaren K. Reichard, MD
Samuel Reynolds, MD
Fausto J. Rodríguez, MD
Karen SantaCruz, MD
Sa A. Wang, MD
Carla S. Wilson, MD, PhD
C. Cameron Yin, MD, PhD
Qian-Yun Zhang, MD, PhD

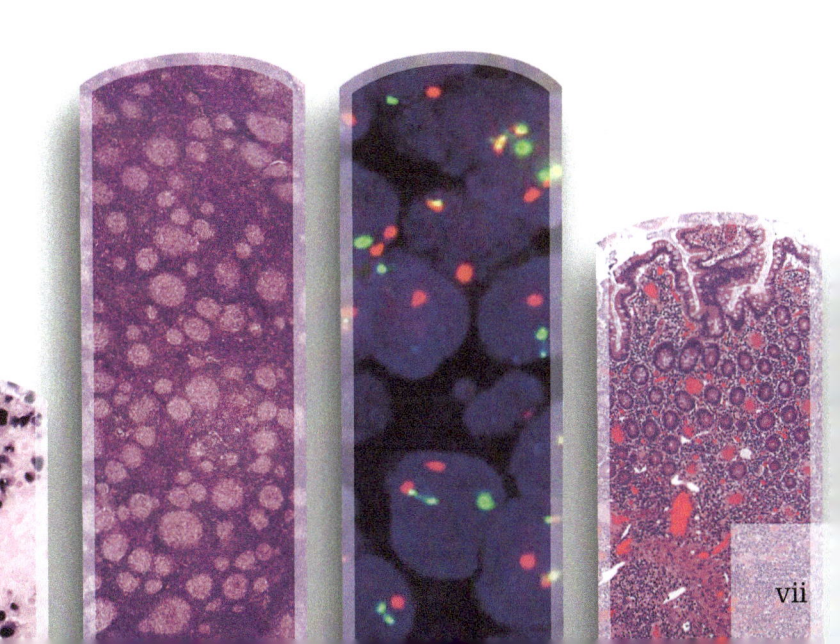

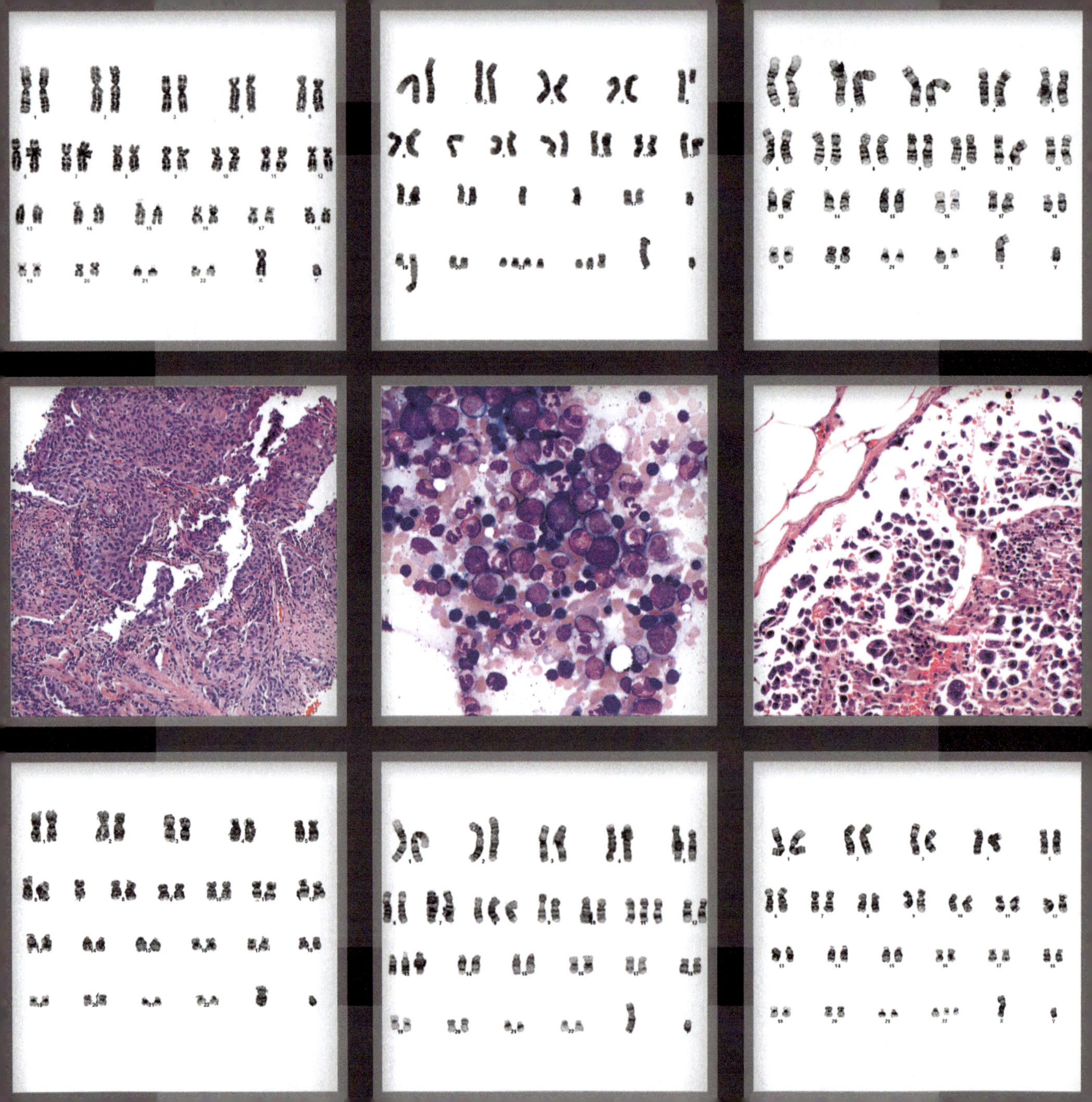

PREFACE

Molecular oncologic pathology is one of the most dynamic fields of medicine and has become an integral part of the field of pathology in particular. Introduction of next-generation sequencing has resulted in the discovery of many clinically actionable somatic mutations in solid tumors and in hematologic malignancies. These discoveries have refined our understanding of molecular pathogenesis of human diseases in general and have led to the discovery of many new molecular targeted therapies, particularly in human cancers. Several of the recently discovered molecular genetic findings have already become critical for the diagnosis of distinct disease entities and are key to personalized medicine. In oncologic pathology, these advancements have dramatically changed the role of the pure morphologic and immunophenotypic-based pathologist to that of a consultant who incorporates molecular genetic results into the pathology report and comprehensively interprets molecular data by creating an integrated report, including the most clinically useful data in the diagnostic line and references to FDA-approved or off-label targeted therapies.

The field of molecular pathology has evolved since the publication of the 2nd edition of *Diagnostic Pathology: Molecular Oncology* in 2020. The aim of the authors in this 3rd edition is to provide the readers with the most updated and current diagnostic resource for both hematopoietic and solid neoplasms. In addition to extensive updates, several new chapters have been added to the 3rd edition of the book, including Clonal Hematopoiesis and Premalignant Clonal Cytopenia and VEXAS Syndrome. The molecular knowledge regarding solid tumors has greatly expanded since the prior edition of this text. Now, nearly every tumor, regardless of rarity, has been analyzed to look for gene alterations that can help us understand the pathogenesis, diagnosis, or treatment of the solid tumor.

The readers may be well aware of new classification proposals, particularly in hematopoietic and CNS tumors. To address preferences of practicing pathologists and oncologists, both the 5th edition of the *WHO Classification of Haematolymphoid Tumours* and the 2022 *International Consensus Classification* (ICC) proposals are applied in all relevant chapters.

This book is intended to keep up with the rapidly evolving practice of pathology in an era of personalized medicine. The 3rd edition of *Diagnostic Pathology: Molecular Oncology* is a detailed, richly illustrated reference covering molecular tests and their clinical applications, along with organ-based chapters on the molecular genetic data relevant to individual disease entities. Focusing on accurate interpretation and diagnosis, as well as appropriate molecular testing, allows the creation of integrated reports that would guide oncologists in making proper treatment decisions.

There is a scarcity of molecular pathology textbooks that are comprehensive but easy to understand. The information covered in this text is cutting edge. Knowledge of the rapidly growing body of information regarding molecular pathology is essential to the understanding of modern-day medicine. We hope that this textbook will be a valuable guide for this purpose.

No book on molecular genetic pathology can be considered complete given the dynamic nature of the field. Therefore, we invite the readers to share their thoughts, and we appreciate any feedback.

Mohammad A. Vasef, MD
Professor, Department of Pathology
Director of MGP Fellowship Program
Medical Director of Molecular Diagnostics
The University of New Mexico Health Sciences Center
TriCore Reference Laboratories

Aaron Auerbach, MD, MPH
Director of Medical Education
Senior Hematopathologist
Joint Pathology Center
Silver Spring, Maryland

x

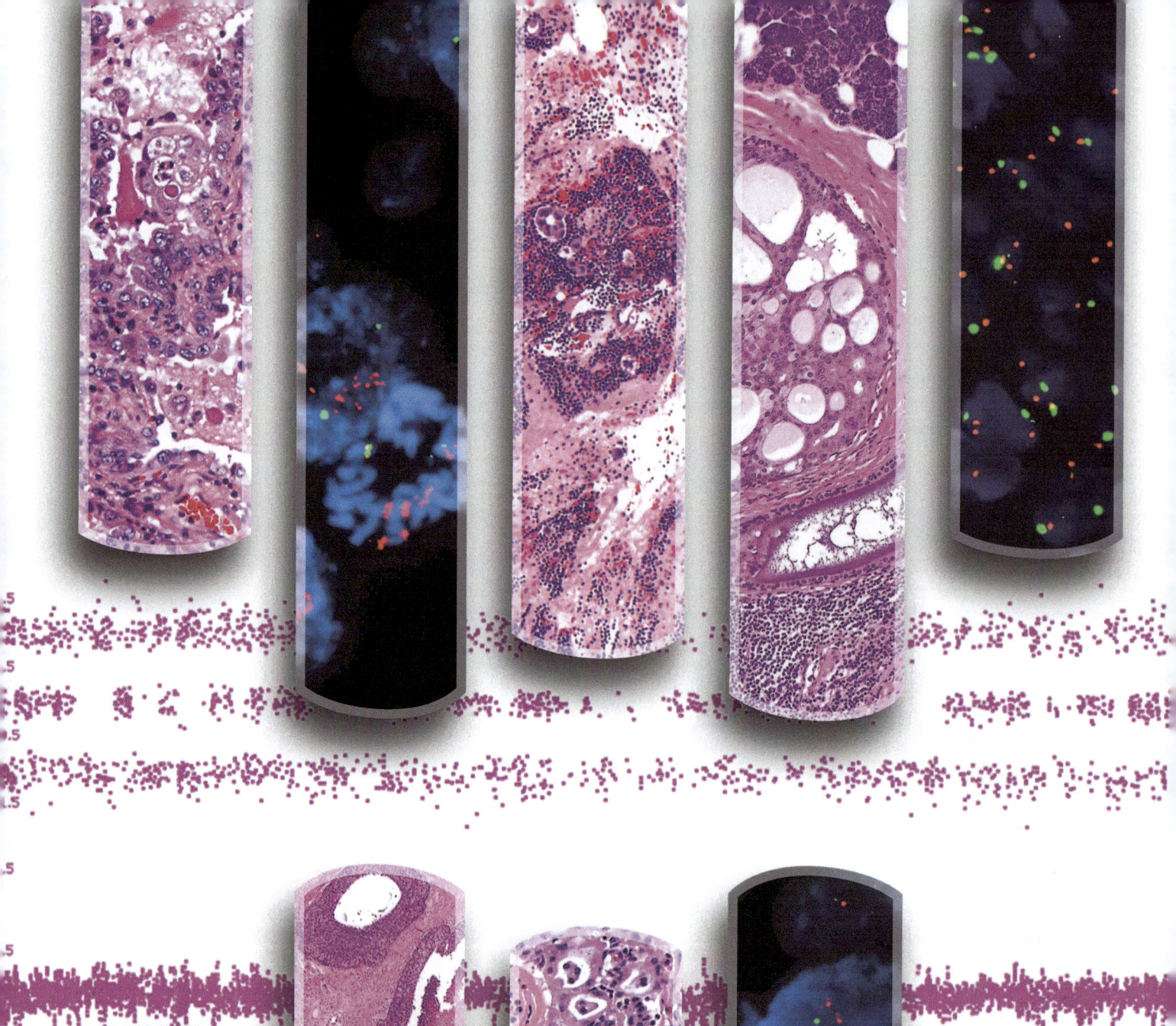

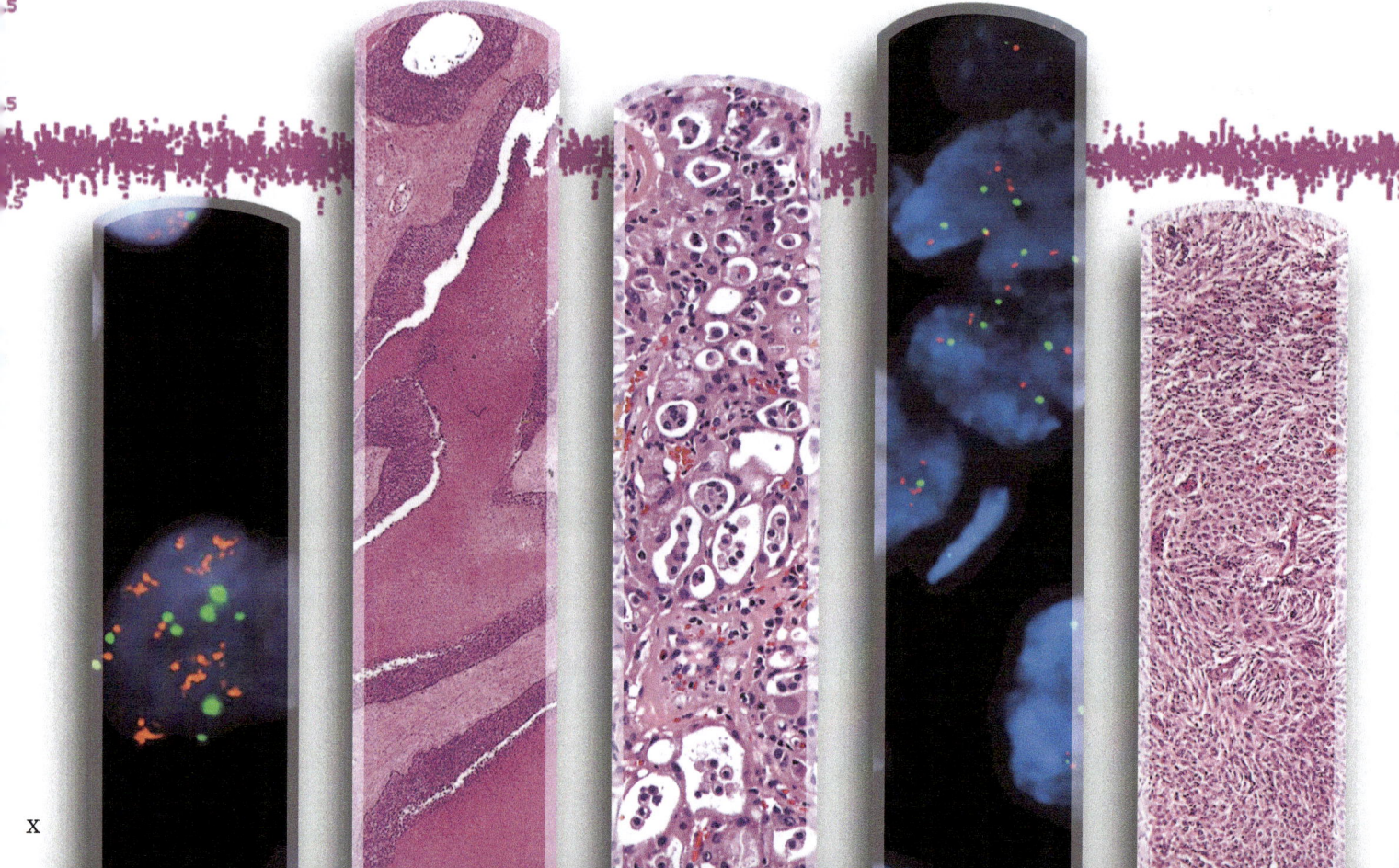

ACKNOWLEDGMENTS

LEAD EDITOR
Arthur G. Gelsinger, MA

LEAD ILLUSTRATOR
Laura C. Wissler, MA

TEXT EDITORS
Rebecca L. Bluth, BA
Nina Themann, BA
Terry W. Ferrell, MS
Megg Morin, BA
Kathryn Watkins, BA
Shannon Kelly, MA

ILLUSTRATIONS
Lane R. Bennion, MS
Richard Coombs, MS

IMAGE EDITORS
Jeffrey J. Marmorstone, BS
Lisa A. M. Steadman, BS

ART DIRECTION AND DESIGN
Cindy Lin, BFA

PRODUCTION EDITORS
Emily C. Fassett, BA
John Pecorelli, BS

AUTHOR ASSISTANT
Meaghan E. Espie

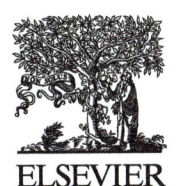

ELSEVIER

xii

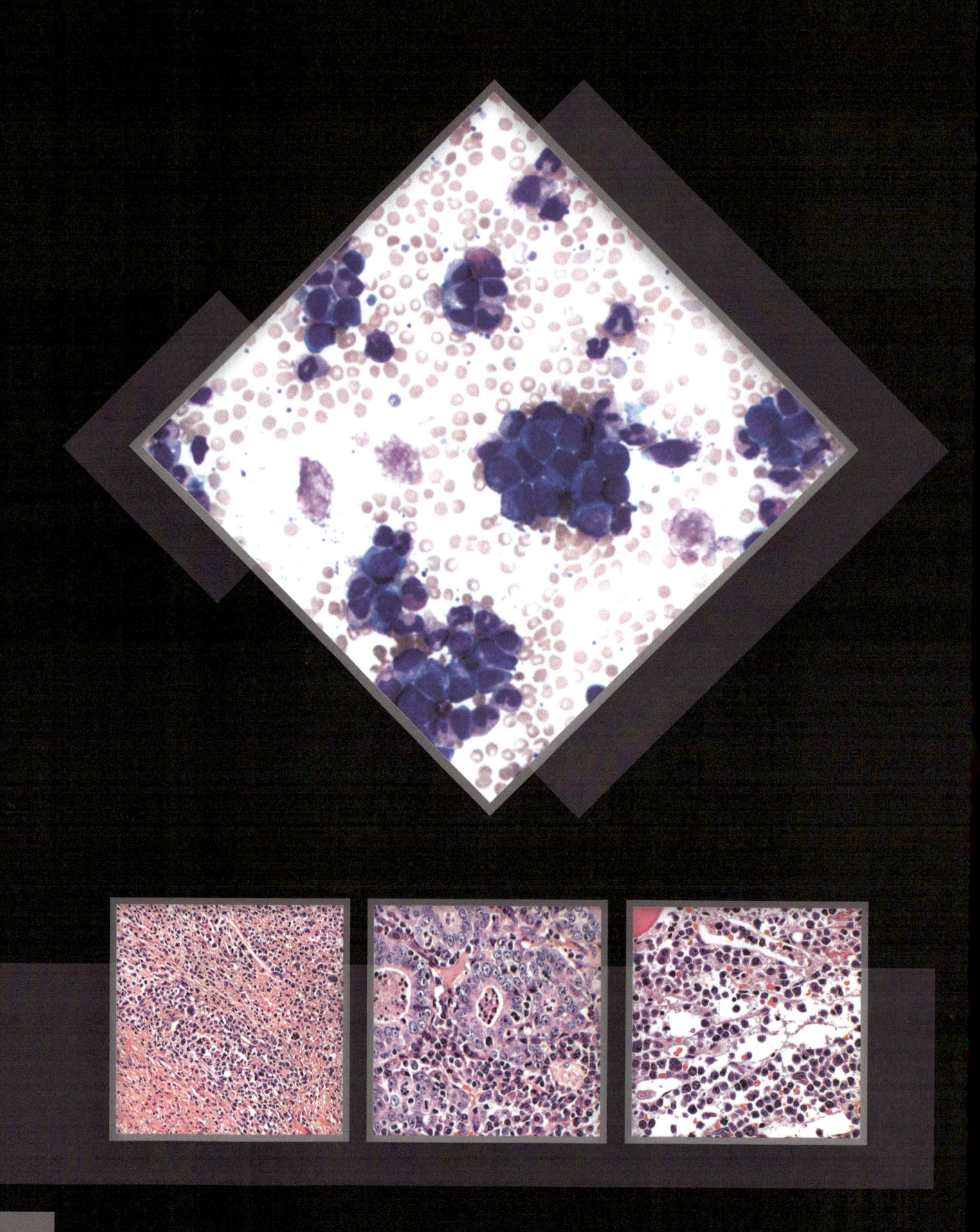

SECTIONS

SECTION 1:
Introduction

SECTION 2:
Common Techniques for Analysis of Alterations in Chromosomes and DNA

SECTION 3:
Molecular Genetic Tests in Hematopoietic Tumors

SECTION 4:
Molecular Genetic Tests in Solid Tumors, Bone and Soft Tissue Tumors, and CNS Tumors

SECTION 5:
Molecular Pathology of Myeloid Neoplasms

SECTION 6:
Molecular Pathology of Lymphoid Neoplasms

SECTION 7:
Molecular Pathology of Dendritic Cell and Histiocytic Neoplasms

SECTION 8:
Molecular Pathology of Solid Tumors

SECTION 9:
Quality Assurance and Regulatory Issues

TABLE OF CONTENTS

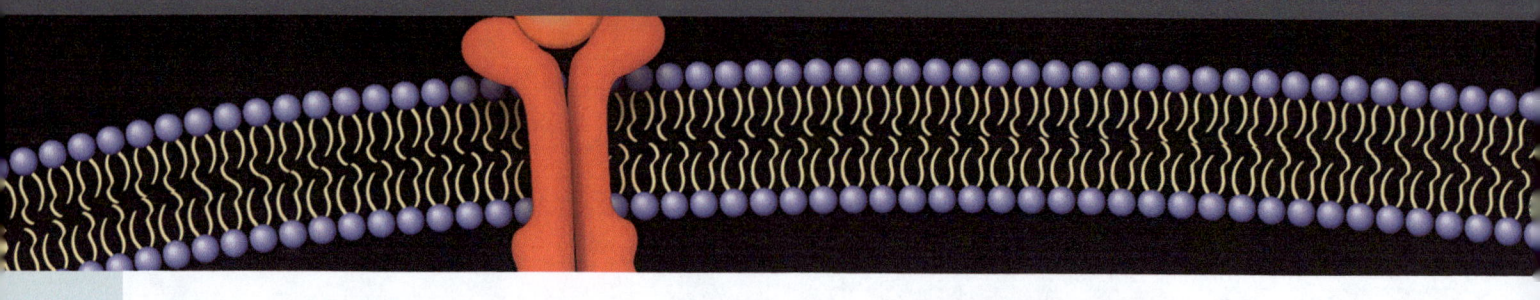

SECTION 1: INTRODUCTION

4 Structure of Chromosomes and Nucleic Acids
    Jeremy C. Wallentine, MD

8 DNA Replication, Transcription, and Translation
    Jeremy C. Wallentine, MD

12 Gene Mutations
    Jeremy C. Wallentine, MD

SECTION 2: COMMON TECHNIQUES FOR ANALYSIS OF ALTERATIONS IN CHROMOSOMES AND DNA

18 Cytogenetics and FISH
    Mohammad A. Vasef, MD and David R. Czuchlewski, MD

22 Chromosomal Microarray
    Mohammad A. Vasef, MD and Sibel Kantarci, PhD

26 Amplification Methods
    Devon Chabot-Richards, MD

30 DNA High-Resolution Melting Curve Analysis
    Amer Mahmoud, MD, FCAP

32 Sequencing Technologies
    Eric Y. Loo, MD and Mohammad A. Vasef, MD

36 High-Throughput Methods in Molecular Pathology
    Rama Gullapalli, MD, PhD

38 DNA Methylation Analysis
    Devon Chabot-Richards, MD

SECTION 3: MOLECULAR GENETIC TESTS IN HEMATOPOIETIC TUMORS

42 *BCR::ABL1* Fusion
    Eric Y. Loo, MD and Mohammad A. Vasef, MD

46 *PML::RARA* Fusion
    Devon Chabot-Richards, MD

48 Reverse Transcription PCR for Myeloid Leukemia Transcripts
    Kristin Hunt Karner, MD

50 *FLT3*, *NPM1*, and *CEBPA* Mutations
    Devon Chabot-Richards, MD

54 *JAK2* Mutations and Rearrangements
    Mohammad A. Vasef, MD

56 *MPL* Mutations
    Eric Y. Loo, MD and David R. Czuchlewski, MD

58 Calreticulin (*CALR*) Mutations
    Eric Y. Loo, MD and Mohammad A. Vasef, MD

60 *CSF3R* Mutations
    Amer Mahmoud, MD, FCAP

62 *SETBP1* Mutations
    Amer Mahmoud, MD, FCAP

64 *KIT* Mutations
    Eric Y. Loo, MD and Mohammad A. Vasef, MD

68 *IDH1* and *IDH2* Mutations
    Eric Y. Loo, MD and David R. Czuchlewski, MD

70 Other Mutations and Gene Panel Testing in Myeloid Neoplasms
    Mohammad A. Vasef, MD and David R. Czuchlewski, MD

72 Immunoglobulin Heavy (*IGH*) Chain Gene Rearrangements
    Mohammad A. Vasef, MD and Anna P. Matynia, MD

76 T-Cell Receptor Gamma (*TRG*) and Delta (*TRD*) Chain Rearrangements
    Mohammad A. Vasef, MD and Anna P. Matynia, MD

80 T-Cell Receptor Beta (*TRB*) Chain Gene Rearrangements
    Mohammad A. Vasef, MD and Anna P. Matynia, MD

84 Southern Blot Analysis of Antigen Receptor Genes
    Mohammad A. Vasef, MD

86 EBV-Associated Human Neoplasms
    Mohammad A. Vasef, MD

94 *MYD88* Mutation
    Giovanni Insuasti-Beltran, MD

96 *NOTCH1* Mutation
    Giovanni Insuasti-Beltran, MD

98 *EZH2* Mutation
    Amer Mahmoud, MD, FCAP

SECTION 4: MOLECULAR GENETIC TESTS IN SOLID TUMORS, BONE AND SOFT TISSUE TUMORS, AND CNS TUMORS

104 *ALK* Rearrangements and Mutations
    Guanghua Wang, MD

106 *ROS1* Rearrangements
    Mohammad A. Vasef, MD and David R. Czuchlewski, MD

108 *RET* Rearrangements
    Eric Y. Loo, MD and David R. Czuchlewski, MD

110 FISH for *MET* Amplifications
    Devon Chabot-Richards, MD

114 FISH for *ERBB2* (HER2) Amplifications
    M. Carmen Frias Kletecka, MD and Kristin Hunt Karner, MD

116 *KRAS* Mutations
    Guanghua Wang, MD

118 *BRAF* Mutations
    Yongjie Zhou, MD, PhD and Guanghua Wang, MD

120 *EGFR* Mutations
    Guanghua Wang, MD

122 Targeted Hotspot Gene Panel Using Massively Parallel Sequencing (Next-Generation Sequencing)
    Mohammad A. Vasef, MD and David R. Czuchlewski, MD

124 Targeted Hotspot Gene Panel Table
    Mohammad A. Vasef, MD and David R. Czuchlewski, MD

TABLE OF CONTENTS

130 **_MGMT_ Promoter Gene Methylation Assay**
Devon Chabot-Richards, MD

SECTION 5: MOLECULAR PATHOLOGY OF MYELOID NEOPLASMS

134 **Molecular Work-Up of Myeloid Neoplasms**
Mohammad A. Vasef, MD and David R. Czuchlewski, MD

MYELOPROLIFERATIVE NEOPLASMS

136 **Chronic Myeloid Leukemia, _BCR::ABL1_-Positive**
Mohammad A. Vasef, MD, Kaaren K. Reichard, MD, and David R. Czuchlewski, MD

144 **Chronic Neutrophilic Leukemia**
Devon Chabot-Richards, MD and David R. Czuchlewski, MD

148 **Polycythemia Vera**
Mohammad A. Vasef, MD and M. Carmen Frias Kletecka, MD

152 **Primary Myelofibrosis**
Devon Chabot-Richards, MD, Kaaren K. Reichard, MD, and Daniel Babu, MD

156 **Essential Thrombocythemia**
Giovanni Insuasti-Beltran, MD

160 **Chronic Eosinophilic Leukemia, NOS**
Devon Chabot-Richards, MD, Kaaren K. Reichard, MD, and Daniel Babu, MD

162 **Myeloproliferative Neoplasm, Unclassifiable**
Devon Chabot-Richards, MD, Kaaren K. Reichard, MD, and Daniel Babu, MD

MASTOCYTOSIS

166 **Mastocytosis**
Mohammad A. Vasef, MD

MYELOID/LYMPHOID NEOPLASMS WITH EOSINOPHILIA AND GENE REARRANGEMENT

174 **Myeloid/Lymphoid Neoplasms With Eosinophilia and Tyrosine Kinase Gene Fusions**
Devon Chabot-Richards, MD and David R. Czuchlewski, MD

PREMALIGNANT CLONAL HEMATOPOIESIS AND CYTOPENIAS

178 **VEXAS Syndrome**
Mohammad A. Vasef, MD and Michael M. Franklin, DO

182 **Clonal Hematopoiesis and Premalignant Clonal Cytopenia**
Mohammad A. Vasef, MD

MYELODYSPLASTIC SYNDROME (MDS)

184 **Overview and Classification of Myelodysplastic Syndrome**
Devon Chabot-Richards, MD, David R. Czuchlewski, MD, and Carla S. Wilson, MD, PhD

188 **Myelodysplastic Syndrome With Mutated _SF3B1_**
Mohammad A. Vasef, MD and Carla S. Wilson, MD, PhD

192 **Myelodysplastic Syndrome, NOS**
Kristin Hunt Karner, MD

200 **Myelodysplastic Syndrome With del(5q)**
Giovanni Insuasti-Beltran, MD

204 **Myelodysplastic Syndrome With _TP53_ Multihit Mutations**
Kristin Hunt Karner, MD

206 **Myelodysplastic Syndrome/Acute Myeloid Leukemia**
Kristin Hunt Karner, MD

208 **Pediatric Myelodysplastic Syndrome and Refractory Cytopenia of Childhood**
Devon Chabot-Richards, MD and Carla S. Wilson, MD, PhD

MYELODYSPLASTIC/MYELOPROLIFERATIVE NEOPLASMS

214 **Overview of Myelodysplastic/Myeloproliferative Neoplasms**
Devon Chabot-Richards, MD

216 **Chronic Myelomonocytic Leukemia**
Kristin Hunt Karner, MD

220 **Atypical Chronic Myeloid Leukemia**
Devon Chabot-Richards, MD

224 **Juvenile Myelomonocytic Leukemia**
Devon Chabot-Richards, MD and Qian-Yun Zhang, MD, PhD

228 **Myelodysplastic/Myeloproliferative Neoplasm, NOS**
Devon Chabot-Richards, MD and Kathryn Foucar, MD

ACUTE MYELOID LEUKEMIA

232 **Overview of Acute Myeloid Leukemia**
Mohammad A. Vasef, MD and Kaaren K. Reichard, MD

240 **Acute Myeloid Leukemia With t(8;21)/_RUNX1::RUNX1T1_**
Devon Chabot-Richards, MD, Kaaren K. Reichard, MD, and David R. Czuchlewski, MD

244 **Acute Myeloid Leukemia With inv(16) or t(16;16)/_CBFB::MYH11_**
Devon Chabot-Richards, MD, Kaaren K. Reichard, MD, and David R. Czuchlewski, MD

248 **Acute Promyelocytic Leukemia With t(15;17)/_PML::RARA_**
Mohammad A. Vasef, MD

254 **Acute Myeloid Leukemia With t(9;11)/_MLLT3::KMT2A_**
Devon Chabot-Richards, MD, Kaaren K. Reichard, MD, and David R. Czuchlewski, MD

258 **Acute Myeloid Leukemia With t(6;9)/_DEK::NUP214_**
Eric Y. Loo, MD and David R. Czuchlewski, MD

260 **Acute Myeloid Leukemia With inv(3) or t(3;3)/_GATA2; MECOM_**
Eric Y. Loo, MD and David R. Czuchlewski, MD

262 **Acute Myeloid Leukemia (Megakaryoblastic) With t(1;22)/_RBM15::MRTFA_**
Eric Y. Loo, MD and David R. Czuchlewski, MD

264 **Acute Myeloid Leukemia With Myelodysplasia-Related Gene Mutations or Cytogenetic Abnormalities**
Kathryn Foucar, MD and Mohammad A. Vasef, MD

TABLE OF CONTENTS

- 270 **Acute Myeloid Leukemia, NOS**
  Kristin Hunt Karner, MD
- 276 **Myeloid Sarcoma**
  Devon Chabot-Richards, MD
- 280 **Myeloid Proliferations Associated With Down Syndrome**
  Eric Y. Loo, MD and David R. Czuchlewski, MD

BLASTIC PLASMACYTOID DENDRITIC CELL NEOPLASM

- 284 **Blastic Plasmacytoid Dendritic Cell Neoplasm**
  Mohammad A. Vasef, MD

SECTION 6: MOLECULAR PATHOLOGY OF LYMPHOID NEOPLASMS

- 292 **Overview of Lymphoid Neoplasms**
  Nadine Aguilera, MD
- 296 **Molecular Work-Up of Lymphoid Neoplasms**
  Mohammad A. Vasef, MD and David R. Czuchlewski, MD

DETERMINATION OF CLONALITY IN B-, T-, AND NK-CELL NEOPLASMS

- 298 **Lymphoma-Associated Chromosomal Translocations**
  Kristin Hunt Karner, MD

PRECURSOR LYMPHOID NEOPLASMS

- 302 **B-Lymphoblastic Leukemia/Lymphoma With Recurrent Genetic Abnormalities**
  Kristin Hunt Karner, MD
- 306 **B-Lymphoblastic Leukemia/Lymphoma, *BCR::ABL1*-Like (Ph-Like ALL)**
  Joanna L. Conant, MD and Mohammad A. Vasef, MD
- 310 **T-Lymphoblastic Leukemia/Lymphoma**
  Mohammad A. Vasef, MD

MATURE B-CELL NEOPLASMS

- 316 **Small Lymphocytic Lymphoma/Chronic Lymphocytic Leukemia**
  Devon Chabot-Richards, MD
- 322 **B-Cell Prolymphocytic Leukemia**
  Aaron Auerbach, MD, MPH
- 326 **Splenic Marginal Zone Lymphoma**
  Aaron Auerbach, MD, MPH and Roberto N. Miranda, MD
- 332 **Hairy Cell Leukemia**
  Mohammad A. Vasef, MD
- 336 **Splenic B-Cell Lymphoma/Leukemia, Unclassifiable**
  Nadine Aguilera, MD
- 344 **Lymphoplasmacytic Lymphoma**
  Aaron Auerbach, MD, MPH
- 350 **Monoclonal Gammopathy of Undetermined Significance**
  Nadine Aguilera, MD
- 354 **Multiple Myeloma (Plasma Cell Myeloma)**
  Nadine Aguilera, MD and Carla S. Wilson, MD, PhD
- 362 **Follicular Lymphoma**
  Aaron Auerbach, MD, MPH, C. Cameron Yin, MD, PhD, and John Schmieg, MD, PhD
- 370 **Mantle Cell Lymphoma**
  Aaron Auerbach, MD, MPH
- 376 **Diffuse Large B-Cell Lymphoma**
  Nadine Aguilera, MD
- 386 **Burkitt Lymphoma**
  Aaron Auerbach, MD, MPH and Carlos Bueso-Ramos, MD, PhD

MATURE T- AND NK-CELL NEOPLASMS

- 394 **T-Cell Prolymphocytic Leukemia**
  Nadine Aguilera, MD
- 398 **Chronic Lymphoproliferative Disorder of NK Cells**
  Nadine Aguilera, MD
- 402 **Aggressive NK-Cell Leukemia**
  Nadine Aguilera, MD
- 406 **Extranodal NK-/T-Cell Lymphoma**
  Aaron Auerbach, MD, MPH and L. Jeffrey Medeiros, MD
- 410 **Adult T-Cell Leukemia/Lymphoma**
  Nadine Aguilera, MD
- 416 **Intestinal T-Cell Lymphoma**
  Aaron Auerbach, MD, MPH and Sa A. Wang, MD
- 424 **Hepatosplenic T-Cell Lymphoma**
  Aaron Auerbach, MD, MPH and Roberto N. Miranda, MD
- 428 **Subcutaneous Panniculitis-Like T-Cell Lymphoma**
  Aaron Auerbach, MD, MPH
- 432 **Mycosis Fungoides/Sézary Syndrome**
  Aaron Auerbach, MD, MPH and Sa A. Wang, MD
- 438 **Primary Cutaneous CD30-Positive T-Cell Lymphoproliferative Disorders**
  Aaron Auerbach, MD, MPH
- 442 **Peripheral T-Cell Lymphoma, NOS**
  Aaron Auerbach, MD, MPH
- 448 **Nodal Follicular Helper T-Cell Lymphoma**
  Aaron Auerbach, MD, MPH
- 456 **Anaplastic Large Cell Lymphoma, ALK-Negative**
  Mohammad A. Vasef, MD
- 462 **Anaplastic Large Cell Lymphoma, ALK-Positive**
  Mohammad A. Vasef, MD

SECTION 7: MOLECULAR PATHOLOGY OF DENDRITIC CELL AND HISTIOCYTIC NEOPLASMS

- 470 **Histiocytic Sarcoma**
  Nadine Aguilera, MD
- 478 **Langerhans Cell Histiocytosis**
  Guanghua Wang, MD
- 484 **Interdigitating Dendritic Cell Sarcoma**
  Aaron Auerbach, MD, MPH and Sa A. Wang, MD
- 488 **Follicular Dendritic Cell Sarcoma**
  Aaron Auerbach, MD, MPH

SECTION 8: MOLECULAR PATHOLOGY OF SOLID TUMORS

HEAD AND NECK, INCLUDING SINONASAL TUMORS AND SALIVARY GLANDS

- 494 **HPV-Associated Head and Neck Carcinomas**
  Thérése Bocklage, MD

TABLE OF CONTENTS

- 500 **Head and Neck Mucosal Squamous Cell Carcinoma, Non-HPV Related**
  Thèrése Bocklage, MD
- 506 **Important Alterations in Non-HPV-Related Head and Neck Squamous Cell Carcinoma**
  Thèrése Bocklage, MD
- 508 **Translocation-Specific Salivary Gland Tumors**
  Thèrése Bocklage, MD
- 518 **Translocation-Specific Salivary Gland Tumors (Continued)**
  Thèrése Bocklage, MD
- 526 **Nasopharyngeal EBV-Related Squamous Cell Carcinoma**
  Thèrése Bocklage, MD
- 530 **Other Head and Neck Tumors**
  Thèrése Bocklage, MD

THYROID

- 538 **Papillary Thyroid Carcinoma**
  Giovanni Insuasti-Beltran, MD
- 542 **Follicular Thyroid Carcinoma**
  Giovanni Insuasti-Beltran, MD
- 546 **Poorly Differentiated Thyroid Carcinoma**
  Von Samedi, MD, PhD
- 550 **Anaplastic Thyroid Carcinoma**
  Von Samedi, MD, PhD
- 554 **Medullary Thyroid Carcinoma**
  Giovanni Insuasti-Beltran, MD

LUNG

- 560 **Adenocarcinoma, Lung**
  Jeremy C. Wallentine, MD
- 568 **Squamous Cell Carcinoma, Lung**
  Jeremy C. Wallentine, MD
- 572 **Small Cell Neuroendocrine Carcinoma**
  M. Carmen Frias Kletecka, MD and Samuel Reynolds, MD
- 576 **Mesothelioma**
  Mohammad A. Vasef, MD and Khalil Sheibani, MD, FCAP

LUMINAL GASTROINTESTINAL TRACT

- 580 **Gastric Adenocarcinoma**
  M. Carmen Frias Kletecka, MD and Joshua Anspach Hanson, MD
- 584 **Colorectal Adenocarcinoma and Precancerous Lesions**
  M. Carmen Frias Kletecka, MD and Joshua Anspach Hanson, MD
- 590 **Gastrointestinal Stromal Tumor**
  M. Carmen Frias Kletecka, MD and Joshua Anspach Hanson, MD

LIVER

- 598 **HNF1A-Inactivated Hepatocellular Adenoma**
  Giovanni Insuasti-Beltran, MD and Joshua Anspach Hanson, MD
- 602 **β-Catenin-Activated Hepatocellular Adenoma**
  Giovanni Insuasti-Beltran, MD and Joshua Anspach Hanson, MD
- 606 **Inflammatory Hepatocellular Adenoma**
  Giovanni Insuasti-Beltran, MD and Joshua Anspach Hanson, MD
- 610 **Hepatocellular Carcinoma**
  Rama Gullapalli, MD, PhD

PANCREATICOBILIARY

- 614 **Pancreatic Ductal Adenocarcinoma**
  Von Samedi, MD, PhD
- 618 **Pancreatic Mucinous Cystic Neoplasm**
  Von Samedi, MD, PhD
- 620 **Pancreatic Intraductal Papillary Mucinous Neoplasm**
  Von Samedi, MD, PhD
- 622 **Cholangiocarcinoma**
  Rama Gullapalli, MD, PhD

TESTIS

- 624 **Testicular Germ Cell Tumors**
  Edgar Fischer, MD, PhD

KIDNEY

- 630 **Clear Cell Renal Cell Carcinoma**
  Edgar Fischer, MD, PhD
- 634 **Chromophobe Renal Cell Carcinoma**
  Edgar Fischer, MD, PhD
- 636 **Papillary Renal Cell Carcinoma**
  Edgar Fischer, MD, PhD
- 638 **TFE3-Rearranged and TFEB-Altered Renal Cell Carcinomas**
  Edgar Fischer, MD, PhD
- 642 **Wilms Tumor**
  Marc Barry, MD
- 648 **Clear Cell Sarcoma of Kidney**
  Marc Barry, MD
- 650 **Oncocytoma**
  Marc Barry, MD
- 652 **Rhabdoid Tumor of Kidney**
  Marc Barry, MD

BLADDER

- 654 **Urothelial Carcinoma**
  Marc Barry, MD

ADRENAL

- 660 **Pheochromocytoma/Paraganglioma**
  M. Carmen Frias Kletecka, MD and Samuel Reynolds, MD
- 666 **Adrenal Cortical Carcinoma**
  M. Carmen Frias Kletecka, MD and Samuel Reynolds, MD
- 672 **Neuroblastoma**
  Giovanni Insuasti-Beltran, MD, Thèrése Bocklage, MD, and Samuel Reynolds, MD
- 680 **Adrenal Cortical Adenoma**
  M. Carmen Frias Kletecka, MD and Samuel Reynolds, MD

PROSTATE

- 684 **Prostatic Adenocarcinoma, Acinar Type and High-Grade Prostatic Intraepithelial Neoplasia**
  Edgar Fischer, MD, PhD

TABLE OF CONTENTS

BREAST

- 688 ADH and DCIS (Dysplastic, Premalignant)
  David G. Hicks, MD
- 694 Ductal Carcinomas
  David G. Hicks, MD
- 700 Lobular Carcinoma
  David G. Hicks, MD
- 706 Invasive Ductal Carcinoma of No Special Type With Medullary Features
  Rania Bakkar, MD
- 710 Metaplastic Breast Carcinoma
  Rania Bakkar, MD
- 716 Phyllodes Tumors
  Rania Bakkar, MD
- 720 Basal-Like and Triple-Negative Breast Carcinomas
  David G. Hicks, MD and Susan C. Lester, MD, PhD

CERVIX/VULVA/VAGINA

- 730 Preneoplastic Conditions, Cervix/Vulva/Vagina
  Nancy Joste, MD
- 734 Squamous Cell Carcinoma, Cervix/Vulva/Vagina
  Nancy Joste, MD
- 738 Adenocarcinoma, Cervix/Vulva/Vagina
  Nancy Joste, MD

UTERUS

- 742 Endometrial Intraepithelial Neoplasia
  Lesley Lomo, MD
- 744 Uterine Endometrioid Carcinoma
  Lesley Lomo, MD
- 748 Uterine Serous Carcinoma
  Lesley Lomo, MD
- 750 Clear Cell Carcinoma, Uterus
  Lesley Lomo, MD
- 754 Uterine Sarcomas
  Thèrése Bocklage, MD

OVARIES/FALLOPIAN TUBE

- 762 Serous Tumors of Ovary and Fallopian Tube
  Rania Bakkar, MD
- 768 Other Surface Epithelial Tumors of Ovary
  Rania Bakkar, MD
- 774 Sex Cord-Stromal Tumors of Ovary
  Rania Bakkar, MD
- 780 Germ Cell Tumor, Ovary
  Rania Bakkar, MD and Aaron Auerbach, MD, MPH

SKIN

- 784 Premalignant Conditions, Skin
  David Cassarino, MD, PhD
- 788 Melanoma
  David Cassarino, MD, PhD
- 792 Squamous Cell Carcinoma, Skin
  David Cassarino, MD, PhD
- 796 Basal Cell Carcinoma, Skin
  David Cassarino, MD, PhD
- 800 Sebaceous Tumors
  David Cassarino, MD, PhD
- 802 Dermatofibroma and Dermatofibrosarcoma Protuberans
  David Cassarino, MD, PhD

BONE

- 804 Overview of Molecular Pathology of Bone and Soft Tissue Tumors
  Thèrése Bocklage, MD
- 810 Osteosarcomas
  Thèrése Bocklage, MD
- 818 Ewing Sarcoma
  Thèrése Bocklage, MD
- 824 Other Small Round Blue Cell Sarcomas
  Thèrése Bocklage, MD
- 832 Giant Cell Tumor of Bone
  Thèrése Bocklage, MD
- 838 Intermediate and Malignant Cartilaginous Tumors of Bone
  Thèrése Bocklage, MD

SOFT TISSUE

- 848 Intermediate and Malignant Myofibroblastic/Fibroblastic Tumors
  Thèrése Bocklage, MD
- 858 Liposarcomas
  Thèrése Bocklage, MD
- 868 Muscle Sarcomas
  Thèrése Bocklage, MD
- 878 Intermediate and Malignant Vascular Tumors
  Thèrése Bocklage, MD
- 886 Malignant Peripheral Nerve Sheath Tumor
  Thèrése Bocklage, MD and David R. Lucas, MD
- 892 Representative Genetic Findings in Bone and Soft Tissue Tumors
  Thèrése Bocklage, MD

SARCOMAS OF UNCERTAIN DIFFERENTIATION

- 898 Rare Sarcomas of Uncertain Differentiation With Specific Molecular Alterations
  Thèrése Bocklage, MD
- 908 Rare Sarcomas of Uncertain Differentiation With Specific Molecular Alterations (Continued)
  Thèrése Bocklage, MD

CNS

- 916 Glioblastoma, IDH Wildtype
  Elisabeth Rushing, MD and Mohammad A. Vasef, MD
- 920 Astrocytoma, IDH-Mutant
  Elisabeth Rushing, MD and Mohammad A. Vasef, MD
- 924 Pilocytic Astrocytoma
  Aaron Auerbach, MD, MPH, Karen SantaCruz, MD, and Elisabeth Rushing, MD

928 **Oligodendroglioma, IDH Mutant, and 1p/19q Codeleted**
Aaron Auerbach, MD, MPH, Karen SantaCruz, MD, and Elisabeth Rushing, MD

932 **Ependymal Tumors**
Mohammad A. Vasef, MD and Fausto J. Rodríguez, MD

938 **Medulloblastoma**
Mohammad A. Vasef, MD and Fausto J. Rodríguez, MD

944 **Choroid Plexus Tumors**
Mohammad A. Vasef, MD and Fausto J. Rodríguez, MD

948 **Meningioma**
Mohammad A. Vasef, MD and Karen SantaCruz, MD

952 **Retinoblastoma**
Mohammad A. Vasef, MD and Fausto J. Rodríguez, MD

SECTION 9: QUALITY ASSURANCE AND REGULATORY ISSUES

958 **Federal Agencies and Regulation of Laboratories**
Amer Mahmoud, MD, FCAP

960 **FDA Regulations**
Yongjie Zhou, MD, PhD

966 **Proficiency Testing and Accreditation**
Amer Mahmoud, MD, FCAP

THIRD EDITION
DIAGNOSTIC PATHOLOGY
MOLECULAR ONCOLOGY

VASEF • AUERBACH

BOCKLAGE • CHABOT-RICHARDS • AGUILERA • KARNER • LOO • KLETECKA

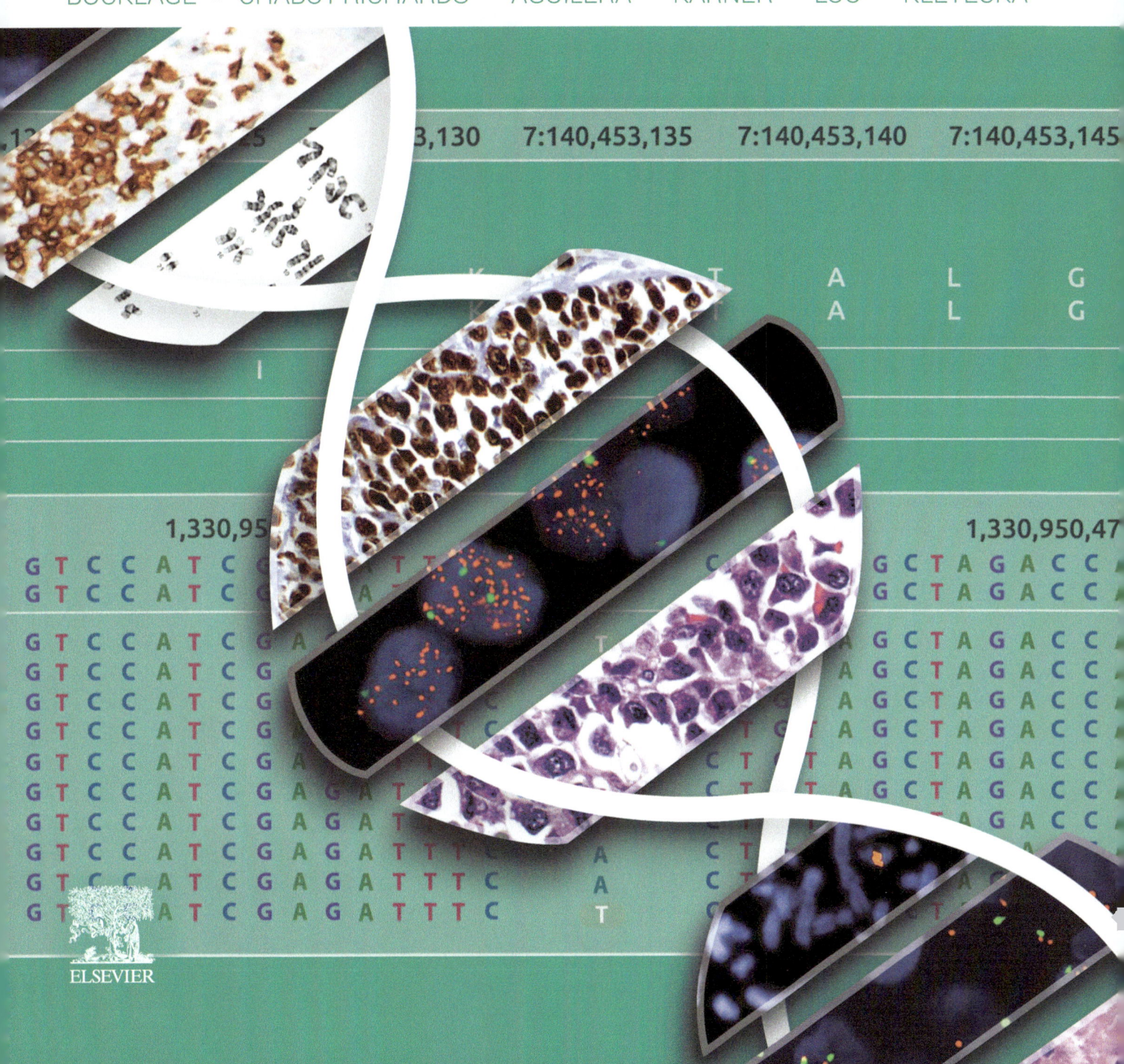

ELSEVIER

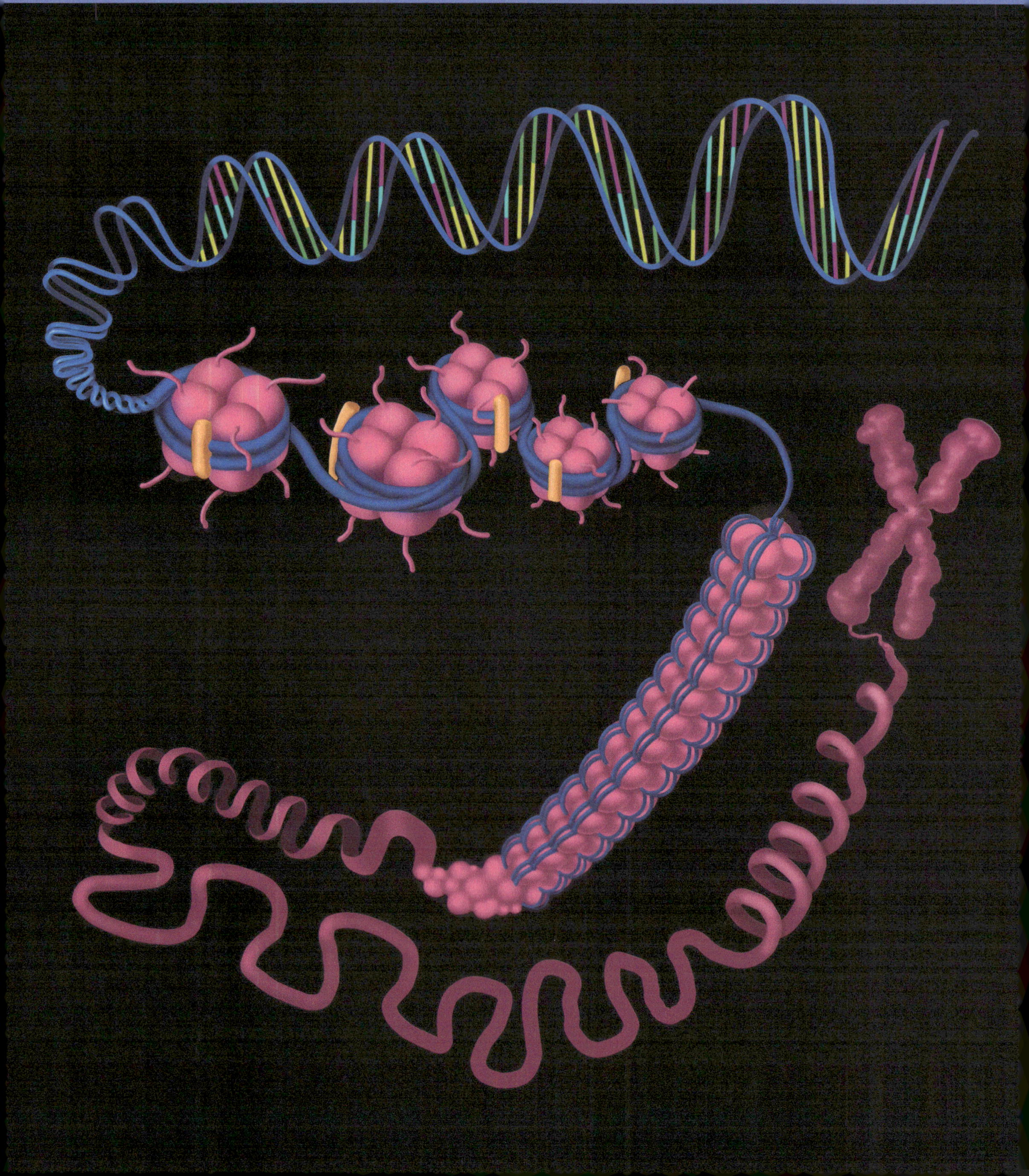

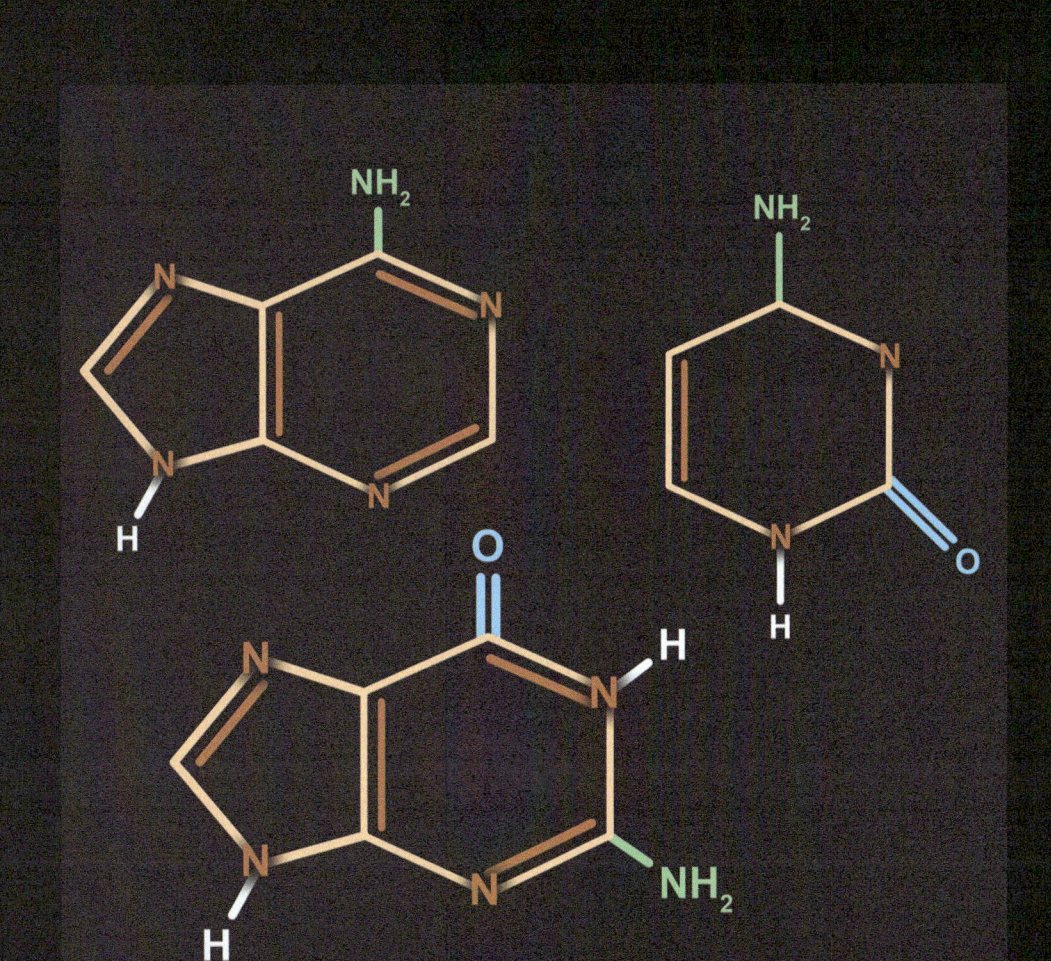

SECTION 1
Introduction

Structure of Chromosomes and Nucleic Acids   4
DNA Replication, Transcription, and Translation   8
Gene Mutations   12

Structure of Chromosomes and Nucleic Acids

CHROMOSOME ORGANIZATION

Overview

- Chromosomes consist of linear double-stranded (ds) DNA complexed with proteins and found in nucleus
- Human genome contains ~ 10^9 base pairs of DNA (3.2×10^9 nucleotides)
- Chromosome number
  - Ploidy
    - Number of homologous chromosome sets in cell [e.g., haploid (1N) = 23 chromosomes; diploid (2N) = 46 chromosomes]
  - Diploid (2N) human genome is contained in 46 chromosomes
    - 22 autosomal chromosomes + 2 sex chromosomes (XX in females or XY in males)
    - ~ 35,000 genes
- Chromosome numerical abnormalities
  - Contribute significantly to genetic disease
  - Autosomal abnormalities are generally more detrimental than sex chromosome abnormalities
  - Polyploidy
    - Refers to cells with extra chromosome set(s) beyond normal set of paired (2N) chromosomes [e.g., haploid (1N) and diploid 2N)]
  - Aneuploidy
    - Refers to abnormal number of chromosomes in cell either by loss or gains of single or multiple chromosomes (e.g., 47,XXY)
    - Monosomy: Type of aneuploidy resulting from loss of 1 parental chromosome (e.g., 45,XY,-7)
    - Trisomy: Type of aneuploidy resulting in gain of 1 parental chromosome (e.g., 47,XY,+21)
  - Mosaic
    - ≥ 2 cell lines derived from single zygote
  - Chimera
    - ≥ 2 cell lines derived from different zygotes

DNA Organization

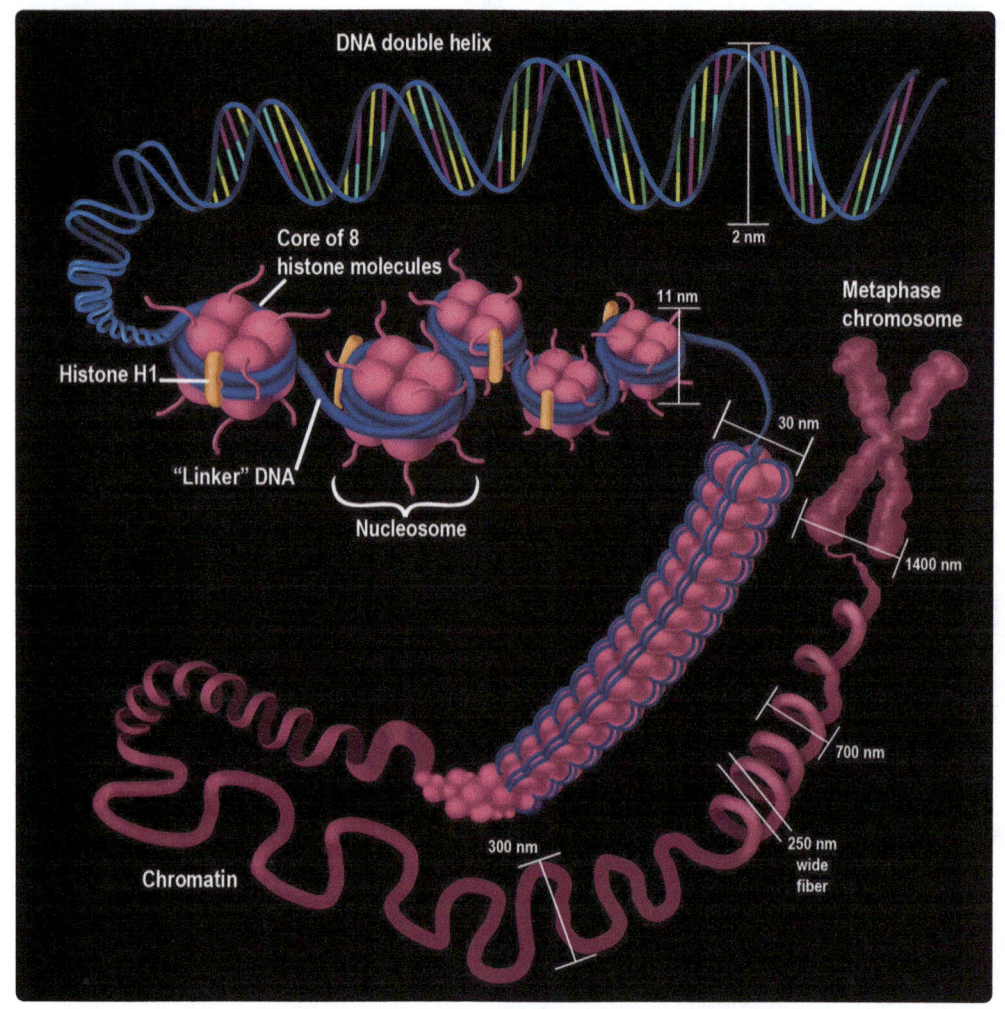

Graphic depicts the organization of DNA complexed with protein followed by highly ordered coiling and supercoiling. The DNA double-helix winds around a complex of 4 basic histone proteins (H2A, H2B, H3, and H4) that form an octamer (2 of each histone). The DNA coils 1.65x around the histone octamer, forming an 11-nm-thick nucleosome filament. Nucleosomes are the fundamental subunits of all eukaryotic chromatin and play an important role in regulating gene expression. Linker DNA is the DNA hanging in between 2 nucleosomes and undergoes additional condensation and coiling to form the 30-nm chromatin fiber, which makes up a chromosome.

Structure of Chromosomes and Nucleic Acids

Chromosomes
- **Chromatin**
  - Form of genetic material that exists during interphase
  - Packaged state of DNA that allows for mitosis, meiosis, and gene expression
  - DNA complexed with protein followed by highly ordered coiling and supercoiling
    - Histones are major chromatin-binding protein
    - Histones H2A, H2B, H3, and H4 form octamers
    - 147 base pairs of dsDNA are coiled in < 2 turns (1.65x) around central core of this histone octamer
    - Coiling forms fundamental unit of DNA packaging (nucleosome)
    - Adjacent nucleosomes are connected by short lengths of linker DNA
    - Nucleosomes are stacked and further coiled (6-8 nucleosomes/turn) into 30-nm fiber (spiral or solenoid arrangement)
    - 30-nm fiber makes up chromosome that resides in nucleus
  - Posttranslational modifications
    - Methylation, phosphorylation, and acetylation of chromatin function to regulate gene expression
    - Modifications allow for different proteins to bind chromatin and subsequently affect chromatin condensation and transcriptional activity
  - Euchromatin
    - Loosely packaged form of DNA
    - Most commonly observed during interphase
    - Represents areas of active transcription (gene expression)
    - Corresponds to light-staining regions in G-banding stain techniques
  - Heterochromatin
    - Tightly packaged form of DNA
    - Represents areas of inactive transcription (nontranscribed DNA)
    - Corresponds to dark-staining regions in G-banding stain techniques
- **Chromosome structure**
  - Each chromosome contains 2 long arms (q), 2 short arms (p), 1 centromere, and multiple telomeres (4 telomeres in each chromosome during metaphase)
  - Centromere
    - Constricted region where duplicated sister chromatids join until anaphase
    - Separates short (p) and long (q) arms
    - Essential for attaching chromosomes to mitotic spindle and for chromosome segregation
  - Telomere
    - Specialized heterochromatic DNA-protein complexes located at ends of chromosomes
    - Protects chromosome ends from deterioration or from fusing with adjacent chromosomes
  - Satellites
    - Small chromosomal segment separated by noncentromeric constriction from remaining chromosome
- **Chromosome categorization and morphology**
  - Numbered (1-22) according to relative size (largest to smallest)
  - Grouped according to centromere position
    - Metacentric: Centromere located at or near middle
    - Submetacentric: Centromere in location that results in clearly unequal lengths of chromosome arms
    - Acrocentric: Centromere located at or near chromosome end

Nucleic Acids
- Both DNA and RNA are large polymers with long linear backbones
  - Linear backbone is composed of alternating residues of phosphate group and 5-carbon sugar
  - Sugars in DNA differ by lack of hydroxyl group at 2' carbon position
  - Sugars in RNA differ by presence of hydroxyl group at 2' carbon position
  - Nitrogenous base is attached to each sugar to form nucleoside
    - Nitrogenous bases of nucleic acid molecule vary
    - Sequence of nitrogenous bases identifies nucleic acid and determines its function
- Nucleotides form when phosphate group attaches to 3' or 5' carbon of nucleoside (nitrogenous base + sugar residue), forming phosphodiester bond
  - Phosphodiester bonds
    - Strong covalent bonds between phosphate groups
    - Connect 5' carbon of 1 nucleoside to 3' carbon of next nucleoside
    - Determines nucleic acid polarity (5' → 3')
  - Nucleic acids are composed of chains of nucleotides
    - Sugar group [ribose (RNA) or deoxyribose (DNA)] + purine or pyrimidine base + phosphate group
- **DNA**
  - Purine or pyrimidine nitrogenous bases attach to and extend from 1st carbon of sugar group
    - Purines [adenine (A) and guanine G)] are composed of 1 joined carbon-nitrogen ring (6- and 5-member rings)
    - Pyrimidines [thymine (T) and cytosine C)] are composed of single 6-member carbon-nitrogen ring
  - Purines (G and A) pair with pyrimidines (C and T) via hydrogen bonds
    - 2 hydrogen bonds form between A and T
    - 3 hydrogen bonds form between G and C
    - Additional hydrogen bond between G and C dramatically increases strength of interaction
- **RNA**
  - In RNA, uracil (U) replaces thymine (T)
  - Normally single stranded
  - 2 RNA molecules may associate transiently to form base pairs
    - Purines (G and A) pair with pyrimidines (C and U) via hydrogen bonds
  - Hydrogen bonds also allow for formation of DNA-RNA duplexes
  - Hydrogen bonds may also form between bases within single RNA or DNA molecule (e.g., hairpin structures)
- **Types of RNA**
  - Messenger RNA (mRNA)
    - Transcribed from DNA template

Structure of Chromosomes and Nucleic Acids

Human Chromosome Groups

Group	Chromosomes	Description
A	1, 2, 3	Largest chromosomes; metacentric (1, 3) and submetacentric (2)
B	4, 5	Large chromosomes; submetacentric; arms vary in size
C	6-12, X	Medium-sized chromosomes; submetacentric
D	13, 14, 15	Medium-sized chromosomes; acrocentric; contain satellites
E	16, 17, 18	Small chromosomes; metacentric (16) and submetacentric (17, 18)
F	19, 20	Small chromosomes; metacentric
G	21, 22, Y	Small chromosomes; 21 and 22 contain satellites

Posttranslational Modification Examples

Modification	Amino Acid(s) Involved	Group Added	Comments
Methylation	Lysine	CH_3	Performed by methylases and reversed by demethylases
Phosphorylation	Tyrosine, threonine, serine	PO_4^-	Performed by kinases and reversed by phosphatases
Hydroxylation	Proline, lysine, aspartate	OH	Modification is common in collagen
Acetylation	Lysine	CH_3CO	Performed by acetylase and reversed by deacetylase
Carboxylation	Glutamine	COOH	Performed by γ-carboxylase
N-glycosylation	Asparagine	Complex carbohydrate	
O-glycosylation	Serine, threonine, hydroxyproline	Complex carbohydrate	

Numerical Chromosome Abnormalities

Abnormality	Example(s)	Type of Ploidy	Comments
Triploidy	69,XXX (triploid syndrome)	Polyploidy	Extremely rare chromosomal disorder
Trisomy	47,XY,+21 (Down syndrome); 47,XY,+18 (Edwards syndrome); 47,XY,+13 (Patau syndrome)	Aneuploidy	Gain of single parental chromosome; chromosome gain indicated by plus sign
Monosomy	45,X (Turner syndrome)	Aneuploidy	Chromosome lost; if somatic, is indicated by minus sign
Mosaicism	47,XXY/46,XY		

- DNA reverse transcribed from mRNA is called cDNA
- Exons encode amino acid sequences in mRNA
- Introns are noncoding sequences that are spliced out of mRNA by exonucleases prior to translation
  o Transfer RNA (tRNA)
    - Adapter molecule that binds and transfers amino acids to site of protein synthesis during translation
  o Ribosomal RNA
    - RNA component of ribosome
    - Ribosome is combination of rRNA and ribosomal proteins involved in translation of mRNA into polypeptides
  o Ribozyme
    - RNA molecule that catalyzes chemical reaction

SELECTED REFERENCES

1. Minchin S et al: Understanding biochemistry: structure and function of nucleic acids. Essays Biochem. 63(4):433-56, 2019
2. Leonard DGB: Molecular Pathology in Clinical Practice. Springer Science, 2016
3. Buckingham L: Molecular Diagnostics: Fundamentals, Methods and Clinical Applications. 2nd ed. F.A. Davis Company, 2012
4. Strachan T et al: Human Molecular Genetics. 4th ed. Garland Science, 2010
5. Cheng L et al: Molecular Genetic Pathology. Humana Press, 2008

Structure of Chromosomes and Nucleic Acids

2-Deoxyribose

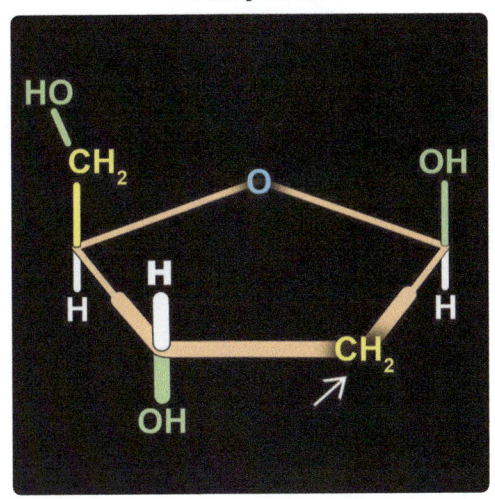

Nitrogen Base

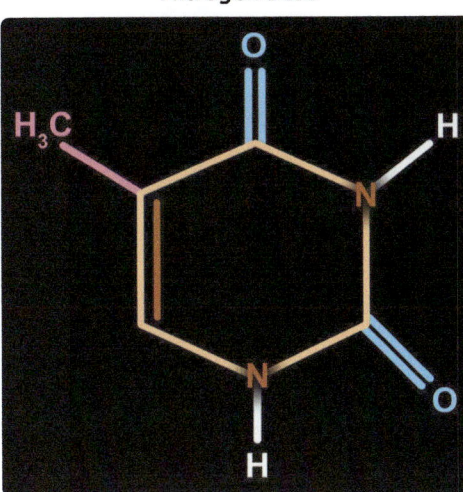

(Left) 2-deoxyribose is the sugar group in DNA. Note there is no oxygen on the 2' carbon ➡ of deoxyribose, while ribose (RNA) contains an oxygen atom that forms a hydroxyl group at the 2' position. **(Right)** There are 4 nitrogen bases in DNA: Adenine (A), guanine (G), thymine (T), and cytosine (C). Adenine and guanine are purines, and thymine and cytosine are pyrimidines. Thymine is a nitrogen base present only in DNA. In RNA, thymine is replaced with uracil.

Phosphate Group

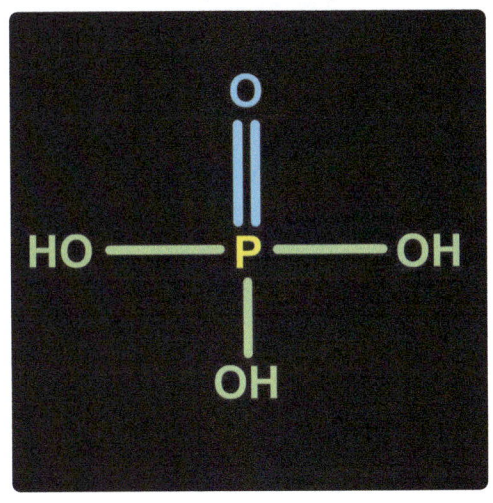

Nitrogen Bases

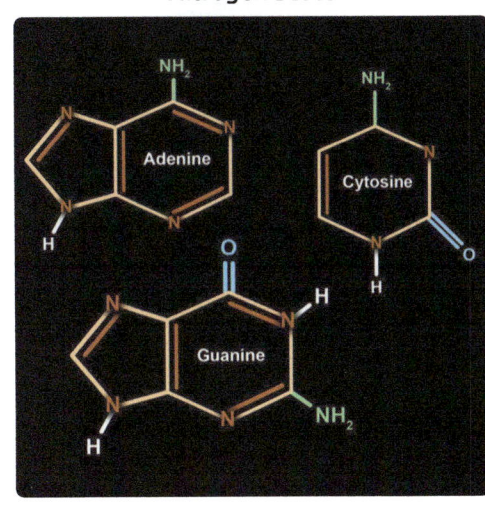

(Left) When a phosphate group is added to a nucleoside, the complex becomes a nucleotide. Nucleotides are the basic building blocks of DNA. **(Right)** Graphic shows the structure of adenine, guanine, and cytosine. Adenine and guanine are purines, and thymine and cytosine are pyrimidines. A nitrogen base, when paired with deoxyribose, forms a nucleoside molecule. When a phosphate group is added to a nucleoside, the complex becomes a nucleotide.

Ribose

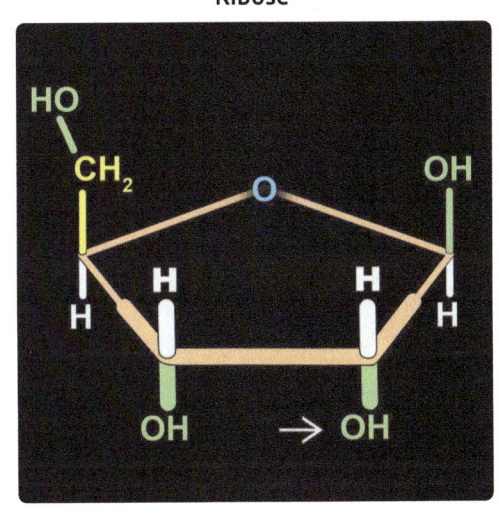

Uracil

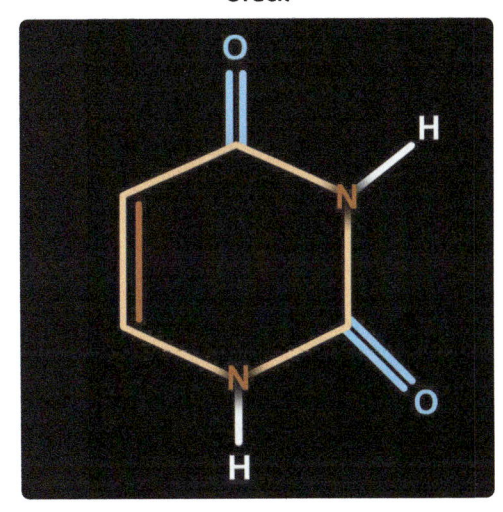

(Left) The 5-carbon sugar in RNA is ribose. Ribose contains a 2' hydroxyl group ➡. Recall deoxyribose, the sugar group of DNA, lacks this hydroxyl group at the 2' position. This difference of 1 oxygen atom is important for the enzymes that recognize DNA and RNA. **(Right)** In RNA, the nitrogen base uracil replaces the nitrogen base thymine, which is only present in DNA. Likewise, uracil is only present in RNA.

Introduction

7

DNA Replication, Transcription, and Translation

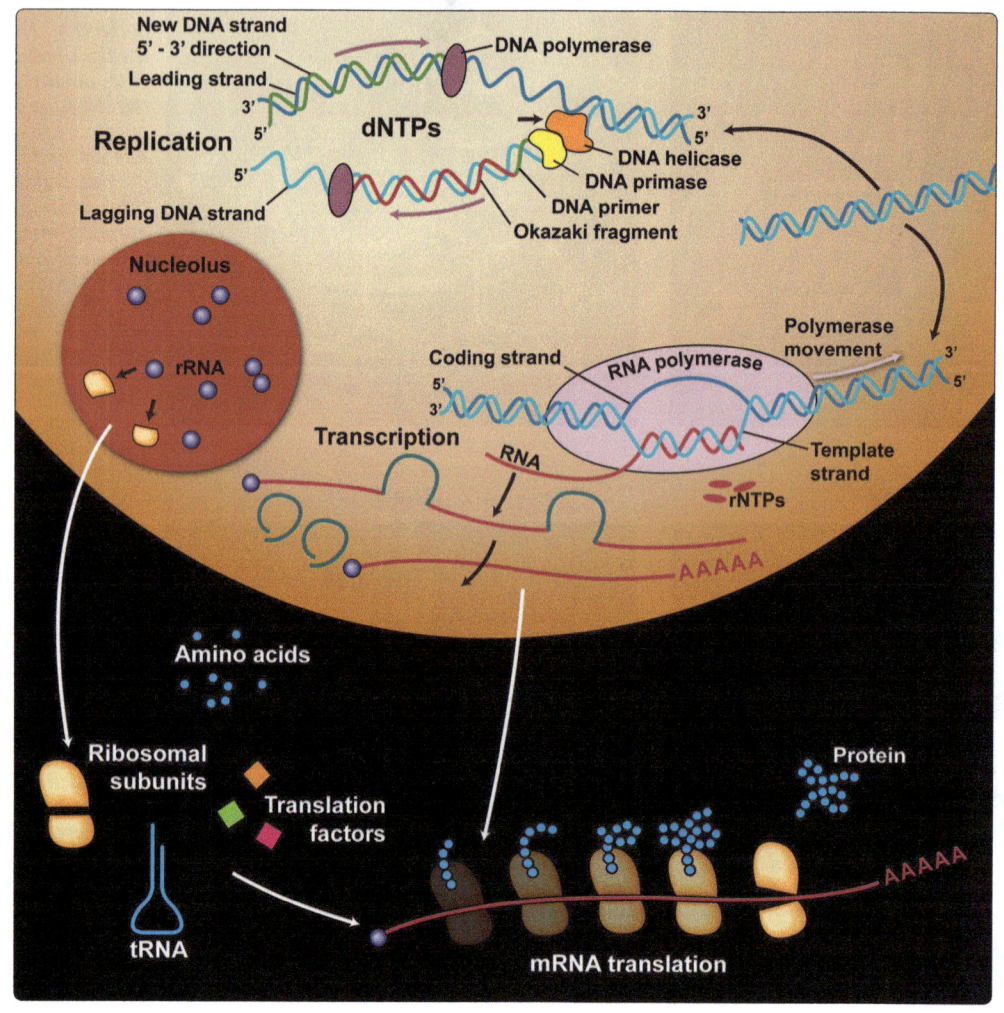

DNA REPLICATION

General Principles
- Exact duplication of double-stranded (ds) DNA takes place prior to cell division
  - Each daughter cell will contain exact replica of parent DNA
- Takes place during synthesis (S) phase of cell cycle
  - Cell cycle consists of G_0, G_1, S, G_2, and M phases
- Replication is semiconservative process
  - Each daughter DNA duplex contains 1 newly synthesized strand and 1 original strand from parent molecule
- **DNA polymerases**
  - Enzymes involved in DNA replication (α, β, γ, δ, and ε)
    - α and δ replicate nuclear DNA
    - β and ε are involved in DNA repair
    - γ replicates mitochondrial DNA
  - Processivity of DNA polymerase enzymes
    - Rate at which 4 nucleotides are polymerized into nucleic acid chain
    - Most have processivity of 1,000 bases per minute
  - Fidelity of DNA polymerase
    - Accuracy in which correct base is incorporated into newly synthesized DNA
  - DNA polymerase error rates
    - Vary from 1 in 1,200 to 1 in 1 million
    - Corrected by DNA proofreading functions
  - DNA repair
    - Usually takes place in G_2 phase of cell cycle
    - Normal healthy cells will pause for this to occur
    - Malignant cells may not pause, and, therefore, replication errors may persist
  - Oncogenesis
    - May result from incorrect bases being incorporated into newly synthesized strand
    - Altered sequence may change protein function

Process Overview
- Dissociation of DNA strands
  - May be accomplished by

DNA Replication, Transcription, and Translation

DNA replication proceeds in a 5' to 3' direction resulting in the synthesis of 2 new daughter strands, each containing 1 newly synthesized strand and 1 original parent strand. Transcription is the process whereby a DNA sequence is converted to a single strand of RNA. Various proteins bind DNA sequence elements in a highly regulated process. RNA polymerase then binds to these bound transcription factors to form the basal transcription apparatus that transcribes in a 5' to 3' direction, synthesizing RNA from 4 nucleotide precursors. Messenger RNA migrates to the cytoplasm where it interacts with ribosomal machinery to initiate translation and polypeptide synthesis.

DNA Replication, Transcription, and Translation

- Chemical or physical conditions, such as alkali or high temperatures (i.e., 95 °C)
- Physiological conditions by numerous enzymes (i.e., helicases, topoisomerases)
- Formation of replication fork
  - Replication is initiated at multiple sites/origins where parental DNA duplex is opened up to form Y-shaped replication fork
  - Initiating proteins, primases, and DNA polymerases bind to original parental strand of DNA (replisome)
  - As replication proceeds, replication fork moves along length of parent DNA strand
- Enzymatic activities generate 2 new nucleic acid strands
  - DNA polymerase α and δ synthesize nucleic acid molecules from nucleotides
  - Strands are complementary (base paired) to original parent DNA strands
    - Semiconservative process
  - Nucleotides are sequentially added according to order of bases in parent strand
    - G:C pairing
    - A:T pairing
  - New "daughter" strand is antiparallel to parent strand
- DNA polymerase can only read parent DNA in 3' to 5' direction and can only synthesize in 5' to 3' direction
- 2 parent strands are designated as leading and lagging strands
  - Leading strand
    - Read by DNA polymerase in 3' to 5' direction
    - New strand of DNA is synthesized continuously in 5' to 3' direction
  - Lagging strand
    - Synthesized in discontinuous manner
    - Replication fork moves in 5' to 3' direction
    - Copied in short stretches forming short DNA fragments (Okazaki fragments)
    - Fragments are joined by ligation into continuous daughter strand that is complementary to parent DNA lagging strand
    - Results in progressive loss of telomeres

DNA TRANSCRIPTION

General Principles

- Process of converting DNA sequence to single strand of RNA
  - Mediated by RNA polymerase
- Transcription requires various proteins (transcription factors) that bind DNA sequence elements in highly regulated process
  - Transcription factors bind DNA sequence elements to form basal transcription apparatus
    - Fixed set of general transcription factors
    - Coactivators and corepressors
    - Gene- or tissue-specific transcription factors
  - Transcription factors help position and guide RNA polymerase
  - Transcription factors recognized by RNA polymerase II include
    - TFIIA
    - TFIIB
    - TFIID
    - TFIIE
    - TFIIF
    - TFIIH
- RNA polymerase requires crucial regulatory DNA sequence elements, such as promoters and enhancers
- Promoter
  - DNA sequence element often located close to and upstream of gene
  - Recognized and bound by transcription factors
  - Promoters recognized by RNA polymerase II
    - TATA (i.e., TATAAA)
    - GC box (i.e., GGGCGG)
    - CAAT box
- Enhancer
  - Recognized by tissue-specific transcription factors
  - Enhance transcriptional activity of specific gene
  - Located at variable distances from transcription initiation sites
- Silencer
  - Similar to enhancer but functions to inhibit transcriptional activity
- RNA polymerases
  - RNA polymerase I
    - Transcribes genes encoding ribosomal RNA
  - RNA polymerase II
    - Transcribes genes encoding proteins (mRNA) and
    - Many functional RNAs (i.e., small nucleolar RNA, microRNA)
  - RNA polymerase III
    - Transcribes genes encoding transfer RNA (tRNA) and
    - 5S ribosomal RNA
- Types of RNA
  - Messenger RNA (mRNA)
    - Transcribed from DNA to carry protein sequence information
  - Transfer RNA (tRNA)
    - Amino acid-specific adapter molecule involved in translation
  - Ribosomal RNA (rRNA)
    - RNA component of ribosome
    - Ribosomes are essential components of protein manufacturing
- Exons
  - Sequences in mRNA that code for protein sequence (coding sequences)
- Introns
  - Noncoding sequences found between exons
  - Spliced out of mRNA by exonucleases prior to translation
- Posttranscription RNA processing
  - RNA splicing
    - Removal of intronic RNA segments
    - Remaining exonic RNA are joined together
    - Process yields overall shorter RNA product
  - 5' capping
    - Following initiation, 7-methylguanosine is linked by 5'-5' phosphodiester bond to first 5' nucleotide
    - Protects RNA transcript from exonuclease activity
    - Facilitates RNA transport from nucleus to cytoplasm

DNA Replication, Transcription, and Translation

- Facilitates RNA splicing and attachment of 40S ribosome subunit during translation
  - 3' polyadenylation
    - Poly(A) polymerase sequentially adds AMP residues to 3' end (~ 200) to produce poly(A) tail
    - Facilitates mRNA transportation, provides stability to mRNA and enhances recognition by ribosomal machinery

Process Overview
- DNA must first be bound by general transcription factors (preinitiation complex)
- RNA polymerase binds to bound transcription factors to form basal transcription apparatus
- Double-stranded DNA bound by RNA polymerase and transcription factors is unwound
  - Unwound segment of DNA acts as template for RNA synthesis
  - Transient double-stranded RNA-DNA hybrid forms with growing RNA strand
- RNA polymerase moves from 3 end of DNA template strand (3'-5') synthesizing RNA from 4 nucleotide precursors
  - ATP
  - CTP
  - GTP
  - UTP
- Elongation proceeds with addition of ribonucleoside monophosphate residues (AMP, CMP, GMP, UMP) to free 3' hydroxyl group at 3' end of growing RNA strand
- Base pairing is identical to that of DNA except that uracil (U) replaces T
- RNA synthesis proceeds in 5' to 3' direction until it reaches stop codon
- AAUAAA sequence signals for 3' cleavage at site 15-30 nucleotides downstream
- RNA processing (i.e., splicing, 5' capping, and 3' polyadenylation)

DNA TRANSLATION

General Principles
- Process of converting sequence information from single strand of mRNA into amino acid sequence
- Messenger RNA migrates to cytoplasm where it interacts with ribosomal machinery to initiate translation and polypeptide synthesis
- Ribosomes
  - Large RNA-protein complexes of ~ 50 different proteins associated with several rRNA molecules
  - Composed of 2 main subunits (eukaryotes)
    - 1 large 60S subunit
    - 1 smaller 40S subunit (eukaryotes)
  - Provide structural framework for polypeptide synthesis
- Transfer RNA (tRNA)
  - Translation relies on tRNA that carries specific amino acid and recognizes corresponding codon in mRNA sequence
  - Collection of tRNA molecules bind to specific amino acid to form amino acid-tRNA complex (aminoacyl tRNA)
  - Each tRNA contains anticodon that allows it to recognize codon in mRNA strand
- Codons
  - Set of 3 bases
  - Convey genetic information to be translated into amino acid sequences
  - Each codon specifies an amino acid

Process Overview
- Messenger RNA
  - Binds to ribosome in cytoplasm
  - Ribosomes recognize 5' cap of mRNA to initiate process
  - Synthesis begins at start codon (AUG)
    - AUG encodes methionine amino acid
    - Establishes reading frame of mRNA
  - Messenger RNA is read in 5' to 3' direction in groups of 3 nucleotides (codons)
- Ribosome
  - Travels down mRNA, 1 codon at a time as amino acids are added
  - Protein translation ends at stop codon
    - Stop codons include UGA, UAG, and UAA
- Protein is manufactured form N (amino)-terminal to C (carboxy)-terminal
- Completed polypeptide then undergoes posttranslational processing
  - Addition of carbohydrate and lipid groups
  - Protein cleavage

Posttranslational Modifications
- Modifications allow for different proteins to bind chromatin and subsequently affect condensation and transcriptional activity
- Examples
  - Phosphorylation (PO_4^-)
    - Targets tyrosine, serine, and threonine via kinases
  - Methylation (CH_3)
    - Targets lysine via methylases
  - Hydroxylation (OH)
    - Targets proline, lysine, aspartic acid
  - Acetylation (CH_3CO)
    - Targets lysine via acetylase
  - Carboxylation (COOH)
    - Targets glutamine via γ-carboxylase
  - Glycosylation (complex carbohydrate)
    - Targets asparagine, serine, threonine, hydroxyproline

SELECTED REFERENCES
1. Mercadante AA et al: Biochemistry, replication and transcription. StatPearls, 2023
2. Lai WKM et al: Understanding nucleosome dynamics and their links to gene expression and DNA replication. Nat Rev Mol Cell Biol. 18(9):548-62, 2017
3. Leonard D, et al: Molecular Pathology in Clinical Practice. 2nd ed. Springer Science, 2016
4. Strachan T et al: Human Molecular Genetics. 4th ed. Garland Science, 2010
5. Cowling VH: Regulation of mRNA cap methylation. Biochem J. 425(2):295-302, 2009
6. Cheng L et al: Molecular Genetic Pathology. Humana Press, 2008

DNA Replication, Transcription, and Translation

Cell Cycle

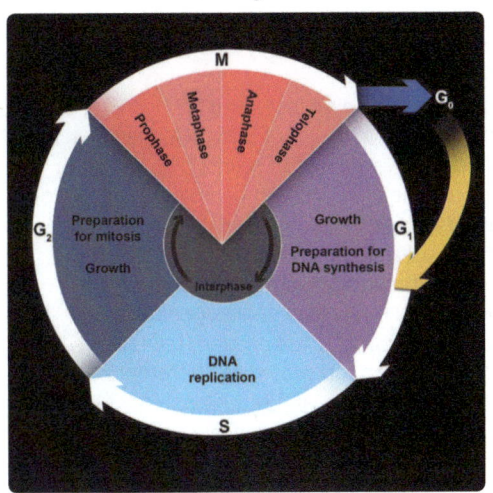

Nucleic Acids

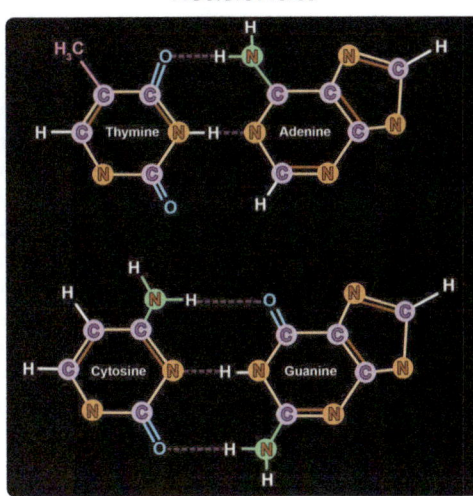

(Left) DNA replication takes place during the synthesis (S) phase of the cell cycle. Checkpoints in G_1 and G_2 ensure that the cell is ready for DNA synthesis and mitosis, respectively. G_0 represents a "postmitotic" phase that fully differentiated, quiescent, or senescent cells enter. **(Right)** Hydrogen bonds form between cytosine and guanine (3) and thymine and adenine (2).

Genetic Code

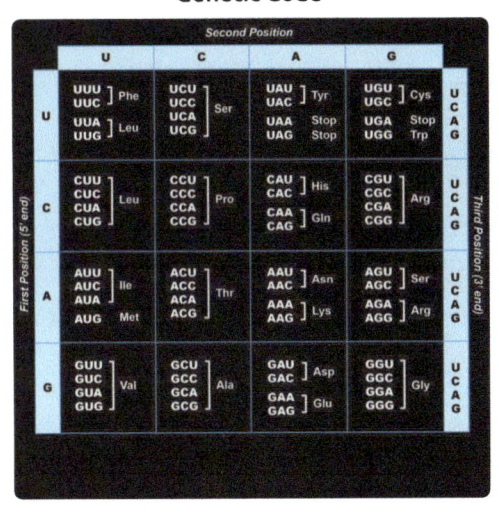

Amino Acid Structures

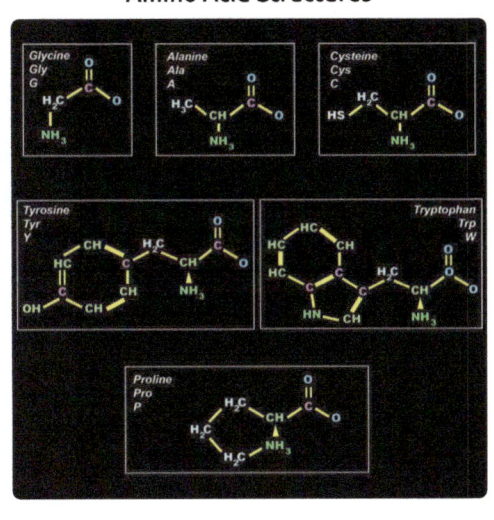

(Left) RNA codon table outlines the fundamental principles of the genetic code. The code defines how sequences of these nucleotide triplets (i.e., codons) specify which amino acid will be added next during protein synthesis. The polypeptide sequence determines the identity, function, and characteristics of the protein. **(Right)** The molecular structure of the amino acids with intermediate-side chains are shown for reference.

Amino Acid Structures

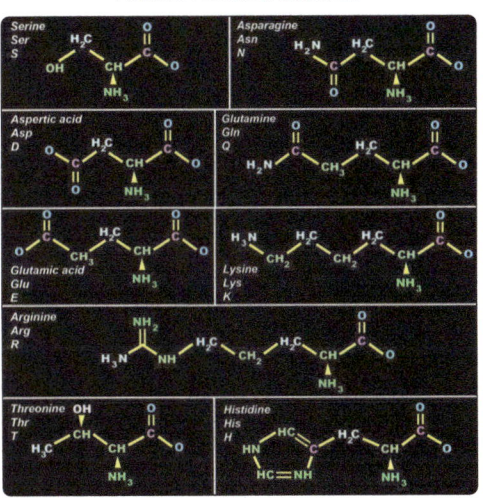

Amino Acid Structures

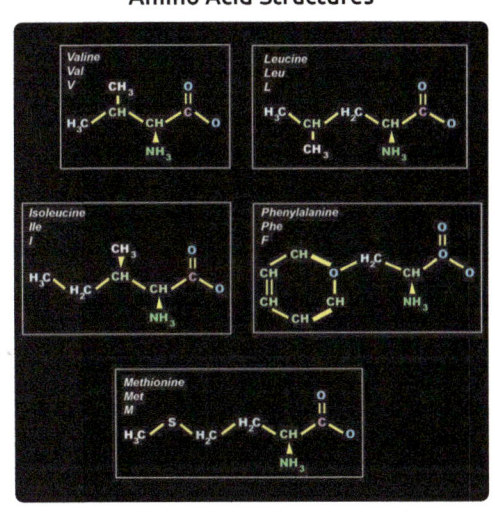

(Left) The molecular structure of the amino acids with hydrophilic side chains are shown for reference. Typically, mutations that result in a substitution of a similar amino acid (i.e., p.Asp > Gln) have less of an impact on protein function as compared to mutations that result in a substitution of a dissimilar amino acid (i.e., p.Gln > Val). **(Right)** The molecular structure of the amino acids with hydrophobic side chains are shown for reference.

Gene Mutations

ETIOLOGY/PATHOGENESIS

Oncogenesis

- Cancer is often multistep process during which cells acquire series of mutations
  - Mutations lead to decreased tumor suppressor gene function &/or increased protooncogene function
  - Results in uncontrolled growth and failure to respond to signals that normally lead to cell death (apoptosis)
  - Rapid growth and uncontrolled cell division may lead to abnormal chromosome segregation and additional changes (genetic instability) in chromosome number (aneuploidy)
- Protooncogenes
  - Cause normal cells to become cancerous when mutated
    - Mutations are typically dominant in nature
  - Oncogene is mutated version of protooncogene
  - \> 40 different human protooncogenes are known
    - ~ 14 protooncogenes are associated with high propensity for cancer
  - Oncogenes arise as result of mutations that increase expression level or activity of protooncogene
    - Point mutations, deletions, or insertions in promoter region of protooncogene may lead to increased transcription
    - Gene amplification events leading to extrachromosomal copies of protooncogene
    - Chromosomal translocation events that relocate protooncogene to new chromosomal site that leads to overexpression
    - Chromosomal translocations that lead to fusion between protooncogene and 2nd gene, which produces fusion protein with oncogenic activity
  - Increased production of these proteins leads to increased cell division, decreased cell differentiation, and inhibition of cell death
    - These characteristics define cancer cells
    - Oncogenes are therefore important targets for cancer therapy
- Tumor suppressor genes

Cell Signaling Steps

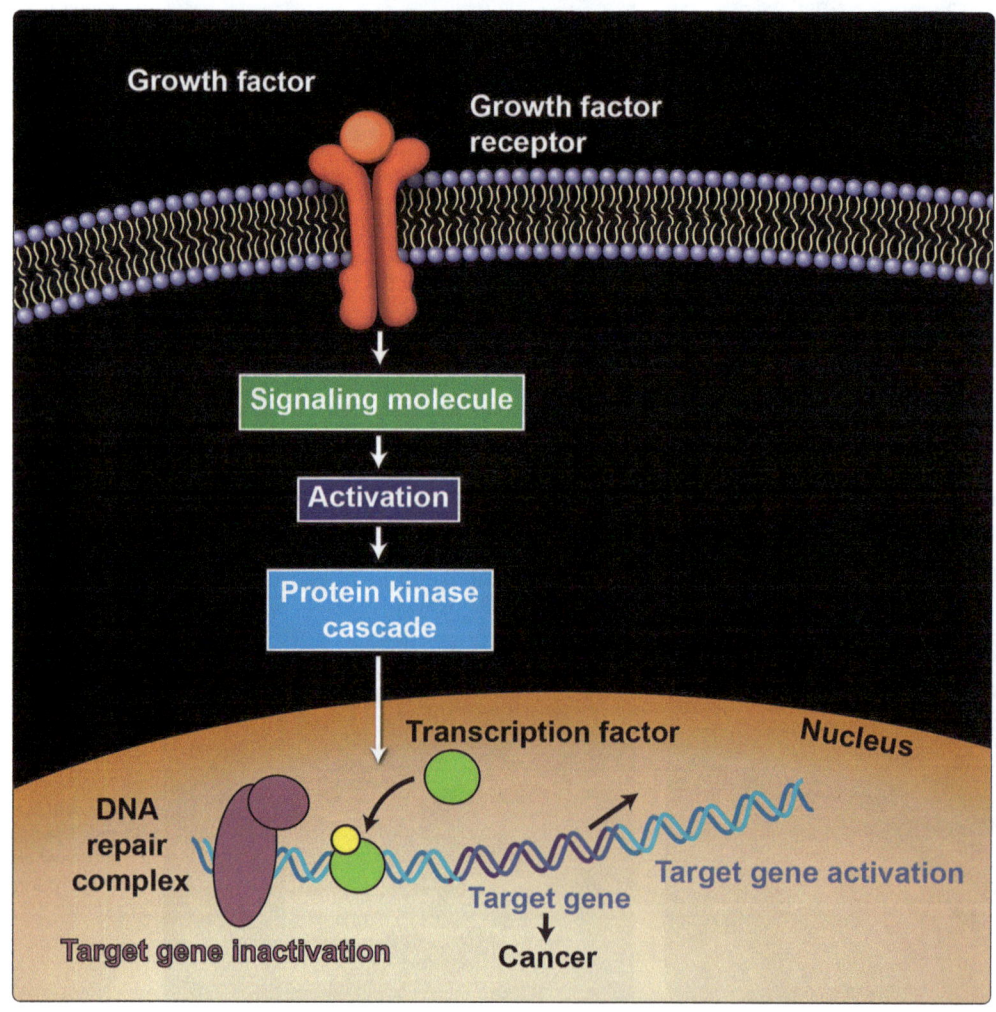

The basic steps of cell signaling are shown to highlight the different mechanisms that are often involved in oncogenesis. Aberrant signaling may occur as a result of growth factor gene amplification, mutations or amplifications (e.g., EGFR, ERBB2), and mutations, methylation, or amplification of genes that encode downstream signaling molecules. Mutations in some signaling molecules may result in constitutive activation (e.g., KRAS, BRAF) or loss of essential negative regulations by deletion or methylation-induced silencing (e.g., PTEN, CDKN2A). Abnormal signaling may thus result in target gene inactivation (e.g., BRCA1, BRCA2) or activation (e.g., CCND1).

Gene Mutations

- o Encode for proteins that repress cell cycle or promote apoptosis
- o Some genes are involved in DNA repair processes
- o Roles may include
  - Repression of genes essential for continuation of cell cycle
  - Coupling of cell cycle to presence of DNA damage
  - Proapoptotic signaling if DNA damage cannot be repaired
  - Cell adhesion proteins that help prevent tumor cells from metastasizing
  - DNA repair proteins (e.g., DNA mismatch repair proteins, *MEN1*- and *BRCA1*/*BRCA2*-encoded proteins)
- o Mutations within tumor suppressor genes result in loss-of-function (recessive in nature)
- o Loss of heterozygosity and "2-hit" hypothesis
  - First proposed by geneticist Alfred Knudson in 1971
  - Both tumor suppressor genes must be mutated in order for particular cell to become cancerous
  - Loss of heterozygosity is phrase often used to describe process that leads to "2nd hit" and results in loss of remaining functional copy of tumor suppressor gene
- o Mutations are often
  - Point mutations or small deletions that disrupt protein function
  - Chromosomal deletions or breaks that delete tumor suppressor gene
  - Somatic recombination during which normal gene copy is replaced with mutant copy
- o At least 30 different tumor suppressor genes have been identified

TERMINOLOGY AND DEFINITIONS

Introduction

- Mutation is thought to imply deleterious genetic sequence variation
  - o This definition is likely overly simplistic
  - o Not all mutations have deleterious effect
- DNA sequence can be altered in various ways
  - o Change in actual sequence
    - Sequence variation
  - o Change in amount of given sequence
    - Copy number variation
  - o Change in position, i.e.,
    - Inversion
    - Translocation
- Gene mutations/sequence alterations have varying effects, depending on where they occur and whether they alter protein function
  - o Where they occur and
  - o Whether they alter protein function
  - o Genetic changes that affect 3rd base in codon are less likely to result in incorporation of incorrect amino acid and therefore rarely alter gene code/protein function
    - Are less likely to result in incorporation of incorrect amino acid
    - Therefore rarely alter gene code/protein function
- Genotype vs. phenotype
  - o Genotype refers to genetic information as it exists in form of nucleic acids
  - o Phenotype refers to how encoded proteins function to create outwardly observable characteristics
  - o Genotypic alterations
    - May or may not result in alterations in phenotype
- Somatic mutations
  - o Acquired mutations that are not inherited from parent and also not passed to offspring
- Germline mutations
  - o Heritable genetic variation/mutation in germ cell (eggs or sperm) lineage
  - o Passed on from parent to offspring
    - Referred to as constitutional mutations in offspring
- Driver mutations
  - o Subset of cancer mutations that provide selective advantage to tumor
    - e.g., *EGFR*, *KRAS*, *EML4::ALK*
  - o Contribute to tumor's growth, progression, and survival (clonal expansion)
  - o Cancer cells rely more heavily on driver mutations than other mutations that are often termed passenger mutations
  - o Driver mutations are more often targets of directed therapy
- Passenger mutations
  - o Typically comprise larger subset of acquired somatic mutations that are not as important to tumor growth and survival
  - o May be associated with clonal expansion because they occur in same genome as driver mutations
  - o Referred to as "hitchhiker" in evolutionary biology
- Polymorphism vs. gene mutations
  - o Numerous single-nucleotide polymorphisms (SNPs) have been identified in human genome
  - o 1 in every 300 nucleotides in human genome is considered polymorphic (i.e., < 1 nucleotide being common in population)
  - o In most cases, SNP has 2 alternative forms (alleles)
    - i.e., A or G at specified nucleotide position
  - o Conceptually, both SNPs and mutations represent variation in genetic sequence
  - o Arbitrary threshold of 1% frequency is widely accepted in making distinction between SNP (polymorphism with frequency of > 1%) and mutation (polymorphism with frequency < 1%)
    - Frequency is thought to be indicative of stability of polymorphism in population
    - High-frequency SNP alleles are not thought to have major consequential phenotypic effects

Types of Mutations

- Missense mutation/substitution
  - o Change in 1 DNA base pair
  - o Results in substitution of 1 amino acid for another
  - o May or may not alter protein function
    - Depends on degree of similarity between amino acids
- Nonsense mutation/substitution
  - o Change in 1 DNA base pair
  - o Results in substitution of 1 amino acid for stop codon

Gene Mutations

- Results in premature termination of translation and truncated protein
  - Truncated protein often function improperly or not at all
- Insertion
  - Addition of ≥ 1 base to original DNA sequence
  - Increases number of DNA bases in gene
  - Protein encoded by gene may not function properly
- Deletion
  - Change in number of DNA bases by removing piece of DNA
  - Small deletions may remove 1 or few base pairs within gene
  - Larger deletions can remove entire gene or several adjacent genes
  - Deleted DNA may alter function of resulting protein(s)
- Duplication
  - Piece of DNA abnormally copied 1 or more times
  - May alter function of resulting protein
- Frameshift
  - Addition or loss of DNA bases that results in change in gene's reading frame
    - Reading frame consists of groups of 3 bases (codon) that each code for 1 amino acid
  - Shifts grouping of these bases and changes overall amino acid code/sequence
  - Resulting protein is usually nonfunctional
    - Insertions, deletions, and duplications can all result in frameshift mutation
    - May result in premature termination if stop codon is formed downstream from mutation
- Repeat expansion
  - Short DNA sequences that are repeated number of times in row, e.g.,
    - Trinucleotide repeat is repeated 3-base pair sequence (e.g., CGT) or
    - Tetranucleotide repeat is repeat of 4-base pair sequence (e.g., CGGT)
    - Increases number of times DNA sequence is repeated
    - Many genes contain these repeats without any alteration in protein function
    - When repeats exceed "normal" range, protein may function improperly or not at all
- Conversion
  - Sequence change where range of nucleotides are replaced by sequence from elsewhere in genome
  - Allelic gene conversion occurs during meiotic recombination
- Deletion/insertion (indel)
  - Sequence change where ≥ 1 nucleotide is replaced by ≥ 1 other nucleotide
  - If only 1 nucleotide is replaced by single other nucleotide, this should be referred to as substitution
- Translocation
  - Chromosome rearrangement between parts of nonhomologous chromosomes
  - 2 chromosomes break, with fragments joining together at "breakpoints"
  - Reciprocal translocation should include description of 1st and 2nd junctions
    - e.g., t(4;X) and t(X;4)
- Transposition
  - Series or range of nucleotides moves from 1 position to another in genome or sequence (i.e., deletion at 1 position is combined with insertion of deleted sequence at another position)

NOMENCLATURE

Introduction

- Consistent and uniform use of nomenclature in management of DNA sequence data is critical for accurate and concise communication of test results and genetic risk assessment
- Unique letter designations
  - Uppercase nucleotide symbols are used when describing DNA (i.e., A, G, C, T)
  - Lowercase nucleotide symbols are used when describing RNA (i.e., a, g, c, u)
  - 3- or 1-letter amino acid codes are used when describing protein/amino acid sequence change (e.g., GLU and E)
    - "Ter" or "*" refers to stop codon
      - "X" was used previously to refer to stop codon
      - Not recommended to be used for stop codon as per Human Genome Society
- Letter designations used to refer to reference sequence
  - Coding DNA: c.
  - Genomic DNA: g.
  - Mitochondrial DNA: m.
  - RNA: r.
  - Noncoding RNA: n.
  - Protein: p.
- Symbols used to describe changes
  - ">" indicates substitution at DNA level
  - "_" indicates range of affected residues, separating 1st and last residue affected
  - "del" indicates deletion
  - "dup" indicates duplication
  - "ins" indicates insertion
  - "inv" indicates inversion
  - "con" indicates conversion
  - "[]" encloses changes from single allele
  - "( )" is used when exact position of change is not known; range of uncertainty is described as precisely as possible and listed between parentheses
- Nucleotide numbering
  - Coding DNA reference sequence (c.)
    - Nucleotide 1 is A of ATG-translation initiation codon
    - There is no nucleotide 0
    - Nucleotide 5' of ATG-translation initiation codon is -1, previous -2, etc.
  - Intronic nucleotides
    - Beginning of intron is denoted by number of last exon in preceding exon followed by plus sign and position of intronic nucleotides (e.g., c.89+1G)
    - End of intron is denoted by number of 1st nucleotide of following exon followed by minus sign preceding upstream intronic nucleotide position (c.89-1T)
    - In middle of intron, plus sign will change to minus sign using these rules
  - Genomic reference sequence

Gene Mutations

- Numbering is arbitrary and starts with 1 at 1st nucleotide of database reference file
- +, -, or other signs are not used
- 3' rule (normalization to 3' end)
  - Applies to variants in stretches of repeated DNA sequences
  - Most 3' position possible is arbitrarily deemed to have been changed
  - e.g., change of 'TTT' to 'TT' is described as g.3del (not g.1del or g.2del)

Nomenclature Examples

- Substitution
  - Designated by ">"
  - Examples
    - c.546A>T describes A to T substitution at nucleotide position 546
    - p.Gln78His describes glutamine to histidine substitution at amino-acid residue 78
    - ">" not used when describing substitution at protein level
- Deletion
  - Designated by "del"
  - Range of deletion indicated by "_"
  - Examples
    - c.546delT, or c.546del describes deletion of T at nucleotide position 546
    - c.586_591del or c.586_591delTGGTCA or c.586_591del6 describes deletion of 6 nucleotides (TGGTCA) starting at nucleotide position 586 to and ending at position 591
- Duplication
  - Designated by "dup"
  - Range of duplication indicated by "_"
  - Examples
    - c.546dupT, or c.546dup describes duplication of a nucleotide (T) at position 546
    - c.586_591dup, or c.586_591dupTGGTCA or c.586_591dup6 describe a duplication of 6 nucleotides (TGGTCA) starting at nucleotide position 586 and ending at position 591
  - Duplications should not be described as insertions
- Insertion
  - Designated by "ins"
  - Range of insertion indicated by "_"
  - Provide inserted sequence
  - Examples
    - c.547_548insT describes insertion of nucleotide T between nucleotides at positions 547 and 548
    - c.1087_1088insTGACGT describes insertion of 6 nucleotides (TGACGT) that occurs between nucleotides at positions 1087 and 1088
  - When insertion is large, inserted sequence can be submitted to database and database accession and version number can be written
- Inversion
  - Designated by "inv"
  - Range of inversion is designated by "_"
  - Example
    - c.547_2032inv 1486 describes sequence of 1,486 nucleotides from nucleotide position 547 to 2032 have been inverted
- Conversion
  - Designated by "con" after indication of 1st and last nucleotides affected by conversion, followed by description of origin of new nucleotides
  - Range of conversion is indicated by "_"
  - Example
    - c.547_658con918_1029 describes conversion replacing nucleotide sequence at position 547 to 658 with new nucleotide sequence originating from position 918 to 1029
    - g.123_678conNG_012232.1:g.9456_10011 describes conversion replacing nucleotides 123 to 678 with nucleotides 9456 to 10011 from sequence as present in GenBank file NG_012232.1
- Translocation
  - Designated by "t"
  - Range indicated by "_"
  - e.g., t(X;4)(p21.2;q35) (c.857+101_857+102)
- Repeated sequences
  - Following format is used when describing repeated sequences: "Position of 1st repeat unit_[number of repeats]"
  - Examples
    - g.123_124[4] describes location of 1st unit of variable sequence (nucleotide position 123 to 124) with number in brackets describing number of repeats present in allele
    - Alternatively, g.123TG[4] describes repeating sequence of TG that repeats 4x where 1st unit (TG) is present at nucleotide position 123_124 in genomic reference sequence
- SNP
  - Database SNP entries designated by "rs"
  - e.g., rs2306220: A>G or g.78654 C>G
- Deletion/insertion
  - Commonly designated as "indel" but may also be designated as "delins"
  - Range indicated by "_"
  - Example
    - c.1166_1177delinsAGT describes deletion that extends from nucleotide position 1166 to 1177 with nucleotides AGT inserted in place of deleted sequence

SELECTED REFERENCES

1. den Dunnen JT: Describing sequence variants using HGVS nomenclature. Methods Mol Biol. 1492:243-51, 2017
2. den Dunnen JT et al: HGVS recommendations for the description of sequence variants: 2016 update. Hum Mutat. 37(6):564-9, 2016
3. HGVS Recommendations for the Description of Sequence Variants: 2016 Update. http://onlinelibrary.wiley.com/doi/10.1002/humu.22981/pdf. Published March 2, 2016. Accessed July 14, 2023
4. Human Genome Variation Society. www.hgvs.org. Updated March 12, 2015. Accessed July 14, 2023
5. Ogino S et al: Standard mutation nomenclature in molecular diagnostics: practical and educational challenges. J Mol Diagn. 2007 Feb;9(1):1-6. Erratum in: J Mol Diagn. 11(5):494, 2009
6. Chial H: Proto-oncogenes to oncogenes to cancer. Nature Education. 1(1):33, 2008
7. Chial H: Tumor suppressor (TS) genes and the two-hit hypothesis. Nature Education. 1(1):177, 2008

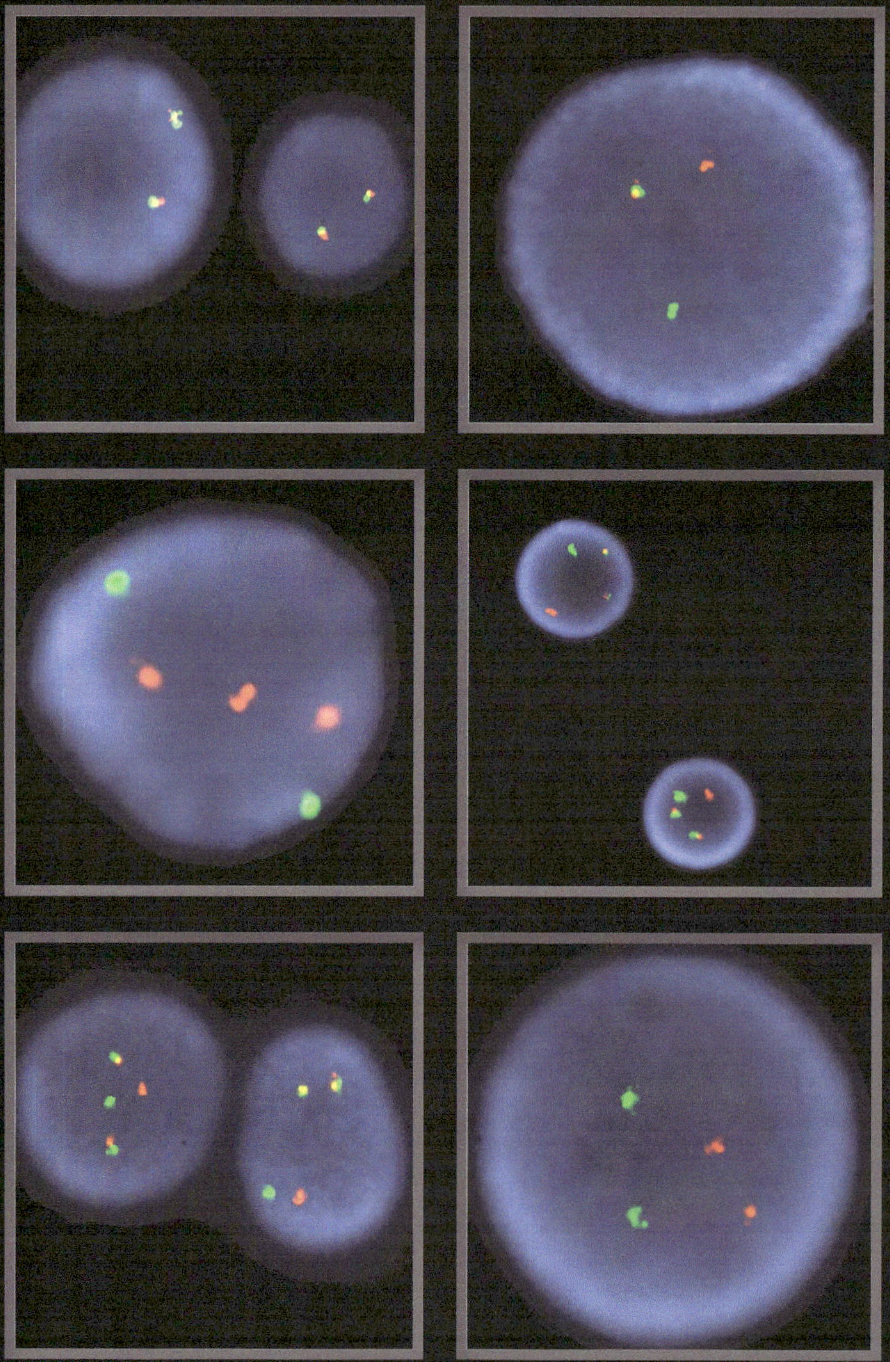

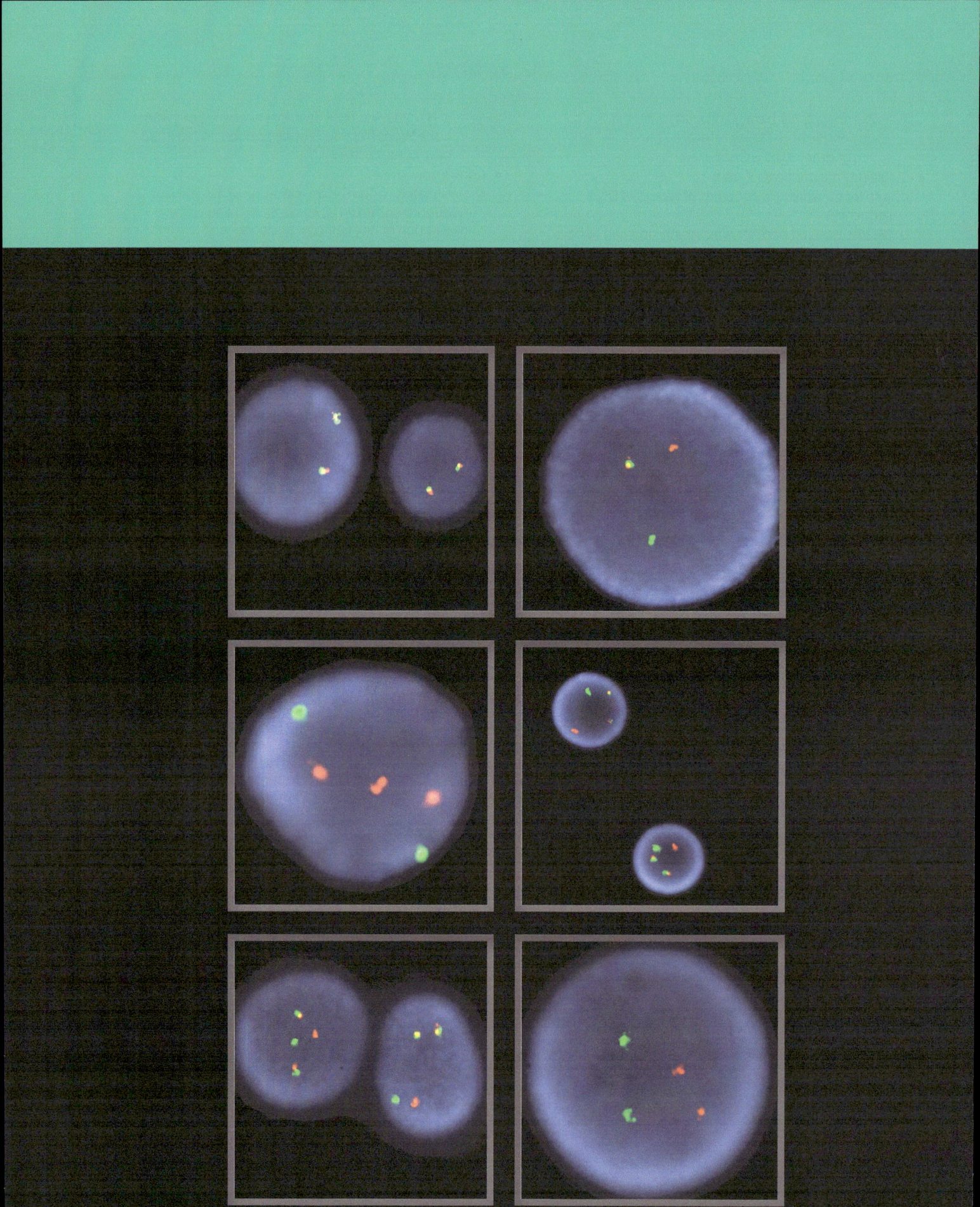

SECTION 2
Common Techniques for Analysis of Alterations in Chromosomes and DNA

Cytogenetics and FISH	18
Chromosomal Microarray	22
Amplification Methods	26
DNA High-Resolution Melting Curve Analysis	30
Sequencing Technologies	32
High-Throughput Methods in Molecular Pathology	36
DNA Methylation Analysis	38

Cytogenetics and FISH

CYTOGENETICS

History

- Historic early explorations
  - 1882: German cytologist Walther Flemming published book describing whole process of mitosis; introduced Aniline staining to observe chromosomes during cell division
  - 1888: German anatomist Wilhelm von Waldeyer-Hartz introduced term chromosome
  - 1902-1903: Walter Sutton and Theodor Boveri proposed chromosomal theory of inheritance
  - 1924: Grigory Andreevich Levitsky coined term karyotype
  - 1959: American pathologist Peter Nowell and research fellow David Hungerford detected tiny chromosome from 2 patients with chronic myeloid leukemia (CML) known as Philadelphia chromosome
    - 1st chromosomal abnormality linked to human neoplasm
- Technical advances
  - 1952: T.C. Hsu discovers that hypotonic solution allows for better separation of chromosomes
    - Serendipitous laboratory error had substituted hypotonic for isotonic solution
  - 1956: Joe Hin Tjio and Albert Levan introduces perfect method for arresting cells in metaphase by using colchicine
    - Permits correct identification of human chromosome number as 46
  - 1960: Peter Nowell discovers that phytohemagglutinin stimulates lymphocytes to divide in culture
    - Allows karyotypes to be produced from normal peripheral blood specimens
  - 1968: Torbjorn Caspersson produced 1st chromosome banding pattern using quinacrine mustard (Q banding)
    - Allows chromosomes and chromosomal regions to be easily identified
  - 1971: Margery Wayne Shaw pioneers Giemsa banding
    - Simpler preparation than fluorescent Q banding; opened era of widespread chromosome analysis
  - 1972: Janet Rowley discovered that Ph chromosome in CML resulted from translocation between long arms of chromosome 9 and 22
    - This finding established cancer as genetic disease
  - 1990s: Optical mapping of genome was originally developed by David Schwartz and his lab at NYU
    - Method has since been integral to assembly process of many large-scale sequencing projects
    - Optical genome mapping (OGM) addresses limitations of existing cytogenetic techniques
      - Offers higher resolution than karyotyping in detecting large-scale structural variants

Sample Requirements

- Living cells are absolutely required for chromosome analysis
  - Cells must be made to divide in culture for successful karyotyping

Technical Procedure

- Living cells are allowed to divide in culture
  - Specific mitogens may be required, depending on specimen type and information desired from study
    - Stem cells, blasts, and many malignant cells have capacity to divide autonomously
    - Terminally differentiated cells (B cells, T cells, and plasma cells) may need stimulation from additional chemicals &/or interleukins in order to divide
- Colchicine is added to culture
  - Inhibits formation of mitotic spindle
  - Dividing cells can no longer progress past metaphase
  - Chromosomes remain in bundled and visible format during this state of "metaphase arrest"
- Hypotonic solution is added to culture
  - Causes water to enter cell and nucleus, which enhances spreading of chromosomes
- Cells are fixed in swollen state
  - Using modified Carnoy solution (3:1 methanol:glacial acetic acid)
- Cells are dropped onto glass slides and stained
  - In situ cultures may also be prepared in similar fashion

Partial Karyotype With t(9;22)

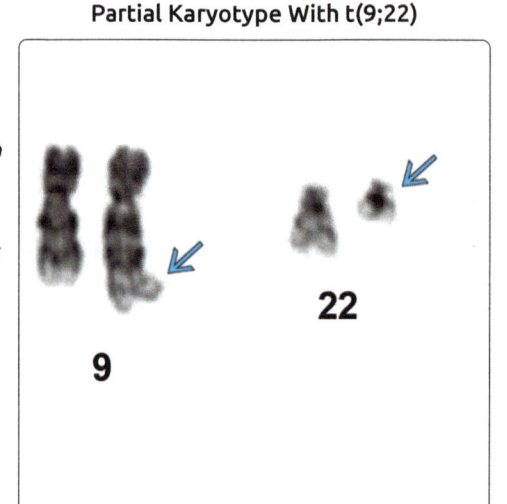

FISH With *BCR::ABL1* Fusion

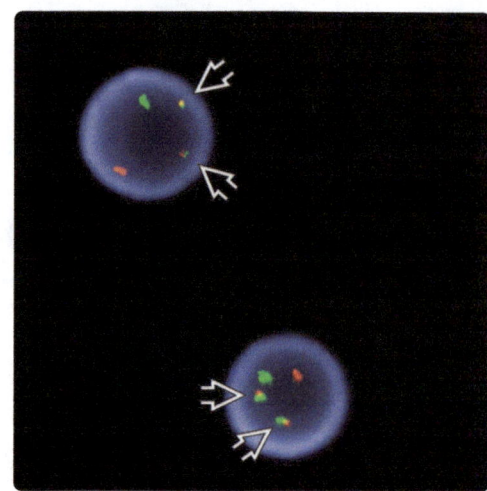

(Left) Partial karyogram shows the t(9;22)(q34;q11.2) associated with BCR::ABL1 fusion ➡. By convention, the abnormal chromosome in each pair is presented on the right side. (Right) FISH for BCR::ABL1 fusion using dual-color, dual-fusion probe shows 2 fusion signals ➡ in each cell. This is a positive result, indicating the presence of BCR::ABL1 fusion.

Cytogenetics and FISH

- Band resolution
  - Number of bands visible depends on sample type and preparation
    - More visible bands yield higher resolution study with greater sensitivity
    - At 450 band resolution (i.e., 450 bands visible in complete karyotype), each band contains ~ 6 Mb of DNA
    - At 850 band resolution, each band would contain ~ 3 Mb of DNA
  - G-banding visual resolution on karyotype is ~ 5-10 Mb in routine practice
    - Abnormalities smaller than this limit will not be detected
- Metaphases are analyzed under light microscope
  - 20 metaphases are analyzed in typical case

Analysis and Nomenclature

- Follows International System for Human Cytogenetic Nomenclature (ISCN) guidelines
- Chromosomal arms
  - Centromere divides each chromosome in short (p) and long (q) arms
- Chromosomal regions
  - Divided into regions, bands, and subbands
  - e.g., 9q34 refers to chromosome 9, long arm, region 3, band 4
    - Said aloud as 9 q three four, not 9 q thirty-four
    - If bands are further divided into subbands, decimal point is used (e.g., 1p31.1)
- Karyotype descriptions
  - Number of chromosomes present is listed 1st, followed by comma
  - Next, sex chromosomes present are listed, followed by comma
  - Finally, any structural &/or numerical abnormalities are listed
  - If ≥ 2 cell lines are present, they are listed individually, separated by "/", and number of counted cells in each cell line is listed in brackets
    - Term idem can be used to indicate abnormalities that 2nd cell line shares with 1st
- Specific terms for structural abnormalities
  - Deletion (del)
    - Part of chromosome is lost
  - Insertion (ins)
    - Part of 1 chromosome is inserted into different area
  - Inversion (inv)
    - Inverted in orientation relative to reference sequence
    - Paracentric inversion affects only 1 chromosomal arm
    - Pericentric inversion involves both p and q arms and thus includes centromere in inverted segment
  - Translocation (t)
    - Exchange of chromosomal regions between 2 different chromosomes
  - Derivative chromosome (der)
    - Structurally rearranged chromosome
  - Marker chromosome (mar)
    - Abnormal chromosome that cannot be identified
  - Ring chromosome (r)
    - Circular configuration with chromosome ends fused

- Criteria for clonality
  - Not every abnormality seen in analysis is considered clonal
    - Random genetic errors may occur during cell culture
  - Clone is defined as
    - 2 cells that share same abnormality, if abnormality is chromosome gain or structural abnormality
    - 3 cells that share same loss of chromosome

Key Types of Clinical Findings

- Aneuploidy
  - Gains or losses of whole chromosomes
  - e.g., Down syndrome, trisomy 21
- Translocations
  - e.g., t(9;22)(q34.1;q11.2)
    - Exchange of chromosomal material between chromosomes 9 and 22 with breakpoints at designated bands on long arms of each
    - Results in *BCR::ABL1* fusion seen in CML and subset of B-lymphoblastic leukemia/lymphoma

Clinical Utility of Cancer Cytogenetics

- For diagnosis
  - Establish neoplastic diagnosis due to presence of clone
    - e.g., monosomy 7 may permit confident diagnosis of myelodysplastic syndrome
  - Establish specific subtype of neoplasm due to cytogenetic abnormality characteristic of that neoplasm
    - e.g., t(8;21)(q21.3;q22.1) permits diagnosis of specific subtype of acute myeloid leukemia
- For prognosis
  - Determine likely behavior of neoplasm based on cytogenetic abnormalities
    - e.g., presence of 17p deletion in chronic lymphocytic leukemia is associated with aggressive disease course
- Identifying residual disease
  - Track presence of neoplasm over time based on presence of previously established clonal abnormalities
- Identifying clonal evolution
  - Detect acquisition of additional cytogenetic abnormalities over time in neoplasm, which may be linked to more aggressive behavior

FLUORESCENCE IN SITU HYBRIDIZATION

History

- Radiolabeled probes were cumbersome and dangerous
- In 1980, fluorescently labeled probe was 1st used
  - Limited by dim fluorescent signal of early probes
- By early 1990s, improved probe labeling technology allowed routine detection of target nucleic acids

Sample Requirements for FISH

- In contrast to chromosome analysis, FISH can be performed on nondividing (interphase) cells, including
  - Fixed cells, paraffin-embedded tissue sections, air-dried smears, touch preparations, or cytospin preparations
- May also be performed on metaphase cells

Technical Procedure

- Pretreatment
  - Includes dehydration of slide with graded ethanol series

Cytogenetics and FISH

Advantages and Disadvantages of Cytogenetics and FISH for Clinical Applications

	Advantages	Disadvantages
Cytogenetics		
	Global look at entire karyotype	Low resolution
		Living cells required for analysis
		Relatively slow (1-2 weeks in average)
		Cryptic abnormalities may not be detected
FISH		
	High resolution	Limited scope (will not detect abnormalities in regions not probed)
	Any cells can be studied, including nonliving, fixed, and paraffin-embedded cells	
	Relatively fast (24-48 hour turnaround time)	
	Many cells can be counted	

- Codenaturation and hybridization
  - Fluorescently labeled probe specific to DNA target sequence is applied
  - Slide is heated to denature double-stranded DNA
  - Slide is incubated for 14-20 hours at temperature permitting hybridization of probe to target DNA
- Final slide preparation
  - Excess probe is washed away
  - Mounting medium with DAPI counterstain is applied
    - DAPI stains DNA at fluorescent wavelength different from that of probe
    - Permits visualization of nuclei under fluorescent microscope

Key Probe Strategies

- Numerical chromosome enumeration probes
  - Hybridize near centromeric region of chromosome
  - Detects presence or absence of specific chromosome
- Dual-color, dual-fusion probes
  - Used to detect specific translocations
    - 2 genes involved in translocations are labeled in different colors (typically red and green)
    - Translocation will result in 2 fused signals
    - Presence of 2 fusion signals in cell is highly specific for translocation in question
- Break-apart probes
  - Used if only 1 gene involved in translocation is known
  - Red and green probes are labeled on either end of gene
    - If there is translocation, red and green signals will become separated
    - Partner gene cannot be identified by this approach

Nomenclature

- Follows International System for Human Cytogenetic Nomenclature (ISCN) guidelines
- Interphase FISH is indicated by "nuc ish"
  - Followed by locus designation for probe, "x," and number of signals seen
  - If signals have become juxtaposed (as with dual-fusion probe), this is indicated with "con" followed by, in brackets, number of cells in which abnormality was seen
    - e.g., FISH in typical new diagnosis of CML could be written as "nuc ish(ABL1x3),(BCRx3),(ABL1 con BCRx2)[162/200]"
- Cases are classified as positive or negative based on established laboratory-specific cutoffs

Clinical Utility of FISH

- For diagnosis
  - e.g., rapid diagnosis of APL by detection of *PML::RARA* fusion
- For prognosis
  - e.g., detection of *TP53* deletion in chronic lymphocytic leukemia
- Detection of residual disease
  - Requires known FISH detectable abnormality
- Noninvasive detection of fetal aneuploidy
  - Successfully performed on fetal nucleated RBCs isolated from maternal blood

SELECTED REFERENCES

1. Balducci E et al: Optical genome mapping refines cytogenetic diagnostics, prognostic stratification and provides new molecular insights in adult MDS/AML patients. Blood Cancer Journal, 2022. https://doi.org/10.1038/s41408-022-00718-1
2. Liehr T: Molecular cytogenetics in the era of chromosomics and cytogenomic approaches. Front Genet. 12:720507, 2021
3. ISCN 2020: An International System for Human Cytogenetic Nomenclature. McGowan-Jordan J, ed. Report of Cytogenetic and Genome Research. Vol 160, No. 7-8, 2020
4. Huber D et al: Fluorescence in situ hybridization (FISH): History, limitations and what to expect from micro-scale FISH? Micro and Nano Engineering, 2018. https://doi.org/10.1016/j.mne.2018.10.006
5. Feng C et al: Non-invasive prenatal diagnosis of chromosomal aneuploidies and microdeletion syndrome using fetal nucleated red blood cells isolated by nanostructure microchips. Theranostics. 8(5):1301-11, 2018
6. Stevens-Kroef M et al: Cytogenetic nomenclature and reporting. Methods Mol Biol. 1541:303-9, 2017
7. Cooley LD et al: Section E6.5-6.8 of the ACMG technical standards and guidelines: chromosome studies of lymph node and solid tumor-acquired chromosomal abnormalities. Genet Med. 18(6):643-8, 2016
8. Campbell LJ: Cytogenetic analysis and reporting. Methods Mol Biol. 730:259-68, 2011

Cytogenetics and FISH

PML::RARA Fusion-Negative FISH

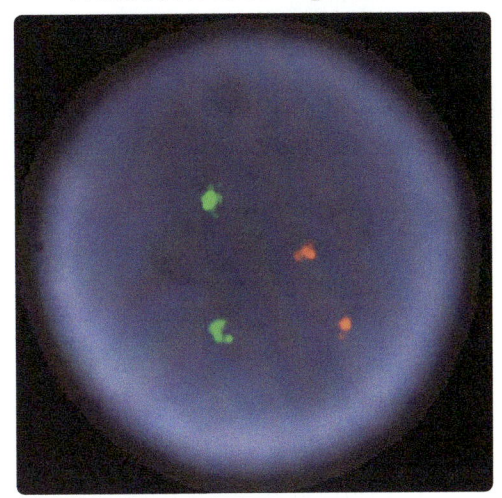

PML::RARA Fusion-Positive FISH

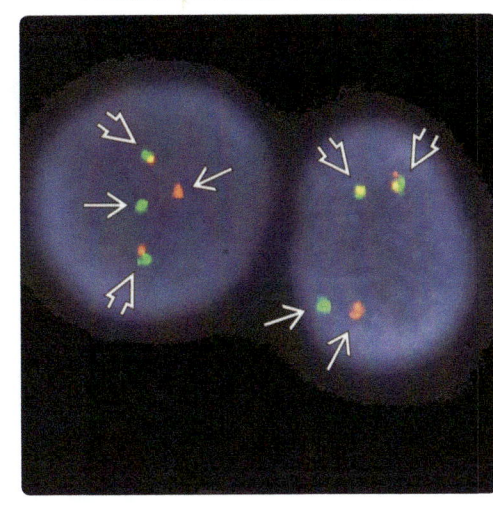

(Left) FISH for PML::RARA fusion using a dual-color, dual-fusion probe shows a negative result. Red and green signals, corresponding to PML and RARA, respectively, remain undisturbed, indicating absence of fusion. (Right) FISH for PML::RARA fusion using a dual-color, dual-fusion probe shows a positive result. Two fusion signals per cell ⇨ indicate the presence of gene fusion. Intact red and green signals ⇨ correspond to the uninvolved alleles.

FISH Break-Apart Probe With Intact CBFB

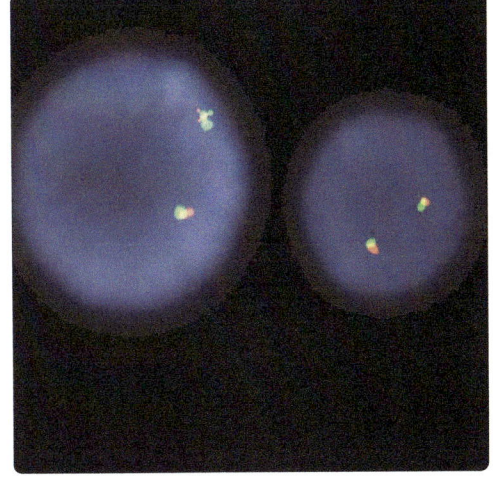

FISH Break-Apart Probe With Rearranged CBFB

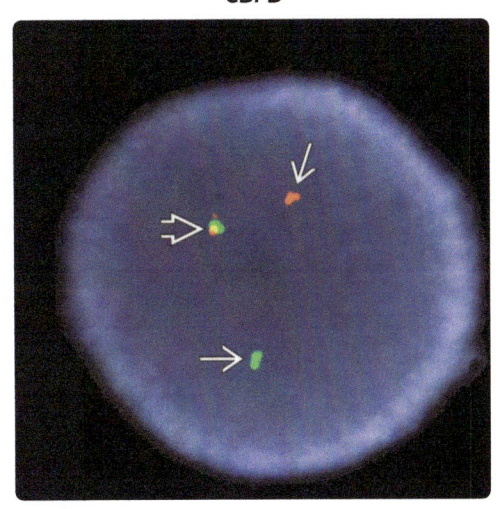

(Left) FISH for CBFB rearrangement using a break-apart probe shows a negative result. Each cell shows 2 fused signals, corresponding to undisturbed alleles of CBFB (each bracketed by red and green probes). (Right) FISH for CBFB rearrangement using a break-apart probe shows a positive result. The separate red and green signals ⇨ indicate rearrangement of 1 allele. The fused signal ⇨ corresponds to the undisturbed 2nd allele.

FISH on Metaphase Preparation

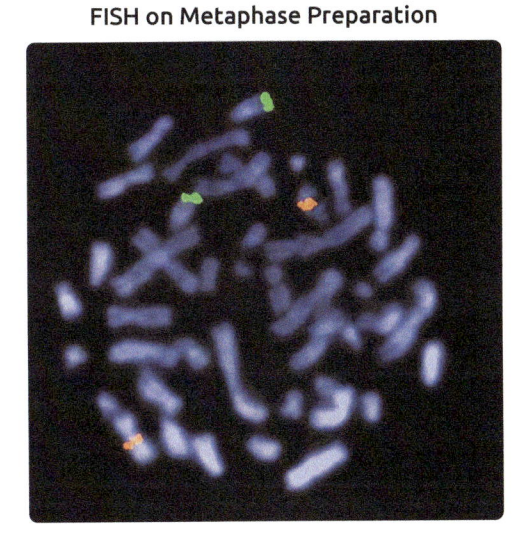

FISH on Blood Sample With Trisomy 21

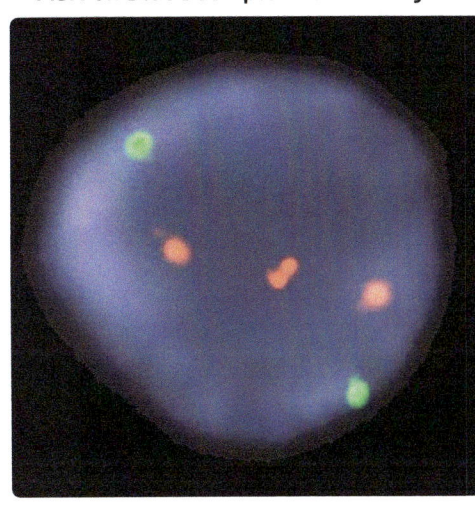

(Left) While clinical FISH assays are most often performed on interphase cells, FISH can also be performed on metaphase preparations. A dual-color, dual-fusion probe for CCND1::IGH fusion was hybridized to this metaphase, showing a normal pattern negative for fusion. (Right) FISH can be used to enumerate chromosomes. Here, 3 red signals indicate trisomy 21 in a patient with Down syndrome. The green probes show a normal pattern for chromosome 13.

Chromosomal Microarray

TERMINOLOGY

Abbreviations
- Chromosomal microarray analysis (CMA)

Definitions
- Molecular cytogenetic method used to analyze genomic copy number variations (CNVs)
  ○ Relative ploidy level of DNA of test sample is compared to reference sample/reference DNA database
  ○ Improved resolution for detection of genomic microdeletions and microduplications compared to conventional cytogenetics and FISH
    – Locus-specific probes used in FISH requires prior knowledge of expected chromosomal aberration
  ○ Prior knowledge of chromosomal aberration is not required in CMA
  ○ No cell culture needed in CMA

Types of Microarrays
- Array-based comparative genomic hybridization (aCGH)
  ○ Detects copy number changes
- Single nucleotide polymorphism (SNP)-based CMA
  ○ Detects copy number changes
  ○ Also detects copy-neutral changes
    – Loss of heterozygosity (LOH)
    – Uniparental disomy (UPD)
    – Identity by descent or consanguinity

METHODS AND TECHNIQUES

Array-Based Comparative Genomic Hybridization
- Microarray platform contains bacterial artificial chromosome (BAC) probes or oligonucleotide probes covering whole genome
  ○ BAC probes are ~ 150 kb in size
    – Evenly spaced at ~ 1-Mb resolution across genome
  ○ Oligonucleotide probes are ~ 45-60 kb in size
    – Average resolution of ~ 30 kb throughout genome
- Test DNA and control DNA labeled with different fluorescent dyes

Comparison of Genomic Resolution in Cytogenetics, FISH, and CMA

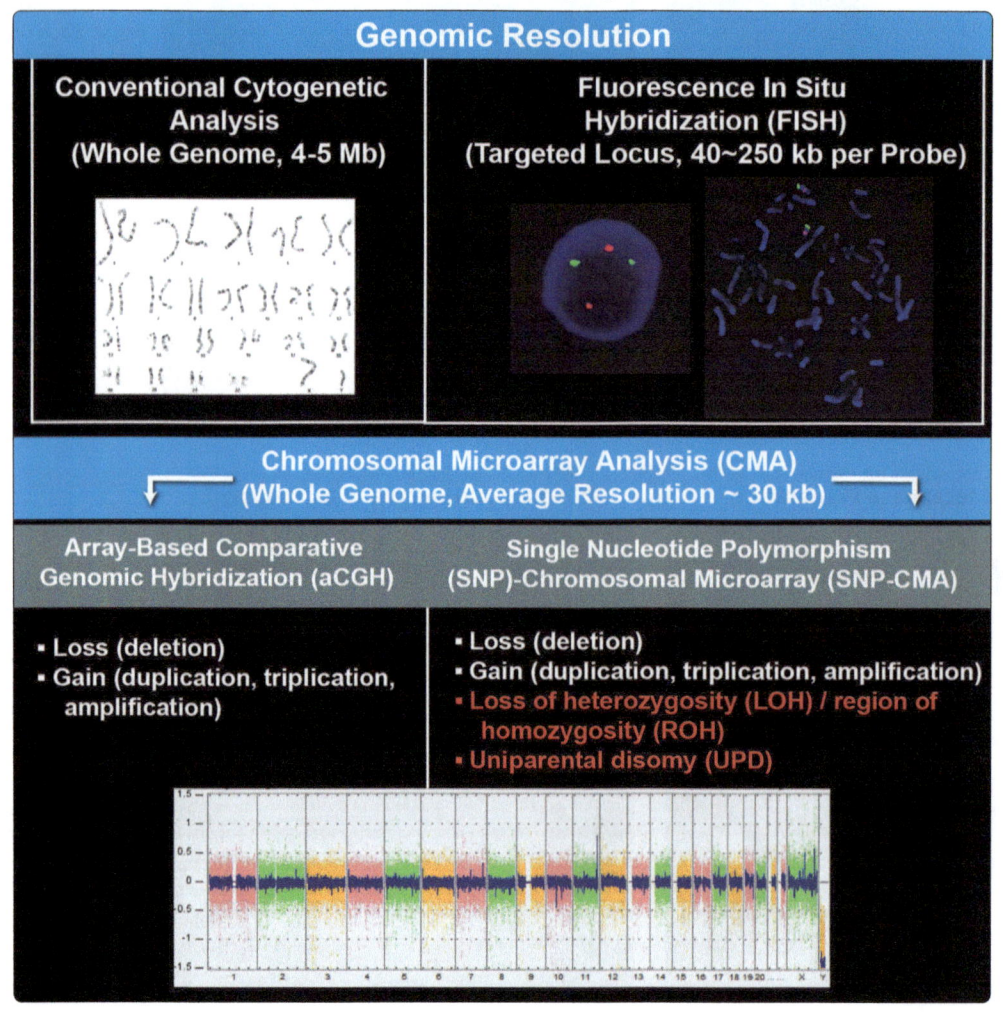

Three different platforms are currently used for chromosomal analysis. Conventional cytogenetic analysis (upper left) detects numerical and structural chromosomal abnormalities with a low resolution of 4-5 Mb. Cryptic and submicroscopic abnormalities will not be detected by this technique. FISH (upper right) detects aberration in only specific chromosomal regions that are targeted by FISH probes with a resolution of ~ 40-250 kb. In contrast, chromosomal microarray analysis (CMA) (lower 1/2) detects submicroscopic genomic copy number variations, which may not be detectable by cytogenetics &/or FISH.

Chromosomal Microarray

- o Cyanin dyes Cy3 and Cy5
- Both test and control DNAs are hybridized to DNA chip
- Relative signal intensity ratio for each individual probe is normalized and converted to log2 ratio
  - o Log2 acts as proxy for copy number
- Signal intensity of test DNA is compared to control DNA
  - o Higher intensity in specific genomic region indicates duplication
  - o Lower intensity in specific genomic region indicates deletion

Single Nucleotide Polymorphism Chromosomal Microarray

- SNP microarray contains both nonpolymorphic copy number probes and SNP probes
  - o Nonpolymorphic copy number probes used to assess copy number changes
  - o SNP probes used to assess both genotype and copy number changes
    - e.g., Affymetrix CytoScan HD array contains ~ 750,000 unique SNPs and 1.9 million nonpolymorphic copy number probes
- Only test DNA is hybridized to DNA array
- Similar to aCGH, relative signal intensity ratio for each individual probe is normalized and converted to log2 ratio
- Signal intensity of test DNA is compared to in silico DNA reference database to determine specific genomic imbalances
- For given SNP with 2 alleles (A or B), data are represented by 3 allelic tracts
  - o AA (homozygous), AB (heterozygous), BB (homozygous)
- SNP genotyping allows detection of copy-neutral changes that are not detectable by aCGH platform

CHROMOSOMAL ABERRATIONS

Aberrations Detected by Array-Based Comparative Genomic Hybridization

- Genomic copy number losses (i.e., deletions)
- Genomic copy number gains (i.e., duplications, triplications, amplifications)

Aberrations Detected by Single Nucleotide Polymorphism Chromosomal Microarray Analysis

- Genomic copy number losses
- Genomic copy number gains
- LOH
- Region of homozygosity (ROH)
- UPD, specially isodisomy

Limitations of Chromosomal Microarray Analysis

- Cannot detect point mutations
- Cannot detect balanced chromosomal rearrangements, including balanced inversions, translocations, insertions
- Low-level mosaicism may not be detected
- Tetraploidy cannot be detected
- CNVs of regions not represented on platform will not be detected
- Cannot detect epigenetic variations, such as methylation

CLINICAL IMPLICATIONS

Constitutional Abnormalities

- Genome-wide detection of clinically significant copy number abnormalities
  - o Chromosomal aneuploidy, microdeletions, microduplications
    - Significantly higher diagnostic yield than conventional karyotype
- Detects UPD of imprinted chromosomes and consanguinity
  - o UPD and consanguinity are not detectable by aCGH
- Cost-effective test for genetic diagnosis of unexplained developmental delay and intellectual disability compared to cytogenetics
  - o Testing of both parents may also be cost-effective when variant of unknown significance is detected in patient

Prenatal Diagnosis

- Common indications for prenatal CMA testing
  - o Advanced maternal age (≥ 35 years at expected delivery)
  - o Enlarged nuchal translucency
  - o Abnormal ultrasound findings
  - o Family history of recurrent pregnancy loss
  - o Abnormal maternal serum screening
  - o Abnormal noninvasive prenatal screening test using cell-free fetal DNA in maternal circulation
  - o Patients with normal fetus undergoing invasive prenatal diagnostic testing (e.g., chorionic villus sampling)
  - o Patients with fetus with ≥ 1 structural abnormality
- DNA is usually obtained from chorionic villus sampling or amniocentesis

Products of Conception (i.e., Fetal Demise or Stillbirth)

- Common chromosomal abnormalities seen in products of conception
  - o Whole-chromosome aneuploidies, including autosomal trisomies and monosomy X
  - o Polyploidies, including triploidy and tetraploidy
- DNA is obtained from fetal &/or placental tissue
- CMA testing eliminates need for cell culture
  - o More complete and faster than fetal chromosomal analysis

Postnatal Diagnosis

- Recommended as 1st-tier diagnostic test for detection of chromosomal imbalances in patients with clinical suspicion for
  - o Autism spectrum disorder
  - o Nonsyndromic developmental delay/intellectual disability
  - o Multiple congenital anomalies
- DNA is usually obtained from peripheral blood lymphocytes

Neoplastic Conditions

- Genome-wide detection of cancer-associated copy number abnormalities
  - o Acquired whole-chromosome aneuploidy
  - o Acquired deletions, duplications, amplifications
  - o Acquired segmental UPD, copy-neutral LOH
- Hematologic malignancies
  - o Chronic lymphocytic leukemia (CLL)

Chromosomal Microarray

- Detects deletions of 6q, 11q, 13q, 17p, and trisomy 12
- SNP array detects both copy number abnormalities and copy-neutral events, such as UPD
- DNA is typically obtained from diagnostic blood, bone marrow aspirate, or fresh lymph node
- Can also be tested on DNA isolated from diagnostic paraffin-embedded fixed tissues
  - Burkitt-like lymphoma with 11q aberration
    - Detects minimal region of proximal gain at 11q23.2-23.3 and terminal losses at 11q24.1-ter
  - Acute myeloid leukemia (AML)
    - Higher detection rate of copy number alterations (CNA) and LOH in AML compared to conventional cytogenetics
    - Useful in cytogenetic (-) and molecular high-risk (-) (intermediate-risk) AML cases
    - Useful in AML cases with unobtainable or inadequate cytogenetics
    - Could prove useful in AML with unusual morphologic and immunophenotypic findings
    - Recommended by some authors for refractory and relapsed AML cases
  - Myelodysplastic syndrome (MDS)
    - Detect monosomy 5, del(5q), monosomy 7, del(7q), +8, del(20q)
    - Detects acquired segmental UPD
    - Detects cryptic chromosomal lesions in MDS
- **Solid tumors**
  - Detects copy number aberrations and copy-neutral LOH
  - Melanoma
    - Deletions of 1p, 3q, 5q, 6q, 9p, 10p, 10q, 11q, 14q
    - Gains of 1q, 6p, 7p, 7q, 8q
    - Helps in differentiating melanoma from benign nevus
  - Prostate cancer
    - Genome-wide LOH may be detected
  - Renal cell carcinoma
    - Deletions of 3p, 1p, 2q, 6q, 9p, monosomy 14, and gains of 5q and 8q
  - Lung and colorectal cancer
    - Targetable CNVs may be detected in cases (-) for pathogenic mutations by NGS
    - Potential benefit with combining CMA and NGS in lung and colorectal cancer
  - DNA isolated from diagnostic paraffin-embedded tissue is suitable for testing

CLINICAL INTERPRETATION

Pathogenic Copy Number Variations
- Clinically significant based on multiple peer-reviewed publications

Copy Number Variations of Uncertain Clinical Significance
- Uncertain, likely pathogenic
  - Described in single case report
  - Compelling genes in CNV interval relevant to patient clinical findings
- Uncertain, likely benign
  - Large CNVs with no genes
  - Described as benign in general population based on small number of cases
- Uncertain
  - Described in multiple contradictory publications &/or in database

Benign
- Known common polymorphism
  - Reported in multiple peer-reviewed publications or curated database

Comparison of CMA With Optical Genome Mapping
- **CMA**
  - Genome-wide detection of clinically significant copy number abnormalities
  - Recommended as 1st-tier clinical diagnostic tool for individuals with developmental disabilities or congenital anomalies
  - Significantly higher diagnostic yield than conventional karyotype
    - Detects chromosomal aneuploidy, microdeletions, and microduplications but not balanced structural variants and orientation of duplicated segments
    - Cost-effective test for genetic diagnosis of unexplained developmental delay and intellectual disability compared to cytogenetics
- **Optical genomic mapping (OGM)**
  - Recently introduced method with potential to become promising cytogenetic tool for prenatal diagnosis, having resolution down to ~ 500 bp
  - Recent studies have shown 100% concordance with CMA findings in detection of pathogenic variants
  - OGM apparently provides additional insight into genomic structure of abnormalities that CMA is unable to provide
  - OGM can provide CNVs as well as balanced and unbalanced chromosomal aberrations, including insertions, inversions, and complex alterations in single test
  - OGM misses detection of whole-arm translocation, telomeric, centromeric, and pseudoautosomal region aberrations

Resources for Interpretation of Copy Number Variations
- Online Mendelian Inheritance in Man (http://www.ncbi.nlm.nih.gov/omim)
- Database of Genomic Variants (DGV) (http://dgv.tcag.ca/dgv/app/home)

SELECTED REFERENCES
1. Barseghyan H et al: Comparative benchmarking of optical genome mapping and chromosomal microarray reveals high technological concordance in CNV identification and structural variant refinement. MedXriv. Preprint. Accessed July 2023. https://doi.org/10.1101/2023.01.21.23284853
2. Liu X et al: Potentials and challenges of chromosomal microarray analysis in prenatal diagnosis. Front Genet. 13:938183, 2022
3. Lee JS et al: Chromosomal microarray with clinical diagnostic utility in children with developmental delay or intellectual disability. Ann Lab Med. 38(5):473-80, 2018
4. Xu X et al: Assessing copy number abnormalities and copy-neutral loss-of-heterozygosity across the genome as best practice in diagnostic evaluation of acute myeloid leukemia: an evidence-based review from the Cancer Genomics Consortium (CGC) myeloid neoplasms working group. Cancer Genet. 228-99:218-35, 2018

Chromosomal Microarray

Normal Copy Number

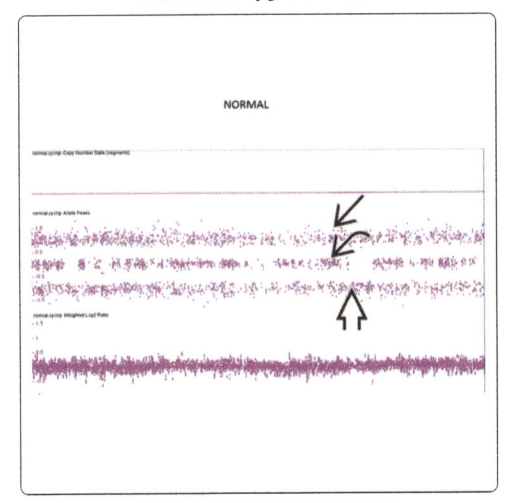

Monosomy X

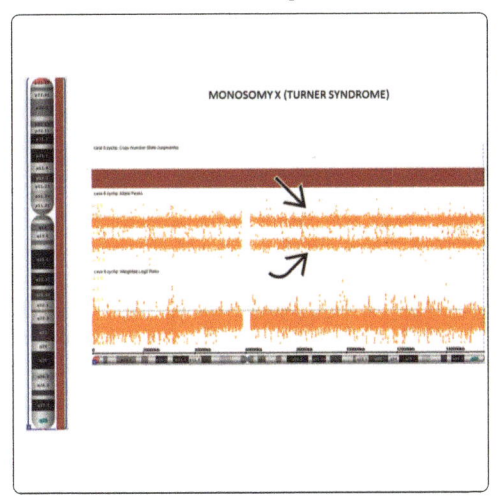

(**Left**) *Microarray using Chromosome Analysis Suite (ChAS) with Affymetrix CytoScan HD array shows normal copy number findings. There are 3 allele difference tracts: Homozygous (AA) ➡, heterozygous (AB) ➡, and homozygous (BB) ➡. The log2 ratio = 0.* (**Right**) *CMA shows monosomy X. Notice there are only 2 allele difference tracts, both of which are hemizygous (A ➡ and B ➡) with a log2 ratio of -0.5 in the entire X chromosome.*

Trisomy 21 (Down Syndrome)

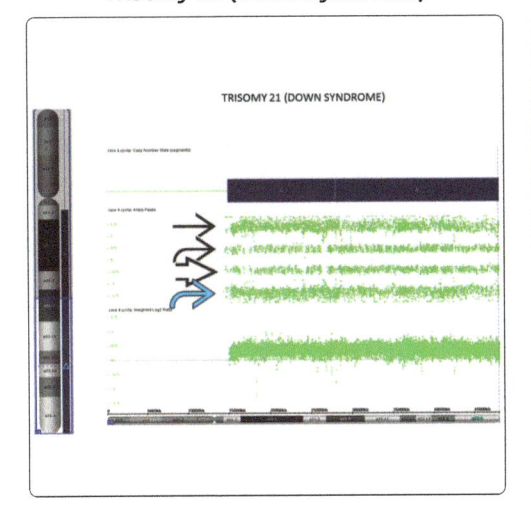

Copy-Neutral Loss of Heterozygosity

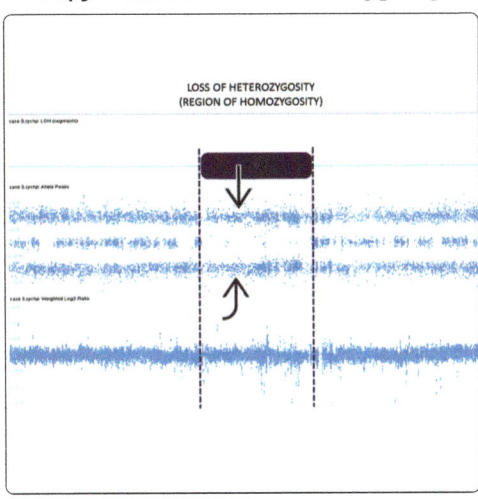

(**Left**) *Microarray shows trisomy 21. Notice 4 allele difference tracts (AAA ➡, AAB ➡, ABB ➡, and BBB ➡) with a log2 ratio > 0.3 in the entire chromosome 21.* (**Right**) *Copy-neutral loss of heterozygosity (cnLOH) is shown. Notice that between the purple dotted lines there are only 2 allele difference tracts (homozygous AA ➡ and homozygous BB ➡). The log2 ratio = 0 (normal copy number findings).*

Duplication

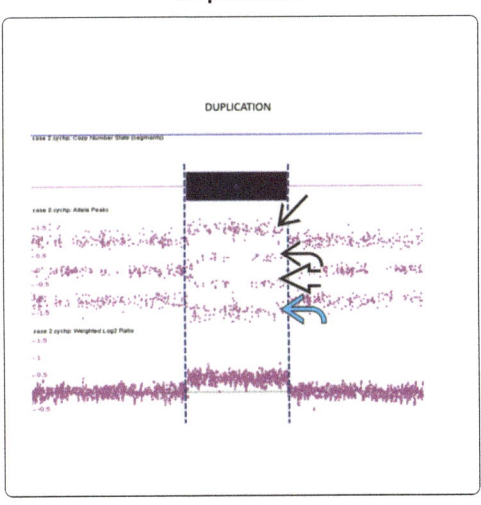

Deletion

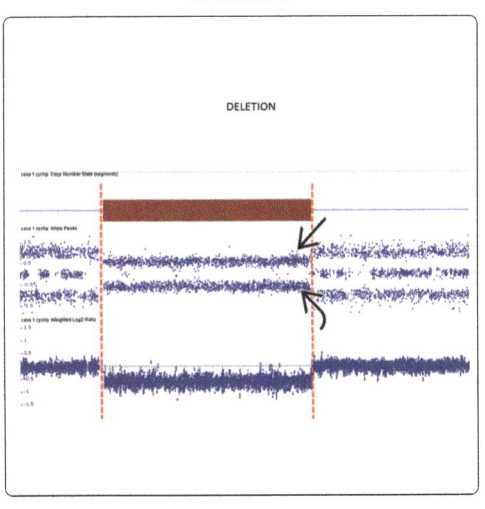

(**Left**) *Microarray illustrates duplication. Four allele difference tracts are seen between the blue dotted lines (AAA ➡, AAB ➡, ABB ➡, and BBB ➡). The log2 ratio is > 0.3.* (**Right**) *Microarray illustrates deletion. There are only 2 allele difference tracts between the red dotted lines. Both A ➡ and B ➡ are hemizygous.*

Amplification Methods

TERMINOLOGY

Definitions

- Target amplification increases amount of nucleic acid of interest
  - Modern molecular methods chiefly rely on polymerase chain reaction (PCR) and modifications of PCR
    - Foundation of molecular pathology
    - Basis of majority of clinical molecular diagnostic testing
  - Much faster than earlier methods, such as Southern blot analysis
  - Can handle high volumes of testing
  - Highly specific
  - Highly sensitive
    - Can detect as few as 10 target molecules per reaction in some situations
    - Produces large quantities of product from rare targets, allowing for analysis
    - Contamination of preamplification areas must be prevented
- Signal amplification increases detection of target without amplifying nucleic acids
  - Less contamination risk
  - Mainly used in infectious disease testing

POLYMERASE CHAIN REACTION

Standard Polymerase Chain Reaction

- Most widely used method of nucleic acid amplification
- Exponentially amplify target sequences of DNA
  - Products of each reaction act as templates in additional reactions
    - Exponentially increases copies of region of interest
  - PCR product amplicons are specific predicted size, bounded by ends of primers used
- Reaction mix includes template DNA, primers, DNA polymerase, deoxynucleotide triphosphates (dNTPs), and reaction buffer

Polymerase Chain Reaction

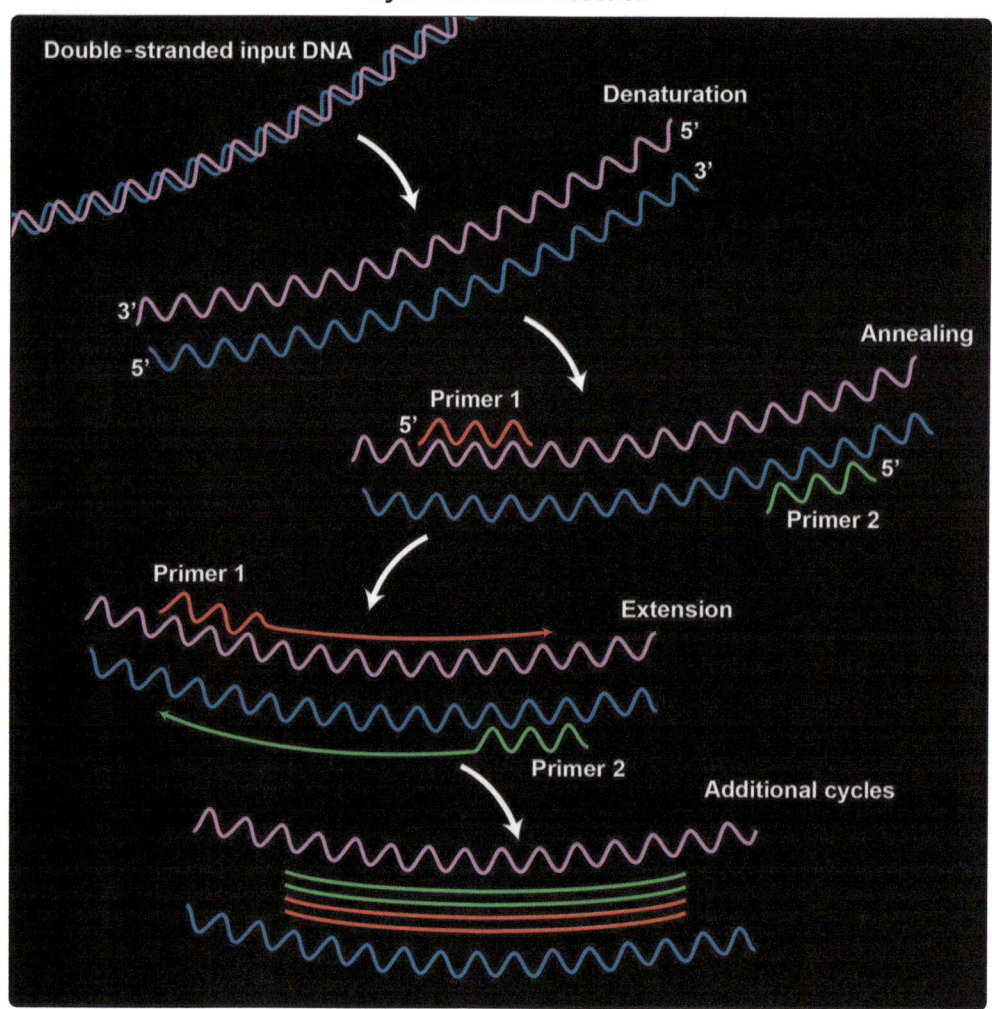

Polymerase chain reaction is shown. First, input DNA is heated and denatured. The reaction is cooled to annealing temperature so that the forward and reverse primers can anneal to the template. The sample is then heated to extension temperature, and DNA polymerase extends the primers. The newly synthesized DNA overlaps the binding site of the opposite primer. This means that the amplicon can act as template for subsequent cycles. The cycle of denaturation, annealing, and extension is repeated many times (thermocycling). The end result is exponentially increased numbers of the target sequence with each product being a predicted size.

Amplification Methods

- Template DNA may be isolated from fresh, frozen, formalin-fixed paraffin-embedded (FFPE), cDNA derived from RNA, and other specimen types
  - Targets are usually short fragments, 200-2,000 bp in length
  - FFPE specimens usually have DNA fragmentation and produce smaller lengths of DNA
  - Amount of template required depends on nature of source and target sequence
- Primers created to target region of interest
  - Primer design is most important factor in PCR sensitivity and specificity
  - Provide specificity of reaction
  - Should target unique sequence
  - Complementary to opposite strands (forward and reverse)
  - Designed so that amplicon produced will include binding site of opposite primer
  - Can be around or overlap area of interest
  - Must not have intraprimer homology, or partially double-stranded (secondary) structures will occur
  - Must not contain regions complementary to other primer, or primers will hybridize (primer dimer)
  - Primer length affects specificity, reaction temperatures, and reaction efficiency
  - Usually 17-30 nucleotides in length
  - Should have 45-55% GC content
  - Usually have G or C at 3' end to improve specificity
  - Annealing temperature should be 5° lower than melting temperature
  - Many internet tools for primer design available
- Heat-stable DNA polymerase required for modern PCR
  - *Thermophilus aquaticus* (*Taq*)-derived polymerase most commonly used
  - 5' to 3' polymerase activity
  - 5' to 3' exonuclease activity
  - Error rate: 1×10^{-4} to 2×10^{-5} errors per base pair
  - Other polymerases are available with lower error rates and 3' to 5' exonuclease activity
  - Improved *Taq* polymerases with modifications to prevent low temperature activity and mispriming and improve specificity are available
- dNTPs (building blocks of DNA) required to synthesize DNA
  - Excess dNTPs leads to decreased specificity
- Reaction buffer controls pH and ion concentrations for optimal performance
  - Optimum pH usually between 8 and 10
  - Magnesium (Mg^{2+}) required for polymerase performance
  - Lower Mg^{2+} increases specificity of primer-template binding
  - Higher Mg^{2+} decreases reaction specificity and inhibits denaturation
  - Mg^{2+} and pH must be optimized for specific primers and desired outcomes
  - Additives, such as bovine serum albumin (BSA) and dimethyl sulfoxide (DMSO), may be included
- Reaction depends on temperature cycling
  - Thermocyclers are used to control temperature cycles
    - Temperatures at each step may be adjusted to alter sensitivity and specificity of reaction
  - Specimen is heated to melting point so DNA becomes single stranded (denaturation stage)
    - Usually ~ 92-94 °C
    - More accurate calculations available
    - Usually ~ 1 minute long
  - Specimen is cooled so that primers and template bind (annealing stage)
    - Annealing stage temperature depends on specific primer length and sequence
    - Temperature can be adjusted to change specificity of binding
    - Cooler temperatures more stringent
    - Warmer temperatures more permissive of mismatched primer-template binding
    - Usually ~ 1 minute long
    - Longer times lead to decreased specificity
  - Specimen is heated to amplification temperature, and synthesis occurs (extension stage)
    - Temperature depends on polymerase, usually 70-80 °C for *Taq* polymerase
    - Usually ~ 2 minutes long
  - Specimen is again heated to melting point (denaturation stage)
    - DNA and primer dissociate
  - Specimen is again cooled to annealing temperature
    - Primers can bind to products of previous amplification step as well as input DNA
  - Specimen is again heated to amplification temperature
    - Results in exponential production of amplicons
  - Steps are repeated many times
    - ≥ 30 cycles may be used
    - Number of cycles depends on required sensitivity and specificity
    - Amount of product depends on starting level of target
    - Increase of 2^n, where n = number of cycles, is expected
    - Production eventually plateaus based on reaction components
- Products can be analyzed using number of methods, including sequence-specific methods
  - Gel electrophoresis
  - Capillary electrophoresis
  - Melting curve analysis
  - Restriction fragment length polymorphism analysis (RFLP)
  - Allele-specific oligonucleotide hybridization (dot-blot analysis)
  - Oligonucleotide ligation (sequence-specific oligonucleotide probe) assay
  - Denaturing gradient gel electrophoresis
  - Temperature gradient gel electrophoresis
  - Heteroduplex analysis
  - Single-strand conformation polymorphism
  - Denaturing high-performance liquid chromatography
  - Protein truncation test
  - Cloning
  - Sequencing

Amplification Methods

- Limitations of PCR
  - Contamination must be stringently prevented
    - Small amounts of DNA contamination lead to exponential amplification
    - Risk reduced by using good laboratory practices, using dedicated equipment, and separating pre- and post-PCR areas
  - Routine tissue processing may prevent amplification
    - Decalcification of bony tissue using solutions containing strong acids significantly induces DNA degradation and prevents amplification of even small targets
    - Formalin fragments DNA and can prevent amplification of large sequence targets
    - Some tissue compounds, such as hemoglobin and urea, act as PCR inhibitors

VARIANTS OF POLYMERASE CHAIN REACTION

Reverse Transcription Polymerase Chain Reaction

- Allows for analysis of RNA through reverse transcription of cDNA
  - Often used for fusion gene analysis
  - Used to evaluate gene expression
  - cDNA is more stable than RNA
  - Extremely sensitive: Even very small input sequences can be amplified
- Template RNA is isolated from cells or tissue and may be total RNA or mRNA
  - RNA is inherently unstable, and RNase is ubiquitous, so careful isolation is required
  - mRNA may have complex secondary structures, which interfere with denaturation
- cDNA primers used
  - Oligo dT primers bind to poly A tail on mRNA
  - Not useful when region of interest is far (> 1 kb) from 3' end of mRNA
  - Gene-specific oligonucleotide primers may be used
- Reverse transcriptase required
  - RNA-dependent DNA polymerase
  - Creates cDNA from RNA template
  - Moloney murine leukemia virus or avian myeloblastosis virus polymerases commonly used
  - Enzymes with both reverse transcriptase and DNA polymerase activity are available
- RNase is added to digest RNA after reverse transcription, leaving only cDNA
- cDNA produced is used as template for conventional-type PCR reactions as described above

Real-Time Polymerase Chain Reaction

- Allows detection and quantification of target DNA molecule
  - Measures gene transcripts when combined with reverse transcription PCR (RT-PCR)
  - Often used for residual disease testing, e.g., in chronic myeloid leukemia (CML)
- Based on detection of fluorescence during PCR
  - Signal increases in direct proportion to amount of product formed
  - Measured during exponential phase
  - Cycle threshold (CT) is set at which fluorescence signal correlates to initial amount of template
  - Higher the input template level, lower the CT
  - Usually compared to amplification level of control gene
- Different types of probes available
  - Intercalating dyes
    - Fluoresce when bound to any double-stranded DNA
    - Signal measure at end of each cycle (annealing stage)
    - Not sequence specific
    - Can bind to primer dimers or nonspecific product
    - Examples include SYBR green and ethidium bromide
- Sequence-specific fluorescent labeled probes
  - More specific to desired product
  - TaqMan probes
    - Short sequences with 5' reporter fluorophore and 3' quencher
    - 5' to 3' exonuclease activity of *Taq* polymerase releases reporter from quencher, allowing fluorescence
    - Fluorescence measured during extension phase
  - Molecular beacon probes
    - Longer sequences with 5' reporter fluorophore and 3' quencher
    - Form hairpin structure when not bound to DNA, bringing ends together and quenching fluorescence
    - Binding to target amplicon by central loop section opens hairpin and separates dyes, leading to fluorescence
    - Fluorescence measured during annealing phase
  - Fluorescence resonance energy transfer (FRET) probes
    - 2 separate probes are used
    - One has donor fluorophore, other has acceptor
    - Usually one is to mutation of interest and other is to nearby sequence
    - When both probes bind, energy is transferred from donor to acceptor, and fluorescence occurs
  - Scorpion primers
    - Type of molecular beacon
    - Extremely sensitive, specific, and rapid
    - Gives stronger signal than other types of probes
    - Contain primer with 5' reporter fluorophore and 3' quencher
    - Primer forms hairpin structure, bringing ends together and quenching fluorescence
    - During PCR, hairpin opens and fluorophore is separated from quencher
    - During annealing step, primer acts as probe and binds to amplicon, separating dyes and leading to fluorescence
  - Duplex scorpion primers
    - Similar to original scorpion primers but with 2 separate complementary primers
    - One is bound to reporter fluorophore and other is bound to quencher
    - Results in lower background
  - Other types of sequence specific probes are available
- Workflow considerations
  - High-throughput test
    - Requires no post-PCR analysis
    - Highly reproducible

Amplification Methods

- Cannot be multiplexed

Multiplex Polymerase Chain Reaction
- PCR using multiple primers that simultaneously amplify several different targets in single reaction
- Used for detection of sequence at multiple sites, as in massively parallel sequencing (NGS)
- Can be multiple sites within 1 gene or region or in multiple genes
- Can be used to amplify control gene, such as housekeeping gene, along with gene or genes of interest
- Reaction conditions can be difficult to optimize
  - Amplification bias is important concern
    - Primers may need to be added in different concentrations
    - Different efficiency of reaction
  - Different primers may have different reaction temperatures
  - Higher risk of primer-dimer formation
  - Higher risk of nonspecific amplification

Droplet Digital Polymerase Chain Reaction
- Utilizes water-oil emulsion droplets that act as partitions to separate nucleic acid molecules
- Sample is partitioned into thousands of droplets and PCR reaction occurs separately in each one
- Allows highly sensitive target detection

Amplification-Refractory Mutation System
- Best for identification of point mutations or single base pair variants
- 3' mismatch between primer and target DNA prevents amplification
  - Primers are designed with base of interest (e.g., single base mutation) at 3' end
  - Production of amplicon indicates presence of base of interest
  - Control primer must also be used to confirm amplification
- Most effective with A to G or G to A mismatches
- Stringent reaction conditions further increase specificity
  - PCR conditions must be carefully optimized
- Can be combined with multiplex PCR to interrogate for multiple bases of interest
- Usually rapid and inexpensive
- Cannot screen for unknown mutations
- a.k.a. allele-specific PCR (ASPCR), PCR amplification of specific alleles (PASA), and sequence-specific primer (SSP) amplification

Nested Polymerase Chain Reaction
- 1st round of PCR performed using standard PCR methods
- 2nd round of PCR then performed using primers internal to 1st set of primers
  - Template enriched for 2nd round of PCR
- Increases overall specificity
  - Noise produced in 1st round of PCR eliminated by 2nd
  - Can be used to find extremely rare target sequences
- Increases overall sensitivity
  - Template is enriched so very low levels of target can be identified
  - Very sensitive to contamination

Restriction Site-Generating Polymerase Chain Reaction
- Artificially creates restriction site that can be recognized by RFLP analysis
- Primers are designed that include site of interest
- Contain mismatch adjacent to site of interest
  - Mismatch incorporated into amplicon
  - Creates novel restriction site
  - Product digested with restriction enzyme and analyzed
- PCR efficiency is decreased due to mismatched base
- Technique not possible for all sequences

Multiplex Ligation-Dependent Probe Amplification
- Utilizes 2 adjacent DNA probes with generic sequences added to ends
  - DNA is denatured and probes bind
- Primers complementary to generic sequences are used
  - 1 primer is fluorescently labeled so that generation of amplicon is measured
- All reactions use same generic primers and, therefore, same PCR parameters
  - 1 reaction can use multiple different-sized probes to different targets with same generic sequence
  - Amplicons are different sizes and can be separated
- Can identify large deletions and copy number changes
  - Mutations in probe-binding area may prevent amplification and appear as deletions

Whole-Exome and Whole-Genome Amplification
- Elimination of amplification bias is essential
  - Primers often tagged with adapter sequences
    - Serve as primers for additional cycles
      - Reduces nonspecific amplification of amplicons
    - May cause amplicons to form hairpin loops
      - Block amplification of amplicons
  - Primers may be randomly generated or degenerate
  - Special enzymes to improve uniformity and decrease nonspecific amplification available

Other Techniques
- Other techniques are more common outside of oncology testing, such as in infectious disease testing
  - Isothermal amplification
  - Transcription mediated amplification
  - Branched DNA amplification

SELECTED REFERENCES
1. Wang X et al: Recent advances and application of whole genome amplification in molecular diagnosis and medicine. MedComm (2020). 3(1):e116, 2022
2. Oliveira BB at al: Isothermal amplification of nucleic acids: the race for the next "gold standard". Front. Sens., 28 September 2021. http://doi.org/10.3389/fsens.2021.752600
3. Green SJ et al: Deconstructing the polymerase chain reaction: understanding and correcting bias associated with primer degeneracies and primer-template mismatches. PLoS One. 10(5):e0128122, 2015
4. Garibyan L et al: Polymerase chain reaction. J Invest Dermatol. 133(3):1-4, 2013
5. Bernard PS et al: Real-time PCR technology for cancer diagnostics. Clin Chem. 48(8):1178-85, 2002
6. O'Leary JJ et al: The polymerase chain reaction in pathology. J Clin Pathol. 50(10):805-10, 1997
7. Rogers BB: Application of the polymerase chain reaction to archival material. Perspect Pediatr Pathol. 16:99-119, 1992

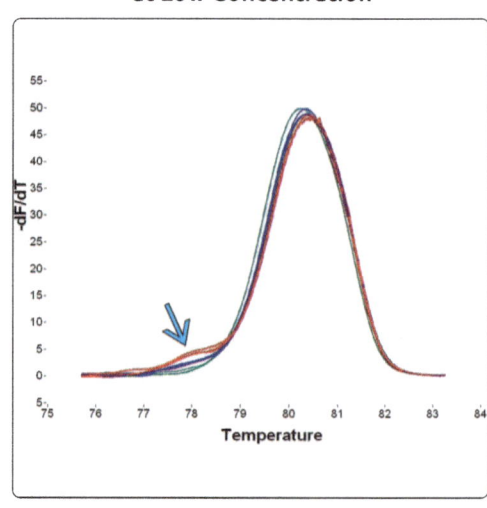

DNA High-Resolution Melting Curve Analysis

TERMINOLOGY

Abbreviations
- High-resolution melting (HRM)

Definitions
- Laboratory technique used to screen for sequence variations, typically in 1 strand of DNA

INTRODUCTION

General Features
- HRM is mainly used as screening tool to identify potential change in sequence (sequence variation)
  - Typically identifies sequence variation in 1 strand of DNA
  - Does not provide information on specific sequence variant or its significance
- Can also be used to detect methylation status (methylation-sensitive HRM)
  - Needs bisulfite DNA digestion prior to amplification and HRM analysis
- Sensitivity of HRM is generally proportional to degree of sequence variation and its percentage
  - In general, detection of sequence variations that are due to deletions or insertions is easier
- Prior PCR amplification of target DNA needed
  - Current instruments can perform both PCR amplification followed by HRM within closed system

PRINCIPLES

Overview
- DNA strands are attached to one another by hydrogen bonds between complementary bases
- Gradual increase in temperature breaks down hydrogen bonds between 2 DNA strands
  - Double-stranded DNA dissociated into 2 separate strands by gradual increase in temperature
    - Fluorescent dye bound to double-stranded DNA
    - When DNA strands dissociate, dye separates from DNA and its fluorescence decreases

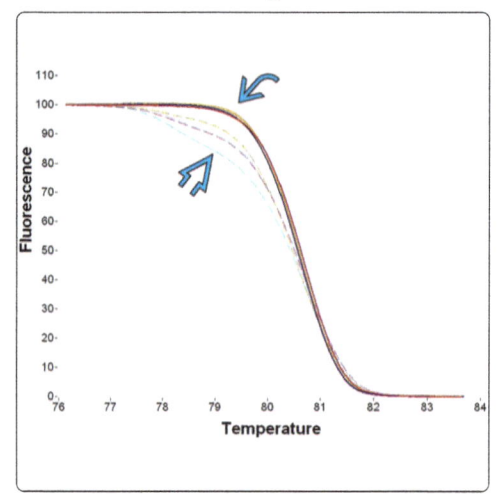

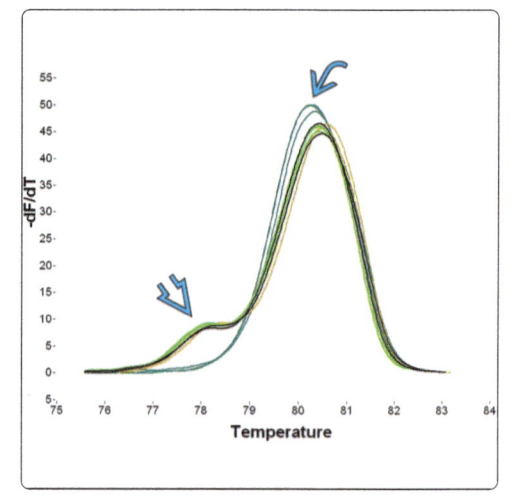

(Left) Melting curves of multiple specimens show those with wildtype DNA ⇨ and those with DNA containing sequence variations ⇨. **(Right)** Derivative of the melting curve easily separates abnormal melting curves of the specimens with sequence variation ⇨ from those that contain wildtype DNA ⇨.

(Left) Melting curve changes are shown as the percentage of DNA containing sequence variation increases in specimen with lowest percentage ⇨ to specimen with highest percentage ⇨. **(Right)** The abnormal-appearing melt ⇨ might represent a sequence variation at low percentage; however, DNA damage induced by formalin fixation can produce similar change. Sequence confirmation must be done in these cases.

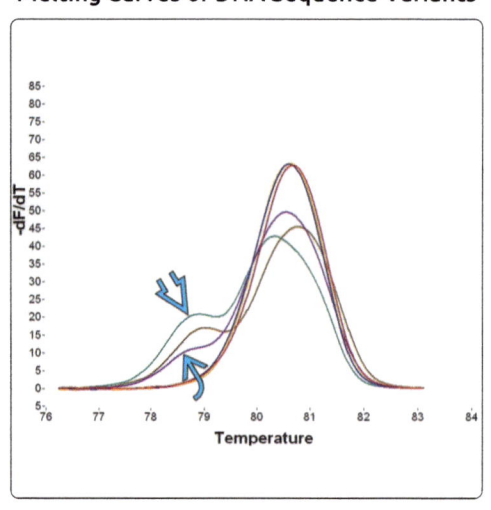

DNA High-Resolution Melting Curve Analysis

- As temperature increases, information on DNA dissociation is gathered through measuring changes in fluorescence activity
  - Curve that reflects changes in fluorescence intensity is called melting curve
- In DNA strands with complete homology in sequences, all nucleotide bases at each position are complementary and are annealed via hydrogen bonds
  - Sequence variation in 1 allele in given position prevents annealing and formation of hydrogen bonds in that position
    - Results in DNA melting at earlier temperature due to lesser numbers of hydrogen bonds to break
    - Shape of melting curve will be different from one generated by completely homologous DNA strands
- Sequence variation will be missed if specimen does not contain wildtype DNA
  - Homozygous variants in high concentration will not be detected
  - Mixing specimen with known wildtype DNA sequence (mixing studies) will enable detection of homozygous mutation in high concentration
- Melting curve analysis is based on comparison between melting curve of test sample and melting curve of known wildtype DNA
  - Deviations of melting curve from known wildtype curve indicate presence of sequence variant
- Temperature at which 50% of double-stranded DNA become single stranded is called melting temperature (Tm)

High Resolution
- Ability of melting method to assess sequence variation at high precision
- Achieved through 2 main improvements
  - Highly controlled temperature transitions and data acquisition
  - Better fluorescent dyes
    - Can be used at concentrations that produce maximum fluorescence intensity

Fluorescent Dyes
- Intercalating dyes bind to double-stranded DNA
  - When bound, they fluoresce brightly; when unbound, they fluoresce at low level
- For HRM application, dyes must be used at saturating concentration without inhibiting PCR to prevent dye molecule redistribution during melting
  - e.g., LCGreen I, LCGreen Plus, EvaGreen, SYTO and Chromofy

Amplicon Sizes
- Smaller the amplicon size, easier to identify smaller sequence variations, such as single-base changes
  - Amplicon size ≤ 50 bp is generally adequate to provide good differentiation for single-base differences
- Amplicons ≥ 300 bp should be avoided

PRE-HRM SPECIMEN PREPARATIONS

DNA Isolation and Amplification
- DNA is isolated from patient specimen
  - Fresh specimen or paraffin-embedded tissue is suitable for analysis
- DNA is amplified through PCR using specific primers that flank sequence of interest
  - Primer design is crucial to avoid risk of primer-dimer formation
  - Primers should produce amplicon size that is appropriate for HRM

CLINICAL IMPLICATIONS

Rapid Screening
- Base changes, best for amplicons ≤ 50 bp
- Insertions/deletions can be detected in larger amplicon sizes
- Sequence confirmation of DNA with abnormal melting curves generally needed

INTERPRETATION OF FINDINGS

Quality Controls
- Must include positive and negative controls and control that contains PCR mix but no DNA template (blank)
- Samples and quality controls should be preferentially run in replicates
  - Can help to ensure reproducibility

Analysis of Results
- Melting curves of test DNA compared to melting curves of known controls in same run
  - Melting curves matching with negative controls are interpreted as negative
    - Homozygous variants in high concentration should be excluded by mixing studies
  - Melting curves not matching with negative controls are interpreted as positive
    - Further sequencing needed in most cases
    - Sequencing defines exact sequence change and its clinical significance
    - Nonpathogenic polymorphisms within amplicon must be excluded
  - In certain circumstances, presumptive diagnosis can be rendered based on analysis of melting curve
    - Laboratory must have fully validated procedure in place for interpretation of given test if bypassing sequencing confirmation
- Potential false-positive results
  - Primer dimers may potentially induce false-positive results
    - Melt is typically seen at unusually early temperature compared with true positive results, which are typically at higher temperature
    - Careful design of primers can help in preventing primer dimer formation

SELECTED REFERENCES

1. Shoute LCT et al: Characterization of the binding interactions between EvaGreen dye and dsDNA. Phys Chem Chem Phys. 20(7):4772-80, 2018
2. Sa'adah N et al: A rapid, accurate and simple screening method for spinal muscular atrophy: high-resolution melting analysis using dried blood spots on filter paper. Clin Lab. 61(5-6):575-80, 2015
3. Er TK et al: High-resolution melting: applications in genetic disorders. Clin Chim Acta. 414:197-201, 2012
4. Wittwer CT: High-resolution DNA melting analysis: advancements and limitations. Hum Mutat. 30(6):857-9, 2009

Sequencing Technologies

TERMINOLOGY

Definitions

- **Sequencing**: Identifying nucleotide order in nucleic acids
- **1st generation**: Generally refers to Sanger sequencing
- **2nd generation**: Includes massively parallel sequencing
  - Library preparation: Preparing sample DNA to become input for sequencing
  - DNA library: Pool of DNA or cDNA fragments with adapters designed to interact with specific sequencing platform, multiplexed samples traceable through indexed adapter sequences
  - Clonal amplification: PCR amplification of individual DNA fragment for sequencing analysis
- **3rd generation**: Includes techniques for long-read DNA sequencing without fragmentation or amplification

SEQUENCING TECHNIQUES

Sanger Sequencing

- **Original methodology**
  - Introduced by Frederick Sanger in mid 1970s
  - Method based on DNA chain termination
  - Polymerase chain reaction (PCR) reaction performed in 4 separate tubes (A, T, C, G)
  - Each tube contains DNA template, primer, polymerase, and all deoxynucleotides (dNTPs)
  - "Chain-terminating" dideoxynucleotides (ddNTPs) added to specific tubes
    - ddNTPs lack critical hydroxyl group, required for addition of subsequent nucleotides
    - ddATP added to tube A, ddTTP to tube T, etc.
    - When polymerase randomly incorporates ddNTP, chain synthesis stops
  - At PCR completion, tubes contain numerous synthesized DNA fragments of variable lengths
    - All fragments have same terminating base at 5' end; determined by ddNTP type in given tube
  - Fragments are separated by size/length in gel electrophoresis
  - Sequence read from bottom to top in sequencing gel radiogram
  - Point and indel mutations detected at ~ 20% sensitivity
- **Semiautomated Sanger methodology**
  - Single-tube PCR with fluorophore-labeled ddNTPs
  - DNA fragments separated by capillary electrophoresis
  - Fluorescence from terminating ddNTP is read and translated into colored peaks
  - Peak tracing order corresponds to DNA sequence
- **Limitations**
  - Low throughput
  - Low sensitivity; limit of detection ~ 15-20%
  - Not cost effective for high numbers of targets
  - Not recommended in samples with low input amounts of starting nucleic acids
  - Low discovery power

Pyrosequencing

- **Methodology overview**
  - Single-stranded DNA template incubated with 4 enzymes and 2 substrates
    - DNA polymerase, ATP sulfurylase, luciferase, apyrase, adenosine 5' phosphosulfate (APS), and luciferin
    - 4 dNTPs sequentially and cyclically added to reaction in predefined dispensation order
  - Pyrophosphate, byproduct of dNTP incorporation, enzymatically converted to light
    - ATP sulfurylase converts pyrophosphate to ATP in presence of APS
    - ATP powers oxidation of luciferin, generating light; intensity recorded in "pyrogram"
    - Apyrase removes unincorporated nucleotides and ATP, prior to addition of next dNTP
  - Light intensity reflects number of dNTPs added
    - Peak associated with 3 nucleotides in tandem is 3x taller than peak seen with single dNTP incorporation
  - Sequence determined by signal peak height review in pyrogram tracing
  - Sequencing method based on DNA synthesis

Images of Sanger Sequencing

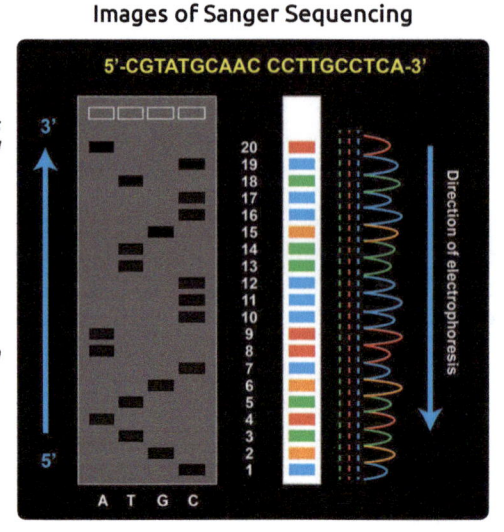

Image of Steps in Pyrosequencing

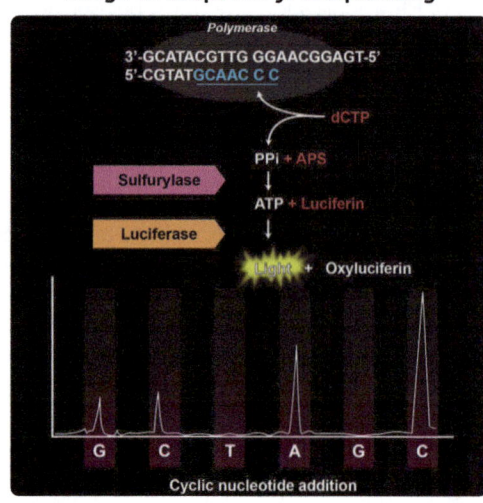

(Left) This schematic image shows original Sanger sequencing using ddNTPs, sequencing gel electrophoresis (left half), and semiautomated Sanger sequencing using fluorescent dyes and capillary electrophoresis (right 1/2). (Right) This image shows the enzymes and substrates employed in DNA sequencing in pyrosequencing platform. The sequence on the pyrogram at the top of the image will be read as GCAACCC.

Sequencing Technologies

- – Developed by Ronaghi and Nyren in 1996, preceding 2nd-generation sequencing
- o Variant detection sensitivity of ~ 5%
- **Limitations**
  - o Read lengths limited by progressively inefficient apyrase degradation
  - o Nucleotide misincorporation errors may occur in homopolymer regions
  - o Requires special instrumentation

Massively Parallel Next-Generation Sequencing
- High throughput fragment sequencing with massively parallel read analysis
  - o Principle driver of "genomics revolution" and accessibility to clinical genetic analysis
  - o Generates hundreds of millions of short sequences in single run, in short period of time, with low per-base cost
  - o Ability to pool different patient samples on same run
  - o Is possible due to technological improvements in microfabrication and high-resolution imaging
  - o General steps include library preparation, clonal amplification, and sequence analysis
- **Library preparation**
  - o Enrichment for target regions; commonly used methods include
    - – Amplicon-based multiplex PCR
      - □ Amplicons simultaneously created in multiplex PCR reaction using primers designed against gene regions of interest
      - □ Amplicons partially digested then adapters/index are ligated to create library
      - □ Requires less input nucleic acid, has fewer steps and lower cost when compared to hybridization capture
    - – Hybridization capture
      - □ Sample nucleic acid is fragmented, followed by ligation of adapters/index
      - □ Oligonucleotide probes then hybridized to fragments with target regions of interest for capture
      - □ Method does not require PCR primer design
      - □ May be more sensitive/better performing than amplicon-based multiplex PCR in mutation detection
  - o Adapter sequence ligation to 5'- and 3'-fragment ends
    - – One adapter often contains primer annealing site
    - – 2nd adapter sequence used to anchor fragment to surface for sequencing
    - – Index/barcode sequence included to tag individual samples for batched specimen runs
      - □ Individual sample data is separated out from pooled/batched sample runs in postsequencing bioinformatic analysis using index/barcode
  - o Size selection optimizes sequencing quality/efficiency
  - o Final library quantification and quality control
    - – All downstream processes depend on library quality
    - – Libraries normalized to ensure uniform representation in pooled/batched testing
- **Clonal amplification**
  - o Introduces amplification-related sequence errors
  - – All polymerases will introduce some sequencing errors; degree of fidelity to template sequence will vary depending on specific polymerase
  - – In-vitro assays lack DNA repair mechanisms that are present in vivo
  - o Multiple DNA libraries can be pooled and sequenced in same run
  - o Library fragments are separated in 3D space, allowing amplification/identification of unique clonal PCR products
    - – Fragments separated and then attached to platform-dependent solid substrate
- **Sequencing chemistry**
  - o Various methods may be used to detect integration of complementary nucleotide
  - o Common methods include optical detection of fluorophore-labeled nucleotides and semiconductor sequencing via measurement of pH changes resulting from release of H+ ions generated as byproduct of nucleotide addition
- **Sequence analysis**
  - o Bioinformatic processing of sequencing data generates multiple files
  - o Demultiplexed data from sequencer are often stored as FASTQ file
    - – Text file of unaligned reads with 4 lines of data per sequence: Sequence identifier, sequence, comments, and quality scores
  - o Sample sequence is aligned to known reference, creating SAM, BAM, or CRAM file
    - – Sequence alignment map (SAM)
      - □ Text file containing alignment information of various sequences that are mapped against reference sequences
      - □ More readable by humans, given text file formatting
    - – Binary alignment map file (BAM) and compressed reference-oriented alignment map (CRAM)
      - □ Compressed form of SAM files
      - □ Binary format, which is not readable by humans
      - □ Smaller and more efficient for software to manipulate; reduces costs of computation and storage
    - – Single-end read: Fragment sequenced in only 1 direction
    - – Paired-end reads: Fragment sequenced from both 5' and 3' end
      - □ Improves accuracy and alignment across regions with repetitive sequences
      - □ Facilitates detection of genomic rearrangements and novel transcripts
  - o Variant calling annotates changes in sequence as compared to reference genome, creating VCF file
    - – Variant call format (VCF): Text file output of bioinformatics pipeline for storing sequence variation and annotations
  - o Bioinformatic software tools are available for sequence analysis and parsing variant implications
- **Clinical applications**
  - o Whole-genome sequencing (WGS): Entire genome is sequenced, including coding and noncoding regions

Sequencing Technologies

Select Next-Generation Sequencing Platforms

Sequencing Platform	MiSeq	NextSeq 550	NovaSeq	Ion S5
Manufacturer	Illumina	Illumina	Illumina	Ion Torrent/Thermo Fisher
Maximum output	15 Gb	120 Gb	6000 Gb	50 Gb
Maximum read length	2 x 300 bp	2 x 150 bp	2 x 250 bp	600 bp

Sequencing Technologies: Representative Examples

	Reversible Chain Termination Sequencing	H(+) Ion Semiconductor Sequencing	Single-Molecule, Real-Time Sequencing	Nanopore-Based Sequencing
Systems	Illumina, Inc	Ion Torrent/Thermo Fisher	Pacific Biosciences	Oxford Nanopore
Applications	2nd gen; WGS, WES, targeted sequencing, many LDT and some FDA-approved tests	2nd gen; mostly targeted sequencing, many LDT and some FDA-approved tests	3rd gen; mostly research use only at present	3rd gen; mostly research use only at present
Amplification method	Amplification on solid-phase flow cell	Amplification on nanobead in emulsion	N/A; single-molecule analysis	N/A; single-molecule analysis
Notes	Current market leader for clinical NGS technology	Decreased read accuracy in homopolymer tracts	Read lengths can exceed 10 KB, kinetic data permits detection of DNA methylation	Fast run times, long read lengths, possible decentralized sequencing
Error rates	< 0.01%	~ 1%	~ 5% overall	~ 5% overall

- o Whole-exome sequencing (WES): Evaluation of only coding regions, less complicated than WGS
- o Targeted sequencing (focused gene panel): Evaluation of specific regions with known clinical relevance
  - – Numerous offerings by many CLIA laboratories in USA; include various panels for oncologic and constitutional disorders
- o Detection of copy number variation
  - – Derived from read depth sequencing information as compared to reference
- o Discovery of gene fusions and characterization of novel splice isoforms
  - – Derived from paired-end RNA-based sequencing
- o Minimal residual disease analysis in oncology
  - – Most commonly in lymphoid and plasma cell neoplasms
  - – Tracking performed on previously identified patient's clonally rearranged B- or T-cell receptor gene sequence

3rd-Generation Sequencing
- a.k.a. long-read sequencing
  - o Emerging technology with multiple potential clinical applications
  - o Generates reads of thousands to millions of bases in length
- May overcome some limitations associated with short-read (2nd-generation) sequencing
  - o Short reads more often have sequence coverage gaps in genome, limiting variant detection
  - o Long reads may resolve complicated structural variants in challenging regions of human genome
    - – Structural variants, nucleotide repeat expansion, transposable elements, pseudogenes, and complex genomic regions may be captured
  - o May soon permit routine assembly of diploid genomes and telomere-to-telomere assemblies

- Can bypass clonal amplification step required for massively parallel sequencing
  - o Significantly shortens DNA preparation time and may have longer average read lengths
  - o Provides continuous real-time sequencing on single molecule of DNA
- Single-molecule real-time (SMRT) sequencing
  - o DNA polymerization occurs in nanostructure well arrays called zero-mode waveguides
  - o Sequence determined by monitoring incorporation of fluorescent dNTPs
- Nanopore sequencing
  - o Protein nanopores are set within electrically resistant polymer membrane, across which voltage is applied
  - o Processing enzyme denatures dsDNA and shunts ssDNA through nanopore; causes distinctive current disruptions that permit sequence identification
- Limitations include low throughput, error rate corrections, and higher per-base cost

SELECTED REFERENCES

1. Shivaprasad H et al: Applications of long-read sequencing technology in clinical genomics. Advances in Molecular Pathology. 5(1):85-108, 2022
2. Quenez O et al: Detection of copy-number variations from NGS data using read depth information: a diagnostic performance evaluation. Eur J Hum Genet. 29(1):99-109, 2021
3. Goodwin S et al: Coming of age: ten years of next-generation sequencing technologies. Nat Rev Genet. 17(6):333-51, 2016
4. Heather JM et al: The sequence of sequencers: the history of sequencing DNA. Genomics. 107(1):1-8, 2016
5. Aziz N et al: College of American Pathologists' laboratory standards for next-generation sequencing clinical tests. Arch Pathol Lab Med. 139(4):481-93, 2015
6. Shendure J et al: Next-generation DNA sequencing. Nat Biotechnol. 26(10):1135-45, 2008
7. Ronaghi M et al: A sequencing method based on real-time pyrophosphate. Science. 281(5375):363, 365, 1998
8. Sanger F et al: DNA sequencing with chain-terminating inhibitors. Proc Natl Acad Sci U S A. 74(12):5463-7, 1977

Sequencing Technologies

General NGS Workflow Overview

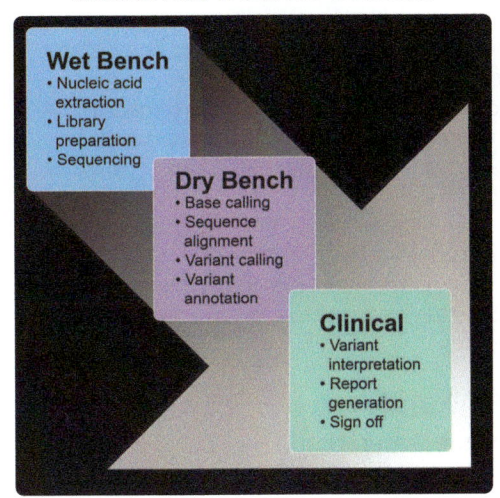

Wet Bench
- Nucleic acid extraction
- Library preparation
- Sequencing

Dry Bench
- Base calling
- Sequence alignment
- Variant calling
- Variant annotation

Clinical
- Variant interpretation
- Report generation
- Sign off

Target Enrichment During Library Preparation

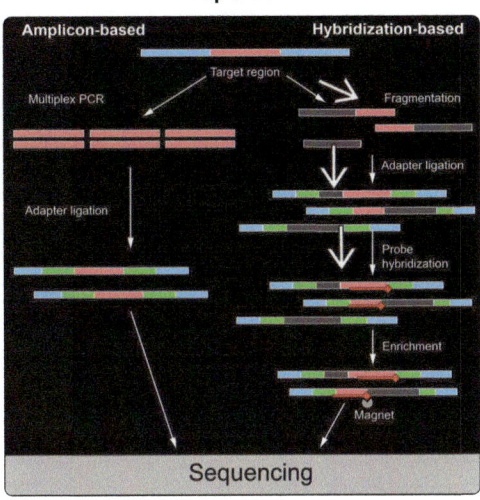

Amplicon-based | Hybridization-based
Multiplex PCR — Target region — Fragmentation
Adapter ligation
Probe hybridization
Enrichment
Magnet
Sequencing

(Left) The significant technical portions of all next-generation sequencing (NGS) assays are generally broken into a "wet-bench" portion (biochemical performance of the assay) and a "dry-bench" portion (data analytics of the generated sequences). **(Right)** Amplicon-based target enrichment is usually used for variant detection. Hybridization capture involves sample fragmentation, followed by enzymatic repair of the ends of the molecules with ligation of platform-specific adapters. This method does not require multiplex PCR primer design.

Solid-Phase Bridge Amplification

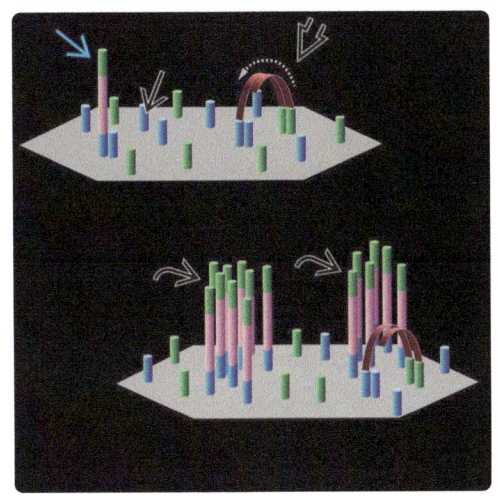

Cyclic Reversible Termination

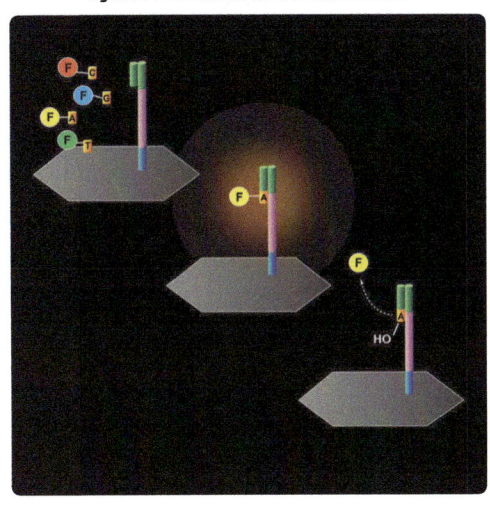

(Left) Free templates hybridize to slide-bound adapters. Nearby bound primers permit bridge PCR amplification. After several rounds of amplification, clonal template clusters are generated. **(Right)** All 4 individually labeled and 3'-blocked dNTPs are added. After a dNTP is added and unbound dNTPs are removed, the surface clusters are imaged to identify the incorporated dNTPs. The fluorophore(F)/blocking group are removed and a new cycle can begin.

Emulsion On-Bead Amplification

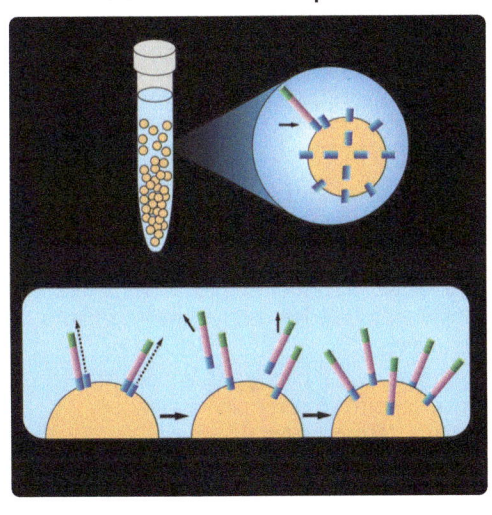

Ion-Semiconductor Sequencing

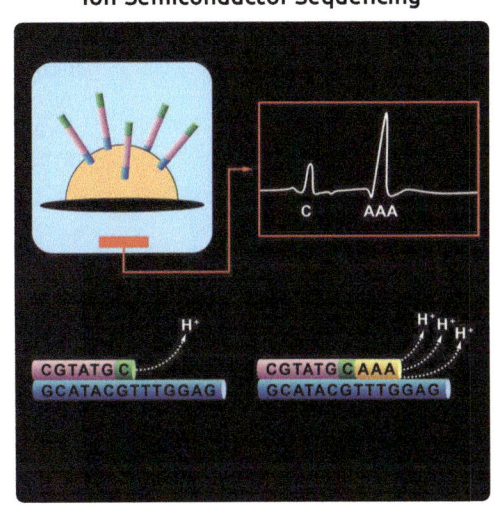

CGTATG C / CGTATG CAAA
GCATACGTTTGGAG / GCATACGTTTGGAG

(Left) Micelles are generated with a sequencing bead with bound primers, template, dNTPs, and polymerase. Templates hybridize and are amplified on the bead. The complementary strand dissociates, leaving bead-bound ssDNA templates. **(Right)** Beads are loaded into millions of wells on a sequencing chip; each well is an ultrasensitive pH meter. Hydrogen ions are released when nucleotides are incorporated during DNA synthesis. The pH change is relatively proportional to the number of nucleotides added.

High-Throughput Methods in Molecular Pathology

TERMINOLOGY

Definitions
- Use of computational software algorithms to analyze and interpret DNA, RNA, and epigenomic sequence data from next-generation sequencing (NGS)

NGS BIOINFORMATICS

Introduction
- NGS (a.k.a. massively parallel sequencing) is now mature laboratory technique to generate DNA, RNA, and epigenetic sequencing data in high-throughput manner
  - Data is generated on single instrument platform without need for multiple instruments for each individual technique (e.g., DNA vs. RNA vs. epigenetics)
- NGS assays are of increasing importance in diagnostic areas, such as hematopathology, solid tumor diagnostics, molecular microbiology/virology, and HLA laboratories
- NGS assays have enormously improved our understanding of human biology
- Obstacles to adoption of NGS technology within clinical laboratory include need for specialized expertise and training, lack of bioinformatics resources, instrumentation costs, and large amounts of data generated

Operating Systems
- Choices of operating systems (OS) include
  - Windows OS-based systems
  - Linux-based systems
- If dedicated bioinformatics personnel are available, Linux-based systems are optimal choice due to high customizability of analysis
  - Disadvantages of Linux
    - Steep learning curve
    - Use of command line interface and need for programming skills
  - Majority of bioinformatics software is open source, based on Linux platform
- For small- to medium-sized laboratory, Windows-based systems are appropriate
  - Does not need significant bioinformatics overhead
  - Advantages of using Windows include familiarity with OS, even for regular lab personnel without background in bioinformatics
  - Disadvantages
    - Lack of open-source software for Windows (high recurring costs)
    - Lack of easy customizability
- MacOS is often used as "bridge" into Linux distribution, such as Ubuntu, which can be simultaneously installed on Mac computer along with MacOS
  - Minimal bioinformatics software is specifically designed for MacOS

COMPUTATIONAL HARDWARE

Hardware Choices
- Important issue for small- to medium-sized laboratories starting out with clinical NGS
- Targeted DNA-seq panels do not require large amounts of computational power for analytical purposes
- Clinical exome or whole-genome sequencing requires dedicated computational resources and bioinformatics expertise
- Other assays, such as RNA-seq and Chip-seq, require large amounts of computational resources as well
- For small- to medium-sized lab considering targeted DNA-seq assays, optimal workstation configuration would be multicore processor with 12-16 cores, 2-4 TB of hard disk space, and 64 GB of RAM as minimum configuration
- Depending on number of samples run in lab, need for computational power may be higher
- Installation of 2 analytical computers to run in parallel and analyze NGS data is preferred to ensure redundancy of data analytic workflow

NGS DATA ANALYSIS

Step 1: Sequence Generation
- Primary genomic sequence is data generated from instrument
- In all NGS platforms, extensive preprocessing of raw signal is performed to ensure highest signal quality sequencing data
- Multiple steps for sequencing data generation include raw signal analysis, base calling, quality score generation, demultiplexing of different sample reads, and finally, generating sequence data file
- Data generated from instrument is FASTQ file, which contains raw sequencing data and quality scores associated with each base call
- FASTQ data are imported manually for further analysis onto local computer or cloud for further analysis

Step 2: Sequence Alignment
- FASTQ raw data are "cleaned up," including trimming at ends of raw reads, eliminating low-quality score data, duplicate read removal, and elimination of very short reads
- Each of individual reads from raw FASTQ file are then aligned against reference human genome database
  - This alignment process is most important step for clinical targeted DNA-seq analysis
- In targeted DNA-seq, each location of target is sequenced many times over, resulting in multiple reads at each genomic location
  - All of these reads are aligned multiple times at each location, and resulting sequence data are then visualized in form of "pileup" diagram

Step 3: Variant Detection and Annotation
- After read alignment, downstream software is used to identify various DNA sequence variants, such as germline single-nucleotide polymorphism (SNP) variants, somatic SNP variants, insertions, deletions, copy number variants, and structural variants
- Variant calling is done by comparing sequenced reads to reference human genome to determine nucleotide locations, which are different from reference
- Sequencing errors, which are common in NGS, are overcome by sequencing genomic region multiple times to create final "read depth"
  - Read depth is average number of times any given location is sequenced

High-Throughput Methods in Molecular Pathology

- Read depth of 1,000x indicates that any given location in target sequence has been sequenced 1,000x over on average
  - Higher percentages of tumor cells in NGS samples provide more reliable results compared to low tumor percentages
- Once sequence variant is identified, it needs to be annotated to determine true nature of detected variant
- Annotation in high-throughput sequencing is performed by comparing variant against population frequency data in different databases, such as 1,000 Genomes Project, NHLBI Cohort, and dbSNP Project
  - Variant identified in database at population frequency level of ≥ 1% may be considered to be true benign variant
  - Various cancer-specific variant databases exist (e.g., COSMIC), against which detected variant can be compared
  - Various software prediction algorithms, such as SIFT and PolyPhen, utilize nucleotide and amino acid level changes in variant to assess likely pathogenicity of variant
    - Reliability of such predictions has not been comprehensively proven

BIOINFORMATICS ANALYSIS

Quality Control

- NGS read generation is inherently error-prone process that depends on sequencing platform being used (e.g., Illumina vs. Ion Torrent)
- Various steps in bioinformatics pipeline can contribute to error process, including read filtering, alignment step, and others
- Increase in read depth of sequencing can minimize NGS false-positives and false-negatives
  - For purpose of clinical NGS, read depth of 400-500x coverage may be used as lab-established threshold to ensure accuracy of clinical variant detection
  - Individual labs need to set sensitivity limits for detection of variants during assay validation process
    - Sensitivity limit of 5% mutant allele frequency for single-position variants and 10% for insertion/deletion variants represents conservative and reasonable approach

NGS BIOINFORMATICS

Storage Issues

- Important to assess clinical volumes to estimate future data storage requirements well in advance of implementing assay
- Compliance with HIPAA regulations
  - Important to estimate data storage needs in secure, HIPAA compliant manner without revealing any direct patient identifiers
    - Local network access storage (NAS) solutions may be implemented for cheap price
- Important to make both on-site and off-site data backups for future retrieval of data
- Close coordination with local IT infrastructure experts is crucial requirement to ensure smooth implementation of NGS data storage process
- Retrospective, ad hoc solutions for data storage are likely to result in roadblocks for smooth implementation of clinical NGS over time

COMMONLY USED SOFTWARE FOR NGS ANALYSIS

Windows-Based Software

- Commercial solutions that are integrated from end-to-end for NGS workflow
- Major disadvantage of Windows-based software may be recurring pricing costs associated with NGS software solutions
- Capable of performing multiple steps of bioinformatics pipeline, including read alignment, single-nucleotide variant detection, indel detection, variant annotation, and visualization on single platform
  - e.g., NextGENe from SoftGenetics, Avadis NGS, CLCBio Genomics Workbench, DNAstar platform

Linux-Based Software

- Mostly open-source software created and provided by individual research groups
  - Bowtie2 (alignment), BWA (alignment), Novoalign (alignment), SOAP (alignment), GATK (SNV, indel calling), SAMtools (SNV, indel calling), VarScan (SNV, indel calling), SomaticSniper (SNV, indel for somatic samples), ExomeCNV (copy number calling), BreakDancer (structural variant calling), PINDEL (structural variant calling)
- Free of cost; represents latest state-of-art in terms of algorithmic development
- Drawbacks include uneven levels of documentation, need to use command line interface to run programs, and requirement for specialized technical expertise

Cloud-Based Software Solutions

- Newer developments in this space include availability of cloud-based IT solutions for NGS bioinformatics
- Cloud-based NGS solutions comprise approach known as "software-as-a-service" (SaaS)
- Some commercial NGS cloud vendors include PieranDx, Roche, Agilent, GenomOncology, and Sunquest
- Institutional IT security concerns must be carefully reviewed before implementing NGS cloud-based solutions
- Cloud-based solutions can provide storage as well as analytical capabilities for institutions with limited local bioinformatics expertise

SELECTED REFERENCES

1. Henriksen RA et al: NGSNGS: next-generation simulator for next-generation sequencing data. Bioinformatics. 39(1), 2023
2. Roy-Chowdhuri S et al: Big data from small samples: informatics of next-generation sequencing in cytopathology. Cancer Cytopathol. 125(4):236-44, 2017
3. Roy S et al: Next-generation sequencing informatics: challenges and strategies for implementation in a clinical environment. Arch Pathol Lab Med. 140(9):958-75, 2016
4. Oliver GR et al: Bioinformatics for clinical next generation sequencing. Clin Chem. 61(1):124-35, 2015
5. Gullapalli RR et al: Next generation sequencing in clinical medicine: challenges and lessons for pathology and biomedical informatics. J Pathol Inform. 3:40, 2012

DNA Methylation Analysis

TERMINOLOGY

Definitions

- Epigenetic modification of promoter DNA regulates gene expression
  - Methyl groups are added enzymatically at carbon 5 position by DNA methyltransferase on cytosine bases followed by guanosine (CpG dinucleotides)
  - Promoter regions of genes may contain many CpG dinucleotides, called CpG islands
    - 40% of gene promoters contain CpG islands
  - Methylation of promoter region leads to decreased gene transcription and expression
    - Methylated CpG sites bind methylated CpG binding proteins 1 and 2 (MECP1/MECP2)
    - MECP decreases transcription through transcription repression domain
    - MECP proteins bind other factors that cause chromatin condensation and block transcription
    - MECP proteins block binding of transcription factors
- Methylation functions in regulation of specific genes, genomic imprinting, and X-chromosome inactivation
- Aberrant methylation is associated with imprinting disorders, X-linked recessive disorders, some trinucleotide repeat disorders, defects in gene expression regulation, and cancer
  - Likely plays role in all human neoplasia
    - Genome-wide changes in methylation occur in cancer
    - Identification of abnormal genomic methylation patterns (e.g., in serum) may indicate presence of neoplastic process
  - Associated with many other types of disease, including neurological disorders, such as autism and dementia
- Methylation assays distinguish methylated from nonmethylated DNA
  - Results vary between methods and laboratories
  - Cutoffs for positivity are not standardized

METHODOLOGY

Nonbisulfite-Dependent Methods

- Restriction endonuclease digestion
  - Genomic DNA incubated with methylation-specific enzymes
  - *Hpa*II and *Msp*I enzymes commonly used
    - *Hpa*II cannot cleave DNA at its recognition sequence CCGG if 5-methyl group is present (methylation sensitive)
    - *Msp*I cleaves DNA irrespective of presence of methyl group at this position (methylation insensitive)
  - Digestion products analyzed
    - Gel electrophoresis detects size of fragments
    - Array hybridization measures relative fluorescent signal intensities of digested and control DNA
    - NGS compares libraries constructed from digested DNA and randomly fragmented DNA
  - Can be used to analyze methylation in large regions of DNA, including whole genome
  - High rate of false-positive results due to incomplete digestion
- Affinity enrichment
  - Methylated DNA is purified
    - Methylated DNA immunoprecipitation (MeDIP) uses antibodies specific for methylated cytosine
    - Methyl-CpG binding domain-based capture (MBDCap) uses methyl-binding proteins
  - Product hybridized to array or analyzed using NGS techniques
  - Used in research settings for whole-genome analysis
- Electrochemical assays
  - Methylated cytosine shows differential adsorption to gold
  - Can be used to measure genome-wide methylation

Bisulfite Conversion Methods

- Most common method of measuring methylation status
- Genomic DNA is isolated and treated with sodium bisulfite

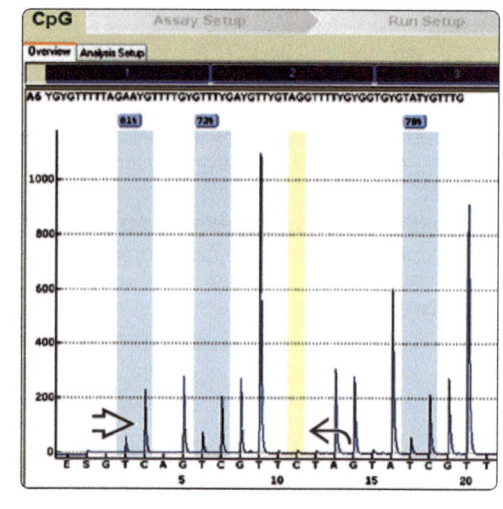

(Left) *Pyrosequencing study shows substantial conversion of cytosine (C) to thymine (T) at C followed by guanine (CpG, blue bars) following bisulfite treatment, indicating unmethylated DNA.* **(Right)** *Pyrosequencing study shows significant residual C, indicating methylation of CpG sites. A C not followed by a G is included as a control and shows no remaining C, as this site cannot be methylated.*

Pyrosequencing of Unmethylated DNA

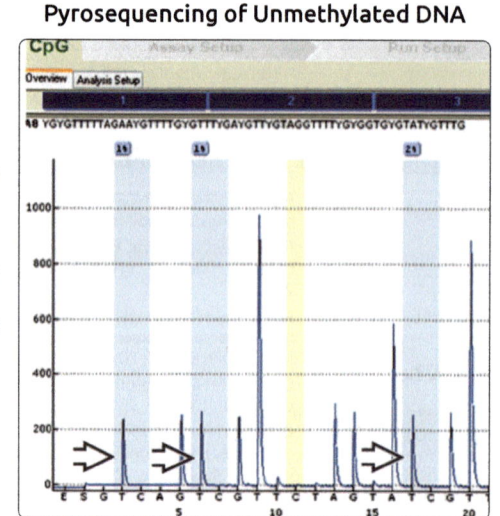

Pyrosequencing of Methylated DNA

DNA Methylation Analysis

- Bisulfite causes chemical conversion of unmethylated cytosines to uracil
  - Uracil will be replaced by thymine during PCR
  - 5-methyl-cytosine is protected from conversion
    - Replaced by cytosine during PCR

Measurement of Bisulfite Conversion

- Restriction endonuclease digestion
  - Cleave amplified DNA at uracil-guanosine sequences
  - Do not cleave cytosine-guanosine sequences
  - Size of resulting fragments is measured
- Methylation-specific PCR
  - Uses primers containing 1-3 CpG sites with 3' specificity for cytosines converted to uracil and separate set with 3' specificity for nonconverted sequence
    - Presence of amplicon in each reaction is measured, e.g., with gel electrophoresis
- Real-time methylation-specific PCR can quantitate methylation level
  - Utilizes probe specific to nonconverted sequence with attached fluorophore and quencher
  - During PCR, probe is degraded, resulting in separation of fluorophore and quencher
  - Resulting fluorescence is quantified
  - Results expressed as methylation index (MI): Ratio of amplification of methylated DNA to control gene
- Sequencing of products with methylation nonspecific primers
  - Amplified DNA is sequenced using polymerase that is to recognize uracil
  - Ratio of cytosine to thymine at each potential conversion site is measured
  - Multiple sequencing methods available
    - Sanger sequencing
    - Pyrosequencing
    - NGS (includes options for targeted as well as whole-genome methylation assessment)
- Melting curve analysis
  - Methylated DNA has higher melting temperature than unmethylated DNA
    - Higher GC content due to preservation of cytosine
  - May be difficult to interpret if methylation is heterogeneous

CLINICAL IMPLICATIONS

Diagnostic and Screening Use

- Gene-specific hypermethylation
  - Promoter methylation prevents normal transcription of tumor suppressor genes
    - *RASSF1A* in lung, bladder, and breast cancers
    - *MLH1* and *SEPTIN9* in colon cancer
    - *RB1* in retinoblastoma
    - *SHOX* in lung cancer
    - *BRCA1* in breast cancer
    - *MGMT* in glioma and colon cancer
    - *CDKN2A* in bladder cancer and lung cancer
    - *GSTP1* in prostate cancer
  - Commercially available assays for epigenetic biomarkers
- Genome-wide hypomethylation
  - Occurs to some degree in all tumors
    - May be used for screening and risk stratification
  - Leads to genomic instability
    - Increased crossover events between normally methylated areas
    - Activation of cryptic promoters disrupts normal gene transcription
  - Hypomethylation of oncogenes can result in activation
    - *RRAS* in gastric cancer
- Identify cell types by identifying gene methylation patterns
  - Can aid in identifying cell of origin, tumor type in cancers
- Human androgen receptor assay (HUMARA)
  - Used to demonstrate clonality in female patients
  - Determines methylation of human androgen receptor gene
    - Gene contains hypervariable CAG repeat that is usually heterozygous
    - Utilizes methylation-sensitive restriction enzymes to digest unmethylated alleles
    - Methylated maternal: Paternal ratio of > 3:1 or < 1:3 indicates nonrandom X chromosome inactivation
  - Other genes may be analyzed to determine X chromosome inactivation, but are not widely used

Prognostic and Predictive Use

- Methylation of specific gene promoters has prognostic significance
- Hypermethylation of microRNA is associated with disease progression
  - miR-34b/associated with metastasis
- Methylation status of specific gene promoters predicts chemotherapy response
  - Promoter methylation of *MGMT* DNA repair gene predicts response to alkylating therapy in high-grade gliomas
- Small molecule inhibitors of epigenetic regulators
  - Reverse epigenetic alterations
  - DNA methyltransferase (DNMT) inhibitors
    - Nucleoside analogues that irreversibly bind DNMT
    - Used in myeloid malignancies, such as MDS and AML
    - Include azacitidine and decitabine
    - Others in clinical trials
    - Trials in other cancers
  - Histone deacetylase inhibitors
    - Used in lymphoid malignancies, such as T-cell lymphoma
    - Vorinostat and romidepsin
    - Others in clinical trials
  - Other inhibitors in clinical trials
    - Histone methyltransferase
    - Histone acetyltransferase
    - Histone demethylase
- Use in measurable residual disease testing being explored
  - Identify cancer associated methylation patterns in circulating tumor DNA

SELECTED REFERENCES

1. Chen K et al: Individualized dynamic methylation-based analysis of cell-free DNA in postoperative monitoring of lung cancer. BMC Med. 21(1):255, 2023
2. Galbraith K et al: Clinical utility of whole-genome DNA methylation profiling as a primary molecular diagnostic assay for central nervous system tumors-A prospective study and guidelines for clinical testing. Neurooncol Adv. 5(1):vdad076, 2023

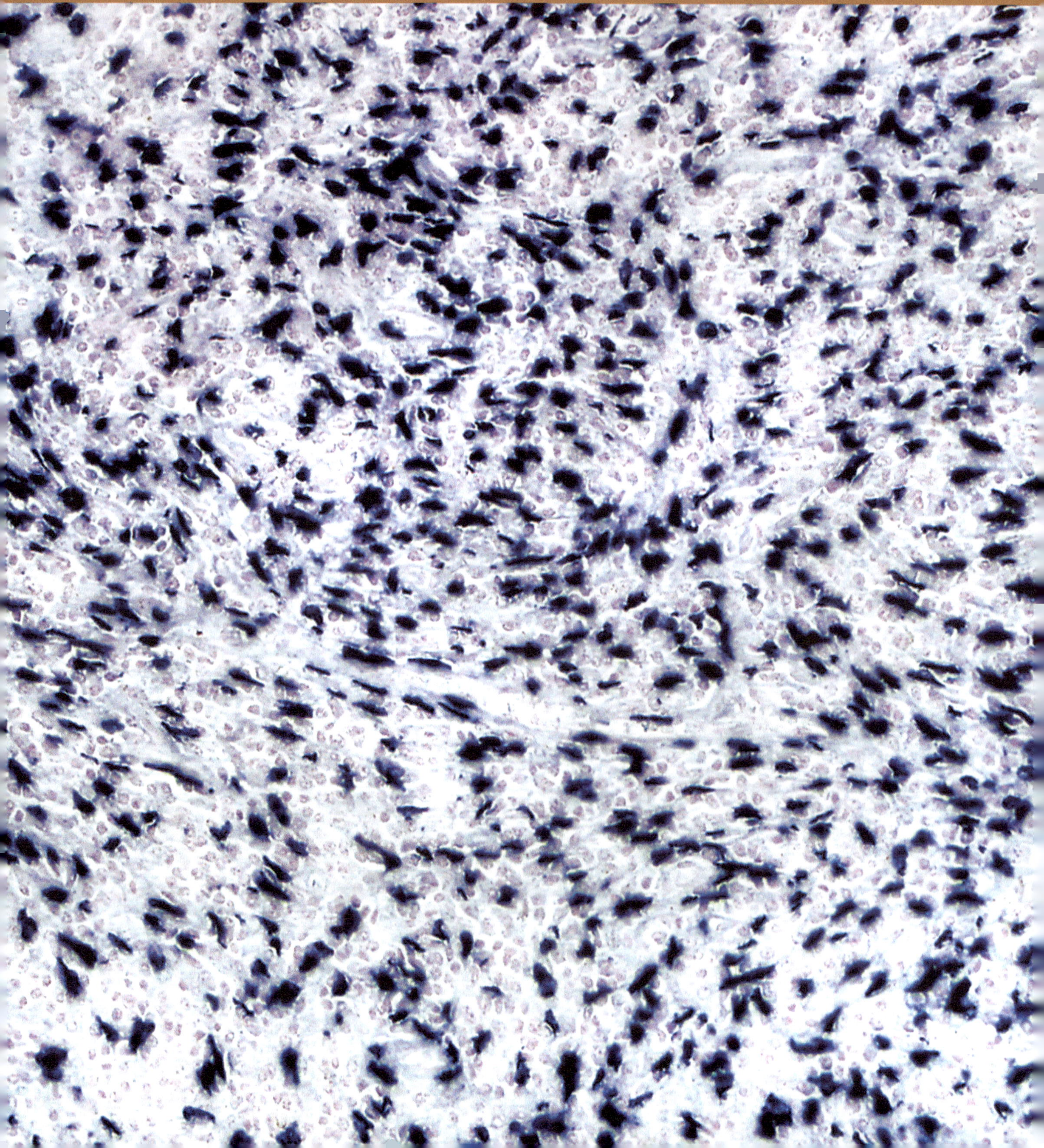

SECTION 3
Molecular Genetic Tests in Hematopoietic Tumors

BCR::ABL1 Fusion	42
PML::RARA Fusion	46
Reverse Transcription PCR for Myeloid Leukemia Transcripts	48
FLT3, *NPM1*, and *CEBPA* Mutations	50
JAK2 Mutations and Rearrangements	54
MPL Mutations	56
Calreticulin (*CALR*) Mutations	58
CSF3R Mutations	60
SETBP1 Mutations	62
KIT Mutations	64
IDH1 and *IDH2* Mutations	68
Other Mutations and Gene Panel Testing in Myeloid Neoplasms	70
Immunoglobulin Heavy (*IGH*) Chain Gene Rearrangements	72
T-Cell Receptor Gamma (*TRG*) and Delta (*TRD*) Chain Rearrangements	76
T-Cell Receptor Beta (*TRB*) Chain Gene Rearrangements	80
Southern Blot Analysis of Antigen Receptor Genes	84
EBV-Associated Human Neoplasms	86
MYD88 Mutation	94
NOTCH1 Mutation	96
EZH2 Mutation	98

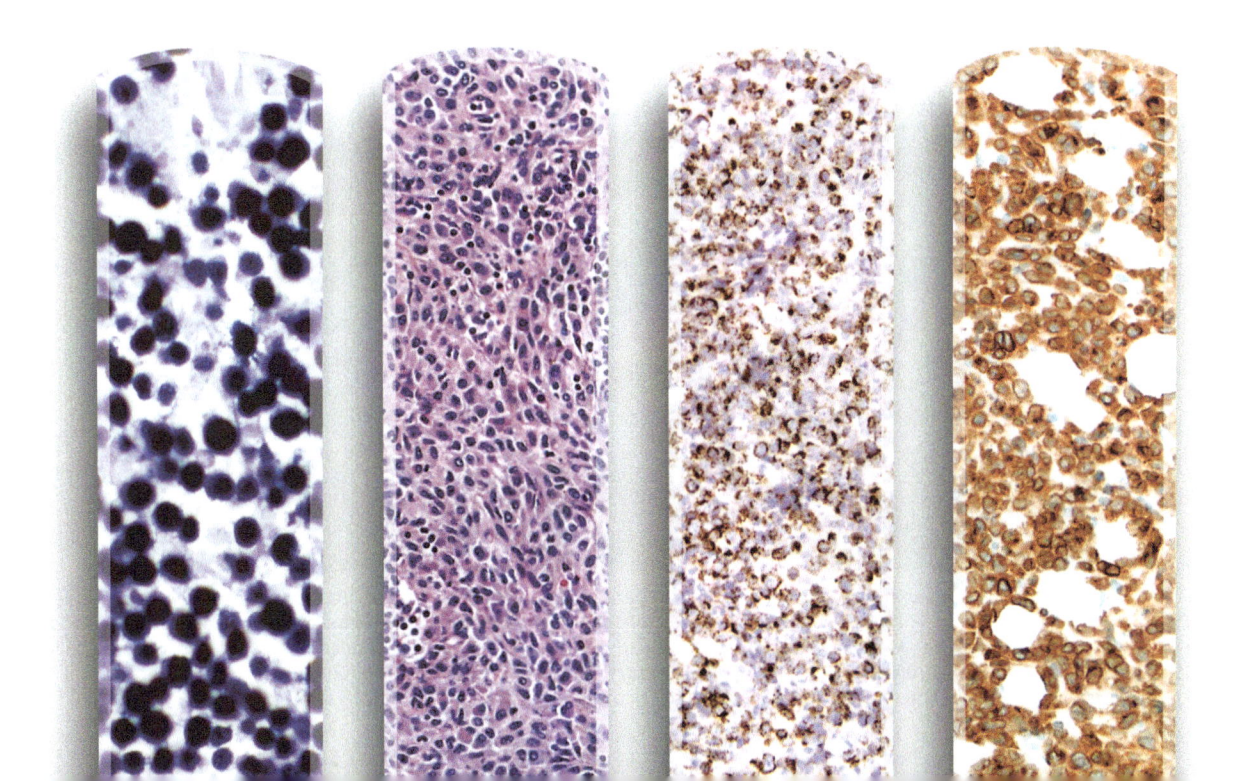

BCR::ABL1 Fusion

TERMINOLOGY

Synonyms
- Philadelphia (Ph) chromosome
  - Terminology extensively used for *BCR::ABL1* fusion

Definitions
- *BCR::ABL1* fusion due to reciprocal translocation involving long arms of chromosomes 9 and 22

Historical View
- 1960: Discovered and named Ph-chromosome by Nowell and Hungerford
  - Called aberrant acrocentric chromosome 22 in 7 patients with chronic myeloid leukemia (CML)
  - 1st recurrent chromosomal abnormality linked to human malignancy
- 1973: Janet Rowley utilized chromosomal banding techniques to demonstrate underlying t(9;22)(q34.1;q11.2)
- 1998: Imatinib (Gleevec) targeted therapy introduced
- 2001: Imatinib approved as 1st-line therapy for CML
  - 2nd- (dasatinib, nilotinib, bosutinib) and 3rd- (ponatinib) generation tyrosine kinase inhibitor (TKI) therapies also available
  - Allosteric inhibitors of *BCR::ABL1* kinase activity (asciminib) and plant alkaloid derived pharmaceuticals (omacetaxine) are other approved treatments

Normal Function of *BCR*
- Localizes to chromosome 22q11.2
- Protein with regulatory activities toward small GTP-binding proteins through GTPase activity modulation, including RAC1
- Amino terminus contains intrinsic kinase activity

Normal Function of *ABL1*
- Localizes to chromosome 9q34.1
- Protooncogene involved in variety of cellular processes, including cell division, adhesion, differentiation, and stress responses

BCR::ABL1 Fusion

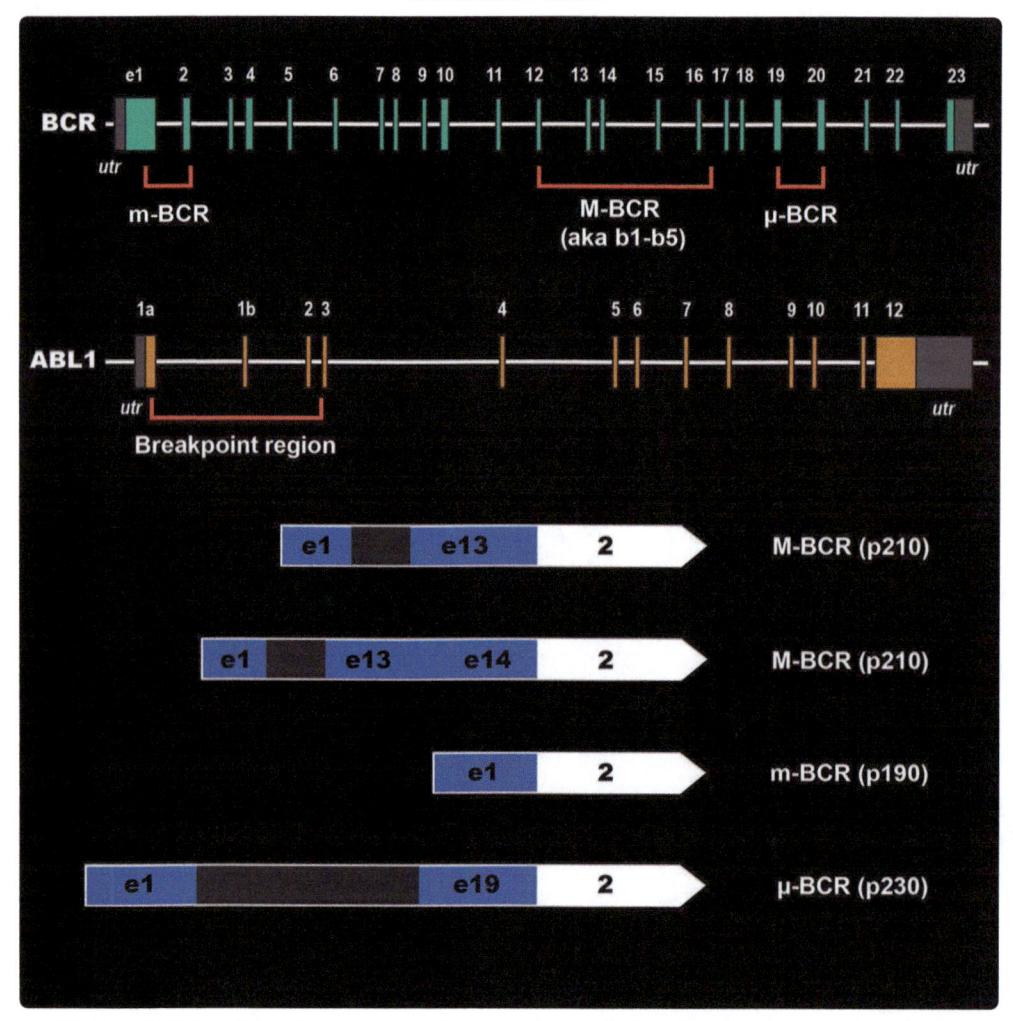

Genomic structure of BCR and ABL1 and their fusion gene products are shown. The breakpoint in ABL1 is relatively constant between exons 1 and 2. In contrast, there are 3 breakpoints in BCR that include major, minor, and μ breakpoint cluster regions abbreviated as M-BCR, m-BCR, and μ-BCR, respectively. M-BCR spans exons 12-16 (a.k.a. b1-b5) of BCR gene and results in 2 mRNA transcripts of e13a2 or e14a2, both encoding p210 fusion protein. m-BCR occurs upstream of M-BCR between exons 1 and 2, resulting in e1a2 transcripts that encode p190 fusion protein. Less common μ-BCR results in e19-a2 transcripts, encoding p230 fusion protein.

BCR::ABL1 Fusion

- Encodes cytoplasmic and nuclear nonreceptor tyrosine kinase

ETIOLOGY/PATHOGENESIS

t(9;22)(q34.1;q11.2)

- Reciprocal translocation following breakpoints within *BCR* and *ABL1* loci
  o Encodes oncogenic *BCR::ABL1* fusion protein
  o Translocation is balanced in majority of cases
  o Loss of portion of reciprocal *ABL1::BCR* found in derivative chromosome 9 in ~ 10% of CML cases
- t(9;22)(q34.1;q11.2) fuses 3' sequences from *ABL1* to 5' sequences from *BCR*
- *ABL1* breakpoint typically between exons 1-2 (a2)
  o Rare *ABL1* breakpoints occur between exons 2-3 (a3)
  o Known a3 fusions include e13a3, e14a3, and e1a3
- *BCR* with at least 3 different breakpoint regions
  o Major breakpoint cluster region (M-BCR)
    – Breakpoints occur in region spanning exon 12-16 (a.k.a. exons b1-b5)
      □ Mostly between exons 13-14 or exons 14-15
    – Fusions with *ABL1 a2* lead to mRNA products referred to as e13a2 or e14a2
      □ Result in 210 kDa fusion protein (p210)
  o Minor breakpoint cluster region (m-BCR)
    – Arise 5' of M-BCR between exons 1-2 (e1)
    – Fusion with *ABL1 a2* results in e1a2 transcripts
      □ Results in 190 kDa fusion protein (p190)
  o Micro breakpoint cluster region (μ-BCR)
    – Rare *BCR* breakpoint between exons 17-20
    – Results in 230 kDa fusion protein (p230)

CLINICAL IMPLICATIONS

Chronic Myeloid Leukemia

- *BCR::ABL1* is required to diagnose CML
  o FISH &/or RT-PCR must be performed in suspected cases with negative cytogenetics
    – FISH &/or RT-PCR may identify cryptic fusions missed by conventional karyotyping
    – Very rare cryptic fusions may also be missed by FISH but can be detected by RT-PCR
- Multipotent hematopoietic progenitor is affected
  o Fusion gene present in all stages of granulocytic, erythroid, and megakaryocytic lineages
- Major breakpoint cluster region (M-BCR, p210 transcripts) involved in ~ 99% of CML cases
- Primary fusion involving minor breakpoint cluster region (m-BCR, p190 transcripts) in only 1% of CML
- > 90% of cases with p210 will have low-level p190 transcripts detectable at initial diagnosis
  o Low-level p190 due to alternative splicing of *BCR*
- Primary micro breakpoint cluster region fusions (μ-BCR, p230 transcripts) are rare
  o Cases with p230 show prominent mature neutrophilia &/or conspicuous thrombocytosis

B-Lymphoblastic Leukemia/Lymphoma

- ~ 25% of adult B-ALL cases are *BCR::ABL1*-positive
  o ~ 60% of Ph(+) cases involve m-BCR (p190)
  o Remaining 40% involve M-BCR (p210)
- ~ 2-4% of childhood B-ALL are *BCR::ABL1*-positive
  o ~ 90% of cases involve m-BCR (p190)
- WHO 5th edition classification for B-ALL with *BCR::ABL1* is unchanged from prior edition
- International Consensus Classification (ICC) system divides *BCR::ABL1*-positive ALL into 2 biologically distinct subsets
  o One subset is biologically closer to CML presenting in lymphoid blast phase
    – Distinguished by detection of *BCR::ABL1* fusion in both leukemic lymphoblasts and non-ALL lymphocytes/granulocytes
      □ Suggests multipotent hematopoietic progenitor is affected by *BCR::ABL1* fusion
      □ This subset is distinguished on basis of FISH analysis and is not identifiable by *BCR::ABL1* fusion transcript analysis
      □ May require cell sorting or granulocyte enrichment step prior to FISH to obtain sufficient cells for analysis
      □ Will demonstrate higher *BCR::ABL1* fusion levels than *IGH/TCR* rearrangements when monitoring for minimal residual disease (MRD)
  o 2nd subset is closer to more conventional lymphoblastic leukemia/lymphoma
    – *BCR::ABL1* fusion is present only in lymphoblasts

Acute Myeloid Leukemia With *BCR::ABL1*

- Rare acute myeloid leukemia (AML) subtype (< 1%) recognized by both WHO 5th edition and ICC systems
  o De novo AML with no evidence of prior CML
  o Most cases involve M-BCR (p210)
  o ≥ 20% blasts required for diagnosis by both WHO and ICC
  o Variable anemia and thrombocytopenia
  o Lower peripheral blood basophilia (usually < 2%)

Mixed Phenotype Acute Leukemia With *BCR::ABL1*

- p190 transcript is more common than p210 transcript
- If p210 transcript detected, CML in mixed blast crisis should be considered; especially if 2 distinct myeloid and lymphoid blast populations are present

METHODS OF DETECTION

Conventional Cytogenetics

- Detects t(9;22)(q34.1;q11.2) in ~ 95% of cases
  o Presumptive evidence for *BCR::ABL1* fusion gene
- Also identifies variant t(9;22) translocations as well as other chromosomal aberrancies if present
- Cryptic translocations are not detected
- Inappropriate for disease monitoring; low detection sensitivity (~ 5%)
  o Not useful for MRD detection

FISH

- Identifies *BCR::ABL1* fusion in > 95% of cases
  o Detects most cryptic rearrangements
  o Rare cryptic rearrangements may be missed
- More sensitive than conventional cytogenetics but insufficient for MRD or early relapse detection
- Cannot differentiate between various fusion transcripts

BCR::ABL1 Fusion

Quantitative Real-Time PCR

- Reliably determines type of *BCR::ABL1* transcript
- More accurately quantifies *BCR::ABL1* transcripts
- Standard for monitoring treatment response, MRD, and early relapse detection
- International Scale was developed to standardize inter-laboratory quantitative reporting of transcript levels
- Basic principles for quantitative real-time PCR
  - RNA extraction from fresh blood, bone marrow, or other involved sites
  - Reverse transcription to convert RNA to cDNA
  - Real-time PCR amplification using primer sets to cover desired *BCR::ABL1* fusions
  - Small probes of ~ 25 bases in length
    - Many laboratories in USA use "European network probes" complementary to portion of *ABL1* sequences in proximity of fusion with *BCR*
  - Simultaneous PCR amplification of internal control gene, such as *ABL1*, *B2M*, *GUSB*, or other genes
  - Inclusion of serially diluted positive cell line/plasmid controls

Digital Droplet PCR

- May be feasible alternate to quantitative real-time PCR
- Returns absolute quantification, which may also be expressed as percentage on IS

DISEASE MONITORING IN CML AND PH(+) B-ALL

Detection of Minimal Residual Disease and Treatment Response in Chronic Myeloid Leukemia

- Quantitative real-time PCR is recommended at diagnosis and for monitoring
- Level of *BCR::ABL1* transcripts can be expressed using 2 different methods
  - Ratio of *BCR::ABL1* to *ABL1* internal control gene (or other selected internal control gene) method
    - Ratios of ≥ 0.1 are typically present at diagnosis and indicate high copy numbers of transcripts
    - Major molecular response (MMR) is defined as *BCR::ABL1* to *ABL1* ratio with ≥ 3 log reduction from baseline
  - Disease burden as determined by International Standard (IS) method
    - Transcript levels at initial diagnosis set as 100% IS
    - Major molecular response (≥ 3 log reduction, MR3.0) defined as IS value of ≤ 0.1%
    - Ongoing lack of consensus regarding levels for deep molecular response (DMR)
      - MR4.0 (IS ≤ 0.01%) and MR4.5 (IS ≤ 0.0032%) both in use
      - Achieving and maintaining DMR required for consideration of discontinuing TKI therapy
- Peripheral blood is suitable for monitoring disease
  - *BCR::ABL1* transcripts are present in all myeloid lineages, including in segmented neutrophils
- Bone marrow specimen is not typically needed for disease monitoring

Detection of Treatment Response and Early Relapse in Ph(+) ALL

- Quantitative real-time PCR is recommended test for disease monitoring
  - Therapeutic aim is complete molecular response with attainment of negativity for *BCR::ABL1* transcripts
    - Detection of low-level *BCR::ABL1* transcripts following complete molecular response predicts recurrent disease at early molecular relapse stage
    - IS reporting is not applicable to Ph(+) B-ALL
- Bone marrow preferred for disease monitoring in Ph(+) B-ALL
  - In contrast to CML, *BCR::ABL1* transcripts may be limited to B lymphoblasts
  - Peripheral blood has low detection sensitivity for patients in morphologic remission

BCR::ABL1-RESISTANT MUTATIONS

Mutations in *ABL1* Kinase Domain

- Most common cause of acquired tyrosine kinase inhibitor (TKI) resistance
- > 80 mutations reported, mostly single nucleotide substitutions
  - Mutations at G250, Y253, E255, T315, M351, F359, and H396 codons account for ~ 60% of all mutations
  - T315I/A and mutations in codon F317 and V299 associated with dasatinib resistance
  - Y253H, E255K/V, T315I, and F359C/V/I mutations are associated with nilotinib resistance
  - L248V, G250E, V299L, T315I, F317L, and F359C mutations are associated with bosutinib resistance
  - Ponatinib (3rd-generation kinase inhibitor), asciminib (allosteric inhibitor), and omacetaxine may be used in some treatment-resistant CML cases with any mutations, including T315I
- Analysis of RNA required to ensure *ABL1* kinase domain mutation is within fusion transcript

SELECTED REFERENCES

1. Alaggio R et al: The 5th edition of the World Health Organization classification of haematolymphoid tumours: lymphoid neoplasms. Leukemia. 36(7):1720-48, 2022
2. Arber DA et al: International Consensus Classification of myeloid neoplasms and acute leukemia: integrating morphological, clinical, and genomic data. Blood. 140(11):1200-8, 2022
3. Khoury JD et al: The 5th edition of the World Health Organization classification of haematolymphoid tumours: myeloid and histiocytic/dendritic neoplasms. Leukemia. 36(7):1703-19, 2022
4. Sweet K et al: NCCN and ELN: What do the guidelines tell us? Best Pract Res Clin Haematol. 29(3):264-70, 2016
5. Soverini S et al: Mutations in the BCR-ABL1 kinase domain and elsewhere in chronic myeloid leukemia. Clin Lymphoma Myeloma Leuk. 15 Suppl:S120-8, 2015
6. Oehler VG: Update on current monitoring recommendations in chronic myeloid leukemia: practical points for clinical practice. Hematology Am Soc Hematol Educ Program. 2013:176-83, 2013
7. Hughes T et al: Monitoring CML patients responding to treatment with tyrosine kinase inhibitors: review and recommendations for harmonizing current methodology for detecting BCR-ABL transcripts and kinase domain mutations and for expressing results. Blood. 108(1):28-37, 2006
8. Gabert J et al: Standardization and quality control studies of 'real-time' quantitative reverse transcriptase polymerase chain reaction of fusion gene transcripts for residual disease detection in leukemia - a Europe Against Cancer program. Leukemia. 17(12):2318-57, 2003
9. Hughes TP et al: Frequency of major molecular responses to imatinib or interferon alfa plus cytarabine in newly diagnosed chronic myeloid leukemia. N Engl J Med. 349(15):1423-32, 2003

BCR::ABL1 Fusion

Karyotype of CML With t(9;22)

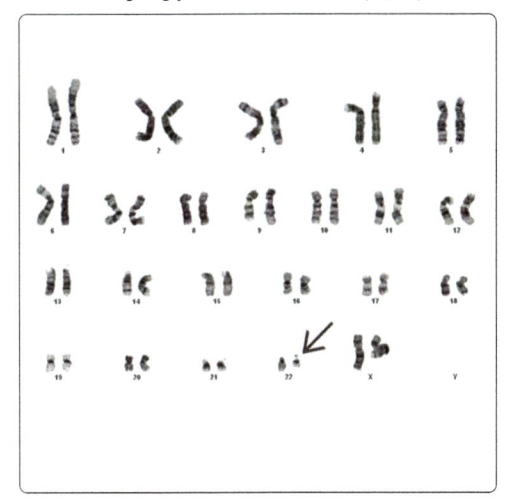

FISH Using BCR and ABL1 Targeted Probes

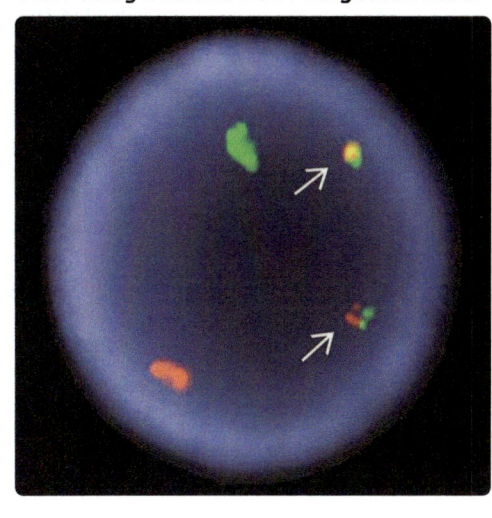

(Left) Conventional cytogenetics show the short derivative chromosome 22 (Philadelphia chromosome) ➡ in a patient with new diagnosis of chronic myeloid leukemia (CML). The underlying cytogenetic abnormality is a reciprocal translocation between the long arms of chromosomes 9 and 22 with fusion of the BCR::ABL1 genes at the molecular level. (Right) Interphase FISH using dual-color, dual-fusion probes shows 2 fused signals ➡, confirming BCR::ABL1 fusion.

RT-qPCR of BCR::ABL1 Transcripts at CML Initial Diagnosis

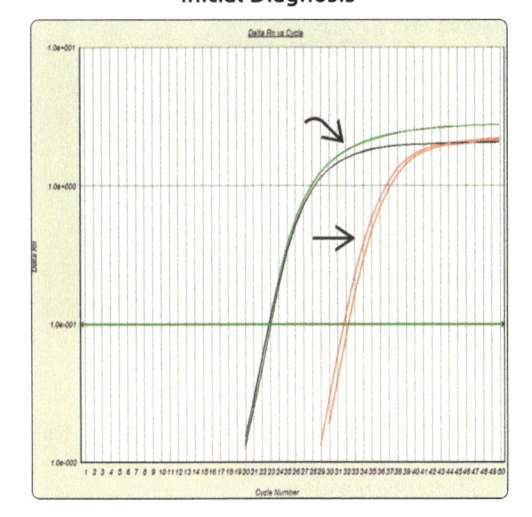

Posttherapy RT-qPCR for BCR::ABL1 Disease Monitoring

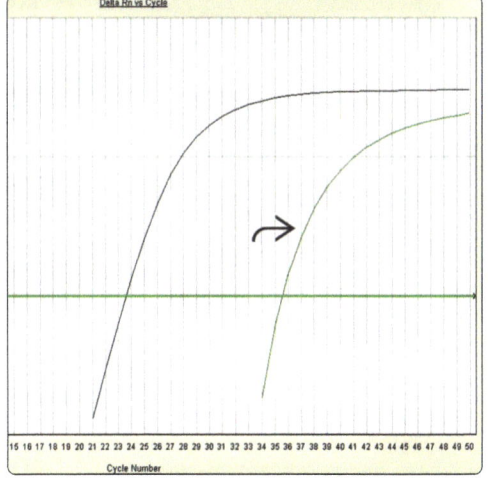

(Left) Quantitative RT-PCR shows high copies of b2a2-type BCR::ABL1 transcripts (green curves ➡) in a patient with CML. The black curve represents amplification of an internal control gene. Note simultaneous presence of low copy numbers of e1a2 transcripts ➡ due to alternative splicing of BCR gene. (Right) Quantitative RT-PCR post imatinib therapy in a CML patient shows > 3 log reduction in BCR::ABL1 transcripts ➡, consistent with major molecular response.

e1/a2 (p190) Type of BCR::ABL1 Detected by RT-qPCR in Child With Ph(+) B-ALL

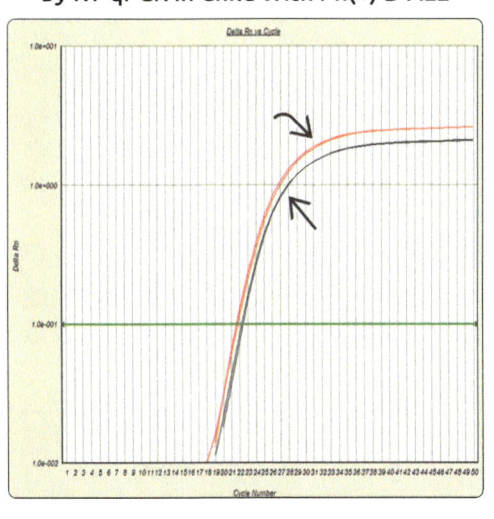

Sanger Sequencing Trace of BCR::ABL1 Resistant-Associated Mutation (E459V)

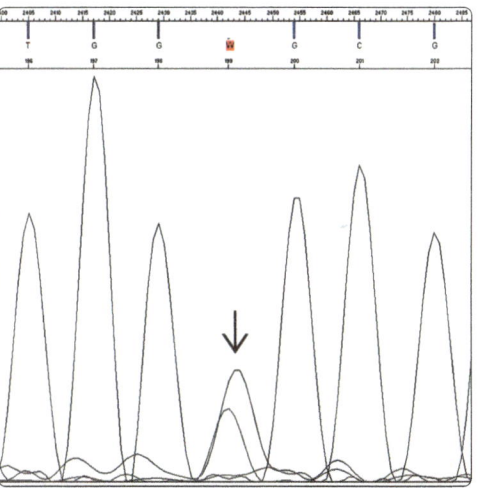

(Left) Quantitative RT-PCR performed on bone marrow from a child with Ph(+) B-ALL shows high copies of e1a2-type BCR::ABL1 transcripts (red amplification curves ➡). The black curves represent amplification of an internal control gene ➡. (Right) BCR::ABL1 mutational analysis of blood from a patient with acquired resistance to imatinib tyrosine kinase inhibitor shows a GAG>GTG point mutation in codon 459 of the ABL1 kinase gene, corresponding to p.E459V ➡.

PML::RARA Fusion

TERMINOLOGY

Definitions

- *PML::RARA* fusion due to reciprocal translocation involving long arms of chromosomes 15 and 17, leading to acute promyelocytic leukemia (APL)
  - t(15;17)(q24.1;q21.2)

Normal Function of *RARA*

- Official name: Retinoic acid receptor alpha
- HGNC ID: 9864
- Chromosomal location: 17q21.2
- Gene family: Nuclear hormone receptors
  - 17 exons with 2 isoforms differing in N-terminal domain
- Regulates gene transcription
  - Binds DNA and regulates genes involved in differentiation, apoptosis, and granulopoiesis
- Present in most tissue types
  - Localizes to cell nucleus

Normal Function of *PML*

- Official name: PML nuclear body scaffold
- HGNC ID: 9113
- Chromosomal location: 15q24.1
- Gene family: Tripartite motif containing RING finger proteins
  - Contains 10 exons; undergoes extensive alternative splicing
  - 3 domains mediate protein interactions and are included in all isoforms
    - RING finger domain
    - 2 B-box zinc finger domains
    - Coiled-coil region
- Transcription factor
- Tumor suppressor
  - Regulates *TP53*
  - Functions in cell death
    - Regulates apoptosis induced by FAS ligand and tumor necrosis factor α

ETIOLOGY/PATHOGENESIS

t(15;17)(q24.1;q21.2)

- Reciprocal translocation following breakpoints at *PML* and *RARA* loci
- Results in novel fusion gene on chromosome 15
- Hallmark of APL

PML::RARA Fusion

- 3 categories of *PML::RARA* fusion transcripts detected
- Consistent breakpoints in intron 2 of *RARA*
- Heterogeneous breakpoints in *PML* lead to different transcript sizes
  - Long form
    - bcr-1
    - 50-60% of APL
    - Breakpoint in *PML* intron 6
    - Results in *PML* exon 6 to *RARA* exon 3 fusion
  - Variable form
    - bcr-2
    - 5% of APL
    - Breakpoint in *PML* exon 6
      - Breakpoints occur at different points in exon, leading to variable length
    - Results in partial *PML* exon 6 and *RARA* exon 3 fusion
  - Short form
    - bcr-3
    - 35-45% of APL
    - Breakpoint in *PML* intron 3
    - Results in *PML* exon 3 to *RARA* exon 3 fusion
  - Alternative splicing of long and variable form transcripts gives further heterogeneity
- Fusion gene prevents normal DNA transcription
  - Binds to nuclear corepressor (NCOR)-histone deacetylase complex and enhances histone deacetylase function
    - Leads to aberrant chromatin deacetylation
    - Prevents gene transcription
  - Blocks differentiation of myeloid cells
  - Gives survival advantage to cell

PML and RARA Breakpoints

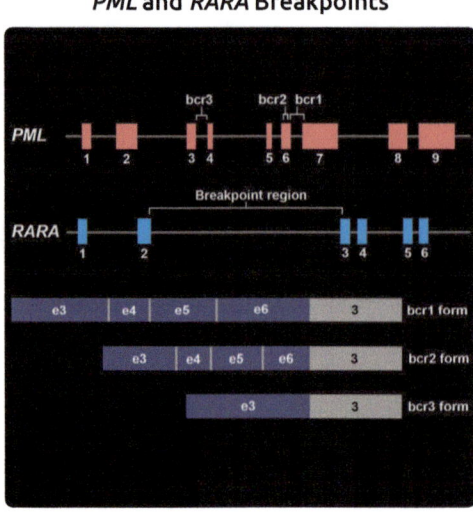

RT-PCR for *PML::RARA* Transcripts

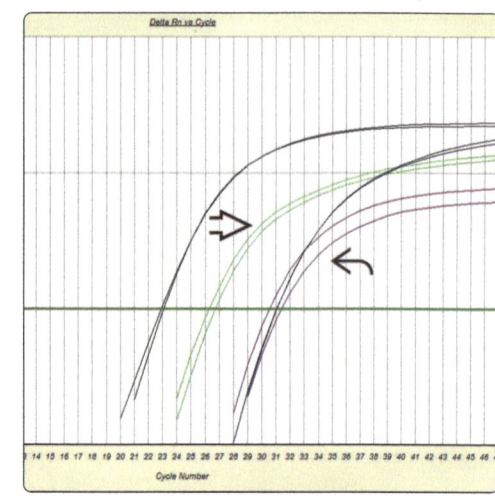

(Left) Graphic shows PML and RARA with the breakpoints and associated fusion genes. PML has 3 main breakpoint clusters, and the breakpoints in RARA are clustered in intron 2, leading to 3 common fusion transcripts. (Right) Quantitative RT-PCR identifies the bcr1 form of transcript ➡. Patients with bcr1 also show a lower level of bcr3 (due to alternative splicing) and bcr2 ➡, as the bcr1 transcript contains the priming sites for the bcr2 primer.

PML::RARA Fusion

- o Has dominant negative function, suppressing normal retinoic acid receptor function
- Critical in leukemogenesis but not sufficient to cause leukemia without other genetic alterations
  - o *FLT3*, *WT1*, *NRAS*, and *KRAS* are most commonly mutated
  - o Additional cytogenetic abnormalities, such as +8 and -7q

CLINICAL IMPLICATIONS

Acute Promyelocytic Leukemia

- Distinct subtype of acute myeloid leukemia (AML)
- Defined by t(15;17)(q24.1;q21.2)/*PML::RARA*
  - o Variant translocations involving *RARA* also implicated
- Increased blasts and abnormal promyelocytes
- Associated with disseminated intravascular coagulation
- Treatment with all-trans retinoic acid (ATRA), arsenic trioxide (ATO), and chemotherapy results in remission in majority of cases
  - o ATRA and ATO induce fusion protein degradation

COMMON METHODS OF DETECTION

Quantitative Real-Time RT-PCR

- General information
  - o Detects RNA transcripts rather than DNA
    - Useful for study of fusion gene transcripts
    - Useful for translocations, as RNA transcript is shorter than DNA
    - Useful in APL, as introns predominate in breakpoint region
  - o Accurately quantifies *PML::RARA* transcripts
    - Sensitive assay for monitoring treatment response, measurable residual disease (MRD), early relapse detection
  - o Reliably determines type of *PML::RARA* transcripts
    - Can identify cases with cryptic translocations
  - o RNA is isolated from blood or bone marrow
- Recommended method for monitoring
  - o Reverse transcribed to produce cDNA
  - o cDNA amplified with standard PCR using control primer set for *ABL1* (internal control gene) and 3 different primer sets for *PML::RARA*
  - o bcr-1 forward primer anneals at 3' end of exon 6
    - Amplifies bcr-1 and low percentage of bcr-2
  - o bcr-2 forward primer sits at beginning of exon 6
    - Multiple bcr-2 variable primers exist
    - bcr-2 breakpoints result in different length transcripts
    - Transcripts can be large (~ 300 bp)
    - No single standard curve is practically possible due to size variation
    - In cases with bcr-2, selection of most appropriate primer improves assay sensitivity
  - o bcr-3 forward primer anneals exon 3
  - o Common reverse primer is used for all transcripts
- Real-time quantitation
  - o Based on detection of fluorescent signal during amplification
    - Signal increases as PCR product is formed
    - Measurement of signal occurs during amplification
  - o Fixed threshold is used to define background
    - Cycle threshold (Ct) is point where reaction fluorescence exceeds threshold
  - o Sequence-specific probes commonly used
    - Fusion transcript probe fluorescence compared to signal from control gene
    - *ABL1* commonly used as internal control gene

Next-Generation Sequencing

- RNA fusion sequencing can identify various translocations and specific breakpoints
- Can screen for additional genetic changes
  - o Majority of cases have ≥ 1 somatic mutations
- Limited utility for rapid diagnosis due to long turnaround times

Karyotype

- Can identify usual t(15;17) fusion as well as fusions with other partners or complex fusions
- Can identify additional cytogenetic abnormalities that may have prognostic impact
  - o Additional abnormalities present in 40% of APL
- Not sensitive for MRD monitoring
- Unable to detect cryptic translocations, such as microinsertions

Fluorescence In Situ Hybridization

- Use targeted probes to detect fusion
  - o Break-apart probes can identify variable translocations
- More sensitive than karyotype but insufficient for MRD monitoring
- More sensitive for microinsertions
  - o Some small insertions still may be missed
  - o Cryptic translocations account for 2-4% of APL
- Provides rapid genetic confirmation of APL

DISEASE MONITORING IN ACUTE PROMYELOCYTIC LEUKEMIA

Minimal Residual Disease and Treatment Response in Acute Promyelocytic Leukemia

- Quantitative real-time PCR recommended at diagnosis
  - o Identifies different types of transcripts
    - May allow selection of more sensitive primers, e.g., if bcr-2 is involved
- Tested again at end of consolidation therapy
  - o Most clinical labs have sensitivity level of ~ 10^{-4}
    - Negative test constitutes major molecular response
  - o Testing prior to end of consolidation less useful, as differentiated cells still carry translocation post treatment
  - o Positive result requires confirmation to prove relapse
    - 2nd sample run in 2-4 weeks
    - Bone marrow testing more sensitive than blood
- Monitor high-risk patients every 3 months for 2 years
  - o Testing in same laboratory recommended
- Testing at suspicion of relapse

SELECTED REFERENCES

1. Scott S et al: Assessment of acute myeloid leukemia molecular measurable residual disease testing in an interlaboratory study. Blood Adv. 7(14):3686-94, 2023

Reverse Transcription PCR for Myeloid Leukemia Transcripts

RUNX1::RUNX1T1

Definition and Etiology/Pathogenesis

- Previously known as *AML1-ETO*
- *RUNX1* is component of core-binding factor (CBF) (α-subunit)
  o CBF transcription factor is essential component of normal hematopoiesis
- Pathologic fusion gene binds DNA as negative competitor with normal *RUNX1* product
  o Results in transcriptional repression of normal target genes
  o Impairs normal hematopoiesis
  o Is not sufficient by itself to cause leukemia in mouse models
    – Need additional mutations to incite leukemia
- Can dimerize with CBF β-subunit
- Altered transcriptional regulation of target genes downstream of *RUNX1*
- Structure of *RUNX1::RUNX1T1* fusion product
  o *RUNX1* on chromosome 21 with 12 exons
    – Breakpoints are clustered in intron 5
  o *RUNX1T1* on chromosome 8 with 20 exons
    – Breakpoints clustered in introns 1a and 1b
  o Coding region of *RUNX1T1* fused to *RUNX1* N-terminus containing DNA-binding domain
    – Fusion product is same regardless of breakpoint variations

Acute Myeloid Leukemia With Recurrent Genetic Abnormality t(8;21)(q21.3;q22.12); RUNX1::RUNX1T1

- Incidence
  o 5-12% of de novo adult acute myeloid leukemia (AML)
  o More common in pediatric population (~ 10-13%)
- Other features
  o Complex karyotype common
  o Concurrent *KIT* (20-40%) &/or *FLT3* ITD (up to 16%) mutations common
  o Associated with maturation morphology
  o Does not require ≥ 20% blasts if genetic abnormality is present
  o May present with myeloid sarcoma
- Prognosis
  o Good response to chemotherapy
    – Relapse still seen in up to 35%, although up to 60% are salvageable
  o *KIT* or *FLT3* ITD mutation negatively affects prognosis

Testing

- Quantitative RT-PCR is available for this fusion gene transcript
  o Consistently detected in patients with t(8;21) AML
    – *RUNX1* breakpoint consistently in intron 5
    – *RUNX1T1* breakpoints upstream of exon 2, clustered in introns 1a and 1b
    – Despite *RUNX1T1* breakpoint variation, all results in single type of fusion gene transcript
  o Especially useful for minimal residual disease (MRD) monitoring
    – Sensitivity up to 1 copy in 100,000
    – Copy number > 500 in bone marrow or > 100 in peripheral blood predictive of relapse
    – Unlike inv(16), low-level MRD is still compatible with durable remission
    – Normalized ratio and copy number are generated using reference gene
- Alternative methods
  o Conventional karyotyping
    – Usually detectable
    – Lower assay sensitivity; not good for minimal residual disease testing
  o FISH
    – Usually count 200 cells, so not good for MRD testing
    – Excellent for rapid diagnosis

CBFB::MYH11

Definition and Etiology/Pathogenesis

- *MYH11* codes for smooth muscle myosin heavy chain

RUNX1::RUNX1T1 Fusion

RUNX1::RUNX1T1 t(8;21)

RUNX1 (21q22) | RUNX1T1 (8q22)

2 3 4 5 | 2 3 4

1057 275

5' Forward primer — Probe — 3' Reverse primer

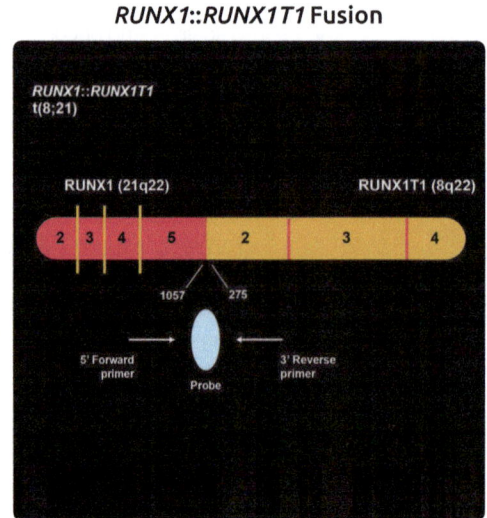

CBFB::MYH11 Fusion Subtypes

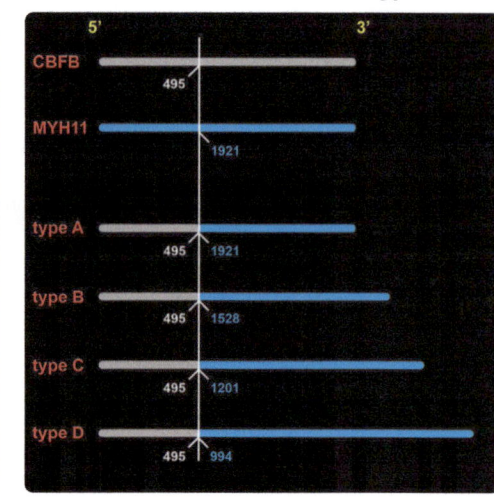

5' 3'

CBFB — 495
MYH11 — 1921
type A — 495 | 1921
type B — 495 | 1528
type C — 495 | 1201
type D — 495 | 994

(Left) RUNX1::RUNX1T1 fusion is depicted. The RUNX1 breakpoint consistently occurs within intron 5, and the RUNX1T1 breakpoint occurs upstream of exon 2, resulting in a single type of transcript. (Right) CBFB::MYH11 has multiple transcript subtypes, with types A-D illustrated here. ~ 85% of patients have type A, with types D and E (not shown) representing ~ 5% each. Other subtypes are uncommon.

Reverse Transcription PCR for Myeloid Leukemia Transcripts

- *CBFB* codes for CBF-β, subunit of heterodimer transcription factor
    - CBFB protein binds RUNX proteins (RUNX 1, 2, or 3) and stabilizes its interaction with DNA
    - CBFB protein may also prevent ubiquitin-mediated degradation of RUNX protein
- Fusion gene is formed
    - Same chromosomal breakpoints for inv(16) and t(16;16)
    - Several breakpoints are possible, leading to several subtypes of fusion gene
    - Fusion protein binds with greater affinity to RUNX1 protein
        - Suppresses normal function through multiple mechanisms, including sequestration and active repression
        - Blocks differentiation of myeloid leukemic cells
    - This fusion is insufficient by itself to cause leukemogenesis
        - As with *RUNX1::RUNX1T1*, other mutations are required to incite leukemogenesis
- Both *RUNX1::RUNX1T1* and *CBFB::MYH11* are included in category known as CBF group of AML because they each include subunit of CBF in fusion gene product

Acute Myeloid Leukemia With Recurring Genetic Abnormality inv(16)(p13.1q22) or t(16;16)(p13.1;q22)

- Incidence
    - 5-9% of cases of AML
    - Usually younger patients
- Other features
    - Majority have inv(16) rather than t(16;16)
    - Monocytic and granulocytic differentiation
    - Abnormal eosinophils
    - Myeloid sarcomas (extramedullary presentation) more frequent
- Prognosis
    - Generally favorable
        - Relapse occurs in up to 35%, although up to 60% are salvageable
    - Prognosis is same for inv(16) and for t(16;16)
    - Worse prognosis with concurrent *KIT* mutations

Testing

- Quantitative RT-PCR is available for this fusion gene transcript
    - At least 10 different fusion gene transcripts have been reported
        - > 85% have type A transcript
        - ~ 5% each have types D and E
        - Most assays just assess for types A, D, and E
        - Other types are uncommon
    - Useful in detection of minimal residual disease
        - Sensitivity up to 1 copy in 100,000
        - Copy number > 50 in bone marrow or > 10 in peripheral blood is predictive of relapse
        - Relapse at much lower MRD levels than t(8;21) AML
- Alternative methods
    - Chromosomal karyotyping
        - Lower sensitivity; not good for MRD detection
        - Occasionally negative in cryptic cases
        - Subtle rearrangement may be overlooked in suboptimal metaphase preparations
        - Secondary abnormalities are common, seen in ~ 40% of cases
        - +22 is fairly specific to this type of AML
    - FISH
        - Good method for detecting cryptic inversions or translocations
        - Will detect subtypes other than A, D, and E
        - Fairly rapid diagnosis
        - Not good for minimal residual disease testing

OTHERS

Other Gene Fusion Transcripts

- Have been detected by RT-PCR in research setting but are not commonly available as commercial tests
    - Entities in AML with defining genetic abnormalities
        - *DEK::NUP214*
        - *RBM15::MRTFA*
        - *KMT2A::MLLT3*
        - Other *KMT2A* rearrangements
        - *NUP98* rearrangements
    - Recognized fusion gene transcripts but not included in AML with defining genetic abnormalities
        - *KAT6A::CREBBP*
        - *MYB::GATA1*
        - *MNX1::ETV6*

SELECTED REFERENCES

1. Weinberg OK et al: The International Consensus Classification of acute myeloid leukemia. Virchows Arch. 482(1):27-37, 2023
2. Al-Harbi S et al: An update on the molecular pathogenesis and potential therapeutic targeting of AML with t(8;21)(q22;q22.1);RUNX1-RUNX1T1. Blood Adv. 4(1):229-38, 2020
3. Ishikawa Y et al: Prospective evaluation of prognostic impact of KIT mutations on acute myeloid leukemia with RUNX1-RUNX1T1 and CBFB-MYH11. Blood Adv. 4(1):66-75, 2020
4. Duployez N et al: Minimal residual disease monitoring in t(8;21) acute myeloid leukemia based on RUNX1-RUNX1T1 fusion quantification on genomic DNA. Am J Hematol. 89(6):610-5, 2014
5. Krauth MT et al: High number of additional genetic lesions in acute myeloid leukemia with t(8;21)/RUNX1-RUNX1T1: frequency and impact on clinical outcome. Leukemia. 28(7):1449-58, 2014
6. Park SH et al: Effects of c-KIT mutations on expression of the RUNX1/RUNX1T1 fusion transcript in t(8;21)-positive acute myeloid leukemia patients. Leuk Res. 37(7):784-9, 2013
7. Eghtedar A et al: Characteristics of translocation (16;16)(p13;q22) acute myeloid leukemia. Am J Hematol. 87(3):317-8, 2012
8. Yang JJ et al: Detection of RUNX1-MECOM fusion gene and t(3;21) in a very elderly patient having acute myeloid leukemia with myelodysplasia-related changes. Ann Lab Med. 32(5):362-5, 2012
9. Yin JA et al: Minimal residual disease monitoring by quantitative RT-PCR in core binding factor AML allows risk stratification and predicts relapse: results of the United Kingdom MRC AML-15 trial. Blood. 120(14):2826-35, 2012
10. Sun X et al: Comparative analysis of genes regulated in acute myelomonocytic leukemia with and without inv(16)(p13q22) using microarray techniques, real-time PCR, immunohistochemistry, and flow cytometry immunophenotyping. Mod Pathol. 20(8):811-20, 2007
11. Huang G et al: Molecular basis for a dominant inactivation of RUNX1/AML1 by the leukemogenic inversion 16 chimera. Blood. 103(8):3200-7, 2004
12. van der Reijden BA et al: RT-PCR diagnosis of patients with acute nonlymphocytic leukemia and inv(16)(p13q22) and identification of new alternative splicing in CBFB-MYH11 transcripts. Blood. 86(1):277-82, 1995

FLT3, NPM1, and CEBPA Mutations

TERMINOLOGY

Definitions

- *FLT3*
  - Official name: Fms-related tyrosine kinase 3
  - HGNC ID: 3765
  - Chromosomal location: 13q12.2
  - Preferred protein name: Receptor-type tyrosine-protein kinase FLT3
- *NPM1*
  - Official name: Nucleophosmin 1
  - HGNC ID: 7910
  - Chromosomal location: 5q35.1
  - Preferred protein name: Nucleophosmin
- *CEBPA*
  - Official name: CCAAT enhancer binding protein alpha
  - HGNC ID: 1833
  - Chromosomal location: 19q13.11
  - Preferred protein name: CCAAT/enhancer-binding protein alpha

GENE FUNCTION

Fms-Related Tyrosine Kinase 3 (*FLT3*)

- Type III receptor tyrosine kinase
  - 5 immunoglobulin-like domains in extracellular region
  - Transmembrane domain
  - Juxtamembrane domain
  - Split tyrosine kinase domain with 2 variable-length insertions by hydrophobic enterokinase sequence
- Binds FLT3 ligand (FL)
  - Constitutively expressed by bone marrow fibroblasts
  - 1 FL binds 2 receptors, bringing them into close proximity
  - Transphosphorylation occurs and results in activation of receptor tyrosine kinase
  - Following binding, ligand is rapidly degraded
- Phosphorylation and activation of downstream signaling cascades
  - PI3K-Akt pathway
    - Blocks apoptosis
    - Increases proliferation
  - Ras-MAP kinase pathway
    - Increases transcription and proliferation
- Expressed by hematopoietic progenitor cells in bone marrow, thymus, and lymph nodes
  - Regulates transcription, proliferation, differentiation, and apoptosis
    - Decreases time in G1 phase of cell cycle
  - Important for B- and T-lymphocyte development
    - Works with IL-7 to induce proliferation of early B-cell progenitors and pro-B cells
    - Synergizes with IL-3 to accelerate B-cell development
  - Regulator of dendritic cell development and activity
    - Generates both classic and plasmacytoid dendritic cells
    - Regulates dendritic cell-mediated NK-cell activation
  - Induces monocyte differentiation
  - Does not play role in megakaryocyte development
- Activity regulated by cytokines
  - TNF-α downregulates activity
  - TGF-β downregulates activity

Nucleophosmin (*NPM1*)

- Nucleolar phosphoprotein
  - N-terminal homooligomerization domain
    - Leads to formation of NPM1 dimers and hexamers
  - Heterodimerization domain
    - Forms dimers of NPM with other proteins, including nucleolin and ARF
  - C-terminal nucleic acid binding domain
    - Allows interaction with ribosomal processing RNA
- Nucleus-cytoplasm shuttling protein
  - Regulates ribosomal protein assembly and transport
  - Controls centrosome duplication
  - Regulates tumor suppressor pathways, such as TP53 and ARF
    - Stabilizes TP53
    - Prevents proteasomal degradation of TP53
  - Regulates stability of nuclear proteins

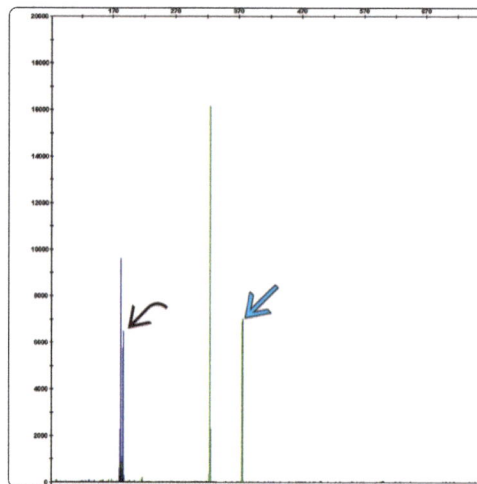

(Left) Electropherogram of PCR products from a patient with AML shows wildtype FLT3 ⇨ and mutated NPM1 with 4 base insertion ↷. The wildtype FLT3/mutated NPM1 genotype is associated with improved prognosis. **(Right)** Electropherogram of PCR products of FLT3 and NPM1 shows FLT3 ITD mutation ⇨ as well as NPM1 mutation ↷. The FLT3 ITD mutation is associated with worse prognosis, regardless of NPM1 status.

Mutated *NPM1*

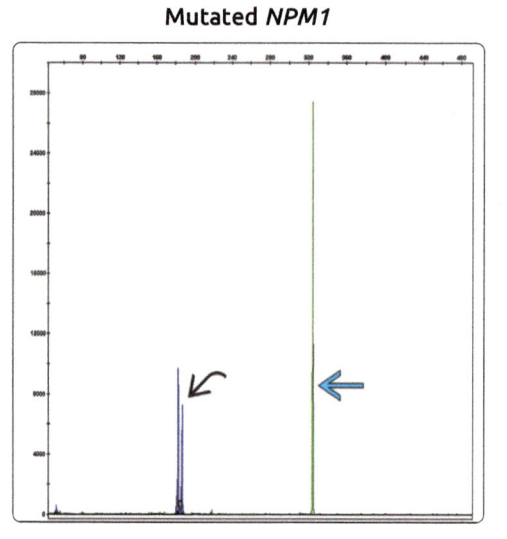

Concurrent *NPM1* and *FLT3* ITD Mutations

FLT3, NPM1, and CEBPA Mutations

- Inhibits caspase-activated DNase
- Prevents apoptosis

CCAAT/Enhancer-Binding Protein Alpha (CEBPA)
- Basic region leucine zipper (bZIP) transcription regulator
  - Forms homo- or heterodimers with other bZIP proteins
    - Can bind coactivators or corepressors
  - Dimerized protein binds promoter region of numerous genes
- 2 possible start sites
  - Major translational start site produces 42 kDa protein (p42)
  - Internal downstream start site produces 30 kDa protein (p30)
    - p30 lacks N-terminal transactivation domain
    - Has altered transcriptional activity
    - p30 can heterodimerize with p42, preventing normal transcriptional activating function
  - Ratio of p42 to p30 is dependent on mTOR activity
  - Rarely, extended 46 kDa protein may be produced from upstream start site
- Expressed in hepatocytes, adipocytes, type II pneumocytes, and granulocytes
  - Involved in granulocyte differentiation and maturation
    - Induces transcription of regulatory proteins required for lineage maturation
    - CEBPA expression increases as cells mature
    - CEBPA-deleted mice show markedly reduced neutrophils and monocytes with elevated platelets and lymphocytes
    - Decreased CEBPA expression is associated with increased monocytes
  - Expression downregulates cell cycle progression

GENE MUTATIONS

FLT3 Mutations
- Most common type of mutation is 6-30 bp internal tandem duplication (ITD) insertions
  - ITD sizes from 3 to > 400 bases have been described
    - Most common length is 20-60 bp
  - Inframe mutations
  - Involve exons 14 and 15 in juxtamembrane domain
    - Occasionally occur in tyrosine kinase domain
  - Interfere with inhibitory function of juxtamembrane domain
    - Receptor shows ligand-independent dimerization
    - Results in production of constitutively active tyrosine kinase
    - Activates downstream RAS, MAPK, and STAT5 signaling
    - Leads to proliferation and cell survival
  - STAT5 signaling is unique to mutated receptor
- Point mutations
  - Kinase domain activation loop (TKD) mutations in exon 20 are most common
    - Results in constitutive phosphorylation and activation
    - Promotes signaling through different pathways than ITD-type FLT3 mutations
    - Oncogenic potential and prognostic significance is not well established
  - Juxtamembrane domain mutations have also been described

NPM1 Mutation
- Most common type of mutation is 4 bp insertion in exon 12
  - Point mutations and deletions have also been described
  - Mutation leads to frameshift, altering C-terminal region of protein
- Mutations are heterozygous, occurring on only 1 allele
  - May have dominant negative effect
  - Normal NPM forms dimers with mutant form
- Mutations disrupt nucleolar localization signal or create export signal
  - Mutated NPM1 is found in cytoplasm rather than nucleus
- NPM1 mutation alone not sufficient for leukemogenesis
- NPM1 translocations
  - Occurs in several hematologic malignancies
    - NPM1::ALK in anaplastic large cell lymphoma
    - NPM1::RARA in acute myeloid leukemia (AML) with variant RARA translocation

CEBPA Mutation
- N-terminus mutation
  - Nonsense or frameshift mutation
  - Mutation occurs between major translational start site and downstream start site
    - Only transcription of shorter (p30) protein isoform can occur
  - Shorter protein has dominant negative effect due to heterodimer formation
  - Germline mutations are commonly N-terminus mutations
  - N-terminus mutations do not meet criteria for AML with in-frame bZIP CEBPA mutations
- C-terminus mutation
  - In-frame insertion or deletion or nonsense mutation
  - Located in basic leucine zipper domain
  - Reduces DNA binding and homo- and heterodimerization
    - Normal transcription promoter functions do not occur
  - Mutated protein still binds NF-κB
    - Induces BCL2 and inhibits apoptosis
  - Associated with favorable prognosis
  - Diagnostic of AML with in-frame bZIP CEBPA mutations
    - Subset of cases have biallelic mutations typically involving both regions
      - Each allele harbors different mutation
      - No wildtype protein is produced
      - Biallelic mutations show distinct gene expression signature
      - Different mutations have synergistic effect in leukemogenesis
      - No difference in prognosis between biallelic mutations and in-frame bZIP mutation only
    - Gene expression may also be dysregulated by other genes or epigenetic modification
- Germline mutations occur in familial myeloid neoplasm susceptibility syndromes
  - Constitutional N-terminal mutation
    - C-terminal mutation occurs as "2nd hit" leading to leukemogenesis

FLT3, NPM1, and CEBPA Mutations

- Patients with N-terminal *CEBPA* mutations should undergo further work-up to evaluate for germline mutation

CLINICAL IMPLICATIONS

Acute Myeloid Leukemia

- Most common acute leukemia in adults
  - Outcomes are poor
    - 5-year survival < 50% overall
    - 5-year survival < 20% in patients > 60 years of age
  - Diagnosis and risk stratification relies on identification of cytogenetic and molecular abnormalities
    - AML with mutated *NPM1* and AML with in-frame bZIP *CEBPA* mutations represent specific AML entities in ICC and WHO classifications
      □ Prognosis may be further refined by identification of *FLT3* mutations
    - AML with normal cytogenetics show variable prognosis
      □ Prognosis may be refined by identification of *FLT3*, *NPM1*, and *CEBPA* mutations

Clinical Significance of *FLT3* Mutations

- Most common mutation in hematologic malignancy
- *FLT3* mutations occur in 20-30% of AML
  - More common in cases with normal karyotype
    - Detected in ~ 30-35% of AML cases with normal karyotype
  - Rare in infant AML
  - Most common in older adults
  - Associated with higher WBC counts at diagnosis
  - Found in 5-10% of myelodysplastic syndrome cases
  - 5-10% of chronic myeloid leukemia cases, particularly in accelerated and blast phase
  - Often seen concurrently in cases with *NPM1* mutation
- Considered high-risk abnormality
  - Associated with increased relapse
  - No difference in treatment response rate
  - Shorter overall survival
  - Length of ITD does not correlate with prognostic impact
  - ITD in tyrosine kinase domain is associated with particularly poor outcomes
- High mutant:wildtype ratio (allelic ratio) is associated with worse outcomes
  - Patients with *FLT3* ITD high allelic ratio may significantly benefit from allogeneic stem cell transplantation in 1st clinical remission
- Prognostic significance of point mutations in tyrosine kinase domain (TKD) is not well established
- Treatment implications
  - FLT3 tyrosine kinase inhibitors offer targeted therapy
    - Best studied in *FLT3* ITD mutations but also recommended with TKD mutations
  - Allogeneic hematopoietic stem cell transplant in 1st remission is recommended in cases with high *FLT3* ITD allelic ratio

Clinical Significance of *NPM1* Mutation

- AML with mutated *NPM1* represents diagnostic entity in ICC and WHO classifications
  - Can be diagnosed with ≥ 10% blasts in ICC and WHO
  - Cases with < 10% blasts with mutation should be monitored very closely for progression
- Occurs in 25-35% of adult AML
  - 45-64% of cases with normal karyotype
  - 2-8% of pediatric AML
  - More common in women
  - Associated with higher WBC count and blast count
  - Associated with anemia and thrombocytopenia
  - Associated with monocytic differentiation
    - 80-90% of acute monocytic leukemia have *NPM1* mutation
  - Associated with dysplastic features in 25% of cases
    - Presence does not impact prognosis
  - Associated with tissue involvement
    - May involve gums, lymph nodes, or skin
  - AML with *NPM1* mutation also harbors *FLT3*-ITD mutation in 40% of cases
    - *NPM1* mutation precedes *FLT3* mutation
    - These cases are more genetically stable in disease progression
  - Other common secondary mutations include *DNMT3A*, *IDH2*, *KRAS*, *NRAS*
  - *NPM1* and *CEBPA* mutations are mutually exclusive
- Considered favorable risk abnormality
  - Good response to induction therapy
  - Cases with normal karyotype and absence of *FLT3*-ITD have favorable prognosis
    - Associated with better overall and disease-free survival and lower cumulative incidence of relapse
      □ Also associated with improved prognosis in cytogenetically abnormal cases
    - Prognosis similar to core-binding factor leukemias in younger patients
  - Coexisting *FLT3* mutation overrides positive effects of *NPM1* mutation
    - These cases have intermediate prognosis between *NPM1*-only mutated and *FLT3*-only mutated cases
- Cases with *NPM1* mutation often also have del 9q
- Treatment implications
  - *NPM1*-mutated AML without *FLT3* mutations is not treated with allogeneic bone marrow transplant in 1st remission
  - Older patients with *NPM1* mutations may receive attenuated chemotherapy regimens
- *NPM1* mutations offer target for measurable residual disease testing

Clinical Significance of *CEBPA* Mutation

- AML with in-frame bZIP *CEBPA* mutation (ICC)/AML with *CEBPA* mutation (WHO) represents distinct diagnostic entity
- Requires mutation in C-terminal bZIP region
  - 5-11% of adult AML
  - 5% of pediatric AML
  - 10-18% of cases with normal karyotype
  - N-terminal mutations should be further worked up for possibility of germline mutation with predisposition to develop AML
  - Associated with higher blast counts
  - Associated with higher hemoglobin levels and lower platelet levels than other AML

FLT3, NPM1, and CEBPA Mutations

- AML with *CEBPA* mutation can be diagnosed with ≥ 10% blasts in ICC classification
  - ≥ 20% required for WHO
- Rarely involves extramedullary tissues
- AML with *CEBPA* mutation also harbors *FLT3* mutation in 22-33% of cases
- *CEBPA* and *NPM1* mutations usually mutually exclusive
- 5-10% of N-terminal mutations are germline and associated with increased risk of early AML
  - Median age at diagnosis: 24.5 years
- Treatment implications
  - AML with *CEBPA* mutation is not treated with allogeneic bone marrow transplant in 1st remission
  - Associated with greater chemosensitivity
- Epigenetic silencing of *CEBPA* is associated with worse outcome

TESTING FOR *FLT3*, *NPM1*, AND *CEBPA* MUTATIONS

FLT3 Mutation Testing

- Exons 14 and 15 harboring ITD are amplified and PCR product is analyzed
  - Amplification by labeled primer followed by fragment analysis by capillary electrophoresis for sizing
    - Both shorter wildtype peak and longer mutated peaks due to ITD are present in mutated cases
  - Direct sequencing by Sanger sequencing can demonstrate presence of duplicated sequence
  - Quantitative RT-PCR using patient-specific primers encompassing ITD is sensitive and may be useful for minimal residual disease testing
  - Next-generation sequencing can be used to identify ITD
    - Software with high sensitivity for insertions is recommended
      - Longer ITDs may not be recognized by standard analysis pipeline
      - May give inaccurate mutant:wildtype allele ratios
    - Deep sequencing is highly sensitive and can be used for MRD
  - Reporting should include *FLT3* ITD allelic ratio in all mutated cases for prognostication
- TKD may be sequenced to identify point mutations in exon 20

NPM1 Mutation Testing

- Region that harbors insertion mutation, including exon 12, is amplified and PCR product is analyzed
  - Amplification by labeled primer followed by fragment analysis by capillary electrophoresis for sizing of amplified products
    - Both shorter wildtype peak and longer mutated peak due to insertion are present in mutated cases
  - Direct sequencing by Sanger sequencing can demonstrate presence of duplicated sequence
  - Quantitative RT-PCR using mixture of primers targeting different insertion types is sensitive and may be useful for minimal residual disease testing
  - Next-generation sequencing can be used to identify insertions
    - RT-PCR is highly sensitive and can be used for disease monitoring and MRD detection
- Identification of cytoplasmic localization can serve as surrogate indicator of gene mutation
  - Immunohistochemical, cytochemical, and immunofluorescent studies are available
    - These tests may be difficult to interpret, and nucleic acid-based molecular testing is preferred

CEBPA Mutation Testing

- Coding sequence is amplified, and product is analyzed
  - Direct sequencing by Sanger sequencing can identify mutations
  - Next-generation sequencing can be used to identify mutations
    - *CEBPA* has high GC content, which may lead to decreased sequencing and lower analytic sensitivity

PREDICTIVE TESTING SUMMARY

Test Interpretation

- Prognostic significance clearest in cytogenetically normal AML
- *FLT3* ITD and TKD mutations associated with unfavorable outcome
  - *FLT3* tyrosine kinase inhibitors are available
- *NPM1* mutation associated with favorable outcome in absence of *FLT3*-ITD mutations
  - AML with both *FLT3* and *NPM1* mutations may have intermediate outcome
- In-frame bZIP *CEBPA* mutation associated with favorable outcome in AML

SELECTED REFERENCES

1. Kurzer JH et al: Updates in molecular genetics of acute myeloid leukemia. Semin Diagn Pathol. 40(3):140-51, 2023
2. Miyashita N et al: Prognostic impact of FLT3-ITD, NPM1 mutation and CEBPA bZIP domain mutation in cytogenetically normal acute myeloid leukemia: a Hokkaido Leukemia Net study. Int J Hematol. 118(1):36-46, 2023
3. Mrózek K et al: Outcome prediction by the 2022 European LeukemiaNet genetic-risk classification for adults with acute myeloid leukemia: an Alliance study. Leukemia. 37(4):788-98, 2023
4. Weinberg OK et al: The International Consensus Classification of acute myeloid leukemia. Virchows Arch. 482(1):27-37, 2023
5. Arber DA et al: International Consensus Classification of myeloid neoplasms and acute leukemia: integrating morphological, clinical, and genomic data. Blood. 140(11):1200-28, 2022
6. Khoury JD et al: The 5th edition of the World Health Organization classification of haematolymphoid tumours: myeloid and histiocytic/dendritic neoplasms. Leukemia. 36(7):1703-19, 2022
7. Wakita S et al: Prognostic impact of CEBPA bZIP domain mutation in acute myeloid leukemia. Blood Adv. 6(1):238-47, 2022
8. Tarlock K et al: CEBPA-bZip mutations are associated with favorable prognosis in de novo AML: a report from the Children's Oncology Group. Blood. 138(13):1137-47, 2021
9. Höllein A et al: NPM1 mutated AML can relapse with wild-type NPM1: persistent clonal hematopoiesis can drive relapse. Blood Adv. 2(22):3118-25, 2018
10. Kunchala P et al: When the good go bad: mutant NPM1 in acute myeloid leukemia. Blood Rev. 32(3):167-83, 2018
11. Mack EKM et al: Comprehensive genetic diagnosis of acute myeloid leukemia by next generation sequencing. Haematologica. 104(1):e9-12, 2018

JAK2 Mutations and Rearrangements

TERMINOLOGY

Definitions

- Official name: Janus kinase 2
- Official symbol: JAK2
- HGNC ID: 6192
- Genomic position: Ch9: 4,984,390-5,129,948 (GRCh38.p14)
- Chromosomal location: 9p24.1
- Number of exons: 28
- Alias: JTK10

ETIOLOGY/PATHOGENESIS

Normal Function of JAK2

- Encodes JAK2 tyrosine kinase protein involved in subset of cytokine receptor signaling pathway
  o Possess N-terminal FERM (band 4.1, ezrin, radixin, moesin-homology), SRC homology-2 (SH2)-like, pseudokinase (JH2), and C-terminal (JH1) domains
    – N-terminal domain is associated with binding to cytokine receptors
    – SH2 domain that binds STAT transcription factors
    – JH1 is activated via transphosphorylation of tandem tyrosines in activation loop
    – JH2 has autoinhibitory activity and regulates activity of JH1
  o Involved mainly in JAK-STAT signaling pathway
    – Also interacts with RAS/MAPK, PI3K, and AKT downstream pathways
  o JAK2 is downstream target of pleiotropic cytokine IL6
    – Dysregulation of IL6/JAK2/STAT3 signaling pathways produces increased cellular proliferation
  o Constitutively associated with prolactin receptor
  o Required for response to γ-interferon
  o Lack of JAK2 expression in mice leads to embryonic lethality due to absence of definitive erythropoiesis

Abnormal Function of Altered JAK2

- JAK2 V617F mutation
  o Point mutation in exon 14 of pseudokinase domain
    – Substitution of G to T at 1849 position (c.1849G>T)
    – 1849G>T leads to substitution of valine for phenylalanine (V617F)
    – p.V617F destabilizes fold of domain that leads to constitutive activation of JAK2
    – Mutation involves myeloid lineages and is absent in lymphocytes
  o Consequences of JAK2 V617F mutation
    – Gain-of-function somatic mutation
    – Constitutive activation of STAT-mediated transcription in absence of EPO ligand
    – Also activates ERK/MAPK and PI3/AKT pathways in absence of alternative cytokine stimulation
  o Most common mutation BCR::ABL1-negative myeloproliferative neoplasms (MPNs), including polycythemia vera (PV), essential thrombocythemia (ET), and primary myelofibrosis (PMF)
- JAK2 exon 12 mutations
  o Mutations involve region adjacent to start of pseudokinase domain from codons 536 to 547
    – Uncommon, except in JAK2 V617F-negative PV
    – Present in ~ 3% of PV cases
    – About 40 different mutations reported
    – Mutations include deletions, duplications/insertions, and nonsynonymous base substitutions
  o Common mutations
    – N542-E543del
    – E543-D544del
    – F537-K539delinsL
    – R541-E543delinsK
    – K539L, F537I, L545V
  o JAK2 exon 12 mutations appear to result specifically in erythrocytosis phenotype
  o Can also occur in patients with myelodysplastic/MPN with SF3B1 mutation and thrombocytosis
  o Patients with JAK2 exon 12-mutated PV show significantly longer overall survival than patients with JAK2 V617F-mutated PV
- JAK2 rearrangements
  o PCM1::JAK2 fusion

JAK2 V617F Mutation Detected by Allelic Discrimination Real-Time PCR

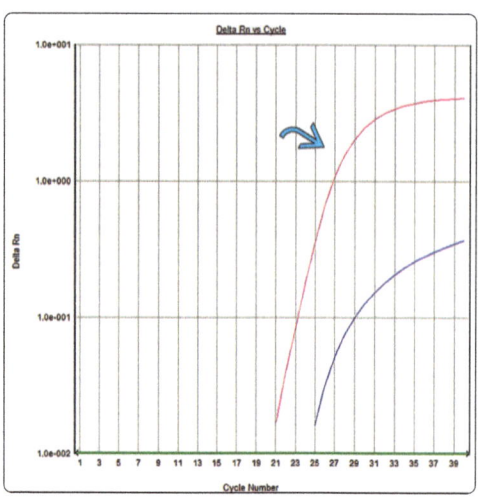

JAK2 Exon 12 Mutation Detected by Sanger Sequencing

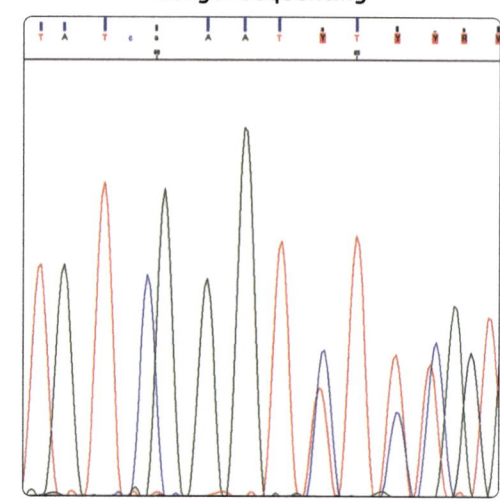

(Left) Analysis of JAK2 exon 14 using allelic discrimination real-time PCR shows a JAK2 V617F mutation (amplification curve in red) ➡ with high mutated allele burden in a patient with polycythemia vera (PV). (Right) Sanger sequencing of JAK2 exon 12 performed on blood sample from a patient with JAK2 V617F-negative PV demonstrates a mixed sequence corresponding to the codons E543 and E544 deletion.

JAK2 Mutations and Rearrangements

- Results from t(8;9)(p22;p24.1) translocation
- Most cases present with MPN
- Some cases show overlap MPN and myelodysplastic syndrome (MPN/MDS)
- Also occurs in subset of BCR::ABL1-like (Ph-like) B-lymphoblastic leukemia (B-ALL)
- Rarely reported in T-lymphoblastic leukemia
○ ETV6::JAK2 fusion
- Results from t(9;12)(p24.1;p13.2) translocation
- Present in subset of BCR::ABL1-like B-ALL
- Rarely reported in MDS
○ BCR::JAK2 fusion
- Results from t(9;22)(p24.1;q11.23) translocation
- Present in subset of BCR::ABL1-like B-ALL
- Reported in MDS/MPN
- Crucial to distinguish from t(9;22)(q34;q11.2); BCR::ABL1
- Resistant to imatinib
○ SSBP2::JAK2 fusion
- Results from t(5;9)(q14.1;p24.1) translocation
- Present in subset of BCR::ABL1-like B-ALL
○ STRN3::JAK2 fusion
- Results from t(9;14)(p24.1;q12) translocation
- Present in subset of BCR::ABL1-like, B-ALL
○ PAX5::JAK2 fusion
- Results from t(9;9)(p13.2;p24.1) translocation
- Occurs in subset of BCR::ABL1-like B-ALL
○ JAK2::PABPC1 fusion
- Reported in subset of ALK(-) anaplastic large cell lymphoma

CLINICAL IMPLICATIONS

Nonchronic Myeloid Leukemia Myeloproliferative Neoplasms
- PV
  ○ JAK2 V617F in ~ 95% of cases
  ○ JAK2 exon 12 mutations in ~ 3% of cases
- ET
  ○ JAK2 V617F in ~ 50% of cases
  ○ Most JAK2 V617F-negative cases harbor either CALR or MPL mutation
  ○ JAK2 exon 12 mutations are typically absent in ET
- PMF
  ○ JAK2 V617F in ~ 60% of cases
  ○ Most JAK2 V617F-negative PMF cases harbor CALR or MPL mutation
  ○ JAK2 mutations typically mutually exclusive with mutations in CALR and MPL genes
- JAK2 mutations not reported in healthy individuals
- Additional recurrent somatic mutations in other genes that may modulate disease progression in MPNs
  ○ TET2, ASXL1, DNMT3A, CBL, SH2B3, IDH1, IDH2, EZH2, TP53, SRSF2

Other Myeloid Neoplasms
- MDS/MPN with SF3B1 mutation and thrombocytosis
  ○ JAK2 V617F is detected in ~ 50% of cases
- Chronic myelomonocytic leukemia (CMML)
  ○ JAK2 V617F reported in small subset of cases
- Acute myeloid leukemia (AML) and MDS
  ○ Sporadic reports of JAK2 V617F(+) MDS and AML cases

Neoplasms With JAK2 Fusion
- Small numbers of cases with MPN, MPN/MDS, and subset of B-ALL
  ○ Leads to constitutive activation of JAK2-STAT signaling pathways
  ○ Possible response to JAK2 inhibitors with some but not all JAK2 gene fusions
- B-ALL with PAX5::JAK2 fusion
  ○ Does not result in constitutive activation of JAK2-STAT
- Classic Hodgkin lymphoma
  ○ 2 isolated case reports with SEC31A::JAK2 fusion

JAK2 Inhibitors
- JAK2 inhibitor ruxolitinib approved by FDA in 2011
  ○ Indicated in treatment of high-risk PMF, post-PV and post-ET myelofibrosis
  ○ Has broad anticytokine effect
  ○ Significantly reduces constitutional symptoms
  ○ Reduces splenomegaly

Suggested Testing Algorithm
- JAK2 V617F with reflex to JAK2 exon 12 mutations in suspected cases of PV
- JAK2 V617F with reflex to CALR and MPL mutations in suspected cases of ET and PMF

Molecular Diagnostic Techniques
- Sanger sequencing
  ○ Method used in original reports of JAK2 V617F
- Pyrosequencing
  ○ Sequence based on synthesis in real time with no need to post PCR analysis procedure
- Allele-specific PCR (amplification refractory mutation system)
  ○ Detects JAK2 V617F with 1-2% sensitivity
- Quantitative real-time PCR
  ○ Can quantify mutated allele burden
  ○ May need granulocyte enrichment for reliable quantification
- DNA melting curve assay
  ○ Cost-effective method for screening of JAK2 exon 12
  ○ Useful method to detect presence of point mutations and indels
- Next-generation sequencing (NGS)
  ○ Powerful technique with ability to simultaneously detect additional mutations in targeted panel

SELECTED REFERENCES

1. Luque Paz D et al: Genetic basis and molecular profiling in myeloproliferative neoplasms. Blood. 141(16):1909-21, 2023
2. Fitzpatrick MJ et al: JAK2 rearrangements are a recurrent alteration in CD30+ systemic T-cell lymphomas with anaplastic morphology. Am J Surg Pathol. 45(7):895-904, 2021
3. Tefferi A et al: JAK2 exon 12 mutated polycythemia vera: Mayo-Careggi MPN Alliance study of 33 consecutive cases and comparison with JAK2V617F mutated disease. Am J Hematol. 93(4):E93-6, 2018
4. Reshmi SC et al: Targetable kinase gene fusions in high-risk B-ALL: a study from the Children's Oncology Group. Blood. 129(25):3352-61, 2017
5. Silvennoinen O et al: Molecular insights into regulation of JAK2 in myeloproliferative neoplasms. Blood. 125(22):3388-92, 2015

MPL Mutations

TERMINOLOGY

Definitions

- Official name: MPL protooncogene, thrombopoietin receptor
- Official symbol: *MPL*
- HGNC ID: 7217
- Gene locus: 1p34.2
- RefSeq: NG 007525.1
- Genomic position
  o Ch1: 43,337,818-43,354,466 (GRCh38.p14)
- Number of exons: 12
- Aliases: MPLV, TPOR, C-MPL, CD110, THCYT2, THPOR

MPL FUNCTION

Encodes Thrombopoietin Receptor

- Thrombopoietin receptor (TPO-R) may alternatively be called c-Mpl
  o Protein is also designated as CD110
  o Major protein isoform includes all exons
    – Alternative transcripts described, including potentially soluble form that lacks exons 9 and 10
- TPO binding induces TPO-R receptor dimerization, activating JAK-STAT signaling cascade
- Primary regulator of megakaryopoiesis and platelet production
  o Its ligand (TPO) produced primarily by liver with smaller amounts made in kidney and bone marrow
  o Receptor present on platelets, megakaryocytes, and hematopoietic stem cells
    – Binding to platelet-based receptors removes TPO from circulation; receptor-ligand complex is internalized and degraded
  o TPO and TPO-R primarily function to control platelet numbers rather than maturation
    – Both TPO and TPO-R knockout mice are viable but have 90% reduction in platelet counts
    – Platelets produced in absence of TPO and TPO-R are morphologically and functionally normal
- TPO-R also important in maintaining regenerative capacity of stem cells
  o c-Mpl knockout mice show markedly reduced numbers and repopulating capacity of CD34(+) hematopoietic stem cells
    – Deficiencies are not limited to megakaryocytic lineage
  o Common myeloid progenitor cell expresses TPO-R but not IL7R
  o Common lymphoid progenitor cell expresses IL7R but not TPO-R

Significant Somatic Variants

- Somatically acquired cytokine-independent activating mutations mostly in exon 10
  o These affect protein juxtamembrane domain
  o Mutation results in constitutive activation of JAK-STAT signaling pathway
    – Single-base substitutions most commonly described
    – Rare activating insertion/deletion mutations have also been described
  o Amino acid 515, tryptophan (W515), most commonly involved
    – 80-90% of significant variants occur at this codon in myeloproliferative neoplasms
    – ~ 70% have tryptophan replaced by leucine: *MPL*, c.1544G>T, p.W515L
    – ~ 10% have tryptophan replaced by lysine: *MPL*, c.1543-1544delinsAA, p.W515K
  o Other uncommon amino acid replacements at codon 515 have been described in myeloproliferative neoplasms
    – p.W515R (accounts for ~ 7% of codon 515 mutations)
    – p.W515S (accounts for ~ 3% of codon 515 mutations)
    – p.W515A (accounts for ~ 3% of codon 515 mutations)
  o *MPL* p.S505N may be found as sporadic mutation in rare myeloproliferative neoplasm cases
    – Many 2nd-site mutations can enhance constitutive signaling by canonical exon 10 mutation
- Activating *MPL* mutations outside of exon 10 have also been described

(Left) Next-generation sequencing (NGS) of *MPL* exon 10 reveals the presence of p.W515L mutation. The c.1544G>T alteration is visualized ➡. This is the most common type of *MPL* mutation in myeloproliferative neoplasms. **(Right)** Pyrosequencing of *MPL* reveals the presence of p.W515K mutation (bottom panel). This is the 2nd most common type of *MPL* mutation in myeloproliferative neoplasms.

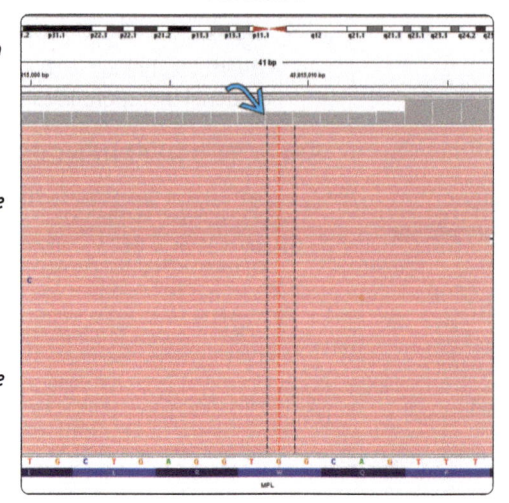

Sequencing Pileup of *MPL* p.W515L Mutation

Pyrosequencing of *MPL* p.W515K Mutation

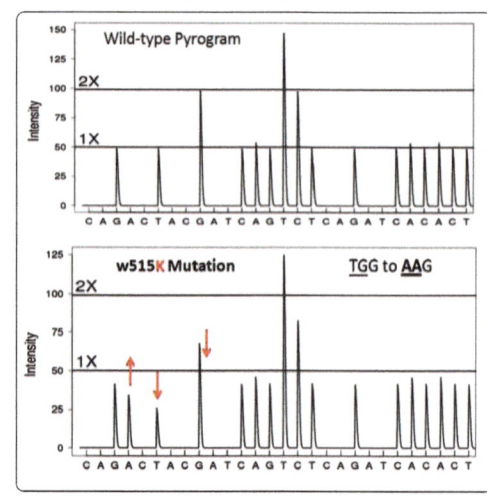

MPL Mutations

- May be found in ~ 10% of so-called "triple-negative" essential thrombocythemia and primary myelofibrosis cases
  - Mutations may be present in exons 3-6 and 12
  - Triple-negative cases are negative for *JAK2* p.V617F, *CALR* exon 9, and *MPL* exon 10 mutations

Significant Germline Variants

- Familial *MPL* p.S505N mutation has been associated with inherited thrombocythemia
  - Autosomal dominant disease
  - Associated with high thrombotic risk
  - Splenomegaly and progression to marrow fibrosis are common
- *MPL* c.1238G>T, p.K39N
  - Known informally as *MPL* Baltimore
  - Found in ~ 7% in Black Americans
  - Associated with higher platelet counts than wildtype controls
- *MPL* loss-of-function mutations found in congenital amegakaryocytic thrombocytopenia (CAMT)
  - Autosomal recessive disease
  - Unlike activating mutations, variety of CAMT-associated mutations may be located throughout gene
  - Transfusion-dependent thrombocytopenia
  - Absent or near-absent megakaryocytes
  - Frequent progression to multilineage bone marrow failure
  - Other organ dysfunction due to hemorrhagic events

Methods of Detection

- Variety of sequencing modalities may be used
  - Sanger sequencing, pyrosequencing, and next-generation sequencing (NGS) are all commonly used methods
  - Present assays are mostly targeted to exon 10
  - Evaluation of other exons may become more common with gene panel-based NGS testing
- Bone marrow or peripheral blood are suitable for evaluation
  - Bone marrow specimens may have higher detection sensitivity

CLINICAL IMPLICATIONS

Diagnosis in *BCR::ABL1*-Negative Myeloproliferative Neoplasms

- Presence of activating *MPL* mutation is major diagnostic criteria for diagnosis of essential thrombocythemia (ET) and primary myelofibrosis (PMF)
  - *MPL* mutation is present in 1-3% of ET
    - ET cases are more likely to show either *JAK2* V617F mutation (50-55%) or *CALR* mutation (23-32%)
  - *MPL* mutation is present in 5-10% of primary myelofibrosis (PMF)
    - PMF cases are more likely to show either *JAK2* V617F mutation (55-60%) or *CALR* mutation (25-35%)
  - ~ 10% of triple-negative ET and PMF cases will carry activating mutations in *MPL* outside of exon 10
    - Generally, triple-negative cases of PMF show decreased survival and greater propensity to blast transformation
    - Triple-negative patients with non-exon-10 mutated *MPL* may have better clinical course
- *MPL* mutations are not seen in polycythemia vera (PV)
  - Identification of *MPL* mutation generally excludes diagnosis of PV
- *MPL* mutations are not specifically diagnostic for ET or PMF, and morphologic evaluation is important in resolving diagnosis
  - ET typically shows
    - Increased platelets > 450 x 10^9/L
    - Normocellular to modestly hypercellular bone marrow
    - Atypical megakaryocytes with "staghorn" hypersegmented nuclei
  - PMF typically shows
    - Hypercellular bone marrow
    - Granulocytic and megakaryocytic proliferation
    - Tightly clustered, bizarre megakaryocytes with increased nuclear:cytoplasmic ratio
    - Reticulin fibrosis (in fibrotic stage of disease)
- Somatically acquired activating mutations in *MPL*, *CALR*, and *JAK2* p.V617F are typically mutually exclusive in myeloproliferative neoplasms

Molecular Approach to *MPL* Analysis

- *BCR::ABL1* fusion must be ruled out to exclude chronic myeloid leukemia (CML)
  - CML may present with striking thrombocytosis
- Suspected polycythemia vera should be tested for *JAK2* p.V617F and other non-V617F mutations (e.g., exon 12 mutations)
- If diagnosis of ET or PMF is favored, recommend evaluating for *JAK2* p.V617F, *CALR* exon 9, and *MPL* exon 10 mutations
  - These mutations are typically mutually exclusive, thus stepwise reflexive testing may be used
    - Based on frequency, best order is *JAK2* p.V617F > *CALR* > *MPL*
  - Single NGS multitarget panel analysis is also common workflow

SELECTED REFERENCES

1. Bridgford JL et al: Novel drivers and modifiers of MPL-dependent oncogenic transformation identified by deep mutational scanning. Blood. 135(4):287-92, 2020
2. Milosevic Feenstra JD et al: Whole-exome sequencing identifies novel MPL and JAK2 mutations in triple-negative myeloproliferative neoplasms. Blood. 127(3):325-32, 2016
3. Tefferi A et al: Long-term survival and blast transformation in molecularly annotated essential thrombocythemia, polycythemia vera, and myelofibrosis. Blood. 124(16):2507-13; quiz 2615, 2014
4. Ma W et al: MPL mutation profile in JAK2 mutation-negative patients with myeloproliferative disorders. Diagn Mol Pathol. 20(1):34-9, 2011
5. Tefferi A: Novel mutations and their functional and clinical relevance in myeloproliferative neoplasms: JAK2, MPL, TET2, ASXL1, CBL, IDH and IKZF1. Leukemia. 24(6):1128-38, 2010
6. Pardanani AD et al: MPL515 mutations in myeloproliferative and other myeloid disorders: a study of 1182 patients. Blood. 108(10):3472-6, 2006
7. Akashi K et al: A clonogenic common myeloid progenitor that gives rise to all myeloid lineages. Nature. 404(6774):193-7, 2000
8. Kimura S et al: Hematopoietic stem cell deficiencies in mice lacking c-Mpl, the receptor for thrombopoietin. Proc Natl Acad Sci U S A. 95(3):1195-200, 1998
9. Murone M et al: Hematopoietic deficiencies in c-mpl and TPO knockout mice. Stem Cells. 16(1):1-6, 1998
10. Fielder PJ et al: Regulation of thrombopoietin levels by c-mpl-mediated binding to platelets. Blood. 87(6):2154-61, 1996

Calreticulin (*CALR*) Mutations

TERMINOLOGY

Definitions
- Official name: Calreticulin
- Official symbol: *CALR*
- HGNC ID: 1455
- Gene locus: 19p13.13
- RefSeq: NG_029662.1
- Genomic position
  - Ch19: 12,938,609-12,944,489 (GRCh38.p14)
- Number of exons: 9

CALR FUNCTION

Encodes Calreticulin Protein
- Multifunctional protein
  - Highly conserved protein folding chaperone
  - Calcium-binding; helps regulate intracellular free calcium homeostasis
  - Regulation of steroid-mediated gene transcription
- Localizes primarily in endoplasmic reticulum (ER) but also found in cytoplasm and nucleus

Homozygous *CALR* Knockout Mouse
- Embryonically lethal at day 18 or earlier
- Embryos show marked decrease in ventricular wall thickness and develop omphalocele
  - Calreticulin is essential for early stages of cardiogenesis

CALR MUTATIONS

Somatically Acquired Driver Mutation
- Associated with myeloproliferative neoplasms (MPNs)
  - Detected in ~ 30% of both essential thrombocythemia (ET) and primary myelofibrosis (PMF)
  - *CALR*, *JAK2*, and *MPL* mutations generally considered mutually exclusive events
    - Co-mutation events uncommon but reported
  - *CALR* mutations are usually absent in polycythemia vera
- *CALR* mutations in familial cases of ET and PMF are also somatically acquired mutations
- Mutations are detected in patient-derived, flow-sorted, highly enriched hematopoietic stem cells, common myeloid progenitors, granulocyte-macrophage progenitors, and megakaryocyte-erythroid progenitors
  - Indicating that mutations occur in multipotent progenitor capable of generating both myeloid and erythroid progeny
    - *CALR* mutations are not detected in T lymphocytes

Common Somatic Mutations
- Clinically relevant mutations limited to exon 9
  - > 50 different mutations reported
  - All are insertion/deletions causing -1/+2 bp shift to novel reading frame
- 2 most common variant types
  - Type 1 mutation
    - 52-bp deletion (c.1092_1143del, p.L367fs*46) found in ~ 53% of cases
    - Incurs loss of Ca2+ binding sites, compared to type 2 mutants
      - Depleted ER Ca2+ activates IRE1α/XBP1 pathway of unfolded protein response
  - Type 2 mutation
    - 5-bp insertion (c.1154_1155insTTGTC, p.K385fs*47)
- Less common mutations
  - 2-bp insertion
  - 1-bp deletion
  - 8-bp deletion
  - Other rare variants also reported

Abnormal Activation of Signaling Pathways
- All frameshifts lead to same novel C-terminal protein sequence
- *CALR*-mutant protein chaperone abnormally interacts with thrombopoietin receptor (TPOR) in ER
  - TPOR coupled with mutant-*CALR* exported to cell surface
  - Physical interaction leads to constitutive cytokine-independent activation of TPOR signaling
    - TPOR signaling mediated by JAK-STAT pathway

Atypical and Pleomorphic Megakaryocytes

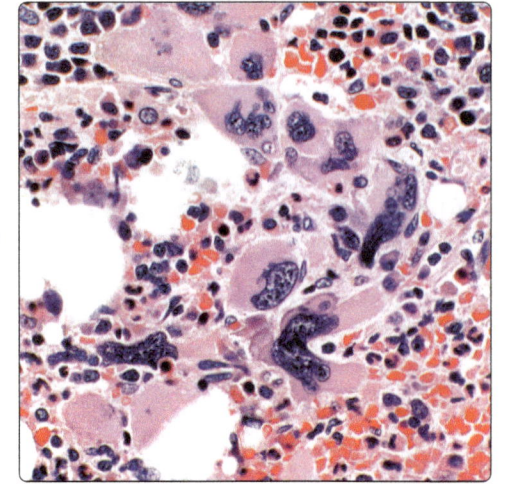

Electropherogram of Mutated *CALR*

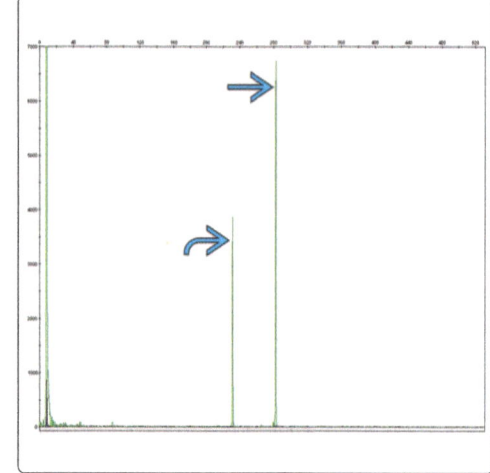

(Left) Bone marrow core biopsy from a patient with primary myelofibrosis shows aggregates of highly atypical and pleomorphic megakaryocytes. (Right) Electropherogram of PCR-amplified product of CALR exon 9 from a patient with primary myelofibrosis shows a mutated peak ➔ corresponding to a 52-bp deletion and a taller wildtype peak ➔.

Calreticulin (CALR) Mutations

- *CALR* mutations also shown to activate MAPK and PI3K/AKT signaling pathways

Constitutional Disorders

- *CALR* allele may be lost along with several other genes in rare 19p13.13 deletion syndrome
  - 19p13.13 microdeletion is not inherited but arises during formation of gametes or in early fetal development
  - Features may include macrocephaly, moderate intellectual disability, delayed speech, vision impairment, hypotonia, and poor coordination

TESTING METHODS FOR DETECTION

Gene Sequencing

- Whole-exome sequencing was used in discovery of *CALR* mutations in *JAK2* and *MPL* nonmutated MPNs
- Sequencing (targeted or gene panel) methods are common
  - Most comprehensive method for assessment of sequence mutations
  - Some larger indels could be missed with earlier types of bioinformatic data analysis

Fragment Sizing Analysis

- Targeted PCR amplification of exon 9 followed by fragment sizing by capillary electrophoresis
- Changes in amplicon size compared to wildtype indicate *CALR* mutation
- Type of *CALR* mutation may determined by difference in sizes of wildtype vs. mutant peak

CLINICAL IMPLICATIONS

Essential Thrombocythemia With *CALR* Mutation

- Affected individuals are relatively younger than those with *JAK2* mutation
- Characterized by markedly elevated platelet counts
- Lower hemoglobin level and WBC count compared to *JAK2*-mutated cases
- Relatively low risk of thrombosis
  - Much lower than *JAK2*-mutated ET cases
  - Cytoreduction may be preferred over antiplatelet therapy in symptomatic patients
  - Genotype does not alter treatment algorithms for high-risk pregnancies
- Increased risk of progression to myelofibrosis compared to *JAK2*-mutated cases
- Longer overall survival compared to *JAK2*-mutated cases

Primary Myelofibrosis With *CALR* Mutation

- Longer overall survival compared to PMF cases with *JAK2* or *MPL* mutations
  - Type 1 mutations associated with superior survival than type 2 *CALR* mutations
- Presence of *CALR* mutation attenuates, but does not fully overcome, unfavorable prognosis seen in PMF with mutated *ASXL1*

General Significance in Myeloid Neoplasms

- Potential target for signaling pathway blockade
  - Ruxolitinib (JAK signaling inhibitor) has been used in treatment of *CALR*-mutant MPNs
  - MAPK, PI3K/AKT, and ATR-CHK1 signaling pathways identified as potential therapeutic targets in *CALR*-mutant MPNs
  - Pharmacologic inhibition of IRE1α/XBP1 signaling reported to induce cell death in *CALR* type 1 but not type 2 mutants
- Compared to *JAK2*-mutant cases, *CALR*-mutant MPN shows decreased responsiveness to interferon therapy
- *CALR* mutation is detected in subset of myelodysplastic/MPNs with *SF3B1* mutation and thrombocytosis
  - *CALR*-mutated cases are generally wildtype for *JAK2* and *MPL*
- Uncommon in acute myeloid leukemia
- Rarely reported in myelodysplastic syndrome (< 1%)
- *CALR* exon 9 frameshift alterations not reported in normal individuals
  - 3-bp inframe *CALR* mutation has been reported in one individual with no evidence of MPN

Myeloproliferative Neoplasms Wildtype for *CALR*, *JAK2*, and *MPL*

- ~ 8-9% of PMF cases lack mutations in *JAK2*, *MPL*, and *CALR* genes (triple negative)
  - Reported median survival of only 2.5 years in one study
  - Triple-negative PMF cases show very poor prognosis
  - *CALR* wildtype/*ASXL1*-mutated genotype showed most detrimental mutation profile in one study
- Triple-negative ET is not homogeneous entity

SELECTED REFERENCES

1. Ibarra J et al: Type I but not type II calreticulin mutations activate the IRE1α/XBP1 pathway of the unfolded protein response to drive myeloproliferative neoplasms. Blood Cancer Discov. 3(4):298-315, 2022
2. Alvarez-Larrán A et al: Unmet clinical needs in the management of CALR-mutated essential thrombocythaemia: a consensus-based proposal from the European LeukemiaNet. Lancet Haematol. 8(9):e658-65, 2021
3. Jia R et al: High-throughput drug screening identifies the ATR-CHK1 pathway as a therapeutic vulnerability of CALR mutated hematopoietic cells. Blood Cancer J. 11(7):137, 2021
4. Czech J et al: JAK2V617F but not CALR mutations confer increased molecular responses to interferon-α via JAK1/STAT1 activation. Leukemia. 33(4):995-1010, 2018
5. Fu C et al: AKT activation is a feature of CALR mutant myeloproliferative neoplasms. Leukemia. 33(1):271-4, 2018
6. Araki M et al: Activation of the thrombopoietin receptor by mutant calreticulin in CALR-mutant myeloproliferative neoplasms. Blood. 94(3):286-90, 2016
7. Tefferi A et al: Long-term survival and blast transformation in molecularly annotated essential thrombocythemia, polycythemia vera, and myelofibrosis. Blood. 124(16):2507-13; quiz 2615, 2014
8. Tefferi A et al: CALR and ASXL1 mutations-based molecular prognostication in primary myelofibrosis: an international study of 570 patients. Leukemia. 28(7):1494-500, 2014
9. Tefferi A et al: CALR vs JAK2 vs MPL-mutated or triple-negative myelofibrosis: clinical, cytogenetic and molecular comparisons. Leukemia. 28(7):1472-7, 2014
10. Tefferi A et al: The prognostic advantage of calreticulin mutations in myelofibrosis might be confined to type 1 or type 1-like CALR variants. Blood. 124(15):2465-6, 2014
11. Klampfl T et al: Somatic mutations of calreticulin in myeloproliferative neoplasms. N Engl J Med. 369(25):2379-90, 2013

CSF3R Mutations

TERMINOLOGY

Definitions
- Official name: Colony-stimulating factor 3 receptor (granulocyte)
- Official symbol: *CSF3R*
- HGNC ID: 2439
- Chromosomal location: 1p34.3
- Genomic coordinates: 1:36,466,043-36,483,314
- Number of exons: 18

Synonyms
- Colony-stimulating factor 3, granulocyte colony-stimulating factor

EPIDEMIOLOGY

Incidence
- *CSF3R* mutations have been found in following neoplasms
  - Chronic neutrophilic leukemia (80-100%)
  - Atypical chronic myeloid leukemia (aCML) (0-40%)
  - Severe congenital neutropenia (~ 33%)
  - Chronic myelomonocytic leukemia (~ 4-7%)
  - Other (< 5%): Myelodysplastic syndromes, acute myeloid leukemia
- T618I is most common mutation

ETIOLOGY/PATHOGENESIS

Granulocyte Colony-Stimulating Factor
- Secreted glycoprotein that interacts with specific cell surface receptor
  - 2 polypeptide types composed of 177 and 180 amino acids, respectively, encoded by same gene
- Produced by macrophages stimulated by endotoxin
- Binds to cell surface receptor on granulocytic cells
  - Stimulates proliferation and differentiation of granulocytes from their progenitor cells
- Filgrastim (analog of G-CSF) is used clinically to stimulate neutrophil production in patients with neutropenia

CSF3R Protein
- Cell surface protein receptor
  - Contains extracellular, transmembrane, and cytoplasmic domains
  - Predominantly expressed by progenitor and mature neutrophilic granulocytes
- Ligand is G-CSF
- Regulates granulocyte differentiation
  - Distal region of cytoplasmic domain
- Increases granulocytic proliferative capacity
  - Proximal region of cytoplasmic domain
- Signals through JAK-STAT pathway and SRC family kinase pathway

CSF3R Mutations
- 2 main types of activating *CSF3R* mutations
  - Membrane proximal mutations
    - Point mutations that affect extracellular domain of receptor
    - Result in constitutive activation of receptor independent of its ligand
    - Downstream signaling through JAK-STAT pathway is preferentially activated
    - Patients with membrane proximal mutations may be candidates for treatment with JAK kinase inhibitors, such as ruxolitinib, with response rates estimated at ~ 30%
  - Truncation mutations
    - Nonsense or frameshift mutations
    - Lead to premature truncation of cytoplasmic tail of receptor
    - Result in constitutive overexpression of receptor and ligand hypersensitivity
    - Downstream signaling mediators, including SRC family kinases (SFKs) and TNK2, are preferentially activated
    - Patients with truncation mutations may be candidates for treatment with SCR inhibitors, such as dasatinib
  - Both mutation types can occur in same patient (compound mutations)
    - Can occur on same *CSF3R* allele with no order for sequential acquisition of mutations
  - Mutations reportedly occur in exons 14 to 17 of *CSF3R*

CLINICAL IMPLICATIONS

Chronic Neutrophilic Leukemia
- Myeloproliferative neoplasm characterized by sustained peripheral blood and bone marrow neutrophilia and hepatosplenomegaly
  - No *BCR::ABL1* fusion
  - Reactive causes of neutrophilia are excluded
- *CSF3R* mutations are found in majority of cases
  - Most common is T618I in membrane proximal domain due to point mutation in codon 618: ACC>ATC
  - ~ 1/2 of cases also have *SETBP1* mutations, which tend to accelerate leukemia progression
- No correlation with age, sex, leukocyte count, or survival
- One case of congenital chronic neutrophilic leukemia (CNL) due to germline T618I mutation has been reported

Atypical Chronic Myeloid Leukemia
- Leukemic neoplasm with overlap myelodysplastic and myeloproliferative features at diagnosis
  - Principal involvement of neutrophil lineage with leukocytosis
  - No *BCR::ABL1* fusion
- Conflicting data regarding prevalence of *CSF3R* mutations in this neoplasm
  - Initially thought to occur in significant number of cases
  - Later data suggests that rate of mutation is low if strict WHO and ICC criteria are used to establish diagnosis
- *CSF3R* mutations have been used as disease-specific marker to monitor patients after bone marrow transplant in 1 report
- t(1;9)(p34;q34); *CSF3R::SPTAN1*
  - Reported in patient with acute chronic neutrophilic leukemia (aCNL)
  - Involves C-terminus of *CSF3R*, suggesting pattern of truncation mutation, but does not respond to SCR inhibitors

CSF3R Mutations

Chronic Myelomonocytic Leukemia
- Mutations are rare can be different from those seen in CNL and aCNL
  - P733T mutation reported to be most common in one study
  - T618I mutation may define proliferative chronic myelomonocytic leukemia (CMML) subtype enriched in *ASXL1* mutations with adverse outcomes

Severe Congenital Neutropenia
- Group of disorders presenting with marked neutropenia at or near birth
  - Decreased bone marrow myeloid cell production
    - Increased propensity for infection because of resulting neutropenia and various causes of reactive neutropenia
- Activating somatic mutations acquired during course of disease
  - Mutations similar to those seen in CNL
  - Associated with transformation to myelodysplasia or acute myeloid leukemia (AML)
  - *RUNX1* mutations are also frequently detected at time of AML transformation, suggesting cooperativity between *RUNX1* and *CSF3R* mutations in progression to AML
- Biallelic inherited loss-of-function mutations have been reported in families with SCN (OMIM: 617014)
  - Autosomal recessive inheritance
  - These mutations are different from activating mutations seen in cases of severe congenital neutropenia (SCN) that evolve into AML
  - These patients do not respond to G-CSF therapy but may respond to GM-CSF

Hereditary Neutrophilia
- Lifelong neutrophilia with benign clinical course
- Inherited as autosomal dominant
- Due to activating T640N mutation of *CSF3R*
  - Seen in patients meeting ICC and WHO criteria for CNL, raising possibility of congenital origin in subset of cases

TESTING

Sequencing
- Gold standard for mutation detection
- Can be performed by Sanger sequencing, pyrosequencing, or next-generation sequencing
- Selective sequencing of hot spots within gene may be performed
  - Membrane proximal mutations in exon 14
  - Truncation mutations in exons 15-17

High-Resolution DNA Melting Curve Analysis
- Screen for mutation within hot spots region of gene
  - Amplified DNA of interest should not exceed 300 base pairs or include prevalent single nucleotide polymorphism (SNP)
  - Amplification of DNA regions that might potentially harbor SNP must be avoided
  - Positive results should be confirmed by sequencing

Specimen
- Fresh whole blood or bone marrow sample, preferentially in EDTA
- Formalin-fixed, paraffin-embedded tissue from extramedullary sites infiltrated by neoplastic cells

SELECTED REFERENCES
1. Guastafierro V et al: CSF3R-mutant chronic myelomonocytic leukemia is a distinct clinically subset with abysmal prognosis: a case report and systematic review of the literature. Leuk Lymphoma. 1-8, 2023
2. Carratt SA et al: Mutated SETBP1 activates transcription of Myc programs to accelerate CSF3R-driven myeloproliferative neoplasms. Blood. 140(6):644-58, 2022
3. Dao KT et al: Efficacy of ruxolitinib in patients with chronic neutrophilic leukemia and atypical chronic myeloid leukemia. J Clin Oncol. 38(10):1006-18, 2020
4. Elliott MA et al: Chronic neutrophilic leukemia: 2018 update on diagnosis, molecular genetics and management. Am J Hematol. 93(4):578-87, 2018
5. Druhan LJ et al: Chronic neutrophilic leukemia in a child with a CSF3R T618I germ line mutation. Blood. 128(16):2097-9, 2016
6. Gotlib J et al: The new genetics of chronic neutrophilic leukemia and atypical CML: implications for diagnosis and treatment. Blood. 122(10):1707-11, 2013
7. Maxson JE et al: Oncogenic CSF3R mutations in chronic neutrophilic leukemia and atypical CML. N Engl J Med. 368(19):1781-90, 2013

High-Resolution Melting Curve

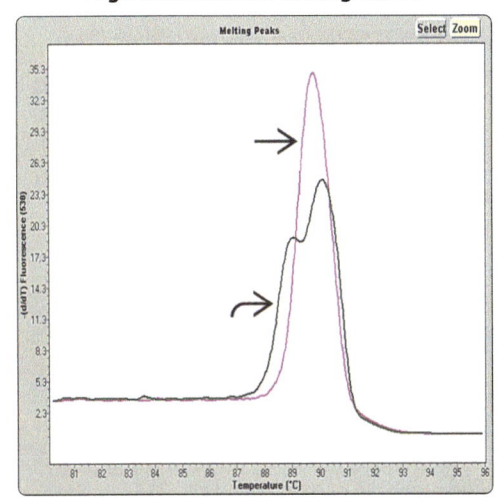

Sanger Sequencing

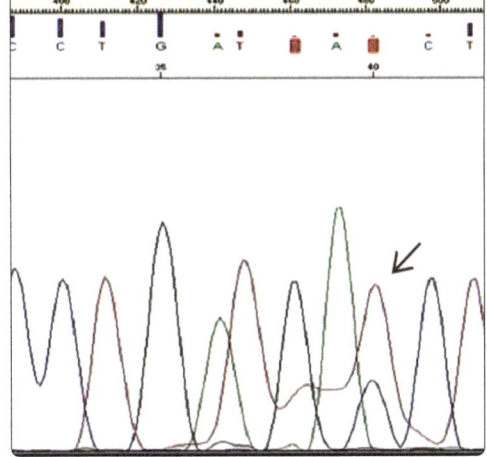

(Left) *High-resolution melting curve of PCR-amplified DNA product from a case of chronic neutrophilic leukemia (CNL) harboring CSF3R mutation shows an abnormal shouldering ➡ compared to wildtype DNA melting curve ➡.* (Right) *Sanger sequencing trace shows the most common CSF3R mutation. There is a C>T base substitution in codon 618 of CSF3R that corresponds to T618I ➡.*

SETBP1 Mutations

TERMINOLOGY

Definitions
- Official name: SET binding protein 1
- Official symbol: SETBP1
- HGNC ID: 15573
- Chromosomal location: 18q12.3
- Genomic coordinates (GRCh38): 18:44,680,073-45,068,510
- Number of exons: 15
- Aliases: SEB, MRD29

EPIDEMIOLOGY

Incidence
- Somatic mutations of SETBP1 have been found in
  - 25% of chronic neutrophilic leukemia (CNL)
  - 24% of atypical chronic myeloid leukemia (aCML)
  - 17% of secondary acute myeloid leukemia (sAML)
  - 4-15% of chronic myelomonocytic leukemia (CMML)
  - 10% of myelodysplastic/myeloproliferative neoplasms, unclassifiable (MDS/MPN-U)
  - 5% of myelodysplastic syndromes (MDS)
  - < 5% of other myeloid malignancies
- Germline mutations of SETBP1 are found in Schinzel-Giedion midface retraction syndrome and SETBP1 haploinsufficiency disorder

ETIOLOGY/PATHOGENESIS

SET Protein
- Nuclear protooncogene with multiple functions
  - Inhibits acetylation of nucleosomes, especially histone H4 by histone acetylases
  - Involved in apoptosis, transcription, nucleosome assembly, and histone chaperoning
- Main function of SET is to inhibit protein phosphatase 2A (PP2A)
  - PP2A has tumor suppressor effect by counteracting kinase-driven intracellular signaling pathways
  - Inhibition of PP2A by SET promotes tumor growth
- SET is stabilized by binding to SETBP1 protein

SETBP1 Protein
- Nuclear protein involved in DNA replication
- Consists of 1,596 amino acids
- Contains several motifs, including SKI homologous region and SET-binding domain
  - SKI homologous region is thought to be involved in protein degradation
  - Most of reported SETBP1 mutations occur in SKI homologous region
    - Mutations cause changes of highly conserved amino acids within this region
- Binding of SETBP1 to SET protein stabilizes latter, enhancing its protooncogenic effect
- ~ 27% of AMLs overexpress SETBP1 protein

SETBP1 Mutations
- Missense mutations in codons 858-871
  - Most common ones are p.E858K, p.D868N, p.S869G, p.G870S, and p.I871T
- All reported mutations are heterozygous
- All are gain-of-function mutations
  - Mutations result in decreased degradation of protein, which is functional equivalent of overexpression

CLINICAL IMPLICATIONS

Atypical Chronic Myeloid Leukemia, BCR::ABL1-Negative
- Myeloid neoplasm with overlapping myelodysplastic and myeloproliferative features at diagnosis
  - Characterized by leukocytosis with dysplastic granulocytic lineage
  - No BCR::ABL1 fusion
- SETBP1 mutations are detected in subset of cases
  - Majority (92%) of mutations in codons 858 and 871
  - Identical to those seen in Schinzel-Giedion syndrome
  - Associated with higher WBC counts and poorer prognosis
  - No differences between mutated and nonmutated cases with regard to age, sex, number of blasts, hemoglobin level, or platelet counts

Chronic Myelomonocytic Leukemia
- Leukemic disorder with myelodysplastic and myeloproliferative features at diagnosis
  - Persistent peripheral blood monocytosis
  - Dysplasia involving 1 or more myeloid lineages
    - If no dysplasia, secondary causes of monocytosis must be excluded or molecular genetic abnormality must be present
  - No BCR::ABL1 fusion or PDGFRA or PDGFRB rearrangements
- SETBP1 mutations are similar to those in aCML
  - Presence of SETBP1 mutation in patient with monocytosis rules out reactive condition
  - Associated with poorer prognosis

Myelodysplastic Syndrome
- Hematopoietic stem cell diseases characterized by
  - Cytopenias
  - Dysplasia in 1 or more major myeloid cell lines
  - Ineffective hematopoiesis
  - Increased risk of development of AML
- SETBP1 mutations are thought to play role in disease progression
  - Coincide with increased leukemic blasts
  - Associated with other genetic abnormalities that are known to occur with disease progression, e.g.,
    - -7/del(7q)
    - Isochromosome 17q [i(17)(q10)]
  - Drive leukemic transformation in ASXL1-mutated MDS

Acute Myeloid Leukemia
- 2 types of SETBP1 alterations have been reported in AML
  - Point mutations similar to those occurring in aCML
    - Most cases are sAML
    - Mostly evolves from underlying myelodysplastic syndrome
    - SETBP1 mutations acquired at time of leukemic evolution and absent at initial presentation
    - Associated with advanced age and del 7q
  - Overexpression of SETBP1 protein

SETBP1 Mutations

- Primary AML cases account for most SETBP1 overexpressing cases
- Associated with decreased survival in patients > 60 years of age
- t(12;18)(p13;q12) involving *SETBP1* and *ETV6* has been shown to be one mechanism for *SETBP1* overexpression

Schinzel-Giedion Syndrome

- Rare congenital disorder characterized by multiple malformations due to aberrant bone formation
- Patients harbor *SETBP1* mutations
- Most patients die in neonatal period
  - Patients who survive develop tumors of neuroepithelial origin

SETBP1 Haploinsufficiency Disorder

- Very rare autosomal disorder typically caused by de novo *SETBP1* mutation (OMIM: 616078)
- Characterized by hypotonia, mild motor developmental delay, intellectual disabilities, speech and language disorder, behavioral problems, refractive errors, and strabismus

Other Myeloid Malignancies

- While some studies indicate that *SETBP1* mutations in CNL do not seem to be associated with poorer prognosis, other studies suggest that coexistence of *SETBP1* and *CSF3R* mutations may be associated with worse outcome and possible resistance to JAK inhibitor therapy
- *SETBP1* mutations have been reported at low frequency (< 5%) in other myeloid malignancies
  - Juvenile myelomonocytic leukemia
  - Pediatric myelodysplastic syndrome

TESTING

Sequencing

- Gold standard for mutation detection
  - Sanger sequencing, pyrosequencing, or next-generation sequencing
- Selective sequencing of exon 4 harboring common mutations

High-Resolution DNA Melting Curve Analysis

- Can be used to screen for hotspot mutations of *SETBP1*
  - Amplified DNA of interest should not exceed 300 base pairs
  - Positive results should be confirmed by sequencing
  - Amplification of DNA regions that might potentially harbor single nucleotide polymorphism must be avoided

Specimen

- Fresh whole blood or bone marrow sample, preferentially collected in EDTA
- Formalin-fixed, paraffin-embedded tissue from extramedullary sites infiltrated by neoplastic cells also acceptable

SELECTED REFERENCES

1. Wang H et al: Identification of a novel de novo mutation of SETBP1 and new findings of SETBP1 in tumorgenesis. Orphanet J Rare Dis. 18(1):107, 2023
2. Carratt SA et al: Mutated SETBP1 activates transcription of Myc programs to accelerate CSF3R-driven myeloproliferative neoplasms. Blood. 140(6):644-58, 2022
3. Szuber N et al: Chronic neutrophilic leukemia: 2022 update on diagnosis, genomic landscape, prognosis, and management. Am J Hematol. 97(4):491-505, 2022
4. Acuna-Hidalgo R et al: Overlapping SETBP1 gain-of-function mutations in Schinzel-Giedion syndrome and hematologic malignancies. PLoS Genet. 13(3):e1006683, 2017
5. Shou LH et al: Prognostic significance of SETBP1 mutations in myelodysplastic syndromes, chronic myelomonocytic leukemia, and chronic neutrophilic leukemia: A meta-analysis. PLoS One. 12(2):e0171608, 2017
6. Inoue D et al: SETBP1 mutations drive leukemic transformation in ASXL1-mutated MDS. Leukemia. 29(4):847-57, 2015
7. Patnaik MM et al: ASXL1 and SETBP1 mutations and their prognostic contribution in chronic myelomonocytic leukemia: a two-center study of 466 patients. Leukemia. 28(11):2206-12, 2014

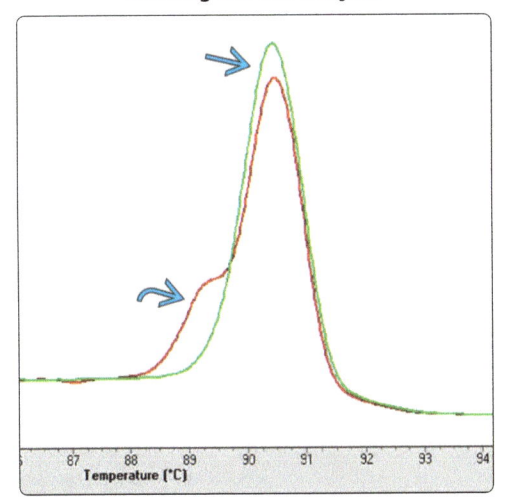

Melting Curve Analysis

Sanger Sequencing

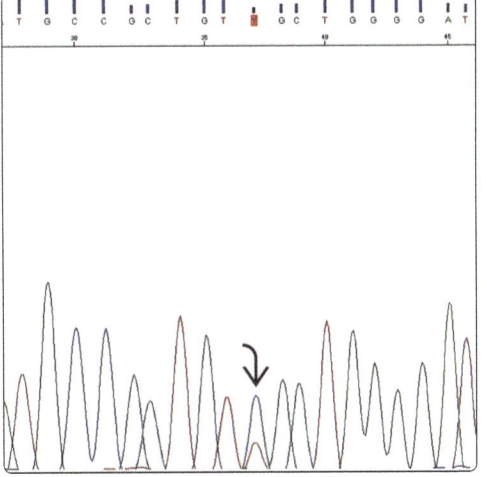

(Left) *This case of BCR::ABL1-negative atypical chronic myeloid leukemia (aCML) with mutant SETBP1 shows an abnormal DNA melting curve (red) ➡ compared to a wildtype DNA melting curve (green) ➡.* (Right) *Sanger sequencing of the same case of aCML with an abnormal melting curve identifies a D868N mutation in SETBP1 gene ➡.*

KIT Mutations

TERMINOLOGY

Definitions

- *KIT*
  - Official name: KIT protooncogene receptor tyrosine kinase
    - Previous name: Feline sarcoma viral oncogene homolog v-kit
  - HGNC ID: 6342
  - Gene locus: 4q12
  - Genomic position
    - Ch4: 54,657,957-54,740,715 (GRCh38.p14)
    - Number of exons: 21
  - RefSeq: NG_007456.1
  - Aliases: PBT, SCFR, C-kit, CD117, and MASTC
- *KITLG*
  - Official name: KIT ligand
  - HGNC ID: 6343
  - Gene locus: 12q21.32
  - Genomic position
    - Ch12: 88,492,793-88,580,471
    - Number of exons: 10
  - RefSeq: NG_012098.2
  - Aliases: MGF (mast cell growth factor), SCF (stem cell factor), SF, SLF, Kitl, KL-1, DFNA69, DCUA, SHEP7, FPHH, and FPH2

KIT Function

- Encodes type III receptor tyrosine kinase
  - Formerly known as PDGF (platelet-derived growth factor) receptor family
    - Other proteins in this category include PDGFRA, PDGFRB, CSF1R, and FLT3
  - 145 kDa protein (976 amino acids)
    - Monomer in absence of bound ligand
    - Homodimer in presence of ligand with further oligomerization forming heterotetramer
    - Extracellular portion contains 5 immunoglobulin-like domains (positions 26-524)
    - Hydrophobic transmembrane domain with 21 amino acids (positions 525-545)
    - Intracellular portion with 2 tyrosine kinase domains separated by kinase insert region (positions 546-976)
- KIT protein normal function
  - Expressed in hematopoietic stem cells
    - Expression lost with cell differentiation
  - Linked to proliferation, survival, and migration of melanocytes from neural crest during embryogenesis
  - Necessary for successful gametogenesis through PIK3/AKT in mTOR pathway
  - Important for development of interstitial cells of Cajal in gastrointestinal tract
  - Associated with migration of neural stem cells to sites of injury in brain
  - Associated with spatial learning function in hippocampus
  - Involved in maintenance of vasculature and regulatory functions in angiogenesis
  - Possible role in maintaining integrity of lung tissue
- Role of KIT in signaling pathways
  - Effector ligand is KITLG (KIT ligand)
    - In utero acts in germ cell and neural cell development, hematopoiesis, and cell migration
    - In adults, has pleiotropic effects with broad expression across multiple tissue types and continued requirement in hematopoiesis
  - Activation of KIT signaling pathway
    - Results in phosphorylation of numerous proteins, including PIK3R1, PLCG1, SH2B2, and CBL
    - Promotes phosphorylation of many other protein phosphatases and transcription factors
  - KITLG binding activates several downstream signaling pathways, including
    - PI3K/AKT/mTOR
    - RAS/RAF/MEK/ERK
    - STAT3
  - Associated pathways are involved in mediation of progrowth, prosurvival, and migration signaling

KIT Exons and Protein Domains

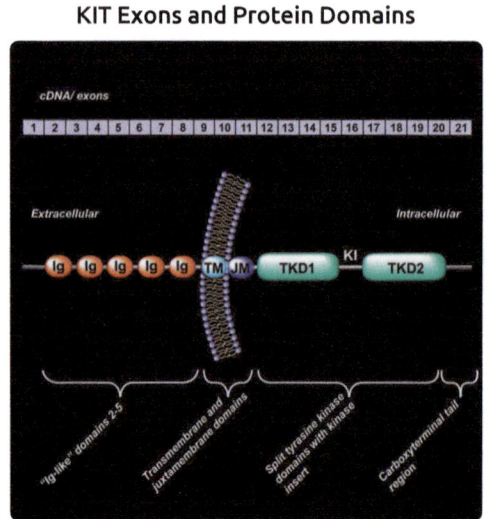

KIT Gene Sequencing

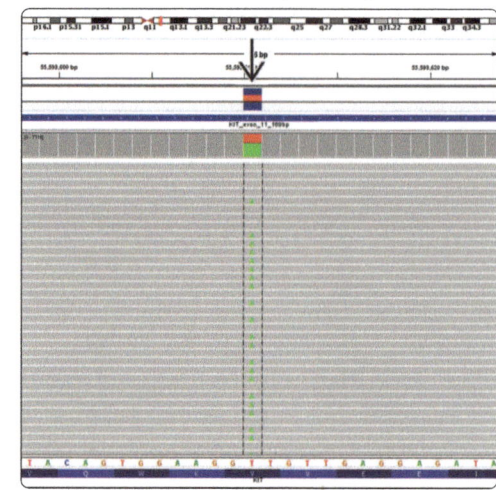

(Left) *KIT tyrosine kinase receptor is composed of 5 Ig-like extracellular domains, a juxtamembrane autoinhibitory domain, and 2 intracellular kinase domains against corresponding encoding exons.* (Right) *Next-generation sequencing (NGS) gene pileup derived from a patient with gastrointestinal stromal tumor (GIST) shows a KIT exon 11 missense mutation, resulting in p.V599D* ➔.

KIT Mutations

KIT Mutations
- Variety of mutations are described throughout *KIT*
- Oncogenic gain-of-function mutations
  - Generally disrupt protein autoinhibitory mechanisms
  - Commonly affected regions include
    - Exon 8 (extracellular dimerization motif) and 9-10 (transmembrane region)
      - Regions are involved in dimer interactions and stabilization
    - Exon 11 juxtamembrane domain
      - Key autoregulatory domain that stabilizes inactive protein conformation
    - Exons 17-18 kinase domain 2
      - Includes activation loop of kinase domain
- Loss-of-function mutations found in many regions, including exons 2-6, 11, 12-14, and 17-19

Diseases Associated With *KIT* Somatic Mutations
- **Gastrointestinal stromal tumor (GIST)**
  - Activating *KIT* mutations in ~ 80% of cases; 5-10% have *PDGFRA* alteration
    - Exon 11 mutations in ~ 70%
    - Exon 9 mutations in ~ 10-15%
    - Less common mutations in exons 10, 13, 14, and 17
    - GIST lacking *KIT* and *PDGFRA* mutation often has SDH deficiency
  - Presence and type of *KIT* and *PDGFRA* alterations not strongly correlated with prognosis or biologic potential of individual cases
  - Tumor mutation status linked to imatinib response rates
    - Exon 11 mutation associated with better response rates and survival (median progression-free and overall) compared to exon 9 mutations or nonmutated *KIT*
    - Exon 9 mutations have lower response rates and progression-free survival than exon 11 mutated cases at 400 mg daily
    - Higher dosing (e.g., 400 mg 2x daily) in exon 9 mutated cases associated with better progression-free survival
    - Cases with exon 11 deletions benefit from longer duration of therapy
  - Exon 11 deletions and exon 9 duplications associated with worse disease-free survival
  - Prior to targeted kinase inhibitor therapy, metastatic GIST was refractory to existing therapy
    - Patients may acquire imatinib resistance due to 2nd mutation in primary mutant KIT allele
    - Exon 17 mutations may confer resistance to tyrosine kinase inhibitors, including sunitinib
- **Melanoma**
  - *KIT* activating mutations found with variable incidence
    - ~ 10-15% in mucosal- and acral-based melanomas
    - ~ 2-3% in cases arising in chronic sun-damaged skin
    - Typically absent in uveal melanomas and melanomas arising in non-sun-damaged skin
  - *KIT* mutations mutually exclusive of *BRAF*, *NRAS*, and other driver mutations
  - Mutations typically involve exons 11, 13, and 17
  - Mutations found to cluster in 4 hotspots
    - L576 and W557-V560 of exon 11
    - K642 of exon 13
    - D816-A829 of exon 17
  - Mutations generally confer imatinib sensitivity
    - Exon 17 mutations (e.g., D816V and A829P) are associated with resistance to imatinib
    - Minimal or no sensitivity with KIT amplification
- **Systemic mastocytosis (SM)**
  - High-sensitivity, quantitative, PCR-based assays preferred
    - Next-generation sequencing (NGS) panel testing may not be sufficiently sensitive
    - Neoplastic cell yield from blood may be lower; marrow preferable for testing, if available
      - Testing in skin or other solid tissue may be considered if marrow mast-cell burden is low
  - *KIT* exon 17 D816V occurs in > 90% of SM
    - Presence of D816V mutation is WHO-defined minor criterion for diagnosis
    - Mutations possible in non-mast-cell component of SM associated with hematologic malignancies
    - *KIT* mutations are detected in ~ 75% of cutaneous mastocytosis with only ~ 1/3 harboring D816V
  - Less common (< 5-10%) mutations may include V560G, D815K, D816Y, D816F, D816H, and D820G
  - *KIT* D816 mutations are resistant to imatinib at clinically achievable doses
    - May reflect favored active protein conformation, to which imatinib cannot bind
    - Nilotinib may be effective in some cases, including those with *KIT* D816V mutation
  - Rare cases with juxtamembrane domain *KIT* mutations may respond to imatinib
  - Midostaurin may be effective in mastocytosis harboring *KIT* D816V mutation
  - Well-differentiated SM (rare variant) often lacks D816V and has mutations in exons 10-11
    - Exon 10-11 mutations may increase potential for responsiveness to imatinib
- **Childhood-onset mastocytosis**
  - Seen with germline or acquired activating *KIT* mutations
  - ~ 40% harbor exon 17 alterations at codon D816
  - Other rare mutations associated with familial mastocytosis include
    - F522C
    - A533D
    - R634W (reported in 3 siblings with urticaria pigmentosa)
- **Core-binding factor (CBF) acute myeloid leukemia (AML)**
  - *KIT* mutations found in ~ 20-30% of CBF AML
    - AML with t(8;21)(q22;q22)
    - AML with inv(16)(p13q22)/t(16;16)(p13;q22)
  - *KIT* mutations in CBF AML
    - No impact on complete remission (CR)
    - Higher incidence of relapse and decreased overall survival in *KIT*-mutated AML with t(8;21)
      - Prognostic associations less clear in AML with inv(16)/t(16;16)
    - Frequently involve exon 17 codon D816 (e.g., D816V, D816Y, D816H, etc.)
      - Other exon 17 codons less frequently involved
    - Infrequent mutations involve *KIT* exon 8

KIT Mutations

KIT Mutations in Gastrointestinal Stromal Tumor, Melanoma, Core-Binding Factor Acute Myeloid Leukemia, Mastocytosis, and Germ Cell Tumors

Disease Association/Prevalence	KIT Domain	Mutation Types	Involved Exon	Imatinib Sensitivity
GIST (~ 85%)	Dimerization motif	Point mutations, indels, duplications	Exon 11 (~ 70%)	Highest sensitivity
	Dimerization motif	Common 6bp (TGCCTA) duplication (A502_Y503)	Exon 9 (~ 10-15%)	Intermediate sensitivity
Melanoma (2-20%)	Juxtamembrane domain	Point mutations in codon 576, 557-560	Exon 11	Imatinib sensitive
	TK domain 1	Point mutations in codon 642	Exon 13	K642E appears imatinib sensitive
	TK domain 2	Point mutations in codons 816-829	Exon 17	Imatinib resistant
Systemic mastocytosis (> 90%)	TK domain 2	Point mutations mainly in codon 816	Exon 17	Imatinib resistant
Core-binding factor AML (~ 20-30%)	TK domain 2	Point mutations in codon 816	Exon 17	Imatinib resistant
	Extracellular domain	Inframe insertions or deletions	Exon 8	Imatinib sensitive per some studies
Germ cell tumors (~ 8%)	TK domain 2	Point mutations in codon 816	Exon 17	Imatinib resistant

AML = acute myeloid leukemia; GIST = gastrointestinal stromal tumor.

- ☐ Mutations in exon 8 include inframe indels
- Rare alterations also reported in exons 10 and 11
- Concurrent KIT + FLT3 mutations seen in ~ 6% of cases
- KIT mutations are typically absent in KRAS- or NRAS-mutated cases
- Minimal residual disease (MRD) status stronger prognostic/risk factor for CBF-AML risk (AML clinical practice guidelines, NCCN, 2.2022)

- **Germ cell tumors**
  - Activating KIT mutations in ~ 8% of germ cell tumors
    - Mutations arise in juxtamembrane domain, tyrosine kinase 2 domain, and tyrosine kinase 1 domain
    - Majority arise in seminomas/dysgerminomas
      - ☐ KIT-mutated seminoma has distinct DNA methylation and immune infiltration profiles
    - Also described in extragonadal sites, such as mediastinum
  - Focal amplifications of KIT also described
  - KIT mutations do not appear to be increased risk factor for bilateral gonadal involvement

Disease Associated With Germline Mutations
- Piebaldism (partial albinism)
  - Loss-of-function mutations
  - Autosomal dominant inheritance pattern
  - Defective melanocytes migration characterized by congenital areas of unpigmented skin and hair
  - Other genes may also modify expressed phenotype

Detection Methods
- Sequencing modalities commonly used
  - High-sensitivity, allele-specific oligonucleotide (ASO)-PCR, digital droplet PCR, etc.
  - NGS
    - Less sensitive than ASO-PCR but can interrogate multiple exon targets at once
    - Limitations in identifying larger deletions
- Nonsequencing molecular techniques, such as allelic discrimination assays, fragment analysis, or high-resolution melting curve analysis may be used
  - Further direct sequencing may be required to identify specific mutations
  - These may target only specific variants and may not exclude other KIT alteration
- No correlation between immunohistochemical expression of CD117 and KIT mutations

SELECTED REFERENCES
1. Pollyea DA et al: NCCN guidelines insights: acute myeloid leukemia, version 2.2021. J Natl Compr Canc Netw. 19(1):16-27, 2021
2. Badr P et al: Detection of KIT mutations in core binding factor acute myeloid leukemia. Leuk Res Rep. 10:20-5, 2018
3. Bishop KS et al: Epigenetic regulation of gene expression induced by butyrate in colorectal cancer: involvement of microRNA. Genet Epigenet. 9:1179237X17729900, 2017
4. Joensuu H et al: Effect of KIT and PDGFRA mutations on survival in patients with gastrointestinal stromal tumors treated with adjuvant imatinib: an exploratory analysis of a randomized clinical trial. JAMA Oncol. 3(5):602-9, 2017
5. Fletcher JA: KIT Oncogenic mutations: biologic insights, therapeutic advances, and future directions. Cancer Res. 76(21):6140-2, 2016
6. Álvarez-Twose I et al: Clinical, immunophenotypic, and molecular characteristics of well-differentiated systemic mastocytosis. J Allergy Clin Immunol. 137(1):168-78.e1, 2016
7. Rossi S et al: KIT, PDGFRA, and BRAF mutational spectrum impacts on the natural history of imatinib-naive localized GIST: a population-based study. Am J Surg Pathol. 39(7):922-30, 2015
8. Paschka P et al: Secondary genetic lesions in acute myeloid leukemia with inv(16) or t(16;16): a study of the German-Austrian AML Study Group (AMLSG). Blood. 121(1):170-7, 2013
9. Alvarez-Twose I et al: Complete response after imatinib mesylate therapy in a patient with well-differentiated systemic mastocytosis. J Clin Oncol. 30(12):e126-9, 2012

KIT Mutations

Gastrointestinal Stromal Tumor Histology

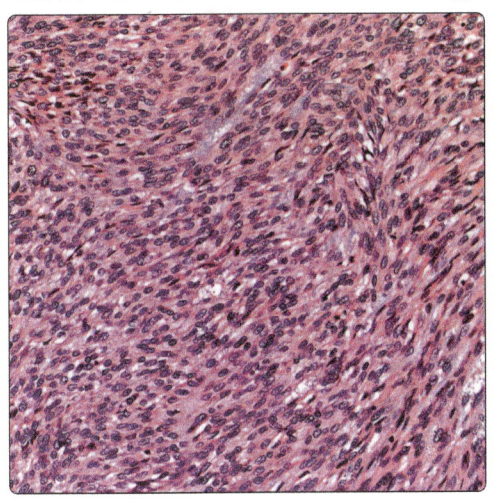

Sequencing of KIT Exon 11 Mutation

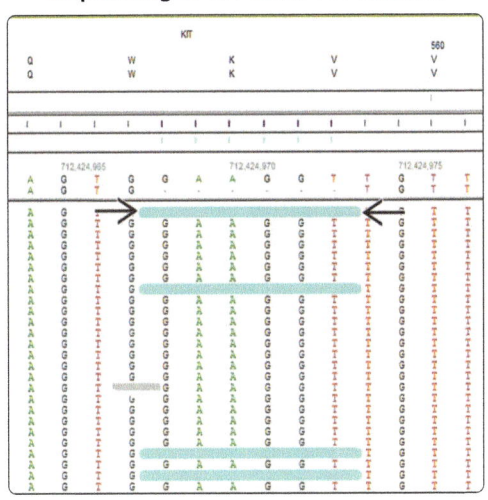

(Left) *GIST shows numerous oval to spindled tumor cells with a storiform growth pattern.* **(Right)** *NGS sequence pileup from a GIST allows visualization of a GAAGGT ➡ 6 bp deletion in KIT exon 11. A variety of KIT exon 11 insertions and deletions are found in GIST and are generally responsive to imatinib therapy.*

Systemic Mastocytosis Histology

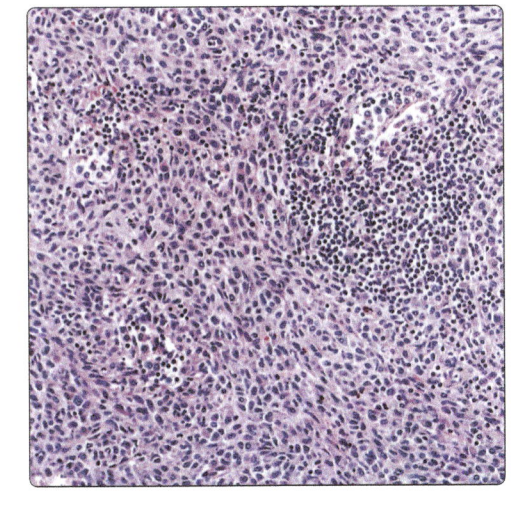

Pyrosequencing of KIT Mutation

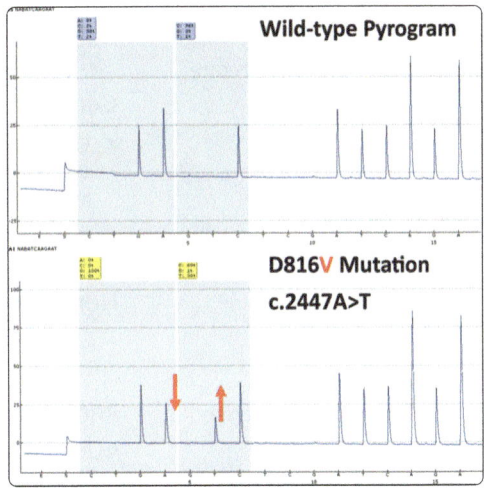

(Left) *Extensive axillary lymph node involvement by systemic mastocytosis is shown. Tryptase and aberrant CD25 expression by immunohistochemistry (not shown) confirmed the diagnosis.* **(Right)** *Pyrosequencing of KIT exon 17 performed on DNA extracted from a case of nodal systemic mastocytosis shows an A to T base substitution in codon 816. The resulting p.D816V mutation confers resistance to imatinib therapy.*

Acute Myeloid Leukemia With t(8;21) Cytology

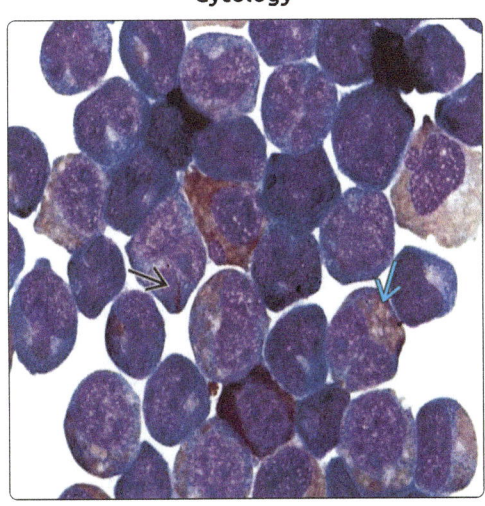

Dual-Color Dual-Fusion Probes for t(8;21)

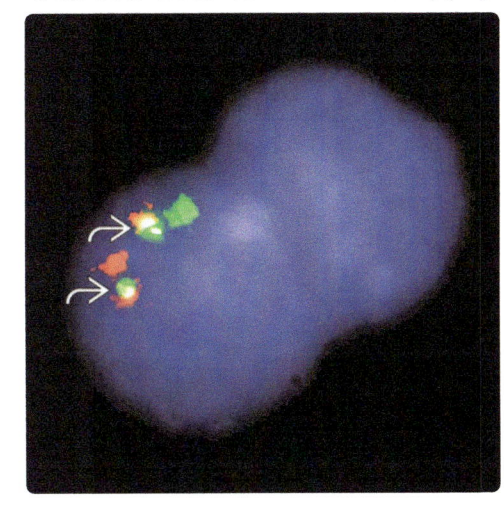

(Left) *Wright-stained bone marrow aspirate shows increased myeloblasts in a case of acute myeloid leukemia (AML) with t(8;21). The blasts show characteristic Auer rods ➡ and chunky, paranuclear, salmon-colored granules ➡.* **(Right)** *Interphase FISH analysis on a leukemic myeloblast using probes directed to RUNX1 and RUNX1T1 demonstrates 2 fusion signals ➡ corresponding to t(8;21)(q22;q22). KIT mutation correlates with decreased overall survival in this subtype of AML.*

IDH1 and IDH2 Mutations

TERMINOLOGY

Definitions

- *IDH1*
  - Official name: Isocitrate dehydrogenase [NADP(+)] 1, cytosolic
  - HGNC ID: 5382
  - Gene locus: 2q34
    - Chr2: 208,236,227-208,255,071 (GRCh38.p14)
  - RefSeq: NG_023319.2
  - Number of exons: 12 (first 2 exons are untranslated)
- *IDH2*
  - Official name: Isocitrate dehydrogenase [NADP(+)] 2, mitochondrial
  - HGNC ID: 5383
  - Gene locus: 15q26.1
    - Chr15: 90,083,045-90,102,468 (GRCh38.p14)
  - RefSeq: NG_023302.1
  - Number of exons: 12

NORMAL GENE FUNCTION

Encode Isocitrate Dehydrogenase Enzymes

- Catalyzes decarboxylation of isocitrate to α-ketoglutarate (a.k.a. 2-oxoglutarate, 2-OG)
- 5 human isocitrate dehydrogenase (IDH) isoforms described
  - IDH1 and IDH2 are NADP(+) dependent
  - Other IDH isoenzymes are NAD(+) dependent
- *IDH1* localizes to cytoplasm and peroxisomes
- *IDH2* localizes to mitochondria
- Necessary for metabolism and energy production

SOMATIC *IDH1* AND *IDH2* MUTATIONS

Typically Heterozygous Gain-of-Function Missense Mutations

- Usually occur at 1 of 3 highly conserved arginine residues
- Mutant converts isocitrate to R-2-hydroxyglutarate (R-2-HG)
- R-2-HG is oncometabolite that mediates transforming effect of mutant IDH
- Some epigenetic regulators are 2-OG dependent and inhibited by r-2-HG (e.g., TET and KDM protein families)
  - R-2-HG accumulation observed in both acute myeloid leukemia (AML) and in glial neoplasms
  - AML associated with *IDH1/IDH2* mutation is characterized by global promoter hypermethylation
- Mutation leads to impaired 2-OG production, elevated cellular R-2-HG, and wide-ranging alterations to metabolism and redox homeostasis

Common Mutations

- *IDH1* mutations often involve exon 2, codon 132
  - c.395G>A p.R132H
  - c.394C>T p.R132C
  - c.394C>G p.R132G
- *IDH2* mutations often involve exon 4, codons 140 or 172
  - c.515G>A p.R172K
  - c.515G>T p.R172M
  - c.419G>A p.R140Q

METHODS OF DETECTION OF *IDH1* AND *IDH2* MUTATIONS

Gene Sequencing

- Whole-exome approach often used for initial associative discovery in tumors, but targeted sequencing preferred in most clinical settings
  - Variety of sequencing modalities are available (e.g., Sanger, pyrosequencing, massively parallel, etc.)

Nonsequencing Molecular Methods

- Other approaches, such as allelic discrimination assays or high-resolution melting curve analysis, may be used

Immunohistochemical Staining

- Mutation-specific antibodies for variety of specific IDH1/IDH2 variants are available
- Only informative for specifically targeted variant; other variants will be missed

---

(Left) Next-generation sequencing pileup shows an IDH1 p.R132C missense mutation ➤. (Right) Wildtype IDH catalyzes the oxidative decarboxylation of isocitrate to α-ketoglutarate, but mutant IDH further reduces α-ketoglutarate to a structurally similar oncometabolite 2-hydroxyglutarate.

IDH1 Exon 2 Mutation

IDH1/IDH2: Substrate and Products

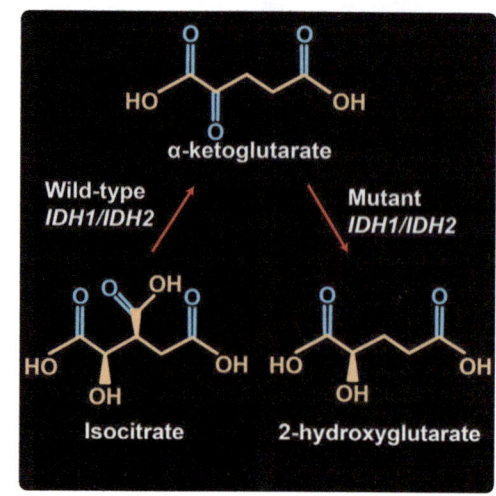

IDH1 and IDH2 Mutations

CLINICAL IMPLICATIONS OF IDH1 AND IDH2 MUTATIONS

Targeted Inhibitor Therapies

- Ivosidenib and enasidenib are oral small-molecule inhibitors of mutant *IDH1* and *IDH2*, respectively
  - Ivosidenib FDA approved in AML and cholangiocarcinoma
  - Enasidenib FDA approved in relapsed/refractory AML
  - Promising treatments in ~ 10% of cases of *IDH*-mutated myelodysplasia
  - Evaluation is ongoing for usage in other cancers
    - May qualify for clinical trials in other tumor types
- PARP inhibitors may have utility in *IDH*-mutant tumors due to impaired PARP1-mediated DNA repair

Gliomas

- Diagnostic value
  - Define grade 4 *IDH*-mutant astrocytomas
    - True 1° glioblastomas are *IDH*-wildtype
    - *IDH*-mutant grade 4 astrocytoma behavior still not as severe as IDH wildtype glioblastoma
  - Define WHO grades 2 and 3 astrocytomas and oligodendrogliomas
    - ATRX deficiency paired with *IDH* mutation is typical of astrocytoma
    - Oligodendrogliomas defined as tumors that have 1p/19q codeletion and *IDH* mutation (unless molecular data are not available and cannot be obtained)
      □ *IDH*-mutant gliomas without loss of ATRX should be considered for 1p/19q testing, even if not oligodendroglial by histology
      □ If *IDH*-wildtype, then 1p/19q testing is unnecessary, and tumors should not be regarded as 1p/19q codeleted
    - Anaplastic gliomas subdivided by *IDH* mutation status
    - Presence of mutation can differentiate grade 2 diffusely infiltrative glioma from gliosis
  - True grade 1 noninfiltrative gliomas (pilocytic astrocytoma, ganglioglioma) are *IDH*-wildtype
- Prognostic value
  - Associated with relatively favorable prognosis compared to *IDH*-wildtype cases
    - Associated with survival benefit for patient treated with radiation or alkylating-agent chemotherapy
  - Associated with MGMT promoter methylation
  - Grade II-III gliomas
    - *IDH*-mutant, 1p/19q-codeletion group has best prognosis
    - *IDH*-wildtype has worst prognosis
  - *IDH1* single nucleotide variant (G>A polymorphism) at p.G105 (rs11554137) associated with adverse outcomes in malignant glioma

Myeloid Neoplasms

- *IDH1* mutated in 6-9% of AML and in 8-16% of normal-karyotype cases
  - Associated with worse outcomes in normal-karyotype AML with favorable or intermediate-risk disease
  - Implication in co-occurrence with other gene mutations is still poorly defined
  - Association of *IDH1* c.315C>T (p.Gly105=) synonymous SNP with survival in adult AML in recent studies
    - Previous studies claimed negative impact on survival
    - More recent studies have shown no significant negative impact
- *IDH2* mutated in 8-12% of AML and up to ~ 19% in normal-karyotype cases
  - Essentially mutually exclusive from *IDH1* mutation
  - Reports on prognostic value in AML have been inconsistent
- *IDH1/IDH2* mutation with < 5% incidence in myelodysplasia
  - Associated with worse prognosis and higher rate of transformation to AML
- Rare in myeloproliferative neoplasms at diagnosis, but in ~ 20% of cases at blast phase

Angioimmunoblastic T-Cell Lymphoma

- *IDH2* mutations (principally at codon R172) detected in up to 20-45% of angioimmunoblastic T-cell lymphomas
- Preliminarily associated with higher response rates to epigenetic modifier therapy

Conventional Central and Periosteal Cartilaginous Tumors

- Seen in ~ 56% of cartilaginous tumors but not in other mesenchymal tumors
- No histologic or clinical differences found with mutant vs. wildtype tumors
- Osteochondromas and 2° peripheral chondrosarcomas are *IDH*-wildtype and instead show *EXT1/EXT2* mutations

Cholangiocarcinoma

- Identified in 10-23% of intrahepatic but < 1% of extrahepatic cholangiocarcinoma
- *IDH1* mutation may be poor prognostic marker in extrahepatic cholangiocarcinoma
- Mutations not generally seen in gallbladder or other gastrointestinal cancers
- No histologic or clinical differences found with mutant vs. wildtype tumors

Other Neoplasms

- Mutations are also identified in variety other cancers (e.g., thyroid carcinoma, prostate carcinoma, colorectal carcinoma, etc.)

Constitutional Disorders

- Mutations also detected in constitutional disorders, such as Maffucci syndrome, Ollier disease, and 2-hydroxyglutaric aciduria

SELECTED REFERENCES

1. Corley EM et al: Impact of IDH1 c.315C>T SNP on outcomes in acute myeloid leukemia: a propensity score-adjusted cohort study. Front Oncol. 12:804961, 2022
2. Hvinden IC et al: Metabolic adaptations in cancers expressing isocitrate dehydrogenase mutations. Cell Rep Med. 2(12):100469, 2021
3. DiNardo CD et al: Durable remissions with ivosidenib in IDH1-mutated relapsed or refractory AML. N Engl J Med. 378(25):2386-98, 2018
4. Ruzzenente A et al: Cholangiocarcinoma heterogeneity revealed by multigene mutational profiling: clinical and prognostic relevance in surgically resected patients. Ann Surg Oncol. 23(5):1699-707, 2016

Other Mutations and Gene Panel Testing in Myeloid Neoplasms

CLINICAL IMPLICATIONS

Mutational Landscape of Acute Myeloid Leukemia

- Large-scale next-generation sequencing (NGS) studies have identified most commonly mutated genes in de novo acute myeloid leukemia (AML)
- Cases of AML show relatively few mutations
  o Much lower mutational burden than solid tumors
- Some 237 genes are recurrently mutated
- ~ 26 genes have been found to be mutated at significant frequency (i.e., > 1%)

Biological Categories of Acute Myeloid Leukemia Mutations

- AML gene mutations may be grouped into several categories based on cellular function of encoded proteins
  o Cell signaling (59%)
    – FLT3, KRAS, NRAS, KIT
  o DNA methylation (44%)
    – TET2, DNMT3A, IDH1, IDH2
  o Chromatin modification (30%)
    – ASXL1, KMT2A, EZH2
  o NPM1, representing its own subcategory (27%)
  o Transcription factors (22%)
    – CEBPA, RUNX1, SETBP1, BCOR, BCORL1, ETV6
  o Tumor suppressor genes (16%)
    – TP53, WT1, PHF6
  o Spliceosome component (14%)
    – SF3B1, SRSF2, U2AF1, ZRSR2
  o Cohesin complex (13%)
    – SMC1A, STAG2, RAD21
- Most frequently mutated genes in AML include
  o NPM1, FLT3, CEBPA, DNMT3A, IDH1, IDH2, TET2, ASXL1, RUNX1, TP53, and KIT

Genes Required for AML Diagnosis and Risk Stratification

- ASXL1, BCOR, CEBPA, DDX41, EZH2, FLT3 ITD, FLT3 TKD, IDH1, IDH2, NPM1, RUNX1, SF3B1, SRSF2, STAG2, TP53, U2AF1, ZRSR2

Additional Genes Recommended to Test at Acute Myeloid Leukemia Diagnosis and For Use in Disease Monitoring

- ANKRD26, BCORL1, BRAF, CALR, CBL, CSF3R, DNMT3A, ETV6, GATA2, JAK2, KIT, KRAS, MPL, NRAS, NF1, PHF6, PPM1D, PTPN11, RAD21, SETBP1, TET2, WT1
  o Testing for NPM1, FLT3, CEBPA, and, in some cases, KIT is standard of care
- Extended testing for additional genes is now offered by many molecular diagnostic laboratories on routine basis
  o Multiple genes are simultaneously assessed via NGS panels
- Additional genes are assessed in broader myeloid gene panels by some laboratories
- Several systems have been proposed for risk-stratifying patients based on these results
  o Widespread implementation and acceptance into consensus guidelines
- Some NGS assays can also differentiate clonal from subclonal mutations
- Relatively high sensitivity of some NGS panels, especially at deep coverage, may facilitate minimal residual disease monitoring
- Some myeloid-associated mutations may be seen in blood and bone marrow of older individuals without evidence of overt myeloid malignancy
  o Somatic mutations in DNMT3A, ASXL1, and TET2 seen in ~ 2% of peripheral blood samples in large screening study
    – May represent clonal hematopoiesis of indeterminate potential (CHIP) with variant allele frequency of ≥ 2%
    – More common in older patients and presents risk for progression to overt hematologic malignancy
  o Thus, clinical and pathologic correlation remains critical

Extended Multigene Panel in MPN and Mastocytosis

- ASXL1, CALR, CBL, CSF3R, DNMT3A, EZH2, IDH1, IDH2, JAK2, KIT, KRAS, MPL, NRAS, PTPN11, RUNX1, SETBP1, SF3B1, SH2B3, SRSF2, TET2, U2AF1, ZRSR2

Blood Smear of Acute Myeloid Leukemia

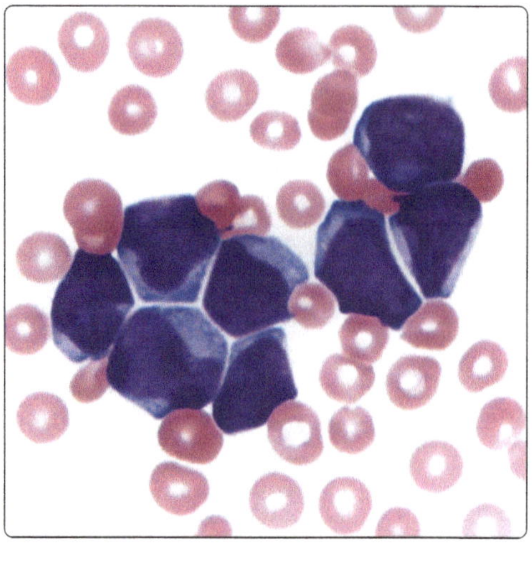

NGS Pile-Up of IDH1 Mutation

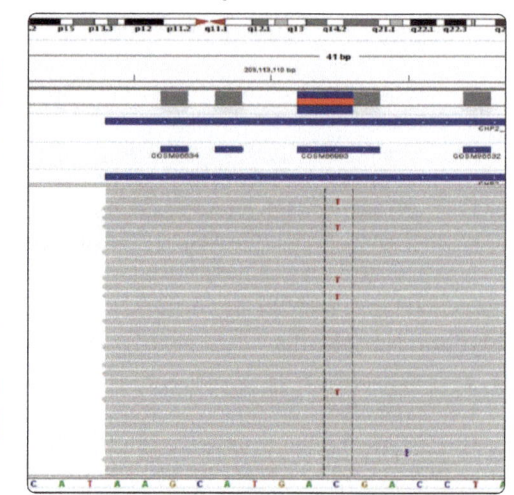

(Left) This patient with acute myeloid leukemia (AML) and a normal karyotype with FLT3 and NPM1 mutations relapsed 5 months after diagnosis. Extended molecular analysis could alter risk stratification in such cases. (Right) Next-generation sequencing (NGS) identifies IDH1 mutation in this case of AML. NGS permits simultaneous assessment for mutations in multiple relevant genes in AML.

Other Mutations and Gene Panel Testing in Myeloid Neoplasms

Frequently Mutated Genes in De Novo Acute Myeloid Leukemia

Gene	Approximate Frequency of Mutation in De Novo Acute Myeloid Leukemia	Biologic Role of Encoded Protein
FLT3	27-37%	Cell signaling
NPM1	27.5-29%	Phosphoprotein, shuttles between cytoplasm and nucleus
DNMT3A	23-28.5%	DNA methylation
TET2	8-14.5%	DNA methylation
CEBPA	9-9.5%	Transcription factor
IDH2	8-10%	DNA methylation (via neomorphic enzyme activity)
NRAS	7.5-10%	Cell signaling
IDH1	7-9.5%	DNA methylation (via neomorphic enzyme activity)
RUNX1	5-10.5%	Transcription factor
WT1	6.5-8%	Tumor suppressor
KIT	5-6%	Cell signaling
TP53	2-9%	Tumor suppressor
KMT2A (formerly MLL)-PTD	5%	Chromatin modification
PTPN11	4.5%	Cell signaling
U2AF1	4%	Spliceosome
SMC1A	3.5%	Cohesin complex
SMC3	3.5%	Cohesin complex
BRINP3	3%	Negative regulation of cell cycle
PHF6	3%	Tumor suppressor
STAG2	3%	Cohesin complex
KRAS	2-4%	Cell signaling
ASXL1	3%	Chromatin modification
RAD21	2.5%	Cohesin complex
PTEN	2%	Cell signaling
HNRNPK	1.5%	Spliceosome
EZH2	0-2%	Chromatin modification

All genes found by TCGA to be recurrently mutated at significant frequency by whole-genome or whole-exome sequencing are listed. When a range of frequency is given, it reflects the independent findings of each study. From the Cancer Genome Atlas (TCGA) Research Network and Patel JP et al.

Extended Multigene Testing in MDS/MPN and Cytopenia

- *ASXL1, BCOR, BCORL1, CBL, CEBPA, CSF3R, DDX41, DNMT3A, ETV6, ETNK1, EZH2, FLT3* ITD, *FLT3* TKD, *GATA2, GNB1, IDH1, IDH2, JAK2, KIT, KRAS, KMT2A*-PTD, *NF1, NPM1, NRAS, PHF6, PPM1D, PRPF8, PTPN11, RAD21, RUNX1, SAMD9, SAMD9L, SETBP1, SF3B1, SRSF2, STAG2, TET2, TP53, U2AF1, UBA1, WT1, ZRSR2*
- Most frequently mutated genes in MDS include
  - *ASXL1, BCOR, DNMT3A, EZH2, IDH1, IDH2, NRAS, RUNX1, SF3B1, SRSF2, STAG2, TET2, U2AF1,* and *ZRSR2*
    - *SF3B1* mutations associated with ring sideroblasts
    - *DNMT3A, TET2,* and *ASXL1* are often present in preleukemic stem or progenitor cells
      - Occur early in leukemogenesis
    - Mutations in genes, such as *ASXL1, TET2,* and *DNMT3A,* and, less frequently, splicing factor genes, such as *SF3B1* and *SRSF2*, can also occur in older healthy individuals as clonal hematopoiesis without evidence of MDS
    - MDS-associated somatic mutations alone are **not** considered diagnostic of MDS
- Most frequently mutated genes in nonchronic myeloid leukemia and MPN
  - *JAK2, CALR, MPL*
  - *ASXL1* and *TP53* mutations in MPN predict poor overall survival
- Most frequently mutated genes in MDS/MPN
  - *ASXL1, CBL, SRSF2, SF3B1, EZH2, IDH1, IDH2, TP53, CALR*
    - *SF3B1* more common in MDS/MPN with ring sideroblasts and thrombocytosis (MDS/MPN with *SF3B1* mutation and thrombocytosis)
      - *JAK2, CALR,* and *MPL* mutations can be seen in MDS/MPN with *SF3B1* mutation and thrombocytosis and in MDS/MPN with ring sideroblasts and thrombocytosis

SELECTED REFERENCES

1. Duncavage EJ et al: Genomic profiling for clinical decision making in myeloid neoplasms and acute leukemia. Blood. 140(21):2228-47, 2022
2. Alonso CM et al: Clinical utility of a next-generation sequencing panel for acute myeloid leukemia diagnostics. J Mol Diagn. 21(2):228-40, 2019

Immunoglobulin Heavy (*IGH*) Chain Gene Rearrangements

TERMINOLOGY

Definitions

- Immunoglobulin heavy locus (*IGH*)
  - Chromosomal location: 14q32.33
  - Genomic position
    - Ch14: 105,586,437-106,879,844
  - Includes variable (VH), diversity (DH), joining (JH), and constant (CH) gene segments
- Immunoglobulin kappa (*IGK*) and lambda (*IGL*) loci
  - Chromosomal location: 2p11.2 and 22q11.22, respectively
  - Include variable (V), joining (J), and constant (C) gene segments
  - *IGK* also includes immunoglobulin kappa deleting element (IGKDE)

IMMUNOGLOBULIN STRUCTURE

Immunoglobulin Heavy Chain

- Y-shaped molecule composed of 2 heavy and 2 light chains connected by disulfide bonds
  - Fragment antigen-binding (Fab) portion at tip of Ig molecule contains antigen-binding site
  - Fragment crystallizable (Fc) portion interacts with complement system and Fc receptors on certain cells
- 5 different types of heavy chains exist: α, δ, ε, γ, and μ
  - Heavy chain type corresponds to specific class of Ig: IgA, IgD, IgE, IgG, and IgM
  - Consist of variable and constant regions
  - Variable region is encoded by VH, DH, and JH gene segments
    - Includes conserved sequences that constitute 4 framework regions (FR1, FR2, FR3, and FR4)
    - Between FRs are 3 hypervariable complementarity determining regions (CDR1, CDR2, and CDR3) involved in antigen binding
    - CDR3 is most variable region
  - Constant region is encoded by CH segment

Immunoglobulin Light Chains

- Light chains include κ and λ
- Similar structure to heavy chain except
  - Variable region encoded by *IGK* or *IGL* V and J gene segments
  - No D segments in *IGK* and *IGL*
  - Shorter constant region
- Steps involved in generation of diversity are similar in both BCR and T-cell receptor (TCR)
  - Somatic hypermutations are unique to Ig genes

OVERVIEW OF B-CELL DEVELOPMENT

Antigen-Independent Stages

- Occur in bone marrow, progress through *IGH* and *IGK*/*IGL* rearrangements, and lead to surface BCR assembly
- *IGH*, *IGK*, and *IGL* are in germline configuration in hematopoietic stem cells
- Early and late progenitor B cells (pro B cells)
  - *IGH* undergoes DH to JH rearrangement followed by VH to DH-JH rearrangement
- Large precursor B cells (pre B cells)
  - Express surface pre B-cell receptor composed of μ heavy chain and surrogate light chain
  - Successful assembly triggers allelic exclusion to prevent *IGH* rearrangements on 2nd allele
  - Nonproductive rearrangements of both *IGH* alleles lead to cell death
- Small precursor B cells (pre B cells)
  - *IGK* undergoes Vκ to Jκ rearrangement
  - If *IGK* rearrangements are unproductive on both alleles, then *IGL* undergoes rearrangements
- Immature B cells
  - Assemble BCR composed of μ heavy chain (IgM), and κ or λ light chain on cell surface
- Mature naive B cells
  - Enter peripheral circulation and migrate to secondary lymphoid tissues
  - Express surface IgM and IgD through alternative splicing

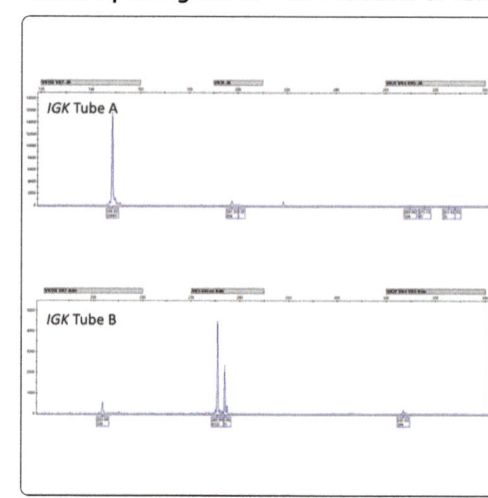

(Left) *B-cell clonality assay by PCR and capillary electrophoresis shows monoclonal IGH rearrangements. Each reaction has generated a single dominant amplicon size.*
(Right) *Electrophoregram shows a prominent clonal IGK peak consistent with clonal population. X axis = amplicon size. Y axis = fluorescence.*

Electrophoregram of PCR Products of *IGH*

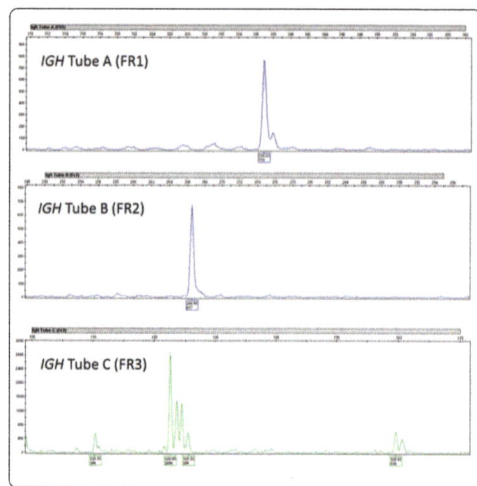

IGH Tube A (FR1)

IGH Tube B (FR2)

IGH Tube C (FR3)

Electrophoregram of PCR Products of *IGK*

IGK Tube A

IGK Tube B

Immunoglobulin Heavy (IGH) Chain Gene Rearrangements

Antigen-Dependent Stages
- T-cell independent B-cell reaction in paracortex
  - Some antigens may activate B cells directly without T-cell cooperation in paracortex of lymph node; consequently, mature naive B cells transform into proliferating extrafollicular B blasts
    - Their progeny can mature into short-lived plasma cells secreting low-affinity IgM
    - No memory B cells are generated
- T-cell dependent B-cell reaction in germinal center
  - Proliferating blasts migrate to primary follicles, form germinal centers (GC), and become centroblasts
    - Selected cells with BCRs to specific antigen present in GC survive and continue to proliferate
  - Centroblasts undergo **somatic hypermutations (SHM)** that introduce point mutations in variable regions of heavy and light chains
  - Centroblasts mature into nonproliferating centrocytes and then undergo selection process
    - Cells capable of producing high-affinity Ig are "rescued" from apoptosis
    - **Affinity maturation** is direct result of SHM and selection process
  - Subset of centrocytes undergo **class switch recombination (CSR)** to produce IgG, IgA, or, rarely, IgE, instead of IgM
    - CSR changes Ig functional characteristics but does not affect antigen specificity
  - Differentiation into effector cells (post-GC step)
    - Memory B cells are detectable in peripheral blood and marginal zone of lymphoid tissues and include IgM and class-switched subsets
    - Long-lived plasma cells secrete Ig of all classes and can be found in lymph node medulla, splenic cords, and bone marrow
  - In adults, new B cells are continuously produced in bone marrow

IGH REARRANGEMENTS

Overview
- Sequence of somatic recombination events occurring at pro B-cell stages in B-cell lineage precursors
  - Joins gene segments that are spatially separated in germline configuration
- General order of Ig gene rearrangements
  - *IGH* 1st followed by *IGK*, followed by *IGL* if rearranged *IGK* in both alleles is nonproductive

IGH Locus
- *IGH* variable region gene cluster contains comparable number of V segments to *IGK*, *IGL*, *TRA*, and *TRB* loci
  - Numbers of V segments vary between individuals
  - Of ~ 123-139 VH segments, only 46-52 are functional
    - Belong to 7 V families based on homology
    - Several VH segments are considered pseudogenes
- Additionally, *IGH* locus contains 26 DH segments, 9 JH segments, and 11 CH segments

Recombination Process
- Requires many enzymes and other proteins
  - Enzymes expressed only in developing lymphocytes
    - RAG1 and RAG2 encoded by recombination activating genes are key components
    - Terminal deoxynucleotidyl transferase (TdT)
- Recombination proceeds in regulated stepwise fashion
  - Begins with RAG complex recognizing and cutting DNA at recombination signal sequences (RSS)
    - RSS located immediately downstream of VH segments, at both sides of DH segments and upstream of JH segments
    - RSS are composed of conserved heptamer, 12 or 23 bp spacer, and conserved nonamer sequences
    - Segments with RSS having 12 bp and 23 bp spacers (12/23 rule) are usually joined (to prevent nonproductive rearrangements, e.g., VH to VH)
  - Next step involves formation of hairpin structure (stem loop) at ends of coding segments
    - Blunt ends of RSS are ligated together into circular DNA containing all intervening sequences
  - Other proteins bind to and open hairpin at random site to yield single-stranded DNA ends
    - Palindromic (P) nucleotides originate from complementary strand of hairpin that is asymmetrically opened
    - Exonuclease and TdT randomly cleave and add nontemplated nucleotides (N), resulting in junctional diversity
  - Finally, DNA ligase joins rearranging gene segments
  - DH to JH rearrangement is followed by VH to DH-JH rearrangement to form recombined complete VDJ
    - Repertoire of inherited gene segments accounts for Ig combinatorial diversity
    - **Combinatorial and junctional diversity** together create essentially limitless repertoire of variable region sequences
- Transcription step is followed by RNA splicing, leading to joining of V region to neighboring C segment
  - Alternative RNA splicing results in expression of μ or δ heavy chains
    - Class-switch recombination is required for α, ε, and γ heavy chain expression
  - Switch from membrane-bound to soluble Ig also occurs at RNA processing step via alternate splicing
- Translation and Ig assembly are final steps
- All Ig and TCR gene rearrangements follow similar steps and use same enzymes and cellular machinery
  - Rearranged *IGK*/*IGL* have reduced junctional diversity compared to *IGH*

Other Related Processes
- Both SHM and CSR also result in somatic changes to germline sequence of Ig genes
- Utilize different enzymes and cellular mechanisms
  - Activation-induced cytidine deaminase is important enzyme in this process

CLONALITY TESTING

General Comments
- Clonality does not equal malignancy
  - Benign and reactive conditions can produce clonal patterns due to antigen-driven lymphocyte expansions
- Clonal rearrangements are not lineage specific

Immunoglobulin Heavy (IGH) Chain Gene Rearrangements

- o B-cell malignancies (especially of B-cell precursors) often have clonal T-cell receptor gene rearrangements
- o T-cell malignancies can have clonal Ig gene rearrangements
- Results of clonality testing should always be interpreted within appropriate clinical context and in conjunction with morphologic findings

Antibody-Based Methods

- Based on evaluation of light chain restriction in B cells &/or plasma cells
  - o Ratio of κ to λ is calculated/estimated
    - Results outside of established normal range are indicative of clonality
- Flow cytometry (FC), in situ hybridization (ISH), and immunohistochemistry (IHC) can be used
  - o Several limitations exist
    - Fresh tissue requirement for FC, inability to evaluate light chain restriction in majority of B cells by IHC/ISH

Nucleic Acid-Based Methods

- Southern blot hybridization
  - o Used to be gold standard for clonality analysis in old days, now largely replaced by PCR-based approaches
  - o Based on principle that antigen receptor gene rearrangements alter restriction-digested DNA fragments compared with germline DNA
    - Genes with significant combinatorial diversity, such as IGH, IGK, and TRB, are suitable targets for analysis
  - o Requires significant amount of high-quality DNA
  - o Sensitivity of this method is ~ 5-10%
  - o Individual gene rearrangements are not detected unless they are overrepresented at ≥ 5% in background lymphoid cells
    - Polyclonal sample appears as germline bands only
    - Clonal rearrangements appear as novel bands
- PCR-based approaches
  - o Current gold standard for clonality analysis
  - o Based on principle that somatic Ig gene rearrangements bring V, (D), and J segments together, enabling their PCR amplification
    - Each rearrangement is unique in length and sequence due to combinatorial and junctional diversity
    - IGH and IGK are usually tested
    - Testing IGL adds little to overall ability to detect clonal rearrangements and is not widely used
  - o Can be performed on variety of specimen types, including formalin-fixed, paraffin-embedded tissue
    - Tissues exposed to strong acid-based decalcification solutions are not suitable for PCR amplification
    - Tissues exposed to heparin-based decalcification solution are suitable for PCR amplification
  - o PCR protocol
  - o Genomic DNA is extracted and IGH and IGK CDR3 regions are PCR amplified
    - BIOMED-2 (from European BIOMED-2 collaborative study) primer strategy is most commonly used
      - □ Commercial kits are available (e.g., IGH + IGK B-cell clonality assay from Invivoscribe)
    - For IGH, primers targeting multiple VH families within FR1, 2, and 3 plus single consensus primer for JH segment (3 separate reactions) are used

- □ SHM can interfere with primers binding
- IGK tube A includes 6 Vκ primers plus 2 Jκ primers
- IGK tube B includes 6 Vκ primers and Jκ-Cκ intron primer plus 1 IGKDE primer (to detect rearrangements involving IGKDE)
  - □ Not affected by SHM (main advantage)
- o Fractionation by capillary electrophoresis (CE)
  - One of PCR primers requires fluorescent labeling
  - Separates amplicons based on length only
  - Conventional gel electrophoresis can also be used as alternative, but it is more labor intensive and time consuming with lesser resolution
- o Interpretation should be assay and specimen specific
  - Polyclonal B cells generate normal (Gaussian) distribution of amplicon of different sizes
  - Clonal B cells produce 1 or 2 prominent amplicons within diminished polyclonal background
- o Generally not suitable for minimal residual disease (MRD) monitoring, unless specific primers for patient-specific clone are designed
- Next-generation sequencing approaches
  - o High throughput sequencing may identifies MRD deeper than conventional clinical cutoff of 0.01 by flow cytometry
  - o High specificity attributable to resolution of rearrangements by size and sequence
  - o High sensitivity suitable for MRD monitoring
  - o Claimed to have lower false-negative rate compared to flow cytometry
- IGH rearrangements analysis using RNA sequencing (RNAseq)
  - o Patient's specific IGH rearrangements is identified in initial presentation for MRD monitoring in lymphoblastic leukemia patients
  - o RNAseq data is generated using antigen receptor research tool (ARResT): http://bat.infspire.org
    - Tool is built within EuroClonality NGS Working Group
  - o RNAseq data is analyzed using ARResT to interrogate and identify possible MRD markers
  - o Similar strategy can be employed for disease monitoring in other lymphomas and multiple myeloma

SELECTED REFERENCES

1. van der Velden VHJ et al: Immunoglobulin/T-cell receptor gene rearrangement analysis using RNA-Seq. Methods Mol Biol. 2453:61-77, 2022
2. Wood B et al: Measurable residual disease detection by high-throughput sequencing improves risk stratification for pediatric B-ALL. Blood. 131(12):1350-9, 2018
3. Gazzola A et al: The evolution of clonality testing in the diagnosis and monitoring of hematological malignancies. Ther Adv Hematol. 5(2):35-47, 2014
4. Grundy GJ et al: One ring to bring them all–the role of Ku in mammalian non-homologous end joining. DNA Repair (Amst). 17:30-8, 2014
5. Langerak AW et al: EuroClonality/BIOMED-2 guidelines for interpretation and reporting of Ig/TCR clonality testing in suspected lymphoproliferations. Leukemia. 26(10):2159-71, 2012
6. Spagnolo L et al: Three-dimensional structure of the human DNA-PKcs/Ku70/Ku80 complex assembled on DNA and its implications for DNA DSB repair. Mol Cell. 22(4):511-9, 2006
7. van Dongen JJ et al: Design and standardization of PCR primers and protocols for detection of clonal immunoglobulin and T-cell receptor gene recombinations in suspect lymphoproliferations: report of the BIOMED-2 Concerted Action BMH4-CT98-3936. Leukemia. 17(12):2257-317, 2003

Immunoglobulin Heavy (*IGH*) Chain Gene Rearrangements

Germline Configuration and Steps Involved in *IGH* Rearrangement

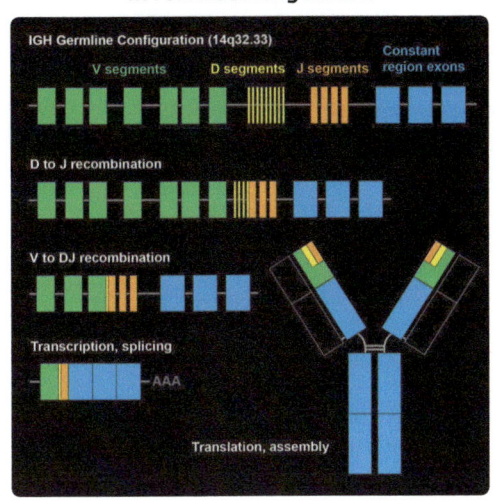

Southern Blot Analysis of *IGH*

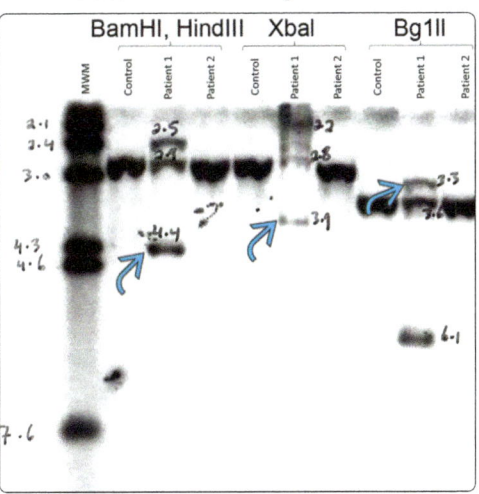

(Left) Graph illustrates the germline configuration of IGH and steps involved in rearrangements of D, J, and V segments. **(Right)** Southern blot analysis of IGH on DNA extracted from fresh diagnostic tissue is shown. Germline bands present in DNA from patient 2 indicate polyclonal population. Nongermline bands in patient 1 represent clonal IGH gene rearrangements. MWM = molecular weight marker. BamHI, HindIII, XbaI, and Bg1II = restriction enzymes.

Electrophoregram of Polyclonal B Cells

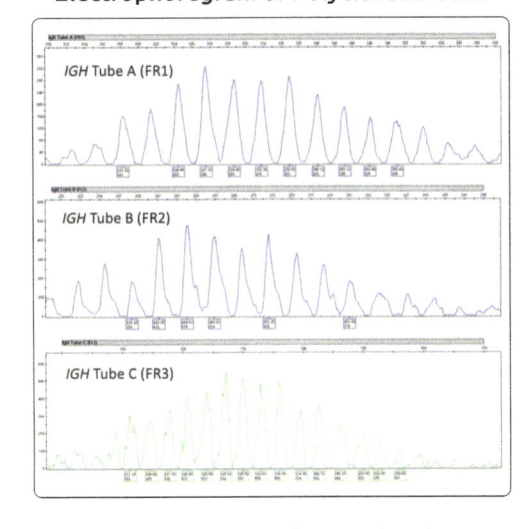

Electrophoregram of PCR Products of *IGK*

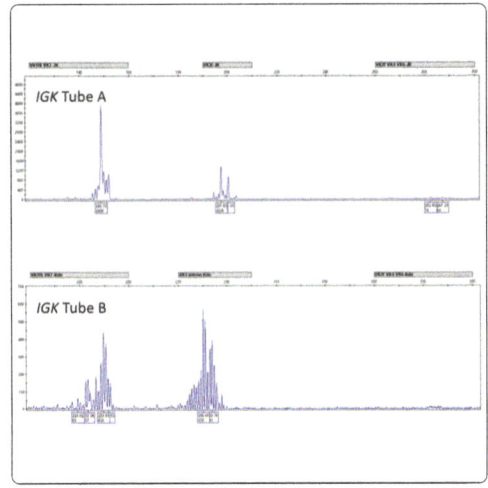

(Left) Electrophoregram shows B-cell clonality assay by PCR and capillary electrophoresis. There is no evidence of monoclonal IGH rearrangement. Each reaction has generated a normal (Gaussian) distribution of amplicon sizes. **(Right)** Electrophoregram analysis of IGK from a patient with atypical lymphoid proliferation shows no definitive clonal lymphoid population. X axis = amplicon size. Y axis = fluorescence.

Electrophoregram of Monoclonal *IGH* Rearrangement

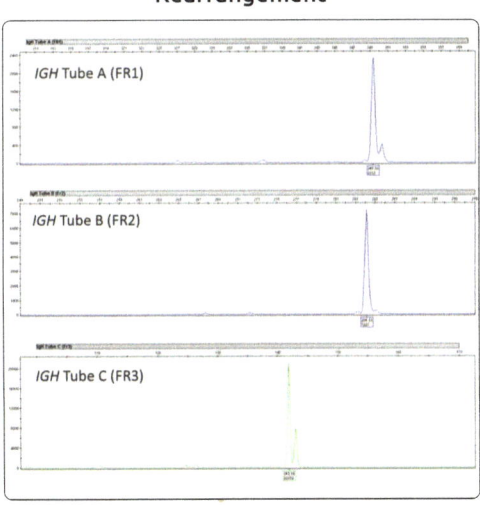

Electrophoregram of Monoclonal *IGK* Rearrangement

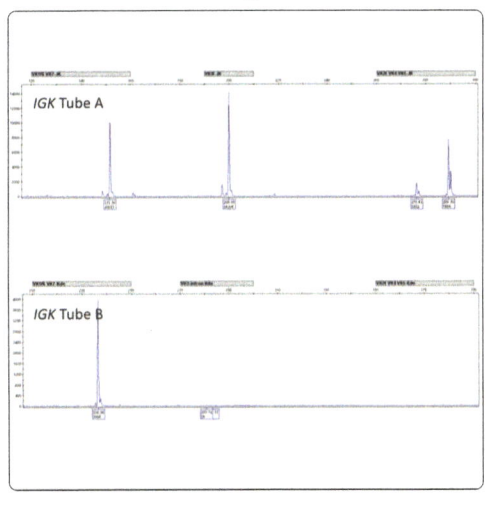

(Left) B-cell clonality assay by PCR and capillary electrophoresis shows a prominent peak in each reaction, consistent with monoclonal IGH rearrangement. **(Right)** Capillary electrophoresis of PCR-amplified products of IGK shows a prominent peak in each reaction, supportive of a clonal lymphoid population. X axis = amplicon size. Y axis = fluorescence.

Molecular Genetic Tests in Hematopoietic Tumors

T-Cell Receptor Gamma (*TRG*) and Delta (*TRD*) Chain Rearrangements

TERMINOLOGY

Definitions

- T-cell receptor (TCR) gamma locus (*TRG*)
  o HGNC ID: 12271
  o Chromosomal location: 7p14.1
  o Includes
    – Variable (Vγ) segments
    – Joining (Jγ) segments
    – Constant (Cγ) segments
- TCR delta locus (*TRD*)
  o HGNC ID: 12252
  o Chromosomal location: 14q11.2
    – Located within TCR alpha (*TRA*) locus
  o Includes
    – Variable (Vδ) segments
    – Joining (Jδ) segments
    – Diversity (Dδ) segments
    – Constant (Cδ) segments

TCR STRUCTURE

Background

- T cells play major role in cell-mediated immunity
- Cell surface molecule responsible for recognizing antigens presented to T cells in context of major histocompatibility complex (MHC) molecules
- TCRs serve primary antigen recognition function in adaptive immune response
- TCRs composed of 2 different protein chains (heterodimer) connected by disulfide bond
  o αβ T cells
    – Account for majority of T cells
    – Express TCR composed of α and β chains
  o γδ T cells
    – Account for minority of T cells in circulation
    – Dominant T-cell subset found in epithelial tissues (gastrointestinal tract and skin)
    – Express TCR composed of γ and δ chains
    – Can recognize antigens that are not associated with MHC molecules
- Each chain (α, β, γ, or δ) is composed of
  o 2 extracellular domains that include variable and constant regions
  o Transmembrane domain
  o Short cytoplasmic tail
- V, D, and J segments in *TRD* and *TRB*
- Only V and J segments in *TRG* and *TRA*
  o Conserved sequences within variable region constitute framework regions (FRs)
  o Hypervariable complementarity determining regions (CDRs)
    – Involved in antigen binding and are interspersed with FRs
    – CDR3 is most variable region
- Extracellular constant region, transmembrane domain, and cytoplasmic tail are encoded by C gene segment
- TCR couples with other signaling molecules to achieve signal propagation due to short cytoplasmic tail
- Resultant octameric protein complex is known as **TCR complex** and consists of
  o TCR αβ or γδ heterodimer
  o 3 dimeric signaling modules, including
    – CD3 δ/ε, CD3 γ/ε, and CD247 ζ/ζ
    – These associated invariant molecules are also necessary for transport of TCR to cell membrane
- Signal originating from TCR complex is enhanced by
  o Simultaneous binding of MHC molecules on antigen presenting cells to specific TCR coreceptors on T cells
    – CD4 is specific for MHC class II
    – CD8 is specific for MHC class I

TRG REARRANGEMENTS

Overview

- Sequence of somatic recombination events
  o Occur at early stage of T-cell development in both αβ and γδ T-cell lineage precursors

Capillary Electrophoresis of Monoclonal *TRG* Rearrangement

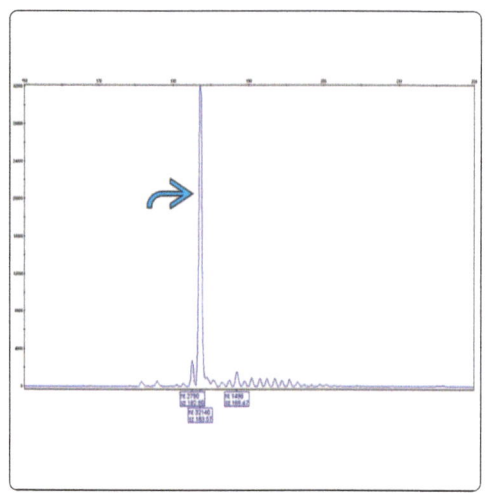

Capillary Electrophoresis of Polyclonal *TRG* Rearrangement

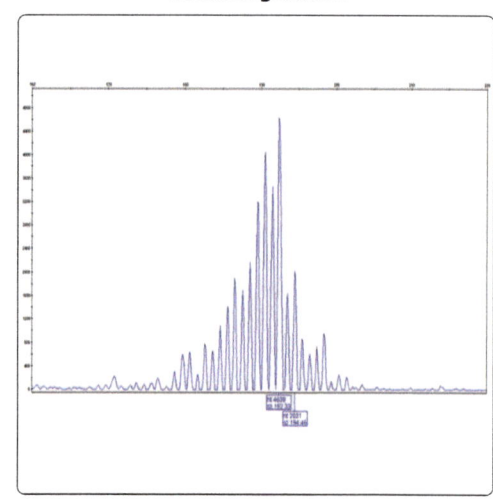

(Left) Monoclonal *TRG* rearrangement is detected by PCR and capillary electrophoresis. A single prominent amplicon ➲ is present in a minimal polyclonal background. X axis = amplicon size. Y axis = fluorescence. **(Right)** Electrophoregram shows no evidence of monoclonal *TRG* rearrangement. Normal distribution of amplicons of different sizes is generated. X axis = amplicon size. Y axis = fluorescence.

T-Cell Receptor Gamma (*TRG*) and Delta (*TRD*) Chain Rearrangements

- o Joins gene segments that are spatially separated in germline configuration
- General order of TCR gene rearrangements
  - o *TRD*, *TRG*, *TRB*, followed by *TRA*
  - o Sequence of rearrangements is not obligate
    - Not all αβ T-cells have rearranged *TRG*

TRG
- Located at 7p14.1
- ~ 128 kb in size
- *TRG* variable region gene cluster contains
  - o Comparable number of V segments to *TRD*
  - o Far simpler compared to *TRB*, *TRA*, *IGH*, *IGK*, and *IGL* genes
  - o Includes 14 Vγ gene segments, 10 of which can undergo rearrangement
    - Only 6 Vγ-rearranged gene segments are functional
  - o Rearranging Vγ gene segments can be grouped into 4 families based on sequence homology
    - VγI family is largest and includes Vγ2, Vγ3, Vγ4, Vγ5, Vγ7, and Vγ8 gene segments
    - Remaining 3 are single-member families that include Vγ9, Vγ10, and Vγ11
  - o Exceptionally, Vγ12 is rearranged, which is rarely targeted in diagnostic PCR strategies
  - o Several Vγ gene segments are designated as pseudogenes
- *TRG* Jγ-Cγ clusters
  - o 1st cluster includes 3 Jγ (all functional) and 1 Cγ gene segment
  - o 2nd cluster includes 2 Jγ (both functional and highly homologous to Jγ segments in 1st cluster) and 1 Cγ gene segment
- *TRG* shows limited **combinatorial diversity** due to restricted germline repertoire in comparison to *TRB*
- **Junctional activity** is also limited
  - o Relatively few nucleotide additions
  - o Restricted to single Vγ-Jγ junction

Recombination Process
- *TRG* rearrangements follow similar steps
  - o Use same enzymes and cellular machinery as other TCR and immunoglobulin gene rearrangements
- Consist of single step of Vγ to Jγ rearrangement
- *TRG* rearrangements occurring in healthy individuals are characterized by nonrandom distribution of Vγ and Jγ gene segments
  - o γδ T-cells can demonstrate "canonical" *TRG* rearrangements
    - Most commonly involves Vγ9 and Jγ1.2 segments
    - Occurs in ~ 1% of peripheral blood T lymphocytes
    - Corresponds to accumulation of γδ T cells in aging individuals
- Steps involved in generation of diversity are similar in both TCR and B-cell receptor

CLONALITY TESTING

General Comments
- Clonality does not equal malignancy
  - o Benign and reactive conditions can produce clonal patterns due to antigen-driven lymphocyte expansions
- Clonal rearrangements are not lineage specific
  - o B-cell malignancies, especially of B-cell precursor origin, often have clonal TCR rearrangements
  - o T-cell malignancies can also have clonal immunoglobulin gene rearrangements
- Results of clonality testing should always be interpreted within appropriate clinical context and in conjunction with morphologic findings
- Rationales for using *TRG* as target for clonality assessment
  - o Restricted *TRG* germline repertoire with very limited number of Vγ and Jγ segments
    - Makes PCR assay design easier
    - May make interpretation difficult (i.e., distinction between clonal and polyclonal PCR products)
  - o *TRG* is rearranged at early stage of T lymphoid development in both αβ and γδ T-lineage precursors
    - *TRG* is retained during subsequent *TRB* and *TRA* rearrangements; therefore, TRG still detectable in malignancies of αβ T-cell origin
  - o In contrast, *TRD* is deleted during subsequent *TRA* rearrangement in αβ T-cell precursors
    - TRD testing is essentially not practical for clonality assessment
- *TRG* rearrangements testing is usually sufficient approach in T-cell clonality assessment
  - o Addition of *TRB* rearrangement analysis may improve clinical sensitivity in certain cases

Nucleic Acid-Based Methods
- **PCR-based approaches**
  - o Current gold standard for clonality analysis
  - o Based on principle that somatic TCR gene rearrangements bring V, (D), and J segments together enabling their PCR amplification
    - No PCR product is generated if germline configuration is retained
  - o Each rearrangement is unique in length and sequence as result of combinatorial and junctional diversity
  - o Can be performed on variety of specimen types, including formalin-fixed, paraffin-embedded (FFPE) tissue
- **Protocol**
  - o Genomic DNA is extracted and CDR3 region is PCR amplified
    - BIOMED-2 (from European BIOMED-2 collaborative study) primer strategy is assay used in some laboratories
      - □ Commercial kits are available (e.g., T-cell receptor gamma gene clonality assay from Invivoscribe)
      - □ 2 multiplex tube design that allows detection of vast majority of clonal *TRG* rearrangements
      - □ Each tube targets 2 Vγ families and 4 Jγ segments
      - □ Jγ1.2 segment, which is rarely involved in clonal rearrangements, is excluded from this strategy to minimize false-positive results due to presence of canonical Vγ9-Jγ1.2 rearrangements
      - □ Tube A contains VγI family and Vγ10 primers plus Jγ1.1/2.1 and Jγ1.3/2.3 primers
      - □ Tube B contains Vγ9 and Vγ11 primers plus Jγ1.1/2.1 and Jγ1.3/2.3 primers
    - Greiner et al primer strategy is used as alternative by other laboratories

T-Cell Receptor Gamma (*TRG*) and Delta (*TRD*) Chain Rearrangements

- □ Single multiplex tube design allows detection of vast majority of clonal *TRG* rearrangements
- □ All 4 Vγ families are targeted using 5 forward primers [specific for Vγ2 (also amplifies Vγ4-8), Vγ3, Vγ9, Vγ10, and Vγ11]
- □ All 5 Jγ segments are targeted using 3 reverse primers (specific for Jγ1.1/2.1, Jγ1.2, Jγ1.3/2.3)
- □ Additionally, multiplex tube can be split into separate PCR reactions to identify which Vγ family is involved in clonal rearrangement
- □ Clonality is assigned based on results from multiplex reaction
- o Fractionation by capillary electrophoresis (CE)
  - One of PCR primes requires fluorescent labeling
  - Separates amplicons based on length only
    - □ No sequence is evaluated
  - Conventional gel electrophoresis can also be used as alternative to CE
    - □ More labor intensive and time consuming
    - □ Low resolution
- o Generally not suitable for minimal residual disease (MRD) monitoring, unless specific primers are designed to detect patient-specific clone within polyclonal background

Diagnostic Interpretation

- Interpretation should be assay and specimen specific, and based on in-house validation procedure
  - o Polyclonal T cells typically generate a bell-shaped (Gaussian) distribution of different sized amplicons
  - o Multiple but limited numbers of peaks represent either oligoclonal T-cell expansion or few T cells in specimen
    - Specimens with scant T cells may result in pseudoclonality
  - o Clonal T cells produce 1 or 2 prominent peaks (uni- or biallelic rearrangements) within diminished polyclonal background
  - o Various strategies for calling clonal results have been proposed
    - Ratio of clonal peak height to height of polyclonal background with cutoff of ≥ 2.0 is often used
    - In general, height of 3rd tallest peak is considered as height of polyclonal background
- Next-generation sequencing (NGS) approaches
  - o Currently used in clinical practice
    - Genomic DNA is extracted and enriched for rearranged *TRG* sequences by PCR amplification
    - Library preparation is followed by pooling multiple samples and sequencing step
    - Analysis is performed by custom software package
      - □ Reads are assigned Vγ and Jγ gene segments based on sequence comparison with ImMunoGeneTics information system (IMGT) reference database
      - □ Following additional computing steps, clusters containing same types of reads (based on Vγ, Jγ, and junction sequence, i.e., same types of rearrangements) are generated
      - □ Reads belonging to each cluster are counted and expressed as percent of total reads
      - □ Clonal samples contain 1 or 2 predominant clusters when compared to background (3rd most common cluster is considered background)
      - □ Polyclonal sample does not contain predominant cluster, and significant proportion of clusters contain only single read
      - □ Cutoff for calling results clonal in 1st-time samples is set to match sensitivity of PCR followed by CE method
- Advantages of NGS-based approach
  - o High specificity attributable to resolution of rearrangements not only by size but also by sequence
  - o Sensitivity for detection of clonal rearrangement in 1st-time sample is similar to one obtained from PCR/CE approach
  - o High sensitivity is achieved in follow-up specimens owing to known patient-specific junction sequence and Vγ and Jγ gene segments used
    - Highly suitable for disease monitoring and MRD detection
- Caveats of NGS-based approach
  - o NGS will not eliminate all interpretation problems
  - o Specimens with paucity of T cells may produce limited diversity in NGS data as well as in other PCR-based strategies
    - May results in false-positive diagnosis
- T-cell receptor gene rearrangements analysis using RNA sequencing (RNAseq) in T-lymphoblastic leukemia
  - o Patient's specific T-cell receptor gene rearrangement is identified at initial presentation for follow-up MRD detection
  - o RNAseq data is generated using antigen receptor research tool (ARResT): http://bat.infspire.org
    - ARResT is built within EuroClonality NGS working Group
  - o RNAseq data is analyzed using ARResT to interrogate and identify possible markers for MRD detection
  - o This strategy can likely be employed for disease monitoring in other subtypes of lymphoid malignancies and multiple myeloma

SELECTED REFERENCES

1. van der Velden VHJ et al: Immunoglobulin/T-cell receptor gene rearrangement analysis using RNA-Seq. Methods Mol Biol. 2453:61-77, 2022
2. Mahe E et al: T cell clonality assessment: past, present and future. J Clin Pathol. 71(3):195-200, 2018
3. Sufficool KE et al: T-cell clonality assessment by next-generation sequencing improves detection sensitivity in mycosis fungoides. J Am Acad Dermatol. 73(2):228-36, 2015
4. Gazzola A et al: The evolution of clonality testing in the diagnosis and monitoring of hematological malignancies. Ther Adv Hematol. 5(2):35-47, 2014
5. Greiner TC: Clinical use of next-generation sequencing of TRG gene rearrangements has arrived. Am J Clin Pathol. 141(3):302-4, 2014
6. Schumacher JA et al: A comparison of deep sequencing of TCRG rearrangements vs traditional capillary electrophoresis for assessment of clonality in T-cell lymphoproliferative disorders. Am J Clin Pathol. 141(3):348-59, 2014
7. Greiner TC et al: Effectiveness of capillary electrophoresis using fluorescent-labeled primers in detecting T-cell receptor gamma gene rearrangements. J Mol Diagn. 2002 Aug;4(3):137-43. Erratum in: J Mol Diagn. 5(3):195, 2003
8. van Dongen JJ et al: Design and standardization of PCR primers and protocols for detection of clonal immunoglobulin and T-cell receptor gene recombinations in suspect lymphoproliferations: report of the BIOMED-2 Concerted Action BMH4-CT98-3936. Leukemia. 17(12):2257-317, 2003
9. Li N et al: New insights into the applicability of T-cell receptor gamma gene rearrangement analysis in cutaneous T-cell lymphoma. J Cutan Pathol. 28(8):412-8, 2001

T-Cell Receptor Gamma (*TRG*) and Delta (*TRD*) Chain Rearrangements

Capillary Electrophoresis of Biallelic Clonal *TRG* Rearrangement

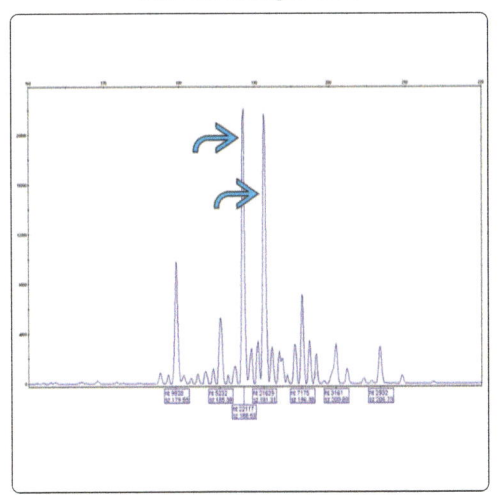

Capillary Electrophoresis of Oligoclonal *TRG* Rearrangement

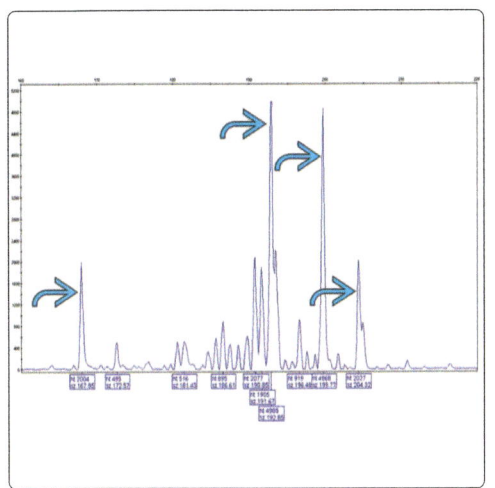

(Left) Monoclonal TRG rearrangement is detected by PCR and capillary electrophoresis. Two distinct prominent amplicons ⇨ are consistent with biallelic clonal TRG rearrangement. X axis = amplicon size. Y axis = fluorescence. **(Right)** Oligoclonal pattern is detected by PCR and capillary electrophoresis. More than 3 distinct peaks ⇨ are visible that meet criteria for oligoclonality. X axis = amplicon size. Y axis = fluorescence.

NGS Analysis of *TRG* Clusters

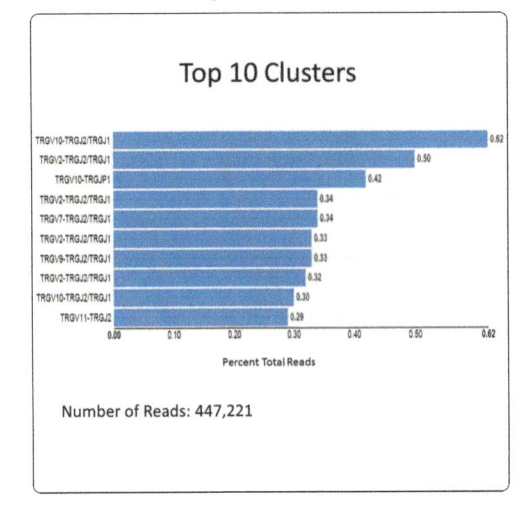

NGS Read Length Distribution of Polyclonal *TRG* Rearrangements

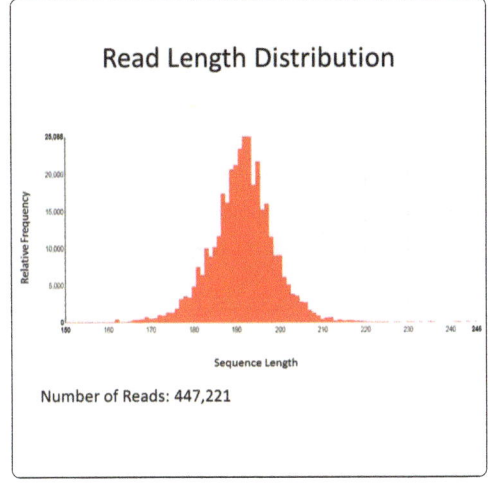

(Left) Next-generation sequencing (NGS) analysis shows no evidence of monoclonal TRG rearrangement. The 10 most prevalent clusters are displayed. There is a lack of predominant cluster type. **(Right)** Read length distribution shows no evidence of monoclonal TRG rearrangement by NGS analysis. Data shows normal distribution of read lengths derived from polyclonal T-cell population.

NGS Analysis of Monoclonal *TRG* Clusters

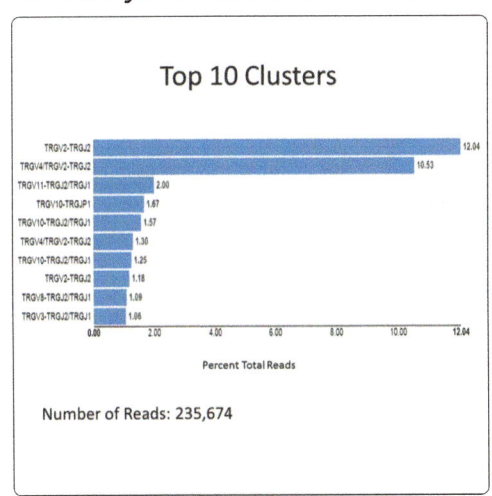

NGS Read Length Distribution With Clonal *TRG* Rearrangement

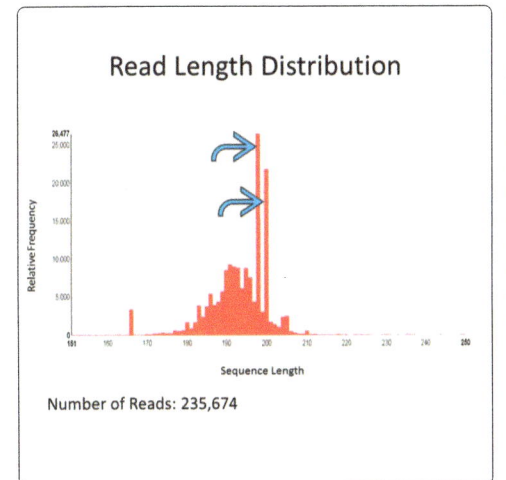

(Left) NGS shows clonal TRG rearrangement. The 10 most prevalent clusters are displayed, 2 of which are present at significantly higher read frequency compared to background (3rd cluster). **(Right)** Read length distribution shows clonal TRG rearrangement detected by NGS. Data shows predominance of 2 distinct read lengths ⇨ over background, consistent with clonal T-cell population.

T-Cell Receptor Beta (*TRB*) Chain Gene Rearrangements

TERMINOLOGY

Definitions

- T-cell receptor beta locus (*TRB*)
  - Chromosomal location: 7q34
  - Includes
    - Variable (Vβ) segments
    - Diversity (Dβ) segments
    - Constant (C) segments
    - Joining (Jβ) segments

T-CELL DEVELOPMENT OVERVIEW

Antigen-Independent T-Cell Differentiation

- **Prothymocyte stage**
  - T cells originate from common lymphoid progenitors in bone marrow
    - T cells then migrate to thymus
  - Subsequent stages of development occur in thymus
- **Thymocyte stage**
  - Earliest thymic precursors
    - Can differentiate into T or NK cells
    - Thymic microenvironment and Notch signaling
      - Crucial for proper T-cell development
  - T-cell receptor delta (*TRD*) and T-cell receptor gamma (*TRG*)
    - 1st T-cell receptor genes that undergo somatic rearrangements during T-cell development
    - T cells then go through several stages of maturation in thymus
- **CD4/CD8 double-negative** subcapsular thymocytes
  - Lack expression of T-cell receptor (TCR) complex and CD3 (a.k.a. triple-negative cells)
  - Give rise to 2 T-cell subtypes
    - γδ and αβ T-cells
  - Early double-negative thymocytes undergo *TRB* Dβ to Jβ rearrangement
  - Late double-negative thymocytes undergo *TRB* Vβ to Dβ-Jβ rearrangement
  - Expression of pre-TCR (composed of β chain and surrogate α chain) occurs subsequent to *TRB* rearrangements
  - Pre-TCR-expressing cells undergo several cycles of proliferation
- **CD4/CD8 double-positive** cortical thymocytes [CD4(+)/CD8(+)]
  - Comprise vast majority of thymocytes
  - Initially continue to express pre-TCR
  - Early double-positive thymocytes then undergo *TRA* Vα to Jα rearrangement
  - Next, subset of resting double-positive thymocytes begin to express low levels of TCR α/β and undergo selection process
  - Thymocytes with strong reactivity with self major histocompatibility complex (MHC) molecules on thymic epithelial cells are **positively selected**
    - Most thymocytes (~ 97%) fail selection process and undergo apoptosis within thymus
  - Interaction with MHC class I and II molecules is essential for development of CD8(+) and CD4(+) T-cells, respectively
  - Thymocytes with antiself specificity (self-reacting clones)
    - Bind to self-antigens presented by thymic dendritic cells (in context of MHC molecules)
    - Die by apoptosis in process of **negative selection**
  - T cells that pass selection process migrate to thymic medulla
- **CD4 or CD8 single-positive** medullary thymocytes
  - After maturation is complete, these cells are exported from thymus as mature naive T cells expressing either CD4(+) or CD8(+)
  - Mature naive T-cells are present in circulation and in paracortical region of lymph nodes
    - Main function of mature naive T-cells is surveillance

Antigen Dependent T-Cell Differentiation

- Occurs in
  - Lymph node paracortex
  - Periarteriolar lymphoid sheath of spleen
  - Other extranodal sites

Electropherogram of Monoclonal *TRB* Rearrangements

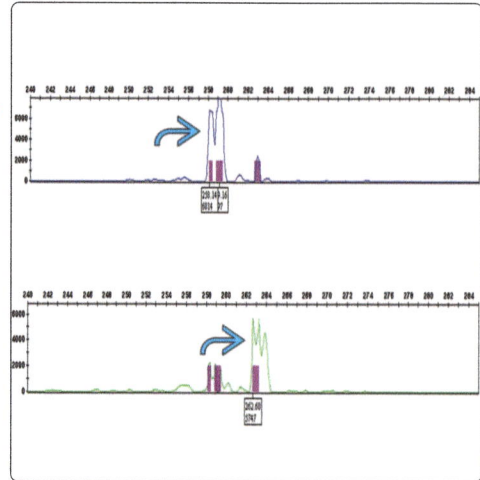

Electropherogram of Polyclonal *TRB* Rearrangements

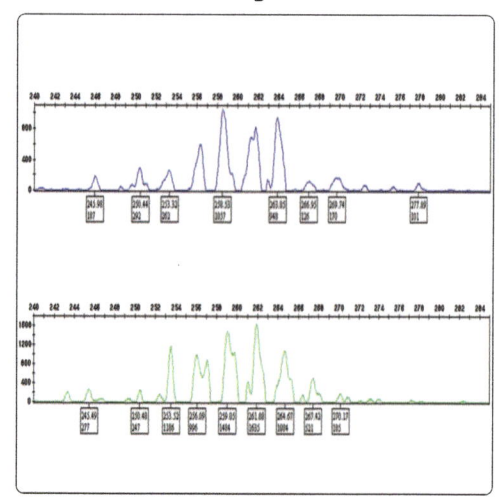

(Left) Monoclonal TRB rearrangement is detected by PCR and capillary electrophoresis. A single prominent-height amplicon ⇗ is seen with minimal polyclonal background. X axis = amplicon size. Y axis = fluorescence. (Right) No evidence of monoclonal TRB rearrangement is shown by PCR and capillary electrophoresis. Gaussian distribution of amplicon sizes is seen. X axis = amplicon size. Y axis = fluorescence.

T-Cell Receptor Beta (*TRB*) Chain Gene Rearrangements

- Interaction of TCR complex with MHC molecules on surface of antigen presenting cells (APC) is required for T-cell activation in response to antigen
    - As part of this process, TCR coreceptors CD4 or CD8 on T cells bind to MHC class II or I molecules on APC, respectively
    - Mature T cells transform to T immunoblasts
    - Types of T cells originated from T immunoblasts
        – Antigen-specific effector T cells
        – Memory T cells of either CD4(+) or CD8(+)
    - Effector CD4(+) and CD8(+) T cells typically act as T helper and T suppressor cells, respectively
    - Both subsets can be cytotoxic (provided that antigen is displayed in appropriate MHC class context)
    - Different subsets of specialized CD4(+) effector T cells are now recognized
        – T helper 1 (Th1), Th2, and Th17 are involved mainly in cytokine production
        – Follicular T helper cells play role in B-cell response
        – T regulatory (T-reg) cells limit expansion of immune response
- In adults, T-cell numbers are generally maintained through division of mature T cells outside of central lymphoid organs (thymus)

TRB REARRANGEMENTS

Overview

- Sequence of somatic recombination events occurring at double-negative thymocyte stage in αβ T-cell lineage precursors
    - Joins gene segments that are spatially separated in germline configuration
- General order of TCR gene rearrangements
    - *TRD*, *TRG*, and *TRB*, followed by *TRA*
    - Not all αβ T-cells have rearranged *TRG*; therefore, above sequence of rearrangements is not obligate

TRB Locus

- Located at 7q34 and ~ 685 kb in size
- *TRB* variable region gene cluster contains comparable number of V segments to *IGH*, *IGK*, *IGL*, and *TRA* loci but is far more complex than *TRD* and *TRG* loci
    - Includes ~ 65 Vβ gene segments belonging to 34 families
        – 39-47 Vβ gene segments (23 families) are functional
        – 10-16 Vβ gene segments are designated as pseudogenes
    - All but 1 Vβ gene segments are located upstream of 2 Dβ-Jβ-Cβ clusters
- *TRB* Dβ-Jβ-Cβ clusters
    - 1st cluster includes 1 Dβ, 6 Jβ (all functional), and 1 Cβ gene segments
    - 2nd cluster includes 1 Dβ, 7 Jβ (also all functional), and 1 Cβ gene segments
    - In comparison with *IGH* locus, both clusters combined contain more J segments but significantly fewer D segments
    - In contrast to *IGH*, constant-region gene cluster encoding several C segments is responsible for different functional properties of corresponding immunoglobulins; *TRB* Cβ1 and Cβ2 gene segments are functionally indistinguishable

- *TRB* shows extensive **combinatorial diversity** owing to broad germline-encoded repertoire of available gene segments
- **Junctional diversity** is also significant at both Dβ-Jβ and Vβ-Dβ junctions

Recombination Process

- *TRB* rearrangements follow similar steps and use same enzymes and cellular machinery as other TCR and immunoglobulin gene rearrangements
- Consists of 2 consecutive steps: Dβ to Jβ rearrangement, followed by Vβ to Dβ-Jβ rearrangement
    - Dβ1 segment may join either Jβ1 or Jβ2 segments; however, Dβ2 can only join Jβ2 segments
- Owing to presence of 2 consecutive Dβ-Jβ-Cβ clusters, 2 Dβ-Jβ rearrangements can be detected on 1 allele, however
    - Only 1 of them can progress to complete Vβ-Dβ-Jβ rearrangement
- *TRB* rearrangements occurring in healthy individuals are characterized by nonrandom distribution of Vβ and Jβ gene segments
    - Some Vβ families are more commonly rearranged than others (e.g., Vβ1-Vβ5 rearranged cells are common in peripheral blood T cells)
    - Jβ2 cluster is used more frequently than Jβ1 cluster

CLONALITY TESTING

General Comments

- Clonality does not equal malignancy
    - Benign conditions can produce clonal patterns due to antigen-driven lymphocyte expansions
- Clonal rearrangements are not lineage specific
    - B-cell malignancies (especially of B-cell precursors) often have clonal TCR gene rearrangements
    - T-cell malignancies can also have clonal immunoglobulin gene rearrangements
- Results of clonality testing always should be interpreted within appropriate clinical context and in conjunction with morphologic findings
- Rationales for using *TRB* locus as target for clonality assessment
    - Extensive combinatorial diversity in conjunction with significant junctional diversity provide background for highly specific detection of clonal populations
        – Polymerase chain reaction (PCR) assay design is more challenging due to extensive combinatorial diversity
    - Targeting solely *TRG* rearrangements is usually sufficient approach in T-cell clonality assessment
        – Complementing it with *TRB* rearrangement analysis can improve clinical sensitivity and be valuable in certain cases
- Commercially available monoclonal antibodies specific to various TCR Vβ regions
    - Alternative to nucleic acid-based assays for detection of clonality

Nucleic Acid-Based Methods

- **Southern blot hybridization**
    - Used to be gold standard for clonality analysis, now largely replaced by PCR-based approaches

T-Cell Receptor Beta (*TRB*) Chain Gene Rearrangements

- Based on principle that antigen receptor gene rearrangements alter restriction-digested DNA fragments compared with germline DNA
  - Genes with significant combinatorial diversity, such as *IGH*, *IGK*, and *TRB* are suitable targets
- Requires significant amount of high-quality intact DNA
- Sensitivity of this method is ~ 5-10%
- Individual gene rearrangements are not detected unless they are overrepresented at ≥ 5% in background lymphoid cells
  - Polyclonal sample appears as germline bands only
  - Clonal rearrangements appear as novel bands
  - At least 2 nongermline bands required to reliably diagnose clonal *TRB* rearrangement
    - DNA polymorphism may lead to nongermline band that could be confused with clonal population
- **PCR-based approaches**
  - Current gold standard for clonality analysis
  - Based on principle that somatic *TCR* rearrangements bring V, (D), and J segments together, enabling their PCR amplification
    - No PCR product is generated if germline configuration is retained
  - Each rearrangement is unique in length and sequence due to combinatorial and junctional diversity
  - Can be performed on variety of specimen types, including formalin-fixed, paraffin-embedded tissue
- **Protocol**
  - Genomic DNA is extracted and CDR3 region (as most variable) is PCR amplified
    - BIOMED-2 (from European BIOMED-2 collaborative study) primer strategy is most commonly used
      - Commercial kits are available (e.g., *TRB* Gene Clonality Assay from Invivoscribe)
      - 3 multiplex tubes design allows detection of vast majority of complete and incomplete clonal *TRB* rearrangements
  - Fractionation by capillary electrophoresis (CE)
    - One of PCR primes requires fluorescent labeling
    - Separates amplicons based on length only
      - No sequence is evaluated
    - Conventional gel electrophoresis can also be used as alternative, but it is more labor intensive and time consuming with much lower resolution
  - Interpretation should be assay and specimen specific and based on in-house validation procedure
    - Polyclonal T cells generate gaussian (bell-shaped) distribution of amplicon sizes
    - Multiple peaks represent either oligoclonal T-cell expansion or few T cells in specimen
    - Clonal T cells produce 1 or 2 prominent peaks within diminished polyclonal background
    - Various strategies for calling clonal results have been proposed
  - Generally not suitable for minimal residual disease (MRD) monitoring, unless specific primers are designed to detect patient-specific clone
- **Next-generation sequencing (NGS) approaches**
  - Used for risk stratification mainly in pediatric and young adult patients with acute lymphoblastic leukemia (ALL) post chemotherapy and hematopoietic stem cell transplant
    - Highly sensitive minimal residual disease (MRD) detection of specific *IGH* or T-cell receptor gene rearrangements
      - Detects blasts at levels ≤ 10^{-6} cells
  - High specificity attributable to resolution of rearrangements not only by size but also by sequence

Antibody-Based Methods

- **TCR Vβ analysis by flow cytometry**
  - Valid alternative to nucleic acid-based methods
    - Fresh tissue requirement is major drawback
    - Ability to separately interrogate populations of interest based on phenotype is main advantage
  - Principles of method
    - Monoclonal antibodies (mAb) to specific TCR Vβ regions are commercially available (e.g., IOTest Beta Mark Kit from Beckman Coulter)
      - Polyclonal T cells express diverse TCR Vβ and stain with mixture of mAbs
      - Monoclonal T cells stain with single mAb type (specific to TCR Vβ expressed by these T-cells)
      - Alternatively, if specific Vβ expressed by monoclonal T-cells is not covered, significant population of T cells will not stain at all
  - Utilizes innovative staining strategy combining 3 mAb with only 2 fluorophores in single vial, thereby minimizing number of vials needed
    - 1st and 2nd mAb are FITC or PE-conjugated, respectively, and 3rd mAb is conjugated with mixture of both fluorophores
    - 8 vials with mAb corresponding to 24 different specificities (covering ~ 70% of normal human TCR Vβ repertoire) are generally used
  - Monoclonal antibodies for additional T-cell markers, such as CD3, CD4, and CD8, conjugated to 3rd fluorophore can be used for gating purposes

Chimeric Antigen Receptor-Modified T Cells

- CAR-modified T cells have been developed targeting antigens, including
  - CD30, CD37, TRB constant region 1 (TRBC1), and CD1A
- Anti-Vβ8 CAR-modified T cells can recognize and kill Vβ8(+) malignant T-cells while sparing malignant or healthy Vβ8-negative T cells
- In vitro studies have demonstrated promising results in selective CAR-modified T-cell therapy to eradicate T-cell malignancies

SELECTED REFERENCES

1. Li F et al: T cell receptor β-chain-targeting chimeric antigen receptor T cells against T cell malignancies. Nat Commun. 13(1):4334, 2022
2. Pulsipher MA et al: Next-generation sequencing of minimal residual disease for predicting relapse after tisagenlecleucel in children and young adults with acute lymphoblastic leukemia. Blood Cancer Discov. 3(1):66-81, 2022
3. Toor AA et al: On the organization of human T-cell receptor loci: log-periodic distribution of T-cell receptor gene segments. J R Soc Interface. 13(114):20150911, 2016

T-Cell Receptor Beta (*TRB*) Chain Gene Rearrangements

Southern Blot Analysis of *TRB*

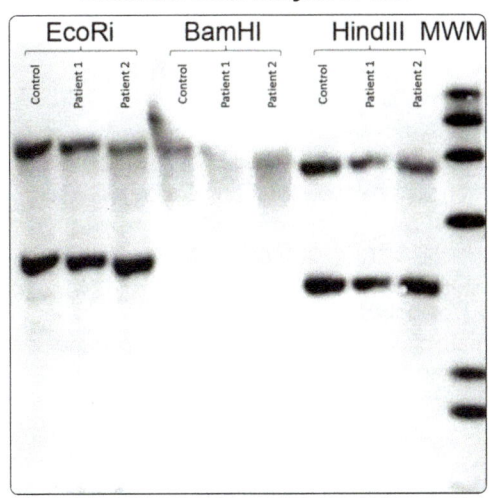

Southern Blot Analysis of *TRB*

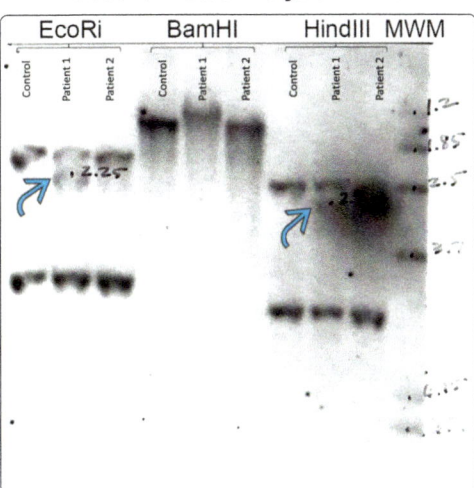

(Left) T-cell clonality assay by southern blot analysis is shown. Three reactions with different restriction enzymes are analyzed for each sample. The *TRB* gene is in germline configuration in the control sample and in both patients. MWM = molecular weight marker. EcoRI, BamHI, and HindIII = restriction enzymes. **(Right)** T-cell clonality assay by southern blot analysis is shown. Nongermline bands in patient 1 represent clonal *TRB* rearrangements.

CD4 vs. CD7 Flow Cytometry

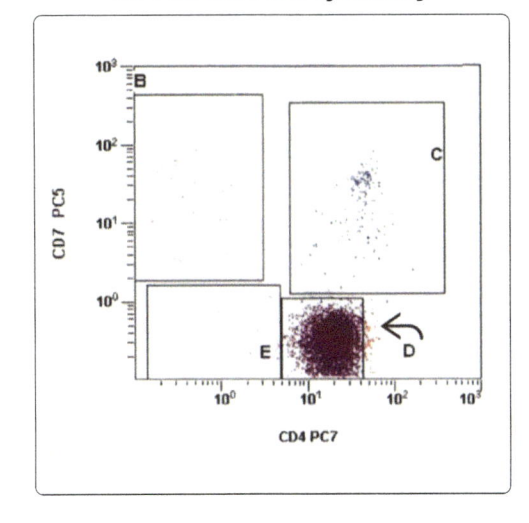

TCR Vβ Flow Cytometry

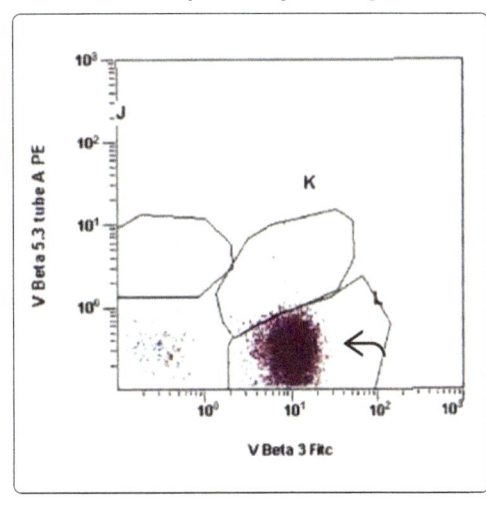

(Left) Flow cytometric analysis shows a phenotypically abnormal T-cell population expressing CD3 (not shown) and CD4 with aberrant loss of CD7. **(Right)** T-cell clonality assay by TCR Vβ flow cytometric analysis shows an atypical T-cell population with overexpression of TCR Vβ 3, consistent with a monoclonal T-cell population. Analysis of the other TCR Vβ markers (not shown) confirmed Vβ 3 restriction.

CD4 vs. CD7 Flow Cytometry

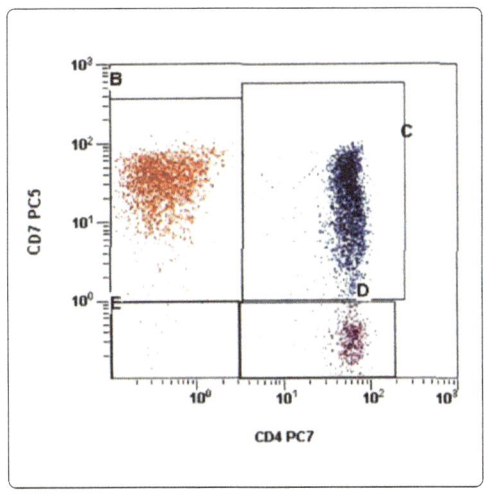

TCR Vβ Flow Cytometry

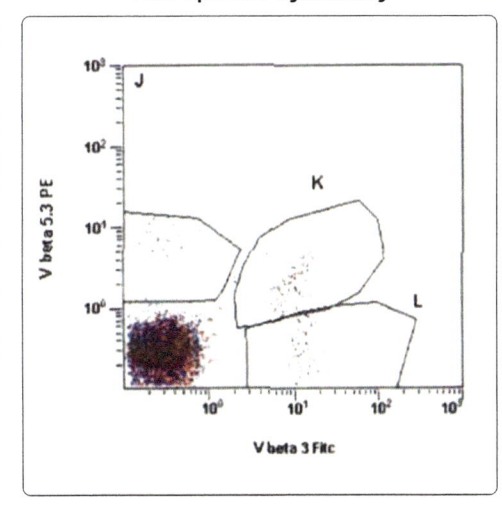

(Left) Flow cytometric analysis of this peripheral blood sample shows phenotypically normal T cells [CD3(+), not shown] that include CD4(+) and CD4(-) [presumed CD8(+)] T subsets. **(Right)** T-cell clonality assay for TCR Vβ by flow cytometric analysis shows T cells with TCR Vβ expression patterns within normal limits (i.e., no single Vβ marker predominates). The histogram is a representative scatter plot of flow cytometric analysis.

Southern Blot Analysis of Antigen Receptor Genes

TERMINOLOGY

Abbreviations
- Southern blot (SB)

Definitions
- Analysis of restriction fragment length polymorphism
- Transfer of electrophoretically separated DNA fragments to filter membrane followed by detection of DNA fragment of interest by specific probe hybridization
  - Technique of transfer of DNA fragments onto filter membrane invented by Edwin Southern in 1973
- SB technique was extensively used in past for analysis of clonality in non-Hodgkin lymphomas
- Currently, PCR has replaced SB in assessment of clonality in non-Hodgkin lymphomas

STEPS IN SOUTHERN BLOT ANALYSIS

DNA Preparation
- Extraction and purification of intact genomic DNA from fresh specimen
  - ~ 10 μg of DNA is required for routine SB analysis
    - Can use as little as 200 ng if high concentration of gene of interest present, such as in plasmid DNA

DNA Digestion
- Restriction enzymes are used to cut intact DNA
  - Restriction enzymes are bacterial-derived
  - Cut DNA at specific sequences known as restriction sites
    - Restriction sites are typically short sequences of 4-8 bp
    - Restriction sites are frequently palindromes
      - Identical sequence on both strands when read from 5' to 3' on both strands
      - Example of palindrome restriction site recognized by enzyme EcoRI: GAATTC
- DNA fragments produced by specific restriction enzyme produce reproducible set of DNA fragments
- Mutations, indels, or rearrangements may alter size of DNA fragments produced within gene
  - Alterations in size pattern of DNA fragments called RFLP

Bone Marrow Core Biopsy

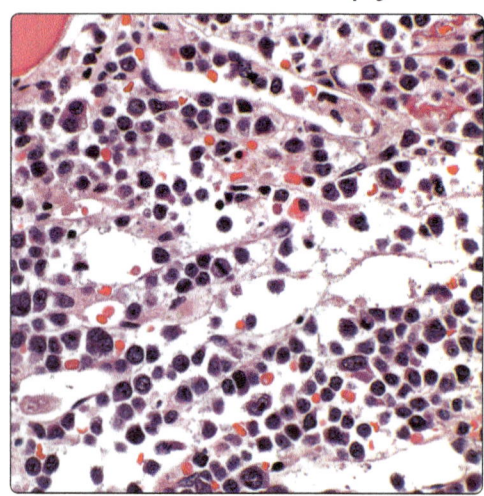

Southern Blot Analysis of IGH

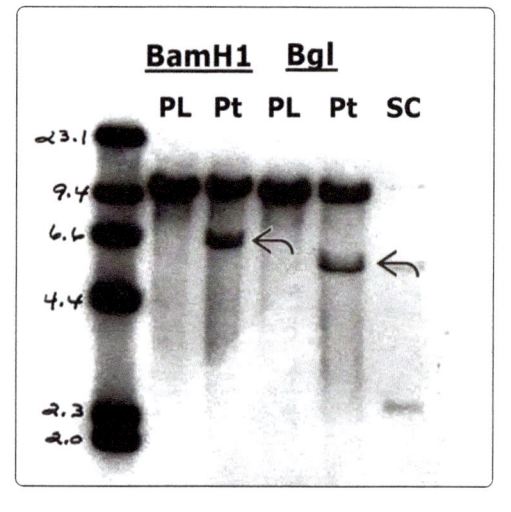

(Left) Bone marrow biopsy from a patient with prior liver transplantation shows a highly atypical lymphoid infiltrate with plasmacytoid differentiation. Flow cytometry was inconclusive for light chain restriction. (Right) Southern blot analysis of IGH performed on bone marrow aspirate of a patient with posttransplant lymphoproliferative disorder shows nongermline bands ⇨ in BamHI and Bgl lanes, supportive of a clonal process.

H&E-Stained Splenic Section

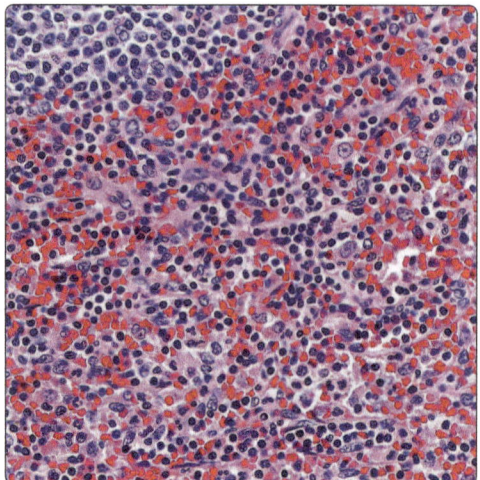

Southern Blot Analysis of TRB

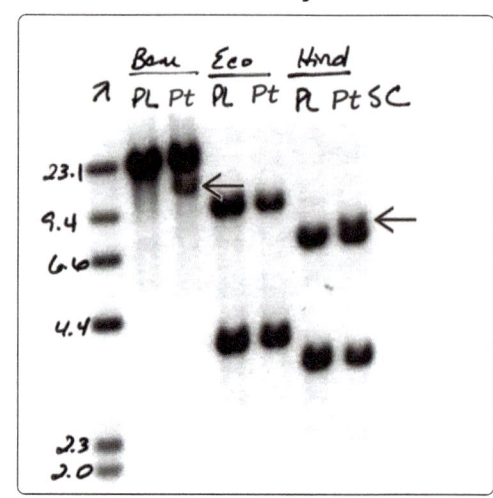

(Left) H&E of the spleen shows expansion of red pulp by a mixed lymphoid infiltrate, including a subset of large atypical and pleomorphic lymphoid cells. Concurrent flow cytometric analysis revealed increased T cells without aberrant antigen expression. (Right) Southern blot analysis of fresh splenic tissue with inconclusive flow cytometry shows nongermline bands ⇨ in BamHI and EcoRI lanes, supportive of a clonal T-cell receptor β (TRB) gene rearrangement.

Southern Blot Analysis of Antigen Receptor Genes

Gel Electrophoresis of DNA Fragments
- Agarose gel functions as sieve that allows separation of DNA fragments
- Negatively charged DNA fragments facilitate their movement through electric field
- DNA fragments are fractionated according to their sizes
- Gel should be adequately covered by buffer
- High voltage should be avoided to prevent melting of agarose gel
- Fragments ranging from 200 bp to 20 kb are typically separated on agarose gel
- Analysis of DNA fragments > 20 kb should be done by pulsed-field electrophoresis
- Fragments < 200 bp can be reliably analyzed using polyacrylamide gel

Transfer of DNA onto Nylon or Nitrocellulose Membrane
- Diluted solution of hydrochloric acid is applied to gel before transfer to hydrolyze larger DNA fragments
- DNA must be denatured before transfer
  - Treatment of gel with alkaline denatures DNA
- Upward capillary action of buffer transfers DNA fragments from gel onto nylon or nitrocellulose membrane

Stabilization of Transferred DNA on Membrane
- DNA must be stabilized on membrane before probe hybridization
  - Transferred DNA will firmly adhere to and be stabilized on membrane after baking membrane at 80° C in oven for ~ 2 hours
  - DNA can also be stabilized by exposing nylon membrane to UV light
    - UV light induces crosslink between nucleic acids and amine groups on membrane

DNA Hybridization
- Hybridization probes
  - Single-stranded specific DNA fragment complementary to target DNA on membrane
  - Probe is labeled with isotopic 32P or nonisotopic systems, such as chemiluminescence
  - Membrane is washed after completion of hybridization to remove unused and nonspecifically bound probes

Interpretation of Southern Blot Analysis of Antigen Receptor Genes
- Radioactive hybridized probes are visualized after exposure to x-ray film and appear as dark bands
- For analysis of antigen receptor genes (ARGs), patient's DNA sample is digested in parallel with germline DNA sample
- Locations of bands in patient's sample are compared to germline DNA bands
  - Polyclonal or reactive lymphoid population
    - Numerous different VDJ rearrangements present, but individual rearrangements are too small to be detected as visible nongermline bands
  - Monoclonal B-cell or T-cell population
    - All neoplastic cells are derived from single transformed cell
    - Identical gene rearrangements are present in all neoplastic cells
    - Restriction fragments containing identical gene rearrangements are detected as novel (nongermline) band(s)
    - Presence of nongermline bands in patient's sample indicate monoclonal ARG rearrangement
  - Nongermline bands are often of lower molecular sizes compared to germline bands
  - Nongermline bands are sometimes of higher molecular sizes compared to germline bands
  - Known DNA polymorphic region in EcoRI restriction digest exists
    - Thus, presence of nongermline band in only EcoRI restriction digest must not be interpreted as evidence for clonality
- At least 2 nongermline bands in 1 digest or 1 nongermline band in 2 different digests are required to establish diagnosis of clonal T-cell receptor β (*TRB*) gene rearrangement

Southern Blot vs. PCR in Assessment of Clonality in Lymphoid Proliferations
- Advantages of SB in assessment of clonality
  - Considered to be gold standard for assessment of clonality in lymphoid neoplasms
  - Fewer false-negative results compared with PCR
- Disadvantages of SB in assessment of clonality
  - Requires relatively large amounts of fresh, intact DNA
  - Lower sensitivity (~ 5%) compared to PCR, which has much higher sensitivity
  - High cost and labor intensive
  - Long turnaround time of ~ 10-14 days

Other Applications of RFLP Analysis
- DNA fingerprinting
  - Analysis of variable number of tandem repeats (VNTRs)
    - VNTRs are repeat sequences of 20-100 bp
    - Each individual has unique numbers of VNTRs at single locus
    - Restriction fragments produce unique pattern in given individual
  - Analysis of VNTRs on samples collected as evidence at crime scene identifies suspects
- Paternity
  - Analysis of VNTRs loci to determine paternity
- Genetic diversity
  - Analysis of RFLP to study evolution and migration of wild life
  - Also used to study breeding patterns in animal population
- Genome mapping and genetic disease analysis

SELECTED REFERENCES
1. Green MR et al: Southern blotting. Cold Spring Harb Protoc. 2021(7), 2021
2. Shah NJ: Southern, Western and Northern Blotting. In: Raj G et al: Introduction to Basics of Pharmacology and Toxicology. Springer, 2019
3. Brown T: Southern blotting. Curr Protoc Immunol. Chapter 10:Unit 10.6A, 2001
4. Southern EM: Detection of specific sequences among DNA fragments separated by gel electrophoresis. J Mol Biol. 98(3):503-17, 1975

EBV-Associated Human Neoplasms

TERMINOLOGY

Abbreviations
- Epstein-Barr virus (EBV)

Definitions
- Lymphoid and nonlymphoid human neoplasms associated with monoclonal episomal EBV

EBV STRUCTURE AND GENOME

EBV Virion
- Double-stranded DNA virus
  o 172 kb in length
  o Wrapped in protein capsid
  o Contains variable numbers of homologous tandem 500-bp repeats (TRs) at each terminus
  o Linear termini are joined in host cells to form episomal (circular) forms
    – Episomal forms are present in EBV-infected tumor cells and cell lines
  o Variability in numbers of TRs generates episomes with variable numbers of TRs
  o EBV-associated monoclonal cell lines or tumors
    – Identical-sized EBV episome in all cells
    – Digestion with restriction enzymes generate homogeneously sized terminal fragments
  o EBV-associated polyclonal processes
    – Different-sized EBV linear forms are present
    – Restriction enzyme digestion generates heterogeneously sized terminal fragments
    – Terminal fragments will differ from each other with increments of 500 bp

BIOLOGY OF EBV INFECTION

EBV Lytic Infection
- Primary EBV infection
  o ~ 95% of adults are infected by EBV
  o Asymptomatic in children
  o Present as infectious mononucleosis in adults
  o Primary infection results in lytic (productive) lifecycle
  o EBV DNA is linear in lytic cycle
  o EBV infects both B cells and epithelial cells
    – Epithelial cells are likely major site of EBV lytic cycle
    – Short lytic infection cycle will follow latent EBV infection in B cells
    – EBV is episomal (circular) in latently infected cells
    – EBV latent infection persists for host's lifetime and cannot be eradicated

EBV Latent Infection
- Viral DNA is not usually integrated into host chromosome
- Viral DNA is present as extrachromosomal episome within nucleus of host cells
- Latent virus may become reactivated in certain circumstances
- EBV-associated tumors
  o Episomal EBV is present in every tumor cell
  o Viral RNAs and proteins are also present in tumor cells
  o 1st EBV RNAs identified are designated as EBER (EBV-encoded RNA)
    – EBERs are noncoding RNAs
    – EBERs are abundant with up to 1 million copies present in infected cell
    – High abundance of EBERs have made EBER stain superb marker to detect EBV
  o EBV is clonal in EBV-associated neoplasms
    – Viral clonality can be demonstrated by analysis of restriction enzyme-digested EBV DNA terminal repeats fragments
    – Detection of clonal EBV episomes in tumor suggests that malignant cells are also clonal
- Latency patterns in EBV-associated neoplasms
  o Latency pattern I
    – EBNA1, EBER1, and EBER2 are expressed
  o Latency pattern II
    – EBNA1, LMP1, LMP2, EBER1, and EBER2 are expressed
  o Latency pattern III

Gastric Adenocarcinoma

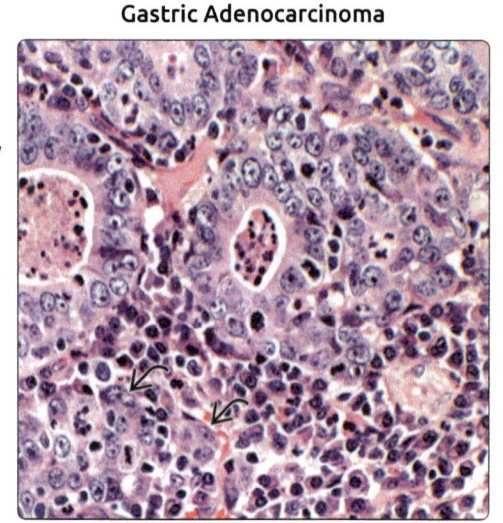

EBER(+) Gastric Adenocarcinoma

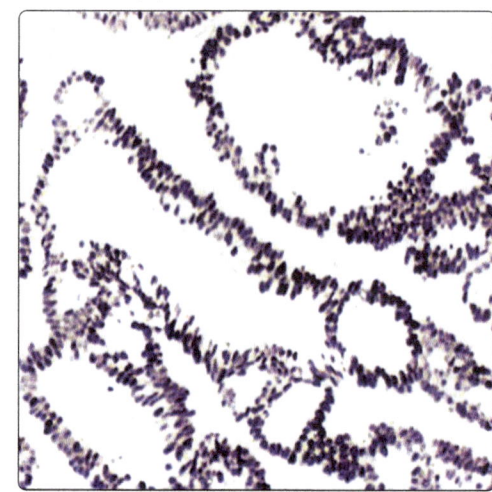

(Left) EBV(+) gastric carcinoma shows glandular differentiation as well as a poorly cohesive cluster of tumor cells ➲ within a stroma rich in plasma cells and lymphocytes. (Right) In situ hybridization using EBV-encoded RNA (EBER) probes shows abundantly transcribed EBER localized to nuclei of neoplastic cells in this EBV-associated gastric carcinoma.

EBV-Associated Human Neoplasms

– EBNA1, EBNA2, EBNA3, LMP1, LMP2, EBER1, and EBER2 are all expressed

EBV-ASSOCIATED LYMPHOMAS

Burkitt Lymphoma
- EBV is present in almost all endemic Burkitt lymphoma, ~ 10-20% of sporadic Burkitt lymphoma, and ~ 40% of HIV-related Burkitt lymphoma
- Restricted pattern of expression of latency proteins limited to EBNA1 and EBERs (latency pattern I)
- Expression of EBNA1 is crucial in maintenance and replication of EBV genome

EBV(+) Diffuse Large B-Cell Lymphoma, Not Otherwise Specified
- In patients without known immunodeficiency or prior lymphoma
- Majority present with extranodal disease
- Latency pattern III, including expression of EBNA2
- Other EBV(+) well-defined lymphoma categories are excluded

Plasmablastic Lymphoma
- Diffuse proliferation of large, immunoblastic-appearing cells with prominent nucleoli
- High incidence in HIV patients
- Occurs predominantly in oral cavity and other extranodal sites
- Expression of CD138 and (-) or weak expression of CD20, PAX5, and CD45
- Very high proliferation rate with Ki-67 index (> 90%)
- EBV(+) in vast majority of cases

Lymphomatoid Granulomatosis
- Angiocentric and angiodestructive B-cell proliferation with predominance of T cells
- Lung is most common site of involvement
- Other extranodal sites of involvement include CNS, kidney, liver, and skin
- Neoplastic B cells vary in numbers and are EBV(+)
- Spectrum of histologic grade depending on proportion of EBV(+) B cells
  - < 5 EBV(+) B cells per HPF in grade 1
  - 5-20 EBV(+) B cells per HPF in grade 2
  - > 20 EBV(+) B cells per HPF in grade 3
  - Cases with sheets of EBV(+) large B cells should be classified as diffuse large B-cell lymphoma (DLBCL)

Diffuse Large B-Cell Lymphoma Associated With Chronic Inflammation
- Develops in patients with longstanding history of pyothorax following induction of pneumothorax for treatment of tuberculosis
- EBV(+) DLBCL that occur in context of longstanding chronic inflammation
- Pyothorax-associated DLBCL accounts for > 90% of cases
- Other sites of involvement include bone, joint, and periarticular soft tissue
- Aggressive lymphoma with 5-year survival of ~ 20-35% in pyothorax-associated DLBCL

Fibrin-Associated Diffuse Large B-Cell Lymphoma
- Subtype of DLBCL associated with chronic inflammation (in ICC)
- Fibrin-associated large B-cell lymphoma (new entity in WHO-HAEM5)
- Localized, microscopic DLBCL found incidentally in fibrinous material
  - Within wall of pseudocysts in spleen, adrenal gland, paratesticular region
  - Also reported within cardiac fibrin thrombus, subdural hematoma, synthetic tube graft
- Does not form mass and not associated with systemic disease
- All EBV(+) with highly favorable clinical course

EBV(+) Mucocutaneous Ulcer
- Upgraded from provisional to distinct entity in ICC
- Included in "Lymphoid proliferation and lymphoma associated with immune deficiency and dysregulation" in WHO-HAEM5
- Present in age-related or iatrogenic immunosuppression
- Involves mucosal or cutaneous sites
  - Most common site is oral cavity
- Dense, polymorphic infiltrate beneath ulcer with B-cell lineage Hodgkin and Reed-Sternberg-like cells
  - CD20, PAX5, OCT2, MUM1, and EBER (+)
  - CD10 and BCL6 (-)
- Indolent course
  - Spontaneous regression in some cases

Hydroa Vacciniforme Lymphoproliferative Disorder
- Listed under "Clinical spectrum of chronic active EBV disease (CAEBVD)" in WHO-HAEM5
  - Varies from indolent "Severe mosquito bite allergy and hydroa vaccinform LPD classic form to systemic disease with fever, organomegaly and adenopathy"
- Listed as entity in ICC
  - 2 forms recognized: Classic and systemic
    - Classic form is indolent, but systemic form is severe with fever, adenopathy, and liver involvement and more common in Asian and Latin Americans
- Typically occurs in children
  - Highly favorable clinical course
  - Vesicles and crust formation on sun-exposed areas of skin
  - Dermal infiltrate of predominantly small lymphoid cells
  - Majority of cases show CD8(+) T-cell immunophenotype
  - ~ 30% of cases show NK-cell immunophenotype with expression of CD56
  - Clonal expansion of γ/δ T cells detectable in peripheral blood in most cases
  - Lymphoid cells are EBV(+), often CD30(+)
  - May resolves spontaneously
    - Can progress to to systemic form with severe and extensive skin lesions, fever, hepatosplenomegaly, and lymphadenopathy
  - Clonal rearrangements of T-cell receptor genes in most cases

EBV-Associated Human Neoplasms

Classic Hodgkin Lymphoma
- EBV is detected in subset of classic Hodgkin lymphoma (CHL)
  - ~ 75% of mixed-cellularity subtype CHL
  - Up to 40% of nodular sclerosis subtype CHL
  - ~ 100% in CHL arising in HIV-infected patients
- EBV is detectable only in Hodgkin and Reed-Sternberg (HRS) cells and absent in background cells
  - Exclusive localization of EBV to only neoplastic cells of CHL supports role in pathogenesis
- EBV-infected HRS cells show latency pattern II
  - EBERs, LMP1, LMP2A, and EBNA1 are expressed

Posttransplant Lymphoproliferative Disorder
- Lymphoproliferative disorders following allogeneic hematopoietic stem cell or solid organ transplantation
- Develops as result of immunosuppression
- Histologic categories of PTLD (in ICC)
  - Nondestructive PTLD
    - Plasmacytic hyperplasia; infectious mononucleosis; florid follicular hyperplasia
  - Polymorphic PTLD
  - Monomorphic PTLD
  - CHL PTLD
- Histologic categories of PTLD (in WHO-HAEM5)
  - Hyperplasias
    - Plasma-cell hyperplasia, mononucleosis-like hyperplasia, follicular hyperplasia
  - Polymorphic lymphoproliferative disorder
  - Lymphoma (classify as immunocompetent patients)
  - CHL PTLD
    - Includes viral association in report
      - EBV(+/-), HHV8 (+/-)
- ~ 80% of PTLD cases are EBV associated
  - Early PTLD (≤ 1 year post transplant) almost 100% EBV associated
  - Decreased cytotoxic T cells induced by immunosuppression play significant role in development of PTLD
  - EBV(+) PTLD shows latency pattern III
    - EBNA1, EBNA2, EBNA3, LMP1, LMP2, and EBERs are expressed
- ~ 20% of PTLD EBV(-)
  - Typically develops > 5 years after transplant
  - Unclear underlying etiology

Extranodal NK-/T-Cell Lymphoma, Nasal Type (in ICC)
- Qualifier "nasal type" has been dropped in WHO-HAEM5
- Angiocentric and angiodestructive neoplasm with aggressive clinical course
  - Majority are true NK cell origin
  - Less frequently derived from cytotoxic T cells
- Strong association with EBV, regardless of ethnicity
  - Mechanism of infection of T cells by EBV is not entirely clear
  - Latency pattern II has been reported
    - EBNA1, LMP1, LMP2, and EBER are expressed
  - 30-bp deletion present in *LMP1* in most cases

EBV-Associated Lymphomas in HIV(+) Patients
- Lymphomas are 2nd most common malignancy in HIV(+) patients
- Incidence is significantly decreased since introduction of antiretroviral therapy
- Majority of lymphomas are high grade and B-cell origin
- Lymphomas that are more often seen in HIV setting
  - Primary effusion lymphoma (PEL)
    - Distinct type of lymphoma that involves body cavities without tumor mass formation
    - Unclear lineage by immunophenotype, including lack of B-cell antigens, but monoclonal *IGH* rearrangements present
    - Predominantly HHV-8 associated
    - Both EBV and HHV-8 detected in > 50% of cases
  - Plasmablastic lymphoma
    - Aggressive lymphoma with immunoblastic morphology
    - Most frequently involve oral cavity but can present in other extranodal sites
    - Immunophenotype of plasma cells with expression of CD138, CD38, and MUM1 but weakly (+) or (-) for CD20, PAX5, and CD45
    - Clonal *IGH* rearrangements
- Lymphoma subtypes that usually occur in immunocompetent patients
  - Burkitt lymphoma
    - Accounts for ~ 30% of HIV-associated lymphoma
    - EBV is detected in ~ 50% of cases
  - DLBCL
    - Accounts for ~ 30% of HIV-associated lymphoma
    - ~ 30% of cases are EBV associated
    - Most cases exhibit centroblastic or immunoblastic morphology
  - Primary central nervous system (CNS) lymphoma
    - Accounts for ~ 25% of HIV-associated lymphomas
    - Almost all cases are EBV-associated
    - Typically express all EBV latency pattern III

EBV-Associated Smooth Muscle Tumors in AIDS Patients
- Occurs in advanced stage of HIV infection with low CD4 count
- Cranial and spinal epidural are common sites of involvement
- Typically multifocal with different EBV clones in different sites

EBV(+) NONLYMPHOID NEOPLASMS

Nasopharyngeal Carcinoma
- Derived from nasopharyngeal epithelium
  - Arises in Rosenmüller fossa in most cases
  - High incidence in Southern China and Hong Kong
- EBV and nasopharyngeal carcinoma (NPC)
  - Virtually all NPC EBV associated, including keratinizing subtypes when sensitive detection methods are used
  - EBV likely plays key role in pathogenesis of NPC
    - EBV is localized to neoplastic cells and is absent in background nonneoplastic cells

EBV-Associated Human Neoplasms

- – EBV is also present in precancerous tissue, including carcinoma in situ and dysplastic epithelium adjacent to invasive carcinoma
  - o EBV is clonal in NPC by Southern blot analysis
    - – Further supports important role of EBV in pathogenesis of NPC
- EBV serology in NPC
  - o Elevated IgG and IgA against viral capsid antigen (VCA) and diffuse component of early antigen (EA)
    - – Elevated IgA against VCA is most specific for NPC
    - – Detected in > 80% of NPC cases
    - – Serologic testing of these antibodies may prove useful as screening method
  - o Elevated IgG against EBV replication activator (ZEBRA)
    - – Present in ~ 25% of IgA VCA(-) NPC cases
  - o Positive serology for EBV infection does not provide direct evidence for presence of EBV in tumor cells

Gastric Carcinoma

- Frequency of EBV-associated gastric carcinoma varies across globe
- EBV detected in ~ 9% of gastric carcinoma per The Cancer Genome Atlas (TCGA) project
  - o ~ 65% of EBV(+) cases involve males
  - o All EBV(+) tumors clustered together in unsupervised clustering of CpG methylation on unpaired tumor samples
    - – Extreme CpG island-methylator phenotype is evident in all EBV-associated gastric carcinoma distinct from those with MSI subtype
    - – Higher prevalence of DNA hypermethylation than any cancers reported by TCGA
  - o All EBV(+) gastric tumors show *CDKN2A* promoter hypermethylation
  - o EBV(+) tumors lack *MLH1* promoter hypermethylation in contrast to MSI-associated tumors
  - o *PIK3CA* mutations in 80% of EBV(+) gastric carcinoma
    - – PI(3) kinase inhibition may warrant further evaluation in EBV(+) gastric carcinomas
  - o *ARID1A* mutations in 55%
  - o *BCOR* mutations in 23%
  - o *TP53* mutations are rare
  - o Highly transcribed EBV viral mRNAs and miRNAs fell within BAMH1A restriction region of viral genome

Lymphoepithelioma-Like Salivary Gland Carcinoma

- Very rare undifferentiated carcinoma of salivary gland with abundant lymphoid stroma
- Relatively higher incidence among Eskimos of Alaska, Greenland, and China
- EBV detected by EBER stain in virtually all cases

Inflammatory Pseudotumor-Like Follicular Dendritic Cell Sarcoma of Liver and Spleen

- Uncommon neoplasm of unknown etiology
- Only sporadic case reports and small case series
  - o Encapsulated and well-circumscribed tumors on gross and radiologic examination
  - o Abundant background lymphocytes and plasma cells with at least focal follicular dendritic cell proliferation
  - o Expression of 1 or more follicular dendritic cell markers, such as CD21, CD35, and CD23
  - o Low malignant potential with recurrence reported in subset of cases
- Virtually all reported cases in liver and spleen are EBV-associated
  - o EBV is localized to follicular dendritic cells and is absent in background lymphocytes and plasma cells
  - o EBV is clonal by Southern blot analysis
    - – Clonal EBV detected in these cases supports neoplastic nature of these tumors
  - o Inflammatory pseudotumors and follicular dendritic cell sarcomas in other locations are EBV(-)

DETECTION OF EBV BY MOLECULAR TECHNIQUES

Nucleic Acid Hybridization Techniques

- In situ hybridization for EBER
  - o Most sensitive method for detection of EBV in latently infected cells
  - o Ability to precisely localize virus in infected tumor cells
- Southern blot techniques
  - o Analysis of restriction enzyme-digested EBV DNA terminal repeats fragments
    - – Ability to determine clonality of EBV-infected tumor cells
    - – Fresh tissues with intact genomic DNA required

PCR Analysis of EBV DNA

- Highly sensitive for detection of EBV DNA
  - o Not useful for disease-specific purposes given ubiquitous nature of virus
  - o Useful in detection of presumably oncogenic EBV *LMP1* with 30 bp deletion

SELECTED REFERENCES

1. Falini B et al: A comparison of the International Consensus and 5th World Health Organization classifications of mature B-cell lymphomas. Leukemia. 37(1):18-34, 2023
2. Quintanilla-Martinez L et al: New concepts in EBV-associated B, T, and NK cell lymphoproliferative disorders. Virchows Arch. 482(1):227-44, 2023
3. Alaggio R et al: The 5th edition of the World Health Organization Classification of Haematolymphoid Tumours: lymphoid neoplasms. Leukemia. 36(7):1720-48, 2022
4. Campo E et al: The International Consensus Classification of Mature Lymphoid Neoplasms: a report from the Clinical Advisory Committee. Blood. 140(11):1229-53, 2022
5. Markouli M et al: Recent advances in adult post-transplant lymphoproliferative disorder. Cancers (Basel). 14(23):5949, 2022
6. Rezk SA et al: Epstein-Barr virus (EBV)-associated lymphoid proliferations, a 2018 update. Hum Pathol. 79:18-41, 2018
7. Coleman CB et al: Epstein-Barr virus type 2 latently infects T cells, inducing an atypical activation characterized by expression of lymphotactic cytokines. J Virol. 89(4):2301-12, 2015
8. Cancer Genome Atlas Research Network: comprehensive molecular characterization of gastric adenocarcinoma. Nature. 513(7517):202-9, 2014
9. Boroumand N et al: Microscopic diffuse large B-cell lymphoma (DLBCL) occurring in pseudocysts: do these tumors belong to the category of DLBCL associated with chronic inflammation? Am J Surg Pathol. 36(7):1074-80, 2012
10. Rosenbaum L et al: Epstein-Barr virus-associated inflammatory pseudotumor of the spleen: report of two cases and review of the literature. J Hematop. 2(2):127-31, 2009
11. Rezk SA et al: Epstein-Barr virus-associated lymphoproliferative disorders. Hum Pathol. 38(9):1293-304, 2007

EBV-Associated Human Neoplasms

T-/NK-Cell Lymphoma

(Left) *Extranodal NK-/T-cell lymphoma, nasal type, shows highly atypical neoplastic cells with anaplastic morphology and adjacent coagulative necrosis. Angiocentric and angiodestructive foci can also be present in this aggressive neoplasm.* (Right) *CD3 shows cytoplasmic expression in this NK-/T-cell lymphoma, nasal type. By flow cytometry, the neoplastic cells lacked surface CD3 antigen.*

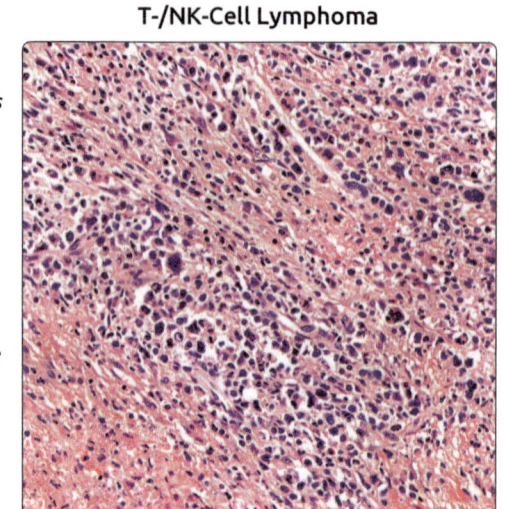

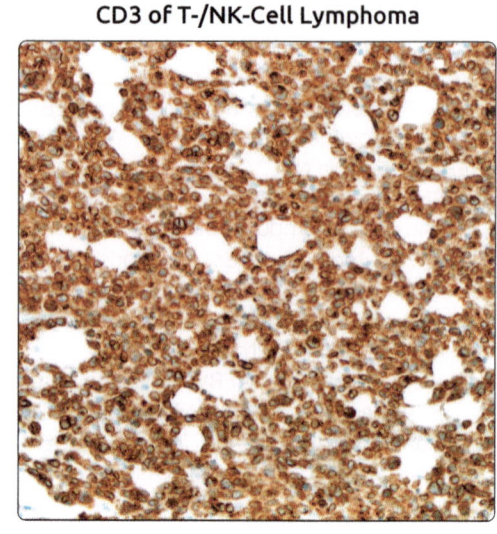

CD3 of T-/NK-Cell Lymphoma

TIA1 of T-/NK-Cell Lymphoma

(Left) *TIA1 highlights cytotoxic molecules within cytoplasm of the neoplastic cells in this NK-/T-cell lymphoma, nasal type. The neoplastic cells lacked CD4, CD5, and CD8 antigens.* (Right) *CD56 shows expression by neoplastic NK-/T-cells with moderate intensity. CD56 is a useful marker for NK cells but is not specific and can also be seen in some peripheral T-cell lymphomas.*

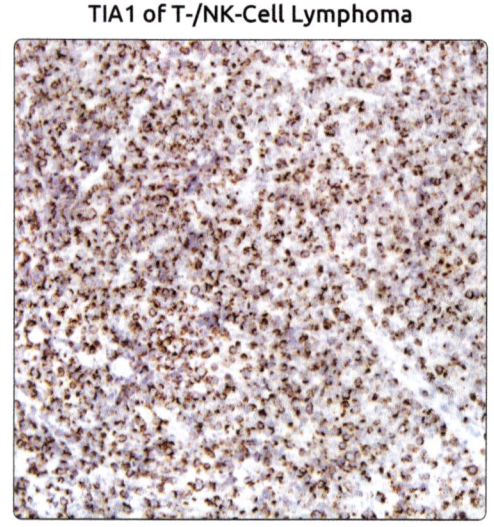

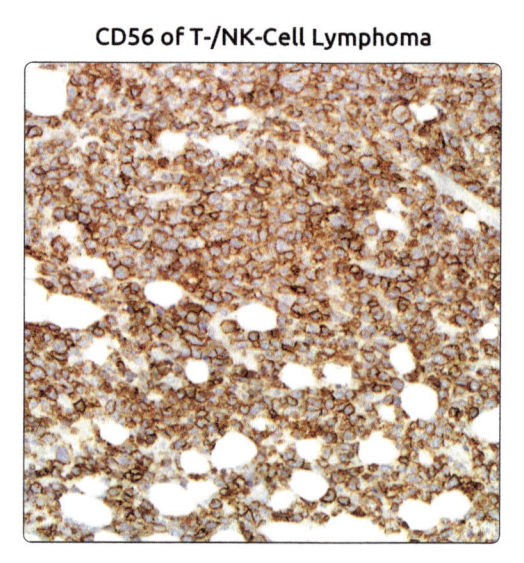

CD56 of T-/NK-Cell Lymphoma

EBER of T-/NK-Cell Lymphoma

(Left) *In situ hybridization for EBER shows abundantly transcribed EBER within nuclei of the neoplastic cells in this NK-/T-cell lymphoma, nasal type. EBER is consistently positive in this neoplasm.* (Right) *Southern blot analysis of EBV DNA terminal repeat region shows a clonal band ⇒ in the sample. PCR analysis of T-cell receptor genes was germline. Detection of clonal EBV is indirect evidence of clonality of EBV-infected tumor cells.*

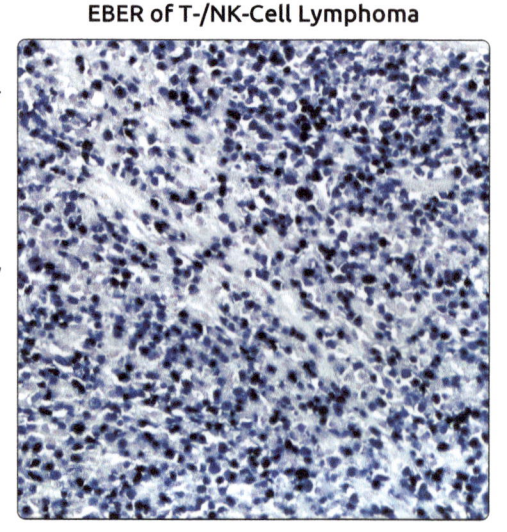

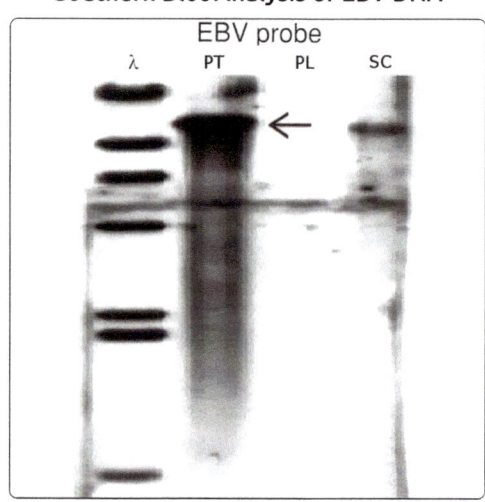

Southern Blot Analysis of EBV DNA

EBV-Associated Human Neoplasms

Lymphoid Cells Infiltrating Skeletal Muscle

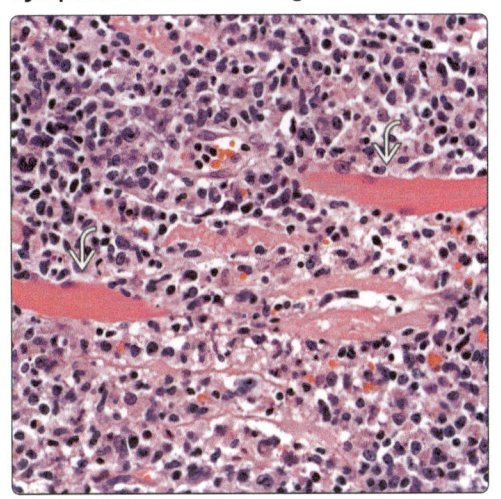

CD20 of Neoplastic Cells

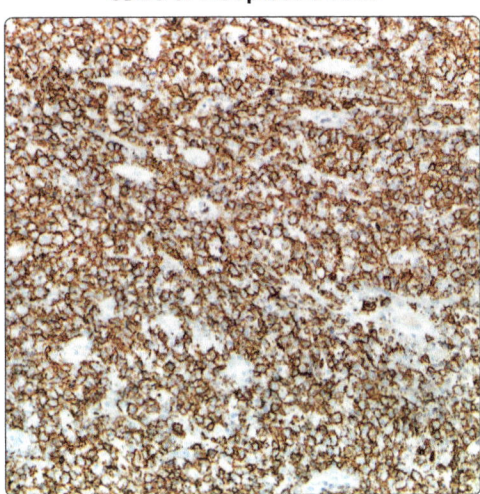

(Left) *A large soft tissue mass excised from a patient with history of kidney transplant shows highly atypical and large, pleomorphic, lymphoid-appearing cells infiltrating skeletal muscle bundles ⇒, consistent with monomorphic posttransplant lymphoproliferative disorder (PTLD).* (Right) *CD20 shows bright and uniform expression by neoplastic cells, supportive of monomorphic PTLD, diffuse large B-cell lymphoma (DLBCL) subtype.*

Plasmacytoid-Appearing Cells

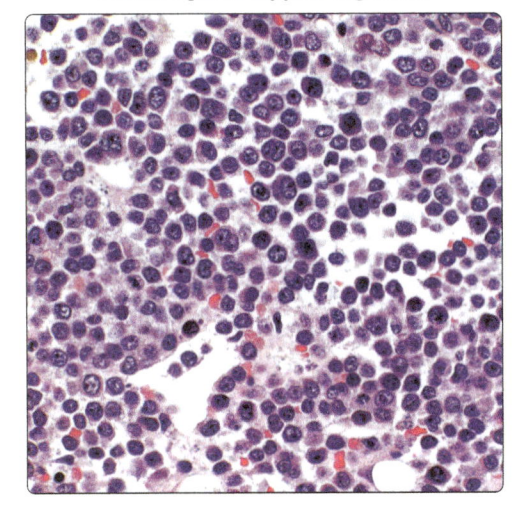

EBER of Neoplastic Cells

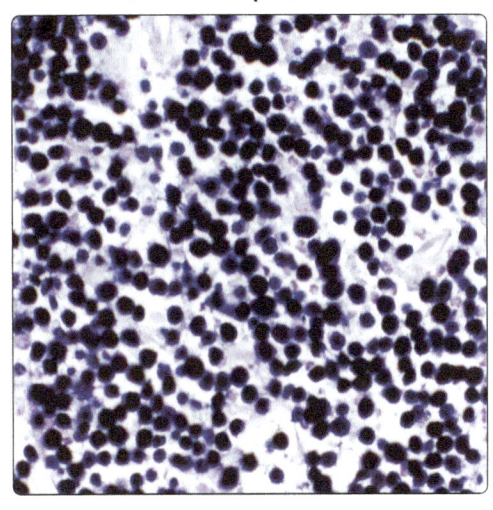

(Left) *Bone marrow biopsy from a patient with history of heart transplantation shows sheets of large, plasmacytoid-appearing cells with moderate amphophilic cytoplasm. Flow cytometry revealed monoclonal plasma cell population, diagnostic of monomorphic PTLD, plasma cell myeloma type.* (Right) *In situ hybridization using EBER probes shows strong and uniform nuclear expression of EBER by neoplastic cells.*

Plasma Cell Hyperplasia

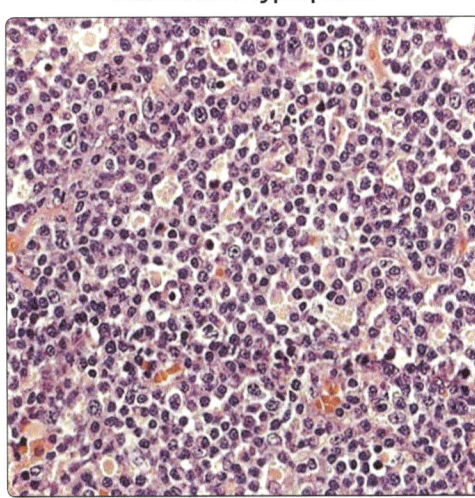

Southern Blot Analysis of EBV DNA

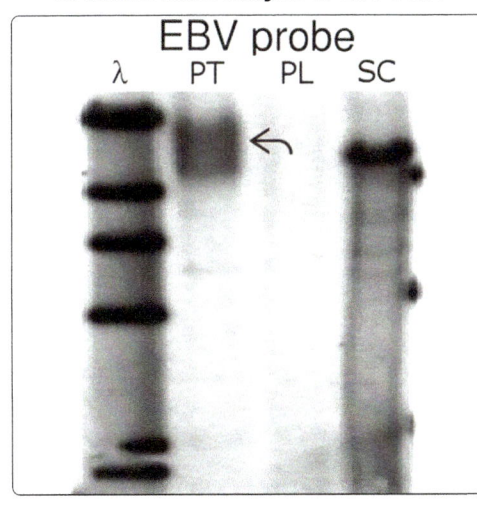

(Left) *Cervical lymph node biopsy from a patient with liver transplant shows an early lesion of PTLD characterized by plasma cell hyperplasia with intermixed, scattered, intermediate lymphoid cells and large, immunoblastic-appearing cells.* (Right) *Southern blot analysis of EBV DNA terminal repeat region performed on fresh lymph node tissue shows a smear ⇒, consistent with polyclonal EBV. Early PTLD regressed in this patient upon reduction of immunosuppression.*

EBV-Associated Human Neoplasms

Wright-Stained Bone Marrow Aspirate of Reed-Sternberg Cells

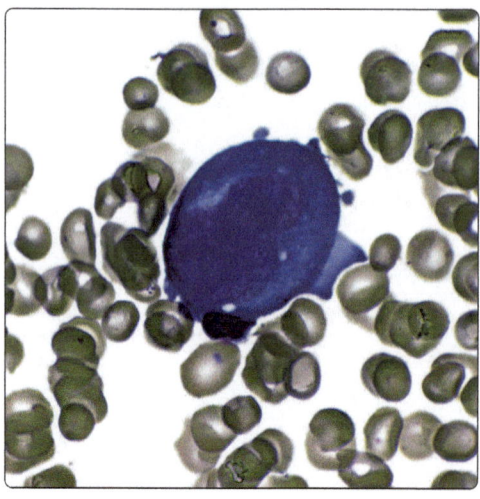

Hodgkin and Reed-Sternberg Cells

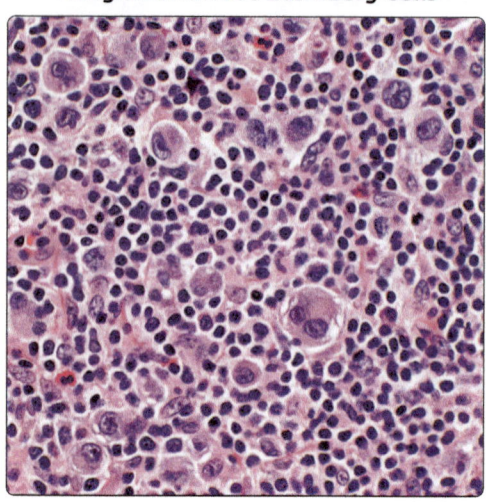

(Left) Wright-stained bone marrow aspirate smear from a patient with recent diagnosis of classic Hodgkin lymphoma shows a mononuclear variant of Reed-Sternberg (RS) cells. Detection of RS cells in marrow aspirate is exceedingly rare due to associated fibrosis. (Right) Lymph node biopsy shows scattered Hodgkin and Reed-Sternberg (HRS) cells in a polymorphous background, including small lymphocytes, occasional histiocytes, and eosinophils.

CD30 of Hodgkin and Reed-Sternberg Cells

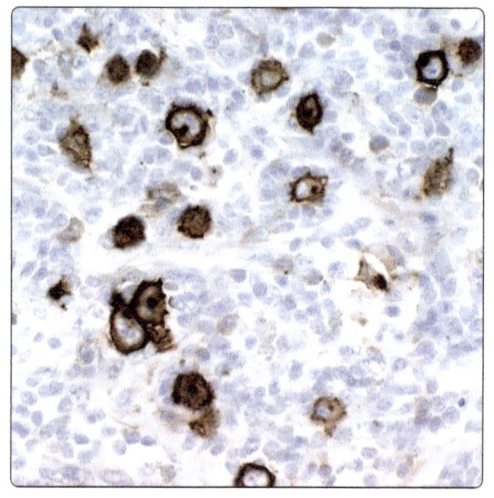

CD15 of Hodgkin and Reed-Sternberg Cells

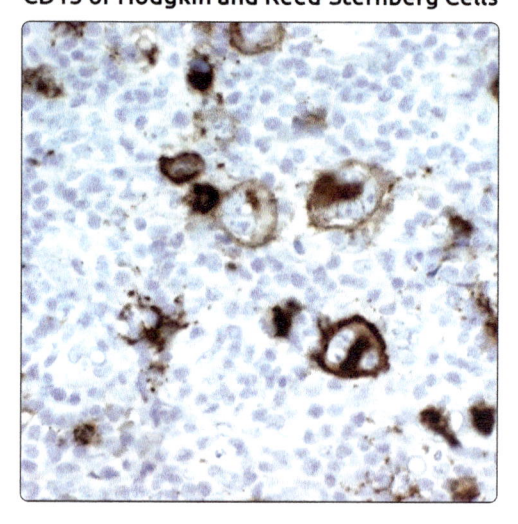

(Left) CD30 highlights HRS cells with a bright membranous and Golgi pattern of expression. The HRS cells were negative for CD45. (Right) Variable expression of CD15 by HRS cells with membranous and Golgi patterns is shown. This finding, in conjunction with expression of CD30 and lack of CD45, supports the diagnosis of classic Hodgkin lymphoma.

CD30/PAX5 Dual Stain of Hodgkin and Reed-Sternberg Cells

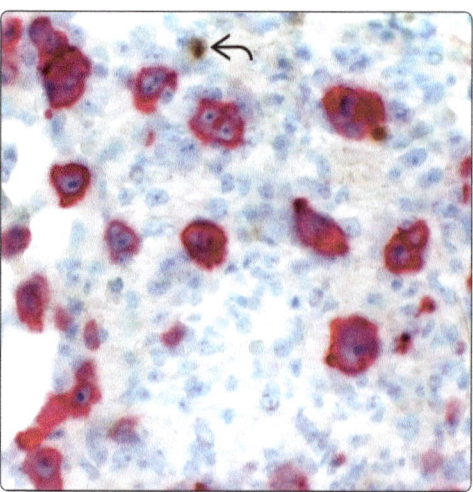

EBER of EBV-Infected Hodgkin and Reed-Sternberg Cells

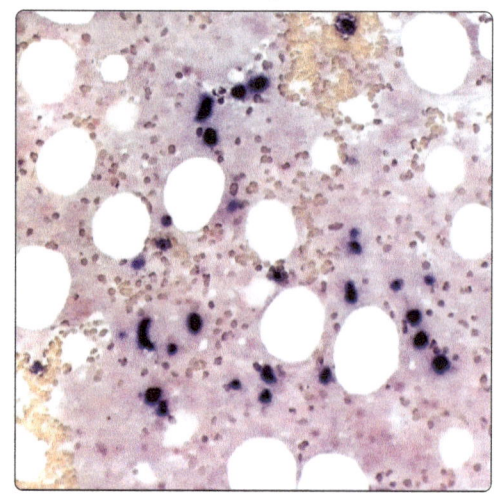

(Left) Dual CD30 and PAX5 show very weak to negative nuclear expression of PAX5 (brown) and bright expression of CD30 (purple) by HRS cells. Note the bright expression of PAX5 by rare background small B cells ⮕. (Right) In situ hybridization for EBER performed on bone marrow involved by classic Hodgkin lymphoma highlights EBV-infected HRS cells. The background small lymphocytes are EBV(-).

EBV-Associated Human Neoplasms

Nasopharyngeal Carcinoma

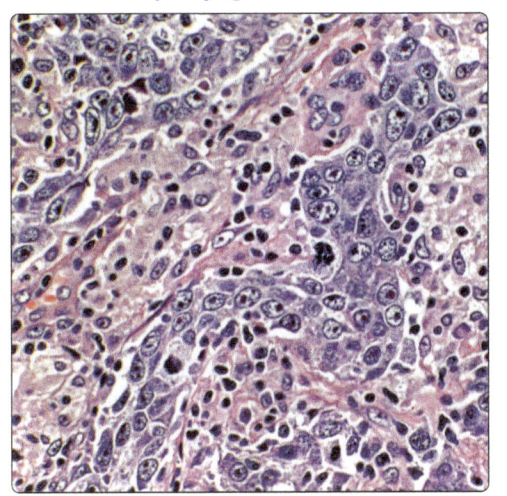

CAM5.2 of Nasopharyngeal Carcinoma

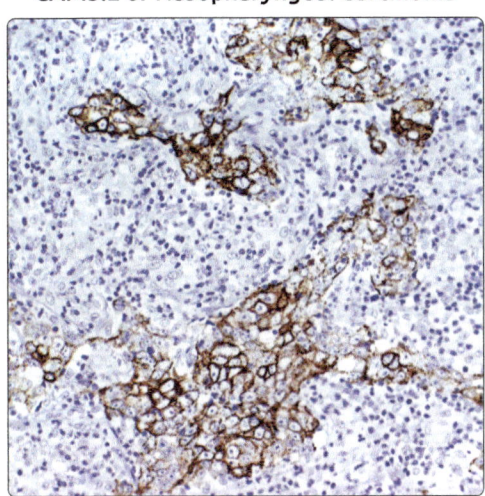

(Left) *Nasopharyngeal carcinoma shows undifferentiated carcinoma cells with a high rate of mitotic activity within a stroma rich in small lymphocytes.* **(Right)** *CAM5.2 highlights syncytial aggregates as well as occasional singly distributed undifferentiated nasopharyngeal carcinoma cells in an intense background of small lymphocytes.*

EBER of Nasopharyngeal Carcinoma

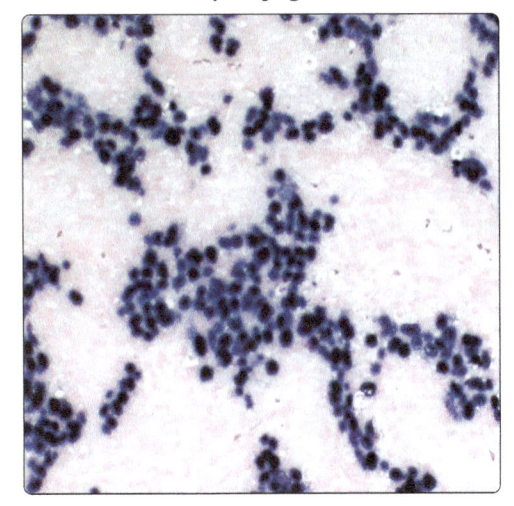

Encapsulated Splenic Mass

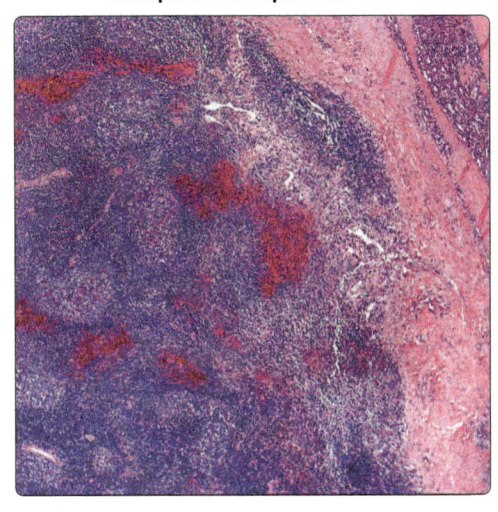

(Left) *In situ hybridization for EBER shows highly transcribed EBERs in the nuclei of metastatic nasopharyngeal carcinoma in a cervical lymph node. EBV is detected in virtually all nasopharyngeal carcinomas, including well-differentiated keratinizing types, by the highly sensitive EBER stain.* **(Right)** *Splenic mass shows an encapsulated, highly lymphocyte-rich, inflammatory pseudotumor-like follicular dendritic cell (FDC) sarcoma.*

Follicular Dendritic Cell Sarcoma

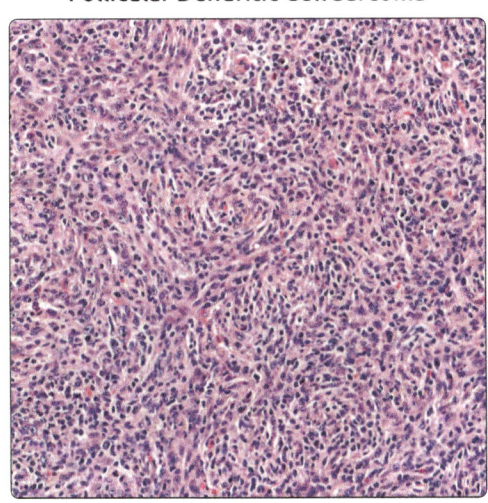

EBER of Follicular Dendritic Cell Sarcoma

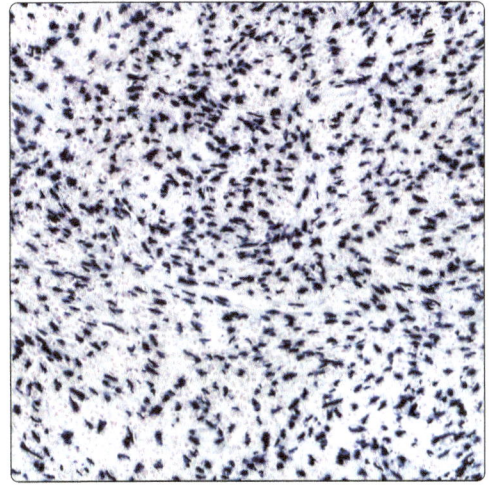

(Left) *Inflammatory pseudotumor-like FDC sarcoma of the spleen shows a focus of spindle-shaped FDCs with a storiform pattern in a background of numerous small lymphocytes and plasma cells.* **(Right)** *EBER shows abundantly transcribed EBERs exclusively localized to spindle-shaped FDCs in inflammatory pseudotumor-like FDC sarcoma of the spleen and liver. EBER is absent in background lymphocytes, plasma cells, and in FDC sarcomas in other locations.*

MYD88 Mutation

TERMINOLOGY

Definitions

- Official name: Innate immune signal transduction adaptor
  - Previous name: Myeloid differentiation primary response 88
- Official symbol: MYD88
- HGNC ID: 7562
- Chromosomal location: 3p22.2
- Molecular location: Base pairs 38,138, 661 to 38, 143, 022 (GRCh38 assembly)
- Number of exons: 5

MOLECULAR FEATURES

MYD88

- Encodes cytosolic adapter protein (MYD88 protein)
  - Critical signal transducer in interleukin-1 receptor (IL-1R) and toll-like receptor (TLR) signaling pathways
    - Upon activation, promotes phosphorylation of interleukin-1 receptor-associated kinases (IRAK)
    - Subsequent activation of nuclear factor κ-light chain enhancer of activated B cells (NF-κB) transcription factors (e.g., p50, p65)
    - Alternative signaling through activation of mitogen-activated protein kinases (MAPK), phosphatidylinositide 3-kinase-AKT (PI3K/AKT), and interferon regulatory factors 3, 5, and 7
  - Overall increased nuclear prosurvival signals
  - MYD88 protein structure
    - N-terminal end (death domain)
    - Central portion (intermediate domain that enables interactions with IRAK kinase family of proteins)
    - C-terminal end [toll interleukin 1 receptor (TIR) domain]
- Cellular functions
  - Regulation of proinflammatory genes
  - Important role in adaptive and innate immune responses
  - Control of important proliferation/survival pathways

MYD88 Mutations

- Most common mutation in MYD88
  - Single nucleotide change of thymine to cytosine (T>C) in exon 5
  - Results in switch of leucine to proline at amino acid position 265 (L265P)
  - HGVS nomenclature: NM_002468.4 (MYD88): c.794T>C (p.Leu265Pro)
- Overexpression of MYD88 protein secondary to L265P mutation will cause activation of NF-κB
  - Increased Bruton tyrosine kinase (BTK) phosphorylation
  - Increased IRAK1/IRAK4 recruitment and signaling
  - Activation and phosphorylation of TRAF6 and TAK1
- Additional concomitant loss of TNFAIP3 tumor suppressor gene (encoding for A20 protein) acts as enhancing 2nd genetic alteration
- Results in increased cellular growth and survival
  - Increased production of IL-6 and CXCL10 leading to upregulation of JAK/STAT pathway
- Numerous additional low-frequency (< 1%) mutations have been also described

CLINICAL IMPLICATIONS

MYD88 L265P Mutation and B-Cell Lymphomas

- One of most recurrent mutations in hematologic malignancies, found in ~ 20% of all lymphomas
  - Important oncogenic pathway in lymphomagenesis
- Present in significant number of B-cell non-Hodgkin lymphomas
- Most important and frequent association with lymphoplasmacytic lymphoma (LPL)/Waldenström macroglobulinemia (WM)
  - Very high prevalence of this mutation in numerous published studies (85-100%)
  - Concurrent CXCR4 mutations
    - Confers resistance to Ibrutinib therapy in LPL
- Frequent genomic abnormality in diffuse large B-cell lymphomas (DLBCL) of activated B-cell-like (ABC) origin (C5/MCD subgroups by gene expression profiling)

Lymphoplasmacytic Lymphoma

Pyrosequencing

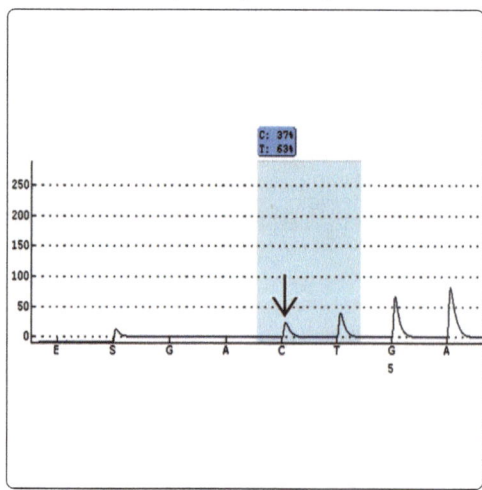

(Left) Bone marrow aspirate smear involved by lymphoplasmacytic lymphoma (LPL) shows a spectrum of small lymphocytes, plasmacytoid lymphocytes, and plasma cells, including a Dutcher body ➡. Mast cells ➡ are also often increased. (Right) Pyrogram demonstrates the presence of the L265P mutation due to substitution of a T for a C ➡ in codon 265 of the MYD88 gene in a patient with history of LPL.

MYD88 Mutation

- Primary DLBCL of central nervous system (70%)
- Primary cutaneous DLBCL, leg type (60%)
- Testicular DLBCL (75%)
- DLBCL, not otherwise specified (NOS), ABC subtype (25%)
- Rarely detected in DLBCL of germinal center B-cell-like subtype
- Low prevalence in other B-cell lymphomas, including
  - Marginal zone B-cell lymphoma (uncommon)
  - Chronic lymphocytic leukemia/small lymphocytic lymphoma (CLL/SLL)
  - Burkitt lymphoma
- Presence of *MYD88* L265P mutation serves as useful tool to differentiate LPL/WM from other low-grade B-cell lymphomas
- Prognostic significance of *MYD88*-mutated monoclonal gammopathy of unknown significance (MGUS)
  - IgM subtype mutated MGUS cases have been associated with higher risk of disease progression and disease burden
    - Typically exhibit higher levels of IgM
    - Usually have lower levels of IgG and IgA
    - Higher incidence of Bence-Jones proteinuria
- Potential for targeted therapies by blocking of associated cellular pathways
  - Most successful target BTK
  - BTK inhibitor Ibrutinib reduces binding strength of BTK to *MYD88* L265P and increases cellular apoptosis
    - In DLBCL, ABC type presence of *MYD88* mutations alone confers resistance to Ibrutinib; however, sensitivity is increased with concomitant *CD79A* or *CD79B* mutations
    - In LPL/WM, mutation confers sensitivity to Ibrutinib

TESTING FOR *MYD88* L265P MUTATION

Testing Strategies

- Varies depending on desired level of sensitivity and specificity
- Most strategies are PCR based
- Selection of appropriate tissue sample for molecular testing
  - Fresh diagnostic specimen is desired
  - Formalin-fixed, paraffin-embedded diagnostic tissue is acceptable
  - Frequent PCR failure in decalcified bone marrow core biopsies when strong acid is used for decalcification
  - EDTA-based decalcified bone marrow biopsy could be acceptable for PCR-based testing

Sanger Sequencing

- a.k.a. traditional or 1st-generation sequencing
- Sequence by chain termination
  - Based on selective incorporation of chain-terminating dideoxynucleotides (ddNTPs)
  - Addition of label (dye) to ddNTPs allows for fluorescent detection and reading of sequences
- Sensitivity
  - ~ 15-20% detection of heterozygous mutated alleles

Pyrosequencing

- Sequence by synthesis method
- Relies on detection of pyrophosphate released upon incorporation of nucleotides
  - Light is emitted after incorporation of complementary nucleotide and sequentially detected to identify specific sequence
- Limitation due to short DNA reads
- Sensitivity
  - ~ 10% detection sensitivity for heterozygous mutated alleles

Allele-Specific PCR

- a.k.a. amplification refractory mutation system (ARMS)
  - 1 primer includes desired mutational sequence (matched primer)
  - Mismatched primer will not initiate replication, while matched primer will
    - Therefore, generation of amplified products will indicate presence of targeted genotype
- High level of sensitivity (Ideal testing method)
  - ~ 0.1% detection of mutated alleles

Next-Generation Sequencing

- Newer and most advanced technology for sequencing
  - Massive parallel sequencing
  - Decreased costs of sequencing, while improving coverage
  - *MYD88* mutation testing is usually included as part of panel
  - May miss up to 1/3 of mutated cases

DIAGNOSTIC CHECKLIST

Clinically Relevant Pathologic Pearls

- *MYD88* mutations play very important role in lymphomagenesis via upregulation of JAK/STAT pathway
- Mutations are frequently detected in
  - LPL/WM
  - DLBCL of ABC origin (C5/MCD subtypes by GEP)
    - Primary DLBCL of central nervous system
    - Primary cutaneous DLBCL, leg type
    - Testicular DLBCL
    - DLBCL, NOS, ABC subtype
- *MYD88* mutations are uncommon in marginal zone lymphoma (MZL) and CLL/SLL
- Detection of *MYD88* mutation is helpful in distinction of LPL/WM from MZL with plasmacytic differentiation

SELECTED REFERENCES

1. Falini B et al: A comparison of the International Consensus and 5th World Health Organization classifications of mature B-cell lymphomas. Leukemia. 37(1):18-34, 2023
2. Alcoceba M et al: MYD88 mutations: transforming the landscape of IgM monoclonal gammopathies. Int J Mol Sci. 23(10), 2022
3. Chapuy B et al: Molecular subtypes of diffuse large B cell lymphoma are associated with distinct pathogenic mechanisms and outcomes. Nat Med. 24(5):679-90, 2018
4. Schmitz R et al: Genetics and pathogenesis of diffuse large B-cell lymphoma. N Engl J Med. 378(15):1396-407, 2018
5. Wang YL: MYD88 Mutations and sensitivity to ibrutinib therapy. J Mol Diagn. 20(2):264-6, 2018
6. Weber ANR et al: Oncogenic MYD88 mutations in lymphoma: novel insights and therapeutic possibilities. Cancer Immunol Immunother. 67(11):1797-807, 2018
7. Wenzl K et al: Loss of TNFAIP3 enhances MYD88L265P-driven signaling in non-Hodgkin lymphoma. Blood Cancer J. 8(10):97, 2018

NOTCH1 Mutation

TERMINOLOGY

Definitions
- Official name: Notch receptor 1
- Official symbol: NOTCH1
- HGNC ID: 7881
- Chromosomal location: 9q34.3
- RefSeq: NG_007458.1
- Number of exons: 34
- Aliases: hN1 (homolog notch 1), TAN1 (translocation-associated notch 1)

NOTCH1 FUNCTIONS

Characteristics of Encoded NOTCH1 Protein
- Transmembrane protein receptor
- Upon activation, intracellular domain is cleaved, released, and translocated to nucleus to interact with specific DNA-binding proteins to activate transcription of target genes
  - Most prominent nuclear targets include helix-loop factors of Hes and Hey families
- Additional noncanonical signaling pathways are also involved

NOTCH1 Protein Structure
- Extracellular domain subunit (NECD)
  - Consist of multiple epidermal growth factor (EGF)-like repeats
  - Cystine-rich Lin 12 NOTCH repeats
- Negative regulatory unit (NRR)
  - Regulates receptor activation
  - 3 Lin 12/Notch repeats (LNRs)
  - HD
- Transmembrane subunit
- Intracellular domain subunit (NICD)
  - RBP-Jkappa-associated module (RAM) domain
  - Ankyrin repeat domain
  - NOTCH cysteine response domain
  - Transcriptional activation domain (TAD)
  - Proline, glutamine, serine, and threonine (PEST)-rich domain

Cellular Functions
- Critical functions in cellular homeostasis, including cell differentiation, proliferation, and survival
- Notch signaling is involved in important biological functions, including embryonic development, neurogenesis, angiogenesis, and hematopoiesis
- Due to many diverse functions of NOTCH1 protein, gene is considered to act as oncogene in some instances and tumor suppressor gene in others

NOTCH1 MUTATIONS

Activating Mutations
- Most NOTCH1 mutations seen in hematologic disorders lead to constitutive activation of Notch signaling (oncogene function)
- Majority of activating mutations cluster in 2 regions
  - Heterodimerization domain (HD)
    - Leads to ligand-independent cleavage of NOTCH receptor
    - Most are missense mutations and inframe insertions/deletions (indels)
  - PEST-rich domain
    - Leads to reduced degradation of NOTCH1 intracellular domain
    - Most mutations are missense, nonsense, and frameshift mutations

Loss-of-Function Mutations
- Most commonly present in solid tumors, particularly head and neck squamous cell carcinomas (HNSCC)
- Its presence highlights importance of NOTCH1 as tumor-suppressor gene
- Mutations mainly present in EGF-like region and ankyrin domain
  - Most mutations are missense, nonsense, and indels resulting in truncated NOTCH1 protein that lacks domains important for transcriptional activity

---

High-Resolution Melting Curve Analysis

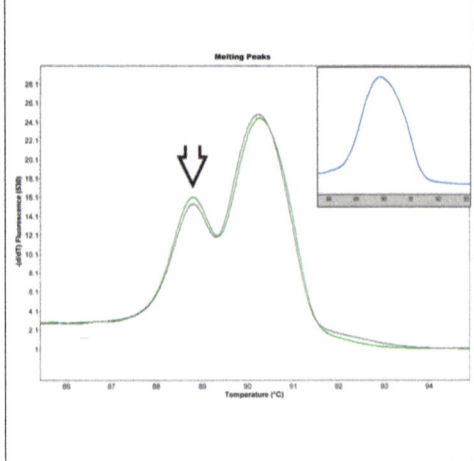

Sanger Sequencing

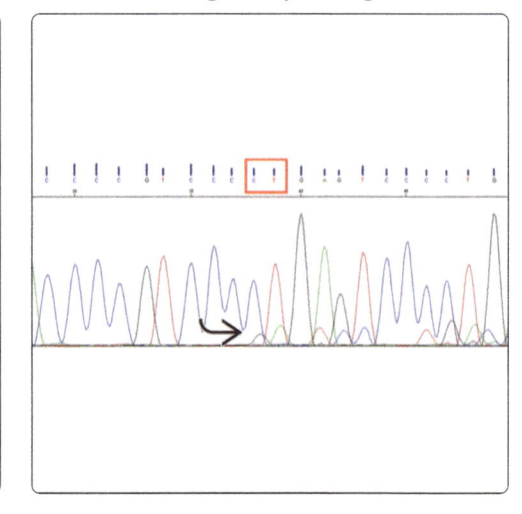

(Left) High-resolution melting curve of PCR-amplified products of DNA extracted from a chronic lymphocytic leukemia/small lymphocytic lymphoma (CLL/SLL) case shows a NOTCH1 mutation evident by an abnormal shouldering ⇨ compared to wildtype DNA melting curve (inset). (Right) Sanger sequencing trace shows the most common NOTCH1 mutation (c.7541_7542delCT) seen in CLL/SLL, resulting in a 2 base pair (CT) deletion ➢.

NOTCH1 Mutation

Other Mutations and Alterations
- Additional less frequent mechanisms have been reported that lead to increased *NOTCH1* expression in cancer cells
  - Mutations other than stop codon in PEST-rich domain
    - Leads to reduced CDC4/Fbw7-mediated degradation and stabilization of intracellular domain

CLINICAL IMPLICATIONS

T-Lymphoblastic Leukemia/Lymphoma
- Neoplasm of lymphoblasts committed to T-cell lineage
- Accounts for ~ 15% of newly diagnosed acute lymphoblastic leukemia (ALL) cases (most commonly seen in pediatric populations)
- *NOTCH1*-activating mutations are found in 70-80% of cases
  - Most mutations are located in HD domain
  - Numerous missense, nonsense, and frameshift mutations
- Most studies suggest favorable long-term prognosis, decreased relapses, and increased overall survival in *NOTCH1*-mutated cases

Chronic Lymphocytic Leukemia/Small Lymphocytic Lymphoma
- Most common leukemia in adults
- B-cell neoplasm composed of small, round, mature lymphoid cells
- *NOTCH1* mutations present in 15-25% of cases at diagnosis
- Most mutations located in C-terminal PEST (exons 33-34) and TAD domains
  - Most frequently (~ 80%) occurring mutation is c.7541_7542delCT (P2514R)
    - Increases stability and defective degradation of NOTCH1 protein
  - Mutations are typically associated with unmutated variable region of immunoglobulin heavy chain
  - Mutations are usually associated with expression of ZAP70 and CD38 expression
  - Also associated with trisomy 12
- Usually seen (20-40%) with refractory/relapsed disease, Richter transformation, and overall worse outcomes

Head and Neck Squamous Cell Carcinoma
- 6th most common cancer in world
- *NOTCH1* mutations have been identified in ~ 15-20% of HNSCC
  - 2nd most frequently mutated gene after *TP53*
  - Most mutations are loss-of-function mutations leading to protein truncation and functional downregulation (missense, nonsense, indels)
  - Mutations are mainly located in N-terminal EGF-like ligand binding domain
    - Alters NOTCH1 protein N-terminal to transmembrane region
  - *NOTCH1* is considered to play bimodal role as tumor suppressor and oncogene
  - Recent studies have associated *NOTCH1*-mutated HNSCC cases with HPV(-) status and more aggressive disease with shorter overall and disease-free survival

Other Tumors
- Activating mutations also described in non-small cell lung cancer, adenoid cystic carcinoma, breast cancer
- Other B-cell lymphomas and T-cell lymphomas, including
  - Mantle cell lymphoma, follicular lymphoma, diffuse large B-cell lymphoma (DLBCL), and adult T-cell leukemia lymphoma
    - *NOTCH1* mutations is independently associated with poor complete response and progression-free survival in DLBCL per some studies
- Loss-of-function mutations reported in chronic myelomonocytic leukemia (CMML), small cell lung cancer, esophageal squamous cell carcinoma, bladder cancer, and some subtypes of breast cancer
  - Clinical implications of *NOTCH1* mutations in these tumors remain under investigation

TESTING

High-Resolution DNA Melting Curve Analysis
- Can be used as screening method for hot spot mutations
- Regions with high numbers of single nucleotide polymorphisms (SNPs) should be avoided
- Sequencing studies are needed to determine specific mutation type

Sequencing
- Common techniques include Sanger sequencing, next-generation sequencing (NGS), and pyrosequencing
- Can be done as standalone test or as part of larger panel

DIAGNOSTIC CHECKLIST

Clinically Relevant Pathologic Pearls
- *NOTCH1* mutations can function as oncogene or tumor suppressor gene
- Important associations with
  - T-lymphoblastic leukemia/lymphoma (T-ALL)
    - More favorable outcome
  - Chronic lymphocytic leukemia/small lymphocytic lymphoma (CLL/SLL)
    - Associated with trisomy 12
    - More aggressive disease
  - HNSCC
    - HPV(-) cases
    - More aggressive disease

SELECTED REFERENCES
1. Pozzo F et al: Multiple mechanisms of NOTCH1 activation in chronic lymphocytic leukemia: NOTCH1 mutations and beyond. Cancers (Basel). 14(12), 2022
2. Farah CS: Molecular landscape of head and neck cancer and implications for therapy. Ann Transl Med. 9(10):915, 2021
3. Li Z et al: Clinical features and prognostic significance of NOTCH1 mutations in diffuse large B-cell lymphoma. Front Oncol. 11:746577, 2021
4. Katoh M et al: Precision medicine for human cancers with Notch signaling dysregulation (Review). Int J Mol Med. 45(2):279-97, 2020
5. Sharif A et al: Notch transduction in non-small cell lung cancer. Int J Mol Sci. 21(16), 2020
6. Chiang MY et al: Oncogenic notch signaling in T-cell and B-cell lymphoproliferative disorders. Curr Opin Hematol. 23(4):362-70, 2016
7. Stilgenbauer S et al: Gene mutations and treatment outcome in chronic lymphocytic leukemia: results from the CLL8 trial. Blood. 123(21):3247-54, 2014

EZH2 Mutation

TERMINOLOGY

Definitions

- Official name: Enhancer of zeste 2 polycomb repressive complex 2 subunit
- Official symbol: *EZH2*
- HGNC ID: 3527
- Chromosomal location: 7q36.1
- Genomic coordinates (GRCh38):Ch7:148,807,383-148,884,291
- Number of exons: 26
- Aliases: *ENX1, KMT6, KMT6A*

NORMAL *EZH2* FUNCTION

Encodes EZH2 Protein

- Member of polycomb-group (PcG) family, which functions as gene silencers
- Enzyme that methylates lysine 27 of histone H3 (H3K27)
  - SET is catalytic domain of EZH2, and it transfers up to 3 methyl groups
  - Functions as part of complex containing other proteins, including EED, SUZ12, and RBBP7
  - Histone methylation leads to more condensed chromatin state and transcriptional repression
  - Removal of methyl group by demethylases, such as UTX and JMJD3, reverses action of EZH2
- Plays role in hematopoietic and central nervous system development

SOMATIC *EZH2* MUTATIONS

Gain-of-Function Mutations

- Seen in lymphomas
  - *EZH2* functions as oncogene in lymphomas
- Almost all are missense mutations occurring at codon 646
  - Result in replacement of single tyrosine (Tyr646) in SET domain of *EZH2*
- Mutations in codons 682 and 692 have been reported in follicular lymphomas (FLs) and diffuse large B-cell lymphoma (DLBCL), such as A692V and A682G
- All mutations are heterozygous

Loss-of-Function Mutations

- Are seen in myeloid neoplasms and T-acute lymphoblastic leukemia (T-ALL)
  - *EZH2* functions as tumor suppressor gene in myeloid neoplasia
- > 50 different mutations reported
- Mutations are either missense or truncating
  - Missense mutations involve evolutionary highly conserved residues that are located in domain II and CXC-SET domains
  - Truncating mutations are dispersed throughout gene
    - Include both nonsense and frameshift due to deletions or insertions
    - 1 mutation is reported at splice site
- Can be homozygous, hemizygous, or heterozygous
- Loss of function of *EZH2* in myeloid neoplasms can also occur due to del(7q) or -7

EPIDEMIOLOGY

Incidence

- Gain-of-function mutations in lymphomas
  - ~ 22% in DLBCL
  - 7-27% in FL
- Loss-of-function mutations in myeloid malignancies and lymphoid leukemias
  - ~ 12% in myelodysplastic syndromes/myeloproliferative neoplasms (MDS/MPN)
  - 3-7% in MDS
  - ~ 6% in MPN
  - < 2% in acute myeloid leukemia (AML)
  - ~ 18% in T-ALL
- Increased expression of *EZH2* has been found in many solid tumors
  - Broad range of incidence reported

(Left) Diffuse large B-cell lymphoma (DLBCL) with mutant EZH2 shows an abnormal melting curve (red) compared to wildtype (yellow). (Right) Sanger sequencing of the same case shows Y646H mutation ➔ (TAC to CAC). DLBCL was of germinal center B-cell (GCB) subtype.

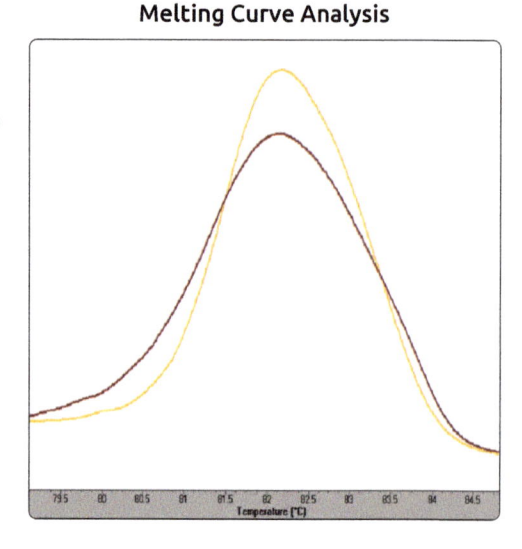

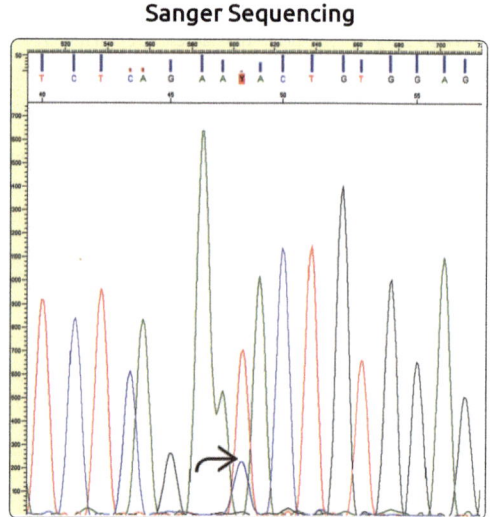

EZH2 Mutation

METHOD OF DETECTION

Whole-Exome Sequencing
- Considered for myeloid neoplasms
  - Typically performed using massively parallel sequencing (next-generation sequencing)
  - All coding exons of gene should be sequenced
  - Tumor percentage should be at least 2x of sensitivity limit of detection for heterozygous mutations
- Can be performed on formalin-fixed, paraffin-embedded tissue or fresh tissue

Targeted Sequencing
- Can be performed by Sanger sequencing, pyrosequencing, or next-generation sequencing
- For cases of DLBCL and FL, selective sequencing of codon 646 is sufficient
  - All mutations are heterozygous
  - Tumor percentage in specimen should be at least 2x of sensitivity limit of assay

High-Resolution Melting Curve Analysis
- Inexpensive screening method to detect codon 646 mutations in FL and DLBCL
  - Amplified DNA of interest should not exceed 300 bp
  - Amplification of DNA regions that might potentially harbor single-nucleotide polymorphism (SNP) must be avoided
  - Positive cases demonstrate abnormal melting curve when compared to wildtype
    - Positive results should be confirmed by sequencing

Immunohistochemistry
- Performed on formalin-fixed, paraffin-embedded tissue
- Used to detect EZH2 protein overexpression
  - Positive nuclear staining indicates EZH2 overexpression
  - Results are reported as positive or negative for solid tumors in majority of published studies with no minimal requirement for percentage of positive cells
- Positive prognostic impact of EZH2 overexpression in DLBCL
  - Requires ≥ 70% positivity among tumor cells

Fluorescence In Situ Hybridization
- Available for formalin-fixed, paraffin-embedded tissue
- Detects gene amplification

CLINICAL IMPLICATIONS

Diffuse Large B-Cell Lymphoma
- Most common form of non-Hodgkin lymphoma (NHL)
- Can be classified according to cell of origin into 2 major broad categories
  - Germinal center B-cell (GCB) type
    - Associated with better prognosis
    - Frequently show t(14;18)
  - Activated B-cell type
    - Associated with worse prognosis
  - Cell of origin determination in DLBCL is done by gene expression profiling (GEP)
    - Panel of antibodies by immunohistochemistry can be used as alternative or surrogate marker for GEP
- *EZH2* mutations in DLBCL are almost exclusively seen in GCB subtype of DLBCL
  - Rarely, *EZH2* mutation may be seen in non-GCB subtype of DLBCL in setting of immunodeficiency
  - Mutations are rare or absent in GCB subtype of primary DLBCL of central nervous system
- Overexpression of EZH2 in absence of mutation occurs in both GCB and activated B-cell (ABC) subtypes of DLBCLs
  - High levels of expression (≥ 70%) are associated with superior overall survival
    - Highest survival rate in ABC subtype with EZH2 overexpression
- No correlation between *EZH2* mutation and EZH2 protein overexpression

Follicular Lymphoma
- 2nd most common type of NHL
- Neoplasm of follicle center B cells that usually has at least partially follicular growth pattern
- Majority of cases demonstrate t(14;18), resulting in *IGH::BCL2* fusion
- *EZH2* mutation is early event in FL
  - In 20% of mutant cases, mutation is only detected in subset of neoplastic cells (subclonal mutation)

Other Lymphoid Malignancies
- Natural killer/T-cell lymphoma (NK-/T-cell lymphoma)
  - Predominantly extranodal lymphoma showing NK-cell &/or cytotoxic T-cell phenotype
    - Angiodestructive and angiocentric patterns
    - Prominent necrosis
    - Strong association with Epstein-Barr virus (EBV)
  - EZH2 protein is overexpressed in majority of NK-/T-cell lymphomas
    - Overexpression is associated with poorer outcome
- T-lymphoblastic leukemia/lymphoma
  - Neoplasm of lymphoblasts committed to T-cell lineage
    - Blasts are small to medium-sized cells with scant cytoplasm and dispersed chromatin
    - Blasts are detected in peripheral blood &/or bone marrow
  - Early T-cell precursor ALL is distinct subtype
    - Arise from neoplastic cells with very early arrest in T-cell differentiation
    - Show higher prevalence of mutations associated with myeloid neoplasms
    - Associated with particularly poor prognosis
  - *EZH2* mutations are common in T-ALL, including early T-ALL
  - *EZH2* mutations are frequently seen concurrently with *NOTCH1* mutations
- Burkitt lymphoma (BL)
  - B-cell lymphoma with extremely short doubling time often presenting in extranodal sites
    - Characterized by translocation involving *MYC* at 8q24
  - Divided into 3 broad categories
    - Endemic: Equatorial Africa, mainly in children
    - Sporadic: Throughout world in children and adults
    - Immunodeficiency associated, mainly seen in patients with HIV

EZH2 Mutation

- *EZH2* mutations similar to those seen in DLBCL have been reported in BL associated with immunodeficiency

EZH2 Mutations in Myeloid Neoplasms
- Generally associated with worse outcome
  - Mutations can be homozygous, hemizygous, or heterozygous
    - Homozygous mutations might be associated with poorer survival than heterozygous
- In general, cases that contain karyotypically visible abnormalities of chromosome 7, including del(7q) or -7, are mostly negative for *EZH2* mutations
- Cases with karyotypically invisible abnormalities of chromosome 7 (unipaternal disomy for 7q or 7q36 microdeletion) are frequently associated with *EZH2* mutations

EZH2 Mutations in Specific Categories of Myeloid Neoplasms
- Myelodysplastic syndromes
  - Group of clonal hematopoietic stem cell diseases characterized by
    - Cytopenias
    - Dysplasia in ≥ 1 of myeloid cell lines
    - Ineffective hematopoiesis
    - Increased risk of development of AML
  - Revised International Prognostic Scoring System (IPSS-R) is used to predict prognosis
    - Incorporates severity of cytopenias, bone marrow blasts percentage, and cytogenetic abnormalities
  - *EZH2* mutations are present in subset of cases
    - Associated with worse outcome if present, even in patients with favorable IPSS-R
    - Lower risk patients with myelodysplastic syndromes who have *EZH2* mutations may require more aggressive treatment than would be predicted by IPSS-R
- MDS/MPN
  - Clonal myeloid neoplasms that at time of initial presentation are associated with some findings that support diagnosis of MDS and other findings more consistent with MPN
  - *EZH2* mutations are present in 10% of cases
    - Frequently cooccur with *TET2* (58%), *RUNX1* (40%), and *ASXL1* (34%) mutations
    - Associated with poorer outcome
- Primary myelofibrosis
  - Clonal MPN characterized by proliferation of predominantly megakaryocytes and granulocytes in bone marrow
    - Associated with reactive deposition of fibrous tissue and extramedullary hematopoiesis in fibrotic phase of disease
    - Most patients have splenomegaly
    - Most cases demonstrate mutations in *JAK2*, *MPL*, or *CALR*
  - *EZH2* mutation is associated with significantly higher leukocyte count, blast count, and larger spleen at diagnosis
- AML
  - Group of relatively well-defined hematopoietic neoplasms involving precursor cells committed to myeloid lineage
  - Classified into 4 major groups
    - AML with recurrent genetic abnormalities
    - AML with myelodysplasia-related changes
    - Therapy-related myeloid neoplasms
    - AML, not otherwise specified
  - *EZH2* mutations have been reported in small minority of cases
    - More common in male patients
    - Associated with lower blast percentage (21-30%) in bone marrow
    - No influence on achieving complete remission or overall survival

EZH2 Protein Overexpression in Solid Tumors
- Overexpression of EZH2 was first described in several nonhematological malignancies
  - Steadily increases as disease progression takes place, which is particularly notable in breast cancer
  - Associated with poorer outcome
- MYC overexpression parallels overexpression of EZH2 and is known to induce EZH2 expression
  - Binds directly to promoter region of *EZH2* and activates its transcription
- *EZH2* inhibition might be promising therapeutic target in solid tumors
- No correlation between EZH2 protein overexpression and presence of *EZH2* mutation
- Specific examples and implications
  - Breast carcinoma
    - Invasive ductal carcinoma
    - Invasive lobular carcinoma
      - Associated with poor response to tamoxifen therapy in metastatic breast carcinoma
      - Correlates with higher rate of locoregional recurrence in inflammatory breast carcinoma after radiotherapy
  - Central nervous system tumors
    - Glioblastoma multiforme
      - May contribute to temozolomide therapy resistance in glioblastomas
    - Childhood ependymoma
  - Endocrine tumors
    - Medullary and anaplastic thyroid carcinoma, parathyroid adenoma and carcinoma
  - Female patient genital tract tumors
    - Cervical intraepithelial neoplasia (CIN) and invasive squamous cell carcinoma
    - Endometrial carcinoma
    - Ovarian serous carcinoma
      - Overexpression of EZH2 contributes to acquired cisplatinum resistance in ovarian cancer
  - Genitourinary tumors
    - Prostate adenocarcinoma
      - Associated with adverse outcome and may confer poor response to immunotherapy
    - Bladder and upper tract urothelial carcinoma
    - Renal cell carcinoma
  - Gastrointestinal tumors

EZH2 Mutation

- Esophageal squamous cell carcinoma
- Gastric carcinoma
  - Positively correlates with tumor size, lymphatic invasion and TNM stage, and poor disease-free survival and overall survival of patients
  - Combined inhibition of EZH2 and EGFR produces synergic effect on tumor growth inhibition
- Colon adenocarcinoma
  - Inhibition of EZH2 may enhance efficacy of EGFR inhibitor therapy in colon cancer
- Gallbladder carcinoma
  - EZH2 overexpression is seen in ~ 50% of gallbladder carcinomas and is associated with poor differentiation, lymph node metastasis, and invasion
- Cholangiocarcinoma
  - IHC for EZH2 can help differentiate cholangiocarcinoma (positive) from ductular reaction and bile duct adenoma (negative)
- Pancreatic intraductal mucinous neoplasm
- Hepatic carcinoma
  - IHC for EZH2 can help differentiate malignant hepatic (positive) from benign hepatic (negative) tumors
  - EZH2 inhibition has been shown to make hepatocellular carcinoma cells more sensitive to sorafenib
- Lung cancer
  - Adenocarcinoma
    - IHC for EZH2 can help differentiate malignant neoplasms (positive) in pleural effusion cytology from reactive mesothelial cells (negative)
- Oral cavity tumors
  - Squamous cell carcinoma
    - Overexpression of EZH2 as evaluated by IHC predicts progression to invasive squamous cell carcinoma in premalignant lesions presenting as leukoplakia
- Skin cancer
  - Squamous cell carcinoma
    - IHC for EZH2 can help differentiate squamous cell carcinoma (positive) from actinic keratosis (negative)
- Soft tissue tumors
  - Embryonal rhabdomyosarcoma
  - Synovial sarcoma

EZH2 Inhibition

- Role of EZH2 inhibition in cancer therapy is currently being investigated in numerous clinical trials
  - Malignancies include but are not limited to: DLBCL, mantle cell lymphoma, prostate cancer, mesothelioma, urothelial carcinoma, and rhabdoid tumors
  - Evaluation of combination therapy with EZH2 inhibitors and other therapies, including immunotherapy, conventional chemotherapy, and targeted therapies, are also currently underway
- 3 main mechanisms for EZH2 inhibition
  - Inhibition of methyltransferase enzymatic activity mainly through small molecular competitive inhibitors
    - Examples: Tazemetostat, GSK126, CPI-1205
  - Breaking down PRC2 structure
    - Examples: Astemizole, SAH-EZH2, AZD9291
  - Triggering EZH2 degradation
    - Examples: GNA022, ANCR, FBW7
- Tazemetostat (EPZ-6438) is only EZH2 inhibitor that is currently approved by FDA
  - Oral pyridine-based competitive inhibitor of SAM pocket of EZH2 SET domain, inhibiting both wildtype and mutant forms of EZH2
  - Highly selective for EZH2 with 35x increased potency relative to EZH1
  - Approved by FDA for following indications
    - Relapsed or refractory FL positive for EZH2 mutation and patient who received at least 2 lines of systemic therapy or have no alternative treatment options
    - Patients 16 years or older with metastatic or locally advanced epithelioid sarcoma not eligible for complete resection
- Resistance to EZH2 inhibitor therapy
  - EZH2 W113C mutation in lymphoma confers resistance to Tazemetostat

SELECTED REFERENCES

1. Chu L et al: EZH2 W113C is a gain-of-function mutation in B-cell lymphoma enabling both PRC2 methyltransferase activation and tazemetostat resistance. J Biol Chem. 299(4):103073, 2023
2. Du TQ et al: EZH2 as a prognostic factor and its immune implication with molecular characterization in prostate cancer: an integrated multi-omics in silico analysis. Biomolecules. 12(11):1617, 2022
3. Straining R et al: Tazemetostat: EZH2 inhibitor. J Adv Pract Oncol. 13(2):158-63, 2022
4. Duan R et al: EZH2: a novel target for cancer treatment. J Hematol Oncol. 13(1):104, 2020
5. Yan L et al: Genetic alteration of histone lysine methyltransferases and their significance in renal cell carcinoma. PeerJ. 7:e6396, 2019
6. Fioravanti R et al: Six years (2012-2018) of researches on catalytic EZH2 inhibitors: the boom of the 2-pyridone compounds. Chem Rec. 18(12):1818-32, 2018
7. Gulati N et al: Enhancer of zeste homolog 2 (EZH2) inhibitors. Leuk Lymphoma. 59(7):1574-85, 2018
8. Fan TY et al: Inhibition of EZH2 reverses chemotherapeutic drug TMZ chemosensitivity in glioblastoma. Int J Clin Exp Pathol. 7(10):6662-70, 2014
9. Katona BW et al: EZH2 inhibition enhances the efficacy of an EGFR inhibitor in suppressing colon cancer cells. Cancer Biol Ther. 15(12):1677-87, 2014
10. Lee HJ et al: Polycomb protein EZH2 expression in diffuse large B-cell lymphoma is associated with better prognosis in patients treated with rituximab, cyclophosphamide, doxorubicin, vincristine and prednisone. Leuk Lymphoma. 55(9):2056-63, 2014
11. Sasaki M et al: Immunostaining for polycomb group protein EZH2 and senescent marker p16INK4a may be useful to differentiate cholangiolocellular carcinoma from ductular reaction and bile duct adenoma. Am J Surg Pathol. 38(3):364-9, 2014
12. Bödör C et al: EZH2 mutations are frequent and represent an early event in follicular lymphoma. Blood. 122(18):3165-8, 2013

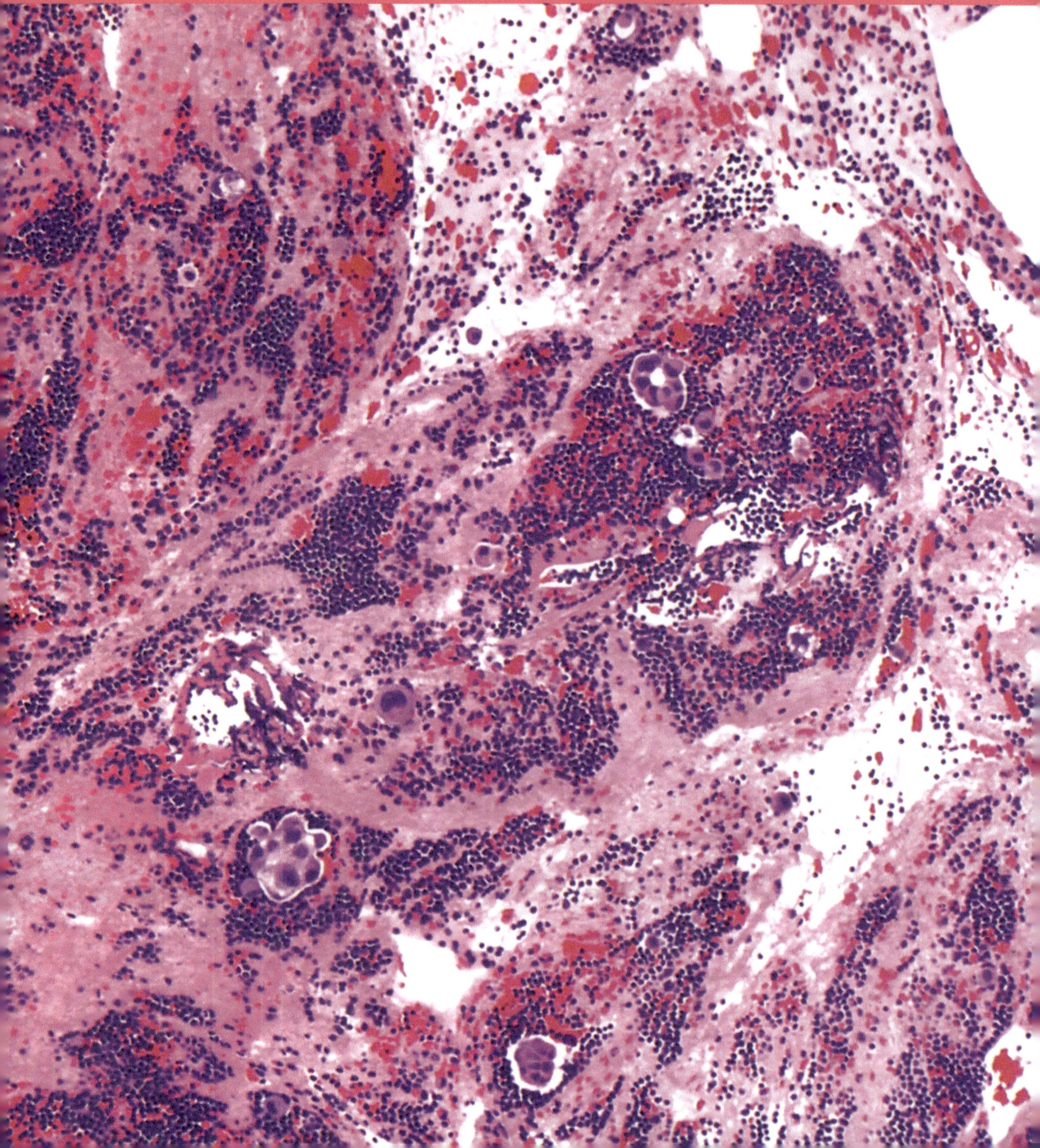

SECTION 4
Molecular Genetic Tests in Solid Tumors, Bone and Soft Tissue Tumors, and CNS Tumors

ALK Rearrangements and Mutations	104
ROS1 Rearrangements	106
RET Rearrangements	108
FISH for *MET* Amplifications	110
FISH for *ERBB2* (HER2) Amplifications	114
KRAS Mutations	116
BRAF Mutations	118
EGFR Mutations	120
Targeted Hotspot Gene Panel Using Massively Parallel Sequencing (Next-Generation Sequencing)	122
Targeted Hotspot Gene Panel Table	124
MGMT Promoter Gene Methylation Assay	130

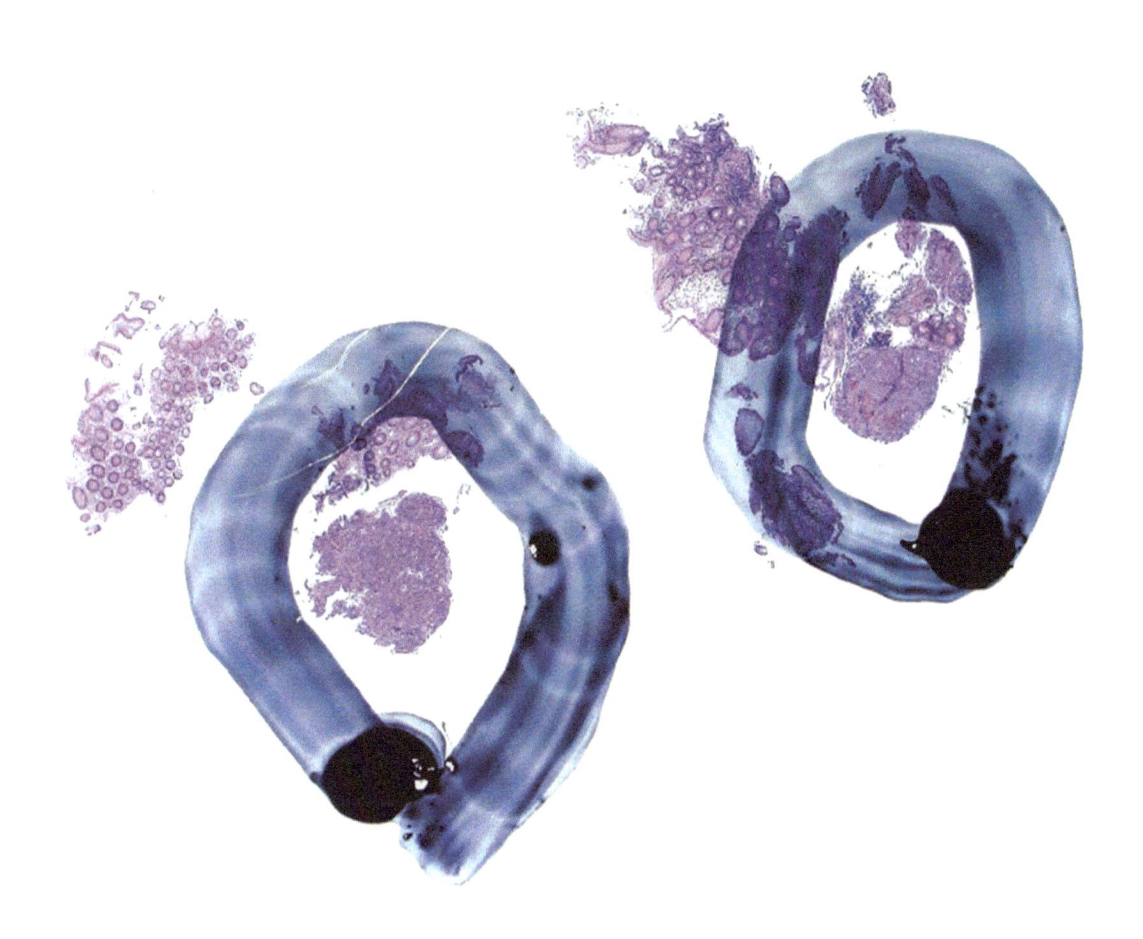

ALK Rearrangements and Mutations

TERMINOLOGY

Definitions

- Official name: *ALK* receptor tyrosine kinase
  - Previous name: Anaplastic lymphoma kinase (Ki-1)
- Official symbol: *ALK*
- HGNC ID: 427
- Chromosomal location: 2p23.2-p23.1
- Number of exons: 29
- Size: 1,620 amino acids with MW of 177 kDa

MOLECULAR FEATURES

Normal Functions of *ALK*

- Encodes ALK receptor tyrosine kinase
  - Member of insulin receptor superfamily
  - ALKAL1 and ALKAL2 identified as ALK ligands
- ALK receptor tyrosine kinase functions
  - Binding of ligand induces homodimerization of ALK and leads to downstream activations of 4 different pathways
    - RAS/RAF/MEK/ERK, JAK/STAT, PLC-Y, and PI3K/AKT
    - Lead to cell proliferation and mediate cell survival
  - Act early in development to help regulate proliferation of nerve cells

ALK Alterations

- Chromosomal translocations main type of *ALK* alterations
  - > 90 *ALK*-related translocations identified
  - C-terminus of ALK protein fuses with N-terminus portion of partner protein
    - ALK fusion proteins lead to ligand-independent constitutive activation of key pathways involved in oncogenesis and tumor progression
  - t(2;5)(p23;q35)/*NPM1*::*ALK* was 1st translocation involving *ALK* identified in anaplastic large cell lymphoma (ALCL) in 1994
- *ALK* gain-of-function mutations
  - Activating mutations of *ALK* are primarily seen in neuroblastomas, both familial and sporadic
  - Mutations are primarily point mutations in kinase domain of *ALK*
  - Few reports in anaplastic thyroid carcinoma and lung cancer
  - Mutations are also frequently acquired in kinase domain within *ALK* fusion gene leading to resistance to tyrosine kinase inhibitors (TKIs)
- *ALK* amplification
  - Reported in various malignancies, including neuroblastoma, non-small cell lung cancer (NSCLC), rhabdomyosarcoma

CLINICAL IMPLICATIONS

Anaplastic Large Cell Lymphoma, ALK(+)

- Translocations involving *ALK* are frequent in ALCL, ALK(+)
  - t(2;5)(p23;q35)/*NPM1*::*ALK* in ~ 75-80% of cases
  - t(1;2)(q21;p23)/*TPM3*::*ALK* in 12-18% of cases
  - Other fusions at lower frequency (< 2%) include t(2;22)(p23;q12)/*MYH9*::*ALK*, inv(2)(p23;q35)/*ATIC*::*ALK*, t(2;17)(p23;q23)/*CLTC*::*ALK*, t(2;3)(p23;q12)/*TFG*::*ALK*, and (X;2)(q12;p23)/*MSN*::*ALK*
- ALCL, ALK(+) has more favorable prognosis than ALCL, ALK(-)

Large B-Cell Lymphoma, ALK(+)

- Accounts for < 1% of diffuse large B-cell lymphoma (DLBCL) cases
- t(2;17)(p23;q23)/*CLTC*::*ALK* in ~ 70%
- t(2;5)(p23;q35)/*NPM1*::*ALK* in 10%
- Cytoplasmic granular ALK immunohistochemical staining in cases with t(2;17)/*CLTC*::*ALK*

Non-Small Cell Lung Cancer

- *ALK* rearrangement
  - ~ 2-7% of NSCLC have *ALK* rearrangement; ~ 19 different fusion partners identified, including
    - inv(2)(p21;p23)/*EML4*::*ALK*, t(2;7)(p23;q11.23)/*HIP1*::*ALK*, t(2;10)(p23;p11)/*KIF5B*::*ALK*, and t(2;14)(p23;q32)/*KLC1*::*ALK* reported

---

Domain Structure of Human *ALK*

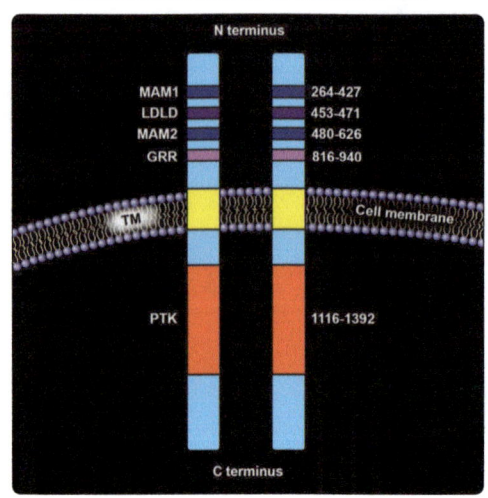

ALK Dual-Color Break-Apart FISH Assay

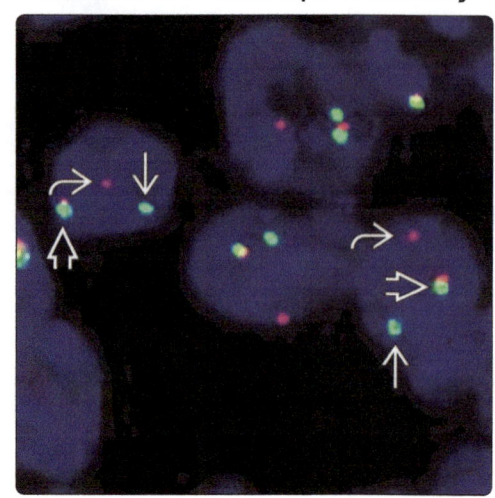

(Left) ALK is composed of an extracellular region, a transmembrane domain (TM), and an intracellular region. Protein tyrosine kinase (PTK) is in the intracellular region. MAM domain: Meprin, A5 protein and receptor protein tyrosine phosphatase mu; LDLa motif: Low-density lipoprotein class a; GRR: Glycine-rich region. **(Right)** FISH assay shows positive ALK rearrangement characterized by 1 green ➡ and 1 red ➡ fluorescent signal. Yellow signal ➡ represents intact ALK gene.

ALK Rearrangements and Mutations

- □ *EML4*::*ALK* most common *ALK* fusion type in NSCLC
- □ Multiple variants: Same cytoplasmic portion of *ALK* joins with different truncated *EML4*
  - *ALK*-rearranged NSCLC is typically seen in adenocarcinoma with signet-ring or acinar histology in nonsmokers and younger patients
  - Mutually exclusive of *EGFR* or *KRAS* mutations
  - *ALK*-rearranged NSCLC are highly sensitive to therapy with ALK TKI
  - 1st-generation ALK TKI, crizotinib, 1st targeted therapy in *ALK*-rearranged NSCLC
  - Resistance to ALK inhibitors occur due to mutations in kinase domain of *ALK* fusion gene
    – Resistance-associated variants include L1196M, F1174L, L1198F, G1202R, G1206Y, G1269A, L1152R, and C1156Y
    – 2nd-generation ALK TKIs: Ceritinib, alectinib, brigatinib, indicated for tumors with acquired resistance to crizotinib
    – 3rd-generation ALK TKI, lorlatinib, indicated for acquired resistance to earlier generation ALK TKIs
- Amplification of *ALK*
  - 10% of NSCLC show *ALK* amplification; 63% of NSCLC have *ALK* copy number gains
  - *ALK* amplification is not involved in mRNA production and protein production
    – May not play role in pathogenesis of NSCLC or indicate specific clinical application

Inflammatory Myofibroblastic Tumor
- *ALK* rearrangements reported in 36-50%
  - *TPM3*::*ALK*, *RANBP2*::*ALK*, *CARS1*::*ALK*, *TPM4*::*ALK*, *ATIC*::*ALK*, *SEC31A*::*ALK*, *CLTC*::*ALK*
- Rare cases of *ALK* amplification without *ALK* rearrangement were reported

Familial and Sporadic Neuroblastomas
- *ALK* is major familial neuroblastoma predisposition gene
- Germline and somatic activating mutations in *ALK* tyrosine kinase domain linked to hereditary and acquired neuroblastomas
  - 50% of familial neuroblastoma cases with germline mutations
    – R1275Q, G1128A, R1192P, I1250T
  - 6-12% of sporadic neuroblastomas show acquired *ALK* mutations
    – R1275Q, T1151M, I1171N, D1091N, F1174C, F1174I, F1174L, F1174V, F1245C, F1245L, F1245V, Y1278S
  - R1275Q found in both familial and sporadic neuroblastomas
- *ALK* amplification in neuroblastomas
  - ~ 23% of sporadic neuroblastomas show gain of 2p region, including *ALK* locus
  - ~ 3% show high-level focal amplification of *ALK*
  - Presence of aberrant *ALK* copy number status is highly associated with aggressive clinical phenotype

Anaplastic Thyroid Carcinoma
- ~ 10% of anaplastic thyroid carcinoma patients harbor activating mutations in *ALK*, such as L1198F, G1201E

ALK-Rearranged Renal Cell Carcinoma
- *ALK* fusions identified: *VCL*::*ALK*, *TPM3*::*ALK*, *EML4*::*ALK*, *STRN*::*ALK*, *HOOK1*::*ALK*, *PLEKHA7*::*ALK*, *CLIP1*::*ALK*, *KIF5B*::*ALK*, and *KIAA1217*::*ALK*
  - Fusion proteins constitutively drive downstream growth promoting pathways
  - *VCL*::*ALK*-affected young patients with sickle cell trait with distinctive histologic features
  - Other *ALK*-rearranged renal cell carcinomas show heterogeneous histologic features
- Some metastatic diseases show dramatic responses to ALK TKI

ALK Fusion in Colorectal Adenocarcinomas
- *ALK* fusions identified: *CAD*::*ALK*, *DIAPH2*::*ALK*, *EML4*::*ALK*, *LOC101929227*::*ALK*, *SLMAP*::*ALK*, *SPTBN1*::*ALK*, and *STRN*::*ALK*
- Rare (< 1% of colorectal adenocarcinomas)

TESTING FOR *ALK* ALTERATIONS

Fluorescence In Situ Hybridization
- Dual-color break-apart probe strategy
- Red and green signals become separated if rearrangement present
- Detects virtually all *ALK* rearrangements
- Cannot identify *ALK* fusion partner, but knowing partner is usually not clinically relevant
- Recommend by CAP/IASLC/AMP guideline to determine eligibility for ALK inhibitors

Next-Generation Sequencing
- *ALK* rearrangements can be detected by NGS
  - Commonly included in commercially available NGS panels
  - Widely used in molecular diagnostics laboratories
- Activating point mutations in *ALK* can be detected by NGS with broad coverage

Immunohistochemistry
- Equivalent alternative to FISH for *ALK* testing for targeted therapy in NSCLC, recommended in CAP/IASLC/AMP guideline
  - Strong granular cytoplasmic staining ± membrane accentuation
  - Ventana ALK (D5F3) CDx assay, FDA-approved diagnostics
- Commonly used for diagnostic purposes for ALCL, ALK(+), inflammatory myofibroblastic tumor, and *ALK*(+) large B-cell lymphoma

SELECTED REFERENCES

1. Cooper AJ et al: Third-generation EGFR and ALK inhibitors: mechanisms of resistance and management. Nat Rev Clin Oncol. 19(8):499-514, 2022
2. Tan AC et al: Targeted therapies for lung cancer patients with oncogenic driver molecular alterations. J Clin Oncol. 40(6):611-25, 2022
3. Reshetnyak AV et al: Mechanism for the activation of the anaplastic lymphoma kinase receptor. Nature. 600(7887):153-7, 2021
4. Trpkov K et al: Novel, emerging and provisional renal entities: the Genitourinary Pathology Society (GUPS) update on renal neoplasia. Mod Pathol. 34(6):1167-84, 2021
5. Lasota J et al: Colorectal adenocarcinomas harboring ALK fusion genes: a clinicopathologic and molecular genetic study of 12 cases and review of the literature. Am J Surg Pathol. 44(9):1224-34, 2020

ROS1 Rearrangements

TERMINOLOGY

Definitions

- Official name: ROS protooncogene 1, receptor tyrosine kinase
- Official symbol: *ROS1*
- HGNC ID: 10261
- Gene locus: 6q22.1
- Genomic position
  - Ch6: 117,287,353-117,425,942 (GRCh38.p14)
- RefSeq: NG_033929.1
- Number of exons: 46
- Size: 137.9 kb

ETIOLOGY/PATHOGENESIS

Normal Function of *ROS1*

- Encodes cell surface receptor tyrosine kinase
  - Insulin receptor subfamily
- "Orphan receptor" without known ligand
- Activation gives rise to signaling through multiple pathways, including MAPK and PI3K
  - Also leads to modification of cytoskeletal proteins
- Mice without *ROS1* are healthy, though males are infertile

Abnormal Function of *ROS1* Fusion Gene

- *ROS1* rearrangement leads to fusion gene
  - Joins C-terminal (intracellular tyrosine kinase domain) of *ROS1* to N-terminal portion of partner gene
    - ROS1 tyrosine kinase domain is entirely retained in fusion protein
    - *ROS1* breakpoints occur 5' to exons 32, 34, 35, or 36
  - Partner genes include
    - *SLC34A2, CD74, EZR, TPM3, SDC4, GOPC, TFG, YWHAE, LIMA1, MSN, LRIG3, KDELR2, CCDC6, CEP85L, TMEM106B, TPD52L1, CLTC, SLC6A17, CEP72, ZCCHC8, SLMAP, WNK1, KMT2C,* and *RBPMS*
  - Activates ROS1 signaling in absence of ligand, leading to tumor cell growth and proliferation

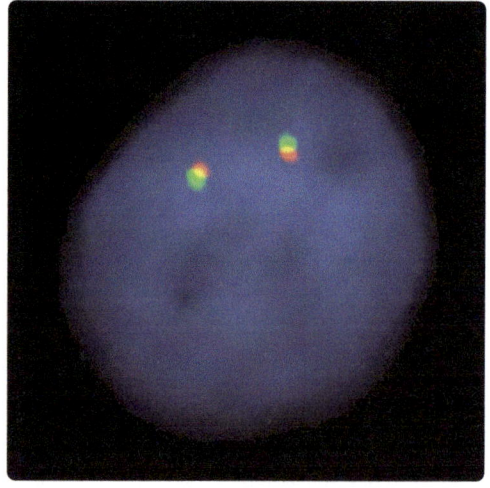

(Left) This case of lung adenocarcinoma is positive for ROS1 rearrangement using dual-color, break-apart FISH probes, as indicated by the separate red and green signals ➔ in each cell. **(Right)** In this case, there is no evidence of ROS1 rearrangement using dual-color, break-apart FISH probes. ROS1 FISH is performed to identify cases sensitive to crizotinib therapy.

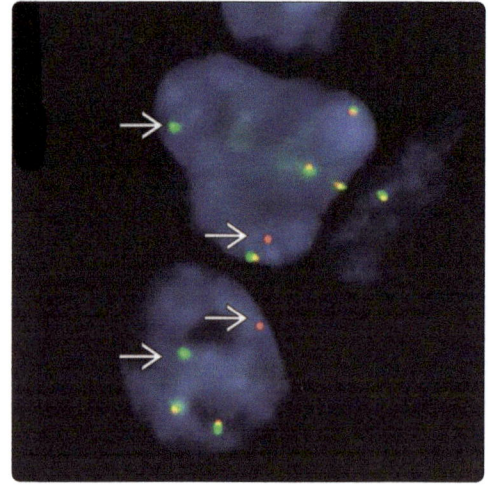

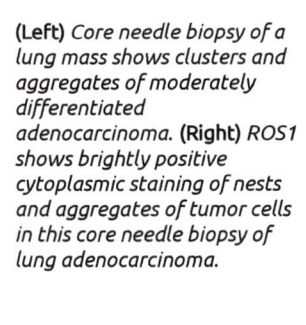

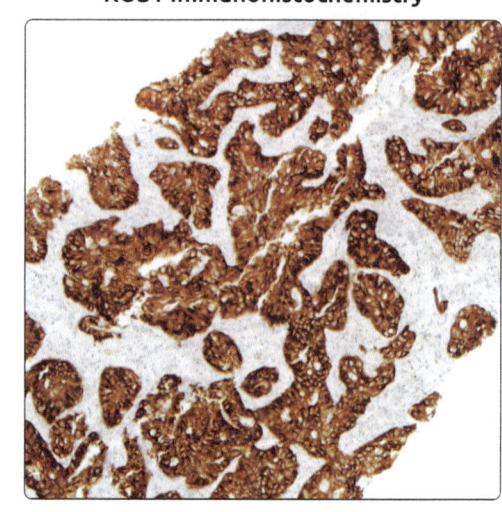

(Left) Core needle biopsy of a lung mass shows clusters and aggregates of moderately differentiated adenocarcinoma. **(Right)** ROS1 shows brightly positive cytoplasmic staining of nests and aggregates of tumor cells in this core needle biopsy of lung adenocarcinoma.

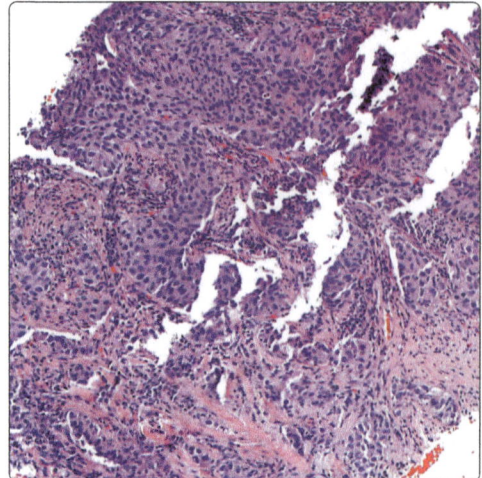

ROS1 Rearrangements

CLINICAL IMPLICATIONS

ROS1 Fusion Genes in Non-Small Cell Lung Cancer
- ROS1 rearrangements are driver oncogenic events
- Occur in ~ 1-2% of non-small cell lung cancer (NSCLC)
  - Generally mutually exclusive with other major driver mutations in NSCLC, such as ALK rearrangement
    - However, rare cases with concomitant ROS1 rearrangement and EGFR mutation have been reported
- More common in
  - Female patients
  - Young patients
  - Never smokers
  - Adenocarcinoma histology
- Epidemiologic distribution is similar to that of ALK-rearranged NSCLC
- In absence of targeted therapy, no inherent survival difference between ROS1-positive and ROS1-negative NSCLC

ROS1 Fusion Genes in Other Malignancies
- ROS1 fusions were 1st identified in glioblastoma cell line
- CEP85L::ROS1 fusion is subsequently reported in adult patients with glioblastoma
- ROS1 fusions have also been documented in
  - Cholangiocarcinoma
  - Inflammatory myofibroblastic tumor
  - Gastric adenocarcinoma
  - Ovarian tumor of low malignant potential
  - Angiosarcoma
  - Colorectal carcinoma
  - Epithelioid hemangioendothelioma
  - Spitzoid melanoma

Targeted Therapy for ROS1
- Crizotinib
  - Efficacy and safety were demonstrated in phase 1 crizotinib study
    - Objective response rate of 72%
    - Median progression-free survival of ~ 19 months
  - Approved by FDA in 2016 for ROS1-rearranged NSCLC
  - Resistance to crizotinib develops in subset of ROS1-rearranged cases
    - Results in disease progression on therapy
    - ROS1 G2032R variant is most common resistance-associated mutation
    - Other crizotinib resistance mutations include
      - D2033N, L2155S, S1986Y/F, L2026M, L1951R, and G2101A
- Inhibitors with potential activity against crizotinib resistance mutations
  - Lorlatinib is highly potent inhibitor with robust CNS penetration and in vitro activity against several crizotinib-resistant mutations
  - Cabozantinib is multitargeted tyrosine kinase inhibitor with activity against ROS1 resistance mutations, including G2032R and D2033N
  - Ceritinib has activity against L2026M resistance mutation but not G2032R or D2033N mutations
  - Brigatinib has in vitro activity against L2026M but not other resistance-associated mutations

Testing for ROS1 Fusion
- RT-PCR
  - Can be challenging due to large number of partner genes, each of which would necessitate additional primers
- ROS1 IHC
  - Effective screening tool with high sensitivity and variable specificity
  - Great advantage over FISH in samples with paucity of tumor cells or abundance of nonneoplastic cells
  - Cost-effective method for screening of lung cancer samples for ROS1 rearrangements
  - Weak expression may be seen in nonneoplastic type II pneumocytes and alveolar macrophages
  - Confirmation of IHC-positive and indeterminate cases by FISH or molecular methods is recommended
- Next-generation sequencing
  - Possible role for fusion gene detection but evolving in application to clinical practice
- FISH
  - Simple and straightforward approach to identifying ROS1 rearrangement
    - Used to determine eligibility for ROS1-targeted therapy
  - Break-apart probe strategy
    - Red and green signals straddle ROS1 breakpoints
    - If rearrangement occurs, red and green signals become separated
    - Does not identify partner gene, but this information has no established clinical relevance

ROS1 Point Mutations
- Acquired crizotinib resistance mutations in ROS1 may be seen (e.g., G2032R, L2155S)
- In addition, ROS1 mutations are seen in other tumors, including melanoma, colorectal carcinoma, endometrial carcinoma, and gastric carcinoma
  - Functional significance of these mutations is unknown
- Direct sequencing analysis, not FISH, would be necessary to detect these point mutations

SELECTED REFERENCES

1. Begum P et al: Crizotinib-resistant ROS1 G2101A mutation associated with sensitivity to lorlatinib in ROS1-rearranged NSCLC: case report. JTO Clin Res Rep. 3(9):100376, 2022
2. Gendarme S et al: ROS-1 fusions in non-small-cell lung cancer: evidence to date. Curr Oncol. 29(2):641-58, 2022
3. Ou SI et al: A catalog of 5' fusion partners in ROS1-positive NSCLC circa 2020. JTO Clin Res Rep. 1(3):100048, 2020
4. Sehgal K et al: Targeting ROS1 rearrangements in non-small cell lung cancer with crizotinib and other kinase inhibitors. Transl Cancer Res. 7(Suppl 7):S779-86, 2018
5. Sgambato A et al: Targeted therapies in non-small cell lung cancer: a focus on ALK/ROS1 tyrosine kinase inhibitors. Expert Rev Anticancer Ther. 18(1):71-80, 2018
6. Lin JJ et al: ROS1 Fusions rarely overlap with other oncogenic drivers in non-small cell lung cancer. J Thorac Oncol. 12(5):872-7, 2017
7. Lin JJ et al: Recent advances in targeting ROS1 in lung cancer. J Thorac Oncol. 12(11):1611-25, 2017
8. Bubendorf L et al: Testing for ROS1 in non-small cell lung cancer: a review with recommendations. Virchows Arch. 469(5):489-503, 2016

RET Rearrangements

TERMINOLOGY

Definitions
- Official name: Ret protooncogene
  - RET stands for "rearranged during transfection"
- Official symbol: RET
- HGNC ID: 9967
- Gene locus: 10q11.21
  - Chr10: 43,077,069-43,130,351 (GRCh38.p14)
- Number of exons: 20

ETIOLOGY/PATHOGENESIS

Normal Function of RET
- Encodes transmembrane receptor tyrosine kinase
  - Activates MAPK- and AKT-signaling pathways; important for cell differentiation, growth, migration, and survival
  - Receptor for glial cell-derived neurotrophic factor family ligands
    - Glial-derived neurotrophic factor (GDNF)
    - Neurturin (NRTN)
    - Artemin (ARTN)
    - Persephin (PSPN)
  - Ligand binding stimulates receptor dimerization, transphosphorylation of kinase domains, and activation of signaling
- Important in development of nervous system, intestine, kidneys, and organs derived from neural crest
- Required for survival and proliferation of undifferentiated spermatogonia
- Isoforms generated by alternative 3' splicing may exert different cellular effects

Abnormal Function of RET Fusion Gene
- Somatic rearrangements involve 3' region of RET, including tyrosine kinase domain and 5' region of partner genes
  - RET breakpoints commonly involve intron 11, less often introns 7 and 10
  - > 35 partner genes described
- Downstream pathway activation via multiple means, including ligand-independent activation of RET kinase, increased expression of RET, or altered fusion partner function
- RET fusions and MAPK-signaling pathway alterations are mutually exclusive

CLINICAL IMPLICATIONS

RET Rearrangements in Non-Small Cell Lung Cancer
- ~ 1-2% incidence in non-small cell lung cancer (NSCLC), particularly adenocarcinoma
- Common RET fusion partner genes
  - KIF5B
  - NCOA4
  - CCDC6
- Associated with responsiveness to oral RET tyrosine kinase inhibitor therapy, regardless of fusion partner
- Rearrangement correlates with never-smoking status, younger age, more advanced disease stage, and coexistence of other genomic alterations
- RET rearrangements are mutually exclusive with mutations in other major driver oncogenes, including ALK, EGFR, and KRAS
- Mechanism of acquired resistance to EGFR small molecule inhibitors therapy

RET Rearrangements in Papillary Thyroid Carcinoma
- Incidence of RET rearrangement is 10-20% in papillary thyroid carcinoma
  - Incidence may be higher if more sensitive detection techniques are used
  - Studies show significant geographic variation
  - Mutually exclusive with BRAF, HRAS, NRAS, and KRAS mutations
- Common RET partner genes in papillary thyroid carcinoma
  - CCDC6
  - NCOA4
- Less common RET partner fusion gene in papillary thyroid carcinoma
  - PRKAR1A

FISH Positive for RET Rearrangement

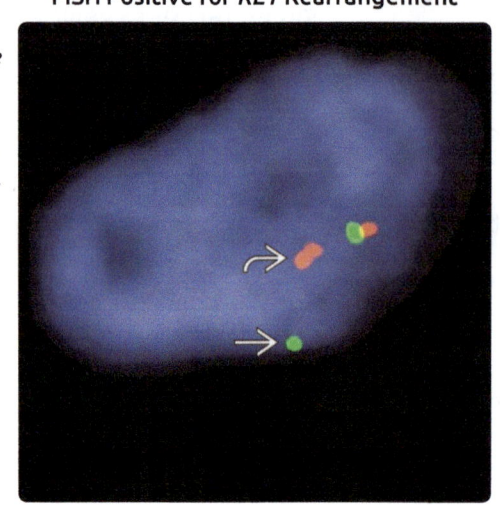

FISH Negative for RET Rearrangement

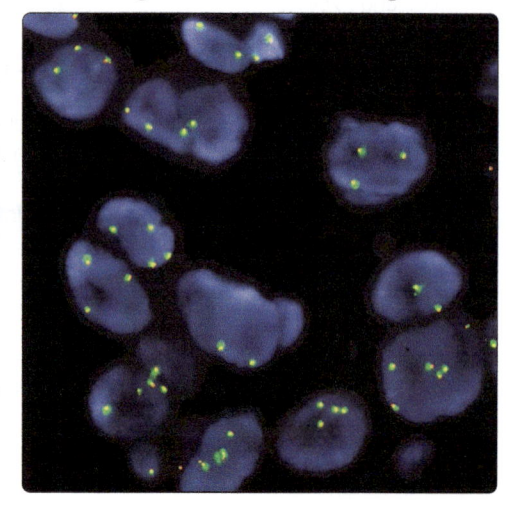

(Left) FISH with dual-color break-apart probes in this case of lung adenocarcinoma shows a rearrangement of RET, as indicated by the separate red ➔ and green ➔ signals. (Right) FISH with dual-color break-apart probes in this case of lung adenocarcinoma shows no evidence of RET rearrangement. Note that extra copies of the RET locus are present, though no rearrangement is seen.

RET Rearrangements

Selected RET Fusion Partner Genes in Non-Small Cell Lung Cancer and Papillary Thyroid Cancer

Non-Small Cell Lung Cancer	Papillary Thyroid Cancer
CCDC6	CCDC6 (PTC1)
CUX1	PRKAR1A (PTC2)
EML4	NCOA4 (PTC3, fused to exon 12 of RET)
ERC1	NCOA4 (PTC4, fused to exon 11 of RET)
KIAA1217	GOLGA5 (PTC5)
RELCH (KIAA1468)	TRIM24 (PTC6)
KIF5B	TRIM33 (PTC7)
NCOA4	KTN1 (PTC8)
PARD3	RELCH (PTC9)
PRKAR1A	ERC1 (PTC10)
TRIM33	HOOK3, PCM1, TRIM27, and others have also been described

Partner genes were originally identified in context of papillary thyroid carcinoma, and these fusions were often designated as RET::PTC.

- RET rearrangements in papillary thyroid carcinoma have strong association with radiation exposure
- Impact on prognosis is controversial and may depend on specific partner gene
- Detection of RET rearrangement can assist in diagnosis
- Selpercatinib or pralsetinib are FDA-approved targeted inhibitors

RET Fusion Genes Reported in Other Malignancies

- Salivary gland intraductal carcinoma (~ 47% of cases)
- Lung carcinosarcoma (~ 15% of cases)
- Spitz tumors and spitzoid melanoma
- Breast cancer (~ 0.2% of cases)
- Secondary acute myeloid leukemia

Testing for RET Fusion

- Next-generation sequencing (NGS)
  - RNA-based NGS can detect fusions with high specificity
  - More efficient than single-target assays for fusion gene detection
  - NGS may also permit determination of fusion partner gene and sequence alterations
- FISH
  - Commonly use break-apart probe strategy
    - Red and green signals straddle RET breakpoints
    - If rearrangement occurs, red and green signals become separated
    - Does not identify fusion partner gene
  - May underdetect some fusions
- Targeted RT-PCR
  - Detection limited to utilized primers
    - Fusion partners that have developed primers may be identified
    - Will not detect fusions with novel partners
- Immunohistochemistry
  - RET protein overexpressed by IHC in many RET-rearranged cases but unreliable for rearrangement detection

RET Mutations

- Direct sequencing is necessary to detect sequence alterations
- Germline RET mutations
  - Activating mutations cause multiple endocrine neoplasia (MEN) types 2A, 2B, and familial medullary thyroid carcinoma
    - Typically gain-of-function point mutations
  - Loss-of-function mutations cause Hirschsprung disease
- Somatic RET mutations
  - Common in sporadic medullary thyroid carcinoma

Targeted Therapies

- Multikinase inhibitors with RET activity explored in tumors with activating RET alterations
  - Modest efficacy but many off-target adverse effects (rash, hypertension, diarrhea)
- Selective RET inhibitors (pralsetinib and selpercatinib) now available
  - May have improved efficacy and more favorable toxicity profile

SELECTED REFERENCES

1. Regua AT et al: RET signaling pathway and RET inhibitors in human cancer. Front Oncol. 12:932353, 2022
2. Wang C et al: RET fusions as primary oncogenic drivers and secondary acquired resistance to EGFR tyrosine kinase inhibitors in patients with non-small-cell lung cancer. J Transl Med. 20(1):390, 2022
3. Santoro M et al: RET gene fusions in malignancies of the thyroid and other tissues. Genes (Basel). 11(4):424, 2020
4. Ferrara R et al: Clinical and translational implications of RET rearrangements in non-small cell lung cancer. J Thorac Oncol. 13(1):27-45, 2018
5. Kato S et al: RET aberrations in diverse cancers: next-generation sequencing of 4,871 patients. Clin Cancer Res. 23(8):1988-97, 2017
6. Sabari JK et al: Targeting RET-rearranged lung cancers with multikinase inhibitors. Oncoscience. 4(3-4):23-4, 2017
7. Lee MS et al: Identification of a novel partner gene, KIAA1217, fused to RET: functional characterization and inhibitor sensitivity of two isoforms in lung adenocarcinoma. Oncotarget. 7(24):36101-14, 2016
8. Ou SH et al: Will the requirement by the US FDA to simultaneously co-develop companion diagnostics (CDx) delay the approval of receptor tyrosine kinase inhibitors for RTK-rearranged (ROS1-, RET-, AXL-, PDGFR-α-, NTRK1-) non-small cell lung cancer globally? Front Oncol. 4:58, 2014

FISH for *MET* Amplifications

TERMINOLOGY

Definitions
- Official name: *MET* protooncogene, receptor tyrosine kinase
- HGNC ID: 7029
- Chromosomal location: 7q31.2
- Number of exons: 22
- Preferred protein name: Hepatocyte growth factor receptor

ETIOLOGY/PATHOGENESIS

MET Protooncogene
- Widely expressed throughout variety of tissue types
  - Most highly expressed in liver and placenta
  - Expressed primarily in epithelial cells
- Dimeric receptor tyrosine kinase
  - Gene produces single-chain precursor protein
  - Precursor is cleaved to produce short α-chain and longer β-chain
    - 2 chains form disulfide-linked heterodimer
    - α-chain is extracellular and includes semaphorin (sema) ligand-binding domain
    - β-chain is transmembrane and cytoplasmic and includes inhibitory juxtamembrane region that inhibits MET kinase activity and leads to receptor degradation, intracellular tyrosine kinase domain, and docking site that recruits downstream signaling pathways
  - Binds hepatocyte growth factor (HGF)
    - HGF is paracrine growth factor with effects on many cell types, including epithelial cells, endothelial cells, and hematopoietic cells
    - HGF binding causes dimerization and phosphorylation of tyrosine kinase domain
- Signaling pathways activated following HGF binding
  - PI3K/Akt pathway
    - Important for cell spreading and motility
  - RA/MAP kinase pathway
    - Controls cell proliferation and motility
  - STAT and NF-κB pathway
    - Induces MET-dependent formation of branched tubules
- Signaling cascades lead to invasive growth program
  - Cells dissociate and become motile, stimulating migration
  - Cells invade new environment
  - Cells proliferate and stimulate angiogenesis
  - Cells form branched tubule structures
  - Apoptosis is inhibited throughout this process
- Signaling is important part of embryological development
  - Plays role in gastrulation, epithelial morphogenesis, angiogenesis, myoblast migration, bone remodeling, and nerve sprouting
- Signaling is normal in wound healing in adulthood
  - Leads to cell proliferation and migration to edges of wounds to regenerate damaged tissue
  - HGF (ligand) expression is upregulated by interleukin-1 and interleukin-6 cytokines
- MET expression is increased following liver, kidney, or heart injury
  - Plays role in liver regeneration

Aberrant MET Signaling
- Overexpression
  - Can occur through *MET* amplification or epigenetic changes
    - Significance of overexpression in absence of amplification is not clear
  - Can also occur through multiple copies (polysomy) of chromosome 7
  - MET overexpression leads to increased signaling and tumorigenesis and metastasis
    - Activation in carcinomas usually occurs in paracrine fashion
    - Tumors with overexpression of MET also show ligand-independent activation of tyrosine kinase
- *MET* mutations
  - Missense mutations in kinase, juxtamembrane, and ligand-binding domains have been identified

Non-Small Cell Lung Carcinoma

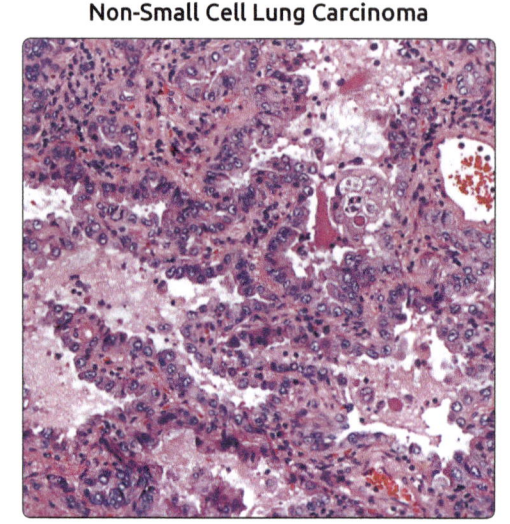

FISH for *MET*

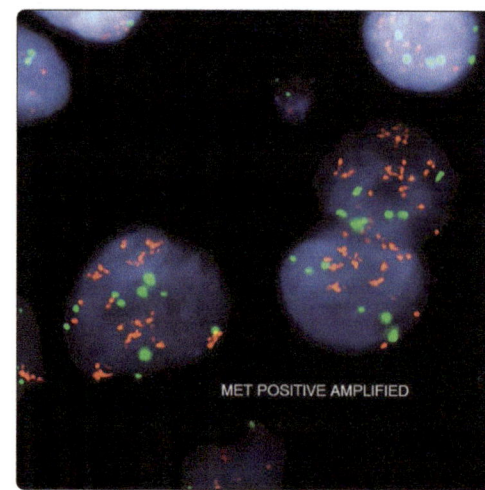

(Left) Excisional biopsy of a lung mass shows involvement by non-small cell lung carcinoma (NSCLC). EGFR mutation analysis was negative, and FISH showed no rearrangements of ALK or ROS1. (Right) FISH for MET shows a MET signal (red) to chromosome 7 centromere signal (green) ratio of > 2, consistent with MET amplification in NSCLC. The tumor responded to MET inhibitor.

FISH for *MET* Amplifications

- Germline mutations in ligand-binding (sema) domain have been described
- Lung tumors tend to include mutations in extracellular and juxtamembrane domains
- Other tumors more commonly include mutations in kinase domain
  o May lead to MET autophosphorylation and constitutive activation of signaling cascades
  o May be tested for, particularly as part of next-generation sequencing panels
- *MET* exon 14 skipping mutations
  o Alterations leading to aberrant splicing with exon 14 skipping
    - Exon 14 includes juxtamembrane domain
  o Occur in cases ± *MET* overexpression
  o Decreased ubiquitination and protein degradation
    - Leads to increased signaling
- *MET* translocations
  o Unusual finding in lung cancer
  o Clinical significance is unclear
- Constitutive kinase activation
  o Increases autocrine or paracrine HGF stimulation

CLINICAL IMPLICATIONS

MET Overexpression in Tumors

- *MET* originally identified in human osteosarcoma cell line
- Overexpression described in many neoplasms, including pancreas, lung, liver, and gastric carcinomas; leiomyosarcoma and osteosarcoma; glioblastoma; and hematologic malignancies, such as multiple myeloma and acute myeloid leukemia
  o MET protein overexpression correlates with poor prognosis in many tumor types
    - Plays role in metastasis and shows greater expression in metastatic than in primary lesions
- Role of *MET* in lung cancer tumorigenesis is well described
  o Can be primary oncogenic driver mutation or occur later in tumor development
  o Mice given MET inhibitors and exposed to tobacco smoke develop fewer lung tumors
  o MET expression is greatest along invasive front of non-small cell lung cancer (NSCLC)
  o 1-6% of NSCLC shows *MET* amplification
    - Average copy number is higher in squamous cell cancers
    - Very high copy number correlates with high-grade tumors
  o 3-4% of NSCLC show *MET* exon 14 skipping mutations
- *MET* amplification
  o Occurs secondary to treatment with anti-EGFR tyrosine kinase inhibitors (TKIs)
    - Patients with resistance to EGFR inhibitors are more likely to have *MET* amplification than those with EGFR inhibitor-sensitive tumors
    - 15-20% of patients with resistance to EGFR inhibitors have *MET* amplification
    - *MET* amplification leads to EGFR-independent activation of PI3K/AKT pathway
  o *MET* amplification is independent predictive factor of poor outcomes in lung cancer
    - Correlates with high-grade and advanced stage of disease
    - Event-free survival in *MET*-amplified cases is 25.8-38.0 months, compared to 47.5-51.0 months in wildtype cases, irrespective of grade and stage
    - Correlates with greater numbers of metastatic sites than nonamplified cases
    - Increased MET activity has also been associated with more aggressive disease in prostate, breast, gastroesophageal, and renal tumors
- *MET* amplification can be sole abnormality or may occur in association with other oncogene mutations
  o Mutations in *KRAS* and *EGFR* can be present
  o Higher prevalence of *BRAF* mutation and *PTEN* loss compared to non-*MET*-amplified tumors

MET Amplification and Chemotherapy

- *MET* amplification testing is primarily performed in NSCLC
  o Lung cancer is leading cause of cancer-related death in USA
  o Median survival with standard 1st-line chemotherapy is 10 months
    - Targeted therapies are sought to improve outcomes
- Targeted anti-MET chemotherapeutic agents have been developed primarily for NSCLC
- Tumors with *MET* alterations are sensitive to MET inhibitors
  o 29% overall response in patients with *MET* amplification
  o 41% overall response in patients with exon 14 skipping mutations
  o Selective MET TKIs
    - Decrease MET phosphorylation and downstream signaling
    - Decrease vascular growth factors and lead to decreased angiogenesis
    - Increased apoptosis of tumor cells and decrease of premalignant lesions also occur
    - Treated tumors show inhibition of growth
    - Phase II clinical trials show significant increase in progression-free survival (PFS) and overall survival (OS) in patients treated with anti-MET TKI tivantinib combined with erlotinib
    - Phase III trial showed improvement of PFS but not OS in random patients; however, OS may be improved in patients with MET-amplified tumors
    - ALK inhibitor crizotinib also shows activity as MET inhibitor
  o MET inhibitors in combination with other chemotherapeutic agents
    - Greater effects in combination with other chemotherapeutic agents
    - Synergistic effect with anti-EGFR TKIs
    - MET inhibitors can restore sensitivity to anti-EGFR TKIs
    - Inhibition of both MET and EGFR leads to improved clinical outcomes
    - Additive effect with ALK and VEGFA inhibitors
    - Combination regimens show increased inhibition of tumor growth
  o Acquired resistance during therapy with MET inhibitors
    - May result from resistance-associated point mutation in tyrosine kinase domain

FISH for *MET* Amplifications

- May also result from TGF-α overexpression that can activate alternate EGFR signaling pathways
  - Anti-HGF monoclonal antibodies
    - Currently in phase I/II clinical trials
  - Anti-HGFR antibodies
    - Blocks ligand binding and prevents receptor dimerization
    - Currently in phases II and III clinical trials

TESTING FOR *MET* AMPLIFICATION

Lung Cancer Testing Algorithms

- *MET* amplification is usually performed as part of series or panel of molecular and genetic tests in NSCLC
  - *EGFR* exon 18-21 mutation testing is priority
  - *ALK* rearrangement by FISH as reflex test in *EGFR* wildtype cases
  - *ROS1* fusions in cases with wildtype *EGFR* and no *ALK* rearrangement
  - *RET* fusion FISH assay typically performed in cases with wildtype *EGFR* and no rearrangement of *ALK* or *ROS1*
  - *KRAS* mutation is mutually exclusive of *EGFR* mutation and *ALK* rearrangements in most cases
  - *BRAF* mutation is rare in NSCLC
  - *ERBB2* (HER2) mutations and amplification occur in NSCLC with low frequency
  - Other gene alterations may occur in NSCLC

FISH for *MET* Amplification

- Preferred testing modality
  - NGS approaches often less sensitive
- Performed on formalin-fixed, paraffin-embedded tissue
- Utilizes 2 probes
  - 1 probe covering entire *MET* locus at 7q31.2
    - Marker of *MET* copy number
  - 1 additional hybridizes to α-satellite DNA at centromere of chromosome 7 (CEP7)
    - Marker of chromosome 7 aneusomy
- Number of signals for each probe per cell is counted
  - Absolute number of *MET* signals per cell is recorded
  - Number of *MET* signals in relation to CEP7 signals is recorded
  - Amplification, identified by increased *MET* signals, may be focal or patchy within tumor
- Interpretation of *MET* FISH results
  - Not well standardized
  - Cells with normal numbers of chromosome 7 and *MET* will show 2 signals for each probe
  - Ratio of *MET* signals to CEP7 signals of ≥ 2 is defined as positive for *MET* amplification
    - Ratios between 1.8 and 2.0 should be interpreted with caution
    - Additional cells may be counted in these cases
  - In general, average of ≥ 5 *MET* signals per cell is present in *MET*-amplified cases
    - Patients with mean *MET* copy number per cell > 5 have worse survival outcomes
    - Some centers use higher cut-off
  - Ratio may correlate better with poor prognosis than mean *MET* copy number

Other Methods

- Comparative genomic hybridization
  - Not cost effective compared to FISH analysis
- PCR
  - Can offer qualitative as well as quantitative results for gene copy number
  - Difficult to isolate pure tumor specimens
  - Results are affected by intermixed normal epithelial cells, inflammatory cells, and fibroblasts
  - Can identify mutations and exon 14 skipping alterations
- IHC
  - Anti-MET monoclonal antibodies are available
  - Evaluates MET protein expression
  - Correlates well with FISH results
    - Protein overexpression is highly associated with high-level amplification
    - Intermediate protein expression shows weaker correlation with amplification results
  - Correlation with clinical outcomes not well established

PREDICTIVE CANCER TESTING SUMMARY

Test Interpretation

- *MET*:CEP7 ratio < 2: Nonamplified
- *MET*:CEP7 ratio ≥ 2: Amplified
- Average number of *MET* signals < 5: Nonamplified
- Average number of *MET* signals ≥ 5: Amplified

Treatment Implications

- Tumors with *MET* amplification show increased sensitivity to TKIs with activity against MET protein, such as crizotinib and MET-specific TKIs
  - *MET* amplification is also associated with resistance to EGFR inhibitors
- Absence of *MET* amplification provides no evidence of increased sensitivity to MET inhibitors

SELECTED REFERENCES

1. Al Jaberi M et al: Latest updates on MET targeted therapy for EXON 14 mutations in lung cancer. Oncotarget. 14:514, 2023
2. Brea E et al: Targeted therapy for non-small cell lung cancer: first line and beyond. Hematol Oncol Clin North Am. 37(3):575-94, 2023
3. Ding C et al: Clinicopathological characteristics of non-small cell lung cancer (NSCLC) patients with c-MET exon 14 skipping mutation, MET overexpression and amplification. BMC Pulm Med. 23(1):240, 2023
4. Heydt C et al: Overview of molecular detection technologies for MET in lung cancer. Cancers (Basel). 15(11):2932, 2023
5. Mazieres J et al: MET exon 14 skipping in NSCLC: a systematic literature review of epidemiology, clinical characteristics, and outcomes. Clin Lung Cancer. 24(6):483-97, 2023
6. Spagnolo CC et al: Targeting MET in non-small cell lung cancer (NSCLC): a new old story? Int J Mol Sci. 24(12):10119, 2023
7. Michaels E et al: Meeting an un-MET need: targeting MET in non-small cell lung cancer. Front Oncol. 12:1004198, 2022
8. Socinski MA et al: MET exon 14 skipping mutations in non-small-cell lung cancer: an overview of biology, clinical outcomes, and testing considerations. JCO Precis Oncol. 5, 2021
9. Wolf J et al: Capmatinib in MET exon 14-mutated or MET-amplified non-small-cell lung cancer. N Engl J Med. 383(10):944-57, 2020
10. Fang L et al: MET amplification assessed using optimized FISH reporting criteria predicts early distant metastasis in patients with non-small cell lung cancer. Oncotarget. 9(16):12959-70, 2018
11. Drilon A et al: Targeting MET in lung cancer: will expectations finally be MET? J Thorac Oncol. 12(1):15-26, 2017

FISH for *MET* Amplifications

Ample Tumor Burden for Testing

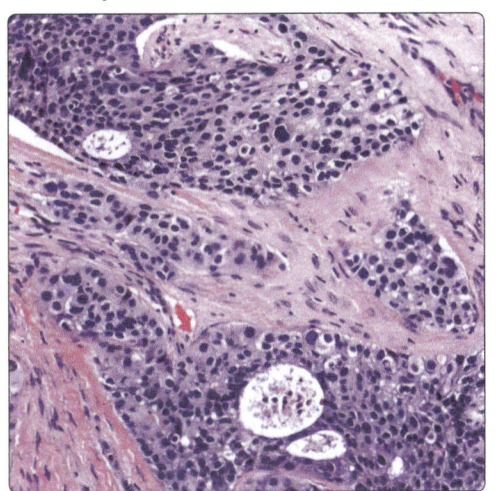

Adenocarcinoma

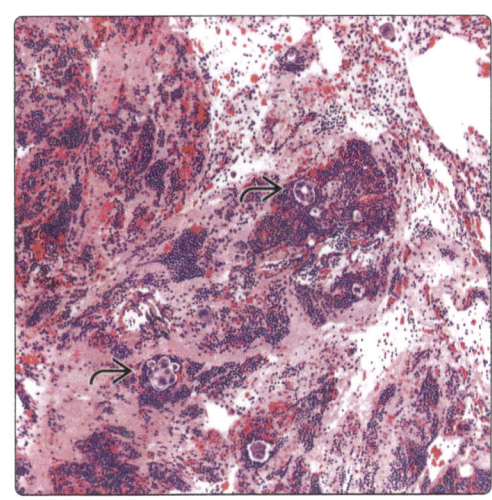

(Left) Lung biopsy specimen shows ample tumor burden for testing for MET amplification by FISH. (Right) Although this FNA cell block of a pleural effusion is clearly diagnostic for adenocarcinoma ⇨, there are significant numbers of admixed inflammatory cells. FISH for MET may still be used, as the tumor cells are large enough for easy identification by fluorescent microscopy.

Positive FISH for *MET*

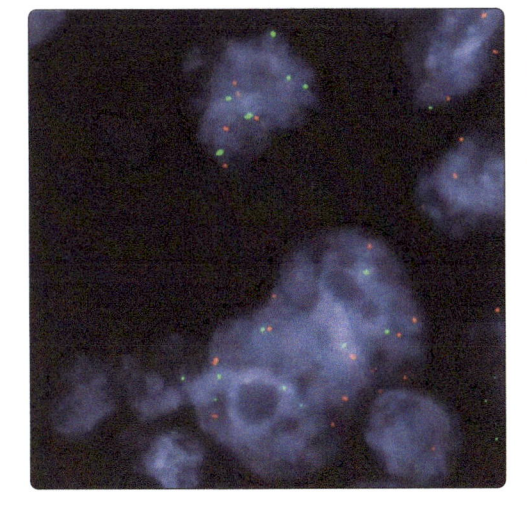

Negative FISH for *MET*

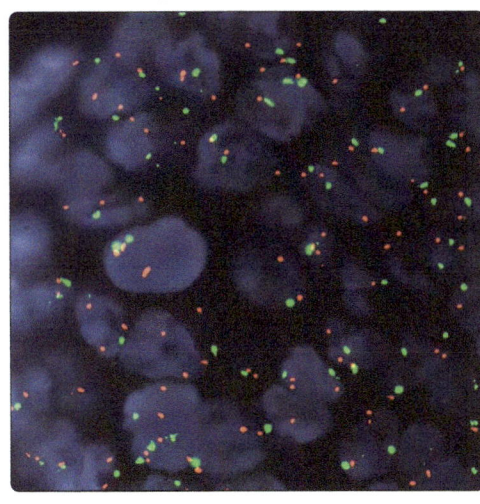

(Left) FISH for MET (red) and centromere of chromosome 7 (green) is positive for MET amplification in this case of lung adenocarcinoma with > 5 copies of MET signals per neoplastic cell. (Right) FISH performed on lung NSCLC is negative for MET amplification. There is an average of 2 signals for MET (red) and 2 signals for centromere of chromosome 7 (green) per cell.

Chromosome 7

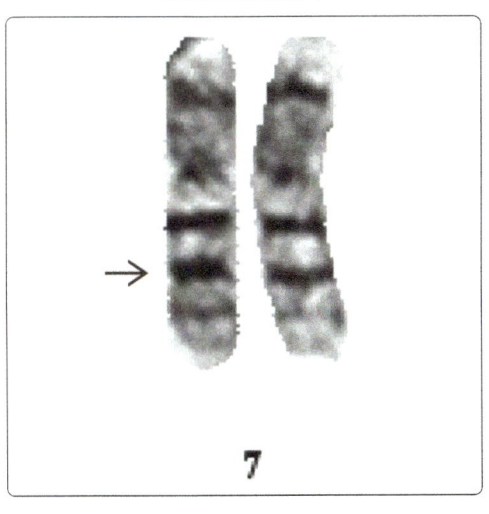

Metaphase FISH for *MET*

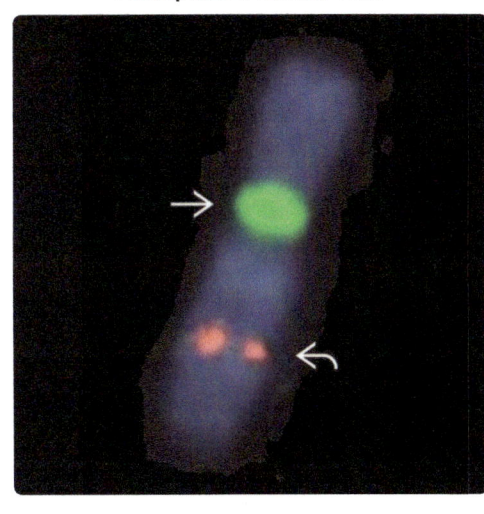

(Left) Partial karyogram shows chromosome 7 with MET location at 7q31.2 ⇨. (Right) Metaphase FISH shows green centromeric probe ⇨ and red MET probe ⇨ located at 7q31.2. Most commercial FISH probes for MET span a 270- to 450-kb area around MET. There is no evidence for MET amplification in this metaphase FISH analysis.

FISH for *ERBB2* (HER2) Amplifications

TERMINOLOGY

Definitions
- Official name: erb-b2 receptor tyrosine kinase 2
  - a.k.a. HER2
    - Terminology used extensively and interchangeably
- Official symbol: *ERBB2*

EPIDEMIOLOGY

Incidence
- *ERBB2* amplification in breast cancer
  - ~ 30% of invasive breast cancer
  - Correlates with poor prognosis
  - Important to evaluate for anti-ERBB2 therapy
- Other malignancies with *ERBB2* amplifications
  - Gastric and gastroesophageal carcinoma (9-38%), colorectal cancer (~ 3% and 5-15% in RAS/RAF-negative tumors), gallbladder (5-10%), cholangiocarcinoma (5-15%), uterine serous carcinoma (25-30%), invasive bladder cancer (~ 9%)

ETIOLOGY/PATHOGENESIS

Normal *ERBB2* Function
- Part of epidermal growth factor receptor (EGFR) family
- Tyrosine kinase receptor involved in growth signaling
- No known ligand-binding domain of its own
  - Binds to other EGFR family members to form heterodimer

Overexpression of *ERBB2* in Cancer
- Usually result of gene amplification
- Can lead to oncogenic transformation

CLINICAL IMPLICATIONS

Treatment
- Patients with amplified *ERBB2* or 3+ IHC-positive tumors can benefit from *ERBB2*-targeted specific therapies
  - Trastuzumab (Herceptin)
    - Monoclonal antibody against *ERBB2*
    - Significantly improves outcome in *ERBB2*(+) cancers
- New indication for trastuzumab-deruxtecan
  - Based on DESTINY-Breast04 phase III trial
  - Patients with nonamplified *ERBB2* by FISH and 1+ or 2+ IHC-positive breast cancer treated with trastuzumab-deruxtecan showed significant improvement in survival
  - Patients with IHC 0 score were not included in trial and thus not eligible

Guidelines
- 2018 American Society of Clinical Oncology-College of American Pathologists (ASCO-CAP) recommendations to determine *ERBB2* status for all newly diagnosed invasive breast cancer and subsequent metastatic disease
  - IHC or ISH methods acceptable
    - If results are equivocal, reflex testing using alternate method should be performed
  - Testing must be performed in CAP-accredited laboratory
    - Preferably use FDA-approved IHC, brightfield ISH, or FISH
  - Optimal specimen handling
    - Slice at 5- to 10-mm intervals
    - Fix in 10% neutral buffered formalin for 6-72 hours
  - Results important to determine appropriate therapy
    - Anti-ERBB2 therapy should **not** be used with negative or equivocal results or while waiting for result
- 2023 ASCO-CAP guideline update
  - 2018 ASCO-CAP recommendations for *ERBB2* testing are affirmed
  - Acknowledges new indication for trastuzumab-deruxtecan
    - Recommends pathologists make best practice efforts to distinguish IHC 0 from 1+ results
    - Recommends adding comment provided by ASCO-CAP to all HER2 test reports
- National Comprehensive Cancer Network (NCCN) *ERBB2* testing recommendations for patients with following
  - Metastatic colorectal cancer with no *RAS/RAF* mutations
  - Advanced gastroesophageal or gastric adenocarcinoma

***ERBB2* Amplification**

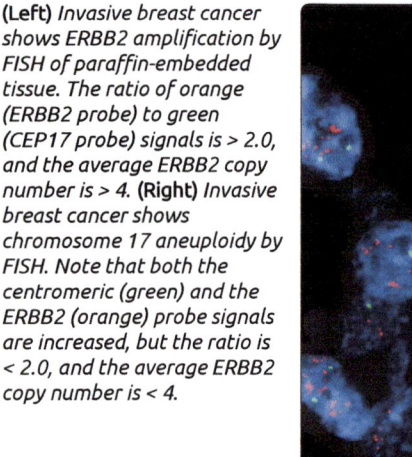

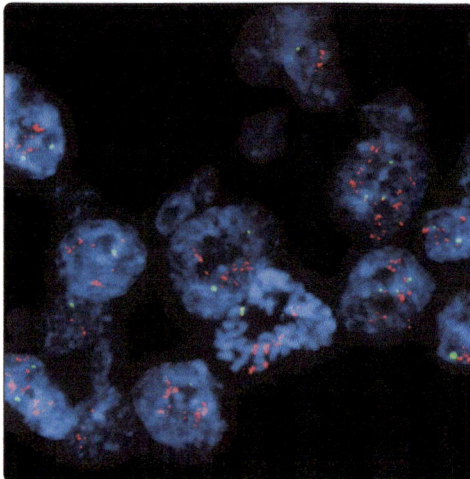

Aneuploidy in Breast Cancer

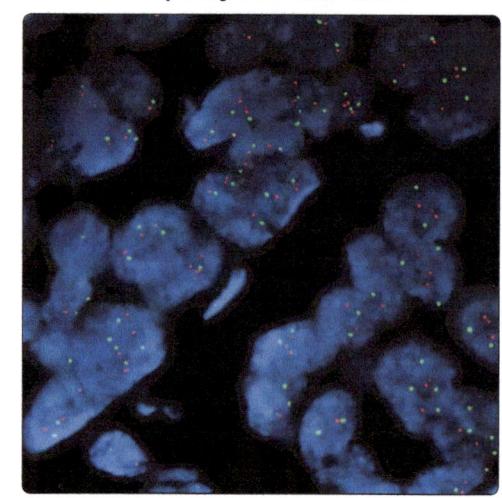

(Left) *Invasive breast cancer shows ERBB2 amplification by FISH of paraffin-embedded tissue. The ratio of orange (ERBB2 probe) to green (CEP17 probe) signals is > 2.0, and the average ERBB2 copy number is > 4.* (Right) *Invasive breast cancer shows chromosome 17 aneuploidy by FISH. Note that both the centromeric (green) and the ERBB2 (orange) probe signals are increased, but the ratio is < 2.0, and the average ERBB2 copy number is < 4.*

FISH for *ERBB2* (HER2) Amplifications

- Unresectable or metastatic gallbladder cancer or cholangiocarcinoma
- Advanced-stage or recurrent serous endometrial carcinoma or carcinosarcoma

PREDICTIVE CANCER TESTING SUMMARY

Test Interpretation
- *ERBB2* IHC on tumor tissue
  - Graded from 0-3+
  - 0 = no staining, or incomplete/barely perceptible in ≤ 10% of tumor cells
    - Interpreted as negative
  - 1+ = barely perceptible, incomplete membrane staining in > 10% of tumor cells
    - Interpreted as negative
  - 2+ = weak to moderate complete membrane staining in > 10% of tumor cells
    - Interpreted as equivocal
    - 2+ criteria were redefined in 2018 ASCO/CAP update
    - Reflex to ISH using same specimen **or** with new specimen can repeat IHC or reflex to ISH
  - 3+ = complete, intense membrane staining in > 10% cells
    - Interpreted as positive
- *ERBB2* FISH reflex testing should be performed on IHC 2+ (equivocal) cases
  - Single-probe assays (*ERBB2* only) require average of ≥ 6 signals per cell to be called positive
  - Dual-signal assay (*ERBB2*/CEP17) requires ratio > 2.0 to be deemed positive result
    - If ratio is < 2.0 but *ERBB2* signal number is still > 6, this is also considered positive
    - If ratio is < 2.0 with ERBB2 copy number between 4.0 and 6.0, this is considered equivocal and requires reflex testing to alternate method

Pathology Review of Concurrent H&E
- Important to avoid inclusion of adjacent in situ carcinoma lesions during FISH read

General Issues
- Repeat testing should be performed
  - On relapse in patients with previously *ERBB2*(-) tumors
  - On excision specimen in patients with *ERBB2*(-) core needle biopsy specimen
- Testing must be reported as **indeterminate** if technical issues preclude diagnosis
  - Inadequate specimen handling
  - Significant artifacts, including crush and edge artifacts
  - Failed analytical testing demonstrated by failed controls
  - Report as indeterminate and request another specimen

FISH METHOD FOR *ERBB2* AMPLIFICATION

Methodology
- Paraffin-embedded, formalin-fixed tumor tissue sections
- Fluorescent DNA probe binds to sequence in *ERBB2* region at 17q12
- Used with chromosome 17 centromeric probe (CEP17)
- Ratio of *ERBB2* signals to CEP17 signals is calculated
- Chromogenic ISH (CISH) is alternative
  - Can correlate better with morphology

Single-Probe ISH Assay
- Positive if ≥ 6.0 signals/cell
- If ≥ 4.0 but < 6.0 signals per cell, need concurrent IHC evaluation
  - Positive if IHC 3+ or dual-probe ISH group 1
  - Negative if IHC 0-2+ or dual-probe ISH group 5
- If < 4.0 signals/cell, considered negative

Dual-Probe ISH Assay
- *HER2*:CEP17 ratio ≥ 2.0
  - **Group 1**: Average *HER2* copy number ≥ 4.0 signals/cell
    - Considered ISH positive and *HER2*(+)
  - **Group 2**: Average *HER2* copy number < 4.0 signals/cell
    - Reflex back to IHC from same tissue
    - If IHC is 2+, recount ISH
      - If same ISH results are obtained, this is considered *HER2*(-) with comment (unclear benefit of trastuzumab in small sample size clinical trial)
    - If IHC is 0-2+, considered *HER2*(-)
    - If IHC is 3+, considered *HER2*(+)
- *HER2*:CEP17 ratio < 2.0
  - **Group 3**: Average *HER2* copy number ≥ 6.0 signals/cell
    - Reflex back to IHC from same tissue
    - If IHC is 2+, recount ISH
      - If same ISH results obtained, considered *HER2*(+)
    - If IHC is 0-1+, considered *HER2*(-)
    - If IHC is 2-3+, considered *HER2*(+)
  - **Group 4**: Average *HER2* copy number ≥ 4.0 and < 6.0 signals/cell
    - Reflex back to IHC from same tissue
    - If IHC is 2+, recount ISH
      - If same ISH results are obtained, considered *HER2*(-) with comment (unclear benefit of trastuzumab)
    - If IHC is 0-2+, considered *HER2*(-)
    - If IHC is 3+, considered *HER2*(+)
  - **Group 5**: Average *HER2* copy number < 4.0 signals/cell
    - Considered ISH negative and *HER2*(-)

OTHER METHODS FOR EVALUATION OF *ERBB2* STATUS

Quantitative Real-Time PCR
- Emerging alternate method can be used in cases (~ 5%) where FISH fails

Next-Generation Sequencing
- For cases with limited available diagnostic tissue or when patient is unable to undergo traditional biopsy

SELECTED REFERENCES

1. Abu-Rustum N et al: Uterine neoplasms, version 1.2023, NCCN Clinical Practice Guidelines in Oncology. J Natl Compr Canc Netw. 21(2):181-209, 2023
2. Wolff AC et al: Human epidermal growth factor receptor 2 testing in breast cancer: American Society of Clinical Oncology-College of American Pathologists guideline update. Arch Pathol Lab Med. 147(9):991-2, 2023
3. National Comprehensive Cancer Network (NCCN): NCCN clinical practice guidelines in oncology. Accessed July 26, 2023. https://www.nccn.org/guidelines/category_1
4. Wolff AC et al: Human epidermal growth factor receptor 2 testing in breast cancer: American Society of Clinical Oncology/College of American Pathologists clinical practice guideline focused update. J Clin Oncol. 36(20):2105-22, 2018

KRAS Mutations

TERMINOLOGY

Definitions
- Official name: KRAS protooncogene, GTPase
- Official symbol: *KRAS*
- HGNC ID: 6407
- Chromosome location: 12p12.1
- Genomic location: Chr12:25,205,246-25,250,929 (GRCh38.p14)
- Size: 2 isoforms, KRAS4A:189 amino acids; KRAS4B:188 amino acids
- Number of exons: 7
- Aliases: KRAS2, v-Ki-ras2 Kirsten rat sarcoma 2 viral oncogene homolog

MOLECULAR FEATURES

Structure and Tissue Expressions of KRAS Protein
- Structural features of KRAS protein
  - N-terminal portion (amino acid 1-164): Highly conserved G domain, including catalytic domain with P loop, switch I, and switch II domain
    - Forms basis of biological functionality of KRAS protein
  - C-terminal portion (amino acid 165-188): Hypervariable region with membrane anchoring function
- KRAS4A is weakly expressed in normal human cells
- KRAS4B is much more highly expressed in normal human cells; dominant form

Functions of KRAS Protein
- Small intracellular GTPase, mainly in GDP-bound ("off" or "inactive") state
- Activated when GTP is bound (Ras-GTP)
- Inactivated when guanosine diphosphate is bound (Ras-GDP)
- KRAS functions in signal transduction cascades initiated by epidermal growth factor receptor (EGFR), platelet-derived growth factor receptor, hepatocyte growth factor receptor, insulin-like growth factor receptor
- Activated KRAS activates RAL, RAF/MEK/ERK, and PI3K/AKT pathways
  - Involving proliferation, differentiation, apoptosis suppression, angiogenesis, cytoskeletal organization, vesicle trafficking, and calcium signaling
- *KRAS* gene alterations lead to oncogenesis and developmental disorders

Classification
- Ras (rat sarcoma) protein is prototypical member of Ras superfamily of proteins
- 3 Ras genes (*HRAS*, *KRAS*, and *NRAS*)
- All Ras protein family members belong to class of small guanosine triphosphate hydrolase (GTPase)

KRAS Alterations
- Mutations
  - Somatic mutations
    - 66 of 188 *KRAS* codons may harbor at least 1 mutation
    - > 99% of alterations are simple substitution missense mutations
    - Majority of mutations associated with cancer occur at 3 hotspots
      □ G12 is most common mutation site (~ 83%)
      □ G13 is 2nd most common mutation site (~ 14%)
      □ Q61 is 3rd most common mutation site (~ 2%)
      □ Frequency of hotspot mutations in KRAS proteins varies depending on tissue of origin
    - These mutations result in constitutive activation of KRAS proteins and subsequent oncogenesis
  - Germline mutations
    - Many germline mutations, including K5E, V14I, Q22R/E, P34L/R/Q, I36M, T58I, G60R, N116S, D153V, and F156I/L
    - Most are gain-of-function mutations but are less activated than oncogenic KRAS proteins, such as G12D
- Amplification
  - Can induce downstream activation of RAF/ERK pathway
  - Occurs much more often in metastatic cancers than in primary cancers
  - Significantly correlates with poor prognosis
  - Essentially confers resistance to anti-EGFR antibody treatment in colorectal carcinoma (CRC)

Structure of KRAS Protein With Germline and Somatic Mutations

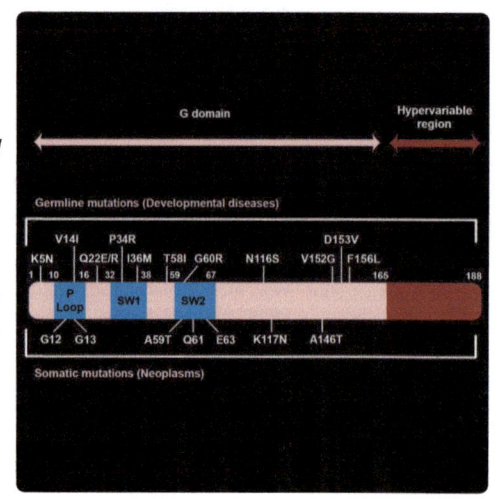

Pyrogram of *KRAS* c.35G>T (G12V) and c.38G>A (G13D) Mutations

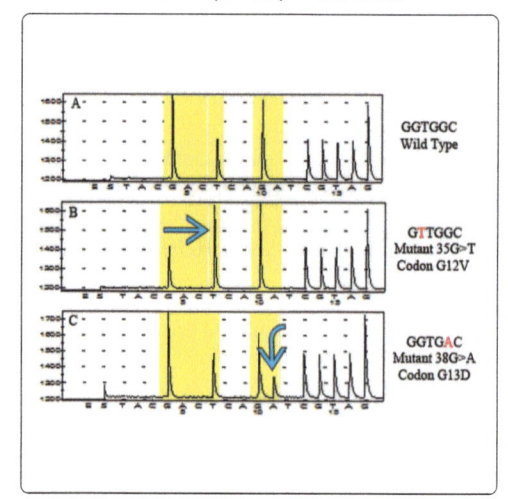

(Left) *KRAS* is a small GTPase composed of a G domain (P loop, switch I, and switch II) and a hypervariable region. *KRAS* gene may harbor germline mutations associated with developmental disorders and somatic oncogenic mutations associated with cancer. (Right) *KRAS* mutation analysis by pyrosequencing shows wildtype DNA sequence of codon 12 and 13 at the top. The middle panel shows mutation c.35G>T (p.G12V) ➔, and the bottom panel shows mutation c.38G>A (p.G13D) ➔.

KRAS Mutations

- Top malignancies with *KRAS* amplification include non-small cell lung cancer (NSCLC) (1.6-15%), adenocarcinoma of gastroesophageal junction (9.4-26%), gastric adenocarcinoma (4.7%), malignant female reproductive system neoplasms (1.8%), head and neck squamous cell carcinoma (1%), and CRC (0.9%)
- *KRAS* fusion
  - Rare
  - *UBE2L3::KRAS* fusion reported in prostatic cancer
  - *MRPS35::KRAS*, *TMBIM4::KRAS*, and *C12orf4::KRAS* fusions reported in NSCLC

CLINICAL IMPLICATIONS

Pancreatic Ductal Adenocarcinoma
- Highest prevalence of *KRAS* mutations is detected in pancreatic carcinomas
- > 90% of pancreatic ductal carcinomas harbor *KRAS* mutations
- G12D is most common mutation
- Tobacco exposure has been associated with *KRAS* mutations and pancreatic carcinoma

Colorectal Carcinoma
- 2nd-highest prevalence of *KRAS* mutations
- ~ 50% of cases harbor *KRAS* mutations
- *KRAS* mutations found in both colonic adenomas and carcinomas but with much lower frequency in adenomas
- Codon 12 is most common mutation site of *KRAS* in CRC
  - G12D is most common mutation
  - Other codon 12 mutations include G12V, G12C, G12A, G12S, and G12R
- *KRAS* mutation is most important predictor of resistance to anti-EGFR monoclonal antibodies cetuximab or panitumumab in CRC
- *KRAS* mutations in CRC confer more aggressive phenotype with reduced survival rates

Lung Non-Small Cell Carcinoma
- 10-30% of lung carcinomas harbor *KRAS* mutations
  - More frequent in adenocarcinomas than in squamous carcinomas
  - G12C is most common *KRAS* mutation in lung carcinoma and conveys poor prognosis
- History of smoking is associated with *KRAS* mutations in lung cancer and conveys poor prognosis
  - *KRAS* mutations in lung cancer essentially confer resistance to EGFR tyrosine kinase inhibitor (TKI) therapy
  - Sotorasib is approved in 2021 for treatment of NSCLC harboring *KRAS* G12C mutation

Biliary Tract Cancer
- 20-50% of cholangiocarcinomas harbor *KRAS* mutations
  - Codon 12 is most common site
- Considered early molecular event from epithelial dysplasia to carcinoma
- *KRAS* mutation has been associated with shorter overall survival in some studies

Developmental Disorders
- Strength &/or duration of signaling through RAS/RAF/MEK/ERK pathway regulate developmental programs
- *KRAS* mutations that cause developmental disorders encode proteins with aberrant biochemical and functional properties
  - Most mutations encode gain-of-function proteins but are less activated than oncogenic KRAS proteins
  - Most germline mutations not associated with cancers
- At least 13 *KRAS* germline mutations have been reported in RASopathy, group of developmental disorders
- Cardiofaciocutaneous syndrome
  - ~ 4% of cases harbor germline *KRAS* mutations
- Noonan syndrome
  - 2-4% of cases harbor germline *KRAS* mutations

DETECTION OF *KRAS* MUTATIONS

Next-Generation Sequencing
- Highly accurate due to much higher degree of sequence coverage
- Mutations occurring in *KRAS* are typically included in targeted NGS panels, widely used in molecular diagnostics laboratories

Pyrosequencing
- Simple, robust, and sensitive method with detection limit of ~ 5% mutant alleles
- Very efficient method to detect *KRAS* mutations

Digital PCR
- Can accurately detect and quantify low nucleic acid targets
- Highly sensitive and accurate in detection of pathogenic mutations

Allele-Specific Real-Time PCR
- Simple, high sensitivity and specificity
- Low-cost and fast diagnostic tool for accurate detection of *KRAS* mutations

Sanger Sequencing
- Can detect all mutated base pairs, small insertions, and deletions
- Disadvantage: Low sensitivity, 20-40% of tumor purity of sample needed for reliable detection
  - Not commonly used for routine clinical service for *KRAS* mutation detection due to low assay sensitivity

SELECTED REFERENCES

1. Nussinov R et al: How can same-gene mutations promote both cancer and developmental disorders? Sci Adv. 8(2):eabm2059, 2022
2. Punekar SR et al: The current state of the art and future trends in RAS-targeted cancer therapies. Nat Rev Clin Oncol. 19(10):637-55, 2022
3. Skoulidis F et al: Sotorasib for lung cancers with KRAS p.G12C mutation. N Engl J Med. 384(25):2371-81, 2021
4. Lindeman NI et al: Updated molecular testing guideline for the selection of lung cancer patients for treatment with targeted tyrosine kinase inhibitors: guideline from the College of American Pathologists, the International Association for the Study of Lung Cancer, and the Association for Molecular Pathology. J Mol Diagn. 20(2):129-59, 2018
5. Ryan MB et al: Therapeutic strategies to target RAS-mutant cancers. Nat Rev Clin Oncol. 15(11):709-20, 2018

BRAF Mutations

TERMINOLOGY

Definitions

- Official name: B-Raf protooncogene, serine/threonine kinase
- Official symbol: BRAF
- HGNC ID: 1097
- Chromosomal location: 7q34
- Genomic location: Chr7:140,713,328-140,924,929 (GRCh38/hg38)
- Size: 766 amino acids
- Number of exons: 24
- Aliases: BRAF1, RAFB1, protooncogene B-RAF

STRUCTURE AND FUNCTIONS OF BRAF PROTEIN

Structure

- BRAF protein is serine/threonine kinase
- Composed of 3 conserved regions (CR)
  - CR1 and CR2 are regulatory domains
  - CR3 contains catalytic protein kinase domain

Functions

- Member of rapidly accelerated fibrosarcoma (RAF) kinase family of serine/threonine kinases (ARAF, BRAF, CRAF) involved in RAS/RAF/MEK/ERK pathway
  - Activated RAS proteins induce dimerization of RAF proteins, leading to cascade of kinase activation from MEK1/MEK2 to ERK1/ERK2, subsequently causing changes in gene expression
- Enzymatic activity of BRAF proteins in cytoplasm is tightly controlled in normal cells

BRAF GENE ALTERATIONS

BRAF Somatic Missense Mutations

- Class I mutations (mutations in codon V600, independent of both upstream RAS activation and need for dimerization)
  - Most commonly identified BRAF mutations in human cancers
  - BRAF c.1799T>A, p.V600E mutation, 80-90% of all V600 codon mutations
  - c.1798_1799delGTinsAA, p.V600K in 5-12%
  - c.1798_1799delGTinsAG, p.V600R in ~ 5%
  - c.1799_1800delTGinsAT, p.V600D in ~ 1%
  - c.1798G>A, p.V600M in < 1%
- Class II mutations (non-V600 mutations, inducing constitutive activation via Ras-independent dimerization)
  - Substitutions at BRAF activation segment
    - K601E, K601N, K601T, L597Q
  - Substitutions within P loop
    - G464, G469A, G469V, G469R
- Class III mutations (non-V600 mutations, lack or possess low kinase activity; increase signaling via enhanced RAS binding and enhancement of CRAF activation)
  - G466V, G466E, N581S, D594N, D594G, G596D

Fusions

- Function similarly to class II BRAF mutants
- C-terminal portion of BRAF is fused in-frame with another protein at N-terminus
- BRAF fusions cause autophosphorylation due to loss of regulatory domain of BRAF protein resulting in constitutively active BRAF dimers
- Found in various neoplasms, such as
  - AGAP3::BRAF, AGK::BRAF, AKAP9::BRAF, and ZNF767P::BRAF in melanoma
  - AGK::BRAF, AKAP9::BRAF, KIAA1549::BRAF, and CCDC6::BRAF in glioma
  - ZC3HAV1::BRAF, AGTRAP::BRAF, and MKRN1::BRAF in GI tract carcinomas
  - SND1::BRAF and MYRIP::BRAF in pancreatic carcinoma
  - BTF3L4::BRAF, NUP214::BRAF, ARMC10::BRAF, and NUP214::BRAF in lung carcinoma
  - KLHL7::BRAF, RBMS3::BRAF, and TANK::BRAF in thyroid carcinoma
  - MKRN1::BRAF in head and neck carcinoma
  - NUB1::BRAF and SLC45A3::BRAF in prostate cancer
  - KIAA1549::BRAF in metastatic breast carcinoma
  - MIGA1::BRAF fusion in Langerhans cell histiocytosis

Structure of BRAF Protein With Mutations

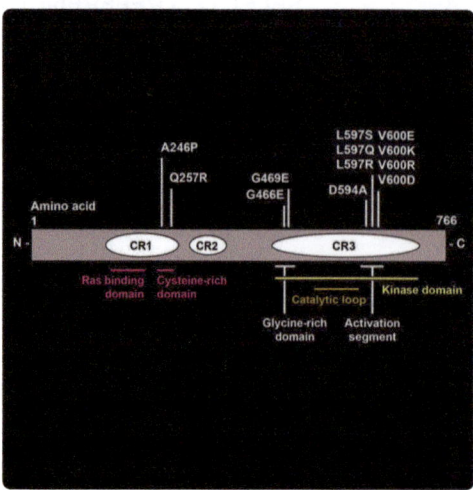

Pyrogram of BRAF V600E Mutation

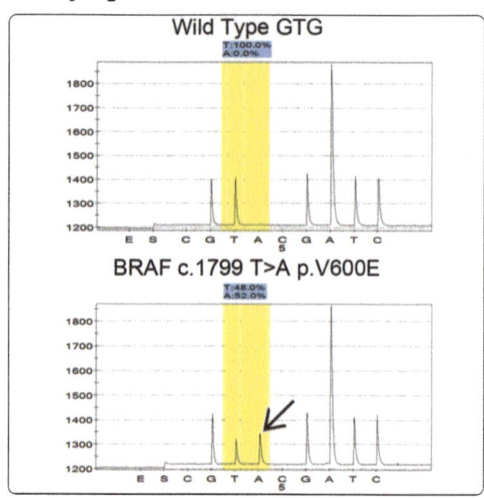

(Left) BRAF is a cytoplasmic serine/threonine kinase. There are 3 conserved regions (CR) among human RAF genes. V600 mutations are at CR3. Other somatic and 2 germline mutations at CR1 are also illustrated. (Right) The top diagram shows wildtype BRAF with GTG detected at the V600 codon by pyrosequencing. The bottom diagram shows c. 1799T>A, p.V600E ➡, which occurs due to a T>A base substitution.

BRAF Mutations

BRAF Germline Mutations
- Involved in developmental disorders and include
  - A246P, Q257R, G469E, L485F, K499E, E501K, and N581D, among others

CLINICAL IMPLICATIONS

Melanoma
- BRAF somatic missense mutations are most common oncogenic driver in melanoma
  - Detected in ~ 60% of melanomas
- BRAF inhibitors
  - Small molecule that binds mutated BRAF and renders BRAF protein inactivation
  - FDA-approved inhibitors: Vemurafenib, dabrafenib, trametinib, cobimetinib, atezolizumab
  - Resistance to BRAF inhibitors
    - Develops in almost all patients, usually within 1 year
    - Thought to be due to alternative survival pathways, including PDGFR, NRAS, and HGF

Colorectal Carcinoma
- BRAF mutations occurs in 6-15% of colorectal carcinoma (CRC)
- Sporadic CRC with microsatellite instability high (MSI-H) vs. hereditary nonpolyposis colorectal carcinoma (HNPCC)
  - Majority of sporadic CRC with MSI-H have BRAF mutation
  - HNPCC patients almost never have BRAF mutation
  - Testing BRAF V600E status can avoid expense of full gene sequencing for mismatch repair genes
- Resistance to EGFR-targeted therapy by cetuximab and panitumumab is common in CRC with BRAF mutations
- FDA has approved cetuximab + encorafenib for metastatic CRC with BRAF V600E mutation

Papillary Thyroid Carcinoma
- BRAF V600E mutation is most common genetic alteration
  - ~ 69% have V600E mutation; mainly in classic variant, rare in other variants
  - V600E is virtually absent in follicular, Hürthle cell carcinoma, medullary thyroid carcinomas, and in benign thyroid tumors
  - Recurrence, lymph node metastases, extrathyroidal extension, and advanced stage are common in tumors with BRAF V600E mutation

Non-Small Cell Lung Cancer
- 1-4% have BRAF somatic mutations
- Types of BRAF mutations
  - V600E in ~ 50%, G469A in 39%, and D594G in 11%
- BRAF mutations are mutually exclusive with KRAS and EGFR mutations

Hairy Cell Leukemia
- Nearly 100% of patients carry BRAF V600E mutation
- BRAF V600E typically negative in other B-cell lymphomas, including
  - Splenic marginal zone lymphoma
  - Hairy cell leukemia variant
  - Splenic red pulp small B-cell lymphoma

Langerhans Cell Histiocytosis
- BRAF V600E mutation found in ~ 60%
- Increased risk of initial treatment failure in patients with this mutation
- Associated with 2x increased risk for recurrence or relapse
- Other isolated case reports of rare types of BRAF mutations
  - BRAF exon 12 in-frame deletion, MIGA1::BRAF fusion

Glioma
- BRAF mutations are significant driver of disease in both pediatric and adult gliomas
- BRAF V600E is associated with improved survival overall in adults with glioma
- FDA-approved dabrafenib with trametinib for pediatric patients with low-grade glioma with BRAF V600E

Cardiofaciocutaneous Syndrome, LEOPARD Syndrome, and Noonan Syndrome
- All linked to gene alterations in RAS/RAF/MEK/ERK signaling pathway
- Different germline BRAF mutations
  - 35-75% in cardiofaciocutaneous syndrome
  - Up to 17% in LEOPARD syndrome
  - ~ 2% in Noonan syndrome

DETECTION TECHNIQUES

Next-Generation Sequencing
- Highly accurate due to much higher degree of sequence coverage
- Most of BRAF mutations are covered in targeted NGS panels

Pyrosequencing
- Efficient method to detect BRAF mutations; commonly used in molecular diagnostics laboratories
  - Simple, robust, and sensitive method with detection limit of ~ 5% mutant alleles

Digital PCR
- Can accurately detect and quantify low nucleic acid targets
- High sensitivity and specificity

Allele-Specific Real-Time PCR
- Simple; high sensitivity and specificity
- Low-cost and fast diagnostic tool for accurate detection of BRAF mutations

Immunohistochemistry
- BRAF V600E mutation-specific antibody (VE1) is targeted to BRAF V600E protein
  - Has high concordance with DNA-based methods detecting BRAF V600E

SELECTED REFERENCES
1. Elez E et al: Seeking therapeutic synergy in BRAF mutant colorectal cancer. Nat Med. 29(2):307-8, 2023
2. Moran JMT et al: Identification of fusions with potential clinical significance in melanoma. Mod Pathol. 35(12):1837-47, 2022
3. Poulikakos PI et al: Molecular pathways and mechanisms of BRAF in cancer therapy. Clin Cancer Res. 28(21):4618-28, 2022
4. Zanwar S et al: Clinical and therapeutic implications of BRAF fusions in histiocytic disorders. Blood Cancer J. 12(6):97, 2022
5. Kopetz S et al: Encorafenib, binimetinib, and cetuximab in BRAF V600E-mutated colorectal cancer. N Engl J Med. 381(17):1632-43, 2019

EGFR Mutations

TERMINOLOGY

Definitions

- Official name: Epidermal growth factor receptor
- Official symbol: *EGFR*
- HGNC ID: 3236
- Chromosomal location: 7p11.2
- Genomic location: Chr7:55,019,017-55,211,628 (GRCh38/hg38)
- Number of exons: 28
- Aliases: Receptor tyrosine-protein kinase ErbB-1, ERBB1, ERBB, ERRP, HER1

STRUCTURE AND FUNCTIONS OF EGFR PROTEIN

EGFR Structure

- Plasma transmembrane glycoprotein composed of
  - Extracellular ligand-binding domains with 2 cysteine-rich regions
  - Single transmembrane helix domain
  - Intracellular region containing tyrosine kinase domain and autophosphorylation regions
- Ligands of EGFR
  - 7 ligands binding EGFR
    - Epidermal growth factor (EGF), transforming growth factor alpha (TGFA), heparin-binding EGF-like growth factor (HB-EGF), amphiregulin (AR), betacellulin (BTC), epiregulin (EPR), and epigen
  - In general, EGFR ligands are synthesized as type 1 transmembrane precursors that undergo extracellular domain cleavage to release soluble ligands

EGFR Functions

- Binding of ligand to extracellular domain results in activation of *EGFR* pathway
- Activation of downstream pathways leads to cell proliferation, differentiation, migration/motility, adhesion, protection from apoptosis, and transformation

EGFR ALTERATIONS

Extracellular Domain Mutations

- *EGFR* variant III: Most common type of extracellular domain mutation
  - Deletion of exons 2-7 of *EGFR* in extracellular domain
  - Renders mutant receptor incapable of binding any known ligands
  - Displays low-level constitutive EGFR activity
  - Drives tumor progression and correlates with poor prognosis
  - Mainly occur in glioblastoma multiforme (GBM) (~ 60%)
  - Rarely occur in epithelial neoplasms, including breast, prostate, ovarian, and non-small cell lung carcinoma (NSCLC)
- Deletion of amino acids 521-603 in extracellular domain: Much less common than *EGFR* variant III

Intracellular Kinase Domain Mutations

- Most are activating mutations affecting exons 18-21
- Mutations result in constitutive activation of EGFR protein and subsequent oncogenesis
- Majority of mutations show enhanced sensitivity to 1st-generation tyrosine kinase inhibitors (TKIs)
- Found in NSCLC with adenocarcinoma histology
  - ~ 10-15% of NSCLC patients in western nations harbor *EGFR* mutations
  - ~ 40% of NSCLC in Asian populations harbor *EGFR* mutations
  - More common in female patients who are nonsmokers or light smokers
- Specific *EGFR* mutations in tyrosine kinase domain
  - Exon 18 mutations
    - Account for ~ 5% of *EGFR* mutations
    - Relatively common mutations include G719C, G719S, and G719A; less common mutations include V689M, E709K, E709Q, and N700D
  - Exon 19 mutations
    - Deletion mutations, 9-18 bp deletions in exon 19

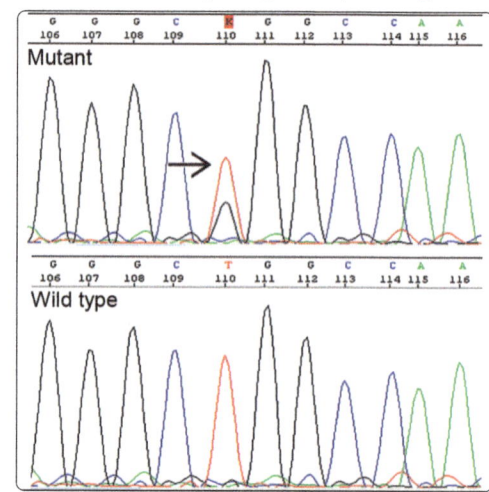

(Left) Exons 2-16 encode the extracellular domains, exon 17 encodes the transmembrane domain (TM), exons 18-21 encode the tyrosine kinase domain, and exons 25-28 encode the autophosphorylation domain. Mutations in exons 18-21 are associated with sensitivity or resistance to tyrosine kinase inhibitors (TKIs). **(Right)** Chromatogram shows mutation of c.2573T>G (p.L858R) ➡ in exon 21 of the EGFR gene. p.L858R mutation accounts for 40-45% of all EGFR mutations with sensitivity to TKI treatment.

Structure of *EGFR* With Mutations

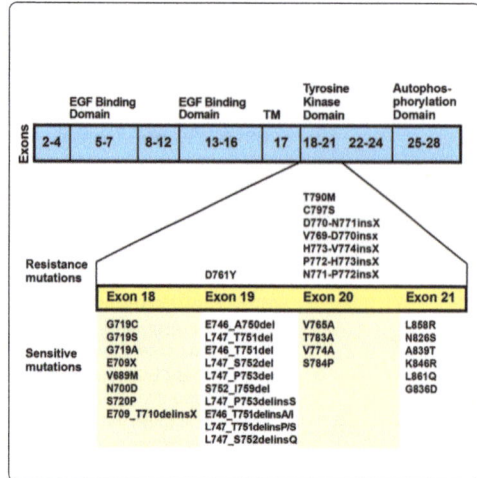

Exons	2-4	5-7	8-12	13-16	17	18-21	22-24	25-28
	EGF Binding Domain		EGF Binding Domain		TM	Tyrosine Kinase Domain		Autophosphorylation Domain

	Exon 18	Exon 19	Exon 20	Exon 21
Resistance mutations	D761Y		T790M C797S D770-N771insX V769-D770insX H773-V774insX P772-H773insX N771-P772insX	
Sensitive mutations	G719C G719S G719A E709X V689M N700D S720P E709_T710delinsX	E746_A750del L747_T751del L747_T751del L747_P753del L747_P753delinsS E746_T751delinsA/I L747_T751delinsP/S L747_S752delinsQ	V765A T783A V774A S784P	L858R N826S A839T K846R L861Q G836D

EGFR c.2573T>G (p.L858R) Mutation Detected by Sanger Sequencing

EGFR Mutations

- □ Account for ~ 45% of *EGFR* mutations; most frequent is p.E746_A750del
- – D761Y (< 1%) is associated with resistance to TKIs
- o Exon 20 mutations
  - – T790M
    - □ Confers resistance to 1st- and 2nd-generation TKIs
    - □ Accounts for ~ 50% of resistance-associated mutations to TKIs
    - □ Develops post EGFR TKI treatment in NSCLC
    - □ Can also be primary event before drug exposure
  - – Exon 20 in-frame insertion mutations
    - □ Heterogeneous in-frame insertions of 1-7 amino acids within D761-C775 in exon 20
    - □ Results in constitutive activation of EGFR protein
    - □ Associated with de novo resistance to targeted EGFR inhibitors and correlated with poor prognosis
    - □ e.g., D770-N771insX, V769-D770insX, H773-V774insX, P772-H773insX, N771-P772insX
- o Exon 21 mutations
  - – Account for 40-45% of *EGFR* mutations
  - – L858R is most common point mutation in *EGFR*
- *EGFR* mutations in exons 18, 19, 20, and 21 are mutually exclusive with *KRAS* and *BRAF* mutations

EGFR Amplification

- CNS tumors
  - o Glioblastoma, IDH-wildtype
    - – ~ 50% of tumors show *EGFR* amplification
    - – Present solely in IDH-wildtype gliomas (26%) and *TERT*-mutated gliomas (27%)
  - o Diffuse pediatric type high-grade glioma, IDH-wildtype
    - – *EGFR* amplification occurs in ~ 50% patients
- Lung cancer
  - o *EGFR* amplification is more prevalent in squamous cell carcinoma than adenocarcinoma
  - o NSCLC with *EGFR* amplification may respond to TKIs
- Breast cancer
  - o ~ 6% show *EGFR* amplification
  - o *EGFR* amplification can coexist with *ERRB2* (HER2) amplification
  - o Metaplastic breast carcinoma has highest *EGFR* amplification rate (~ 70%)
- Ovarian cancer
  - o *EGFR* amplification and high polysomy present in 20% of primary and recurrent ovarian carcinomas
  - o *EGFR* mutation is extremely rare in ovarian cancer
- Gastroesophageal adenocarcinoma
  - o *EGFR*-amplified tumors are associated with higher stage, more poorly differentiated histology, increased vascular invasion, and potentially shorter survival
- Metastatic colorectal carcinoma (mCRC)
  - o EGFR amplification occurs in ~ 1% of mCRC
  - o Most *EGFR*-amplified tumors are microsatellite stable and HER2 nonamplified

EGFR Small Molecule Inhibitors

- 1st-generation EGFR TKIs include erlotinib and gefitinib
- 2nd-generation EGFR TKIs include neratinib, dacomitinib, and afatinib
- 3rd-generation EGFR TKIs include rociletinib and osimertinib
- *EGFR* mutation testing should be used to select patients for EGFR-targeted TKI therapy

Anti-EGFR Monoclonal Antibodies for Chemotherapy-Refectory Metastatic Colorectal Carcinoma

- Cetuximab (Erbitux) and panitumumab (Vectibix)
- Resistance to EGFR blockade in mCRC with constitutive activation mutation in *KRAS*, *NRAS*, or *BRAF*
- Recommend testing *KRAS*, *NRAS*, and *BRAF* mutation status before treatment
- Mutation status of *EGFR* catalytic domain does not correlate with disease response with anti-EGFR monoclonal antibodies

DETECTION OF *EGFR* GENE ALTERATIONS

Detection of Gene Mutations

- **Next-generation sequencing (NGS)**
  - o *EGFR* mutations are typically included in targeted gene panel; commonly used in clinical laboratories
  - o Highly sensitive and accurate when adequate sequencing depth of coverage present
- **Sanger sequencing**
  - o Used in some clinical laboratories to detect *EGFR* mutations
  - o Can reliably detect many possible mutations
  - o Less sensitive compared to NGS
    - – Requires 20-25% mutant alleles in background of wildtype alleles for reliable detection of mutations

Detection of *EGFR* Amplification

- Fluorescence in situ hybridization (FISH)
  - o Standard method for detecting *EGFR* amplification
  - o Detects *EGFR* gene copy number gain, high degrees of polysomy
- Digital PCR (dPCR)
  - o Can accurately detect and quantify low nucleic acid targets
  - o Highly sensitive and high specificity
- NGS
  - o Can be used to detect *EGFR* amplification
  - o Commonly included in targeted solid tumor panels
- Immunohistochemistry
  - o Used to detect EGFR protein overexpression

SELECTED REFERENCES

1. Cooper AJ et al: Third-generation EGFR and ALK inhibitors: mechanisms of resistance and management. Nat Rev Clin Oncol. 19(8):499-514, 2022
2. Passaro A et al: Recent advances on the role of EGFR tyrosine kinase inhibitors in the management of NSCLC with uncommon, non exon 20 insertions, EGFR mutations. J Thorac Oncol. 16(5):764-73, 2021
3. Uribe ML et al: EGFR in cancer: signaling mechanisms, drugs, and acquired resistance. Cancers (Basel). 13(11):2748, 2021
4. Kato S et al: Revisiting epidermal growth factor receptor (EGFR) amplification as a target for anti-EGFR therapy: analysis of cell-free circulating tumor DNA in patients with advanced malignancies. JCO Precis Oncol. 3, 2019
5. Vyse S et al: Targeting EGFR exon 20 insertion mutations in non-small cell lung cancer. Signal Transduct Target Ther. 4:5, 2019
6. Neilsen BK et al: Comprehensive genetic alteration profiling in primary and recurrent glioblastoma. J Neurooncol. 142(1):111-8, 2019

Targeted Hotspot Gene Panel Using Massively Parallel Sequencing (Next-Generation Sequencing)

TERMINOLOGY

Definitions
- Hotspot: Region within genome that is commonly mutated, giving rise to specific clinically significant phenotype

BASIC ASPECTS OF HOTSPOT GENE PANELS

Next-Generation Sequencing
- a.k.a. massively parallel sequencing
- Permits amplification and sequencing of many regions simultaneously

General NGS Procedure
- Sample preparation
  o Assessment of adequacy and quality of submitted sample is 1st step in clinical NGS analysis
  o Tumor content in hematologic specimen may require separate analysis, such as flow cytometry
  o Solid tumor samples require microscopic review by certified pathologist before accepted for NGS testing
    – Microscopic review used to assess adequacy and mark tumor areas for macrodissection
    – Includes assessment for required tumor percentage as determined during validation in given lab
- Library preparation
  o Generates DNA or cDNA of specific size range
    – Amplicon-based library preparation
      □ Multiplex PCR amplification to enrich target sequences
    – Ligation-based library preparation
      □ Uses long biotinylated oligonucleotide probes
- Sequencing
  o Sequencing by synthesis or ion semiconductor-based sequencing
  o All fragments sequenced simultaneously
- Data analysis
  o Bioinformatic pipeline
    – Base calling, read alignment, variant identification, and variant annotation and variant identification
    – Annotate clinical significance of detected variants

Scope of Sequencing
- Hotspot panels represent middle ground between single-gene and whole-exome sequencing
- Allows cost-effective analysis by concentrating on specific mutations felt to be most common &/or most clinically significant

Common Platforms
- Ion torrent
  o Generates sequence by measuring change in pH when H⁺ is released from incorporated bases (ion semiconductor-based)
  o Susceptible to noise calls in homopolymer tracts
  o Personal Genome Machine (PGM) vs. Ion Proton systems for sequencing capacity
- Illumina
  o Generates sequence by reversible dye termination (sequencing by synthesis)

Source of Hotspot Panels
- Several panels commercially available
- Laboratories often create custom hotspot panels

Panels for Specific Clinical Settings
- Panels for hematologic malignancies often have different genes than panels designed for solid tumors
- Panels for specific inherited conditions
  o May include multiple genes that can cause single phenotype
  o May include groups of genes that, when mutated, cause clinically overlapping or similar phenotypes
  o Can greatly simplify genetic work-up and avoid lengthy "diagnostic odysseys"

HOTSPOT GENES

Commonly Mutated Genes
- Common tumor suppressor genes and oncogenes
- May or may not have associated targeted therapeutic options
- e.g., *TP53*, *RB1*

NGS Pile-Up of *TP53* Mutation

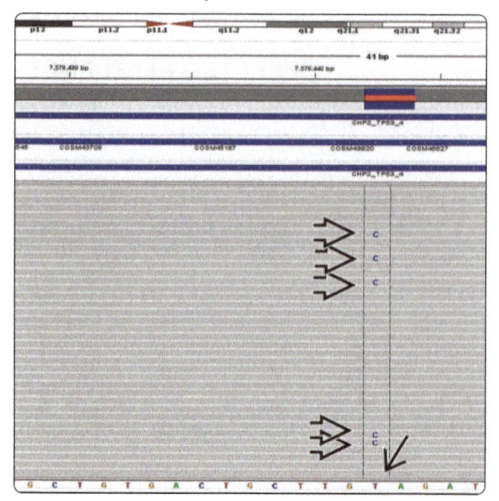

Circled Tumor Foci for Macrodissection

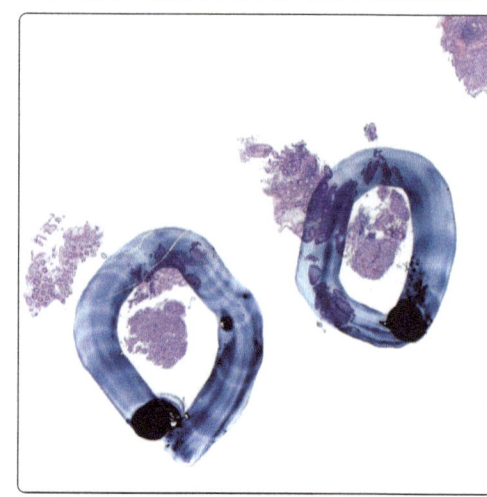

(Left) Hotspot next-generation sequencing (NGS) panel reveals a TP53 mutation, as identified by the C detected in multiple reads ➡ rather than the wildtype T ➡. (Right) A pathologist has circled small fragments of tumor for macrodissection prior to NGS hotspot analysis. Small biopsies with scant tumor are a challenge for molecular analysis.

Targeted Hotspot Gene Panel Using Massively Parallel Sequencing (Next-Generation Sequencing)

Genes Mutated in Specific Neoplasms
- May or may not have associated targeted therapeutic options but could theoretically assist in diagnosis and subclassification
  - e.g., *GNA11* (uveal melanoma), *MPL* (essential thrombocythemia, primary myelofibrosis)

Genes for Targeted Therapy
- NGS panels offer more extensive coverage than achieved with standalone single-gene assays
- With increasing demands for testing for multiple genes via both sequencing and FISH, NGS panels may optimize yield from scant tumor samples
- e.g., *EGFR*, *KRAS*, *NRAS*, *BRAF*

TECHNICAL AND INTERPRETIVE CHALLENGES

Validation
- Challenging due to number of mutated genes/targets
- Extensive and costly validation is necessary to fulfill CLIA requirements
- Some reference standards for NGS are commercially available
  - "Cocktails" that combine many different mutations in single sample

Size of Panel
- Optimal number of genes to include is moving target
- Must achieve balance between cost and practical benefit

Biopsy Specimen Quality
- Tissue obtained for molecular analysis is often very small with scant tumor cells
- Macrodissection is typically employed to maximize specimen yield

Variant Annotation
- Must distinguish between somatic mutation and possible rare population polymorphisms [single nucleotide polymorphism (SNP)]
  - Useful databases include dbSNP, COSMIC, ClinVar, and cBioPortal, but these are not exhaustive or error free
- Must attempt to distinguish between "driver" and "passenger" somatic mutations
  - Software tools for functional prediction (e.g., PolyPhen-2) of impact of variant on protein function are sometimes contradictory or otherwise unhelpful
  - Extensive literature and database searches are often necessary
- Many genes on somatic cancer hotspot panels are also affected by germline mutations
  - e.g., *TP53* in Li-Fraumeni syndrome
  - Hotspot panels run on tumor tissue alone usually cannot reliably differentiate between somatic and germline variants

Reporting
- 4-tier system proposed to categorize somatic sequence variants
  - Tier I: Variants with strong clinical significance
  - Tier II: Variants of potential clinical significance
  - Tier III: Variants of unknown clinical significance
  - Tier IV: Benign or likely benign variants
- Reports should include information about clinical trials and targeted therapy
- Some reports are voluminous and challenging for clinicians to utilize

LIMITS OF HOTSPOT APPROACH

Coverage
- While these assays are intended to cover most common &/or most significant mutations, pathogenic mutations outside of target regions will not be identified
  - Even for genes included in assay, some exons may be excluded
  - Other clinically significant genes may not be included

Large-Scale Genetic Changes
- Hotspot panels may not identify medium- to large-scale genetic changes
  - Larger insertions or deletions may not be identified
- Insertions or deletions of small to intermediate size are typically detectable
- Additional types of genetic changes may be detected on some panels
  - Translocations and fusion genes
  - Changes in copy number (including gene amplification or deletion)
    - These alterations require specialized analytic &/or bioinformatic approaches

Analytic Sensitivity
- Largely function of depth of coverage
- Common limit of detection is in range of 5% mutated alleles in wildtype background
- For certain mutations (e.g., *JAK2* V617F), clinically recommended limit of detection may be lower than achieved by typical hotspot panel

Clinical Applicability
- Some mutations identified via hotspot panels are not clearly actionable
  - May lack FDA-approved targeted therapy
  - FDA-approved drug may exist for different indication, mutation, or tumor type
  - Preclinical data may exist to support personalized therapy for some targets, but clinical data may be lacking
- Patients may be eligible for clinical trials, depending on trial availability

SELECTED REFERENCES

1. Pervez MT et al: A comprehensive review of performance of next-generation sequencing platforms. Biomed Res Int. 2022:3457806, 2022
2. Hu T et al: Next-generation sequencing technologies: an overview. Hum Immunol. 82(11):801-11, 2021
3. Zhong Y et al: Application of next generation sequencing in laboratory medicine. Ann Lab Med. 41(1):25-43, 2021
4. Roy S et al: Standards and guidelines for validating next-generation sequencing bioinformatics pipelines: a joint recommendation of the Association for Molecular Pathology and the College of American Pathologists. J Mol Diagn. 20(1):4-27, 2018
5. Williams HL et al: Validation of the Oncomine™ focus panel for next-generation sequencing of clinical tumour samples. Virchows Arch. 473(4):489-503, 2018

Targeted Hotspot Gene Panel Table

Features of Genes Commonly Included on Cancer Hotspot NGS Panels

Gene	Function	Most Common Class of Mutation*	Key Tumor Types	Germline Syndrome**	Comments
ABL1	Tyrosine kinase	(Rearranged)	CML, ALL, AML		ABL1 kinase domain mutations may arise during tyrosine kinase inhibitor therapy for CML
AKT1	Serine threonine kinase	Substitution missense	Breast, colorectal, ovarian, NSCLC	Cowden syndrome, Cowden-like syndrome	Participates in PI3K/AKT/mTOR pathway; possible role for mTOR or AKT inhibitors
ALK	Receptor tyrosine kinase	(Rearranged, many partner genes)	ALCL, NSCLC, sporadic neuroblastoma, inflammatory myofibroblastic tumor	Familial neuroblastoma	Rearrangement leading to ALK fusion is much more common and clinically significant than point mutations; crizotinib is FDA-approved for ALK-rearranged metastatic NSCLC; limited data on ALK inhibitors for activating point mutations; acquired ALK mutations during crizotinib therapy have been documented to confer drug resistance
APC	Wnt signaling antagonist	Substitution nonsense	Colorectal, pancreatic, desmoid, hepatoblastoma, glioma, other CNS	Familial adenomatous polyposis, Turcot syndrome	Somatic APC mutations are present in most sporadic colorectal tumors; > 60% of somatic mutations in APC occur between codons 1286 and 1513; small molecule inhibitors that inhibit Wnt signaling are under investigation (e.g., ICG-001)
ATM	Serine-threonine (pI3/pI4 kinase)	Substitution missense	Melanoma, colorectal, papillary thyroid, borderline ovarian, NSCLC, cholangiocarcinoma, pilocytic astrocytoma, mantle cell lymphoma	Ataxia-telangiectasia	Clinical studies, including PI3K/ATM inhibitor KU-59403, BKM120, and BYL719; suggested that ATM-deficient tumors may be inherently more radiosensitive, ATM inhibitors block DNA repair and enhance radiotherapy effects
BRAF	Serine/threonine kinase	Substitution missense	Hairy cell leukemia, melanoma, colorectal, papillary thyroid, borderline ovarian, NSCLC, cholangiocarcinoma, pilocytic astrocytoma	Noonan syndrome, LEOPARD syndrome, cardiofaciocutaneous syndrome	Involved in MAP kinase signaling; FDA-approved vemurafenib for melanoma with BRAF V600E, dabrafenib with V600 mutant metastatic melanoma, and trametinib (MEK inhibitor) for unresectable or metastatic melanoma with V600E or V600K; BRAF mutations are associated with sporadic colon cancer and are therefore useful in work-up for Lynch syndrome
CDH1	Cadherin (cell-cell adhesion glycoprotein)	Substitution missense	Lobular breast, gastric	Hereditary diffuse gastric carcinoma	E-cadherin maintains overall state of adhesion between epithelial cells; loss is thought to promote invasiveness and metastasis
CDKN2A	Cell cycle G1 control	(Varied)	Melanoma, multiple other tumor types	Familial multiple melanoma, pancreatic cancer	p16-INK4a isoform acts as tumor suppressor by inhibiting CDK4/6 kinase; alternative P14ARF isoform acts as tumor suppressor by sequestering MDM2 and stabilizing TP53; mostly in vitro studies have assessed effect of CDK inhibitors
CSF1R	Receptor for colony-stimulating factor 1	Substitution missense	MDS, AML, CMML, lung carcinoma, colon carcinoma, endometrial adenocarcinoma	Hereditary diffuse leukoencephalopathy with axonal spheroids	CSF1R is normally expressed predominantly in committed monocytes and macrophages
CTNNB1	Present in adherens	Substitution	Colorectal, ovarian,	Intellectual disability,	β-catenin functions downstream in

Targeted Hotspot Gene Panel Table

Features of Genes Commonly Included on Cancer Hotspot NGS Panels (Continued)

Gene	Function	Most Common Class of Mutation*	Key Tumor Types	Germline Syndrome**	Comments
	junctions between cells; anchors actin cytoskeleton; binds APC; binds TCF/LEF transcription factors	missense	hepatoblastoma, pleomorphic salivary gland adenoma, hepatocellular carcinoma, medulloblastoma, pilomatricoma, melanoma, other tumor types	autosomal dominant 19 (OMIM 615075: Neurodevelopmental disorder with spastic diplegia and visual defects)	Wnt signaling pathway; β-catenin translocates to nucleus and transactivates genes related to cell proliferation and apoptosis inhibition; CTNNB1 mutations stabilize β-catenin and promote this transactivation
EGFR	Tyrosine kinase	Substitution missense; exon 19 deletions	Glioma, lung adenocarcinoma	Inflammatory skin and bowel disease, neonatal, 2 (OMIM 616069: Caused by homozygous mutation of EGFR), inherited lung cancer syndrome due to germline EGFR T790M mutation	Epidermal growth factor receptor; exon 19 deletions and exon 21 L858R constitute ~ 85% of all EGFR mutations in NSCLC; afatinib and erlotinib are FDA approved for 1st-line treatment in metastatic NSCLC with these EGFR mutations; "EGFRvIII-type" deletions seen in glioblastoma
ERBB2 (HER2)	Tyrosine kinase; binds, stabilizes, and enhances signaling from other ligand-bound epidermal growth factor receptor-type receptors	(Amplification)	Breast, gastric, ovarian, NSCLC, colon, other tumor types	Germline mutations associated with increase risk of myeloproliferative neoplasms	Protein product is better known as HER2; gene amplification in breast and gastric cancer and few other tumors indicates enhanced sensitivity to HER2-targeted therapy, such as trastuzumab (and pertuzumab and lapatinib in combination therapy in some cases); there is developing interest in targeted therapy for ERBB2 (HER2) point mutations and small indels
ERBB4	Tyrosine kinase, epidermal growth factor receptor subfamily	Substitution missense	Melanoma, gastric, colorectal	Amyotrophic lateral sclerosis 19 (OMIM 615515)	ERBB4 mutations predict sensitivity to lapatinib (dual tyrosine kinase inhibitor) in melanoma
EZH2	Polycomb group family; methylates histone H3	Dependent on type of neoplasm	DLBCL, follicular lymphoma (missense, gain of function); myeloid malignancies (loss of function); T-ALL (loss of function)	EZH2-related overgrowth/Weaver syndrome	Polycomb group family members form protein complexes that maintain epigenetic silencing of genes over successive cell generations; tazemetostat is FDA-approved EZH2 inhibitor for follicular lymphoma and epithelioid sarcoma
FBXW7	Tumor suppressor, participates in phosphorylation-dependent ubiquitination	Substitution missense	Colorectal, endometrial, T-ALL, squamous cell cancer of head and neck, liver, ovarian	Germline mutations lead to neurodevelopmental syndrome	Binds several protooncoproteins, including cyclin-E, and targets them for degradation; limited early clinical experience with mTOR inhibitors
FGFR1	Tyrosine kinase	(Rearranged)	Pilocytic astrocytoma, rarely reported in other tumors	Encephalocraniocutaneous lipomatosis; Pfeiffer syndrome, Jackson-Weiss syndrome, Hartsfield syndrome, hypogonadotropic hypogonadism 2 ± anosmia, osteoglophonic dysplasia, trigonocephaly 1	Binds both acidic and basic fibroblast growth factors and is involved in limb induction; FGFR1 rearrangement is defining feature of myeloid and lymphoid neoplasms with FGFR1 rearrangements (WHO 2016), which is unresponsive to most tyrosine kinase inhibitors (PKC412 successful in 1 case); preclinical studies of small molecular inhibitors; amplification also occurs in solid tumors; rare fusion seen in NSCLC
FGFR2	Tyrosine kinase	Substitution missense	Endometrial, melanoma, NSCLC, colon, esophageal	Various craniosynostosis syndromes including Pfeiffer, bent bone	High-affinity receptor for acidic, basic, &/or keratinocyte fibroblast growth factor; clinical trials of several

Targeted Hotspot Gene Panel Table

Features of Genes Commonly Included on Cancer Hotspot NGS Panels (Continued)

Gene	Function	Most Common Class of Mutation*	Key Tumor Types	Germline Syndrome**	Comments
			squamous cell	dysplasia, Apert, and others	small molecule inhibitors; amplification also occurs in solid tumors
FGFR3	Tyrosine kinase	Substitution missense	Bladder, colon, lung, breast cancers, glioblastoma, multiple myeloma, T-cell lymphoma	Achondroplasia, Crouzon syndrome with acanthosis nigricans, Muenke syndrome, others	Binds acidic and basic fibroblast growth factors, plays role in bone development and maintenance; recent use of BGJ398 in early clinical trial for FGFR3-mutated bladder cancer; rare fusion seen in NSCLC
FLT3	Tyrosine kinase	Insertion inframe (ITD)	AML, ALL		Poor prognostic factor in AML; tyrosine kinase domain point mutation is less common
GNA11	G protein subunit-α 11	Substitution missense	Uveal melanoma, lung adenocarcinoma, colon carcinoma, breast cancer	Hypocalcemia, autosomal dominant 2 (OMIM 615361), hypocalciuric hypercalcemia type II	Highly homologous to GNAQ; either GNA11 or GNAQ mutations are present in most uveal melanomas; GNA11 mutations are not present in extraocular melanomas; preclinical work using combination of PKC and MEK inhibitors
GNAS	G protein subunit	Substitution missense	Lung, carcinoma, colon cancer, breast cancer, pituitary adenoma	McCune-Albright syndrome, ACTH-independent macronodular adrenal hyperplasia, progressive osseous heteroplasia, pseudohypoparathyroidism, pseudopseudohypoparathyroidism	Better response to octreotide in GNAS-mutated pituitary adenomas in some studies
GNAQ	G protein subunit	Substitution missense	Uveal melanoma, lung adenocarcinoma, colon carcinoma, endometrial endometrioid carcinoma	Sturge-Weber syndrome (mosaic); capillary malformation 1, somatic, mosaic	Highly homologous to GNA11; either GNA11 or GNAQ mutations are present in most uveal melanomas; GNA11 mutations are rare in extraocular melanomas; preclinical work using combination of PKC and MEK inhibitors
HNF1A	Transcription factor	Substitution missense	Hepatic adenoma	Maturity-onset diabetes of young, type 3	Required for expression of certain liver-specific genes
HRAS	Ras GTPase	Substitution missense	Bladder, breast, thyroid, lung, breast	Costello syndrome	Most common mutations affect codons 12, 13, and 61; participates in MAPK signaling cascade; possible role for MEK inhibitors
IDH1	Isocitrate dehydrogenase	Substitution missense	Low-grade gliomas, secondary high-grade glioblastoma, AML, angioimmunoblastic T-cell lymphoma, cartilaginous tumors, cholangiocarcinoma	Maffucci syndrome, Ollier disease, 2-hydroxyglutaric aciduria	Catalyzes conversion of isocitrate to α-ketoglutarate; mutation confers neomorphic enzyme activity, leading it to produce 2-hydroxyglutarate, which in turn inhibits normal epigenetic regulation; better prognosis in IDH1-mutated gliomas; conflicting data on prognostic significance of IDH1 mutations in AML; ivosidenib approved by FDA for relapsed/refractory AML with mutated IDH1
IDH2	Isocitrate dehydrogenase	Substitution missense	Low-grade gliomas, secondary high-grade glioblastoma, AML, angioimmunoblastic T-cell lymphoma, cartilaginous tumors, cholangiocarcinoma		Catalyzes conversion of isocitrate to α-ketoglutarate; mutation confers neomorphic enzyme activity, leading it to produce 2-hydroxyglutarate, which in turn inhibits normal epigenetic regulation; better prognosis in IDH2-mutated gliomas; conflicting data on prognostic

Targeted Hotspot Gene Panel Table

Features of Genes Commonly Included on Cancer Hotspot NGS Panels (Continued)

Gene	Function	Most Common Class of Mutation*	Key Tumor Types	Germline Syndrome**	Comments
					significance of *IDH2* mutations in AML; enasidenib is approved by FDA for treatment of relapsed/refractory *IDH2*-mutated AML
JAK2	Tyrosine kinase	Substitution missense	Myeloid neoplasms (especially MPN, including virtually all PV)	Rare report of familial thrombocythemia (OMIM 614521)	Highly useful in diagnosis and subtyping of MPN
JAK3	Tyrosine kinase	Substitution missense	Acute megakaryoblastic leukemia, ETP-ALL, T-PLL, T-ALL, lung carcinoma, colon cancer, breast cancer	SCID, autosomal recessive, T-cell-negative, B cell-positive, NK cell-negative type	Important in transducing signals from binding of interleukins; specific JAK3 inhibitor tofacitinib is FDA approved for treatment of rheumatoid arthritis
KDR	Tyrosine kinase	Substitution missense	NSCLC, melanoma, colorectal, glioblastoma, angiosarcoma	Infantile capillary hemangioma	Encodes receptor for VEGFA; preclinical and early clinical investigation of multikinase inhibitors; *KDR* amplification may also be seen
KIT	Tyrosine kinase	Substitution missense	GIST, AML, mastocytosis, mucosal melanoma	Familial GIST, familial mastocytosis	Mutations occur mostly in exons 8, 9, 11, 13, 17, and 18; imatinib for many *KIT*-mutated neoplasms, but efficacy (and dose) depends on specific malignancy and site/type of mutation; secondary mutations in GIST acquired during imatinib treatment correspond to resistance; codon 816 mutation is minor criterion for diagnosis of systemic mastocytosis; *KIT* mutation refines prognostic expectations in core-binding factor AML
KRAS	Ras GTPase	Substitution missense	Pancreatic, colorectal, NSCLC, thyroid, AML, other tumor types	Noonan syndrome 3	Most common mutations affect codons 12, 13, and 61; presence of codon 12 or 13 mutation in metastatic colon cancer indicates lack of efficacy of anti-EGFR monoclonal antibody therapy
MET	Tyrosine kinase	Substitution missense	NSCLC, colon cancer, cutaneous melanoma, papillary renal, head and neck squamous cell carcinoma	Familial papillary renal carcinoma 1	Encodes hepatocyte growth factor receptor; recognized role for crizotinib (or perhaps other tyrosine kinase inhibitors) in *MET*-amplified tumors; *MET* amplification is mode of resistance to EGFR inhibitor therapy in *EGFR*-mutated NSCLC
MLH1	DNA mismatch repair	Substitution missense	Colorectal, endometrial, ovarian, CNS	Lynch syndrome	Somatic *MLH1* mutations do occur in cases of sporadic MSI-high tumors, though *MLH1* promoter hypermethylation is more typical clinical laboratory finding, predictive biomarker for immunotherapy
MPL	Thrombopoietin receptor	Substitution missense	MPN	Familial thrombocytosis; congenital amegakaryocytic thrombocytopenia	Mutations usually at codon 515; useful in diagnosis and subtyping of MPN (present in ET and PMF)
NOTCH1	Notch signaling protein	Substitution missense	T-ALL, colon, lung, and breast cancers	Adams-Oliver syndrome 5 (OMIM 616028)	Named for strain of *Drosophila* with wing notches; cell surface receptor binds ligands, upon which cytoplasmic portion detaches and translocates to nucleus; clinical trials of NOTCH inhibition using γ-

Targeted Hotspot Gene Panel Table

Features of Genes Commonly Included on Cancer Hotspot NGS Panels (Continued)

Gene	Function	Most Common Class of Mutation*	Key Tumor Types	Germline Syndrome**	Comments
					secretase inhibitors under investigation
NPM1	Phosphoprotein, shuttles between cytoplasm and nucleus	Insertion frameshift (rearrangement)	AML	Dyskeratosis congenita	Most common is 4 bp insertion in exon 12, leading to loss of nuclear localization signal; useful for refining prognostic expectations in AML (normal karyotype with NPM1 mutation but no FLT3 mutation is good risk disease)
NRAS	Ras GTPase	Substitution missense	Melanoma, AML, colorectal, NSCLC, JMML	Noonan syndrome	Most common mutations affect codons 12, 13, and 61; partial response to MEK inhibitor in melanoma
PDGFRA	Tyrosine kinase	Substitution missense (rearrangement)	GIST, lung, colon, glioblastoma	Hereditary inflammatory fibroid polyps and multiple heterogeneous gastrointestinal mesenchymal tumors reported	Encodes platelet-derived growth factor receptor; mutations in exons 12, 14, and 18 are seen in GIST and are sensitive to imatinib (exception: D842V, T674I); rearrangement is defining feature of myeloid and lymphoid neoplasms with PDGFRA rearrangement and is also seen in glioblastoma
PIK3CA	Catalytic subunit of phosphatidylinositol 3-kinase	Substitution missense	Breast, colorectal, gastric, glioblastoma, NSCLC, ovarian, hepatocellular, endometrial	Cowden syndrome, Clove syndrome, CLAPO (overgrowth syndrome)	Key hotspots are E542K, E545K, and H1047R; participates in PI3K/AKT/mTOR pathway; possible role for mTOR inhibitors
PTEN	Phosphatidylinositol -3,4,5-trisphosphate 3-phosphatase	Substitution missense	Glioma, prostate, colon, breast, endometrial, lung	Cowden syndrome, Lhermitte-Duclos syndrome	Converts PIP3 to PIP2, which inhibits PI3K-dependent activation of AKT; possible role for AKT and mTOR inhibitors
PTPN11	Tyrosine phosphatase	Substitution missense	JMML, AML, MDS	Noonan syndrome 1, LEOPARD syndrome 1, metachondromatosis	Intracellular signal transducer, activates RAS/MAPK pathway and negatively regulates JAK/STAT signaling; small-molecule PTPN11 (SHP2) inhibitors exist
RB1	Key cell cycle regulator	Substitution nonsense	Retinoblastoma, sarcoma, breast, small cell lung carcinoma	Familial retinoblastoma, retinoblastoma, trilateral	Phosphorylated by cyclin-dependent kinases, upon which transcription factor E2F is released to activate transcription of S-phase genes
RET	Tyrosine kinase	Substitution missense (rearrangement)	Medullary thyroid, pheochromocytoma	MEN2a/2b, familial medullary thyroid carcinoma, Hirschsprung disease	Receptor for glial cell line-derived neurotrophic factors, important for neural development; RET rearrangements seen in papillary thyroid carcinoma (termed RET/PTC) and NSCLC; several multikinase inhibitors have anti-RET activity (e.g., sunitinib, sorafenib, cabozantinib, vandetanib, ponatinib, lenvatinib); many general trials of multikinase inhibitors in papillary thyroid carcinoma and NSCLC; patients with RET-rearranged NSCLC have responded to cabozantinib, and this agent also shows specific benefit in medullary thyroid carcinoma with RET mutations
SMAD4	Signal transduction protein	Substitution missense	Colorectal, pancreatic, small intestine	Juvenile polyposis/hereditary hemorrhagic telangiectasia,	TGFB signaling causes activation of SMADs, which then bind specific target genes to regulate

Targeted Hotspot Gene Panel Table

Features of Genes Commonly Included on Cancer Hotspot NGS Panels (Continued)

Gene	Function	Most Common Class of Mutation*	Key Tumor Types	Germline Syndrome**	Comments
				juvenile intestinal polyposis, Myhre syndrome	transcription
SMARCB1	Chromatin remodeling protein	Deletion frameshift	Malignant rhabdoid	Rhabdoid predisposition syndrome 1, Coffin-Siris syndrome 3, schwannomatosis-1	Corresponds to INI1 protein assessed by immunohistochemistry
SMO	G protein-coupled receptor	Substitution missense	Lung adenocarcinoma, basal cell and squamous carcinoma, medulloblastoma		Binding of hedgehog ligand to PTCH1 releases inhibition of SMO, which activates GLI zinc finger transcription factor; vismodegib is FDA-approved SMO inhibitor for metastatic basal cell carcinoma (but not limited to SMO-mutated cases)
SRC	Tyrosine kinase	Substitution missense	Colon, gastric, breast, lung		Interacts with diverse array of proteins, mediating cross-talk between normally distinct signaling pathways; dasatinib is known to inhibit SRC in cell lines
STK11	Serine/threonine kinase	Substitution missense	NSCLC, pancreatic	Peutz-Jeghers syndrome	Regulates cell division, assists cell polarization, regulates cellular energy utilization (by activating adenine monophosphate-activated protein kinase), promotes apoptosis; loss of STK11 leads to loss of suppression of mTOR signaling; rare case of treatment response with mTOR inhibitor
TP53	Transcription factor	Substitution missense	Breast, colorectal, lung, sarcoma, adrenocortical, glioma, many other tumor types	Li-Fraumeni syndrome	"Guardian of genome" tasked with responding to DNA damage by upregulating expression of genes related to cell cycle arrest and apoptosis; mutated in ~ 50% of malignancies
VHL	Oxygen-sensing pathway	Substitution missense	Renal (clear cell), hemangioma, pheochromocytoma	von Hippel-Lindau syndrome, familial erythrocytosis-2	RCC with VHL mutation may be more sensitive to VEGFA-targeted therapy, though responses are also seen in non-VHL-mutated cases
WT1	Transcription factor	Substitution, missense, nonsense, frameshift deletions (rearrangement)	Kidney cancers, lung cancer, breast carcinoma, colon carcinoma, AML, ALL, desmoplastic small round cell tumor	Wilms tumor-aniridia-genitourinary malformation-retardation, Denys-Drash syndrome	WT1 functions as both tumor suppressor and oncogene, it is implicated in the regulation of cell survival, proliferation, and differentiation

While the information in this table was correct at the time of this writing, genetic knowledge and targeted therapy strategies evolve rapidly, and the reader should obtain up-to-date information for clinical applications. Details regarding targeted therapy are given for informational purposes only, and treatment decisions should be based on all available clinical information by the responsible physician.* Mutation class derived from COSMIC data and excludes rearrangements and amplification. [If rearrangement or amplification are felt to be the most clinically significant for a given gene, they are listed in this column in parentheses; next-generation sequencing (NGS) panels will not routinely detect these changes.]** Cancer Hotspot NGS panels are not intended for detection of germline mutations. However, for purposes of complete clinicopathologic correlation, the pathologist should be aware that many genes on these panels are mutated in inherited syndromes, including cancer predisposition syndromes.

CML = chronic myeloid leukemia; ALL = acute lymphoblastic leukemia/lymphoma; NSCLC = non-small cell lung carcinoma; MDS = myelodysplastic syndrome; AML = acute myeloid leukemia; CMML = chronic myelomonocytic leukemia; DLBCL = diffuse large B-cell lymphoma; MPN = myeloproliferative neoplasm; ETP = early T-cell precursor; PLL = prolymphocytic leukemia; GIST = gastrointestinal stromal tumor; PV = polycythemia vera; ET = essential thrombocythemia; PMF = primary myelofibrosis; JMML = juvenile myelomonocytic leukemia; MEN = multiple endocrine neoplasia; SCID = severe combined immunodeficiency; ITD = internal tandem duplication; ALCL = anaplastic large cell lymphoma; COSMIC = catalogue of somatic mutations in cancer; T-ALL = T-cell acute lymphoblastic lymphoma; MSI = microsatellite instability.

MGMT Promoter Gene Methylation Assay

TERMINOLOGY

Definitions
- Official name: O-6-methylguanine-DNA methyltransferase
- Official symbol: *MGMT*
- HGNC ID: 7059
- Chromosomal location: 10q26.3
- Preferred protein name: Methylated-DNA-protein-cysteine methyltransferase
  - Alternative protein names: Methylguanine-DNA methyltransferase, O-6-methylguanine-DNA-alkyltransferase, O-6-methylguanine-DNA methyltransferase, 6-O-methylguanine-DNA methyltransferase

Function of *MGMT*
- DNA repair gene
  - Protects against cytotoxic and mutagenic alkyl adducts to O-6-guanine residues in DNA
    - Chemical carcinogens (including N-nitrosamines, aflatoxins, aromatic amines, and polycyclic aromatic hydrocarbons) cause creation of DNA alkyl adducts
    - Alkyl adducts also occur naturally in vivo at low rate
  - Recognizes alkyl adducts and removes them from DNA by transfer of alkyl group to internal cysteine acceptor site
    - Also repairs O-6 ethylguanine and O-4 methylthymine
    - Following transfer of alkyl group, alkylated MGMT is degraded
    - Expression of MGMT is induced by DNA damage, glucocorticoids, cyclic AMP, and protein kinase C

Methylation of *MGMT* Promoter
- Promoter region includes at least 97 CpG sequences, constituting CpG island
- Epigenetic modification of promoter region of gene decreases gene transcription
  - Methylated CpG sites bind methylated CpG binding proteins 1 and 2 (MECP1/MECP2)
    - MECP proteins decrease transcription directly through transcription repression domain
    - MECP proteins bind other factors that cause chromatin condensation and block transcription
    - MECP proteins block binding of transcription factors
- Methyl groups are added to cytosines followed by guanines (CpG dinucleotides)
  - CpG islands are DNA regions with many cytosine-guanine linear sequence pairs in 5' to 3' direction
  - CpG islands are often found in promoter region of genes, where transcription machinery binds
- Associated with several cancer types

CLINICAL IMPLICATIONS

Loss of *MGMT* Expression in Tumors
- Loss of *MGMT* expression has been described in many neoplasms, including gliomas, lymphomas, breast and prostate cancer, germ cell tumors, and retinoblastoma
  - Typically results from *MGMT* promoter hypermethylation, which is predictive marker in high-grade gliomas (GBM)
    - GBM is most common primary brain tumor in adults
    - Treatment includes surgery, radiation therapy, and chemotherapy
    - Median survival with standard of care treatment is 14.6 months
    - Methylated MGMT promoter region correlates with improved survival in gliomas treated with alkylating agents
  - Percentage of GBM with epigenetic methylation of *MGMT* promoter regions varies by grade and methylation detection method

MGMT Promoter Methylation and Survival in High-Grade Gliomas
- *MGMT* methylation status is essential part of work-up for high-grade gliomas
  - Evidence suggests methylation may correlate with response in low-grade tumor as well
- *MGMT* promoter methylation is well characterized as predictive factor in GBM

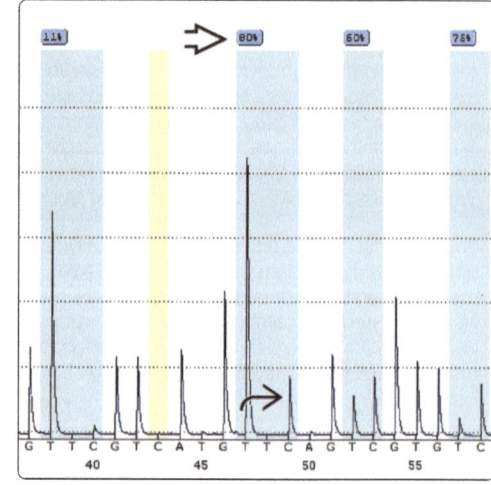

(Left) *Glioblastoma* is characterized by hypercellularity with cellular atypia, karyorrhexis, endothelial proliferation, and pseudopalisading necrosis. (Right) *Pyrogram* shows the methylation percentages at CpG sites (highlighted in light blue columns) in this case of glioblastoma. The presence of cytosine indicates the amount of methylation at each CpG site.

Glioblastoma

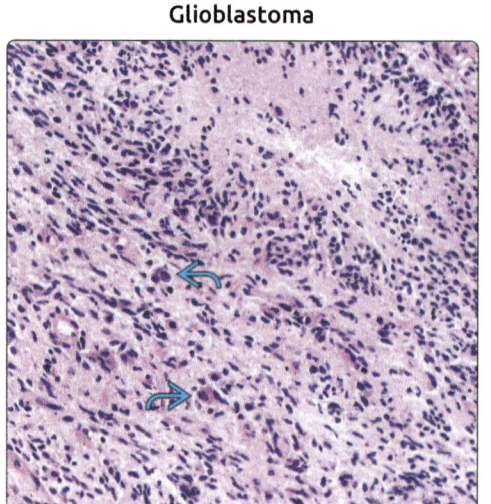

Methylation Analysis by Pyrosequencing

MGMT Promoter Gene Methylation Assay

- *MGMT* methylation is associated with increased overall survival in patients treated with radiotherapy and chemotherapy
  - Patients with hypermethylated *MGMT* promoter show survival rates of 49% and 14% at 2 years and 5 years when treated with temozolomide and radiotherapy
  - Patients with unmethylated *MGMT* promoter show survival rates of 15% and 8% at 2 years and 5 years with same treatment
- *MGMT* methylation status used for risk stratification in clinical trials
- Methylation is associated with *IDH* mutations and genome-wide epigenetic changes

MGMT Promoter Methylation and GBM Treatment

- Temozolomide and lomustine are alkylating agents that cross blood-brain barrier and are standard of care for treatment of high-grade glioma
  - Causes cell death by creating O-6 methylguanine adducts
  - Methylguanine preferentially pairs with thymine rather than cytosine, creating mismatch
    - Mismatch repair genes attempt to repair mismatch, but methylguanine continues to pair with thymine, causing futile cycle of mismatch repair
    - After several futile attempts to repair, cell eventually undergoes apoptosis
- **Methylated MGMT promoter region**
  - Results in suppression of *MGMT* expression in tumor cells
    - Decreases function of mismatch repair genes and increases incidence of acquired mutations
    - Leads to unrepaired alkylated guanine residues in tumor cells
    - Promotes apoptosis of tumor cells
- **Nonmethylated MGMT promoter region**
  - Results in expression of *MGMT* in tumor cells
    - Removes alkyl group
    - Allows mismatch repair proteins to successfully repair G:T mismatches
    - Promotes tumor cell survival
    - Results in resistance to treatment with alkylating agents, such as temozolomide
- **MGMT methylation status is used to guide treatment**
  - Patients with methylated *MGMT* promoter region have improved outcomes with temozolomide
  - Difference in response is particularly marked in patients > 65 years of age
  - Methylation status greater predictor of treatment response than other tumor or patient factors

TESTING METHODS

Bisulfite Conversion Dependent

- Most common method of assessment of methylation status
- Genomic tumor DNA is isolated and treated with sodium bisulfite
- Bisulfite causes chemical conversion of all unmethylated cytosines to uracil
  - Uracil will be replaced by thymine during PCR
- 5-methyl-cytosine is protected from conversion by bisulfite
  - 5-methyl-cytosine will be replaced by cytosine during PCR
- Bisulfite-treated DNA is amplified using primers to CpG island, including part of promoter region and exon 1
  - This region contains 98 CpG methylation sites
  - Most assays target limited number of sites
    - Methylation may be heterogeneous, and studies targeting very limited numbers of sites may give misleading results
  - Average level of methylation over tested sites is used to determine if statistically significant level of methylation is present above background
    - These CpG sites are unmethylated in normal tissue
  - Cut-offs are not well defined or standardized
    - Presence of methylation at or above validated cut-off for positive correlates with improved survival with alkylating chemotherapy compared to unmethylated tumors
    - By pyrosequencing, 1/2 of all high-grade gliomas have methylation of *MGMT* promoter regions
  - Alternative analysis involves determining normal methylation levels at individual CpG sites
    - Anything above normal is considered positive at particular site

Measuring Rate of Conversion

- Methylation-specific pyrosequencing
  - Amplified DNA is sequenced
  - Ratio of cytosine to thymine at each potential conversion site is measured
  - Best correlation with prognosis
- Methylation-specific PCR (MS-PCR)
  - 2 different primer sets are used
    - Methylated primer pair is specific for nonconverted sequence
    - Nonmethylated primer pair is specific for sequences with cytosine residues converted to uracil
  - Agarose gel electrophoresis is performed to visualize presence of PCR products
- Real-time MS-PCR
  - Utilizes probe specific to nonconverted sequence with attached fluorophore and quencher
  - Resulting fluorescence is quantified
  - Results are expressed as methylation index (MI): Ratio of amplification of methylated *MGMT* to control gene
- Methylation-specific high-resolution melting curve
  - Following bisulfite conversion, methylated and nonmethylated sequences have different melting points

SELECTED REFERENCES

1. Ashkan K et al: MGMT promoter methylation: prognostication beyond treatment response. J Pers Med. 13(6):999, 2023
2. Kinslow CJ et al: Association of MGMT promotor methylation with survival in low-grade and anaplastic gliomas after alkylating chemotherapy. JAMA Oncol. 9(7):919-27, 2023
3. Torre M et al: The predictive value of partial MGMT promoter methylation for IDH-wild-type glioblastoma patients. Neurooncol Pract. 10(2):126-31, 2023
4. Brandner S et al: MGMT promoter methylation testing to predict overall survival in people with glioblastoma treated with temozolomide: a comprehensive meta-analysis based on a Cochrane Systematic Review. Neuro Oncol. 23(9):1457-69, 2021

SECTION 5
Molecular Pathology of Myeloid Neoplasms

Molecular Work-Up of Myeloid Neoplasms	134

Myeloproliferative Neoplasms

Chronic Myeloid Leukemia, *BCR::ABL1*-Positive	136
Chronic Neutrophilic Leukemia	144
Polycythemia Vera	148
Primary Myelofibrosis	152
Essential Thrombocythemia	156
Chronic Eosinophilic Leukemia, NOS	160
Myeloproliferative Neoplasm, Unclassifiable	162

Mastocytosis

Mastocytosis	166

Myeloid/Lymphoid Neoplasms With Eosinophilia and Gene Rearrangement

Myeloid/Lymphoid Neoplasms With Eosinophilia and Tyrosine Kinase Gene Fusions	174

Premalignant Clonal Hematopoiesis and Cytopenias

VEXAS Syndrome	178
Clonal Hematopoiesis and Premalignant Clonal Cytopenia	182

Myelodysplastic Syndrome (MDS)

Overview and Classification of Myelodysplastic Syndrome	184
Myelodysplastic Syndrome With Mutated *SF3B1*	188
Myelodysplastic Syndrome, NOS	192
Myelodysplastic Syndrome With del(5q)	200
Myelodysplastic Syndrome With *TP53* Multihit Mutations	204
Myelodysplastic Syndrome/Acute Myeloid Leukemia	206
Pediatric Myelodysplastic Syndrome and Refractory Cytopenia of Childhood	208

Myelodysplastic/Myeloproliferative Neoplasms

Overview of Myelodysplastic/Myeloproliferative Neoplasms	214
Chronic Myelomonocytic Leukemia	216
Atypical Chronic Myeloid Leukemia	220
Juvenile Myelomonocytic Leukemia	224
Myelodysplastic/Myeloproliferative Neoplasm, NOS	228

Acute Myeloid Leukemia

Overview of Acute Myeloid Leukemia	232
Acute Myeloid Leukemia With t(8;21)/*RUNX1::RUNX1T1*	240
Acute Myeloid Leukemia With inv(16) or t(16;16)/*CBFB::MYH11*	244
Acute Promyelocytic Leukemia With t(15;17)/*PML::RARA*	248
Acute Myeloid Leukemia With t(9;11)/*MLLT3::KMT2A*	254
Acute Myeloid Leukemia With t(6;9)/*DEK::NUP214*	258
Acute Myeloid Leukemia With inv(3) or t(3;3)/*GATA2; MECOM*	260
Acute Myeloid Leukemia (Megakaryoblastic) With t(1;22)/*RBM15::MRTFA*	262
Acute Myeloid Leukemia With Myelodysplasia-Related Gene Mutations or Cytogenetic Abnormalities	264
Acute Myeloid Leukemia, NOS	270
Myeloid Sarcoma	276
Myeloid Proliferations Associated With Down Syndrome	280

Blastic Plasmacytoid Dendritic Cell Neoplasm

Blastic Plasmacytoid Dendritic Cell Neoplasm	284

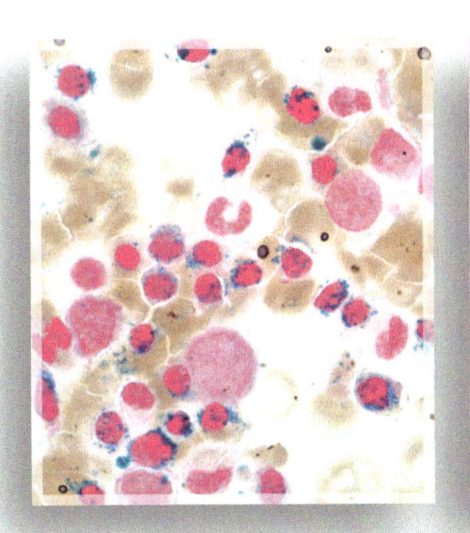

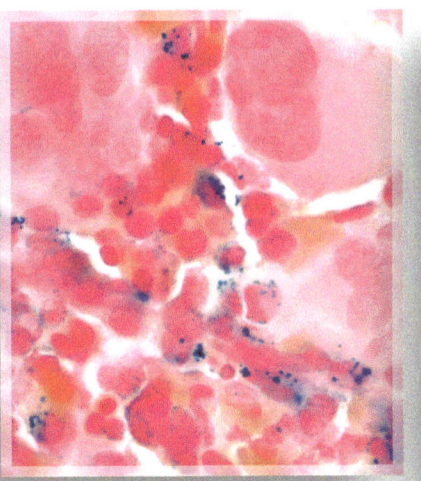

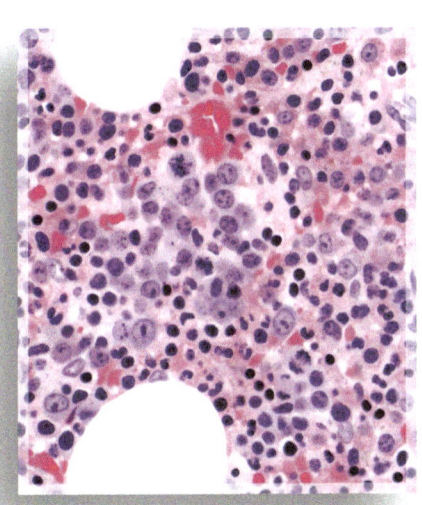

Molecular Work-Up of Myeloid Neoplasms

MOLECULAR/GENETIC TECHNIQUES COMMONLY USED

Chromosome Analysis (Karyotype)
- Reveals large-scale structural changes in genome
- Clonal cytogenetic abnormalities often correlate with clonal hematopoiesis
- Karyotype derived from unstimulated bone marrow culture will typically reflect myeloid stem cells or blasts

FISH
- Uses fluorescently labeled probes to identify presence, absence, or rearrangement of specific genomic regions
- Important findings in myeloid neoplasms
  - Numerical abnormalities
  - Translocations
  - Deletions

PCR-Based Analysis
- Numerous types of molecular assays derive from common technique of PCR
- Identifies gene mutations (via sequencing or other detection methods)
- RT-PCR identifies and quantifies presence of fusion transcripts

Next-Generation Sequencing
- Enables simultaneous assessment of many genes
- Significantly mutated genes identified in myeloid neoplasms by next-generation sequencing (NGS) technology
  - *ASXL1, BCOR, CALR, CBL, CEBPA, CSF3R, DNMT3A, EZH2, FLT3, IDH1, IDH2, JAK2, KIT, KRAS, MPL, NRAS, NPM1, RUNX1, SETBP1, SF3B1, SRSF2, TET2, TP53, U2AF1,* and *WT1*
- Clinical utility of NGS myeloid gene panel assessment
  - May improve diagnosis
  - May help in therapeutic decisions
  - May provide prognostic information

- *DNMT3A, ASXL1, TET2, SF3B1,* and *SRSF2* are also associated with clonal hematopoiesis in apparently healthy older individuals

PURPOSES OF MOLECULAR ANALYSIS IN MYELOID NEOPLASMS

Establish Diagnosis
- Detection of specific abnormalities may establish presence of myeloid neoplasm
  - e.g., monosomy 7 and myelodysplastic syndrome

Establish Subtype of Myeloid Neoplasm
- Even if diagnosis of myeloid neoplasia is known, certain molecular findings may establish presence of specific subtype of myeloid neoplasm
  - e.g., acute promyelocytic leukemia with t(1;17); acute myeloid leukemia (AML) with mutated *TP53*, etc.

Establish Prognosis
- Certain molecular findings may refine prognostic expectations for patient
  - e.g., *KIT* mutation in AML with t(8;21)

LIMITATIONS OF TECHNIQUES

Karyotype
- Myeloid neoplasms not infrequently have normal karyotype
- Some changes may be cryptic (invisible) on karyotype
  - Some are routinely cryptic or submicroscopic
    - e.g., *PDGFRA::FIP1L1* rearrangement
- Recently introduced optical genome mapping platform appears promising in refining chromosomal aberrations with high resolution compared to conventional karyotype

FISH
- Will only identify specific abnormalities targeted with given probe set

PCR
- Will only identify specific abnormalities targeted by given primer pair

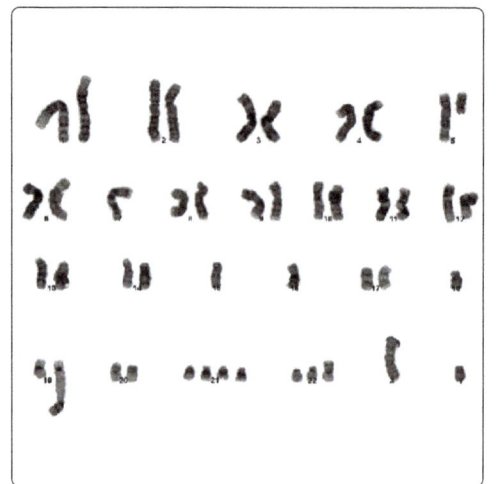

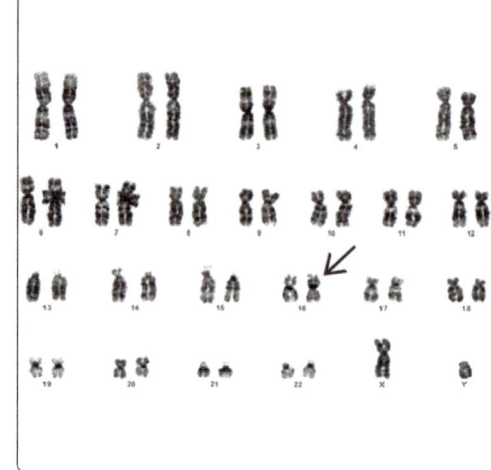

(Left) Highly complex karyotype, including monosomy 7 and deletion of 5q, is associated with a very poor prognosis in this patient with acute myeloid leukemia. (Right) Chromosome analysis of acute myeloid leukemia reveals inv(16)(p13.1q22) ➡. This finding is diagnostic of a specific subtype of acute myeloid leukemia and indicates a relatively good prognosis.

Molecular Work-Up of Myeloid Neoplasms

Global Approach to Cytogenetic and Molecular Testing in Myeloid Neoplasms (With Key Examples)

Purpose of Molecular Study	Utility of Karyotype	Utility of FISH	Utility of Molecular Genetic Analysis
Myelodysplastic Syndrome			
Establish diagnosis	Yes: WHO-HAEM5 and ICC-defined, MDS-associated cytogenetic abnormalities (e.g., monosomy 7, 5q-, etc.)	Yes: FISH MDS panel is useful when cytogenetic analysis fails or is not available	Yes: NGS panels identify MDS-related gene mutations (e.g., *SF3B1*, *SRSF2*, *U2AF1*)
Establish subtype	Yes: Karyotype is necessary to define cases of MDS with isolated del(5q)	Maybe: Deletion of 5q can be documented, but it cannot be shown to be isolated by FISH	No: There is overlap between MDS subcategories regarding specific mutated genes
Prognosis	Yes: Karyotype is critical for clinical risk stratification, according to R-IPSS	Yes: FISH MDS panel can identify abnormalities used in clinical risk stratification, according to R-IPSS	Yes: Gene mutations may provide prognostic information beyond R-IPSS and are incorporated in IPSS-M
Myeloproliferative Neoplasms			
Establish subtype	Yes: t(9;22)(q34;q11) is prerequisite for diagnosis of CML by karyotype, FISH, or RT-PCR	Yes: *BCR::ABL1* fusion is prerequisite for diagnosis of CML by either FISH, karyotype, or RT-PCR	Yes: Specific mutation, such as *JAK2* V617F, *JAK2* exon 12, *CALR*, *MPL*, and *CSF3R*; RT-PCR for *BCR::ABL1* transcripts
Prognosis	Sometimes: e.g., clonal evolution in CML	No	Yes: e.g., *CALR* and *ASXL1* mutations in PMF; RT-PCR for change in *BCR::BL1* transcript level over time
Acute Myeloid Leukemia			
Establish diagnosis	Yes: Certain karyotypic findings establish diagnosis of AML regardless of blast count [e.g., t(15;17)], per WHO-HAEM5, and with ≥ 10% blasts per ICC	Yes: Certain FISH abnormalities establish diagnosis of AML [e.g., t(15;17) regardless of blast count (WHO-HAEM5)] or with ≥ 10% blasts per ICC	Yes: Fusion transcripts by RT-PCR can diagnose certain types of AML (e.g., APL)
Establish subtype	Yes: Many subtypes of AML defined by cytogenetic findings [e.g., inv(16)], myelodysplasia-related cytogenetic abnormalities or gene mutations	Yes: e.g., *PML::RARA* fusion in APL	Yes: e.g., *PML::RARA* transcripts in APL; AML with mutated *NPM1* or in-frame bZIP *CEBPA* mutation
Prognosis	Yes: Karyotype is critical for risk assessment	Yes: Certain FISH abnormalities define better risk disease	Yes: Numerous examples (e.g., *FLT3*, *NPM1*, *KIT*); RT-PCR for change in transcript level over time in certain types (e.g., APL)
Myeloid Neoplasms With Eosinophilia and Tyrosine Kinase Gene Fusions (PDGFA, PDGFRB, FGFR1, and PCM1::JAK2)			
Establish diagnosis and subtype	Yes: Karyotype detects typical *PDGFRB*, *FGFR1* rearrangements and *PCM1::JAK2*, *ETV6::ABL1*, *ETV6::JAK2*, and *BCR::JAK2*	Yes: Necessary to detect *PDGFRA* rearrangement, which is cryptic on karyotype; often via *CHIC2* deletion	Uncertain due to rarity of these entities
Myelodysplastic/Myeloproliferative Neoplasms			
Establish diagnosis	Yes: Clonal cytogenetic abnormality is necessary for diagnosis of CMML if diagnostic dysplasia is not present and monocytosis is of recent onset/reactive causes not yet excluded	Yes: FISH MDS panel will show abnormalities in some cases of CMML (especially +8)	Maybe: *TET2*, *ASXL1*, and *SRSF2* mutations are common in CMML but not included in formal criteria for diagnosis as of yet
Prognosis	Yes: Cytogenetic findings (including monosomal karyotype) have prognostic significance in CMML	Yes: FISH MDS panel is useful when routine cytogenetic analysis yields poor or incomplete study	Yes: *ASXL1* mutations prognostic in CMML

Chronic Myeloid Leukemia, *BCR::ABL1*-Positive

KEY FACTS

TERMINOLOGY
- Chronic myeloid leukemia (CML), *BCR::ABL1*-positive
  - Myeloproliferative neoplasm subtype that harbors *BCR::ABL1*
  - t(9;22)(q34;q11) or variant translocations result in *BCR::ABL1*
    - BCR::ABL1 oncoprotein promotes growth and proliferation through downstream signaling pathways
  - Abnormal derivative chromosome 22 historically known as Philadelphia chromosome

ETIOLOGY/PATHOGENESIS
- Major (M) *BCR::ABL1* transcript form is expected in CML
  - e13-a2 or e14-a2
  - Encoded protein is p210
- *BCR::ABL1* not specific for CML
  - Seen in subset of acute lymphoblastic leukemia and rarely in de novo acute myeloid leukemia
  - *BCR::ABL1* subtypes include e13-a2/e14-a2, e1-a2, and other rare fusions

CLINICAL ISSUES
- 10-year survival rate 80-90% with tyrosine kinase-targeted therapy

ANCILLARY TESTS
- Karyotype, FISH, or RT-PCR required to confirm t(9;22)(q34;q11) or *BCR::ABL1*
- Quantitative RT-PCR necessary for minimal residual disease monitoring
  - International scale (IS) established in 2005
  - Major molecular response is ≤ 0.1% *BCR::ABL1* transcript levels by IS or ≥ 3-log decrease (1,000x) from baseline levels determined at diagnosis
  - Essential to monitor patients even after good response
- *BCR::ABL1* kinase domain mutation analysis may be necessary to detect acquired mutations that decrease effectiveness of tyrosine kinase inhibitor therapy

Left-Shifted Neutrophilia and Basophilia

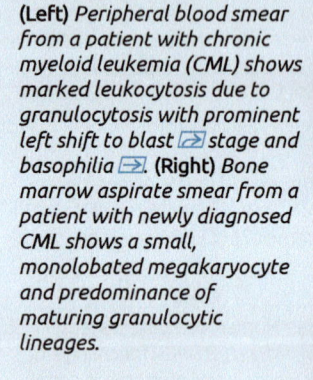

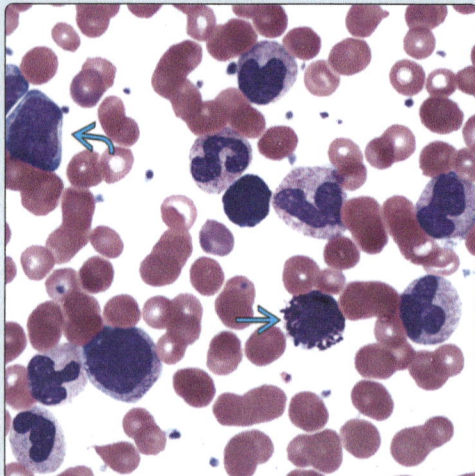

Small Monolobated Megakaryocyte

(Left) Peripheral blood smear from a patient with chronic myeloid leukemia (CML) shows marked leukocytosis due to granulocytosis with prominent left shift to blast ➡ stage and basophilia ➡. (Right) Bone marrow aspirate smear from a patient with newly diagnosed CML shows a small, monolobated megakaryocyte and predominance of maturing granulocytic lineages.

Small Hypolobated Megakaryocytes

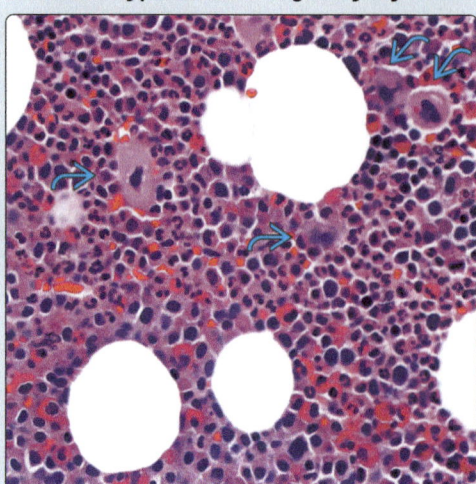

9;22 Translocation

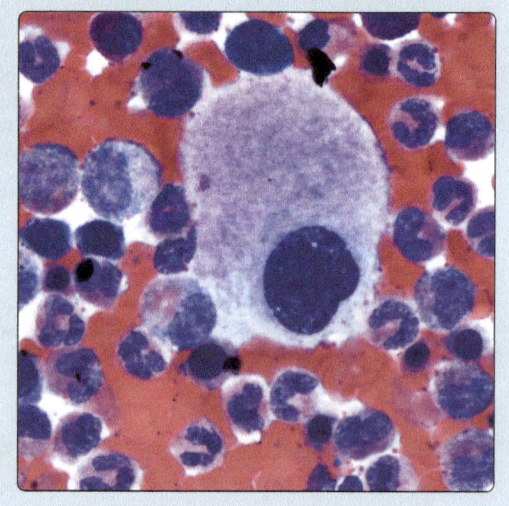

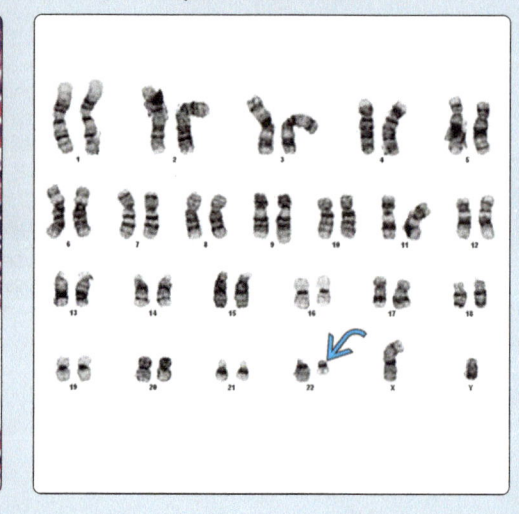

(Left) Bone marrow clot section from a CML patient shows hypercellular marrow with marked granulocytic hyperplasia and frequent small, hypolobated megakaryocytes ➡. (Right) Karyotype of an older man shows reciprocal translocation involving long arms of chromosomes 9 and 22, characteristic of CML. The short chromosome 22 that harbors the BCR::ABL1 fusion is historically called the Philadelphia chromosome ➡.

Chronic Myeloid Leukemia, BCR::ABL1-Positive

TERMINOLOGY

Abbreviations
- Chronic myeloid leukemia (CML), BCR::ABL1-positive

Definitions
- Myeloproliferative neoplasm subtype that harbors BCR::ABL1
  o Results from t(9;22)(q34;q11) or variant translocations
    - Abnormal derivative chromosome 22 is historically known as Philadelphia chromosome
- BCR
  o Official name: BCR activator of RhoGEF and GTPase
  o HGNC ID: 1014
  o Gene locus: 22q11.23
- ABL1
  o Official name: ABL protooncogene 1, nonreceptor tyrosine kinase
  o HGNC ID: 76
  o Gene locus: 9q34.12

CLASSIFICATION

WHO-HAEM5 vs. ICC
- Similar diagnostic criteria in both classifications
- Accelerated phase (AP) omitted in WHO-HAEM5
  o Essentially replaced by "high-risk chronic phase" designation
    - Resistance due to ABL1 kinase mutations &/or emergence of additional cytogenetic abnormalities and development of blast phase (BP) represent key disease attributes per WHO-HAEM5
- AP retained in ICC
  o Defined by 10-19% blood or bone marrow blasts, > 20% basophilia, or identification of additional clonal cytogenetic abnormalities
  o Prior WHO 2017 criteria for AP (such as thrombocytopenia unrelated to therapy, or therapy-resistant thrombocytosis &/or splenomegaly) discarded by current ICC CML working group
  o Additionally, failure to achieve complete hematological response, development of resistance to sequential tyrosine kinase inhibitors (TKIs), or emergence of > 2 BCR::ABL1 mutations has also been eliminated as AP criteria
- > 5% lymphoblasts in blood or bone marrow defines lymphoid blast phase in ICC
- < 10% lymphoblasts in blood or bone marrow considered for lymphoid BP diagnosis in WHO-HAEM5

ETIOLOGY/PATHOGENESIS

Normal Function of BCR Protein
- Incompletely understood, despite in-depth study of abnormal BCR::ABL1 fusion protein
- BCR protein has
  o Autophosphorylation activity
  o Transphosphorylation activity
  o Serine/threonine kinase activity
  o GTPase-activating activity

Normal Function of ABL1 Protein
- Nonreceptor tyrosine kinase
- Involved in cell division, adhesion, differentiation, and response to stress

Abnormal BCR::ABL1 Fusion Oncoprotein
- Derived from fusion of 5' region of BCR with 3' region of ABL1
  o ABL1 breakpoint can occur anywhere within large span of 200-300 kb
  o Major BCR breakpoint regions (M) occur between BCR exons 13 and 14 and between exons 14 and 15
    - Results in 2 most common BCR::ABL1 isoforms: e13-a2 or e14-a2 (historically referred to as b2a2 and b3a2)
      □ Translated fusion protein is known as p210 form
  o Minor BCR breakpoint region (m) falls downstream of exon 1
    - Results in transcript with fusion of exon 1 of BCR to exon 2 of ABL1 (e1-a2 form transcript)
      □ Translated fusion protein is known as p190 form
  o Rare micro-BCR breakpoint region is downstream of exon 19
    - Results in transcript with fusion of exon 19 of BCR to exon 2 of ABL1 (e19-a2 form transcript)
      □ Translated fusion protein is known as p230 form
- BCR::ABL1 fusion disrupts regulated functioning of ABL1 protein
  o Activity of abnormal BCR::ABL1 kinase is highly dependent on coiled-coil domain derived from BCR that permits oligomerization
- BCR::ABL1 fusion not specific for CML
  o Seen in subset of acute lymphoblastic leukemia and rarely in de novo acute myeloid leukemia (AML)

Molecular Correlates of Disease Progression in CML
- CML progression is typically associated with clonal evolution
- Up to 80% of CML cases with disease progression harbor additional chromosomal abnormalities, including
  o Monosomy 7, +8, i(17q), +17, +19, +21, duplicate Philadelphia chromosome
- CML progression to advanced disease shares biological features associated with resistance to tyrosine kinase inhibitor TKI therapy
- Genes reported to be altered in transformed CML
  o TP53, RB1, MYC, CDKN2A, TET2, CBL, ASXL1, IDH1, and IDH2

CLINICAL ISSUES

Epidemiology
- Incidence
  o 1-2 cases per 100,000 people per year
- Age
  o Median at diagnosis: 50-70 years, but may occur at any age

Presentation
- Splenomegaly, weight loss, fatigue, night sweats
- Prominent left-shifted neutrophilia and basophilia

Chronic Myeloid Leukemia, BCR::ABL1-Positive

Treatment

- Drugs
  - Historically, nontargeted therapies utilized
    - Radiation, busulfan, hydroxyurea, interferon-α
  - Currently, targeted therapies with TKIs
  - 1st-generation TKI (imatinib) or 2nd-generation TKIs (dasatinib, nilotinib) are frontline treatment options
    - TKIs potently interfere with interaction between BCR::ABL1 protein and ATP
      □ Block cellular proliferation of malignant clone
    - Many patients respond to standard oral dose of imatinib (400 mg/day), but some require more potent 2nd-generation TKIs
    - Some patients do not achieve adequate levels of response due to resistance
  - Rate of transformation to AP or BP reported lower in patients who received dasatinib vs. imatinib
  - 2nd-generation TKIs overcome most of ABL1 kinase mutations that confer resistance to imatinib except T315I variant
  - Ponatinib is 3rd-generation TKI that shows activity against CML with T315I mutation
- Allogeneic stem cell transplantation (ASCT)
  - Indicated in ~ 2% of patients who become resistant to many TKIs

Prognosis

- Prior to TKI-targeted therapies, median survival ranged 3-6 years
- With TKIs, prognosis determined by rate of hematologic, cytogenetic, and molecular response
  - 8-year survival with imatinib therapy is 93% (for CML-related death)
- Mechanisms of relapse/resistance
  - BCR::ABL1 kinase domain mutations
- 3 classically defined phases of disease
  - Chronic phase: < 5% blasts
  - AP and BP
    - Represent disease progression
    - Generally refractory to therapy
  - Blast phase: ≥ 20% blasts; myeloid lineage in 75-80%, lymphoid blasts lineage in 20-25% (predominantly B-lineage)
- Moderate/marked reticulin fibrosis in chronic phase reported to be associated with worse prognosis

MICROSCOPIC

Key Microscopic Features

- Peripheral blood (chronic phase)
  - Granulocytic leukocytosis with prominent left shift
  - Blasts < 5%, basophilia, often eosinophilia
  - Preserved/elevated platelet count
- Bone marrow (chronic disease)
  - Hypercellular, blasts < 5%
  - Granulocytic lineage predominates with myeloid:erythroid ratio > 10:1
  - Minimal dysplasia in granulocytes and erythroid lineages
  - Usually increased megakaryocytes
    - Distinctive megakaryocytic morphology; small and monolobulated
  - No clusters of blasts
  - May see increased reticulin fibrosis

ANCILLARY TESTS

Flow Cytometry

- Useful in blast lineage determination in AP/BP
- If concern for lymphoblasts, immunophenotyping is warranted

Genetic Testing

- Conventional chromosomal analysis
  - t(9;22)(q34;q11) or BCR::ABL1 fusion by FISH or RT-PCR is required for diagnosis
  - Derivative chromosome 22, which is historically termed Philadelphia chromosome, harbors BCR::ABL1
  - BCR::ABL1 reportedly cryptic on karyotype in ~ 5% of cases
    - FISH or RT-PCR can detect cryptic rearrangements
- t(9;22)(q34;q11) is not specific for CML
  - May be seen in lymphoblastic leukemia and rare cases of de novo AML
- Clonal evolution in AP/BP
  - Typically associated with additional cytogenetic aberrations, including monosomy 7, +8, i(17q), +19, +21, and additional Philadelphia chromosome

Quantitative RT-PCR for BCR::ABL1 Transcripts

- mRNA as target nucleic acid-based assay used for detection
- Common strategy is to employ 2 separate reactions: 1 to detect e13-a2/e14-a2 transcript and 1 to detect e1-a2 transcript
- Other rare isoforms can also be targeted
  - Some labs include reaction to detect e19-a2
- Transcripts of BCR::ABL1 are normalized to endogenous control transcript and expressed as ratio
- Can be used to establish presence of BCR::ABL1 fusion at diagnosis
  - FISH and karyotype can also serve this purpose
- Quantitative RT-PCR is necessary for high-sensitivity studies for MRD detection and disease monitoring

International Scale Reporting

- Raw BCR::ABL1 transcript ratios are inconsistent and problematic
  - Different labs use different endogenous controls
- International scale (IS) established in 2005
  - Anchored to baseline BCR::ABL1 expression level from landmark IRIS trial (100% IS)
  - Most labs are now reporting on IS
  - Permits comparison of BCR::ABL1 results between different laboratories
- Labs convert their own unique BCR::ABL1 results to IS by running commercially available IS reference standards

Major Molecular Response

- Major molecular response (MMR) is value of 0.1% on IS or 3-log decrease (1,000x) from baseline levels at diagnosis
  - MMR is critical goal of CML treatment
  - MMR within first 12-18 months of imatinib or other TKI therapy predicts long-term disease remission status

Chronic Myeloid Leukemia, *BCR::ABL1*-Positive

Characteristic Types of *BCR::ABL1* Fusion

Breakpoints	Transcript Generated	Fusion Protein Size	Disease Association
Major (M)			
	e13-a2 or e14-a2 (previously known as b2-a2 and b3-a2)	p210 (210 kDa)	CML (nearly all cases)
	e13-a2 or e14-a2 (previously known as b2-a2 and b3-a2)	p210 (210 kDa)	Adult Ph+ B-ALL (~ 30-40%)
	e13-a2 or e14-a2 (previously known as b2-a2 and b3-a2)	p210 (210 kDa)	Pediatric Ph+ B-ALL (~ 10%)
Minor (m)			
	e1-a2	p190	CML (rare cases, associated with monocytic proliferation)
	e1-a2	p190	Adult Ph+ B-ALL (~ 60-70%)
	e1-a2	p190	Pediatric Ph+ B-ALL (~ 90%)
Micro (μ)			
	e19-a2	p230	CML (very rare cases, associated with neutrophilia and thrombocytosis)

B-ALL = B-acute lymphoblastic leukemia; CML = chronic myeloid leukemia; Ph = Philadelphia chromosome.

- Complete molecular response is absence of *BCR::ABL1* transcript as measured by assay of sufficient sensitivity (> 4.5 logs below baseline level)
- Transcript ratio should fall predictably over time in patient on treatment
  - Achieving MMR by 12 months of treatment is optimal
  - Many milestones have been established during this time to guide treatment decisions
    - *BCR::ABL1* transcripts at > 10% IS at 6 months would be considered treatment failure

Minimal Residual Disease Monitoring by Quantitative RT-PCR

- Standard of care to monitor patients even after good response
  - Rising transcript level may signal
    - Disease progression
    - Need for *ABL1* kinase domain mutation analysis
    - Need for change in TKI treatment

BCR::ABL1 Kinase Domain Mutation Analysis

- Sequencing to detect acquired mutations in *BCR::ABL1* kinase domain that decrease effectiveness of TKI therapy
- These mutations arise in response to drug therapy
  - Mutations that occur at contact point of imatinib and *BCR::ABL1* kinase
    - e.g., T315I
  - Mutations that affect conformation of kinase; imatinib cannot bind
    - Mutations in P loop: M244V, E255K/V, etc.
    - Mutations in activation loop: H396R/H396P
- 40-90% of patients resistant to imatinib have demonstrable mutation
  - T315I mutation has been unresponsive to 1st- and 2nd-generation TKIs but responsive to 3rd-generation TKIs (ponatinib, omacetaxine, and asciminib)

DIFFERENTIAL DIAGNOSIS

Leukemoid Reaction
- Normal genetics, in contrast to *BCR::ABL1* fusion seen in CML

Myeloproliferative Neoplasm, *BCR::ABL1*-Negative
- Key feature distinguishing from CML is lack of *BCR::ABL1*
  - *JAK2* V617F mutation identified in
    - > 95% of polycythemia vera and in ~ 50% of essential thrombocythemia and primary myelofibrosis
    - Not seen in classic CML
  - Also *JAK2* exon 12, *CALR*, and *MPL* mutations are detected in specific subsets of these diseases
  - Chronic neutrophilic leukemia
    - Most cases harbor *CSF3R* mutation

Atypical Chronic Myelogenous Leukemia, *BCR::ABL1*-Negative
- No relationship to CML
- Dysplasia prominent
- *BCR::ABL1*-negative by definition
- Recurrent *SETBP1* mutations in subset of cases

Acute Myeloid Leukemia With *BCR::ABL1*
- De novo AML without prior or after therapy evidence of CML
- Can be challenging to separate from BP of CML

SELECTED REFERENCES

1. Gianelli U et al: International Consensus Classification of myeloid and lymphoid neoplasms: myeloproliferative neoplasms. Virchows Arch. 482(1):53-68, 2023
2. Khoury JD et al: The 5th edition of the World Health Organization classification of haematolymphoid tumours: myeloid and histiocytic/dendritic neoplasms. Leukemia. 36(7):1703-19, 2022
3. Jabbour E et al: Chronic myeloid leukemia: 2018 update on diagnosis, therapy and monitoring. Am J Hematol. 93(3):442-59, 2018
4. Baccarani M et al: European LeukemiaNet recommendations for the management of chronic myeloid leukemia: 2013. Blood. 122(6):872-84, 2013

Chronic Myeloid Leukemia, *BCR::ABL1*-Positive

Cell Clumping

Classic Cellular Features

(Left) Peripheral blood shows marked leukocytosis with shift to immaturity in the granulocytic series with < 2% blasts. Characteristic clumping of cells ⇨ is easily recognized at low power in CML. **(Right)** Peripheral blood shows the classic cellular features of CML, including granulocytic leukocytosis with left shift, rare myeloid blasts ⇨, myelocyte bulge ⇨, and prominent basophilia, suggestive of disease progression. Granulocytes lack dysplastic features.

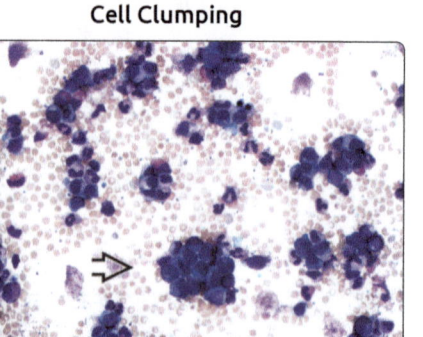

Classic Cellular Features

Circulating Nucleated Red Blood Cells

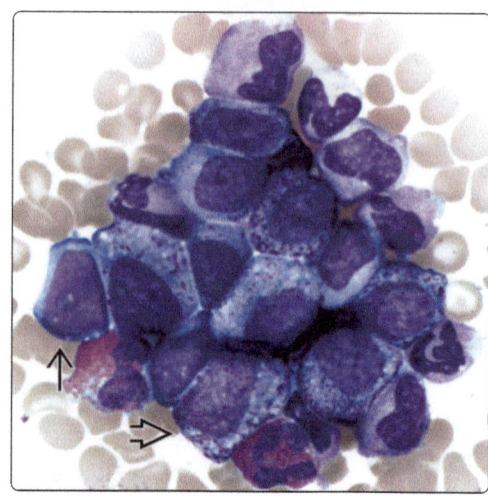

(Left) Peripheral blood at high power shows the classic cellular features of CML, including granulocytic predominance with left shift, basophilia ⇨, and no overt granulocytic dysplasia. **(Right)** Peripheral blood in CML may occasionally show a leukoerythroblastic blood picture with circulating nucleated red blood cells ⇨.

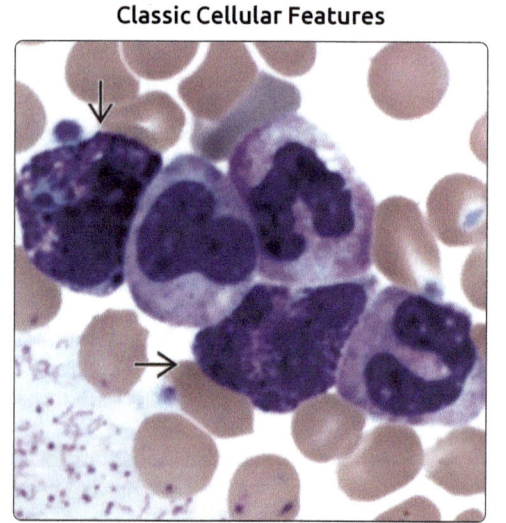

Megakaryocytic Cytoplasm

Circulating Blasts

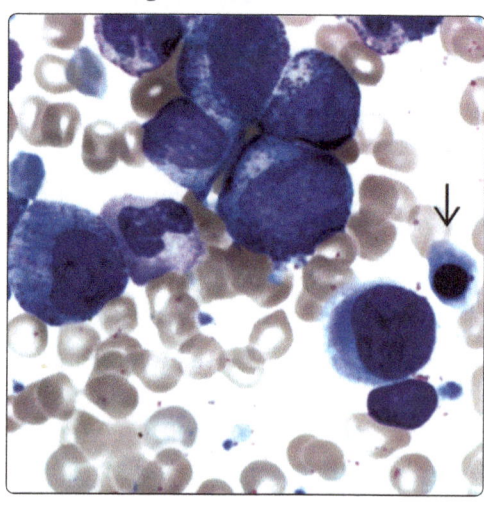

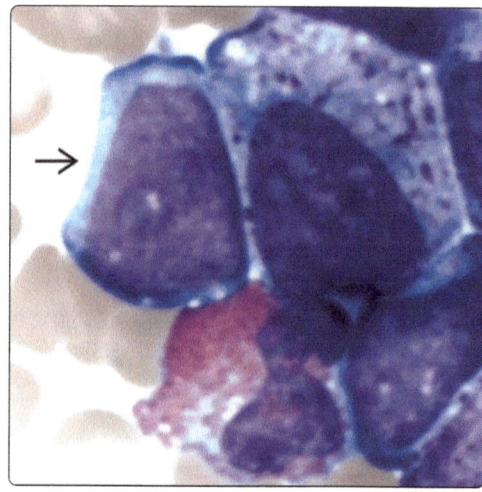

(Left) Peripheral blood in CML may show large, abnormal platelets. Here, a large fragment of megakaryocytic cytoplasm with obvious platelet budding at the perimeter is shown. **(Right)** In chronic-phase CML, circulating blasts ⇨ comprise < 5% of total blood and bone marrow nucleated cells. As a stem cell disorder, the blasts contain *BCR::ABL1*, as do all bone marrow cellular progeny.

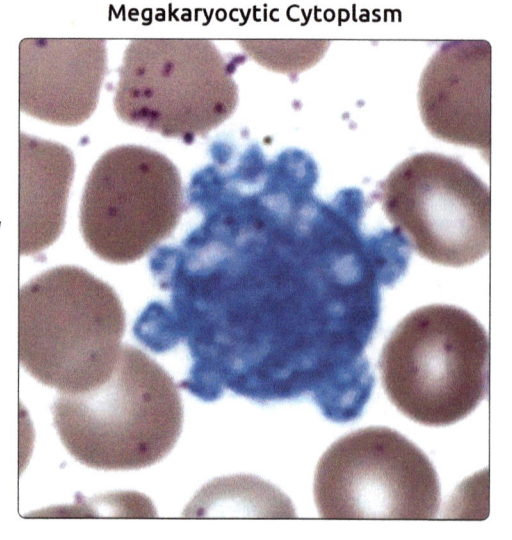

Chronic Myeloid Leukemia, *BCR::ABL1*-Positive

Philadelphia Chromosome

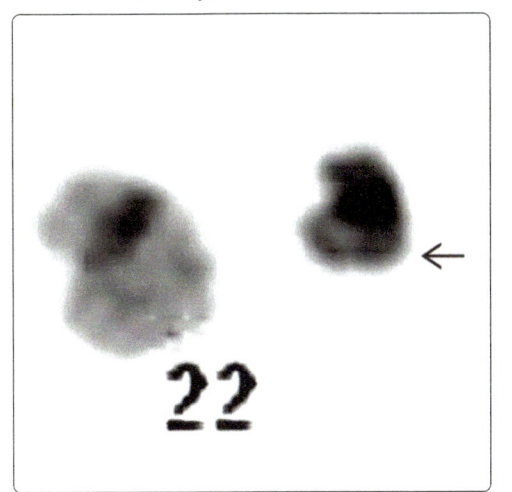

Small Lobulated Megakaryocytes

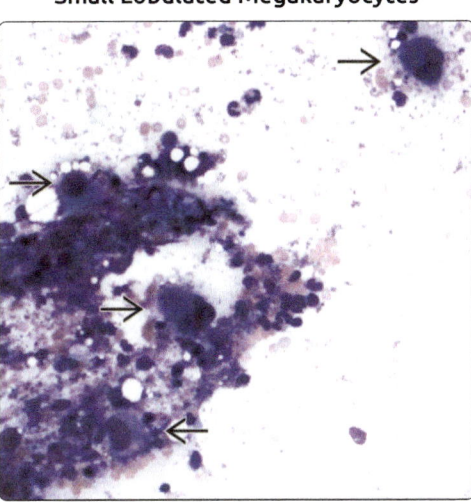

(Left) *GTW-banded chromosomes show the typical shortened chromosome 22 ➔, a.k.a. Philadelphia chromosome. This chromosome results in BCR::ABL1 fusion at the molecular genetic level.* **(Right)** *Bone marrow aspirate smear shows 4 small, singly lobulated megakaryocytes ➔, which are characteristic for CML. This megakaryocytic appearance is unique among myeloproliferative neoplasms.*

Sea Blue Histiocyte

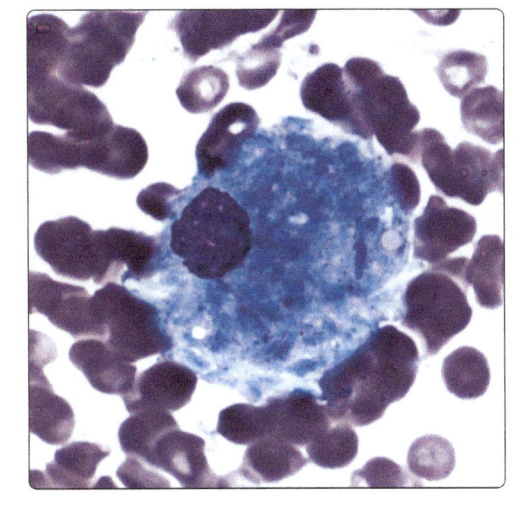

Small Monolobated Megakaryocytes

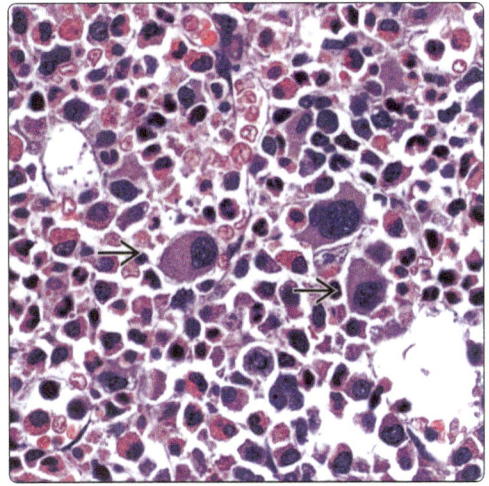

(Left) *Bone marrow aspirate smear shows a sea blue histiocyte in CML. These cells are commonly seen due to the marked cell turnover.* **(Right)** *Bone marrow core biopsy in CML shows hypercellular marrow dominated by granulocytes and precursors. Megakaryocytes are present, unclustered in typical chronic phase, and often show a small, monolobulated appearance ➔.*

Monolobulated Megakaryocytes

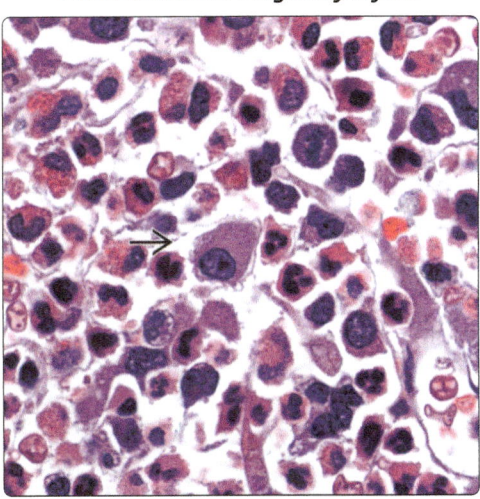

Reticulin Histochemistry

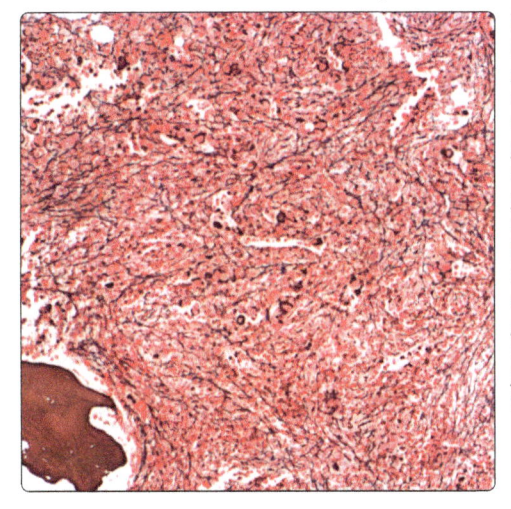

(Left) *Bone marrow core biopsy in CML shows granulocytic predominance and monolobulated megakaryocytes ➔ at high power. Additionally, this field also shows an increased population of eosinophils, which is not uncommon.* **(Right)** *Reticulin-stained bone marrow core biopsy shows moderate fibrosis in chronic-phase CML at presentation. Some reports suggest that fibrosis may be associated with a worse prognosis.*

Chronic Myeloid Leukemia, *BCR::ABL1*-Positive

Basophil Population on Flow Histogram

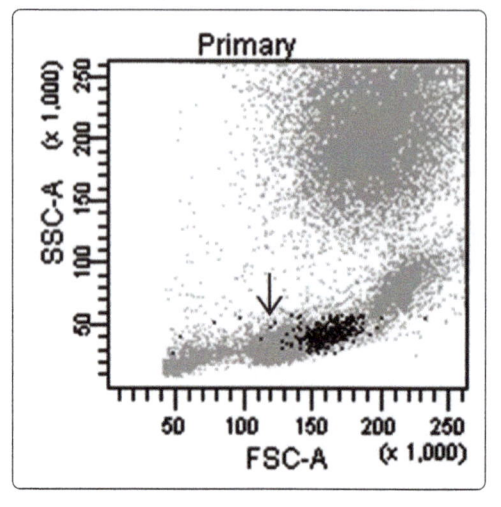

CD33(+)Basophils on Flow Histogram

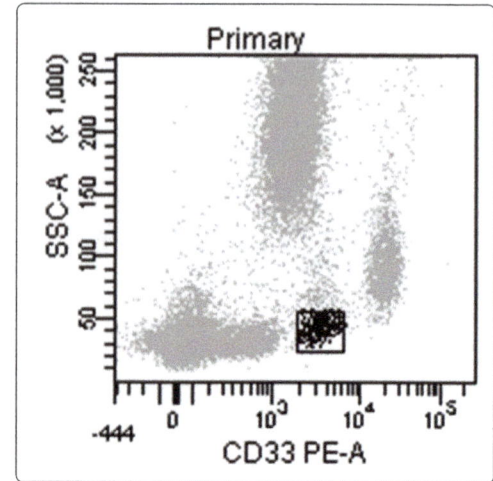

(Left) *Flow cytometric analysis shows typical lymphoid ⇾, monocyte, and granulocyte populations based on forward and side-angle light scatter properties in CML (chronic phase). Basophils (black) often form a conspicuous population, which are low on side scatter (SSC) but slightly larger than lymphocytes on forward scatter (FSC).* (Right) *Flow cytometry in chronic-phase CML identifies the conspicuous CD33-positive basophil population (seen in black), which is characteristic of this disease.*

Philadelphia Chromosome

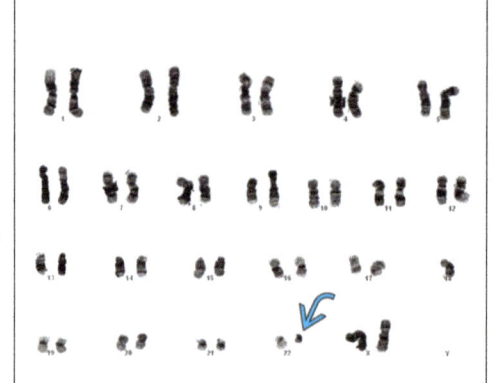

FISH: *BCR::ABL1* Fusion

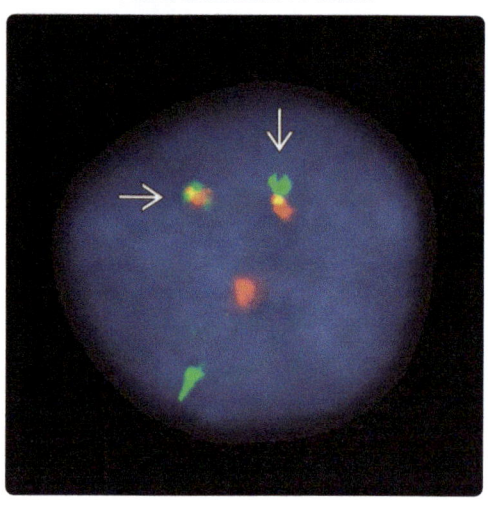

(Left) *Karyogram shows the classic derivative chromosome 22 (Philadelphia) in CML ⇾. This reciprocal translocation involves 9q34 and 22q11 juxtaposing the ABL1 and BCR genes at the molecular level.* (Right) *Using a dual-color, dual-fusion probe strategy, FISH shows a classic abnormal cell in CML, demonstrating the presence of a BCR::ABL1 fusion. Abnormal fusion signals confirming the positive results ⇾.*

Quantitative RT-PCR for *BCR::ABL1* transcripts

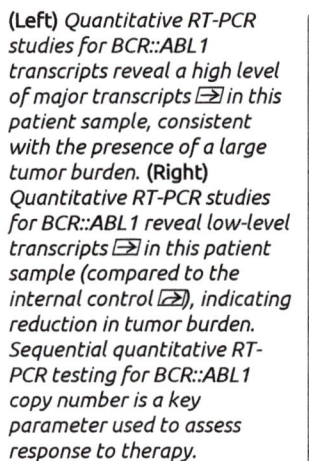

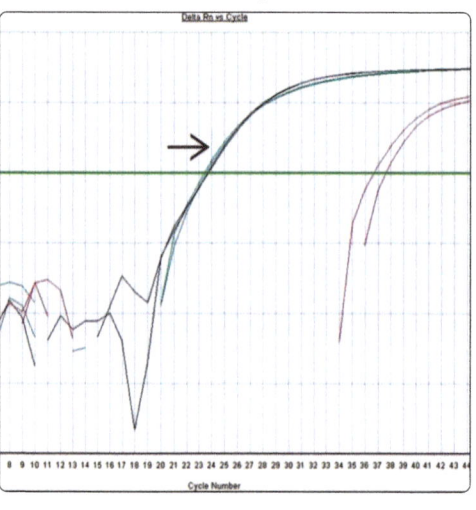

Quantitative RT-PCR for *BCR::ABL1*

(Left) *Quantitative RT-PCR studies for BCR::ABL1 transcripts reveal a high level of major transcripts ⇾ in this patient sample, consistent with the presence of a large tumor burden.* (Right) *Quantitative RT-PCR studies for BCR::ABL1 reveal low-level transcripts ⇾ in this patient sample (compared to the internal control ⇾), indicating reduction in tumor burden. Sequential quantitative RT-PCR testing for BCR::ABL1 copy number is a key parameter used to assess response to therapy.*

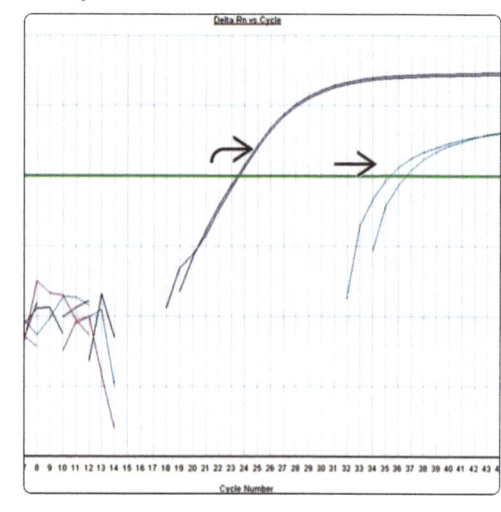

Chronic Myeloid Leukemia, *BCR::ABL1*-Positive

Accelerated-Phase CML

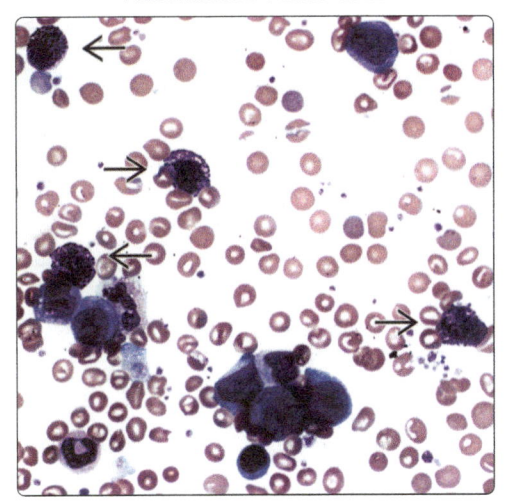

Lymphoid Blast Crisis of CML

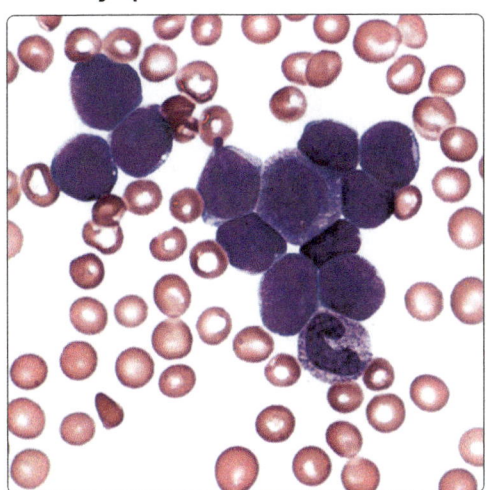

(Left) Peripheral blood demonstrates accelerated-phase CML at disease presentation, characterized by prominent basophilia ➔ (23% of the circulating leukocytes). (Right) Peripheral blood shows lymphoid blast crisis in a patient diagnosed with CML 8 years before the current presentation. Flow cytometry demonstrated the lineage of the blasts as B-lymphoblast. Blast crisis is of lymphoid lineage (B- or T-) ~ 15-20% of the time.

Increased Circulating CD34(+) Blasts

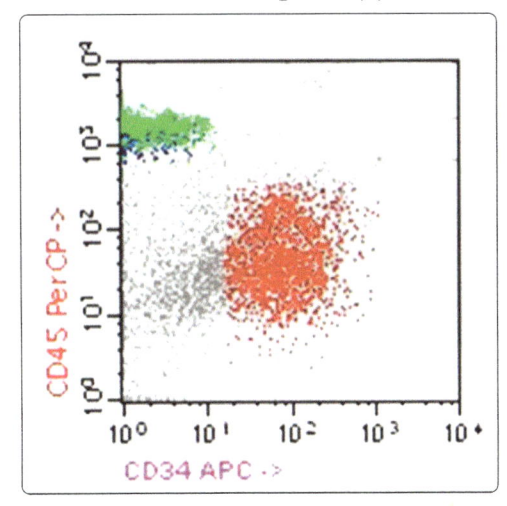

Lymphoblast Population

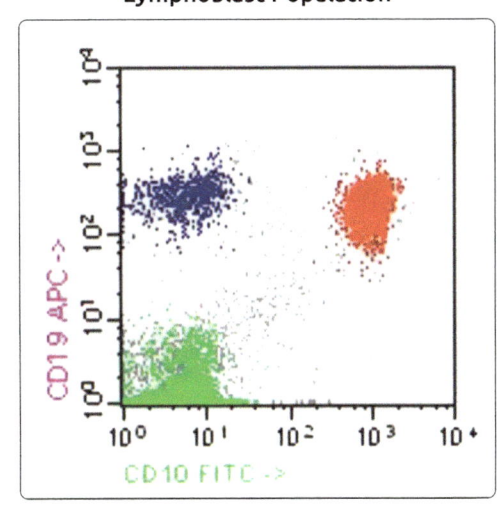

(Left) Flow cytometric analysis of peripheral blood reveals an increased weak CD45(+), CD34(+) blast population in a case of accelerated-phase CML (red). CD34 positivity is not a substitute for the true blast count, as not all blasts are CD34(+). (Right) Flow cytometric analysis shows a B-lymphoblastic population positive for CD19 and bright CD10 (red) in blast phase of CML.

Clonal Evolution With Double Philadelphia Chromosomes

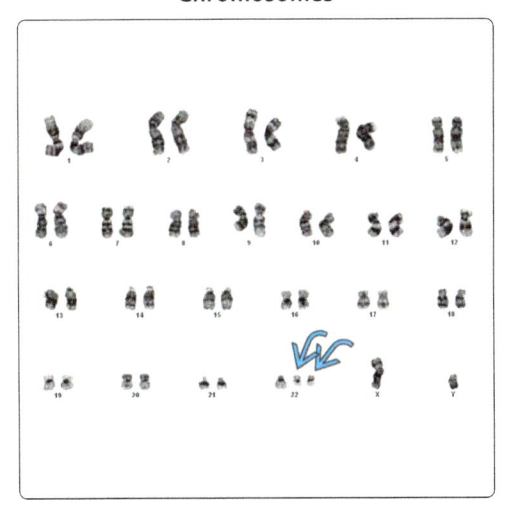

Clusters of CD31(+) Small Megakaryocytes

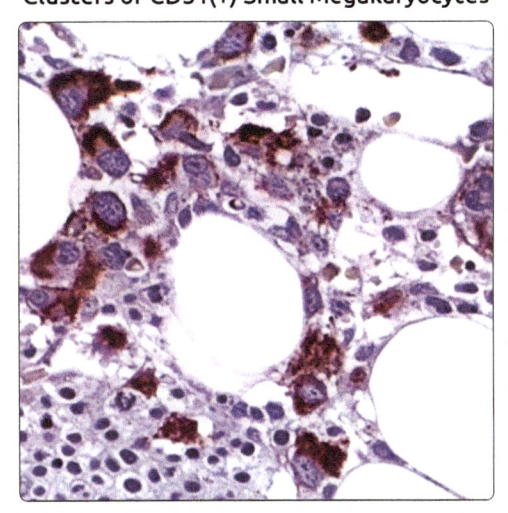

(Left) Karyogram demonstrates clonal evolution in CML with the presence of an additional Philadelphia chromosome ➔. Typical cytogenetic findings in clonal evolution include additional Philadelphia chromosome (as shown), +8, isochromosome 17q, and +19 among other cytogenetic aberrations. (Right) Immunohistochemistry for CD31 shows a marked increase and clustering of abnormal, small megakaryocytes in a CML case.

Chronic Neutrophilic Leukemia

KEY FACTS

ETIOLOGY/PATHOGENESIS
- *CSF3R* mutation testing required part of work-up
  - *CSF3R* membrane proximal mutations
    - Leads to ligand independent receptor signaling
  - *CSF3R* exon 17 truncating mutations affecting cytoplasmic tail
    - Cytoplasmic tail region involved in maturation signaling and suppression of proliferation
    - Mutation prevents degradation, leading to increased cell surface expression
    - Activates SRC-TNK2 tyrosine kinase pathway
- *CSF3R* encodes cell surface receptor for granulocyte colony-stimulating factor
  - Major cytokine regulator of neutrophil production

CLINICAL ISSUES
- Prognosis variable with possible disease progression
- Early interest in targeted therapy for some patients based on *CSF3R* mutation

MICROSCOPIC
- PB neutrophilia; blasts < 1%
- WBC: ≥ 25 x 10⁹/L ± *CSF3R* mutations (WHO-HAEM5)
- WBC: ≥ 13 x 10⁹/L in *CSF3R*-mutated cases (ICC)
- BM hypercellular; granulocytic predominance; blasts < 5%
- No dysplasia, overt basophilia, or monocytosis

ANCILLARY TESTS
- Genetics
  - *CSF3R* mutation in most cases
    - T618I most common
  - Additional common mutations include
    - *ASXL1*, *SETBP1*, *TET2*, *SRSF2*, and *U2AF1*
      - *ASXL1* mutation associated with adverse outcomes
  - Cytogenetics most often normal
    - Most common abnormality is del(20q); others include +8, +9, +21, del(11q), and loss of 17

Neutrophilic Leukocytosis

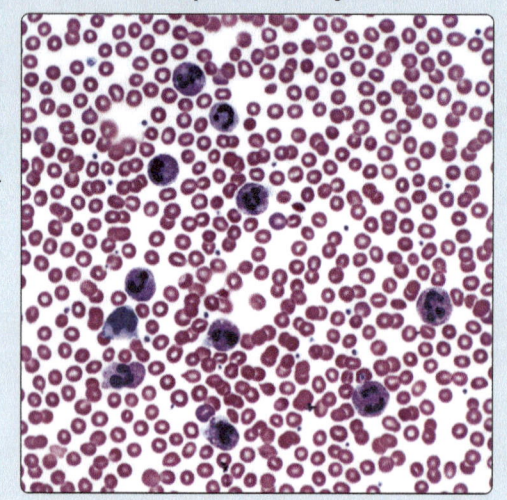

Melting Curve Analysis for *CSF3R* Mutation

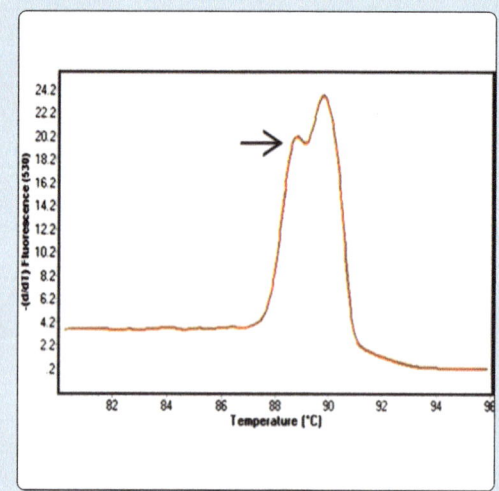

(Left) Peripheral blood smear shows typical neutrophilic leukocytosis with minimal left shift in this case of chronic neutrophilic leukemia (CNL). (Right) *CSF3R* T618I mutation is identified in this case of CNL by high-resolution melting curve analysis. The shoulder peak ➡ on the left indicates the presence of the mutation.

Granulocytic Predominance

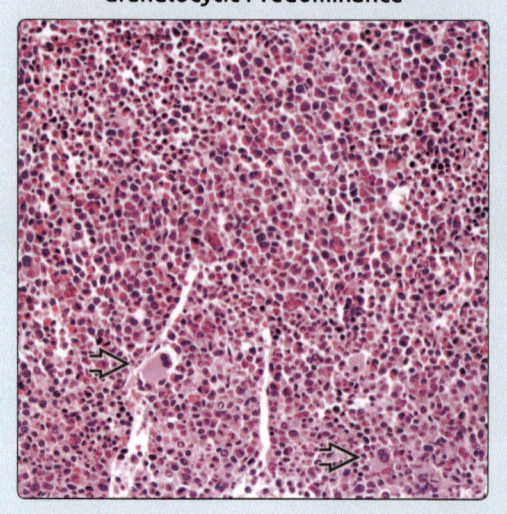

Typical Appearance

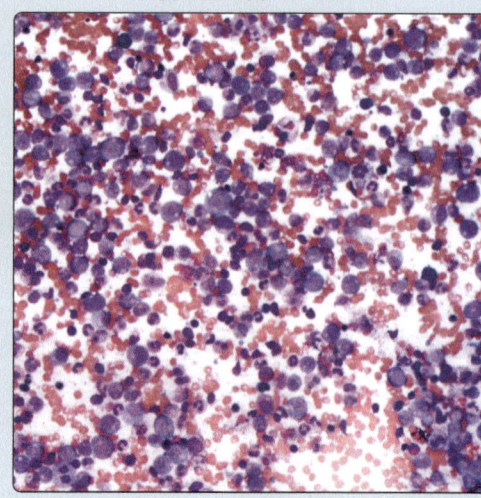

(Left) Bone marrow core biopsy highlights massive granulocytic predominance with complete maturation in this case of CNL. Intermixed megakaryocytes ➡ are morphologically normal. No foci or large collections of blasts are present. (Right) Bone marrow aspirate smear shows typical findings of CNL: Hypercellularity, prominent granulocytic proliferation, no significant erythroid, granulocytic, or megakaryocytic dysplasia, and < 5% blasts.

Chronic Neutrophilic Leukemia

TERMINOLOGY

Abbreviations
- Chronic neutrophilic leukemia (CNL)
- International Consensus Classification (ICC)
- World Health Organization, 5th edition (WHO-HAEM5)

Definitions
- Myeloproliferative neoplasm (MPN) manifesting predominantly in granulocytic lineage
- Persistent peripheral blood (PB) neutrophilia and bone marrow (BM) granulocytic proliferation
- *CSF3R* mutation is present in most cases and is valuable clonal marker
  o Official name: Colony-stimulating factor (G-CSF) 3 receptor
  o HGNC ID: 2439
- Reactive neutrophilia and other MPNs must be excluded in cases lacking *CSF3R* mutation

CLASSIFICATION

ICC vs. WHO-HAEM5
- Similar requirements for WBC and degree of left shift (e.g., neutrophils and bands ≥ 80% of WBC), BM findings and exclusionary criteria in both classifications
  o *CSF3R* mutation analysis to establish clonality
  o Sustained unexplained neutrophilia ≥ 3 months and splenomegaly
- Key difference between ICC and WHO-HAEM5 is in WBC cutoff
  o ICC: WBC ≥ 13 x 10⁹/L sufficient for diagnosis in *CSF3R*-mutated cases
  o ICC: WBC ≥ 25 x 10⁹/L required for diagnosis in *CSF3R*-unmutated cases
  o WHO-HAEM5: WBC ≥ 25 x 10⁹/L required for diagnosis in both *CSF3R*-mutated and unmutated cases
- Accelerated and blast phases as defined by ICC: 10-19% and ≥ 20% blasts, respectively

ETIOLOGY/PATHOGENESIS

CSF3R Mutation
- Normal function of *CSF3R*
  o Chromosomal location 1p34.3
  o Encodes cell surface receptor for granulocyte G-CSF
  o G-CSF is major cytokine regulator of neutrophil production
    – CSF3R protein is major intermediary of stimulus for BM to produce neutrophils
    – Binding of G-CSF induces dimerization and activation
      □ Predominantly via JAK/STAT pathway
      □ Additional signaling via PI3K/AKT and MAPK/ERK pathways
  o Proximal region involved in signaling that induces cell division
  o Cytoplasmic tail region involved in maturation signaling and suppression of proliferation
  o *CSF3R* mutations are activating, leading to overactive drive to produce neutrophils
- Types of *CSF3R* mutation
  o *CSF3R* membrane proximal mutations
    – Commonly seen in CNL
    – Key mutation in exon 14 membrane proximal region is T618I, seen in > 80% of cases
    – Leads to ligand independent receptor signaling by CSF3R dimers
      □ Activates JAK/STAT pathway
      □ Induces proliferation and survival signals
    – May occur alone or in conjunction with truncating C terminal cytoplasmic tail mutation
      □ 25% of cases carry compound mutations
  o *CSF3R* exon 17 truncating mutations affecting cytoplasmic tail
    – Prevent degradation, leading to increased cell surface expression
    – Activates SRC-TNK2 tyrosine kinase pathway
      □ Results in increased/unregulated stimulus to produce neutrophils
    – Most common is D771fs
    – Usually accompanied by proximal membrane mutation
    – Acquired truncating mutations in cytoplasmic tail are also seen in severe congenital neutropenia
- *CSF3R* mutations in other myeloid neoplasms
  o Not specific for CNL; other neoplasms, particularly atypical chronic myeloid leukemia (aCML), can have *CSF3R* mutations

CLINICAL ISSUES

Epidemiology
- Incidence: 0.1 cases per million
- Median age: 67 years
  o Can rarely occur in children
- Male predominance (70% of cases)

Presentation
- Neutrophilia, hepatosplenomegaly, fatigue
- Majority of patients asymptomatic

Laboratory Tests
- CBC, PB and BM examination
- Molecular analysis for *CSF3R* mutation
- Cytogenetics

Treatment
- Not well defined
  o Options, depending on symptomatology, include
    – Watchful waiting for indolent cases
    – Cytoreductive agents (e.g., hydroxyurea)
    – Toxic chemotherapy in progressive or symptomatic cases
    – Allogeneic stem cell transplant in rare cases
      □ Only curative therapy

Prognosis
- Heterogeneous
- May be indolent
- Presence of additional mutations
  o May affect prognosis and treatment response
  o *SETBP1*, *ASXL1* mutations associated with shortened overall survival
- Disease progression

Chronic Neutrophilic Leukemia

- o Progressive neutrophilia refractory to therapy
- o Progressive splenomegaly
- o Refractory thrombocytopenia with bleeding complications
- o Cytogenetic clonal evolution
- o Myelodysplasia may develop
- o Rare leukemic transformation
- Survival ranges from < 1 year to > 20 years

MOLECULAR

Cytogenetics

- 90% of cases are cytogenetically normal
- Most common abnormality is del(20q); others include +8, +9, +21, del(11q), and loss of 17
- Clonal evolution with disease progression
- Absence of recurrent genetic abnormality defining another myeloid disorder
  - o Lacks t(9;22)(q34;q11.2); BCR::ABL1
  - o Other alterations associated with myeloid/lymphoid neoplasm with eosinophilia and tyrosine kinase gene fusion

Molecular Genetics

- *CSF3R* mutation
  - o Present in most cases
    - Prevalence ranges from 80-100% in different case series
  - o Critical region for examination includes membrane proximal region coded by exon 14
    - *CSF3R* T618I mutation is most common mutation
- Additional common mutations
  - o *ASXL1*, *SETBP1*, *TET2*, *SRSF2*, *U2AF1*
  - o *ASXL1* mutation associated with adverse outcomes
    - Seen in 70-80% of cases
    - Associated with thrombocytopenia
  - o *TET2* mutation associated with dysplasia
  - o *SETBP1* mutation associated with increased hemoglobin

MICROSCOPIC

Peripheral Blood

- WBC ≥ 13 x 10^9/L in cases with *CSF3R* mutation in ICC; ≥ 25 x 10^9/L in cases without *CSF3R* mutation in ICC and all cases in WHO-HAEM5
  - o Segmented neutrophils and bands ≥ 80% (ICC)
  - o Neutrophil precursors constitute < 5% but could be up to 10% of WBC (WHO-HAEM5)
- Toxic changes with prominent granules may be seen
  - o Must exclude reactive conditions
- Absence of significant dysplasia
- No significant basophilia
- No significant monocytosis (< 10% of WBC in ICC)
- Variable anemia and thrombocytopenia

Bone Marrow

- Hypercellular; granulocytic predominance; blasts < 5%
- Markedly increased myeloid:erythroid ratio
- No significant dysplasia
- Reticulin fibrosis is uncommon

DIFFERENTIAL DIAGNOSIS

Atypical Chronic Myeloid Leukemia

- Myelodysplastic/myeloproliferative neoplasm with neutrophilia
- Unlike CNL, aCML shows significant dysplasia

CSF3R Mutation in Neoplasms Other Than CNL and aCML

- *CSF3R* mutations also described in very rare cases of
  - o CMML, de novo AML, and early T-cell precursor acute lymphoblastic leukemia/lymphoma

Somatic *CSF3R* Mutations in Patient With Severe Congenital Neutropenia

- Acquired *CSF3R* mutations are seen in patients with inherited severe congenital neutropenia
- May be present for years before progression to AML

Germline *CSF3R* Mutation

- Rare familial cases of hereditary neutrophilia with germline *CSF3R* T617N mutation

Chronic Myeloid Leukemia

- PB neutrophilia with left shift and basophilia
- Cytogenetics reveal t(9;22)q34;q11.2); BCR::ABL1
- Cases of CML with variant *BCR* breakpoint may show striking neutrophilic predominance
  - o *BCR::ABL1* e19-a2 fusion variant
    - Leads to variant p230 form of chimeric protein
  - o Key feature is presence of Philadelphia chromosome
    - *BCR::ABL1* fusion by FISH &/or t(9;22) on karyotype

Other Myeloproliferative Neoplasms

- Generally lack significant neutrophilia (mild neutrophilia may be present in some cases of primary myelofibrosis)
- Distinguished from CNL by highly characteristic PB and BM findings

DIAGNOSTIC CHECKLIST

Pathologic Interpretation Pearls

- Sustained, unexplained neutrophilia
- Should exclude alternative causes of neutrophilia
- Molecular detection of *CSF3R* mutations is critical component of CNL work-up
  - o Permits demonstration of clonality in most cases
- No significant blasts in PB or BM

SELECTED REFERENCES

1. Gianelli U et al: International Consensus Classification of myeloid and lymphoid neoplasms: myeloproliferative neoplasms. Virchows Arch. 482(1):53-68, 2023
2. Thiele J et al: The International Consensus Classification of myeloid neoplasms and acute leukemias: myeloproliferative neoplasms. Am J Hematol. 98(1):166-79, 2023
3. Khoury JD et al: The 5th edition of the World Health Organization classification of haematolymphoid tumours: myeloid and histiocytic/dendritic neoplasms. Leukemia. 36(7):1703-19, 2022
4. Szuber N et al: Chronic neutrophilic leukemia: 2022 update on diagnosis, genomic landscape, prognosis, and management. Am J Hematol. 97(4):491-505, 2022
5. Thomopoulos TP et al: Chronic neutrophilic leukemia: a comprehensive review of clinical characteristics, genetic landscape and management. Front Oncol. 12:891961, 2022

Chronic Neutrophilic Leukemia

Granulocytic Leukocytosis

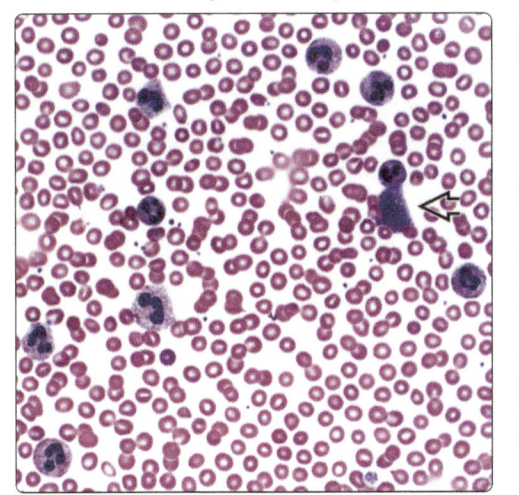

Toxic Changes

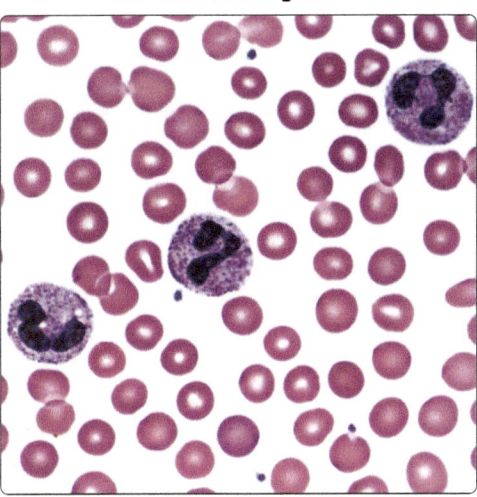

(Left) Peripheral blood shows granulocytic leukocytosis with a rare myelocyte ⇨. Platelet and red cell counts are within normal range. No dysplasia is identified. (Right) Peripheral blood shows the occasional finding of toxic changes in CNL. These neutrophils contain prominent eosinophilic granules and rare Döhle bodies. Immature granulocytes comprise < 10% of WBC.

Granulocytic Predominance

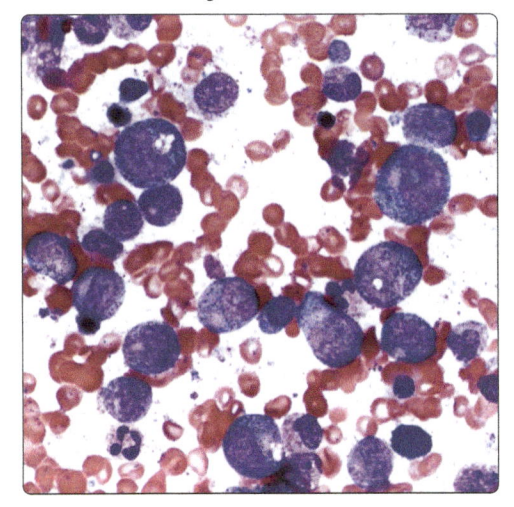

Marked Hypercellularity

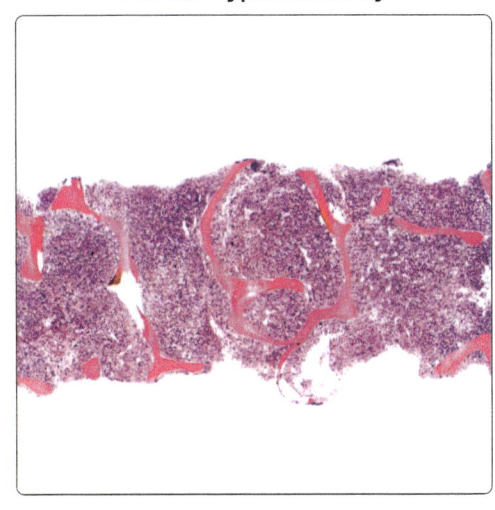

(Left) Bone marrow aspirate shows granulocytic predominance with left shift. These cells are predominantly promyelocytes and myelocytes. (Right) Bone marrow core biopsy shows marked hypercellularity. Note that the bony trabeculae are not overtly abnormal. Reticulin stain showed no significant fibrosis.

MPO Immunohistochemistry

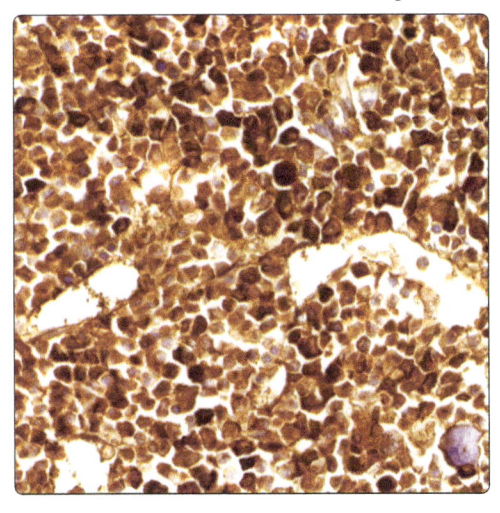

Sanger Sequencing for *CSF3R* Mutation

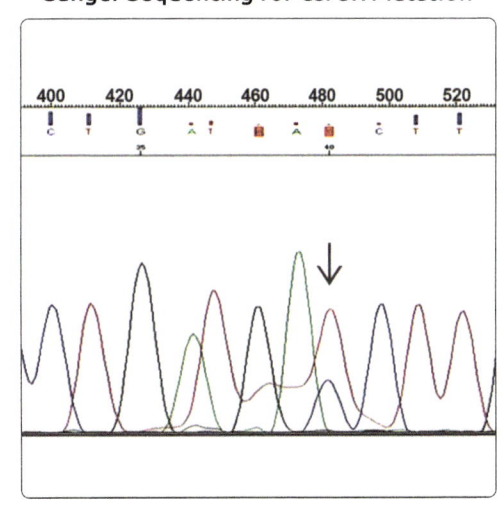

(Left) MPO shows the expected, striking predominance of reactive granulocytes in the bone marrow in this case of CNL. (Right) Sanger sequencing identifies a CSF3R T618I mutation ⇨ in this case of CNL. This is considered a "membrane proximal" mutation and is the most common CSF3R mutation in CNL. The identification of CSF3R mutation establishes the presence of a clonal process and assists in the diagnosis of CNL.

Molecular Pathology of Myeloid Neoplasms

Polycythemia Vera

KEY FACTS

TERMINOLOGY

- Polycythemia vera (PV): Myeloproliferative neoplasm characterized by
  - Increased, unregulated erythropoiesis
  - Bone marrow with panmyelosis
- 2022 International Consensus Classification (ICC) diagnostic criteria for PV
  - Major criteria
    - Hgb > 16.5 g/dL in men, > 16 g/dL in women or Hct > 49% in men, > 48% in women or RBC mass > 25% above mean normal predicted value
    - Hypercellular for age bone marrow with panmyelosis
    - Presence of JAK2 V617F or JAK2 exon 12 mutations
  - Minor criteria
    - Subnormal serum EPO level
  - Diagnosis of PV requires either all 3 major criteria or first 2 major criteria + minor criterion
- World Health Organization, 5th edition (WHO-HAEM5)
  - Diagnostic criteria for PV is essentially similar but not entirely identical
  - Option of increased red cell mass as diagnostic criterion has been removed in WHO-HAEM5
- Clinical phases of PV
  - Prepolycythemic phase with mild erythrocytosis
  - Polycythemic phase with pronounced red cell mass
  - Spent phase and postpolycythemic myelofibrosis

ETIOLOGY/PATHOGENESIS

- Acquired JAK2 gain-of-function mutations in almost all cases

MOLECULAR

- JAK2 V617F in > 95% of cases
- JAK2 exon 12 mutations in 3-4% of cases
- Gene mutations with adverse effect on survival
  - ASXL1, SRSF2, IDH2, EZH2, RUNX1, TP53

Blood Smear

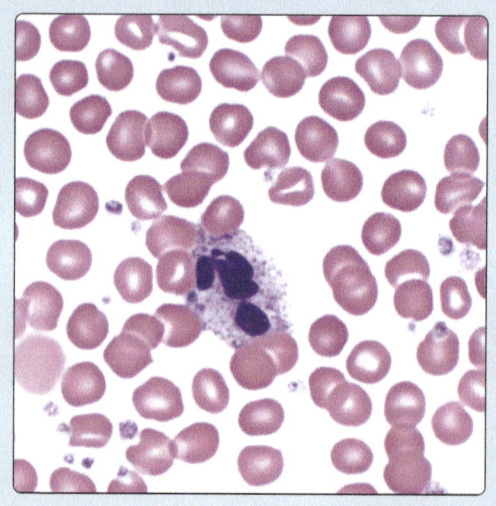

JAK2 V617F-Mutated Polycythemia Vera

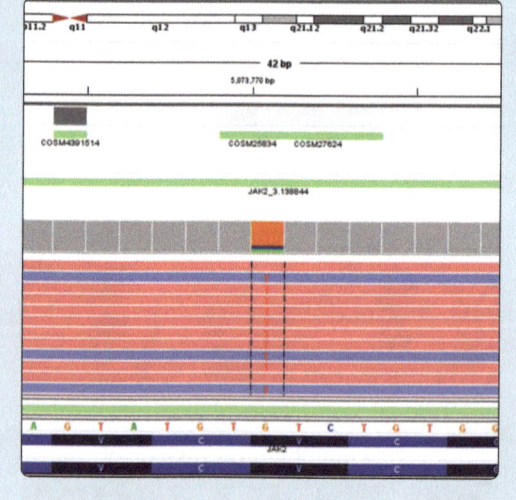

(Left) Peripheral blood smear from a patient with the polycythemic phase of polycythemia vera (PV) shows mild erythrocytosis and thrombocytosis. Additional studies showed a low serum erythropoietin (EPO) level. (Right) NGS analysis of JAK2 exon 14 shows a c.1849 G>T substitution mutation resulting in a JAK2 V617F mutation in a patient with erythrocytosis and low serum EPO level.

IDH1 R132C Mutation

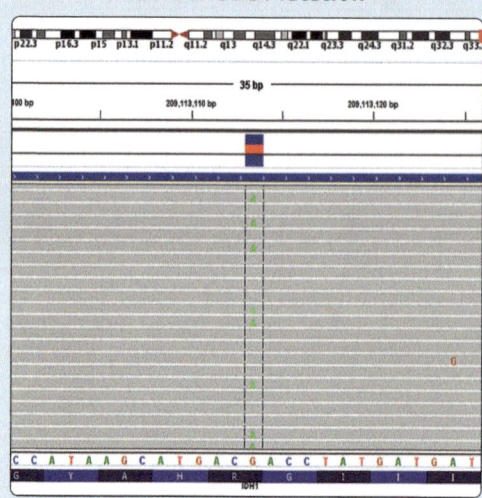

Acute Myeloid Leukemia Transformation

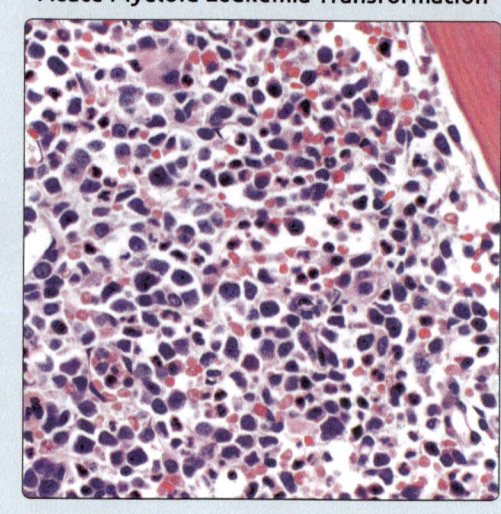

(Left) NGS pile-up of IDH1 exon 2 shows a G>A substitution in codon 132 of IDH1 corresponding to R132C mutation. This mutation was detected in a patient with postpolycythemic myelofibrosis. However, this mutation is not specific and can be seen in other myeloid neoplasms. (Right) Bone marrow core biopsy from a patient with longstanding history of PV shows a prominent population of blasts diagnostic of the blast transformation phase of PV.

Polycythemia Vera

TERMINOLOGY

Abbreviations
- Polycythemia vera (PV)

Definitions
- Classic myeloproliferative neoplasm (MPN) characterized by
  - Unregulated erythropoiesis and marrow panmyelosis
  - *JAK2* mutations in almost all cases
- **2022 International Consensus Classification (ICC) diagnostic criteria for PV**
  - Major criteria
    - Hgb > 16.5 g/dL in men, > 16 g/dL in women **or** Hct > 49% in men, > 48% in women **or** RBC mass > 25% above mean normal predicted value
    - Hypercellular for age bone marrow with panmyelosis
    - Presence of *JAK2* V617F or *JAK2* exon 12 mutations
      - Recommend using highly sensitive assays for *JAK2* V617F
      - Consider searching for noncanonical *JAK2* mutations in exons 12-15 in negative cases
  - Minor criteria
    - Decreased/subnormal serum erythropoietin (EPO) level
  - Diagnosis of PV requires either all 3 major criteria or first 2 major criteria + minor criterion
    - Bone marrow biopsy recommended for purposes of establishing baseline (including assessment of fibrosis) and to obtain cytogenetics information
- **World Health Organization, 5th edition (WHO-HAEM5)**
  - Diagnostic criteria for PV is essentially similar but not entirely identical
    - Option of increased red cell mass as diagnostic criterion has been removed in WHO-HAEM5
- **Clinical phases of PV**
  - Prepolycythemic phase with mild erythrocytosis
  - Polycythemic phase with pronounced red cell mass
  - Spent phase and postpolycythemic myelofibrosis
    - Bone marrow fibrosis
    - Cytopenias due to ineffective hematopiesis
    - Normalization of RBC mass followed by decrease in erythropoiesis
    - Progressive splenomegaly
    - Extramedullary hematopoiesis
- **Diagnostic criteria for post-PV myelofibrosis**
  - Requires previous established diagnosis of PV and bone marrow fibrosis 2 or 3 on scale of 0-3

ETIOLOGY/PATHOGENESIS

Underlying Cause of PV
- Underlying etiology is not clear in majority of cases

JAK2 Gene Mutations
- Acquired *JAK2* mutations in almost all cases
  - *JAK2* V617F somatic mutation in > 95% of cases
  - *JAK2* exon 12 mutation in 3-4% of cases
- *JAK2* mutations promote erythrocytosis and increase granulopoiesis and megakaryopoiesis in PV

CLINICAL ISSUES

Epidemiology
- Incidence
  - ~ 1-3 per 100,000 per year in North America and Europe
- Age
  - Median at diagnosis: ~ 60 years

Presentation
- Common symptoms of PV
  - Nonspecific symptoms, including headaches, fatigue, dizziness, sweating, pruritus, and erythromelalgia
  - May present with deep venous or arterial thrombotic events, myocardial ischemia, or stroke
  - PV should be considered in patients with portal or splenic vein thrombosis or Budd-Chiari syndrome
  - Hepatosplenomegaly, ruddy cyanosis, and hypertension may be present on physical exam
- Laboratory findings
  - Low/subnormal serum EPO level
  - Endogenous erythroid colony formation
  - *JAK2* V617F or *JAK2* exon 12 mutations

Treatment
- Risk-adapted treatment algorithm
  - Low-risk PV (age < 60 years, no thrombosis history)
    - Low-dose aspirin and phlebotomy
  - High-risk PV (age > 60 years &/or thrombosis history)
    - Low-dose aspirin, phlebotomy, and hydroxyurea or interferon-α
- Targeted therapy with JAK2 inhibitors
  - Ruxolitinib therapy for cytoreductive therapy-resistant or intolerant patients with severe constitutional symptoms, pruritus, and marked splenomegaly may benefit
  - ≥ 50% reduction in splenic size in ~ 50% of patients
- Allogeneic stem cell transplantation
  - Potentially curative in post-PV myelofibrosis

Prognosis
- Risk factors for survival include age > 60 years, leukocytosis, venous thrombosis, and abnormal karyotype
  - Median survival: ~ 23 years in absence of advanced age and leukocytosis
  - Median survival: ~ 9 years when both advanced age and leukocytosis are present

MOLECULAR

Gene Mutations
- *JAK2* c.1849G>T, p.V617F mutation
  - Acquired gain-of-function mutation in > 95% of PV
    - Mutations are typically homozygous or hemizygous
  - *JAK2* V617F is not specific for PV
    - Also seen in ~ 40-60% of essential thrombocythemia (ET) and primary myelofibrosis (PMF)
- *JAK2* exon 12 mutations
  - Commonly seen in *JAK2* V617F-negative cases of PV
    - ~ 4% frequency among all PV cases
    - Usually predominant erythropoiesis, subnormal EPO level, and younger age at diagnosis
    - Include point mutations, double mutations, deletions, and insertions

Polycythemia Vera

- Increased allele burden does not effect survival
- *TET2* mutations
  - Reported in ~ 10-18% of PV
- Additional mutations with adverse effect on survival
  - *ASXL1, SRSF2, IDH2, EZH2*
    - Adverse effect appears to be independent of conventional prognostic models
- Mutational profile of post-PV acute myeloid leukemia (AML) transformation
  - 2.5% incidence of AML transformation of PV at 10-year follow-up
    - Mutational profile of post-PV AML differs from de novo AML
    - Frequently occurring mutations in post-PV AML include *ASXL1, SRSF2, IDH1, IDH2, SH2B3, NRAS, RUNX1*, and *TP53*
    - *TP53* is most frequently mutated gene detected in ~ 50% of post-PV AML cases with VAF > 50%
      □ Subclonal *TP53* mutations with low VAF detected by deep NGS in subset of MPN at diagnosis
      □ However, majority of these patients with subclonal *TP53* mutations remain stable at follow-up
- *MPL* and *CALR* mutations are typically absent in PV

Cytogenetics

- Cytogenetic abnormalities
  - Present in 15-20% of patients with PV and post-PV myelofibrosis
  - Include +8, +9, del(20q), del(13q), del(9p), and complex karyotype
  - May contribute to worsening prognosis

MICROSCOPIC

Blood and Bone Marrow Findings

- Prepolycythemic and polycythemic phase
  - Peripheral blood
    - Normochromic, normocytic erythrocytosis
    - Neutrophilia without significant immature forms or blasts
    - Basophilia may be present in rare cases
    - Thrombocytosis in ~ 15% of cases
  - Bone marrow
    - Typically hypercellular for age
    - Panmyelosis but with more prominent erythroid and megakaryocytic lineages
    - Normal-appearing erythropoiesis and granulopoiesis with complete maturation
    - Pleomorphic megakaryocytes with hyperlobated nuclei may be present
    - Loose clusters of megakaryocytes may be seen
    - Reticulin fibrosis is typically absent or minimal
- Postpolycythemic myelofibrosis
  - Peripheral blood
    - Leukoerythroblastic reaction
    - Anemia may be present
  - Bone marrow
    - Typically hypocellular but can be variable
    - Significant reticulin and collagen fibrosis
    - Prominent sinusoidal dilatation with intrasinusoidal hematopoiesis
    - Clustering of megakaryocytes with atypical and hyperchromatic forms
    - Osteosclerosis typically present in late stage

Diagnostic Criteria for Post-PV Myelofibrosis

- Required criteria
  - Documented prior diagnosis of WHO-/ICC-defined PV
  - Bone marrow fibrosis grades 2-3 (on 0-3 scale)
- Additional criteria (2 are required)
  - Anemia or sustained need of either phlebotomy (in absence of cytoreductive therapy) or cytoreductive treatment for erythrocytosis
  - Leukoerythroblastic peripheral blood picture
  - Increasing splenomegaly: Either increase in palpable splenomegaly of > 5 cm from baseline (distance from left costal margin) or appearance of newly palpable splenomegaly
  - Development of > 1 of 3 constitutional symptoms: 10% weight loss in 6 months, night sweats, unexplained fever (> 37.5 °C)

ANCILLARY TESTS

Histochemistry

- Reticulin and collagen histochemical stains
  - Should be performed routinely
  - Increased reticulin fibrosis at presentation associated with increased risk of progression to myelofibrotic phase

Genetic Testing

- *JAK2* V617F testing should be done in all suspected cases
- *JAK2* exon 12 in all *JAK2* V617F-negative cases

DIFFERENTIAL DIAGNOSIS

Secondary Polycythemia

- Hypoxia driven due to cardiac or pulmonary disease, high-altitude habitat, smoking, etc.
- Oxygen independent due to drugs (androgen, EPO, etc.)
- Congenital due to EPO receptor mutation or high-oxygen-affinity hemoglobinopathy
- All secondary polycythemias lack *JAK2* mutations

Chronic Myeloid Leukemia

- Absence of *BCR::ABL1* and presence of *JAK2* mutation separate PV from chronic myeloid leukemia

Essential Thrombocythemia

- Prepolycythemic PV with thrombocytosis may mimic ET
- Bone marrow panmyelosis and subnormal EPO level can prove useful in separating PV from ET

Primary Myelofibrosis

- Post-PV myelofibrosis may show bone marrow morphology indistinguishable from PMF
- Prior documented diagnosis of PV helps to separate post-PV myelofibrosis from PMF

SELECTED REFERENCES

1. Gianelli U et al: International Consensus Classification of myeloid and lymphoid neoplasms: myeloproliferative neoplasms. Virchows Arch. 482(1):53-68, 2023
2. Harrison CN et al: Polycythaemia vera. In: WHO Classification of Tumours Editorial Board. Haematolymphoid tumours. IARC, 2022

Polycythemia Vera

Blood Smear With Leukoerythroblastic Picture

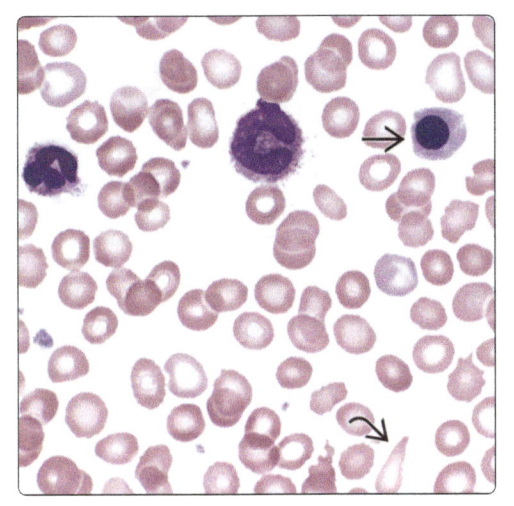

Bone Marrow Aspirate

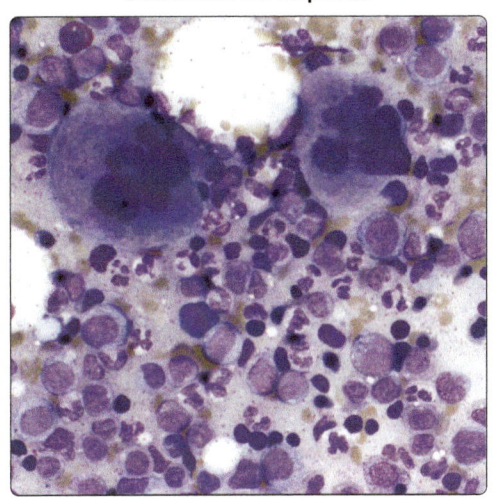

(Left) Wright-stained peripheral blood from a patient with PV shows a leukoerythroblastic picture, including anisopoikilocytosis with teardrop forms ⇘ and circulating nucleated RBCs ➞. The leukoerythroblastic picture in this setting suggests increased marrow fibrosis. (Right) Bone marrow aspirate smear from a patient in the polycythemic phase of PV shows increased trilineage hematopoiesis (panmyelosis) and hyperlobulated megakaryocytes.

Bone Marrow Core Biopsy

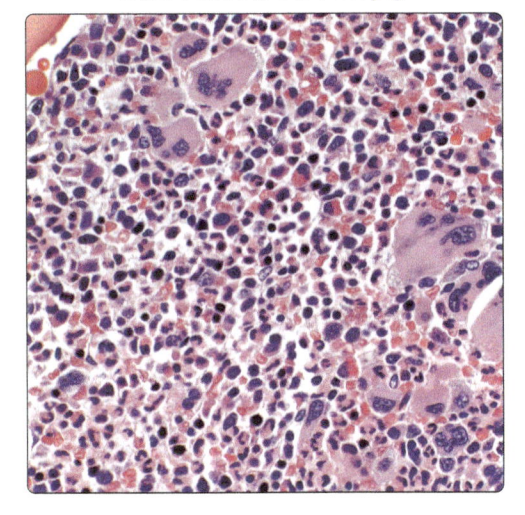

Postpolycythemic Myelofibrosis

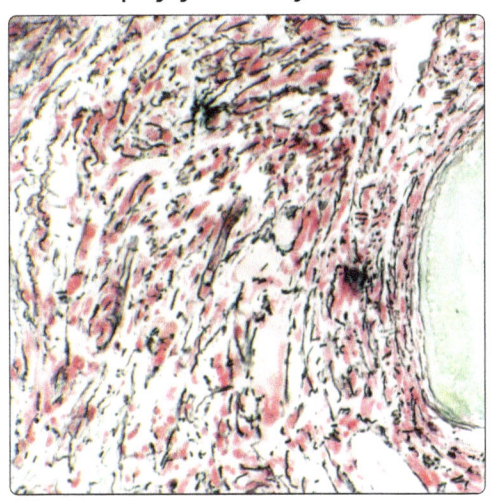

(Left) Bone marrow core biopsy from a patient in the polycythemic phase of PV shows markedly hypercellular marrow with panmyelosis and loose clusters of pleomorphic-appearing megakaryocytes. (Right) Reticulin stain performed on marrow trephine biopsy from a patient with documented history of PV shows moderate to marked increase in reticulin fibrosis, consistent with progression to postpolycythemic myelofibrosis.

High-Resolution Melting Curve of *JAK2* Exon 12 PCR-Amplified Products

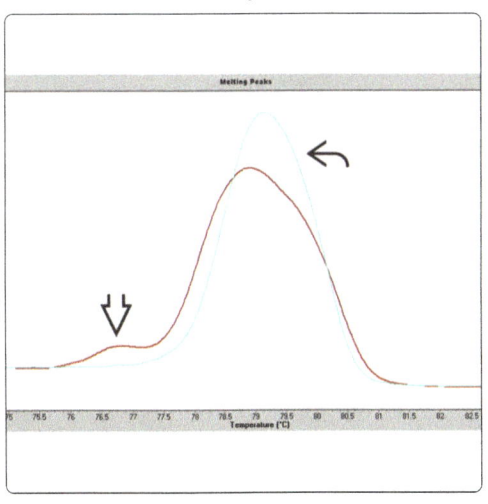

Sanger Sequencing of *JAK2* Exon 12

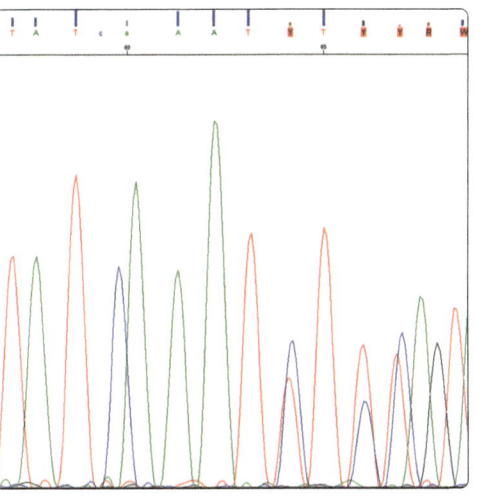

(Left) High-resolution melting curve analysis of PCR-amplified DNA from a PV patient harboring JAK2 exon 12 mutation reveals an abnormal shouldering ➞ compared to wildtype DNA melting curve ⇘, consistent with exon 12 mutation. (Right) Sanger sequencing of JAK2 exon 12 performed on blood sample from a patient with JAK2 V617F-negative PV shows 6 bp deletion involving codons E543 and D544. The mixed sequences on the sequence traces correspond to the end of the 6 bp deletion.

Molecular Pathology of Myeloid Neoplasms

151

Primary Myelofibrosis

KEY FACTS

TERMINOLOGY
- Primary myelofibrosis (PMF)
- Megakaryocytic and granulocytic proliferation with ultimate bone marrow fibrosis

CLINICAL ISSUES
- Median survival for pre-PMF: 15 years
- Median survival for PMF with overt fibrosis: 6-7 years

MICROSCOPIC
- Anemia
- Variable thrombocytosis
- Variable granulocytic leukocytosis
- Marked erythroid anisopoikilocytosis, including dacrocytes (teardrop forms)

ANCILLARY TESTS
- Algorithmic approach useful
- Initial testing for JAK2 V617F mutation
  - JAK2 mutations in 50-60%
- If negative, follow with CALR and MPL testing
  - CALR mutations in 20-35%
    - Associated with better outcomes than CALR-negative cases
  - MPL mutations in 5%
- Mutations in other genes may be identified by NGS targeted myeloid gene panels
  - Provide additional information in JAK2/CALR/MPL wildtype (triple-negative) cases
  - Provide prognostic information
    - High-risk mutations include ASXL1, SRSF2, IDH1, IDH2, and EZH2
- Recurrent karyotypic abnormalities have prognostic significance
  - Unfavorable abnormalities: +8, -7/7q-, i(17q), inv(3), -5/5q-, 12p-, 11q23 rearrangement, complex karyotype, monosomal karyotype
  - Favorable abnormalities: 20q-, 13q-, +9

Fibrotic Stage

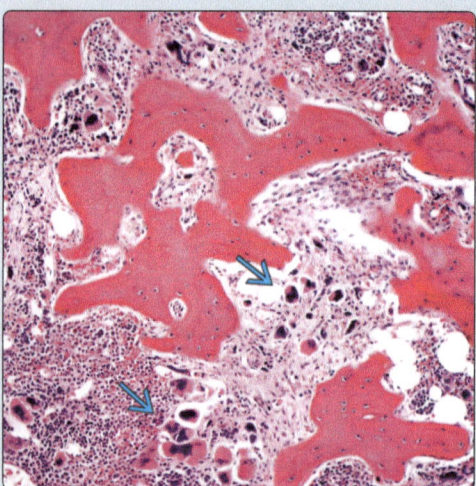

Trisomy 8

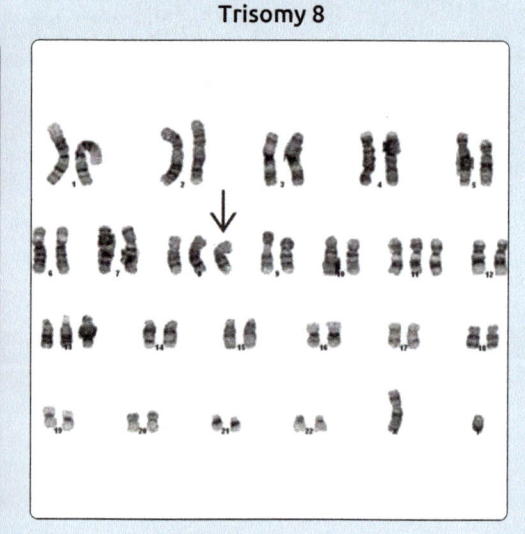

(Left) Marked osteosclerosis, myelofibrosis, and megakaryocytic pleomorphism are hallmark histologic features of primary myelofibrosis (PMF). Megakaryocytes range from small to large and are hyperchromatic and clustered ➡. (Right) Karyogram shows multiple abnormalities, including trisomy 8 ➡. Trisomy 8 is not specific for a particular type of myeloid neoplasm but is one of the more common findings in PMF.

JAK2 Testing

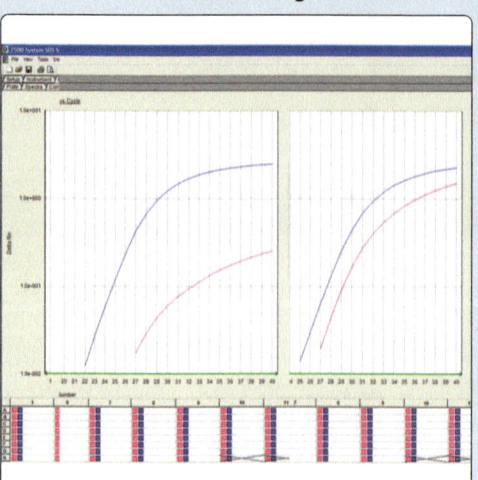

MPL Mutation

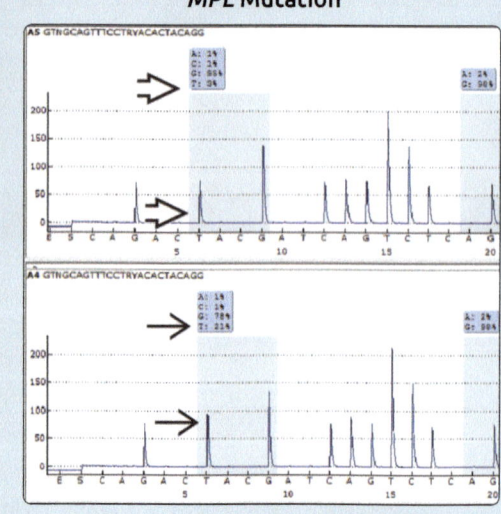

(Left) Semiquantitative JAK2 testing is shown by allelic discrimination using labeled probes. The wildtype sample on the left shows greater separation between the wildtype (blue) and mutant (pink) amplification curve compared to the mutated sample on the right. (Right) Pyrogram shows the common W515L mutation in codon 515 of MPL. The mutated case in the lower image shows increased percentage of T at position 6 ➡ compared to the wildtype sample ➡.

Primary Myelofibrosis

TERMINOLOGY

Abbreviations
- Primary myelofibrosis (PMF)

Definitions
- Myeloproliferative neoplasm (MPN)
- Clonal stem cell disorder
- Manifests as megakaryocytic and granulocytic proliferations with ultimate fibrosis

PMF, Early/Prefibrotic Stage (Pre-PMF) Diagnostic Criteria
- Requires all 3 major and 1 minor
- Major criteria
  o Megakaryocytic proliferation and atypia, BM fibrosis grade < 2, hypercellularity, granulocytic proliferation, often with decreased erythropoiesis
  o JAK2, CALR, or MPL mutation **or** presence of another clonal marker **or** absence of marrow reactive reticulin fibrosis
  o Diagnostic criteria for BCR::ABL1-positive chronic myeloid leukemia, polycythemia vera, essential thrombocythemia, myelodysplastic syndromes, or other myeloid neoplasia are not met
- Minor criteria
  o Anemia not attributed to comorbid condition
  o Leukocytosis ≥ 11 x 10^9/L
  o Palpable splenomegaly
  o Lactate dehydrogenase level above normal

PMF, Overt Fibrotic Stage Diagnostic Criteria
- Requires all 3 major and 1 minor
- Major criteria same as for prefibrotic PMF
- Minor criteria same as prefibrotic PMF except for addition of "leukoerythroblastosis" as another minor criterion

CLASSIFICATION

ICC and WHO-HAEM5 Comparison (Prefibrotic PMF and PMF With Overt Fibrosis)
- Essentially same major and minor criteria and exclusions
  o ICC defines dense megakaryocyte clustering as > 6 megakaryocytes with no other intervening BM cells
  o ICC indicates that minor criteria must be confirmed 2 consecutive times
  o ICC indicates that megakaryocytes in PMF show greater degree of atypia than seen in other MPN
  o ICC provides criteria to distinguish PMF with monocytosis from chronic myelomonocytic leukemia (CMML)

CLINICAL ISSUES

Epidemiology
- Incidence
  o ~ 0.4/100,000 in United States
- Age
  o Median at diagnosis: 67 years

Presentation
- Splenomegaly
- Constitutional symptoms

Treatment
- Only potential cure is allogeneic stem cell transplantation
- Drug therapy
  o Hydroxyurea
    – Decrease leukocytosis, thrombocytosis, and splenomegaly
  o Thalidomide/lenalidomide and steroids
  o Molecular-targeted therapy
    – JAK2 inhibitors

Prognosis
- Median survival for pre-PMF: 15 years
- Median survival for PMF with overt fibrosis: 6-7 years
- Prognostic stratification
  o International Prognostic Scoring System
    – Age: > 65 years; hemoglobin < 10 g/dL; leukocyte count > 25 x 10^9/L; circulating blasts ≥ 1%; constitutional symptoms
    – Dynamic International Prognostic Scoring System (DIPSS) used during disease course
    – DIPSS-plus incorporates additional factors
      □ Platelet count < 100 x 10^9/L, transfusion requirement, unfavorable karyotype
  o Mutation-enhanced International Prognostic Scoring System (MIPSS)
    – Incorporates clinical and laboratory findings with molecular and cytogenetic abnormalities
    – ASXL1, SRSF2, EZH2, U2AF1, IDH1, and IDH2 defined as high-risk mutations
    – Absence of CALR type 1 mutation associated with increased risk
  o Genetically inspired prognostic scoring system (GIPSS) only involves mutations and karyotype

MOLECULAR

Cytogenetics
- Recurrent abnormalities have prognostic significance
  o Normal karyotype in 57% of cases
    – Favorable prognostic factor
    – Associated with higher hemoglobin, WBC, platelet count
    – More common in pre-PMF
  o 20q-, most common abnormality in 24% of cases
    – Favorable prognostic factor
    – Associated with lower leukocyte count and thrombocytopenia
  o 13q- in 19% of cases
    – Favorable prognostic factor
    – Associated with CALR mutations
    – Associated with thrombocytosis
  o Trisomy 8 in 11% of cases
    – Unfavorable prognostic factor
    – Associated with leukopenia
    – Lower incidence of constitutional symptoms
  o Trisomy 9 in 10% of cases
    – Favorable prognostic factor
  o Abnormalities of chromosome 1 in 10% of cases
    – Includes duplications, translocations, and other aberrations
    – Favorable prognostic factor

Primary Myelofibrosis

- Other unfavorable cytogenetic abnormalities
  - -7/7q-, iso17q [i(17q)], inv(3), -5/5q-, 12p-, 11q23 rearrangement
  - Complex karyotype
  - Monosomal karyotype

Molecular Genetics

- *JAK2* mutations
  - Found in 50-60% of PMF
  - Exon 14 V617F is most common mutation
    - Associated with intermediate prognosis
    - Associated with increased risk of thrombosis compared to *CALR* mutation
  - Exon 12 mutations are not seen in PMF
- *CALR* exon 9 frameshift mutations
  - Found in 20-35% of PMF
    - 88% of *JAK2*- and *MPL*-negative cases
    - Type 1: 52-bp deletion most common in PMF
    - Leads to use of alternate reading frame
    - Generates novel C-terminal peptide sequence
  - Associated with lower WBC count and higher platelet count than *JAK2*-mutated PMF
  - Type 1 deletion mutation is associated with longer overall survival than *JAK2*- and *MPL*-mutated PMF
  - Favorable prognostic factor
    - Improved survival compared to *JAK2*-mutated and triple-negative cases
    - Lower risk of thrombosis compared to *JAK2*-mutated cases
    - 18-year overall survival rate
- *MPL* mutations
  - Found in 5% of PMF
  - Codon 515 is common location
  - Associated with intermediate prognosis
  - Higher risk of thrombosis than *CALR*-mutated cases
- *JAK2*, *CALR*, and *MPL* wildtype cases (triple negative)
  - Accounts for 10% of PMF cases
  - Unfavorable prognostic factor
    - 3-year overall survival rate
    - Inferior leukemia-free survival compared to *JAK2*- and *CALR*-mutated cases
  - Mutations may be identified in combination with each other or more common mutations
    - *TET2* mutation seen in 17%
    - *SRSF2* mutation seen in 14%
      - □ Inferior overall and leukemia-free survival
    - *ASXL1* mutation seen in 13%
      - □ Associated with aggressive disease, shorter survival
    - *DNMT3A* mutation seen in 6%
    - *EZH2* mutation seen in 6%
    - *IDH1* or *IDH2* mutation seen in 4%
      - □ Inferior leukemia-free survival
    - *CHEK2* mutation seen in 3%
    - *TP53* mutation associated with leukemic transformation and aggressive disease

MICROSCOPIC

Peripheral Blood

- Early/prefibrotic phase
  - Anemia, variable thrombocytosis
  - Variable granulocytic leukocytosis
- Fibrotic phase
  - Leukoerythroblastosis with marked erythroid anisopoikilocytosis, including teardrop forms
  - Circulating micromegakaryocytes, megakaryocytic nuclei
  - Variable circulating blasts

Bone Marrow

- Early/prefibrotic phase
  - Fibrosis may be absent/minimal
  - Hypercellular, granulocytic predominance, blasts < 5%
  - Megakaryocytic atypia
- Fibrotic phase
  - Marked reticulin &/or collagen fibrosis
  - Dilated sinuses, intrasinusoidal hematopoiesis, osteosclerosis
  - Focal hypocellularity admixed with foci of intact hematopoiesis
  - Marked megakaryocytic atypia, including cloud-shaped, hyperlobated, and hyperchromatic forms
    - May form large sheets and tight clusters
  - Increased blasts
    - 10-19%: Accelerated-phase disease
    - ≥ 20%: Blast phase (transformation to acute leukemia)

ANCILLARY TESTS

Genetic Testing

- Initial testing for *JAK2*, *CALR*, and *MPL*
- Panels for genes associated with myeloid neoplasms
  - Prove clonality in *JAK2*/*CALR*/*MPL* triple-negative cases
  - Provide prognostic information

DIFFERENTIAL DIAGNOSIS

Other MPN

- Essential thrombocythemia (ET)
  - Manifestations largely restricted to megakaryocytes
- Polycythemia vera (PV)
  - Post-PV myelofibrosis histologically mimics PMF

Chronic Myeloid Leukemia

- *BCR::ABL1* fusion present

SELECTED REFERENCES

1. Al-Ghamdi YA et al: Triple-negative primary myelofibrosis: a bone marrow pathology group study. Mod Pathol. 36(3):100016, 2023
2. Gianelli U et al: International Consensus Classification of myeloid and lymphoid neoplasms: myeloproliferative neoplasms. Virchows Arch. 482(1):53-68, 2023
3. How J et al: Biology and therapeutic targeting of molecular mechanisms in MPNs. Blood. 141(16):1922-33, 2023
4. Kuo MC et al: Comparison of clinical and molecular features between patients with essential thrombocythemia and early/prefibrotic primary myelofibrosis presenting with thrombocytosis in Taiwan. Am J Clin Pathol. 159(5):474-83, 2023
5. Maslah N et al: Clonal architecture evolution in myeloproliferative neoplasms: from a driver mutation to a complex heterogeneous mutational and phenotypic landscape. Leukemia. 37(5):957-63, 2023
6. Luque Paz D et al: Genetic basis and molecular profiling in myeloproliferative neoplasms. Blood. 141(16):1909-21, 2023
7. Khoury JD et al: The 5th edition of the World Health Organization classification of haematolymphoid tumours: myeloid and histiocytic/dendritic neoplasms. Leukemia. 36(7):1703-19, 2022

Primary Myelofibrosis

Karyotypic Abnormalities

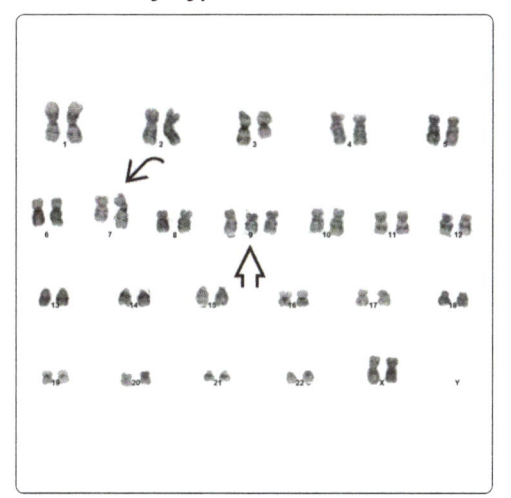

Leukoerythroblastic Blood Picture

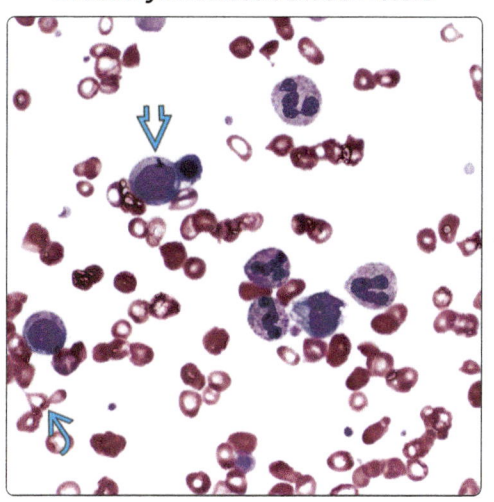

(Left) Karyotype from a patient with PMF shows 47,XX,der(1;7)(q10;q10),del(3)(q21),+9,add(10)(q22). Gain of 1q [from the unbalanced translocation t(1;7) ⇨] and trisomy 9 ⇨ are common in PMF and associated with a favorable prognosis. (Right) Fibrotic-phase PMF is typically characterized by anemia and a leukoerythroblastic blood picture with dacrocytes ⇨. Circulating blasts may be evident ⇨ but constitute < 20% of leukocytes.

Bone Marrow Findings

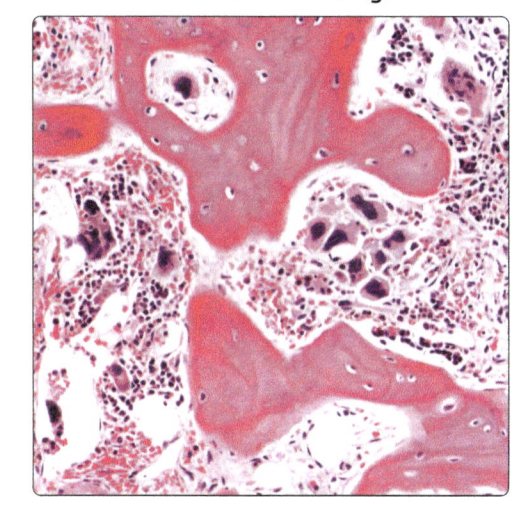

Bone Marrow Findings

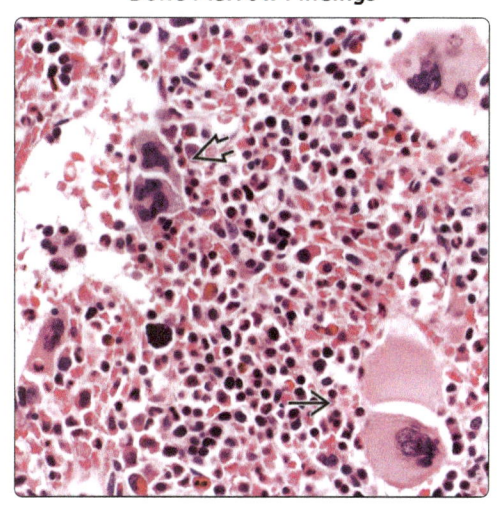

(Left) Typical bone marrow features of PMF include osteosclerosis, megakaryocytic atypia with clustering and bizarre nuclei, dilated sinuses, and intrasinusoidal hematopoiesis. Varying degrees of reticulin fibrosis are present. (Right) Marked megakaryocytic atypia with clustering ⇨ is an early feature of PMF. Megakaryocytes range from small to large and exhibit bizarre and hyperchromatic nuclear features. Intrasinusoidal hematopoiesis is often identified ⇨.

Fibrotic Stage

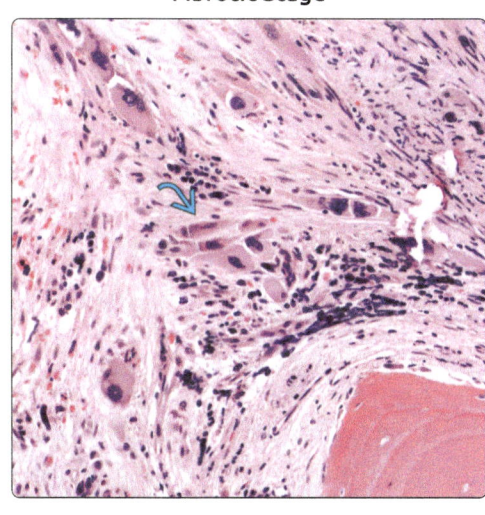

Grade 3 Reticulin Fibrosis

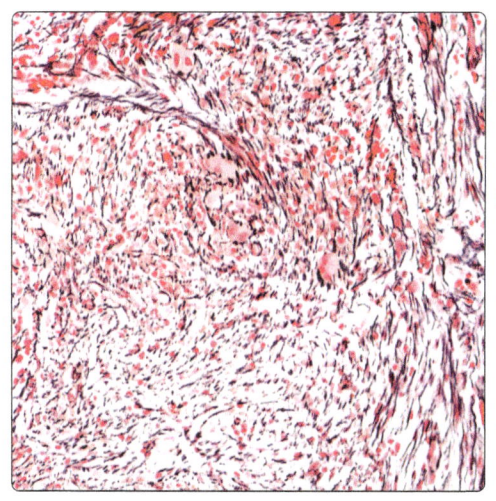

(Left) End-stage PMF shows marked reticulin &/or collagen fibrosis in hypocellular foci within the bone marrow and a "streaming effect." Residual abnormal megakaryocytes with tight clustering remain ⇨. (Right) Grade 3 (0-3 range) reticulin fibrosis is shown here in an advanced case of PMF. Significant fibrosis can be seen in progressed phases of essential thrombocythemia and polycythemia vera, but this is rare. Concurrent collagen fibrosis may be evident in core biopsies with marked reticulin fibrosis.

Molecular Pathology of Myeloid Neoplasms

155

Essential Thrombocythemia

KEY FACTS

TERMINOLOGY
- Essential thrombocythemia (ET): Myeloproliferative neoplasm restricted to proliferation of megakaryocytic lineage
- BCR::ABL1-positive chronic myeloid leukemia, polycythemia vera, primary myelofibrosis, and other myeloid neoplasms should be excluded

CLINICAL ISSUES
- Increased risk of thrombosis &/or hemorrhagic events

MOLECULAR
- JAK2 V617F mutation
  - Present in 50-60% of cases
- CALR mutations
  - Present in ~ 15-25% of cases
- MPL mutations
  - Present in < 5% of cases with W515L mutation being most common
- Mutations are mutually exclusive and are not specific for ET
- "Triple-negative" cases (cases without identifiable mutations in JAK2, CALR, and MPL) account for ~ 15-20% of ET cases

MICROSCOPIC
- Peripheral blood
  - Platelet count ≥ 450 x 10⁹/L with platelet anisocytosis
  - No significant leukoerythroblastosis or increased blasts
  - White and red cell morphology mostly unremarkable
  - Dysplastic features (e.g., platelet hypogranulation) are not typical
- Bone marrow
  - Striking megakaryocytic proliferation with large, hyperlobulated forms
    - Highly atypical or bizarre forms are not characteristic of ET
  - Normal or mildly hypercellular marrow with < 5% blasts and absent or only minimal fibrosis

Thrombocytosis With Anisocytosis

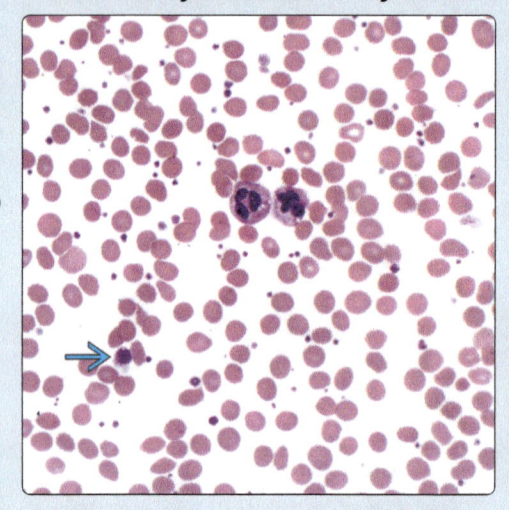

Hyperlobulated Megakaryocytes

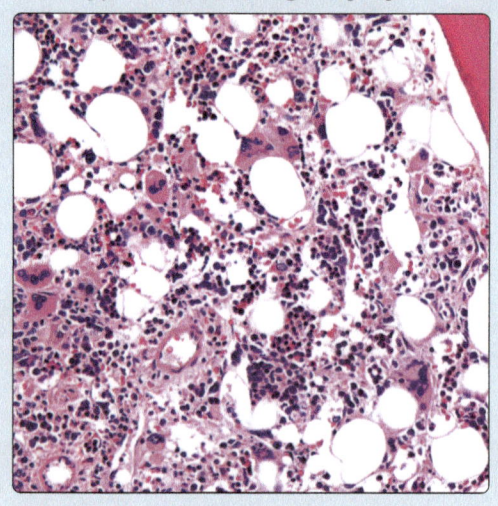

(Left) Blood smear shows thrombocytosis with anisocytosis, including large forms ➡. WBC count and differential, as well as RBCs, are usually normal in classic cases of essential thrombocythemia (ET). (Right) Bone marrow from a patient with ET shows increased, enlarged, hyperlobulated megakaryocytes with loose clustering. There is no significant myeloid or erythroid proliferation.

Large to Giant Megakaryocytes

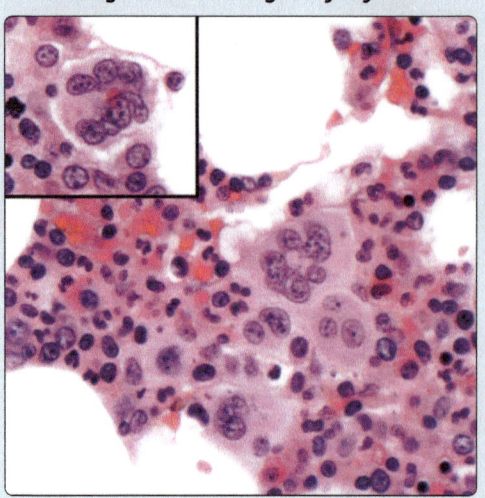

Allelic Discrimination Real-Time PCR

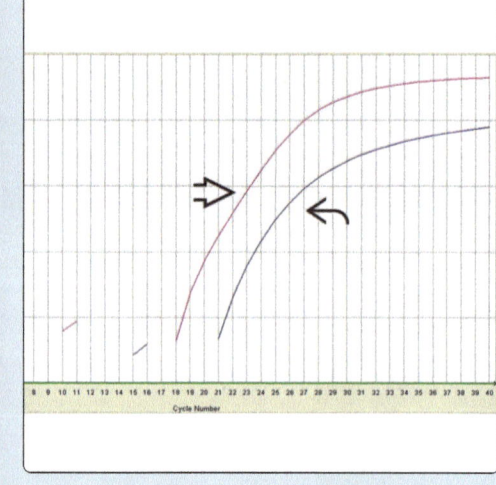

(Left) Megakaryocytes show large to giant forms with abundant, mature cytoplasm and deeply lobated and hypersegmented (staghorn-like) nuclei. (Right) PCR shows the presence of JAK2 V617F mutation ➡ in this case of ET. The blue amplification curve represents the wildtype allele ➡.

Essential Thrombocythemia

TERMINOLOGY

Abbreviations
- Essential thrombocythemia (ET)

Synonyms
- Primary thrombocytosis (obsolete)
- Essential thrombocytosis (obsolete)

Definitions
- Clonal myeloid neoplasm characterized by hematologic and morphologic alterations primarily restricted to megakaryocytic lineage
- Defined as myeloproliferative neoplasm (MPN), per revised WHO 5th edition (HAEM5) and 2022 International Consensus Classification (ICC)
- *BCR::ABL1*-positive chronic myeloid leukemia, polycythemia vera (PV), primary myelofibrosis (MF), and other myeloid neoplasms should be excluded

ETIOLOGY/PATHOGENESIS

Sporadic Essential Thrombocythemia
- Most common genetic alterations include somatic mutations in *JAK2*, *CALR*, or *MPL*
  - *JAK2* (Janus kinase 2), *CALR*, and *MPL* mutations are mutually exclusive in vast majority of cases
- In general, mutations result in dysregulation and activation of JAK-STAT signaling pathway
  - JAK-STAT signaling pathway activation promotes myeloproliferation via cytokine overproduction

Hereditary Thrombocythemia
- Rare heterogeneous disorders with spectrum of genetic mutations
- *THPO* (thrombopoietin) germline mutations
  - Associated with hereditary thrombocythemia type 1 (THCYT1)
    - G > C transversion in splice donor site at position 1+ of intron 3
    - 1-bp deletion in 5' untranslated region (UTR) at nucleotide position 3252 (3252delG)
    - G516T located in 5' UTR
- *MPL* (thrombopoietin receptor) germline mutations
  - Associated with thrombocythemia type 2 (THCYT2), including K39N, P106L, and S505N variants
- *JAK2* germline mutations
  - Associated with thrombocythemia type 3 (THCYT3), including V617I and R564Q variants
  - Only THCYT3 cases are considered neoplastic and have low but elevated risk to develop MF &/or acute leukemia

CLINICAL ISSUES

Epidemiology
- 1.5-3/100,000 cases per year
- Most cases occur in patients 50-60 years of age

Site
- Peripheral blood and bone marrow

Presentation
- Most patients are asymptomatic, and thrombocytosis is discovered incidentally
- Common associated symptoms
  - Vascular occlusion with transient ischemic attacks and digital ischemia
  - Thrombosis with particular involvement of hepatic/splenic veins
  - Hemorrhage, mainly mucosal bleeding
- Persistent thrombocytosis, defined as platelet count ≥ 450 x 10⁹/L
- Mild splenomegaly (15-20%) and hepatomegaly (rare)

Treatment
- Primarily aimed to prevent thrombohemorrhagic complications
- Risk-adapted treatment approach
  - Based on age, thrombosis history, presence of *JAK2* V617F mutation, and cardiovascular risk
  - Includes observation, low-dose aspirin, and hydroxyurea

Prognosis
- Indolent process
  - Strictly WHO-/ICC-defined ET has very good prognosis
  - 15-year survival ~ 80%
  - Risk of transformation to acute myeloid leukemia (AML) or MF is < 5%
- Main morbidity results from thrombosis and hemorrhagic events

MOLECULAR

Cytogenetics
- Abnormal karyotype seen in ~ 5-10% of cases
  - Most common abnormalities include trisomy 8, abnormalities of 9q or trisomy 9, and deletion of 20q

Molecular Genetics
- *JAK2* mutations
  - *JAK2* located at 9p24.1
  - Critical role in JAK-STAT signaling pathway
    - JAK2 signaling via class I cytokine receptors critically regulates normal myelopoiesis
  - Mutations lead to constitutive activation of JAK signaling pathway and lead to enhanced cell proliferation, differentiation, and survival
  - *JAK2* V617F mutation
    - G > T base substitution results in replacement of valine by phenylalanine in codon 617 position of exon 14 (V617F)
    - Most common mutation, present in ~ 50-60% of ET cases
      - Associated with older age, higher hemoglobin levels, mild leukocytosis, and lower platelet count
    - Usually lower allele burden compared to other *JAK2* V617F-mutated MPNs
  - Mutation has clinical predictive value
    - Increased risk of arterial thrombosis
    - Lower risk of transformation to MF
  - *JAK2* exon 12 mutations are extremely rare in ET
- *CALR* mutations
  - *CALR* (calreticulin) located at 19p13.13

- Encodes for multifunctional calcium-binding protein chaperone located in endoplasmic reticulum
- Mutations present in ~ 15-25% of ET cases
- Most common mutations include exon 9 frameshift indels with 2 common variants
  - Type 1 variant (p.L367fs*46) results in 52-bp deletion
  - Type 2 variant (p.K385fs*47) results in 5-bp, TTGTC insertion (preferentially associated with ET)
- Mutations associated with younger age, higher platelet counts, lower hemoglobin level and leukocyte count, and relatively low risk of thrombosis

- *MPL* mutations
  - *MPL* located at 1p34.2
  - Encodes for thrombopoietin receptor protein
    - Mutations result in thrombopoietin-independent activation of JAK2-STAT signaling pathway
  - Activating mutations reported in < 5% of ET cases
    - Most mutations occur in exon 10, at tryptophan 515 (W515L)
  - Other less frequent mutations include W515K and S505N
    - S505N can be seen as both germline and acquired mutation in hereditary THCYT1 as well as in sporadic cases of ET, respectively
  - Mutations associated with older age, female sex, lower hemoglobin level, and higher platelet count

- Other mutations
  - *TET2* and *ASXL1* are most frequent additional gene mutations
  - Mutations associated with decreased overall survival include *SH2B3*, *SF3B1*, *U2AF1*, *IDH2*, *EZH2*, and *TP53*
    - *TP53* mutations and increased karyotypic complexity usually associated with progression to more aggressive stages

MICROSCOPIC

Peripheral Blood
- Variable thrombocytosis with increased anisocytosis
- Circulating megakaryocytes can be seen, including
  - Nuclear fragments and micromegakaryocytes
- Dysplastic features (e.g., platelet hypogranulation) are not typical
- Granulocytes and erythrocytes are usually within normal parameters
  - Leukoerythroblastosis should not be present
  - Increased circulating blasts are extremely unusual

Bone Marrow
- Usually normocellular or mildly hypercellular for age
- Megakaryocytes display distinctive abnormalities
  - Markedly increased in number with predominance of large to giant forms
  - Hyperlobulated nuclei (staghorn-like) with ample cytoplasm and overall preserved maturation
    - Highly atypical or bizarre forms are not characteristic of ET
  - Distributed mostly individually, although focal loose clusters can be seen
    - Intrasinusoidal and perisinusoidal with frequent emperipolesis of neutrophils may be seen
- Remaining myelopoiesis and erythropoiesis are generally unremarkable
- Blasts usually < 5%
- Absent or minimal reticulin fibrosis
- Normal or near-normal iron stores

DIFFERENTIAL DIAGNOSIS

Reactive Thrombocytosis
- Causes are diverse and can include
  - Iron deficiency anemia (platelet count usually < 550 x 10^9/L)
  - Acute infection
  - Acute stress (trauma, surgery)
  - Chronic infections/inflammatory conditions
  - Post splenectomy
  - Occult malignancies
- Usually clinically explained

Other Myeloproliferative Neoplasms
- Chronic myeloid leukemia with thrombocytosis
  - Presence of *BCR::ABL1*
- Primary MF
  - In early prefibrotic stages, may display significant morphologic overlap with ET
  - Megakaryocytic morphology can be useful to discriminate from ET
  - Molecular genetic overlap with ET, including *JAK2*, *CALR*, and *MPL* mutations
  - Fibrosis and osteosclerotic changes uncommon in ET
- PV
  - Erythrocytosis (may not be present in prodromal phase)
  - Subnormal serum erythropoietin level
  - Bone marrow panmyelosis
  - Loose collections of pleomorphic megakaryocytes

Myelodysplastic Syndromes With Thrombocytosis
- Myelodysplastic syndrome with isolated del(5q)
  - Characteristic small, hypolobated megakaryocytes
  - Interstitial deletion of chromosome 5 (q31-q33) as sole abnormality

Myelodysplastic/Myeloproliferative Neoplasm With Ring Sideroblasts and Thrombocytosis
- Anemia with erythroid dysplasia and ≥ 15% ring sideroblasts or *SF3B1* mutation with > 10% VAF
- Persistent thrombocytosis (≥ 450 x 10^9/L)
- *SF3B1* mutations (60-90%)
  - Often (> 60%) found in association with *JAK2* V617F mutation and less commonly (< 10%) with *CALR* or *MPL* mutations

SELECTED REFERENCES

1. Gianelli U et al: International Consensus Classification of myeloid and lymphoid neoplasms: myeloproliferative neoplasms. Virchows Arch. 482(1):53-68, 2023
2. Puglianini OC et al: Essential thrombocythemia and post-essential thrombocythemia myelofibrosis: updates on diagnosis, clinical aspects, and management. Lab Med. 54(1):13-22, 2023
3. Khoury JD et al: The 5th edition of the World Health Organization classification of haematolymphoid tumours: myeloid and histiocytic/dendritic neoplasms. Leukemia. 36(7):1703-19, 2022

Essential Thrombocythemia

Molecular Pathology of Myeloid Neoplasms

Peripheral Thrombocytosis

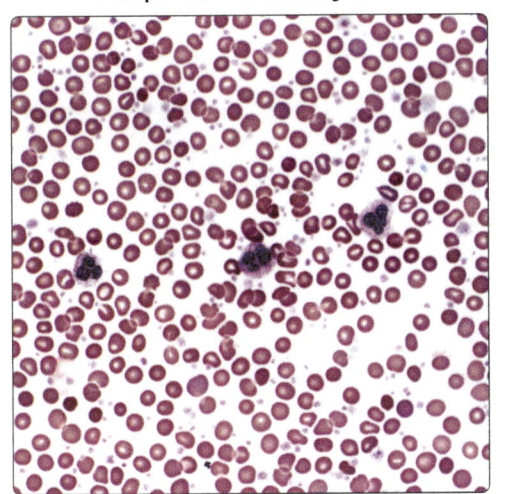

Increased Number of Megakaryocytes

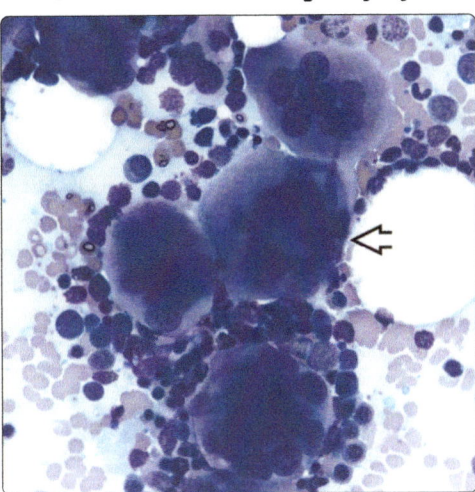

(Left) ET shows peripheral thrombocytosis, as expected, and normal WBC and RBC numbers and morphology. In this example, the platelets are variably hypogranular. (From DP: Blood & Bone Marrow.) (Right) Bone marrow aspirate smear from a patient with ET shows an increased number of megakaryocytes with very large, hyperlobulated forms and loose clustering ⇨.

CALR Type 1 Mutation

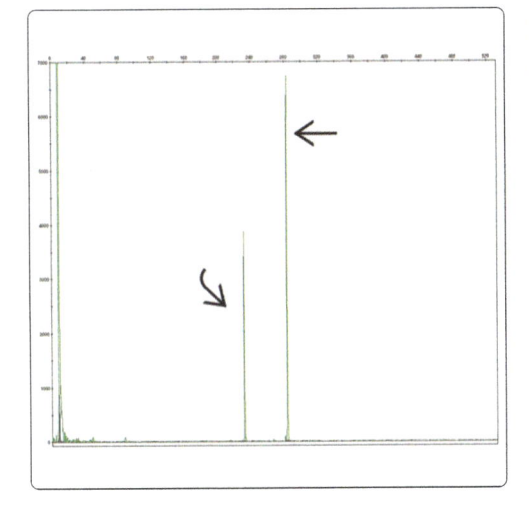

CALR Type 2 Mutation

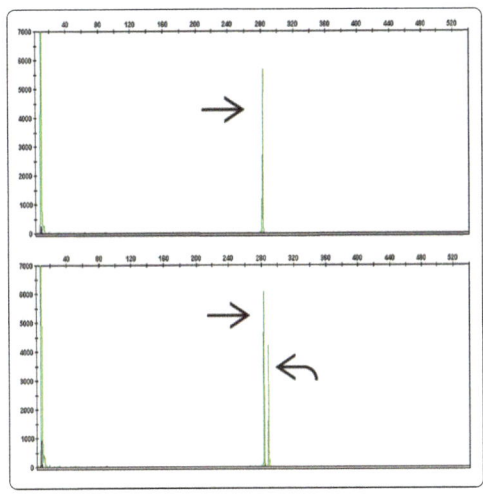

(Left) Electropherogram of PCR-amplified DNA from exon 9 of the CALR gene shows a mutated peak ⇨ corresponding to a 52-bp deletion and a taller wildtype peak ⇨. A 52-bp deletion in exon 9 of the CALR gene is the most common CALR mutation. (Right) Electropherogram shows a 5-bp insertion mutation ⇨ in the CALR gene. The taller peak in this composite image corresponds to the wildtype peaks ⇨. This mutation is the 2nd most common CALR mutation.

Pyrosequencing of Wildtype MPL

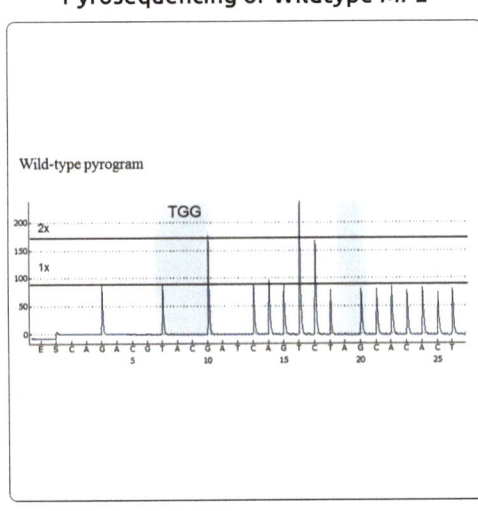

Pyrosequencing of Mutated MPL

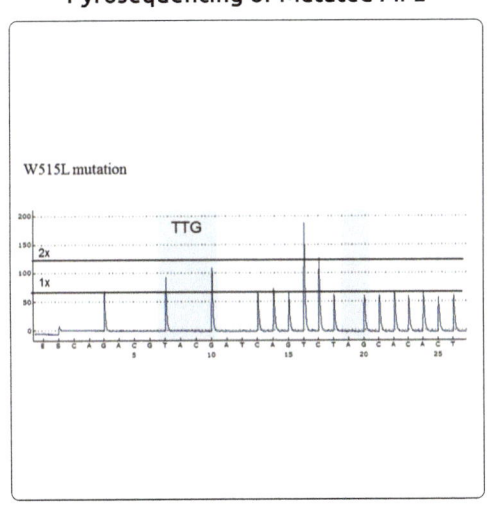

(Left) Pyrosequencing of the MPL gene performed on peripheral blood from a patient with ET shows the normal TGG sequence at codon 515 (wildtype). (Right) Pyrosequencing of the MPL gene performed on DNA extracted from peripheral blood of a patient with ET shows the presence of a TTG sequence instead of the normal TGG at codon 515, corresponding to the p.W515L mutation. This is the most common MPL mutation in cases of ET.

159

Chronic Eosinophilic Leukemia, NOS

KEY FACTS

CLASSIFICATION
- ICC and WHO-HAEM5 have similar diagnostic criteria

MICROSCOPIC
- Peripheral blood (PB) and bone marrow (BM)
  - Eosinophilia; ≥ 1.5 x 10⁹/L and eosinophils ≥ 10% of WBC, sustained and unexplained
  - Blasts < 20%; confirmed clonality (cytogenetic abnormality or myeloid-associated gene mutation)
    - Abnormal bone marrow morphology supportive of chronic eosinophilic leukemia (CEL) and exclusion of other causes of eosinophilia sufficient in **absence** of confirmed clonality (ICC)
  - Absence of lymphoma or other myeloid neoplasm

ANCILLARY TESTS
- Cytogenetics helpful to demonstrate clonal genetic abnormality, exclude abnormalities associated with other diagnoses
- High-throughput sequencing (NGS) for myeloid-associated genes
  - *ASXL1*, *TET2*, *EZH2*, *SETBP1*, *CBL*, and *NOTCH1* most common mutations
- Exclude T-cell clone by T-cell receptor gene rearrangement studies

TOP DIFFERENTIAL DIAGNOSES
- Reactive eosinophilia
- Other myeloid neoplasms
  - Myeloid neoplasms with eosinophilia and tyrosine kinase rearrangement
  - AML with inv(16) and abnormal eosinophils
  - Chronic myeloid leukemia, *BCR::ABL1*-positive
  - Other MPNs (PV, ET, PMF)
  - Myelodysplastic syndrome; MDS/MPN
- Idiopathic hypereosinophilic syndrome
- Hypereosinophilic syndrome

Peripheral Blood Eosinophilia

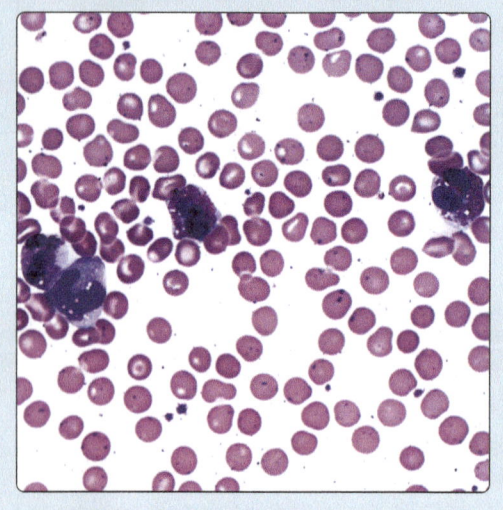

Monosomy 7

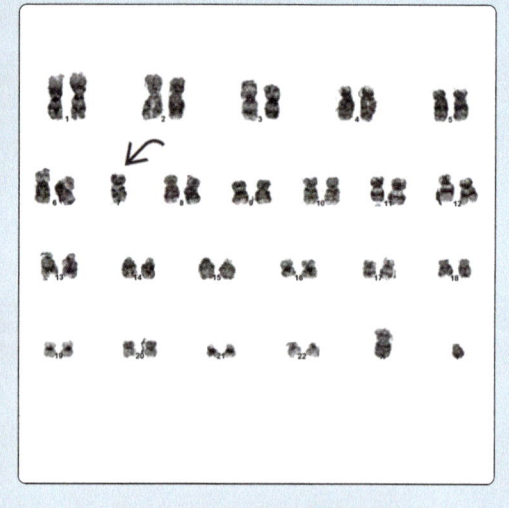

(Left) Peripheral blood smear shows increased eosinophils in a patient with chronic eosinophilic leukemia (CEL). The eosinophils may or may not (as in this image) exhibit atypical cytologic features. (Right) Karyotype from a patient with CEL, not otherwise specified (NOS) shows monosomy 7 ➡, a myeloid neoplasm-associated abnormality that can be seen as a clonal abnormality in rare cases of CEL, NOS.

Normal Trilineage Hematopoiesis

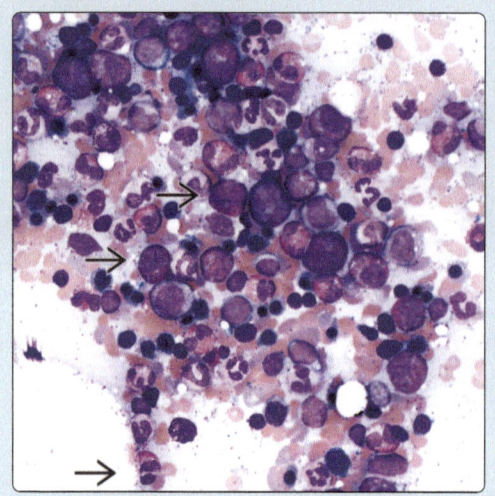

Bone Marrow Eosinophilia

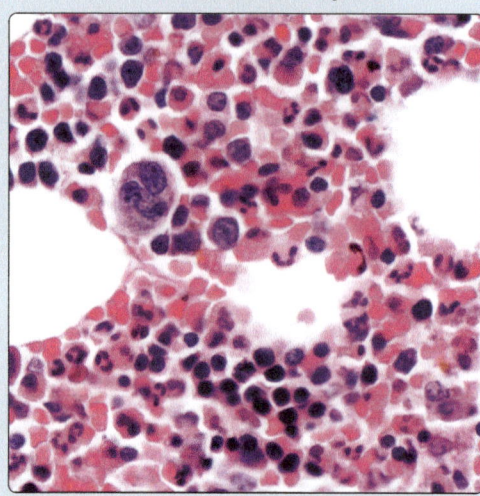

(Left) Intact erythropoiesis and granulopoiesis are seen in this bone marrow (BM) aspirate from a patient with CEL. There is no significant dysplasia, increase in blasts, or increased/abnormal mast cells. Eosinophils are at all stages of maturation ➡. (Right) BM core biopsy from a patient with CEL shows increased eosinophils in a background of trilineage hematopoiesis.

Chronic Eosinophilic Leukemia, NOS

TERMINOLOGY

Abbreviations
- Chronic eosinophilic leukemia, not otherwise specified (CEL, NOS)

Definitions
- Clonal hematopoietic myeloproliferative neoplasm
  - Sustained proliferation of eosinophils and precursors
  - Exclusion of other neoplastic or reactive conditions

CLASSIFICATION

International Consensus Classification
- CEL, NOS
  - Eosinophilia ≥ 1.5 x 10⁹/L and eosinophils ≥ 10% of WBC
  - Confirmed clonality
    - In absence of clonal abnormality, sustained eosinophilia and bone marrow (BM) findings of CEL suffice for diagnosis, as long as other causes of persistent eosinophilia have been excluded
  - Abnormal BM morphology or increased peripheral blood (PB)/BM blasts
    - Blasts < 20%

WHO 5th Edition
- CEL
  - Eosinophilia ≥ 1.5 x 19⁹/L, sustained for at least 4 weeks
  - Abnormal BM morphology, blasts < 20%
  - Confirmed clonality

CLINICAL ISSUES

Site
- PB and BM
- Peripheral tissues with end-organ damage

Presentation
- May be asymptomatic
- Symptomatic
  - Due to eosinophil-mediated end-organ damage

Treatment
- Hydroxyurea, corticosteroids, or interferon-α
- Eosinophil-targeted therapies being developed

MICROSCOPIC

Peripheral Blood
- Eosinophilia ≥ 1.5 x 10⁹/L and ≥ 10% of WBC (ICC)
- Abnormal eosinophil cytology
- Blasts < 20%

Bone Marrow
- Usually hypercellular with eosinophilia
- Blasts may be slightly increased but < 20%
- May have dyspoiesis
- Charcot-Leyden crystals may be observed
- Fibrosis due to release of eosinophil granules

ANCILLARY TESTS

Genetic Testing
- *JAK2*, *CALR*, and *MPL* mutation testing to evaluate for associated myeloproliferative neoplasms
- T-cell receptor gene rearrangement to exclude T-cell clone
- High-throughput sequencing for myeloid-associated genes
  - *ASXL1*, *TET2*, *EZH2*, *SETBP1*, *CBL*, and *NOTCH1* most common
  - Mutations may support clonality when variant allele frequency ≥ 10%
    - Patients with diagnosis of idiopathic hypereosinophilic syndrome with these mutations show similar survival to patients with CEL, NOS
    - Must be aware of possibility of clonal hematopoiesis of indeterminate potential

Cytogenetics
- Document clonality
- Common abnormalities are myeloid neoplasm associated
  - Most common are +8, t(10;11)(p14;q21), and t(7;12)(q11;p11)
  - Others include -7 or del(7q), -5 or del(5q), del(20q), i(17q), and -13 or del(13q)
  - Caution required, as reactive eosinophilia may be present in other myeloid neoplasms
- Exclude abnormality diagnostic of different neoplasm
  - AML with inv(16)(p13q22) or t(16;16)(p13;q22) may have overlapping morphologic features
  - *FIP1L1::PDGFRA* fusion is cytogenetically cryptic and requires FISH testing

DIFFERENTIAL DIAGNOSIS

Reactive (Secondary) Eosinophilia
- Due to underlying clonal, nonmyeloid neoplasm
  - T-cell lymphoma
  - Acute lymphoblastic leukemia
  - Hodgkin lymphoma
- Due to reactive condition

Myeloid/Lymphoid Neoplasms With Eosinophilia and Tyrosine Kinase Fusion
- Fusions involving *PDGFRA*, *PDGFRB*, *FGFR1*, or *ETV6::ABL1*, *PCM1::JAK2*, *FLT3*

Idiopathic Hypereosinophilic Syndrome
- Persistent, unexplained eosinophilia ≥ 6 months **with** associated end-organ damage
- PB blasts < 2% and BM blasts < 5%
- Normal BM morphology except for increased normal-appearing eosinophils
- **No** clonal genetic abnormality but may have CHIP by molecular assessment

Hypereosinophilia of Uncertain Significance
- Nonclonal eosinophilia with **no** end-organ damage

SELECTED REFERENCES

1. Gianelli U et al: International Consensus Classification of myeloid and lymphoid neoplasms: myeloproliferative neoplasms. Virchows Arch. 482(1):53-68, 2023

Myeloproliferative Neoplasm, Unclassifiable

KEY FACTS

TERMINOLOGY
- Definition
  - Myeloproliferative neoplasm, unclassifiable (MPN-U)
  - Clonal hematopoietic neoplasm
  - Features not sufficient to render more specific MPN diagnosis

MOLECULAR
- *JAK2*, *CALR*, or *MPL* mutation often present
- *TET2* mutation more common in MPN-U than other MPNs
- Triple-negative cases
  - MPN-U is more likely to be negative for *JAK2*, *CALR*, and *MPL* mutations than other MPNs

MICROSCOPIC
- Early phase of disease
  - Thrombocytosis
  - Mild neutrophilic leukocytosis
  - Blasts < 10%
  - Hypercellular bone marrow
  - Abnormal megakaryocytic proliferation
  - Minimal fibrosis
- Late phase of disease
  - Leukoerythroblastosis
  - Blast percentage increased
  - Marked fibrosis

ANCILLARY TESTS
- Conventional cytogenetics and FISH
  - Exclude alterations diagnostic in other entities
- Identification of *JAK2*, *CALR*, or *MPL* mutation confirms diagnosis of MPN
- Molecular testing can identify other clonal abnormalities, provide prognostic information, and guide management

TOP DIFFERENTIAL DIAGNOSES
- Specific MPN subtype
- Reactive conditions

Thrombocytosis and Increased Anisopoikilocytosis

Osteosclerosis

(Left) Peripheral blood smear from a patient with myeloproliferative neoplasm, unclassifiable (MPN-U) shows thrombocytosis and increased anisopoikilocytosis with elliptocytes. (Right) Bone marrow biopsy shows osteosclerosis and megakaryocytic proliferation in a patient with MPN-U.

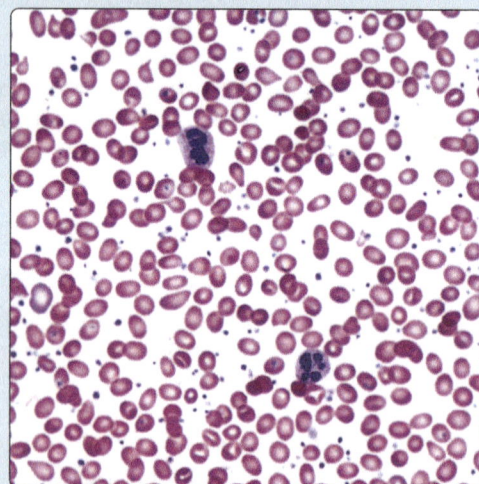

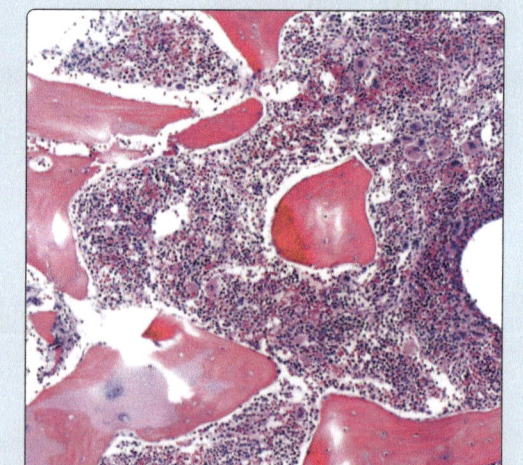

Osteosclerosis

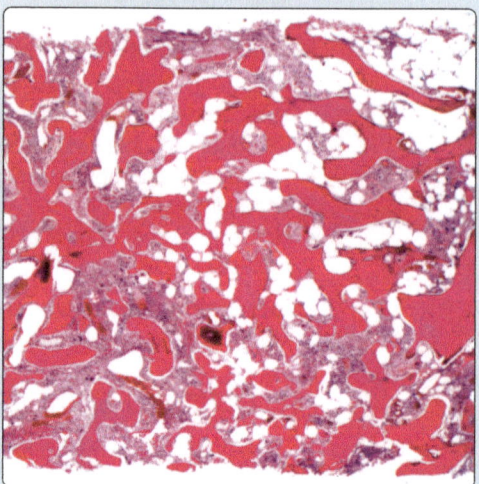

Megakaryocyte Proliferation

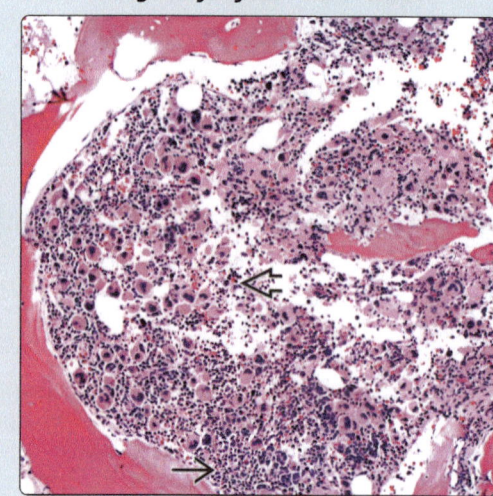

(Left) Bone marrow core biopsy shows dramatic osteosclerosis at presentation of MPN. Marked fibrosis is nearly always present and often precludes identification of the particular underlying MPN. Chronic myeloid leukemia is excluded by the absence of BCR::ABL1 fusion. (Right) Bone marrow core biopsy shows marked megakaryocytic proliferation ⇨ in a patient presenting with MPN-U. The bone is not osteosclerotic, and background hematopoiesis is evident ⇨.

Myeloproliferative Neoplasm, Unclassifiable

TERMINOLOGY

Abbreviations
- Myeloproliferative neoplasm, unclassifiable (MPN-U) [International Consensus Classification (ICC)]
- MPN, not otherwise specified (MPN-NOS) [WHO 5th edition (WHO-HAEM5)]

Definitions
- Clonal hematopoietic neoplasm
- Diagnostic criteria for MPN are met
- Do not fit criteria for any specific MPN category
  - May represent early disease presentation prior to development of distinct diagnostic features
  - May represent end-stage disease, precluding recognition of more specific underlying MPN
  - Diagnostic features may be obscured by concurrent inflammatory or neoplastic disorder
  - Detailed clinical and laboratory history may aid more specific categorization
- If diagnostic criteria for specific MPN met later in patient course, should be reclassified as specific entity

CLASSIFICATION

ICC and WHO-HAEM5
- Many similarities in terms of diagnostic criteria for MPN-U/MPN-NOS
- Similar exclusionary criteria and genetic testing recommendations

ETIOLOGY/PATHOGENESIS

Myeloproliferative Neoplasm-Associated Mutations
- Mutations in *JAK2*, *CALR*, and *MPL* are considered driver mutations in MPN
  - May not be initiating somatic mutation in disease development
    - Not all MPN-U carry these mutations
  - Presence of other mutations may alter disease presentation, leading to classification as MPN-U
  - *TET2* mutation has been shown to precede *JAK2* mutation in some cases
    - Order of mutations may alter disease characteristics

CLINICAL ISSUES

Presentation
- Similar to other MPN
  - Accounts for 5-10% of MPN
- Early disease
  - Increase in platelet, erythroid, or granulocytic lineage
  - Unexplained thrombotic events
- Late-stage disease
  - Leukoerythroblastosis and cytopenias
  - Marked hepatosplenomegaly
  - Increased blasts
  - Bone marrow (BM) failure
    - Marked reticulin fibrosis, may have collagen fibrosis

MOLECULAR

Cytogenetics
- Normal cytogenetics in most cases, but frequency of abnormalities increases with increasing disease stage
- No specific cytogenetic abnormalities
- Testing required to exclude entity-defining alterations
  - FISH may be useful to evaluate for cryptic abnormalities
- Most frequent abnormalities
  - del(20q)
  - del(13q)
  - Trisomy 8
  - Trisomy 9
  - Chromosome 1 abnormalities

Molecular Genetics
- *JAK2* mutation
  - *JAK2* V617F mutation seen in 20% of MPN-U
    - Presence of *JAK2* exon 12 mutation should raise suspicion of polycythemia vera (PV)
  - Associated with higher WBC count
  - Associated with splenomegaly
- *CALR* mutation
  - Seen in ~ 37% of MPN-U
- *MPL* mutation
  - Exon 10 mutations
  - Rare in MPN-U
- Triple-negative cases
  - MPN-U is more likely to be negative for *JAK2*, *CALR*, and *MPL* mutations than other MPNs
  - Other mutations can confirm clonality but may also represent clonal hematopoiesis of indeterminate potential (CHIP)
    - Very low variant allele frequency may suggest CHIP
- *TET2* mutations
  - *TET2* encodes for enzyme that converts 5-methylcytosine to 5-hydroxymethylcytosine
    - May lead to loss of DNA methylation
    - Mutation leads to myeloproliferation
  - Nonsense or frameshift mutations common
    - Exons 4 and 12 most common locations
  - Often seen in combination with other mutations
    - Higher frequency in cases with *JAK2* V617F mutation
  - More common in MPN-U than in other MPNs
    - Presence of *TET2* mutation significantly associated with MPN-U diagnosis
    - Leads to monocytic differentiation, which may affect morphology and prevent more specific classification
    - May be associated with evolution of MPN-U to myelodysplastic/MPN
  - Associated with lower platelet count
  - May be associated with increased monocytes
  - Associated with older age
- *ASXL1* mutations
  - Associated with normal cytogenetics
  - Associated with older age
  - Prognostic significance not clear in MPN-U
    - Poor prognostic indicator in primary myelofibrosis (PMF)
- *IDH1*/*IDH2* mutations

Myeloproliferative Neoplasm, Unclassifiable

- o May be identified with progressive disease
- *EZH2* mutation
  - o Prognostic significance not clear in MPN-U
  - o Associated with high risk of leukemic evolution in PMF

MICROSCOPIC

Peripheral Blood Microscopic Features

- Early phase of disease
  - o Thrombocytosis
  - o Mild neutrophilic leukocytosis common
  - o Blasts < 10%
  - o Normal hemoglobin or mild anemia
- Late phase of disease
  - o Leukoerythroblastosis
    - Left shift in granulocytes
    - Variable blast percentage
    - Teardrop-shaped red blood cells (dacrocytes)
    - Nucleated red blood cells

Bone Marrow Microscopic Features

- Early phase of disease
  - o Hypercellular
  - o Abnormal megakaryocytic proliferation
  - o No significant reticulin fibrosis
  - o Myelodysplastic features unusual
  - o Occasional predominance of granulocytic or erythroid lineage
- Late-stage disease
  - o Marked reticulin &/or collagen fibrosis
  - o Accelerated stage of MPN-U
    - 10-19% peripheral blood (PB) &/or BM blasts
  - o Blast transformation of underlying MPN-U
    - ≥ 20% PB &/or BM blasts

ANCILLARY TESTS

Immunohistochemistry

- Useful to assess BM cellular elements and architecture
  - o Particularly if unable to obtain aspirate
  - o CD34 identifies CD34-positive blasts
  - o CD117 highlights blasts as well as immature erythroids and mast cells
  - o CD42b and CD61 stain megakaryocytes

Flow Cytometry

- Quantify blast percentages
- Useful to identify aberrant phenotype

Genetic Testing

- Identification of *JAK2*, *CALR*, or *MPL* mutation confirms diagnosis of MPN
- *TET2* mutation associated with MPN-U
  - o Not sufficient for definitive diagnosis
- High-throughput (next-generation) myeloid gene panel sequencing
  - o Provides additional diagnostic and prognostic information
  - o Detects clonal markers in other genes
- Rule out abnormalities diagnostic of other myeloid neoplasms

DIFFERENTIAL DIAGNOSIS

Specific Type of Myeloproliferative Neoplasm

- Essential thrombocythemia (ET)
- PV
- PMF
- Chronic myeloid leukemia (CML)
  - o t(9;22)(q34;q11.2), *BCR::ABL1* present

Myelodysplastic/Myeloproliferative Neoplasm

- Myelodysplastic features, cytopenias, monocytosis

Reactive Condition

- Collagen vascular disease/autoimmune disease
- Medication effect
- BM recovery/regeneration after toxic insult

DIAGNOSTIC CHECKLIST

Pathologic Interpretation Pearls

- Unexplained cytoses
- BM hypercellularity
- Abnormal megakaryocytic proliferation
- Variable granulocytic and erythroid proliferation
- Clonal cytogenetic abnormality
- Mutation in MPN-associated gene (*JAK2*, *CALR*, or *MPL*) often present

REPORTING

Key Features

- Utilize ICC or WHO-HAEM5 classification criteria
- Specify reason case does not meet criteria for specific subtype

Defer Diagnosis of Myeloproliferative Neoplasm, Unclassifiable

- If clinical, laboratory, or morphologic findings are suboptimal/inadequate
  - o Request additional testing/pathologic material as needed
- If patient received therapies that could alter BM pathology (erythropoietin, thrombopoietin, granulocyte colony-stimulating factor)
  - o Repeat evaluation after treatment for underlying reactive or neoplastic disorder

SELECTED REFERENCES

1. Gianelli U et al: International Consensus Classification of myeloid and lymphoid neoplasms: myeloproliferative neoplasms. Virchows Arch. 482(1):53-68, 2023
2. Thiele J et al: The International Consensus Classification of myeloid neoplasms and acute leukemias: myeloproliferative neoplasms. Am J Hematol. 98(1):166-79, 2023
3. Khoury JD et al: The 5th edition of the World Health Organization classification of haematolymphoid tumours: myeloid and histiocytic/dendritic neoplasms. Leukemia. 36(7):1703-19, 2022
4. Maddali M et al: Molecular characterization of triple-negative myeloproliferative neoplasms by next-generation sequencing. Ann Hematol. 101(9):1987-2000, 2022
5. Deschamps P et al: Clinicopathological characterisation of myeloproliferative neoplasm-unclassifiable (MPN-U): a retrospective analysis from a large UK tertiary referral centre. Br J Haematol. 193(4):792-7, 2021
6. Lee J et al: Genomic heterogeneity in myeloproliferative neoplasms and applications to clinical practice. Blood Rev. 42:100708, 2020

Myeloproliferative Neoplasm, Unclassifiable

CALR 52-bp Deletion

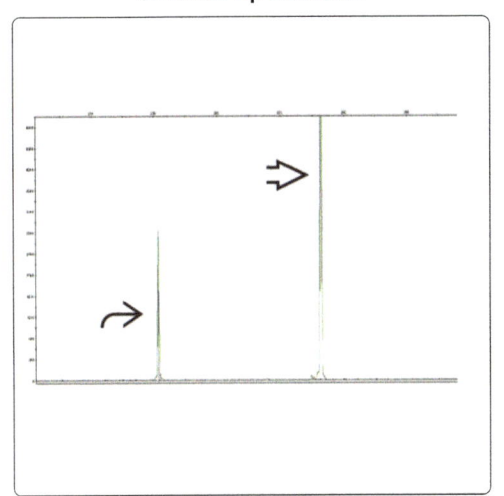

Thrombocytosis

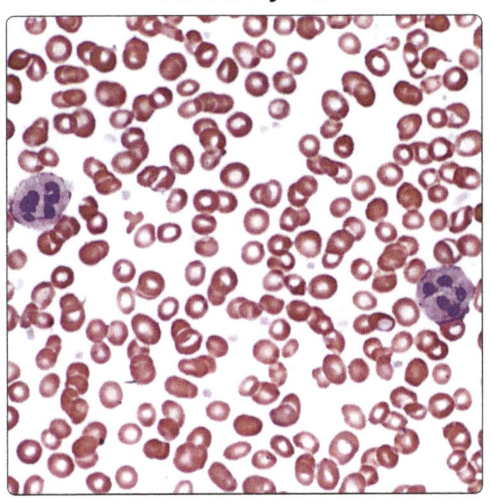

(Left) *Fragment length analysis shows a 52-base pair deletion (type 1 mutation) ➤ in CALR compared to the wildtype peak ➤. This is the most frequent type of CALR mutation. JAK2, CALR, and MPL are frequently identified driver mutations in MPN.* **(Right)** *Peripheral blood smear from a patient with MPN-U who presented with thrombocytosis shows no significant leukocytosis, dysplasia, or erythrocytosis.*

Dysmegakaryopoiesis

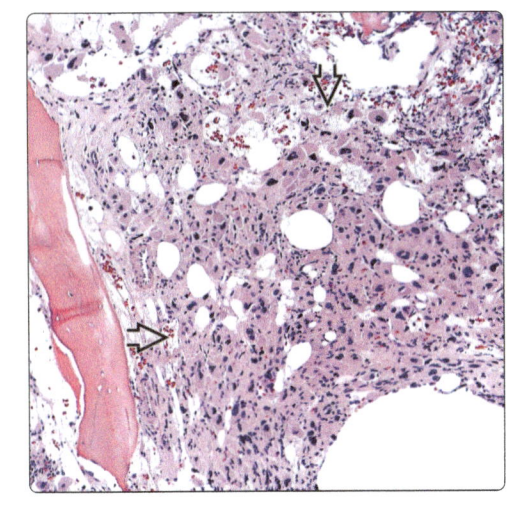

Mild Increase in Blasts

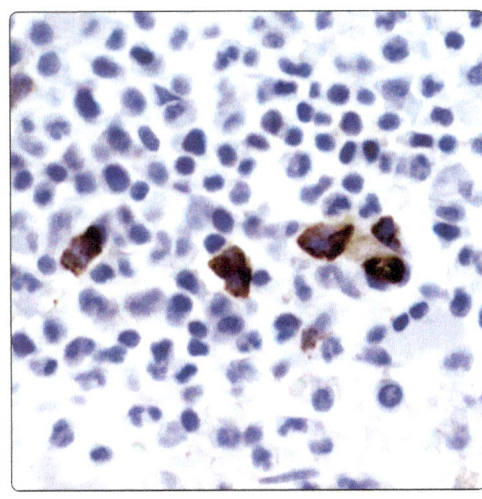

(Left) *Bone marrow biopsy shows a marked increase in bizarre and dysplastic megakaryocytes ➤ in a patient who presented with late-stage MPN. Given the lack of features specific for a particular MPN, the case was diagnosed as MPN-U.* **(Right)** *CD34 shows a mild increase in CD34-positive bone marrow blasts in a patient with late-stage MPN-U. Advanced-stage disease is associated with additional cytogenetic and molecular abnormalities.*

Hypercellular Marrow

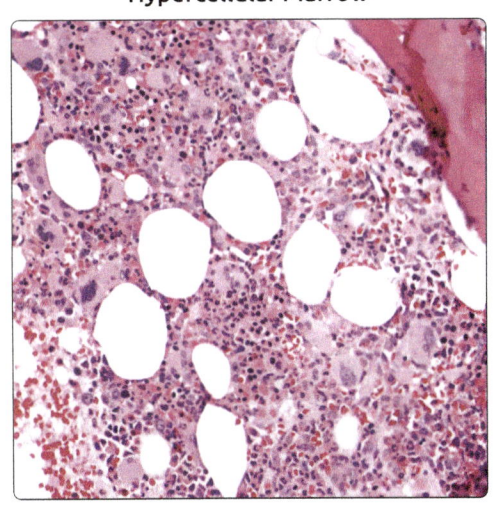

Increased Reticulin Fibrosis

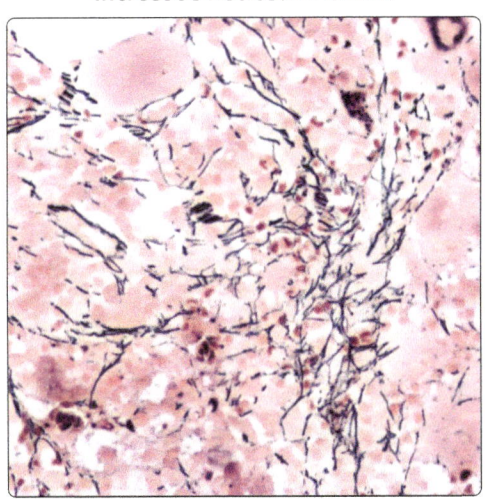

(Left) *Bone marrow core biopsy shows hypercellular marrow with abnormal megakaryocytic proliferation. There is no evidence of erythrocytosis or osteosclerosis, and BCR::ABL1 was negative, warranting a diagnosis of MPN-U.* **(Right)** *Reticulin shows moderate increased fibrosis in a patient with MPN. Reticulin fibrosis is not specific and can be seen in later stages of all MPNs.*

Molecular Pathology of Myeloid Neoplasms

Mastocytosis

KEY FACTS

TERMINOLOGY
- Proliferation of clonal mast cells in ≥ 1 organ system
- Heterogeneous, ranging from skin lesion that may regress to highly aggressive disease with multiorgan failure

CLASSIFICATION
- Cutaneous mastocytosis (CM)
- Systemic mastocytosis (SM)
  - Indolent SM (ISM)
  - Smoldering SM
  - Aggressive SM
  - SM with associated hematologic neoplasm
- Mast cell leukemia
- Mast cell sarcoma

ETIOLOGY/PATHOGENESIS
- Mast cells are derived from multipotent hematopoietic progenitor cells
- *KIT* mutation results in constitutive activation of KIT tyrosine kinase signaling pathway
- *KIT* D816V is most common mutation
- Other mutations in advanced SM include those commonly seen in myeloid neoplasms
  - *TET2*, *SRSF2*, *ASXL1*, *RUNX1*, *NRAS*, *KRAS*, and *IDH2*

CLINICAL ISSUES
- Symptoms secondary to uncontrolled proliferation of mast cells in marrow, CNS, GI tract, and other organs
- Symptoms due to release of mediators by mast cells
- Variable clinical course depending on subtype of mastocytosis

ANCILLARY TESTS
- Reactive and neoplastic mast cells express tryptase, CD117, CD33, and CD43
- Neoplastic mast cells aberrantly coexpress CD25 ± CD2

Mast Cells

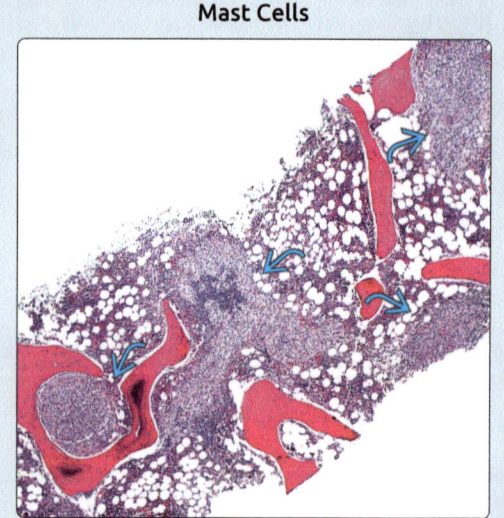

CD25 Immunohistochemistry

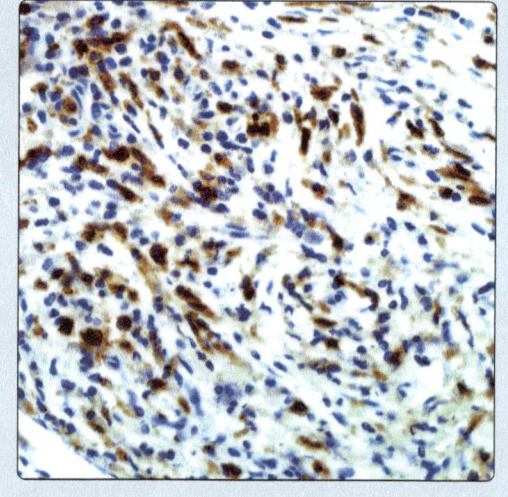

(Left) Bone marrow core biopsy shows multifocal compact aggregates of pale-staining mast cells ➡ with paratrabecular and interstitial distributions and background trilineage hematopoiesis. (Right) CD25 performed on bone marrow biopsy shows aberrant coexpression by spindled mast cells. The neoplastic mast cells in this case were scattered within a background rich in plasma cells and eosinophils.

Atypical Mast Cells and Myeloid Blasts

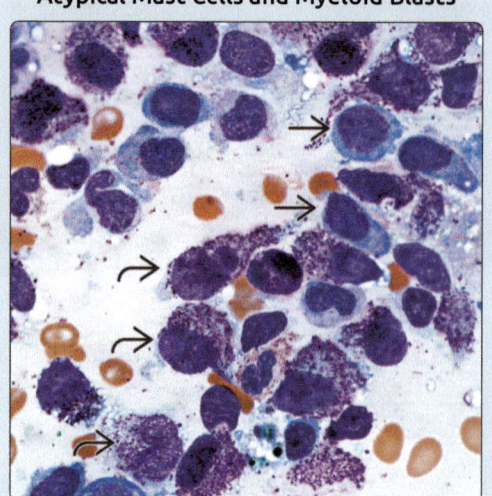

Next-Generation Sequencing Pileup of *KIT* Exon 17 Mutation

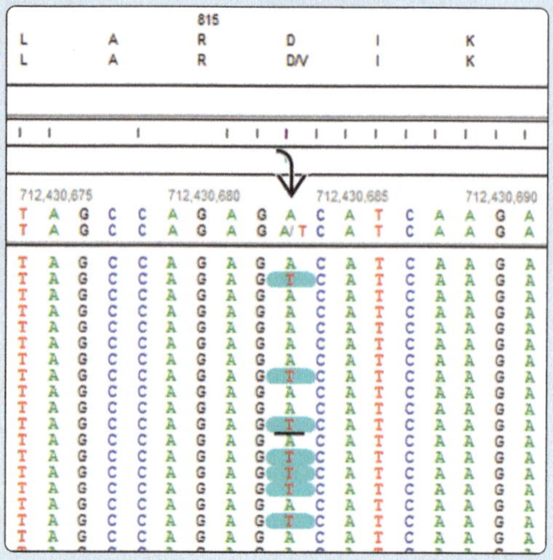

(Left) Wright-stained bone marrow aspirate smear from a patient with systemic mastocytosis (SM) and concurrent acute myeloid leukemia shows increased blasts ➡ and immature mast cells ➡. (Right) Sequence analysis using NGS on DNA extracted from bone marrow aspirate of a patient with SM shows an exon 17 *KIT* mutation corresponding to D816V ➡.

Mastocytosis

TERMINOLOGY

Definitions
- Proliferation of clonal mast cells in ≥ 1 organ system with heterogeneous clinical presentation
  - Ranges from indolent to aggressive

CLASSIFICATION

Essentially Similar Subtypes in Both WHO-HAEM5 and ICC
- Cutaneous mastocytosis (CM)
  - Maculopapular CM (ICC); urticaria pigmentosa/maculopapular pigmentosa (WHO-HAEM5)
  - Diffuse CM
  - Cutaneous mastocytoma
- Systemic mastocytosis (SM)
  - Indolent SM (ISM)
  - Bone marrow mastocytosis
    - Clinico-pathologic variant of ISM in ICC but SM subtype in WHO-HAEM5
  - Smoldering SM
  - Aggressive SM
  - Systemic mastocytosis with associated **myeloid** neoplasm (ICC); systemic mastocytosis with associated **hematologic** neoplasm (WHO-HAEM5)
    - Co-occurring lymphoid or plasma cell neoplasms are rare and clonally unrelated per ICC
- Mast cell leukemia
- Mast cell sarcoma

ETIOLOGY/PATHOGENESIS

Cell of Origin
- Mast cells are derived from multipotent hematopoietic progenitor cells
  - Differentiation is induced following binding of growth factor to KIT receptor
  - 4 defined stages of maturation
    - Nongranulated tryptase-positive blast
    - Metachromatic blast
    - Promastocytes with bi- or multilobated nuclei
    - Mature mast cells with abundant metachromatic intracytoplasmic granules

KIT Mutations
- KIT plays key role in regulation of mast cell biology
- Virtually all subtypes of mastocytosis harbor activating *KIT* mutation
  - Activating somatic gain-of-function point mutations typically involve codon 816 of exon 17 of *KIT*
  - *KIT* D816V is most common mutation in mastocytosis
  - *KIT* D816Y/H in small subset of cases
- *KIT* mutations result in constitutive activation of KIT tyrosine kinase signaling pathway
- Rare familial mastocytosis with germline mutation of *KIT* has been reported
- Other gene mutations detected in advanced systemic mastocytosis
  - *TET2*, *SRSF2*, *ASXL1*, *RUNX1*, *NRAS*, *KRAS*, and *IDH2*

Symptoms of Mastocytosis
- Symptoms due to release of mediators by mast cells
  - Mast cells release proinflammatory and vasoactive mediators triggered by stimulated IgE
  - Symptoms may range from mild to severe and life-threatening
  - Symptoms include flushing, syncope, severe headache, diarrhea, bone pain, or hypotensive shock
- **B findings** (burden of disease)
  - > 30% mast cell infiltrate in bone marrow and serum tryptase > 200 ng/mL
  - Cytopenia (not meeting criteria for C finding) or cytosis
    - Reactive causes are excluded, and criteria for other myeloid neoplasms are not met
  - Hepatomegaly with intact liver function, or splenomegaly without hypersplenism, &/or lymphadenopathy (> 1 cm in size) on palpation or imaging
  - *KIT* D816V mutation with variant allele frequency (VAF) ≥ 10% qualifies as B finding (WHO-HAEM5)
- Symptoms secondary to uncontrolled proliferation of mast cells in bone marrow, CNS, skeletal system, GI tract, and other organs
  - C findings
    - Bone marrow dysfunction due to neoplastic mast cell infiltrate with ≥ 1 cytopenia (absolute neutrophil < 1 x 10^9/L, Hgb < 10g/dL, &/or platelet < 100 x 10^9/L
    - Palpable hepatomegaly with impairment of liver function, ascites, &/or portal hypertension
    - Palpable splenomegaly with hypersplenism
    - Skeletal involvement with large osteolytic lesions ± pathologic fracture
    - Malabsorption with weight loss due to GI mast cell infiltration

Refined Diagnostic Criteria for Systemic Mastocytosis
- Major criterion
  - Multifocal, dense infiltrate of tryptase &/or CD117 (+) mast cells (≥ 15 mast cells in aggregate) in sections of bone marrow &/or other extracutaneous organs
    - In absence of *KIT* mutation in cases with eosinophilia, tyrosine kinase fusions associated with myeloid/lymphoid neoplasms with eosinophilia must be excluded
- Minor criteria
  - > 25% of mast cells are spindle-shaped or exhibit cytologically atypical, immature morphology in bone marrow biopsy or in sections of other extracutaneous organs
  - Mast cells aberrantly coexpress CD25, CD2, &/or CD30 in addition to mast cell markers
  - *KIT* D816V or other activating *KIT* mutation detected in bone marrow, blood, or extracutaneous organs
  - Persistent serum tryptase level > 20 ng/mL, except for SM with associated myeloid in which elevated serum tryptase does not count as SM minor criterion
- Diagnosis of SM requires presence of major criterion or, in its absence, presence of at least 3 minor criteria

Mastocytosis

Cutaneous Mastocytosis
- Increased mast cells in skin lesions &/or presence of activating *KIT* mutation
- Patients may experience mast cell mediator-related symptoms, including
  o Pruritus, flushing, headache, diarrhea, abdominal pain, and even anaphylaxis
- 3 subtypes are distinguished
  o Maculopapular with 2 variants (monomorphic and polymorphic)
    – Polymorphic variant almost exclusively seen in children
- Diffuse subtype shows mast cell infiltration of entire skin along with edema and accentuation of skin folds (peau d' orange)
  o Blisters typically present, and mast cell mediator-related symptoms can be severe
- Mastocytoma subtype presents as single brown lesion, which may blister
  o Up to 3 typical mastocytoma lesions may still be regarded as mastocytoma, multicentric
  o Presence of > 4 lesions would favor diagnosis of maculopapular CM
- *KIT* mutation analysis recommended in difficult cases
- May regress spontaneously

Systemic Mastocytosis
- Defined by presence of major criterion **or** presence of at least 3 minor criteria
- Includes several different subtypes, ranging from indolent to aggressive

Indolent Systemic Mastocytosis
- Mast cell burden is only modestly increased
- Most patients present with either skin lesions or mast cell-related symptoms
- Spleen, liver, or GI tract may also show mast cell infiltrate
- No C findings and no associated hematologic neoplasm

Bone Marrow Mastocytosis
- Recognized as clinicopathologic variant of ISM (ICC)
- Defined by isolated and limited bone marrow involvement by ISM
  o Absence of skin lesions and tryptase level < 125 ng/mL
  o Strong association with severe anaphylaxis on sting of bee, wasp, or other Hymenoptera insects
- Standalone SM subtype (WHO-HAEM5)
- Associated osteopenia/osteoporosis and bone marrow fibrosis

Smoldering Systemic Mastocytosis
- High mast cell burden
- ≥ 2 B findings; no C findings

Aggressive Systemic Mastocytosis
- ≥ 1 C finding indicating end-organ damage
  o Lytic bony lesions with occasional pathologic fracture
- Hepatomegaly with abnormal liver function
- Must exclude mast cell leukemia and SM with associated hematologic/myeloid malignancy

Systemic Mastocytosis With Associated Hematologic Neoplasm
- ~ 10-20% of patients with SM present with associated hematologic neoplasm
  o May be diagnosed before, concurrently, or after diagnosis of SM
  o Includes any myeloid malignancy and rarely lymphoid neoplasm
    – Lymphoid or plasma cell neoplasms excluded from this category in 2022 ICC
- Myeloid neoplasm may mask SM, which may become evident after chemotherapy

Mast Cell Leukemia
- Accounts for < 6% of SM
  o Rapidly fatal with median survival of 2-31 months
- ≥ 20% atypical immature mast cells in bone marrow aspirate
- ≥ 10% circulating mast cells
- < 10% circulating mast cells in aleukemic variant
- Diffuse and compact infiltrate of mast cells in marrow trephine biopsy

Mast Cell Sarcoma
- Extremely rare with only few published cases
- Usually presents in unusual locations for mastocytosis, such as larynx, colon, or intracranial sites
- Rapidly progressive disease

CLINICAL ISSUES

Epidemiology
- Age
  o CM most often present in children
  o SM typically present in adults but can occur at any age

Site
- Skin is most common site of involvement in mastocytosis
- Bone marrow is always involved in SM
  o Bone marrow biopsy is extremely helpful to confirm or rule out diagnosis of SM
- Spleen, lymph nodes, liver, and GI tract can be involved in SM

Treatment
- No curative treatment is available for mastocytosis
  o Treatment is directed toward symptoms in each individual patient
- Treatment of patients with mediator-related symptoms
  o Administration of drugs that target mediators
    – Histamine-2 (H1) antagonists, steroids
  o Administration of epinephrine in patients with anaphylactic episodes
- Treatment of ASM and mast cell leukemia
  o Midostaurin
    – FDA approved for treatment of advanced SM
    – Effective against *KIT* D816V-mutated SM
    – 60% overall response rate
  o Avapritinib (selective inhibitor of *KIT* D816V)
    – Approved by FDA in 2021 for treatment of advanced SM and by European Medicines Agency in 2022 for advanced SM after prior systemic therapy

Mastocytosis

- – 36% overall complete remission among 69 patients in recent study
- o Dasatinib
  - – Blocks *KIT* D816V activity in ASM with 37% overall response rate
- o Imatinib
  - – Effective in ASM without *KIT* D816V mutation
- o Cytoreductive drugs
  - – α-interferon (IFN-α) with glucocorticoids
    - □ Major clinical response in only ~ 20% of ASM and mast cell leukemia
  - – Cladribine (2CdA) reduces mast cell burden in ASM
  - – Intensive chemotherapy is reserved for ASM and mast cell leukemia with rapidly progressive disease
- o Many other investigative drugs in clinical trials
  - – mTOR and PI3K inhibitors, multikinase inhibitors, anti-CD30 antibody
- Treatment of SM with associated hematologic neoplasm
  - o Treatment directed against hematologic neoplasm
  - o Separate treatment directed against SM

Prognosis

- CM and ISM
  - o Indolent course for many years and even decades
- ASM, mast cell leukemia, and SM with associated hematologic neoplasm
  - o Aggressive clinical course with often fatal outcome
- Mast cell sarcoma
  - o Rapidly progressive disease with dissemination

MOLECULAR

Molecular Genetics

- *KIT* mutations present in all subtypes of mastocytosis
- Mutations result in gain-of-function activity
  - o Mutations typically involve tyrosine kinase domain in adults with mastocytosis
  - o Mutations involve extracellular domain in 1/2 of children with mastocytosis
- *KIT* exon 17 mutations
  - o *KIT* D816V mutation in ~ 80% of mastocytosis
  - o Less common mutations include D816Y, D816H, D816F, D815K, V560G, D820G, and insVI815-816
- Germline *KIT* mutations are rarely reported in familial mastocytosis
- Mutations in other genes frequently occur in advanced SM
  - o *TET2*, *SRSF2*, *ASXL1*, *RUNX1*, *NRAS*, *KRAS*, and *IDH2*
    - – Often precede *KIT* D816V mutation
    - – *KIT* D816V mutation may act as phenotypic modifier toward mast cell differentiation in these cases

MICROSCOPIC

Histologic Features

- Patterns of mast cell infiltrate in bone marrow
  - o Multifocal, dense perivascular and paratrabecular aggregates of mast cells
  - o Diffuse and singly distributed interstitial mast cell infiltrate
    - – May be seen in mast cell hyperplasia
    - – Can also be seen with associated myeloid neoplasm

Cytologic Features

- Cytologic features of neoplastic mast cells
  - o Oval to spindle forms with eccentric nuclei, elongated cytoplasmic tail, and decreased to absent granules
  - o Multilobated (promastocytes) or bilobed forms with less cytoplasmic granules than reactive mast cells
  - o Blast forms show high N:C ratio, immature chromatin, visible nucleoli, and variable granules
- Cytomorphologic features of neoplastic mast cells on H&E-stained sections
  - o Oval to spindle nuclei and abundant pale to hypogranular cytoplasm

ANCILLARY TESTS

Immunohistochemistry

- Reactive and neoplastic mast cells express tryptase, CD117, CD33, and CD43
  - o Expression of tryptase or CD117 not specific for mast cells
- Neoplastic mast cells aberrantly coexpress CD25 ± CD2
- Expression of CD30 in subsets of ASM and mast cell leukemia

Flow Cytometry

- Mast cells express bright CD117 and moderate CD45 on flow cytometry
  - o Aberrant coexpression of CD25 in neoplastic mast cells
- Mast cell percentage are often underestimated by flow cytometry
- Additional markers, including CD34, should be assessed to exclude concurrent hematologic neoplasm

DIFFERENTIAL DIAGNOSIS

Mast Cell Hyperplasia

- Reactive without compact aggregate formation
- No cytologic atypia
- No aberrant coexpression of CD25

Mast Cell Activation Syndrome

- Condition associated with mast cell degranulation
- Associated with cell mediator release

Myeloid/Lymphoid Neoplasm With Eosinophilia and Tyrosine Kinase Fusion

- Often show significant mast cell proliferation in bone marrow
- Mast cells are spindled and may mimic SM
- Presence of *FIP1L1::PDGFRA* or other TK fusions separate them from SM

SELECTED REFERENCES

1. Leguit RJ et al: The International Consensus Classification of mastocytosis and related entities. Virchows Arch. 482(1):99-112, 2023
2. Gotlib J et al: Avapritinib for advanced systemic mastocytosis. Blood. 140(15):1667-73, 2022
3. Khoury JD et al: The 5th edition of the World Health Organization classification of haematolymphoid tumours: myeloid and histiocytic/dendritic neoplasms. Leukemia. 36(7):1703-19, 2022
4. Sciumè M et al: Target therapies for systemic mastocytosis: an update. Pharmaceuticals (Basel). 15(6):738, 2022

Mastocytosis

(Left) Bone marrow core biopsy of SM shows large aggregates of abnormal mast cells with oval to spindled and irregular nuclei and abundant clear cytoplasm. **(Right)** CD30 shows bright expression in this case of mast cell leukemia. The neoplastic mast cells expressed CD117 and tryptase but lacked aberrant coexpression of CD25 and were negative for KIT D816V mutation.

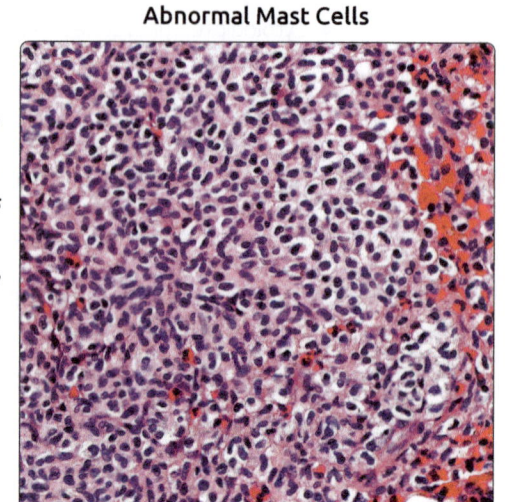

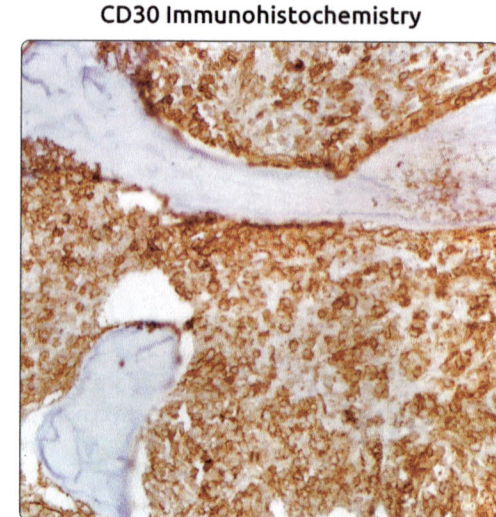

Abnormal Mast Cells

CD30 Immunohistochemistry

(Left) Bone marrow trephine biopsy of SM shows a loose aggregate of predominantly spindle-shaped mast cells ⇨ associated with thin sclerotic fibers. **(Right)** Bone marrow biopsy of SM shows a subtle population of spindled mast cells masked by an abundant infiltrate of eosinophils. The neoplastic mast cells in this case were highlighted by tryptase and CD25. FISH analysis revealed no rearrangement of tyrosine kinases.

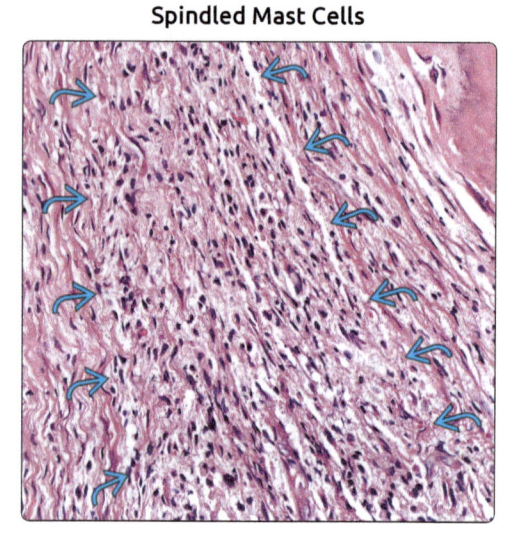

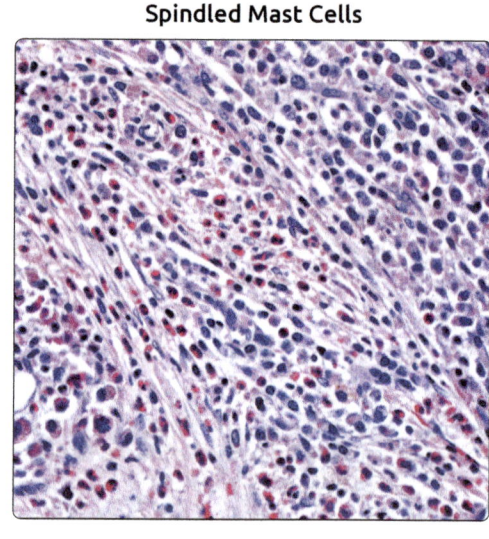

Spindled Mast Cells

Spindled Mast Cells

(Left) Tryptase highlights an interstitial, ill-defined aggregate of mast cells with cytoplasmic and granular patterns of staining. **(Right)** CD25 shows aberrant coexpression by the interstitial aggregate of mast cells, supporting the neoplastic nature of the mast cell proliferation. Reactive mast cells do not express CD25.

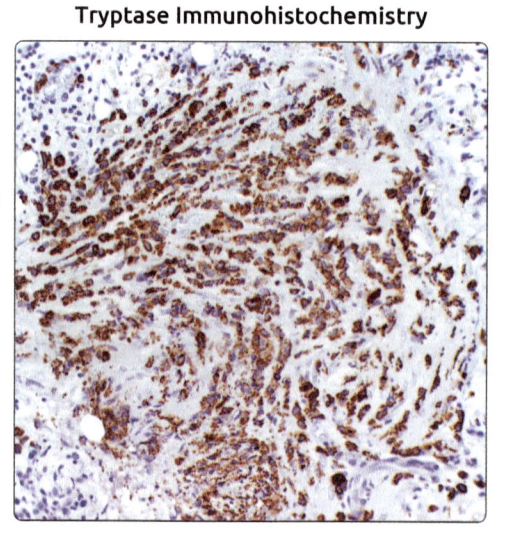

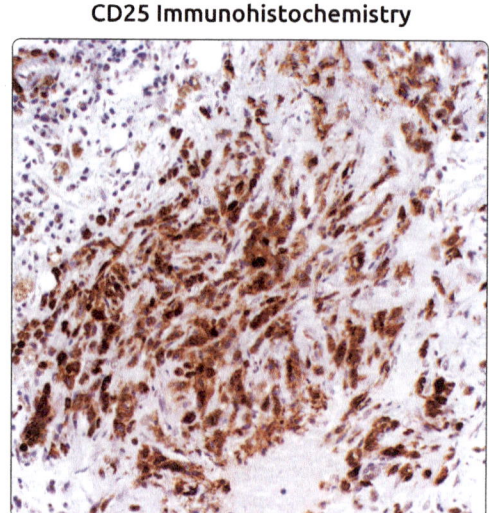

Tryptase Immunohistochemistry

CD25 Immunohistochemistry

Mastocytosis

Molecular Pathology of Myeloid Neoplasms

Splenic White Pulp

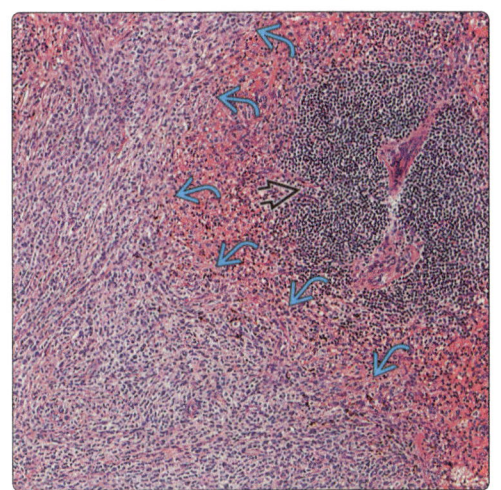

Splenic White Pulp

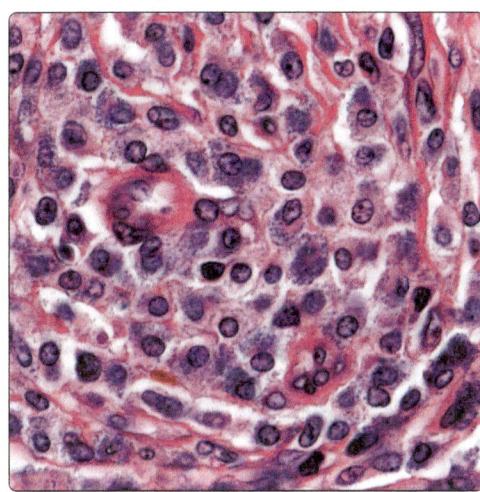

(Left) Spleen from a patient with SM shows sheets of pale-staining abnormal mast cells ⊞ in splenic red pulp surrounding an attenuated splenic white pulp ⇒. **(Right)** Splenic red pulp shows compact sheets of abnormal mast cells with oval nuclei and abundant cytoplasm with intracytoplasmic faint basophilic small granules. Background fibrosis is also present.

CD117 Immunohistochemistry

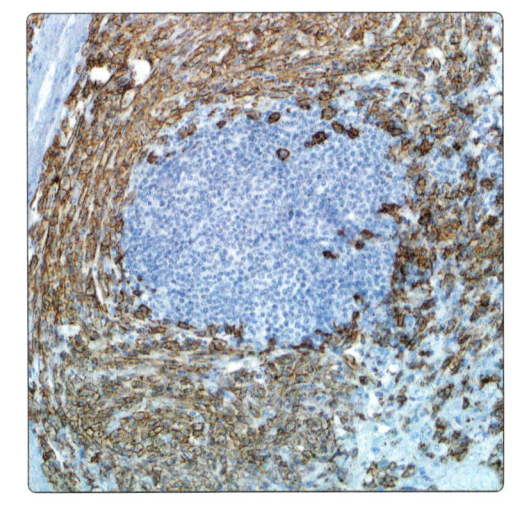

Tryptase Immunohistochemistry

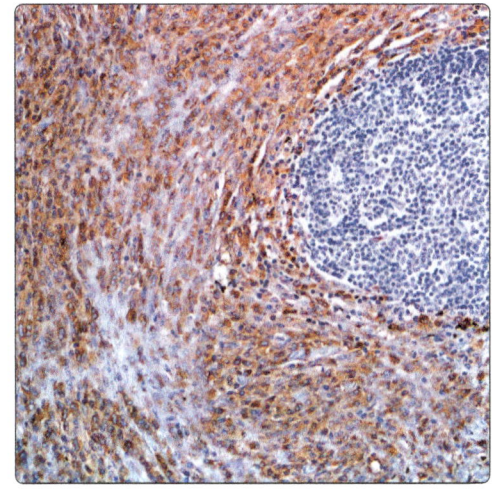

(Left) CD117 shows bright expression by sheets of neoplastic mast cells within the splenic red pulp. CD117 is expressed by both reactive and neoplastic mast cells. **(Right)** Tryptase highlights sheets of neoplastic mast cells within splenic red pulp with cytoplasmic and granular patterns of staining. The tryptase-positive mast cells surround an uninvolved splenic white pulp.

CD25 Immunohistochemistry

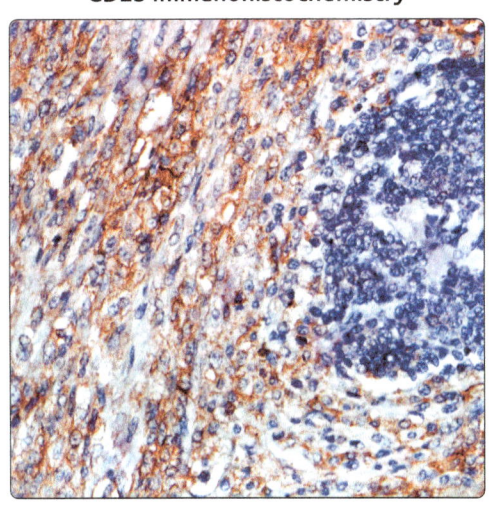

Pyrogram of *KIT* Codon 816

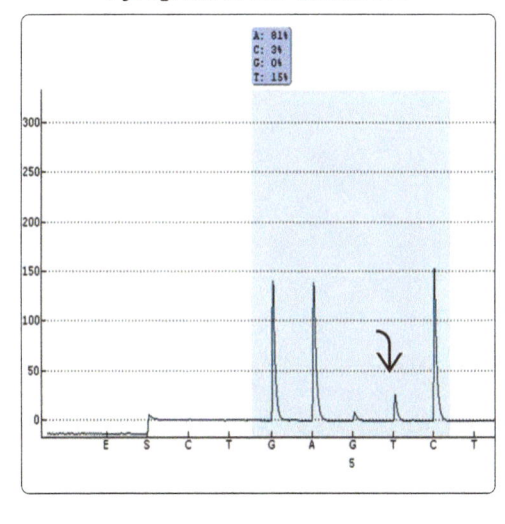

(Left) CD25 shows aberrant coexpression by mast cells. Aberrant coexpression of this antigen supports the neoplastic nature of this mast cell proliferation. Reactive mast cell proliferations do not coexpress CD25. **(Right)** DNA sequence analysis using pyrosequencing on DNA extracted from diagnostic splenic tissue scraped from unstained sections shows a GAC > GTC ⊞ mutation in codon 816 of the KIT gene corresponding to D816V.

Mastocytosis

Immature Mast Cell in Peripheral Blood Smear

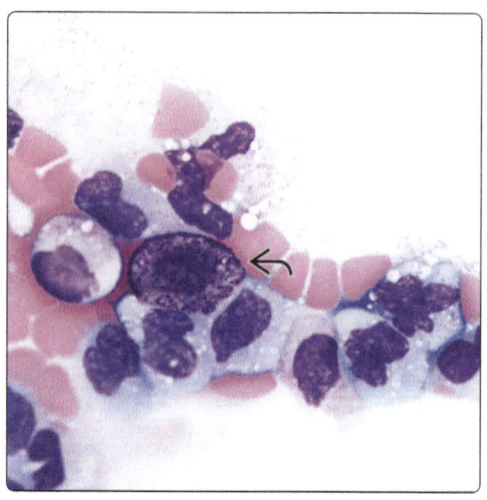

Osteosclerosis

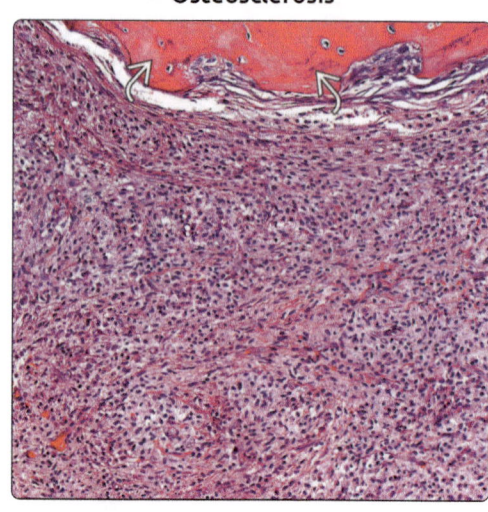

(Left) Wright-stained peripheral blood smear from a patient with mast cell leukemia shows a poorly granulated, circulating mast cell ⇨ at the "feather edge" of this blood smear preparation. (Right) Concurrent bone marrow biopsy shows confluent sheets of neoplastic mast cells with virtual replacement of marrow space with significantly decreased to absent trilineage hematopoiesis. Adjacent trabecular bone shows osteosclerosis ⇨.

Abnormal Mast Cells

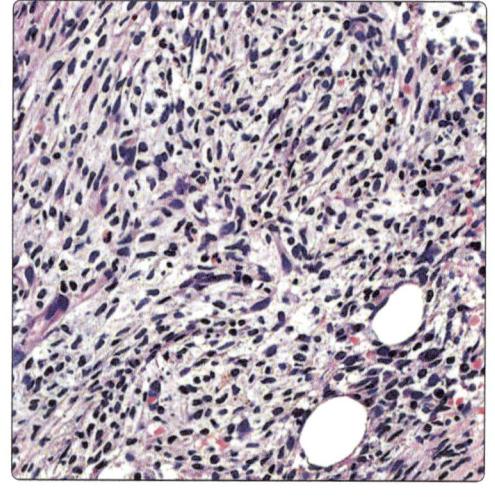

CD117 Immunohistochemistry

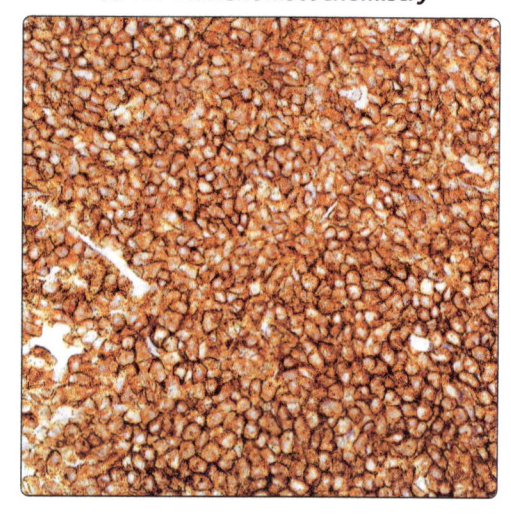

(Left) Bone marrow core biopsy shows sheets of abnormal mast cells with oval to spindle nuclei and abundant clear cytoplasm. The marrow fat cells and trilineage hematopoiesis are markedly reduced. (Right) CD117 antibody shows bright expression by confluent sheets of mast cells. The mast cell proliferation was also positive for tryptase and aberrantly coexpressed CD25.

Preservation of Nodal Architecture

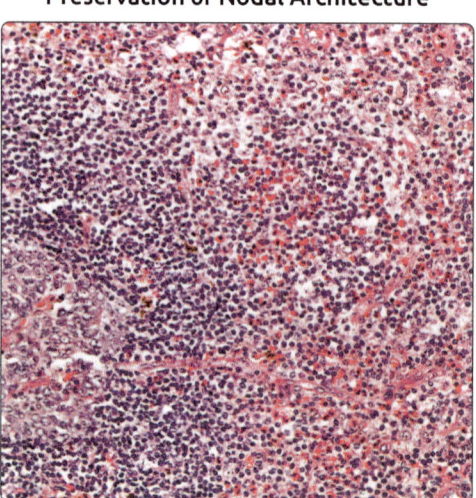

Tryptase Immunohistochemistry

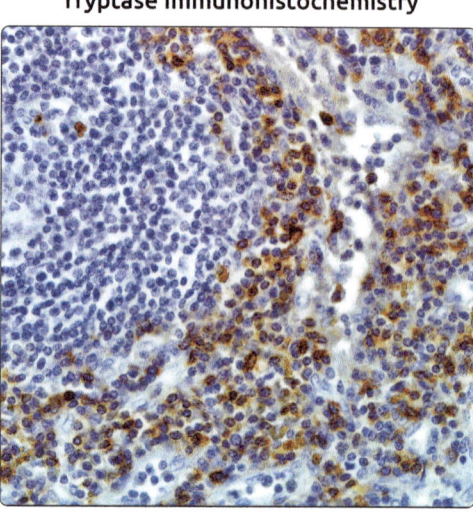

(Left) Incidental lymph node from a patient with mast cell leukemia shows preservation of nodal architecture except for mild interfollicular expansion with scattered pale-staining cells intermixed with a prominent population of eosinophils. (Right) Tryptase highlights subtle infiltrate of positive mast cells. Mast cell infiltrate can be easily overlooked when abundant eosinophils are present.

Mastocytosis

Circulating Blast and Promastocyte

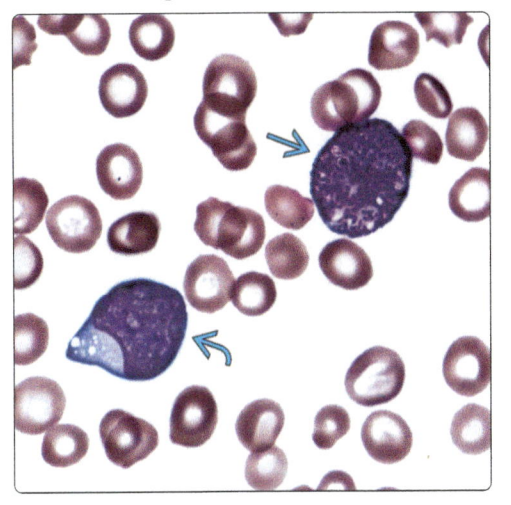

Poorly Granulated Mast Cells and Increased Blasts

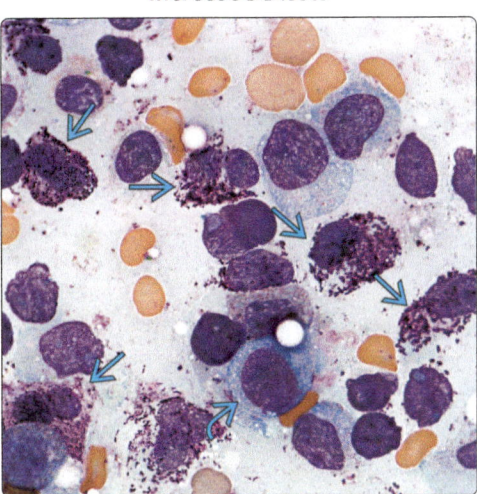

(Left) Wright-stained peripheral blood smear from a patient with concurrent acute myeloid leukemia and mast cell leukemia shows anemia, profound thrombocytopenia, a circulating blast ⮕, and a circulating abnormal mast cell with poor granulation (promastocyte) ⮕. (Right) Concurrent Wright-stained bone marrow aspirate smear shows numerous poorly granulated mast cells ⮕ and increased blasts ⮕. Blasts expressed CD34 and CD33, consistent with acute myeloid leukemia.

Abundant Pale Cytoplasm

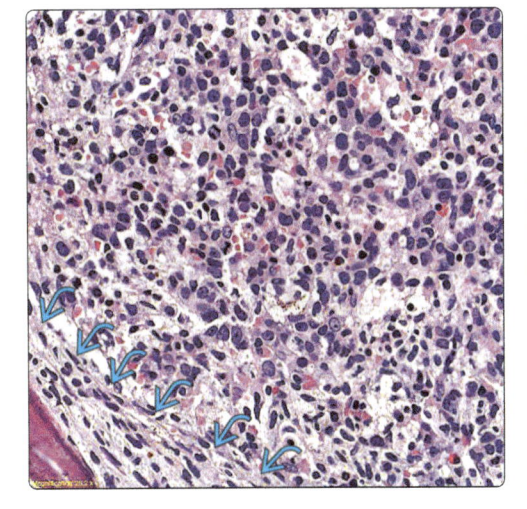

CD117 Immunohistochemistry

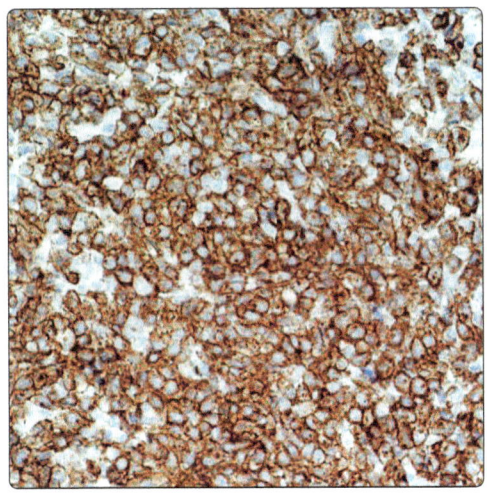

(Left) Bone marrow core biopsy shows sheets of blasts with a high N:C ratio and immature nuclei. In addition, a paratrabecular aggregate of spindled mast cells is seen with abundant pale cytoplasm ⮕. Trilineage hematopoiesis is markedly decreased. (Right) CD117 shows sheets of myeloid blasts as well as mast cells. CD117 does not discriminate between CD117(+) blasts and mast cells.

Tryptase Immunohistochemistry

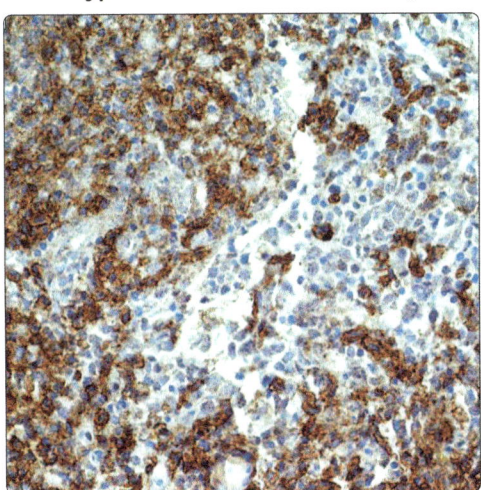

CD34 Immunohistochemistry

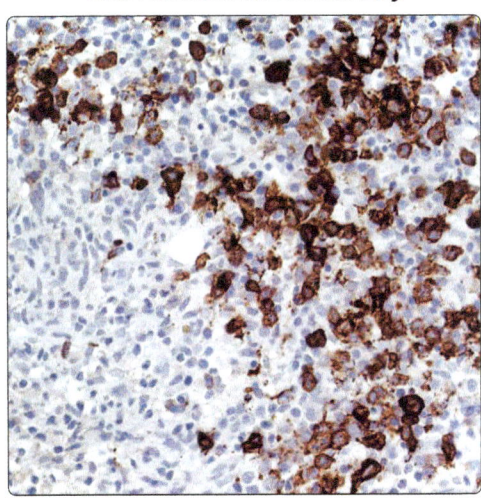

(Left) Tryptase highlights a significant increase in mast cells intermixed with negative myeloid blasts in this portion of bone marrow involved by concurrent acute myeloid leukemia and mast cell leukemia. (Right) CD34 antibody shows increased positive blasts in the same portion of bone marrow with a mirror image-like distribution.

Myeloid/Lymphoid Neoplasms With Eosinophilia and Tyrosine Kinase Gene Fusions

TERMINOLOGY

Definitions

- Neoplasms driven by fusion and subsequent constitutive activation of tyrosine kinase genes
  o PDGFRA, PDGFRB, FGFR1, ETV6::ABL1, FLT3, and JAK2
  o Other fusions
  o Originate from pluripotent stem cells
    – May show lymphoid &/or myeloid differentiation
    – Can show similar presentation to diverse acute and chronic hematopoietic neoplasms
  o Often associated with eosinophilia
  o Response to treatment with tyrosine kinase inhibitors
    – Most associated with PDGFRA and PDGFRB alterations

Classifications

- ICC and WHO-HAEM5
  o Identical categories of M/LN-eo in both classifications

ETIOLOGY/PATHOGENESIS

Fusion Gene Formation

- Driver genes encode tyrosine kinases
- Rearrangements generate fusion genes, leading to constitutive activation of kinase signaling

CLINICAL IMPLICATIONS

General Clinical Implications

- Rearrangements of these genes are diagnostic
- Heterogeneous group of diseases that often feature eosinophilia
  o Eosinophilia not required for diagnosis
  o Includes acute and chronic myeloid and lymphoid processes
- Important to identify due to potential response to treatment with tyrosine kinase inhibitors (TKIs)

PDGFRA Rearrangement

- Diagnostic feature of myeloid/lymphoid neoplasms with eosinophilia and PDGFRA rearrangement
  o Most common alteration is small (800 kb) interstitial deletion (including CHIC2) creating FIP1L1::PDGFRA fusion
    – Other rare reported PDGFRA fusion variants
      □ KIF5B, CDK5RAP2, STRN, ETV6, BCR, TNKS2, and FOXP1
  o PDGFRA mutations (rather than rearrangements), which may be seen in diverse neoplasms, are not encompassed by this diagnosis
  o Diagnosis requires high index of suspicion for cases of eosinophilia, as rearrangements are cryptic on karyotype
- PDGFRA encodes platelet-derived growth factor receptor α
- M:F = 17:1
- Most commonly presents as chronic eosinophilic leukemia
  o Rarely presents as acute myeloid leukemia or T-lymphoblastic leukemia
  o Symptoms due to eosinophil infiltration and cytokine release
    – Fatigue, pruritus, organ involvement, including respiratory, cardiac, skin, CNS, and GI tract
  o Can transform to acute leukemia
- Often associated with increased mast cells
  o May show atypical features similar to those seen in systemic mastocytosis
- Most patients have splenomegaly
- Prognosis is favorable in absence of cytokine-associated end-organ damage
- Treatment with imatinib highly successful and can lead to complete remission
  o Some patients may develop resistance to imatinib
    – Most often secondary to D842V or T674I mutation within ATP-binding domain of PDGFRA
    – Treatment with alternative TKIs, such as ponatinib, may be effective
    – Allogeneic stem cell transplantation may be considered

PDGFRB Rearrangement

- Diagnostic feature of myeloid/lymphoid neoplasms with eosinophilia and PDGFRB rearrangement

(Left) FISH for FIP1L1::PDGFRA fusion shows a normal pattern (absence of rearrangement). Aqua, orange, and green probes show 2 tricolor fusion signals. (Right) FISH for FIP1L1::PDGFRA fusion shows an abnormal pattern (presence of rearrangement). The CHIC2 probe (orange) is missing ➡, indicating FIP1L1::PDGFRA fusion due to interstitial CHIC2 region deletion.

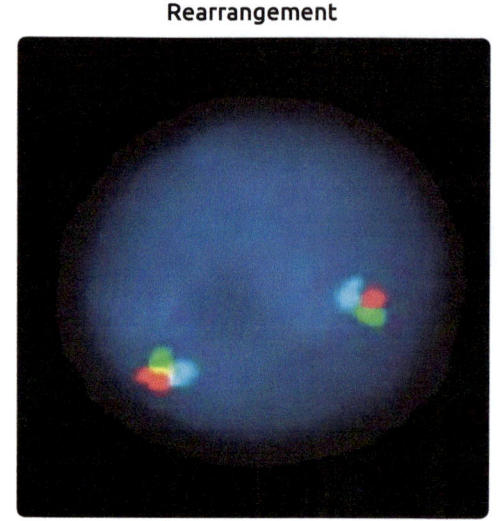

Negative FISH for FIP1L1::PDGFRA Rearrangement

Positive FISH for FIP1L1::PDGFRA Rearrangement

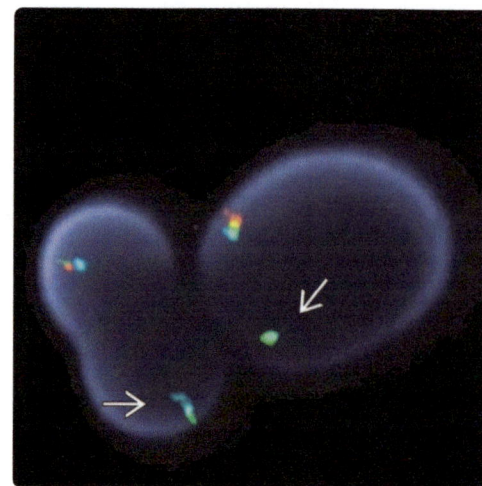

Myeloid/Lymphoid Neoplasms With Eosinophilia and Tyrosine Kinase Gene Fusions

- o > 30 fusion partner genes
  - Most common is *ETV6::PDGFRB*
  - Other fusion partner genes include *DIAPH1*, *BCR*, *AFAP1L1*, *SART3*, and *G3BP1*
- o Excludes fusions associated with *BCR::ABL1*-like B-lymphoblastic leukemia (B-ALL)
  - Partners include *EBF1*, *SSBP2*, *TNIP1*, *ZEB2*, and *ATF7IP*
  - Cases with other fusion partners presenting as typical B-ALL should also be assigned to *BCR::ABL1*-like category
- *PDGFRB* encodes platelet-derived growth factor receptor β
- M:F = 2:1
- Most commonly presents with monocytosis resembling chronic myelomonocytic leukemia
  - o More rarely presents as atypical chronic myeloid leukemia, chronic eosinophilic leukemia, or myeloproliferative neoplasm
  - o Presentation varies with fusion partner
  - o Can transform to acute leukemia
- May be associated with increased mast cells
- May lack eosinophilia
- Most patients have splenomegaly
- More aggressive disease with median survival < 2 years in absence of TKI therapy
- Treatment with TKIs highly successful

FGFR1 Rearrangement

- Diagnostic feature of myeloid/lymphoid neoplasms with eosinophilia and *FGFR1* rearrangement
- a.k.a. 8p11 myeloproliferative syndrome in past (obsolete terminology)
- Many fusion partners
  - o *ZMYM2* fusion partner in ~ 50% of cases
    - Frequently presents with T-lymphoblastic lymphoma component admixed with perivascular myeloblasts termed "bilineal lymphoma"
  - o Other partners include *BCR*, *CEP110*, *CEP43*, *CNTRL*, *CPSF6*, *CUX1*, *FGFR1OP2*, *LRRFIP1*, *MYO18A*, *NUP98*, *SQSTM1*, *TFG*, *TPR*, *TRIM24*
- M:F = 1.5:1
- Most commonly presents as myeloproliferative neoplasm
  - o Can transform to acute leukemia
  - o May present as acute myeloid leukemia, acute T- or B-ALL, or mixed-phenotype acute leukemia
    - Thought to represent transformation of undiagnosed chronic neoplasm
- Can present as lymphoma
- Poor prognosis
  - o High incidence of transformation
- Resistant to 1st-line TKIs in vivo
  - o Some evidence of response to alternative inhibitors and *FGFR1*-specific inhibitors

PCM1::JAK2 Fusion

- Diagnostic feature of myeloid/lymphoid neoplasms with eosinophilia and *PCM1::JAK2* (ICC)
  - o *ETV6* and *BCR* partner genes are considered genetic variants of *PCM1::JAK2* (ICC)
  - o *ETV6::JAK2* may present as B-lymphoid blasts phase features overlapping with B-ALL, *BCR::ABL1*-like
  - o *BCR::JAK2* may present with MDS with proliferative features or B-ALL with *BCR::ABL1*-like features
- M:F = 27:5
- Most commonly presents as myeloproliferative neoplasm or myelodysplastic/myeloproliferative neoplasm
  - o Often presents with hepatosplenomegaly
- Variable prognosis
  - o May show aggressive disease and transformation
- Some response to JAK inhibitors, such as ruxolitinib
- Fusions of *JAK2* with partners genes listed below are common in de novo *BCR::ABL1*-like B-ALL
  - o *STRN3*, *PAX5*, *SSBP2*, *RFX3*, *USP25*, and *ZNF274*
- De novo B-ALL with *PCM1::JAK2* and no apparent myeloid/myeloproliferative component or eosinophilia may be best classified as *BCR::ABL1*-like B-ALL (WHO-HAEM5)

Other Tyrosine Kinase Fusions

- *ETV6::ABL1*
  - o Seen most commonly in pediatric patients, including infants
  - o Eosinophilia less common
  - o Cases with pure lymphoid leukemia presentation should be categorized as *BCR::ABL1*-like B-ALL or T-ALL
  - o Variable response to TKI therapy with alternative inhibitors showing greater response
- *FLT3* rearrangements
  - o Variable partners, most commonly *ETV6*
  - o Often present with monocytic features
  - o Variable response to TKI therapy

Clinical Presentation

- Eosinophilia
  - o Characteristically present in these neoplasms but may not be seen in all cases
- Variable disease phenotype
  - o Includes presentation with features of
    - Chronic eosinophilic leukemia
    - Acute myeloid leukemia
    - Lymphoblastic leukemia/lymphoma
    - Chronic myelomonocytic leukemia
    - Mixed phenotype acute leukemia
    - Other myeloid or immature lymphoid neoplasms
- Gene-defined entities
  - o Regardless of clinical presentation, defining rearrangement is key diagnostic finding

TESTING FOR *PDGFRA*, *PDGFRB*, *FGFR1*, AND *PCM1::JAK2*

Karyotype vs. FISH/RT-PCR

- Karyotype will **not** detect typical *PDGFRA* rearrangement
  - o FISH or RT-PCR is necessary for this purpose
- Karyotype will detect typical *PDGFRB*, *FGFR1* translocations and *PCM1::JAK2*
  - o FISH is indicated to confirm these rearrangements
  - o RT-PCR may help identify exact fusion partners
- RT-PCR may be used in measurable residual disease testing

Myeloid/Lymphoid Neoplasms With Eosinophilia and Tyrosine Kinase Gene Fusions

DETECTION OF *PDGFRA* REARRANGEMENT

Common *FIP1L1::PDGFRA* Fusion
- Fusion of *PDGFRA* with *FIP1L1* is characteristic type of *PDGFRA* rearrangement
- Occurs due to small interstitial deletion at 4q12
  - Because of small size of deletion, this change is **not** visible on routine karyotyping
  - FISH or RT-PCR is necessary to identify rearrangement
    - Both are clinically available
- 1 popular FISH strategy uses 3 probes, 1 of which hybridizes at or near *CHIC2* (in deleted region), with others flanking *PDGFRA* and *FIP1L1*
- Probe pattern for negative case is tricolor fusion signal, indicating presence of *PDGFRA*, *CHIC2*, and *FIP1L1*
- Probe pattern for positive case is fusion of *PDGFRA-* and *FIP1L1*-specific signals only, without intervening *CHIC2*-specific signal
  - Indicates deletion of region between *PDGFRA* and *FIP1L1* with loss of *CHIC2*, resulting in fusion between *PDGFRA* and *FIP1L1*
    - Though this test is sometimes referred to as "*CHIC2* deletion," *CHIC2* is irrelevant bystander in formation of pathogenic *FIP1L1::PDGFRA* fusion
- Alternate strategy utilizes break-apart probe encompassing *FIP1L1* and *PDGFRA*

Other Rare *PDGFRA* Rearrangements
- Rare translocations involving *PDGFRA* have also been described with other partner genes
  - *KIF5B*, *CDK5RAP2*, *STRN*, *ETV6*, and *BCR*
- These reciprocal translocations are typically detected on routine karyotyping
  - Would also generally give rise to abnormal variant FISH patterns with tricolor *FIP1L1/CHIC2/PDGFRA* probe set
- RT-PCR for specific *FIP1L1::PDGFRA* fusion would be negative in case of these alternative partners

DETECTION OF *PDGFRB* REARRANGEMENT

Common *ETV6::PDGFRB* Fusion
- Fusion of *PDGFRB* with *ETV6* is most common type of *PDGFRB* rearrangement

Alternative *PDGFRB* Rearrangements
- \> 30 reciprocal translocation partners are also seen

Karyotyping for *PDGFRB* Rearrangements
- *PDGFRB* rearrangements are typically detected on routine karyotyping
- Of note, not all t(5;12)(q32;p13) translocations involve *PDGFRB* &/or *ETV6*
  - FISH is recommended to confirm presence of *PDGFRB* rearrangement in cases with 5q32 abnormality

FISH for *PDGFRB* Rearrangements
- Break-apart probe strategy is commonly employed
  - Useful for confirming *PDGFRB* rearrangement
  - May be used when karyotype cannot be performed
- Rare cases with positive karyotype or molecular analysis may be negative by FISH
- Very rare cases of karyotypically cryptic *PDGFRB* rearrangements (detectable only by FISH) are also described

DETECTION OF *FGFR1* REARRANGEMENT

Karyotyping for *FGFR1* Rearrangement
- Most common translocation is with *ZMYM2* at 13q12.1
- At least 13 other reciprocal translocation partner genes have also been described for *FGFR1*
  - However, not all 8p11 translocations involve *FGFR1*
    - In particular, *KAT6A* at 8p11 is also rearranged in some myeloid neoplasms
    - Thus, FISH may be indicated for confirmation

FISH for *FGFR1* Rearrangement
- Break-apart probe strategy is commonly employed
- Useful for confirming presence of *FGFR1* rearrangement in cases with 8p11 abnormality

DETECTION OF *PCM1::JAK2*

Karyotyping for *PCM1::JAK2*
- Associated with t(8;9)(p22;p24.1)
- Other *JAK2* fusion partners include *ETV6*, *BCR*

FISH for *PCM1::JAK2*
- Dual-fusion probe strategy is commonly employed
  - Break-apart probes for *PCM1* or *JAK2* are not adequate for confirmation of this diagnosis

ADDITIONAL TESTING

Cytogenetics
- Presence of complex karyotype in any of these diseases may confer worse prognosis

Molecular Testing
- Large NGS panels may be helpful
  - Myeloid gene panels should be considered, particularly in cases with myeloid lineage presentations
  - Most commonly mutated genes include *ASXL1*, *DNMT3A*, and *TET2*
    - May represent background clonal hematopoiesis of indeterminate potential in some cases
    - Have been demonstrated in rearranged cells in some patients
  - May help with prognostic stratification
- Neoplasms with *FGFR1* rearrangement show high incidence of additional mutations
  - *RUNX1* mutations are seen in 83%
  - May play role in poor prognosis in these diseases

SELECTED REFERENCES

1. Tzankov A et al: Updates on eosinophilic disorders. Virchows Arch. 482(1):85-97, 2023
2. Shomali W et al: World Health Organization-defined eosinophilic disorders: 2022 update on diagnosis, risk stratification, and management. Am J Hematol. 97(1):129-48, 2022
3. Pozdnyakova O et al: Myeloid/lymphoid neoplasms associated with eosinophilia and rearrangements of PDGFRA, PDGFRB, or FGFR1 or with PCM1-JAK2. Am J Clin Pathol. 155(2):160-78, 2021
4. Wang SA: The diagnostic work-up of hypereosinophilia. Pathobiology. 86(1):39-52, 2019

Myeloid/Lymphoid Neoplasms With Eosinophilia and Tyrosine Kinase Gene Fusions

Eosinophils and Eosinophil Precursors

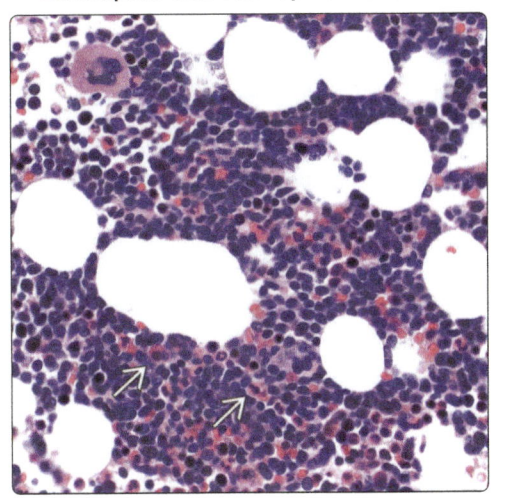

Rearrangement Involving 5q *PDGFRB* Region

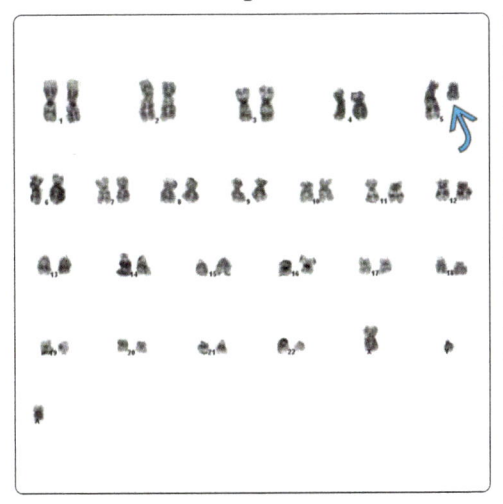

(Left) Bone marrow biopsy shows sheets of blasts with increased intermixed eosinophils and eosinophil precursors ➡. Cytogenetics and FISH confirmed rearrangement of PDGFRB. (Right) Karyotype from a patient with hematopoietic neoplasm shows a rearrangement involving the long arm of chromosome 5 ➡, concerning for PDGFRB rearrangement.

Positive FISH for *PDGFRB* Rearrangement

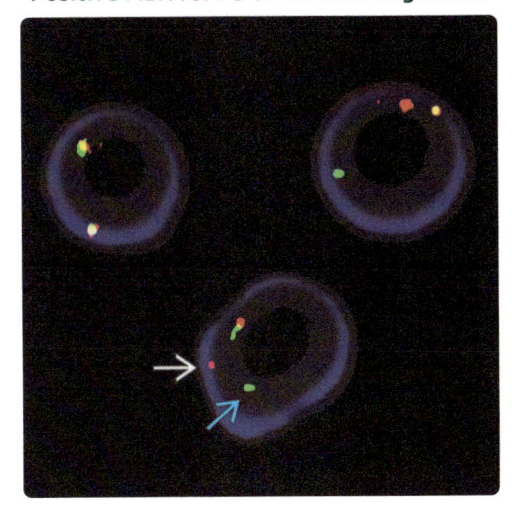

Negative FISH for *PDGFRB* Rearrangement

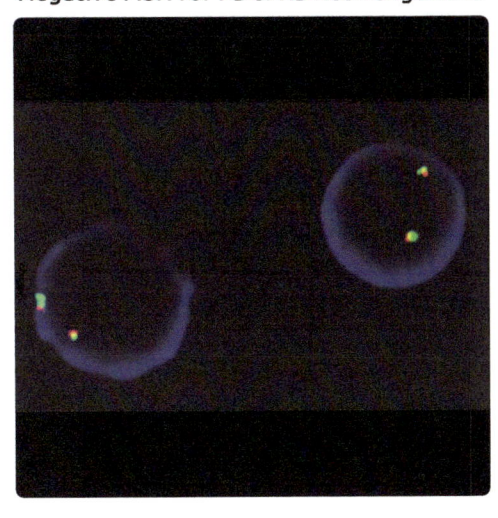

(Left) Break-apart FISH for PDGFRB was performed to confirm involvement. The study shows separation of the red ➡ and green ➡ signals, supportive of rearrangement involving this locus. (Right) FISH for PDGFRB locus shows a normal pattern (absence of rearrangement). Red and green probes show 2 overlapping fusion signals.

Anemia and Eosinophilia

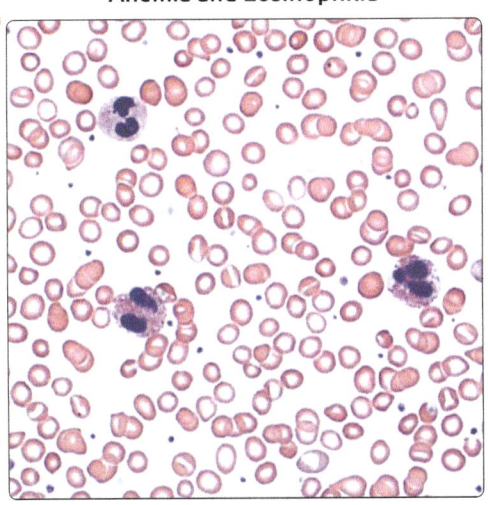

PCM1::JAK2 Fusion

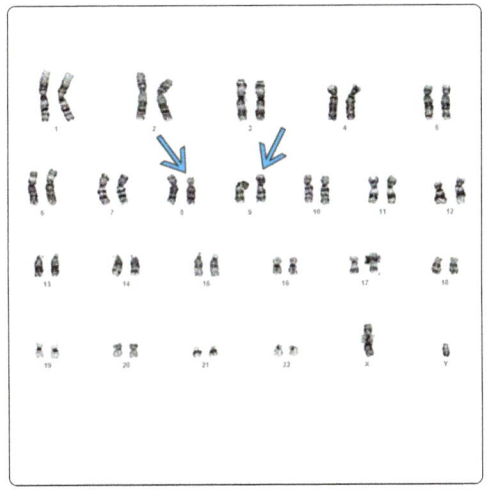

(Left) Peripheral blood smear from a 52-year-old man shows anemia and eosinophilia. FISH was positive for PDGFRA rearrangement. These patients may present with symptoms related to eosinophilia, including endomyocardial fibrosis. (Right) Karyotype from a patient with anemia and leukocytosis shows t(8;9)(p22;p24) ➡, consistent with PCM1::JAK2 fusion. (Courtesy D. Babu, MD.)

VEXAS Syndrome

KEY FACTS

TERMINOLOGY

- VEXAS (**v**acuoles, E1 **e**nzyme, **x**-linked, **a**utoinflammatory, **s**omatic) syndrome
- Acquired monogenic progressive systemic autoinflammatory disease
- Caused by somatic mutations in *UBA1* in hematopoietic progenitor cells
- Increased risk of myelodysplasia and other hematopoietic neoplasm

ETIOLOGY/PATHOGENESIS

- *UBA1* codes for ubiquitin-activating enzyme
  - Marks cellular proteins for ubiquitin-dependent protein degradation
- Most common *UBA1* mutations involve codon 41 and include M41T, M41V, and M41L variants
- Specific variant of *UBA1* mutation may affect phenotypic spectrum of disease

CLINICAL ISSUES

- Progressive, recurrent episodes of systemic and organ-specific inflammation, often refractive to multiple therapies
- Cytopenias become more pronounced over time
  - Transfusion-dependent cytopenias are associated with decreased survival
  - Leukopenia-induced immunosuppressed status may develop
- Hypercoagulable state carries risk of thromboembolism
- Related hematologic malignancies may develop and may require chemotherapy

DIAGNOSTIC CHECKLIST

- Patients are predominantly men > 50 years of age
- Progressive, multisystem autoinflammation
- Macrocytic anemia and other cytopenias
- Thromboembolic disease
- Concurrent myelodysplasia or other hematopoietic neoplasm may be present

Macrocytic Anemia and Thrombocytopenia

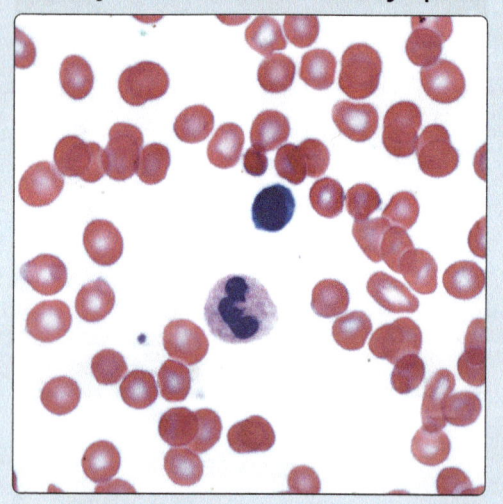

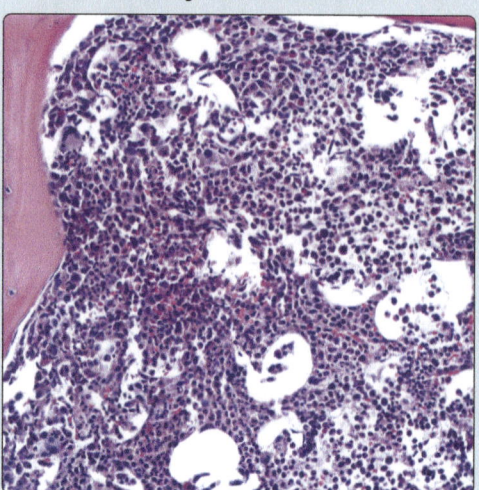

Cytoplasmic Vacuoles

(Left) Wright-stained peripheral blood smear in an older patient with cytopenias shows macrocytic anemia and thrombocytopenia. (Right) Bone marrow aspirate smear shows cytoplasmic vacuoles in myeloid ➡ and erythroid ➡ precursors. In VEXAS syndrome, vacuoles can also be seen in the cytoplasm of megakaryocytes and plasma cells.

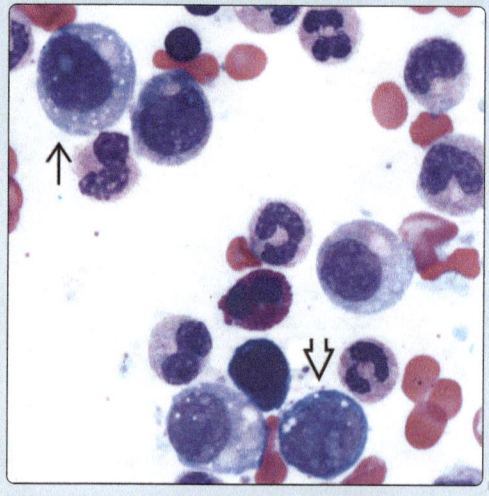

Hypercellular Bone Marrow With Myeloid Granulocytic Predominance

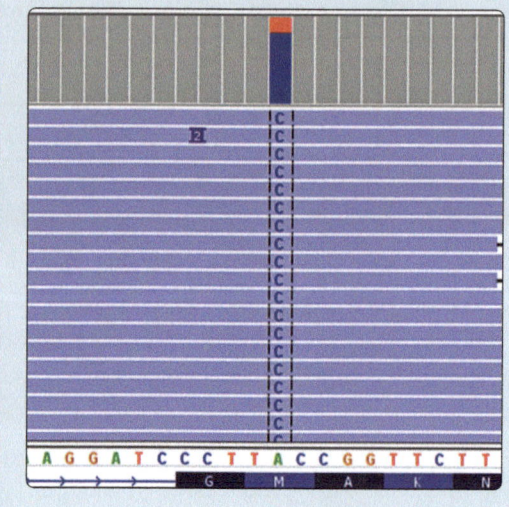

UBA1 Mutational Analysis by NGS

(Left) Bone marrow core biopsy from a patient with UBA1 mutation and clinical characteristics of VEXAS syndrome shows a markedly hypercellular for age marrow with myeloid hyperplasia and erythroid hypoplasia. (Right) NGS pile-up shows a T>C base substitution in UBA1 (Ch X: 47058451) corresponding to a M41T missense mutation. (Courtesy R. Press, MD, PhD.)

VEXAS Syndrome

TERMINOLOGY

Abbreviations
- VEXAS (**v**acuoles, E1 **e**nzyme, **x**-linked, **a**utoinflammatory, **s**omatic) syndrome

Definitions
- Acquired monogenic progressive systemic autoinflammatory disease
- Caused by somatic mutations in *UBA1* in hematopoietic progenitor cells
- Increased risk of myelodysplasia and hematopoietic neoplasm

CLASSIFICATION

WHO-HAEM5 vs. ICC
- Not currently recognized distinct entity in either classification

ETIOLOGY/PATHOGENESIS

UBA1
- Official name: Ubiquitin-like modifier activating enzyme 1
- HGNC ID: 12469
- Gene locus: Xp11.3
- Genomic position
  - ChX: 47,190,847-47,215,128 (GRCh38)
  - Number of exons: 32

Normal Function of *UBA1*
- Encodes E1-activating enzyme (UBA1b)
  - Catalyzes 1st step in ubiquitin conjugation
  - Responsible for > 90% of activation of ubiquitin
- Marks cellular proteins for ubiquitin-dependent protein degradation

UBA1-Acquired Mutations
- Responsible for VEXAS syndrome
- Result in decreased expression of functional UBA1b protein
- Predominantly found in myeloid lineages and absent in lymphoid lineages
  - Propagation of mutant alleles through positive selection pressure in myeloid, erythroid, and megakaryocytic lineages
    - Increased variant allele frequencies seen in these cell types
  - Negative selection pressure of mutant alleles is seen in lymphocytes due to incompatibility with survival
    - Evident clinically with development of lymphopenia
    - Lymphocytes present will demonstrate wildtype alleles
- Most common *UBA1* mutations involve codon 41 and include
  - M41T, M41V, and M41L variants
- Other less common reported mutations
  - G40L and S56F
- Specific variant of *UBA1* mutation may affect phenotypic spectrum of disease

UBA1 Germline Mutations
- Associated with X-linked infantile spinal muscular atrophy

CLINICAL ISSUES

Epidemiology
- Age: > 50 years
- Sex: Male predominance due to *UBA1* mutation on X chromosome
  - Can present in females with monosomy X
- Incidence: ~ 1 in 10,000

Presentation
- Intermittent fevers, fatigue, myalgias
- Inflammatory symptoms affecting cartilage, joints, skin, lungs, and blood vessels
  - Ear, nose, and airway chondritis
  - Arthritis
  - Cutaneous and mucosal lesions
  - Pleural effusion
  - Pulmonary embolism and unprovoked deep vein thrombosis
- Multiple autoinflammatory syndromes
  - Sweet syndrome
  - Relapsing polychondritis
  - Polyarteritis nodosa
- Progressive cytopenias
  - Macrocytic anemia
  - Lymphopenia
  - Monocytopenia
  - Thrombocytopenia
- Concurrent hematopoietic neoplasms
  - Myelodysplastic syndrome (MDS)
  - Clonal cytopenia of undetermined significance (CCUS)
  - Plasma cell neoplasm
  - Chronic lymphocytic leukemia (CLL)/monoclonal B-cell lymphocytosis (MBL)
- Thromboembolic disease
  - Venous thrombosis is most common and recurrent

Treatment
- Autoimmune disease
  - Often requires high-dose corticosteroids despite addition of novel agents, such as JAK inhibitors, TNF-α inhibitors, IL-1 inhibitors, and IL-6 inhibitors
- Hematologic malignancies
  - Often require chemotherapy
- Supportive therapy
  - Subset of patients will develop transfusion-dependent anemia &/or thrombocytopenia
  - Anticoagulation for thrombotic complications
  - Antibiotics for infections due to immunosuppressed status
- Allogeneic stem cell transplant
  - Only treatment with curative intent

Prognosis
- Progressive, recurrent episodes of systemic and organ-specific inflammation, often refractory to multiple therapies
  - Steroid therapy successful in treatment of autoinflammation, but extended use limited by toxicity
  - Novel agents, including JAK-inhibitors, provide response in some patients
- Cytopenias become more pronounced over time

VEXAS Syndrome

- Transfusion-dependent cytopenias are associated with decreased survival
- Leukopenia-induced immunosuppressed status may develop
- Hypercoagulable state carries risk of thromboembolism
  - Recurrent episodes and often early events preceding diagnosis
- Related hematologic malignancies may develop and require chemotherapy
- M41V genotype is associated with decreased survival
  - Produces lower levels of residual UBA1b protein and is associated with more severe disease

MICROSCOPIC

Histologic Features

- Peripheral blood
  - Macrocytic anemia (most common)
  - Thrombocytopenia
  - Lymphopenia
- Bone marrow
  - Vacuoles in cytoplasm of blasts, myeloid and erythroid precursors
    - May also be seen in plasma cells and megakaryocytes, while absent in lymphocytes
  - Hypercellular bone marrow with myeloid hyperplasia
  - Erythroid hypoplasia
  - May demonstrate concurrent hematolymphoid neoplasm
    - Low-grade MDS
    - Plasma cell neoplasm
    - CCUS
  - Dyspoiesis in myeloid, erythroid precursors, and megakaryocytes is often appreciated in cases not meeting criteria for MDS
  - Other findings may include
    - Mild reticulin fibrosis
    - Mildly increased polytypic plasma cells
    - Blasts < 5%

ANCILLARY TESTS

Immunohistochemistry

- CD34
  - Highlights blasts, usually < 5%
- MPO
  - Stains increased myeloid precursors
- CD71
  - Demonstrates erythroid hypoplasia
- CD138
  - May show mildly increased plasma cells

Flow Cytometry

- Evaluation of blasts and myeloid progenitor cells for evidence of immunophenotypic aberrancy
- Evaluation of lymphocytes and plasma cell population for identifying monotypic populations

In Situ Hybridization

- Kappa/Lambda
  - Evaluation for light chains expression among plasma cells to rule out plasma cell neoplasm

Conventional Cytogenetics

- Useful to assess for possibility of recurrent cytogenetic abnormalities

Molecular Testing (Next-Generation Sequencing)

- Virtually all cases demonstrate *UBA1* mutation, predominantly involving codon 41
  - M41T, M41V, and M41L variants
    - M41T is most frequently identified
    - M41V is associated with decreased survival
- Other less commonly identified *UBA1* mutations
  - G40L and S56F
- Screening of VEXAS patients with myeloid gene panel may identify additional mutations associated with MDS
  - *DNMT3A*, *TET2*, *ASXL1*, among others

DIFFERENTIAL DIAGNOSIS

Hematolymphoid Neoplasm

- Concurrent with VEXAS or independent
  - MDS often presents with cytopenias, hypercellular bone marrow, and dysplasia

Nutritional Deficiency

- Folate/B12 deficiency can present with macrocytic anemia
- Copper/zinc deficiency can lead to cytoplasmic vacuoles in myeloid and erythroid precursors

Sideroblastic Anemia

- Cytoplasmic vacuoles can be seen in acquired sideroblastic anemia
- Ring sideroblasts are present
- *UBA1* mutation is absent

DIAGNOSTIC CHECKLIST

Clinically Relevant Pathologic Features

- Patients are predominantly men > 50 years of age
- Progressive, multisystem autoinflammation
- Macrocytic anemia and other cytopenias
- Thromboembolic disease
- Hematopoietic neoplasm

Pathologic Interpretation Pearls

- *UBA1* somatic mutation
- Myeloid and erythroid precursors with cytoplasmic vacuoles
- Macrocytic anemia
- May have concurrent hematologic malignancy

SELECTED REFERENCES

1. Al-Hakim A et al: An update on VEXAS syndrome. Expert Rev Clin Immunol. 19(2):203-15, 2023
2. Kucharz EJ: VEXAS syndrome: a newly discovered systemic rheumatic disorder. Reumatologia. 61(2):123-9, 2023
3. Vitale A et al: VEXAS a new paradigm for adult-onset monogenic autoinflammatory diseases. Intern Emerg Med. 18(3):711-22, 2023
4. Muratore F et al: VEXAS syndrome: a case series from a single-center cohort of Italian patients with vasculitis. Arthritis Rheumatol. 74(4):665-70, 2022
5. Poulter JA et al: Novel somatic mutations in UBA1 as a cause of VEXAS syndrome. Blood. 137(26):3676-81, 2021

VEXAS Syndrome

Hypercellular Marrow With Granulocytic Hyperplasia

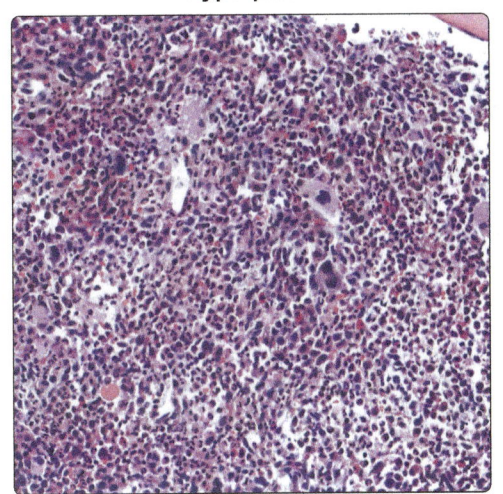

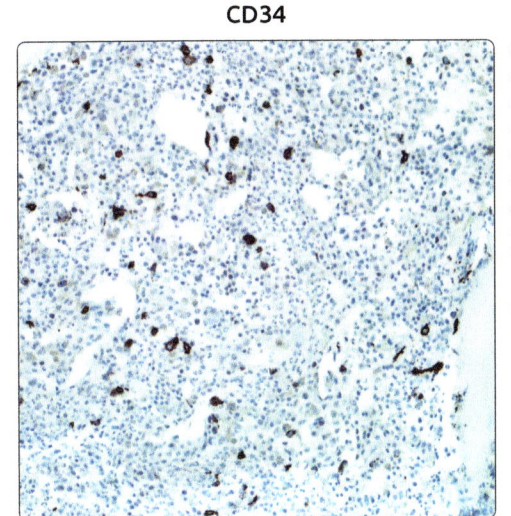

CD34

(Left) Bone marrow core biopsy shows hypercellular marrow with trilineage hematopoiesis and increased myeloid:erythroid ratio. The marrow space is predominantly occupied by maturing myeloid precursors. **(Right)** Blasts may be mildly increased in VEXAS syndrome, but usually make up < 5% of total marrow cellularity, even in a very hypercellular marrow, as seen here.

Vacuoles in Precursors and Increased Plasma Cells

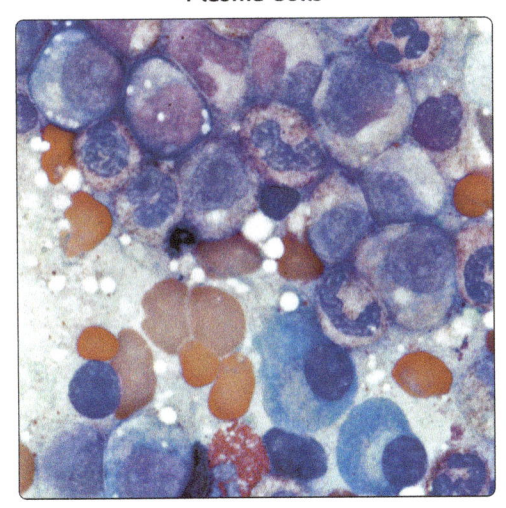

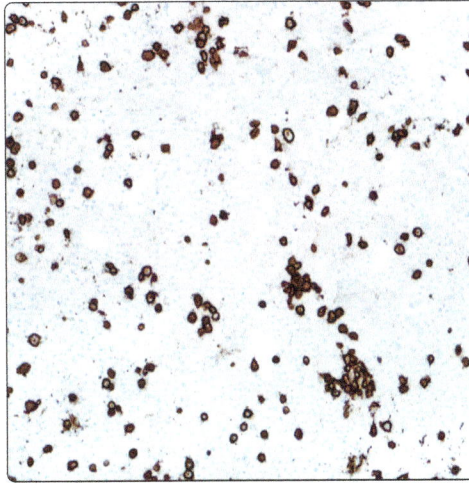

CD138

(Left) Bone marrow aspirate smear shows predominance of maturing myeloid cells. Cytoplasmic vacuoles are present within some of the granulocytic precursors. In addition, there are mildly increased plasma cells also present. **(Right)** Bone marrow core biopsy from a patient with VEXAS syndrome shows plasma cells that are mildly increased in number, arranged in both small clusters and scattered singe cells, prompting further evaluation with in situ hybridization for kappa and lambda light chains.

Kappa In Situ Hybridization

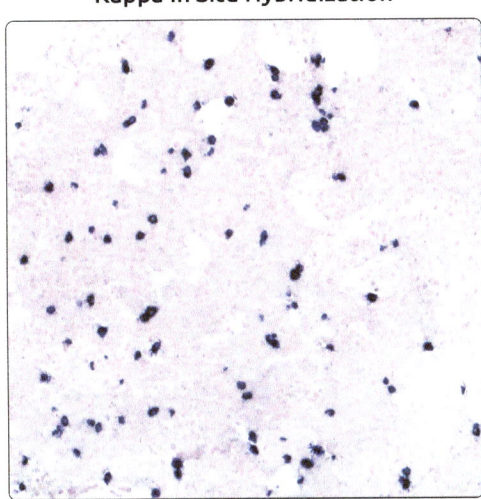

Lambda In Situ Hybridization

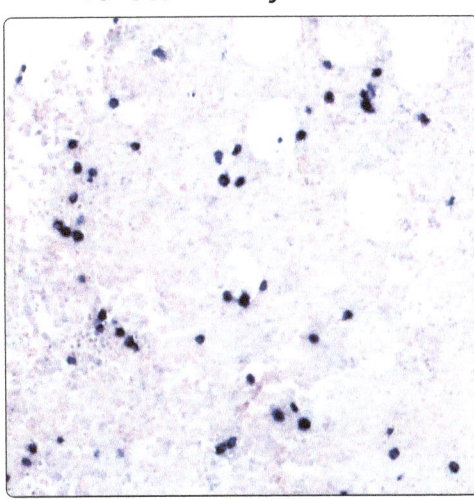

(Left) In situ hybridization highlights scattered κ-light chain expressing plasma cells. **(Right)** In situ hybridization in the same case highlights lambda-expressing plasma cells with a kappa:lambda ratio of ~ 2:1. Staining for light chains is recommended in patients with VEXAS syndrome, given that some may have associated plasma cell neoplasm.

Clonal Hematopoiesis and Premalignant Clonal Cytopenia

KEY FACTS

TERMINOLOGY

- **Clonal hematopoiesis of indeterminate potential (CHIP)**
  - Detected in blood or bone marrow at variant allele fraction (VAF) of ≥ 2% or non-myelodysplastic syndrome (MDS) defining clonal cytogenetic abnormality
  - Absence of unexplained cytopenia
  - Clonal evolution of CHIP to myeloid neoplasm is comparable to MGUS to multiple myeloma
- **Clonal cytopenia of undetermined significance (CCUS)**
  - Main premalignant clonal cytopenia
  - Mutations in ≥ 1 myeloid-associated genes (VAF ≥ 2%) accompanied by persistent cytopenia(s) (≥ 4 months)
  - > 50% risk of progression to myeloid neoplasm within 5 years
- **Idiopathic cytopenia of undetermined significance (ICUS)**
  - Unexplained cytopenia with no dysplasia
  - Similar to CCUS but with no clonality and no MDS-related gene mutation
- **Clonal monocytosis of undetermined significance (CMUS)**
  - Clonal hematopoiesis and monocytosis not fulfilling criteria for diagnosis of CMML
  - CCUS with monocytosis ≥ 10% of WBC and > 0.5 x 10⁹/L
- **Paroxysmal nocturnal hemoglobinuria (PNH)**
  - Clonal cytopenia associated with somatic mutations in *PIGA* in hematopoietic cells
  - Mutations leads to loss of GPI-anchored proteins on surface of erythrocytes, resulting in hemolytic anemia
- **Aplastic anemia (AA)**
  - Genetic abnormalities detected in ~ 50% of patients with acquired AA
  - Mutated genes in AA involve genes commonly mutated in myeloid malignancies
- **VEXAS syndrome**
  - Autoinflammatory syndrome with *UBA1* somatic mutation
  - Autoimmune manifestation

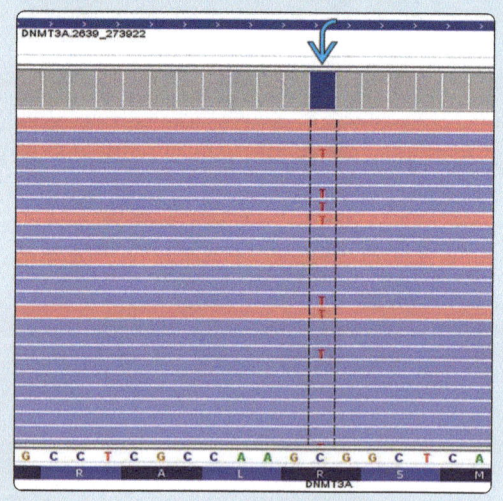

(Left) Peripheral blood smear from a 61-year-old woman with unexplained, persistent thrombocytopenia and anemia is shown. Morphologic examination of bone marrow aspirate and biopsy revealed no significant dysplasia or increased blasts. **(Right)** Next-generation sequencing pile-up shows a c.2645G>A p.R882H missense mutation in DNMT3A ➡. The patient had unexplained, persistent bicytopenia. The finding is consistent with clonal cytopenia of undetermined significance.

Peripheral Blood With Cytopenias

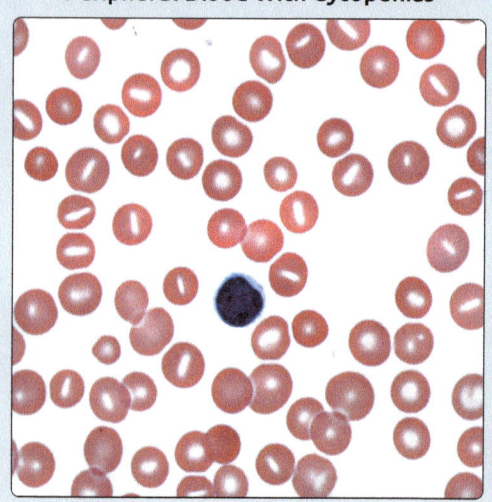

DNMT3A pR882H Missense Mutation

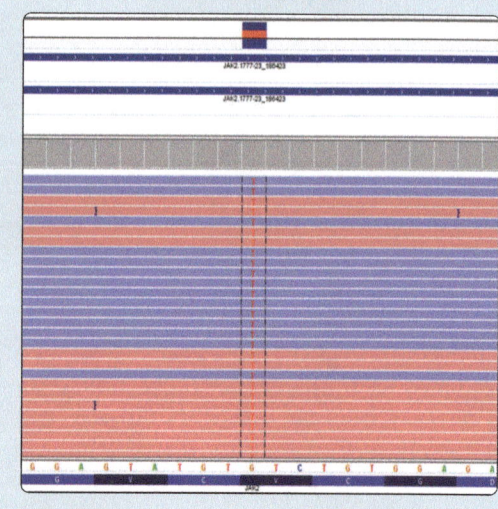

(Left) Next-generation sequencing pile-up of TET2 shows a C to T base substitution in codon 591, resulting in Q591* nonsense mutation ➡. The patient presented with unexplained cytopenia. **(Right)** Next-generation sequencing pile-up of JAK2 exon 14 reveals a c. > missense mutation at borderline variant allele frequency of 2% in a patient with portal vein thrombosis and unremarkable CBC indices, consistent with clonal hematopoiesis of indeterminant significance.

TET2 Q591* Nonsense Mutation

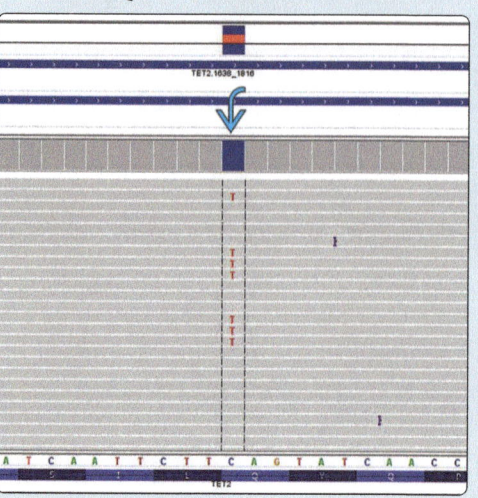

JAK2 V617F Mutation

Clonal Hematopoiesis and Premalignant Clonal Cytopenia

TERMINOLOGY

Abbreviations
- Clonal hematopoiesis of indeterminate potential (CHIP)
- Clonal cytopenia of undetermined significance (CCUS)
- Idiopathic cytopenia of undetermined significance (ICUS)
- Clonal monocytosis of undetermined significance (CMUS)
- Paroxysmal nocturnal hemoglobinuria (PNH)
- Aplastic anemia (AA) with somatic mutations

Definitions
- CHIP
  - Clonal hematopoiesis harboring somatic mutations in myeloid-associated genes
    - Detected in blood or bone marrow (BM) at variant allele fraction (VAF) of ≥ 2% or non-myelodysplastic syndrome (MDS) defining clonal cytogenetic abnormality
    - Most common affected genes include
      - *DNMT3A*, *TET2*, and *ASXL1* with VAF of ~ 10%
      - Minimal dysplasia (< 10% of given lineage)
    - Significance of variants detected at < 2% unclear
    - No known hematopoietic disorder
    - Absence of unexplained cytopenia
    - Relatively common in older individuals
    - Risk of progression to MDS, acute myeloid leukemia (AML), myeloproliferative neoplasm (MPN), or chronic myelomonocytic leukemia (CMML) ~ 0.5-1.0%
    - Clonal evolution of CHIP to myeloid neoplasm is comparable to MGUS to multiple myeloma
    - Increased morbidity and mortality due to other causes, mainly cardiovascular disease
- CCUS
  - Main premalignant clonal cytopenia
  - Mutations in ≥ 1 myeloid-associated genes (VAF ≥ 2%) accompanied by persistent cytopenia(s) (≥ 4 months)
    - Acquired cytopenia defined as persistent anemia (Hgb < 12 g/dL in females and < 13g/dL in males), neutropenia (absolute neutrophil count < 1.8 x 10⁹/L), or thrombocytopenia (platelets < 150 x 10⁹/L)
    - 8-36% of cytopenia(s) represent CCUS
    - Cytopenia(s) due to morbid conditions must be excluded
  - BM examination is required to
    - Categorize clonal cytopenia as CCUS by exclusion of morphologic dysplasia &/or increased blasts
  - Risk of CCUS progression to myeloid neoplasm
    - Progression to myeloid neoplasm occurs in > 50% of cases within 5 years
    - 14x more likely to develop myeloid neoplasm in CCUS in 16 months
  - Progression to myeloid neoplasms depends on
    - Numbers of genes mutated
    - VAF of individual mutations
    - Genes mutated
      - Mutations in spliceosome and epigenetic modifier genes in combination with other mutated genes confer higher risk of progression to myeloid neoplasms
  - Patients with higher-risk CCUS mutations show prognosis comparable to patients diagnosed with lower risk MDS
    - However, currently morphologic dysplasia is required for separating MDS from CCUS
- ICUS
  - Unexplained cytopenia with no dysplasia
  - Similar to CCUS but with no clonality and no MDS-related gene mutation
- CMUS
  - Clonal hematopoiesis and monocytosis not fulfilling criteria for diagnosis of CMML
  - CCUS with monocytosis ≥ 10% of leukocytes and > 0.5 x 10⁹/L
    - May have high potential to progress to overt CMML
    - Recognized as CMML precursor in International Consensus Classification (ICC)
- PNH
  - Clonal cytopenia associated with somatic mutations in *PIGA* in hematopoietic cells
    - Mutations lead to loss of GPI-anchored proteins on surface of erythrocytes, resulting in hemolytic anemia
    - PNH may progress to MDS
- AA
  - Genetic abnormalities detected in ~ 50% of patients with acquired AA
  - Mutated genes in AA involve genes commonly mutated in myeloid malignancies, including
    - *DNMT3A*, *ASXL1*, *BCOR*, *BCORL1*, and *PIGA*
  - Mutations exhibit distinct chronological profiles and clinical impacts
    - High frequency and overrepresentation of mutations in *BCOR*, *BCORL1*, and *PIGA*, and 6p uniparental disomy (UPD) are unique to AA
    - Predict better response to immunosuppressive therapy and significantly better clinical outcome
    - Tend to disappear or show stable clone size
  - Mutations in *DNMT3A*, *ASXL1*, and other genes are likely to increase their clone size
    - Associated with faster progression to MDS/AML
    - Detection of these mutations may predict clonal evolution in AA
- Hypoplastic MDS ± small PNH clone
  - May mimic PNH &/or AA
    - Significant dysplasia in granulocytic and megakaryocytic lineages are typical of MDS
    - Isolated erythroid dysplasia is typical of PNH as well AA
- VEXAS syndrome
  - Autoinflammatory syndrome characterized by
    - Autoimmune manifestations
    - Somatic mutations in *UBA1*
  - Vacuoles in BM precursor cells, including erythroid and myeloid lineages

SELECTED REFERENCES

1. Ahmad H et al: Clonal hematopoiesis and its impact on human health. Annu Rev Med. 74:249-60, 2023
2. Hasserjian RP et al: The International Consensus Classification of myelodysplastic syndromes and related entities. Virchows Arch. 482(1):39-51, 2023

Overview and Classification of Myelodysplastic Syndrome

TERMINOLOGY

Definitions

- Myelodysplastic syndromes (MDS) are molecularly heterogeneous group of entities that have
  - Variable degrees of ineffective hematopoiesis
    - Simultaneous proliferation and apoptosis of hematopoietic cells
    - < 20% blasts
  - Peripheral blood with unexplained and persistent cytopenia(s)
    - < 0.5 x 10⁹/L monocytes
    - < 20% blasts
  - Dysplasia in ≥ 10% of cells in ≥ 1 myeloid lineages
  - Increased risk of acute myeloid leukemia

Classifications

- **International Consensus Classification (ICC)**
  - MDS cases with defining cytogenetic or molecular criteria along with blast percentage and cytopenias, no requirement for dysplasia
    - MDS with mutated *SF3B1* (≥ 10% VAF)
      - < 5% BM blasts and < 5% PB blasts, without *RUNX1* or multihit *TP53* mutation, any cytogenetic abnormality except isolated del(5q), -7/del(7q), abnormality of 3q26.2, or complex karyotype
    - MDS with del(5q)
      - < 5% BM blasts and < 5% PB blasts, thrombocytosis allowed, del(5q) with up to 1 additional abnormality except -7/del(7q), any mutations except multihit *TP53*
    - MDS, NOS with single or multilineage dysplasia
      - < 2% PB blasts or < 5% BM blasts, any cytogenetic except not meeting criteria for MDS-del(5q), any mutation except multihit *TP53* and not meeting criteria for MDS-*SF3B1*
    - MDS, NOS without dysplasia
      - < 2% PB blasts or < 5% BM blasts, no dysplasia-7/del(7q) or complex cytogenetics, any mutations except multihit *TP53* or *SF3B1* (≥ 10% VAF)
    - MDS with excess blasts (MDS-EB)
      - Dysplasia often in ≥ 1 lineage, 2-9% PB or 5-9% BM blasts or Auer rods, any cytogenetics, any mutations except multihit *TP53*
    - MDS with mutated *TP53*
      - 0-9% PB/BM blasts, multihit *TP53* mutations, or *TP53* mutation with VAF > 10% and complex karyotype and often with loss of 17p
    - MDS/AML with mutated *TP53*
      - 10-19% BM or PB blasts with any somatic *TP53* mutation with VAF ≥ 10%
    - MDS/AML, NOS
      - Dysplasia in ≥ 1 lineages, 10-19% BM or PB blasts, any cytogenetics except AML defining, any mutations except *NPM1*, bZIP *CEBPA*, or *TP53*
    - Pediatric cases (< 18 years of age) with 10-19% blasts classified as MDS with excess blasts (MDS-EB)
    - MDS/AML with myelodysplasia-related gene mutation
      - 10-19% blasts, and mutations in *ASXL1*, *BCOR*, *EZH2*, *RUNX1*, *SF3B1*, *SRSF2*, *STAG2*, *U2AF1*, *ZRSR2* (VAF ≥ 2%)
    - MDS/AML with myelodysplasia-related cytogenetic abnormalities
      - 10-19% blasts, and del(5q), -7, del(7q), or complex karyotype with ≥ 3 independent abnormalities, excluding -Y
- **WHO 5th Edition (WHO-HEN5)**
  - Myelodysplastic neoplasms with defining genetic abnormalities
    - MDS with low blasts and 5q deletion
      - Anemia, megakaryocytic dysplasia, < 2% PB and < 5% BM blasts, 1 additional cytogenetic abnormality allowed, except any abnormality of chromosome 7, no *TP53* mutation
    - MDS with low blasts and *SF3B1* mutation
      - ≥ 1 cytopenia, erythroid dysplasia, < 2% PB and < 5% BM blasts, absence of del(5q), monosomy 7 or complex karyotype
    - MDS with biallelic *TP53* inactivation

Dysplastic Neutrophils

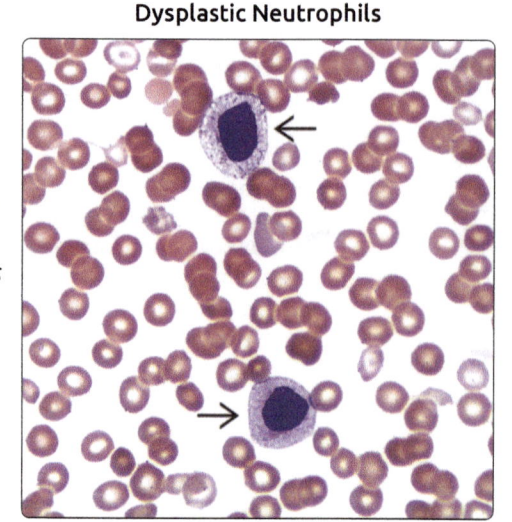

Increased Blasts

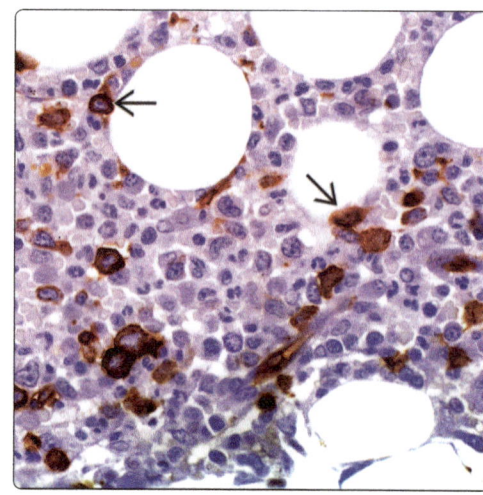

(Left) Dysplastic neutrophils ➡ in this case of myelodysplastic syndrome (MDS) have hyposegmented nuclei. (Right) Bone marrow core biopsy shows an uneven distribution of CD34(+) blasts ➡ that are slightly increased (~ 5%), fulfilling minimum criteria for a diagnosis of MDS with excess blasts.

Overview and Classification of Myelodysplastic Syndrome

- < 20% blasts in PB and BM, usually complex cytogenetics, ≥ 2 *TP53* mutations, or 1 mutation with TP53 copy number loss or copy neutral loss of heterozygosity
- Myelodysplastic neoplasms, morphologically defined
  - MDS with low blasts in cases with ≥ 1 cytopenia and dysplasia with < 2% PB and < 5% BM blasts
    - ≥1 cytopenia and dysplasia, < 2% PB and < 5% BM blasts
  - MDS, hypoplastic in cases with ≥ 1 cytopenias and dysplasia of myeloid &/or megakaryocytic lineages with < 2% PB and < 5% BM blasts and hypocellular BM
    - ≥ 1 cytopenia and dysplasia in myeloid &/or megakaryocytic lineages, < 2% PB and < 5% BM blasts, and hypocellular BM
  - MDS with increased blasts (MDS-IB)
    - ≥ 1 cytopenia and dysplasia, 2-4% PB or 5-9% BM blasts (MDS-IB1)
    - ≥ 1 cytopenia and dysplasia, 5-19% PB or 10-19% BM blasts, or Auer rods (MDS-IB2)
  - MDS with increased blasts and fibrosis (MDS-f)
    - BM fibrosis (grade 2 or 3), 2-19% PB blasts, 5-19%, increased megakaryocytes with prominent dysplasia
    - IHC recommended to highlight increased CD34(+) blasts

EPIDEMIOLOGY

Age Range
- Median: 70 years in Western countries
  - Annual incidence of > 30 per 100,000 among those > 70 years of age

ETIOLOGY/PATHOGENESIS

Histogenesis
- MDS-associated mutations affect genes related to distinct biological functions
  - Spliceosome
    - *SF3B1*, *SRSF2*, *ZRSR2*, *U2AF1*, etc.
  - DNA methylation: *TET2, DNMT3A, IDH1, IDH2*
  - Transcription factors: *RUNX1, BCOR*
  - Chromatin modification: *ASXL1, EZH2*
  - Cell signaling/kinases: *NRAS, KRAS*
  - Cohesin complex: *STAG2*
  - Tumor suppressor genes: *TP53*

CLINICAL IMPLICATIONS

Clinical Risk Factors
- Prognostic factors and risk
  - Revised International Prognostic Scoring System (IPSS-R)
    - Based on number and severity of cytopenias, BM blast percentage, and cytogenetic abnormalities
    - Useful for predicting survival and risk of leukemic transformation for adults
  - WHO Prognostic Scoring System (WPSS)
    - Based on uni- or multilineage dysplasia, BM blast percentage, distinctive cytogenetic findings, and hemoglobin level
  - International Prognostic Scoring System-Molecular (IPSS-M)
    - Continuous index defined as weighted sum of prognostic variables
    - Based on hemoglobin, platelet count, BM blast percentage, IPSS-R cytogenetic category, and type and number of specific somatic gene mutations
      - > 30 genetic alterations included in scoring system, including *TP53* mutations and loss of heterozygosity, *FLT3*-ITD and TKD mutations, and *KMT2A*-PTD

Molecular Genetic Testing in Myelodysplastic Syndrome
- Conventional cytogenetic analysis
  - Requires adequate BM aspirate specimen
  - Essential at diagnosis to establish baseline karyotype
    - 40-60% of patients have clonal abnormality
    - Most common are gains or losses of large chromosome segment (e.g., -5, 5q-, -7, +8)
  - Helpful for diagnosis when persistent cytopenias but insufficient dysplasia or blasts
    - Certain chromosomal abnormalities may be used as presumptive evidence of MDS
      - del(5q), -7, del(7q), or complex karyotype except -Y
  - Essential for risk assessment
  - Karyotypes associated with poor prognosis are seen more frequently in high-grade MDS
    - Complex (> 3 abnormalities) and monosomal karyotype are particularly adverse
- Fluorescence in situ hybridization (FISH)
  - Helpful if insufficient conventional cytogenetic study (i.e., < 20 metaphases)
    - Can perform on BM touch preparations, aspirate smears, or cultured cells
- Molecular analysis
  - Large-panel sequencing is typically used to assess multiple genes simultaneously
  - Most frequently mutated genes include *TET2, SF3B1, ASXL1, SRSF2, U2AF1, DNMT3A, RUNX1, TP53, STAG2, ZRSR2, BCOR*, and *EZH2*
  - Presence of mutations refines prognostic assessment
  - Caution is necessary in assessing clinical significance of these mutations
    - Normal older individuals may harbor somatic mutations without overt myeloid neoplasm
      - Clonal hematopoiesis of indeterminate potential

SELECTED REFERENCES

1. Falini B et al: Comparison of the International Consensus and 5th WHO edition classifications of adult myelodysplastic syndromes and acute myeloid leukemia. Am J Hematol. 98(3):481-92, 2023
2. Hasserjian RP et al: The International Consensus Classification of myelodysplastic syndromes and related entities. Virchows Arch. 482(1):39-51, 2023
3. Cazzola M: Risk stratifying MDS in the time of precision medicine. Hematology Am Soc Hematol Educ Program. 2022(1):375-81, 2022
4. Duncavage EJ et al: Genomic profiling for clinical decision making in myeloid neoplasms and acute leukemia. Blood. 140(21):2228-47, 2022

Overview and Classification of Myelodysplastic Syndrome

Most Frequently Mutated Genes in Myelodysplastic Syndrome

Gene	Approximate Frequency (%)	Biologic Role of Encoded Protein
TET2	24	DNA methylation
SF3B1	22	Spliceosome
ASXL1	19	Chromatin modification
SRSF2	12	Spliceosome
U2AF1	10	Spliceosome
DNMT3A	11	DNA methylation
RUNX1	10	Transcription factor
TP53	8	Tumor suppressor
STAG2	7	Cohesin complex
ZRSR2	5	Spliceosome
BCOR	5	Transcriptional corepressor
EZH2	5	Chromatin modification

Data are computed directly from Haferlach et al and Xu et al, representing 1,140 myelodysplastic syndromes (MDS) patients via next-generation sequencing (NGS) panel sequencing. This table presents only individual genes with a combined average of ≥ 5% in these 2 studies. Many more genes were recurrently mutated at a slightly lower frequency.

Recurring Chromosomal Abnormalities in Myelodysplastic Syndrome

Abnormality	Frequency (%)	Abnormality	Frequency (%)
-7 or del(7q)	10	+8*	10
del(5q)	10	del(20q)*	5-8
i(17q) or t(17p)	3-5	-Y*	5
-13 or del(13q)	3		
del(11q)	3		
del(12p) or t(12p)	3		
del(9q)	1-2		
idic(X)(q13)	1-2		
t(1;3)(p36.3;q21.2)	1		
t(2;11)(p21;q23)	1		
inv(3)(q21q26.2)	1		
t(6;9)(p23;q34)	1		

*This karyotypic abnormality is insufficient alone for a presumptive diagnosis of myelodysplastic syndromes (MDS).

International Prognostic Scoring System (Revised) for Myelodysplastic Syndrome

Variable	0	-0.5	1	1.5	2	3	4
Bone marrow blasts percentage	≤ 2		> 2 to < 5		5-10	> 10	
Hemoglobin g/dL	≥ 10		8 to < 10	< 8			
Platelets 10^9/L	>100	50 to < 100	< 50				
ANC 10^9/L	≥ 0.8	< 0.8					
Cytogenetics	Very good		Good		Intermediate	Poor	Very poor

Very good: -Y, del11q; good: Normal, del(5q), del(12p), del(20q), double including del(5q); intermediate: del(7q), +8, +19, i(17q), any other single/double independent clone; poor: -7, inv(3)/t(3q)/del(3q), double including -7/del(7q), complex with 3 abnormalities; very poor: Complex with > 3 abnormalities.

Overview and Classification of Myelodysplastic Syndrome

Erythroid Dysplasia

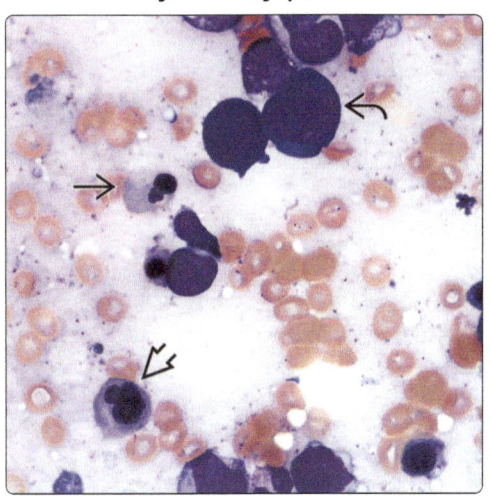

Megakaryocytic Dysplasia

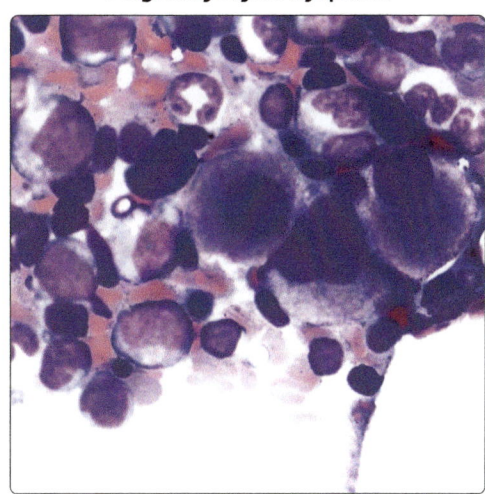

(Left) Bone marrow aspirate smear from an older woman with MDS shows ≥ 10% dysplastic erythroid precursors, as manifested by nuclear budding ➡, hyperlobation ➡, and megaloblastic changes ➡. Although the erythroid lineage is slightly increased, the woman has moderate normochromic normocytic anemia. Anemia in MDS is also commonly macrocytic. (Right) Small, dysplastic megakaryocytes with hypolobated and hyperchromatic nuclei are features of MDS.

Dysplastic Platelets

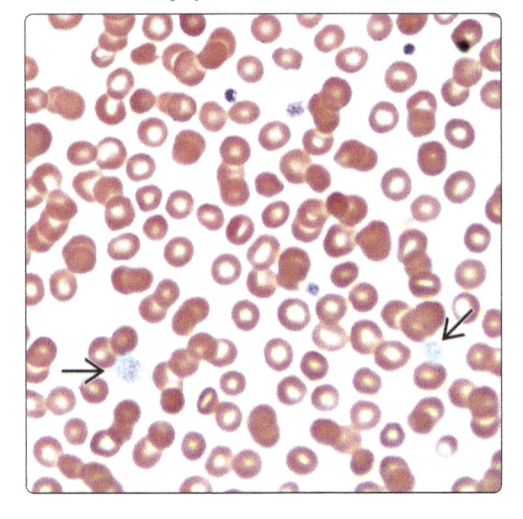

Megakaryocytic Dysplasia

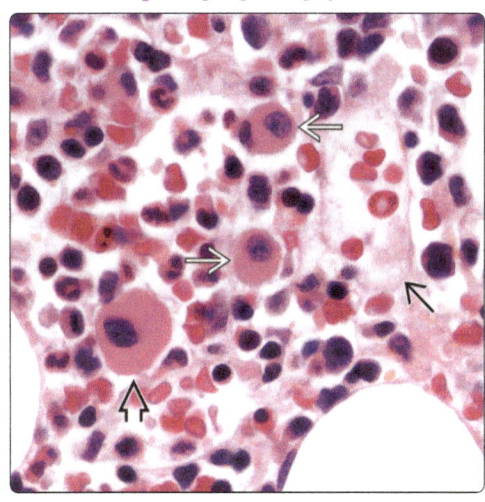

(Left) Large and hypogranular platelets ➡ are another dysplastic finding in MDS blood films. (Right) Higher power examination of bone marrow biopsy shows dysmegakaryopoiesis with monolobated ➡ and small ➡ megakaryocytes. The erythroid and myeloid lineages show complete maturation, and sinuses are patent ➡.

Granulocytic Dysplasia

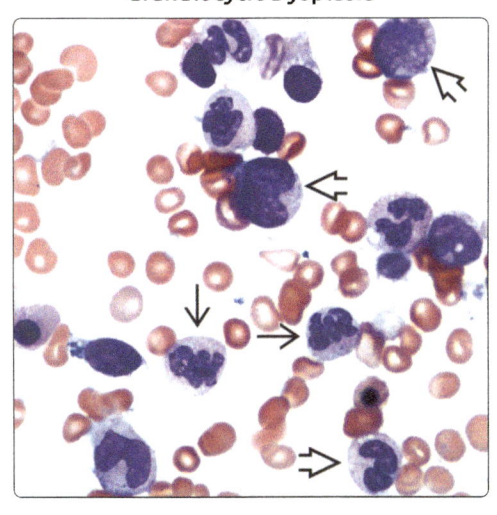

Blasts

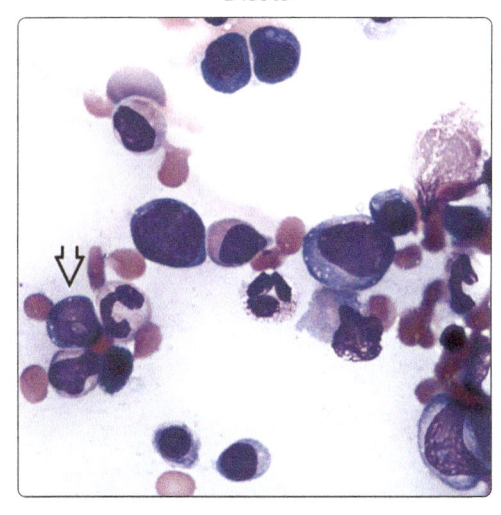

(Left) Dysgranulopoiesis in ≥ 10% of the myeloid lineage is the predominant finding in this case of MDS. Dysplastic features include irregular and abnormal nuclear segmentation ➡ and cytoplasmic hypogranulation ➡. (Right) Blasts in MDS may be small ➡ and are particularly difficult to identify in poorly prepared or suboptimally stained smears. Some cases of MDS with excess blasts may not have prominent dysplastic features.

Molecular Pathology of Myeloid Neoplasms

187

Myelodysplastic Syndrome With Mutated *SF3B1*

KEY FACTS

TERMINOLOGY
- Low-grade myelodysplastic syndrome (MDS) with defining *SF3B1* mutation
- Blasts < 2% in peripheral blood, < 5% in bone marrow, no Auer rods
  - *SF3B1* somatic mutations
    - Variant allele fraction (VAF) ≥ 10% per ICC
    - VAF ≥ 5% per WHO-HAEM5
- Cytopenia involving ≥ 1 lineage
- WHO-HAEM5 only: ≥ 15% ring sideroblasts (RS) fulfills criteria if mutation analysis not available
- Dysplasia not required to make diagnosis per ICC
- RS are not required to make diagnosis per ICC

ETIOLOGY/PATHOGENESIS
- Clonal hematopoietic stem cell disorder
  - *SF3B1* mutation is early event in pathogenesis
- Primary defects of mitochondrial iron metabolism
- Abnormal iron stain in erythroid precursors with formation of RS in most cases

CLINICAL ISSUES
- Often present with moderate anemia; clinical symptoms related to anemia
- Thrombocytopenia (13%), neutropenia (8%)

MOLECULAR
- *SF3B1* somatic mutation
  - K700E and G742D are common hotspot mutations
  - Less common involve K666, H662, and R625 codons
  - Positive predictive value for myeloid neoplasm with RS is 98%
  - *SF3B1* mutations can be seen in other MDS subtypes or MDS/MPN neoplasms with lesser frequency
  - *SF3B1*-mutated MDS lacks mutations associated with congenital sideroblastic anemias
  - *SF3B1* testing typically performed in panel by next-generation sequencing (NGS)

Macrocytic Anemia

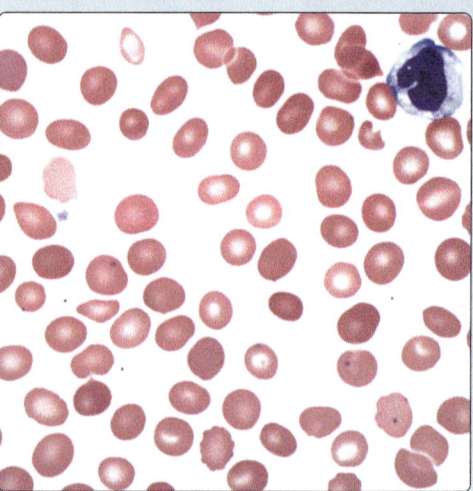

Erythroid Dysplasia

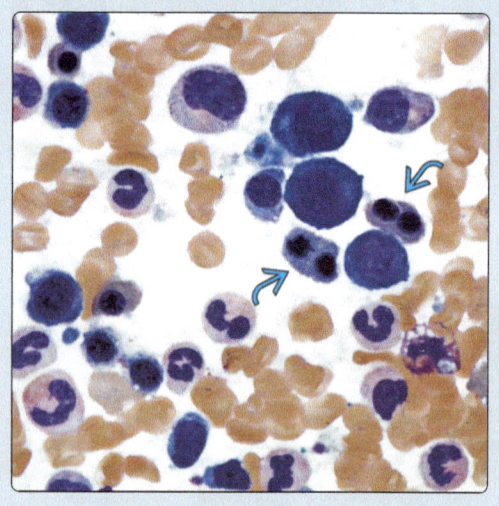

(Left) Peripheral blood smear from a patient with myelodysplastic syndrome (MDS) with mutated SF3B1 shows macrocytic anemia with a dimorphic population of red blood cells and mild thrombocytopenia. (Right) Bone marrow aspirate shows left-shifted erythroid predominance with megaloblastoid change and dysplasia limited to erythroid lineage ⇨.

Ring Sideroblasts

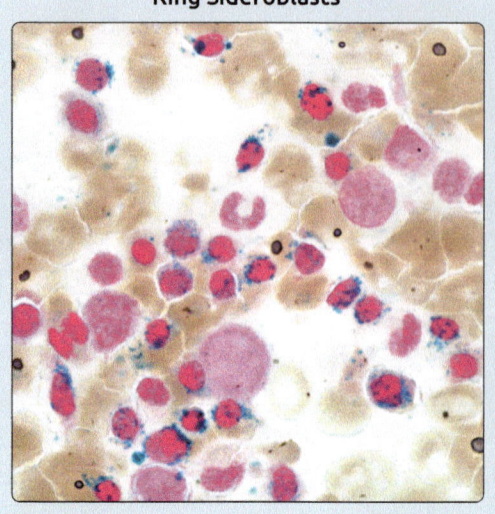

SF3B1 Mutation Analysis by NGS

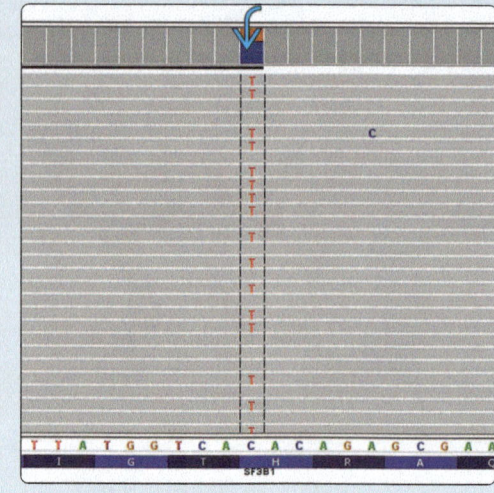

(Left) Iron-stained bone marrow aspirate shows numerous ring sideroblasts (RS) in a case of MDS with mutated SF3B1. Nonneoplastic causes of RS and congenital sideroblastic anemia should always be excluded before diagnosing MDS with mutated SF3B1. (Right) Next-generation sequencing pile-up shows a c.1986C>A (pH662Q) mutation in the SF3B1 gene ⇨. The test was performed on DNA extracted from bone marrow with significant erythroid dysplasia and > 15% RS.

Myelodysplastic Syndrome With Mutated *SF3B1*

TERMINOLOGY

Abbreviations
- Myelodysplastic syndrome with mutated *SF3B1* (MDS-*SF3B1*); International Consensus Classification (ICC)
- Myelodysplastic neoplasm with low blasts and *SF3B1* mutation (MDN-*SF3B1*); WHO 5th edition (WHO-HAEM5)

Synonyms
- MDS with single lineage or multilineage dysplasia (WHO 4th edition)

Definitions
- Low-grade MDS with defining *SF3B1* mutation
  - Blasts < 2% in peripheral blood, < 5% in bone marrow, no Auer rods
  - *SF3B1* mutation
    - Variant allele fraction (VAF) ≥ 10% per ICC
    - VAF ≥ 5% per WHO-HAEM5
  - Cytopenia involving ≥ 1 lineage
    - Hgb < 13 g in males, < 12 g in females
      □ Anemia, if present, is often macrocytic
    - Absolute neutrophil count < 1.8 x 10⁹/L
    - Platelet count < 150 x 10⁹/L
  - Ring sideroblasts (RS) are not required to make diagnosis per ICC
    - WHO-HAEM5 only: ≥ 15% RS fulfills criteria if mutation analysis not available
  - Dysplasia (> 10%) involving ≥ 1 lineage (WHO-HAEM5)
  - Dysplasia not required to make diagnosis per ICC
- Does not meet criteria for other myeloid neoplasm
  - No del(5q), -7/del(7q), complex karyotype, multihit TP53 (VAF ≥ 10%)
  - ICC: No inv(3), abnormal 3q26, or *RUNX1* mutations
  - No cytoses, including
    - WBC ≥ 13 × 10⁹/L, monocytosis (≥ 0.5 × 10⁹/L and ≥ 10% of leukocytes), or platelets ≥ 450 × 10⁹/L

ETIOLOGY/PATHOGENESIS

Molecular Pathogenesis
- Clonal hematopoietic stem cell disorder
- Primary defects of mitochondrial iron metabolism
  - Abnormal iron stain in erythroid precursors with formation of RS in most cases
    - Iron deposited in perinuclear mitochondria in ferritin form
  - Causes intramedullary erythroid apoptosis
- *SF3B1*
  - Official name: Splicing factor 3b, subunit 1
  - Gene locus: 2q33.1
  - Normal function of gene
    - Encodes subunit 1 of splicing factor 3b (SF3b)
    - SF3b together with SF3a and 12S RNA unit forms U2 small nuclear ribonucleoproteins complex (U2 snRNP)
    - SF3b/3a complex binds pre-mRNA and may anchor U2 snRNP to pre-mRNA
    - Critical component of splicing machinery
    - Catalyzes removal of introns from precursor mRNA
    - Alternative splicing results in multiple transcript variants encoding different isoforms
  - *SF3B1* heterozygous knockout mice develop RS
    - Suggests that *SF3B1* haploinsufficiency leads to formation of RS
    - Distinct iron distribution is mediated through splicing patterns in key mitochondrial iron proteins
      □ *SLC25A37* with several splice variants with retained intron is linked to iron distribution
- *SF3B1* somatic mutations
  - Positive predictive value for myeloid neoplasm with RS is 98%
  - Heterozygous substitution
  - Clustered in exons 12-16 of gene
  - *SF3B1* K700E accounts for > 50% of mutations
  - *SF3B1* mutations can be seen in other MDS subtypes or MDS/MPN with lesser frequency
  - *SF3B1* mutations can also be detected in cases of chronic lymphocytic leukemia (CLL)
- ~ 100 genes involved in erythroid differentiation are misspliced, including
  - *ABCB7*, *PPOX*, and *TMEM14C*
- Mutations in other splicing factor genes are mutually exclusive of *SF3B1* mutations, including
  - *SRSF2*, *U2AF1*, and *ZRSR2*
- More common cooccurring mutated genes with *SF3B1* mutations, including
  - *TET2* and *DNMT3A*

CLINICAL ISSUES

Epidemiology
- Incidence
  - MDS-SF3B1 composes 17% of MDS
- Age
  - Older individuals; median: 70-75 years

Presentation
- Often present with moderate anemia
  - Clinical symptoms related to anemia
- Thrombocytopenia (13%), neutropenia (8%)
- Liver and spleen may show iron overload

Laboratory Tests
- Blood counts and smear review
- Bone marrow evaluation, including
  - Iron-stained aspirate smear
    - Count at least 100 nucleated erythroid precursors for RS percentage
    - Count all stages of erythroid precursors
  - Cytogenetic analysis
    - Clonal chromosomal abnormalities in up to 20% of cases
    - Usually involves single chromosome
  - Flow cytometric analysis
    - No significant increase in blasts
    - Aberrant erythroid maturation pattern or phenotype
      □ Lower mean expression of CD71
  - Immunohistochemistry
    - E-cadherin and CD117 highlight left-shifted erythroid lineage
  - Molecular testing

Myelodysplastic Syndrome With Mutated *SF3B1*

- *SF3B1* testing typically included in panel and tested by NGS

Treatment

- Red cell transfusions if symptomatic
  - Contributes to iron overload
  - Iron chelation therapy for systemic iron overload
- Erythropoietin administration
- Drugs modulating TGF-β superfamily ligands
  - Luspatercept abolishes transfusion requirement for many patients
- Lenalidomide; other medications in clinical trials
- Bone marrow transplant in severe cases for eligible patients

Prognosis

- Indolent with median overall survival of 69-108 months
- *SF3B1* mutation is independent predictor of favorable prognosis
  - Not affected by mutation type, VAF percentage, or recurrent mutations in epigenetic regulators
- Very low risk of leukemic evolution

MOLECULAR

Cytogenetics

- No specific chromosomal abnormality
  - Normal karyotype in ~ 80% of cases
  - Chromosomal abnormalities typically include single chromosome aberration
    - Trisomy 8, del(11q), del(20q)

Molecular Genetics

- *SF3B1* mutations
  - Identified by whole-exome sequencing in 2011
  - Linked to formation of RS
  - Heterozygous point mutations clustered in exons 12-16
    - K700E and G742D are common hotspot mutations
    - Less common involve K666, H662, and R625 codons

Gene Expression Profiling

- Overexpression of *ALAS2*
- Overexpression of *FTMT*
- Reduced expression of *ABCB7*
  - *ABCB7* encodes transport protein

MICROSCOPIC

Cytologic Features

- Peripheral blood
  - Blasts account for < 2% in blood
  - Macrocytic or normochromic normocytic anemia
  - May have concurrent neutropenia or thrombocytopenia
- Bone marrow
  - < 5% blasts
  - Increase in erythroid precursors with left shift
    - Often dysplastic, i.e., megaloblastic, abnormal nuclear segmentation, binucleation
    - No significant dysplasia or only mild dysplasia in nonerythroid lineage
- Iron-stained bone marrow aspirate smears
  - Increased iron stores, erythroid iron, RS
  - Sideroblasts: International Working Group definitions
    - Type 1: < 5 siderotic granules in cytoplasm
    - Type 2: ≥ 5 siderotic granules not in perinuclear distribution
    - Type 3: ≥ 5 siderotic granules in perinuclear distribution surrounding ≥ 1/3 of nuclear circumference
      - Only type 3 qualifies as RS

DIFFERENTIAL DIAGNOSIS

Acquired Sideroblastic Anemias

- Nonneoplastic causes of sideroblastic anemias
  - Drug induced (e.g., isoniazid), toxin exposure (lead, benzene, alcohol), zinc-induced copper deficiency

Congenital Sideroblastic Anemia

- Nonsyndromic congenital sideroblastic anemias (CSA)
  - X-linked due to germline mutation of *ALAS2*
  - *SLC25A38* mutation resulting in SLC25A38 transporter deficiency
  - *GLRX5* mutation resulting in glutaredoxin 5 deficiency
- Syndromic CSA
  - X-linked with ataxia
    - Germline mutations in *ABCB7*
  - Myopathy, lactic acidosis, and sideroblastic anemia
    - Germline mutations in *PUS1* and *YARS2*
  - Thiamine-responsive megaloblastic anemia
    - Germline mutations in *SLC19A2*
- *SF3B1*-mutated MDS lacks mutations associated with CSA

Other Myeloid Neoplasms

- Clonal cytopenia of undetermined significance (CCUS)
  - *SF3B1* mutation VAF ≥ 2% (ICC) and ≤ 5% (WHO)
- Genetic abnormalities that supersede *SF3B1* mutation in MDS classification
  - 20% of MDS with del(5q) have *SF3B1* mutation
  - MDS with mutated TP53 multihit mutations
  - MDS, not otherwise specified
    - MDS with RS and wildtype *SF3B1* (ICC)
    - *SF3B1* mutation with concurrent *RUNX1* mutation, -7, del(7q), or complex karyotype
- MDS/MPN with *SF3B1* mutation and thrombocytosis (ICC)
  - *SF3B1* mutation in 80-90%; *JAK2* mutation in 50-60%
    - Rarely *MPL* or *CALR* mutations
- CMML with *SF3B1* mutation

SELECTED REFERENCES

1. Hasserjian RP et al: The International Consensus Classification of myelodysplastic syndromes and related entities. Virchows Arch. 82(1):39-51, 2023
2. Zhang Y et al: Impact of the International Consensus Classification of myelodysplastic syndromes. Br J Haematol. 201(3):443-8, 2023
3. Cazzola M: Risk stratifying MDS in the time of precision medicine. Hematology Am Soc Hematol Educ Program. 2022(1):375-81, 2022
4. Clough CA et al: Coordinated missplicing of TMEM14C and ABCB7 causes ring sideroblast formation in SF3B1-mutant myelodysplastic syndrome. Blood. 139(13):2038-49, 2022
5. Khoury JD et al: The 5th edition of the World Health Organization Classification of Haematolymphoid Tumours: myeloid and histiocytic/dendritic neoplasms. Leukemia. 36(7):1703-19, 2022
6. Patnaik MM et al: Refractory anemia with ring sideroblasts (RARS) and RARS with thrombocytosis (RARS-T) - "2019 update on diagnosis, risk-stratification, and management". Am J Hematol. 94(4):475-88, 2019

Myelodysplastic Syndrome With Mutated *SF3B1*

Erythroid Dysplasia

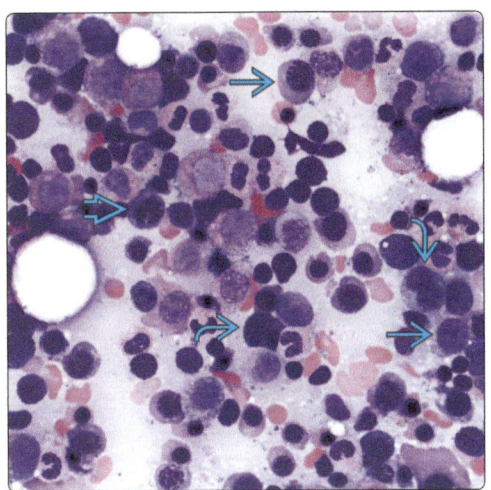

Erythroid Hyperplasia

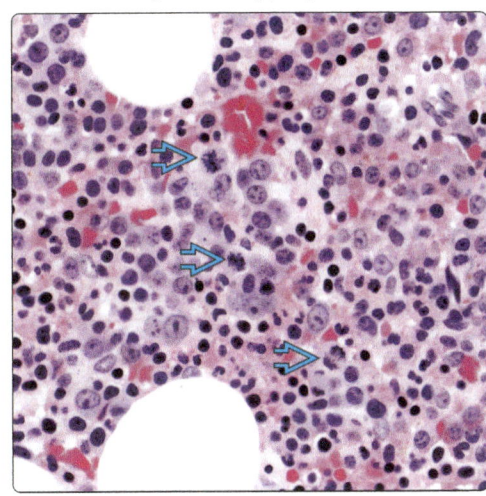

(Left) Bone marrow aspirate smear from a patient with MDS-SF3B1 shows increased erythroid precursors. Dysplasia is limited to the erythroid lineage, as evidenced here with megaloblastoid changes, binucleation ⇨, karyorrhexis ⇨, and asynchronous nuclear to cytoplasmic maturation ⇨. (Right) Bone marrow biopsy shows hypercellular marrow with erythroid predominance. There is left-shifted erythropoiesis and increased mitotic activity ⇨.

Macrocytic Anemia and Thrombocytosis

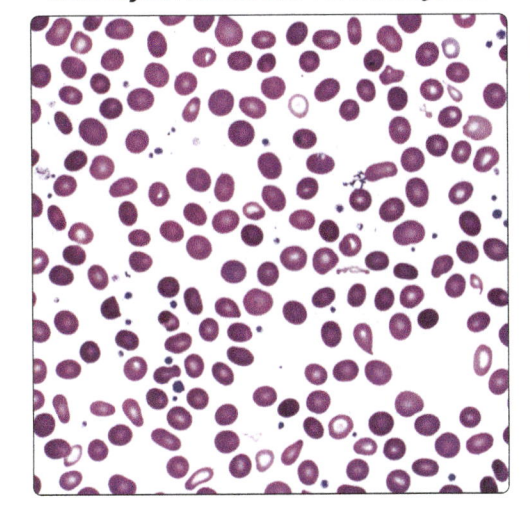

Increased Atypical Megakaryocytes

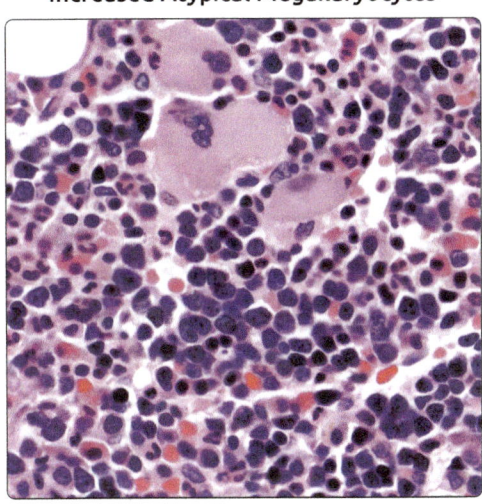

(Left) Peripheral blood smear from a 73-year-old with myelodysplastic/myeloproliferative neoplasm with RS and thrombocytosis (MDS/MPNRS-T) shows macrocytic anemia and thrombocytosis. The red cells are dimorphic with small, hypochromic and macrocytic cells. Prominent anisopoikilocytosis is present. (Right) Hypercellular bone marrow from a patient with MDS/MPN-RS-T shows an M:E ratio of 0.5:1.0 with increased atypical megakaryocytes. The megakaryocytes form loose clusters.

Large Megakaryocytes

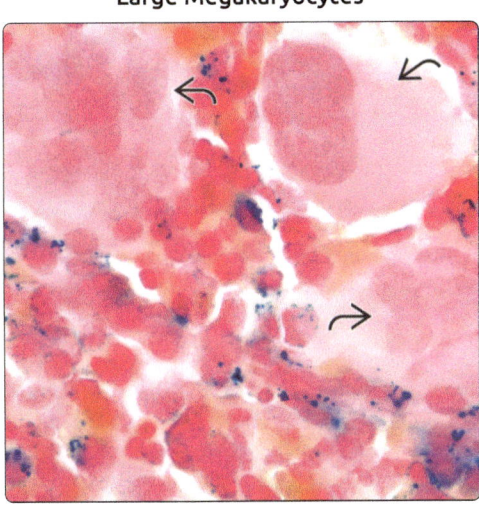

PCR-Based Allelic Discrimination Analysis of *JAK2* V617F

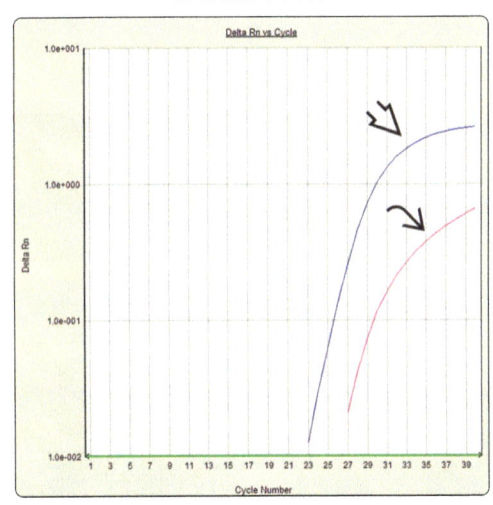

(Left) Perls Prussian blue iron stain of bone marrow aspirate from the same patient shows increased storage iron and scattered RS. Large megakaryocytes ⇨ are present in the background. (Right) Allelic discrimination real-time PCR shows a JAK2 V617F mutation ⇨ in a patient with MDS/MPN-RS-T. The blue amplification curve represents the wildtype allele ⇨.

Myelodysplastic Syndrome, NOS

KEY FACTS

TERMINOLOGY
- Diagnostic criteria of MDS, NOS (ICC)
  - At least 1 cytopenia; no cytosis
  - Morphology
    - Without dysplasia: ≤ 10% dysplasia in any lineage
    - Single-lineage dysplasia: ≥ 10% dysplasia in 1 lineage
    - Multilineage dysplasia: > 10% dysplasia in 2 or 3 lineage
  - < 2% blasts in blood, < 5% blasts in marrow; no Auer rods
  - Cytogenetics
    - Without dysplasia: -7/del(7q) or complex karyotype
    - With single lineage/multilineage dysplasia: Does not meet cytogenetic criteria for MDS-del(5q)
  - Molecular genetics: No multihit *TP53* (VAF ≥ 10%) or *SF3B1* mutation (≥ 10%) without *RUNX1* mutation
- MDS with low blasts (MDS-LB) would be equivalent of MDS-NOS (with SLD or with MLD) in WHO-HAEM5
  - Definition of lineage dysplasia is optional (WHO-HAEM5)

MOLECULAR
- Clonal chromosomal cytogenetic abnormalities in ~ 50%
  - Strongly correlated with prognosis
- Gene mutations assessed by myeloid gene panels
  - Mutations detected in 70-90% of MDS cases
  - Include mutations in *TET2*, *DNMT3A*, *ASXL1*, *RUNX1*, *SRSF2*, *STAG2*, and *CBL*
- FISH panels focus on chromosomes 5, 7, 8, 20

TOP DIFFERENTIAL DIAGNOSES
- Other MDS categories
  - Genetic correlation essential
- VEXAS syndrome
- Paroxysmal nocturnal hemoglobinuria
- Reactive (nonneoplastic) causes
  - Drugs/medications
  - Nutritional deficiencies
  - Autoimmune diseases

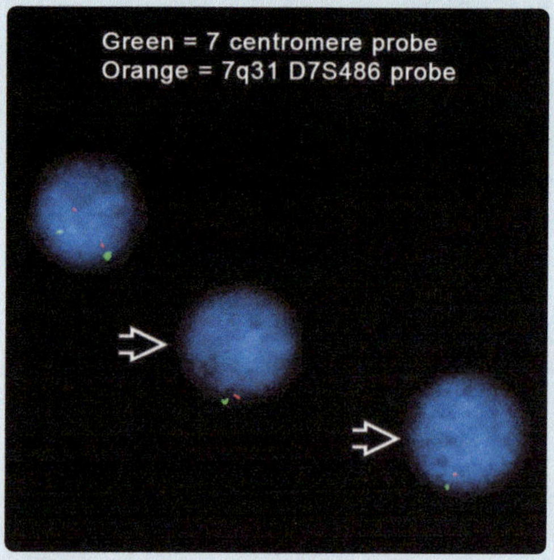

(Left) Peripheral blood smear shows hypogranular neutrophils ➡ and a dimorphic red cell population with prominent anisopoikilocytosis and hypochromic red blood cells. (From DP: Blood & Bone Marrow.) (Right) FISH testing of bone marrow shows monosomy 7 (loss of 1 green and 1 orange probe signal) ➡ in this patient with myelodysplastic syndrome, NOS with multilineage dysplasia (MDS-NOS-MLD). Monosomy 7 is associated with a poorer prognosis.

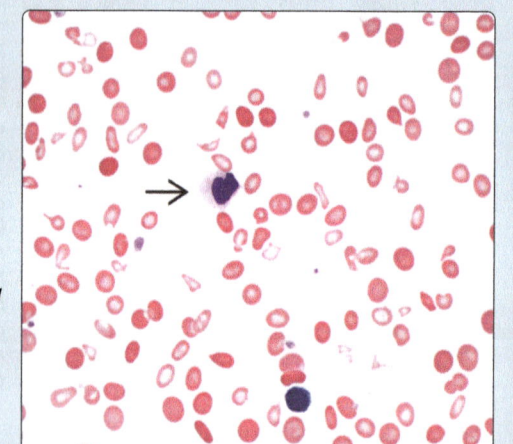

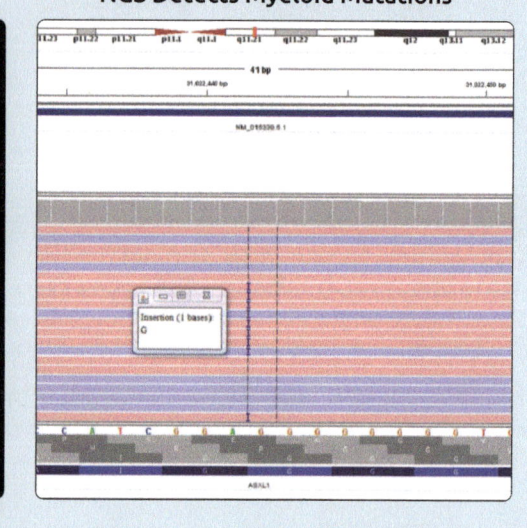

(Left) Common spliceosome mutations lead to aberrant splicing of target genes, which in turn has various negative downstream effects in MDS. (Adapted from Pellagatti et al: Blood 2018.) (Right) *ASXL1* frameshift mutation on chromosome 20 (c.1934dup, p.Gly646fs) is commonly seen in MDS and other myeloid malignancies. Somatic *ASXL1* mutations are identified in 15-23% of MDS. Next-generation sequencing (NGS) result is shown on IGV software.

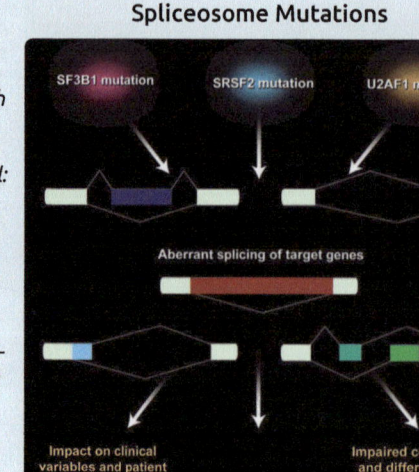

Myelodysplastic Syndrome, NOS

TERMINOLOGY

Abbreviations
- Myelodysplastic syndrome with multilineage dysplasia (MDS-NOS-MLD)
- Myelodysplastic syndrome with single-lineage dysplasia (MDS-NOS-SLD)

Synonyms
- Myelodysplastic neoplasms with low blasts (WHO-HAEM5)

Definitions
- Diagnostic criteria of MDS, NOS (ICC)
  - At least 1 cytopenia; no cytosis
  - Morphology
    – Without dysplasia: ≤ 10% dysplasia in any lineage
    – Single-lineage dysplasia: ≥ 10% dysplasia in 1 lineage
    – Multilineage dysplasia: > 10% dysplasia in 2 or 3 lineage
  - < 2% blasts in blood, < 5% blasts in marrow; no Auer rods
  - Cytogenetics
    – Without dysplasia: -7/del(7q) or complex karyotype
    – With single-lineage/multilineage dysplasia: Does not meet cytogenetic criteria for MDS-del(5q)
  - Molecular genetics: No multihit *TP53* (VAF ≥ 10%) or *SF3B1* mutation (≥ 10%) without *RUNX1* mutation
- MDS with low blasts (MDS-LB) would be equivalent of MDS-NOS in WHO-HAEM5
  - Definition of lineage dysplasia is optional (WHO-HAEM5)

CLASSIFICATION

ICC vs. WHO-HAEM5
- 3 subcategories in MDS, NOS (ICC)
  - Without dysplasia, with single lineage, and with multilineage dysplasia
- MDS with low blasts (MDS-LB) would be equivalent in WHO-HAEM5
  - Distinction between single-lineage and multilineage dysplasia is optional in WHO-HAEM5

ETIOLOGY/PATHOGENESIS

Environmental Exposure
- Industrial solvents
  - Benzene
  - Insecticides, pesticides
- Cigarette smoking
- Radiation

Genetic Predisposition
- Acquired clonal hematopoietic mutations increase with age
  - Increased number of mutations and mutational burden increase risk of transformation to hematologic malignancy

CLINICAL ISSUES

Epidemiology
- Incidence
  - MDS-NOS accounts for ~ 50% of MDS cases
    – 15-20% MDS-SLD
    – 30% MDS-MLD
- Age
  - Typically seen in older individuals
    – Median: 65-70 years of age

Presentation
- Single or multiple cytopenias by definition
  - Anemia
    – Most common cytopenia
    – Often macrocytic but can be normocytic or microcytic
    – Fatigue, pallor
  - Thrombocytopenia
    – Bleeding, purpura, easy bruising
  - Neutropenia
    – Infections

Treatment
- Options, risks, complications
  - Based on severity of disease and ability to tolerate treatment
    – Age
    – Risk (based on karyotype, degree of cytopenia and dysplasia)
    – Performance status, comorbidities
- Drugs
  - Hypomethylating agents
    – Azacytidine
    – Decitabine
  - Immunomodulatory agents
    – Antithymocyte globulin
  - Multiagent therapy
  - Many new agents in clinical trials
    – For low-risk MDS
      □ Luspatercept
      □ Roxadustat
      □ Imetelstat
      □ Pexmetinib
      □ Romiplostin
      □ Eltrombopag
  - Supportive therapy
    – For lower grade, lower risk disease with fewer symptoms
    – Erythropoiesis-stimulating agents
      □ Most cases respond
    – Corticosteroids
    – Transfusions
- Allogeneic stem cell transplant
  - Only curative strategy
  - Generally reserved for younger patients with excellent performance status

Prognosis
- Revised International Prognostic Scoring System (IPSS-R)
  - Defined by
    – Percentage of blasts
    – Number and severity of cytopenias
    – Cytogenetic abnormalities
      □ Very poor prognosis with complex karyotype
    – Age
- Other prognostic models
  - World Health Organization prognostic scoring system (WPSS)

Myelodysplastic Syndrome, NOS

- Global MD Anderson prognostic scoring system (MDAPSS)
- Also emphasize cytogenetics, bone marrow blast percentage and cytopenias
- Molecular mutations still have not made it into most prognostication scoring systems
- Fibrosis is independent poor prognosticator
  - Should be considered in transplant candidacy
- MDS-NOS
  - Median survival: 66 months
  - Very low rate of progression to acute myeloid leukemia (AML)
- MDS, NOS, hypoplastic
  - Significantly worse than aplastic anemia
  - Better prognosis than other MDS subtypes (even when using IPSS-R)
  - May have good response to immunosuppressive therapy

MOLECULAR

Cytogenetics
- In ~ 50% of cases, clonal chromosomal cytogenetic abnormalities
- Strongly correlated with prognosis

Fluorescence In Situ Hybridization
- FISH panels commonly include evaluation of aberrations in chromosomes 5, 7, 8, and 20

Array Comparative Genomic Hybridization
- High-resolution techniques reveal cryptic changes beyond those detected by conventional cytogenetics
  - Similar regions and genes to conventional karyotyping
- Cannot detect balanced chromosomal translocations

Molecular Genetics
- Single-nucleotide polymorphism (SNP) arrays
  - Higher resolution than conventional methods
    - Reveals abnormalities in up to 75% of MDS patients
  - May distinguish hypocellular MDS from aplastic anemia
  - Cannot detect balanced chromosomal translocations
  - May miss minor clones
- Gene mutations
  - Detected in up to 90% of MDS cases
  - Lower grade disease may have fewer mutations
  - *DNMT3A* mutations
  - *TET2* mutations
    - High response rate with azacytidine
  - *ASXL1* mutations
    - Associated with poorer prognosis
    - ~ 20% of MDS
  - *RUNX1* mutations
    - Associated with progression to AML
    - Seen in 10% of MDS
  - *NRAS* mutation
    - Codon 12 mutation most common
  - *EZH2* mutations
    - Seen in 5% of MDS
  - Spliceosome genes
    - Mutated in 50-60% of MDS
    - *SRSF2, U2AF1, ZRSR2*
    - *SRSF2, U2AF1* usually in higher grade
      - Poorer prognosis
      - High risk of evolution to AML
  - Hypoplastic MDS mutations may differ
    - Germline mutations of *GATA2, DDX41,* or *FANCA* or telomerase complex genes
      - Genetic predisposition to bone marrow failure in this subset
      - Do not respond to immunosuppressive therapy
      - Suspect with younger patients, family history

MICROSCOPIC

Histologic Features
- Hypercellular bone marrow
  - Due to ineffective hematopoiesis in clonal stem cells
  - Some cases are normocellular or even hypocellular
  - Hypocellular MDS has significant hypocellularity compared to age-matched controls
    - < 30% of normal cellularity in patients < 70 years of age
    - < 20% cellularity in patients > 70 years of age
- Dysplasia
  - On biopsy sections, megakaryocyte dysplasia is most prominent
    - Separation of nuclear lobes
    - Micromegakaryocytes with small, monolobated nuclei
- Abnormal bone marrow architecture
  - Abnormal localization of immature precursors (ALIP)
  - Increased megakaryocytes with occasional clustering
  - Disruption of erythroid colony architecture
- Fibrosis occasionally present
  - Important to assess due to prognostic implications
- Iron assessment (Prussian blue stain)
  - Increased storage iron in histiocytes

Cytologic Features
- At least 10% of cells should be dysplastic in at least 1 or ≥ 2 lineages to assess for presence of SLD or MLD
  - Erythroid lineage
    - Cytoplasmic vacuoles
      - Also seen in copper deficiency
    - Internuclear chromatin bridging
    - Nuclear budding
    - Multinucleation
    - Megaloblastoid nuclei
    - Presence of ring sideroblasts in absence of *SF3B1* or any genetic exclusionary features is qualified for MDS, NOS category
  - Granulocytic lineages
    - Hypogranulation
    - Nuclear hyposegmentation
  - Megakaryocytic lineage
    - Hypolobated or monolobated nuclei
    - Separated nuclear lobes
    - Micromegakaryocytes

Peripheral Blood
- Usually anemia, sometimes with neutropenia or thrombocytopenia

Myelodysplastic Syndrome, NOS

- o Usually normochromic normocytic, sometimes macrocytic
- Neutropenia
- Thrombocytopenia
- Blasts must be < 2% in peripheral blood
- Anisopoikilocytosis highly variable
- Neutrophil dysplasia
  - o Including hypolobated and hypogranular forms
  - o Dysplasia is often easier to see in blood than bone marrow

ANCILLARY TESTS

Immunohistochemistry
- CD34, CD117 helpful in highlighting myeloblasts/immature precursors on biopsy sections

Flow Cytometry
- Can detect percentage and phenotype of myeloblasts
- Often shows abnormal maturation pattern in myeloid lineage

In Situ Hybridization
- Rapid turnaround time but seldom adds new information in addition to karyotype
- Useful if fresh specimen not available or karyotype fails
- Seldom adds new information to karyotype

Genetic Testing
- Next-generation sequencing myeloid mutation panel
  - o Detects gene mutations in 70-90% of MDS cases

DIFFERENTIAL DIAGNOSIS

Reactive (Nonneoplastic) Causes of Cytopenias and Cytologic Dysplasia
- Nutritional deficiencies
  - o Vitamin B12, folate
  - o Copper deficiency
    - Ring sideroblasts common
- Heavy metal poisoning
- Drugs/medications
  - o Methotrexate
  - o Tacrolimus
  - o Other immunomodulatory and antimetabolite agents
  - o Antineoplastic chemotherapy regimens
  - o Growth factor therapy, including erythropoietin
- Autoimmune/collagen vascular diseases

Congenital Hematologic Disorders
- Chromosomal breakage syndromes
  - o Fanconi anemia
  - o Ataxia telangiectasia
  - o Bloom syndrome
  - o Xeroderma pigmentosum
- Shwachman-Diamond syndrome
- Dyskeratosis congenita
- Kostmann disease
  - o One of severe congenital neutropenia causes
- Congenital dyserythropoietic anemia

Myelodysplastic Syndrome and Acute Myeloid Leukemia, Post Cytotoxic Exposure
- Must have history of cancer with radiation or chemotherapy, including alkylating agent or topoisomerase II inhibitor

Other Subtypes of Myelodysplastic Syndrome
- Need to exclude subtypes with specific, defining genetic abnormalities

Aplastic Anemia
- In differential diagnosis with hypoplastic MDS
- Erythroid dysplasia common in both, but hypoplastic MDS also may have myeloid, megakaryocytic dysplasia

Paroxysmal Nocturnal Hemoglobinuria
- Subset of MDS may have concurrent small PNH clones by flow cytometry
- PNH typically shows isolated erythroid dysplasia
- Presence of significant dysplasia, including in granulocytic and megakaryocytic lineages, &/or MDS-defining genetic abnormalities useful in separating MDS form PNH

VEXAS Syndrome
- Distinction is important due to low incidence of progression to MDS
- Significant myeloid and erythroid vacuolization
- Recurrent *UBA1* mutation in VEXAS
- Acquisition of additional genetic aberrations may qualify diagnosis of MDS in setting of VEXAS

DIAGNOSTIC CHECKLIST

Pathologic Interpretation Pearls
- Must have ≥ 1 peripheral blood cytopenias
- Dysplasia must be in > 10% of cells of specific lineage for establishing SLD and MLD categories
  - o Unless there is MDS-defining cytogenetic abnormality (MDS-NOS, without dysplasia)
- Blasts must be < 2% in blood and < 5% in BM
- Rule out category defining genetic abnormalities (e.g., *SF3B1*, *TP53* mutations, etc.)
- Monocytes < 1 x 10^9 in peripheral blood

SELECTED REFERENCES

1. Falini B et al: Comparison of the International Consensus and 5th WHO edition classifications of adult myelodysplastic syndromes and acute myeloid leukemia. Am J Hematol. 98(3):481-92, 2023
2. Hoff FW et al: Molecular drivers of myelodysplastic neoplasms (MDS)-classification and prognostic relevance. Cells. 12(4), 2023
3. Hasserjian RP et al: The International Consensus Classification of myelodysplastic syndromes and related entities. Virchows Arch. 482(1):39-51, 2023
4. Jain AG et al: Myelodysplastic syndromes with bone marrow fibrosis: an update. Ann Lab Med. 42(3):299-305, 2022
5. Khoury JD et al: The 5th edition of the World Health Organization classification of haematolymphoid tumours: myeloid and histiocytic/dendritic neoplasms. Leukemia. 36(7):1703-19, 2022
6. Chiereghin C et al: The genetics of myelodysplastic syndromes: Clinical Relevance. Genes (Basel). 12(8), 2021
7. Scalzulli E et al: Therapeutic strategies in low and high-risk MDS: what does the future have to offer? Blood Rev. 45:100689, 2021
8. Gangat N et al: Mutations and prognosis in myelodysplastic syndromes: karyotype-adjusted analysis of targeted sequencing in 300 consecutive cases and development of a genetic risk model. Am J Hematol. 93(5):691-7, 2018

Myelodysplastic Syndrome, NOS

Pancytopenia With Erythroid Dysplasia

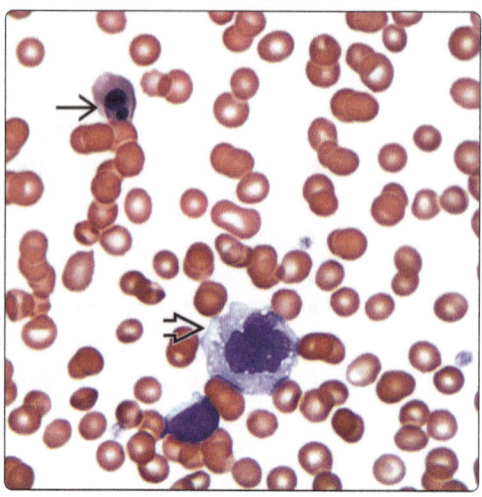

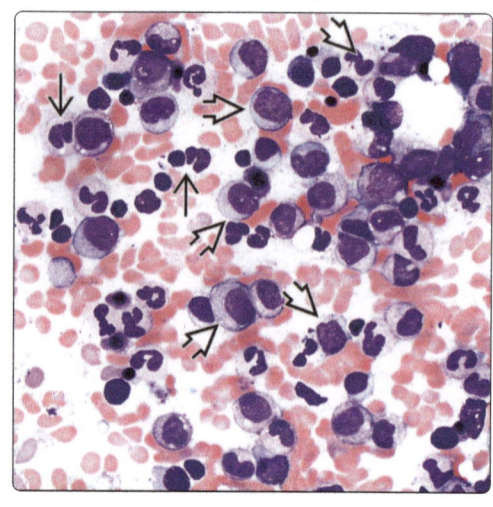

(Left) Peripheral blood smear from a 76-year-old woman with pancytopenia is shown. Rare circulating nucleated red blood cells with nuclear budding ⇒ are present. Only a few monocytes ⇒ are evident with irregularly shaped nuclei. (From DP: Blood & Bone Marrow.) **(Right)** Bone marrow shows myeloid dysplasia with cytoplasmic hypogranulation ⇒ in both granulocytic precursors and neutrophils. Occasional pseudo-Pelger-Huët nuclei ⇒ are also seen. (From DP: Blood & Bone Marrow.)

Granulocytic Dysplasia

Megakaryocytic Dysplasia

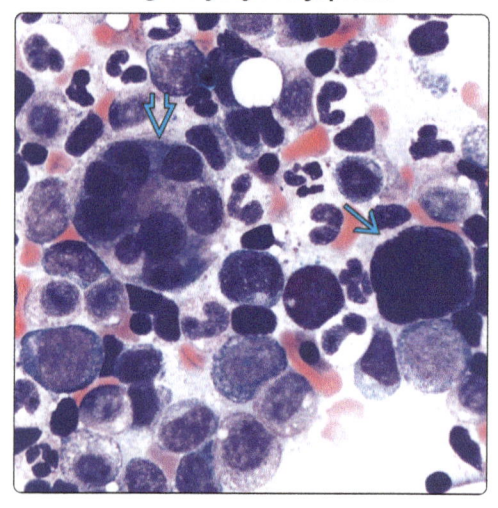

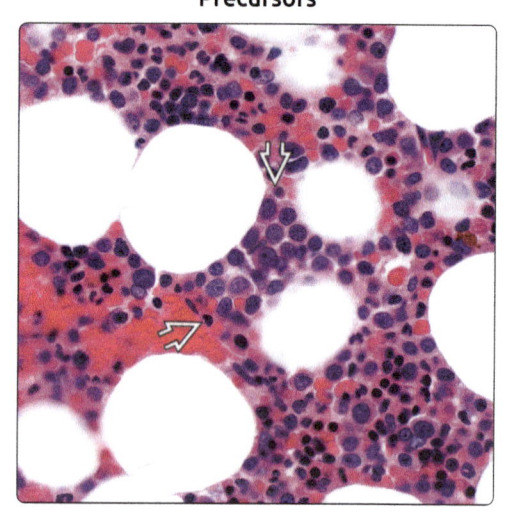

(Left) Dysplasia is also evident in the megakaryocytic lineage. Many megakaryocytes are small and hyperchromatic (micromegakaryocytes) ⇒, although some are larger with separate nuclei ⇒. (From DP: Blood & Bone Marrow.) **(Right)** Hypercellular marrow shows architectural distortion with abnormal localization of immature myeloid precursors (ALIP) ⇒. (From DP: Blood & Bone Marrow.)

Abnormal Localization of Immature Precursors

Limitations of FISH

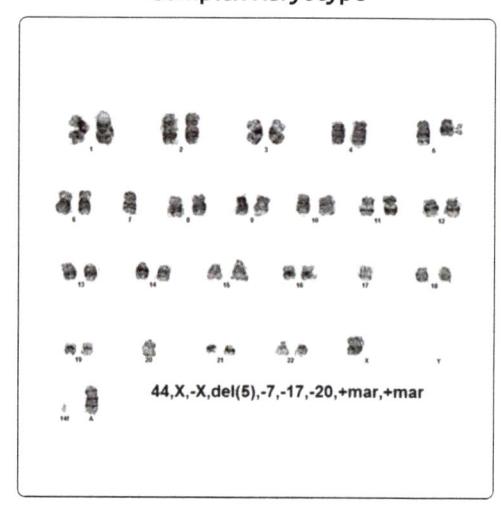

(Left) The information gained by FISH is limited by the probe set used. In this case of a patient with complex karyotype, only trisomy 8 and del(20q) are detected ⇒. Trisomy 8 is indicated by 3 green signals and del(20q) by the loss of 1 orange signal. **(Right)** Complex karyotype is defined by ≥ 3 cytogenetic abnormalities, as is seen in this karyogram of bone marrow. Complex karyotypes are associated with poor prognosis.

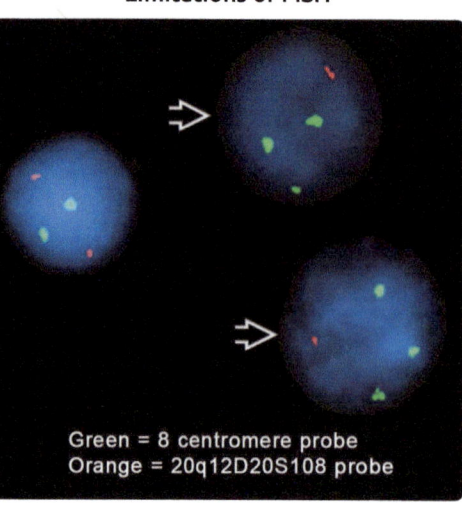

Green = 8 centromere probe
Orange = 20q12D20S108 probe

Complex Karyotype

44,X,-X,del(5),-7,-17,-20,+mar,+mar

Myelodysplastic Syndrome, NOS

Erythroid Dysplasia

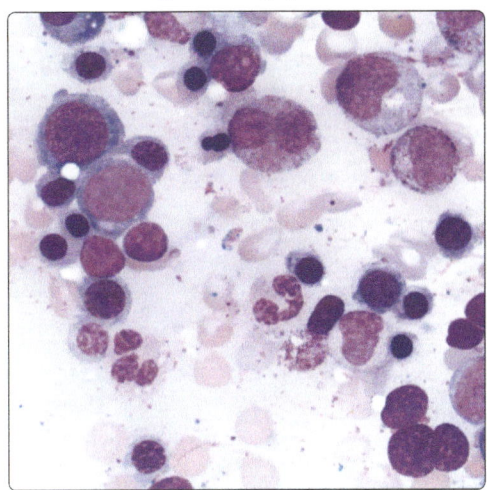

Disrupted Erythroid Colony Formation

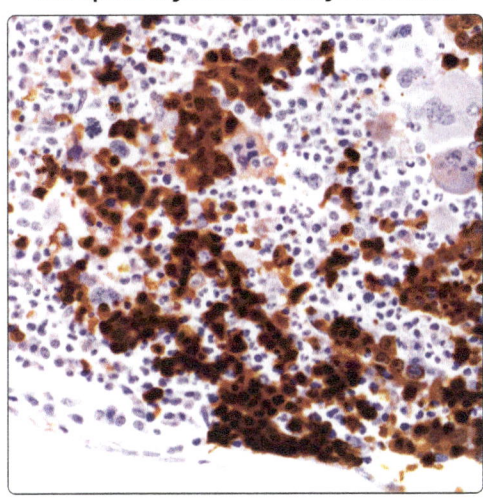

(Left) Myelodysplastic syndrome with single-lineage dysplasia (MDS-NOS, SLD) in a 52-year-old man shows typical features in the bone marrow aspirate smear, including megaloblastoid changes and mild dysplasia limited to erythroid lineage. (Right) Hemoglobin A shows disruption of normal erythroid colony formation and abnormal localization of erythroid precursors adjacent to bony trabeculae in this patient with MDS-NOS.

del(5q) With 5q Deletion

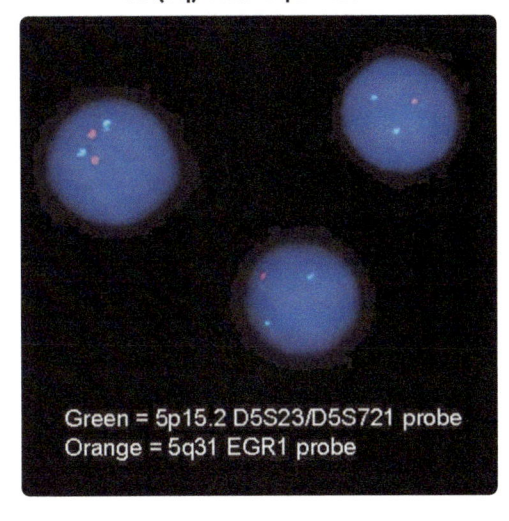

Green = 5p15.2 D5S23/D5S721 probe
Orange = 5q31 EGR1 probe

Karyotype With Isolated del(20q)

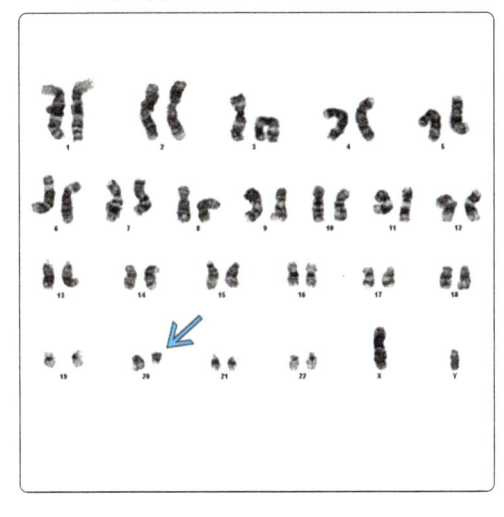

(Left) Cytogenetic abnormalities can be seen in up to 50% of MDS cases. del(5q), pictured here, can be seen in MDS with isolated 5q or concurrent with other MDS-related cytogenetic abnormalities. (Right) This case of MDS-NOS had an isolated del(20q) ➡ in 7 of 20 metaphases examined, confirming a clonal abnormality considered to be favorable by IPSS-R. If the bone marrow lacks significant dysplasia, only -7/7q or complex karyotype will qualify as MDS without dysplasia.

Dysplastic Megakaryocytes

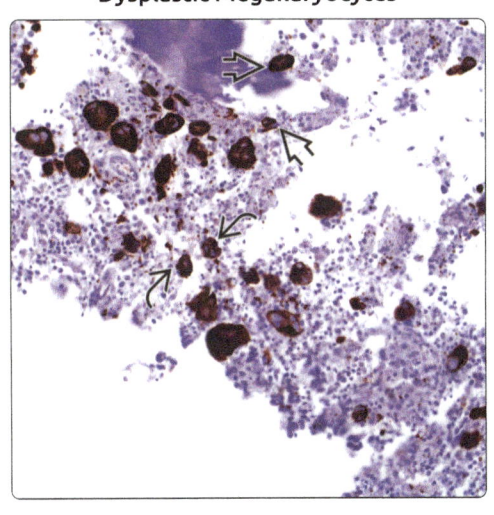

Increased Storage Iron

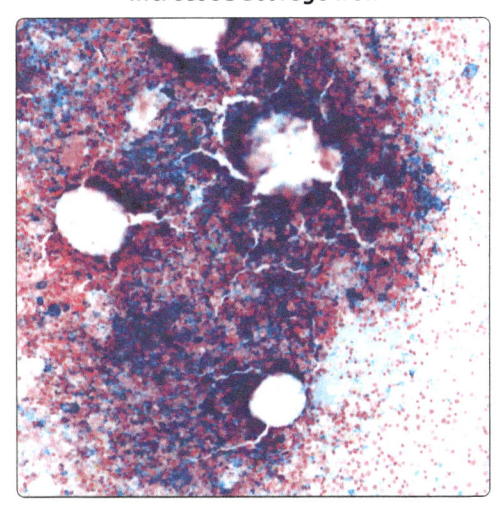

(Left) CD42b highlights increased megakaryocytes with many small forms ➡. Some of the megakaryocytes are abnormally localized adjacent to bony trabeculae ➡. (From DP: Blood & Bone Marrow.) (Right) A marked increase in storage iron is seen in this iron-stained aspirate smear from a man with MDS-NOS. If there are ring sideroblasts, molecular studies for SF3B1 mutations should be performed as this would change the classification. (From DP: Blood & Bone Marrow.)

Molecular Pathology of Myeloid Neoplasms

Myelodysplastic Syndrome, NOS

Single-Lineage (Erythroid) Dysplasia

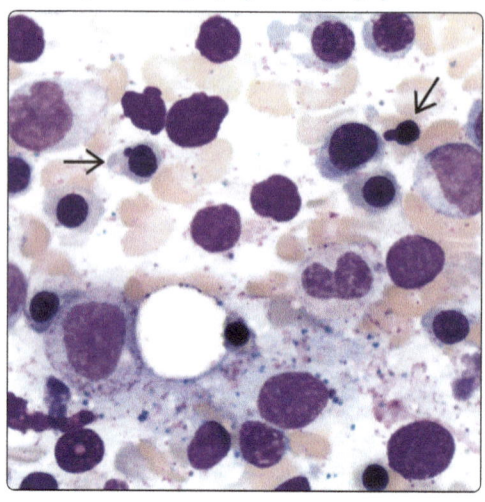

MDS-LB-SLD Lacks Ring Sideroblasts

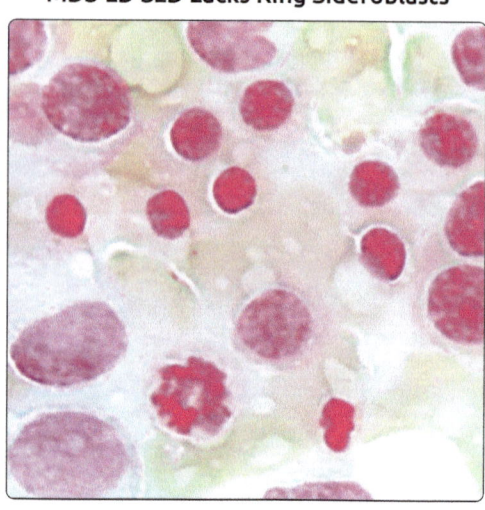

(Left) Dysplasia must be present in at least 10% of any one lineage without qualifying cytogenetics. Common erythroid dysplastic features include nuclear budding, binucleation, and other nuclear irregularities. They are often seen in the more mature erythroid precursors ➡. (Right) Iron stain of bone marrow aspirate smear shows decreased sideroblastic iron. Erythroid iron incorporation may vary, but by definition, there should be no SF3B1 mutation to qualify for MDS-NOS.

MDS-LB With Erythroid Hyperplasia

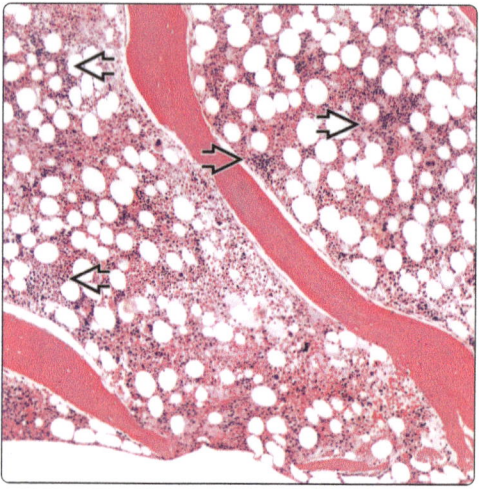

Dysplasia Isolated to Single Lineage

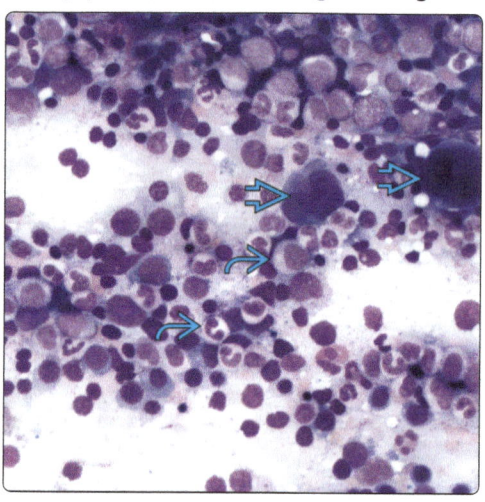

(Left) Core biopsy shows hypercellular bone marrow. In MDS-NOS, the marrow is often hypercellular relative to the patient's age and in many cases shows increased proliferation of the erythroid lineage. Erythroid colonies ➡ are easily identified. (Right) In MDS-NOS-SLD, only 1 lineage should have significant (> 10%) dysplasia. In this case with anemia and erythroid dysplasia (the most common presentation), note the normal morphology in the megakaryocytes ➡ and myeloid granulocytic lineage ➡.

Monosomy 7 in MDS

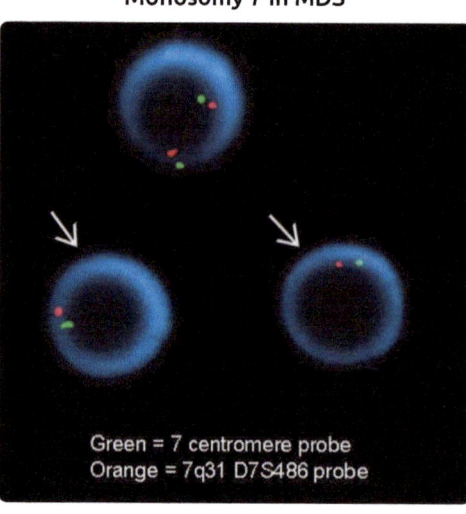

Karyotype Corroborates FISH Findings

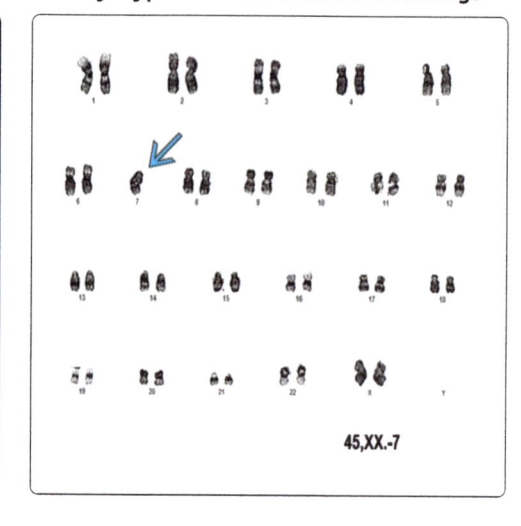

(Left) FISH shows a high percentage of cells with monosomy 7, one of the more common cytogenetic abnormalities in MDS. Note the loss of 1 copy of both the centromeric and 7q31 region probes in 2 of the 3 cells ➡. (Right) Chromosomal analysis should be used to confirm monosomy 7 ➡ if suspected from abnormal FISH results. This karyogram shows the loss of 1 copy of chromosome 7, corroborating the FISH findings.

Green = 7 centromere probe
Orange = 7q31 D7S486 probe

45,XX,-7

Myelodysplastic Syndrome, NOS

Differential Diagnoses: Megaloblastic Anemia

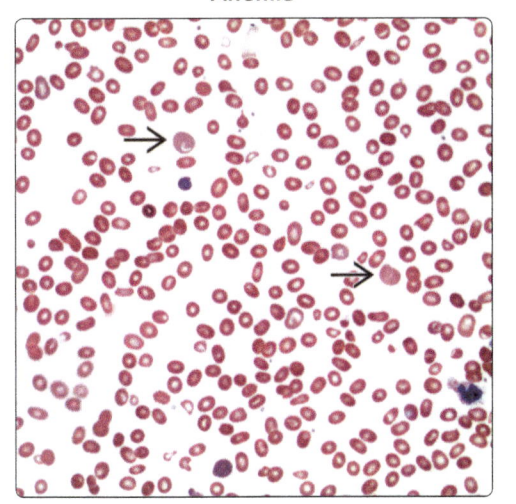

Differential Diagnosis: Folate Deficiency

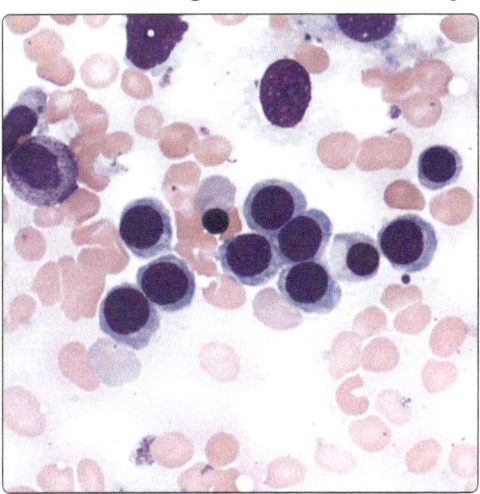

(Left) Peripheral blood smear from a patient with vitamin B12 deficiency shows macrocytic anemia with significant anisopoikilocytosis and occasional megalocytes ➡. (Right) Bone marrow aspirate smear from a patient with folate deficiency shows characteristic features of erythroid hyperplasia with megaloblastic changes. Note the sieve-like lacy chromatin pattern in the nuclei of erythroid precursors.

Dysplasia in Megaloblastic Anemia

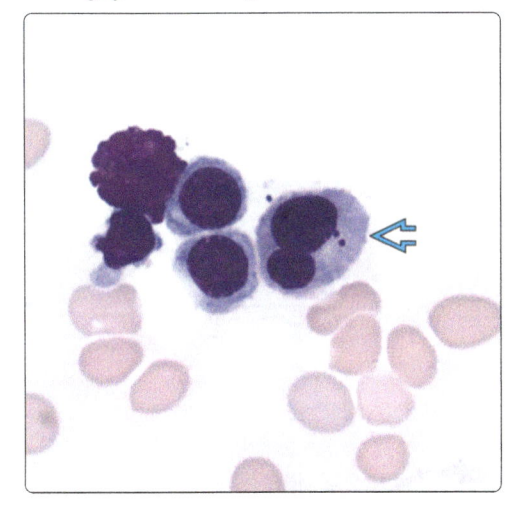

Megaloblastic Anemia

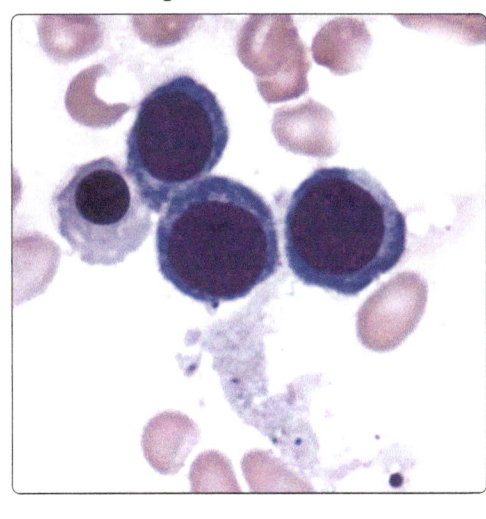

(Left) Erythroid series can show mild dysplastic features in patients with folate or vitamin B12 deficiency. Note the binucleated erythroid cell ⇦. (Right) Megaloblastic features include fine, lacy chromatin, seen in early erythroid precursors. This is caused by a defect in DNA synthesis that interferes with cellular proliferation and maturation, while the cytoplasmic components remain relatively unaffected, resulting in nuclear-cytoplasmic dyssynchrony.

Folate Deficiency

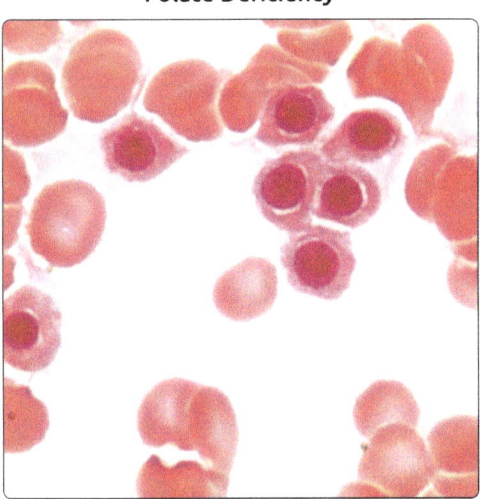

Folate Deficiency

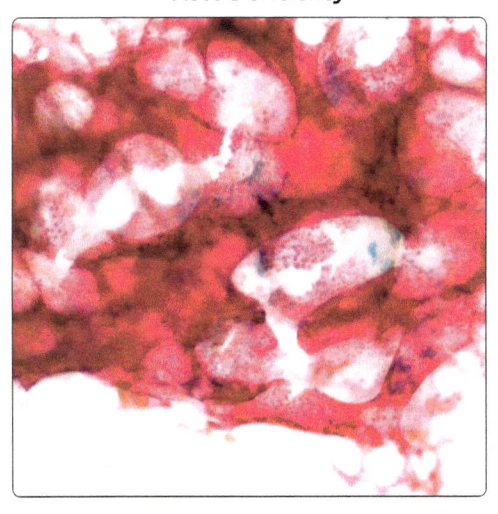

(Left) Iron stain of bone marrow aspirate smear from a patient with folate deficiency shows an absence of any ring sideroblasts. (Right) Evaluation of thicker particles in the same bone marrow aspirate smear shows adequate but not significantly increased amounts of storage iron in the macrophages in this patient with folate deficiency. Patients with anemia of chronic disease or myelodysplastic syndromes may have increased storage iron.

Molecular Pathology of Myeloid Neoplasms

199

Myelodysplastic Syndrome With del(5q)

KEY FACTS

TERMINOLOGY
- MDS with del(5q) (2022 ICC)
- MDS with low blasts and isolated 5q deletion (WHO-HAEM5)

ETIOLOGY/PATHOGENESIS
- Heterozygous interstitial deletion of 5q
  - Haploinsufficiency of deleted genes plays critical role in molecular pathogenesis
  - Deleted region includes ~ 44 genes
  - Commonly and invariably involve q32-33.1 designated as commonly deleted region 1
  - Significant genes and miRNAs affected
    - *CSNK1A1*
      - Important target for lenalidomide
      - CK1A1 is targeted for degradation via ubiquitination by lenalidomide
      - Degradation of CK1A1 leads to activation of TP53 and consequent cell cycle arrest and apoptosis
    - *RPS14*
      - Allelic deletion is mainly responsible for ineffective erythropoiesis
      - Deficiency leads to erythroid maturation block and increased TP53-dependent apoptosis
    - *G3BP1*
      - Encodes DNA unwinding enzyme that binds specifically to Ras-GTPase activating protein
      - Initiates signal transduction cascades, including NFκB
      - Haploinsufficiency results in downstream NF-κB activation
  - Other important genes implicated
    - *TNIP1*, *ANXA6*, *SPARC*, *RBM22*, *EGR1*, *TCOF1*

CLINICAL ISSUES
- Most symptoms are related to anemia, usually macrocytic
- Platelets are increased or normal
- Thrombocytosis seen in 30-50% of cases
- Thrombocytopenia is uncommon
- Significant clinical response to lenalidomide
- Overall good prognosis
  - Transformation to acute myeloid leukemia in < 10% of cases
- Decreased overall survival and resistance to lenalidomide in cases with *TP53* mutations

MICROSCOPIC
- Peripheral blood
  - Macrocytic anemia
  - Normal or increased platelets
  - Blasts < 2%
- Bone marrow
  - Normocellular to hypercellular
  - Megakaryocytic proliferation with increased small, hypolobated forms
  - Blasts < 5%

ANCILLARY TESTS
- Conventional cytogenetics
  - Deletion 5q in isolation or 1 other abnormality (excluding monosomy 7 or deletion 7q)
- FISH
  - May be useful
  - Does not detect other abnormalities
- Molecular testing
  - Mutations in *JAK2* or *MPL* detected in ~ 5% and 4%, respectively
  - *TP53* mutations, if present, cannot be biallelic or multihit
    - Associated with inferior outcomes
  - Other uncommon but reported mutations include *ASXL1*, *TET2*, *SF3B1*, *RUNX1*, and *WT1*

TOP DIFFERENTIAL DIAGNOSES
- Other subtypes of MDS
- MDS, not otherwise specified with single or multilineage dysplasia

Macrocytic Anemia and Thrombocytosis

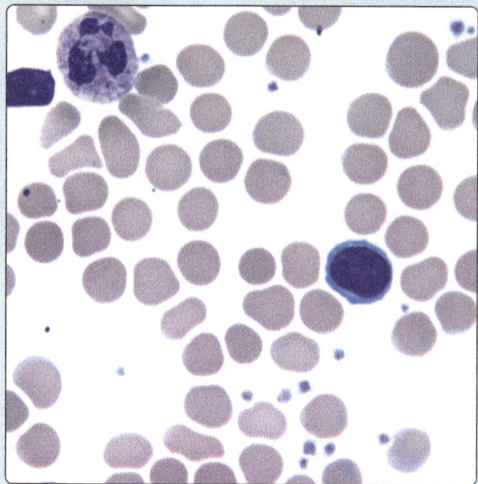

Hypolobated Megakaryocyte

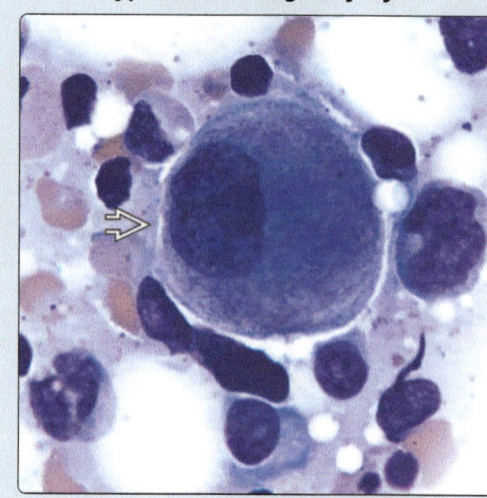

(Left) Peripheral blood from a patient with myelodysplastic syndrome (MDS) with del(5q) shows macrocytic anemia and thrombocytosis. (Right) Bone marrow aspirate shows an atypical small, hypolobated megakaryocyte ➡, characteristic of MDS with del(5q). No increased blasts or other features of dyspoiesis are present in this case.

Myelodysplastic Syndrome With del(5q)

TERMINOLOGY

Abbreviations
- MDS with deletion 5q [MDS-del(5q)]

Synonyms
- Myelodysplastic syndrome with isolated del(5q)

Definitions
- Distinct WHO/ICC-defined category of MDS characterized by anemia (usually macrocytic) ± other cytopenias &/or thrombocytosis
- Interstitial deletion of chromosome 5q involving heterozygous deletion at q32-33 either in isolation or with 1 other cytogenetic abnormality other than monosomy 7 or del(7q)
- Myeloblasts < 5% in bone marrow and < 2% in peripheral blood

CLASSIFICATION

ICC vs. WHO-HAEM5
- MDS with del(5q) (2022 ICC)
- MDS with low blasts and isolated 5q deletion (WHO-HAEM5)
- Similar diagnostic criteria in both 2022 ICC and WHO-HAEM5
  - Blasts < 2% in peripheral blood and < 5% in bone marrow
  - 5q deletion alone or with 1 additional abnormality except -7/del7(q)

ETIOLOGY/PATHOGENESIS

Heterozygous Interstitial Deletion of 5q
- Haploinsufficiency of deleted genes plays critical role in molecular pathogenesis
- Deleted region includes ~ 44 genes
- Commonly and invariably involve q32-q33.1 designated as commonly deleted region 1 (CDR1)
- Significant genes and miRNAs affected
  - *CSNK1A1*
    - Important target for lenalidomide
    - Encodes for casein kinase 1A1 (CK1A1) protein
    - Heterozygous loss contributes to clonal advantage of 5q minus cells
      - Via WNT/β-catenin pathway deregulation
    - CK1A1 is targeted for degradation via ubiquitination by lenalidomide
    - Degradation of CK1A1 leads to activation of TP53 and consequent cell cycle arrest and apoptosis
  - *RPS14*
    - Allelic deletion is mainly responsible for ineffective erythropoiesis
      - Deficiency leads to block of erythroid maturation and increased TP53-dependent apoptosis
  - Other altered genes implicated in pathogenesis of MDS with isolated del(5q)
    - *TNIP1, G3BP1, ANXA6, SPARC, RBM22, EGR1, TCOF1*

CLINICAL ISSUES

Epidemiology
- Strongly associated with female sex
- ~ 60-70 years of age

Presentation
- Most symptoms related to anemia, usually macrocytic
- Platelets are increased or normal
  - Thrombocytosis seen in 30-50% of cases
  - Thrombocytopenia is uncommon

Treatment
- Significant clinical response to lenalidomide

Prognosis
- Median overall survival: 66-145 months
- < 10% incidence of transformation to AML
- Worse outcomes associated with male sex, older age, neutropenia, and *SF3B1* mutations

MOLECULAR

Cytogenetics
- Detects interstitial deletion of long arm of chromosome 5 (5q32-33)
- 1 additional cytogenetic abnormality can be present, except for monosomy 7 or del(7q)

Molecular Genetics
- *JAK2* V617F and *MPL* W515L mutations may be present and do not alter prognosis
- *TP53* mutations
  - If present, cannot be biallelic or multihit
  - Associated with resistance to lenalidomide, increased risk of transformation, and decreased overall survival

MICROSCOPIC

Peripheral Blood
- Typically macrocytic anemia
- Normal platelet or thrombocytosis
- White cells are usually unremarkable
- Blasts account for < 2%

Bone Marrow
- Cellularity is usually normal or increased
- Erythroid hypoplasia is frequent
- Hypolobated micromegakaryocytes
- Dysplasia in myeloid or erythroid lineages is uncommon
- Blasts not increased (< 5%)

DIFFERENTIAL DIAGNOSIS

Other Subtypes of Myelodysplastic Syndrome
- MDS, not otherwise specified with single lineage or multilineage dysplasia
  - Multilineage dysplasia is uncommon in MDS with del(5q)

SELECTED REFERENCES

1. Hasserjian RP et al: The International Consensus Classification of myelodysplastic syndromes and related entities. Virchows Arch. 482(1):39-51, 2023
2. Arber DA et al: International Consensus Classification of myeloid neoplasms and acute leukemia: integrating morphological, clinical, and genomic data. Blood. 40(11):1200-28, 2022
3. Khoury JD et al: The 5th edition of the World Health Organization Classification of haematolymphoid tumours: myeloid and histiocytic/dendritic neoplasms. Leukemia. 36(7):1703-19, 2022

Myelodysplastic Syndrome With del(5q)

Hypolobated Megakaryocytes

Intact Erythropoiesis and Granulopoiesis

(Left) Bone marrow aspirate shows small, hypolobated megakaryocytes in a case of MDS with del(5q) ⇒. This abnormal megakaryocytic morphology is characteristic of MDS with del(5q) but not specific. (From DP: Blood & Bone Marrow.) (Right) Bone marrow aspirate shows intact erythropoiesis and granulopoiesis in a case of MDS with del(5q). While some cases may show dyserythropoiesis, granulocytic dysplasia or increased blasts (≥ 5%) are absent. (From DP: Blood & Bone Marrow.)

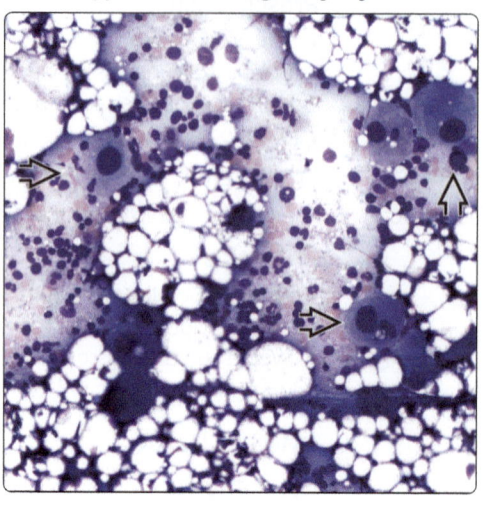

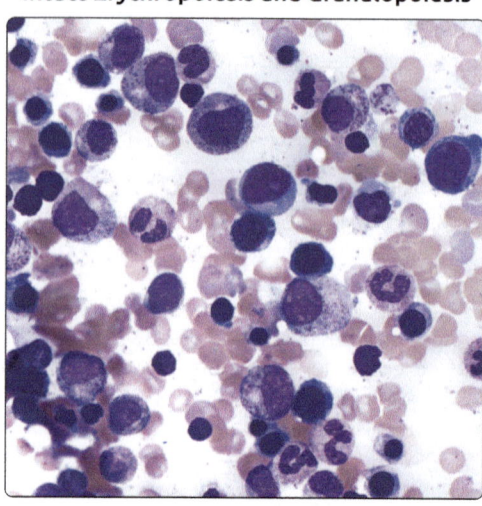

Hypolobated Micromegakaryocytes and Mild Dyserythropoiesis

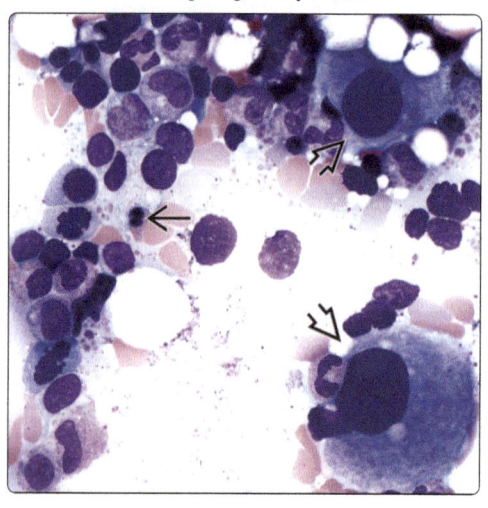

Normocellular Marrow

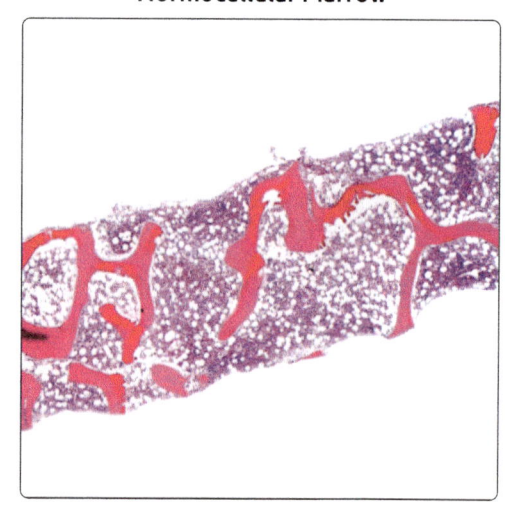

(Left) Bone marrow aspirate shows hypolobated micromegakaryocytes ⇒ and mild dyserythropoiesis ⇒ in a case of MDS with del(5q). The granulocytic lineage is intact. (From DP: Blood & Bone Marrow.) (Right) Bone marrow core biopsy from a 55-year-old patient with MDS with del(5q) shows normocellular marrow. (From DP: Blood & Bone Marrow.)

Hypolobated Megakaryocytes

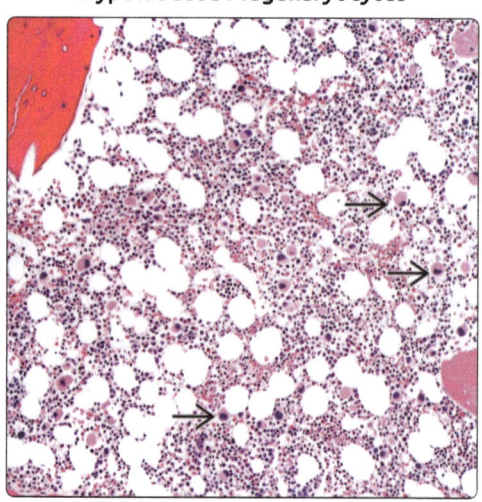

Variably Sized Megakaryocytes

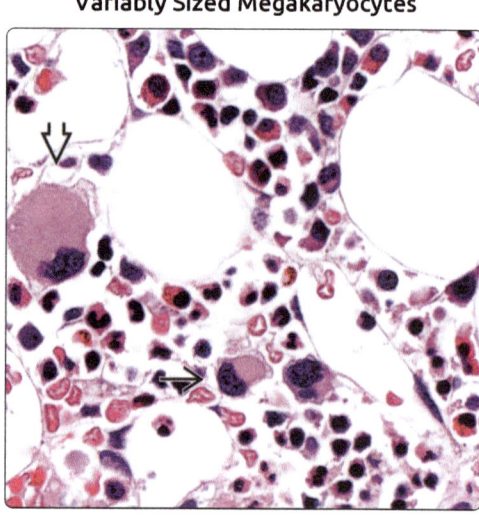

(Left) Bone marrow core biopsy shows intact trilineage hematopoiesis with characteristic abnormal small, hypolobated megakaryocytes ⇒. No significant fibrosis or increased immature cells are seen. (From DP: Blood & Bone Marrow.) (Right) Bone marrow core biopsy from a patient with MDS with del(5q) shows some variability in size of the abnormal megakaryocytes, ranging from small ⇒ to relatively large ⇒. (From DP: Blood & Bone Marrow.)

Myelodysplastic Syndrome With del(5q)

Micromegakaryocytes

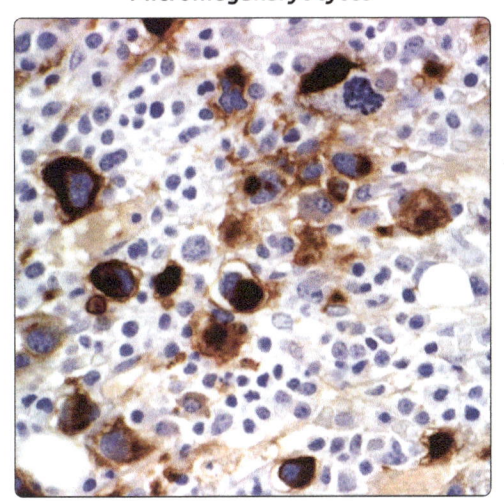

Aggregates of Dysplastic Megakaryocytes

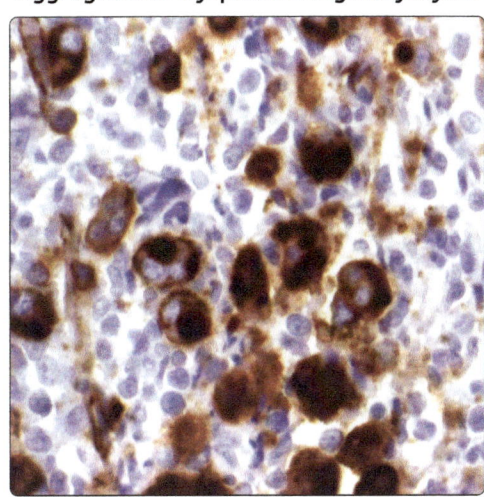

(Left) CD42b highlights micromegakaryocytes in this case of MDS with del(5q). Often, CD42b reveals more megakaryocytes than are appreciated on H&E. (From DP: Blood & Bone Marrow.) (Right) CD61 is a useful marker of megakaryocytic differentiation, including immature forms. This case of MDS with del(5q) shows increased and loosely clustered aggregates of dysplastic megakaryocytes. (From DP: Blood & Bone Marrow.)

Neoangiogenesis and Rare Blast

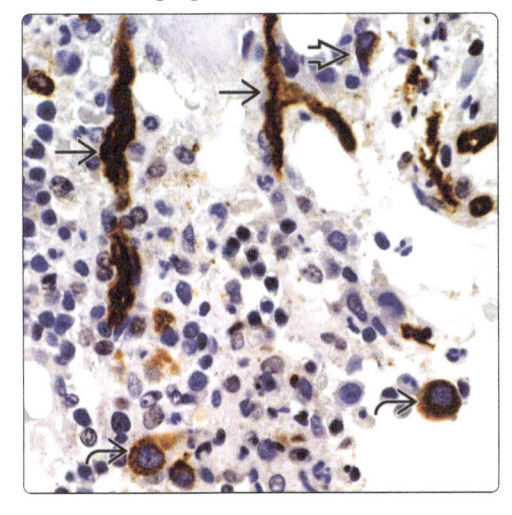

PCR for *JAK2* Exon 14 Mutation Analysis

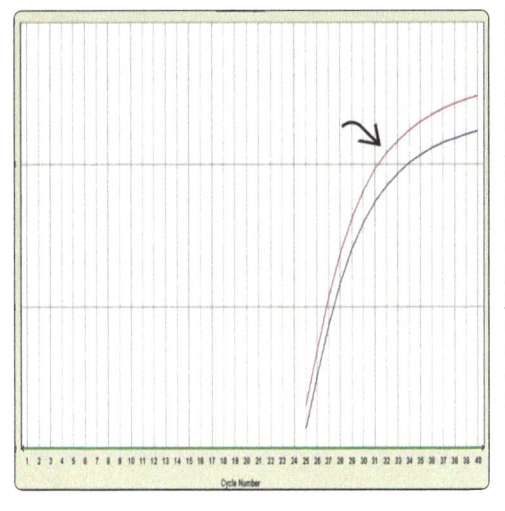

(Left) CD34 shows neoangiogenesis ➡ and a rare blast ➡ in this case of MDS with del(5q). Abnormal megakaryocytes show strong positivity ➡, as reported in the literature. (From DP: Blood & Bone Marrow.) (Right) PCR analysis of JAK2 exon 14 using an allelic discrimination assay performed on peripheral blood from a patient with MDS with del(5q) shows a JAK2 V617F mutation ➡. JAK2 mutations are detectable in ~ 5% of MDS with isolated del(5q).

FISH of Interphase Nuclei

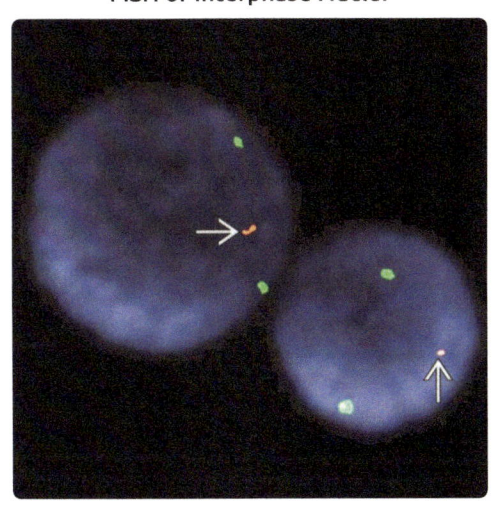

Conventional Cytogenetics

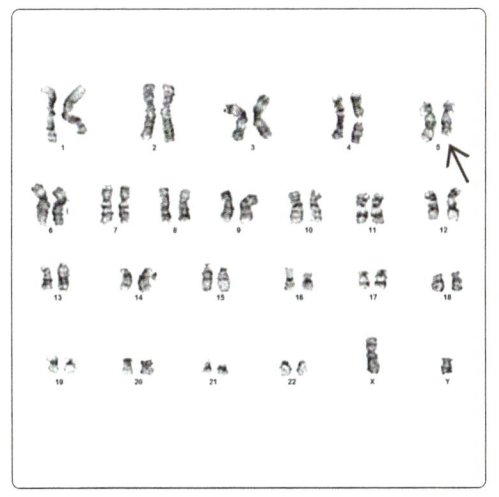

(Left) FISH for 5q shows 2 interphase nuclei, each with an abnormal pattern. Each nucleus shows a single orange signal ➡ instead of 2 normal signals, consistent with loss of 5q. (From DP: Blood & Bone Marrow.) (Right) Karyogram shows deletion of the 5q32-33 region ➡ as the only abnormal finding. In the proper clinical and morphologic setting, this would be diagnostic for MDS with isolated del(5q).

Myelodysplastic Syndrome With *TP53* Multihit Mutations

KEY FACTS

TERMINOLOGY
- MDS with mutated *TP53* (ICC)
- Myelodysplastic neoplasm with biallelic *TP53* inactivation (WHO-HAEM5)
- Multihit/biallelic status generally determined by
  - ≥ 2 distinct *TP53* mutations [each with variant allele fraction (VAF) > 10%] **or** 1 mutation associated with either cytogenetic deletion of 17p, VAF > 50%, or copy neutral loss of heterozygosity (LOH) at 17p *TP53* locus (ICC)

ETIOLOGY/PATHOGENESIS
- Minority of cases are hereditary
  - Li-Fraumeni syndrome (germline *TP53* mutations)

CLINICAL ISSUES
- Prognosis
  - High risk of transformation and death, independent of Revised International Prognostic Scoring System (IPSS-R) and treatment, even with allogeneic stem cell transplant

MOLECULAR
- Most common inactivating mutations are within DNA binding domain
- Typically accompanied by complex karyotype

ANCILLARY TESTS
- Immunohistochemistry
  - p53 accumulation (increased nuclear p53 staining) in many cases
  - Good screening tool but not specific

DIAGNOSTIC CHECKLIST
- Must include sequencing-based assay to make this diagnosis

Circulating Blasts and Dysplastic Neutrophils

Dysplastic Megakaryocytes

(Left) Peripheral blood smear from a 74-year-old man with pancyopenia shows circulating blasts ➡ and dysplastic neutrophils ➡ with atypical nuclear lobulation and hypogranular cytoplasm. (From DP3: Blood and Bone Marrow.) (Right) Bone marrow biopsy shows hypercellularity with numerous dysplastic megakaryocytes ➡ with nuclear hypolobation. The myeloid lineage is left shifted with hypolobated mature neutrophils present ➡. (From DP3: Blood and Bone Marrow.)

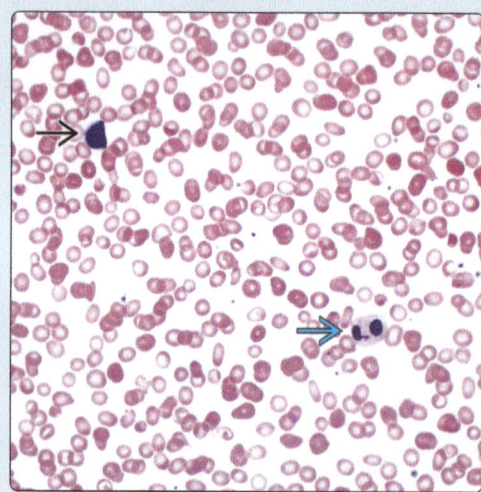

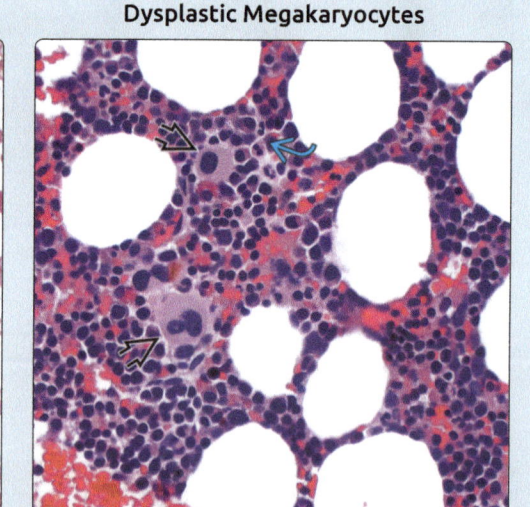

p53 Immunohistochemistry

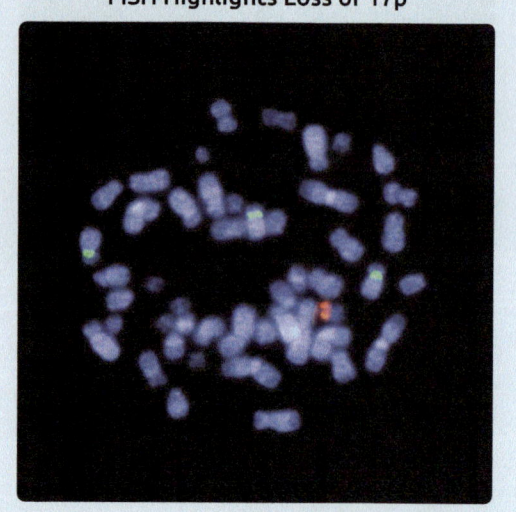

FISH Highlights Loss of 17p

(Left) p53 shows strong nuclear positivity in numerous cells in bone marrow. This finding raises suspicion for TP53 mutation. (From DP3: Blood and Bone Marrow.) (Right) Metaphase FISH preparation shows only 1 red signal for TP53, indicating loss of one 17p region, including the loss of TP53. Note that there are 3 green signals, indicating trisomy of chromosome 8. (From DP3: Blood and Bone Marrow.)

Myelodysplastic Syndrome With *TP53* Multihit Mutations

TERMINOLOGY

Synonyms
- MDS with mutated *TP53* (MDS-*TP53*) (ICC)
- MDS/AML with mutated *TP53* (ICC)

Definitions
- New genetic subtype of MDS with multihit *TP53* mutation
  - Cytopenia(s)
  - 0-9% blasts (ICC)
    - In ICC classification, if 10-19% blasts, classified as MDS/AML with mutated *TP53*
  - < 20% blasts (WHO-HAEM5)
  - ≥ 2 distinct *TP53* mutations (each with VAF > 10%) **or** 1 mutation associated with either cytogenetic deletion of 17p, VAF > 50%, or copy neutral loss of heterozygosity (LOH) at 17p *TP53* locus (ICC)
  - In absence of LOH information, presence of single *TP53* mutation at VAF ≥ 10% in context of any complex karyotype is considered equivalent to multihit *TP53*

CLASSIFICATION

ICC vs. WHO-HAEM5
- MDS with mutated *TP53* (ICC)
- MDS with biallelic *TP53* inactivation (WHO-HAEM5)

ETIOLOGY/PATHOGENESIS

Environmental Exposure
- DNA-damaging agents
  - Chemotherapy
  - Radiation

Hereditary
- Li-Fraumeni syndrome (germline *TP53* mutations)
- Bone marrow failure syndromes

CLINICAL ISSUES

Epidemiology
- ~ 10% of all MDS

Presentation
- Related to cytopenia(s)
  - Anemia
  - Thrombocytopenia
  - Neutropenia

Prognosis
- High risk of transformation and death, independent of Revised International Prognostic Scoring System (IPSS-R) and treatment, even with transplant

MOLECULAR

Cytogenetics
- Typically accompanied by complex karyotype, which often includes
  - del(5q), 17p LOH, -7/del(7q), -18
  - Monosomal karyotype

Molecular Genetics
- *TP53* mutations
  - Variable; best detected by various sequencing methods
  - Most often in DNA binding domain, inactivating
  - Copy number status can be detected by FISH probe
    - Also by array CGH or massively parallel sequencing methods
    - 17p13.1 deletion is not sufficient to confirm *TP53* copy number loss
    - Variant allele fraction on massively parallel sequencing > 49% is presumptive evidence of biallelic status
    - ≥ 2 mutations can be assumed to act as biallelic (in trans)

MICROSCOPIC

Bone Marrow Findings
- Nonspecific but more aggressive features
  - May have higher blast percentage
  - Fibrosis may be more common

ANCILLARY TESTS

Immunohistochemistry
- p53 accumulation (increased nuclear p53 staining) in many cases
  - Good screening tool but not specific
  - Cases with truncation types of mutations may have virtual absence of p53

DIFFERENTIAL DIAGNOSIS

Acute Myeloid Leukemia
- Distinguish by blast count and any other defining/recurrent genetic abnormalities

Acute Erythroid Leukemia
- ICC includes this entity within AML with mutated *TP53*
- WHO-HAEM5 still considers this as distinct entity
  - > 80% cells of erythroid lineage
  - > 30% erythroblasts/pronormoblasts

DIAGNOSTIC CHECKLIST

Pathologic Interpretation Pearls
- Sequencing studies (often massively parallel sequencing myeloid panels) are essential to make this diagnosis
  - Additional studies to determine copy number/loss of heterozygosity may also be necessary
- p53 IHC can be used as screening tool
  - Patterns are not entirely specific but high expression or complete absence of expression is suggestive
  - Follow with confirmatory genetic testing

SELECTED REFERENCES

1. Hasserjian RP et al: The International Consensus Classification of myelodysplastic syndromes and related entities. Virchows Arch. 482(1):39-51, 2023
2. Arber DA et al: International Consensus Classification of myeloid Neoplasms and acute leukemia: integrating morphological, clinical, and genomic data. Blood. 140(11):1200-28, 2022
3. Khoury JD et al: The 5th edition of the World Health Organization Classification of haematolymphoid umours: myeloid and histiocytic/dendritic neoplasms. Leukemia. 36(7):1703-19, 2022
4. Tashakori M et al: TP53 copy number and protein expression inform mutation status across risk categories in acute myeloid leukemia. Blood. 140(1):58-72, 2022

Myelodysplastic Syndrome/Acute Myeloid Leukemia

KEY FACTS

TERMINOLOGY
- Myelodysplastic syndrome (MDS) with increased blasts 2 (MDS-IB-2) in WHO-HAEM5 is essentially equivalent to MDS/acute myeloid leukemia (AML) definition in ICC

CLASSIFICATION
- MDS/AML (ICC only)
  - Genetic profile more important than arbitrary blast count
- Not recognized as entity in WHO-HAEM5

CLINICAL ISSUES
- Can be managed as MDS or AML as appropriate
- New "hybrid" classification allows for earlier intervention in what were previously high-risk MDS cases that behaved similarly to AML
- Prognosis similar to AML

ANCILLARY TESTS
- Genetic/molecular testing
  - Both increase in numbers of mutated genes and increase in variant allele fraction are seen with worsening disease and progression to AML

TOP DIFFERENTIAL DIAGNOSES
- AML with recurrent genetic abnormality
  - Cytogenetic and molecular testing at presentation are essential in proper classification, prognostication, and treatment
- Myeloproliferative neoplasms in accelerated phase
- Chronic myelomonocytic leukemia

DIAGNOSTIC CHECKLIST
- Clinical features and molecular profile help predict biologic subtype and course of disease
- Cytogenetic analysis required to exclude AML-defining cytogenetic abnormalities

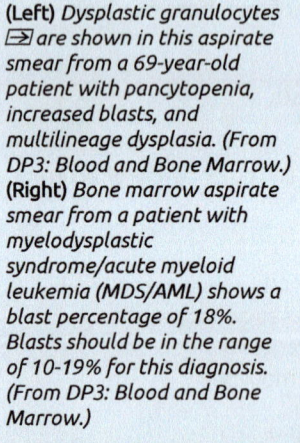

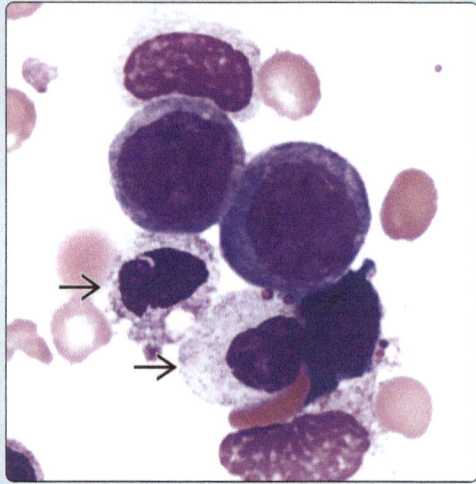

Dysplastic Granulocytes
(Left) Dysplastic granulocytes ➡ are shown in this aspirate smear from a 69-year-old patient with pancytopenia, increased blasts, and multilineage dysplasia. (From DP3: Blood and Bone Marrow.)

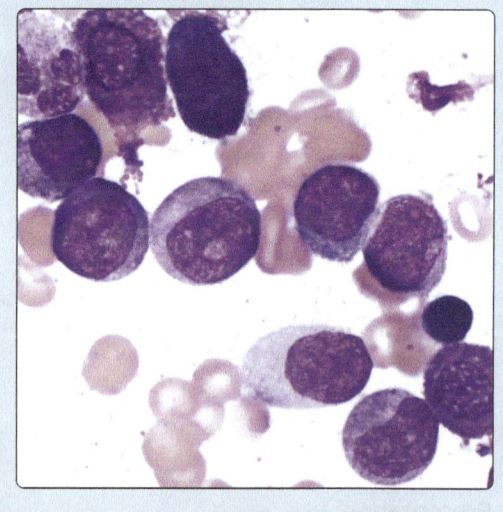

Increased Blasts
(Right) Bone marrow aspirate smear from a patient with myelodysplastic syndrome/acute myeloid leukemia (MDS/AML) shows a blast percentage of 18%. Blasts should be in the range of 10-19% for this diagnosis. (From DP3: Blood and Bone Marrow.)

Hypercellular Bone Marrow
(Left) Bone marrow core biopsy from a patient with MDS/AML shows marked hypercellularity. All lineages are present but abnormal. Note the increased immature precursors as well as erythroid ➡ and megakaryocytic ➡ dysplasia. (From DP3: Blood and Bone Marrow.)

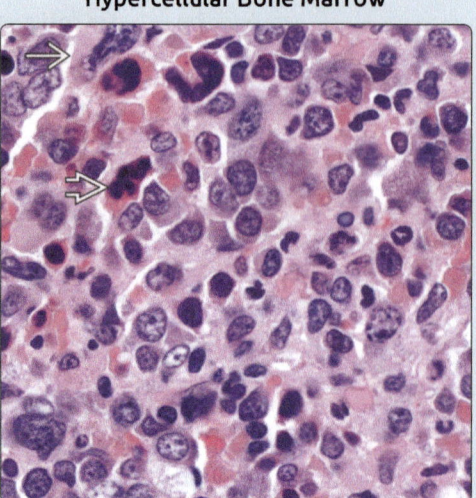

CD34 Immunohistochemistry
(Right) CD34 can be especially useful when aspirates or touch preps are inadequate for cytologic evaluation. Although blasts are not always CD34(+), in this case, blasts are increased and seen in clusters. (From DP3: Blood and Bone Marrow.)

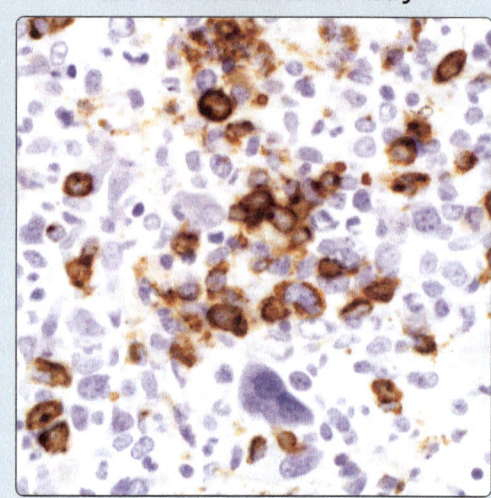

Myelodysplastic Syndrome/Acute Myeloid Leukemia

TERMINOLOGY

Abbreviations
- Myelodysplastic syndrome/acute myeloid leukemia (MDS/AML)

Synonyms
- Previously MDS with excess blasts (MDS-EB-2)

Definitions
- ≥ 1 cytopenias
- Dysplasia in ≥ 1 lineages
- 10-19% blasts in peripheral blood (PB) or bone marrow (BM)
- Must exclude AML cases with defining genetic abnormality
- Does not apply to pediatric population

CLASSIFICATION

ICC Only
- Genetic profile more important than arbitrary blast count
- MDS/AML terminology not used in WHO-HAEM5 classification
- MDS with increased blasts 2 (MDS-IB-2) in WHO-HAEM5 is essentially equivalent to MDS/AML definition in ICC

ETIOLOGY/PATHOGENESIS

Genetics
- Acquisition of somatic mutations leads to expansion of hematopoietic clones; further mutations lead to transformation to malignancy

CLINICAL ISSUES

Epidemiology
- Age
  - Older individuals

Presentation
- Cytopenias

Treatment
- Can be managed as MDS or AML as appropriate
- New "hybrid" classification allows for earlier intervention in what were previously high-risk MDS cases that behaved similarly to AML

Prognosis
- Similar to AML
- Median survival: 1.3 years
- Influenced by comorbidities

MICROSCOPIC

Histologic Features
- Marrow cellularity is often increased but can be normal or even decreased

Cytologic Features
- Dysplasia typically present in at least 1 lineage
  - Neutrophils often bilobed, monolobated, &/or hypogranular
  - Erythroid lineage often shows nuclear budding or other nuclear irregularities
  - Megakaryocytes may be small and monolobated or have separated lobes
- Blasts
  - Percentage should be 10-19% in PB or in BM aspirate smear

Peripheral Blood
- ≥ 1 cytopenias required

ANCILLARY TESTS

Immunohistochemistry
- CD34 on core biopsy can be helpful if aspirate smears are inadequate

Genetic Testing
- Increases in variant allele fraction (VAF) of mutated genes and number of genes mutated are seen with worsening disease and progression to AML

DIFFERENTIAL DIAGNOSIS

Acute Myeloid Leukemia With Recurrent Genetic Abnormality
- Cytogenetic and molecular testing at presentation are essential in proper classification, prognostication, and treatment

Myeloproliferative Neoplasms in Accelerated Phase
- Also have 10-19% blasts, but have MPN features
  - Cytoses are often present; should not be seen in MDS
  - Megakaryocytes have MPN-like features rather than dysplasia
    - May have "staghorn," cloud-like, or balloon-like morphology
    - Often large and hypersegmented

Chronic Myelomonocytic Leukemia-2
- PB monocytosis
- Myeloproliferative components, such as other cytoses
- BM increase in monocytes, promonocytes, and monoblasts (10-19%)

DIAGNOSTIC CHECKLIST

Clinically Relevant Pathologic Features
- Clinical features and molecular profile help predict biologic subtype and course of disease
- MDS/AML designation opens treatment options to include AML-appropriate modalities

Pathologic Interpretation Pearls
- Cytogenetic and molecular correlation is essential for appropriate classification

SELECTED REFERENCES

1. Hasserjian RP et al: The International Consensus Classification of myelodysplastic syndromes and related entities. Virchows Arch. 482(1):39-51, 2023

Pediatric Myelodysplastic Syndrome and Refractory Cytopenia of Childhood

KEY FACTS

TERMINOLOGY
- Refractory cytopenia of childhood (RCC)/childhood myelodysplastic syndrome (MDS)-low blasts
  - Persistent cytopenia(s) during childhood
  - < 2% blasts in peripheral blood (PB)
  - < 5% blasts in bone marrow (BM)
- Classify as MDS-EB (ICC) or cMDS-IB (WHO-HAEM5) if 2-19% PB or 5-19% BM blasts present

CLINICAL ISSUES
- Pediatric MDS
  - RCC is most common subtype
- Prognosis
  - Monosomy 7 or complex karyotype has highest risk for disease progression
  - Trisomy 8 or normal karyotype have long, stable course

MOLECULAR
- Monosomy 7 is most common karyotypic abnormality
- Somatic mutations may help support diagnosis of childhood MDS
- Testing for germline predisposition is warranted

MICROSCOPIC
- Minimal diagnostic criteria required
  - Dysplastic changes in 2 lineages (erythroid, granulocytic, megakaryocytic) or ≥ 10% dysplasia in single lineage
- 80% of RCC cases hypocellular
- CD34 helps to identify blasts and subtype of MDS
- CD61 or CD41 helpful to identify micromegakaryocytes

TOP DIFFERENTIAL DIAGNOSES
- Myeloid neoplasms, post cytotoxic &/or radiation therapy
- Acquired aplastic anemia
- Acquired BM failure disorders
- Low-blast-count acute myeloid leukemia
- Reactive disorders with cytologic dysplasia

Pseudo-Pelger Huët Neutrophil

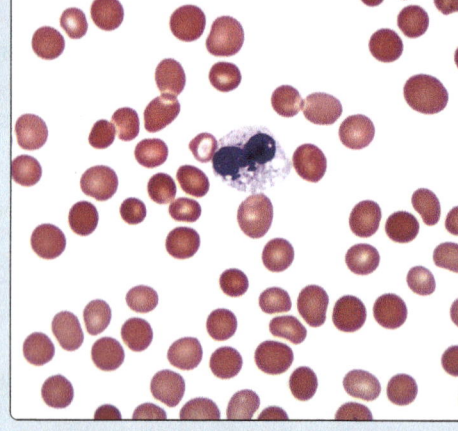

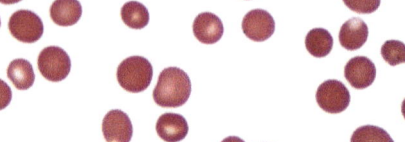

Hypocellular Bone Marrow

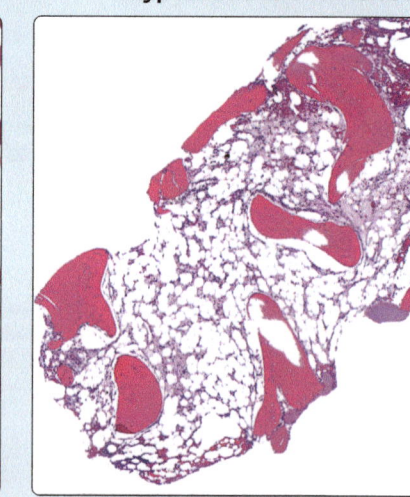

(Left) Peripheral blood in this patient with refractory cytopenia of childhood (RCC) is pancytopenic with circulating neutrophils with dysplastic features, including cytoplasmic hypogranulation and a pseudo-Pelger Huët nuclear anomaly. (Right) Trephine biopsy sections are markedly hypocellular (~ 5% cellularity) and show severe trilineage hypoplasia in RCC. Differentiating RCC from aplastic anemia in this type of case is difficult.

Monosomy 7 by FISH

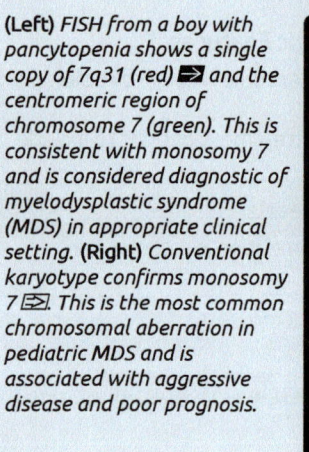

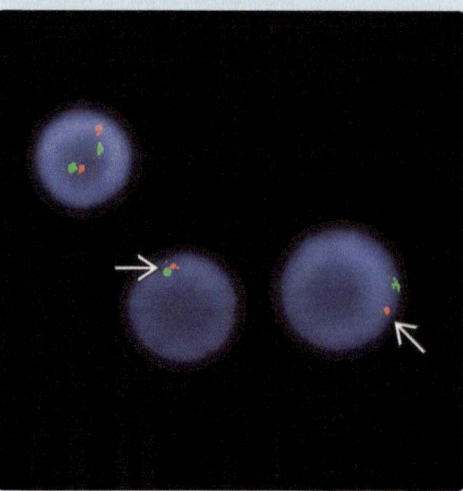

Karyotype With Monosomy 7

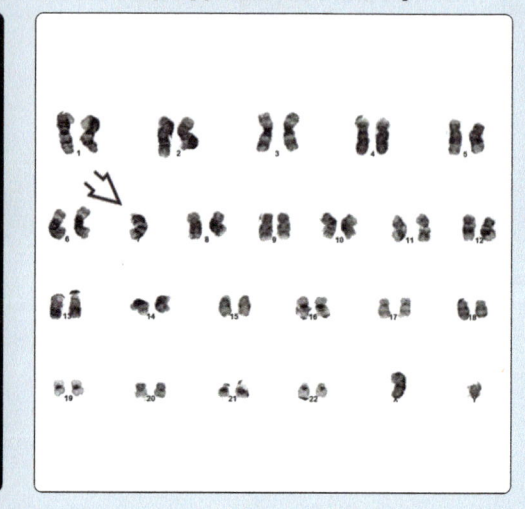

(Left) FISH from a boy with pancytopenia shows a single copy of 7q31 (red) ➡ and the centromeric region of chromosome 7 (green). This is consistent with monosomy 7 and is considered diagnostic of myelodysplastic syndrome (MDS) in appropriate clinical setting. (Right) Conventional karyotype confirms monosomy 7 ➡. This is the most common chromosomal aberration in pediatric MDS and is associated with aggressive disease and poor prognosis.

Pediatric Myelodysplastic Syndrome and Refractory Cytopenia of Childhood

TERMINOLOGY

Abbreviations
- Myelodysplastic syndrome (MDS)
- Refractory cytopenia of childhood (RCC)
- Childhood myelodysplastic syndrome with low blasts (cMDS-LB)
- Childhood myelodysplastic syndrome with increased blasts (cMDS-IB)

Synonyms
- Refractory anemia of childhood

Definitions
- Pediatric MDS
  o Children and adolescents (< 18 years of age)
  o < 2% blasts in peripheral blood (PB)
  o < 5% blasts in bone marrow (BM)
  o No marrow fibrosis
  o No genetic alteration diagnostic of specific disorder
  o No previous cytotoxic chemotherapy or radiation therapy
- Clonal stem cell disorder
  o Ineffective hematopoiesis
  o Cytopenias
  o Dysplasia in ≥ 1 lineages

CLASSIFICATION

ICC
- RCC
  o Persistent cytopenia(s) during childhood
    – Criteria for cytopenia based on age-adjusted reference ranges
    – Often ≥ 2 refractory cytopenias
      □ Thrombocytopenia and neutropenia most common; isolated anemia rare
  o Dysplasia in ≥ 2 lineages or ≥ 10% in single lineage
  o Blasts < 2% in PB, < 5% in BM
  o Histomorphologic pattern is defining
    – ~ 80% have hypocellular BM with patchy distribution of hematopoiesis
      □ Predominantly erythropoiesis; other lineages markedly decreased
- Pediatric MDS, not otherwise specified (NOS)
  o Does not have histomorphologic pattern of RCC
  o Includes cases without cytopenias &/or dysplasia if
    – Monosomy 7 or del(7q) detected
  o Includes progression to MDS or early manifestation (RCC) in individuals with
    – Genetic predisposition or BM failure syndromes
      □ Guidelines for progression to MDS depend on clinical judgment with
      □ Gain of MDS-defining or pathogenic genetic alterations or
      □ Changes in degree of cytopenias, BM cellularity, dysplasia
- Classify into adult-type MDS category if
  o MDS with excess blasts (EB)
    – Blasts: 2-19% in PB or 5-19% in BM or Auer rods
  o MDS with mutated *SF3B1* or del(5q)
    – Exceedingly rare in children

WHO 5th Edition
- Childhood MDS with low blasts
  o Cytopenia of ≥ 1 lineages
  o Dysplastic changes in ≥ 1 lineages, in ≥ 10% of cells
  o < 5% BM blasts, < 2% PB blasts
  o With 1 of following criteria
    – Detection of clonal cytogenetic &/or molecular abnormality
    – Exclusion of other causes of cytopenia
    – Meeting morphologic criteria for cMDS-LB, hypocellular
      □ Erythropoiesis patchy with left shift and increased mitoses
      □ Granulopoiesis markedly decreased with left shift
      □ Megakaryopoiesis markedly decreased
- cMDS-IB
  o Cytopenia of 1 or more lineages
  o Dysplastic changes in ≥ 1 lineages, in ≥ 10% of cells
  o 5-19% BM blasts &/or 2-19% PB blasts
  o Exclusion of Down syndrome, juvenile myelomonocytic leukemia, and acute myeloid leukemia (AML) with defining genetic abnormalities

ETIOLOGY/PATHOGENESIS

Genetic Alterations
- Significantly different than adult MDS
- RAS/MAPK pathway mutations most common
- Somatic aberrations in *SETBP1*, *RUNX1*
- Lack recurrent epigenetic regulator gene mutations
- Spliceosome complex gene, *TET2*, or *DNMT3A* mutations are rare
- Some germline mutations predispose to MDS at young age: *GATA2*, *SAMD9*, *SAMD9L*

Germline Predisposition or Immune Dysregulation
- Increase risk of MDS
- BM insufficiency and chromosomal instability impart selective advantage to clones that promote cell proliferation
  o MDS clones suppress normal hematopoiesis
  o Acquire additional somatic mutations over time

CLINICAL ISSUES

Epidemiology
- Incidence
  o Rare disease
    – < 5% of hematopoietic neoplasms in children < 14 years of age
    – RCC is most common subtype, 50% of pediatric MDS
- Age
  o All infants and children

Presentation
- Initial presentation of cytopenia(s)
  o Thrombocytopenia is most common
    – 75% of patients
  o Neutropenia is 2nd most common
    – 50% of patients

Pediatric Myelodysplastic Syndrome and Refractory Cytopenia of Childhood

- Subset with concurrent anemia
- Isolated anemia is uncommon
- Most common symptoms related to cytopenias
  - Malaise
  - Bleeding
  - Fever
  - Infection
- Many patients are asymptomatic at diagnosis
  - ~ 20% of RCC cases

Laboratory Tests
- CBC and smear review
- BM biopsy with flow cytometry, cytogenetics, and molecular testing
- Cultures and serologies to exclude infections
- Molecular testing for underlying germline predisposition mutations
- Specialized testing for BM failure syndromes
  - Chromosome breakage studies, telomere length, telomerase activity

Treatment
- Careful observation in early disease
  - Severe cytopenia(s)
- Supportive care for symptoms
  - Antibiotics for infection
  - Transfusion for symptomatic or significant cytopenias
- Immunosuppressive therapy
  - For some cases with early BM failure
  - 63% response at 6 months of treatment
  - More effective if small paroxysmal nocturnal hemoglobinuria (PNH) clone present
  - Remain at risk for clonal evolution and relapse
- Hematopoietic stem cell transplantation
  - Reduced intensity conditioning regimens used
  - Only curative therapy
    - Indicated early for cases of RCC with monosomy 7 or complex karyotypes
    - Indicated with severe symptoms (transfusion dependence, infections)
    - May be performed in other situations if suitable donor is available
  - Must exclude germline predisposition syndrome if family members are evaluated as marrow donors

Prognosis
- RCC
  - Multilineage dysplasia associated with increased risk of progression
  - Disease often stable for months to years
- Cytogenetic findings have prognostic significance
  - Complex karyotype is strongest independent marker of poor prognosis
    - Also have worse outcomes following BM transplant
  - Monosomy 7 associated with disease progression
    - Median time to progression: 1.9 years
    - Children with monosomy 7 and *SAMD9L* mutation may have spontaneous resolution
  - Normal karyotype and trisomy 8 associated with stable disease

MOLECULAR
Cytogenetics
- Identification of MDS-associated abnormality
  - Helps to establish diagnosis
  - Provides prognostic information
- Normal karyotype
  - Seen in 60-67% of cases
  - Associated with stable clinical course
  - Associated with increased presence of small PNH clones
- Monosomy 7
  - Most common abnormality, seen in 30%
  - Associated with poor prognosis
  - More common in patients with normal or increased BM cellularity
    - May be transient in patients with *SAMD9*- and *SAMD9L*-related MDS
- Trisomy 8
  - Associated with stable clinical course
  - May represent mosaic germline abnormality
- Trisomy 21
  - Evaluation needed to exclude Down syndrome
    - Constitutional trisomy 21 indicates Down syndrome-related process
      - MDS in Down syndrome is not included in childhood MDS category
  - Somatic trisomy may be seen in childhood MDS
- Complex karyotype
  - ≥ 3 abnormalities with at least 1 structural aberration
  - Associated with poor prognosis
  - 2-year survival 14%
  - More common in patients with multilineage dysplasia
  - Monosomal karyotype not meeting criteria for complex karyotype does not have prognostic significance
  - Clonal evolution generally associated with clinical disease progression
- Isolated del(5q) extremely rare
- Gains of 1q reported in subset of patients
  - Caution required, as this is common finding in Fanconi anemia
- Exclude AML with recurrent cytogenetic abnormality
- Specialized tests to exclude underlying congenital syndromes
  - Chromosome breakage study

FISH
- Multiprobe panels for changes associated with MDS should be performed
  - Especially if conventional cytogenetic evaluation is inadequate
- Can be performed on BM touch preparations or aspirate smears
  - Useful for hypocellular specimens

Molecular Testing
- For somatic and germline predisposition mutations
- Somatic mutations may help support diagnosis of childhood MDS
  - Mutations may have prognostic significance
  - Increasing numbers of mutations associated with more severe disease

Pediatric Myelodysplastic Syndrome and Refractory Cytopenia of Childhood

- o RAS pathway mutations more common with high blast count
- o *SETBP1* mutation associated with loss of chromosome 7
- 20% of RCC have germline predisposition mutations
  - o Common germline mutations include *RUNX1*, *GATA2*, *CEBPA*, *SAMD9*, and *SAMD9L*
  - o May require mutation testing on blood and fibroblasts to demonstrate somatic vs. germline

MICROSCOPIC

Peripheral Blood

- Similar to findings in adult MDS in most cases
- Blasts
  - o < 2% in RCC
  - o BM blasts > 5% but < 20% in MDS-EB
- Anemia
  - o 50% of RCC have hemoglobin level < 10 g/dL
    - Most commonly macrocytic
    - Anisopoikilocytosis
    - Dimorphic red cell population possible
- Neutropenia
  - o ≥ 10% neutrophils with dysplasia
    - Hypogranulation or abnormal granulation
    - Pseudo-Pelger-Huët nuclei
    - Giant bands
    - Dysplasia helps to distinguish childhood MDS from aplastic anemia
  - o 25% of RCC have marked neutropenia
    - May have insufficient neutrophils to evaluate for dysplasia
    - Evaluation of buffy coat specimen helps for identification of dysplastic neutrophils
- Thrombocytopenia
  - o 75% of RCC
  - o Occasional large and giant platelets

Bone Marrow

- Minimal diagnostic criteria required
  - o Dysplastic changes in 2 lineages (erythroid, granulocytic, megakaryocytic) or ≥ 10% dysplasia in single lineage
  - o Ring sideroblasts are extremely rare
- RCC and cMDS-LB
  - o < 5% myeloblasts
  - o Hypocellular in ~ 80% of cases
    - Often 5-10% of normal age cellularity
    - Erythroids show impaired maturation
    - Usually few clusters of ≥ 10 erythroid precursors
    - Increased proerythroblasts
    - Erythroid precursors have increased number of mitoses
    - Left-shifted and markedly decreased granulopoiesis
    - Promyelocytes specifically decreased
    - Megakaryocytes are usually very low in number or absent
    - Identification of micromegakaryocytes strongly supports diagnosis
    - Lymphocytes, plasma cells, and mast cells may be increased
    - No increase in fibrosis
  - o Normocellular or hypercellular
    - Often left-shifted erythroid hyperplasia
    - Mild to moderately decreased granulopoiesis
    - Decreased, adequate, or increased dysplastic megakaryocytes
- cMDS-IB
  - o Increased blasts or Auer rods
    - Includes all types of blasts or equivalents: Myeloblasts, monoblasts, promonocytes, megakaryoblasts
    - 5-19% blasts
  - o Often multilineage dysplasia

ANCILLARY TESTS

Immunohistochemistry

- CD34 is important to evaluate for subtle blast population
  - o MDS subtype may be difficult to ascertain in hypocellular BM
  - o Clusters of blasts should not be present in RCC
- CD61 or CD41 for detection of megakaryocytes
  - o Megakaryocytes are often decreased and difficult to visualize in hypocellular BM
    - Helpful in detecting dysplastic and small megakaryocytes
    - Identification of micromegakaryocytes aids in confirming diagnosis of MDS, especially RCC

Flow Cytometry

- Quantify myeloblasts
- Identify small PNH clones
  - o Seen in 41% of childhood MDS
  - o More common in association with normal karyotype
  - o Overt PNH is rare
- Identify aberrant phenotypic antigen expression
  - o Aids in diagnosis
  - o CD7 expression by myeloblasts correlates with poor outcomes
  - o CD56 expression by myeloblasts seen in some cases of MDS but not aplastic anemia
  - o CD56 expression by monocytes seen in 20%
  - o Abnormal pattern of CD16 and CD13 expression in granulocytes may be seen
  - o Presence of abnormal antigen expression increases with disease progression

DIFFERENTIAL DIAGNOSIS

Myeloid Neoplasm, Post Therapy

- Occurs after chemotherapy or radiation therapy

Acquired Aplastic Anemia

- Megaloblastic or dysplastic features not typical at presentation
- BM is hypocellular with increased adipocytes
  - o No increase in blasts
  - o Lacks erythroid islands
    - Possible single small focus with < 10 cells showing maturation
    - Increased erythroblasts
  - o Absent or markedly decreased granulocytic myelopoiesis
    - No significant dysplasia
    - Few small foci or scattered cells show maturation
  - o Absent or markedly decreased megakaryocytes

Pediatric Myelodysplastic Syndrome and Refractory Cytopenia of Childhood

- No significant dysplasia or "micromegakaryocytes"
  - Small lymphoid aggregates or increased dispersed lymphocytes common
    - Associated mast cells
- May have morphologic features similar to RCC after immunosuppressive therapy
- Subset of aplastic anemia patients demonstrate clonal cytogenetic abnormalities
- Subset of patients progress to MDS

Acquired Bone Marrow Failure Disorders
- PNH
  - Flow cytometric analysis for PNH clones is diagnostic
    - Small PNH clones may be seen in aplastic anemia and low-grade MDS with ultrasensitive testing
    - Some studies suggest better response to immunosuppressive therapy if small PNH clones present
- Aplastic anemia during hematologic recovery

Low-Blast-Count Acute Myeloid Leukemia
- Cytogenetic, FISH, or molecular identification of AML-defining genetic abnormality is required
  - Diagnostic of AML, irrespective of blast percentage
- Auer rods in blasts more commonly seen in AML than in MDS

Reactive Disorders With Cytologic Dysplasia
- Nutritional deficiencies
  - Vitamin B12 or folate deficiency
  - Copper deficiency
- Medication or toxin effect
- Autoimmune disorders
  - Systemic lupus erythematosus
  - Autoimmune lymphoproliferative disorders
    - FAS deficiency
- Rheumatic diseases
- Metabolic disorders
  - Mevalonate kinase deficiency
- Infections
  - Cytomegalovirus
  - Varicella
  - Epstein-Barr virus
  - Hepatitis viruses
  - Parvovirus B19
  - HIV

DIAGNOSTIC CHECKLIST

Clinically Relevant Pathologic Features
- BM specimens in RCC are often hypocellular
  - Distinction from aplastic anemia or congenital BM failure syndromes may be difficult
    - Clinical correlation is essential
    - Specialized testing to evaluate for congenital syndrome is warranted
    - Aplastic anemia and congenital BM failure syndromes may progress to MDS
  - BM evaluation
    - IHC (CD34, CD117) useful for blast identification and MDS classification
    - Step sections of trephine biopsy help to identify micromegakaryocytes
    - IHC for megakaryocytes aids in detecting dysplastic megakaryocytes
- Children with MDS may have slowly progressive disease
- Ring sideroblasts are rare in childhood MDS
  - Consider mitochondrial disorder or disorder of heme synthesis

Pathologic Interpretation Pearls
- Assessment for neutrophil and megakaryocytic dysplasia is essential
- Diagnosis of RCC may be made when dysplasia is identified in ≥ 10% of cells in single lineage
  - Lesser degree of dysplasia in at least 2 lineages will also qualify for diagnosis
    - Erythroid, neutrophilic myeloid, &/or megakaryocytic dysplasia
    - Follow closely with repeat BM evaluations before definitive diagnosis is rendered if normal karyotype
    - Provide data to refute other differential diagnostic considerations
- BM touch preparations are particularly helpful in RCC
  - Many cases have hypocellular BM
    - Aspirate material is often insufficient for adequate morphologic &/or conventional cytogenetic evaluation
  - FISH studies can be performed to evaluate for MDS-related cytogenetic abnormalities
- Hematogones are often decreased in low-grade MDS

SELECTED REFERENCES

1. Rudelius M et al: The International Consensus Classification (ICC) of hematologic neoplasms with germline predisposition, pediatric myelodysplastic syndrome, and juvenile myelomonocytic leukemia. Virchows Arch. 482(1):113-30, 2023
2. Avagyan S et al: Lessons from pediatric MDS: approaches to germline predisposition to hematologic malignancies. Front Oncol. 12:813149, 2022
3. Gao J et al: The effect of decitabine-combined minimally myelosuppressive regimen bridged allo-HSCT on the outcomes of pediatric MDS from 10years' experience of a single center. BMC Pediatr. 22(1):312, 2022
4. Khoury JD et al: The 5th edition of the World Health Organization classification of haematolymphoid tumours: myeloid and histiocytic/dendritic neoplasms. Leukemia. 36(7):1703-19, 2022
5. Tsang MMC et al: Spontaneous resolution of refractory cytopenia of childhood with monosomy 7 in an infant without an identifiable genetic cause. Pediatr Blood Cancer. 69(10):e29654, 2022
6. Patel SS: Pediatric myelodysplastic syndromes. Clin Lab Med. 41(3):517-28, 2021
7. Marchesi RF et al: Clinical impact of dysplastic changes in acquired aplastic anemia: a systematic study of bone marrow biopsies in children and adults. Ann Diagn Pathol. 45:151459, 2020
8. Nakano TA et al: Diagnosis and treatment of pediatric myelodysplastic syndromes: a survey of the North American Pediatric Aplastic Anemia Consortium. Pediatr Blood Cancer. 67(10):e28652, 2020
9. Galaverna F et al: Myelodysplastic syndromes in children. Curr Opin Oncol. 30(6):402-8, 2018
10. Wlodarski MW et al: Monosomy 7 in pediatric myelodysplastic syndromes. Hematol Oncol Clin North Am. 32(4):729-43, 2018
11. Aalbers AM et al: Bone marrow immunophenotyping by flow cytometry in refractory cytopenia of childhood. Haematologica. 100(3):315-23, 2015
12. Collin M et al: Haematopoietic and immune defects associated with GATA2 mutation. Br J Haematol. 169(2):173-87, 2015
13. Hasegawa D et al: Clinical characteristics and treatment outcome in 65 cases with refractory cytopenia of childhood defined according to the WHO 2008 classification. Br J Haematol. 166(5):758-66, 2014

Pediatric Myelodysplastic Syndrome and Refractory Cytopenia of Childhood

Dysplastic Neutrophils

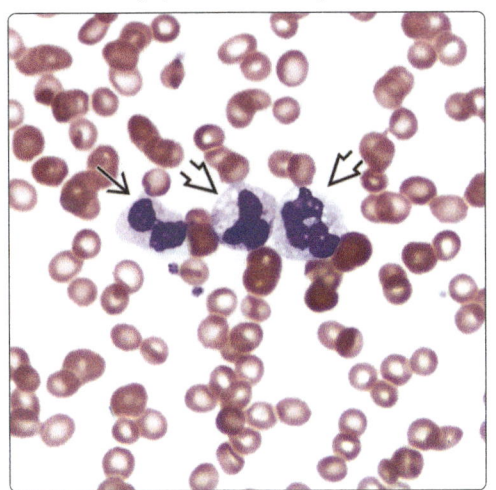

Transformation to Acute Myeloid Leukemia

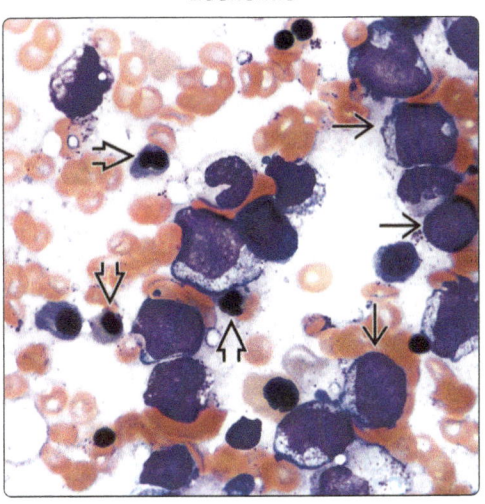

(Left) Peripheral blood in pediatric MDS may have dysplastic neutrophils, including cytoplasmic hypogranulation pseudo-Pelger-Huët nuclei ⇒, and abnormal nuclear segmentation ⇒. (Right) Aspirate smears are cellular with sufficient blasts ⇒ (~ 25%) to be diagnostic of transformation from RCC to acute myeloid leukemia in this child's bone marrow. Background dyserythropoiesis ⇒ and decreased myeloid maturation are evident.

Hypocellular Bone Marrow

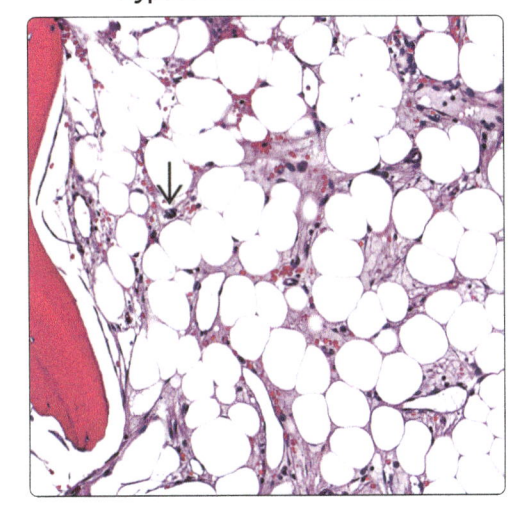

CD34 Immunohistochemistry

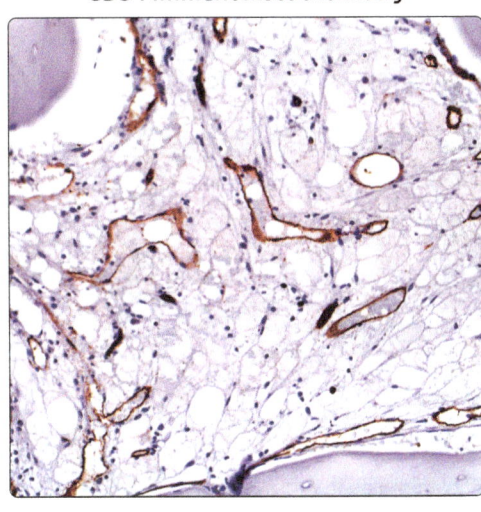

(Left) Core biopsy shows markedly hypocellular bone marrow (~ 5% cellularity) with no clusters of blasts identified. Megakaryocytes are decreased with micromegakaryocytes ⇒ present, supporting a diagnosis of pediatric MDS. (Right) CD34 highlights the vasculature and shows no significant CD34(+) blast population. Stains for megakaryocytes are also useful to identify micromegakaryocytes.

Trisomy 8

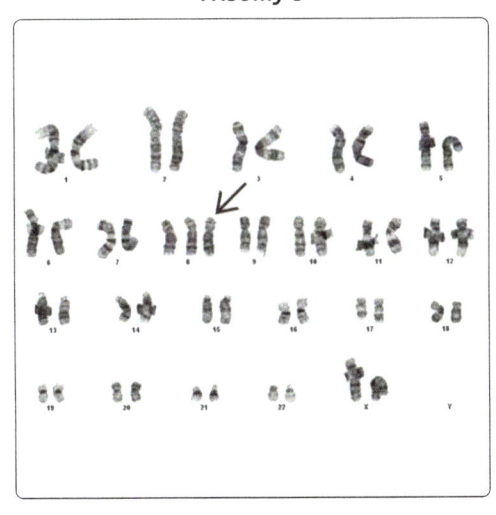

Trisomy 8 by FISH

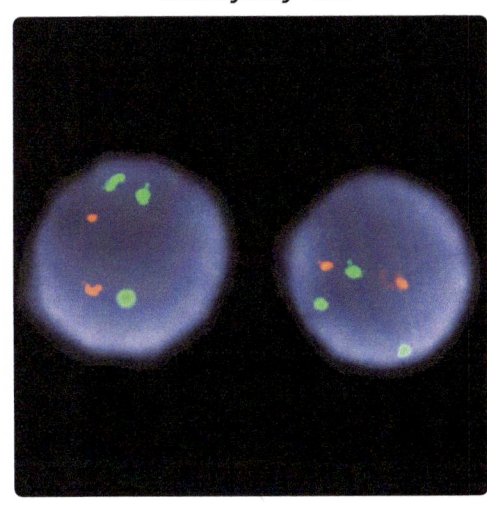

(Left) Conventional cytogenetic study from a 4-year-old girl with relatively stable cytopenias shows trisomy 8 ⇒. This is a recurrent abnormality in MDS and is associated with a long, stable course similar to the identification of a normal karyotype. (Right) FISH analysis of an aspirate smear shows trisomy 8 with the 3 copies of chromosome 8 (CEP8 signals) shown in green. The 2 red signals represent normal 20q12 chromosomal regions.

213

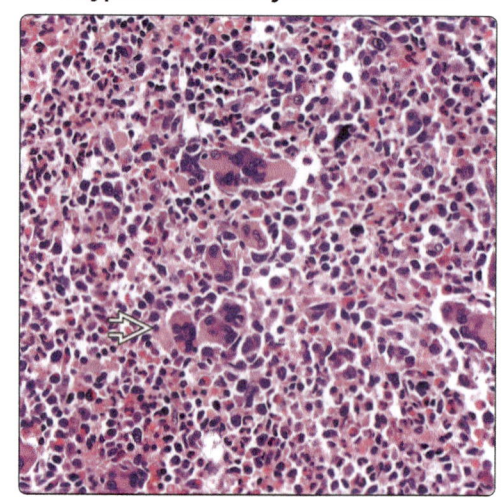

Overview of Myelodysplastic/Myeloproliferative Neoplasms

TERMINOLOGY

Abbreviations
- Myelodysplastic/myeloproliferative neoplasms (MDS/MPN)

Definitions
- De novo clonal chronic myeloid neoplasm characterized by hybrid myelodysplastic and myeloproliferative features manifested by at least 1 cytopenia and at least 1 cytosis in blood
- Maturation is intact; mature cells predominate
- Blasts and blast equivalents are < 20% in blood and bone marrow

Classifications
- **International Consensus Classification (ICC)**
  - Chronic myelomonocytic leukemia (CMML)
    – Myelodysplastic and myeloproliferative subtypes based on WBC count < or > 13.0 x 10⁹/L
    – CMML types 1 and 2 based on blast percentages in blood and bone marrow
      □ Monocyte count ≥ 0.5 x 10⁹/L, WBC ≥ 10%, and increased blasts or morphologic dysplasia or abnormal immunophenotype c/w CMML would be required for diagnosis in cases without evidence of clonality
  - Atypical chronic myeloid leukemia (aCML)
  - MDS/MPN with *SF3B1* mutation and thrombocytosis (MDS/MPN-*SF3B1*-T)
  - MDS/MPN with ring sideroblasts and thrombocytosis, not otherwise specified (MDS/MPN-RS-T, NOS)
  - MDS/MPN, NOS
  - MDS/MPN with iso(17q) (provisional entity)
- **WHO 5th edition (WHO-HAEM5)**
  - CMML
    – Myelodysplastic and myeloproliferative subtypes based on WBC < or > 13.0 x 10⁹/L
    – CMML types 1 and 2 based on blast percentages in blood and bone marrow
    – Monocyte count ≥ 0.5 x 10⁹/L and ≥ 10% WBC for clonality-confirmed cases
  - MDS/MPN with neutrophilia (MDS/MPN-N)
  - MDS/MPN-*SF3B1*-T
    – ≥ 15% ring sideroblasts meets diagnostic criteria in absence of *SF3B1* mutation
  - MDS/MPN-NOS
- **MDS/MPN classifications in ICC and WHO-HAEM5 largely similar**
  - aCML (ICC) and MDS/MPN with neutrophilia (WHO-HAEM5) are essentially same entity with similar diagnostic criteria
  - Ring sideroblasts ≥ 15% substitutes for *SF3B1* mutation for MDS/MPN-*SF3B1*-T in WHO-HAEM5 only
  - Both systems have removed juvenile myelomonocytic leukemia from MDS/MPN group

ETIOLOGY/PATHOGENESIS

Cytogenetic Findings
- No specific cytogenetic abnormalities in MDS/MPN
  - Abnormalities associated with myeloid neoplasms are seen
  - Clonal abnormalities present in up to 40% of CMML
  - Clonal abnormalities present in up to 80% of aCML
  - Clonal abnormalities present in up to 10% of MDS/MPN-*SF3B1*-T
- Diagnosis requires **absence** of *BCR::ABL1, PDGFRA, PDGFRB, FGFR1, JAK2, FLT3,* and *ETV6::ABL1* rearrangements, isolated del(5q), inv3(q21.3q26.2), and acute myeloid leukemia (AML)-defining translocations, including AML with t(8;21) or inv(16)
  - All of these genetic aberrations are pathogenetically linked to other types of myeloid neoplasms

Molecular Findings
- Next-generation sequencing panels often most cost-effective way to screen for mutations
- CMML
  - Somatic mutations in 90% of cases
  - *TET2* mutations in ~ 50% of cases
  - *SRSF2* mutations in 30-50% of cases
  - *ASXL1* mutations in 40-50% of cases

Chronic Myelomonocytic Leukemia

Atypical Chronic Myeloid Leukemia

(Left) Peripheral blood from a patient with chronic myelomonocytic leukemia (CMML) shows monocytosis and dysplastic neutrophils ⮕. There is also anemia present. TET2, SRSF2, and ASXL1 mutations are common in CMML. (Right) Bone marrow biopsy from a patient with atypical chronic myeloid leukemia (aCML) shows hypercellularity with increased granulocytes and megakaryocytes with clustering and dysplasia ⮕. SETBP1 and ETNK1 mutations were detected in this case of aCML.

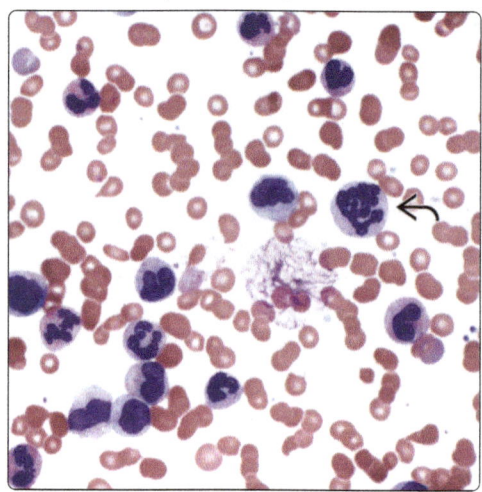

Overview of Myelodysplastic/Myeloproliferative Neoplasms

- aCML (ICC) or MDS/MPN-N (WHO-HAEM5)
  - *SETBP1* mutations in > 30% of cases
    - Not specific but can support diagnosis of aCML
  - *ETNK1* mutations in ~ 9% of cases
    - Not specific but can support diagnosis of aCML
  - *CSF3R* mutations rarely reported
    - Identification should prompt consideration of chronic neutrophilic leukemia
- MDS/MPN-*SF3B1*-T
  - *SF3B1* mutations
    - Associated with presence of bone marrow-ring sideroblasts
  - *JAK2* mutations in 50-80% of cases
- MDS/MPN-NOS
  - *TET2* mutations in 30% of cases
  - *JAK2* mutations in ~ 19% of cases
    - Often associated with other mutations
  - *SETBP1* mutations in ~ 10% of cases
  - Identification of *ASXL1*, *SRSF2*, or *CSF3R* mutations should prompt exploration of alternative diagnosis

EPIDEMIOLOGY

Sex
- Clear-cut male predominance in CMML
- No significant sex predominance in aCML

Incidence
- All MDS/MPN subtypes are rare
- CMML most common

Age
- MDS/MPNs predominantly affect older adults; incidence increases with age

Presentation
- Generally older adults who manifest with gradual symptoms of progressive cytopenias (notably anemia) and splenomegaly
- Splenomegaly is common in all types of MDS/MPN
- Abnormal myelomonocytic infiltrates can be apparent in skin, lymph nodes, or mucosal sites

Laboratory Tests
- CBC with differential and morphologic review
  - Confirm hybrid cytosis/cytopenia picture
  - Assess all lineages for dysplasia
  - Determine percent of blasts/blast equivalents
  - Determine absolute neutrophil, monocyte, eosinophil, and basophil counts
- Many other tests to exclude nonneoplastic causes for blood abnormalities, assess for cell turnover

Ancillary Tests
- Cytogenetic/molecular genetic testing
  - Assess for clonality
  - Isochromosome 17q defines MDS/MPN with iso(17q); provisional subtype in ICC
  - Mutations, such as *SF3B1* that defines MDS/MPN-*SF3B1*-T, often with concurrent *JAK2* mutation
  - Mutations that support diagnosis, such as *SETBP1* in aCML (ICC)/MDS/MPN-N (WHO-HAEM5)

MICROSCOPIC

Blood
- Dysplasia in at least 1 lineage for cases **without** confirmed clonality by cytogenetic or molecular testing in ICC
  - Dysplasia ≥ 10% required in WHO-HAEM5
- Atypical, absolute monocytosis (≥ 10% of WBC) in CMML
- Neutrophilia with left shift and prominent dysplastic changes in aCML or MDS/MPN-N
- Blasts/blast equivalents < 20%

Bone Marrow
- Hypercellular in all MDS/MPN subtypes
- Increased megakaryocytes with variable dysplasia
- Dysplasia in at least 1 lineage for cases without confirmation of clonality in ICC, for all cases in WHO-HAEM5
- Prominent myelomonocytic cells in CMML
- Blasts/blast equivalents < 20%
- ≥ 15% ring sideroblasts in MDS/MPN-RS-T, NOS
  - Hyperlobated MPN-like megakaryocytes in MDS/MPN-*SF3B1*-T

DIAGNOSTIC CHECKLIST

Clinicopathologic Interpretation Pearls
- Diagnosis of MDS/MPD is dependent upon careful clinical assessment and morphologic review
- Clinical information is essential in confirming de novo presentation of MDS/MPN
- Transformations of either MDS or MPN should **not** be included within MDS/MPN categories
- Many nonneoplastic disorders can exhibit hybrid cytopenias and cytoses
- Appropriate testing essential to exclude nonneoplastic disorders, such as chronic infections, collagen vascular diseases
- Knowledge of recent chemotherapy or cytokine therapy, notably granulocyte-colony-stimulating factor (G-CSF) therapy, is essential
  - Recombinant G-CSF can increase blasts and induce prominent granulocytic hyperplasia
- Myeloid neoplasms arising in setting of prior chemotherapy &/or radiation therapy are classified as myeloid neoplasms, post cytotoxic therapy
- Molecular genetic testing can identify recurrent mutations found in MDS/MPN
- Cytogenetics may show abnormalities associated with myeloid neoplasms

SELECTED REFERENCES

1. Prakash S et al: Advances in myelodysplastic/myeloproliferative neoplasms. Virchows Arch. 482(1):69-83, 2023
2. Arber DA et al: International Consensus Classification of myeloid neoplasms and acute leukemia: integrating morphological, clinical, and genomic data. Blood. 140(11):1200-28, 2022
3. Kanagal-Shamanna R et al: Myelodysplastic/myeloproliferative neoplasms-unclassifiable with isolated isochromosome 17q represents a distinct clinico-biologic subset: a multi-institutional collaborative study from the Bone Marrow Pathology Group. Mod Pathol. 35(4):470-9, 2022
4. Khoury JD et al: The 5th edition of the World Health Organization classification of haematolymphoid tumours: myeloid and histiocytic/dendritic neoplasms. Leukemia. 36(7):1703-19, 2022

Chronic Myelomonocytic Leukemia

KEY FACTS

TERMINOLOGY
- Myelodysplastic/myeloproliferative neoplasm
- Specific diagnostic criteria for chronic myelomonocytic leukemia (CMML)
  o Persistent peripheral blood monocytosis ≥ 0.5 x 10⁹/L with appropriate molecular profile
  o No *BCR::ABL1* fusion product
  o No *PDGFRA*, *PDGFRB*, *FGFR1*, or *PCM1::JAK2* rearrangement
  o < 20% blasts/promonocytes in blood or bone marrow
  o Dysplasia in ≥ 1 myeloid lineages
  o Can diagnose without dysplasia if clonal cytogenetic/molecular abnormality is present or if monocytosis has persisted for > 3 months and reactive causes are excluded

CLINICAL ISSUES
- Up to 30% of cases progress to acute myeloid leukemia

MOLECULAR
- Most cases have at least 1 of following genes mutated
  o *TET2*, *ASXL1*, RAS gene family (i.e., *KRAS*, *NRAS*), *SRSF2*

MICROSCOPIC
- CMML-1
  o Blasts (including promonocytes) up to 5% in peripheral blood or up to 10% in bone marrow
- CMML-2
  o Blasts (including promonocytes) 5-19% in peripheral blood or 10-19% in bone marrow
  o If Auer rods are present, automatically upgraded to CMML-2 regardless of blast count
- Some cases show nodular collections of plasmacytoid dendritic cells

DIAGNOSTIC CHECKLIST
- Cytochemical assessment of NSE is rapid and efficient means of documenting monocytic lineage

Peripheral Blood Monocytosis

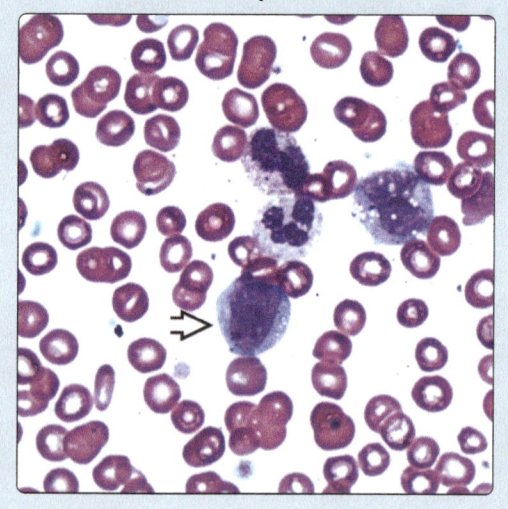

(Left) *Peripheral blood in chronic myelomonocytic leukemia (CMML) shows monocytosis > 1 x 10⁹/L (or > 0.5 x 10⁹/L with appropriate molecular profile) and usually > 10% of white blood cells. Dysplastic neutrophils ➡ are also common.* (Right) *Blasts ➡ and promonocytes may be commonly seen in the peripheral blood in CMML but by definition must be < 20%. The distinction between promonocytes and atypical monocytes can be very difficult.*

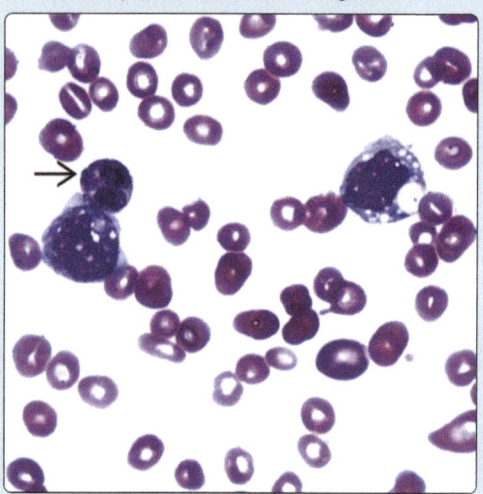

Blasts in Peripheral Blood

Common Primary Mutations in Chronic Myelomonocytic Leukemia

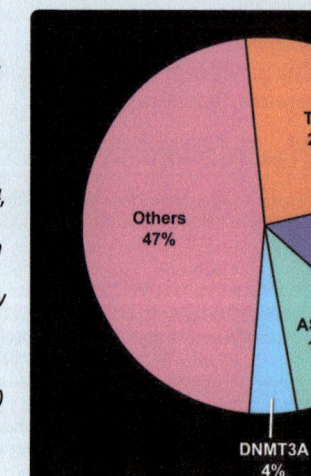

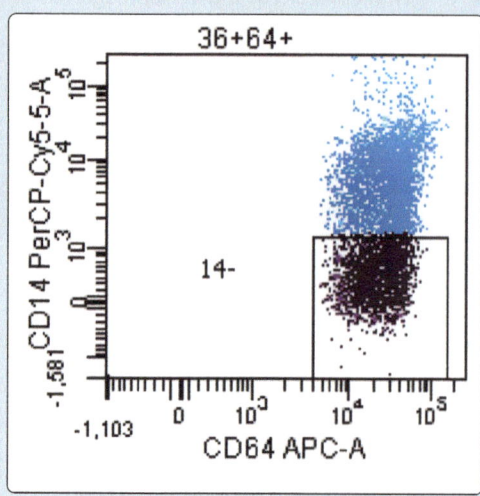

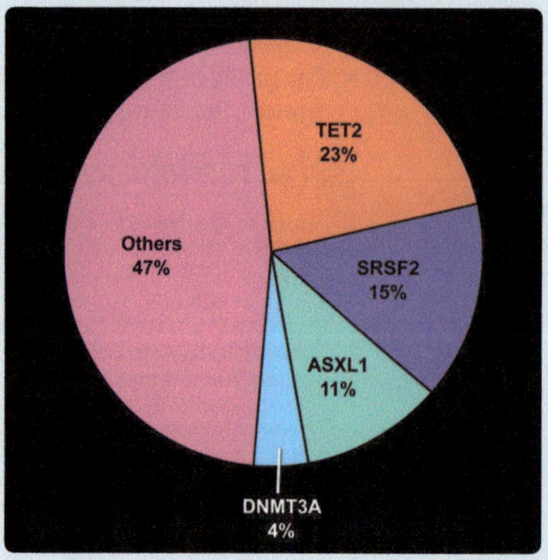

(Left) *Graph shows frequencies of the most common ancestral mutations by gene in CMML. (Adapted from Patel et al, Leukemia 2017.)* (Right) *Monocytic lineage cells in CMML frequently show loss of CD14, as highlighted by the population in purple. This can be seen as an immunophenotypic aberrancy or in an immature monocyte population and alone is not diagnostically specific. (From DP: Blood and Bone Marrow.)*

- Others 47%
- TET2 23%
- SRSF2 15%
- ASXL1 11%
- DNMT3A 4%

Aberrant Loss of CD14

Chronic Myelomonocytic Leukemia

TERMINOLOGY

Abbreviations
- Chronic myelomonocytic leukemia (CMML)

Definitions
- Myelodysplastic/myeloproliferative neoplasm (MDS/MPN)
  o Combines features of both myelodysplastic syndrome and myeloproliferative neoplasms
- Peripheral blood with persistent absolute (≥ 0.5 x 10⁹/L monocytes) and relative (≥ 10%) monocytosis
- Dysplasia in ≥ 1 myeloid lineage
  o If absent, CMML can still be diagnosed if all other criteria are met and clonal cytogenetic or molecular abnormality, or monocytosis persists > 3 months, and other reactive causes have been excluded
- Other myeloid malignancies must be excluded
  o No *BCR::ABL1* fusion
  o No *PDGFRA*, *PDGFRB*, *FGFR1*, or *PCM1::JAK2* rearrangements
  o Blasts < 20%
- CMML-1
  o Blasts < 5% in peripheral blood
  o Blasts < 10% in bone marrow
- CMML-2
  o Blasts 5-19% in peripheral blood
  o Blasts 10-19% in bone marrow, or
  o Auer rods present
- Both ICC and WHO 5th edition include myelodysplastic (MD-CMML) and myeloproliferative (MP-CMML) subgroups

ETIOLOGY/PATHOGENESIS

Environmental Exposure
- Etiology largely unknown
- Possible causes
  o Occupational and environmental carcinogens

CLINICAL ISSUES

Epidemiology
- Incidence
  o Estimated at 0.4 per 100,000
- Age
  o Median: 65-75 years
- Sex
  o Male predominance

Site
- In addition to peripheral blood and bone marrow involvement, tissue-based leukemic infiltrates may occur

Presentation
- Leukocytosis in majority
  o Hepatomegaly and splenomegaly more common in those with leukocytosis

Treatment
- Drugs
  o Hypomethylating agents
    - Response rate 40-50%
    - Complete remission rates 7-17%
- Transplantation
  o Allogeneic stem cell transplantation is only curative option at this time

Prognosis
- Highly variable due to heterogeneity of disease
  o Survival ranges from 1 month to > 100 months
  o Median survival: 20-40 months
  o ~ 15-30% of cases progress to acute myeloid leukemia (AML)
- Parameters affecting outcome
  o Blast percentage
  o Cytogenetic abnormalities
  o WBC count
  o Severity of CBC abnormalities
  o Molecular profile
  o Fibrosis

MOLECULAR

Molecular Genetics
- Molecular abnormalities found in ~ 90% of cases
  o Most cases have at least 1 of following genes mutated
    - *TET2*, *ASXL1*, *SRSF2*, RAS pathway
  o Key mutated genes per WHO 5th edition
    - *ASXL1*, *SRSF2*, *EZH2*, *BCOR*, *U2AF1*, *SF3B1*, *ZRSR2*
- *ASXL1* mutations
  o Frequency: ~ 40-50%
  o Poor prognosis with frameshift mutations
- *TET2* mutations
  o Frequency: ~ 60%
  o Unclear prognostic value
- *SRSF2* mutations
  o Frequency: ~ 50%; hotspot P95 codon
- *KRAS* and *NRAS* mutations
  o Frequency: ~ 30%
  o Myeloproliferative phenotype
- *JAK2* V617F mutation
  o Present in ~ 10% but not specific
- *RUNX1* mutations
  o Frequency: 20%
  o Poor prognostic indicator
- *SETBP1* mutations
  o Frequency: 15%; poor prognostic indicator
- *CBL* mutations
  o Frequency: 15%
- *SF3B1* mutations
  o Frequency: 5-10%

MICROSCOPIC

Peripheral Blood
- Monocytosis
  o Peripheral blood persistent absolute (≥ 0.5 x 10⁹/L) and relative (≥ 10%) monocytosis
  o Blasts and promonocytes must be < 20%
- Other CBC changes are variable
  o Neutrophilia or neutropenia
    - Dysgranulopoiesis is common
  o Some cases also show mild basophilia or eosinophilia
  o Anemia is common

Chronic Myelomonocytic Leukemia

- Platelet counts are variable
  - Abnormal, large platelets are common

Bone Marrow
- Usually hypercellular
  - Granulocytic proliferation common
  - Monocytic proliferation may require special stains or immunohistochemistry to detect
    - α-naphthyl acetate esterase
    - α-naphthyl butyrate esterase
    - CD14, CD68, CD163, lysozyme
- Dysplasia
  - Dysgranulopoiesis is typical
  - Dyserythropoiesis in > 50%
    - Megaloblastic changes
    - Nuclear budding, blebbing, abnormal nuclear contours
    - Ring sideroblasts
  - Megakaryocyte dysplasia is very common
    - Abnormal nuclear lobation
- Reticulin fibrosis in ~ 30%
- Plasmacytoid dendritic cell nodules in ~ 20%
- Further subclassified by blast and "blast equivalent" percentage
  - Blast equivalents include promonocytes
    - Intermediate immature form between monoblast and mature monocyte
    - Nucleus is not round but slightly folded or creased

ANCILLARY TESTS

Flow Cytometry
- Expression of myelomonocytic antigens CD33, CD13
- Expression of monocytic antigens CD14, CD68, CD64
- Aberrant phenotype
  - Usually ≥ 2 of following
    - Decreased CD14 (immaturity)
    - CD56 overexpression
    - CD2 aberrant expression
    - Abnormal decreased expression of HLA-DR, CD13, CD15, CD64, or CD36
    - Abnormal side scatter on neutrophils

Genetic Testing
- Karyotypic abnormalities found in 30% of patients but not specific for CMML
  - High risk
    - Trisomy 8
    - -7/del(7q)
    - Complex karyotype
  - Low risk
    - Loss of Y or normal karyotype
  - Intermediate risk
    - All other cytogenetic abnormalities
- By definition, CMML must not have certain cytogenetic abnormalities or rearrangements
  - BCR::ABL1
  - PDGFRA, PDGFRB, FGFR1, or PCM1::JAK2 rearrangements
- > 90% of patients have detectable somatic mutations
- Typical molecular profile by massive parallel sequencing
  - Usually multiple of TET2, ASXL1, SRSF2, or RAS pathway

DIFFERENTIAL DIAGNOSIS

Reactive Monocytosis
- Lacks significant dysplasia
- Normal cytogenetics
- Possible causes
  - Chronic infections
  - Collagen vascular diseases
  - Sarcoidosis
  - Compensatory monocytosis in setting of neutropenia of unrelated etiology
  - Splenectomy

Chronic Myeloid Leukemia, BCR::ABL1-Positive
- CML with p190 form of fusion protein may show significant monocytosis, mimicking CMML

Myeloid Neoplasms With Eosinophilia and Rearrangements of PDGFRA, PDGFRB, FGFR1, or PCM1::JAK2
- Cases with PDGFRB rearrangement are especially associated with CMML-like appearance

Atypical Chronic Myeloid Leukemia, BCR::ABL1-Negative
- Monocytes represent < 10% of cells

Acute Myelomonocytic Leukemia
- Blast and promonocyte percentage critical

Systemic Mastocytosis
- CMML is most common neoplasm seen in conjunction with systemic mastocytosis

DIAGNOSTIC CHECKLIST

Pathologic Interpretation Pearls
- Use cytogenetic and molecular studies to exclude other myeloid neoplasms
  - Must rule out BCR::ABL1, PDGFRA, PDGFRB, FGFR1, and PCM1::JAK2 rearrangements
  - Clonal cytogenetic abnormality also helps establish diagnosis of malignancy rather than reactive monocytosis
- Careful morphologic assessment of monocytic cells in CMML is critical
  - Must distinguish mature monocytes from promonocytes that would potentially change diagnosis to AML

SELECTED REFERENCES

1. Prakash S et al: Advances in myelodysplastic/myeloproliferative neoplasms. Virchows Arch. 482(1):69-83, 2023
2. Arber DA et al: International Consensus Classification of myeloid neoplasms and acute leukemia: integrating morphological, clinical, and genomic data. Blood. 140(11):1200-28, 2022
3. Khoury JD et al: The 5th edition of the World Health Organization Classification of haematolymphoid tumours: myeloid and histiocytic/dendritic neoplasms. Leukemia. 36(7):1703-19, 2022
4. Patnaik MM et al: Chronic myelomonocytic leukemia: 2022 update on diagnosis, risk stratification, and management. Am J Hematol. 97(3):352-72, 2022

Chronic Myelomonocytic Leukemia

Monocytic Infiltrate in Bone Marrow

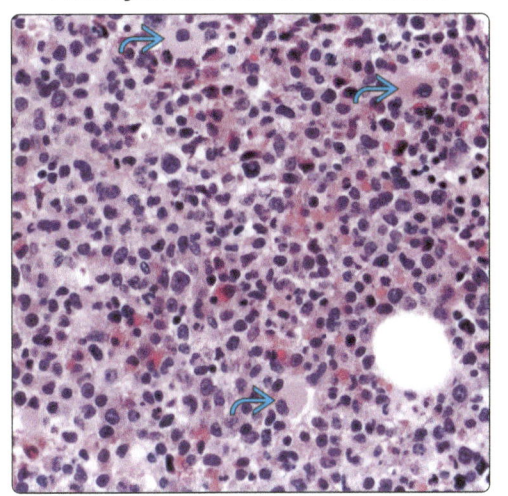

Bone Marrow Fibrosis

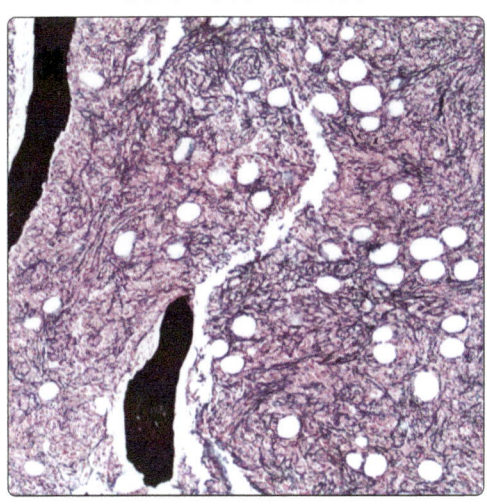

(Left) *Bone marrow core biopsy from a patient with CMML shows hypercellular marrow with predominance of monocytes and granulocytes. The monocytes have delicate, folded nuclei. Megakaryocytes ⇨ may be dysplastic (small and monolobated in this case) or have a myeloproliferative type of morphology.* (Right) *Reticulin stain of bone marrow core biopsy shows significant fibrosis. Mild to moderate fibrosis can be seen in up to 30% of patients with CMML and has been associated with a worse prognosis.*

Trisomy 8

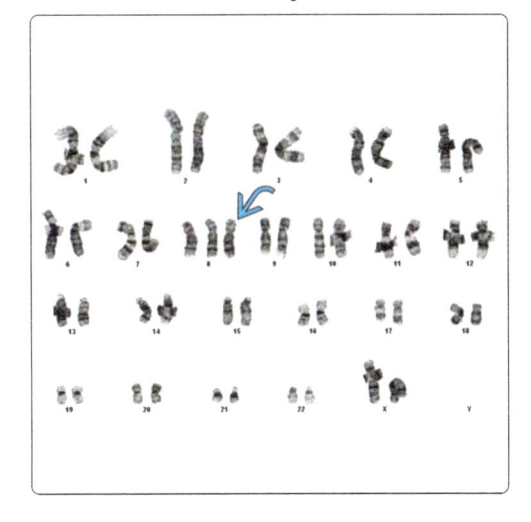

Plasmacytoid Dendritic Cell Nodule

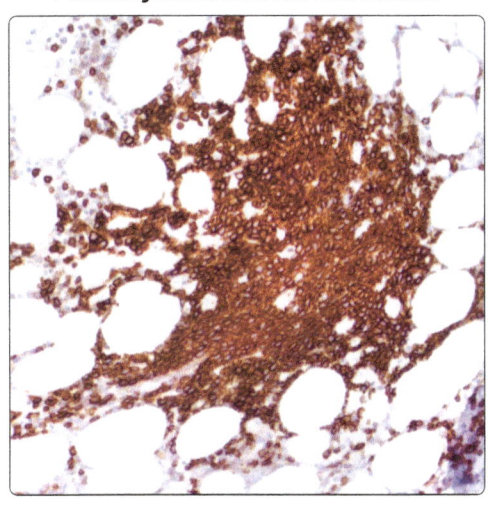

(Left) *CMML must be differentiated from reactive monocytosis. Detection of a clonal cytogenetic or molecular abnormality (as illustrated here by trisomy 8 ⇨) will exclude a reactive process.* (Right) *CD123 highlights a distinct nodular collection of plasmacytoid dendritic cells in this case of CMML.*

Differential Diagnosis: Chronic Myeloid Leukemia With p190

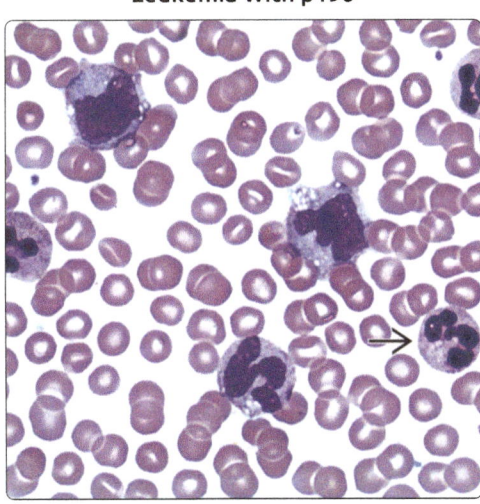

Differential Diagnosis: Chronic Myeloid Leukemia With p190

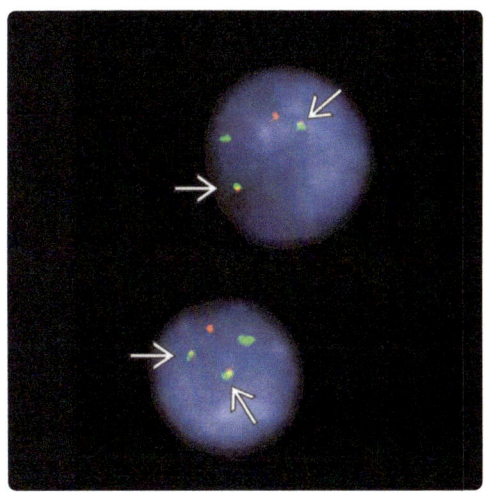

(Left) *Cases of chronic myeloid leukemia (CML) with the p190 fusion gene product may have significant monocytosis, as depicted, mimicking CMML. Note the absence of dysplasia in neutrophils ⇨* (Right) *FISH documents the presence of BCR::ABL1 fusion ⇨. This translocation must be excluded before a diagnosis of CMML is established. Alternative methods include chromosomal karyotyping or RT-PCR.*

Atypical Chronic Myeloid Leukemia

KEY FACTS

TERMINOLOGY
- Atypical chronic myeloid leukemia (aCML) (ICC)
- Myelodysplastic/myeloproliferative neoplasm with neutrophilia (WHO-HAEM5)

CLINICAL ISSUES
- Patients usually present with symptoms related to anemia, thrombocytopenia, or hepatosplenomegaly
- Overall poor prognosis; mean survival: 14-30 months
  - 15-40% of aCML transforms to acute myeloid leukemia (AML)

MOLECULAR
- *SETBP1* mutation
  - ~ 24-31% of cases
  - Associated with higher WBC counts
  - Presence desirable to support diagnosis according to ICC and WHO-HAEM5
- *ETNK1* mutation
  - ~ 13-15% of cases
  - Presence desirable to support diagnosis according to WHO-HAEM5
- *ASXL1* mutation
  - ~ 65-90% of cases
  - Presence desirable to support diagnosis of aCML according to ICC
- Next-generation sequencing (NGS) myeloid gene panel testing recommended for diagnosis and prognosis

MICROSCOPIC
- Leukocytosis with WBC > 13 x 10^9/L
- Neutrophil precursors, including promyelocytes, myelocytes, and metamyelocytes, compose ≥ 10-20% of WBC
- Prominent dysgranulopoiesis
- Anemia and thrombocytopenia common
- < 20% blasts in peripheral blood and bone marrow

Leukocytosis

Dysplastic Neutrophils

(Left) Peripheral blood smear from a patient with atypical chronic myeloid leukemia (aCML) shows leukocytosis with predominance of neutrophils with left shift. There is dysplasia among neutrophils, including hypogranular forms. (Right) Wright stain of peripheral blood from a patient with aCML shows dysplastic features of the neutrophils, including frequent hypolobation of nuclei at high power.

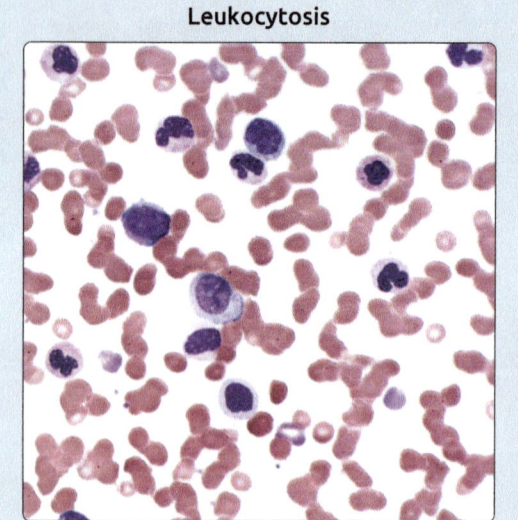

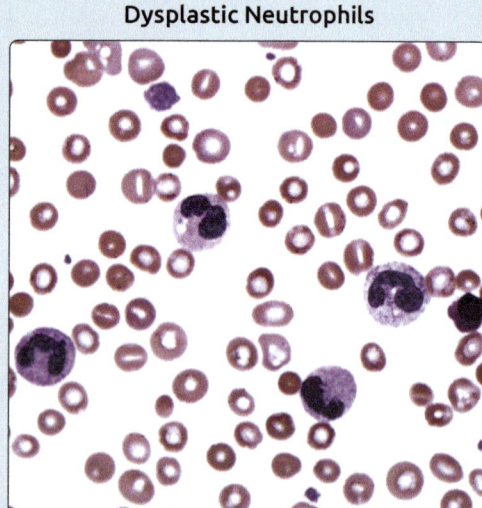

Granulocytic Dysplasia

Hypercellular Marrow

(Left) Bone marrow aspirate from a patient with aCML shows granulocytic dysplasia with hypolobation and hypogranulation. (Right) Bone marrow core biopsy from a patient with aCML shows hypercellular marrow with granulocytic hyperplasia. The megakaryocytes show mild dysplasia with hypolobation and small-sized forms.

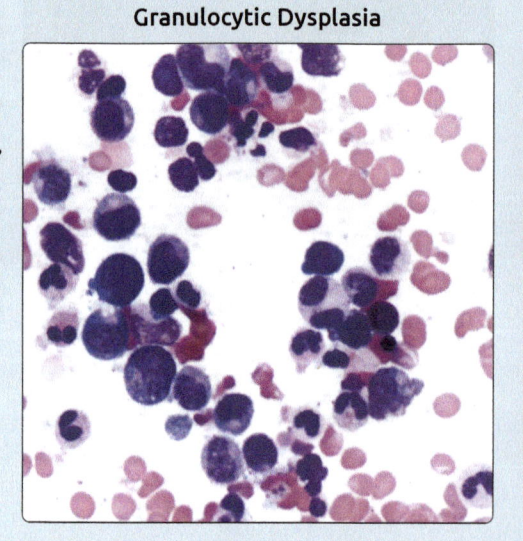

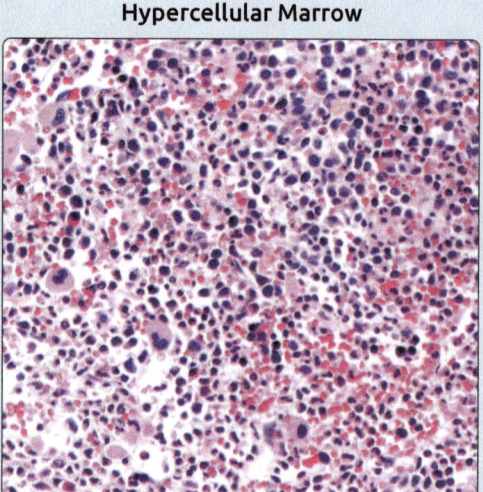

Atypical Chronic Myeloid Leukemia

TERMINOLOGY

Abbreviations
- Atypical chronic myeloid leukemia (aCML)

Definitions
- Myelodysplastic/myeloproliferative neoplasm (MDS/MPN) with sustained peripheral blood neutrophilia and neutrophilic left shift

CLASSIFICATION

ICC vs. WHO-HAEM5
- Atypical chronic myeloid leukemia (ICC)
- MDS/MPN with neutrophilia (WHO-HAEM5)

Essentially Similar Diagnostic Criteria for "Atypical CML" in ICC and "MDS/MPN With Neutrophilia" in WHO-HAEM5
- Leukocytosis ≥ 13 X 10^9/L, due to increased neutrophils and precursors (promyelocytes, myelocytes, and metamyelocytes) with latter constituting ≥ 10% of leukocytes
- Cytopenia with same threshold as for MDS (ICC)
- Blasts < 20% in blood and bone marrow
- Dysgranulopoiesis (abnormal hyposegmented &/or hypersegmented neutrophils ± abnormal chromatin clumping)
- No eosinophilia; eosinophils < 10% of peripheral blood leukocytes
- Requires exclusion of *BCR::ABL1* fusion, including cryptic rearrangement &/or alternative *BCR::ABL1* transcripts
  o Morphologic criteria is important to distinguish this entity from chronic neutrophilic leukemia, CMML, and MDS/MPN, NOS (WHO-HAEM5)
  o No or minimal absolute monocytosis; monocytes < 10% of peripheral blood leukocytes (ICC)
- Hypercellular bone marrow with granulocytic proliferation with granulocytic dysplasia ± dysplasia and erythroid and megakaryocytic lineages
- No *BCR::ABL1* or genetic abnormalities of myeloid/lymphoid neoplasms with eosinophilia and tyrosine kinase gene fusions
- Diagnosis supported by
  o Presence of *SETBP1* in association with ASXL1 (ICC) and absence of MPN associated driver mutation (ICC)
  o Presence of *SETBP1* &/or *ETNK1* mutations and absence of mutations in *JAK2*, *CALR*, *MPL*, and *CSF3R* (WHO-HAEM5)

CLINICAL ISSUES

Epidemiology
- Incidence
  o Rare: < 5% of myeloid neoplasms
- Age
  o Tends to occur in older patients
    – Median at diagnosis: Early 70s

Presentation
- Anemia, thrombocytopenia, leukocytosis
- Splenomegaly in 75%; hepatomegaly

Treatment
- Treatment not uniform, response rates are poor
  o In some series, patients were given acute myeloid leukemia (AML)-like intensive treatment; in other series, patients treated conservatively
- Hydroxyurea controls leukocytosis and splenomegaly
- Bone marrow transplantation only curative treatment
  o More effective in chronic-phase disease
- Targeted therapies may be considered based on specific mutation profiles

Prognosis
- Overall poor; mean survival: 10-25 months
  o Careful application of diagnostic criteria required for correct prognosis
  o Outcomes significantly worse than MDS/MPN, NOS
- Factors associated with adverse prognosis
  o Age > 65 years
  o WBC > 50 x 10^9/L at presentation
- Up to 40% of aCML transforms to AML
  o Median time to transformation: 11 months
  o Respond poorly to chemotherapy

MOLECULAR

Cytogenetics
- Clonal abnormalities in 40% of cases
  o Single abnormality in 1/3 of cases
  o Complex karyotype (> 3 abnormalities) in 8% of cases
    – Associated with poorer survival
- Most common abnormalities are nonspecific myeloid neoplasm associated
  o Trisomy 8, isochromosome 17q, -7 or del(7q), del(20q), del(13q), trisomy 9

Molecular Genetics
- Mutations in multiple genes common
- *SETBP1* mutation
  o ~ 24-31% of cases
  o Presence desirable to support diagnosis of aCML according to ICC and WHO-HAEM5
  o Mutation likely occurs later in clonal evolution in most cases and include
    – D868N (most common)
    – Other recurrent mutations include E858K, S869G, and I871T
  o Associated with -7 and i(17q) abnormalities
  o Associated with higher WBC counts and lower hemoglobin and platelet counts
  o Not specific to aCML
    – Less commonly seen in CMML and CNL
  o Associated with better prognosis
- *ASXL1* mutation
  o ~ 65-90% of cases
  o Presence desirable to support diagnosis of aCML according to ICC
  o Mutation likely occurs early in clonal evolution in most cases
  o Not specific
  o Mutation commonly seen with coexisting *SETBP1* mutation

Atypical Chronic Myeloid Leukemia

- o Prognostic significance in aCML has not been demonstrated
  - Likely due to very high incidence in aCML
  - Associated with shorter time to progression in other myeloid neoplasms
- *ETNK1* mutation
  - o ~ 13-15% of cases
  - o Presence desirable to support diagnosis of MDS/MPN-N according to WHO-HAEM5
  - o Mutation likely occurs early in clonal evolution in most cases
  - o Missense mutations in kinase domain
    - N244S most common
    - Result in decreased intracellular phosphoethanolamine
  - o Mutations also seen in CMML but rare in other myeloid neoplasms
    - Identification supports diagnosis of aCML if CMML excluded
- *DNMT3A* mutation in ~ 10% of cases
- *SRSF2* mutation in ~ 58% of cases
  - o Associated with better prognosis
- *KRAS* or *NRAS* mutation in 10-35% of cases
  - o Not specific
  - o Associated with disease progression and shorter overall survival
- *EZH2* mutation in ~ 24% of cases
- *CBL* mutation in 8% of cases
  - o Associated with uniparental disomy of 11q
    - Homozygous mutation
  - o Mutation associated with *SETBP1* mutation
- *CSF3R* mutation
  - o Exclude diagnosis of MDS/MPN with neutrophilia according to WHO-HAEM5 criteria
  - o Initial studies described incidence of near 40%, but if strict diagnostic criteria are applied, incidence is near 0%
  - o Much more associated with chronic neutrophilic leukemia
- *JAK2*, *CALR*, and *MPL* mutations should exclude diagnosis of aCML according to ICC and WHO

MICROSCOPIC

Histologic Features

- Peripheral blood
  - o Leukocytosis with WBC > 13 x 10⁹/L
    - Median: 40.8 x 10⁹/L
    - Most patients have WBC > 40 x 10⁹/L
  - o Neutrophil precursors, including promyelocytes, myelocytes, and metamyelocytes, compose ≥ 10-20% of WBC (median: 17%)
  - o Prominent dysgranulopoiesis
  - o Minimal absolute basophilia; < 2% of leukocytes
  - o Eosinophils account for < 10% of leukocytes
  - o Absent or minimal monocytosis; < 10% of leukocytes
  - o < 20% blasts in peripheral blood and bone marrow
  - o Cytopenia
    - Anemia and thrombocytopenia common
- Bone marrow
  - o Hypercellular marrow
  - o May have increased blasts but < 20%
  - o Prominent dysgranulopoiesis similar to peripheral blood
  - o Dyserythropoiesis in 1/2 of cases
  - o Dysmegakaryopoiesis common, including small or micromegakaryocytes and hypolobated forms
  - o Increased reticulin fibrosis in subset of cases
- Immunophenotype
  - o Neutrophils and precursors positive for MPO, CD33, CD13, CD15; immature forms positive for CD117
    - May see aberrant patterns of antigen expression

ANCILLARY TESTS

Genetic Testing

- Large next-generation sequencing (NGS) panels for myeloid-associated genes recommended for diagnosis and prognosis
- *SETBP1*, *ASXL1*, and *ETNK1* mutations strongly associated with diagnosis of aCML
- *JAK2*, *CALR*, *MPL*, and *CSF3R* mutations should strongly suggest alternate diagnosis
- May be used to demonstrate clonality
- Has prognostic significance

DIFFERENTIAL DIAGNOSIS

Chronic Myeloid Leukemia, *BCR::ABL1* (+)

- Harbor t(9;22)/*BCR::ABL1* by routine cytogenetic karyotype, FISH, or PCR studies
- No significant dysplasia in chronic phase

Chronic Neutrophilic Leukemia

- Leukocytosis due to mature neutrophilia
  - o < 10% immature granulocytes
- Dysplasia not present
- Positive for *CSF3R* mutation

Chronic Myelomonocytic Leukemia

- Significant absolute monocytosis, usually > 10% of WBC
- Shows similar mutation profile to aCML

MDS/MPN-U

- Distinction important for correct prognostication
- Disease does not meet criteria for more specific diagnosis
- Often associated with lower WBC count than aCML

Myelodysplastic Syndrome

- Dysplasia in ≥ 1 lineages
- Lacks leukocytosis
- Cytopenias predominate

SELECTED REFERENCES

1. Patnaik MM et al: Atypical chronic myeloid leukemia and myelodysplastic/myeloproliferative neoplasm, not otherwise specified: 2023 update on diagnosis, risk stratification, and management. Am J Hematol. 98(4):681-9, 2023
2. Sun Y et al: Molecular genetics and management of World Health Organization defined atypical chronic myeloid leukemia. Ann Hematol. 102(4):777-85, 2023
3. Prakash S et al: Advances in myelodysplastic/myeloproliferative neoplasms. Virchows Arch. 482(1):69-83, 2023
4. Arber DA et al: International Consensus Classification of myeloid neoplasms and acute leukemia: integrating morphological, clinical, and genomic data. Blood. 140(11):1200-28, 2022
5. Khoury JD et al: The 5th edition of the World Health Organization Classification of haematolymphoid tumours: myeloid and histiocytic/dendritic neoplasms. Leukemia. 36(7):1703-19, 2022

Atypical Chronic Myeloid Leukemia

Leukocytosis

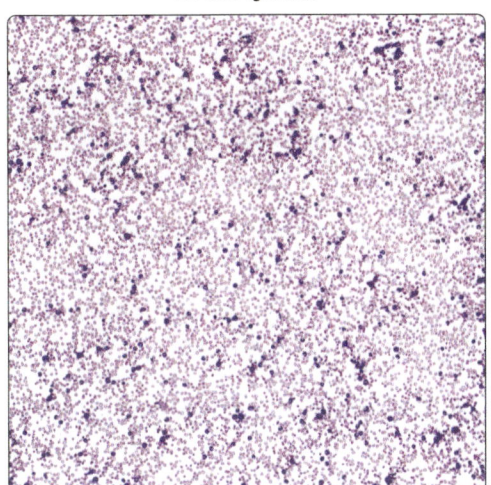

Increased Granulocytes With Dysplasia

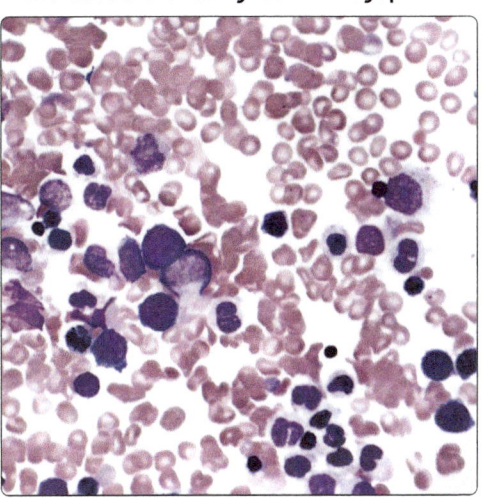

(Left) Wright stain of peripheral blood from a patient with aCML shows leukocytosis on low-power view. *(Right)* Aspirate smear from a patient with aCML shows increased granulocytes with dysplasia, including cytoplasmic hypogranulation and hypolobation.

Dysgranulopoiesis

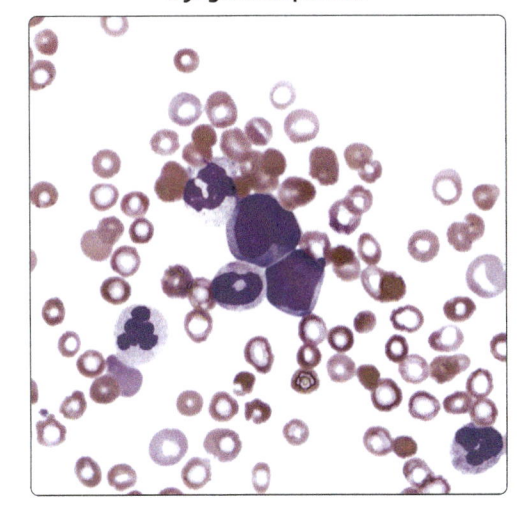

Dysgranulopoiesis

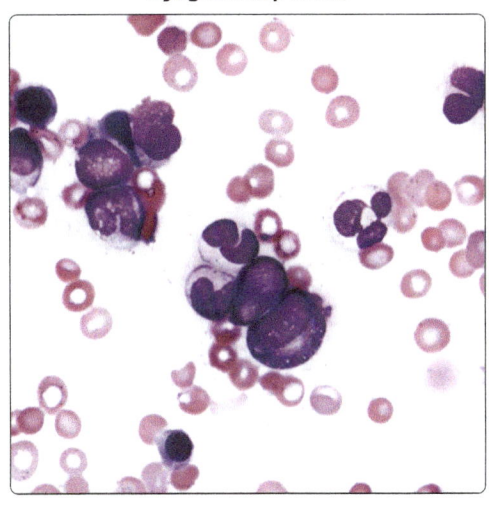

(Left) Wright stain of bone marrow aspirate smear from a patient with aCML shows a blast and dysplastic granulocytic lineages. *(Right)* Wright stain of bone marrow aspirate smear from a patient with aCML shows abundant granulocytes and precursors. Neutrophils show abnormal nuclear hypolobation.

Chronic Myeloid Leukemia

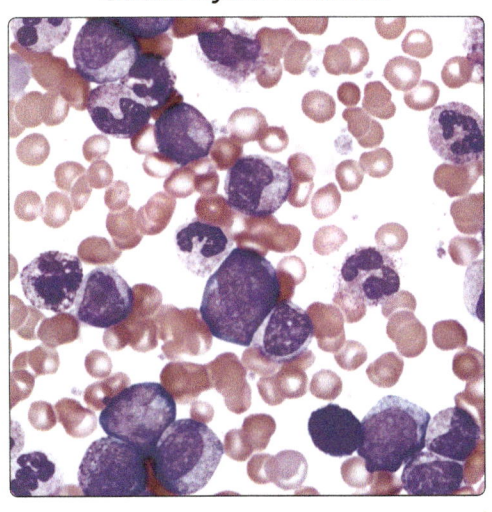

Chronic Myelomonocytic Leukemia

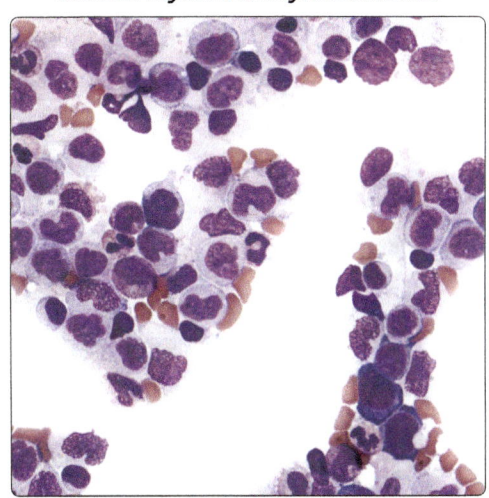

(Left) Peripheral blood from a patient with CML shows leukocytosis, left shift, occasional blasts, basophilia, and large platelets. Unlike aCML, there is no significant dysplasia. *(Right)* Bone marrow aspirate smear from a patient with chronic myelomonocytic leukemia (CMML) shows increased monocytes and monocytic precursors. There is significant overlap in the mutation profiles of aCML and CMML, so proper classification relies on morphologic and clinical findings.

Molecular Pathology of Myeloid Neoplasms

Juvenile Myelomonocytic Leukemia

KEY FACTS

TERMINOLOGY
- Clonal hematopoietic disorder of childhood characterized by proliferation of myelomonocytic cells
- Associated with RAS pathway mutations
  - 3 subtypes based on somatic or germline mutations

CLASSIFICATION
- Both ICC and WHO-HAEM5 removed JMML from MDS/MPN category
- ICC assigns JMML to pediatric &/or germline mutation-associated disorders
- WHO-HAEM5 assigns JMML to myeloproliferative neoplasms
- ICC separates cases into JMML or JMML-like based on presence of RAS pathway mutation; WHO-HAEM5 includes these cases in JMML
- ICC has separate category of Noonan syndrome-associated myeloproliferative disorder; WHO-HAEM5 includes these cases in JMML

ETIOLOGY/PATHOGENESIS
- Constitutive activation of RAS pathway and cell proliferation

CLINICAL ISSUES
- Resistant to essentially all chemotherapy
- Allogeneic hematopoietic SCT is only curative option
- Hypermethylation status, gene expression profile, and *SETBP1* mutation status important for prognosis

MOLECULAR
- Gain-of-function mutations in RAS/MAPK signaling pathway
- 30% have somatic *NRAS* or *KRAS* mutation
- 20-30% have *PTPN11* mutation
- Loss of *NF1* tumor suppressor gene function leads to activation of RAS signaling pathway
- 10-15% of patients have *CBL* mutation or deletion
- 35-40% of cases have abnormal karyotype
- Monosomy 7 seen in 25%

(Left) *Peripheral blood from an 11-month-old boy with hepatosplenomegaly, leukocytosis, and monocytosis who was diagnosed with juvenile myelomonocytic leukemia (JMML) shows an immature monocyte ⮕.* (Right) *Conventional cytogenetics shows monosomy 7 ⮕. This finding is seen in 25% of patients with JMML.*

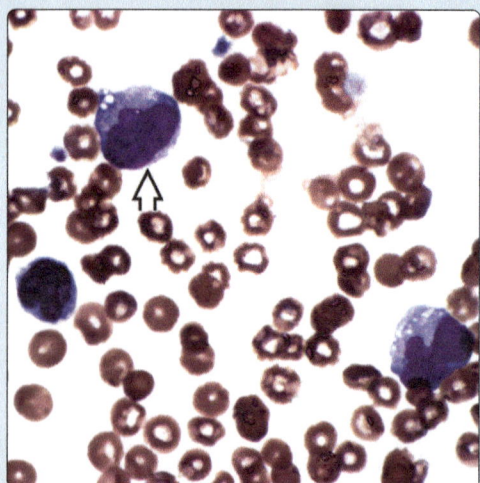

Immature Monocyte

Monosomy 7

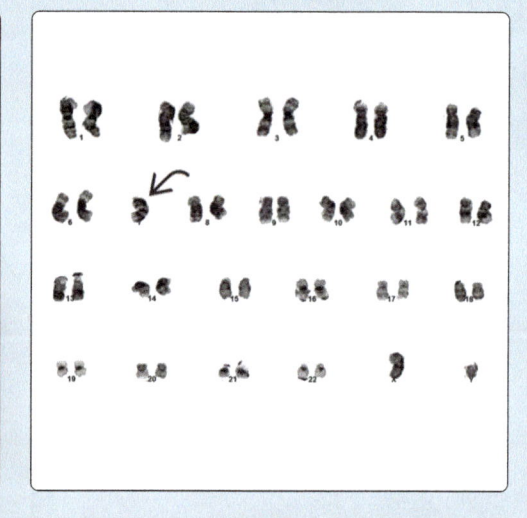

(Left) *Blood from a 5-month-old girl with JMML shows dysplastic neutrophils ⮕ as well as an immature cell ⮕.* (Right) *Bone marrow biopsy from a child with JMML shows trilineage hematopoiesis, occasional hypolobulated megakaryocytes, and left-shifted myeloid and erythroid precursors.*

Dysplastic Neutrophils

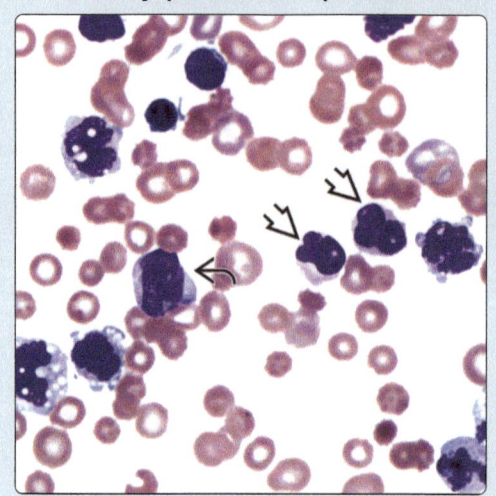

Bone Marrow Findings

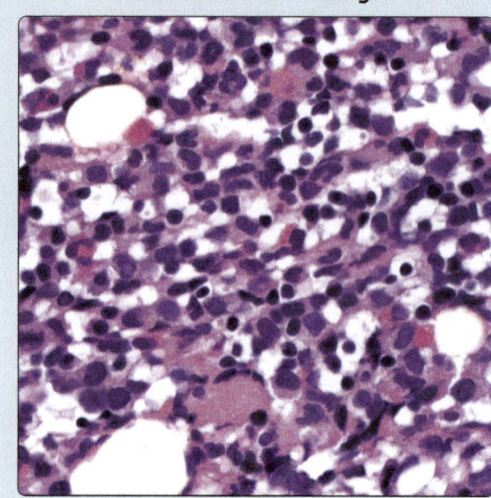

Juvenile Myelomonocytic Leukemia

TERMINOLOGY

Abbreviations
- Juvenile myelomonocytic leukemia (JMML)
- Neurofibromatosis type 1 (NF1)

Definitions
- JMML
  - Myeloid neoplasm with leukocytosis, anemia, and thrombocytopenia
  - Rare, aggressive clonal hematopoietic disorder of childhood characterized by proliferation of myelomonocytic cells
  - Canonical RAS pathway gene mutation required for diagnosis
    - NF1, CBL, PTPN11, KRAS, NRAS, RRAS
- JMML-like
  - Neoplasm with clinical and hematologic features resembling JMML without mutation in RAS pathway
- Noonan syndrome-associated myeloproliferative disorder
  - Transient disease with self-limiting course
  - Diagnosis of Noonan syndrome
    - Germline mutation in PTPN11, KRAS, NRAS, or RIT1
  - Clinical and hematologic features resembling JMML
  - May rarely have monosomy 7

CLASSIFICATION

ICC Diagnostic Criteria for JMML
- Clinical and hematologic features
  - Required features
    - Blast percentage in blood and bone marrow < 20%
    - Absence of BCR::ABL1
  - Typically present but not required
    - Peripheral blood monocytes ≥ 1 x 10⁹/L
      - Not reached in ~ 7% of cases
    - Splenomegaly
      - Not present in ~ 3% of cases
  - Genetic features (1 finding required)
    - Somatic mutation in PTPN11, KRAS, NRAS, or RRAS
    - NF1 germline mutation and loss of heterozygosity of NF1 or clinical diagnosis of NF1
    - Germline CBL mutation and loss of heterozygosity of CBL

ICC Diagnostic Criteria for JMML-Like Neoplasms
- Clinical and hematologic features of JMML
- Genetic features
  - No RAS pathway mutations
  - Includes cases with rearrangements in ALK, ROS1, FIP1L1::RARA, and CCDC88C::FLT3
  - Excludes cases with cytogenetic findings of other myeloid neoplasia or myeloid/lymphoid neoplasms with eosinophilia and tyrosine kinase gene fusions

WHO-HAEM5 Diagnostic Criteria for JMML
- Included under MPN
- Clinical and hematologic features (all required)
  - Peripheral blood monocytes ≥ 1 x 10⁹/L
  - Blast and promonocyte percentage in blood and bone marrow < 20%
  - Clinical evidence of organ involvement (splenomegaly)
  - No BCR::ABL1 fusion
  - No KMT2A rearrangement
- Genetic features (1 finding required, if none present, other criteria must be met)
  - Mutation in RAS pathway
    - Somatic mutation in PTPN11, KRAS, or NRAS
    - Somatic or germline NF1 mutation and loss of heterozygosity or compound heterozygosity of NF1
    - Somatic or germline CBL mutation and loss of heterozygosity of CBL
  - Noncanonical RAS pathway variant or fusions causing activation of genes upstream of RAS pathway
    - Includes ALK, PDGFRB, ROS1, and others
- Other criteria
  - If genetic features are not identified or testing is not available
    - ≥ 2 of following
      - Increased hemoglobin F for age
      - Circulating myeloid and erythroid precursors
      - Thrombocytopenia with hypercellular marrow, often with decreased megakaryocytes ± dysplasia
      - Hypersensitivity to GM-CSF as tested in clonogenic assays in methylcellulose or by measuring STAT5 phosphorylation in absence or with low dose of exogenous GM-CSF

ETIOLOGY/PATHOGENESIS

Pathogenesis
- Mutations in RAS/MAPK signaling pathway characteristic
  - Cause constitutive activation of RAS pathway and cell proliferation
  - Gain-of-function mutations in RAS/MAPK signaling pathway seen in 90% of patients
  - 30% have somatic NRAS or KRAS mutation
    - Causes accumulation of activated protein
  - 20-30% have PTPN11 mutation
    - Mutation causes dysregulation of RAS pathway
  - 10-15% have CBL mutation
    - Normally functions in degradation of tyrosine kinase receptors
    - Loss leads to increased RAS pathway signaling
  - Mutations lead to increased sensitivity to granulocyte colony-stimulating factors
    - RAS/MAPK and JAK/STAT pathways are responsible for GM-CSF signaling
    - Small doses of GM-CSF lead to aberrant increase in STAT5 phosphorylation

CLINICAL ISSUES

Epidemiology
- 1.3 per 1 million children 0-14 years of age per year
- 75% in children < 3 years of age; median age: 2 years
  - Ranges from 1 month to adolescence
- M:F = 2.5:1

Presentation
- Constitutional symptoms may mimic viral infections
- Symptoms related to anemia and thrombocytopenia
  - Pallor
- Hepatosplenomegaly in 97%

Juvenile Myelomonocytic Leukemia

- Lymphadenopathy in 76%
- Maculopapular rash
- Café au lait spots and neurofibromas in patients with NF1
  - JMML may be 1st presenting feature of NF1
- Short stature, macrocephaly, dysmorphic facies, and cardiac defects in patients with Noonan syndrome

Laboratory Tests
- CBC shows leukocytosis due to monocytosis, thrombocytopenia, and anemia
- In vitro granulocyte-macrophage colony-stimulating factor (GM-CSF) hypersensitivity of myeloid progenitors
- Increased fetal hemoglobin (HbF)
  - Patients with monosomy 7 may have normal HbF
- Phosphospecific flow cytometry showing STAT5 hyperphosphorylation in myeloid cells

Treatment
- JMML and JMML-like neoplasms
  - Patients with germline *CBL* mutations often experience spontaneous remission
  - All other JMML cases resistant to essentially all chemotherapy
    - Azacitidine has been shown to induce remission in some cases
  - Stem cell transplantation (SCT) is only curative option
    - Recommended early in disease with *PTPN11*, *KRAS*, or *NF1* mutation
    - Curative in ~ 50% of cases
      - Graft vs. leukemia effect is instrumental in cure
      - Immunosuppression following transplant should be rapidly decreased
    - Disease recurrence is primary cause of treatment failure post SCT
      - 2nd transplants successful in up to 50% of relapsed patients
  - Targeted therapies being developed
    - GM-CSF pathway inhibitors
      - JAK2 inhibitors
    - RAS-MAPK pathway inhibitors
      - Farnesyltransferase, bisphosphonates
      - In future, specific mutation types may guide targeted therapies
    - Other pathway inhibitors
      - MEK, RAF, PI3K, AKT, mTOR
      - Kinase inhibitors
      - ALK inhibitors
    - Alternate targetable mutations may be identified in individual patients
- Noonan syndrome-associated myeloproliferative disorders
  - Typically self-limiting and do not require treatment
  - Rarely follow JMML-like course

Prognosis
- JMML and JMML-like neoplasms
  - 5-year event-free survival after SCT is ~ 50%
    - Relapse occurs in 40%
      - Usually within 2-4 months of transplant
  - Median survival without SCT is 1 year
  - Age > 2 years at diagnosis, high fetal hemoglobin (HbF), and low platelet count correlate with worse prognosis
  - Patients with *PTPN11* mutation show reduced overall survival and increased risk of relapse following SCT
  - Increasing numbers of secondary mutations correlates with poor prognosis
    - Patients with secondary *SETBP1* or *JAK3* mutation have worse prognosis
  - Increased methylation of key genes corresponds to decreased progression-free and overall survival
    - *BMP4*, *CALCA*, *CDKN2A*, and *RARB*
    - Associated with mutations in genes controlling epigenetic modification, such as *ASXL1* and *EZH2*
- Noonan syndrome-associated myeloproliferative disorder
  - Self-limiting disease in most cases
  - Presence of secondary somatic mutations may correlate with cases that follow JMML-like course

Association With Syndromes
- 10-15% of JMML occurs in children with NF1
  - Due to germline mutation of *NF1*
  - May be presenting symptom of NF1
- Children with Noonan syndrome and Noonan syndrome-like disorder are at increased risk of associated myeloproliferative disorder
- Children with JMML or similar neoplasms and their families may benefit from consultation with pediatric geneticist

MOLECULAR

Cytogenetics
- 35-40% of cases have abnormal karyotype
  - Monosomy 7 seen in 25%

Molecular Genetics
- JMML
  - Gain-of-function mutations in RAS/MAPK signaling pathway seen in 75-80% of patients
    - 30% have somatic *NRAS* or *KRAS* mutation
      - Mutation causes accumulation of activated protein
    - 35% have somatic *PTPN11* mutation
      - Encodes SHP-2 RAS regulatory protein
      - Have strong SHP-2 activation effect
    - Loss of *NF1* tumor suppressor gene function leads to activation of RAS signaling pathway
      - Normally functions to restrict RAS activation
      - Germline in NF or somatic
      - 15-20% of JMML without NF have *NF1* mutation or deletion
    - 10-15% of patients have *CBL* mutation
      - Uniparental isodisomy of mutated allele common
      - Codon Y371 is common hotspot site of mutation
      - Codes for ubiquitin ligase regulator Grb2-SOS
      - Normally functions in degradation of tyrosine kinase receptors
      - Loss leads to increased RAS pathway signaling
  - RAS pathway activated by GM-CSF receptor signaling
    - Leads to in vivo GM-CSF hypersensitivity
  - Secondary mutations in *SETBP1* or *JAK3* in 17% of cases
    - Associated with poor outcomes
    - May be involved in disease progression
- Noonan syndrome-associated myeloproliferative disorder

Juvenile Myelomonocytic Leukemia

- Associated with germline *PTPN11*, *KRAS*, *NRAS*, or *RIT1* mutations
  - Can cause JMML-like myeloproliferative disorder with spontaneous regression
  - Seen in 1st weeks to months of life
  - Resolves over months to years without treatment
  - Associated *PTPN11* mutations have intermediate gain-of-function effect

MICROSCOPIC

Histologic Features
- Blood
  - Leukocytosis
    - Monocytes ≥ 1 x 10⁹/L
      - Immature monocytes present
      - May show dysplasia, including nuclear atypia
    - Neutrophilia with some immature forms (left shift)
      - Granulocytes may show dysplasia, including nuclear hypolobation and hypogranulation
    - Eosinophilia and basophilia may be present
  - Blasts must be < 20%; usually blasts are < 5%
    - Monocyte precursors (monoblasts and promonocytes) should be included in blast percentage
  - Nucleated RBCs often present
  - Thrombocytopenia often present
    - May be severe
- Bone marrow
  - Bone marrow findings are nonspecific
  - Hypercellular with myeloid hyperplasia
  - Minimal dysgranulopoiesis, including pseudo-Pelger-Huët forms or hypogranularity
  - Monocytic lineage accounts for 5-10% of all cells
    - Monocytes often lower than in peripheral blood
  - Blasts often elevated but must be < 20%
  - Nonspecific erythroid findings
    - Erythroid cells may show megaloblastic changes
  - Megakaryocytes may be reduced or, less often, increased and dysplastic
  - Reticulin fibrosis may be present

ANCILLARY TESTS

Genetic Testing
- Testing for RAS pathway mutations required for diagnosis
  - May be of use in minimal residual disease monitoring
- High-throughput sequencing for genes mutated in myeloid malignancies
  - Important for prognosis
- Hypermethylation studies
  - Patients with high methylation scores may be considered for SCT early in treatment

Cytogenetics
- 35% of cases have abnormal karyotype
  - Most common abnormality is monosomy 7, seen in 25%
    - Associated with *KRAS* mutated cases
    - Monosomy 7 in Noonan syndrome-associated myeloproliferative disorder may be transient

DIFFERENTIAL DIAGNOSIS

Viral Infection
- CMV, EBV, parvovirus, HHV6 may cause myeloproliferation
- Negative for *RAS*, *NF1*, *PTPN11*, or *CBL* mutations

Acute Myeloid Leukemia
- > 20% blasts in blood or bone marrow
  - ≥ 10% in cases with recurrent genetic abnormalities, as per ICC
- Cytogenetic studies may show AML-associated specific abnormality

Immunodeficiency
- Wiskott-Aldrich syndrome
  - *WAS* mutation positive or WASP protein deficient
  - Negative for *RAS* pathway mutations
- Leukocyte adhesion defect

RAS-Associated Lymphoproliferative Disease
- Transient disease with self-limiting course
  - Associated with spontaneous regression
- Leukopenia with lymphadenopathy and autoimmune manifestations
- Clinical and hematologic findings can be similar to JMML
- Somatic mutation in *KRAS* or *NRAS*
  - Gain-of-function mutations causing lymphocyte apoptosis
- Monosomy 7 may be identified and may be transient

SELECTED REFERENCES

1. Rudelius M et al: The International Consensus Classification (ICC) of hematologic neoplasms with germline predisposition, pediatric myelodysplastic syndrome, and juvenile myelomonocytic leukemia. Virchows Arch. 482(1):113-30, 2023
2. Pabari R et al: The clinical landscape of NRAS-mutated juvenile myelomonocytic leukemia-like myeloproliferation includes children with Costello syndrome. J Pediatr Hematol Oncol. 45(3):e401-5, 2023
3. Behnert A et al: Exploring the genetic and epigenetic origins of juvenile myelomonocytic leukemia using newborn screening samples. Leukemia. 36(1):279-82, 2022
4. De Vos N et al: Targeted therapy in juvenile myelomonocytic leukemia: where are we now? Pediatr Blood Cancer. 69(11):e29930, 2022
5. Fiñana C et al: Genomic and epigenomic landscape of juvenile myelomonocytic leukemia. Cancers (Basel). 14(5), 2022
6. Khoury JD et al: The 5th edition of the World Health Organization classification of haematolymphoid tumours: myeloid and histiocytic/dendritic neoplasms. Leukemia. 36(7):1703-19, 2022
7. Leguit RJ et al: EAHP 2020 workshop proceedings, pediatric myeloid neoplasms. Virchows Arch. 481(4):621-46, 2022
8. Wintering A et al: Therapy-related myeloid neoplasms resembling juvenile myelomonocytic leukemia: a case series and review of the literature. Pediatr Blood Cancer. 69(5):e29499, 2022
9. Frisanco Oliveira A et al: Immunophenotypic characteristics of juvenile myelomonocytic leukaemia and their relation with the molecular subgroups of the disease. Br J Haematol. 192(1):129-36, 2021
10. Niemeyer CM: JMML genomics and decisions. Hematology Am Soc Hematol Educ Program. 2018(1):307-12, 2018
11. Hasle H: Myelodysplastic and myeloproliferative disorders of childhood. Hematology Am Soc Hematol Educ Program. 2016(1):598-604, 2016
12. Chang TY et al: Bedside to bench in juvenile myelomonocytic leukemia: insights into leukemogenesis from a rare pediatric leukemia. Blood. 124(16):2487-97, 2014

Myelodysplastic/Myeloproliferative Neoplasm, NOS

KEY FACTS

TERMINOLOGY
- Myelodysplastic/myeloproliferative neoplasm, not otherwise specified (MDS/MPN, NOS)
  - De novo presentation
  - Hybrid myelodysplastic and myeloproliferative features at presentation
    - At least 1 cytopenia in blood
    - At least 1 cytosis in blood
  - Does **not** meet criteria for other MDS/MPN subtypes
  - Does **not** meet criteria for other myeloid neoplasm
  - Many **exclusionary** cytogenetic and molecular findings

CLINICAL ISSUES
- Generally older patients affected
- Nonspecific symptoms related to cytopenias
- Variable splenomegaly

MOLECULAR
- Heterogeneous mutation profile
- *TET2* mutation in 30%

ANCILLARY TESTS
- Large-panel testing for myeloid neoplasms recommended
- May help to demonstrate clonality
  - Myeloid-associated mutations in correct clinicopathologic context support diagnosis
- Key exclusionary role

TOP DIFFERENTIAL DIAGNOSES
- Other myeloid neoplasms, especially MDS and MPN
- Nonneoplastic disorders, especially recent treatment effects, chronic viral infections, and collagen vascular disorders

DIAGNOSTIC CHECKLIST
- Assess for recent G-CSF, chemotherapy, other therapy
  - Recommend repeat evaluation for patients who have recently received G-CSF or chemotherapy
- Diagnosis of exclusion

Neutrophilia and Anemia

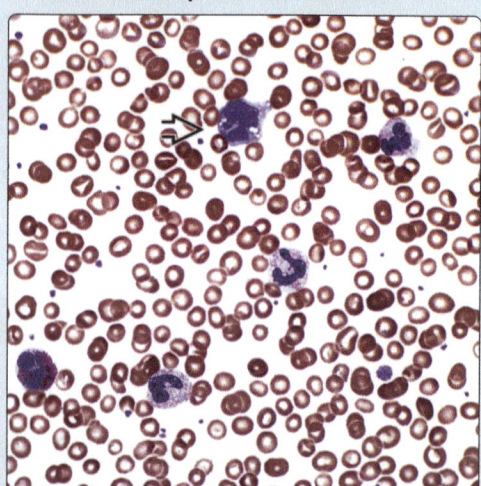

Granulocytic Predominance

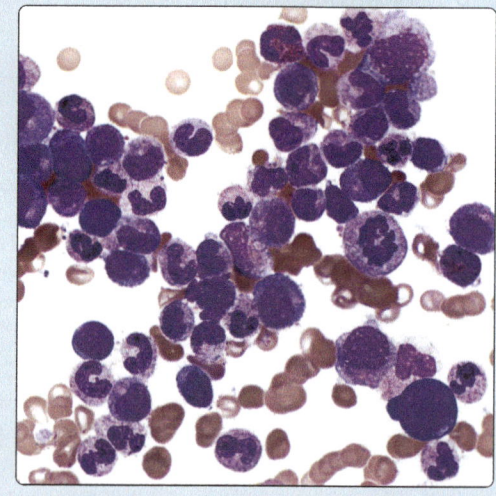

(Left) Peripheral blood smear from a 55-year-old man shows neutrophilia and anemia. Neutrophils show mild dysplastic changes. Monocytes ⇨ are also present. *(Right)* Bone marrow aspirate smear in MDS/MPN-NOS shows striking granulocytic predominance with intact maturation. Mild dysplastic features are noted.

Deletion of 17p by FISH

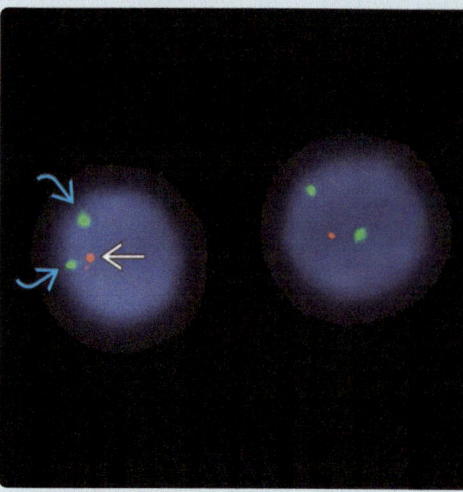

Karyotype With Isochromosome 17q

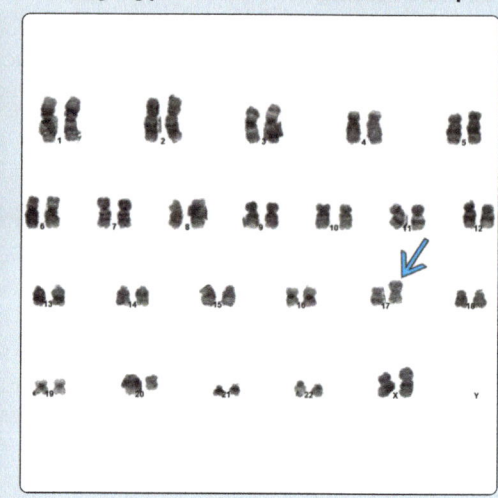

(Left) FISH for 17p on bone marrow from a patient with MDS/MPN-NOS shows 2 signals for the centromere ⇨ but only 1 signal for TP53 locus ⇨, consistent with deletion of the TP53 region. However, multihit TP53 alterations must be excluded since, if present, would be exclusionary. *(Right)* Karyotype from the same patient shows isochromosome 17q ⇨. This causes deletion of TP53 and is associated with dysplastic features. In the ICC, this meets criteria for MDS/MPN with isolated isochromosome 17q.

Myelodysplastic/Myeloproliferative Neoplasm, NOS

TERMINOLOGY

Abbreviations
- Myelodysplastic/myeloproliferative neoplasm, not otherwise specified (MDS/MPN, NOS)

Definitions
- Myeloid neoplasm with mixed myeloproliferative and myelodysplastic features that does not meet criteria for specific subtype
  o Both effective and ineffective hematopoiesis
  o De novo presentation with hybrid dysplastic and proliferative features

CLASSIFICATION

International Consensus Classification
- Neoplasm with MDS/MPN features that does not meet criteria for any specific myeloid neoplasm
- Cytopenia (thresholds similar as for MDS)
- Blasts < 20% in blood and bone marrow
- WBC ≥ 13 x 10⁹/L &/or platelet count ≥ 450 x 10⁹/L
- Presence of clonal marker or exclusion of all other causes (e.g., prior cytotoxic exposure or GCSF therapy and all other primary cause that could explain MDS/MPN features)
- No genetic changes meeting criteria for a specific diagnosis
- Notes that MPN in later stage may simulate MDS/MPN and should not be reclassified
- MDS/MPN with isolated isochromosome (17q) constitute specific subtype

WHO 5th Edition
- Both cytopenias and proliferative features in blood
- Bone marrow with combination of dysplasia and proliferative features
- Not meeting criteria for a specific diagnosis
- Not therapy related
- Notes that MDS can evolve to MDS/MPN-NOS and should be reclassified if proliferative features persist

CLINICAL ISSUES

Epidemiology
- Incidence
  o Rare (~ 1% of myeloid neoplasms)
- Age
  o Median at diagnosis: 70 years
- Sex
  o Male predominance

Presentation
- No distinctive clinical manifestations
- Symptoms from cytopenias
- Variable degree of splenomegaly

Laboratory Tests
- CBC with differential count and morphologic review
  o Document cytosis and cytopenia(s)
    – Platelet count > 450 x 10⁹/L or WBC > 13 x 10⁹/L
  o Confirm < 20% blasts and blast equivalents
  o Assess for dysplasia
- Elevated LDH

Treatment
- General treatment strategies used for other chronic myeloid neoplasms
  o Hydroxyurea commonly used
  o Other chemotherapeutics agents, including
    – Hypomethylating agents
    – Induction chemotherapy
    – Targeted therapies

Prognosis
- Often aggressive with generally poor response to therapy
- Median overall survival: 24 months from diagnosis
- ~ 20% progress to acute myeloid leukemia (AML)

MOLECULAR

Cytogenetics
- Normal karyotype in 65%
- No diagnostic cytogenetic abnormalities
  o Exclude abnormalities diagnostic of specific entities
- Clonal aberrations include those common in myeloid neoplasms
  o Trisomy 8 in ~ 18% of cases
  o Deletion 7 or 7q- in 6% of cases
  o Isochromosome 17q in 1% of cases
    – Constitutes new provisional entity under diagnostic umbrella of MDS/MPN, NOS (ICC)
    – Leukocytosis, basophilia, monocytosis
    – Pseudo-Pelger-Huët abnormality, dysplasia
    – Bone marrow fibrosis
    – Numerous small, hypolobated megakaryocytes
    – *SETBP1* and *SRSF2* mutations are common
  o Complex karyotype
    – 3-12% of cases
  o Other cytogenetic abnormalities
    – 29% of cases

Molecular Genetics
- Diseases in MDS/MPN category show significant overlap in mutation profile
  o Can lead to overlap in diagnostic features, resulting in categorization as MDS/MPN-NOS
  o Mutations **not** considered diagnostic
    – No specific mutations for any subtype
- MDS/MPN-NOS shows heterogeneous mutation profile
  o Genetics used for risk stratification
  o Presence of ≥ 1 mutations associated with worse outcomes with exception of *CALR* mutation
- *TET2*
  o 30% of cases
  o Mutation causes constitutive activation
- *JAK2*
  o 19% of cases
  o Often present with other mutations in MDS/MPN-NOS
- *NPM1*
  o 15% of cases
  o May be associated with dysplastic features
- *RUNX1*
  o 14% of cases
  o Associated with unfavorable prognosis
- *KRAS/NRAS*

Myelodysplastic/Myeloproliferative Neoplasm, NOS

- o 13% of cases
- o Associated with monocytosis
  - Some cases more appropriately classified as chronic myelomonocytic leukemia (CMML)
- *SETBP1*
  - o 10% of cases
  - o Higher WBC count
  - o Lower hemoglobin and platelet count
- *FLT3*
  - o 3% of cases
- *ASXL1*
  - o Rare in MDS/MPN-NOS
    - More common in aCML and CMML
  - o Associated with unfavorable prognosis
- *SRSF2*
  - o Rare in MDS/MPN-NOS
    - More common in CMML
  - o Associated with unfavorable prognosis
- *CSF3R*
  - o Rare in MDS/MPN-NOS
    - *CSF3R* mutation along with mutation in another gene, such as *JAK2* or *SETBP1*
    - Should prompt careful exclusion of MDS/MPN-*SF3B1*-T category of MDS/MPN neoplasm
- *KIT*
  - o Should prompt evaluation for associated mastocytosis

MICROSCOPIC

Blood
- Anemia often present, variable anisopoikilocytosis and macrocytosis
- Thrombocytopenia common
- WBC count
  - o Leukocytosis common
  - o Granulocytic dysplasia usually present
- Circulating blasts < 20%

Bone Marrow
- Hypercellular
- Myeloid lineage predominance
  - o Variable dysplasia, should be present in at least 1 lineage
  - o Blasts/blast equivalents < 20%
- Increased megakaryocytes
  - o Dysmegakaryopoiesis in > 90% of cases

ANCILLARY TESTS

Genetic Testing
- Large-panel testing for myeloid neoplasms recommended
- May help to demonstrate clonality
  - o Myeloid-associated mutations in correct clinicopathologic context support diagnosis
  - o Certain mutations may indicate more specific diagnosis
    - *SF3B1* mutation should prompt work-up for MDS/MPN with *SF3B1* mutation and thrombocytosis
    - *SRSF2* and *TET2* comutations suggest CMML
    - *CSF3R* mutation alone should prompt suspicion for chronic neutrophilic leukemia
- Cytogenetics/FISH
  - o **Exclude** cases with alternative specific diagnosis

DIFFERENTIAL DIAGNOSIS

Other Myeloid Neoplasms
- Other MDS/MPN
  - o Consider CMML if monocytosis prominent
  - o Consider atypical CML if case shows pronounced granulocytic dysplasia and prominent left shift
  - o If pediatric, consider juvenile myelomonocytic leukemia
  - o Consider MDS/MPN-*SF3B1*-T in cases with *SF3B1* mutation, ring sideroblasts, and thrombocytosis
- MDS
  - o Generally exhibits pure ineffective hematopoiesis picture with single or multilineage cytopenias
  - o MPN features may be seen with disease progression
- MPN
  - o Presence of *BCR::ABL1* will establish diagnosis of CML and exclude MDS/MPN-NOS
  - o MPN generally lacks significant dysplasia at presentation in stable phase
    - Dysplastic features may be seen with transformation
- AML
  - o Careful blast/blast equivalent enumeration
  - o Molecular genetic assessment for AML-defining abnormalities

Nonneoplastic Disorders
- Chronic viral infections
- Collagen vascular disorders
- Granulocyte (macrophage) colony-stimulating factor therapy (G-CSF, GM-CSF)

DIAGNOSTIC CHECKLIST

Pathologic Interpretation Pearls
- Confirm de novo presentation
- Confirm hybrid dysplastic/proliferative features
- Cases of MPN that **transform** into MDS/MPN-like picture are **excluded**
- Assess for recent G-CSF administration, chemotherapy, other therapy
- Recommend repeat evaluation for patients who have recently received these treatments
- Be especially cautious in making definitive diagnosis in patients who have recently received G/GM-CSF
- Delineate blast/blast equivalent percentage in blood and bone marrow
  - o **Include** promonocytes as blast equivalents
  - o **Exclude** promyelocytes, atypical promonocytes, and erythroblasts from blast percentage
- Exclude other MDS/MPN, MDS, MPN, or AML by comprehensive clinical, hematologic, morphologic, and molecular/genetic testing

SELECTED REFERENCES

1. Prakash S et al: Advances in myelodysplastic/myeloproliferative neoplasms. Virchows Arch. 482(1):69-83, 2023
2. Hasserjian RP et al: The International Consensus Classification of myelodysplastic syndromes and related entities. Virchows Arch. 482(1):39-51, 2023
3. Arber DA et al: International Consensus Classification of myeloid neoplasms and acute leukemia: integrating morphological, clinical, and genomic data. Blood. 140(11):1200-28, 2022

Myelodysplastic/Myeloproliferative Neoplasm, NOS

Granulocytic Predominance

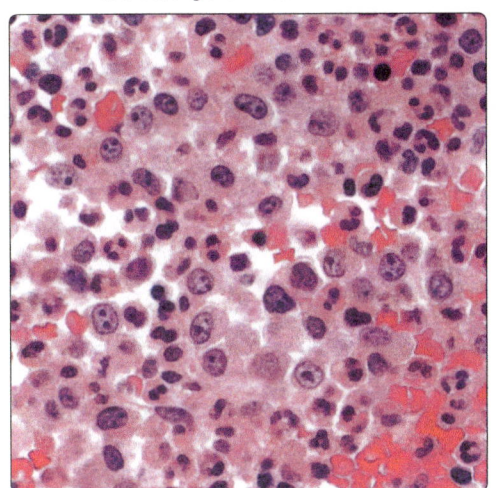

Granulocytic Predominance

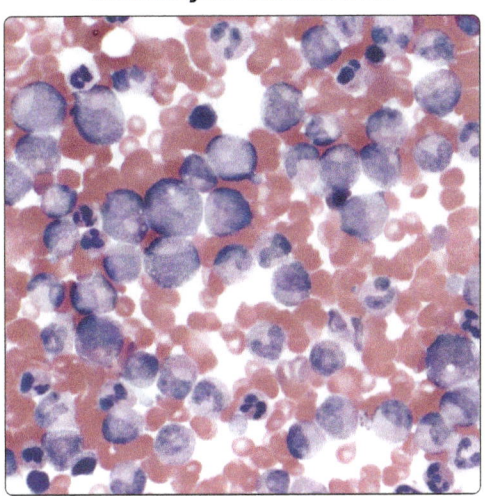

(Left) Bone marrow core biopsy shows hypercellularity with granulocytic predominance and increased immature granulocytes. Erythroid precursors and megakaryocytes are decreased. (Right) Bone aspirate smear in MDS/MPN-NOS shows a granulocytic predominance with left shift. Dysplasia is not significant. Erythroid precursors are markedly decreased.

CD34(+) Blasts

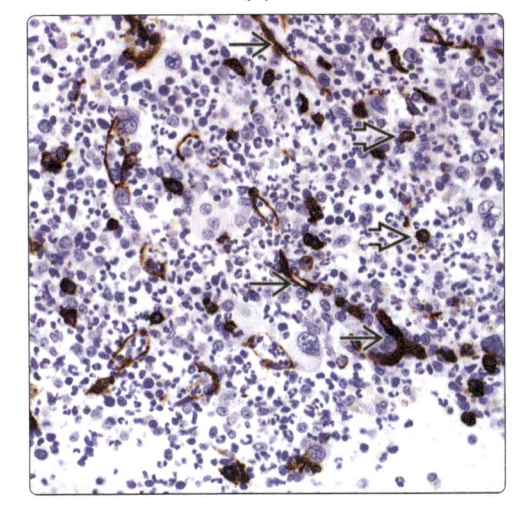

Reticulin Fibrosis

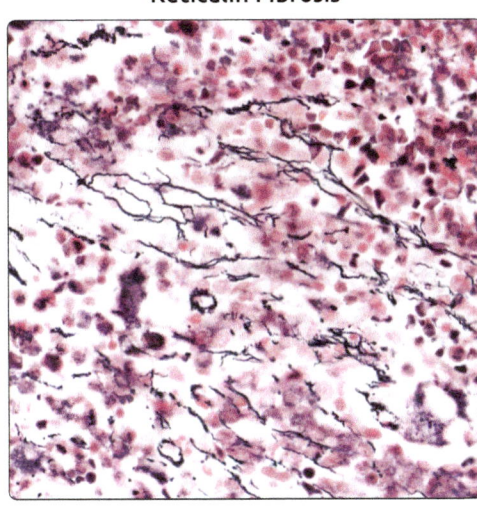

(Left) CD34 in MDS/MPN-NOS shows a mild increase in positive blasts ➡ in conjunction with neoangiogenesis ➡. The blast count is clearly < 20%. Neoangiogenesis is a common finding in many bone marrow neoplasms. (Right) Mildly increased reticulin fibers are evident on this bone marrow core biopsy from a patient with MDS/MPN-NOS. Reticulin fibrosis is sometimes seen in this subtype of MDS/MPN, making distinction from MPN challenging.

Dysplastic Megakaryocytes

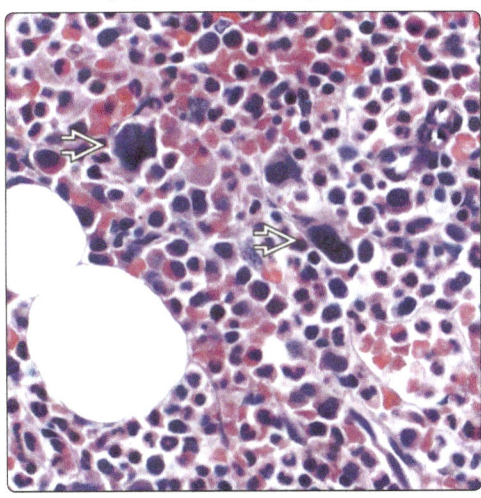

Complex Karyotype

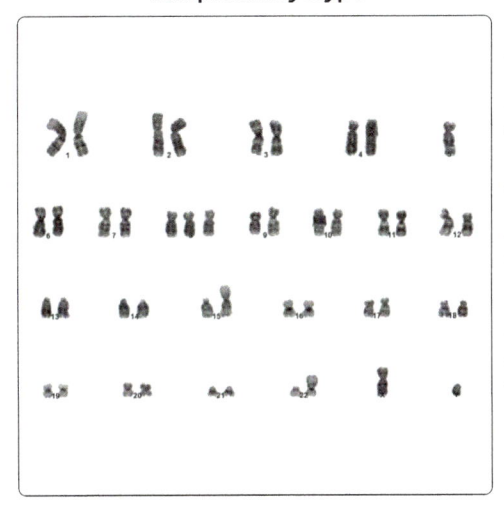

(Left) Bone marrow core biopsy shows hypercellularity and dysplastic megakaryocytes ➡. Aspirate smear showed trilineage dysplasia. This case was positive for JAK2 V617F and CSF3R T618I mutations. The presence of multiple mutations may lead to atypical presentation and classification as MDS/MPN-NOS. (Right) Karyotype from a patient with MDS/MPN-NOS shows numerous abnormalities, including monosomy 5 and trisomy 8, recurrent abnormalities in myeloid disorders.

Overview of Acute Myeloid Leukemia

TERMINOLOGY

Abbreviations
- Acute myeloid leukemia (AML)
- International Consensus Classification (ICC)
- World Health Organization classification, 5th edition (WHO-HAEM5)

Synonyms
- Acute myelogenous leukemia

Definitions
- Clonal hematopoietic stem cell proliferation encompassing heterogeneous group of genetically distinct neoplasms

WHO-HAEM5 and ICC
- AML with recurrent genetic abnormalities in both ICC and WHO-HAEM5
  - Both ICC and WHO-HAEM5 require blasts ≥ 20% in following categories
    - AML with BCR::ABL1
    - AML with myelodysplasia-related cytogenetic abnormalities
    - AML with myelodysplasia-related gene mutation
    - AML, NOS (ICC)/ AML defined by differentiation (WHO-HAEM5)
  - ICC category of AML with mutated TP53 requires ≥ 20% blasts as well
  - In addition, WHO-HAEM5 requires ≥ 20% blasts for AML with CEBPA mutation
  - No blasts cutoff in WHO-HAEM5 for remaining AML subtypes with recurrent genetic abnormalities
  - ICC requires ≥ 10% bone marrow blasts for AML with recurrent genetic abnormalities except for AML with BCR::ABL1 and AML with TP53
  - AML defined by differentiation in WHO-HAEM5 designated as AML, NOS in ICC

Common Examples of AML With Recurrent Genetic Abnormalities
- AML with BCR::ABL1 fusion
  - Included in AML with recurrent genetic abnormalities in both classifications
  - Defined as de novo AML with BCR::ABL1 fusion at initial diagnostic presentation and lack of subsequent evidence of chronic myeloid leukemia (CML)
  - Compared with myeloid blast phase of CML, AML with BCR::ABL1 frequently presents with higher percentage of blasts, lower basophils, and lower incidence of splenomegaly
  - ≥ 20% blasts required by both ICC and WHO-HAEM5
  - Recognition important due to availability of targeted kinase inhibitors
- AML with mutated NPM1
  - Remains unchanged in both WHO-HAEM5 and ICC
  - Usually seen in normal karyotype
    - ~ 10% of cases show chromosomal abnormalities, including +8 and del(9q)
  - Rare cooccurrence of TP53 mutation may be seen
    - Should still be classified as NPM1-mutated AML but annotating TP53 mutation
  - Multilineage dysplasia present in ~ 23% of de novo NPM1-mutated AML
    - No prognostic significance in absence of prior myelodysplastic syndrome (MDS) or myeloproliferative neoplasm (MPN) or MDS-related cytogenetic abnormalities
    - Impact of secondary-type myelodysplasia-related gene mutations on outcome remains controversial
  - Favorable prognosis in absence of FLT3 ITD
  - NPM1 mutation in secondary AML
    - Lack favorable prognosis seen in NPM1-mutated de novo AML cases
- AML with inframe basic leucine zipper region (bZIP) CEBPA mutation (ICC)
  - Only inframe mutations involving bZIP confer favorable outcome irrespective of occurrence as biallelic or monoallelic
  - > 10% blasts required for diagnosis
  - Frequent comutation of GATA2 is seen
  - Concurrent cytogenetic abnormalities are uncommon

Bone Marrow Effacement

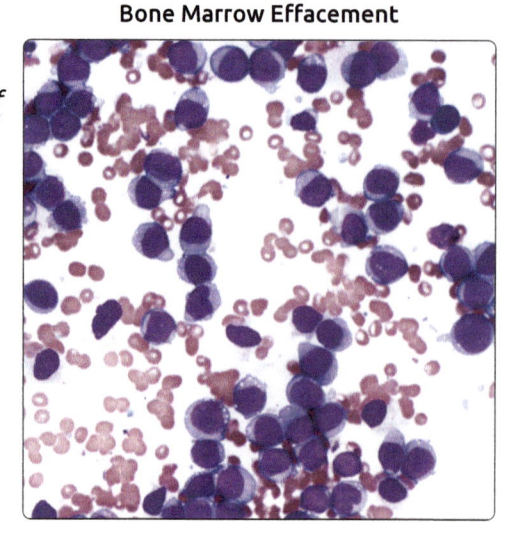

NPM1-Mutated FLT3 Wildtype AML

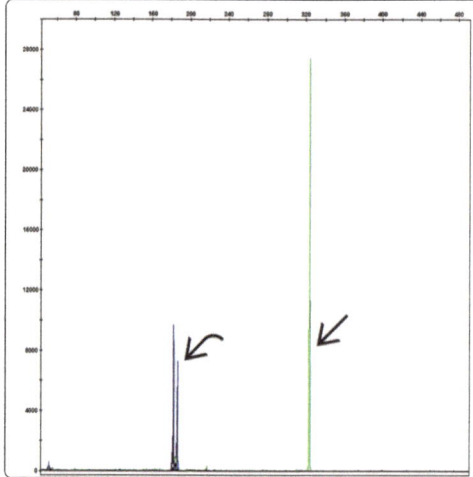

(Left) Acute monoblastic leukemia has effaced the entire bone marrow, typical of the behavior of acute myeloid leukemia (AML) in general. Clinical symptoms reflected this bone marrow failure. (Right) PCR analysis performed on bone marrow aspirate from a patient with newly diagnosed AML shows NPM1 4 base insertion mutation ➡ and wildtype FLT3 ➡, conferring a favorable prognosis.

Overview of Acute Myeloid Leukemia

- o Multilineage dysplasia maybe present in subset of cases
  - No prognostic significance in absence of MDS-related cytogenetic abnormalities
- AML with *CEBPA* mutation (WHO-HAEM5)
  - o Requires presence of biallelic mutations in *CEBPA* or single mutation located in bZIP region
    - 20% blasts required for diagnosis
- AML with mutated *TP53* (ICC)
  - o New distinct entity in ICC but not recognized in WHO-HAEM5
  - o *TP53* pathogenic mutation at VAF of ≥ 10% required ± loss of the *TP53* wildtype allele
  - o Regarded as poor prognostic leukemia
- AML with myelodysplasia-related gene mutation (ICC)
  - o Corresponds to AML, myelodysplasia-related of WHO-HAEM5
  - o Associated mutated genes include
    - *ASXL1*, *BCOR*, *EZH2*, *RUNX1*, *SF3B1*, *SRSF2*, *STAG2*, *U2AF1*, and *ZRSR2*
    - ≥ 20% blasts required by both classifications
    - Poor risk category of AML
- AML with myelodysplasia-related cytogenetic abnormalities (ICC)
  - o Corresponds to AML, myelodysplasia-related in WHO-HAEM5
  - o Associated cytogenetic abnormalities include
    - Complex karyotype or del(5q)/t(5q)/add(5q), -7/del(7q), +8, del(12p)/t(12p)/add(12p), i(17q), -17/add(17p)/del(17p), and del(20q), idic(X)(q13)
  - o ≥ 20% blasts required by both classifications

Familial AML With Germline Predisposition

- Included under separate hematologic neoplasms with germline predisposition

EPIDEMIOLOGY

Age Range

- All ages affected
  - o Median: 63 years
- Overall, proportion of acute leukemias that are AML increases with age
  - o ~ 80% of adult acute leukemias are myeloid
- Some AML subtypes are more prevalent in older adults
  - o AML with myelodysplasia-related gene mutations or myelodysplasia-related cytogenetic abnormalities
- Some AML subtypes are more prevalent in younger age groups
  - o AML with recurring genetic abnormality [e.g., t(15;17)/*PML::RARA*, t(8;21)/*RUNX1::RUNX1T1*, inv(16)/t(16;16)/*CBFB::MYH11*, t(9;11)/*MLLT3::KMT2A*]
  - o AML with t(1;22)/*RBM15::MRTFA* occurs in infants and children < 3 years of age
    - Rare occurrence in young adults have also been reported

Incidence

- Age-adjusted incidence: 3.4 cases per 100,000 individuals
- ~ 20,000 new cases in USA each year

Natural History

- Variable clinical course

- o Clinically aggressive disease in most cases
- o Acute promyelocytic leukemia (APL) can be cured
- o Rare cases may regress spontaneously
  - Neonatal AML with t(8;16)/*KAT6A::CREBBP*
- Prognosis of unfavorable AML subtypes remains poor in older patients and those who are not eligible for allogeneic stem cell transplant

ETIOLOGY/PATHOGENESIS

De novo AML Development

- Somatic driver mutations
  - o Serial acquisition of somatic mutations in hematopoietic stem cells (HSC)
- Down syndrome (sporadic)
  - o 10-20x increased risk for AML
  - o > 500x increased risk for acute megakaryoblastic leukemia

Familial Predisposition Syndromes

- Inherited bone marrow (BM) failure syndromes
  - o Fanconi anemia (FA), dyskeratosis congenita, Diamond-Blackfan anemia, severe congenital neutropenia, Shwachman-Diamond syndrome
- Familial platelet disorder with propensity to AML, familial AML with mutated *CEBPA*, familial AML with *GATA2* mutations

Environmental Exposures

- Radiation, benzene, cytotoxic therapy

Progression of Underlying Hematopoietic Neoplasm

- MDS, MPN, and MDS/MPN overlap neoplasms
  - o Secondary to acquisition of additional genetic mutations

Pathogenesis of Leukemogenesis

- Accumulation of multiple genetic hits
- Class I and II mutations
  - o Class I: Proproliferative signal
    - e.g., *FLT3*, *JAK2*, *KIT*
  - o Class II: Impairment of cellular maturation
    - e.g., *PML::RARA*, *CEBPA*, *RUNX1::RUNX1T1*
- Complex interplay of genetic events contributes to AML pathogenesis
  - o AML genome shows fewer mutations compared to other cancers
    - At least 1 potential driver mutation is detected in each de novo AML based on The Cancer Genome Atlas (TCGA) published data
  - o Virtually all AML cases show at least 1 nonsynonymous mutations in 1 of 9 gene categories, including
    - Transcription factor fusions, *NPM1*, tumor suppressor genes, DNA methylation-related genes, signaling genes, chromatin modifying genes, myeloid transcription factor genes, and spliceosome complex genes
  - o Examples of well-established mutated genes relevant to AML pathogenesis include
    - *FLT3*, *NPM1*, *CEBPA*, *RUNX1*, *IDH1*, and *IDH2*

Overview of Acute Myeloid Leukemia

CLINICAL IMPLICATIONS

Clinical Presentation
- Symptoms related to BM failure
  - Fatigue (anemia), bleeding (thrombocytopenia), infection (neutropenia)
- Extramedullary involvement
  - Skin lesions, gingival hyperplasia, myeloid sarcomas

Clinical Risk Factors
- Prognostic factors and risk
  - Cytogenetics and molecular genetics
  - Prior chemotherapy &/or radiation
  - Underlying hematopoietic neoplasm, e.g., MDS
  - Increasing age (> 60 years), performance status
  - Elevated LDH

Treatment of AML
- Intensive induction therapy
  - 3 days of anthracycline and 7 days of cytarabine (also called "7+3" regimen)
- FDA-approved targeted therapies
  - *FLT3* inhibitors
    - Midostaurin is 1st FDA-approved *FLT3*-targeted therapy in AML
  - *IDH2* inhibitors
    - Enasidenib is oral *IDH2* inhibitor approved by FDA
  - Humanized anti-CD33 antibody (gemtuzumab ozogamicin)
    - Reasonable treatment option in certain AML patients
- Other agents in active clinical trials
  - Guadecitabine (hypomethylating agent)
    - Being studied in phase I and II clinical trials
    - Longer half-life compared to decitabine
  - BCL2 inhibitor (venetoclax)
    - Promising results in phase I/II trial in combination with low-dose cytarabine
  - *IDH1* inhibitors
    - Ivosidenib is 1st *IDH1* inhibitor for patients with *IDH1*-mutated AML
  - Immunotherapy (checkpoint inhibitors)
    - Modest results with PD1 or PDL1 inhibitors in AML
- Intensive chemotherapy followed by autologous transplantation
  - One randomized study showed better RFS and similar OS to conventional consolidation chemotherapy
- Allogeneic HSC transplantation
  - Only curative option in patients with primary refractory disease

DIAGNOSTIC CHECKLIST

Required Elements
- Peripheral blood (PB) &/or BM microscopic examination
- Flow cytometry
- Cytogenetics
- Complete and accurate clinical history
  - Prior therapy, prior hematologic neoplasm
- Molecular genetics
  - *FLT3*, *NPM1*, *CEBPA* mutational analysis required
- Upfront gene panel mutational analysis by next-generation sequencing recommended, including
  - *ASXL1, BCOR, BRINP3, CALR, CBL, CSF3R, DNMT3A, EZH2, FLT3, IDH1, IDH2, JAK2, KIT, KRAS, NPM1, NRAS, PHF6, PTPN11, RAD21, RUNX1, SETBP1, SF3B1, SMC1A, SMC3, SRSF2, STAG2, TET2, TP53, U2AF1, WT1,* and *ZRSR2*

MOLECULAR PATHOLOGY

Cytogenetics
- ~ 50% of AML cases show chromosomal abnormalities
- Favorable risk group
  - AML with t(15;17), t(8;21), inv(16) or t(16;16) cytogenetic abnormalities
- Unfavorable risk
  - Complex cytogenetics (≥ 3), 3q abnormalities, inv(3), del(5q), -5, t(9;22), -17, 11q23 rearrangements excluding 9;11 abnormalities

Acquired Gene Alterations
- *FLT3* ITD mutations
  - Detected in ~ 20% of AML cases
  - Associated with poor prognosis and resistance to standard chemotherapy
  - Testing is recommended in all newly diagnosed AML cases for prognostic and therapeutic decisions
  - *FLT3* ITD mutations are not stable over course of disease
    - Not useful for disease monitoring
- *FLT3* TKD mutations
  - Testing is recommended for *FLT3*-targeted therapy
- *NPM1* mutations
  - Present in ~ 30% of AML
  - More common in cytogenetically normal AML (50-60%)
  - Associated with good prognosis in absence of *FLT3* ITD mutations
  - Are stable over course of disease
    - Useful marker for minimal residual disease detection
- *CEBPA* mutations
  - *CEBPA* mutations detected in ~ 10% of AML
  - Mostly in normal cytogenetic AMLs and in AML with 9q deletion
  - Mutations can be single (50% of mutated case), double (usually biallelic), or homozygous
    - Only inframe bZIP *CEBPA* mutations are associated with favorable prognosis per ICC
- *RUNX1* mutations
  - *RUNX1*-mutated AML has unfavorable prognosis with resistance to chemotherapy
    - Useful as marker for disease monitoring
- *TET2* mutations
  - Detected in ~ 8% of AML, mostly in cytogenetically normal cases
  - Prognostic significance in AML is not entirely clear
- *IDH1* and *IDH2* mutations
  - Detected in ~ 7-8% of AML, mostly in cytogenetically normal cases
  - *IDH1* and *IDH2* mutations are largely absent in AML with recurrent chromosomal translocations
  - *IDH1-* and *IDH2-* targeted therapies available
- *DNMT3A* mutations

Overview of Acute Myeloid Leukemia

- Encodes enzyme that catalyze transfer of methyl group to 5' position of cytosine at CpG dinucleotides
- Typically associated with intermediate cytogenetic profile
- *ASXL1* mutations
  - Associated with adverse prognosis and overall shorter survival
- Many other low-frequency mutations occur in AML

Familial AML Gene Mutations
- Familial *CEBPA*-mutated AML
  - Most individuals inherit frameshift mutation
  - ~ 1% of sporadic AML could be attributed to familial AML with *CEBPA* mutation
- Familial *GATA2*-mutated AML
  - Same mutations lead to different clinical syndromes
    - No genotype-phenotype correlation
- Familial platelet disorder with propensity to MDS/AML
  - Monoallelic *RUNX1* mutation
  - Progression to MDS/AML requires 2nd-hit mutations
- Other mutated genes associated with familial AML include
  - *SRP72, DKC1, DIDO1, DDX41, ETV6, TERT, TERC, ANKRD26,* and *TP53*

MICROSCOPIC

Blasts and Blast Equivalents
- Myeloblasts
  - Cytoplasmic azurophilic granules, Auer rods
- Monoblasts
  - Very fine cytoplasmic azurophilic granules; abundant blue-gray cytoplasm
- Megakaryoblasts
  - May see cytoplasmic blebbing/shedding, but not specific
- Promyelocytes in APL
  - Single or bilobed nuclei, hypo- or hypergranular cytoplasm, may see cytoplasm packed with Auer rods

Peripheral Blood
- Cytopenias
- Circulating blasts/blast equivalents
- Assess erythrocytes for evidence of disseminated intravascular coagulation

Bone Marrow Aspirate
- Requirements
  - Well-stained, adequate specimen
  - If fibrotic or dry tap, assess touch preparations
- Enumerate blasts and assess for dysplasia
- Assess for increased/abnormal-appearing mast cells
  - Mastocytosis may be concurrent

Bone Marrow Core Biopsy
- Identify blasts
  - Utilize immunohistochemistry if needed
    - Not all blasts are CD34(+), particularly APL blasts, megakaryocytic, monocytic, and erythroid blasts
- Assess megakaryocytic dysplasia
- Evaluate for associated concurrent neoplasm

Specialized Testing
- Cytochemical stains

- MPO
  - If positive, confirms myeloid lineage
  - If negative, does not exclude myeloid lineage
  - ~ 5% of acute monoblastic leukemias may show scattered MPO(+) granules
- NSE
  - If positive, confirms monocytic lineage
  - If negative, does not exclude monocytic lineage
- Flow cytometry
  - Should be performed in all new cases of AML
  - Establishes lineage
  - Establishes phenotype "fingerprint" for future monitoring
  - Blast markers
    - CD34: Not all blasts are CD34(+)
    - CD117: Also stains pronormoblasts, mast cells
    - TdT: Stains subset of AML
  - Myeloid markers
    - MPO, CD13, CD33
  - Monocytic markers
    - CD14, CD36/CD64 coexpression, CD163, CD4 (weak), CD33 (bright)
  - Megakaryocytic markers
    - CD31, CD41, CD42b, CD61
  - Erythroid markers
    - Glycophorin A, hemoglobin A, CD71 (not specific), e-cadherin (expressed in erythroblasts and normoblasts)
- IHC
  - Useful if flow cytometry inadequate or not performed
  - In general, fewer antibodies are available compared with flow cytometry
    - Some are unique to IHC, however
    - CD68: Myeloid and monocytic
    - Lysozyme: Monocytic
    - CD31, CD42b: Megakaryocytic lineage
- Cytogenetics
  - Should be performed in all new cases of AML
  - Submit in sodium heparin anticoagulant
  - Diagnostic: e.g., AML with recurring genetic abnormality
  - Prognostic: Favorable, intermediate, and unfavorable risk groups
- FISH
  - Perform as needed, depending on morphologic suspicion and cytogenetic findings
- Molecular genetics
  - *FLT3, NPM1,* and *CEBPA* mutations
  - Upfront AML-associated gene panel mutation analysis by next-generation sequencing recommended

Monitoring of Measurable Residual Disease
- Multiparameter flow cytometry
  - Must distinguish AML cells from normal hematopoietic cells
- Molecular measurable residual disease (MRD) testing
  - Include quantitative PCR (qPCR) and next-generation sequencing
  - Leukemia-related abnormalities suitable for qPCR include *NPM1, BCR::ABL1, CBFB::MYH11, RUNX1::RUNX1T1, KMT2A::MLLT3, PML::RARA,* and others
  - Should reach limit of detection at least 10^{-3}

Overview of Acute Myeloid Leukemia

Comparison of AML Nomenclatures in WHO-HAEM4, WHO-HAEM5, and ICC

WHO-HAEM4	WHO-HAEM5	ICC
Acute promyelocytic leukemia with *PML::RARA*	Acute promyelocytic leukemia with *PML::RARA* fusion	Acute promyelocytic leukemia with t(15;17)(q24.1;q21.2)/*PML::RARA* (≥ 10% blasts)
AML with t(8;21)(q22;q22.1)/*RUNX1::RUNX1T1*	AML with *RUNX1::RUNX1T1* fusion	AML with t(8;21)(q22;q22.1)/*RUNX1::RUNX1T1* (≥ 10% blasts)
AML with inv(16)(p13.1q22)/t(16;16)(p13.1;q22)/*CBFB::MYH11*	AML with *CBFB::MYH11* fusion	AML with inv(16)(p13.1q22)/t(16;16)(p13.1;q22)/*CBFB::MYH11* (≥ 10% blasts)
AML with t(9;11)(p21.3;q23.3)/*MLLT3::KMT2A*	AML with *KMT2A* rearrangements	AML with t(9;11)(p21.3;q23.3)/*MLLT3::KMT2A* (≥ 10% blasts) AML with other *KMT2A* rearrangements (≥ 10% blasts)
AML with t(6;9)(p23;q34.1)/*DEK::NUP214*	AML with *DEK::NUP214* fusion	AML with t(6;9)(p23;q34.1)/*DEK::NUP214* (≥ 10% blasts)
AML with inv(3)(q21.3q26.2) or t(3;3)(q21.3;q26.2)/*GATA2::MECOM*(*EVI1*)	AML with *MECOM* rearrangements AML with other defined genetic alterations (rare fusions)	AML with inv(3)(q21.3q26.2) or t(3;3)(q21.3;q26.2)/*GATA2::MECOM*(*EVI1*) (≥ 10% blasts) AML with other *MECOM* rearrangements (≥ 10% blasts) AML with other rare recurring translocations, including *NUP98* rearrangements and *RBM15::MRTF1*
AML with t(9;22)(q34.1;q11.2)/*BCR::ABL1*	AML with *BCR::ABL1* fusion (≥ 20% blasts)	AML with t(9;22)(q34.1;q11.2)/*BCR::ABL1* (≥ 20% blasts)
AML with mutated *NPM1*	AML with *NPM1* mutation	AML with mutated *NPM1* (≥ 10% blasts)
AML with biallelic mutation of *CEBPA*	AML with *CEBPA* mutation (≥ 20% blasts)	AML with inframe bZIP *CEBPA* mutation (≥ 10% blasts) AML with TP53 (≥ 20% blasts)
AML with mutated *RUNX1*	AML, myelodysplasia related (≥ 20% blasts)	AML with myelodysplasia-related gene mutations (*ASXL1, BCOR, EZH2, RUNX1, SF3B1, SRSF2, STAG2, U2AF1,* or *ZRSR2*) (≥ 20% blasts)
AML with MRC	AML, myelodysplasia related (≥ 20% blasts)	AML with myelodysplasia-related cytogenetic abnormalities (≥ 20% blasts)
AML, NOS	AML defined by differentiation (≥ 20% blasts)	AML, NOS) (≥ 20% blasts)
Myeloid sarcoma	Myeloid sarcoma	Myeloid sarcoma

AML = acute myeloid leukemia; bZIP = basic leucine zipper region; ICC= International Consensus Classification; myelodysplasia-related changes (MRC), not otherwise specified (NOS); WHO-HAEM4 = World Health Organization classification of hematolymphoid tumors, 4th edition; WHO-HAEM5 = World Health Organization classification of hematolymphoid tumors, 5th edition.

Adopted from Falini et al: Am J Hematol, 98: 481-92, 2023.

- Mutations consistent with clonal hematopoiesis (e.g., *ASXL1, DNMT3A, TET2*) should not be considered as MRD

DIFFERENTIAL DIAGNOSIS

Granulocyte Colony-Stimulating Factor Administration
- Blasts may account for ≥ 20% in hypocellular specimen
- Nonclonal transient phenomenon

Blast Phase of Preexisting Myeloid Neoplasms
- Clinical history help to separate from de novo AML

SELECTED REFERENCES

1. Falini B et al: Comparison of the International Consensus and 5th WHO edition classifications of adult myelodysplastic syndromes and acute myeloid leukemia. Am J Hematol. 98(3):481-92, 2023
2. Weinberg OK et al: The International Consensus Classification of acute myeloid leukemia. Virchows Arch. 482(1):27-37, 2023
3. Döhner H et al: Diagnosis and management of AML in adults: 2022 recommendations from an international expert panel on behalf of the ELN. Blood. 140(12):1345-77, 2022
4. Khoury JD et al: The 5th edition of the World Health Organization classification of haematolymphoid tumours: myeloid and histiocytic/dendritic neoplasms. Leukemia. 36(7):1703-19, 2022
5. Click ZR et al: New Food and Drug Administration-approved and emerging novel treatment options for acute myeloid leukemia. Pharmacotherapy. 38(11):1143-54, 2018

Overview of Acute Myeloid Leukemia

Molecular Pathology of Myeloid Neoplasms

Bilobed Forms and Auer Rods

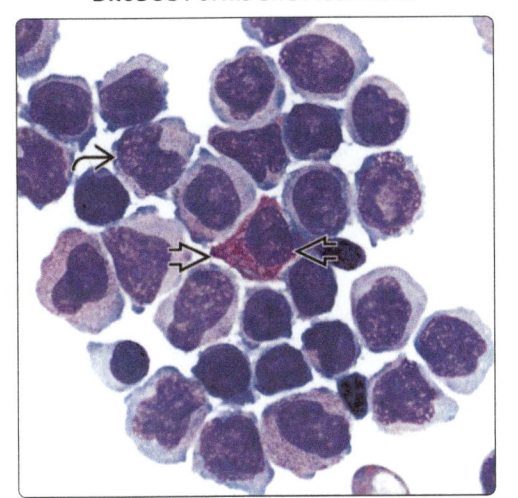

Flow Cytometry of CD13 vs. HLA-DR

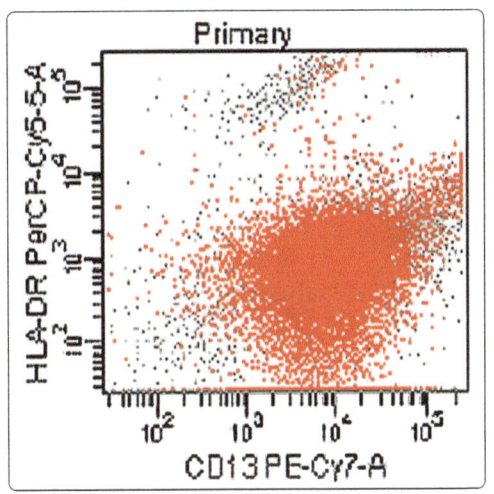

(Left) Cytospin preparation of bone marrow aspirate shows numerous hypogranular blasts with bilobed forms ⇨ and a blast with numerous Auer rods ⇨, highly suggestive of acute promyelocytic leukemia (APL). (Right) Flow cytometric analysis performed on bone marrow aspirate from a patient with acute leukemia with features suspicious for APL shows blasts brightly positive for CD13 and negative for HLA-DR.

PML::RARA-Targeted FISH

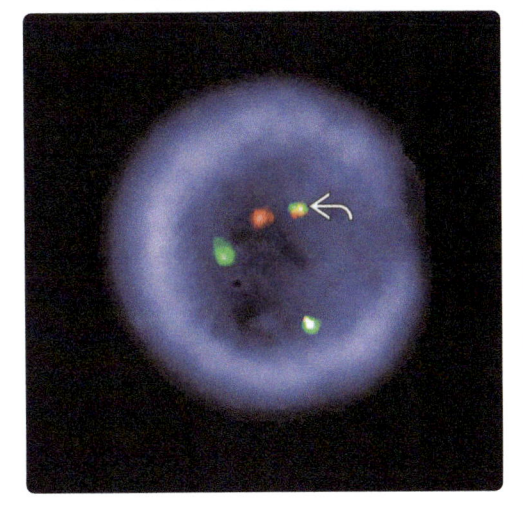

Quantitative RT-PCR for PML::RARA

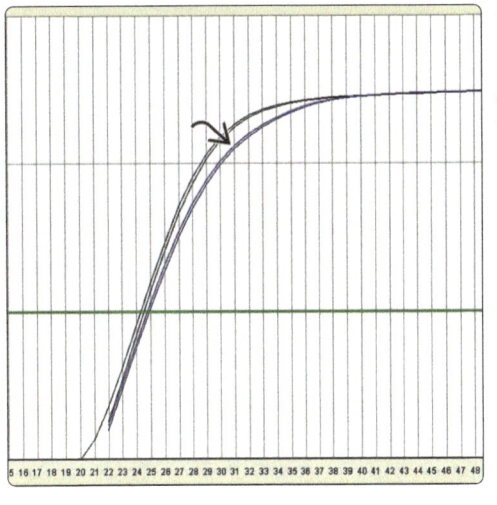

(Left) FISH analysis using targeted probes for PML and RARA shows PML::RARA fusion signal ⇨, supportive of APL. (Right) Quantitative RT-PCR performed on bone marrow aspirate shows high copy numbers of bcr3-type PML::RARA transcripts (blue curves) ⇨, supportive of APL. This assay is valuable for disease monitoring in APL. The amplification curves in black represent an internal control gene.

Quantitative RT-PCR: Complete Molecular Remission

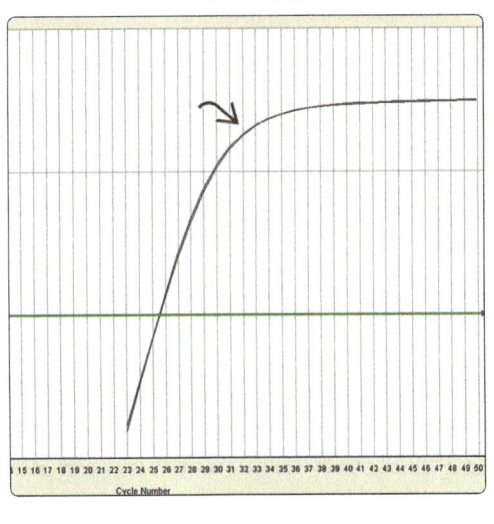

Quantitative RT-PCR for PML::RARA

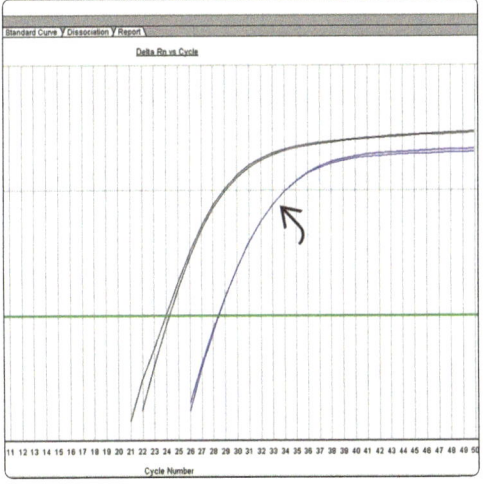

(Left) Quantitative RT-PCR performed on posttreatment bone marrow aspirate from a patient with previously diagnosed APL shows no detectable PML::RARA transcripts, consistent with complete molecular remission. The amplification curves in black ⇨ represent internal control gene. (Right) Quantitative RT-PCR performed on bone marrow aspirate from a patient with APL in morphologic remission detects low copy numbers of bcr3 transcripts ⇨, consistent with early molecular relapse.

Overview of Acute Myeloid Leukemia

MPO Cytochemistry

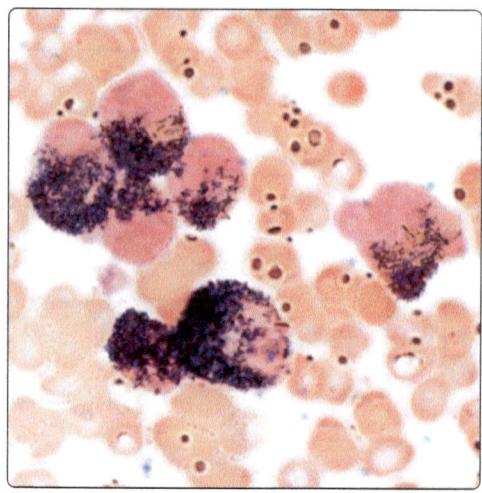

NSE Cytochemistry

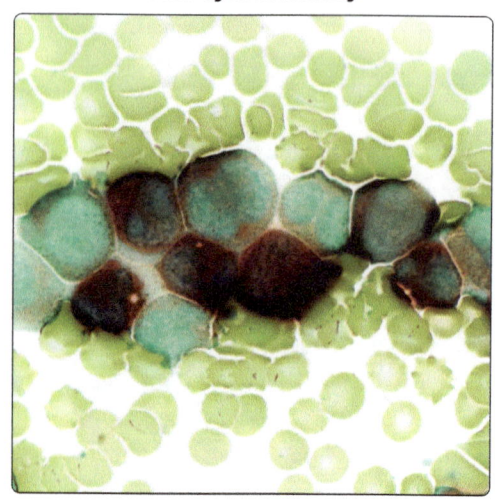

(Left) MPO shows marked, dense cytoplasmic granulation in blast-like cells, confirming diagnosis of APL. In the cytologically hypogranular variant of APL, one may be surprised by the dense MPO positivity. (Right) NSE (brown) highlights monoblasts in this case of AML. Any degree of positivity is sufficient for monocytic differentiation.

Flow Cytometry of CD34 vs. CD33

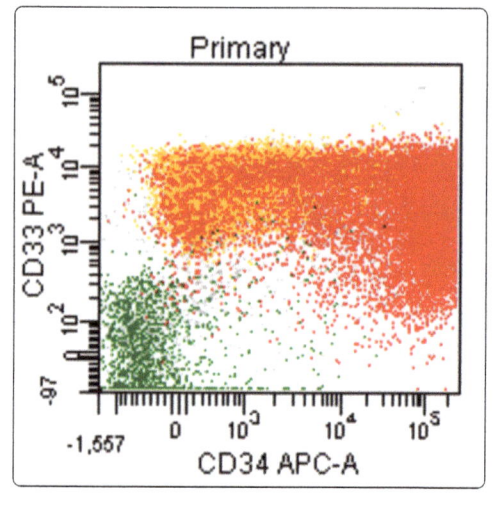

CD34 Immunohistochemistry

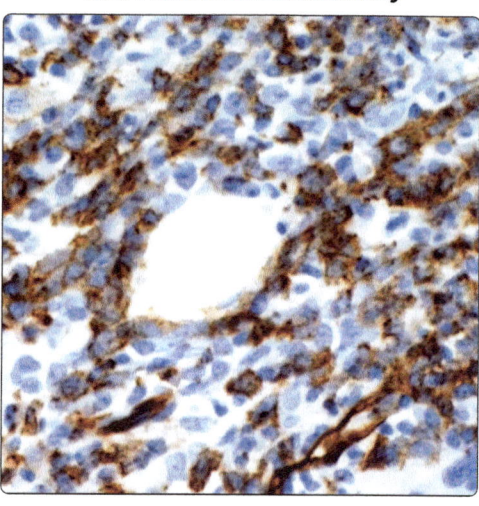

(Left) Flow cytometry is a crucial component of AML work-up, assigning lineage while establishing a phenotype that can be followed subsequently for residual disease testing. Neoplastic cells (red) in this case are myeloid [CD33(+)] and confirmed blasts [CD34(+)]. (Right) On occasion, flow cytometry is suboptimal or not available. IHC stains can verify acute leukemia using lineage-specific and blast markers. CD34 reveals > 20% blasts in this acute leukemia.

Karyotype Showing t(15;17)

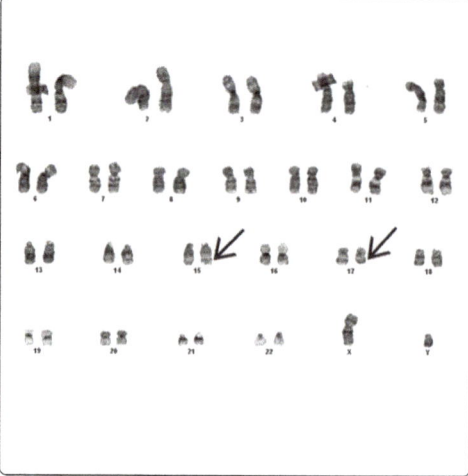

Complex Karyotype of AML

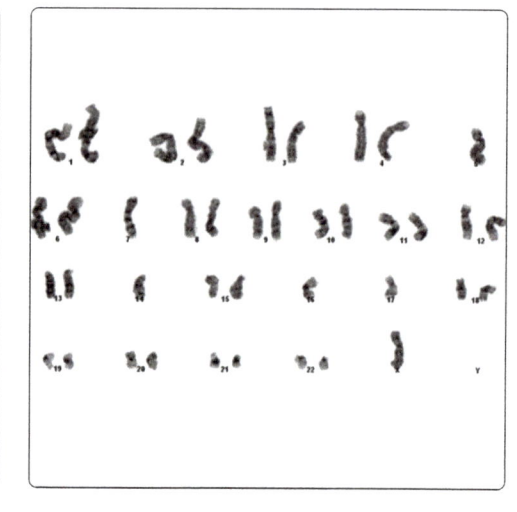

(Left) Conventional cytogenetics is a necessary component of AML work-up. Recurring genetic translocations with prognostic significance may be identified. This karyogram shows t(15;17) ⇨ associated with APL. (Right) Complex karyotype in a case of de novo AML is shown. A complex karyotype is variably defined (usually ≥ 3 abnormalities) and is associated with an unfavorable genetic risk stratification.

Overview of Acute Myeloid Leukemia

Increased Blasts and Eosinophils With Abnormal Granules

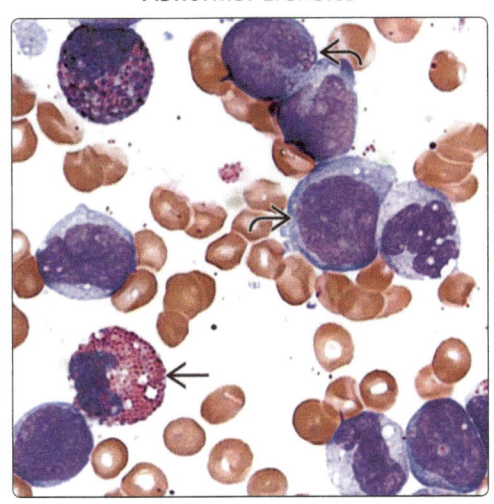

Pyrogram of *KIT* Codon 816

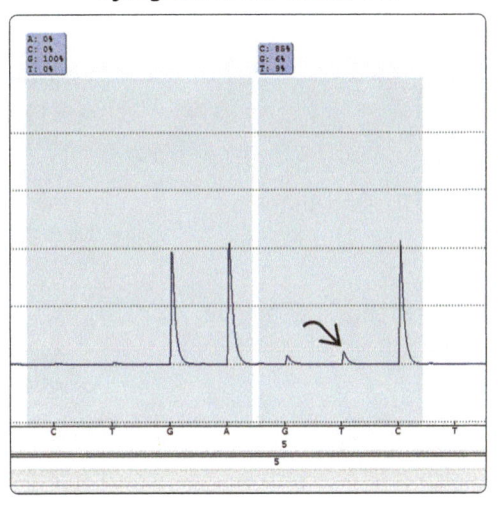

(Left) Bone aspirate smear shows increased blasts ⇒ and eosinophils with abnormal granules ⇒. FISH detected inv(16), diagnostic of a core-binding factor leukemia with inv(16). (Right) Pyrosequencing analysis of KIT performed on bone marrow aspirate from a patient with newly diagnosed AML with inv(16) shows a G>T base substitution ⇒ in codon 816 of exon 17 of KIT, consistent with D816V mutation.

Next-Generation Sequencing Pileup of *IDH1*

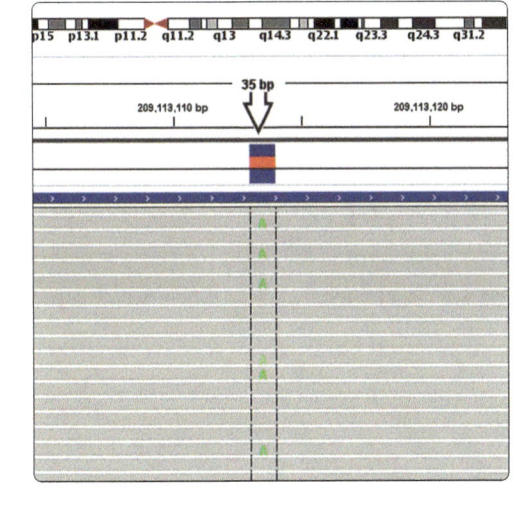

Diffuse Bone Marrow Involvement

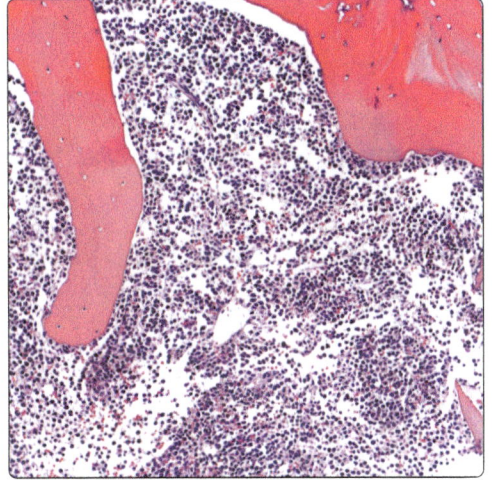

(Left) Next-generation sequencing performed on a diagnostic sample from a cytogenetically normal AML shows a G>A base substitution in codon 132 of IDH1 ⇒, corresponding to R132C mutation. (Right) Bone marrow core biopsy shows AML with diffuse bone marrow involvement, confirmed by flow cytometry. Although the bone is abnormally osteosclerotic, an underlying occult systemic mastocytosis was not appreciated until posttreatment bone marrow was reviewed.

CD117 Immunohistochemistry

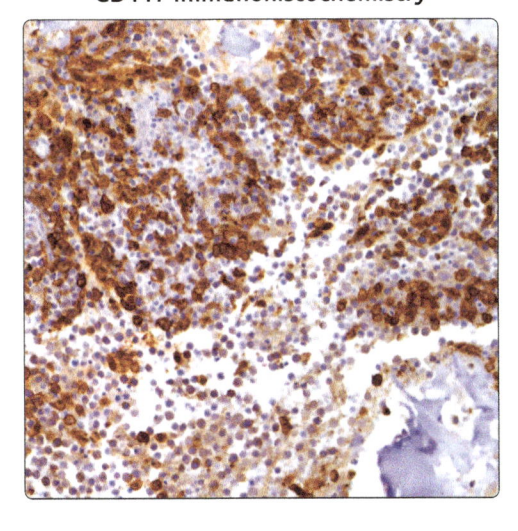

Next-Generation Sequencing Pileup of *KIT* Codon 822

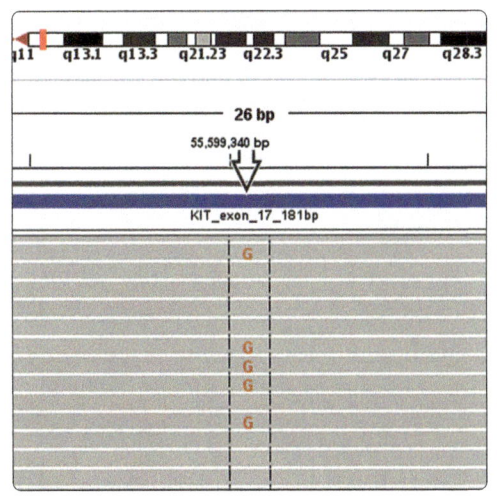

(Left) CD117 shows occult mastocytosis, which was identified after treatment. The compact aggregates of mast cells are strongly CD117 positive, while AML blasts are weakly staining. (Right) Next-generation sequencing of bone marrow clot section from a patient with AML and concurrent occult mastocytosis shows a T>G base substitution in codon 822 of exon 17 of KIT ⇒, corresponding to N822K. KIT exon 17 mutations are common in mastocytosis and in a small subset of AML.

Acute Myeloid Leukemia With t(8;21)/*RUNX1::RUNX1T1*

KEY FACTS

ETIOLOGY/PATHOGENESIS
- *RUNX1::RUNX1T1* fusion due to t(8;21)(q21.3;q22.1)
  - Abnormal protein leads to transcriptional repression
- *KIT* mutations seen in 12-47% of cases

CLINICAL ISSUES
- Favorable risk
  - Presence of mutations, such as *KIT*, associated with worse outcomes in adults

MICROSCOPIC
- Characteristic Auer rods with tapered ends
- Abnormal neutrophilic precursors with salmon-colored granules

ANCILLARY TESTS
- Translocation t(8;21)(q21.3;q22.1) readily detected on conventional cytogenetic analysis
  - Additional abnormalities seen in 70% of cases
- FISH also demonstrates *RUNX1::RUNX1T1* fusion
- RT-RCR for *RUNX1::RUNX1T1* transcripts
  - Consistent in-frame *RUNX1::RUNX1T1* transcript form facilitates assay design
  - > 1 log increase in transcript levels associated with increased relapse risk
  - < 3 log reduction in *RUNX1::RUNX1T1* transcripts in bone marrow at remission is associated with relapse
- Next-generation sequencing (NGS) myeloid gene panels may provide additional prognostic information
  - *KIT* mutations associated with adverse prognosis
  - *KRAS* or *NRAS* mutations in ~ 20%
  - *ASXL1* mutations in 10%
  - *ASXL2* mutations in 20-25%

TOP DIFFERENTIAL DIAGNOSES
- Acute myeloid leukemia, not otherwise specified
  - Lacks t(8;21); *RUNX1::RUNX1T1*

Long Tapered Auer Rod

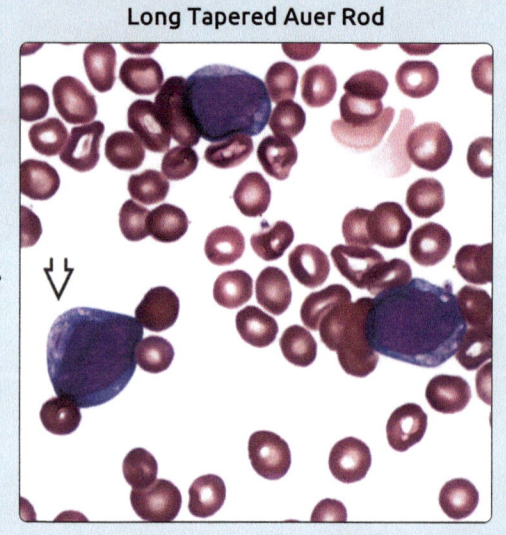

Translocation (8;21)

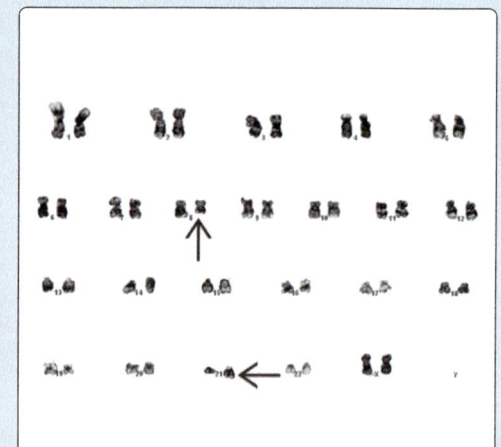

(Left) Peripheral blood smear shows 3 circulating blasts, 1 with a classic, thin Auer rod with tapered ends ⇒ in acute myeloid leukemia (AML) with t(8;21)(q21.3;q22.1). (Right) Karyogram shows the recurring abnormality of t(8;21)(q21.3;q22.1) in this case of de novo AML. Note the abnormal chromosomes ⇒.

Myeloid Blast Population

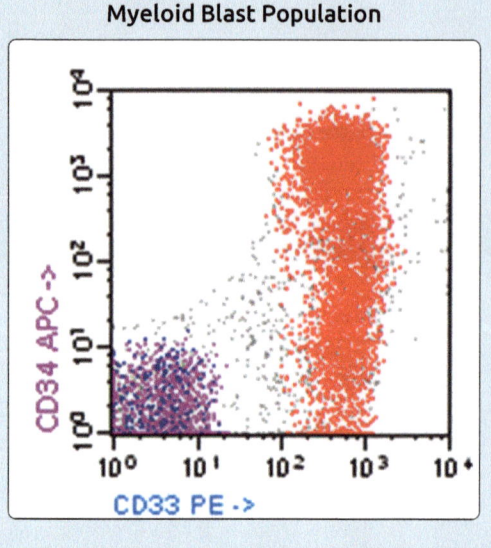

Aberrant Immunophenotype

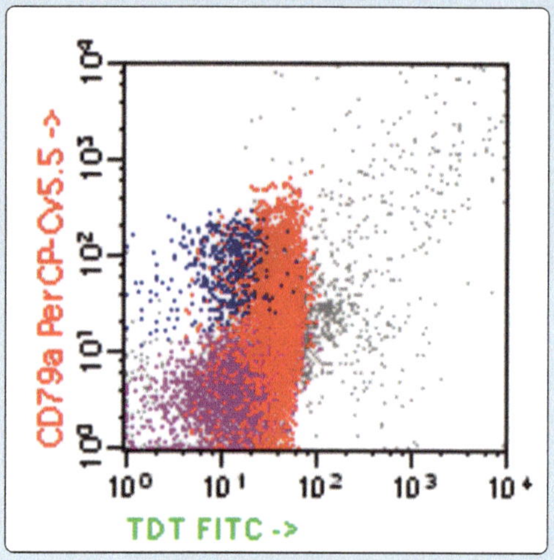

(Left) Flow cytometric analysis shows a prominent population of blasts in this case of newly diagnosed AML with t(8;21) (red). The blasts are recognized by their CD34 positivity (y-axis) and are of myeloid lineage (CD33 positive). (Right) Flow cytometric analysis shows aberrant CD79A (y-axis) and TdT expression in this case of AML with t(8;21). Expression of other B-lineage markers, including CD19 and PAX5, are described in this entity as well. This aberrant antigen profile is a clue to AML with t(8;21).

Acute Myeloid Leukemia With t(8;21)/*RUNX1::RUNX1T1*

TERMINOLOGY

Abbreviations
- Acute myeloid leukemia (AML)

Definitions
- Subtype of AML with recurrent genetic abnormalities characterized by t(8;21) with fusion of *RUNX1* with *RUNX1T1*
  o *RUNX1::RUNX1T1* fusion
    – Results from t(8;21)(q21.3;q22.1)
- *RUNX1*
  o Official name: RUNX family transcription factor 1
  o HGNC ID: 10471
  o Gene locus: 21q22.12
  o Number of exons: 12
- *RUNX1T1*
  o Official name: RUNX1 partner transcriptional corepressor 1
  o HGCN ID: 1535
  o Gene locus: 8q21.3
  o Number of exons: 20

CLASSIFICATION

ICC vs. WHO-HAEM5
- AML with t(8;21)(q21.3;q22.1)/*RUNX1::RUNX1T1* (ICC)
- AML with *RUNX1::RUNX1T1* fusion (WHO-HAEM5)
- ≥ 10% blasts in blood or bone marrow required for diagnosis by ICC
- No blast threshold in WHO-HAEM5

ETIOLOGY/PATHOGENESIS

Normal Function of *RUNX1*
- One of 3 genes that encodes a subunit of core-binding factor (CBF)
- CBF is heterodimeric transcription factor consisting of
  o 1 subunit known as CBFα
    – Encoded by *RUNX1*
    – Binds directly to target DNA
  o 1 subunit known as CBFβ
    – Encoded by *CBFB*
      □ Same gene is involved in AML with inv(16)
    – Does not directly bind DNA
    – Peptide-binding regulatory subunit that influences DNA binding by α subunit
- CBF binds to core sites of enhancers and promoters of genes involved in hematopoiesis
  o Expressed in all hematopoietic cells
  o Targets include GM-CSF promoter
  o Facilitates access by other transcription factors
    – Increases acetylation of histones by histone acetyltransferases
  o Increases transcription of these target genes and promotes hematopoietic differentiation and maturation

Normal Function of *RUNX1T1*
- Encodes CBFβ protein that binds transcription factors and recruits corepressors
  o Results in transcriptional repression at sites bound by transcription factor
  o Expressed in megakaryocytic and erythroid lineages

RUNX1::RUNX1T1 Fusion
- Results from t(8;21)(q21.3;q22)
  o 1st AML reciprocal translocation identified with common banding techniques (1975)
- Chimeric transcript encodes abnormal protein derived from
  o 5'-region of *RUNX1*
    – Contains runt homology domain that recognizes specific DNA sequence for target binding
  o 3'-region of *RUNX1T1*
    – Almost entire RUNX1T1 protein is present in chimeric protein, including regions responsible for corepressor activity
- End result is chimeric protein (RUNX1::RUNX1T1) that can
  o Bind RUNX1 target regions in promoter regions
  o Assemble transcriptional repressor complex at these sites due to RUNX1T1
  o Block transcription of genes that would otherwise be targeted for enhanced expression by normal RUNX1
    – These genes are required for hematopoietic differentiation; block in cellular maturation is created
  o Additional effects via mediation of expression of microRNAs, epigenetic effects, increased proliferation
- "Multihit" model of AML
  o Both class 1 and class 2 mutations are needed for leukemogenesis
    – Class 1 mutations increase proliferation
    – Class 2 mutations impair differentiation or maturation
  o *RUNX1::RUNX1T1* fusion is considered class 2 mutation
  o *KIT* mutations, which are seen in 12-47% of cases, represent cooperating class 1 mutations
    – Other common mutations in AML with t(8;21) include *NRAS*, *ASXL1*, *ASXL2*, *DHX15*, *ZBTB7A*, *EZH2*, *FLT3*, *CBL*, and *KRAS*

CLINICAL ISSUES

Epidemiology
- Incidence: 10-15% of pediatric, 5% of adult AML cases
- Age: Predominates in younger patients (20-40 years)

Presentation
- Abnormal CBC
  o Pancytopenia, anemia, thrombocytopenia, neutropenia
  o Variable WBC and blast count
- Myeloid sarcomas common

Treatment
- Chemotherapy
  o Cytarabine-based regimen
  o Anti-CD33 antibody therapy often used
  o Targeted therapy for specific mutations based on results of molecular testing
    – Avapritinib for *KIT*-mutated cases

Prognosis
- Favorable risk by cytogenetics
  o Specific mutation profile may impact outcome
- Complete remission common
  o Especially with intensive postremission treatment
    – Multiple cycles of high-dose cytarabine

Acute Myeloid Leukemia With t(8;21)/*RUNX1::RUNX1T1*

- Prognostic cytogenetics factors
  - 60-70% of patients harbor additional chromosomal abnormality
    - -Y, -X, +8, +22, hyperdiploidy associated with more favorable outcome
    - del(9q) associated with better overall survival
- *KIT* mutation
  - Found in 12-47% of cases
  - Linked to concurrent systemic mastocytosis
  - Associated with higher risk of relapse and decreased overall survival in adults, especially in cases with variant allele fraction ≥ 25%
  - Occur mostly in exon 17 hotspot regions
    - Most commonly p.D816V
- *FLT3* ITD or TKD mutations
  - Infrequent (~ 15%)
  - Some reports suggest worse prognosis especially with high mutant allele variant, others report no impact
  - Higher mutation burden likely correlates with worse outcomes
- Measurable minimal residual disease (MRD) monitoring
  - MRD can be detected by quantitative RT-PCR
    - Molecular remission predicts durable complete remission
    - \> 1 log increase in transcript levels associated with increased relapse risk
    - < 3 log reduction in *RUNX1::RUNX1T1* transcripts in bone marrow at remission is associated with relapse
    - Absence of *RUNX1::RUNX1T1* fusion may not be necessary for long-term remission

Association With Systemic Mastocytosis

- AML with t(8;21) is most common AML associated with mastocytosis
- *KIT* D816V mutation in both blasts and mast cells may indicate common progenitor

MICROSCOPIC

Key Microscopic Features

- Bone marrow aspirate
  - Increased myeloid blasts
  - Variable blast count
    - Some cases < required 20% (low-blast-count AML)
  - Characteristic Auer rods
    - Thin with tapered ends
    - Usually single within cell
    - Found in blasts and maturing granulocytes
  - Abnormal neutrophilic precursors
    - Numerous pink/salmon-colored granules
    - Granules may abnormally aggregate in discrete region of cytoplasm
    - Dysplastic nuclei with megaloblastoid change and abnormal nuclear segmentation
  - Increased and atypical, spindled mast cells if concurrent systemic mastocytosis present

ANCILLARY TESTS

Immunohistochemistry

- Increased blasts: CD34(+), CD117(+)
  - Express myeloid antigens: CD33 and myeloperoxidase
  - May express B-cell markers: CD19, CD79A, and PAX5
- Associated mast cell disease: Mast cells positive for tryptase, CD117, CD25, and CD2

Flow Cytometry

- Myeloblasts positive for CD34, CD33, CD13, weak CD45, and often aberrant CD19 coexpression
  - Coexpression of CD19 and CD56 is highly associated with AML with t(8;21)
  - CD56 expression is associated with *KIT* mutation

In Situ Hybridization

- FISH for *RUNX1::RUNX1T1*
  - Dual-color, dual-fusion probe
    - Detection sensitivity of ~ 1%
  - Confirmatory of recurring genetic abnormality

Genetic Testing

- RT-RCR for *RUNX1::RUNX1T1* transcripts
  - Breakpoints involve limited set of introns in both genes
    - Consistent in-frame *RUNX1::RUNX1T1* transcript form facilitates assay design
  - Diagnostic if other techniques suboptimal or unavailable
  - Useful for MRD monitoring
- Next-generation sequencing (NGS) myeloid gene panels may provide additional prognostic information
  - Additional mutations identified in majority of cases
  - High mutation burden associated with worse outcome
  - Concurrent mutations in kinase signaling, cohesin, and chromatin modifier genes linked to increased rate of relapse
  - Specific mutations may provide targets for therapy
  - *KIT* mutations in 20-30%
  - *KRAS* or *NRAS* mutations in ~ 20%
    - More common in pediatric cases
    - Less common than in AML with inv16/t(16;16)
  - *ASXL1* mutations in 10%
    - More common in adult cases
  - *ASXL2* mutations in 20-25%
  - *RELN* mutations in 8%
  - *NOTCH1* mutations in 8%

Cytogenetics

- Translocation typically identified by routine karyotype
- Rare, more complex translocations or submicroscopic events involving these breakpoints can occur
  - May require FISH for diagnosis
- 70% of cases show additional cytogenetic abnormalities

SELECTED REFERENCES

1. Weinberg OK et al: The International Consensus Classification of acute myeloid leukemia. Virchows Arch. 482(1):27-37, 2023
2. Scott S et al: Assessment of acute myeloid leukemia molecular measurable residual disease testing in an interlaboratory study. Blood Adv. 7(14):3686-94, 2023
3. Arber DA et al: International Consensus Classification of myeloid neoplasms and acute leukemia: integrating morphological, clinical, and genomic data. Blood. 140(11):1200-28, 2022
4. Khoury JD et al: The 5th edition of the World Health Organization Classification of haematolymphoid tumours: myeloid and histiocytic/dendritic neoplasms. Leukemia. 36(7):1703-19, 2022
5. Al-Harbi S et al: An update on the molecular pathogenesis and potential therapeutic targeting of AML with t(8;21)(q22;q22.1);RUNX1-RUNX1T1. Blood Adv. 4(1):229-38, 2020

Acute Myeloid Leukemia With t(8;21)/*RUNX1::RUNX1T1*

Dysplastic Neutrophils and Circulating Blasts

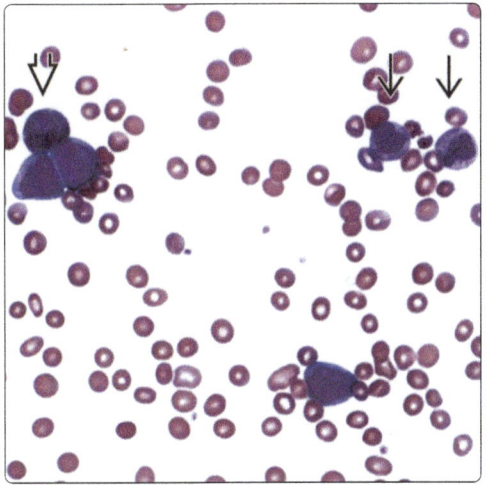

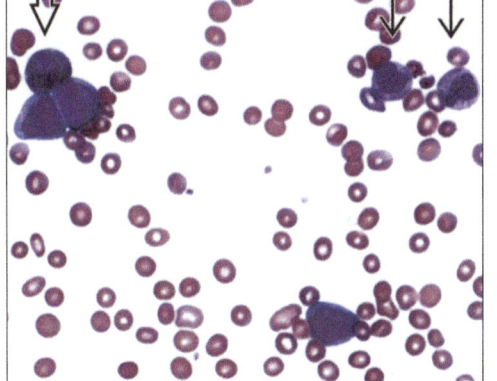

Tapered Auer Rod and Abnormal Granulation

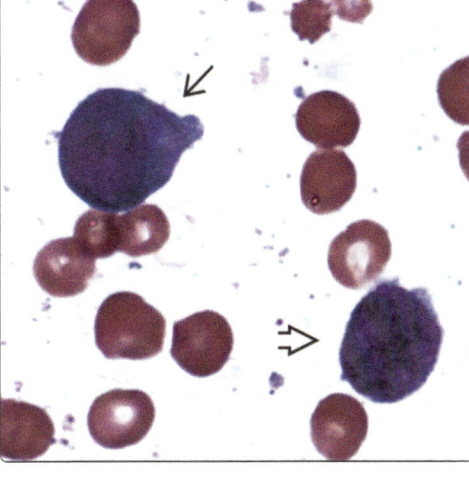

(Left) Blood shows mild leukocytosis consisting of circulating blasts and maturing granulocytes in this case of AML with t(8;21). Many of the granulocytes have an abnormal appearance characterized by abnormal nuclear segmentation ⇨ or cytoplasmic granulation ⇨. (Right) A long, thin Auer rod ⇨ with tapered ends is seen in the cytoplasm of a blast in this case of AML with t(8;21). Also present is a hypergranular neutrophilic precursor with salmon-colored granules ⇨.

Abnormal Granulation and Monocytic Component

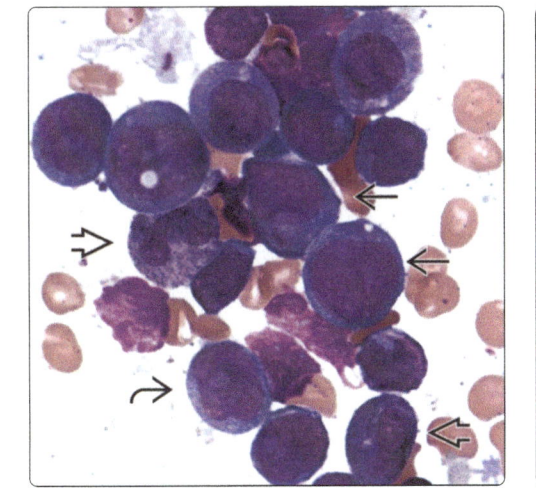

Abnormal Myeloid Maturation

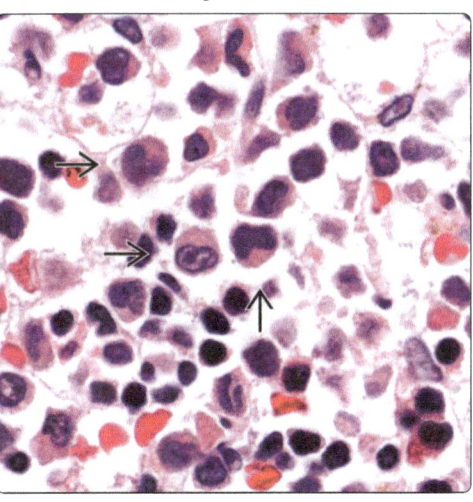

(Left) Bone marrow aspirate smear shows blasts with Auer rods and peripheral cytoplasmic basophilia ⇨. The background granulocytes appear hypergranulated ⇨, and conspicuous immature monocytic cells ⇨ are also seen. (Right) Bone marrow core biopsy shows characteristic myeloid predominance with abnormal myeloid cells showing prominent cytoplasmic granulation and prominent nucleoli ⇨.

Conventional Cytogenetics

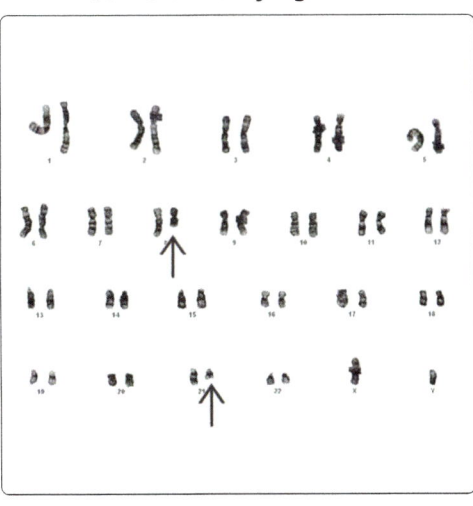

Dual-Color/Dual-Fusion FISH

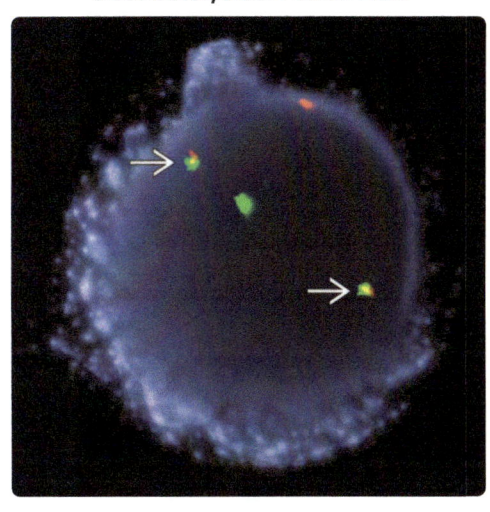

(Left) Karyogram shows t(8;21)(q21.3;q22.1) in this case of AML. The specific genes (RUNX1 and RUNX1T1) are not identified by this technique but are reasonably inferred. Note the abnormal chromosomes ⇨. (Right) FISH is positive for RUNX1::RUNX1T1 fusion in an interphase nucleus from this case of AML with t(8;21). The reciprocal translocation is depicted by 2 fusion (yellow) signals ⇨.

Acute Myeloid Leukemia With inv(16) or t(16;16)/*CBFB::MYH11*

KEY FACTS

ETIOLOGY/PATHOGENESIS

- *CBFB::MYH11* fusion arises as consequence of inv(16)(p13.1q22) or t(16;16)(p13.1;q22)
  - Abnormal chimeric protein impairs normal core-binding factor (CBF) function
  - Functions as aberrant transcriptional repressor at target sites where CBF normally enhances gene expression
  - Impairs *RUNX1* transcription and blocks myeloid differentiation

MICROSCOPIC

- Increased blasts and blast equivalents: Myeloblasts, monoblasts, and promonocytes
- Abnormal eosinophils with mixed eosinophil and basophil-type granules

ANCILLARY TESTS

- Inv(16) may be subtle &/or overlooked on karyotype
- If cytogenetics normal but morphology suggests acute myeloid leukemia (AML) with inv(16), pursue FISH, molecular studies
- RT-PCR for *CBFB::MYH11*
  - Can be used for measurable minimal residual disease monitoring
- Next generation sequencing (NGS) may be useful for further risk stratification
  - *KIT* exon 8 and 17 mutations in 30%
    - Associated with worse prognosis in adults
  - *NRAS* mutations in 30-50%
  - *KRAS* mutations in 10-15%
  - *FLT3* mutations in 14-30%
- Additional chromosomal abnormalities seen in 30-40% of cases
  - +22, +8, and +21
  - Trisomy 22 is more commonly seen in AML inv(16) than in other myeloid neoplasms
- RNA-seq can be used to define rearrangement breakpoints

Bone Marrow Findings

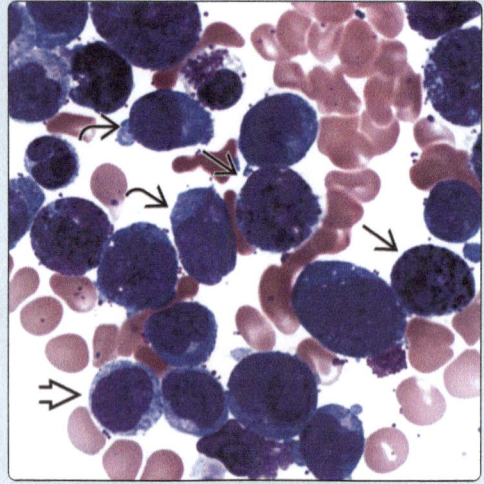

inv(16)

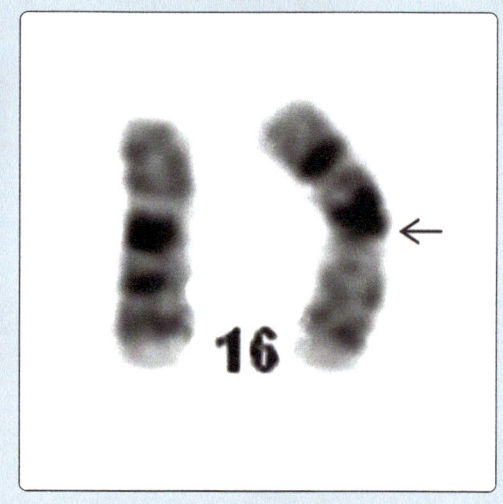

(Left) Bone marrow aspirate smear shows an increased population of blasts ⇨, immature-appearing monocytes ⇨, and abnormal eosinophils ⇨ in this case of acute myeloid leukemia (AML) with inv(16). (Right) Conventional cytogenetic analysis shows classic inv(16) in this case of AML. Abnormal chromosome ⇨ (G-banded partial karyogram) is noted.

FISH Break-Apart Probes

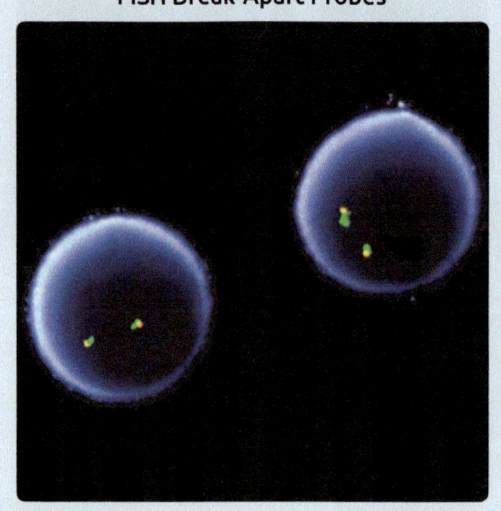

Positive FISH

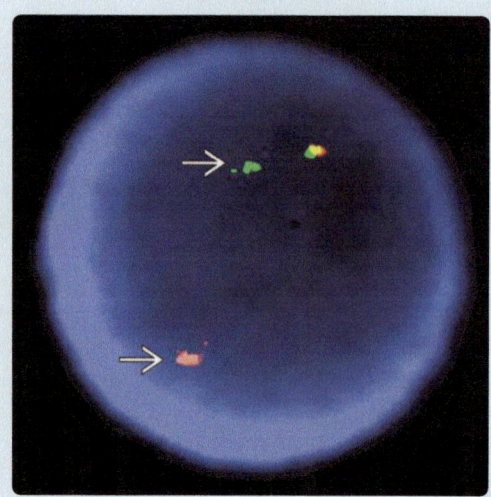

(Left) FISH using break-apart probes shows 2 normal interphase nuclei for CBFB (2 fused/yellow signals) in this case of AML, not otherwise specified. (Right) FISH shows an abnormal signal pattern with break-apart probes for CBFB. The separated orange and green signals ⇨ indicate CBFB rearrangement. This finding, along with morphology, would support a diagnosis of AML with inv(16) or t(16;16).

Acute Myeloid Leukemia With inv(16) or t(16;16)/*CBFB*::*MYH11*

TERMINOLOGY

Synonyms
- Acute myeloid leukemia (AML), inv(16)(p13q22)
- Core-binding factor (CBF) AML (along with AML with *RNX1*::*RUNX1T1* fusion)
- AML, M4Eo (historic FAB classification)

Definitions
- AML with inv(6) or t(16;16) is characterized by fusion of core binding factor beta (*CBFB*) and myosin heavy chain 11 (*MYH11*)
  - ≥ 10% blast threshold in blood or bone marrow (BM) is required for diagnosis by ICC
  - No blast threshold required by WHO-HAEM5
- *CBFB*
  - Official name: Core-binding factor subunit beta
  - HGNC ID: 1539
  - Gene locus: 16q22.1
  - Size: 71.9 kb
  - Number of exons: 6
- *MYH11*
  - Official name: Myosin heavy chain 11
  - HGNC ID: 7569
  - Gene locus: 16p13.11
  - Size: 153.9 kb
  - Number of exons: 43

CLASSIFICATION

ICC vs. WHO-HAEM5
- AML with inv(16)(p13.1q22) or t(16;16)(p13.1;q22)/*CBFB*::*MYH11* (ICC)
- AML with *CBFB*::*MYH11* fusion (WHO-HAEM5)
  - ≥ 10% blast threshold in blood or BM required for diagnosis by ICC
  - No blast threshold required (WHO-HAEM5)

ETIOLOGY/PATHOGENESIS

Normal Function of *MYH11*
- Encodes smooth muscle myosin belonging to myosin heavy chain family
  - Gene product is subunit of hexameric protein composed of 2 heavy chains and 2 pairs of nonidentical light chains
  - Contractile protein that hydrolyzes ATP to generate muscle cell contraction

Normal Function of *CBFB*
- Encodes β subunit of CBF
- CBF is heterodimeric transcription factor consisting of
  - 1 subunit known as CBFα
    - Encoded by multiple genes: *RUNX1*, *RUNX2*, *RUNX3*
    - This subunit binds directly to target DNA
  - 1 subunit known as CBFβ
    - Gene product of *CBFB*
    - This subunit does not directly bind DNA
    - Peptide-binding regulatory subunit that influences DNA binding by α subunit
- CBF binds to core site of enhancers and promoters of genes involved in hematopoiesis
  - Targets include T-cell receptor, cytokine genes
  - Facilitates access by other transcription factors
    - Increases acetylation of histones
  - Increases transcription of these target genes that promotes hematopoietic differentiation and maturation

CBFB::*MYH11* Fusion
- Arises from 2 recurrent cytogenetic events
  - Inversion results from breakage and rejoining of 16p13.1 and 16q22
    - *CBFB* and *MYH11* on same chromosome are fused
  - Translocation t(16;16)(p13.1;q22)
    - Less common than inv(16)(p13.1q22)
    - *CBFB* and *MYH11* on 2 different copies of chromosome 16 are fused
- Chimeric transcript encodes abnormal protein consisting of
  - First 165 residues from N terminus of *CBFB*
  - C-terminal portion of *MYH11*
  - Several different rearrangements involving different exons have been identified
    - Type A most common
      □ > 80% of cases
      □ Fuses exon 5 of *CBFB* to exon 33 of *MYH11*
      □ *KIT* mutations are more common in cases with type A fusion than in other types
    - Types D and E each account for ~ 5% of cases
    - Specific rearrangement does not impact prognosis
- Abnormal chimeric protein
  - Disrupts *CBFB*
  - Impairs normal CBF function
  - Sequesters normal CBFα protein in cytoplasm
  - Functions as aberrant transcriptional repressor at target sites where CBF normally enhances gene expression
    - Impairs *RUNX1* transcription and blocks myeloid differentiation
  - Prevents normal proteolysis of CBF complex
- Multihit model of AML
  - In multihit model of AML pathogenesis, both class 1 and class 2 mutations are needed for leukemogenesis
    - Class 1 mutations increase cellular proliferation
    - Class 2 mutations impair differentiation or maturation
  - *CBFB*::*MYH11* fusion is considered class 2 mutation
  - Development of overt leukemia requires concurrent mutation in gene activating kinase signaling-induced increased cell proliferation
    - *KIT* mutations, which are seen in up to 30% of AML with inv(16)/t(16;16), represent cooperating class 1 mutations
      □ Other common class 1 mutations in AML with inv(16)/t(16;16) include *NRAS*, *FLT3*, and *KRAS*

CLINICAL ISSUES

Epidemiology
- Incidence
  - ~ 6-12% of pediatric AML
  - ~ 5% of adult AML
- Age
  - Median: 40-45 years

Presentation
- Abnormal complete blood count (CBC)

Acute Myeloid Leukemia With inv(16) or t(16;16)/*CBFB*::*MYH11*

- Anemia, neutropenia, and thrombocytopenia may be present
- Variable white blood cell count (WBC)
  - Variable percentage blast count
  - Variable percentage monocytic cells
- Extramedullary involvement (myeloid sarcoma) common
  - May be only disease site

Treatment
- Chemotherapy
  - High dose, cytarabine based, generally
- Anti-CD33 antibody therapy (i.e., gemtuzumab) often used

Prognosis
- Favorable risk
- Complete remission very common
  - Rates reach ~ 90% after standard induction therapy
- Cytogenetics
  - Cooccuring trisomy 8 associated with improved overall survival in some studies
- *KIT* mutation
  - Found in up to 30% of cases
  - Mutations may involve *KIT* exon 17 hotspot regions (e.g., codon 816), but mutations affecting exon 8 are also common
  - Adults with *KIT* mutations have higher risk of relapse and worse survival
    - Impact on prognosis appears less significant than that of *KIT* mutation in setting of AML with t(8;21)
    - May depend on specific mutation
      - Exon 17 mutations associated with worse outcomes, and exon 8 mutations associated with no difference in outcomes in some studies
- *FLT3* ITD and TKD mutations associated with worse outcome but are less common in this subtype of AML
- Measurable residual disease (MRD) monitoring
  - Assessed by quantitative RT-PCR studies
  - Molecular remission predicts durable complete remission
  - Specific findings predictive of continued remission vs. relapse have been identified
    - PCR negativity in at least 1 sample during consolidation therapy may predict better outcome
    - Conversion to PCR positivity during remission may predict morphologic or hematologic relapse

MICROSCOPIC

Key Microscopic Features
- Peripheral blood
  - Generally leukocytosis dominated by blasts and immature-appearing monocytic cells
    - WBC may exceed 100 x 10^9/L in 20% of patients
  - Eosinophils may be mildly increased
    - Morphology variable, classic appearance seen in BM may not be identified in blood
- BM aspirate
  - Blasts and promonocytes typically > 20% of cells
    - Must exceed ≥ 10% threshold as per ICC
  - Strikingly abnormal immature eosinophils
    - Contain large, coarse, dark purple granules in addition to typical eosinophilic granules
  - Mature eosinophils may have dysplastic features, such as hyposegmentation and hypogranulation

ANCILLARY TESTS

Immunohistochemistry
- Increased myeloblasts: CD34(+), CD117(+)
- Monocytic component: CD68(+), CD163(+), lysozyme (+)

Flow Cytometry
- Aberrant antigenic expression common
- Myeloblasts express CD34, CD33, weak CD45, CD117, CD13, and CD2
- Monocytic cells express CD36, CD64, CD33, HLA-DR, moderate CD45, weak CD4, and variable CD14

Genetic Testing
- PCR-based testing
  - Quantitative RT-PCR for *CBFB*::*MYH11* fusion transcript
    - Significant breakpoint heterogeneity complicates assay design and target detection
      - 85% of cases harbor type A fusion
    - May be used for residual disease monitoring
  - RNA-seq to define rearrangement breakpoints
    - Can identify rare rearrangement types
  - Gene mutations
    - Next generation sequencing (NGS) panel testing may be useful for further risk stratification
    - Increasing numbers of mutations, especially multiple kinase mutations, associated with worse outcomes
    - *KIT* mutations in 30-40%
      - Most commonly involve exon 17 hotspot regions, including codon 816
      - Exon 8 mutations also seen
    - *NRAS* mutations in 30-50%
    - *KRAS* mutations in 10-15%
    - *FLT3* mutations in 14-30%
      - Associated with worse prognosis
- Cytogenetic/FISH studies
  - Essential for diagnosis
  - Inversion 16 abnormality is subtle, may be cryptic
  - If cytogenetics normal but morphology suggests AML with inv 16, pursue FISH &/or molecular studies
  - FISH with break-apart probe for *CBFB*
    - Confirmatory of cytogenetic finding inv(16) or t(16;16)
    - Sensitivity of 3-5%
  - Additional chromosomal abnormalities in 40% of cases
    - +22, +8, and +21
    - Hyperdiploidy in 25%

DIAGNOSTIC CHECKLIST

Pathologic Interpretation Pearls
- Increased myeloid blasts, promonocytes, monoblasts, and abnormal eosinophils
- inv(16)(p13.1q22) or t(16;16)(p13.1;q22)/*CBFB*::*MYH11* identified by FISH, cytogenetics, or RT-PCR-based methods

SELECTED REFERENCES

1. Falini B et al: Comparison of the International Consensus and 5th WHO edition classifications of adult myelodysplastic syndromes and acute myeloid leukemia. Am J Hematol. 98(3):481-92, 2023

Acute Myeloid Leukemia With inv(16) or t(16;16)/*CBFB::MYH11*

Immature-Appearing Monocytes and Circulating Blasts

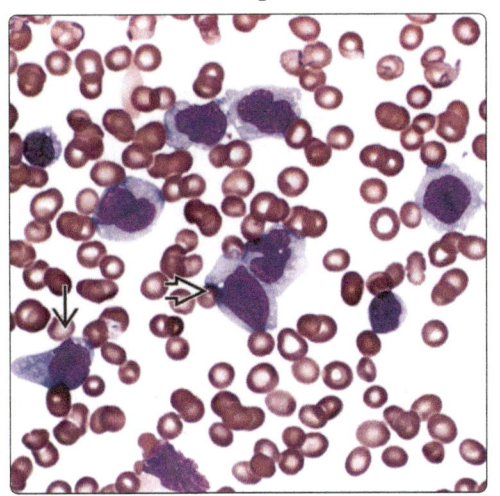

Immature-Appearing Monocytes and Background Eosinophils

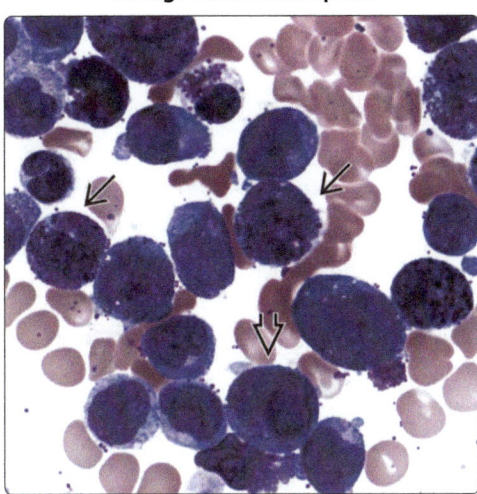

(Left) Peripheral blood shows leukocytosis composed of increased and immature-appearing monocytes ⇨ and circulating blasts ⇨ in this case of AML with inv(16). The monocytes are immature in appearance with more dispersed chromatin and delicate nuclear clefts. **(Right)** Bone marrow aspirate smear shows an increased population of blasts, immature-appearing monocytes ⇨, and background eosinophils ⇨ in this case of AML with inv(16). Promonocytes are counted as blast equivalents.

NSE Immunohistochemistry

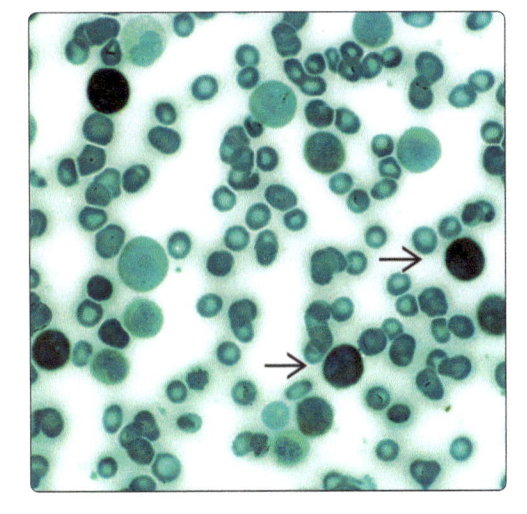

Myeloblast Population

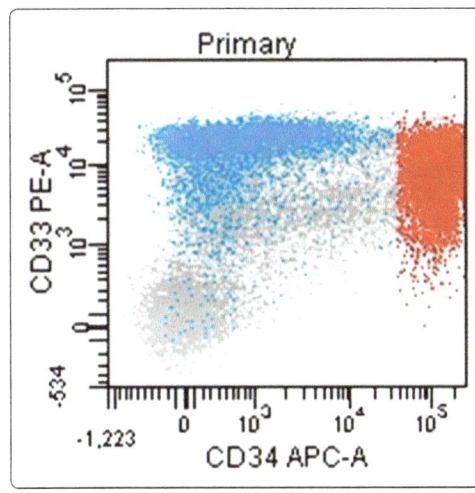

(Left) NSE (a naphthyl butyrate esterase) shows monocytic component of myelomonocytic proliferation ⇨. Such a finding in ≥ 20% of cells indicates monocytic differentiation in AML. **(Right)** Flow cytometric analysis of AML with inv(16) shows increased myeloblast population (red) expressing CD34 and CD33 and increased monocytic population, which is brighter for CD33, and lack of CD34 (cyan).

Increased Monocytes

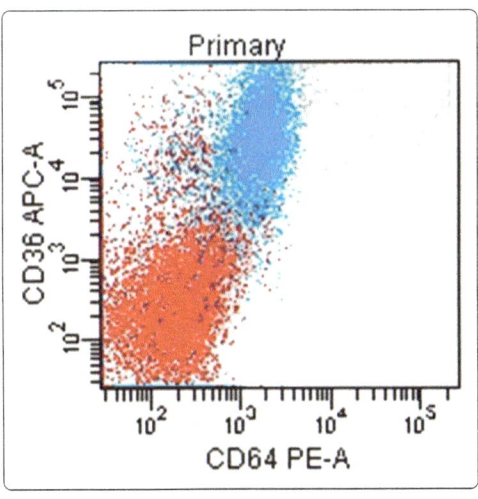

Subtle Inversion 16 on Karyotyping

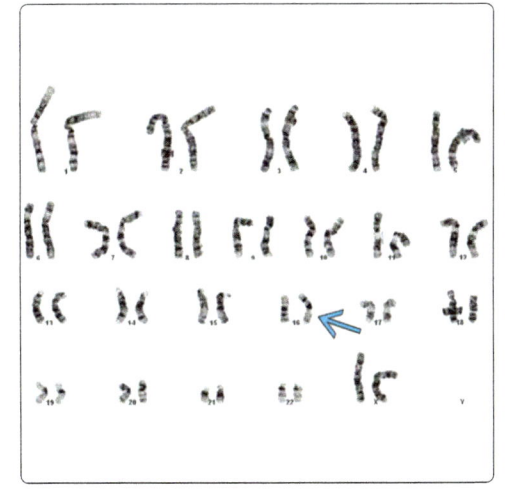

(Left) Flow cytometric analysis shows a population of monocytic cells (cyan) with coexpression of CD36 and CD64. Myeloblasts (red) lack expression of these markers. These findings are common in AML with monocytic differentiation. **(Right)** G-banded karyogram shows inv(16)(p13.1q22) ⇨. This abnormality may be subtle and could be easily overlooked on karyotype.

247

Acute Promyelocytic Leukemia With t(15;17)/*PML::RARA*

KEY FACTS

TERMINOLOGY

- Acute promyelocytic leukemia (APL) with t(15;17)/*PML::RARA*
  - Distinct and unique subtype of acute myeloid leukemia
- International Consensus Classification (ICC) vs. WHO 5th ed (WHO-HAEM5)
  - Both classifications require documentation of *PML::RARA* fusion
  - ICC requires at least 10% abnormal promyelocytes (blast equivalents) vs. no blast percent threshold in WHO-HAEM5
  - ICC does not include specific therapy related neoplasm diagnostic category as WHO-HAEM5 does; ICC rather uses therapy relatedness as qualifier that can be added to any myeloid neoplasm subtype diagnosis
    - APL with t(15;17)/*PML::RARA*, therapy-related (ICC)
    - Prior cytotoxic therapy excludes designation of APL with *PML::RARA* category in WHO-HAEM5

CLINICAL ISSUES

- Life-threatening coagulopathy as main clinical feature
  - Rapid diagnosis crucial to decrease early death rate due to coagulopathy
  - Hypogranular variant typically present with leukocytosis
  - Pediatric patients often present with high-risk features
- All trans retinoic acid (ATRA) as single agent
  - Induces complete remission in up to 90%
  - Majority of patients cured with current molecular targeted therapy
  - More favorable prognosis compared with other AML with recurrent cytogenetic abnormalities
- Mortality during early treatment phase due to ATRA-induced differentiation syndrome
  - Syndrome characterized by fever, hypotension, fluid retention, and pulmonary infiltrates
- No adverse impact when additional cytogenetic abnormalities exist

Blasts on Cytospin Preparation of Bone Marrow

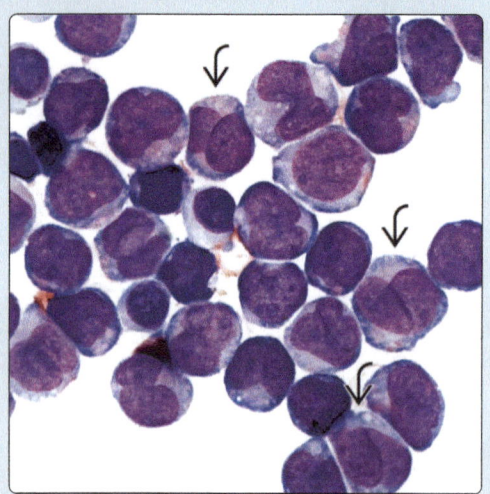

Bright MPO(+) Blasts

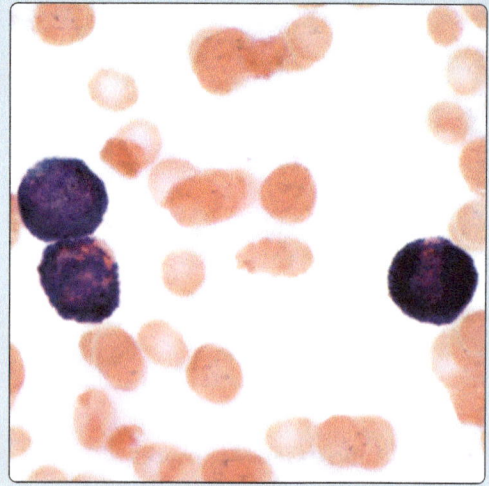

(Left) Wright-stained cytospin preparation of bone marrow aspirate from a patient with hypogranular variant of acute promyelocytic leukemia (APL) shows frequent bilobed blasts (sliding plates) ➡ with hypogranular cytoplasm. (Right) Cytochemical stain for MPO performed on peripheral blood of a patient with hypogranular variant of APL demonstrates strong expression of cytoplasmic MPO despite the submicroscopic nature of the cytoplasmic granules.

FISH Using *PML*- and *RARA*-Targeted Probes Detects *PML::RARA* Fusion

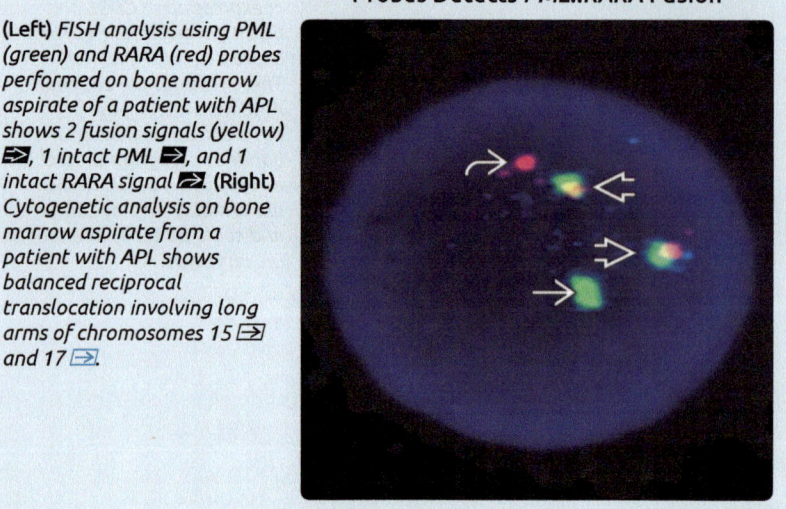

Chromosomal Translocation Between Long Arms of Chromosomes 15 and 17

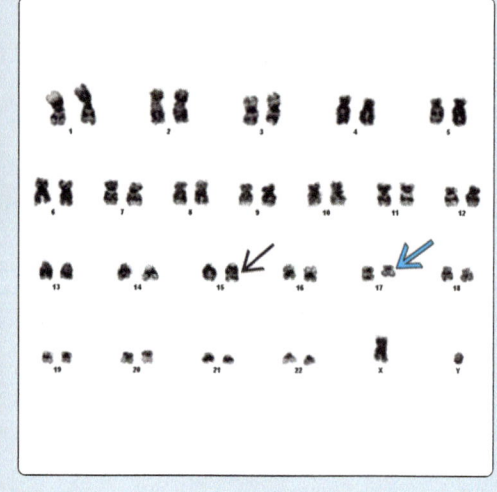

(Left) FISH analysis using PML (green) and RARA (red) probes performed on bone marrow aspirate of a patient with APL shows 2 fusion signals (yellow) ➡, 1 intact PML ➡, and 1 intact RARA signal ➡. (Right) Cytogenetic analysis on bone marrow aspirate from a patient with APL shows balanced reciprocal translocation involving long arms of chromosomes 15 ➡ and 17 ➡.

Acute Promyelocytic Leukemia With t(15;17)/*PML::RARA*

TERMINOLOGY

Abbreviations
- Acute promyelocytic leukemia (APL) with *PML::RARA*

Synonyms
- APL with t(15;17)(q24.1;q21.2)/*PML::RARA* [2022 International Consensus Classification (2022 ICC)]
- APL with *PML::RARA* fusion [WHO 5th ed (WHO-HAEM5)]
- AML-M3 (FAB classification)

Definitions
- Distinct and unique subtype of AML
  - t(15;17)(q24.1;q21.2) with *PML::RARA* fusion is hallmark
  - Increased blasts and abnormal promyelocytes (blast equivalent)
  - Diagnosis requires ≥ 10% blasts/blasts equivalent (ICC)
  - Blockage of maturation at promyelocyte stage
  - Blasts with frequent bilobed nuclei
  - 2 common morphologic variants: Microgranular (hypogranular) and hypergranular (typical)
  - Potentially life-threatening coagulopathy

ETIOLOGY/PATHOGENESIS

Molecular Pathogenesis
- APL driven by balanced (15;17)(q24.1;q21.2) reciprocal translocation
  - Results in fusion of promyelocytic leukemia (*PML*) gene and retinoic acid receptor alpha (*RARA*) gene
    - *PML*: Tumor suppressor gene
    - *RARA*: Promotes cell differentiation and suppresses cell growth
    - Fusion protein results in uncontrolled proliferation and blockage of differentiation at promyelocyte stage

CLINICAL ISSUES

Epidemiology
- Incidence
  - 5-8% of all AML cases; M:F ~ 1:1
  - Higher incidence among Latino population
  - Subset of APL cases are therapy related
    - Post chemotherapy or radiation for prior malignancy

Presentation
- Patients with APL may present with life-threatening coagulopathy as main clinical feature
  - Disseminated intravascular coagulation (DIC) and hyperfibrinolysis
  - Marked thrombocytopenia
- Pediatric patients often present with high-risk features
  - High WBC count &/or hypogranular variant
- t(15;17)(q24.1;q21.2)/*PML::RARA* is hallmark of disease

Treatment
- Rapid diagnosis crucial to decrease early death rate due to coagulopathy
- Treatment of coagulopathy
  - Rapid administration of all trans retinoic acid (ATRA) should begin at 1st suspicion of APL
    - ATRA can reverse coagulopathy and reduce bleeding
    - ATRA can also reduce amounts of blood product consumption
      - No significant harm if given to patient with misdiagnosed APL
  - Administration of cryoprecipitate, fibrinogen, and platelets
    - Maintain fibrinogen level at > 100-150 mg/dL and platelet count at > 50,000/μL until resolution of coagulopathy
  - Fresh frozen plasma if prothrombin time or activated partial thromboplastin time prolonged
- ATRA as single agent
  - Induces complete remission in up to 90%
  - Resistance and subsequent relapse may occur with ATRA monotherapy
  - ATRA may induce differentiation syndrome
    - Characterized by fever, hypotension, fluid retention, and pulmonary infiltrates with early mortality
- ATRA plus anthracycline-based chemotherapy
  - Superior to ATRA alone
  - Complete remission in ~ 90-95%
  - Concurrent administration more effective than sequential therapy
  - Decreases risk of differentiation syndrome
- ATRA plus arsenic trioxide (ATO)
  - Currently standard treatment of APL
  - Eliminates need for traditional cytotoxic chemotherapy
  - Cures almost all patients with low or normal WBC
  - Has minimal toxicity
- Addition of anthracycline may be needed in APL patients with WBC of > 5X10⁹/L after ATRA administration
- Treatment of differentiation syndrome in APL patients
  - Can be controlled with high-dose corticosteroids
    - Give immediately at 1st suspicion of syndrome
  - Prophylactic dexamethasone can reduce morbidity and mortality in ATRA-induced leukocytosis
- Disease monitoring by quantitative real-time PCR (RT-PCR)
  - Sequential assessment for measurable/minimal residual disease (MRD) and early relapse
    - More reliable after completion of consolidation
    - Recommended every 3 months for 36 months in high-risk patients
    - Higher detection sensitivity with analysis of bone marrow compared to peripheral blood
  - Advantages of preemptive therapy in patients with MRD or early molecular relapse
    - Reduced mortality from potential coagulopathy that occurs with clinical relapse
    - Decreased therapy-related toxicity
    - Improved outcome and reduced hospitalization

Prognosis
- Curable in most patients with current therapy
- Overall survival exceeds 90% with ATRA and ATO therapy
  - More favorable prognosis compared with other AML with recurrent cytogenetic abnormalities
    - Early death results from coagulopathy or ATRA-induced differentiation syndrome
  - Inferior event-free survival for cases with complex cytogenetic abnormalities reported

Acute Promyelocytic Leukemia With t(15;17)/*PML::RARA*

- Pediatric patients often present with high-risk features, including high WBC &/or microgranular variant
- Worse survival reported in APL with *FLT3* ITD mutation

MOLECULAR

Cytogenetics

- **t(15;17)(q24.1;q21.2)**
  - Diagnostic hallmark of APL
  - Reciprocal balanced translocation involving long arms of chromosomes 15 and 17
  - Results in fusion of *PML* at 15q24.1 with *RARA* at 17q21.2
  - Novel *PML::RARA* fusion on chromosome 15 encodes PML::RARA fusion oncoprotein
- **Functions of PML::RARA fusion oncoprotein**
  - Critical role in molecular pathogenesis of APL
  - Blockage of differentiation beyond promyelocyte stage
  - Disruption of signaling pathways of both *PML* and *RARA*
- **APL with complex cytogenetics**
  - Complex translocations involve chromosomes 15 and 17 with 1 or 2 additional chromosomes
  - Inferior event-free survival for cases with 2 or more additional cytogenetic abnormalities reported
- **APL with cryptic 15;17 translocation**
  - Cytogenetics fails to detect cryptic translocation
  - FISH usually detects cryptic *PML::RARA* rearrangements
  - FISH may be negative in rare cases with cryptic *PML::RARA* rearrangements
    - RT-PCR would detect these rare cryptic microinsertion missed by FISH
- **APL with secondary cytogenetic abnormalities**
  - Detected in ~ 40% of APL cases
  - Trisomy 8 most common secondary cytogenetic abnormality

In Situ Hybridization

- FISH using *PML*- and *RARA*-targeted probes detects > 95% of *PML::RARA* fusions
- FISH using *RARA* break-apart probes can detect variant *RARA* translocations
  - Rare APL cases with microinsertion may be negative for t(15;17) by cytogenetics and *PML::RARA* fusion by FISH
  - Must perform RT-PCR in all suspected APL cases with negative FISH and cytogenetics

PCR

- RT-PCR detects all 3 types of *PML::RARA* transcripts
  - Breakpoint in *RARA* gene consistently occurs in intron 2
  - Breakpoints in *PML* occur in 3 different loci
    - Intron 6 (bcr1) that results in long-form transcript
    - Exon 6 (bcr2) that results in variable-form transcript
    - Intron 3 (bcr3) that results in short-form transcript
- Quantitative RT-PCR for disease monitoring
  - Most sensitive method for detection of early molecular relapse following molecular remission

Gene Mutations in APL

- *FLT3* ITD mutations detected in ~ 40% of cases
  - Associated with higher WBC, higher risk of relapse, higher rate of hypogranular morphology and short form of *PML::RARA* transcript

- *FLT3* TKD mutations in ~ 12% and *WT1* in ~ 10% of cases
- Other less common mutations reported in APL includes
  - *KRAS*, *NRAS*, *ARID1A*, *ARID1B*, *ASXL1*, *DNMT3A*, and *RUNX1*

MICROSCOPIC

Hypergranular (Typical) APL

- High level of suspicion required to accurately identify this type due to low WBC count
- Marked thrombocytopenia typically present
- Increased blasts with bilobed or convoluted nuclei
- Increased abnormal promyelocytes with abundant large granules (blast equivalent)
- Occasional blasts with numerous Auer rods

Hypogranular (Microgranular) APL

- Frequently high WBC count
- Blasts with frequent bilobed nuclei and absent cytoplasmic granules
- Morphologic overlap with acute monocytic leukemia
- Rare Auer rods detected with extensive search

ANCILLARY TESTS

Histochemistry

- MPO
  - Strongly positive in all leukemic cells in APL, including hypogranular forms
- NSE
  - Weakly positive in ~ 25% of cases

Flow Cytometry

- Bright CD33(+), variably CD13(+)
- CD117(+) in majority of cases
- Absence of CD34 and HLA-DR expression in most cases
- Variable expression of CD34 and CD2 can be seen in
  - APL with hypogranular blasts
  - APL with short-form transcript (bcr3)
- CD64(+) in most cases
- CD56(+) in ~ 20%
- CD15 typically (-)

PCR

- RT-PCR
  - Detects specific forms of *PML::RARA* transcripts
  - Requires high-quality RNA
- Quantitative RT-PCR
  - Assessment of treatment response
  - Minimal/measurable residual disease detection
  - Detection of early relapse

Genetic Testing

- FISH analysis using targeted probes
  - Recommended as initial diagnostic test in all suspected APL cases
    - Rapid turnaround time
    - Detects *PML::RARA* fusion, including most cryptic rearrangements
    - Rare molecularly detectable, small, cryptic *PML::RARA* may be missed on FISH analysis
- Conventional cytogenetic should be done in all cases

Acute Promyelocytic Leukemia With t(15;17)/*PML::RARA*

Acute Promyelocytic Leukemia With Variant *RARA* Fusions

Variant RARA Translocations	Fusion Genes	Microscopic Features	Frequency	Response to ATRA
t(11;17)(q13;q21)	*NUMA1::RARA*	Similar to classic APL with *PML::RARA*	Isolated case reports	Sensitive
t(11;17)(q23;q21)	*ZBTB16::RARA*	Regular nuclei, coarse or fine cytoplasmic granules, absent Auer rods, pelgeroid neutrophils	~ 1% among all APL cases	Resistant
t(5;17)(q35;q21)	*NPM1::RARA*	Similar to classic APL with *PML::RARA*	~ 0.5% among all APL cases	Sensitive
t(17;17)(q21;q21)	*STAT5B::RARA*	Some blasts may resemble hypogranular variant of classic APL with *PML::RARA*	Rare	Resistant
t(X;17)(p11;q21)	*BCOR::RARA*	Promyelocytes with rectangular and round cytoplasmic inclusions	Isolated case reports	Sensitive
t(3;17)(q26;q21)	*TBL1XR1::RARA*	Hypergranular promyelocytes, absent Auer rods	Isolated case reports	Resistant

APL = acute promyelocytic leukemia; ATRA = all trans retinoic acid alpha.

- Detects t(15;17)(q22.1;q21.2) in ~ 90% of cases
- Identifies complex variant translocations involving chromosomes 15 and 17 and ≥ 1 additional chromosomes
- Can detect additional chromosomal aberrations, if present
- Detects *RARA* rearrangements with alternative partners
- Causes of false-negative cytogenetic results
  - Cryptic translocations
  - Microinsertions

DIFFERENTIAL DIAGNOSIS

Acute Monocytic Leukemia
- Monocytic blasts may resemble hypogranular variant of APL
- MPO weak to (-)
- NSE(+)
- Typically CD15(+), HLA-DR(+)
- Absence of *PML::RARA* rearrangements

APL With Variant *RARA* Translocations
- AML with t(11;17)(q13;q21); *NUMA1::RARA*
  - Isolated case reports
  - Absence of *PML::RARA* fusion by FISH and RT-PCR
  - Sensitive to ATRA
- AML with t(5;17)(q35;q21); *NPM1::RARA*
  - Morphologic overlap with APL
  - Prominent hypergranular promyelocytes
  - Auer rods usually not detected
  - Sensitive to ATRA
- AML with t(11;17)(q23;q21); *ZBTB16::RARA*
  - Blasts contain regular nuclei and coarse or fine cytoplasmic granules
  - Auer rods usually absent
  - Increased neutrophils with pelgeroid nuclei
  - Strong MPO reactivity
  - Resistant to ATRA
- AML with t(17;17)(q21.2;q21); *STAT5B::RARA*
  - Blasts may resemble hypogranular type of APL blasts
  - Resistant to ATRA
- AML with t(X;17)(p11;q21); *BCOR::RARA*
  - Isolated case report
  - Abnormal promyelocytes with rectangular cytoplasmic bodies and round inclusions
  - Responds to ATRA per isolated case reports but resistant to ATO

Reactive Increase in Promyelocytes
- Growth factor administration (i.e., GCSF)
- Early marrow recovery post chemotherapy
- Drug-induced maturation arrest (i.e., levamisole-tinted cocaine)

DIAGNOSTIC CHECKLIST

Clinically Relevant Pathologic Features
- APL is medical emergency with risk of early death due to coagulopathy
- Rapid and accurate diagnosis of APL critical
- Presumptive diagnosis of APL should be communicated with clinicians in all suspected cases

Pathologic Interpretation Pearls
- Presumptive diagnosis of APL should be made when morphology and MPO supportive
  - Early administration of ATRA can correct coagulopathy
  - ATRA administration can also reduce blood products consumption
- ATRA responsiveness must be communicated with clinicians in AML cases with variant *RARA* translocations

SELECTED REFERENCES

1. Weinberg OK et al: The International Consensus Classification of acute myeloid leukemia. Virchows Arch. 482(1):27-37, 2023
2. Arber DA et al: International Consensus Classification of myeloid neoplasms and acute leukemia: integrating morphological, clinical, and genomic data. Blood. 140(11):1200-28, 2022
3. Khoury JD et al: The 5th edition of the World Health Organization Classification of Haematolymphoid Tumours: myeloid and histiocytic/dendritic neoplasms. Leukemia. 36(7):1703-19, 2022
4. Liquori A et al: Acute promyelocytic leukemia: a constellation of molecular events around a single PML-RARA fusion gene. Cancers (Basel). 12(3), 2020
5. Fasan A et al: Molecular landscape of acute promyelocytic leukemia at diagnosis and relapse. Haematologica. 102(6):e222-4, 2017
6. Cicconi L et al: Current management of newly diagnosed acute promyelocytic leukemia. Ann Oncol. 27(8):1474-81, 2016
7. Lucena-Araujo AR et al: Internal tandem duplication of the FLT3 gene confers poor overall survival in patients with acute promyelocytic leukemia treated with all-trans retinoic acid and anthracycline-based chemotherapy: an International Consortium on Acute Promyelocytic Leukemia study. Ann Hematol. 93(12):2001-10, 2014

Acute Promyelocytic Leukemia With t(15;17)/*PML::RARA*

Hypergranular (Typical) Variant

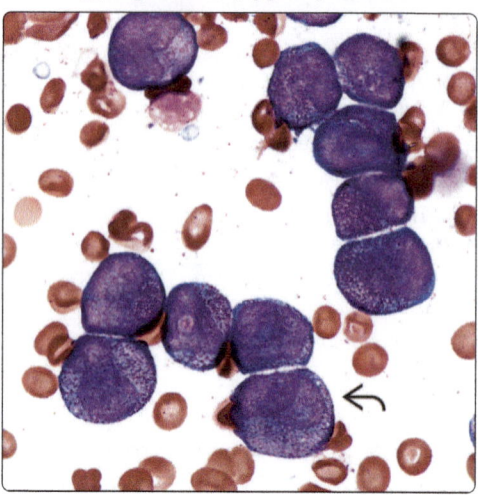

Bundles of Auer Rods in Blasts

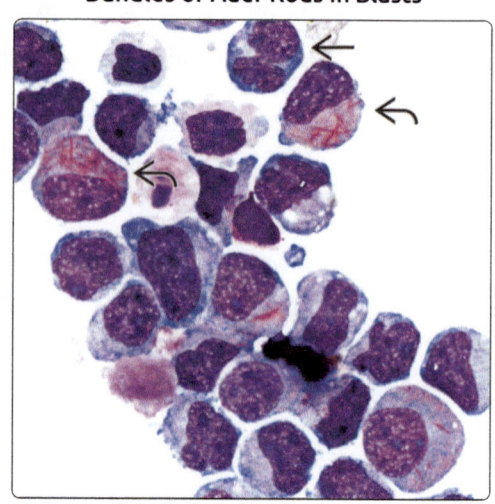

(Left) Wright-stained peripheral blood smear from a patient with hypergranular variant of APL shows anemia and prominent thrombocytopenia as well as many abnormal promyelocytes (blast equivalents) with prominent granules and irregular to occasional bilobed nuclei ➡. (Right) Wright-stained cytospin preparation of bone marrow in APL shows hypogranular blasts with a bilobed form ➡. Intracytoplasmic Auer rods and 2 faggot cells ➡ are also present.

Sheets of Promyelocytes

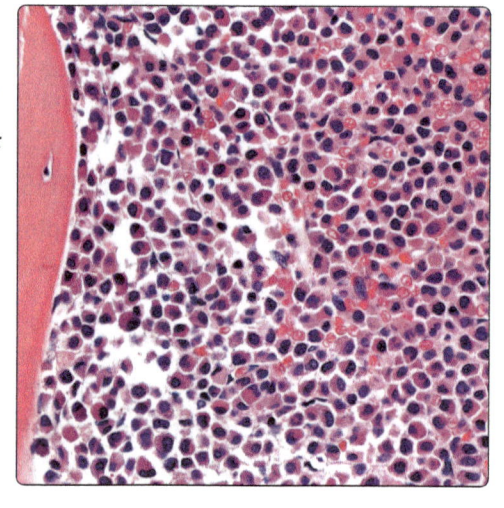

***FLT3* ITD Mutation**

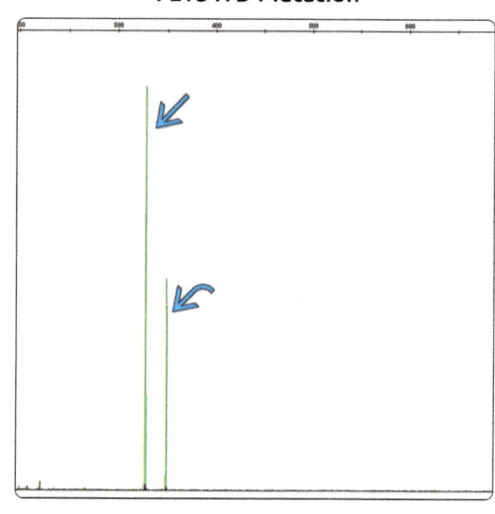

(Left) Trephine biopsy from a patient with hypergranular variant of APL shows markedly decreased trilineage hematopoiesis due to extensive marrow involvement by sheets of abnormal promyelocytes (blast equivalent) with irregular nuclei and pink, granulated cytoplasm. (Right) Electropherogram of PCR products of FLT3 gene amplification shows a FLT3 ITD mutation peak ➡ in this patient with APL. The taller peak represents the FLT3 wildtype allele ➡.

Absence of CD34 Expression

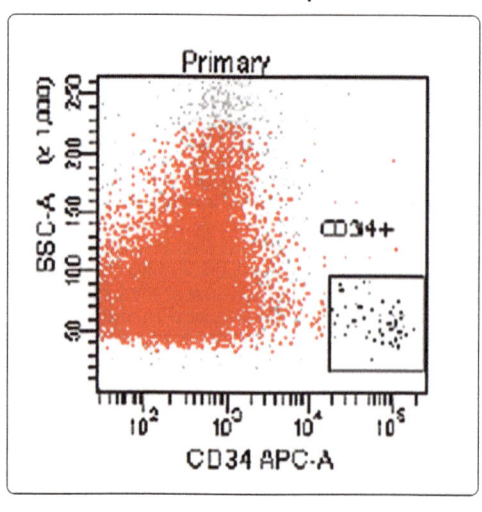

Absence of HLA-DR Expression

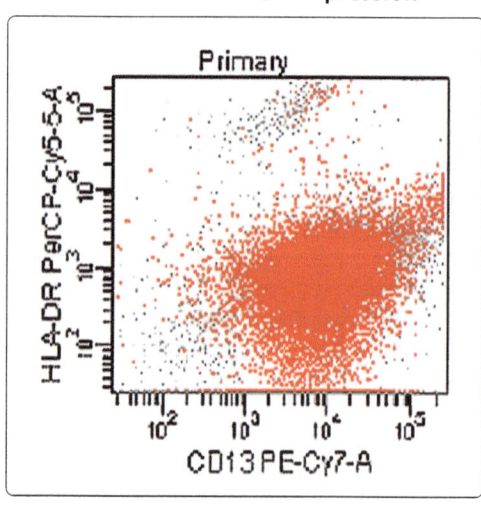

(Left) Flow cytometric analysis on a peripheral blood specimen from a patient with hypogranular variant of APL shows a prominent CD34(-) blast population (red). (Right) Flow cytometric analysis on a peripheral blood specimen from a patient with hypogranular variant of APL shows bright expression of CD13 and lack of expression of HLA-DR by blasts (red). A significant proportion of APL cases typically show lack of HLA-DR and CD34 antigens.

Acute Promyelocytic Leukemia With t(15;17)/*PML::RARA*

Circulating Bilobed Blasts

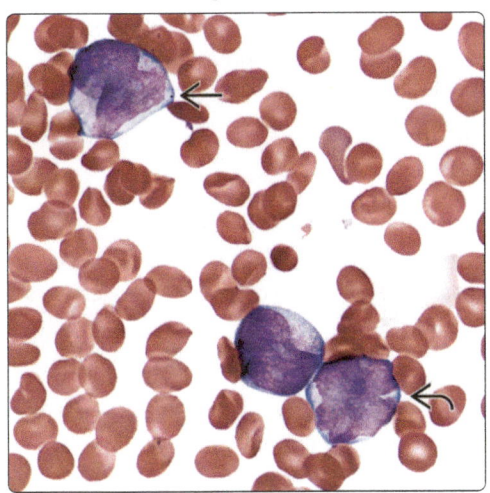

Bilobed Nuclei

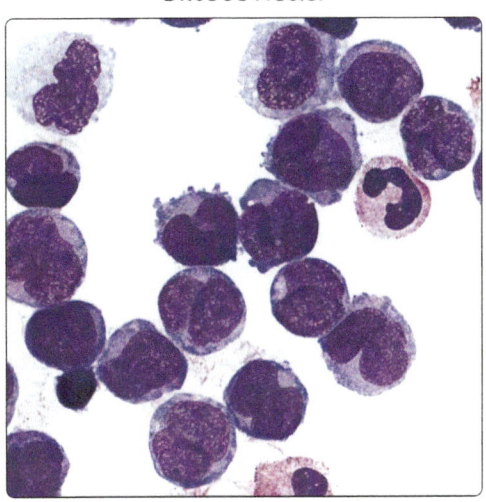

(Left) Wright-stained peripheral blood smear from a patient with APL shows marked thrombocytopenia and 3 circulating blasts with high N:C ratio and bilobed ➡ to lobulated nuclei ➡ mimicking blasts of monocytic lineage. **(Right)** Wright-stained marrow touch preparation of hypogranular variant of APL shows many blasts with bilobed nuclei. The presence of blasts with bilobed nuclei should raise high suspicion for diagnosis of APL.

Bundles of Intracytoplasmic Auer Rods

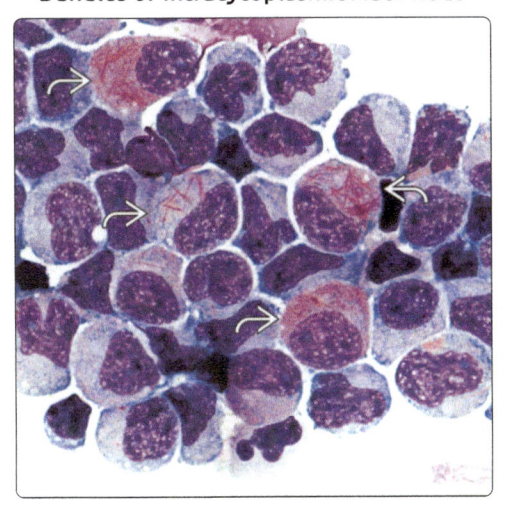

Abnormal Promyelocytes (Blast Equivalents)

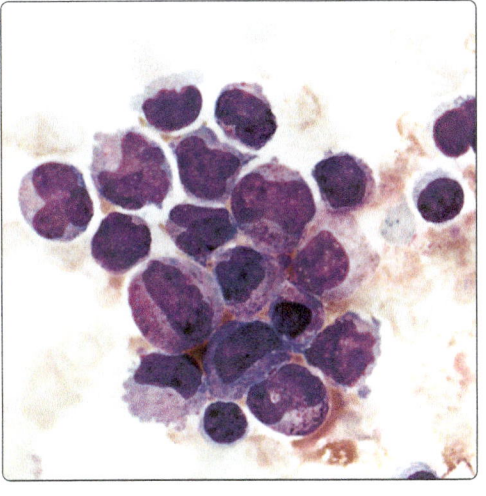

(Left) Cytospin preparation of bone marrow aspirate from a patient with APL shows several blasts with bundles of Auer rods (faggot cells) ➡ that are typically found in most but not all APL cases. **(Right)** Bone marrow aspirate smear from a patient with pancytopenia and FISH-positive PML::RARA fusion shows slightly abnormal promyelocytes with features that may suggest a regenerative bone marrow. The diagnosis of APL should always be considered when abnormal promyelocytes are present.

High Copies of *PML::RARA* Transcripts Detected by Quantitative PCR

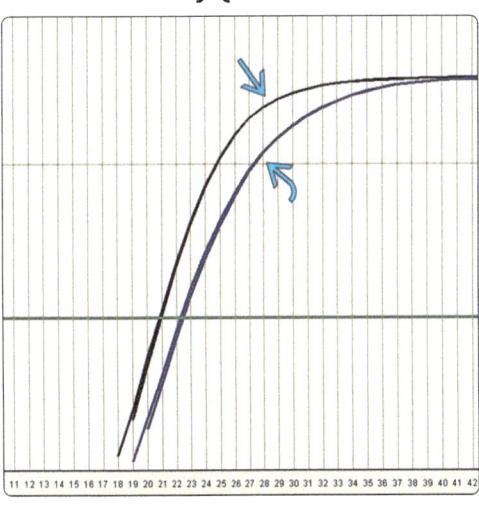

No Detectable *PML::RARA* Transcripts Following Consolidation

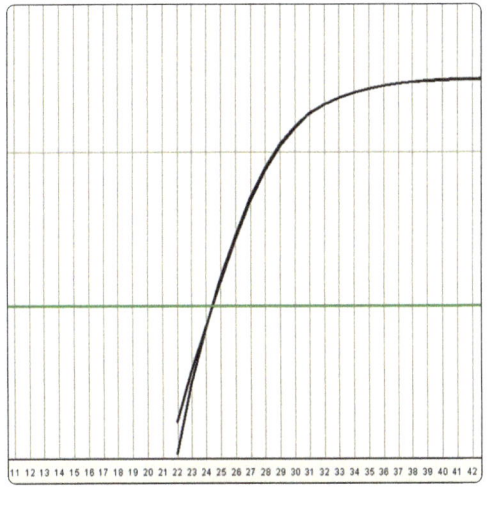

(Left) Quantitative real-time PCR using primers designed to amplify 3 subtypes of PML-RARA transcripts and TaqMan probes shows high copy numbers of PML::RARA short isoform transcripts (blue-colored curves) ➡ in a case of APL at presentation. The black-colored curves represent amplification of ABL1 ➡ internal control gene. **(Right)** Quantitative PCR after 8 weeks treatment of APL shows no PML::RARA transcripts, indicative of complete molecular remission. Black-colored curves represent amplification of control gene.

Acute Myeloid Leukemia With t(9;11)/*MLLT3::KMT2A*

KEY FACTS

TERMINOLOGY
- Acute myeloid leukemia (AML)

ETIOLOGY/PATHOGENESIS
- *KMT2A* is frequent target for rearrangement
  - *MLLT3* is most common, t(9;11)(p21.3;q23.3)
  - ICC specifies 7 *KMT2A*-rearranged subtypes as distinct entities
- Chimeric transcript encodes abnormal protein derived from
  - 5'-region of *KMT2A*, which encodes N-terminal DNA-binding motif
  - 3'-region of respective partner gene
- Fusion protein overrides normal differentiation stimuli

CLINICAL ISSUES
- AML with t(9;11)/*KMT2A::MLLT3* corresponds to intermediate-risk group
- AMLs with other *KMT2A* rearrangements stratified to adverse-risk group

MICROSCOPIC
- ≥ 10% blasts/blast equivalents in peripheral blood &/or bone marrow (BM) required for diagnosis by ICC
- Typically monoblasts and promonocytes

ANCILLARY TESTS
- Cytogenetics
  - Karyotype reveals classic translocation
- FISH also useful to document *KMT2A* rearrangement
  - Partner gene is **not** revealed using break-apart probe
  - Useful in cases with cryptic or complex rearrangements
- Molecular genetics
  - Multiplex RT-PCR approach is recommended due to breakpoint heterogeneity
  - Can be used to monitor minimal residual disease status
- RNA sequencing may determine exact nature of rearrangement or identify partner gene in translocations

Predominance of Monoblasts

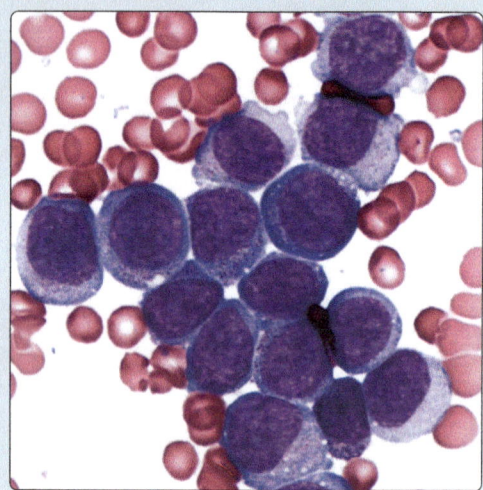

Karyotype With t(9;11)

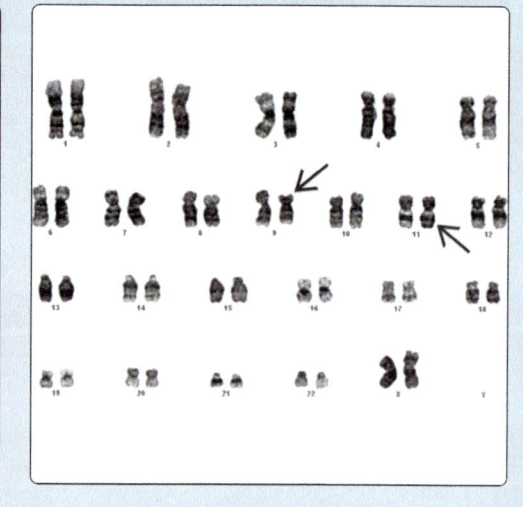

(Left) Bone marrow aspirate smear shows the classic cytology of acute myeloid leukemia (AML) with t(9;11). The cells are monoblasts with an abundant rim of cytoplasm containing MPO(-) azurophilic granules. (Right) Karyogram shows t(9;11)(p21;q23) ➡ in a case of AML with monocytic differentiation. At the molecular level, KMT2A (11q23) and MLLT3 are aberrantly juxtaposed, resulting in a chimeric fusion protein.

Blasts Lack CD34

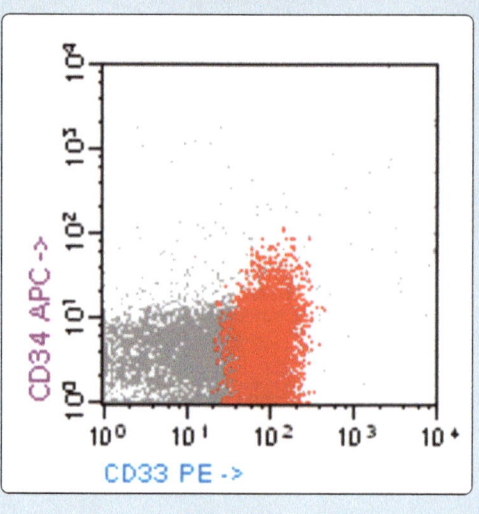

Blasts With Monocytic Differentiation

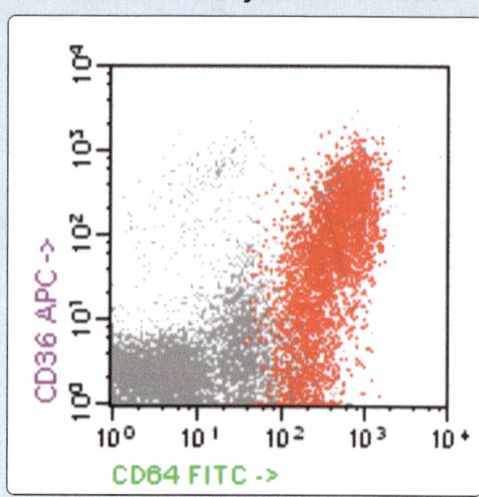

(Left) Flow cytometric analysis in AML with t(9;11) shows a prominent population of monocytic blasts that characteristically express bright CD33 and lack CD34 (red population). The expression of HLA-DR (not shown) is a useful finding to distinguish from acute promyelocytic leukemia. (Right) Flow cytometric analysis in AML with t(9;11) shows a population of neoplastic cells that coexpress CD36 and CD64. This pattern is characteristic of monocytic differentiation (red population).

Acute Myeloid Leukemia With t(9;11)/*MLLT3::KMT2A*

TERMINOLOGY

Abbreviations
- Acute myeloid leukemia (AML)

Synonyms
- AML with t(9;11)(p21;q23) resulting in *MLLT3::KMT2A*

Definitions
- Subtype of AML in which *KMT2A* at 11q23 is rearranged with *MLLT3* at 9p21.3
  - *MLLT3::KMT2A* fusion
    - Results from t(9;11)(p21.3;q23.3)
- AML with other *KMT2A* rearrangements
  - Includes 6 entities with other *KMT2A* partners rearrangements
    - t(4;11)/*AFF1::KMT2A*, t(6;11)/*AFDN::KMT2A*, t(10;11)(p12.3;q23.3)/*MLLT10::KMT2A*, t(10;11)(q21.3;q23.3)/*TET1::KMT2A*, t(11;19)(q23.3;p13.1)/*KMT2A::ELL*, t(11;19)(q23.3;p13.3)/*KMT2A::MLLT1*
- *KMT2A*
  - Official full name: Lysine methyltransferase 2A
  - HGNC_ID: 7132
  - Gene locus: 11q23.3
  - 37 exons
- *MLLT3*
  - Official full name: MLLT3 super elongation complex subunit
  - HGNC_ID: 7136
  - Gene locus: 9p21.3
  - 12 exons
- Morphology and immunophenotype usually indicate monocytic differentiation

CLASSIFICATION

ICC vs WHO-HEAM5
- AML with t(9;11)(p21.3;q23.3)/*MLLT3::KMT2A* (ICC)
- AML with *KMT2A* rearrangement (WHO-HAEM5)
  - ICC requires ≥ 10% blood or bone marrow (BM) blast for diagnosis
  - No blood or BM blast number cutoff required for diagnosis by WHO-HAEM5

ETIOLOGY/PATHOGENESIS

Epidemiology
- May occur at any age
  - ~ 9-12% of pediatric AML, ~ 1-2% of adult AML

Normal Function of *KMT2A*
- Encodes DNA-binding transcriptional coactivator protein
  - Transcription regulatory factor important in embryogenesis and hematopoiesis (e.g., *HOX* homeobox genes)
  - Cleaved into 2 fragments that reassociate and bind to specific multiprotein transcriptional complexes
  - N-terminal "A-T hook" motif binds DNA
    - Directly binds to promoter sequences
  - SET domain has histone H3 lysine 4 (H3K4) methyltransferase activity
  - Leads to chromatin remodeling in epigenetic regulation of gene expression

Normal Function of *MLLT3*
- Participates in regulation of transcription

Abnormal KMT2A Fusion Proteins
- *KMT2A* is frequent target for rearrangement
  - Alterations implicated in leukemogenesis include deletions, duplications, inversions, translocations
  - Arise due to DNA breaks on both participating chromosomes and repair via nonhomologous end-joining DNA repair pathway
  - At least 121 cytogenetically characterized *KMT2A* translocations described
  - > 80 have been well characterized at molecular level with specific partner genes and breakpoints identified
    - *MLLT3* is most common, t(9;11)(p22;q23)
    - ICC specifies 7 *KMT2A* rearranged subtypes as distinct entities
      - In addition to *MLLT3*, includes *AFF1*, *AFDN*, *MLLT10*, *TET1*, *ELL*, and *MLLT1*
- Chimeric transcript encodes abnormal protein derived from
  - 5'-region of *KMT2A*, which encodes N-terminal DNA-binding motif
  - 3'-region of respective partner gene
- Most common *KMT2A* translocation partners all associate with common multiprotein complex
  - Necessary for transcriptional elongation and maintained gene expression
    - Via additional histone modifications and phosphorylation of RNA polymerase
  - Abnormal fusion proteins recruit this complex to *KMT2A* target genes and aberrantly maintain gene expression
  - Leukemia with *KMT2A* rearrangement have distinct gene expression profile
    - Similar to early hematopoietic stem cells
- Multihit model of AML
  - In multihit model of AML pathogenesis, both class 1 and class 2 mutations are needed for leukemogenesis
    - Class 1 mutations increase cellular proliferation
    - Class 2 mutations impair cellular differentiation and maturation
  - *KMT2A* fusions are considered class 2 changes
    - KMT2A fusion proteins override normal differentiation stimuli and enforce continued expression of genes associated with early hematopoiesis
  - Other common molecular alterations in *KMT2A* rearranged cases include *NRAS*, *KRAS*, *PTPN11*, *FLT3* TKD, *SETD2*, *RUNX1*, *TET2*, *PLCG2*, and *ZRSR2*
  - Mutation profiles of *KMT2A* rearranged AML tend to show fewer mutations than other types of AML

CLINICAL ISSUES

Presentation
- Leukocytosis, monocytosis, increased blasts
- Anemia and thrombocytopenia
- May present with disseminated intravascular coagulation
- Extramedullary myeloid sarcoma may be present
  - Gingival or cutaneous leukemic infiltration may be seen

Acute Myeloid Leukemia With t(9;11)/*MLLT3::KMT2A*

Prognosis
- AML with t(9;11)/*KMT2A::MLLT3* corresponds to intermediate-risk group
  - AMLs with other *KMT2A* rearrangements stratified to adverse-risk group
- Measurable residual disease monitoring
  - Early achievement of molecular negativity for *KMT2A::MLLT3* transcripts may portend longer remission status
  - Increasing *KMT2A::MLLT3* transcripts may herald early disease relapse
- Presence of additional mutations may influence prognosis
  - *RAS* pathway mutations associated with worse prognosis

MICROSCOPIC

Morphology
- Peripheral blood
  - Often leukocytosis
  - Anemia, thrombocytopenia
  - Circulating blasts and blast equivalent
    - Usually > 20% of WBC counts
    - Monoblasts with fine chromatin, large round nuclei, prominent nucleoli, and moderate to abundant cytoplasm
  - Promonocytes (blast equivalent)
    - Intermediate to large in size with gently lobulated nuclei with delicate nuclear folding and abundant, lightly basophilic cytoplasm
- BM aspirate smears
  - Usually sheets of monoblasts and promonocytes
  - No significant basophilia or eosinophilia

ANCILLARY TESTS

Flow Cytometry
- Monoblasts and promonocytes
  - CD64, CD36, CD4, CD33 (+), HLA-DR + (variable), CD14 (diminished/lost), and CD13 (variable)
  - CD56 [variable (+)], CD123(+), CD45(+)
- Typical myeloid blasts
  - CD34, CD117, CD13, and CD33; lacks monocyte-associated markers

Immunohistochemistry
- Blasts often (-) for CD34 and CD117
- Monocytic lineage markers
  - CD68(+) (KP1 clone), CD4 [weak (+)], lysozyme (+), CD163(+)
- Myeloid-associated antigens
  - CD33(+), MPO(-), CD13 (variable)

Cytogenetics
- Translocations involving 11q23 are typically readily evident on karyotype
- In rare instances, complex, unusual, or cryptic rearrangements may require further evaluation
  - FISH break-apart strategy for *KMT2A* rearrangement is very helpful in these cases
- Secondary cytogenetic abnormalities are common

FISH for *KMT2A* Rearrangement
- Confirms *KMT2A* rearrangement using break-apart probe
- Detects *KMT2A* rearrangement otherwise masked in complex karyotype or cryptic rearrangement
- Rare *KMT2A* rearrangements (like *KMT2A::USP2*) are not detected by FISH testing
- Partner gene is **not** revealed by break-apart probe
- *KMT2A* rearrangements are **not** specific for AML
- Seen in some acute leukemias of B-cell, T-cell, or ambiguous lineage types

Genetic Testing
- Molecular detection of fusion transcripts
  - RNA sequencing may determine exact nature of rearrangement or identify *KMT2A* partner gene in translocations
  - *KMT2A* partial tandem duplication is seen in myelodysplastic syndromes (MDS) and AML and does not meet criteria for AML with *KMT2A* rearrangement
- RT-PCR for *KMT2A::MLLT3*
  - Not available for all rearrangements
  - Breakpoints occur within large regions in each gene
    - *KMT2A* breakpoints span exons 8-11
    - *MLLT3* breakpoints span exons 4-9
    - Multiplex RT-PCR approach is recommended to accommodate this breakpoint heterogeneity
    - Assay may also include reverse primers to detect additional types of *KMT2A* translocations (e.g., with *AFF1*, *MLLT1*)
    - Because of breakpoint variability and large number of partner genes, negative result may not exclude true *KMT2A* translocation
  - *KMT2A::MLLT3* measurable residual disease testing
    - Detection of transcript after attaining remission may predict early relapse prior to clinical &/or morphologic relapse
    - Assessment of transcript levels while on therapy may aid in disease monitoring
- Gene expression profiling
  - Not routinely used in clinical care
  - Can identify cases with cryptic *KMT2A* rearrangements

DIFFERENTIAL DIAGNOSIS

KMT2A-Rearranged B-Lymphoblastic Leukemia
- Other non-*MLLT3* partner genes (e.g., *AFF1*) more common in this setting, but t(9;11) does occur
- Immunophenotyping will demonstrate B lineage

SELECTED REFERENCES

1. Falini B et al: Comparison of the International Consensus and 5th WHO edition classifications of adult myelodysplastic syndromes and acute myeloid leukemia. Am J Hematol. 98(3):481-92, 2023
2. Yuen KY et al: Mutational landscape and clinical outcome of pediatric acute myeloid leukemia with 11q23/KMT2A rearrangements. Cancer Med. 12(2):1418-30, 2023
3. Arber DA et al: International Consensus Classification of myeloid neoplasms and acute leukemia: integrating morphological, clinical, and genomic data. Blood. 140(11):1200-28, 2022
4. Khoury JD et al: The 5th edition of the World Health Organization Classification of haematolymphoid tumours: myeloid and histiocytic/dendritic neoplasms. Leukemia. 36(7):1703-19, 2022

Acute Myeloid Leukemia With t(9;11)/*MLLT3::KMT2A*

Blasts With Abundant Cytoplasm

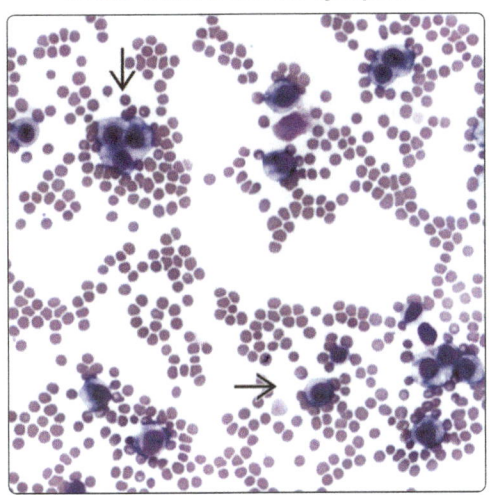

Circulating Monoblasts

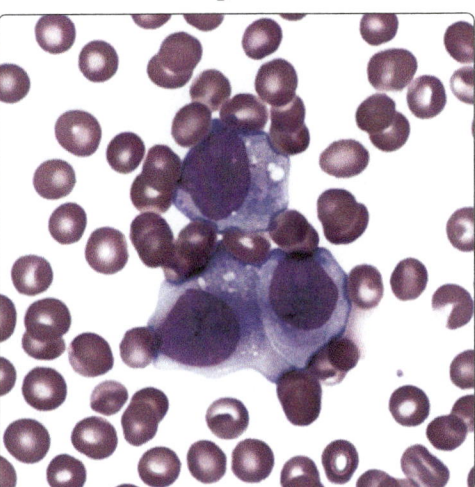

(Left) Peripheral blood smear shows leukocytosis dominated by blasts with abundant cytoplasm ➡ in a newly diagnosed AML with t(9;11). Note the associated findings of bone marrow failure (anemia and thrombocytopenia). (Right) High-power view of blood from a patient with AML with t(9;11) shows characteristic monoblasts: Large-sized with voluminous cytoplasm, occasional vacuoles, and prominent nucleoli. Faint, azurophilic granules can also be appreciated.

Predominance of Monoblasts

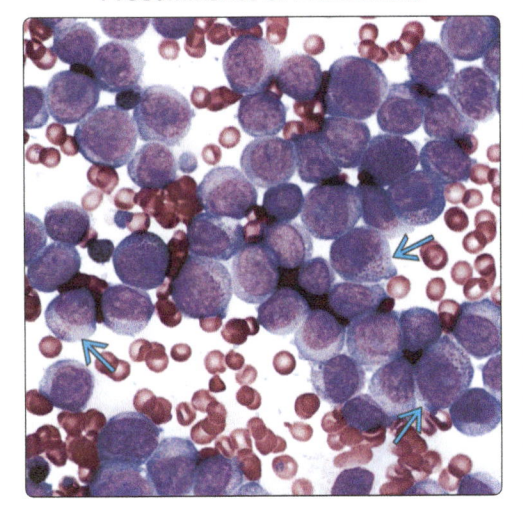

Hypercellular and Effaced Bone Marrow

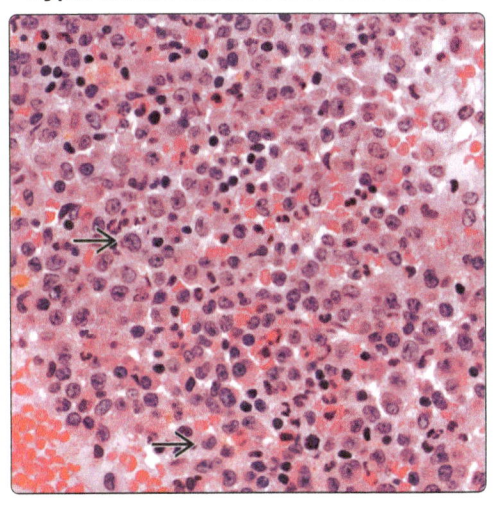

(Left) Bone marrow aspirate smear from a patient with AML with t(9;11) shows > 90% blasts with nearly uniform cytology characteristic of monoblasts (large cells with round nuclei, prominent nucleolus, abundant cytoplasm, and often distinct azurophilic granules ➡). (Right) Bone marrow clot section shows an acute monocytic infiltrate in AML with t(9;11). Some of the cells exhibit round nuclei, while others bear a typical folded nuclear appearance ➡.

Karyotype With t(9;11)

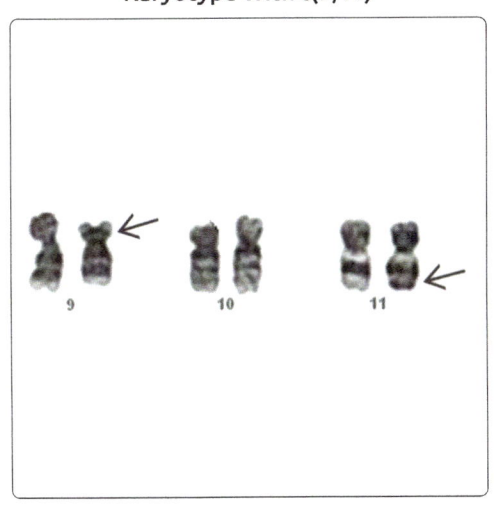

FISH Break-Apart Probe for *KMT2A*

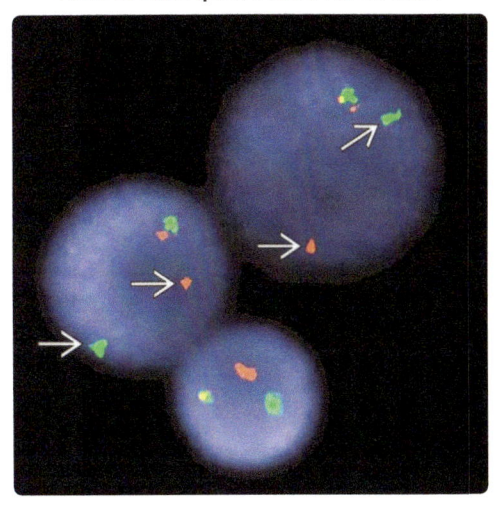

(Left) Partial karyogram shows the t(9;11)(p21;q23) seen in some cases of AML. These AML cases typically show a monocytic component. The KMT2A gene at 11q23.3 is involved. Abnormal chromosomes ➡ are noted. (Right) Three interphase nuclei show KMT2A rearrangement as depicted by the distinct separation of orange and green signals ➡. The normal KMT2A allele is seen as a yellow (green/orange overlap) signal.

Molecular Pathology of Myeloid Neoplasms

Acute Myeloid Leukemia With t(6;9)/*DEK::NUP214*

KEY FACTS

TERMINOLOGY
- Acute myeloid leukemia (AML) with t(6;9)(p22.3;q34.1) resulting in *DEK::NUP214* fusion
- May use to diagnose AML even when blast count is < 20% by WHO 5th edition and ICC systems
  - No diagnostic blast percentage requirement by WHO 5th edition, if present in correct clinicopathologic setting
  - ≥ 10% blasts are required by ICC diagnostic criteria
- Commonly has multilineage dysplasia and basophilia

CLINICAL ISSUES
- Represents ~ 1-2% of all AML; seen in children and adults
- Poor overall prognosis
  - Allogeneic hematopoietic stem cell transplant may improve overall survival

MICROSCOPIC
- Basophilia (≥ 2%) is characteristic; seen in ~ 50-60% of cases
- Multilineage dysplasia (especially erythroid and granulocytic)
- Features of diverse morphologic subtypes may be seen; AML with maturation being most common
- Myeloblasts may be TdT(+) in ~ 50-60% of cases

ANCILLARY TESTS
- t(6;9) translocation is detectable by karyotype but may be cryptic or subtle
  - Karyotype cryptic cases still detectable by FISH or NGS
- Limited numbers of breakpoints facilitate detection of fusion transcript by RT-PCR
  - Achievement RT-PCR negativity is highly associated with better outcome following transplant
- *DEK::NUP214* is associated with *FLT3* internal tandem duplication in ~ 80% of cases
  - *FLT3*-ITD(+) cases found to relapse significantly faster than *FLT3*-ITD(-) cases
    - Addition of inhibitor therapy is beneficial if positive

AML With t(6;9): Bone Marrow Aspirate

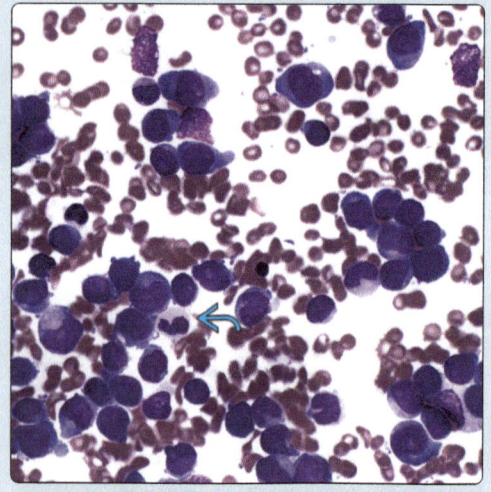

Peripheral Blood Basophilia

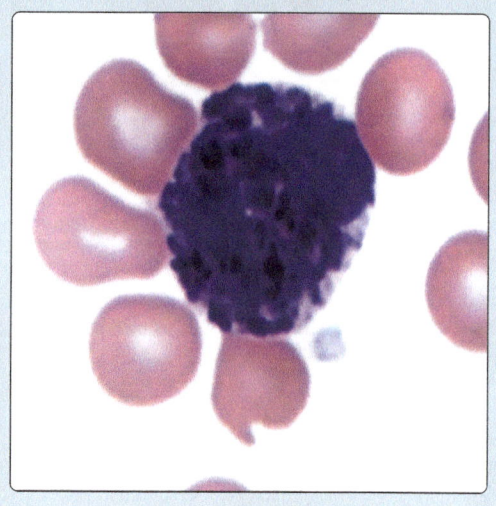

(Left) Bone marrow aspirate smear from a patient with acute myeloid leukemia (AML) with t(6;9); DEK::NUP214 does not show basophilia but demonstrates dyspoiesis. Note dysgranulopoiesis with a hypogranular neutrophil ➡. (Right) Approximately 50% of AML with t(6;9); DEK::NUP214 will have an associated peripheral blood and marrow basophilia. Basophilia is generally an uncommon finding in other AML subtypes.

Karyotype With t(6;9) Rearrangement

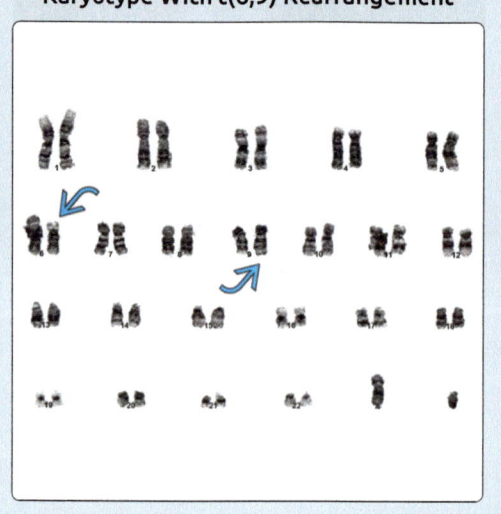

***FLT3*-ITD Mutation Analysis**

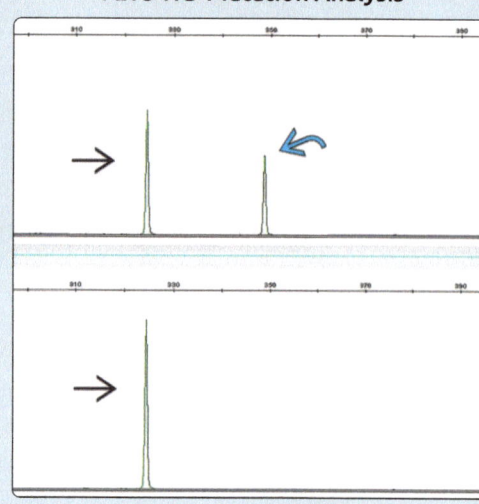

(Left) t(6;9)(p22.3~23;q34.1) translocation is visible on this karyotype ➡ from a patient with DEK::NUP214 fusion. This finding is associated with poor prognosis in AML. (Right) Capillary electrophoresis shows wildtype FLT3 amplicon peak ➡. The extra peak ➡ in the top tracing indicates a FLT3 internal tandem duplication mutation, which is a very common finding in AML with t(6;9); DEK::NUP214.

Acute Myeloid Leukemia With t(6;9)/*DEK::NUP214*

TERMINOLOGY

Abbreviations
- Acute myeloid leukemia (AML)

Synonyms
- AML with t(6;9)(p22.3;q34.1)/*DEK::NUP214* (2022 ICC)
- AML with *DEK::NUP21* fusion (WHO 5th edition)

Definitions
- *DEK* gene (locus: 6p22.3)
  - Official name: DEK protooncogene
- *NUP214* gene (locus: 9q34.13)
  - Official name: Nucleoporin 214
- *DEK::NUP214* fusion is recurrent (or defining) genetic abnormality in AML
  - May use to diagnose AML even when blast count is < 20% by WHO 5th edition and ICC systems
  - ICC blast cutoff criteria for this entity is ≥ 10%
    - Cases with 5-9% marrow blasts categorized as myelodysplastic syndrome with excess blasts but should be monitored especially closely for progression
  - No blast threshold criteria endorsed by WHO system
  - Associated with basophilia and multilineage dysplasia

ETIOLOGY/PATHOGENESIS

Normal Function of *DEK*
- Involved in chromatin organization and in splice site selection during mRNA processing
- In regulating myeloid differentiation, DEK is recruited to chromatin with critical myeloid transcription factor CEBPA to enhance *CSF3R* promoter activation
  - Depletion of DEK reduces G-CSF-mediated granulocytic differentiation in CD34(+) stem cells

Normal Function of *NUP214*
- Encodes cytoplasmic facing protein component of nucleoporin complex
  - Required for proper cell cycle progression and nucleocytoplasmic transport

DEK::NUP214 Fusion
- In-frame fusion of 5' *DEK* to 3' *NUP214*
  - Includes nearly all of DEK protein and ~ 2/3 of NUP214
- Effects of fusion protein still poorly understood
  - Appears to inhibit nuclear export receptor CRM1, disrupting protein export from nucleus
  - Forced expression in cell lines does not seem to block differentiation
  - May induce proliferation through mTOR pathway
  - Cooperating mutations (e.g., *FLT3*) appear to be crucial

CLINICAL ISSUES

Epidemiology
- Represents ~ 1-2% of all AML
- Seen in both children and adults

Prognosis
- Associated with poor prognosis
  - Median survival: ~ 1 year
  - 5-year survival in adults estimated at 9%
- Better overall survival with allogeneic hematopoietic stem cell (HSC) transplant

MOLECULAR

Genetic Findings
- ~ 70-90% have *FLT3* internal tandem duplication (ITD)
  - *FLT3*-ITD(+) cases may relapse faster than *FLT3*-ITD(-) cases, but mutation status has no survival impact
    - Addition of inhibitor therapy is beneficial if positive
- Other diverse secondary genetic mutations may contribute to poor survival outcomes

Genetic Testing
- Limited number of breakpoints facilitates RT-PCR detection of fusion transcript
  - RT-PCR negativity associated with better outcomes following HSC transplant
  - Sampling interval of 2 months has been proposed to detect minimal residual disease and molecular relapse
    - Rapid doubling time of transcript level precedes hematologic relapse
- Translocation may be subtle or cryptic on karyotype
  - Karyotype cryptic cases still detectable by FISH or NGS

MICROSCOPIC

Peripheral Blood and Bone Marrow
- Basophilia (≥ 2%) is characteristic, seen in ~ 50-60% of cases
- Multilineage dysplasia (especially erythroid and granulocytic)
- Features of diverse morphologic subtypes may be seen
  - AML with maturation being most common
- ~ 50-60% of cases show TdT expression in myeloid blasts
  - TdT expression is neither sensitive nor specific for t(6;9)

DIFFERENTIAL DIAGNOSIS

Acute Myeloid Leukemia With Mutated *TP53* or Myelodysplasia-Related Gene Mutations
- Basophilia is uncommon, and t(6;9) should be absent

Myelodysplastic Syndrome With Excess Blasts
- Cases with 5-9% blasts classified as myelodysplastic syndromes (MDS) per ICC criteria
  - Close monitoring and clinical correlation needed
  - MDS with *DEK::NUP214* is prognostically not equivalent to AML with *DEK::NUP214* per some studies
- This designation not present in WHO 5th edition; no lower blast threshold criteria, if present in correct clinicopathologic setting

Chronic Myeloid Leukemia, Blast Phase
- Basophilia is frequent finding
- Basophilia may also be seen in de novo AML with t(9;22)/*BCR::ABL1*

SELECTED REFERENCES

1. Arber DA et al: International Consensus Classification of Myeloid Neoplasms and Acute Leukemia: integrating morphological, clinical, and genomic data. Blood. 140(11):1200-28, 2022
2. Khoury JD et al: The 5th edition of the World Health Organization Classification of Haematolymphoid Tumours: myeloid and histiocytic/dendritic neoplasms. Leukemia. 36(7):1703-19, 2022

Acute Myeloid Leukemia With inv(3) or t(3;3)/*GATA2*; *MECOM*

KEY FACTS

TERMINOLOGY
- Subtype of acute myeloid leukemia (AML) with inv(3) or t(3;3) associated with juxtaposition of *GATA2* enhancer with *MECOM* gene

CLASSIFICATION
- AML subtype associated with *MECOM* gene rearrangement
  - WHO 5th edition recognizes all *MECOM* rearrangements
  - ICC classification only recognizes inv(3)/t(3;3)
    - Others classified as "AML with other *MECOM* rearrangements"
- Abnormalities lead to *MECOM* overexpression
  - Classic inv(3)/t(3;3) also cause *GATA2* haploinsufficiency
- May use to diagnose AML even when blast count is < 20% by WHO 5th edition and ICC classification systems
  - ICC requires ≥ 10% for AML with inv(3)/t(3;3) and with other *MECOM* rearrangements

CLINICAL ISSUES
- ~ 1-2% of all AML; seen mostly in adults
- May arise de novo or from prior myelodysplastic syndromes (MDS)
- Overall poor prognosis with short survival
- Dysgranulopoiesis associated with even worse prognosis

MOLECULAR
- May be cryptic by standard chromosome analysis
  - Karyotype cryptic cases still identifiable by FISH or NGS
- Most cases carry additional cytogenetic aberrancies
  - Monosomal or complex karyotype
- Mutations in RAS receptor pathway genes are found in ~ 98% of cases

MICROSCOPIC
- Multilineage dysplasia
- Characteristically small mono- or bilobated megakaryocytes

Partial Karyogram With t(3;3)

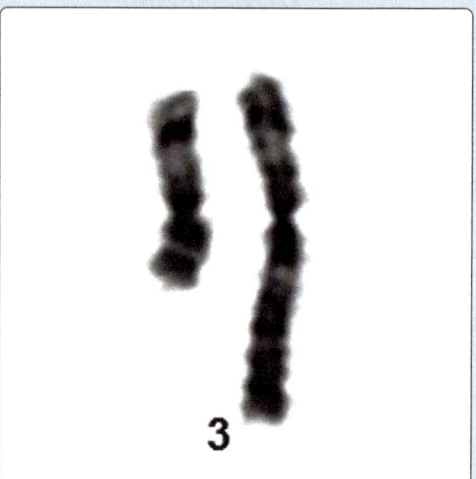

AML With t(3;3): Peripheral Blood Smear

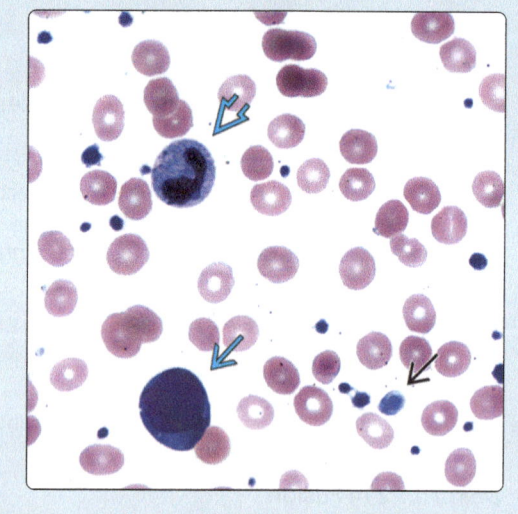

(Left) Partial karyogram from a patient with acute myeloid leukemia (AML) shows chromosome 3 with t(3;3)(q21.3; q26.2) translocation. (Right) Wright-stained peripheral blood from a patient with AML with t(3;3)(q21.3;q26.2) shows a blast ➡, a hypogranular neutrophil ➡, and a large, hypogranular platelet ➡.

AML With t(3;3): Bone Marrow Core

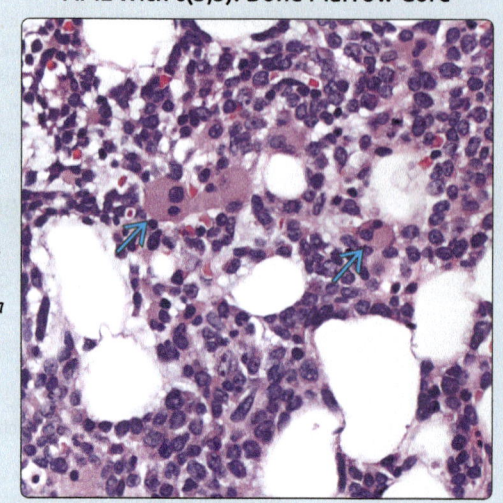

AML With inv(3): Core Biopsy CD42b

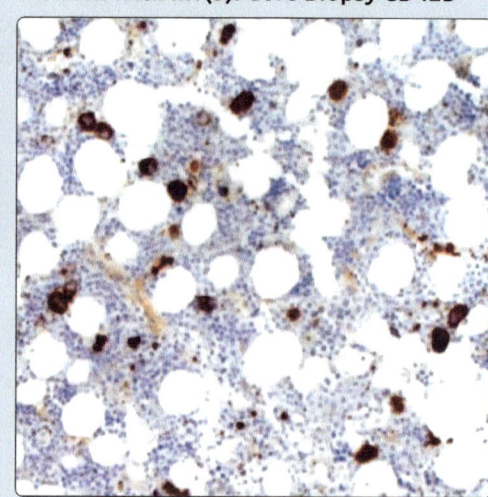

(Left) Bone marrow core biopsy from a patient with AML with t(3;3)(q21.3;q26.2) shows small clusters and scattered, small, mono- and bilobated megakaryocytes ➡ in a background with numerous blasts. (Right) CD42b performed on bone marrow core biopsy highlights the small, hypolobated, and bilobated megakaryocytes in a patient found to have AML with inv(3)(q21.3q26.2).

Acute Myeloid Leukemia With inv(3) or t(3;3)/GATA2; MECOM

TERMINOLOGY

Definitions
- Acute myeloid leukemia (AML) with inv(3) or t(3;3)/GATA2; MECOM (EVI1)
  - Subtype of AML with inv(3) or t(3;3) associated with juxtaposition of GATA2 enhancer with MECOM
- GATA2 (locus: 3q21.3)
  - Official name: GATA binding protein 2
- MECOM (locus: 3q26.2)
  - Official name: MDS1 and EVI1 complex locus
- MECOM rearrangements recognized as recurrent (or defining) genetic abnormality in AML

ICC vs. WHO-HAEM5
- AML with inv(3) or t(3;3) is recognized as distinct AML category by ICC
- ICC blast cutoff requirement for this entity and AML with other MECOM rearrangements is ≥ 10%
  - Cases with 5-9% marrow blasts would be categorized as myelodysplastic syndrome with excess blasts, but should be monitored especially closely for progression
- WHO classification includes this entity along with all other MECOM rearrangements as single category
  - Diagnosis can be made when blast count is < 20% with no minimum blast requirement by WHO-HAEM5
- Other MECOM rearrangements include
  - t(2;3)(p11~23;q26.2)/MECOM::?
  - t(3;8)(q26.2;q24.2)/MYC, MECOM
  - (3;12)(q26.2;p13.2)/ETV6::MECOM
  - t(3;21)(q26.2;q22.1)/MECOM::RUNX1

ETIOLOGY/PATHOGENESIS

Normal Function of GATA2
- Encodes zinc-finger transcription factor
- Functions in development and proliferation of hematopoietic and endocrine cell lines

Normal Function of MECOM
- Encodes zinc-finger transcription factor
- Involved in hematopoiesis, apoptosis, development, cell differentiation, and proliferation
- 19 transcript variants described; different isoforms and chimeric proteins encoded through alternative splicing and distinct transcription sites

Abnormal Function of MECOM Rearrangement
- inv(3) and t(3;3) both relocate distal GATA2 enhancer, leading to aberrant MECOM overexpression and GATA2 haploinsufficiency
  - Breakpoints appear to differ with inv(3) breaks 3' of MECOM and t(3;3) breaks 5' of MECOM
- MECOM drives leukemogenesis via aberrant ERG activation
  - This may be possible target for therapy
- Other rearrangements can cause MECOM overexpression
- High MECOM expression is poor prognostic indicator, independent of 3q26.2 locus rearrangement type

CLINICAL ISSUES

Epidemiology
- Represents ~ 1-2% of all AML
- Seen mostly in adults, shows no sex predilection, and may arise de novo or from myelodysplastic syndromes (MDS)

Prognosis
- Overall poor prognosis with short survival
  - Monosomal or complex karyotype and dysgranulopoiesis associated with even worse prognosis

MOLECULAR

Molecular Genetics
- MECOM rearrangements may be cryptic by karyotype
  - Karyotype cryptic cases still identifiable by FISH or NGS
- Most cases will carry additional cytogenetic aberrancies
  - Often MDS-related, including del(5q), monosomy 7, and complex karyotypes
- Mutations of genes activating RAS receptor pathways are found in ~ 98% of cases and include
  - NRAS, PTPN11, FLT3, KRAS, NF1, CBL, and KIT
- Other comutated genes include GATA2, RUNX1, and SF3B1

MICROSCOPIC

Peripheral Blood
- Dysplastic neutrophils and platelets

Bone Marrow
- Multilineage dysplasia, characteristically with small mono- or bilobated megakaryocytes
- Variably differentiated myeloblasts, including without differentiation, myelomonocytic, or megakaryoblastic

DIFFERENTIAL DIAGNOSIS

Myelodysplastic Syndromes With GATA2; MECOM Rearrangements
- MECOM rearranged cases with 5-9% blasts are classified as MDS per ICC criteria
  - Close patient monitoring and clinical correlation recommended
- No lower blast threshold per WHO 5th edition criteria

Blast Phase of Chronic Myeloid Leukemia
- Chronic myeloid leukemia (CML) may acquire inv(3) or t(3;3) with disease progression
- BCR::ABL1-positive CML cases with acquired inv(3)/t(3;3) would be classified as aggressive phase of CML

SELECTED REFERENCES

1. Schmoellerl J et al: EVI1 drives leukemogenesis through aberrant ERG activation. Blood. 141(5):453-66, 2023
2. Arber DA et al: International Consensus Classification of myeloid neoplasms and acute leukemia: integrating morphological, clinical, and genomic data. Blood. 140(11):1200-28, 2022
3. Gao J et al: Comparison of myeloid neoplasms with nonclassic 3q26.2/MECOM versus classic inv(3)/t(3;3) rearrangements reveals diverse clinicopathologic features, genetic profiles, and molecular mechanisms of MECOM activation. Genes Chromosomes Cancer. 61(2):71-80, 2022
4. Khoury JD et al: The 5th edition of the World Health Organization classification of haematolymphoid tumours: myeloid and histiocytic/dendritic neoplasms. Leukemia. 36(7):1703-19, 2022
5. Paredes R et al: EVI1 protein interaction dynamics: targetable for therapeutic intervention? Exp Hematol. 107:1-8, 2022

Acute Myeloid Leukemia (Megakaryoblastic) With t(1;22)/*RBM15::MRTFA*

KEY FACTS

TERMINOLOGY
- Acute myeloid leukemia (AML) (megakaryoblastic) with t(1;22)(p13.3;q13.1)/*RBM15::MRTFA* fusion
- International Consensus Classification (ICC) vs. WHO 5th edition (WHO-HAEM5) comparison
  - *RMB15::MRTFA* fusion recognized as recurrent (or defining) genetic abnormality in AML by both classification systems
  - ≥ 10% blasts threshold is required for diagnosis in ICC system
  - No minimum blasts threshold is required for diagnosis in WHO-HAEM5

CLINICAL ISSUES
- AML with t(1;22) accounts for < 1% of all AML
- Primarily affects infants and young children
  - Median age at diagnosis: 4 months
  - 80% of cases diagnosed in 1st year of life
- Hepatosplenomegaly &/or bone lesions are common at diagnosis
- Some cases may present as myeloid sarcoma without marrow involvement
- Generally high-risk disease, but intensive therapy may confer good response

MOLECULAR
- t(1;22) translocation typically visible on karyotype, but analysis may be limited by myelofibrosis-related inadequate bone marrow aspirate
  - t(1;22) is often sole karyotypic abnormality
- *RBM15::MRTFA* fusion also detectable via RT-PCR or NGS

MICROSCOPIC
- Blasts are morphologically and immunophenotypically megakaryoblasts
- Marrow typically shows myelofibrosis and micromegakaryocytes without multilineage dysplasia

Circulating Blasts

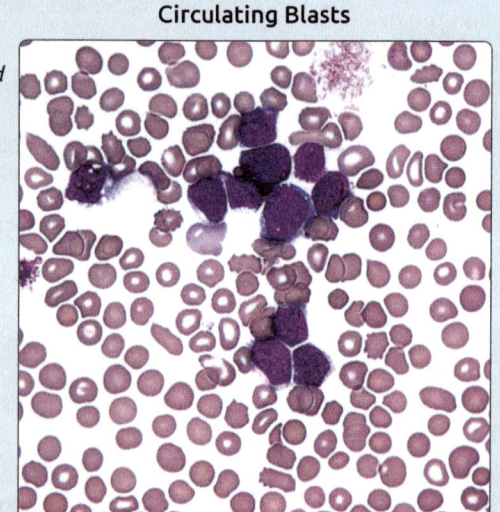

Acute Myeloid Leukemia With t(1;22)

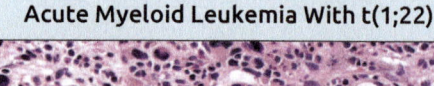

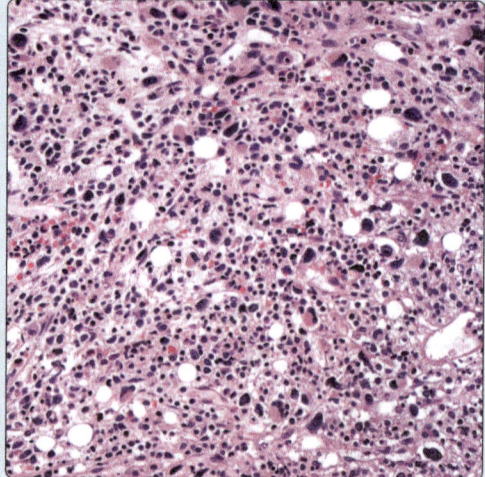

(Left) Circulating blasts are present in the peripheral blood of a 4-week-old boy with Down syndrome. Myeloid leukemia associated with Down syndrome is a major differential diagnostic consideration in megakaryoblastic leukemias of young childhood, including AML with t(1;22). (Right) Megakaryocytic features are seen in fibrotic bone marrow from an infant with AML with t(1;22).

Flow Histogram: CD41a vs. CD42b

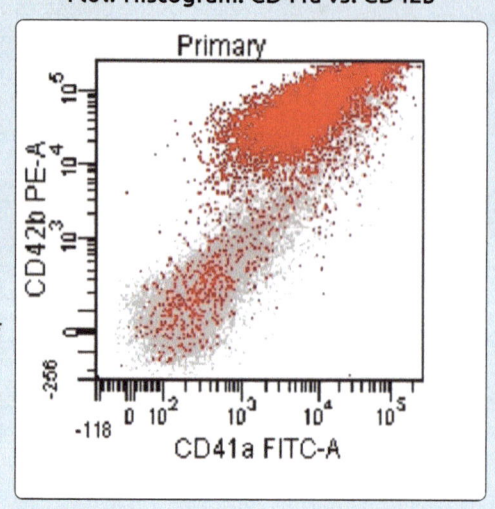

Partial Karyogram With t(1;22)(p13;q13)

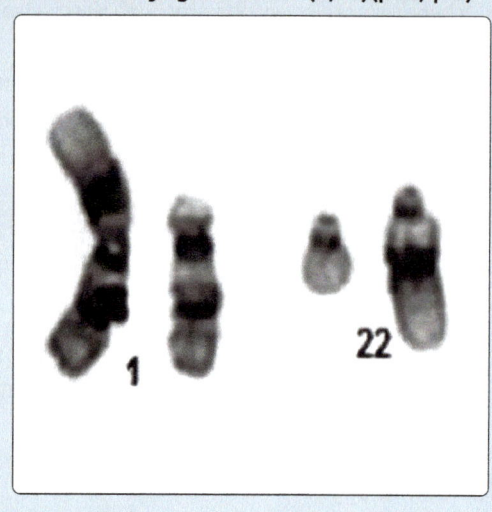

(Left) Flow cytometric analysis shows that the blasts in a case of AML with t(1;22) express megakaryocytic markers CD41a and CD42b. AML with t(1;22) shows megakaryoblastic differentiation. (Right) Partial karyogram from a child with acute myeloid (megakaryoblastic) leukemia shows t(1;22)(p13;q13) translocation, characteristic of RBM15 and MRTFA (MKL1) fusion.

Acute Myeloid Leukemia (Megakaryoblastic) With t(1;22)/*RBM15::MRTFA*

TERMINOLOGY

Definitions
- Acute myeloid leukemia (AML) (megakaryoblastic) with t(1;22)(p13.3;q13.1)/*RBM15::MRTFA* fusion
- *RBM15*
  - Gene locus: 1p13.3
- *MRTFA* (previously MKL1)
  - Gene locus: 22q13.1-q13.2
- ICC vs. WHO-HAEM5 comparison
  - *RMB15::MRTFA* fusion recognized as recurrent (or defining) genetic abnormality in AML by both classification systems
  - ≥ 10% blasts threshold is required for diagnosis in ICC system
  - No minimum blasts threshold is required for diagnosis in WHO-HAEM5

ETIOLOGY/PATHOGENESIS

Normal Function of *RBM15*
- Encoded protein binds to RNA and regulates N6-methyladenosine (m6A) RNA methylation
  - m6A modification involved in RNA splicing, stability, and transcription efficiency
- Expressed at highest levels in hematopoietic stem cells
  - Enforced expression impairs myeloid differentiation; affects Notch signaling by binding to RBPJκ

Normal Function of *MRTFA*
- Interacts with transcription factor myocardin
  - Serve as coactivators of transcription factor serum response factor (SRF)
    - Regulates cytoskeleton during development, morphogenesis, and cell migration

Abnormal Function of *RBM15::MRTFA* Fusion
- Fusion generates chimeric protein containing near full-length coding regions of both genes
- Alters modulation of chromatin organization, *HOX*-induced differentiation, and extracellular signaling pathways

CLINICAL ISSUES

Epidemiology
- Accounts for < 1% of all AML
  - ~ 14% of all non-Down syndrome acute megakaryoblastic leukemias (AMKLs)
- Most commonly in infants; female predominance
  - Median age at diagnosis is 4 months
  - 80% of cases diagnosed in 1st year of life
- Rare congenital presentations have been described

Presentation
- Hepatosplenomegaly &/or bone lesions common
- Some cases may primarily show extramedullary disease/myeloid sarcoma
  - Evaluate for extramedullary disease if bone marrow appears minimally involved

Prognosis
- Higher risk disease when compared to pediatric megakaryoblastic leukemia without t(1;22)
- Intensive AML therapy may confer good response

MICROSCOPIC

Cytomorphologic Features
- Megakaryoblasts by morphology and immunophenotype
  - Nuclear chromatin may be condensed
  - May be cytoplasmic blebbing

Bone Marrow Histology
- Micromegakaryocytes and megakaryoblasts without multilineage dysplasia
- Significant myelofibrosis is often present

ANCILLARY TESTS

Flow Cytometry
- Usually positive: CD36, CD41a, CD42b, CD61
- Usually negative: CD13, CD34, CD45, MPO, HLA-DR

Genetic Testing
- Translocation t(1;22)(p13;q13) visible on karyotype
  - t(1;22) is often sole karyotypic abnormality
  - Additional abnormalities more frequent in patients older than 6 months
- Fusion transcript detection by RT-PCR or next-generation sequencing
  - May prove useful when specimen is scant (dry tap) due to bone marrow fibrosis

DIFFERENTIAL DIAGNOSIS

Myeloid Leukemia Associated With Down Syndrome
- AMKL in infants or children with Down syndrome
  - Negative for t(1;22) translocation
  - *GATA1* mutations are pathognomonic
  - Often show higher frequencies of immature CD34(+)/CD117(+) leukemic cells, compared to other AMKL

Non-Down Syndrome-Associated Acute Megakaryoblastic Leukemia With Novel Fusions
- AMKL with *CBFA2T3::GLIS2* fusion
  - Results from cryptic inversion of chromosome 16
  - Aggressive with poor prognosis
  - Characterized by bright CD56(+), CD45[dim to (-)] and CD38(-) HLA-DR
- AMKL with *NUP98::KDM5A* fusion
  - High-risk disease
  - Often megakaryoblastic, but also seen with monocytic and erythroid phenotypes

SELECTED REFERENCES

1. Weinberg OK et al: The International Consensus Classification of acute myeloid leukemia. Virchows Arch. 482(1):27-37, 2023
2. Khoury JD et al: The 5th edition of the World Health Organization Classification of Haematolymphoid Tumours: Myeloid and Histiocytic/Dendritic Neoplasms. Leukemia. 6(7):1703-19, 2022
3. Hara Y et al: Prognostic impact of specific molecular profiles in pediatric acute megakaryoblastic leukemia in non-Down syndrome. Genes Chromosomes Cancer. 56(5):394-404, 2017

Acute Myeloid Leukemia With Myelodysplasia-Related Gene Mutations or Cytogenetic Abnormalities

KEY FACTS

TERMINOLOGY

- Acute myeloid leukemia (AML) with ≥ 20% blasts in blood or bone marrow
  - **Excludes** AML cases with recurrent genetic abnormalities, AML with *BCR::ABL1*, and AML with mutated *TP53* by ICC criteria
- Cases of AML following chemotherapy &/or radiation therapy often have MDS-related cytogenetic abnormalities or MDS-related gene mutations
- Consequently most cases of AML following chemotherapy &/or radiation therapy fulfill criteria for AML with myelodysplasia-related gene mutation or AML with myelodysplasia-related cytogenetic abnormalities by ICC
  - ICC lists "therapy-related" as diagnosis qualifier appended to any AML category
  - WHO-HAEM5 includes "therapy-related AML" but now renamed as "AML, post cytotoxic therapy" category under secondary myeloid neoplasms

CLASSIFICATION

- AML with myelodysplasia-related gene mutation (ICC)
  - Defined by *ASXL1, BCOR, EZH2, RUNX1, SF3B1, SRSF2, STAG2, ZRSF2* mutations (VAF ≥ 2%)
- AML with myelodysplasia-related cytogenetic (ICC)
  - Complex karyotype (≥ 3 unrelated clonal chromosomal abnormalities in absence of other classification-defining recurrent genetic abnormalities), del(5q)/t(5q), -7/del(7q), +8, del(12p)/t(12p)/add(12p), i(17q), -17/add(17p), or del(17p), del(20q), &/or idic(X)(q13) clonal abnormalities
- AML myelodysplasia-related (WHO-HAEM5)
  - Includes list of gene mutations and cytogenetic abnormalities that are generally similar to ICC except
    - *RUNX1* is not included in WHO-HAEM5 gene mutation list
    - 11q deletion is included in WHO-HAEM5 list but not included in ICC list of cytogenetic abnormalities

Monocytic Blasts

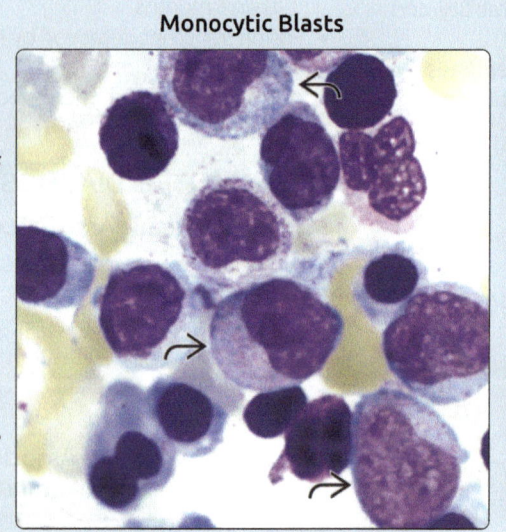

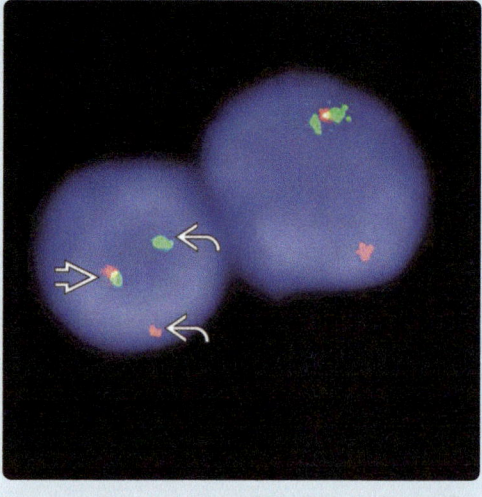

(Left) Bone marrow aspirate shows monocytic blasts. This patient had received topoisomerase II inhibitors for sarcoma therapy. Cytogenetics showed 11q23 rearrangement. The findings are diagnostic of AML with myelodysplasia-related cytogenetics abnormality, therapy-related. (Right) FISH break-apart probe on a bone marrow aspirate of a newly diagnosed acute myeloid leukemia shows a normal fused signal and 2 separate orange and green signals, consistent with 11q23 rearrangement.

FISH Break-Apart Using 11q23 Probes

NGS Showing SRSF2 P95R Mutation

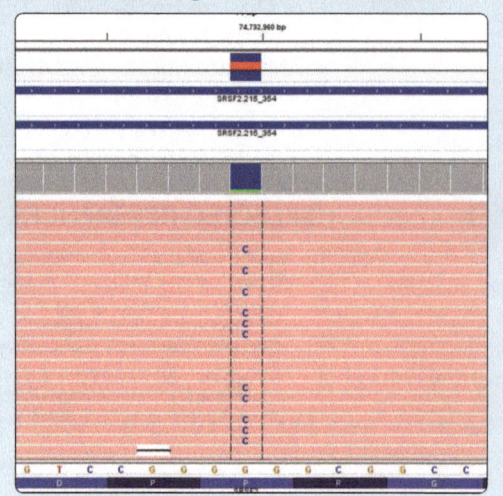

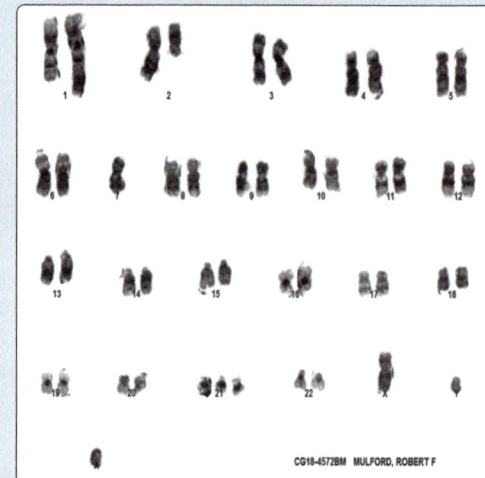

(Left) NGS pileup shows C > G base substitution in codon 95 of SRSF2, consistent with P95R pathogenic variant in newly diagnosed AML supportive of AML with myelodysplasia-related gene mutation. (Right) Karyotype performed on bone marrow with > 20% blasts shows a complex karyotype that includes monosomy of 7, trisomy of 21, t(1;2) translocation, and a marker chromosome supportive of AML with myelodysplasia-related cytogenetic abnormality.

Karyotype With Complex Cytogenetic Abnormality

Acute Myeloid Leukemia With Myelodysplasia-Related Gene Mutations or Cytogenetic Abnormalities

TERMINOLOGY

Abbreviations
- International Consensus Classification (ICC)
- World Health Organization, 5th edition (WHO-HAEM5) classification
- Acute myeloid leukemia with myelodysplasia-related gene mutations (AML-MRGM) (ICC designation)
- Acute myeloid leukemia with myelodysplasia-related cytogenetic abnormalities (AML-MRCA) (ICC designation)
- Acute myeloid leukemia, myelodysplasia-related (AML-MR) (WHO-HAEM5 designation)

Definitions
- AML with ≥ 20% blasts in blood or bone marrow (BM)
  - **Excludes** AML cases with recurrent genetic abnormalities, AML with *BCR::ABL1*, and AML with mutated *TP53* by ICC criteria
  - Cases of AML following chemotherapy &/or radiation therapy often have myelodysplastic syndrome (MDS)-related cytogenetic abnormalities or MDS-related gene mutations
  - Consequently most cases of AML following chemotherapy &/or radiation therapy fulfill criteria for AML-MRGM or AML-MRCA by ICC
    – ICC lists "therapy-related" as diagnosis qualifier appended to any AML category
    – WHO-HAEM5 includes "therapy-related AML" but now renamed as "AML, post cytotoxic therapy" category under secondary myeloid neoplasms
    – Both ICC and WHO-HAEM5 add "therapy-related" or "post cytotoxic therapy" as qualifier to myeloid neoplasm
      □ e.g., AML with *KMT2A* rearrangement, post cytotoxic therapy
  - Morphologic dysplasia is **no** longer defining feature in AML-MRGM, AML-MRCA, or AML-MR (i.e., both ICC and WHO-HAEM5)

CLASSIFICATION

International Consensus Classification
- AML-MRGM
  - Blasts ≥ 20% in blood or BM
  - Defined by *ASXL1, BCOR, EZH2, RUNX1, SF3B1, SRSF2, STAG2, ZRSF2* mutation(s) with variant allele frequency (VAF) ≥ 2%
- AML-MRCA
  - Blasts ≥ 20% in blood or BM
  - Defined by complex karyotype (≥ 3 unrelated clonal chromosomal abnormalities in absence of other classification-defining recurrent genetic abnormalities), del(5q)/t(5q), -7/del(7q), +8, del(12p)/t(12p)/add(12p), i(17q), -17/add(17p), or del(17p), del(20q), &/or idic(X)(q13) clonal abnormalities

World Health Organization, 5th Edition
- AML-MR
  - Blasts ≥ 20% in blood or BM
  - Includes list of gene mutations and cytogenetic abnormalities that are generally similar to ICC except
    – *RUNX1* is not included in WHO-HAEM5 gene mutation list
    – 11q deletion is included in WHO-HAEM5 list but not included in ICC list of cytogenetic abnormalities

ETIOLOGY/PATHOGENESIS

Acquired Genetic Alterations
- Genetic mutations with important role in pathogenesis of AML-MRGM category
  - *SRSF2, SF3B1, U2AF1, ZRSR2, AXSL1, EZH2, RUNX1, BCOR,* and *STAG2* have been shown to be > 95% specific for secondary AML
  - NGS data has been incorporated by European Leukemia Net (ELN) in risk stratification system used in AML management
  - Lower survival rates and higher relapse rates confirmed in patients with chromatin-spliceosome gene mutations including *SRSF2, ASXL1,* and *STAG2*
- Cytogenetic abnormalities involved in pathogenesis of AML-MRCA category
  - Complex karyotype defined by ≥ 3 unrelated clonal abnormalities in absence of AML-defining cytogenetics
  - del(5q)/t(5q)/add(5q), -7/del(7q), +8, del(12p)/t(12p)/add(12p), i(17q), -17/add(17p) or del(17p), del(20q), or idic(X)(q13) clonal abnormalities
    – AML with antecedent MDS or MDS/MPN and de novo AML with MDS-related cytogenetics confers worse prognosis than patients with 2016 WHO category of AML with myelodysplasia-related change based on multilineage dysplasia

Acquired Molecular Genetic Alterations Induced by Exposure to Chemotherapy or Radiation
- Molecular genetic alterations induced by exposure to chemotherapy or radiation
  - Overall similar molecular pathways to those involved in de novo myeloid neoplasms
  - AML arising in setting of cytotoxic exposure or radiation therapy was previously characterized as "therapy-related myeloid neoplasms" in 2016 WHO
  - In 2022 ICC, "therapy-related" is now used as qualifier for disease entities that are primarily defined by their genetic profile
  - WHO-HAEM5 includes therapy-related AML category but is renamed as "AML, post cytotoxic therapy" category of Secondary Myeloid Neoplasms
  - Most patients with AML, post cytotoxic therapy have received both alkylating agents and topoisomerase II inhibitors
  - ~ 20% of post-cytotoxic therapy AML cases show normal cytogenetics
    – These cases may harbor *FLT3, NRAS, KRAS,* &/or *RUNX1* mutations
- Genetic abnormalities induced by alkylating agents or ionizing radiation therapy
  - Exposure to alkylating agents or radiation accounts for ~ 75% of AML, post cytotoxic therapy cases
  - Alkylating agents typically induce centromeric or pericentromeric chromosomal DNA break leading to
    – Monosomy of chromosomes 5 and 7 or loss of 5q &/or 7q or complex karyotype

Acute Myeloid Leukemia With Myelodysplasia-Related Gene Mutations or Cytogenetic Abnormalities

- – May be associated with other chromosomal losses/gains
  - o Latency period of 5-7 years
  - o Usually preceded by MDS phase
- Acquired molecular genetic aberrancies induced by exposure to topoisomerase II inhibitors
  - o Topoisomerase II inhibitors block religation of DNA breaks and lead to recombination of nonhomologous DNA strands
    - – DNA cleavage sites include *KMT2A* at 11q23, *RUNX1* at 21q22, or *RARA* at 17q21
    - – Typically results in balanced translocations, including t(8;21), t(15;17), or inv(16)
  - o Generally present as AML without antecedent MDS
  - o Short latency period of 1-3 years post cytotoxic exposure with abrupt onset of symptoms
- Other cytotoxic agents commonly implicated include
  - o Antimetabolites (thiopurine, fludarabine, etc.), antitubulin agents (e.g., vincristine), and PARP1 inhibitors
- Chemotherapy-driven selection and expansion of preexisting hematopoietic clones in *TP53*, *PPM1D*, *DNMT3A*, *ASXL1*, and *TET2*
  - o Documented as pathogenic pathway in significant percentage of AML, post cytotoxic therapy cases
  - o Tumor clones with at least subsets of these gene mutations confer resistance to chemotherapy
- Pathogenic pathways mostly in pediatric-age AML, post cytotoxic therapy cases
  - o Involves mutations in RAS/MAPK pathway, alterations in *RUNX1* or *TP53*, and *KMT2A* rearrangements
- *TP53* mutations
  - o ~ 35% of AML, post cytotoxic therapy cases harbor *TP53* mutations
  - o Confer resistance to chemotherapy
    - – AML with *TP53* mutations with VAF ≥ 10% is **new distinct AML entity in ICC**
    - – *TP53* mutations are listed among other commonly mutated genes in **AML, post cytotoxic therapy in WHO-HAEM5**
- Other mutated genes in AML, post cytotoxic therapy with variant allele fraction of ≥ 5% include
  - o *NPM1*, *FLT3* ITD, *NRAS*, *KRAS*, *PTPN11*, *TET2*, *DNMT3A*, *IDH1*, *IDH2*, *STAG2*, *RUNX1*, and *ASXL1*

Genetic Predisposition

- Only small proportion of patients exposed to chemotherapy may develop AML
  - o This may suggest underlying genetic predispositions in post-cytotoxic therapy AML development
  - o Inherited germline mutations associated with increased risk of post-cytotoxic therapy development of AML include
    - – Germline mutations in *BRCA1*, *BRCA2*, *BARD1*, *TP53*, *RAD51*, *HLX*, Fanconi anemia genes (*FANCA* and others), *BCL2L10*
  - o Genetic variants in gene-encoding drug metabolizing enzymes
    - – Polymorphisms in genes, such as *NQO1*, that affect drug metabolism
    - – Some studies suggest increased risk of AML development in clonal hematopoiesis in context of cytotoxic therapy

CLINICAL ISSUES

Epidemiology
- Incidence
  - o Common type of AML in older patients
  - o Incidence increases with age

Presentation
- Symptoms often relate to cytopenia(s)
  - o Fatigue
  - o Infection
  - o Bleeding
- Some patients may have history of antecedent chemotherapy, radiation therapy, or immunotherapy
  - o Development of cytopenias in this patient population may indicate that myeloid neoplasm, post cytotoxic therapy has occurred
  - o Therapy-related is diagnosis qualifier in ICC that would be applied to these cases
  - o Therapy-related AML is classified as distinct category renamed as "AML, post cytotoxic therapy" by WHO-HAEM5

Laboratory Tests
- Complete blood count (CBC) with differential and morphologic review
  - o Blast percent determination key
    - – Morphologic blast enumeration is essential
  - o Dysplasia usually present but not required for diagnosis
- IHC
  - o CD34 to assess for CD34(+) blasts percentage and clustering
    - – Especially useful in marrow inaspirable cases
  - o Additional stains of utility include MPO, CD61, CD71, and CD117
- Flow cytometry
  - o Determine lineage of blasts and aberrant antigen expression profile of immature cells
- Cytogenetics
  - o Identifies MRCA
  - o Identifies **exclusionary** recurrent cytogenetic abnormalities that define other AML subtypes
- Molecular genetic testing
  - o NGS myeloid gene panel is essential
    - – Identifies MRGM
    - – Identifies *TP53*, *NPM1*, bZip*CEBPA*, *NUP98* mutations that **exclude** AML-MRGM

Natural History
- Adverse clinical course typical
- Prognosis primarily influenced by karyotypic and genetic abnormalities
  - o In general, patients with chromosome 5 &/or 7 deletions, *TP53* mutations, or complex karyotype have particularly poor outcome

Treatment
- Traditional antileukemic therapy not curative in most patients
- Allogeneic stem cell transplant in selected patients may improve survival
- Novel treatment approaches

Acute Myeloid Leukemia With Myelodysplasia-Related Gene Mutations or Cytogenetic Abnormalities

- o FDA-approved CPX-351 (fixed combination of cytarabine and daunorubicin)
  - Has shown prolonged overall survival in phase 2 clinical trial
  - Improved median overall survival compared to "7 + 3" cohort (9.6 vs. 6 months)
- o Chimeric antigen receptor T-cells (CAR-T) and checkpoint inhibitors

Prognosis

- Both cytogenetic abnormalities and specific gene mutations provide key prognostic information
- Prognosis primarily influenced by karyotypic and genetic abnormalities
- Adverse prognostic factors as per NCCN (National Comprehensive Cancer Network) include
- o Complex karyotype ≥ 3 unrelated chromosomal abnormalities
- o Monosomal karyotype
  - 1 monosomy (excluding loss of X or Y) plus another monosomy or structural chromosomal abnormality
- o Mutations in *RUNX1* or *ASXL1*

MOLECULAR

Cytogenetics

- Karyotype criteria for AML-MRCA
  - o Complex karyotype (≥ 3) unrelated clonal abnormalities, including del(5q)/t(5q)/add(5q), -7/del(7q),+8, del(12p)/t(12p)/add(12p), i(17q),-17/add(17p) or del(17p), del(20q), or idic(X)(q13) clonal abnormalities
  - o Karyotype is key prognostic factor

Mutational Profile of Acute Myeloid Leukemia With Myelodysplasia-Related Gene Mutations

- Qualifying mutations include *ASXL1*, *BCOR*, *EZH2*, *RUNX1*, *SF3B1*, *SRSF2*, *STAG2*, *U2AF1*, and *ZRSR2* with VAF ≥ 2%
- Identify mutations that define other AML subtypes
  - o *TP53*, *NPM1*, *CEBPA*, and *NUP98* mutations define other AML subtypes

MICROSCOPIC

Blood

- Severe anemia, thrombocytopenia, WBC variable
  - o Neutropenia common
  - o Blasts may be > 20%

Bone Marrow

- Variable appearance but often hypercellular with multilineage dysplasia
  - o Blasts ≥ 20%, pronormoblasts excluded
  - o May have fibrosis

ANCILLARY TESTS

Immunohistochemistry

- CD34 highlights positive blasts, but blasts can be CD34(-)
  - o Very useful in inaspirable BM cases

Flow Cytometry

- Assess lineage of immature cell populations
- Assess for aberrant antigen expression profile

Genetic Testing

- Cytogenetics
- Myeloid gene panel, other molecular tests

DIFFERENTIAL DIAGNOSIS

Other Myeloid Neoplasms With ≥ 20% Blasts in Blood or Bone Marrow

- AML with recurrent genetic abnormality
  - o Includes 17 subtypes identified by conventional karyotyping
  - o Includes 4 subtypes defined by gene mutations
  - o Some cases may have > 20% blasts, but diagnostic threshold in ≥ 10% blasts for all except AML with mutated *TP53* and AML with t(9;22)(q34.1;q11.2) *BCR::ABL1*, which both have ≥ 20% threshold
- AML with mutated *TP53*
- AML, not otherwise specified (NOS)
- Myeloproliferative neoplasm in blast phase (≥ 20% blasts required for designation of blast phase)

DIAGNOSTIC CHECKLIST

Pathologic Interpretation Pearls

- AML cases occurring in setting of antecedent chemotherapy/radiation/immunotherapy
  - o Therapy-related is diagnosis qualifier in ICC
    - Example of diagnosis: AML-MRCA, therapy-related (ICC)
  - o Therapy-related neoplasms are retained in separate diagnostic category but renamed as "myeloid neoplasms, post cytotoxic therapy" in WHO-HAEM5
    - As per WHO-HAEM5, Mutational Profile of AML-MRG, these cases would be classified as myeloid neoplasms, post cytotoxic therapy and excluded from AML-MR
- Morphologic blast percentage in blood or BM must be ≥ 20%

SELECTED REFERENCES

1. College of American Pathologists: What's new in AML classification (WHO 2022 vs. International Consensus Classification). Published March 29, 2023. Accessed July 2023. https://www.cap.org/member-resources/articles/whats-new-in-aml-classification-who-2022-vs-international-consensus-classification
2. Falini B et al: Comparison of the International Consensus and 5th WHO edition classifications of adult myelodysplastic syndromes and acute myeloid leukemia. Am J Hematol. 98(3):481-92, 2023
3. Rausch C et al: Validation and refinement of the 2022 European LeukemiaNet genetic risk stratification of acute myeloid leukemia. Leukemia. 37(6):1234-44, 2023
4. Weinberg OK et al: The International Consensus Classification of acute myeloid leukemia. Virchows Arch. 482(1):27-37, 2023
5. Arber DA et al: International Consensus Classification of myeloid neoplasms and acute leukemia: integrating morphological, clinical, and genomic data. Blood. 140(11):1200-28, 2022
6. Döhner H et al: Diagnosis and management of AML in adults: 2022 recommendations from an international expert panel on behalf of the ELN. Blood. 140(12):1345-77, 2022
7. Khoury JD et al: The 5th edition of the World Health Organization Classification of haematolymphoid tumours: myeloid and histiocytic/dendritic neoplasms. Leukemia. 36(7):1703-19, 2022
8. Krauss AC et al: FDA approval summary: (daunorubicin and cytarabine) liposome for injection for the treatment of adults with high-risk acute myeloid leukemia. Clin Cancer Res. 25(9):2685-90, 2019
9. Morton LM et al: Association of chemotherapy for solid tumors with development of therapy-related myelodysplastic syndrome or acute myeloid leukemia in the modern era. JAMA Oncol. 5(3):318-25, 2019

Acute Myeloid Leukemia With Myelodysplasia-Related Gene Mutations or Cytogenetic Abnormalities

Myeloblasts and CLL Cells

Myeloblasts and Residual CLL

(Left) Bone marrow aspirate smear from a patient with AML and posttherapy persistent chronic lymphocytic leukemia (CLL) shows myeloblasts ⇒ and CLL cells ⇒, consistent with AML post cytotoxic therapy/AML, therapy-related. (Right) Bone marrow core biopsy from a patient who developed AML, therapy-related with persistent CLL shows sheets of myeloblasts ⇒ and residual CLL ⇒. The blast percentage was > 20%.

Immature Monocytic Cells and Marked Cytopenias

Increased Myeloblasts

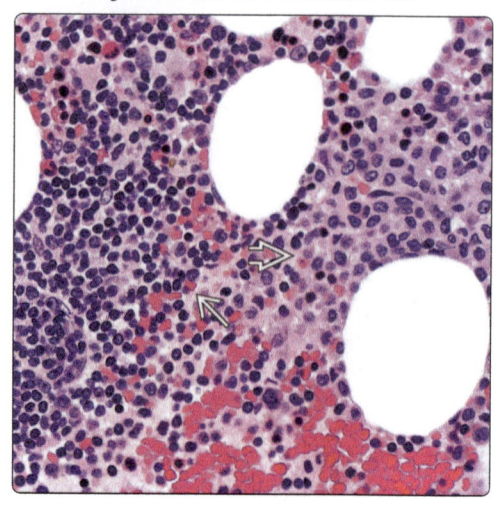

(Left) Blood smear from a young man who developed topoisomerase II-induced myeloid neoplasm shows circulating immature monocytic cells and marked cytopenias. (Right) Bone marrow aspirate smear shows AML, therapy-related that developed after intensive topoisomerase II inhibitor therapy for disseminated Ewing sarcoma. Note the increased myeloblasts ⇒.

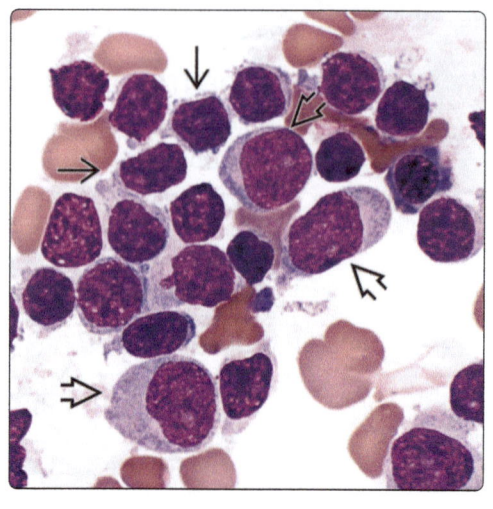

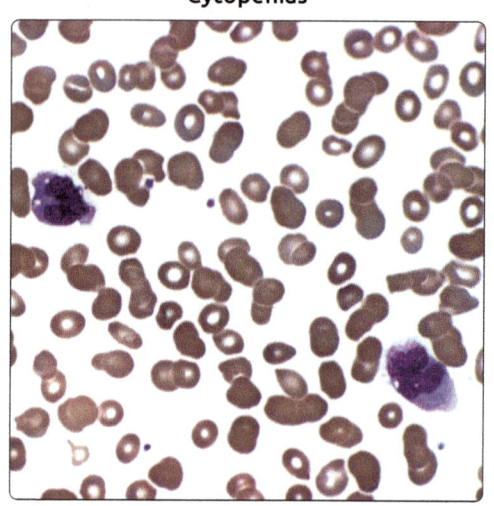

Residual Ewing Sarcoma

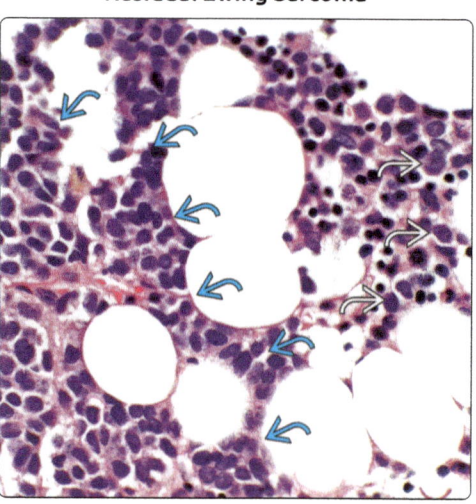

CD117 Immunohistochemistry

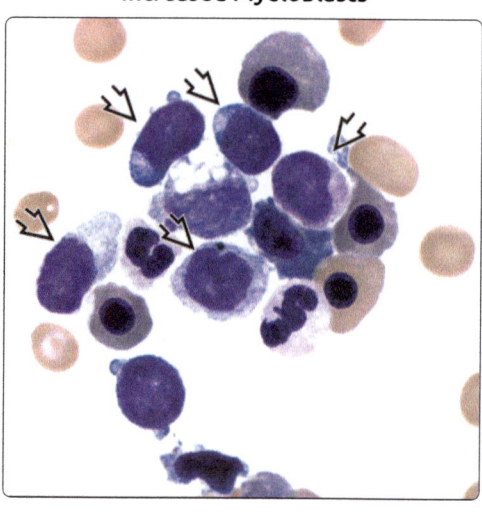

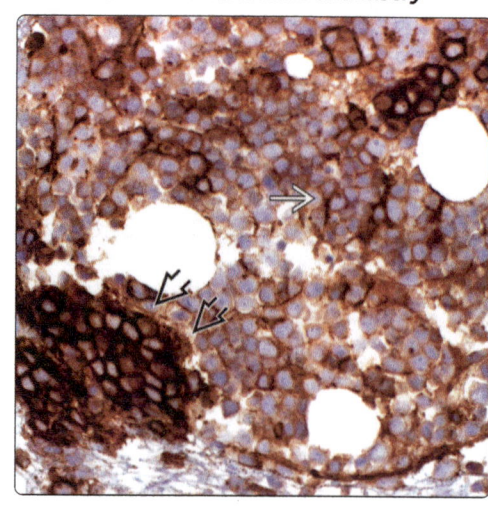

(Left) Bone marrow clot section from a young adult with myeloid neoplasm post intensive topoisomerase II inhibitor therapy shows aggregates of residual Ewing sarcoma ⇒ and increased blasts within residual trilineage hematopoiesis ⇒. (Right) CD117 shows 2 patterns of staining intensity (strong and moderate) in myeloid neoplasm, post cytotoxic therapy in a patient with widespread Ewing sarcoma. Ewing sarcoma cells ⇒ are brightly positive. Leukemic blasts are moderately positive ⇒.

Acute Myeloid Leukemia With Myelodysplasia-Related Gene Mutations or Cytogenetic Abnormalities

FISH Using *EWSR1* and *FLI1* Probes

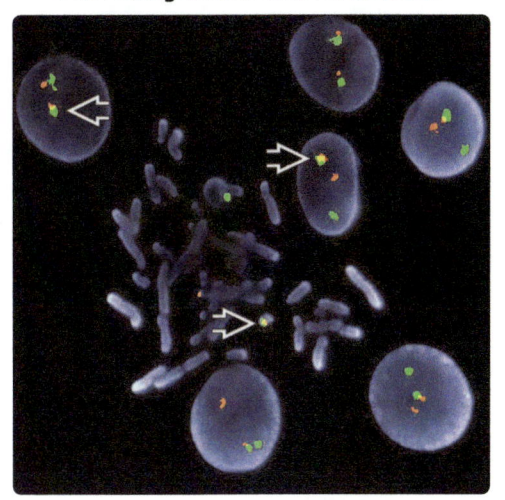

Myeloid Neoplasm Post Cytotoxic Therapy

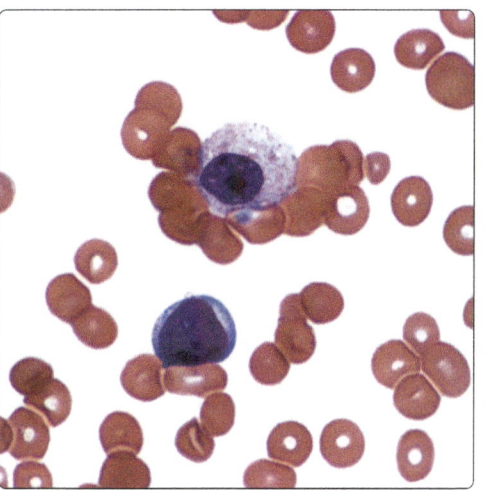

(Left) FISH using *EWSR1* and *FLI1* probes performed on bone marrow from a patient with refractory Ewing sarcoma who developed therapy-related AML shows *EWSR1::FLI1* fusion signals ⇨, consistent with residual Ewing sarcoma. (Right) Peripheral blood smear from a patient with longstanding myeloma who developed profound cytopenias, circulating blasts, and dysplastic neutrophils as a result of myeloid neoplasm post cytotoxic therapy is shown.

Dysplastic Megakaryocytes

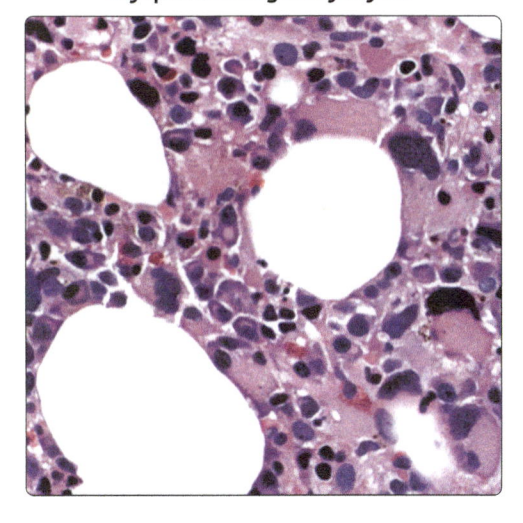

Hemoglobin A Immunohistochemistry

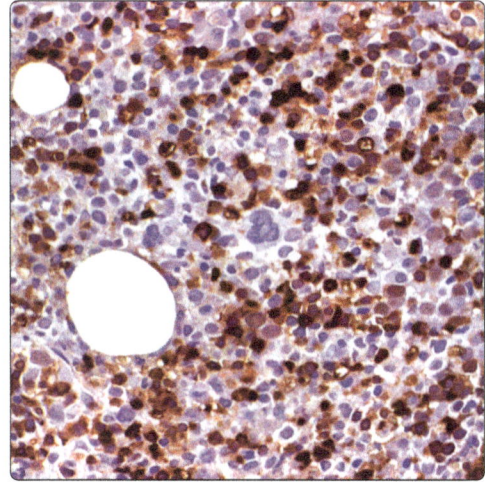

(Left) Bone marrow core biopsy from a patient with multiple myeloma shows myeloid neoplasm, therapy-related with markedly dysplastic megakaryocytes in conjunction with persistent myeloma. (Right) Bone marrow core biopsy stained with hemoglobin A shows loss of normal colony formation in myeloid neoplasm, post cytotoxic therapy in a patient with longstanding myeloma. Normal erythroid precursors would form tight colonies.

Blasts With Erythrophagocytic Activity

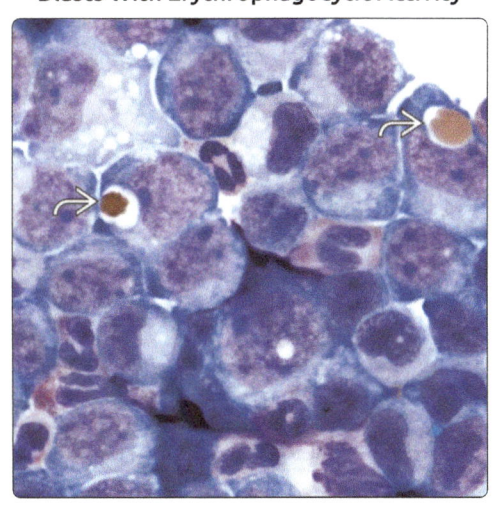

Karyotype With t(8;16)

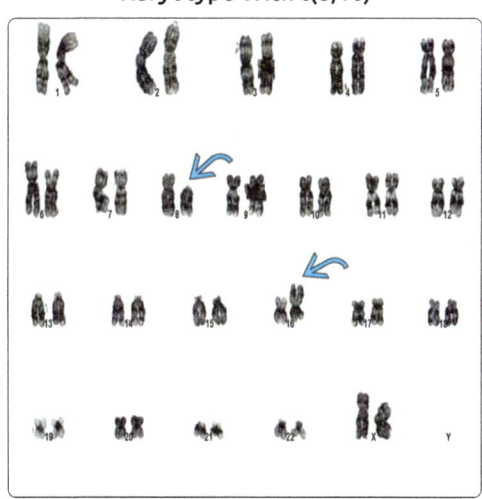

(Left) Cytospin preparation of bone marrow aspirate from a patient with AML, post cytotoxic therapy shows increased monocytic blasts with frequent erythrophagocytosis ⇨. Although not specific, increased erythrophagocytic activity in monocytic blasts may suggest t(8;16). (Right) Karyotype of bone marrow aspirate from a patient with AML, therapy-related shows 8;16 chromosomal translocation ⇨.

Molecular Pathology of Myeloid Neoplasms

Acute Myeloid Leukemia, NOS

KEY FACTS

TERMINOLOGY
- Acute myeloid leukemia (AML) cases that do not fulfill criteria for any genetically defined AML
- ≥ 20% blasts/blast equivalent required for all AML, NOS

CLASSIFICATION
- International Consensus Classification (ICC) vs. WHO 5th edition (WHO-HAEM5)
  - ICC contains smaller number of AML, NOS cases than WHO-HAEM5
    - ICC has greater number of genetically defined entities
    - ICC classifies acute erythroid leukemia as AML with mutated *TP53* because virtually all cases harbor *TP53* mutations
  - WHO-HAEM5 retains AML defined by differentiation categories based on French American British (FAB)/WHO 4th edition
    - AML with minimal differentiation
    - AML without maturation
    - AML with maturation
    - Acute basophilic leukemia
    - Acute myelomonocytic leukemia
    - Acute monoblastic and monocytic leukemia
    - Acute erythroid leukemia
    - Acute megakaryocytic leukemia

CLINICAL ISSUES
- Aggressive disease course with generally poor prognosis
- Common subtypes each comprise ~ 5-10% of AML cases
- Rarer subtypes each comprise < 5% of AML cases

TOP DIFFERENTIAL DIAGNOSES
- Acute lymphoblastic leukemia
- Blast phase of preexisting myeloid neoplasm
- Myelodysplastic syndrome with increased/excess blasts (MDS-IB/EB)
- Chronic myelomonocytic leukemia

Typical Appearance of AML

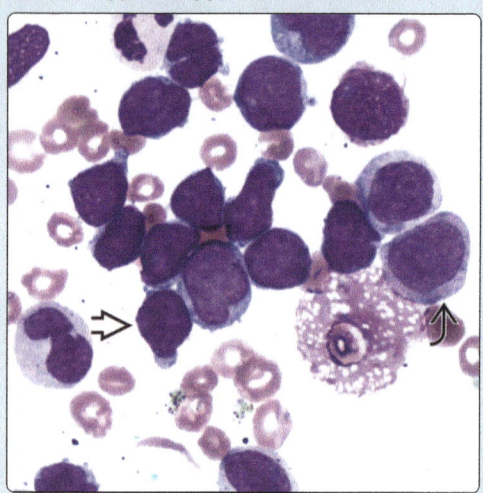

Leukemic Infiltrate in Bone Marrow

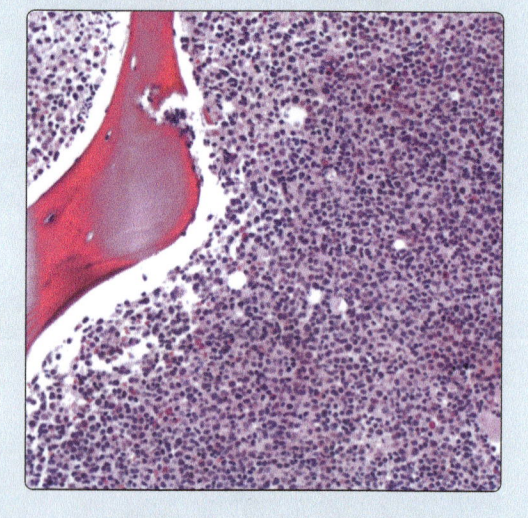

(Left) Typical case of acute myeloid leukemia (AML) shows abundant myeloblasts in peripheral blood. Morphology ranges from large blasts with abundant cytoplasm ⇨ to smaller, lymphoblast-like blasts ⇨. (Right) The bone marrow is nearly 100% cellular with replacement of normal hematopoietic elements by a monotonous infiltrate of myeloblasts with round to irregular nuclei and variable amounts of cytoplasm.

Common Mutations in AML

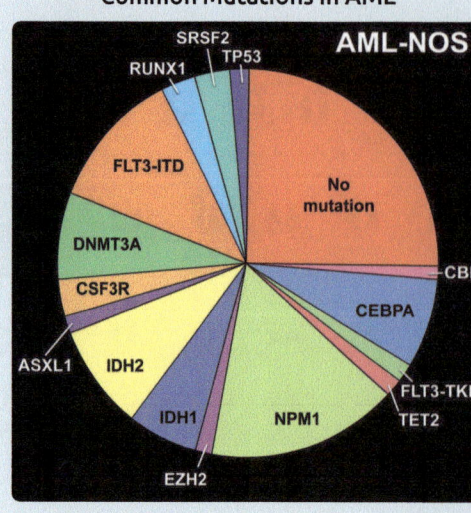

FLT3 ITD Detected by PCR/Fragment Analysis

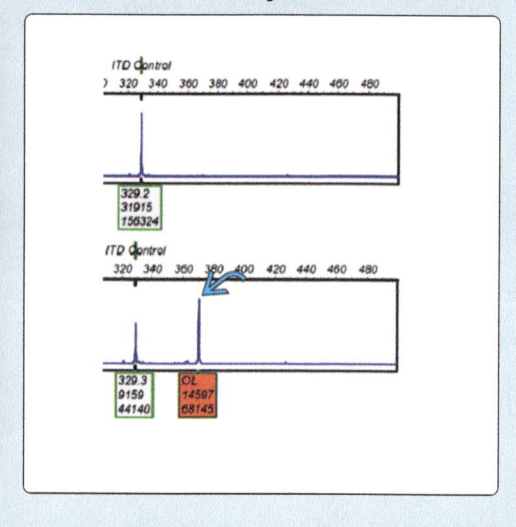

(Left) Graph shows frequencies of the most common mutations by gene in AML, NOS. Mutations in certain genes, including but not limited to NPM1, CEBPA, and TP53, are now considered part of AML with recurrent/defining genetic abnormalities. (Adapted from Ohgami et al, Mod Path 2015.) (Right) FLT3 ITD can be detected by PCR followed by fragment analysis. The top image shows a wildtype FLT3 amplicon, while the bottom image shows both wildtype and FLT3 ITD ⇨.

Acute Myeloid Leukemia, NOS

TERMINOLOGY

Abbreviations
- Acute myeloid leukemia, not otherwise specified (AML, NOS)
- International Consensus Classification (ICC)
- World Health Organization of Hematolymphoid Tumors, 5th edition (WHO-HAEM5)

Synonyms
- Acute myelogenous leukemia

Definitions
- AML cases that do not fulfill criteria for any genetically defined AML
  - ≥ 20% blasts/blast equivalent required for all AML, NOS

ICC vs. WHO-HAEM5
- ICC contains smaller number of AML, NOS cases than WHO-HAEM5
  - ICC has greater number of genetically defined entities
  - ICC classifies acute erythroid leukemia as AML with mutated *TP53* because virtually all cases harbor *TP53* mutations
- WHO-HAEM5 retains AML defined by differentiation categories based on French American British (FAB)/WHO 4th edition
  - AML with minimal differentiation
  - AML without maturation
  - AML with maturation
  - Acute basophilic leukemia
  - Acute myelomonocytic leukemia
  - Acute monocytic leukemia
  - Acute erythroid leukemia
  - Acute megakaryocytic leukemia

CLINICAL ISSUES

Epidemiology
- Incidence
  - Common WHO-HAEM5 subtypes each comprise ~ 5-10% of AML cases
    - AML without maturation
    - AML with maturation
    - Acute myelomonocytic leukemia
  - Remaining WHO-HAEM5 subtypes each comprise < 5% of AML cases
    - AML with minimal differentiation
    - Acute monoblastic and monocytic leukemia
    - Pure erythroid leukemia
    - Acute megakaryoblastic leukemia
    - Acute basophilic leukemia
- Age
  - Any age with slight variation between subtypes

Presentation
- Pancytopenia, including
  - Anemia, neutropenia, and thrombocytopenia

Natural History
- Clinically aggressive disease

Treatment
- Drugs
  - Standard myeloablative chemotherapy regimens
  - Increasing use of targeted regimens
    - Based on mutation profile or expression pattern
- Hematopoietic stem cell transplantation
  - Only potentially curative treatment

Prognosis
- Aggressive disease course with generally poor prognosis
- Some subtypes have especially poor prognosis
  - Pure erythroid leukemia
  - Acute megakaryoblastic leukemia
  - Acute basophilic leukemia

MICROSCOPIC

Acute Myeloid Leukemia With Minimal Differentiation (WHO-HAEM5)
- Blasts are medium-sized, agranular, poorly differentiated, or may be smaller and resemble lymphoblasts with no Auer rods
- Blasts are negative for MPO by cytochemical stain, but small subset may express MPO by IHC &/or flow cytometry
- Early hematopoietic antigens are expressed, including CD34, CD38, and HLA-DR
- Negative for markers of myeloid/monocytic maturation, including v
- Negative for B- and T-cell lymphoid markers
- CD7 is exception, expressed in ~ 40% of cases
- Other typically positive markers include CD13 and CD117
- CD33(+/-), TdT(+/-)

Acute Myeloid Leukemia Without Maturation (WHO-HAEM5)
- High numbers of bone marrow blasts without significant maturation
  - < 10% maturing myeloid granulocytic lineage in bone marrow
  - MPO and Sudan black B cytochemical stains positive (≥ 3% of blasts)
  - Expression of ≥ 1 myeloid antigens, including CD13, CD33, and CD117
  - CD34 and HLA-DR expressed in ~ 70% of cases
  - Negative for CD15 and CD65
  - Generally negative for B- and T-cell-associated antigens
    - Aberrant expression of CD7 in ~ 30% of cases; rarely other reported lymphoid markers, including CD2, CD4, CD19, and CD56

Acute Myeloid Leukemia With Maturation (WHO-HAEM5)
- Must have ≥ 10% maturing cells of granulocytic lineage
- Cells of monocytic lineage < 20% of bone marrow cells
- Blast morphology
  - ± azurophilic granules
  - Auer rods are common
- Immunophenotypic profile
  - Expression of myeloid antigens (≥ 2), including CD13, CD33, CD117, CD11b, CD15, and CD65

Acute Myeloid Leukemia, NOS

- Markers of immaturity may be present in subset, including CD34 and CD117
- HLA-DR is often positive, and CD7 is expressed in 20-30% of cases

Acute Myelomonocytic Leukemia (WHO-HAEM5)

- Has both neutrophil and monocyte precursors
  - Each of these lineages, including mature forms, comprises > 20% of marrow cells
- Separate monoblast/promonocyte and myeloblast populations can be identified
  - MPO and NSE can be helpful in identification
- Immunophenotypic profile
  - At least subset will show monocytic differentiation markers
    - CD14, CD64, CD11b, CD11c, CD4, CD36, CD64 (bright), CD163
  - Variable expression of myeloid antigens, including CD13, CD33, CD65, CD15, and immature markers CD34 and CD117
  - Other markers expressed include HLA-DR in most cases and aberrant CD7 in ~ 30%

Acute Monocytic Leukemia (WHO-HAEM5)

- ≥ 80% of leukemic cells are of monocytic lineage
  - Includes mature monocytes
  - Cytochemical staining pattern
    - Positive for NSE in 80-90% of cases, negative for MPO
- In acute monoblastic leukemia subtype, majority of cells are monoblasts
  - Monoblasts are large with round nucleus, abundant cytoplasm, and can have fine azurophilic granules and vacuoles in cytoplasm
- In acute monocytic leukemia, majority of cells are promonocytes
  - Promonocytes have more irregular and delicately folded nucleus than monoblasts
  - Cytoplasm may be paler and may have more granules and vacuoles than monoblasts
- Neutrophils should be < 20%
- Extramedullary lesions are more common
- Immunophenotypic profile
  - Variable expression of myeloid antigens, including CD13, CD33 (bright), CD15, and CD65
  - At least 2 monocytic differentiation markers present, including CD14, CD4, CD11b, CD11c, CD64 (bright), CD36 (bright), CD68, lysozyme, and CD163
  - Markers of immaturity
    - CD117 is often expressed, but CD34 is expressed in only 30% of cases
    - HLA-DR is expressed in most cases
    - Aberrant expression of CD7 and CD56 common

Acute Erythroid Leukemia (WHO-HAEM5)

- a.k.a. pure erythroid leukemia
- ICC has removed this diagnosis and placed this into AML with mutated *TP53* category
- Proliferation of immature erythroid cells
  - > 80% of marrow cells are of erythroid lineage
  - ≥ 30% immature erythroid cells (proerythroblasts)
  - Erythroblasts contain round nuclei, prominent nucleolus/nucleoli, deeply basophilic cytoplasm, vacuoles
- Immunophenotypic profile
  - Somewhat nonspecific in many cases; can be difficult to prove erythroid lineage
  - More differentiated cases express glycophorin, hemoglobin A
  - E-cadherin is positive in majority of cases
  - Absence of MPO, other myeloid markers
  - Typically negative for CD34 and HLA-DR; may express CD117
  - Nonspecific markers, including CD36 and CD71, are often positive
- Special stains
  - Erythroblasts negative for MPO and Sudan black B
  - Block-like staining with PAS
- *TP53* mutations are typical; if lacking, should question diagnosis

Acute Megakaryoblastic Leukemia (WHO-HAEM5)

- At least 50% of blasts are of megakaryocytic lineage
  - Cases in patients with Down syndrome are excluded and belong to different category
- May see dysplasia in any single lineage or multiple lineages
- May have bone marrow fibrosis, leading to "dry tap"
- Megakaryoblast morphology
  - Medium to large size with basophilic agranular cytoplasm, often with blebbing or pseudopod formation
- Immunophenotypic profile
  - At least one megakaryocytic lineage marker is expressed, including CD41, CD42, and CD61
  - Myeloid markers CD13 and CD33 may be positive
  - Aberrant expression of CD7 in some cases
  - CD36 positive but not specific
  - CD34, HLA-DR, and CD45 often negative
- Cytochemical stains
  - Negative for MPO and Sudan black B
  - NSE may show focal or punctate positivity

Acute Basophilic Leukemia (WHO-HAEM5)

- Medium-sized blasts with high N:C ratio and basophilic cytoplasm with coarse basophilic granules
- Infrequent mature basophils
- Dysplastic erythroid precursors are common
- Immunophenotypic profile includes expression of CD9, CD13, CD33, CD123, CD203c, CD11b, CD34, and CD38
  - Negative to weak CD117; negative for HLA-DR
- Special stains
  - Metachromatic positivity with toluidine blue, diffuse/block-like positivity for PAS, negative for MPO, Sudan black B, and NSE by cytochemical stains

ANCILLARY TESTS

Genetic Testing

- *FLT3* internal tandem duplication (ITD) mutations
  - 20% of AML with minimal differentiation
  - Higher frequency in cytogenetically normal AML (35-45%)
  - Poor prognosis

Acute Myeloid Leukemia, NOS

Common Genetic Mutations and Approximate Frequencies in Acute Myeloid Leukemia

Function	Gene	Approximate Frequency	Prognosis
DNA methylation/epigenetic modulation	DNMT3A	20-30%	Poor
DNA cytosine and posttranslational modification	IDH1	6-8%	Indeterminate
Intracellular signal transduction	KRAS, NRAS	10-25%	Indeterminate
Tyrosine kinase receptor	FLT3 ITD	20-30%	Poor
Tyrosine kinase receptor	FLT3 TKD	5-10%	Indeterminate
Tumor suppressor	TET2	10-30%	Poor

- o FLT3 inhibitors (e.g., midostaurin) addition to standard chemotherapy significantly prolongs overall and event-free survival among patients with FLT3-mutated AML
- DNMT3A mutations
  - o Worse prognosis in those with FLT3 mutations and intermediate-risk AML
- TET2 mutations
  - o Also common in myelodysplastic syndrome, myeloproliferative neoplasms
  - o Poorer prognosis
- IDH1 mutations
  - o Higher frequency in normal karyotype AML
  - o Poorer prognosis
  - o IDH1 inhibitor, olutasidenib, approved in 2022 for treatment of relapsed/refractory AML with susceptible IDH1 mutation
- KRAS and NRAS mutations
  - o Unclear prognostic implications in AML, NOS
- KMT2A (MLL) partial tandem duplication (PTD)
  - o Poor prognosis

Recurrent Genetic Abnormalities Excluding Diagnosis of Acute Myeloid Leukemia, Not Otherwise Specified

- NPM1, CEBPA, and TP53 mutations
  - o Presence of any of these mutations exclude AML, NOS categories in ICC and WHO-HAEM5
- AML with mutated ASXL1, BCOR, EZH2, RUNX1, SF3B1, SRSF2, STAG2, U2AF1, &/or ZRSR2 is now categorized as AML with myelodysplasia-related gene mutations in ICC and WHO-HAEM5
  - o Presence of these mutations exclude AML, NOS categories

Chromosomal Abnormalities Excluding Diagnosis of Acute Myeloid Leukemia, Not Otherwise Specified

- del5(q), -7/del(7q), +8 (ICC only), del(11q) (WHO-HAEM5 only), del(17p), i(17q), -17, idic(X)(q13), del(20q) (ICC only), and complex karyotype (≥ 3 unrelated abnormalities)

DIFFERENTIAL DIAGNOSIS

Acute Undifferentiated Leukemia of Ambiguous Lineage

- Typically express CD34, CD38, and HLA-DR
- Lack of lineage-specific myeloid markers by flow cytometry &/or immunohistochemistry
- Lack of B- and T-cell lineage specific markers by flow cytometry &/or immunohistochemistry
- Lack of MPO and NSE by cytochemistry

Acute Lymphoblastic Leukemia

- Flow cytometric immunophenotyping is essential
  - o Positive for B- or T-cell-lineage specific associated markers
  - o Negative for MPO or monocytic differentiation

Granulocyte Colony-Stimulating Factor Effect

- Administered in certain cases of severe neutropenia
- Blasts can be significantly elevated, especially shortly after administration, in hypocellular marrows
- Transient phenomenon; blasts will mature
- No molecular or cytogenetic abnormalities
- No Auer rods
- Marked toxic granulation of neutrophils and precursors

Blast Phase of Preexisting Myeloid Neoplasm

- Clinical history will be crucial

Myelodysplastic Syndrome With Increased/Excess Blasts (WHO-HAEM5)/MDS/Acute Myeloid Leukemia (ICC)

- Blasts 10-19% in bone marrow, 5-19% in peripheral blood
- Careful blast count on aspirate smear is required

Chronic Myelomonocytic Leukemia

- < 20% blasts or promonocytes in blood and bone marrow

SELECTED REFERENCES

1. Weinberg OK et al: The International Consensus Classification of acute myeloid leukemia. Virchows Arch. 27–37, 2023
2. Arber DA et al: International Consensus Classification of Myeloid Neoplasms and Acute Leukemia: integrating morphological, clinical, and genomic data. Blood. 140(11):1200-28, 2022
3. Khoury JD et al: The 5th edition of the World Health Organization Classification of Haematolymphoid Tumours: myeloid and histiocytic/dendritic neoplasms. Leukemia. 36(7):1703-19, 2022
4. Falini B et al: Comparison of the International Consensus and 5th WHO edition classifications of adult myelodysplastic syndromes and acute myeloid leukemia. Am J Hematol. 98(3):481-92, 2023
5. Sargas C et al: Comparison of the 2022 and 2017 European LeukemiaNet risk classifications in a real-life cohort of the PETHEMA group. Blood Cancer J. 13(1):77, 2023
6. Döhner H et al: Diagnosis and management of AML in adults: 2022 recommendations from an international expert panel on behalf of the ELN. Blood. 140(12):1345-77, 2022
7. Montesinos P et al: Ivosidenib and azacitidine in IDH1-mutated acute myeloid leukemia. N Engl J Med. 386(16):1519-31, 2022

Acute Myeloid Leukemia, NOS

Monocytes, Promonocytes, and Blasts

Promonocytes

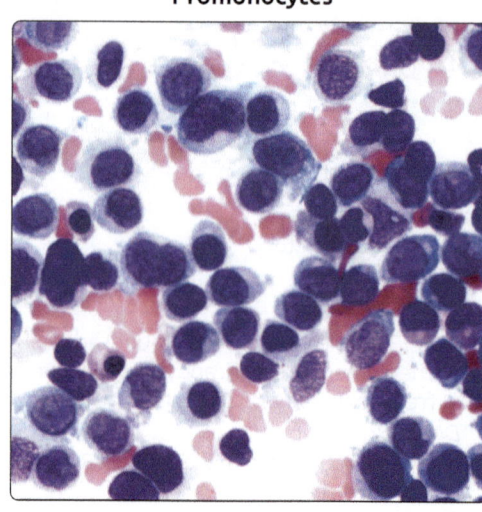

(Left) Blood smear from a 33-year-old man with acute monocytic leukemia shows monocytes ⇨, promonocytes ⇨, and blasts ⇨ as well as anemia and thrombocytopenia. (Right) In this case of AML, the majority of neoplastic cells are promonocytes. These are classified as blast equivalents and have immature chromatin with delicate nuclear folding.

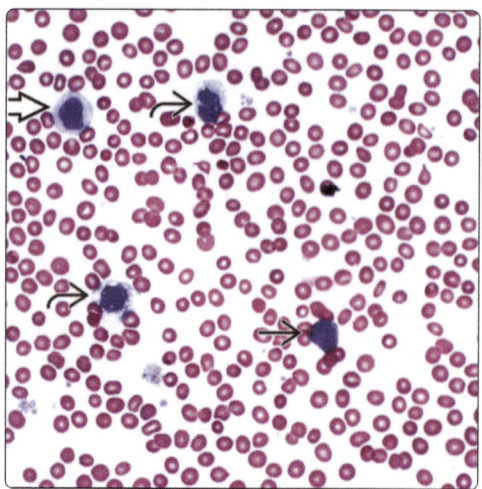

AML Infiltrate in Bone Marrow

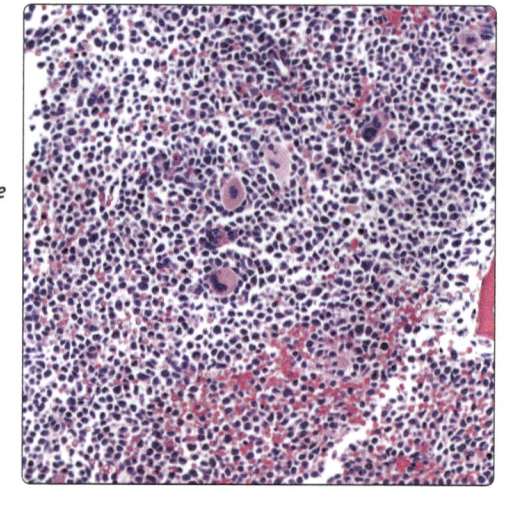

Extramedullary Involvement

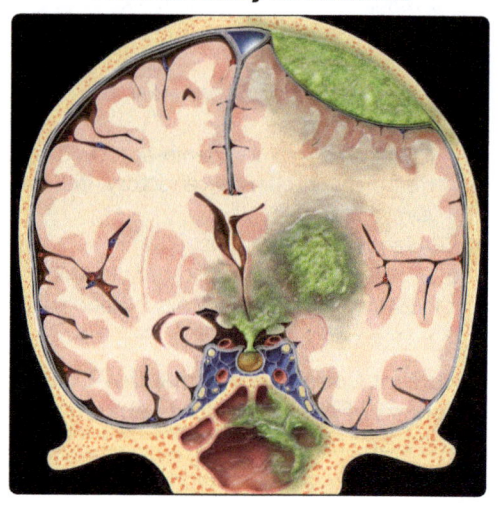

(Left) Core biopsy from a patient with AML is markedly hypercellular with an extensive leukemic infiltrate composed of immature mononuclear cells. Note the preservation of some of the megakaryocytes. (Right) Acute monocytic leukemia is particularly prone to formation of extramedullary masses, such as these brain lesions, historically called chloromas due to their green color on gross examination.

Acute Erythroid Leukemia in Bone Marrow

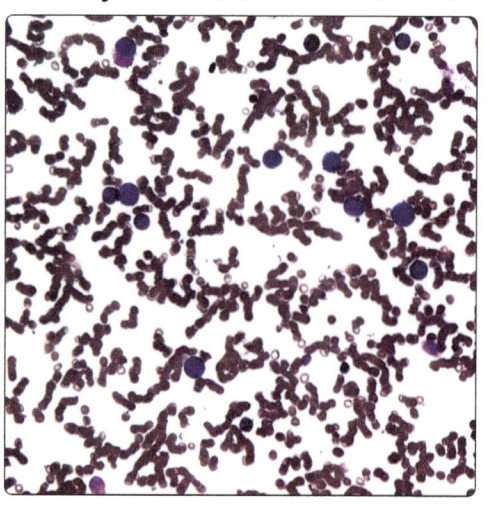

Acute Erythroid Leukemia in Marrow Core

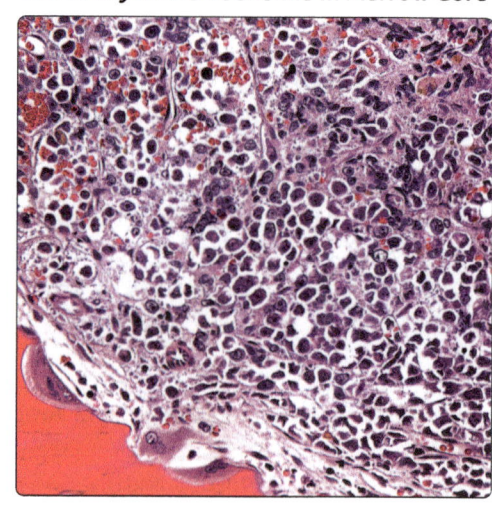

(Left) In this case of acute erythroid leukemia in a 13-month-old, aspirate smear shows a monotonous population of pronormoblasts. There is very little maturation and minimal myeloid component. Per ICC, this is now classified as AML with mutated TP53. (Right) In acute erythroid leukemia, the cells are immature and monotonous with a leukemic pattern of infiltration. They may or may not retain features of erythroid lineage and can be very difficult to diagnose even with immunophenotyping.

Acute Myeloid Leukemia, NOS

Lack of CD34 Expression

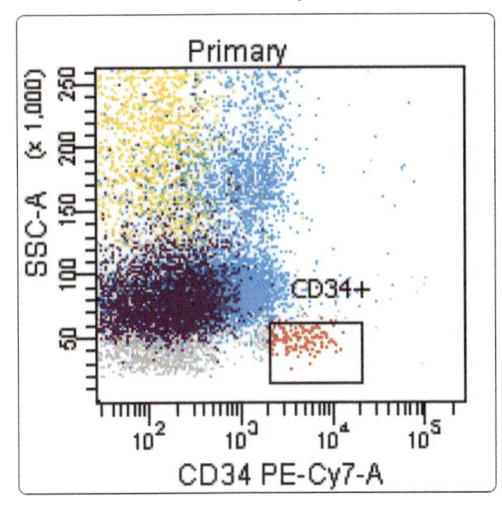

Monocytic Differentiation

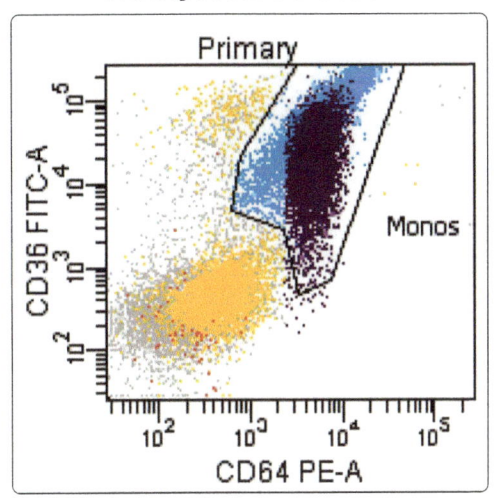

(Left) Many cases of AML do not express certain immature markers, such as CD34. This is often true of cases with monocytic differentiation. The monocytes and blast equivalents are highlighted in blue and purple, respectively. (Right) Coexpression of CD36 and CD64 is very useful in identifying monocytic differentiation. In this case of AML, mature monocytes (blue) and blast equivalents (purple) both show strong expression of CD64 and coexpression of CD36.

AML Without Maturation

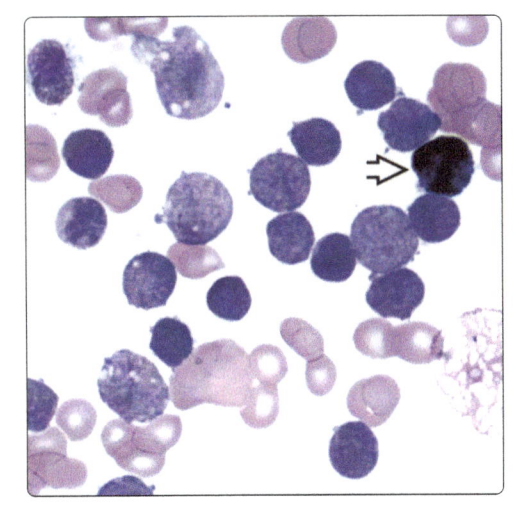

CD117: Core Biopsy

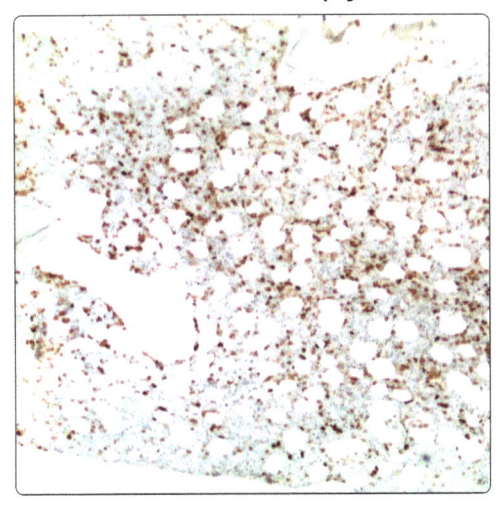

(Left) Some cases of AML, particularly those without maturation, may be negative for Sudan black B (shown) or MPO. Mature neutrophils serve as an internal control ⮕. (Right) Blasts are often positive for CD34 &/or CD117 (shown). CD117 is not specific for blasts and may also be seen on other hematopoietic progenitor cells as well as mast cells. This case of AML had a blast percentage just exceeding 20%. Note the leukemic pattern of infiltration.

AML With Normal Karyotype

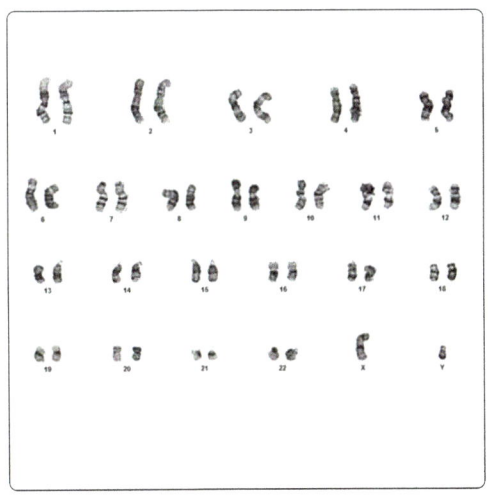

AML in Cerebrospinal Fluid

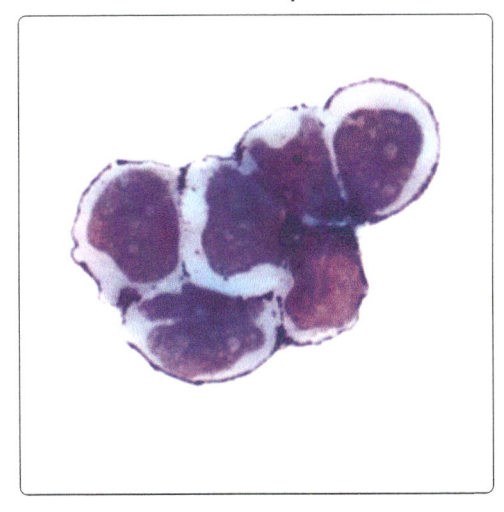

(Left) Normal karyotype is shown in a patient with AML. Normal karyotype is seen in 40-50% of adult AML. AML with normal karyotype is actually a heterogeneous group with the majority having various mutations detectable at the molecular level. (Right) Cerebrospinal fluid cytospin shows a case of AML relapsing in the central nervous system. Cytospin preparations may alter the morphology, often making nuclear contours appear more irregular with prominence of the nucleoli.

Molecular Pathology of Myeloid Neoplasms

275

Myeloid Sarcoma

KEY FACTS

TERMINOLOGY
- Myeloid sarcoma (MS)
  - Mass-producing proliferation of myeloid blasts in site other than bone marrow
  - Diagnosis is equivalent to diagnosis of acute myeloid leukemia (AML)

ETIOLOGY/PATHOGENESIS
- MS may express unique homing and cell-cell interaction proteins compared to bone marrow

MOLECULAR
- Cytogenetics may or may not be concordant between bone marrow AML and MS
  - AML-associated aberrations
  - Myelodysplastic/myeloproliferative neoplasm-associated aberrations
  - Complex karyotype more common in MS than AML
- Gene mutations
  - AML-associated gene mutations, such as *FLT3* and *NPM1*
  - RAS signaling pathway mutations in 85%
  - *FLT3* ITD, *KIT*, *IDH1*, and *IDH2*, among others

MICROSCOPIC
- Disrupts tissue architecture
- May show variable maturation
- Subset show myelomonocytic or monocytic features

ANCILLARY TESTS
- Immunohistochemistry often key in diagnosis
- Often positive for CD34, TdT, CD117, and MPO
  - Lysozyme, CD4, and CD163 expression with monocytic differentiation
- Massively parallel (next-generation) sequencing panels for myeloid-associated mutations
  - Screen for mutations with diagnostic and prognostic significance
  - Identify targetable mutations for therapy

Highly Atypical Cells

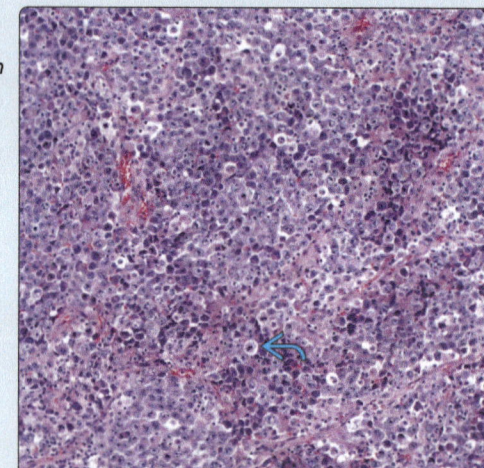

CD33 Immunohistochemistry

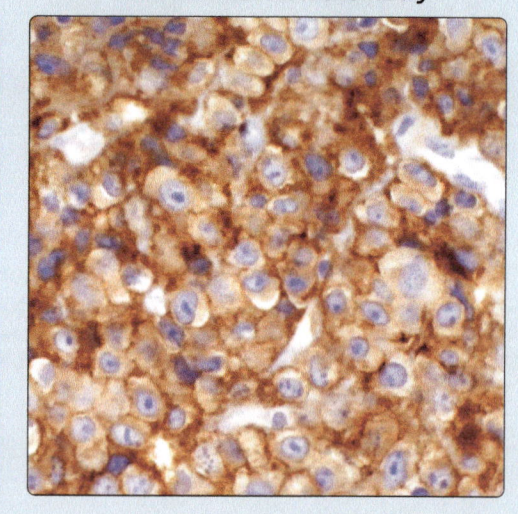

(Left) Myeloid sarcoma (MS) shows poorly differentiated, large, highly atypical cells with hyperchromatic, round nuclei, prominent nucleoli, and moderate cytoplasm with numerous mitoses ➡. (Right) Atypical cells are positive for CD33. Additionally, proliferating cells also expressed MPO and CD34, consistent with myeloblastic proliferation.

FISH for *KMT2A*

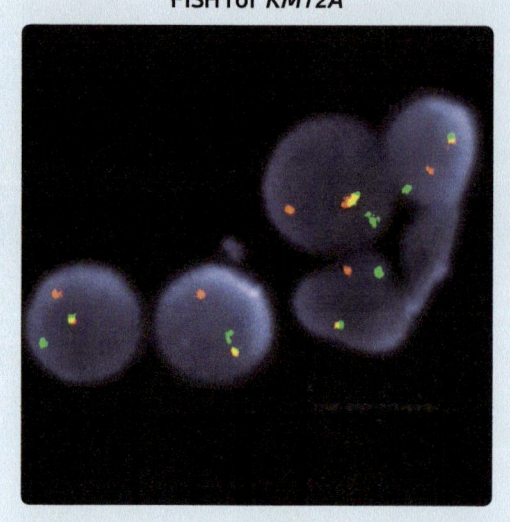

Karyogram With t(11;19)

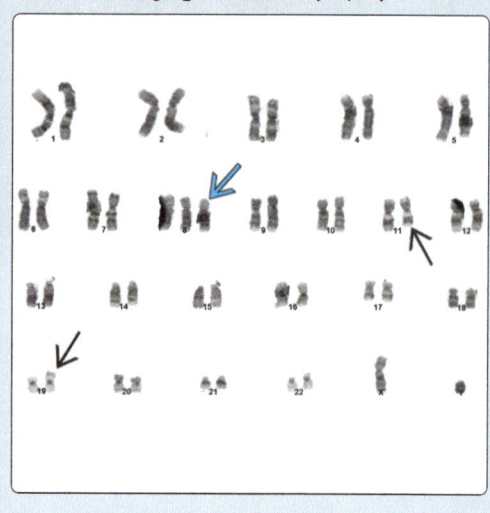

(Left) FISH using break-apart probe shows rearrangement of *KMT2A* (formerly known as MLL) at 11q23. This finding can be associated with MS, particularly involving the skin or breast. (Right) Karyogram shows 11;19 chromosomal translocation ➡, consistent with *KMT2A* rearrangement. This is a common finding in MS. In addition, there is trisomy 8 ➡.

Myeloid Sarcoma

TERMINOLOGY

Abbreviations
- Myeloid sarcoma (MS)

Definitions
- Mass-producing proliferation of myeloid blasts in site other than bone marrow
- Diagnosis is equivalent to diagnosis of acute myeloid leukemia (AML)

CLASSIFICATION

ICC and WHO-HAEM5
- MS is recognized in both ICC and WHO classifications

ETIOLOGY/PATHOGENESIS

Aberrant Myeloblast Localization
- Specific reason for extramedullary homing unclear but cytokines and adhesion molecules may be involved
  - Cytokine receptors, including CCR5, CXCR4, CXCR7, and CX3CR1
    - May cause homing and retention of blasts in skin
  - Matrix metalloproteinases and receptors
    - MMP-9 and MMP-2, promote tissue invasion
  - Adhesion molecules including ITGA7
- MS shares cytogenetics and molecular abnormalities with bone marrow AML

CLINICAL ISSUES

Epidemiology
- Age
  - Wide range
    - More common in older patients
    - Median: 56 years
- Sex
  - Slight male predominance
    - M:F = 1.2:1.0

Site
- Any extramedullary body site can be involved
  - Skin is most common site
  - Other common sites include lymph node, GI tract, soft tissue, and testis
- Rarely presents at multiple sites

Presentation
- Tumor mass

Natural History
- Occurs in 2-9% of AML patients
- May precede diagnosis of AML in ~ 25% of cases
  - May be diagnosed months or years prior to bone marrow involvement
  - May be diagnosed concurrently with AML in 15-35% of cases
  - MS after diagnosis of AML occurs in ~ 50% of cases
    - May represent relapse in extramedullary site
- Rarely presents as blastic transformation of other myeloid neoplasm
- 8-15% of AML patients treated with allogeneic stem cell transplant develop MS
- Rarely occurs as presentation of post cytotoxic therapy myeloid neoplasm

Treatment
- Drugs
  - Conventional AML protocols recommended but show reduced efficacy
    - High rate of progression in patients only receiving localized treatment
  - Targeted therapies
    - Tyrosine kinase inhibitors
    - FLT3 inhibitors
    - Anti-CD33 monoclonal antibody
    - IDH2 inhibitors
  - Immune checkpoint inhibitors
- Radiation
  - Not recommended without systemic chemotherapy
  - May be used in consolidation period
- Bone marrow transplant
  - More often used in relapsed disease
  - 5-year survival rate of ~ 47%

Prognosis
- May be associated with worse prognosis in adults when diagnosed concurrently with AML
- Allogeneic bone marrow transplant may prolong survival

MOLECULAR

Cytogenetics
- Fresh specimen often not available
- Cytogenetics concordant between bone marrow AML and MS in only 71% of cases
  - May show additional abnormalities compared to marrow
  - Suggests common stem cell derivation
- Normal karyotype seen in 50% of cases
- AML-associated aberrations include *KMT2A* rearrangements in ~ 10% of cases
  - Associated with monocytic differentiation
  - Other AML-associated abnormalities may be seen
- t(8;21); *RUNX1::RUNX1T1*
  - Associated with MS in orbital region
  - More common in pediatric cases
- t(15;17); *PML::RARA*
  - Usually associated with relapse of acute promyelocytic leukemia
- Inv(16) or t(16;16); *CBFB::MYH11*
  - Up to 13% of pediatric cases
  - Associated with breast or intestinal disease
    - Monosomy 16 and del 16q may also be seen
- Myeloid neoplasm-associated aberrations
  - Trisomy 8, more common in MS involving skin or breast
  - Monosomy 7, del 5q/monosomy 5, del 20q
  - t(9;22); *BCR::ABL1*
    - In MS arising from chronic myeloid leukemia
- Other abnormalities
  - Trisomy 4, trisomy 11, monosomy 16, del 6q
- Complex karyotype
  - More common in MS than AML

Myeloid Sarcoma

- o May represent clonal evolution

In Situ Hybridization
- FISH may prove useful when fresh specimen not available for karyotype
  - o AML and MDS panel should be performed

Array Comparative Genomic Hybridization
- May be performed on formalin-fixed, paraffin-embedded tissue
- Virtually all cases of MS demonstrate abnormalities
  - o Common losses include 4q21.1-q35.2, 6q16.1-q21, and 12p12.2
  - o Common gains include 8q21.2-q24.3, 8, 11q21-q25, 13q21.32-34, 19, and 21

Molecular Genetics
- AML-associated gene mutations
  - o *FLT3* internal tandem duplication in 15-30%
    - More common with normal karyotype
  - o *NPM1* in 20-30%
    - More frequent with monocytic differentiation
    - Associated with normal karyotype
    - More frequent in cases with skin involvement
  - o Other mutated genes include *FLT3* TKD, *TET2*, *ASXL1*, *EZH2*, *CEBPA*, and RAS pathway genes (e.g., *NRAS*, *KRAS*)
- Myeloproliferative-associated aberrations
  - o *JAK2* mutations seen in MPN-related cases
    - Mutation may be discordant between MS and bone marrow
- Occasionally, patient may have same mutations identified in MS and normal-appearing bone marrow
  - o May represent tissue-based transformation of clonal hematopoiesis

MICROSCOPIC

Histologic Features
- Disrupts tissue architecture
- Diffuse or single file pattern
- May mimic carcinoma

Cytologic Features
- May show variable maturation
  - o Blastic type primarily myeloblasts
  - o Immature type shows some maturation
    - Myeloblasts, promyelocytes
  - o Differentiated type shows more mature forms
    - Promyelocytes, myelocytes, metamyelocytes
- Large subset show myelomonocytic or monocytic features
- Erythroid or megakaryocytic differentiation is rare

ANCILLARY TESTS

Immunohistochemistry
- Varies with differentiation status of cells
- Common positive markers
  - o Markers of immaturity
    - CD34, TdT, CD117
  - o Lineage-associated markers
    - MPO
    - NSE, CD11c, CD14, CD64, CD68, lysozyme, CD163
  - – May express B-cell-associated markers in cases with t(8;21); *RUNX1::RUNX1T1*

Genetic Testing
- Targeted gene mutation testing
  - o *FLT3* and *NPM1* have prognostic significance as in AML
  - o *JAK2*, *CALR*, and *MPL* in MPN-associated cases
- Massively parallel (next-generation) sequencing panels for myeloid-associated mutations
  - o Screen for mutations with diagnostic and prognostic significance
  - o Identify targetable mutations for therapy

DIFFERENTIAL DIAGNOSIS

Lymphoblastic Lymphoma
- Morphology may appear similar to MS
- Lymphoid immunophenotype
  - o Expression of B- or T-lineage-associated markers
  - o No expression of MPO or monocytic markers

Diffuse Large B-Cell Lymphoma
- Common diagnostic dilemma
  - o Typically bright CD45 positive
  - o Expression of CD19, CD20, and CD79A
  - o No expression of MPO or monocytic markers

Mixed Phenotype Acute Leukemia
- Express myeloid/monocytic lineage markers and lymphoid markers
  - o Myeloid/monocytic markers MPO, NSE, CD11c, CD14, CD64, and lysozyme
  - o B-cell markers CD19, CD79A, CD22, and CD10
  - o T-cell marker surface or cytoplasmic CD3

Nonhematopoietic Tumors
- No expression of MPO
- Expression of cytokeratin in carcinoma
- Expression of S100 and Melan-A in melanoma

DIAGNOSTIC CHECKLIST

Pathologic Interpretation Pearls
- High index of suspicion required
  - o Fresh specimen for ancillary testing often not available if hematologic neoplasm not suspected
  - o Immunohistochemistry is crucial to determine lineage
- Cytogenetic and molecular findings are similar to those seen in AML and other myeloid neoplasms

SELECTED REFERENCES

1. Loscocco GG et al: Myeloid sarcoma: more and less than a distinct entity. Ann Hematol. 102(8):1973-84, 2023
2. Ramia de Cap M et al: Myeloid sarcoma: an overview. Semin Diagn Pathol. 40(3):129-39, 2023
3. Ramia de Cap M et al: Myeloid sarcoma with NPM1 mutation may be clinically and genetically distinct from AML with NPM1 mutation: a study from the Bone Marrow Pathology Group. Leuk Lymphoma. 64(5):972-80, 2023
4. Zhang L et al: Myeloid/lymphoid neoplasms associated with eosinophilia and rearrangements of PCM1::JAK2 with erythroblastic sarcoma: a case report and literature review. Haematologica. ePub, 2023

Myeloid Sarcoma

Myeloid Sarcoma in *JAK2*-Positive Myeloproliferative Neoplasm

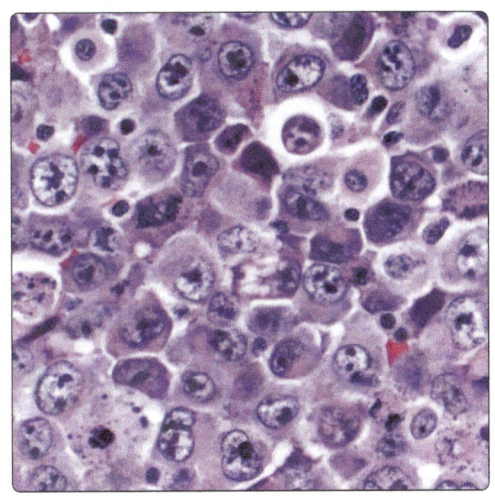

Myeloid Sarcoma in *JAK2*-Positive Myeloproliferative Neoplasm

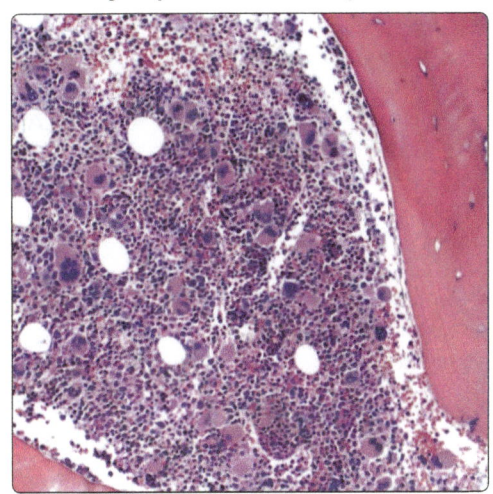

(Left) MS in a patient with history of JAK2-positive myeloproliferative neoplasm is shown. The tumor was also positive for JAK2 V617F mutation. (Right) Bone marrow biopsy from the same case shows features of myeloproliferative neoplasm, including markedly hypercellular marrow with myeloid and megakaryocytic hyperplasia but no evidence of involvement by acute myeloid leukemia (AML). Bone marrow may be negative for involvement by AML in a subset of MS cases.

Complex Karyotype

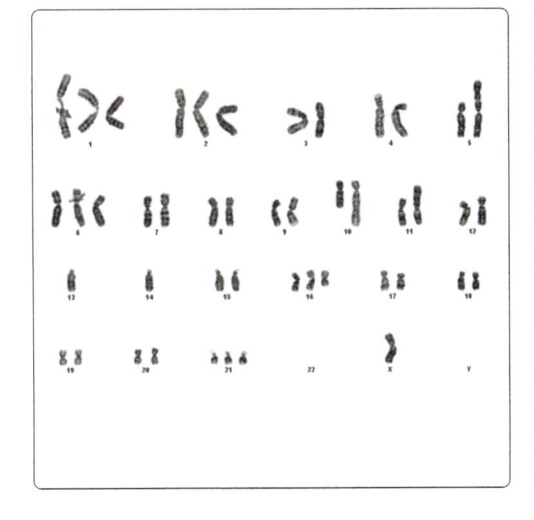

FISH Using *CBFB* Break-Apart Probes

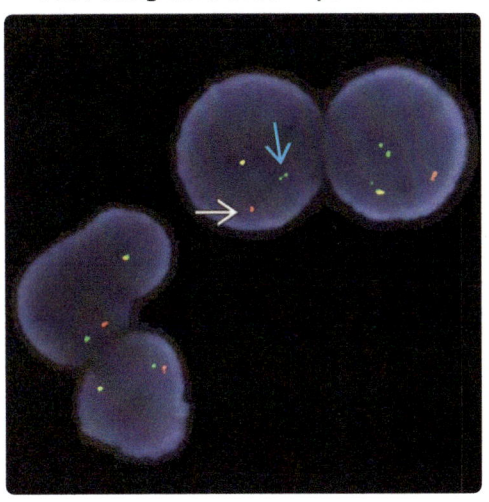

(Left) Complex karyotype from a patient with MS shows with 46X,+1,+2,add(5)(p15),+6,t(9;18)(p10;p10), add(10)(q24),add(11)(p15),-13,-14,+del(16)(q21), and +21,-22,-22. Complex cytogenetics are more common in MS than AML. (Right) FISH shows separate red ➡ and green ➡ signals using dual-color, break-apart probe for CBFB, indicating rearrangement. This pattern can be seen with inv(16)(p13.1q22) or t(16;16), a finding associated with MS of the breast or gastrointestinal tract.

Blastic Morphology

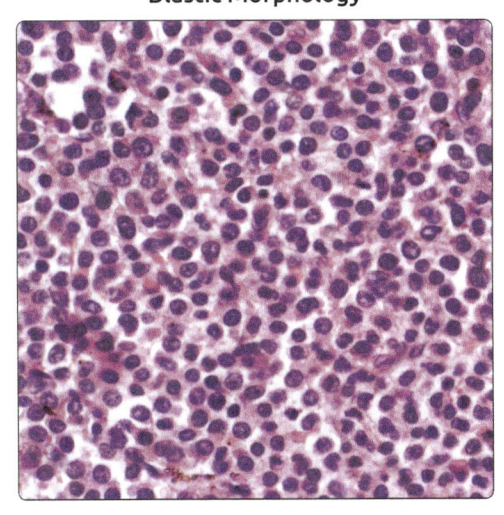

Lysozyme Immunohistochemistry

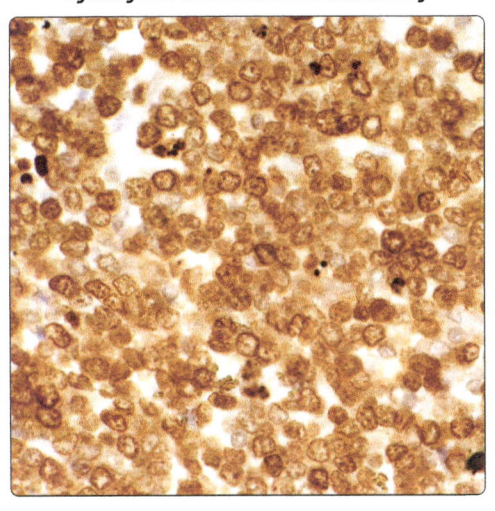

(Left) MS shows an infiltrate composed of immature mononuclear cells, consistent with blastic histologic subtype. However, some MS cases may show differentiation with components of maturing myeloid cells, including promyelocytes, myelocytes, and eosinophils. (Right) MS with a monotonous population of immature cells is brightly positive for lysozyme by immunohistochemistry, supporting monocytic differentiation.

Myeloid Proliferations Associated With Down Syndrome

KEY FACTS

TERMINOLOGY
- Myeloid proliferations associated with Down syndrome (DS) encompass both transient abnormal myelopoiesis (TAM) and myeloid leukemia of DS (ML-DS)
- TAM
  - Abnormal myeloid proliferation resembling acute myeloid leukemia (AML)
  - Confined to first 6 months of age
  - Resolves spontaneously
- ML-DS
  - Often includes prolonged myelodysplasia-like phase, but MDS and overt AML phases are biologically indistinct
  - Differentiation between these phases has no prognostic or therapeutic implications

ETIOLOGY/PATHOGENESIS
- Acquired N-terminal truncating *GATA1* mutations pathognomonic for TAM and ML-DS
  - These *GATA1* mutations are not leukemogenic in absence of trisomy 21
- *GATA1*-mutated TAM clone subsequently acquires additional genetic abnormalities, leading to ML-DS

CLINICAL ISSUES
- Spontaneous remission of TAM is generally expected within 3 months
  - Few patients may suffer life-threatening or fatal complications
- 20-30% of patients with TAM later develop ML-DS
  - Most patients develop ML-DS prior to 5 years of age; onset usually 1-3 years after TAM
- ML-DS usually associated with chemosensitivity and good prognosis

TOP DIFFERENTIAL DIAGNOSES
- "Conventional" AML in setting of DS
- Reactive leukocytosis due to neonatal infection
- AML with t(1;22)(p13.3;q13.1); *RBM15::MRTFA*

Karyotype Showing Trisomy 21

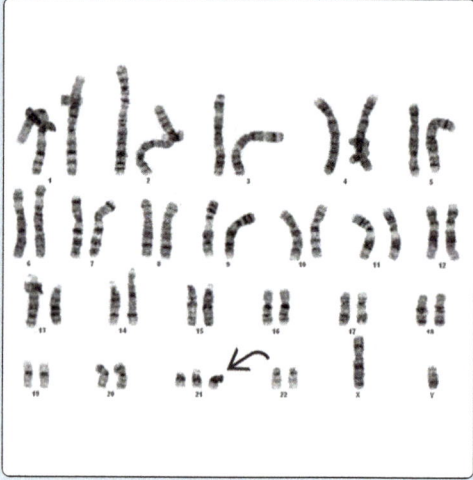

Circulating Blasts in TAM

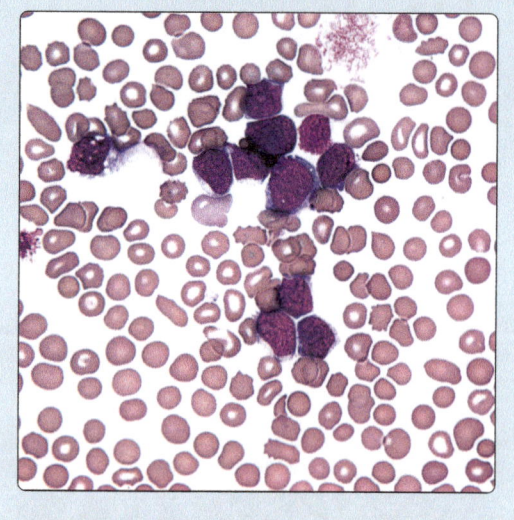

(Left) *Myeloid proliferations in young children with constitutional trisomy 21 ➔ have distinct clinical and biologic behavior. GATA1 mutations are predictably present in this setting.* (Right) *Circulating blasts are present in the peripheral blood of a 4-week-old boy with Down syndrome, consistent with transient abnormal myelopoiesis (TAM). As expected, the TAM in this child spontaneously resolved.*

Megakaryoblast in ML-DS

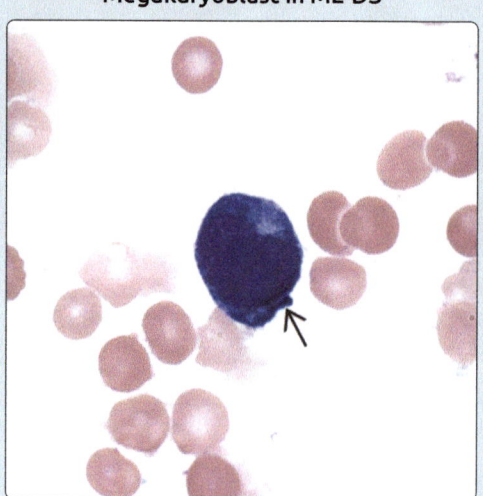

Hypercellular Marrow in ML-DS

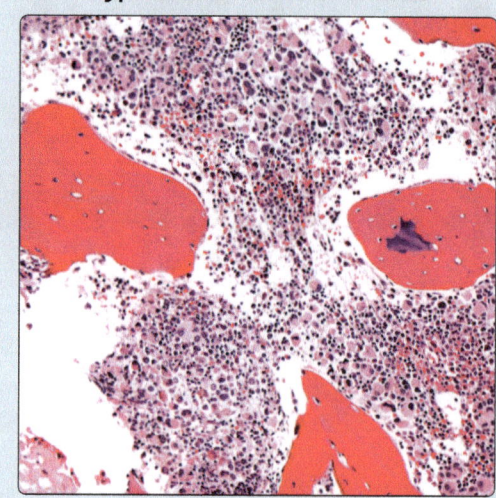

(Left) *Megakaryoblast from a patient with myeloid leukemia of Down syndrome is shown. Characteristic cytologic features include basophilic cytoplasm and cytoplasmic "blebbing" ➔.* (Right) *Hypercellular marrow containing clusters of abnormal megakaryocytes in myeloid leukemia of Down syndrome is shown. The marrow was also fibrotic and showed some bony changes.*

Myeloid Proliferations Associated With Down Syndrome

TERMINOLOGY

Abbreviations
- Down syndrome (DS)
- Myeloid leukemia of Down syndrome (ML-DS)
- Transient abnormal myelopoiesis (TAM)

Definitions
- Down syndrome
  - Constitutional gain of extra copy of chromosome 21
  - Characterized by intellectual disability, distinctive facies, and variety of developmental abnormalities
  - Most patients have trisomy 21, but DS may also arise from chromosomal translocation or mosaicism
    - Mosaic case phenotypes are variable; depend on prominence of trisomic cell subset
    - Mosaic DS-related myeloid proliferations occur rarely
- Myeloid proliferations associated with DS
  - Major category of myeloid neoplasia, recognized by both ICC and WHO 5th edition, includes both TAM and ML-DS
    - Transient abnormal myelopoiesis
      - Transient/self-limited myeloid proliferation resembling acute myeloid leukemia
      - Confined to first 6 months of life
    - Myeloid leukemia of Down syndrome
      - Neoplastic proliferation often with prolonged myelodysplasia-like phase
      - ML-DS includes both dysplastic and leukemic phases regardless of blast percentage
- GATA1
  - Official name: GATA binding protein 1
  - HGNC ID: 4170
  - Gene locus: Xp11.23
    - Chr X: 48,786,590-48,794,311 (GRCh38.p14)
  - Number of exons: 6

ETIOLOGY/PATHOGENESIS

Trisomy 21 and Hematopoiesis
- Trisomy 21 itself causes abnormal fetal hematopoiesis
  - Dysregulated erythroid and megakaryocytic expansion during 2nd trimester liver-based hematopoiesis
    - May precede any acquisition of GATA1 mutation
  - Impairs B-cell lineage development and reduces granulocyte-macrophage progenitors
  - Increased ERG (21q22.2) dosage potential driver
    - Family member of erythroblast transformation-specific transcription factors
- Certain Chr 21 miRNAs may contribute more heavily to preleukemia initiation: miR-99a, miR-125b-2, and miR-155

Normal Function of GATA1
- Belongs to family of transcription factors that can to bind to DNA sequence 5'-[AT]GATA[AG]-3'
- Key regulator of normal erythro- and megakaryopoiesis

Role of GATA1 Mutation in Transient Abnormal Myelopoiesis and Myeloid leukemia of Down Syndrome
- Acquired N-terminal truncating mutations in exons 2 and 3 in essentially all cases of TAM and ML-DS
  - GATA1 mutation with trisomy 21 sufficient to cause TAM
  - Mutations not leukemogenic in absence of trisomy 21
  - GATA1 mutations acquired in prenatal period
- Spontaneous resolution of TAM may relate to physiologic downregulation of fetal hepatic hematopoiesis
- JAK3 mutations may accompany GATA1 mutations
- Leukemia in germline GATA1 patients with acquired trisomy 21 produces ML-DS-like megakaryoblastic phenotype

Etiologic Relationship Between Transient Abnormal Myelopoiesis and Myeloid leukemia of Down Syndrome
- ML-DS blasts are clonally related to preceding TAM blasts
  - Carry identical GATA1 mutation
- Some studies found differences in gene expression profiles between TAM and ML-DS blasts
- Blasts in ML-DS often gain clonal abnormalities in addition to constitutional trisomy 21
  - Trisomy 8 found in 13-44% of cases
  - Monosomy 7 very rare in ML-DS
  - Mutations in following genes additionally implicated
    - CSF2RB p.A455D, CTCF, EZH2, KANSL1, JAK2, JAK3, MPL, SH2B3, and RAS pathway genes
- Epigenetic changes also pivotal in ML-DS progression
  - KDM1A-driven gene signatures activated in ML-DS

CLINICAL ISSUES

Epidemiology
- DS affects ~ 1 in 800 newborns
  - TAM develops in ~ 10% of newborns with DS
    - 20-30% of patients with TAM later develop ML-DS
  - ML-DS develops in 1-2% of patients with DS
    - In vast majority of cases, patients < 5 years old

Presentation
- TAM
  - Increased circulating blasts that may exceed 20%
  - Hepatosplenomegaly
  - Average age at diagnosis: 3-7 days
  - TAM has also been found during fetal development
    - Can cause hydrops fetalis
- ML-DS
  - May present as months-long myelodysplasia-like state with similarities to refractory cytopenia of childhood

Prognosis
- TAM
  - Spontaneous remission is generally expected; few patients may have life-threatening or fatal complications
    - Circulating blasts usually clear within 3 months of diagnosis (average: ~ 5 weeks)
    - 20-30% develop ML-DS in 1-3 years but remaining experience durable remission
  - Findings associated with increased mortality include
    - Extreme leukocytosis
    - Hyperviscosity
    - Hepatosplenomegaly causing respiratory compromise
    - Heart failure
    - Hydrops fetalis
    - Renal or hepatic dysfunction
    - Disseminated intravascular coagulation with bleeding

Myeloid Proliferations Associated With Down Syndrome

- Patients with such risk factors may require leukapheresis or moderately low-dose cytarabine
- ML-DS
  - Good prognosis in young DS patients with *GATA1* mutations
    - 80% overall survival
    - Due in part to enhanced chemosensitivity to cytarabine
      - Cytarabine is metabolized by cytidine deaminase, which has decreased expression in DS
  - Targeted KDM1A (a.k.a. LSD1) and JAK1/2 inhibition may show synergy
  - Relapsed ML-DS has very poor 3-year overall survival
  - Higher risk of late mortality vs. non-DS acute leukemia survivors or DS control patients
    - Risk not attributable to cardiac disease or subsequent malignant neoplasm; causes of premature death in non-DS survivors

MOLECULAR

Cytogenetics
- Karyotype and/or FISH can detect trisomy 21
- May detect other cytogenetically detectable structural abnormalities if exist

PCR/NGS-Based Analysis
- Detect *GATA1* and other gene mutations in suspected TAM or ML-DS
- Assess trisomy 21 mosaicism if *GATA1* mutation detected in phenotypically normal infant with leukemia
- Low-level *GATA1*-mutant clones may be detected by NGS in ~ 20% of DS neonates without evidence of overt TAM

MICROSCOPIC

Transient Abnormal Myelopoiesis
- Peripheral blood
  - Increased blasts; often phenotypically megakaryoblasts
  - Leukocytosis; some cases may have normal WBC counts
  - Thrombocytopenia
- Bone marrow
  - Erythroid and megakaryocyte dysplasia
  - Blast % in marrow may be lower than in peripheral blood

Myeloid Leukemia of Down Syndrome
- Peripheral blood
  - Pronounced dysplasia and macrocytosis seen in early stages, even in absence of circulating megakaryoblasts
- Bone marrow
  - Trilineage dysplasia and increased megakaryoblasts
    - No biological differences between MDS and overt AML phases; diagnostic differentiation considered irrelevant

ANCILLARY TESTS

Immunohistochemistry
- Lack of full-length GATA1 (GATA1f) expression in megakaryocytes is sensitive and specific for TAM and ML-DS

Flow Cytometry
- Similar findings in TAM and ML-DS

- Blasts express CD13, CD33, CD7, CD117, CD36, CD42, and CD61
  - TAM blasts more likely to express CD34, CD56, and CD41 than ML-DS blasts

DIFFERENTIAL DIAGNOSIS

"Conventional" Acute Myeloid Leukemia in Setting of Down Syndrome
- Patients with DS may also develop "conventional" AML
  - Patients usually > 5 years of age at diagnosis
  - *GATA1* mutations are absent

Reactive Leukocytosis With Increased Blasts
- Increased blasts in TAM is generally in excess of left shift associated with infection or inflammation, though overlap may occur
  - *GATA1* mutation supports TAM over reactive leukocytosis
- Few circulating blasts normally found in 98% of newborns with DS (median: 4%) without TAM or *GATA1* mutation

Acute Myeloid Leukemia With t(1;22)(p13.3;q13.1); *RBM15::MRTFA*
- Megakaryoblastic leukemia that presents in infants and young children
  - Features overlap significantly with TAM and ML-DS but pathobiologically separate and distinct entity

DIAGNOSTIC CHECKLIST

Multistep Model of Pathogenesis
- Trisomy 21 disturbs hematopoiesis in fetal liver
- *GATA1* mutation acquisition leads to TAM
- TAM regresses during hematopoietic transition from liver to bone marrow
- *GATA1*-mutated clone acquires additional genetic abnormalities leading to ML-DS

SELECTED REFERENCES

1. Grimm J et al: Combining LSD1 and JAK-STAT inhibition targets Down syndrome-associated myeloid leukemia at its core. Leukemia. 36(7):1926-30, 2022
2. Gupta S et al: Risks of late mortality and morbidity among survivors of childhood acute leukemia with Down syndrome: a population-based cohort study. Cancer. 128(6):1294-301, 2022
3. Hasle H et al: Germline GATA1s-generating mutations predispose to leukemia with acquired trisomy 21 and Down syndrome-like phenotype. Blood. 139(21):3159-65, 2022
4. Boucher AC et al: Clinical and biological aspects of myeloid leukemia in Down syndrome. Leukemia. 35(12):3352-60, 2021
5. Wagenblast E et al: Mapping the cellular origin and early evolution of leukemia in Down syndrome. Science. 373(6551), 2021
6. Labuhn M et al: Mechanisms of progression of myeloid preleukemia to transformed myeloid leukemia in children with Down syndrome. Cancer Cell. 36(2):123-38.e10, 2019
7. Lee WY et al: Loss of full-length GATA1 expression in megakaryocytes is a sensitive and specific immunohistochemical marker for the diagnosis of myeloid proliferative disorder related to Down syndrome. Am J Clin Pathol. 149(4):300-9, 2018
8. Ng AP et al: Early lineage priming by trisomy of Erg leads to myeloproliferation in a Down syndrome model. PLoS Genet. 11(5):e1005211, 2015
9. Bombery M et al: Transient abnormal myelopoiesis in neonates: GATA get the diagnosis. Arch Pathol Lab Med. 138(10):1302-6, 2014
10. Roy A et al: Perturbation of fetal liver hematopoietic stem and progenitor cell development by trisomy 21. Proc Natl Acad Sci U S A. 109(43):17579-84, 2012

Myeloid Proliferations Associated With Down Syndrome

Megakaryoblasts in ML-DS

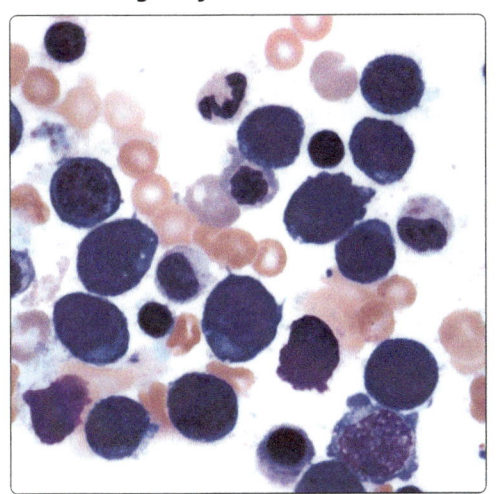

Megakaryoblast With Cytoplasmic Blebs

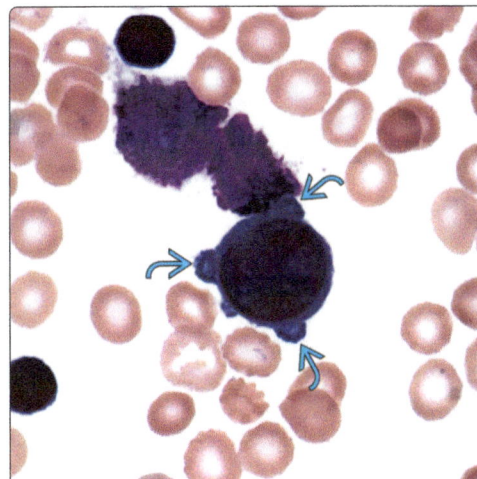

(Left) Bone marrow aspirate from a 1-year-old boy with Down syndrome and prior history of TAM with *GATA1* mutation is shown. Numerous megakaryoblasts are present, consistent with myeloid leukemia of Down syndrome. (Right) Megakaryoblast from a patient with myeloid leukemia of Down syndrome shows characteristic cytologic features, including basophilic cytoplasm and cytoplasmic "blebbing" ⇗.

Blastic Infiltrate With Atypical Megakaryocytes

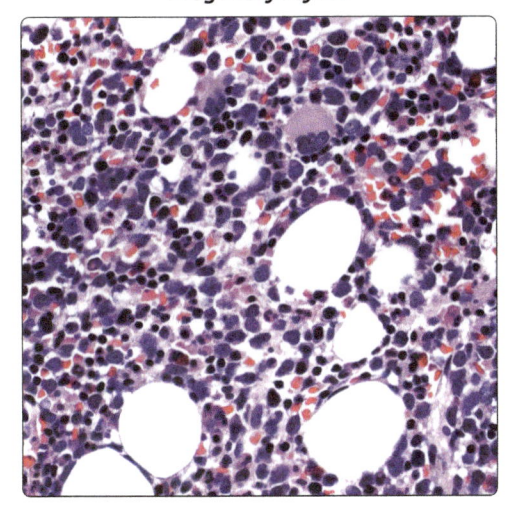

CD117 Immunohistochemistry

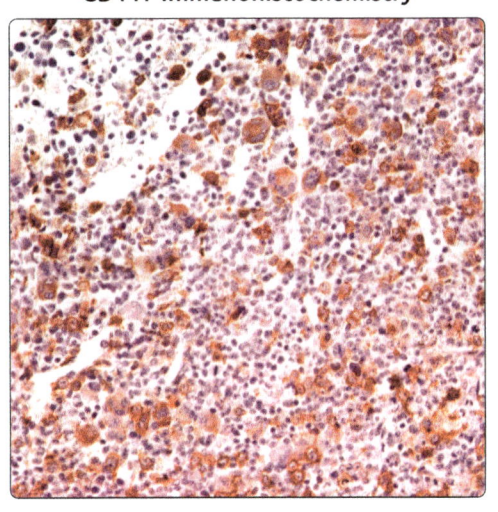

(Left) Bone marrow core biopsy shows a blastic infiltrate with atypical megakaryocytes. The karyotype showed multiple abnormalities in addition to constitutional trisomy 21, including acquired trisomies of chromosomes 8, 14, and 19. (Right) CD117 stains increased blasts and abnormal megakaryocytes. CD117 is a useful marker in this setting, as blasts can be CD34 negative.

CD31 Immunohistochemistry

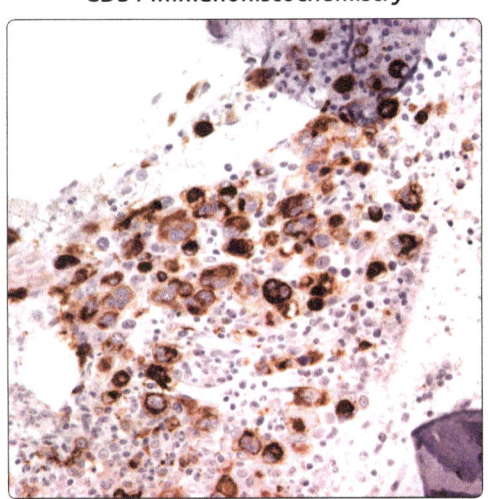

CD42b Immunohistochemistry

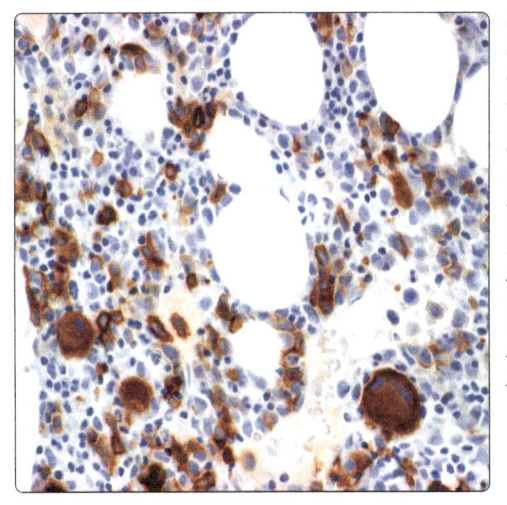

(Left) CD31 highlights atypical megakaryocytes admixed with megakaryoblasts in a 20-month-old child with ML-DS and history of resolved TAM. (Right) CD42b highlights atypical megakaryocytes and megakaryoblasts in a child with myeloid leukemia associated with Down syndrome. In general, patients with myeloid leukemia associated with Down syndrome have a relatively good prognosis.

Blastic Plasmacytoid Dendritic Cell Neoplasm

KEY FACTS

TERMINOLOGY
- Blastic plasmacytoid dendritic cell neoplasm (BPCDCN)
  - Distinct clinicopathologic entity in both WHO HAEM5 and ICC
  - Derived from clonal proliferation of precursor plasmacytoid dendritic cells
  - Aggressive clinical behavior with rapid systemic dissemination

CLINICAL ISSUES
- Most patients present with asymptomatic cutaneous lesions as 1st symptom
- High frequency of bone marrow and blood involvement
- Regional lymph nodes may be involved at presentation
- Dismal prognosis with overall poor therapeutic response

MOLECULAR
- Complex chromosomal aberrations in most cases
- Recurrent mutations identified by NGS
  - *TET2* and *ASXL1* mutations most common
  - Other common mutations include *ZRSR2*, *NRAS*, *CDKN2A*, *SRSF2*, *ATM*, *IKZF1*, and *CHD8*
  - Mutations in genes commonly seen in AML and other myeloid malignancies are also detected in BPCDCN
    – *IDH2*, *RUNX1*, *JAK2*, *NPM1*, *FLT3* ITD, and *DNMT3A*

ANCILLARY TESTS
- Expected positive markers
  - CD123, TCF4, TCL1, CD303, CD304, CD4, and CD56
- Expected negative markers
  - Cytoplasmic and surface CD3, CD19, CD20, CD34, lysozyme, and MPO
- Immunophenotypic diagnostic criteria of BPCDCN (WHO HAEM5)
  - Expression of CD123 and 1 other PCDC marker (TCF4, TCL1, CD303, or CD304) in addition to CD4 &/or CD56

Cutaneous Disease

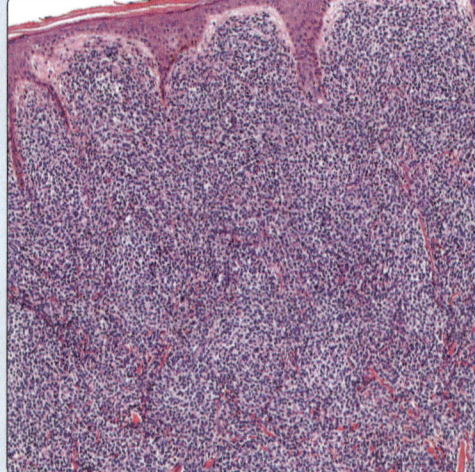

CD123 Expression

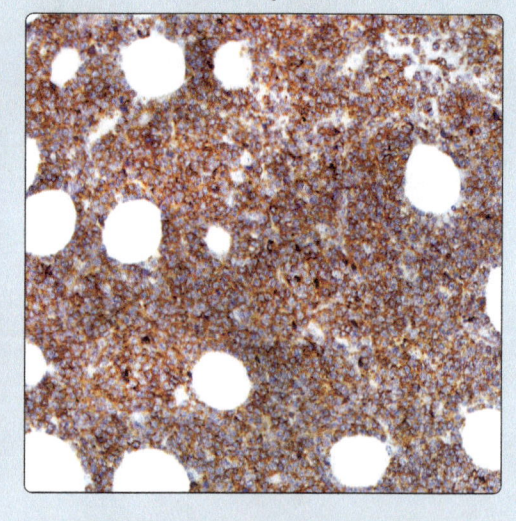

(Left) Skin biopsy from a patient with cutaneous blastic plasmacytoid dendritic cell neoplasm (BPCDCN) shows sheets of monotonous-appearing neoplastic cells with effacement of dermis. Note the intact overlying epidermis. (Right) CD123 shows moderate expression in cutaneous BPCDCN. CD123 is expressed in the vast majority of BPCDCN; however, CD123 is not entirely specific for this tumor. Myeloblasts and rarely lymphoblasts can also express this antigen.

Circulating Neoplastic Cells

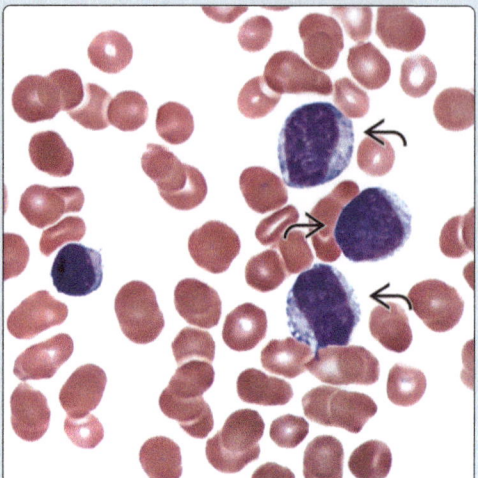

Decreased Trilineage Hematopoiesis

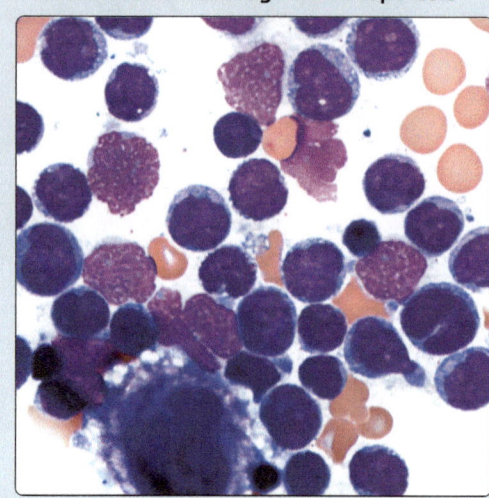

(Left) Blood smear from a patient with leukemic presentation of BPCDCN shows severe thrombocytopenia and circulating blast-like cells. In this example, the circulating neoplastic cells ⇨ resemble lymphoblasts. (Right) Bone marrow aspirate smear from a patient with BPCDCN shows markedly decreased trilineage hematopoiesis and increased blast-like cells with high N:C ratio and scant cytoplasm reminiscent of lymphoblasts.

Blastic Plasmacytoid Dendritic Cell Neoplasm

TERMINOLOGY

Abbreviations
- Blastic plasmacytoid dendritic cell neoplasm (BPCDCN)

Synonyms
- Agranular CD4(+) NK-cell leukemia
- Blastic NK-cell leukemia/lymphoma (not recommended)
- Agranular CD4(+)/CD56(+) hematodermic neoplasm (not recommended)

Definitions
- BPCDCN: Hematologic neoplasm consisting of immature cells
  - Derived from clonal proliferation of precursor plasmacytoid dendritic cells
  - Aggressive clinical behavior with rapid systemic dissemination

CLASSIFICATION

WHO 5th Edition
- Defines BPCDCN as distinct entity under plasmacytoid dendritic cell neoplasms

International Consensus Classification
- Retains similar terminology and immunophenotypic diagnostic criteria as defined in WHO 4th edition

ETIOLOGY/PATHOGENESIS

Pathogenesis
- NF-kB pathway activation
- *ETV6* deletion detected in most cases could represent early pathogenic event
- Copy number losses and complex karyotype
- Mutations in epigenetic regulation genes and genes involved in RNA splicing

CLINICAL ISSUES

Epidemiology
- Age
  - Can present at any age, including childhood, but mainly affects older adults

Presentation
- Most patients initially present with asymptomatic cutaneous lesions
- High frequency of blood and bone marrow involvement
- Cytopenias can occur in patients with leukemic presentation
- Association with antecedent or concurrent myelodysplastic syndrome or myelodysplastic/myeloproliferative neoplasm (MDS/MPN) in 20-30% of cases
- Regional lymph nodes may be involved at presentation
- Some patients may develop BPCDCN following chemotherapy for other malignancies

Treatment
- CD123 targeted therapy
  - Tagraxofusp is CD123-directed cytotoxin consisting of IL3 fused to diphtheria toxin
  - Approved in 2018 by FDA for treatment of BPCDCN in patients ≥ 2 years age
  - Long-term outcomes have confirmed durable efficacy and safety in subset of patients
  - Other agents targeting CD123 available in clinical trials
    - IMGN632 (antibody-drug conjugate) for patients in both front line and refractory settings
    - Anti-CD123 CART-cells
- Venetoclax (BCL2 antagonists)
  - Response has been reported in several patients with refractory/relapsed disease
  - However, benefits of venetoclax monotherapy are often transient, suggesting combination therapy may be preferred
  - Clinical trials studying hypomethylating agents plus venetoclax combinations
- Multiagent chemotherapy
  - Most groups prefer more intensive ALL-based chemotherapy as regimen of choice
  - Encouraging response to intense regimens, such as hyper CVAD, but relatively short-lived
  - Patients with skin-only disease frequently experience relapse with more aggressive systemic disease
    - Localized therapies are considered palliative with very limited use
- Hematopoietic stem cell (HSC) transplantation
  - Allogeneic HSC transplantation
    - Patients may achieve long-term remissions if allografted in complete remission, but rate of relapse is high
  - Autologous HSC transplantation
    - Paucity of published data for selection of patients who may benefit from high-dose therapy followed by autologous HSC transplantation
    - Patients with chemorefractory disease or bone marrow involvement may not achieve durable remission after autologous transplantation

Prognosis
- Dismal prognosis with overall poor therapeutic response
- 3-year overall survival of ~ 40% with allogenic HSC transplantation per data from European Group for Blood and Marrow Transplantation

MOLECULAR

Cytogenetics
- Complex karyotype (≥ 3 chromosomal aberrations) in ~ 30% of cases
- Chromosomal losses are common and include
  - -13, -9, -15, -12p, -6q, -7, -5q, -3
- Chromosomal gains are less common than losses and include
  - +8, +12p, +1, +7, +6q, +20
- Most common recurrent chromosomal structural abnormalities
  - t(6;8)(p21;q24); *RUNX2::MYC*, t(2;8)(p12;q24), t(X;8)(q24;q24), t(3;8)(p25;q24), t(1;6)(q21;q23), t(8;14)(q24;q32); *IGH::MYC*, i(7)(q10), inv(9)(p12q13)
  - *MYC* rearrangements are most common structural abnormalities reported at 12% of total cases

Blastic Plasmacytoid Dendritic Cell Neoplasm

Molecular Genetics
- Recurrent mutations identified by targeted next-generation sequencing (NGS) panel
  - *TET2* and *ASXL1* mutations most common at 53% and 31%, respectively
  - Other common mutations include *ZRSR2*, *NRAS*, *CDKN2A*, *SRSF2*, *ATM*, *IKZF1*, and *CHD8*
  - Mutations in genes commonly seen in acute myeloid leukemia (AML) and other myeloid malignancies are also detected in BPCDCN, including
    – *IDH2*, *RUNX1*, *JAK2*, *NPM1*, *FLT3* ITD, and *DNMT3A*

MICROSCOPIC

Histologic Features
- Skin lesions
  - Predominant dermal infiltrate that spares epidermis
  - Perivascular and periadnexal aggregates of neoplastic cells
  - Extension into subcutaneous adipose tissue may be seen
  - Neoplastic infiltrate is composed of monotonous, medium-sized cells with fine chromatin and moderate amounts of cytoplasm
- Lymph nodes
  - May show partial or diffuse involvement
    – Partial involvement is typically interfollicular
    – Diffuse involvement completely effaces nodal architecture
- Peripheral blood
  - Circulating neoplastic cells resemble leukemic blasts of myeloid or lymphoid origin
- Bone marrow
  - Can be focal with clusters of tumor cells or interstitial infiltrate
  - May be extensively replaced in advanced disease

Cytologic Features
- Blast-like cytomorphology with high N:C ratio
- Resemble lymphoblasts or myeloblasts
- Moderate cytoplasm with microvacuoles uniformly distributed around nucleus (pearl necklace)

ANCILLARY TESTS

Histochemistry
- MPO(-), NSE(-)

Immunohistochemistry
- Expected positive markers
  - CD123, TCF4, TCL1, CD303, CD304, CD4, CD56
- Expected negative markers
  - CD3, CD14, CD19, CD34, lysozyme, MPO
- Immunophenotypic diagnostic criteria of BPCDCN (WHO HAEM5)
  - Expression of CD123 and 1 other PCDC marker (TCF4, TCL1, CD303, or CD304) in addition to CD4 &/or CD56

Flow Cytometry
- Distinct flow cytometric immunophenotyping of BPCDCN
  - Positive for HLA-DR, CD123 (bright), CD4, CD56
  - Negative for MPO, monocytic markers, and B- and T-cell lineage-defining markers
  - Basophils express CD123 but lack HLA-DR
  - Monocytes, some hematopoietic precursors, and AML blasts are positive for both CD123 and HLA-DR, but expression level of CD123 is significantly lower that that of plasmacytoid dendritic cells
  - CD45 is negative or very dim positive

In Situ Hybridization
- EBER is consistently negative

Antigen Receptor Genes
- Immunoglobulin heavy chain gene (*IGH*) is germline
- T-cell receptor genes (*TRB* and *TRG*) are germline

DIFFERENTIAL DIAGNOSIS

Acute Leukemias (Acute Myeloid Leukemia and Acute Lymphocytic Leukemia)
- Morphologic and immunophenotypic overlap in subset of AML cases with BPCDCN
  - TCF4, CD303, &/or TCL1 expression combined with absence of lineage-specific markers usually help to establish diagnosis of BPCDCN
- Mature plasmacytoid dendritic cell (PDC) proliferation in myeloid neoplasms
  - Expression of CD34 along with PDC markers recognized as feature of AML with PDC differentiation
- Features useful in distinguishing lymphoblastic leukemia/lymphoma from BPCDCN
  - Expression of B-cell-associated antigens, including CD19 and CD79A, and uniform expression of TdT in B-lymphoblastic leukemia
  - Expression of T-cell-specific antigen, including cytoplasmic CD3 (cCD3), and variably positivity for other T-cell-associated antigens in T-lymphoblastic leukemia

Aggressive NK-Cell Leukemia
- Strong expression of CD56, similar to BPCDCN
- Virtually always associated with Epstein-Barr virus

Nodules of Plasmacytoid Dendritic Cells
- Can be seen in bone marrow biopsy in chronic myelomonocytic leukemia (CMML)
- Clonally related to the CMML
- CD123 highlights nodules

SELECTED REFERENCES

1. Pemmaraju N et al: North American Blastic Plasmacytoid Dendritic Cell Neoplasm Consortium: position on standards of care and areas of need. Blood. 141(6):567-78, 2023
2. Ohgami RS et al: An analysis of the pathologic features of blastic plasmacytoid dendritic cell neoplasm based on a comprehensive literature database of cases. Arch Pathol Lab Med. 147(7):837-46, 2023
3. Khoury JD et al: The 5th edition of the World Health Organization classification of haematolymphoid tumours: myeloid and histiocytic/dendritic neoplasms. Leukemia. 36(7):1703-19, 2022
4. Wang W et al: Immunophenotypic characterization of reactive and neoplastic plasmacytoid dendritic cells permits establishment of a 10-color flow cytometric panel for initial workup and residual disease evaluation of blastic plasmacytoid dendritic cell neoplasm. Haematologica. 106(4):1047-55, 2021
5. Sumarriva Lezama L et al: An analysis of blastic plasmacytoid dendritic cell neoplasm with translocations involving the MYC locus identifies t(6;8)(p21;q24) as a recurrent cytogenetic abnormality. Histopathology. 73(5):767-76, 2018
6. Wang S et al: Blastic plasmacytoid dendritic cell neoplasm: update on therapy especially novel agents. Ann Hematol. 97(4):563-72, 2018

Blastic Plasmacytoid Dendritic Cell Neoplasm

Cutaneous Disease

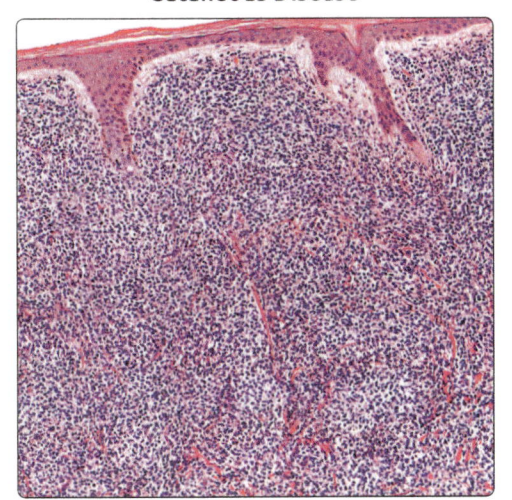

Cutaneous Disease

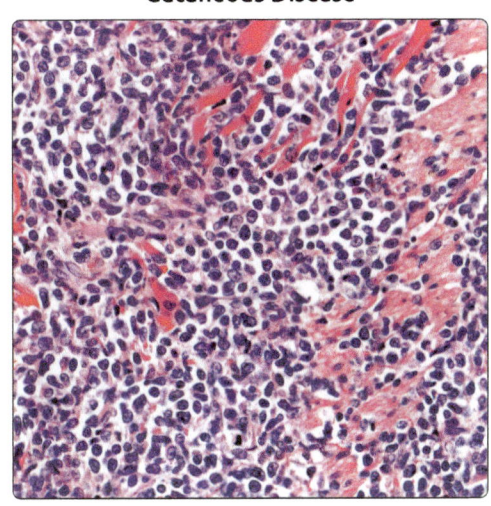

(Left) Skin biopsy from a patient with cutaneous BPCDCN reveals extensive superficial and deep dermal effacement by neoplastic infiltrate. The overlying epidermis is intact. **(Right)** High-power view of dermal infiltrate by BPCDCN shows a diffuse distribution of monotonous-appearing, medium-sized cells with immature nuclei and scant cytoplasm. The neoplastic cells lacked B- and T-cell-associated antigens.

CD4 Expression

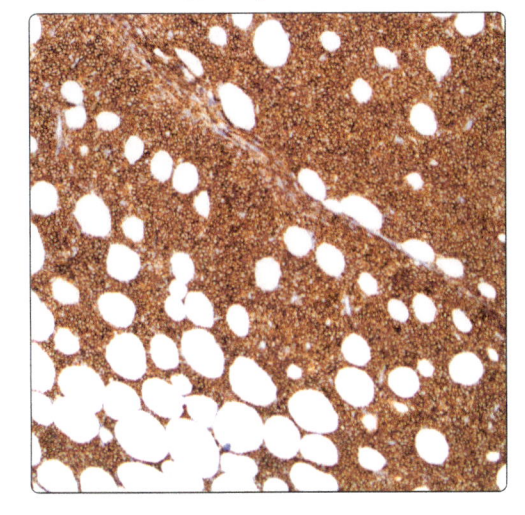

TCL1 Expression

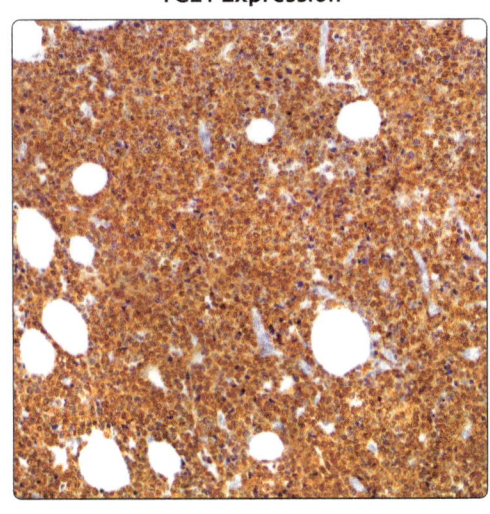

(Left) CD4 shows uniform expression by neoplastic cells of BPCDCN in the deep dermis with extension to subcutaneous tissue. **(Right)** TCL1 shows diffuse nuclear expression by neoplastic cells of BPCDCN within the dermis and subcutaneous tissue in this patient with disseminated disease. The neoplastic cells also expressed CD56.

CD33 Expression

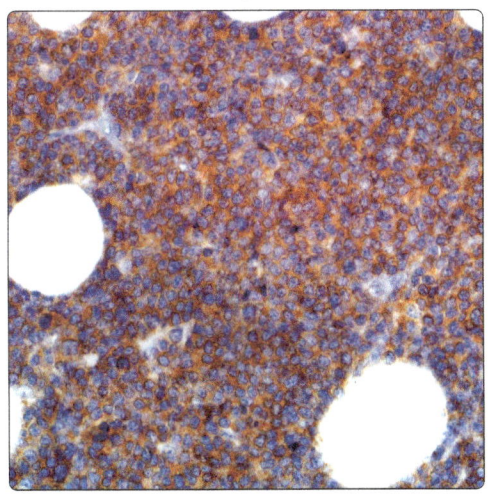

CD123 Expression

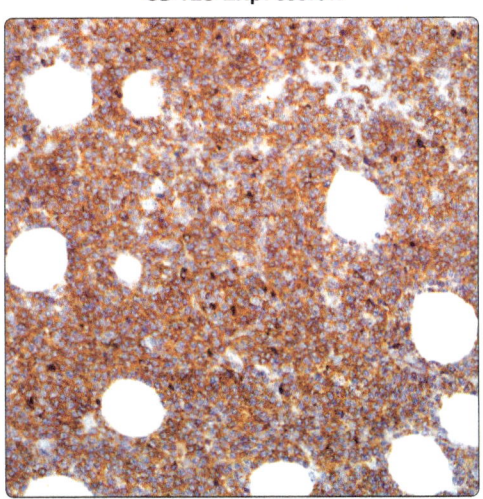

(Left) Dim expression of CD33 by neoplastic cells of BPCDCN is shown. Expression of this myeloid-associated antigen can be seen in subsets of BPCDCN. **(Right)** CD123 shows moderate expression by neoplastic cells in this case of cutaneous BPCDCN. CD123 is typically expressed in BPCDCN; however, it is not entirely specific for this neoplasm. Occasional myeloblasts and, rarely, lymphoblasts may also express this antigen.

Blastic Plasmacytoid Dendritic Cell Neoplasm

(Left) Lymph node from a patient with disseminated BPCDCN shows sheets of neoplastic cells in interfollicular areas surrounding an intact lymphoid follicle with a reactive, polarized germinal center. (Right) CD4 shows moderate expression among neoplastic cells in this lymph node involved by BPCDCN. Bright CD4(+) cells within uninvolved germinal center represent reactive T-helper cells.

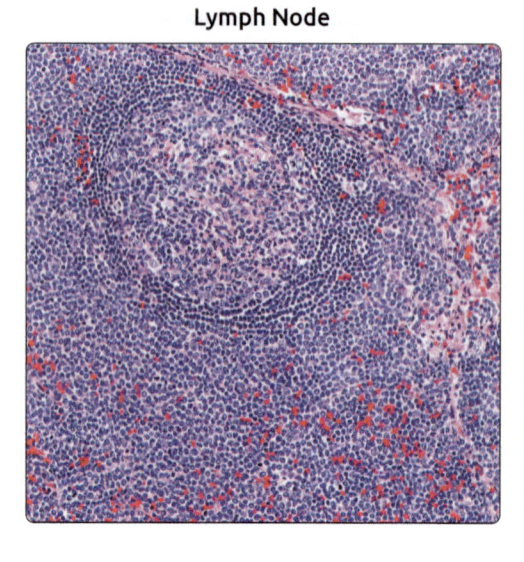

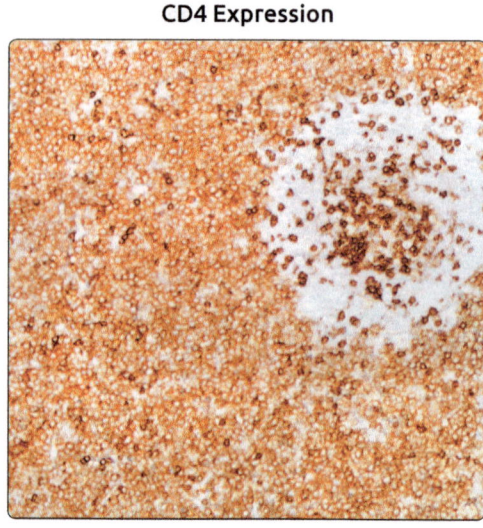

(Left) CD56 shows variable expression among neoplastic cells in this lymph node involved by BPCDCN. Rarely, expression of CD56 may be absent, but the diagnosis of BPCDCN can still be made if the neoplastic cells express CD4, CD123, and TCL1. (Right) Bright expression of CD123 is evident in this lymph node with extensive involvement by BPCDCN. Neoplastic cells also expressed CD4 and TCL1.

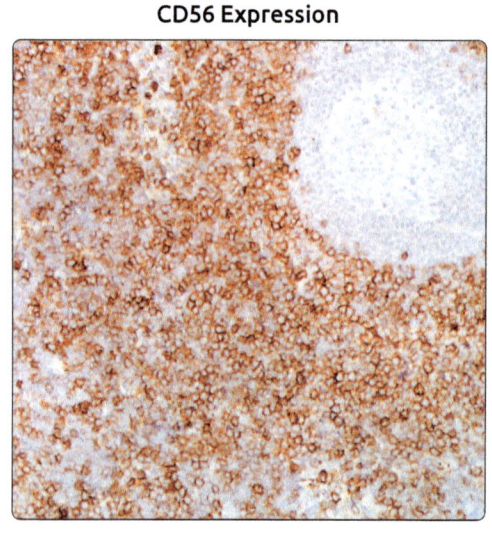

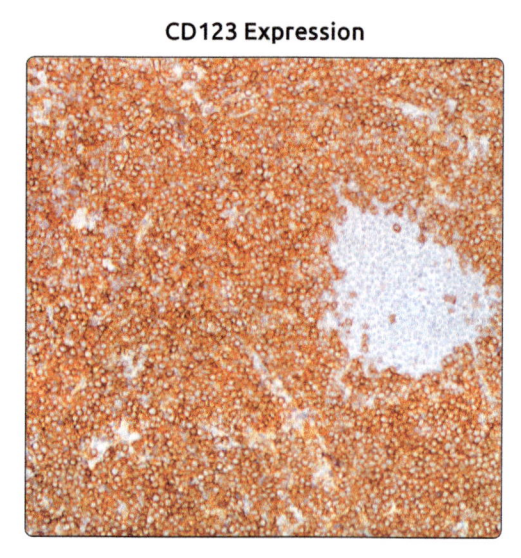

(Left) Moderate nuclear expression of TCL1 is shown in BPCDCN involving lymph node. Bright TCL1(+) cells with reactive germinal center represent nonneoplastic background T cells. (Right) Expression of CD33 is seen in this lymph node involved by BPCDCN. This myeloid-associated antigen is occasionally expressed in BPCDCN. To avoid an erroneous diagnosis of AML, CD33 expression must always be interpreted along with CD4, CD56, CD123, and TCL1 expression.

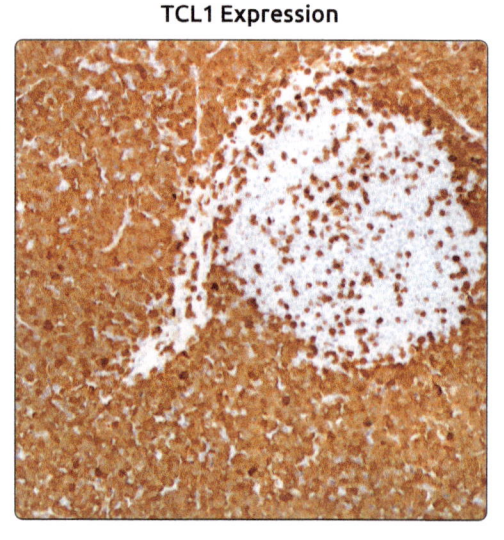

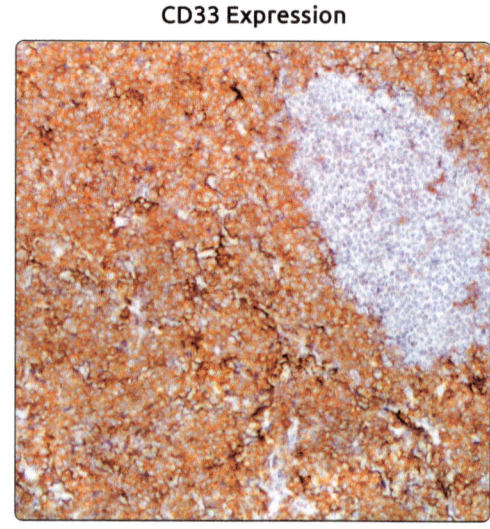

Blastic Plasmacytoid Dendritic Cell Neoplasm

Severe Thrombocytopenia and Blast-Like Cells

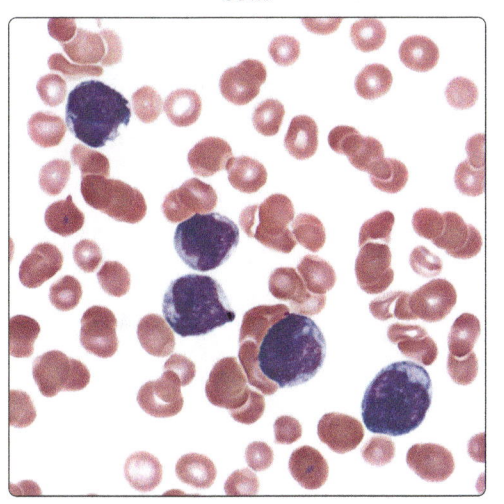

Blasts With High N:C Ratio

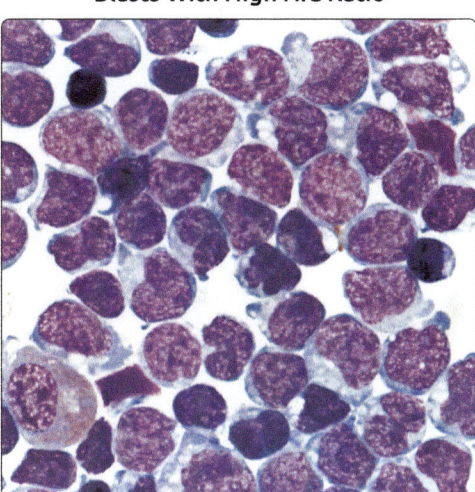

(Left) Wright-stained peripheral blood smear from a patient in leukemic phase of BPCDCN shows severe thrombocytopenia and circulating blast-like cells with irregular to lobated nuclei, immature chromatin, and scant agranular cytoplasm resembling lymphoblasts. (Right) Wright-stained cytospin preparation of marrow aspirate from a patient with BPCDCN shows numerous blasts with high N:C ratio and irregular nuclei with immature chromatin resembling monocytic blasts.

Flow Histogram: CD45

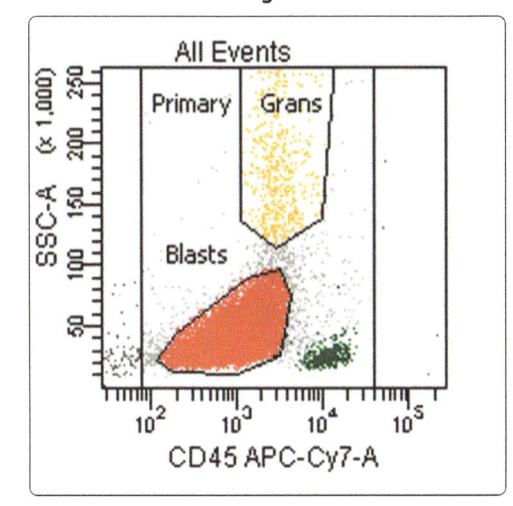

Flow Histogram: CD33 vs. CD34

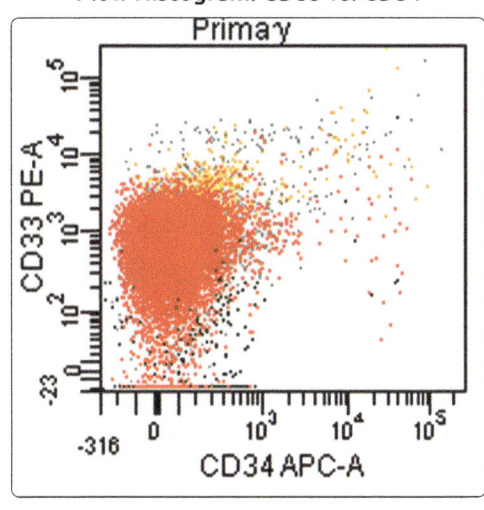

(Left) Flow cytometric analysis of bone marrow from a patient with leukemic presentation of BPCDCN reveals a prominent CD45 dim to negative population that falls in blast gate (red color event). (Right) Flow cytometric immunophenotyping of bone marrow with BPCDCN shows that the blasts are CD34(-) but dim CD33(+). CD33 is occasionally expressed with variable intensity in this neoplasm and needs to be interpreted in a panel to avoid misinterpretation.

Flow Histogram: CD4

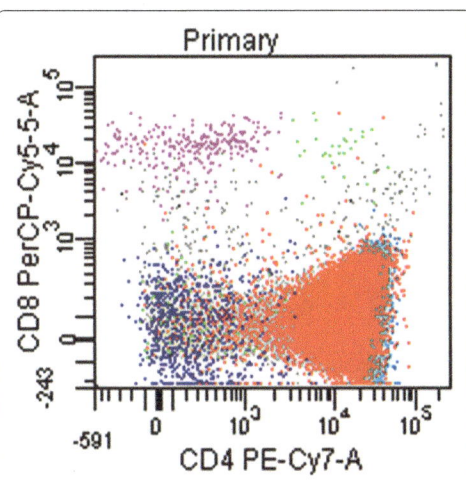

Flow Histogram: CD117 vs. CD56

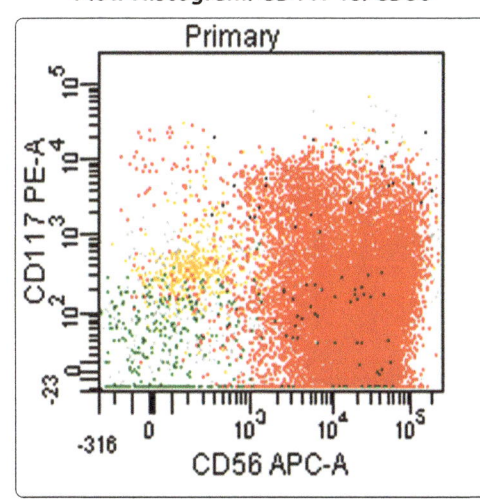

(Left) Bright expression of CD4 is evident in neoplastic cells of BPCDCN in this bone marrow aspirate. CD4 is expressed in almost all BPCDCN; however, CD4 expression is nonspecific, and interpretation should be performed along with a panel of antibodies that includes CD56, CD123, and TCL1. (Right) Bright expression of CD56 is present in this bone marrow aspirate from a case of BPCDCN. CD56 may be absent in BPCDCN, but the diagnosis can still be made if cells are CD4(+), CD123(+), and TCL1(+).

Molecular Pathology of Myeloid Neoplasms

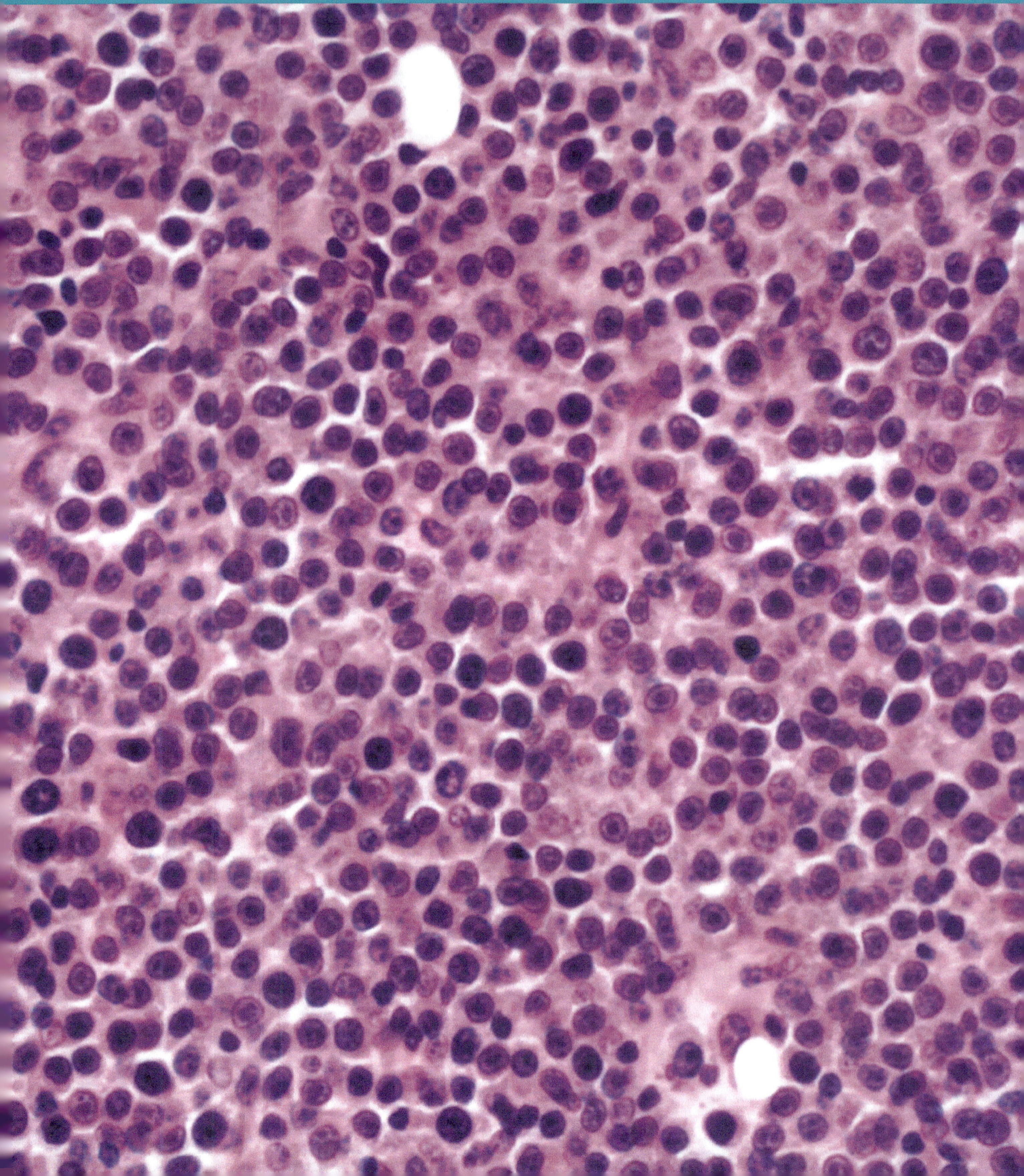

SECTION 6
Molecular Pathology of Lymphoid Neoplasms

Overview of Lymphoid Neoplasms	292
Molecular Work-Up of Lymphoid Neoplasms	296

Determination of Clonality in B-, T-, and NK-Cell Neoplasms

Lymphoma-Associated Chromosomal Translocations	298

Precursor Lymphoid Neoplasms

B-Lymphoblastic Leukemia/Lymphoma With Recurrent Genetic Abnormalities	302
B-Lymphoblastic Leukemia/Lymphoma, *BCR::ABL1*-Like (Ph-Like ALL)	306
T-Lymphoblastic Leukemia/Lymphoma	310

Mature B-Cell Neoplasms

Small Lymphocytic Lymphoma/Chronic Lymphocytic Leukemia	316
B-Cell Prolymphocytic Leukemia	322
Splenic Marginal Zone Lymphoma	326
Hairy Cell Leukemia	332
Splenic B-Cell Lymphoma/Leukemia, Unclassifiable	336
Lymphoplasmacytic Lymphoma	344
Monoclonal Gammopathy of Undetermined Significance	350
Multiple Myeloma (Plasma Cell Myeloma)	354
Follicular Lymphoma	362
Mantle Cell Lymphoma	370
Diffuse Large B-Cell Lymphoma	376
Burkitt Lymphoma	386

Mature T- and NK-Cell Neoplasms

T-Cell Prolymphocytic Leukemia	394
Chronic Lymphoproliferative Disorder of NK Cells	398
Aggressive NK-Cell Leukemia	402
Extranodal NK-/T-Cell Lymphoma	406
Adult T-Cell Leukemia/Lymphoma	410
Intestinal T-Cell Lymphoma	416
Hepatosplenic T-Cell Lymphoma	424
Subcutaneous Panniculitis-Like T-Cell Lymphoma	428
Mycosis Fungoides/Sézary Syndrome	432
Primary Cutaneous CD30-Positive T-Cell Lymphoproliferative Disorders	438
Peripheral T-Cell Lymphoma, NOS	442
Nodal Follicular Helper T-Cell Lymphoma	448
Anaplastic Large Cell Lymphoma, ALK-Negative	456
Anaplastic Large Cell Lymphoma, ALK-Positive	462

Overview of Lymphoid Neoplasms

TERMINOLOGY

Definitions
- B- and T-/NK-cell neoplasms are clonal lymphoid proliferations of mature and immature B cells, T cells, and NK cells at various stages of differentiation
  - Lymphoid neoplasms appear to recapitulate normal stages of B-cell and T-cell development
  - Clonality difficult to document in NK-cell neoplasms

Classifications
- 2 classifications used for diagnosis
  - International Consensus Classification (ICC)
  - World Health Organization (WHO) 5th edition
    - Previous revised 4th edition of WHO may still be used

Abbreviations
- Precursor lymphoid neoplasms
  - B-lymphoblastic leukemia/lymphoma (B-ALL/B-LBL)
    - Clonal neoplasms of immature lymphocytes committed to B-cell lineage
  - T-lymphoblastic leukemia/lymphoma (T-ALL/T-LBL)
    - Clonal neoplasms of immature lymphocytes committed to T-cell lineage
- Mature B-cell lymphoid neoplasms (B-NHL)
  - Heterogeneous group of clonal mature B-cell neoplasms
- Classic Hodgkin lymphoma (CHL)
  - Clonal mature B-cell neoplasms of germinal center origin
- Mature T-cell lymphoid neoplasms (T-NHL)
  - Heterogeneous group of clonal mature T-cell neoplasms

EPIDEMIOLOGY

Age Range
- B-ALL/B-LBL
  - Seen primarily in early childhood with male predominance
  - With increasing age, outcomes decline
  - Infant forms are seen
- T-ALL/T-LBL
  - Peak incidence in preadolescent male children
  - Can be seen in tissue or blood
- T-NHL
  - Disease of older individuals
- B-NHL
  - Wide age range
- Classic HL
  - Young adults commonly

Incidence
- Mature lymphomas
  - B-cell more common than T-cell lymphoma
    - In order of occurrence: Diffuse large B-cell lymphoma, follicular, marginal zone, classic HL, mantle cell, Burkitt, T-cell lymphoma (all types), and nodular lymphocyte-predominant B-cell lymphoma (ICC)
  - Non-HL more common than HL
  - M > F in most subtypes
  - No sex difference in survival
- Precursor B-ALL and T-ALL
  - B-ALL much more common than T-ALL
  - Leukemia is common malignancy in children < 20 years of age; highest in children 1-4 years of age
  - Highest rates of B-ALL in Hispanic patients
    - Difference in rates between Hispanic and non-Hispanic children highest in older age group (> 4 years of age), particularly in adolescents
  - In order of occurrence: Hispanic, non-Hispanic White, Black, and other ethnic groups
  - Slight male predominance

ETIOLOGY/PATHOGENESIS

Histogenesis
- Lymphoid neoplasms are heterogeneous entities derived from common progenitor clones, which mirror complexity of immune system
  - Pathogenesis is also heterogeneous and involves varying genetic abnormalities
- Precursor B- and T-cell neoplasms
  - Chromosomal abnormalities observed in significant number of cases

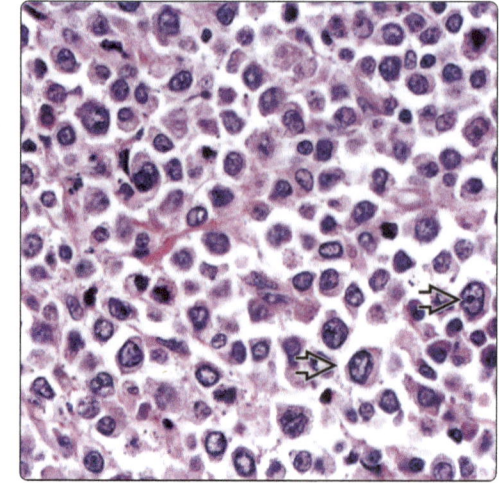

(Left) B-lymphoblastic leukemia/lymphoma involving lymph node is shown. TdT, CD34, CD19, and CD10 are positive by IHC. The cells have fine chromatin ➡, and mitoses are present ➡. Studies including FISH, cytogenetics, and NGS may be used for further characterization. (Right) Diffuse large B-cell lymphoma shows plasmacytoid differentiation ➡. The cells were CD20 positive and CD5 and CD10 negative by IHC. FISH can further classify this lymphoma into GCB or non-GCB subtypes.

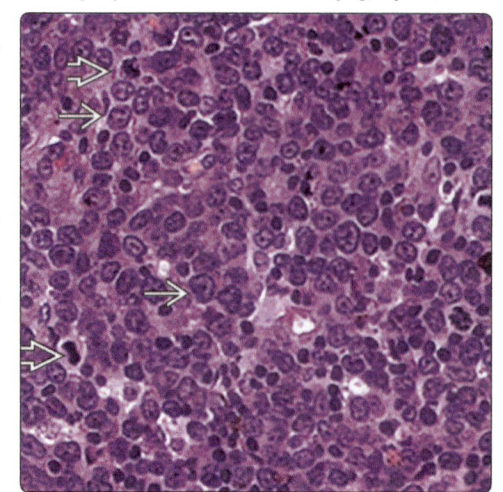

B-Lymphoblastic Leukemia/Lymphoma

Diffuse Large B-Cell Lymphoma, Not Otherwise Specified

Overview of Lymphoid Neoplasms

- Most chromosomal normal cases have other genetic abnormalities
- Epidemiologic studies suggest ALL may begin in utero
- Rarely associated with hereditary cancer syndromes
- B-NHL
  - Many mature B-cell lymphomas have specific translocations
  - Immunocompromise predisposes to B-NHL
  - EBV may play role and often indicates immunodeficiency
- T-NHL
  - Unknown etiology
  - Consistent genetic abnormalities may be seen but are less common than in B-NHL
  - Ethnic groups are predisposed to some forms

CLINICAL IMPLICATIONS

Clinical Presentation
- Precursor T- and B-cell neoplasms are acute and usually aggressive if not treated
- Mature B-cell neoplasms range from indolent to aggressive, depending on classification and genetics
- Mature T-cell neoplasms are usually aggressive with rare exceptions that show indolent behavior

Treatment
- Chemotherapy and, rarely, radiation if localized
- Immunotherapy has become common
- Molecular genetic findings may lead to targeted therapy

MOLECULAR PATHOLOGY

TRG, *TRB*, and *IGH* Rearrangements
- PCR-based studies
- Detect clonality in B- and T-cell mature and precursor neoplasms
- Have become important in diagnosis of mature T- and B-cell neoplasms to confirm clonality
- HL can have clonal gene rearrangement studies, particularly with newer modalities

Fluorescent In Situ Hybridization
- Used to detect translocations and specific cytogenetic abnormalities in both mature and precursor B- and T-cell neoplasms
  - Examples include many small B-cell lymphomas [e.g., mantle cell t(11;14), follicular lymphoma t(14;18)]
- Does not detect all cytogenetic abnormalities
- Different FISH panels can detect most common abnormalities in B- and T-cell neoplasms

Conventional Cytogenetic Studies
- Used for broad cytogenetic screening in both precursor and mature B- and T-cell neoplasms
  - Examples include cases of T-cell lymphoma, B-ALL, and T-ALL that show complex cytogenetics
- Does not detect cryptic genetic findings
- Does not always detect balanced translocations

Polymerase Chain Reaction
- PCR-based tests are often used to detect genetic mutations
  - Examples include *BRAF* mutation for hairy cell leukemia and *STAT3* mutation for T-large granular lymphocyte leukemia

Array Comparative Genomic Hybridization
- Used to detect gains and losses of chromosomes
  - Examples include chronic lymphocytic leukemia/small lymphocytic lymphoma (losses in 6p, 8p, 14q32, 18q and gains in 10p)
- Translocations are not easily detected

DNA Microarray Technology
- Used to detect abnormalities in key cellular pathways
  - Examples include diffuse large B-cell lymphoma, which can be split into activated and germinal center types for prognosis
- Used to interrogate genetic alterations in genome-wide fashion
- Used for broad assessment of classified lymphoid neoplasms

Genomic Sequencing
- Detects mutations and abnormalities that cannot be identified with conventional karyotyping or FISH
- Has changed our understanding of pathogenesis of B- and T-cell neoplasms
  - e.g., *BRAF* V600E mutation in hairy cell leukemia
- Conventional sequencing
  - Sanger sequencing
  - Pyrosequencing

Next-Generation Sequencing
- Analyzes large numbers of genes in panels
  - Genes of interest must be included in panel
- Useful in both mature and precursor lymphoid lesions
- Rapidly becoming cost effective for clinical use
- Key genetic alterations in lymphoid neoplasms
  - T-ALL: *PHF6*, *CNOT3*, *RPL5*, *RPL10*
  - *BCR::ABL1*-like B-ALL: JAK mutations with rearrangements of *CRLF2*, *ABL1*, *ABL2*, *EPOR*, and *PDGFRB*
  - Hypodiploid B-ALL: RAS mutations (*NRAS*, *KRAS*), *NF1*, *PTPN11* in near haploid; *IKZF2*, and *TP53* mutations in low haploid; *TP53* germline
  - Relapsed B-ALL: *CREBBP* mutations, *NT5C2* mutations
  - Diffuse large B-cell lymphoma and non-HL: Gene alterations of *CD79B*/*CD79A*, NF-kB pathway signaling (*CARD11*, *MYD88*), histone modification (*CREBBP*/*EP300*, *EZH2*, *MEF2B*, *KMT2D*/*KMT2C*), *TP53*
  - Splenic marginal zone lymphoma: *NOTCH2*, *KLF2* mutations
  - Mantle cell lymphoma: *NOTCH1*, *BIRC3* mutation
  - CHL: *CIITA* rearrangements
  - Primary mediastinal large B-cell lymphoma: *CIITA* mutation
  - Chronic lymphocytic leukemia: *NOTCH1* mutation, mRNA splicing mutation (*SF3B1*), DNA damage and repair (*ATM*, *POT1*), regulation of apoptosis (*BIRC3*), innate immunity (*MYD88*, *TLR2*)
  - Hairy cell leukemia: *BRAF* mutations

Overview of Lymphoid Neoplasms

Common Genetic Abnormalities and Molecular Tests for Clinical Use

Disease	Common Genetic Abnormalities	Genes Involved	Common Methods of Detection
Mature B-Cell Neoplasms			
Chronic lymphocytic leukemia	11q32 loss; trisomy 12; 13q14 loss; 17p loss	NOTCH1 (most frequent); TP53	FISH, array comparative genomic hybridization (aCGH)
Follicular lymphoma	t(14;18)	BCL2::IGH	FISH
Mantle cell lymphoma	t(11;14)	IGH::CCND1	FISH
Lymphoplasmacytic lymphoma	MYD88 L265P or CXCR4 mutation	MYD88, CXCR4	PCR (pyrosequencing, allele specific PCR), Sanger sequencing, NGS
Marginal zone B-cell lymphoma (MALT lymphoma)	t(11;18), t(14;18), t(3;14)	BIRC3::MALT1; IGH::MALT1; IGH::FOXP1	FISH
High-grade B-cell lymphoma (HGBCL) with MYC, BCL2, &/or BCL6 rearrangements (ICC)	MYC::BCL2 rarely MYC::BCL2::BCL6	MYC, BCL2, BCL6	FISH, break-apart
Diffuse large B-cell lymphoma	t(14;18);t(3;14); t(2;3);t(8;14)	BCL2::IGH, IGH::BCL6; IGL::BCL6; IGK::BCL6; IGH::MYC	FISH, NGS, gene microarray
Burkitt lymphoma	t(8;14);t(2;8);t(8;22)	IGH::MYC; MYC::IGK; MYC::IGL	FISH, conventional karyotype
Multiple myeloma (plasma cell myeloma) (ICC); plasma cell myeloma (WHO)	t(11;14);t(6;14);t(4;14); t(4;16); t(14;20)	IGH::CCND1; IGH::CCND3; IGH::NSD2, IGH::MAF, IGH::MAFB	FISH, conventional karyotyping
Hairy cell leukemia	BRAF V600E mutation	TP53 (rare)	PCR (pyrosequencing, allele-specific PCR), Sanger sequencing
T-large granular lymphocytic leukemia	STAT3 mutation	STAT3 or STAT5B	Gene array, Sanger sequencing
Anaplastic large cell lymphoma	t(2;5), t(1;2), t(2;22), inv(2), t(2;3), t(2;17), t(2;X), .6p25.3 rearrangements	NPM1::ALK; TPM3::ALK; MYH9::ALK; ATIC::ALK; TFG::ALK; CLTC::ALK; MSN::ALK; DUSP22/IRF4	FISH
Chronic lymphoproliferative disorder of NK cells (ICC); NK-cell large granular lymphocytic leukemia (WHO)	STAT3; TET2 and CCL22 mutations (common); TNFAIP3 and JAK3	STAT3 or STAT5B	Gene array, Sanger sequencing
T-prolymphocytic leukemia	inv(14), t(4;14), structural abnormalities of 14q32; t(X;14)	TCL1A or TCL1B or MTCP1	FISH, conventional karyotyping
Hepatosplenic T-cell lymphoma	Isochromosome 7q	STAT5B	FISH, conventional karyotyping
Adult T-cell leukemia/lymphoma	Integrated HTLV-I	CIC or REL	PCR
B-ALL/B-LBL (various subtypes)	t(1;19); t(12;21); t(9;22); t(4;11), hyperdiploid, hypodiploid	TCF3::PBX1; ETV6::RUNX1; BCR::ABL1; KMT2A::AFF1; IGH/IL3	FISH, conventional karyotyping
T-ALL/T-LBL (various subtypes)	1p32 deletion; t(1;14); t(10;14); t(7;10); t(5;14)	STIL::TAL1; TRD::TAL1; TRD::TLX1; TRD::TLX3	FISH, conventional karyotyping

- o Plasma cell myeloma: Multiple targets of mutation (NRAS, KRAS, TP53, CCND1, DIS3, BRAF), signaling, and histone modification
- o Lymphoplasmacytic lymphoma: MYD88, CXCR4 mutations

ANCILLARY TESTS

Flow Cytometry

- Diagnostic tool for immunophenotyping in fresh tissue
- Differentiates subtypes of precursor and mature B- and T-cell lymphoma
- Immunohistochemistry is sometimes necessary to confirm even after flow cytometry

Immunohistochemistry

- Diagnostic tool in paraffin section for immunophenotyping
- Differentiates subtypes of precursor and mature B- and T-cell lymphoma
- Used in cases for which flow cytometry is nonspecific (i.e., classic HL)
- Immunohistochemical surrogate markers (i.e., BCL2, MYC, cyclin-D1) are used but cannot substitute for genetic tests

SELECTED REFERENCES

1. Alaggio R et al: The 5th edition of the World Health Organization classification of haematolymphoid tumours: lymphoid neoplasms. Leukemia. 36(7):1720-48, 2022
2. Campo E et al: The International Consensus Classification of mature lymphoid neoplasms: a report from the Clinical Advisory Committee. Blood. 140(11):1229-53, 2022
3. Morin RD et al: Molecular profiling in diffuse large B-cell lymphoma: why so many types of subtypes? Br J Haematol. 196(4):814-29, 2022
4. Jaffe ES: Diagnosis and classification of lymphoma: impact of technical advances. Semin Hematol. 56(1):30-6, 2019

Overview of Lymphoid Neoplasms

Flow Cytometry for NK-Cell Leukemia

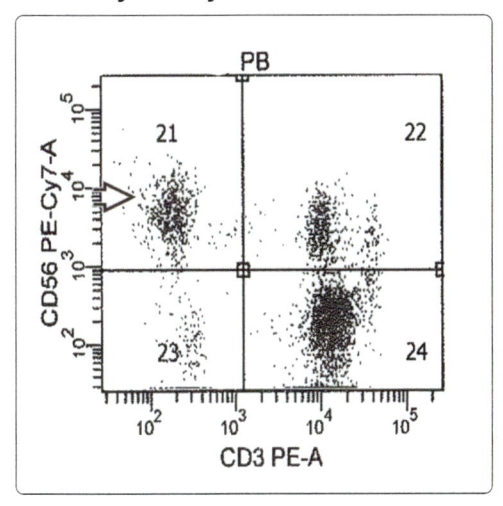

Dual-Fusion FISH Probe for *IGH/CCND1*

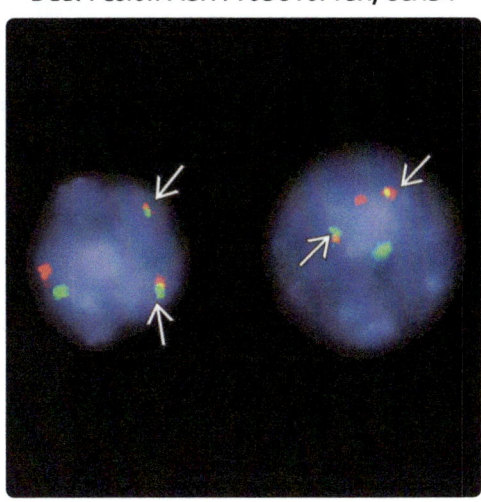

(Left) Flow cytometry for NK-cell leukemia is shown. Note the CD56-positive, CD3-negative cells ➡. Flow cytometry is the optimal clinical study for NK-cell leukemia. PCR detects STAT3 mutations in both chronic NK-cell leukemia and T-large granular lymphocyte leukemia. **(Right)** FISH studies of IgM myeloma show dual fusion for t(11;14) ➡. The probes used were IGH/CCND1 as evidenced by the yellow signals. FISH panels are used clinically for plasma cell myeloma.

t(14;18) Cytogenetic Karyotype

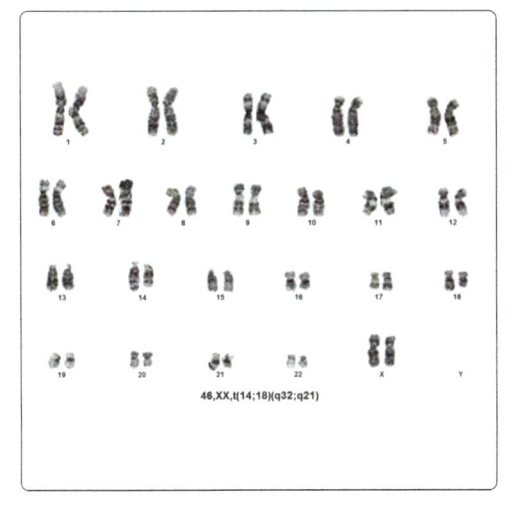

Dual-Fusion FISH Probe for *IGH/BCL2*

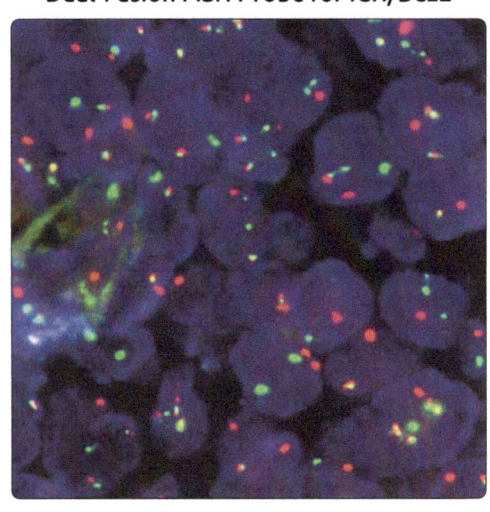

(Left) Conventional cytogenetic testing of a follicular lymphoma shows t(14;18)(q32;q21). This study has been largely replaced by FISH in both paraffin tissue or fresh tissue to diagnose follicular lymphoma. **(Right)** FISH was performed on lymph node with follicular lymphoma using dual-fusion probes for BCL2 (red) and IGH (green). A yellow fusion signal indicates the presence of t(14;18)(q32;q21)/IGH/BCL2.

T-Cell Receptor γ-Gene Rearrangement

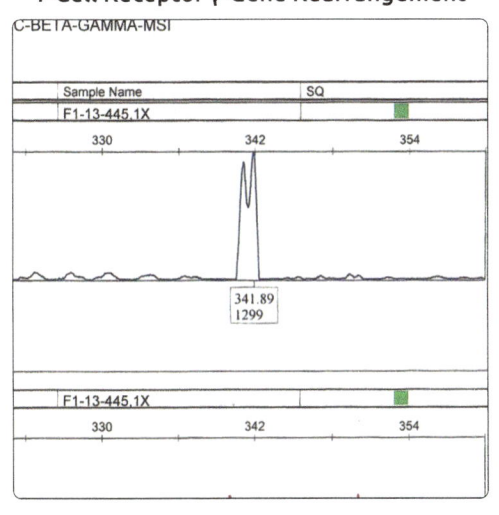

Pyrosequencing for *BRAF* V600E

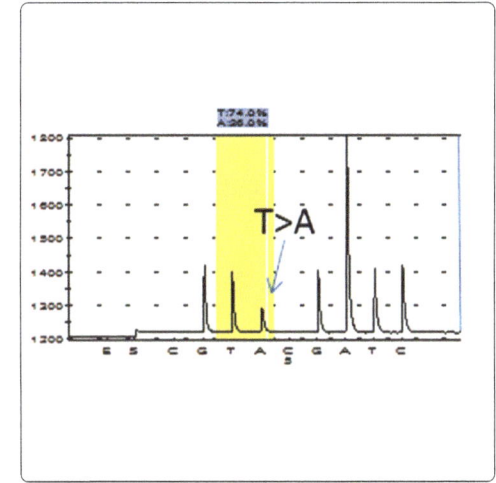

(Left) Dominant monoclonal peak is seen on PCR testing for T-cell receptor γ at position 341. The peak indicates that there is a clonal process. This test supports a diagnosis of T-cell lymphoma. **(Right)** Detection of mutation of BRAF V600 by pyrosequencing, which is common in hairy cell leukemia. The mutation occurs due to T>A change. BRAF mutation, along with morphology and immunophenotype, has helped define hairy cell leukemia.

Molecular Work-Up of Lymphoid Neoplasms

MOLECULAR/GENETIC TECHNIQUES COMMONLY USED

Clonality Testing
- Application of PCR-based molecular analysis unique to work-up of lymphoid neoplasms
- Immunoglobulin molecules and T-cell receptors must recognize vast array of antigens
  - Accomplished by random selection of specific V regions, J regions, and in some cases D regions to join together within individual maturing lymphocytes
- Polyclonal population of lymphocytes is characterized by diversity at these rearranged regions
- Monoclonal population of lymphocytes shows single characteristic arrangement
- PCR using consensus primers generates products that can be sized using capillary or gel electrophoresis
  - Gaussian (bell-shaped) distribution of amplicon sizes in polyclonal lymphoid population
  - Single or double prominent peaks, usually standing out from polyclonal background in monoclonal lymphoid population

FISH
- Used to detect specific chromosomal translocations that can assist in diagnosis and subclassification of lymphoid neoplasms
  - Detection of CCND1::IGH in mantle cell lymphoma
- In most cases, because both partners in translocation are known, dual-color dual fusion probe sets are used
- Break-apart probe strategy can also be used (e.g., MYC break-apart probe) to detect rearrangement with immunoglobulin light chain partners or with heavy chain

Karyotype
- Identifies characteristic chromosomal translocations
  - May also identify abnormalities beyond those seen with usual targeted FISH probes
- Fresh tissue is required
- For most lymphoid neoplasms, stimulation with mitogens is required to induce neoplastic cells to divide

RT-PCR for Gene Fusions
- Available for common gene fusions such as IGH::BCL2
  - More suitable for the purpose of disease monitoring and minimal residual disease detection

Next-Generation Sequencing
- Whole-genome, exome, and targeted sequencing have identified many gene alterations in several subtypes of lymphomas
  - BRAF V600E mutation in hairy cell leukemia
  - MYD88 L265P, CXCR4, and ARID1A mutations in lymphoplasmacytic lymphoma
  - ATM, CCND1, KMT2D, and NOTCH1 mutations in mantle cell lymphoma
  - SF3B1, NOTCH1, TP53, ATM, BIRC3, POT1, and MYD88 mutations in 3-15% of chronic lymphocytic leukemia (CLL)
  - KLF2 and NOTCH2 mutations in splenic marginal zone lymphoma
  - EZH2, ARID1A, MEF2B, EP300, FOXO1, CREBBP, and CARD11 mutation analysis useful in clinical prognostication in follicular lymphoma
  - Other genes mutated in follicular lymphoma include EPHA7, BCL2, BCL6, TNFRSF14, and TNFAIP3
  - STAT3 mutations in T-cell large granular lymphocytic leukemia
  - ATM, TP53, JAK3, JAK1, and STAT5B mutations in T-cell prolymphocytic leukemia
  - PLCG1, PRKCB, VAV1, IRF4, FYN, CARD11, and STAT3 mutations in adult T-cell leukemia/lymphoma
  - SETD2, INO80, ARID1B, and STAT5B mutations in hepatosplenic T-cell lymphoma
  - TET2, IDH2, DNMT3A, and RHOA overlapping mutations and less common FYN, PLCG1, CD28, STAT3, and EP300 mutations in angioimmunoblastic T-cell lymphoma

Detection of Somatic Hypermutation
- Somatic hypermutation is physiologic process in which B cells randomly mutate their immunoglobulin heavy chain variable regions (IGHV) to produce molecule with greater affinity for given antigens

Karyotype of Mantle Cell Lymphoma

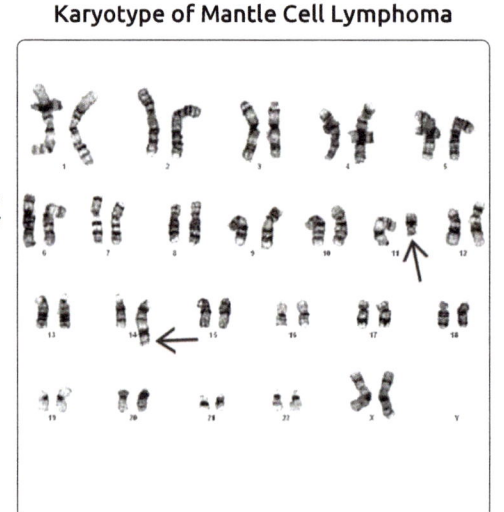

FISH Analysis for CCND1::IGH

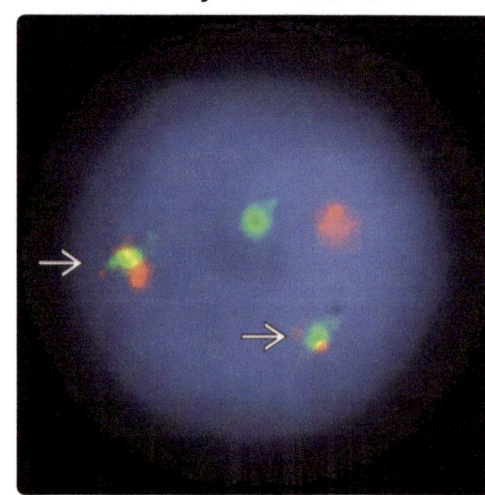

(Left) Karyotype in a case of mantle cell lymphoma shows t(11;14)(q13;q32) associated with fusion between the CCND1 and IGH genes. (Right) FISH using dual-color, dual-fusion probe shows CCND1::IGH fusion in a case of mantle cell lymphoma, as indicated by the presence of 2 fusion signals.

Molecular Work-Up of Lymphoid Neoplasms

- In this assay, heavy chain region sequence is obtained from clonal population and compared to closest germline sequence
  - Significant divergence from best matched germline sequence indicates that B-cell clone has undergone somatic hypermutation

PURPOSES OF MOLECULAR ANALYSIS

Establish Diagnosis
- Detection of specific abnormalities may establish presence of lymphoma
  - e.g., clonal T-cell receptor gene rearrangement may assist in identifying T-cell lymphoma

Establish Subtype of Lymphoma
- Certain molecular findings may help to establish presence of specific subtype of lymphoma
  - e.g., presence of *MYD88* mutation favors diagnosis of lymphoplasmacytic lymphoma

Establish Prognosis
- Certain molecular findings may refine prognostic expectations for patient
  - e.g., *IGHV* somatic hypermutation in CLL

Minimal Residual Disease detection
- Highly sensitive detection of specific *IGH* or T-cell receptor gene rearrangements using NGS
- Currently used in MRD detection in pediatric and young adults with acute lymphoblastic leukemia (ALL)

LIMITATIONS OF TECHNIQUES

Clonality Testing
- Clonal population is not always equivalent to neoplasm
  - Prominent clonal expansion can occur in reactive conditions (e.g., EBV infection)
  - Pseudoclonality can occur when sample has only scant lymphocytes
- Nonclonal population is not always equivalent to benign
  - Primer sets are optimized for broad detection (e.g., using framework regions) but may not bind in some cases
    - Particular problem in post germinal center B-cell lymphomas, in which somatic hypermutation may alter primer binding sites
- Clonal immunoglobulin region and T-cell receptor gene rearrangements may sometimes be detected in T-cell and B-cell lymphomas, respectively
  - May be due to background clonal or subclonal populations (e.g., B-cells in angioimmunoblastic T-cell lymphoma)
  - Rearrangement of T-cell receptor and immunoglobulin regions may occasionally occur in B cells and T cells, respectively known as lineage infidelity

FISH and PCR
- Only identify specific abnormalities targeted with given probe or primer set

Karyotype
- Obtaining karyotype from some types of lymphoma cells is difficult, even with mitogen stimulation
  - e.g., plasma cells in myeloma may not easily divide in culture

UTILITY OF TESTING METHODS FOR KEY LYMPHOID NEOPLASMS

B-Lymphoblastic Leukemia/Lymphoma
- Karyotype, FISH panel, and Ph-like signature testing critical for risk stratified treatment
- Highly sensitive MRD detection using NGS

Chronic Lymphocytic Leukemia
- FISH panel, *IGHV* somatic hypermutation, and *TP53* mutation analysis useful for prognosis

Lymphoplasmacytic Lymphoma
- *MYD88* mutation has relatively high sensitivity and specificity for this diagnosis

Plasma Cell Myeloma
- FISH panel and karyotype critical for risk stratification

Follicular Lymphoma
- Most cases positive for *BCL2::IGH* fusion associated with t(14;18)(q32;q21) by FISH or karyotype

Mantle Cell Lymphoma
- Almost all cases positive for *CCND1::IGH* fusion associated with t(11;14)(q13;q32) by FISH or karyotype

Burkitt Lymphoma
- Characteristic *MYC* rearrangement, most commonly in t(8;14) by FISH or karyotype

High-Grade B-Cell Lymphoma
- Double-/triple-hit lymphoma shows translocation of *MYC* as well as *BCL2* &/or *BCL6*
- Typically detected by FISH, though karyotype would also detect these abnormalities
- Markedly aggressive disease course, poorly responsive to standard therapies

T-Cell Prolymphocytic Leukemia
- Karyotype shows t(14;14)(q11;q32) or t(X;14)(q28;q11)

T-Cell Leukemias and Lymphomas (Multiple Subtypes)
- Clonality testing especially useful in distinguishing neoplastic from reactive T-cell infiltrates

Anaplastic Large Cell Lymphoma
- *ALK* rearrangement [most commonly *NPM1::ALK*, t(2;5)] seen in ALK-positive ALCL by FISH or karyotype
  - Not usually required if ALK is positive by IHC
- ALK-negative ALCL may show rearrangement of *TP63* and *DUSP22* by FISH with prognostic connotations

SELECTED REFERENCES

1. Alaggio R et al: The 5th edition of the World Health Organization classification of haematolymphoid tumours: lymphoid neoplasms. Leukemia. 36(7):1720-48, 2022
2. Campo E et al: The International Consensus Classification of mature lymphoid neoplasms: a report from the Clinical Advisory Committee. Blood. 140(11):1229-53, 2022
3. de Leval L et al: Genomic profiling for clinical decision making in lymphoid neoplasms. Blood. 140(21):2193-227, 2022

Lymphoma-Associated Chromosomal Translocations

TERMINOLOGY

Definitions
- Set of translocations seen in certain types of mostly mature B-cell and also some T-cell lymphomas
  - Some translocations are pathognomonic for specific subtype of lymphoma

T(11;14)(Q13;Q32); CCND1::IGH

Mantle Cell Lymphoma
- Must have *CCND1::IGH* or alternative translocation, by definition
  - Variants include translocations of *CCND1* with immunoglobulin light chains
  - Rare variants involve *CCND2*, *CCND3*, or *CCNE*
- *CCND1::IGH* rearrangement is considered primary genetic event in lymphomagenesis of MCL

Plasma Cell Neoplasms
- Monoclonal gammopathy of undetermined significance (MGUS)
- Plasma cell myeloma/multiple myeloma
  - Seen in ~ 15% of cases
  - Good prognosis in absence of additional genetic abnormalities

Pathogenesis
- Upregulation of cyclin D1 due to placement of *CCND1* next to *IGH* promoter

Prognosis
- Worse in mantle cell lymphoma with accumulation of additional translocations, such as *MYC* rearrangements

Methods of Detection
- FISH cytogenetic method is most sensitive and specific
- Conventional karyotyping also detects t(11;14) in most cases
- Cyclin D1 positivity by IHC generally correlates with 11;14 translocation
  - Some exceptions apply, including weak expression in hairy cell leukemia, which does **not** have this translocation

T(14;18)(Q32;Q21); IGH::BCL2

Follicular Lymphoma
- Incidence
  - *IGH::BCL2* present in up to 90% of low-grade follicular lymphomas
  - Lower incidence in high-grade follicular lymphoma
    - "Follicular large B-cell lymphoma" per WHO-HAEM5 and "follicular lymphoma, grade 3B" per 2022 ICC
  - Pediatric-type follicular lymphoma is usually negative for *IGH::BCL2*
  - Primary cutaneous follicle center lymphoma generally do not exhibit *IGH::BCL2* rearrangements
- Alternative translocations of *BCL2* with immunoglobulin light chains have also been rarely reported

Diffuse Large B-Cell Lymphoma
- Incidence
  - 20-30% of cases
- Usually indicates germinal center B-cell subtype
- May represent transformation of underlying follicular lymphoma

Incidental Finding
- *IGH::BCL2* rearrangement can be found at very low levels by very sensitive RT-PCR methods in blood of healthy individuals
  - Incidence of 25-75% in healthy individuals
    - Usually no increased risk or apparent progression to lymphoma
    - Similarly, can be found in reactive lymph nodes

Prognosis
- *IGH::BCL2* by itself does not appear to change prognosis
- Worse prognosis with additional mutations, such as *MYC* rearrangement

---

Karyotype of Mantle Cell Lymphoma

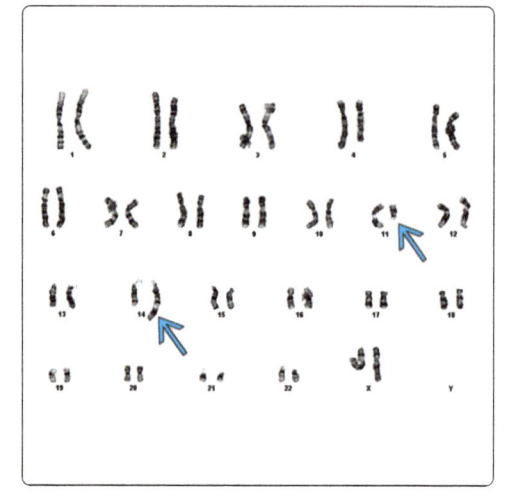

Cyclin-D1 in Hairy Cell Leukemia

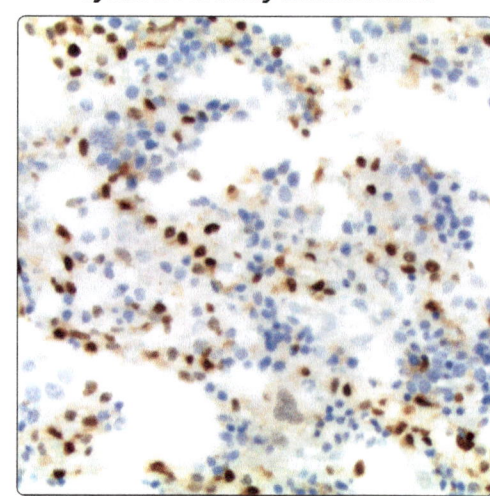

(Left) *In this case of mantle cell lymphoma involving peripheral blood, karyotype shows the t(11;14)(q23;q32) translocation ➡ that fuses CCND1 and IGH and is pathognomonic of this disease.* **(Right)** *This case of hairy cell leukemia shows weak and partial cyclin-D1 expression on bone marrow core biopsy but lacks the CCND1::IGH rearrangement (not shown) typical of mantle cell lymphoma.*

Lymphoma-Associated Chromosomal Translocations

Methods of Detection
- FISH is sensitive and specific
- Gene expression profiling (GEP)
  - DLBCL cases with *BCL2* rearrangement often show germinal center subtype on GEP
  - Not commonly performed except in research setting
- Conventional karyotyping
- RT-PCR (rarely used)

BCL6 REARRANGEMENTS

Follicular Lymphoma
- Incidence: 5-20%
- Often in addition to *IGH*::*BCL2* rearrangement
- More common in high-grade cases
- *BCL6* located at 3q27
- Many partners, including *IGH*, *IGK*, and *IGL*
- ~ 20 nonimmunoglobulin partners, including *MBNL1* and *IL21R*

Diffuse Large B-Cell Lymphoma
- Incidence: Up to 30%
  - Most common translocation in DLBCL

Prognosis
- Unclear, conflicting data

Method of Detection
- FISH break-apart probe is most commonly used strategy

MYC REARRANGEMENTS

Burkitt Lymphoma
- Most cases involve classic t(8;14)(q24;q32) resulting in *MYC*::*IGH* fusion
- Less commonly, *MYC* is fused with *IGK* or *IGL*
- Up to 10% may be negative by FISH methods
  - Case must have otherwise completely typical morphology and immunophenotype to be classified as Burkitt lymphoma

Diffuse Large B-Cell Lymphoma
- Incidence
  - Up to 10%
- Cases have otherwise typical DLBCL morphology and phenotype and do not meet criteria for Burkitt lymphoma or "double-hit" lymphoma

Double-Hit Lymphomas
- Defined by *MYC* translocation plus *BCL2* rearrangement
- High proliferation rate
- Aggressive disease course
- Morphology may resemble Burkitt lymphoma, DLBCL, or "blastic" transformation of follicular lymphoma

Prognosis
- Poor in double-hit lymphomas
- Burkitt lymphoma has aggressive disease course if left untreated, otherwise very chemosensitive
- Correlates with very high proliferation rate

High-Grade B-Cell Lymphoma With *MYC* and *BCL6* Rearrangements
- New provisional entity in ICC

Methods of *MYC* Rearrangement Detection
- Conventional karyotyping
  - Translocations of chromosome 8 with various partners
    - *IGH* on chromosome 14 is partner in 40% of cases of DLBCL
  - Often seen in complex karyotype
- FISH break-apart probe can detect rearrangement of *MYC* with any partner
- Inconsistent correlation with MYC expression by IHC

IRF4 REARRANGEMENTS

Large B-Cell Lymphoma With *IRF4* Rearrangement
- Very rare, mostly in children and young adults
- Can be diffuse or nodular (resembling follicular lymphoma)
  - Distinct entity from pediatric follicular lymphoma
- Waldeyer ring/head and neck primarily involved
- Strong expression of IRF4/MUM1
- Expresses CD10 in ~ 50-60% of cases

Prognosis
- Favorable after chemotherapy

Methods of Detection
- *IRF4*::*IGH* rearrangement detected by FISH in most cases
  - Cryptic (not detectable) by conventional karyotyping
  - Mutually exclusive from *MYC* or *BCL2* rearrangements

T(11;18)(Q22;Q21); *BIRC3*::*MALT1*

Extranodal Marginal Zone Lymphoma of Mucosa-Associated Lymphoid Tissue (MALT Lymphoma)
- *BIRC3*::*MALT1* encodes chimeric protein
- Mainly seen in pulmonary (present in 40%) and gastric (present in 25%) tumors
- Other less common translocations are also associated with MALT lymphomas
  - t(1;14)(p22;q32); *BCL10*::*IGH*
  - t(14;18)(q32;q21); *IGH*::*MALT1*
  - t(3;14)(p13;q32); *FOXP1*::*IGH*

Prognosis
- Presence of this translocation indicates resistance to *Helicobacter pylori* eradication therapy

Methods of Detection
- FISH is reliable method of detection
- Alternative translocations will require specific probe sets or chromosomal analysis

T(9;14)(P13;Q32); *PAX5*::*IGH*

B-Cell Lymphoproliferative Disorders (Not Specific)
- Lymphoplasmacytic lymphoma
- Plasma cell myeloma
- Chronic lymphocytic leukemia/small lymphocytic lymphoma
- Diffuse large B-cell lymphoma
- Follicular lymphoma
- Mantle cell lymphoma

Lymphoma-Associated Chromosomal Translocations

- Splenic marginal zone lymphoma

Pathogenesis
- Similar to other *IGH* (14q32) rearrangements
- Upregulation of *PAX5* by juxtaposition to promoter region of *IGH*
- No fusion gene is created

Prognosis
- No known prognostic relevance

Methods of Detection
- Detectable by conventional cytogenetics
  - Usually accompanied by complex karyotype
- Also detectable by FISH

T(2;5)(P23;Q35); *ALK::NPM1*

ALK(+) Anaplastic Large Cell Lymphoma
- Incidence
  - 10-15% of pediatric/adolescent non-Hodgkin lymphoma (NHL)
  - 3% of adult NHL

Alternative Translocations
- t(1;2)(q21;p23); *TPM3::ALK*
  - Highest incidence after *ALK::NPM1*
  - Seen in almost 15% of ALK(+) ALCL
  - IHC shows diffuse cytoplasmic staining pattern with peripheral intensification
- t(2;17)(p23;q23); *ALK::CLTC*
  - Seen in ALK(+) large B-cell lymphoma
- Many others; all involve *ALK* at 2p23 locus

Prognosis
- No difference between *ALK::NPM1* and alternative translocations
- ALK(+) ALCL patients have better prognosis than ALK(-) ALCL

Methods of Detection
- FISH break-apart probe strategy virtually detects all *ALK* rearrangements
  - Will not determine *ALK* partner genes
- RT-PCR
  - Designed to detect *ALK::NPM1* translocation but will not detect alternative translocations
  - Useful for minimal residual disease evaluation
- Immunohistochemistry
  - ALK is negative in normal tissues (except some CNS neuronal cells)
  - Positive ALK staining generally denotes rearrangement
  - Pattern of staining suggests specific translocation
    - Most common, *ALK::NPM1* shows both nuclear and diffuse cytoplasmic staining
    - Many variants show only diffuse cytoplasmic staining
    - t(2;17)(p23;q23) shows granular cytoplasmic staining
    - t(X;2)(q12;p23) shows membrane staining

DUSP22 REARRANGEMENTS

ALK(-) Anaplastic Large Cell Lymphoma
- *DUSP22* rearrangements at 6p25.3 detected in ~ 30%

Prognosis
- Favorable outcome, comparable to ALK(+) ALCL

Methods of Detection
- *DUSP22/IRF4* (6p25.3) FISH break-apart probe is used
- FISH cannot distinguish between *DUSP22* and *IRF4* rearrangements because of close proximity
  - Not usually issue because *IRF4* rearrangements are not typically encountered in ALCL

TRA REARRANGEMENTS

T-Cell Lymphomas/Leukemias
- Usually occurs as inv(14)(q11q32); *TRA/TRD::TCL1A* or t(14;14)(q11;q32); *TRA/TRD::TCL1A*
  - In 5%, *MTCP1* is partner instead of *TCL1A*
- Most commonly seen in T-cell prolymphocytic leukemia or adult T-cell leukemia/lymphoma
  - Not specific to particular subtype of T-cell lymphoma

Prognosis
- Not well studied

Methods of Detection
- Often detected by conventional karyotyping
- Many labs do not routinely use FISH probes for T-cell receptor genes because of their low incidence

SELECTED REFERENCES

1. Alaggio R et al: The 5th edition of the World Health Organization classification of haematolymphoid tumours: lymphoid neoplasms. Leukemia. 36(7):1720-48, 2022
2. Campo E et al: The International Consensus Classification of mature lymphoid neoplasms: a report from the Clinical Advisory Committee. Blood. 140(11):1229-53, 2022
3. Frauenfeld L et al: Diffuse large B-cell lymphomas in adults with aberrant coexpression of CD10, BCL6, and MUM1 are enriched in IRF4 rearrangements. Blood Adv. 6(7):2361-72, 2022
4. Ohno H et al: t(9;14)(p13;q32)/PAX5-IGH translocation as a secondary cytogenetic abnormality in diffuse large B-cell lymphoma. J Clin Exp Hematop. 61(4):216-20, 2021
5. Odabashian M et al: IGHV sequencing reveals acquired N-glycosylation sites as a clonal and stable event during follicular lymphoma evolution. Blood. 135(11):834-44, 2020
6. Rosenwald A et al: Prognostic significance of MYC rearrangement and translocation partner in diffuse large B-cell lymphoma: a study by the Lunenburg Lymphoma Biomarker Consortium. J Clin Oncol. 37(35):3359-68, 2019
7. Staber PB et al: Consensus criteria for diagnosis, staging, and treatment response assessment of T-cell prolymphocytic leukemia. Blood. 134(14):1132-43, 2019
8. Swerdlow SH et al: WHO Classification of Tumours of Haematopoietic and Lymphoid Tissues. 4th ed. IARC, 2017
9. Pedersen MB et al: DUSP22 and TP63 rearrangements predict outcome of ALK-negative anaplastic large cell lymphoma: a Danish cohort study. Blood. 130(4):554-7, 2017
10. Chisholm KM et al: Expression profiles of MYC protein and MYC gene rearrangement in lymphomas. Am J Surg Pathol. 39(3):294-303, 2015
11. Salaverria I et al: CCND2 rearrangements are the most frequent genetic events in cyclin D1(-) mantle cell lymphoma. Blood. 121(8):1394-402, 2013

Lymphoma-Associated Chromosomal Translocations

FISH for *BIRC3*::*MALT1* Fusion

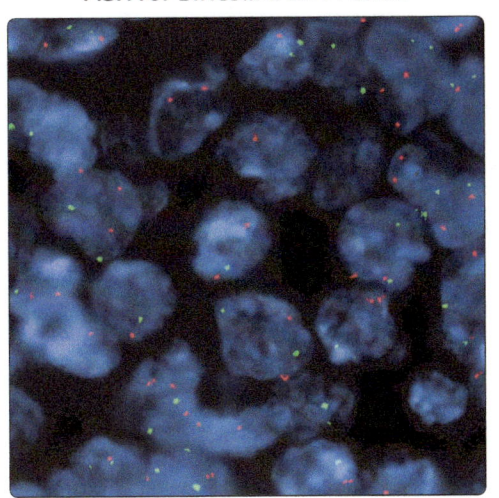

Alternate Translocations in ALK(+) ALCL

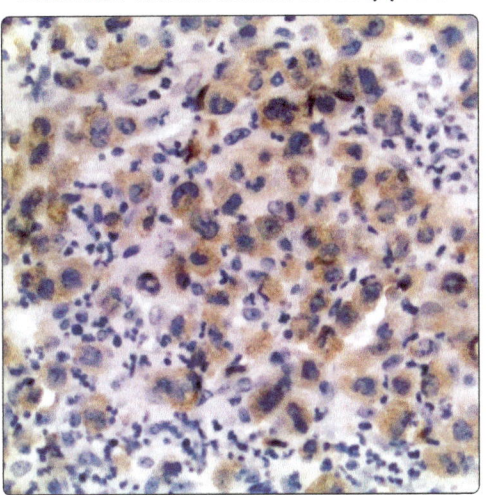

(Left) *FISH of MALT lymphoma is negative for the t(11;18) translocation in this case with a normal pattern of 2 orange and 2 green signals. Interpretation of paraffin sections can be difficult, as signals can be lost due to artifacts of sectioning.* (Right) *ALK(+) anaplastic large cell lymphoma shows ALK staining only in the cytoplasm. Cases with the t(2;5) should also have nuclear staining. Evaluation with FISH (not shown) showed an alternate translocation.*

Double-Hit Lymphoma

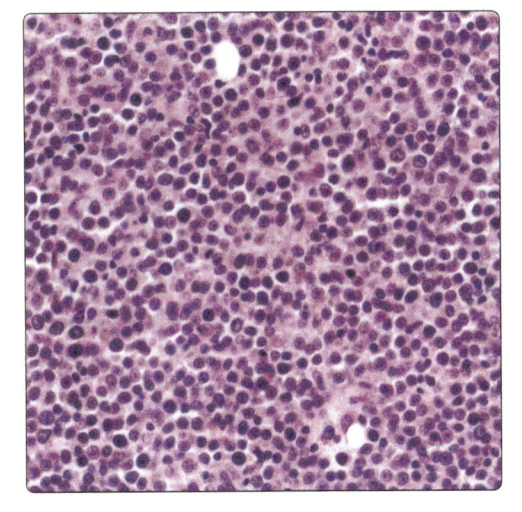

Double-Hit Lymphoma

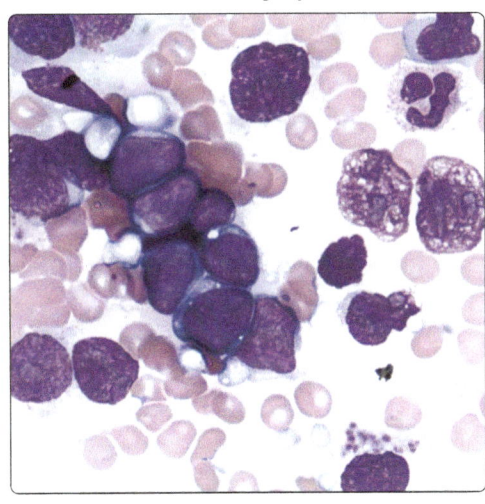

(Left) *"Double-hit" lymphoma extensively involves the bone marrow in this core biopsy. Double-hit lymphomas include rearrangement of MYC along with BCL2 rearrangement. MYC and BCL6 double-hit lymphoma is a provisional category in 2022 ICC.* (Right) *In the same case of double-hit lymphoma, the lymphoma cells are large and blast-like and are frequently seen in clusters. This can be misleading and lead to an erroneous diagnosis of acute leukemia. In this case, flow cytometry identified these as mature B cells.*

Karyotype of Burkitt Lymphoma

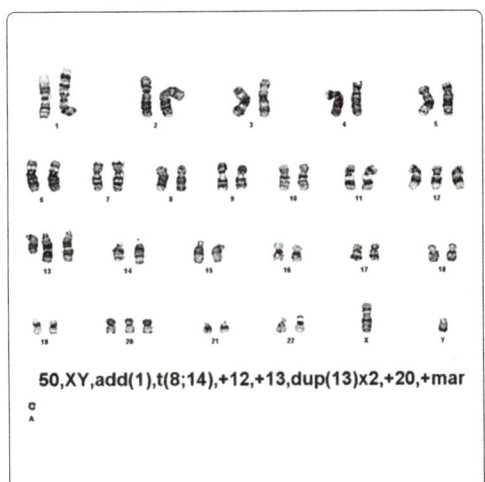

50,XY,add(1),t(8;14),+12,+13,dup(13)x2,+20,+mar

inv(14) in T-Prolymphocytic Leukemia

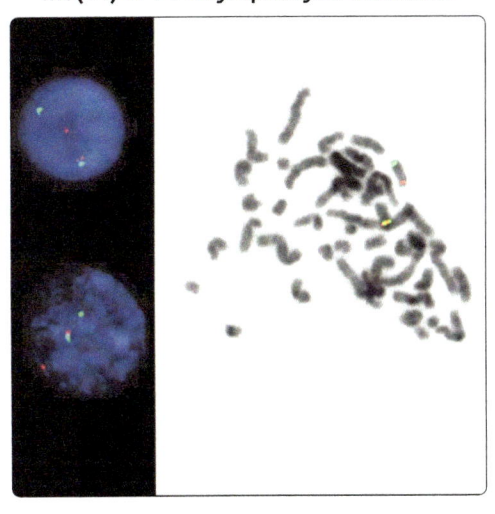

(Left) *This case of Burkitt lymphoma shows the typical t(8;14)(q24;q32) MYC::IGH rearrangement. The complex karyotype, as seen here, can be seen in Burkitt lymphoma.* (Right) *FISH images of the 14q11 TRA/TRD break-apart probe (interphase at left, metaphase at right) show the inv(14)(q11q32) TRA/TRD::TCL1 in a case of T-cell prolymphocytic leukemia. The normal 2-fused-signal pattern has been replaced with 1 fused, 1 orange, and 1 green signal.*

B-Lymphoblastic Leukemia/Lymphoma With Recurrent Genetic Abnormalities

KEY FACTS

TERMINOLOGY
- New variants added, including many provisional

ETIOLOGY/PATHOGENESIS
- High hyperdiploid, *ETV6::RUNX1* most common in pediatric group
- *BCR::ABL1* and *BCR::ABL1*-like most common in adults

CLINICAL ISSUES
- *KMT2A*-rearranged type is most common leukemia in infants < 1 year of age and may occur in utero
  - Frequently has CNS involvement at presentation
- Poor prognosis
  - *BCR::ABL1* and *BCR::ABL1*-like
  - *KMT2A* rearrangements
  - Hypodiploidy
  - iAMP21
  - *TCF3::HLF* rearranged
- Excellent prognosis
  - *ETV6::RUNX1*
  - High hyperdiploidy

MICROSCOPIC
- Most groups have typical lymphoblast morphology
  - Exception is *IL3::IGH*
    - Increased circulating reactive eosinophils
- *KMT2A*-rearranged subtype usually has very high WBC count (> 100 x 10⁹/L)

ANCILLARY TESTS
- Many recurrent genetic abnormalities are detectable by conventional cytogenetics (karyotyping)
- FISH testing is critical in conjunction with karyotyping to detect growing number of cryptic variants
  - *ETV6::RUNX1*
  - Rearrangements associated with *BCR::ABL1*-like variant
  - iAMP21
- Massively parallel sequencing necessary for some variants

Lymphoblasts

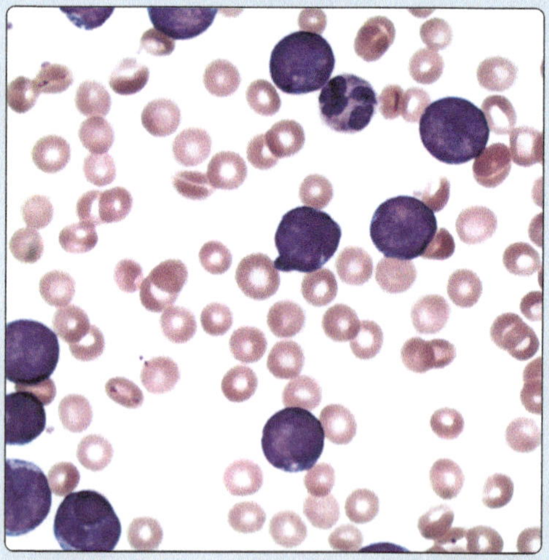

FISH Showing iAMP21

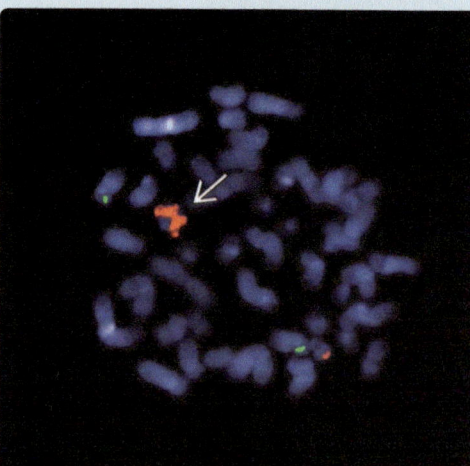

(Left) Peripheral blood smear from a 21-year-old woman shows typical morphology of B-ALL. Cases with recurrent cytogenetic abnormalities usually have typical lymphoblast morphology as well. (Right) Metaphase FISH using probe for RUNX1 shows multiple copies on the ring chromosome ➡, consistent with diagnosis of iAMP21. (From DP3: B&BM.)

JAK2 Rearrangement by FISH

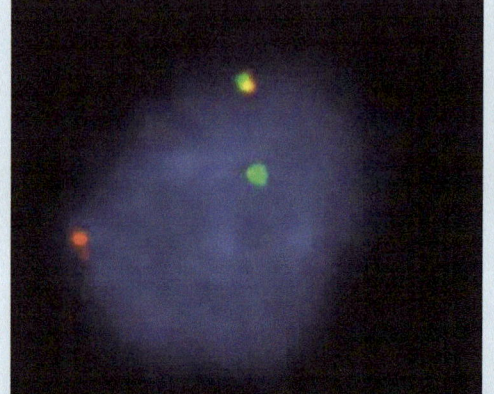

FISH for PDGFRB

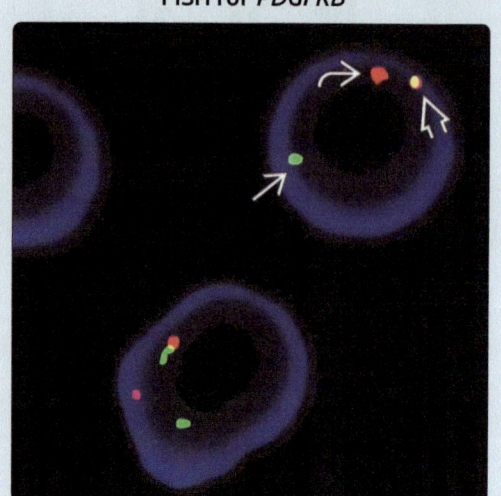

(Left) This patient had a positive BCR::ABL1-like result by genomic study. FISH was performed as a follow-up study, and JAK2 rearrangement was identified. The final diagnosis was B-ALL BCR::ABL1-like. (From DP3: B&BM.) (Right) Break-apart probe for PDGFRB confirms involvement of PDGFRB with cells showing 1 normal fusion signal ➡, 1 red signal ➡, and 1 green signal ➡, indicating translocation. This finding is associated with BCR::ABL1-like acute lymphoblastic leukemia. (From DP3 B&BM.)

B-Lymphoblastic Leukemia/Lymphoma With Recurrent Genetic Abnormalities

TERMINOLOGY

Synonyms
- B acute lymphoblastic leukemia (B-ALL)

Definitions
- B-ALL/LBL with recurrent genetic abnormalities

CLASSIFICATION

ICC vs. WHO-HAEM5
- B-ALL with recurrent genetic abnormalities recognized by both ICC and WHO-HAEM5
  - B-ALL with t(9;22)/*BCR::ABL1* fusion
  - B-ALL with *KMT2A* rearrangement
  - B-ALL with *ETV6::RUNX1*
  - B-ALL, *ETV6::RUNX1*-like
  - B-ALL with hyperdiploidy
  - B-ALL with hypodiploidy (low hypodiploid, near haploid)
  - B-ALL with *IL3::IGH* fusion
  - B-ALL with *TCF3::PBX1* fusion
  - B-ALL, *BCR::ABL1*-like
  - B-ALL with iAMP21
  - B-ALL with *TCF3::HLF* fusion
- ICC new B-ALL entities defined by translocations or gene mutations not listed in WHO-HAEM5
  - B-ALL with *MYC* rearrangements
  - B-ALL with *DUX4* rearrangement
  - B-ALL with *MEF2D* rearrangement
  - B-ALL with *ZNF384* rearrangement
  - B-ALL with *NUTM1* rearrangement
  - B-ALL with *UBTF::ATXN7L3/PAN3*, *CDX2* (CDX2/UBTF)
  - B-ALL with *TCF4::HLF* rearrangement
  - B-ALL with *PAX5* P80R mutation
  - B-ALL with *IKZF1* N159Y mutation
- ICC B-ALL provisional entities
  - B-ALL, *ETV6::RUNX1*-like
  - B-ALL with *PAX5* alteration
  - B-ALL with mutated *ZEB2* (p.H1038R)/*IGH::CEBPE*
  - B-ALL, *ZNF384* rearranged-like
  - B-ALL, *KMT2A* rearranged-like
- ICC recognizes 3 subcategories for B-ALL, *BCR::ABL1*-like
  - ABL1 class rearranged, JAK-STAT activated, and NOS
- ICC further divides hypodiploid B-ALL
  - Low hypodiploid and near haploid

ETIOLOGY/PATHOGENESIS

Genetics
- In many cases, patients are thought to have genetic predisposition
  - Single nucleotide polymorphisms (SNP) in certain genes with increased risk of B-ALL
    - *GATA3*, *ARID5B*, *IKZF1*, *CEBPE*, *CDKN2A*, and *CDKN2B*
  - Rare constitutional Robertsonian t(15;21)(q10;q10) have ~ 3,000x risk of B-ALL with iAMP21

CLINICAL ISSUES

Epidemiology
- Incidence
  - High hyperdiploid B-ALL very common in children (25-35% of B-ALL cases)
  - *ETV6::RUNX1* most common recurrent translocation in childhood B-ALL (~ 25%)
  - *BCR::ABL1*-like B-ALL is especially common in patients with Down syndrome (50-60%)
- Age
  - *BCR::ABL1*-associated and *BCR::ABL1*-like B-ALL are relatively more common in adults
  - *KMT2A*-rearranged type is most common leukemia in infants < 1 year of age and may occur in utero

Presentation
- Bone marrow failure
  - Leukocytosis or leukopenia
- *KMT2A*-rearranged type frequently has CNS involvement at presentation
- *IGH::IL3*-rearranged type may have peripheral blood eosinophilia, eosinophilic infiltrates in organs

Treatment
- Drugs
  - Intensive chemotherapy protocols
  - Tyrosine kinase inhibitors in *BCR::ABL1*-rearranged ALL in addition to standard chemotherapy and in some cases of *BCR::ABL1*-like B-ALL
- Stem cell transplant, CAR-T therapy for high-risk patients

Prognosis
- Poor prognosis specific to these genetic subtypes
  - *BCR::ABL1* B-ALL had historically worst prognosis, both in children and adults
    - Tyrosine kinase inhibitors have significantly improved outcome
    - ICC subcategorizes into with "lymphoid only" and with "multilineage" involvement
  - *BCR::ABL1*-like
  - *KMT2A* rearrangements
  - Hypodiploidy
    - ~ 50% of low-hypodiploid group have germline *TP53* mutations (Li-Fraumeni syndrome)
  - iAMP21
    - Intensive chemotherapy may overcome poor prognosis
  - *TCF3::HLF* rearranged
    - Dismal prognosis
    - CAR-T therapy and BCL2 inhibitors are showing better results
- Intermediate prognosis
  - *TCF3::PBX1* rearranged
    - Dismal prognosis if CNS relapse occur
- Excellent prognosis specific to these genetic subtypes
  - *ETV6::RUNX1* rearrangement
  - High hyperdiploidy

MICROSCOPIC

Peripheral Blood
- *KMT2A*-rearranged subtype usually has very high WBC count (> 100 x 10^9/L)

B-Lymphoblastic Leukemia/Lymphoma With Recurrent Genetic Abnormalities

Bone Marrow
- Most groups have typical lymphoblast morphology with no specific or unique features
  - Exception is B-ALL with *IL3::IGH*
    - Increased circulating eosinophils that are reactive

ANCILLARY TESTS

Flow Cytometry
- B-ALL with *BCR::ABL1*
  - Commonly express myeloid antigens CD13 and CD33
- B-ALL with *KMT2A* rearrangement
  - Pro-B stage markers
    - CD19(+), CD10(-), CD24(-), commonly TdT(-)
    - CD15(+), CD65(+)
- B-ALL with *ETV6::RUNX1*
  - CD19(+), CD10(+), CD34(+), commonly express myeloid antigens including CD13
- B-ALL, *BCR::ABL1*-like
  - Strong surface CRLF2 in cases with *CRLF2* translocations

In Situ Hybridization
- FISH panels part of routine diagnostic testing for B-ALL
  - Necessary to detect cryptic translocations
- *ETV6::RUNX1* FISH
  - Also identifies iAMP21 variant
    - Indicated by amplification of *RUNX1* signal ≥ 5 copies with at least 3 copies being on same chromosome or derivative chromosome
- FISH panel for *BCR::ABL1*-like B-ALL
  - Targets most commonly rearranged genes in this entity
  - *CRLF2* rearrangements in 50% of cases
  - *JAK2* fusion in ~ 7% of cases
  - *EPOR* rearrangements in ~ 5% of cases
  - *CSF1R*
  - *ABL1*, involves partners other than *BCR*
  - *ABL2*
  - *PDGFRB*
    - May confer resistance to induction chemotherapy
    - May be overcome by tyrosine kinase inhibitors

Genetic Testing
- *KMT2A*-rearranged B-ALL
  - > 100 fusion partners reported
  - Rearrangements detectable by standard karyotyping or FISH break-apart probe
- *BCR::ABL1*-like B-ALL
  - Whole-transcriptome analysis gold standard
  - Break-apart FISH probes can be used for most common subgroups
  - DNA/RNA sequencing can detect rarer rearrangements
- *ETV6::RUNX1*-like B-ALL
  - Currently no standard for testing/identification
  - Lacks *ETV6::RUNX1* rearrangement but shares genetic expression profile or *ETV6* with alternative fusion partner
- *TCF3::PBX1* B-ALL
  - Detectable by karyotype, FISH, and molecular methods
- *IGH::IL3* rearranged
  - Potentially detected by karyotype but may be cryptic
  - Massively parallel sequencing assays may identify *IGH::IL3*
- *TCF3::HLF* rearranged
  - Karyotype, FISH, and molecular methods can be used
- Hyperdiploid B-ALL
  - Extra copies of X, 4, 10, 17, 18, and 21 most common
  - High hyperdiploid 51-65 chromosomes
- Hypodiploid B-ALL
  - Most commonly lost include chromosomes 3, 4, 7, 9, 13, 17, and 20 lost in all cases
  - 3 subtypes: Near haploid (24-31 chromosomes), low hypodiploid (32-39 chromosomes), and high hypodiploid (40-43 chromosomes)
- iAMP21
  - Intrachromosomal amplification of chromosome 21
    - Not detectable by standard karyotyping
    - Defined by multiple copies of *RUNX1* probe (amplification)
      - Must have ≥ 5 copies per cell with ≥ 3 copies on single chromosome 21
      - Distinctive SNP array profile can validate FISH result

RT-PCR
- B-ALL with *BCR::ABL1* rearrangement
  - Most pediatric cases have p190 kd fusion protein
  - In adults, ~ 50% have p190 and 50% have p210
  - Minimal residual disease monitoring
    - Assays should have sensitivity of at least 10^{-4}

Gene Expression Profiling
- *BCR::ABL1*-like ALL
  - Reliable screening test to identify ALL cases with *BCR::ABL1*-like signature
  - Often have deletion/mutation of *IKZF1*
  - Frequently have rearrangement of *CRLF2*
  - Some have rearrangements leading to truncation and activation of *EPOR*

DIFFERENTIAL DIAGNOSIS

B-ALL, Not Otherwise Specified
- Cytogenetic evaluation and FISH B-ALL panels, including those for rearrangements associated with *BCR::ABL1*-like variant, are essential

DIAGNOSTIC CHECKLIST

Pathologic Interpretation Pearls
- All cases of B-lymphoblastic leukemia need cytogenetic evaluation
- FISH is necessary to address cryptic translocations
- Recently identified molecular mutations are constantly evolving classification, treatment, and prognosis
  - Alternative ancillary studies, such as massively parallel sequencing or gene expression profiling, will likely become routine in B-ALL initial evaluation

SELECTED REFERENCES

1. Duffield AS et al: International Consensus Classification of acute lymphoblastic leukemia/lymphoma. Virchows Arch. 482(1):11-26, 2023
2. Alaggio R et al: The 5th edition of the World Health Organization classification of haematolymphoid tumours: lymphoid neoplasms. Leukemia. 36(7):1720-48, 2022
3. Tran TH et al: Whole-transcriptome analysis in acute lymphoblastic leukemia: a report from the DFCI ALL Consortium Protocol 16-001. Blood Adv. 6(4):1329-41, 2022

B-Lymphoblastic Leukemia/Lymphoma With Recurrent Genetic Abnormalities

CML Transformed to B-ALL

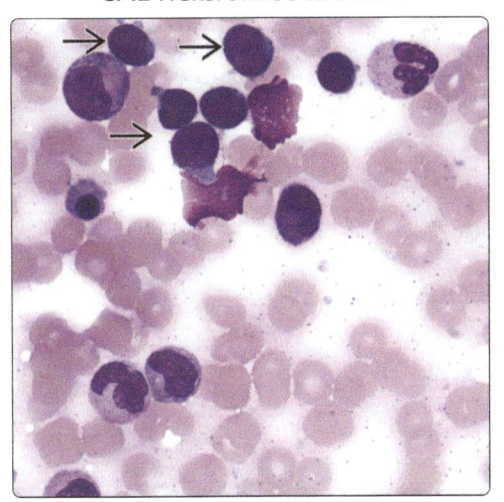

B-ALL With *KMT2A* Rearrangement

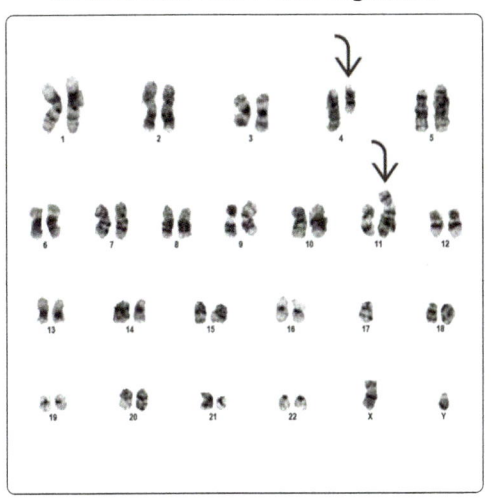

(Left) This case of B-ALL with BCR::ABL1 rearrangement is a transformation of previous chronic myeloid leukemia (CML) in a 55-year-old man. Note the residual myeloid precursors in the background with lymphoblasts ⇒. Not all cases with p210 isoform are transformations from underlying CML. (Right) Karyotype of this patient with B-ALL shows translocation of t(4;11) ⇒, which is typical of the AFF1::KMT2A fusion. (From DP3: B&BM.)

B-ALL With *IGH::IL3* Rearrangement

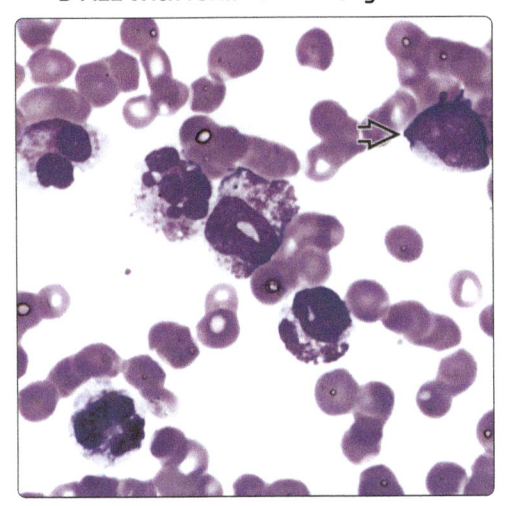

Lymphoblast Morphology

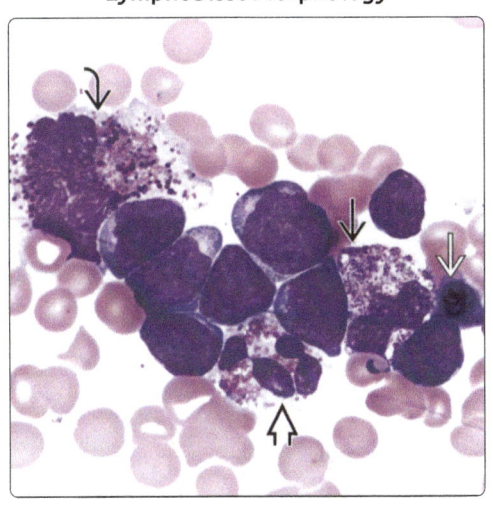

(Left) A lymphoblast ⇒ is accompanied by eosinophilia in peripheral blood from a patient with B-ALL with IGH::IL3 rearrangement, which was identified by routine karyotyping. (From DP3: B&BM.) (Right) Bone marrow aspirate smear from the same patient shows a cluster of blasts surrounded by a mature eosinophil ⇒, an eosinophil precursor with basophilic granules ⇒, a segmented neutrophil ⇒, and an erythroid precursor ⇒. (From DP3: B&BM.)

DNA Index Showing Hyperdiploidy

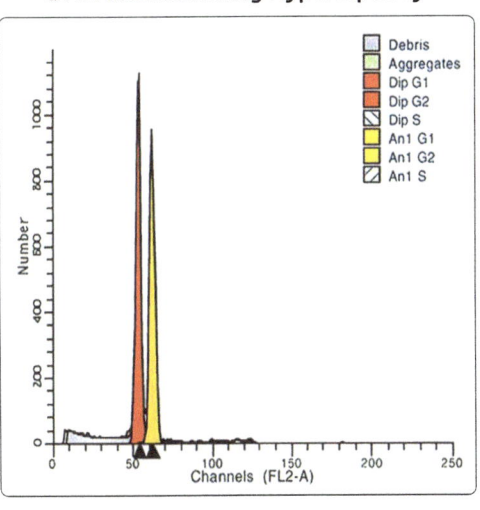

ETV6::RUNX1 Fusion in B-ALL

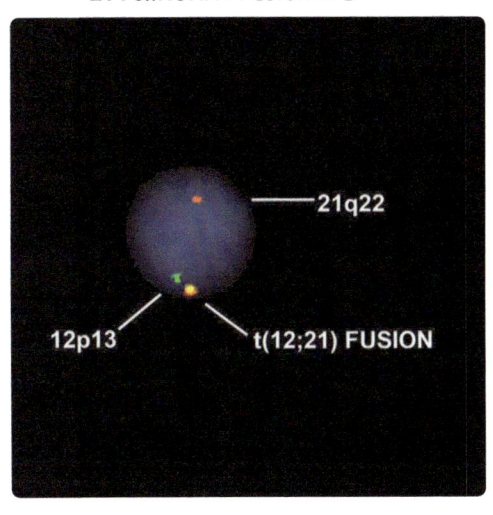

(Left) DNA index of 1.16 (i.e., hyperdiploidy) is calculated as the patient (yellow) with normal (red) DNA content ratio in a mixing study. Conventional karyotyping is used to determine which chromosomes are duplicated. (From DP3: B&BM.) (Right) Dual-color, dual-fusion FISH probes show 1 t(12;21) ETV6::RUNX1 fusion, 1 orange and 1 green signal. One fusion signal is considered positive for ETV6::RUNX1 fusion. (From DP3: B&BM.)

B-Lymphoblastic Leukemia/Lymphoma, *BCR::ABL1*-Like (Ph-Like ALL)

TERMINOLOGY

Abbreviations
- B-acute lymphoblastic leukemia (B-ALL), *BCR::ABL1*-like

Synonyms
- Philadelphia-like or Ph-like ALL
  - Terminology used extensively

Definitions
- ICC: B-ALL, *BCR::ABL1*-like; 3 subtypes
  - JAK-STAT activated cases
  - *ABL1*-class rearranged
  - Not otherwise specified (NOS)
- WHO-HAEM5: B-lymphoblastic leukemia/lymphoma, *BCR::ABL1*-like features
  - No defined subtypes
- 1st described in 2009 based on gene expression profile similar to *BCR::ABL1*-positive B-ALL
- Many different rearrangements and mutations
- Genetic alterations converge on pathways leading to deregulation of kinase signaling
- Genetic alterations often exquisitely sensitive to targeted therapies, including tyrosine kinase inhibitors
- *CRLF2* alterations in 50% of cases ± *JAK* alterations
- *ABL* class fusions
  - *ABL1*, *ABL2*, *CSF1R*, *PDGFRB*, *PDGFRA*
- Other JAK/STAT pathway fusions
  - *JAK2* and *EPOR* rearrangements
- High frequency of *IKZF1* deletions or alterations

EPIDEMIOLOGY

Incidence
- Overall 10-30% of B-ALL
  - 10-15% in children overall
    - Higher incidence in high-risk childhood B-ALL
    - Low incidence in standard-risk childhood B-ALL
  - 20-30% in adolescents and young adults
  - 20-25% in older adults

Algorithm to Identify B-ALL, *BCR::ABL1* Like Using LDA Screen

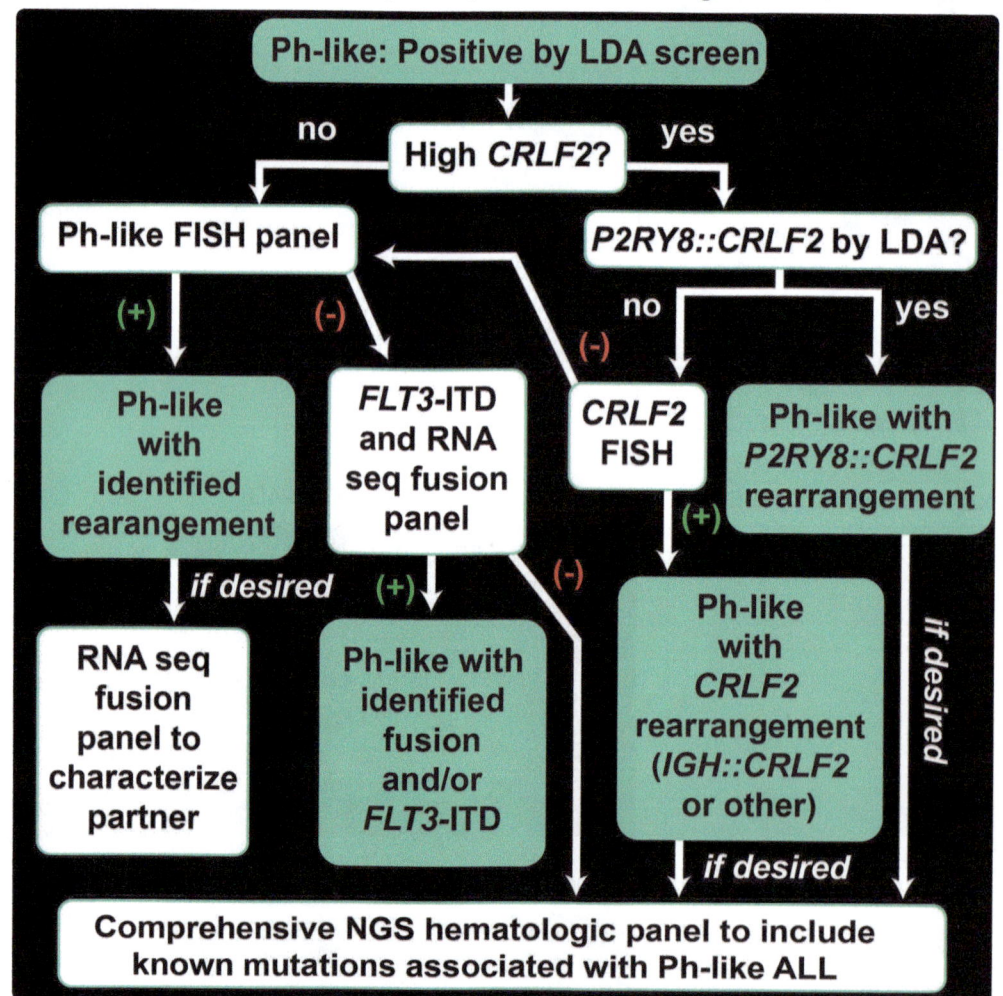

This diagram provides an algorithm for the work-up of suspected B-ALL, BCR::ABL1-like when the low-density array (LDA) sensitive screening assay is available. Cases that are negative by LDA are not Ph-like and therefore do not need additional Ph-like testing.

B-Lymphoblastic Leukemia/Lymphoma, *BCR::ABL1*-Like (Ph-Like ALL)

- 50-60% of B-ALL diagnosed in individuals with Down syndrome have *CRLF2* alterations
- High frequency of *IGH::CRLF2* rearrangements in those of Hispanic and Native American descent

ETIOLOGY/PATHOGENESIS

Cytokine Receptor-Like Factor 2

- Located on pseudoautosomal region 1 (PAR1) of chromosomes Xp22/Yp11
- Encodes type 1 receptor family protein
- CRLF2 monomer pairs with a subunit of IL7R to form heterodimeric thymic stromal lymphopoietin receptor (TSLPR)
  - Leads to activation of JAK/STAT pathway
- *CRLF2* alterations results in overexpression of CRLF2
  - Seen in ~ 50% of Ph-like ALL
  - Responds to targeted therapy with JAK inhibitors, such as ruxolitinib
  - Most common alterations
    - *P2RY8::CRLF2* fusion due to interstitial deletion of PAR1
    - *IGH::CRLF2* fusion due to translocation: t(X;14) or t(Y;14)
  - 30-50% of cases with *CRLF2* rearrangements also harbor *JAK2* point mutations, less commonly other gene mutations
  - Concomitant mutations in *CRLF2* rearranged cases
    - *JAK1, JAK2,* or *JAK3* mutations identified in ~ 50%
    - Ras pathway genes also commonly mutated (*KRAS, NRAS, PTPN11, NF1*)
    - Other less common mutated genes: *KRAS, CRLF2, IKZF1, PAX5, ASXL1, ARID2, LRP1B, ITPKB*
  - Part of "B-ALL, *BCR::ABL1*-like: JAK-STAT activated cases" subtype (ICC)

JAK2 Rearrangements

- 7-10% of of Ph-like ALL demonstrate *JAK2* fusion, more common in young adults and adults
- Translocations or interstitial deletions lead to *JAK2* fusion genes
  - Lead to activation of JAK/STAT pathway
  - Responsive to targeted therapy with JAK inhibitors, such as ruxolitinib
- Part of "B-ALL, *BCR::ABL1*-like: JAK-STAT activated cases" subtype (ICC)

EPOR Rearrangements

- Detected in ~ 5% of cases
- Common partner genes: *IGH, IGK, LAIR1, THADA*
- Leads to overexpression of truncated receptor with loss of negative regulatory domain
- Results in activation of JAK-STAT pathway
- Responsive to targeted therapy with JAK inhibitors, such as ruxolitinib
- Part of "B-ALL, *BCR::ABL1*-like: JAK-STAT activated cases" subtype (ICC)

ABL Class Alterations

- *ABL1, ABL2, CSF1R, PDGFR,* and *PDGFRA* fusions
- Detected in 15-20% of cases
- Responsive to targeted therapy by ABL-class inhibitors, such as imatinib, dasatinib, and nilotinib
- "B-ALL, *BCR::ABL1*-like: *ABL1*-class rearranged" subtype (ICC)

Ras Signaling Mutations

- *KRAS, NRAS, NF1, PTPN11, BRAF, CBL* mutations
- Detected in 6% of cases
- Part of "B-ALL, *BCR::ABL1*-like, NOS" subtype (ICC)

Other Kinase Rearrangements

- *FLT3, FGFR1, NTRK3, PTK2B* rearrangements
- Detected in 5% of cases
- Part of "B-ALL, *BCR::ABL1*-like, NOS" subtype (ICC)

CLINICAL IMPLICATIONS

Clinical Presentation

- ~ 25% of B-ALL patients ≥ 10 years of age
- Associated with significantly higher WBC count at diagnosis (≥ 50,000)
- Higher frequency in NCI-defined high-risk B-ALL
- Lowest frequency in NCI-defined standard-risk B-ALL
- High incidence those of Hispanic and Native American descent, especially with *IGH::CRLF2* fusion

Prognosis and Outcomes

- Associated with increased likelihood of minimal residual disease (MRD) at end of induction
- Higher risk of relapse and death
- CRLF2 rearrangements associated with particularly poor outcome
- Those without *IKZF1* alterations may have better prognosis
- Majority harbor somatic genetic alterations that activate kinase and cytokine receptor signaling pathways
  - Potential response to targeted therapies

MICROSCOPIC

General Features

- Blood
  - Typically high WBC with abundant circulating blasts
  - Blasts may vary in size with spectrum from small to large
  - Blast morphology essentially similar to other WHO subtypes of B-ALL
- Bone marrow
  - Hypercellular with extensive replacement by sheets of lymphoblasts
  - Similar to other WHO subtypes of B-ALL with no characteristic features

Ancillary Tests

- Many different genetic alterations makes diagnosis challenging
- Gene expression profiling (GEP) is considered gold standard
  - Most reliable screening method
  - Currently not widely available as clinical assay
- GEP assay using low-density array (LDA) card
  - Real-time quantitative PCR using customized 384-well microfluidic LDA card
  - 8-gene and 15-gene predictor algorithm identifies Ph-like ALL signature
  - Advantages of GEP assay using LDA card

B-Lymphoblastic Leukemia/Lymphoma, *BCR::ABL1*-Like (Ph-Like ALL)

- Assay used in Children Oncology Group (COG) and adult clinical trials with > 8,000 cases tested
- Accepted as standard screening assay to identify Ph-like ALL in clinical trials
- Relatively inexpensive
- Short turnaround time
    - Requires additional testing to characterize targetable genetic alterations except for cases with *P2RY8::CRLF2* fusion
- Flow cytometry to assess CRLF2 overexpression
    - High CRLF2 expression correlates with *CRLF2* rearrangements
        - CRLF2 antibodies commercially available
        - Relatively inexpensive
        - Rapid turnaround time
    - Only identifies Ph-like ALL cases that harbor *CRLF2* rearrangements (30-50% of cases)
    - Fails to identify non-*CRLF2* rearranged Ph-like cases
- FISH panel to assess for common Ph-like ALL fusions
    - Many fusions are cytogenetically cryptic and will not be identified by karyotype
    - Common FISH panel
        - *ABL1, ABL2, CRLF2, CSF1R, EPOR, JAK2,* and *PDGFRB* break-apart probe sets
        - Relatively fast turnaround time
    - Requires additional testing to identify fusion partners
    - Will miss novel or rare rearrangements that are not tested
- High throughput DNA and RNA sequencing
    - More comprehensive approach to identifying genetic alterations
    - Capable of identifying rare and novel fusions
    - Expensive with longer turnaround time

Targetable Kinase Gene Fusions in Ph-Like ALL

- Data from COG study (Reshmi et al)
    - *ABL1* fusions
        - Fusion partners: *CENPC, ETV6, LSM14A, NUP153, NUP214, RANBP2, RCSD1, ZMIZ1*
    - *ABL2* fusion partners
        - *RCSD1, ZC3HAV1*
    - *CSF1R* fusion partners
        - *SSBP2, TBL1XR1*
    - *PDGFRB* fusion partners
        - *ATF7IP, EBF1, TNIP1, ZMYND8*
    - *LYN* fusion partner
        - *GATAD2A*
    - *JAK2* fusion partners
        - *BCR, PAX5, PCM1, RFX3, USP25, ZNF274*
    - *EPOR* fusion partner
        - *IGH*
    - *NTRK3* fusion partner
        - *ETV6*
    - Majority of fusions involve chromosomal translocations
    - Some fusions arise from interstitial deletions
        - Within 1q24.2-q25.2 (*RCSD1::ABL2*), 5q14.1-q23.2 (*SSBP2::CSF1R*), or 5q32 (*TNIP1::PDGFRB*)
        - Within 9p24.1-p24.2 (*RFX3::JAK2*), 9p13.2-p24.1 (*PAX5::JAK2*), or 9q34.12-q34.13 (*NUP214::ABL1*)
- Data from Dutch/German Pediatric Cohort (Boer et al)
    - Fusions predictive for activated ABL signaling
        - *EBF1::PDGFRB*
        - *SSBP1::CSF1R*
        - *ZMIZ1::ABL1*
        - *FOXP1::ABL1*
        - *RCSD1::ABL2*
    - Fusions predictive for activated JAK2 signaling
        - *PAX5::JAK2*
        - *BCR::JAK2*
        - *TERF2::JAK2*

Diagnostic Checklist

- B-ALL with *BCR::ABL1*-like features (Ph-like ALL) accounts for 10-30% of B-ALL with high-risk features
- Complex range of genomic aberrations
- ~ 80% of cases harbor cytokine receptor or kinase activating alterations
    - Associated with activation of ABL class and JAK-STAT signaling pathways
- Several methodologies to identify
    - Gene expression profiling using low-density array (LDA) card
        - Reflex to downstream FISH, RNA, &/or DNA sequencing to identify possible targetable alterations
    - Flow cytometric analysis for CRLF2 overexpression
        - Will only pick up those that harbor CRLF2 rearrangement (~ 50% of cases)
    - FISH for most common genetic rearrangements
        - Will only pick up those that carry these specific rearrangements
    - High throughput DNA and RNA sequencing
        - More costly with longer turnaround times
- Who to screen
    - Children with high-risk B-ALL
    - Adults
- Screening can be considered in children with standard-risk B-ALL
    - Particularly those with
        - Residual disease at end of induction
        - CNS or testicular involvement
    - Only subset of standard-risk B-ALL harbor targetable mutation

SELECTED REFERENCES

1. Duffield AS et al: International Consensus Classification of acute lymphoblastic leukemia/lymphoma. Virchows Arch. 482(1):11-26, 2023
2. Alaggio R et al: The 5th edition of the World Health Organization classification of haematolymphoid tumours: lymphoid neoplasms. Leukemia. 36(7):1720-48, 2022
3. Harvey RC et al: Clinical diagnostics and treatment strategies for Philadelphia chromosome-like acute lymphoblastic leukemia. Blood Adv. 4(1):218-28, 2020
4. Jain S et al: BCR-ABL1-like B-acute lymphoblastic leukemia/lymphoma: a comprehensive review. Arch Pathol Lab Med. 144(2):150-5, 2020
5. Kotb A et al: Philadelphia-like acute lymphoblastic leukemia: diagnostic dilemma and management perspectives. Exp Hematol. 67:1-9, 2018
6. Boer JM et al: Tyrosine kinase fusion genes in pediatric BCR-ABL1-like acute lymphoblastic leukemia. Oncotarget. 8(3):4618-28, 2017
7. Jain N et al: Ph-like acute lymphoblastic leukemia: a high-risk subtype in adults. Blood. 129(5):572-81, 2017
8. Reshmi SC et al: Targetable kinase gene fusions in high-risk B-ALL: a study from the Children's Oncology Group. Blood. 129(25):3352-61, 2017
9. Roberts KG et al: Targetable kinase-activating lesions in Ph-like acute lymphoblastic leukemia. N Engl J Med. 371(11):1005-15, 2014

B-Lymphoblastic Leukemia/Lymphoma, *BCR::ABL1*-Like (Ph-Like ALL)

Bone Marrow Aspirate

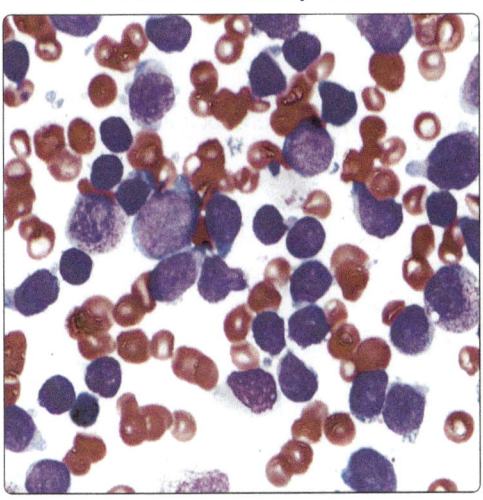

PCR Amplified Curves from LDA Card

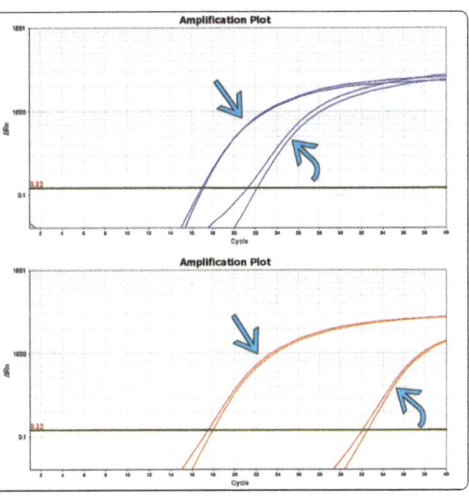

(Left) Wright-stained bone marrow aspirate smear from a 17-year-old with high-risk B-ALL with CNS involvement shows numerous lymphoblasts with fine chromatin and high N:C ratio. LDA screening assay revealed a BCR::ABL1-like signature with high CRLF2 expression. **(Right)** Screening using LDA assay is shown. The upper graph shows a BCR::ABL1-like B-ALL with high expression of CRLF2 ➔ compared to a reference gene ➔. The lower graph shows a negative control with low expression of CRLF2 compared to the reference gene.

Identifying B-ALL, *BCR::ABL1*-Like Without LDA Screen

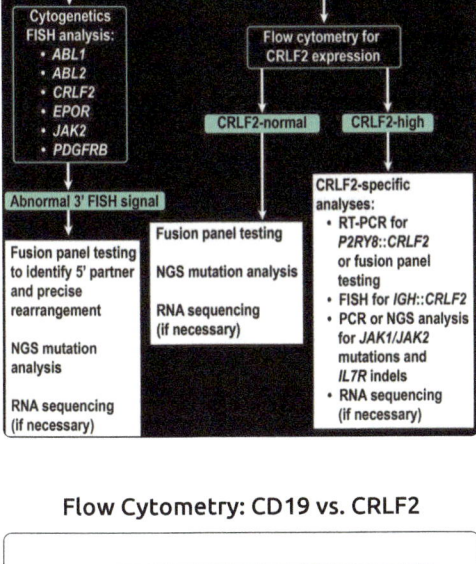

CRLF2 Break-Apart FISH

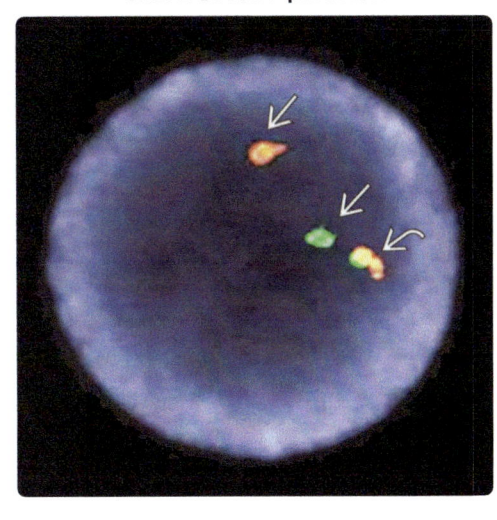

(Left) This diagram provides an algorithm for the work-up of suspected BCR::ABL1-like B-ALL when the LDA sensitive screening assay is not available. (Adapted from Harvey & Tasian, 2020.) **(Right)** FISH using CRLF2 break-apart probe reveals green and red separated signals ➔, consistent with CRLF2 rearrangement, and a fused signal ➔ corresponding to the intact CRLF2.

Flow Cytometry: CD19 vs. CRLF2

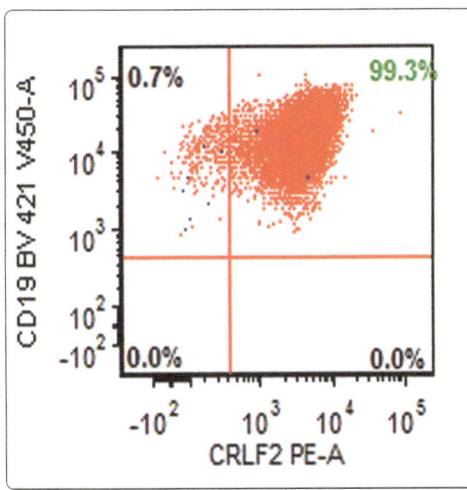

Sanger Sequencing of *JAK2* Codon 694

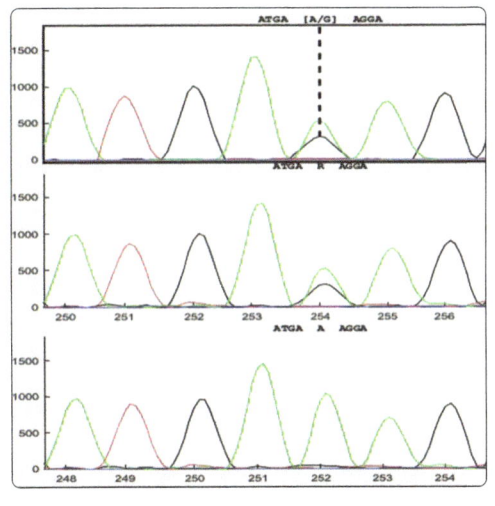

(Left) Histogram of flow cytometric analysis of a bone marrow aspirate from a case of high-risk B-ALL reveals high expression of CRLF2, consistent with BCR::ABL1-like B-ALL. (Courtesy S. Konoplev, MD.) **(Right)** The reverse traces of JAK2 exon 16 Sanger sequencing (upper and middle images) show a T>C substitution in codon 694 of the JAK2 gene corresponding to a F694L mutation in this case of BCR::ABL1-like B-ALL. The lower image represents the wildtype sequence.

T-Lymphoblastic Leukemia/Lymphoma

KEY FACTS

TERMINOLOGY

- **Abbreviations**
  - T-acute lymphoblastic leukemia (T-ALL)/T-lymphoblastic lymphoma (T-LBL)
- **Definitions**
  - T-ALL/T-LBL
    - Neoplasms of lymphoblasts committed to T-cell lineage
    - T-ALL and T-LBL are separated based on number of lymphoblasts in bone marrow
      - T-ALL when > 25% blasts in bone marrow
    - Distinction between leukemia and lymphoma becomes arbitrary when there is mass lesion and increased marrow blasts
  - Early T-cell precursor ALL (ETP-ALL) expresses ≥ 1 myeloid stem cell-associated antigens: CD117, CD34, HLA-DR, CD13, CD33, CD11b, &/or CD65 in ≥ 25% of blasts

MOLECULAR

- **Antigen receptor gene rearrangements**
  - Clonal rearrangements of T-cell receptor (TCR) genes detected in virtually all cases
  - Concurrent clonal rearrangements of immunoglobulin heavy chain (*IGH*) in 20% of cases
- **Cytogenetics**
  - Structural chromosomal abnormalities detected in ~ 50-60% of T-ALL/T-LBL
  - Chromosomal translocation involving TCR gene loci
    - Found in ~ 40% of T-ALL cases

ANCILLARY TESTS

- **Flow cytometry**
  - T lymphoblasts variably express CD1A, CD2, CD3 (surface or cytoplasmic), CD4, CD5, CD7, CD8, and usually TdT
  - CD13 &/or CD33 are expressed in 20-30% of cases

Lymphoblasts in Bone Marrow Aspirate Smear

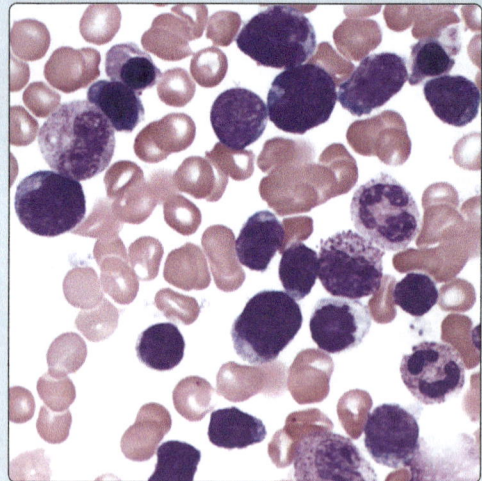

Next-Generation Sequencing Analysis of *IDH2*

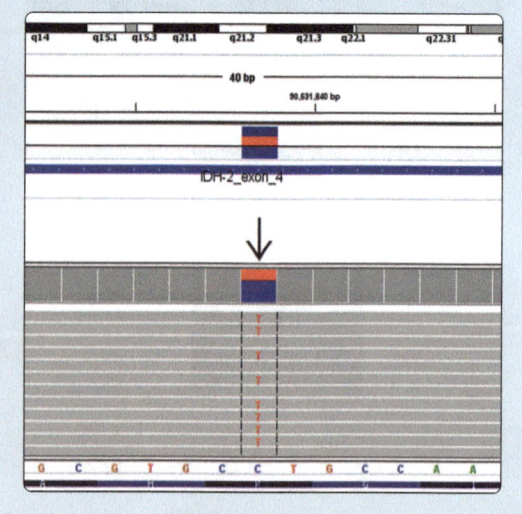

(Left) Bone marrow aspirate smear from a child with precursor T-acute lymphoblastic leukemia (T-ALL) shows variably sized lymphoblasts. Note at least partial preservation of hematopoiesis. (Right) Next-generation sequencing of an early T-cell precursor ALL (ETP-ALL) shows a c.515G>A (R172K) missense mutation ➡ in the IDH2 gene. ETP-ALL may show myeloid-associated gene abnormalities, including IDH2 mutation.

Cytospin Preparation of Pleural Fluid

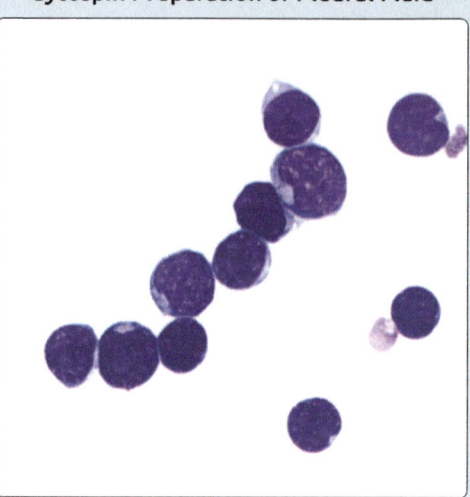

Clonal T-Cell Receptor γ

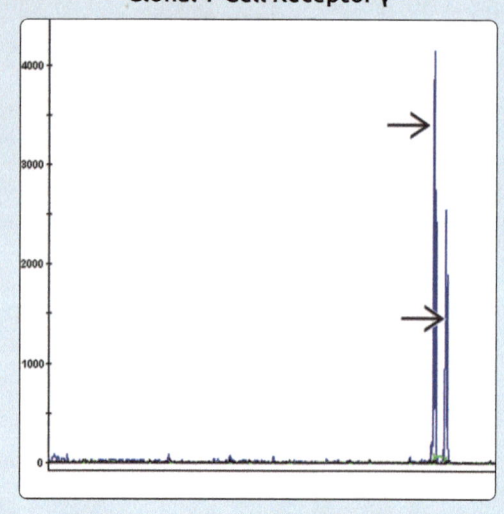

(Left) Cytospin preparation of pleural effusion from a pediatric patient shows lymphoblasts with a spectrum of size and chromatin immaturity. (Right) PCR analysis of T-cell receptor γ chain gene performed on DNA extracted from bone marrow aspirate specimen shows clonal T-cell receptor γ gene rearrangement ➡. This assay cannot be used to determine the lineage due to lineage cross-over commonly seen in ALL/lymphoblastic lymphoma (LBL).

T-Lymphoblastic Leukemia/Lymphoma

TERMINOLOGY

Abbreviations
- T-acute lymphoblastic leukemia (T-ALL)/T-lymphoblastic lymphoma (T-LBL)

Synonyms
- Precursor T-cell neoplasms

Definitions
- T-ALL/T-LBL
  o Neoplasms of lymphoblasts committed to T-cell lineage
  o T-ALL and T-LBL are separated based on number of lymphoblasts in bone marrow
    – T-ALL when > 25% blasts in bone marrow
    – Distinction between leukemia and lymphoma becomes arbitrary when there is mass lesion and increased marrow blasts
- Early T-cell precursor ALL (ETP-ALL)
  o Cases of T-ALL that meet **all** following criteria
    – Absence of expression CD1A and CD8
    – Absence or weak expression of CD5 in < 75% of blasts
    – Expression of ≥ 1 myeloid stem cell-associated antigens, including CD117, CD34, HLA-DR, CD13, CD33, CD11b, &/or CD65 in ≥ 25% of blasts

CLASSIFICATION

ICC of Precursor T-Cell Neoplasms
- T-ALL
- Early T-cell precursor ALL, *BCL11B*-activated (new entity)
- Early T-cell precursor ALL, NOS
- "Near early T-cell precursor"
  o Accounts for subset of ETP-ALL
  o Phenotypically similar to ETP-ALL except for ≥ 75% expression of CD5 on blasts
  o Genetically different from ETP-ALL with enrichment for *TLX3* rearrangements
- Natural killer (NK) cell T-ALL (provisional entity)
- T-ALL provisional entity classified based on aberrant activation of transcription factors genes
  o *TAL1* and *TAL2*
  o *TLX1*
  o *TLX3*
  o HOXA gene cluster
  o *LMO1/LMO2*
  o *NKX2-1*, *NKX2-2*, and *NKX2-5*
  o *SPI1*
  o *OLIG1/OLIG2*

WHO-HAEM5
- T-lymphoblastic leukemia/lymphoma, NOS
- Early T-precursor lymphoblastic leukemia/lymphoma
- Genetically defined provisional entities listed in ICC are not currently recognized in WHO-HAEM5
  o Not sufficient evidence to establish genetically defined T-ALL with clinical relevance per WHO-HAEM5
- NK-lymphoblastic leukemia/lymphoma recognized as provisional entity in ICC is not separately listed in WHO-HAEM5
  o Lack of clear-cut and reliable diagnostic criteria per WHO-HAEM5

CLINICAL ISSUES

Epidemiology
- Incidence
  o T-ALL
    – ~ 15% of all childhood ALL
    – ~ 25% of adult ALL
  o T-LBL
    – ~ 85% of all lymphoblastic lymphomas
    – Can occur at any age

Presentation
- T-ALL
  o Commonly present with high leukocyte count with circulating blasts
  o Bone marrow is always involved
    – Relative sparing of trilineage hematopoiesis in bone marrow compared to B-acute lymphoblastic leukemia (B-ALL)
  o Often concurrent mediastinal or other tissue mass
  o Lymphadenopathy and hepatosplenomegaly common
  o CNS involvement is more common than in T-LBL
- T-LBL
  o Frequently presents with rapidly growing anterior mediastinal mass
    – Pleural &/or pericardial effusions often present
    – Respiratory symptoms and superior vena cava syndrome may be seen
  o Lymph node involvement may be seen
  o Bone marrow involvement at diagnosis in ~ 20% of cases

Prognosis
- Childhood T-ALL
  o Higher risk compared to B-ALL
  o Increased risk of induction failure and early relapse
  o Increased risk of isolated CNS relapse
  o Detectable minimal residual disease (MRD) after therapy is strong adverse prognostic factor
    – Patients may still do well if there is no detectable MRD by day 78
- Adult T-ALL
  o Better prognosis than B-ALL, likely due to low rate of adverse cytogenetic abnormalities in T-ALL
- Pediatric T-LBL
  o Inferior event-free survival with marrow &/or CNS involvement
- Adult T-LBL
  o Longer survival, complete remission (CR) rate, and CR duration in patients with
    – Age < 40 years
    – LDH level < 2x upper limits of normal
    – Absent or single extranodal site of disease
  o Short survival with failure to achieve CR in patients with
    – Age > 40 years
    – LDH level > 2x upper limits of normal
    – Hemoglobin level < 10 g/dL
- ETP-ALL
  o Very poor prognosis reported initially in several studies
  o More recent studies showed no significant difference in outcome with more effective therapy
  o Higher incidence of MRD at end of induction

T-Lymphoblastic Leukemia/Lymphoma

- o Overall survival reported comparable with other pediatric T-ALL in one recent study
- Indolent T-lymphoblastic proliferation
  - o Involve upper aerodigestive tract in most cases
  - o May have multiple recurrences without systemic dissemination

MOLECULAR

Antigen Receptor Gene Rearrangements
- Clonal rearrangements of T-cell receptor (TCR) genes detected in virtually all cases
- Concurrent clonal rearrangements of immunoglobulin heavy chain (*IGH*) in 20% of cases

Recurrent Cytogenetic Abnormalities
- Structural chromosomal abnormalities detected in ~ 50-60% of T-ALL/T-LBL
- Numerical chromosomal abnormalities are rare, but tetraploidy occurs in ~ 5% of cases
- Chromosomal translocation involving TCR gene loci
  - o Found in ~ 40% of T-ALL cases
    - TCR α (*TRA*) and TCR δ (*TRD*) at 14q11
    - TCR β (*TRB*) at 7q34
    - TCR γ (*TRG*) at 7p14
  - o Chromosomal translocations occur due to errors during TCR gene rearrangements
- Translocations result in juxtaposition of transcription factor genes to promoters and enhancers of TCR loci
  - o t(7;10); *TRB::TLX1* and t(10;14); *TLX1::TRA/TRD* in 7-31%
  - o t(5;14); *TLX3::TRA/TRD*, cryptic in 13-20%
  - o inv(7)(p15.q34)/t(7;7)(p15;q34); *HOTTIP::TRB* in 5%
  - o t(1;14); *TAL1::TRD* in 3%
  - o t(1;7); *TAL1::TRB* in 3%
  - o t(7;9); *TRB::TAL2* in 1%
  - o t(7;19); *TRB::LYL1* in 1%
  - o t(14;21); *TRA::OLIG2* in 1%
- Translocations generating fusion genes encoding oncogenic chimeric proteins
  - o t(10;11); *PICALM::MLLT10*, often cryptic in 10%
  - o *STIL::TAL1* fusion gene due to cryptic interstitial deletion of 1p33 in 9-30% of pediatric cases
  - o *KMT2A* (a.k.a. *MLL*) fusion with many partner genes, including *MLLT1*, *AFDN* (a.k.a. *MLLT4*), *MLLT10*, *FOXO4*, and *AFF1* in 8%
  - o t(9;12); *ETV6::JAK2* in < 1%
  - o t(4;11); *NUP98::RAP1GDS1* in < 1%
- *ABL1* rearrangements in T-ALL
  - o t(9;9)(q34;q34); *NUP214::ABL1* in < 6%
  - o Cryptic t(9;14)(q34;q32); *EML1::ABL1* in < 1%
  - o t(9;12); *ETV6::ABL1* in < 1%
  - o t(9;22)(q34;q11); *BCR::ABL1* (very rare)
- *MYC* rearrangements in T-ALL
  - o Occur in ~ 6% of cases
  - o *MYC* translocations occur as secondary abnormality in subclones in ~ 1/2 of cases
  - o *MYC* rearrangements may be associated with induction failure and relapse
- Other rare translocations in T-ALL
  - o t(11;14); *LMO1::TRD* in 2%
  - o t(11;14); *LMO2::TRD* in 3-6%
  - o t(7;11); *TRB::LMO2* in 1%
  - o t(1;7); *LCK::TRB* in < 1%
  - o t(7;9); *TRB::NOTCH1* in < 1%
  - o t(7;12); *TRB::CCND2* in < 1%
  - o t(12;14); *CCND2::TRD* in < 1%

Cryptic Deletions
- Typically leads to loss of tumor suppressor genes
- Cryptic deletions are frequent and may be concomitant with other changes
  - o Deletion of *CDKN2A* at 9p21 is most frequent cryptic deletion found in > 50%
  - o Variable size deletion at chromosome 6q

Somatic Gene Mutation
- *NOTCH1*
  - o Key regulator of T-cell fate
  - o Activating mutations present in ~ 50% of T-ALL
- *FBXW7*
  - o Inactivating mutations present in ~ 30%
  - o Contributes to NOTCH1 signaling pathway activation
- *PHF6*
  - o Mutations present in ~ 40%
- *DNMT3A*
  - o Mutations present in ~ 18%
  - o Associated with poor prognosis
- *RUNX1*
  - o Mutations present in 16-18% of T-ALL
    - Significantly associated with higher age and lower white blood cell count
    - Associated with inferior outcome in subgroup of early T-ALL
- *PTEN*
  - o Mutations present in ~ 10% of T-ALL
- *CDKN2A*
  - o Mutations present in ~ 4% of T-ALL
- *FLT3*
  - o *FLT3* ITD mutation present in ~ 2-5% of T-ALL

Other Reported Mutated Genes
- *JAK1*, *JAK3*, *NRAS* activating mutations
- *NF1*, *EZH2*, *SUZ12*, *EED* inactivating mutations

Gene Mutations in Early T-Cell Precursor ALL
- Mutations identified by next-generation sequencing
  - o Recurrent mutations in myeloid-specific oncogenes, including
    - *IDH1*, *IDH2*, *DNMT3A*, *FLT3*, and *NRAS*
    - Mutations in *IDH1*, *IDH2*, and *DNMT3A* found to be associated with poor prognosis
  - o Loss-of-function mutations in regulators of hematopoietic and lymphoid development
    - *RUNX1*, *IKZF1*, *ETV6*, *GATA3*, and *EP300*

Gene Expression Signatures
- Several gene expression signatures described
  - o *LYL1* signature corresponds to immature prothymocytes
  - o *TLX1* signature corresponds to early cortical thymocytes
  - o *TAL1* signature corresponds to late thymocytes
- ETP-ALL
  - o Strongly enriched for genes expressed in hematopoietic stem cells

T-Lymphoblastic Leukemia/Lymphoma

- Upregulation of *KIT*, *GATA2*, and *CEBPA*
- Overexpression of *LYL1* and *ERG*
- Underexpression of *CD3E*, *CD4*, *CD8A*, *RAG1*, and *ZAP70*
- Enriched for genes expressed in early thymocyte progenitor CD4/CD8 T subsets
  – Identification of ETP-ALL solely by defined immunophenotypic criteria may underestimate number of cases
  – ETP-ALL correlates best with CD1A(-), CD4(-), CD8(-), CD34(+), &/or myeloid markers CD13(+) or CD33(+)

MICROSCOPIC

Blood and Bone Marrow Findings

- Peripheral blood findings in T-ALL
  o Leukocytosis with circulating lymphoblasts
    – Lymphoblasts are small to medium-sized with high N:C ratio in most cases
    – Lymphoblasts can show significant size variation ranging from small to large
    – Small lymphoblasts often contain condensed chromatin with inconspicuous nucleoli
    – Cases with small lymphoblasts may be confused with circulating mature T-cell lymphoma
    – Large lymphoblasts typically contain immature nuclear chromatin and distinct nucleoli
    – Nuclei of lymphoblasts may be round, slightly irregular, or convoluted
    – Cytoplasmic vacuoles may be seen in some cases
    – T lymphoblasts are morphologically indistinguishable from B lymphoblasts
  o Cytopenias may be present
- Bone marrow findings in T-ALL
  o Lymphoblasts in marrow aspirate show morphologic features similar to those found in blood
  o Extensive marrow involvement on core biopsy and clot sections
  o Sheets of blasts with immature nuclear chromatin and numerous mitoses typically seen
  o In contrast to B-lineage ALL, normal trilineage hematopoiesis relatively preserved
- Peripheral blood findings in T-LBL
  o Absent to minimal involvement of peripheral blood
- Bone marrow findings in T-LBL
  o Bone marrow involved in < 20% of cases at diagnosis
  o By definition, blasts account for < 25% of nucleated marrow cells in cases with marrow involvement

ANCILLARY TESTS

Flow Cytometry

- Overview of T-ALL immunophenotype
  o T lymphoblasts usually express TdT
  o T lymphoblasts variably express CD1A, CD2, CD3 (surface or cytoplasmic), CD4, CD5, CD7, and CD8
    – CD7 and cytoplasmic CD3 are most often expressed
    – CD3 is considered lineage specific
    – T lymphoblasts frequently coexpress CD4 and CD8 but could express only 1 of these or neither
    – T lymphoblasts may also coexpress CD10
  o Subset of T-ALL/T-LBL cases also express CD34
  o CD13 &/or CD33 are expressed in 20-30% of cases

DIFFERENTIAL DIAGNOSIS

B-Lymphoblastic Leukemia/Lymphoma

- B lymphoblasts are cytomorphologically similar to T lymphoblasts
- Flow cytometry or immunohistochemistry can easily separate T lymphoblasts from B lymphoblasts

Mature T-Cell Lymphoma

- Subset of T lymphoblasts with mature-appearing morphology may mimic mature T-cell lymphoma
- Angioimmunoblastic T-cell lymphoma may have overlapping immunophenotype, including expression of CD3 and CD10
- Expression of immature markers in T lymphoblasts is useful to separate T lymphoblasts from mature T-cell lymphoma

Myeloid and Lymphoid Neoplasm With Eosinophilia and *FGFR1* Abnormalities

- Previously known as 8p11 myeloproliferative syndrome
- Aggressive neoplasms with eosinophilia, circulating blasts, leukemoid reaction, and myeloproliferative features
- > 20% blasts of either myeloid, mixed, or T lineage in some cases
- Myeloproliferative features and rearrangements of *FGFR1* at 8p11 separates this neoplasm from T-ALL/T-LBL

Indolent T-Lymphoblastic Proliferation

- Rare isolated case reports of indolent T-lymphoblastic proliferation in upper airway
- Often associated with Castleman disease or follicular dendritic cell tumors
- Nonclonal by TCR gene rearrangement studies
- Immunophenotype typically includes expression of CD3 and TdT
  o Aberrant T-cell phenotype may include CD4/CD8 double positive
- No known molecular genetic abnormalities reported
- No cytogenetic aberrancies reported
- Chronic and benign nature
  o No chemotherapy is required
- Important to consider in differential diagnosis of immature T-ALL

SELECTED REFERENCES

1. Müller J et al: How T-lymphoblastic leukemia can be classified based on genetics using standard diagnostic techniques enhanced by whole genome sequencing. Leukemia. 37(1):217-21, 2023
2. Alaggio R et al: The 5th edition of the World Health Organization classification of haematolymphoid tumours: lymphoid neoplasms. Leukemia. 36(7):1720-48, 2022
3. Duffield AS et al: International Consensus Classification of acute lymphoblastic leukemia/lymphoma. Virchows Arch. 482(1):11-26, 2022
4. Weinberg OK et al: Clinical, immunophenotypic and genomic findings of NK lymphoblastic leukemia: a study from the Bone Marrow Pathology Group. Mod Pathol. 34(7):1358-66, 2021
5. Lepretre S et al: Adult T-type lymphoblastic lymphoma: treatment advances and prognostic indicators. Exp Hematol. 51:7-16, 2017

T-Lymphoblastic Leukemia/Lymphoma

Cell Block from Pleural Fluid With T-LBL

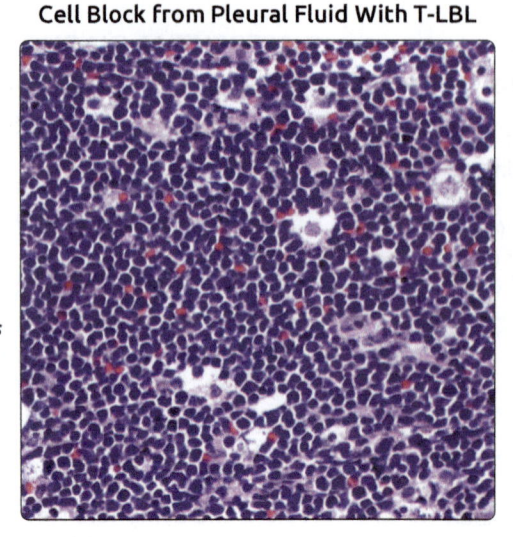

Clot Section of T-ALL

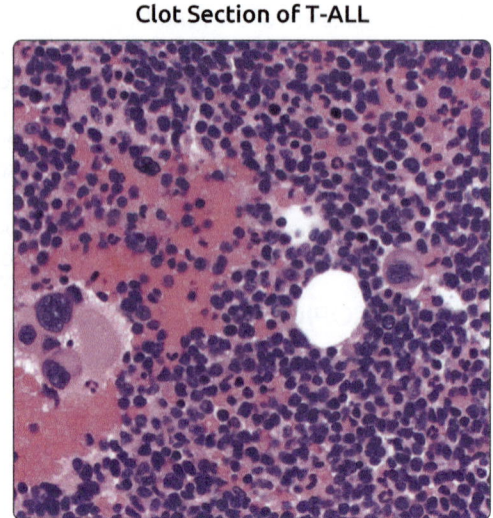

(Left) Cell block from pleural fluid shows sheets of lymphoblasts with scattered tingible body macrophages with starry-sky pattern in a patient with T-LBL. (Right) Bone marrow clot section from a patient with T-ALL shows numerous blasts and at least partially preserved trilineage hematopoiesis. The bone marrow hematopoiesis is typically partially preserved in most T-ALL cases.

CD3 Immunohistochemistry

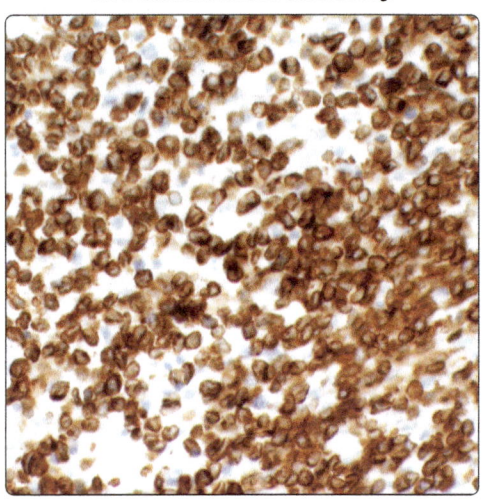

TdT Immunohistochemistry

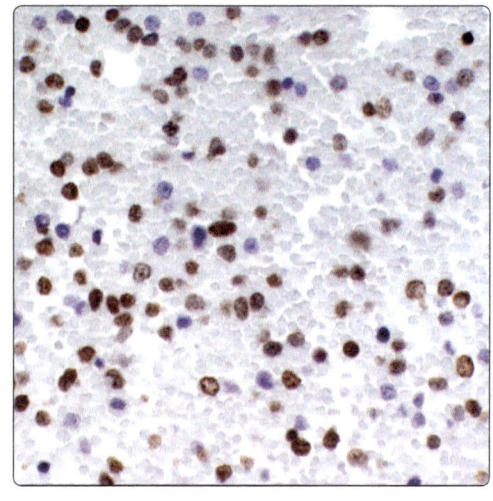

(Left) CD3 of bone marrow trephine biopsy from a pediatric patient with extensive involvement by T-ALL highlights sheets of positive lymphoblasts. (Right) Td on hemodilute bone marrow clot section shows strong nuclear expression by lymphoid blasts. TdT is not lineage specific and is typically expressed in lymphoblasts of both B and T lineages.

B-Acute Lymphoblastic Leukemia in Bone Marrow Core Biopsy

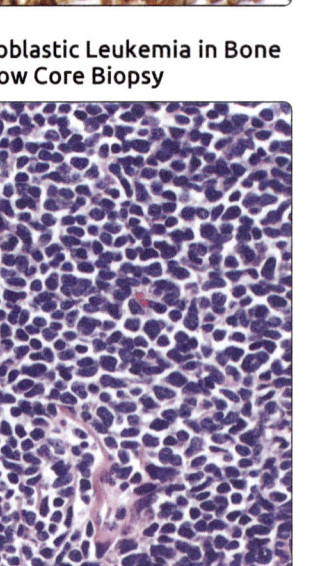

B-Acute Lymphoblastic Leukemia, CD79A Immunohistochemistry

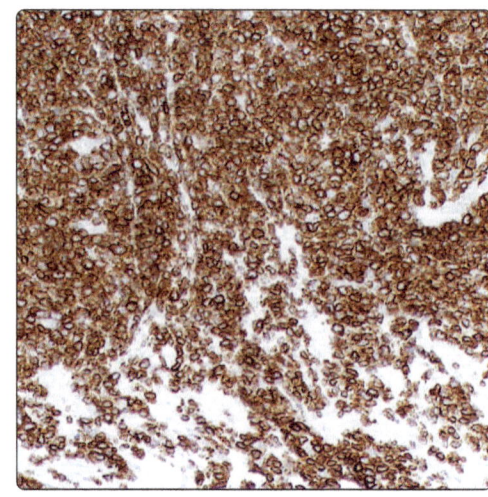

(Left) Bone marrow biopsy from a pediatric patient shows sheets of blasts. Concurrent flow cytometry revealed an immunophenotype diagnostic of B-lymphoblastic leukemia. B and T lymphoblasts are cytomorphologically identical; however, flow cytometry or IHC can easily separate B lymphoblasts from T lymphoblasts. (Right) CD79A highlights sheets of positive lymphoblasts in a pediatric patient with newly diagnosed B-lymphoblastic leukemia.

T-Lymphoblastic Leukemia/Lymphoma

CD1A and cCD3 (+) T-Acute Lymphoblastic Leukemia

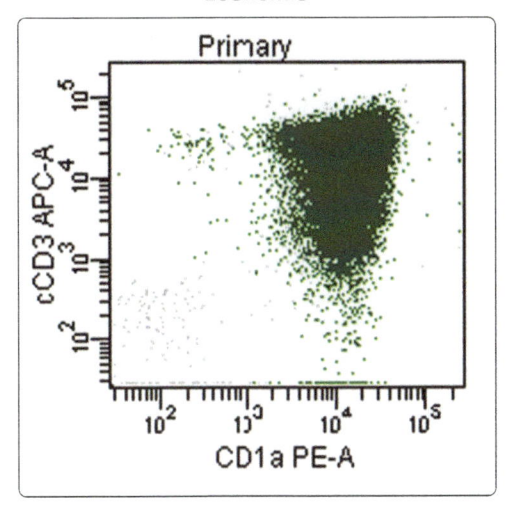

CD10 Expression in T Lymphoblasts

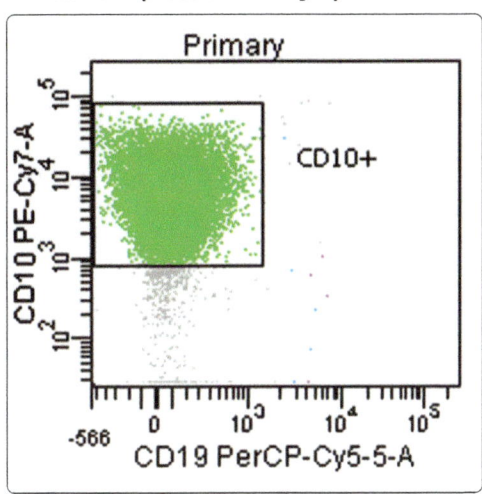

(Left) Flow cytometric analysis performed on bone marrow aspirate from a patient with increased lymphoblasts reveals a distinct cCD3(+) population that also coexpresses CD1A. (Right) Flow cytometric immunophenotyping performed on bone marrow aspirate from a patient with cCD3(+)/CD1A(+) population of lymphoblasts shows coexpression of CD10. Aberrant coexpression of CD10 can be detected in a subset of T-ALL.

CD4/CD8 Double-Positive T Lymphoblasts

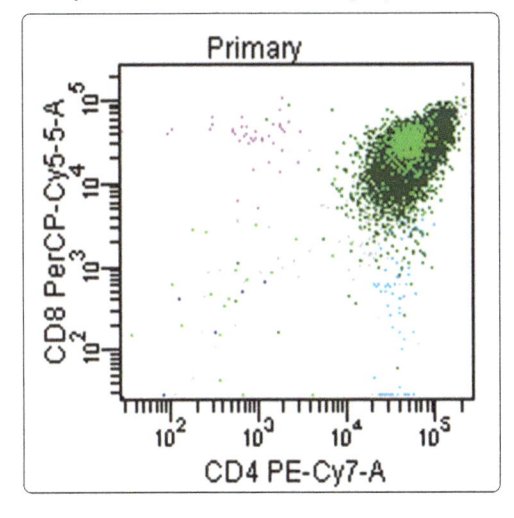

Coexpression of CD2 and TdT

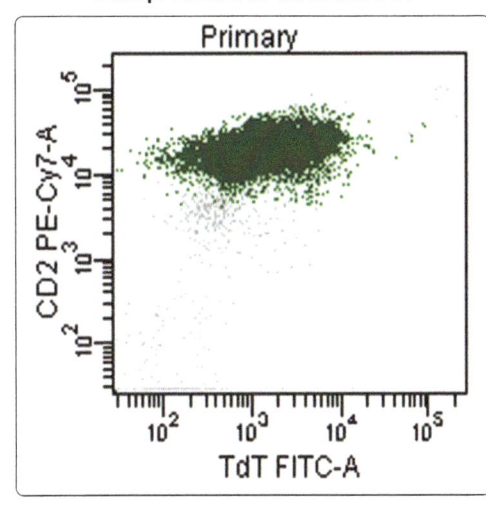

(Left) Flow cytometric analysis using antibodies directed against T-helper-associated antigen CD4 and cytotoxic-associated antigen CD8 shows that the abnormal T-lineage lymphoid population is double positive for CD4 and CD8. (Right) Flow cytometric immunophenotyping shows that the abnormal T-lineage lymphoid population coexpresses CD2 and a subset TdT. Expression of TdT supports the immature nature of the cells.

CD5(+) Population

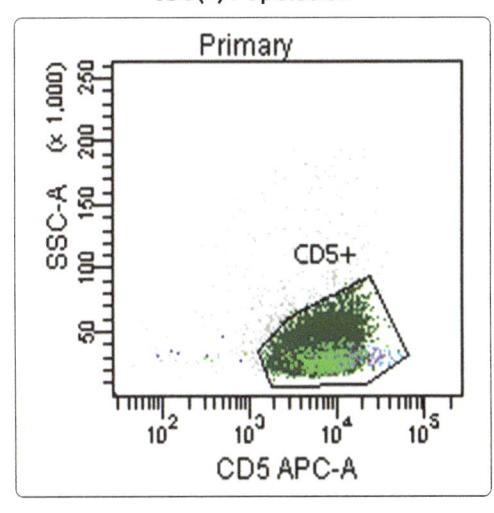

CD7(+) Population

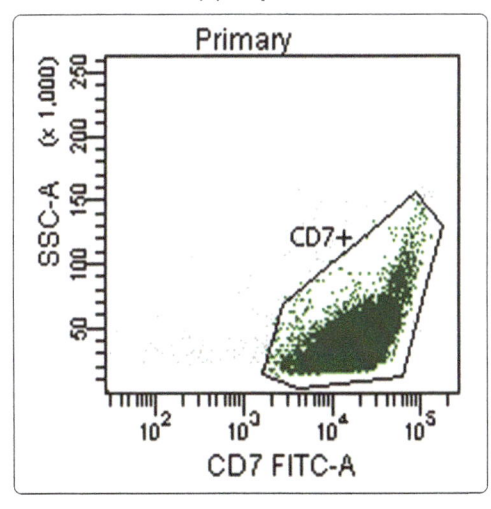

(Left) Flow cytometric analysis shows that the immature and aberrant T-cell population also expresses CD5. However, CD5 is typically negative in ETP-ALL. (Right) Flow cytometric analysis shows that the immature and aberrant T-cell population also expresses CD7. CD7 is not a lineage-specific antigen; however, it is often expressed in both mature and immature T cells.

Small Lymphocytic Lymphoma/Chronic Lymphocytic Leukemia

KEY FACTS

TERMINOLOGY
- Monoclonal B-cell neoplasm with mature, CD5-positive lymphocytes in blood, bone marrow, &/or extramedullary tissues

CLINICAL ISSUES
- Most common leukemia in adults; incidence increases with age
- Treatment decisions depend on *TP53* deletion or *IGHV* mutation status

MOLECULAR
- Important for prognosis and to guide treatment
- Testing at diagnosis should include at minimum assessment of cytogenetic abnormalities, *IGHV* mutational status, and testing for *TP53* mutations
  o Additional testing for other somatic mutations and for BCR stereotypes provide additional information
- Acquired cytogenetic abnormalities seen in 80% of cases
  o Favorable prognosis: 13q14 deletion as sole abnormality
  o Intermediate prognosis: Trisomy 12, normal karyotype
  o Unfavorable prognosis: 11q22-23 deletion, 17p13 deletion
  o Other cytogenetic abnormalities include 6q deletion, 14q deletion, unbalanced translocations, and complex karyotypes
- Immunoglobulin heavy chain variable region (*IGHV*) mutational status
  o > 2% nucleotide difference is hypermutated chronic lymphocytic leukemia (CLL); has better prognosis
  o < 2% nucleotide difference is unmutated CLL; has worse prognosis
- Single gene mutations
  o *TP53*
    – Most important for prognosis and treatment
  o Additional genes of interest include *ATM*, *BIRC3*, *NOTCH1*, *SF3B1*, and *MYC*

Lymphocytosis

(Left) Peripheral blood from a patient with chronic lymphocytic leukemia (CLL) shows lymphocytosis with small, mature, homogeneous lymphocytes with condensed chromatin. (Right) In the bone marrow, CLL often forms small, nonparatrabecular nodules composed of small, mature lymphocytes.

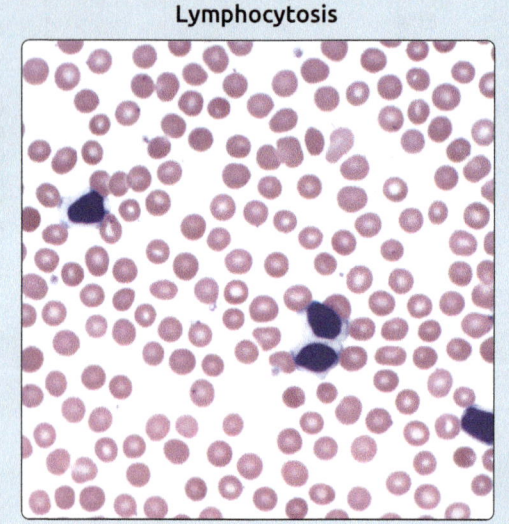

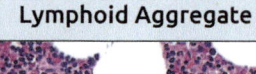

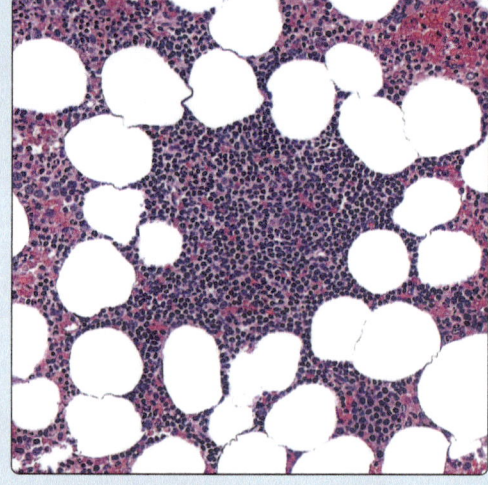

Lymphoid Aggregate

Flow Cytometry Immunophenotype

(Left) Flow cytometry of CLL shows κ-light chain restricted, CD20- and CD19-positive B-cell population with CD5 coexpression. This case shows expression of CD38, an adverse prognostic indicator. (Right) Flow cytometry shows that CLL cells, as identified by CD79A expression (red), are positive for ZAP70, an adverse prognostic indicator. T cells are shown in blue. (Courtesy S. Wenceslao, MD.)

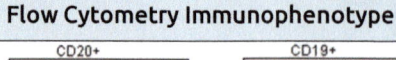

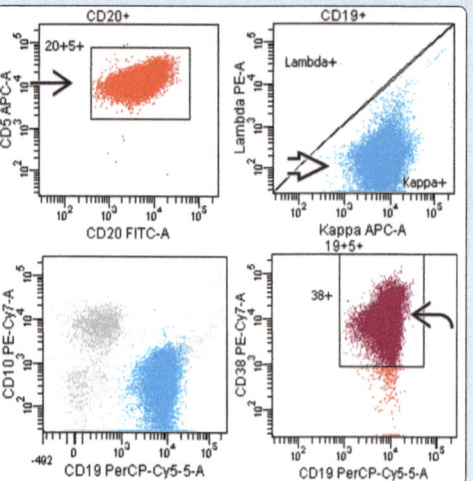

Flow Cytometry for ZAP70

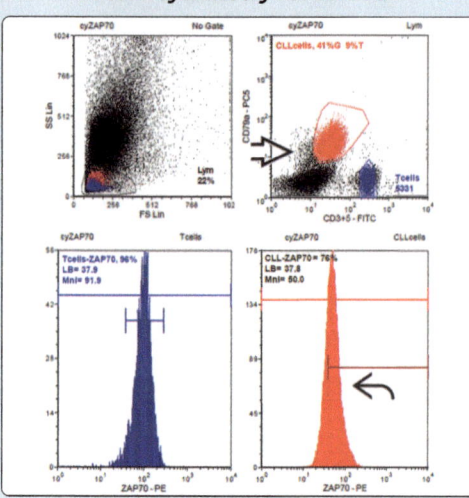

Small Lymphocytic Lymphoma/Chronic Lymphocytic Leukemia

TERMINOLOGY

Abbreviations
- Small lymphocytic lymphoma (SLL)/chronic lymphocytic leukemia (CLL)

Definitions
- B-cell neoplasm of mature, small, round B cells
  - Blood and bone marrow are involved in CLL
  - Primary tissue involvement without significant peripheral blood involvement is termed SLL
    - Tissue shows morphologic and immunophenotypic features of CLL
  - Low-level blood involvement or minimal tissue involvement is termed monoclonal B lymphocytosis (MBL)

CLASSIFICATION

International Consensus Classification and WHO 5th Edition
- CLL
  - ≥ 5 x 10⁹/L monoclonal lymphocytes in blood with CLL immunophenotype
    - Most commonly CD19, CD5, CD20, CD200, CD23 (variable), and dim monotypic light chain
      □ Negative for cyclin-D1, SOX11, and FMC7
    - Prolymphocytes account for ≤ 55% of cells
      □ Increased prolymphocytes may be sign of disease progression
      □ Most often account for ≤ 10%
    - May also involve extramedullary tissues
- SLL
  - Nodal, splenic, or extramedullary involvement with CLL immunophenotype and ≤ 5 x 10⁹/L monoclonal lymphocytes in blood
- MBL
  - Clonal B lymphocytes in peripheral blood < 5 x 10⁹/L
  - Tissue involvement < 1.5-cm, nondistorted architecture with absent proliferation centers

ETIOLOGY/PATHOGENESIS

Cell of Origin
- Derives from mature, antigen-experienced B cells
  - Cells show downregulation of IgM, consistent with exposure to antigen and anergy
  - Gene expression profile similar to that of memory and marginal zone B cells
  - Different B-cell maturation pathways give rise to different subtypes
    - Classic germinal center pathway gives rise to *IGHV*-mutated memory B cells
    - T-cell dependent and independent extrafollicular pathways give rise to *IGHV*-unmutated memory B cells
- Normal adults show low levels of CD5-positive B cells in peripheral blood
- Fetal blood and lymphoid tissue show CD5-positive B cells

Pathogenesis
- Posttranscriptional deletions in small noncoding RNA genes, termed microRNA
  - MicroRNA normally regulate gene expression, function as tumor suppressors
  - Downregulation leads to expression of antiapoptotic proteins
    - Increased BCL2 expression leads to prolonged cell survival

Immunoglobulin Heavy Chain Variable Regions Usage and Stereotyped B-Cell Receptors
- CLL shows preferential usage of certain immunoglobulin heavy chain variable regions (IGHV)
  - Hypermutated CLL is associated with usage of *VH4-34*
  - Unmutated cases are associated with usage of *VH1-69* and *VH4-39*
- Subset of cases show stereotyped B-cell receptors
  - Cases demonstrate highly similar amino acid sequences
  - Seen in 30% of cases
  - Used to define subsets with common clinical and molecular features
- Preferential variable regions usage and stereotyped receptors may indicate role for chronic antigen stimulation in pathogenesis
  - Possible antigens include autoantigens and superantigens, such as *Staphylococcus aureus* protein A and CMV phosphoprotein pUL32
  - Other potential environmental, medical, and occupational risk factors, including radiation exposure, have been proposed

CLINICAL ISSUES

Epidemiology
- Incidence
  - Most common leukemia of adults in Western countries
  - Annual incidence is 4-10 per 100,000 persons
- Age
  - 90% of cases occur > 50 years of age
    - Median at diagnosis: ~ 73 years of age
    - Patients diagnosed < 55 years of age often have more aggressive disease
    - 16.7 cases per 100,000 persons > 65 years of age
- Sex
  - M:F = 1.9:1
- Familial CLL/SLL
  - Most common familial leukemia
  - Family history of CLL or other low-grade lymphoma is significant risk factor for development of CLL
  - Risk of CLL in family members with 1st-degree relative with CLL is ~ 7.5%
  - Familial cases present earlier and are more aggressive

Presentation
- Anemia
- Lymphocytosis
- Generalized lymphadenopathy
- Splenomegaly or other organomegaly
- Fatigue
- Asymptomatic in up to 80% of cases

Natural History
- Often indolent
- Genetic features strongly influence disease course

Small Lymphocytic Lymphoma/Chronic Lymphocytic Leukemia

- Autoimmune complications seen in 4-25%
  - Autoimmune hemolytic anemia
  - Immune thrombocytopenic purpura (ITP)
  - Pure red cell aplasia
  - Autoimmune agranulocytosis
- Immune system impairment
  - Decreased numbers and function of B cells
    - Hypogammaglobulinemia is common
  - Decreased number and function of T cells and NK cells
  - Decreased complement activity
  - Decreased neutrophil and monocyte function

Treatment
- Often held until patient develops progressive or symptomatic disease
- Goal of treatment is complete remission
- Treatment decisions often depend on *TP53* status
  - *TP53* mutation or deletion associated with resistance to chemoimmunotherapy
- Therapeutic options
  - Chemotherapeutic agents
  - Immunotherapy/monoclonal antibodies
  - Targeted therapies
  - BCR pathway and tyrosine kinase inhibitors
- Allogeneic stem cell transplantation may be considered in high-risk or younger patients
- Immunosuppression may be used in patients with autoimmune complications
- Splenectomy may be used in refractory ITP or autoimmune hemolytic anemia

Prognosis
- Overall 10-year median survival
  - With favorable prognostic factors: > 25 years
  - With unfavorable prognostic factors: < 10 years
- ~ 5-10% of cases transform to high-grade lymphoid neoplasm (Richter transformation)
  - Prolymphocytoid transformation (very rare)
- Clinical prognostic factors
  - Rai and Binet staging system
    - Stage determined by extent of disease, cytopenias
  - Unfavorable factors include male sex, age ≥ 60 years, ECOG status > 0, lymphocyte doubling time < 12 months
  - Favorable factors include female sex, age < 60 years
- Laboratory prognostic factors
  - Unfavorable
    - CD49d positive
    - CD38 positive
    - ZAP70 positive
    - Elevated serum free light chain
    - Elevated serum thymidine kinase
    - Elevated β2-microglobulin
    - Unmutated *IGHV*
    - Usage of *IGH*V3-23 or *IGH*V3-21 region irrespective of mutation status
    - Complex karyotype
    - 17p13 (*TP53*) deletion or *TP53* mutation
    - t(14;19)(q32;q13); *IGH::BCL3*
  - Favorable
    - CD38 negative
    - ZAP70 negative
    - Hypermutated *IGHV*
    - 13q14 deletion

MOLECULAR
Cytogenetics
- Acquired cytogenetic abnormalities seen in 80% of cases
  - Not sensitive or specific for diagnosis of CLL
  - Carry implications for disease behavior and prognosis
- 13q14 deletion
  - Most common cytogenetic abnormality (~ 70%)
  - Favorable prognostic factor
  - Monoallelic and biallelic deletion show similar outcomes
  - Associated with shorter time to 1st treatment if seen in > 65% of cells
  - Associated with normal morphology, CD38 negativity, and hypermutated *IGHV*
  - More common with blood and bone marrow involvement than with tissue
  - Genes and microRNA-coding regions involved in 13q14 deletion
    - *DLEU1/DLEU2*
      - NFκB and nuclear factor of activated T cell inhibitors and may function as tumor suppressor genes
    - *RB1* at 13q14 deleted in ~ 40% of cases
    - miR-15a and miR-16-1 expression decreased in 13q14 deletion
      - Correlates with increased BCL2 signaling and inhibition of apoptosis
    - Genes and microRNA may also be silenced through epigenetic changes
  - Pathways involved in alteration of 13q14 region
    - Loss of 13q chromosomal arm
    - Interstitial deletion of 13q14 region
    - Loss of heterozygosity
    - Unbalanced translocations
    - Epigenetic silencing of region
- Trisomy 12
  - 10-20% incidence
  - Effects may be due to gene dosage effect and alter gene expression in other regions
    - Genes located on chromosome 12 that show increased expression
      - *HIP1R*, *CDK4*, and *MYF6*
    - Genes located on chromosome 3 that may show decreased expression
      - *P2RY14* and *CD200*
    - Many cases associated with microdeletion of miR-15a/16-1 cluster on chromosome 13
  - Associated with mutation of *NOTCH1*
    - Higher risk disease
  - Clinically heterogeneous; overall intermediate prognosis
    - Increased risk of Richter transformation
  - Associated with atypical morphology, bright CD20 expression, and increased CD49d expression
  - Associated with tissue involvement
- 11q22-23 deletion
  - 20% incidence
  - Unfavorable prognostic factor

Small Lymphocytic Lymphoma/Chronic Lymphocytic Leukemia

- o Associated with unmutated *IGHV*, high WBC count, splenomegaly, and extramedullary tissue involvement
- o Results in deletion of *ATM* and *BIRC3*
  - *ATM* deletion associated with chromosomal instability
  - *BIRC3* deletion leads to constitutive activation of NFκB signaling pathway
    - □ Associated with aggressive disease and resistance to fludarabine treatment
    - □ Usually mutually exclusive with *TP53* abnormalities
- o Numerous other genes are present in deleted region, including
  - *RDX, FDX1, RAB39A, CUL5, ACAT1, NPAT, ZW10, ZBTB16, CADM1,* and *H2AX*
- o *DDX10* and *CASP10* show decreased expression
- 17p13 deletion
  - o 3-8% incidence at diagnosis
    - Incidence 40% in treatment-refractory CLL
    - Incidence 60% in Richter syndrome
  - o Higher percentage of cells carrying deletion associated with worse outcomes
  - o Genes involved
    - *TP53* tumor suppressor gene
    - Decreased expression of tumor suppressor genes and genes involved in mRNA and protein processing, including *DPH1, GABARAP, GPS2, NCOR1, NLRP1,* and *CAMTA2*
    - Overexpression of *CCND2, NME1,* and *STT3A*
  - o 80% of patients with deletion of 17p13 have mutations in remaining *TP53*
    - *TP53* mutation may cause genomic instability, leading to loss of 17p13
  - o Poor prognostic factor
    - *TP53* loss associated with resistance to alkylating chemotherapy
  - o Associated with presentation in advanced stage, rapidly progressive disease, treatment refractoriness, Richter syndrome, and aberrant immunophenotype with bright CD20, FMC7, and surface immunoglobulin expression
    - Associated with CD38 and ZAP70 expression
    - Associated with unmutated *IGHV*
  - o Mutation testing needed in addition to FISH/karyotype
- Other cytogenetic abnormalities
  - o Complex karyotype (≥ 3 abnormalities)
    - Seen in 40% of cases
    - Associated with high-risk disease
    - Associated with unmutated *IGHV* and CD38 antigen expression
    - High complexity karyotype (≥ 5 abnormalities) is independent marker of poor prognosis
  - o 14q deletion
    - May or may not involve *IGH* at 14q32
    - Associated with typical CLL immunophenotype and unmutated *IGHV*
  - o 6q deletion
    - Associated with high WBC count, splenomegaly, atypical morphology, positive CD38 expression, and intermediate prognosis
  - o Chromosomal translocations
    - May be balanced or unbalanced
    - Many involve *IGH*
      - □ t(14;19)(q32;q13); *IGH::BCL3* CLL has atypical morphology and immunophenotype, associated with trisomy 12 and complex karyotype, and unmutated *IGHV*
    - *MYC* translocations correlate with poor prognostic features, including increased prolymphocytes, 17p deletion, and complex karyotype

Genetic Testing

- *IGHV* mutational status
  - o Somatic mutation of *IGHV* is physiologic process
    - Somatic hypermutation in *IGHV* occurs after antigen exposure
    - Increases B-cell affinity for antigen
  - o Testing aligns sequence of *IGH* variable region to closest *IGH* variable sequences in data base
    - > 2% nucleotide difference is considered mutated CLL
  - o Mutated CLL
    - More indolent behavior and better outcome
  - o Unmutated CLL
    - Greater likelihood of progression, treatment requirement, and shorter survival
  - o Testing also determines V region utilized in *IGH* rearrangement
    - Use of *IGH*V3-23 or *IGH*V3-21 correlates with adverse prognosis regardless of mutation status

Somatic Mutations

- *TP53* mutation
  - o Located at 17p13
  - o Cell cycle regulator, detects DNA damage, causing cell cycle arrest and DNA repair or apoptosis
  - o Testing at diagnosis recommended to guide therapy
    - Complete assessment should include exons 2-11
      - □ At minimum exons 4-10 should be assessed
      - □ Includes DNA binding domain and oligomerization domain
  - o Mutations seen in 16% of CLL cases
    - More common in advanced disease
    - Seen in 90% of cases with *TP53* deletion
  - o Associated with resistance to alkylating agents, presentation in advanced stage, rapidly progressive disease, Richter transformation
- *ATM* mutation
  - o Located at 11q22.3
  - o *ATM* detects DNA damage
  - o Mutations present in 12% of CLL cases
  - o Mutations associated with adverse prognosis
- *BIRC3* mutation
  - o Located at 11q22
  - o *BIRC3* negatively regulates NKκB signaling pathway
  - o Mutations are rare at diagnosis but more common in advanced disease
  - o Mutations associated with aggressive disease and resistance to treatment with fludarabine
- *NOTCH1* mutation
  - o Located at 9q34
  - o Transcription factor that functions in cell differentiation, proliferation, and apoptosis
    - Loss leads to increased MYC expression

319

Small Lymphocytic Lymphoma/Chronic Lymphocytic Leukemia

- o Mutations detected in 10-15% of cases at diagnosis, more common in advanced disease
  - Seen in 30% of Richter transformation
- o Mutations associated with unmutated *IGHV* and increased ZAP70 and CD38 expression, decreased CD20 expression, more aggressive disease, resistance to treatment, Richter transformation, and worse outcomes
  - Often show resistance to rituximab
- o Other Notch pathway mutations show similar clinical course
  - *FBXW7* and *MED12*
- *SF3B1* mutation
  - o Located at 2q33
  - o *SF3B1* encodes part of spliceosome, allowing proper RNA-to-protein translation
  - o Mutations seen in 7-15% of cases at diagnosis, more common in advanced disease
  - o Mutations more common with *IGHV3-21* and possibly *IGHV1-69* usage, mutually exclusive of *IGHV1-2* usage
  - o Mutations associated with aggressive disease, short survival, higher WBC count and higher leukemic cell count, CD38 antigen positivity, and unmutated *IGHV*
  - o Mutations not seen in patients with Richter syndrome
- *MYC* mutations
  - o Located at 8q24
  - o Seen in < 1% of cases
  - o Associated with high-risk disease
  - o Seen with 17p13 deletion, complex karyotype
  - o Associated with increased prolymphocytes
- Other mutated genes include *MYD88* and *POT1*

Chromosomal Microarray

- Increasing numbers of abnormalities by array CGH correlate with worse prognosis
- Gains in 2p, including *MYCN*, *REL*, and *MSH2*
  - o Associated with high-stage disease, unmutated *IGHV*, and Richter transformation
- Gains in 8q
  - o Associated with aggressive disease with negative ZAP70 expression
- Loss in 8p
  - o May predict shorter time from diagnosis to treatment

Gene Expression Profiling

- CLL shows distinct gene expression profile
  - o *IGHV*-mutated and unmutated cases show similar profiles
  - o Profile is similar to memory and marginal zone B cells
  - o CLL cells overexpress oncogenes, such as *LEF1*, and other tumor-related genes
  - o CLL cells underexpress immunoglobulin-related genes, including IgM, IgG3, J chain, and IgA, and genes known to be underexpressed in other tumors
- Can distinguish aggressive from indolent disease
  - o Distinct profiles of lowest stage and highest stage disease

MICROSCOPIC

Peripheral Blood

- Absolute lymphocyte count > 5×10^9/L
- Lymphocytes are monotonous, mature with round nuclei, condensed chromatin, and scant cytoplasm
- Atypical cases are more heterogeneous and may show larger cells with prominent nucleoli or nuclear irregularity or plasmacytoid appearance
  - o Associated with genetic subtypes, including trisomy 12
  - o Prolymphocytes should account for < 55% of cells in CLL
- May have anemia &/or thrombocytopenia

Bone Marrow

- Nonparatrabecular aggregates, growing in nodular, interstitial, diffuse or mixed pattern, and composed mostly of mature lymphocytes

Lymph Node

- Diffuse effacement by small mature lymphocytes
  - o Overall cytology is similar to peripheral blood
    - Proliferation centers containing variable numbers of prolymphocytes with prominent central nucleolus and more abundant cytoplasm and occasional larger transformed cells (paraimmunoblasts)

Transformation

- Prolymphocytoid transformation
  - o Prolymphocytes account for > 55% of lymphocytes
  - o Prolymphocytes are larger lymphoid cells with oval to round central nucleus, abundant blue cytoplasm, and single prominent nucleolus
- Diffuse large B-cell lymphoma
  - o May show mixed appearance with low-grade CLL-like features and large cell areas with atypia and high proliferation rate
- Classic Hodgkin lymphoma

ANCILLARY TESTS

Immunohistochemistry

- Neoplastic cells express CD20, CD79A, CD5, CD23, LEF1

Flow Cytometry

- Neoplastic cells are positive for CD5, CD23, and CD200 and show dim CD20 and surface light chain restriction
- CD38, ZAP70, or CD49d positivity define higher risk group

DIFFERENTIAL DIAGNOSIS

Monoclonal B Lymphocytosis

- Monoclonal B cells in blood account for < 5×10^9/L
- Patients are asymptomatic

Mantle Cell Lymphoma

- Express CD5 antigen similar to CLL
- Associated with t(11;14)(q13;q32); *CCND1::IGH*
- Cyclin-D1 (+), SOX11 (+)

Other B-Cell Lymphomas

- Marginal zone lymphoma may express CD5 in 25% of cases
- Other low-grade lymphomas are most commonly CD5 negative and have distinct clinical, morphologic, and immunophenotypic features

SELECTED REFERENCES

1. Parviz M et al: Prediction of clinical outcome in CLL based on recurrent gene mutations, CLL-IPI variables, and (para)clinical data. Blood Adv. 6(12):3716-28, 2022
2. Ljungström V et al: Prognostic and predictive implications of cytogenetics and genomics. Hematol Oncol Clin North Am. 35(4):703-13, 2021

Small Lymphocytic Lymphoma/Chronic Lymphocytic Leukemia

IGHV Mutational Status

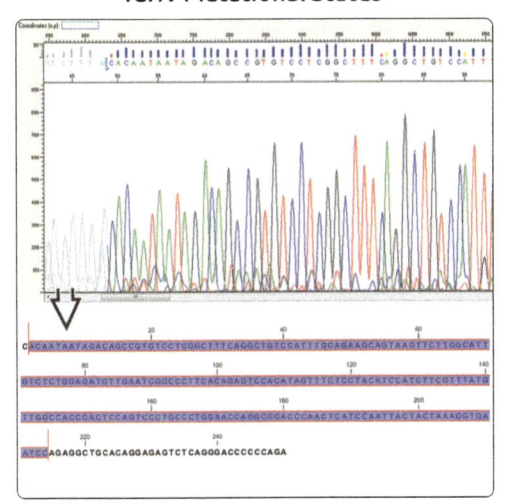

IMGT Database for IGHV

(Left) PCR-amplified products of IGH using primers flanking leader and joining regions is sequenced via Sanger sequencing. The DNA sequence of the variable region ⇒ is selected (highlighted in blue) for comparison to the reference sequence in the database. **(Right)** Compared to the database reference sequence, this case of CLL uses the IGHV3-7*01 region and shows < 98% homology (> 2% difference), consistent with somatic hypermutation of the variable region.

Lymphocytosis

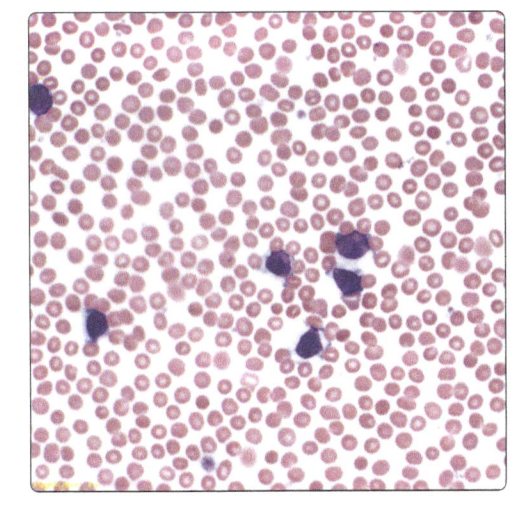

Normal FISH for TP53 and ATM

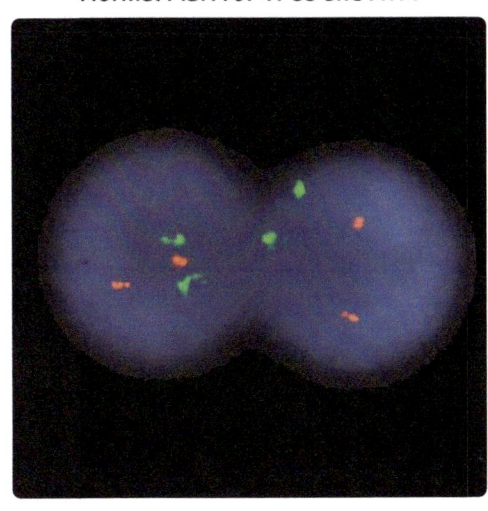

(Left) Peripheral blood shows lymphocytosis with mature lymphocytes. FISH using a standard probe set for prognosis in CLL was performed. **(Right)** FISH probe set shows 2 signals for ATM and 2 signals for TP53, consistent with a normal study.

FISH for Chromosome 12 and 13q

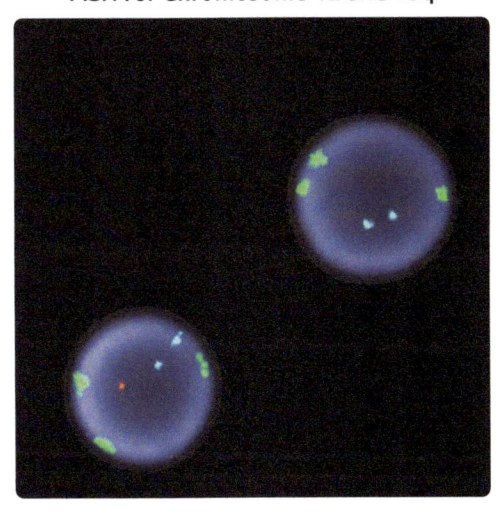

Karyotype in CLL

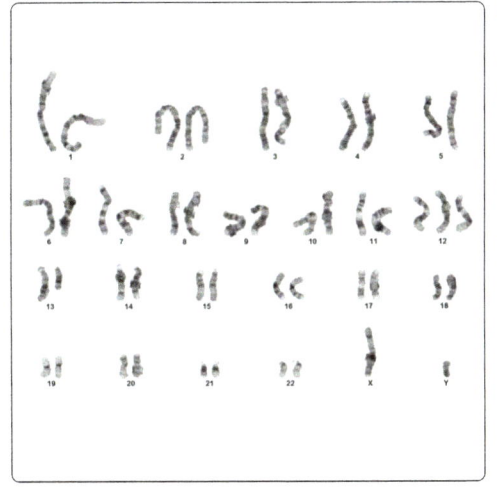

(Left) FISH probe set shows 3 copies of chromosome 12 (green) and loss of 13q14.3 (red), consistent with trisomy 12 and deletion of the 13q14.3 region. Probes directed against 11q22.3 (ATM locus) show 2 intact copies in each cell (aqua). **(Right)** Karyotype from the same case shows trisomy 12 and interstitial deletion of chromosome 13. Also, there is additional material on chromosomes 3 and 17. These additional abnormalities were not detected by the limited FISH panel.

B-Cell Prolymphocytic Leukemia

KEY FACTS

TERMINOLOGY
- Neoplasm composed of prolymphocytes involving peripheral blood, bone marrow, or spleen with > 55% (usually > 90%) prolymphocytes
- No longer entity in WHO; remains entity in ICC

CLINICAL ISSUES
- Massive splenomegaly
- Marked peripheral lymphocytosis
- Aggressive behavior, resistant to treatment

MOLECULAR
- No single defining cytogenetic aberration
- Complex karyotypes in ~ 50%
- *MYC* translocations/gains (*MYC* aberration)
- Deletion 17p or *TP53* mutations may contribute to poor response to treatment
- Clonal immunoglobulin heavy chain (*IGH*) rearrangement
  - *IGH* variable region mutational status, CD38 or ZAP70 expression not related to prognosis

MICROSCOPIC
- Peripheral blood shows marked lymphocytosis with large lymphocytes containing prominent nucleoli
- Spleen with expanded white pulp nodules with white and red pulp infiltration
- Bone marrow shows nodular and interstitial infiltrates

ANCILLARY TESTS
- B-cell markers (+)
- CD5 and CD23 (+) in subset of cases
- Cyclin-D1 (-)
- CD200 only weakly (+) or (-)

TOP DIFFERENTIAL DIAGNOSES
- Small lymphocytic lymphoma/chronic lymphocytic leukemia
- Mantle cell lymphoma

Peripheral Blood

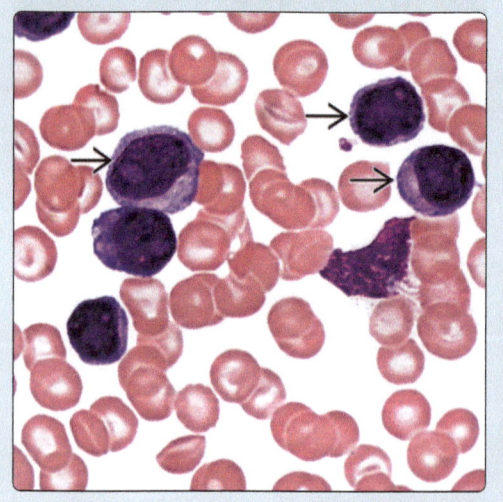

Lymph Node

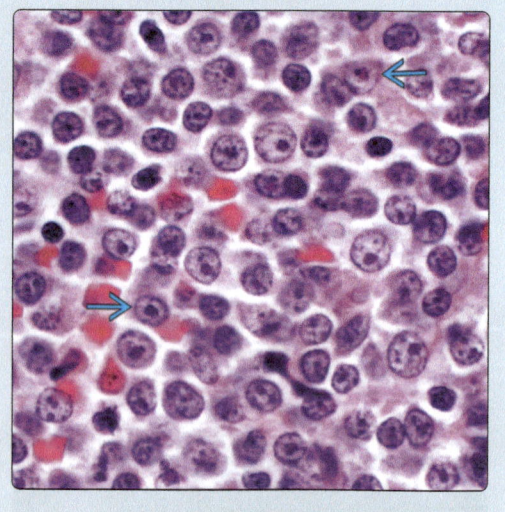

(Left) *Peripheral blood involved by B-cell prolymphocytic leukemia (B-PLL) shows marked leukocytosis consisting of B cells ⇥ with distinct central nucleoli. These cells lacked expression of either CD5 or CD23 by flow cytometry.* (Right) *Lymph node in a patient with B-PLL shows tumor cells that are medium sized, round, and have distinct nucleoli ⇥.*

IGH Rearrangement

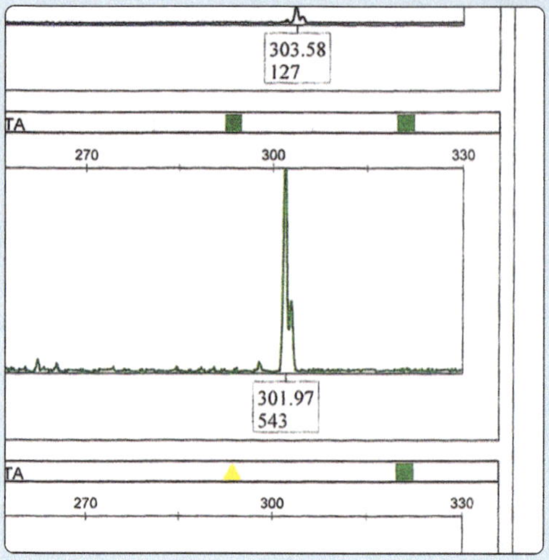

FISH MYC Break-Apart Probe

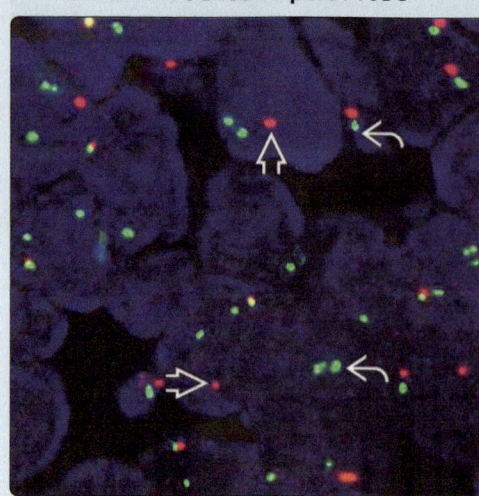

(Left) *PCR test for immunoglobulin heavy (IGH) chain gene rearrangement shows a dominant monoclonal peak at position 301. IGH monoclonality is expected since this is a mature B-cell neoplasm.* (Right) *MYC break-apart probe detects MYC rearrangement in a case of B-PLL. The presence of separated red ⇥ and green ⇥ signals indicates that there has been gene rearrangement at the MYC locus.*

B-Cell Prolymphocytic Leukemia

TERMINOLOGY

Abbreviations
- B-cell prolymphocytic leukemia (B-PLL)

Definitions
- Rare neoplasm composed of mature B cells involving peripheral blood, bone marrow, or spleen with > 55% (usually > 90%) prolymphocytes

ETIOLOGY/PATHOGENESIS

Classification
- International Consensus Classification (ICC)
  - Retains B-PLL as distinct entity
- World Health Organization (WHO) 5th Edition
  - Reclassifies B-PLL into following categories
    - Mantle cell lymphoma, blastoid subtypes (MCL)
    - Progression of chronic lymphocytic leukemia/small lymphocytic lymphoma (CLL/SLL)
    - Splenic B-cell lymphoma with prominent nucleoli (SBLPN)
  - Cases diagnosed as MCL or CLL/SLL have phenotype/genotype of those diseases
  - Remaining cases lumped into SBLPN, which is nonspecific category

CLINICAL ISSUES

Epidemiology
- Incidence
  - Very rare
    - < 0.5% of lymphocytic leukemias
- Age
  - Usually > 60 years
    - Median: 65-69 years
- Sex
  - M = F

Presentation
- Marked lymphocytosis often with massive splenomegaly
  - Lack of lymphadenopathy

Laboratory Tests
- Complete blood count
  - Marked leukocytosis (median: 150 x 10^9/L)
    - Characteristic of disease
    - Rapidly rising white blood cell count (WBC)
  - Variable cytopenias
    - Anemia and thrombocytopenia in 50%

Natural History
- Usually aggressive in nature

Treatment
- Due to rarity of disease and lack of randomized clinical trials, treatment is not standardized
- Some use chronic lymphocytic leukemia (CLL) guidelines/therapies
- Watch and wait can be used for asymptomatic B-PLL
- Combination chemotherapy with rituximab commonly employed
  - Cyclophosphamide, doxorubicin, vincristine, and prednisone (CHOP)
  - Alemtuzumab and BCR inhibitors (ibrutinib)
  - BTKi7-10 and PI3Ki11 as possible future therapies
- Splenectomy may improve symptoms
- Splenic radiation is used in some cases if splenectomy cannot be performed
- Allogeneic stem cell transplantation is only curative therapy for eligible patients

Prognosis
- Poor
  - Aggressive clinical course and resistance to treatment
- Median survival: 3 years
  - MYC aberration and del17p has worse outcome with median OS < 2 years

MACROSCOPIC

General Features
- Splenomegaly with prominent white pulp

MOLECULAR

Molecular Diversity
- B-PLL has shown remarkable biological molecular heterogeneity
- Limits classification by molecular alterations as specific entity

Molecular Genetics
- *MYC* aberrations
  - *MYC* translocations and gains are frequent
  - t(8;14); *MYC/IGH*, t(2;8); *IGK/MYC* and t(8;22); *MYC/IGL* have all been reported
  - More frequently detected in Burkitt lymphoma and diffuse large B-cell lymphoma
- *TP53* mutations/deletions
  - Found in 50% of cases
  - Located at 17p13.1
  - Cell cycle regulator, detects DNA damage
  - May contribute to poor response to treatment
- *ATM* mutations
  - Located at 11q22.3
  - *ATM* detects DNA damage
  - Detected in > 50% of cases of PLL

Cytogenetics
- No single defining cytogenetic aberration
  - Complex karyotypes
    - ~ 50% of cases
  - *MYC* translocations
    - Sole abnormality or part of complex karyotype
  - Deletion 17p
    - ~ 50% of cases
    - Associated with *TP53* mutations
  - Del 13q14 in 27%, del 11q23 less common
  - Trisomy 12 is very rare

In Situ Hybridization
- Detects *CMYC* rearrangement
  - Often use *CMYC* break-apart probes

B-Cell Prolymphocytic Leukemia

- o Amplification of *MYC* by FISH also reported
- No t(11;14)(q13;q32); *CCND1::IGH*
  - o Cases with t(11;14)(q13;q32) reclassified as mantle cell lymphoma

Polymerase Chain Reaction
- Clonal immunoglobulin heavy chain (*IGH*) gene rearrangement
  - o Can have mutated or unmutated immunoglobulin heavy chain variable region (IGHV)
  - o No clear association between IGHV mutation, ZAP70, or CD38 expression and prognosis, unlike CLL
- *BRAF* V600E mutation detected at very low frequency

Gene Expression Profiling
- Different genetic signatures between PLL and CLL support that PLL is distinctive leukemia that could be classified separately
- Shows increased *MYC* expression in B-PLL as compared to CLL

MICROSCOPIC

Histologic Features
- Blood with prolymphocytes > 55% of lymphoid cells
  - o Number of prolymphocytes may exceed 90% of lymphocytes
- Spleen
  - o Expansion of white pulp and red pulp with cells with central eosinophilic nucleolus
- Bone marrow
  - o Nodular/interstitial infiltrates of prolymphocytes
  - o Hypercellular marrow
  - o Lack of other hematopoietic cells
- Lymph node
  - o Only very rarely demonstrates infiltrates of prolymphocytes
  - o Diffuse or vaguely nodular infiltrates of cells with prominent central nucleoli
  - o No proliferation centers

Cytologic Features
- Prolymphocytes
  - o Medium to large in size with prominent central nucleoli
    - 2x size of normal lymphocyte
  - o Round to oval nuclei; ample, basophilic cytoplasm; and perinuclear condensed chromatin
  - o Cytoplasm may be more abundant than in CLL

ANCILLARY TESTS

Immunohistochemistry
- B-cell markers (+)
  - o CD20, CD19, CD22, CD79a
- CD5(+) in 25% of cases
- CD23(+) in 15% of cases
  - o CD5(+) and CD23(+) cases are more commonly seen in CLL with PLL transformation
- CD200 only weakly (+) or (-)
- FMC7(+), CD43(+/-)
- High proliferation index (Ki-67)
- CD38(+) in 57% and ZAP70(+) in ~ 50% of cases
  - o No definitive prognostic value
  - o Not related to mutational status of immunoglobulin genes
- Cyclin-D1 (-)
- Strongly express surface IgM(+/-)

DIFFERENTIAL DIAGNOSIS

Small Lymphocytic Lymphoma/Chronic Lymphocytic Leukemia
- Lower absolute lymphocyte count compared to PLL
- History of CLL precludes diagnosis of PLL
- Prolymphocytoid transformation of SLL/CLL shows increased prolymphocytes in peripheral blood and usually is CD23(+) and CD5(+)
- CLL can have mix of both small lymphocytes and prolymphocytes rather than only prolymphocytes
- Immunohistochemistry shows B-cell phenotype with CD5(+), CD23(+), FMC7(-), CD10(-), and surface immunoglobulin (weak)
- Trisomy 12; del 13q, 11q, or 17p may present

Mantle Cell Lymphoma
- Leukemic variant may have prominent nucleoli and (commonly) very high WBCs
  - o Misclassified in past as PLL
- CD5(+), cyclin-D1 (+), and SOX11(+)
  - o Cyclin-D1 and SOX11 should be (-) in PLL
- t(11;14)(q13;q32); *CCND1::IGH* detected by cytogenetics and FISH
  - o Not found in PLL
- Some believe that B-PLL is subtype of mantle cell lymphoma

Splenic Marginal Zone Lymphoma
- Can show similar appearance to B-PLL if peripheralized
- Small lymphocytes, sometimes with abundant cytoplasm
- May show polar villi
- B-cell phenotype with CD5(-), CD10(-), and CD23(-)
- Deletion of 7q in ~ 70%

DIAGNOSTIC CHECKLIST

Clinically Relevant Pathologic Features
- Prolymphocytes in peripheral blood > 55% of lymphoid cells

Pathologic Interpretation Pearls
- Prolymphocytes are oval to round B cells with ample cytoplasm and prominent central nucleoli

SELECTED REFERENCES

1. Algrin C et al: Retrospective analysis of a cohort of 41 de novo B-cell prolymphocytic leukemia patients: impact of genetics and targeted therapies (a FILO study). Haematologica. 108(6):1691-6, 2023, 2022
2. El Hussein S et al: B-prolymphocytic leukemia: is it time to retire this entity? Ann Diagn Pathol. 54:151790, 2021
3. Chapiro E et al: Genetic characterization of B-cell prolymphocytic leukemia: a prognostic model involving MYC and TP53. Blood. 134(21):1821-31, 2019
4. Damlaj M et al: Ibrutinib therapy is effective in B-cell prolymphocytic leukemia exhibiting MYC aberrations. Leuk Lymphoma. 59(3):739-42, 2018
5. Collignon A et al: Prolymphocytic leukemia: new insights in diagnosis and in treatment. Curr Oncol Rep. 19(4):29, 2017

B-Cell Prolymphocytic Leukemia

Peripheral Blood

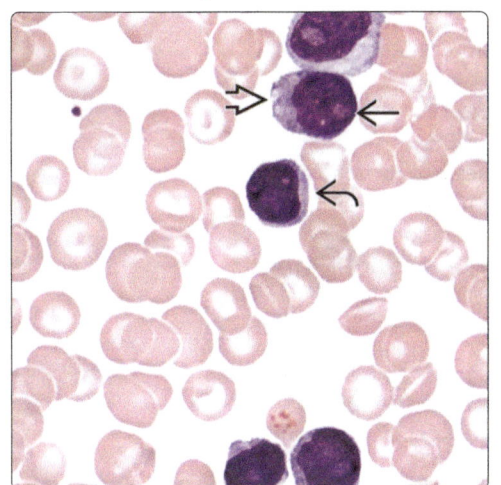

Spleen

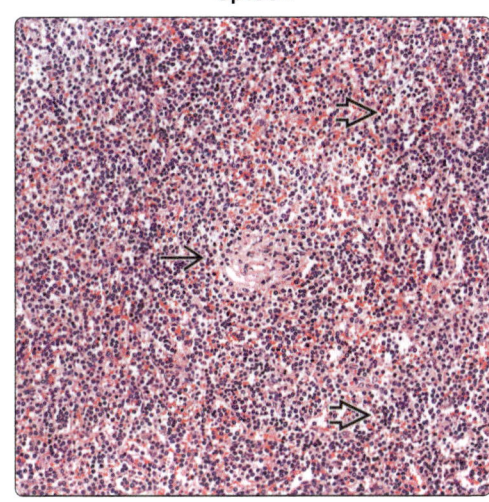

(Left) Peripheral blood shows numerous prolymphocytes with prominent central nucleoli ➔, round to oval nuclei ➔, and ample cytoplasm ➔. (Right) Spleen involved by B-PLL shows extensive red pulp ➔ infiltration, leaving only remnants of white pulp ➔ around an arteriole.

Neoplastic B Cells

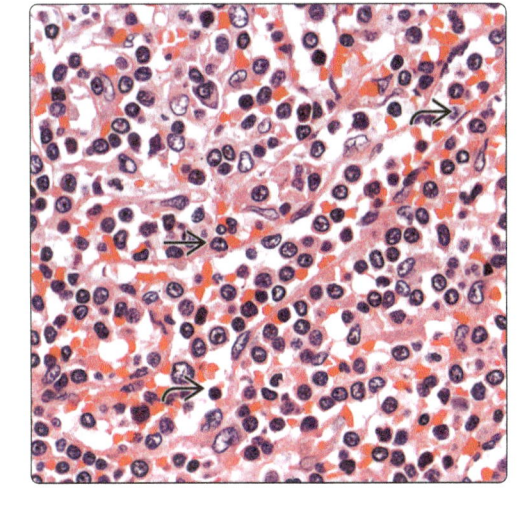

Lymph Node

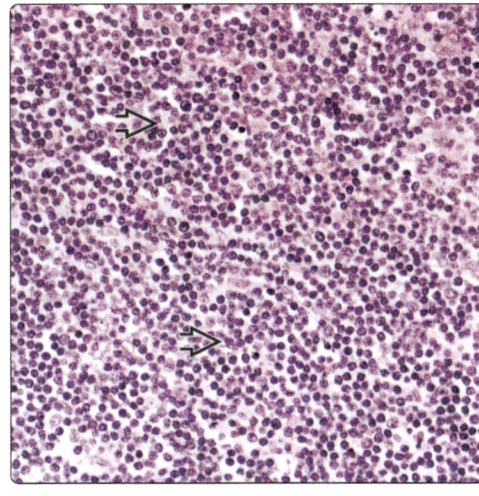

(Left) Neoplastic B cells are shown expanding cords ➔ and sinuses ➔. Neoplastic lymphocytes are intermediate in size and many have distinct nucleoli. (Right) Lymph node effaced by B-PLL shows monotonous sheets of medium-sized B cells ➔.

Bone Marrow

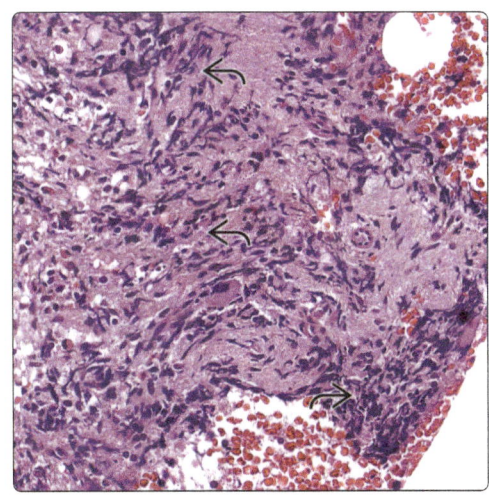

CD5

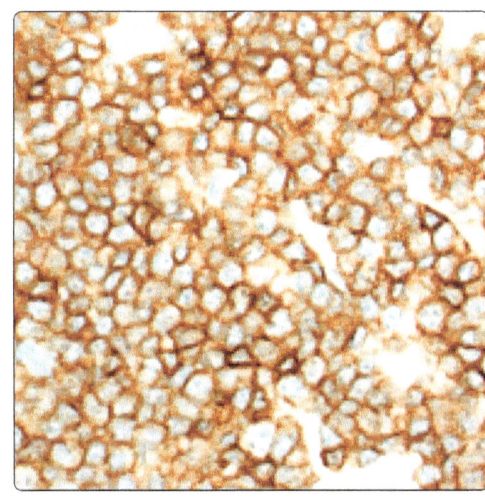

(Left) In this example of bone marrow involvement by B-PLL, the B cells ➔ are seen scattered or clustered in small aggregates. There is considerable crush artifact. (Right) This case of B-PLL is immunoreactive for CD5. CD5 and CD23 are positive in a subset of cases. CD5 is expressed in ~ 25% of these tumors.

Splenic Marginal Zone Lymphoma

KEY FACTS

TERMINOLOGY
- B-cell neoplasm composed of small lymphocytes arising in spleen, thought to be from marginal zone

CLINICAL ISSUES
- Splenomegaly
- Peripheral blood lymphocytosis with villous cytoplasmic projections
- Cytopenias

MOLECULAR
- Deletion 7q
  - Most frequent cytogenetic abnormality
  - Found in ~ 30%
  - Specific chromosomal translocations have not been consistently identified
- Immunoglobulin heavy and light chain genes are clonally rearranged
  - *IGVH1-2*04* in ~ 30%
  - *IGH* gene variable region hypermutated in some and unmutated in others
- *KLF2* inactivating mutations
  - Found in ~ 20%
- *NOTCH2* mutations
  - Found in ~ 40%
  - Not in other B-cell lymphomas
- 2 genetic pathways of SMZL (NNK and DMT)
  - NNK has alterations of NF-κB pathway
  - DMT has alterations in DNA damage response genes and TLR signaling genes (e.g., *MYD88*)

MICROSCOPIC
- Monophasic or biphasic clusters of small B cells replace white pulp and infiltrate red pulp

ANCILLARY TESTS
- Phenotype is nonspecific

Typical Biphasic Pattern

Deletion of 7q

(Left) Splenic marginal zone lymphoma (SMZL) expands the white pulp in a typical biphasic pattern with dark centers ➡ and pale peripheral zones ➡. There is also secondary red pulp ➡ involvement. (Right) Karyotype shows loss of the long arm of chromosome 7 in SMZL. Deletion of 7q is the most frequent cytogenetic abnormality in this lymphoma. (Courtesy L. Nguyen, CG, CM.)

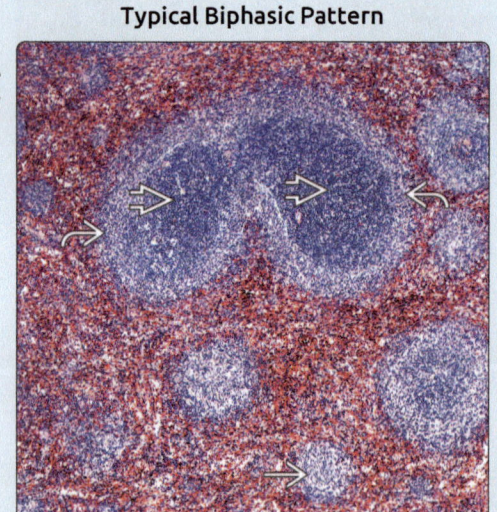

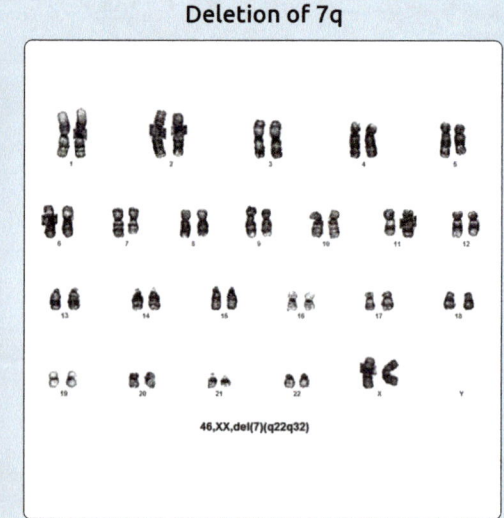

Low-Power View

CD20

(Left) Low-power view shows splenic marginal zone expanding the white pulp ➡. There is only a small amount of red pulp remaining, but scattered, small clusters of SMZL are seen in the red pulp ➡. (Right) CD20 is diffusely positive for SMZL. The phenotype is not specific but can be readily diagnosed in splenic B-cell lymphoma, which does not show the phenotype of another type of lymphoma, and blood with polar cytoplasmic projections.

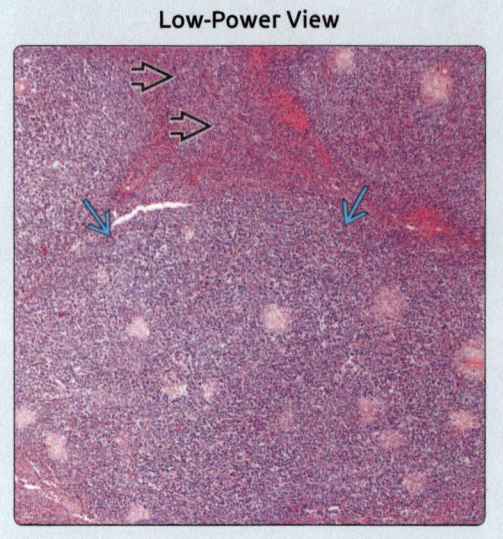

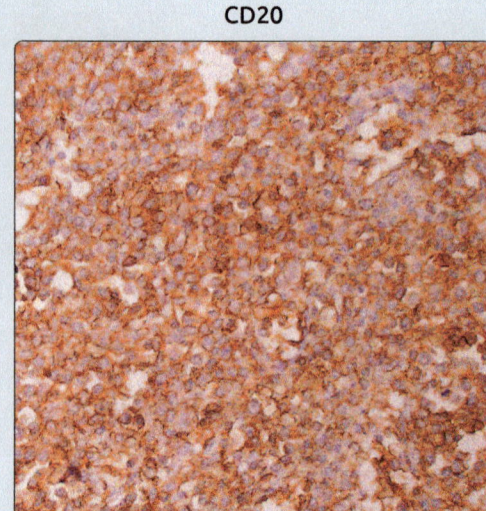

Splenic Marginal Zone Lymphoma

TERMINOLOGY

Abbreviations
- Splenic marginal zone lymphoma (SMZL)

Synonyms
- Splenic B-cell marginal zone lymphoma
- Splenic lymphoma with circulating villous lymphocytes

Definitions
- B-cell neoplasm composed of small lymphocytes primarily arising in spleen, thought to be derived from marginal zone B cells, often with villous lymphocytes in blood

CLINICAL ISSUES

Epidemiology
- Incidence
  - < 2% of lymphoid neoplasms
- Age
  - Middle-aged to older patients
- Sex
  - No sex predilection

Presentation
- Splenomegaly
  - Enlarged splenic hilar lymph nodes
    - Other lymph nodes usually not involved
- Peripheral blood
  - Lymphocytosis
    - So-called polar villous lymphocytes
    - Absolute lymphocytosis in ~ 60% of patients
    - Often initial finding
  - Cytopenias
    - Thrombocytopenia (~ 20%) or anemia (~ 30%)
  - International Consensus Classification (ICC) specifies that SMZL cannot be diagnosed on bone marrow or peripheral blood involvement alone and that splenic involvement by clinical, imaging, or morphology should be assessed
- Bone marrow involved in ~ 80% of patients
- Autoimmune findings in ~ 20% of patients
- Monoclonal serum protein in 1/3 of patients

Treatment
- Watchful waiting for patients with favorable prognostic indicators
- Splenectomy in symptomatic patients who are fit for surgery
- Rituximab is becoming 1st-line treatment
- Interferon-α plus ribavirin used for HCV-related SMZL

Prognosis
- Clinical course is indolent
- Transformation to large cell lymphoma in ~ 10% of cases
  - Prolymphocytoid transformation in blood can occur
- Adverse clinical prognostic factors
  - Hb < 12 g/dL or abnormal lactate dehydrogenase level
  - Albumin < 3.5 g/dL or large tumor size
  - Poor general health status
- Molecular factors associated with unfavorable outcome
  - Complex karyotype, 14q aberrations
  - *TP53* deletions, *NOTCH2* and *PLK1* mutations
  - Unmutated *IGH* variable region gene

MACROSCOPIC

General Features
- Micronodular growth pattern with numerous miliary small white nodules

MOLECULAR

Cytogenetics
- ~ 70% have abnormal karyotype
  - Loss of long arm of chromosome 7 (deletion 7q31-32)
    - Detected in ~ 30% of cases
      - Most frequent cytogenetic abnormality
    - Probably fundamental to pathogenesis of tumor
    - Not found in other B-cell lymphoproliferative disorders
    - No genes have been identified as target of deletion
  - Specific chromosomal translocations have not been consistently identified
    - But translocations involving 7q21, 8q, 1q, 2p11-12, or 14q 32 occur
    - Translocation of *CDK6* at 7q21 in small subset of cases
    - Translocations of *MALT1* not seen in SMZL
  - Trisomy 3 and trisomy 18 detected in 1/4 of cases
    - Also detected in nodal MZL and extranodal MZL
    - Only rarely seen in other B-cell lymphomas
  - Deletion of 6q and gains of 12q (~ 20%) can also be seen in some cases
- Complex karyotype in ~ 20%

In Situ Hybridization
- Also can detect deletion 7q

Polymerase Chain Reaction
- Immunoglobulin heavy and light chain genes are clonally rearranged
- Some SMZL have *IGH* variable region somatic hypermutation, and some are not mutated
  - SMZL with unmutated *IGH* variable region have higher prevalence of del (7q31)
  - SMZL with hypermutated *IGH* variable region may have more favorable prognosis
- Selective use of immunoglobulin heavy chain variable region 1-2*04 allele
  - Found in ~ 30% of patients
  - Suggests that antigenic stimulation is part of pathogenesis of disease
  - These cases often have unmutated immunoglobulin variable region genes

Array Comparative Genomic Hybridization
- Gains in 3q, 5q, 9q, 12q, 13q, 16p, and 20q
- Loss of 7q, 6q, 14q, and 17p

Molecular Genetics
- 2 genetic pathways of SMZL (NNK and DMT)
  - NNK [4-(N-methyl-N-nitrosoamino)-1-(3-pyridyl)-1-butanone]
    - 60% of cases
    - Alterations of NF-κB pathway

Splenic Marginal Zone Lymphoma

- Genes involved include *TNFAIP3*, *TRAF3*, *BIRC3*, *NOTCH2*, *NOTCH1*, *SPEN*, and *KLF2*
- NNK-SMZL enriched in IGHV1-2*04 usage and del 7q31-32, whereas DMT-SMZL lacks both
  o DMT [differentially methylated targets]
  – 30% of cases
  – Alterations in DNA damage response genes (e.g., *TP53*, *ATM*), MAPK (e.g., *BRAF*) and TLR signaling genes (e.g., *MYD88*)
- *KLF2* inactivating mutations in ~ 20% of cases
  o Only rarely identified in other B-cell lymphomas
  o Cases with *KLF2* mutations also showed 7q deletion and *IGH* variable allele 1-2*04 usage
  o Regulator of both NOTCH and NF-κB signaling
- Cases without *KLF2* mutations
  o *MYD88* and *TP53* mutations often present
  o *MYD88* L265P mutations found in only ~ 5% of SMZL
  – *MYD88* mutations detected in ~ 90% of lymphoplasmacytic lymphoma (LPL)
  – *MYD88* testing is helpful in differential diagnosis of SMZL and LPL

Gene Expression Profiling

- Signatures suggest activation of NF-κB, CD40 signaling, interleukins, inflammatory pathways, memory B-cell-related pathways, and B-cell receptor signaling pathways
- Deregulated expression of lymphoma oncogenes, such as *RHOH* and *TCL1A*

MicroRNA

- Overexpressed microRNA
  o miR-21, miR-34a, miR-100, miR-155, miR-146a, and miR-193b
- Underexpressed microRNA
  o miR-139, miR-345, miR-125a, miR-126, miR-377, miR-27b, and miR-145
- SMZL with 7q deletion
  o miR593, miR-129, miR-182, miR-96, miR-183, miR-335, miR-29a, and miR-29b1 are all underexpressed
  o 7q deletion likely underlies reduced expression of these miRNA
- SMZL and nodal marginal zone lymphoma express different groups of miRNAs, supporting that these 2 diseases are different entities

MICROSCOPIC

Histologic Features

- Spleen
  o Monophasic or biphasic pattern of small lymphocytes replacing white pulp and secondarily infiltrating red pulp
  o Biphasic pattern shows dark inner white pulp and pale outer white pulp
  – Biphasic pattern may mimic mantle zone and marginal zones of normal white pulp
  – Both components are part of neoplastic process
  – Germinal centers and mantle zones usually effaced but may be present
    □ Germinal centers often may be colonized
  – Scattered larger cells with nucleoli also present
  o Red pulp infiltrated with diffuse involvement of splenic sinuses and cords
  – Epithelioid histiocytes in red pulp
- Lymph nodes
  o Splenic hilar lymph nodes often involved
  o Typically, partially replaced by SMZL and show dilated sinuses
- Peripheral blood
  o Lymphocytes are small and often display polar cytoplasmic projections (villous lymphocytes)
- Bone marrow
  o Often interstitial and intrasinusoidal infiltrates of small B cells with scant to moderate pale cytoplasm
  – Can be nodular or more diffuse rarely
  o Similar morphology as in spleen
  o Rarely show expanded marginal zones around reactive germinal centers

Cytologic Features

- Lymphocytes usually small in size with round to slightly irregular contours, coarse chromatin, and minimal cytoplasm
  o Small, medium, and larger lymphocytes with pale cytoplasm in marginal zones
  o Monocytoid cells have increased clear cytoplasm
  o Plasmacytoid differentiation in subset of cells; can be marked
  o Mitotic figures are rare

Predominant Cell/Compartment Type

- Marginal zone B cell

ANCILLARY TESTS

Immunohistochemistry

- CD19(+), CD20(+), CD79a(+), PAX5(+), CD3(-), BCL2(+)
  o FMC7(+), CD27(+), CD38(dim), IgM(+), IgD(+)
- Cyclin-D1 (-), CD10(-), BCL6(-), annexin-A1 (-)
- CD103(-), SOX11(-), LEF1(-)
- Rare cases express CD123, CD5, CD25, CD43, CD200, and DBA44
- Any reactive germinal centers are CD10(+) and BCL2(-) and have high Ki-67 index
- Bone marrow lymphoid aggregates
  o Follicular dendritic cell meshworks highlighted with CD21, CD23, or CD35
  – ~ 30-50% of neoplastic lymphocytes are dim (+) for CD21 or CD35

Flow Cytometry

- Monotypic surface immunoglobulin light chain
  o IgM(+)
  o Usually IgD(+)
- CD19(+), CD20(+), CD22(+), CD79a(+), CD79b(+)
- CD11c(+), CD5(+) in ~ 20% of cases
- CD103 rarely (+), CD10(-), BCL6(-)

DIFFERENTIAL DIAGNOSIS

Splenic Diffuse Red Pulp Small B-Cell Lymphoma

- Similar morphology, phenotype, and clinical characteristics to SMZL
- Cannot reliably be differentiated on bone marrow and blood

Splenic Marginal Zone Lymphoma

- Splenic diffuse red pulp small B-cell lymphoma (SDRPL) usually has interstitial and intrasinusoidal growth pattern in bone marrow, whereas SMZL has more nodular infiltrates
- Splenectomy or possibly splenic biopsy needed
    - SDRPL usually has atrophic white pulp, unlike SMZL, and diffuse involvement on red pulp
    - Predominant red pulp involvement with effacement of white pulp, unlike SMZL, which primarily involves white pulp
- Homogeneously beefy-red cut surface without miliary-like nodularity
- Peripheral blood smear may show villous lymphocytes
- DBA.44(+), IgG(+/-), IgD(-)
- CD5(-), CD11c(-), CD25(-), CD103(-)
- SDRPL and SMZL have different Toll-like receptor patterns, which may be able to separate them diagnostically
- *CCND3* mutations reported in SDRPL and not in SMZL
- *BCOR* alterations in ~ 25% of SDRPL but < 10% of SMZL

Splenic B-Cell Lymphoma/Leukemia With Prominent Nucleoli

- Includes entities that currently cannot be separated into biologically meaningful entities
    - e.g., hairy cell leukemia (HCL) variant and CD5(-) B prolymphocytic leukemia
- Medium to large-sized atypical lymphoid cells with distinct single nucleolus, poorly defined cytoplasmic projections reminiscent of hairy cells, nonspecific phenotype
- Spleen involves red pulp; marrow is intrasinusoidal
- Cases can resemble HCL, but probably unrelated
    - CD103(+) in ~ 70%; CD25(-), annexin-A1 (-)
- May have complex karyotypes involving 14q32 and 8q24, deletion 17p, and trisomy 12 reported but no *BRAF* V600E mutations
- Deletion 7q favors SMZL

Nodal or Extranodal Marginal Zone Lymphoma (Mucosa-Associated Lymphoid Tissue Lymphoma)

- Deletion 7q in SMZL and not in mucosa-associated lymphoid tissue (MALT) lymphoma
- t(11;18) *BIRC3::MALT1* detected in MALT lymphoma but not in SMZL
- Gene expression profiles differ in SMZL and MALT lymphoma
- By definition, splenic involvement excludes diagnosis of nodal marginal zone lymphoma
- Splenomegaly and lymphocytosis are uncommon in patients with MALT lymphoma

Splenic Follicular or Marginal Zone Hyperplasia

- No deletion 7q
- No clonal *IGH* rearrangement
- No aberrant B-cell immunophenotype by flow cytometry
- Immunohistochemistry reveals preserved BCL6(+) or CD10(+) lymphocytes
    - No disruption of germinal centers by infiltrating marginal zone lymphocytes
- Spleen may be of normal size but can also weigh up to 1,000 g
- White pulp displays germinal centers, mantle, and marginal zones
    - Triphasic pattern (as compared with biphasic pattern of SMZL)
- Red pulp is well preserved with only rare lymphocytes in sinuses or splenic cords

Chronic Lymphocytic Leukemia/Small Lymphocytic Lymphoma

- Expansion of white pulp by small lymphocytes with round to oval nuclei, clumped chromatin, and scant cytoplasm
    - Proliferation centers, when present, support diagnosis
    - No evidence of biphasic pattern
- Red pulp involvement is common and often extensive
- LEF1(+), CD5(+), CD23(+), CD22 (dim -/+), FMC7(-)

Mantle Cell Lymphoma

- t(11;14)(q13;q32) by classic cytogenetics, FISH, or RT-PCR
    - This translocation is not seen in SMZL
- Expansion of white pulp by centrocytes
    - Residual germinal centers uncommon
- No villous lymphocytes in peripheral blood
- CD5(+), FMC7(+), CD23(-), cyclin-D1 (+), SOX11(+)
    - CD23 rarely (dim +) when assessed by flow cytometry

Follicular Lymphoma

- t(14;18)(q32;q21) is detected in follicular lymphoma but not in SMZL
- Follicles can enlarge and coalesce to form large, grossly visible masses
- Neoplastic lymphocytes are centrocytes and centroblasts
- Expresses germinal center markers CD10(+) and BCL6(+), unlike SMZL
- In peripheral blood, lymphocytes are cleaved with minimal cytoplasm ("buttock" cells)

Lymphoplasmacytic Lymphoma/Waldenström Macroglobulinemia

- Can be difficult to distinguish from SMZL in patients with serum paraprotein and bone marrow involvement
- *MYD88* L265P mutations can help differentiate lymphoplasmacytic lymphoma (LPL)/Waldenström macroglobulinemia (WM) from SMZL
    - Mutations found in most cases of LPL/WM but only ~ 3-15% of SMZL
- del 6q favors WM; del 7q and gains of 3q favor SMZL
- Periarteriolar aggregates of small lymphocytes, plasmacytoid lymphocytes, and plasma cells
- Absence of marginal zone differentiation

Hairy Cell Leukemia

- *BRAF* V600E mutations detected in ~ 100% of HCL but not in SMZL
- Patients present with splenomegaly and usually pancytopenia; monocytopenia is very common
- Red pulp involvement with effacement of white pulp
- Red cell "lakes" and "pseudosinuses" represent areas of disruption of sheets of tumor cells
- Indented nuclei with abundant clear cytoplasm
- TRAP(+) by cytochemistry or immunohistochemistry
- CD11c (bright +), CD22 (bright +), CD25(+), CD103(+), FMC7(+)
- DBA.44(+), annexin-A1 (+) by immunohistochemistry
- Currently rare to obtain splenectomy specimens with HCL

Splenic Marginal Zone Lymphoma

Immunohistochemistry

Antibody	Reactivity	Staining Pattern	Comment
IgM	Positive	Cell membrane	> 90% of cases are positive
IgD	Positive	Cell membrane	~ 50% of cases are positive
CD20	Positive	Cell membrane	Bright expression by neoplastic cells
PAX5	Positive	Nuclear	
BCL2	Positive	Cell membrane and cytoplasm	Negative in residual germinal center cells
Ki-67	Positive	Nuclear	Low proliferation rate; positive cells usually at marginal zone
DBA44	Positive	Cytoplasmic	~ 50% of cases are positive
CD5	Negative	Cell membrane	~ 20% of cases are positive; usually faint reactivity
CD23	Negative	Not applicable	Positive in follicular dendritic cell meshworks; if positive, consider chronic lymphocytic leukemia (CLL)
CD43	Negative	Not applicable	If positive, consider CLL or mantle cell lymphoma (MCL)
Cyclin-D1	Negative	Not applicable	If positive, consider MCL
Annexin-A1	Negative	Not applicable	If positive, consider hairy cell leukemia
CD10	Negative	Not applicable	If positive, consider follicular lymphoma
BCL6	Negative	Not applicable	Positive in residual GC cells; may be positive in transformed splenic marginal zone lymphoma

Most Common Molecular Changes in B-Cell Lymphomas

Type of Lymphoma/Leukemia	Molecular Change
Splenic marginal zone lymphoma	Deletion 7q
Extranodal marginal zone lymphoma	t(11;18)(q22;q21) BIRC3::MALT1
Lymphoplasmacytic lymphoma/Waldenström macroglobulinemia	MYD88 L265P mutations; only rarely detected in SMZL
Follicular lymphoma	t(14;18)(q32;q21) IGH::BCL2
Mantle cell lymphoma	t(11;14)(q13;q32) CCND1::IGH
Hairy cell leukemia	BRAF V600E mutation

Molecular Findings in SMZL, SDRPL, HCL, and SBLPN

Molecular Finding	SMZL	SDRPL	HCL	SBLPN
del(7q)	~ 40%	~ 25%	~ 20%	~ 20%
NOTCH2 alterations	~ 20%	2%	None	None
KLF2 alterations	20%	2%	15%	None
CCND3 alterations	0	25%	0	Undetermined
BRAF V600E alterations	< 1%	< 10%	≥ 95%	Undetermined

SMZL = splenic marginal zone lymphoma; SDRPL = splenic diffuse red pulp small B-cell lymphoma; HCL = hairy cell leukemia; SBLPN = splenic B-cell lymphoma/leukemia with prominent nucleoli.

o Diagnosis can be made confidently based on peripheral blood, bone marrow, and immunophenotypic features

DIAGNOSTIC CHECKLIST

Pathologic Interpretation Pearls

- Deletion 7q is main molecular abnormality
- Nodular expansion of white pulp by small B-cell lymphoma with biphasic appearance

SELECTED REFERENCES

1. Alderuccio JP et al: NOTCH signaling in the pathogenesis of splenic marginal zone lymphoma-opportunities for therapy. Leuk Lymphoma. 63(2):279-90, 2022
2. Bonfiglio F et al: Genetic and phenotypic attributes of splenic marginal zone lymphoma. Blood. 139(5):732-47, 2022

Splenic Marginal Zone Lymphoma

Medium-Power View

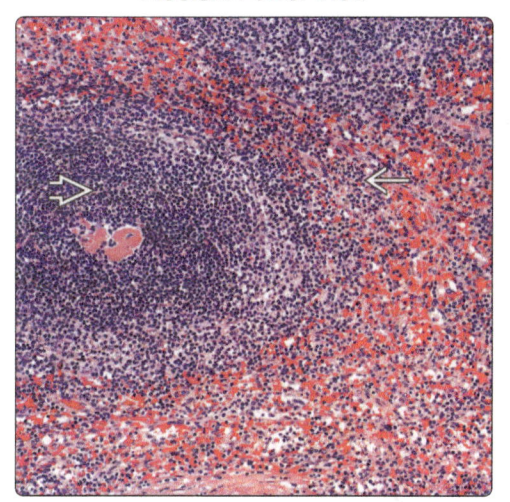

High-Power View

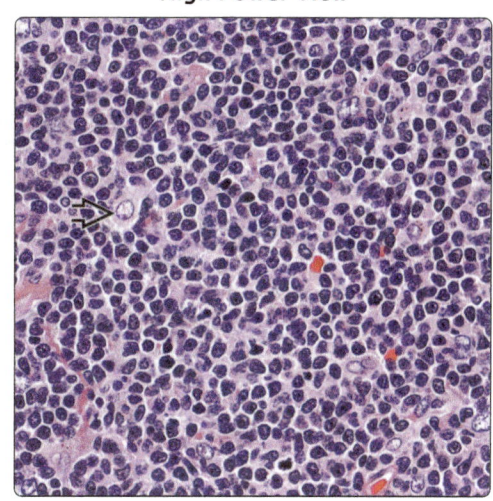

(Left) Medium-power view shows SMZL expanding the white pulp ➡ in a biphasic pattern. The center is dark, while the peripheral marginal zone is pale. In addition, there is secondary red pulp ➡ involvement. (Right) High-power view shows central white pulp in SMZL. Most of the lymphocytes are small, round to slightly irregular, and hyperchromatic. Scattered histiocytes ➡ are noted.

White Pulp and Red Pulp

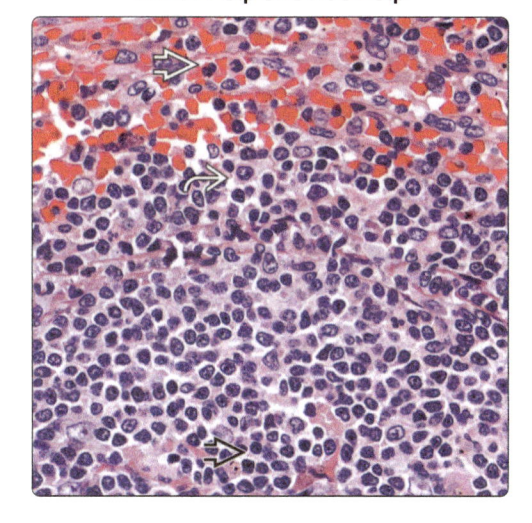

CD20

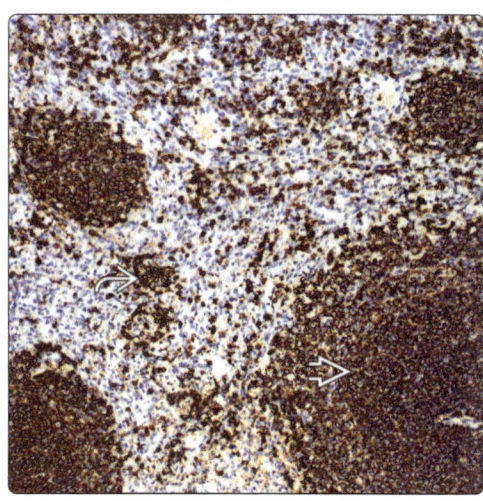

(Left) White pulp shows a biphasic pattern with small lymphocytes ➡ surrounded by marginal zone lymphocytes with pale cytoplasm ➡. Red pulp ➡ is noted at the top of the field. (Right) CD20 highlights B cells in the white pulp ➡ as well as secondary involvement of the red pulp ➡ noted as small lymphoid aggregates.

Peripheral Blood

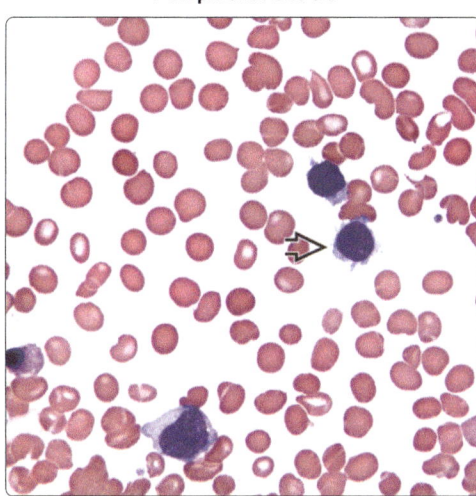

***IGH* Rearrangement**

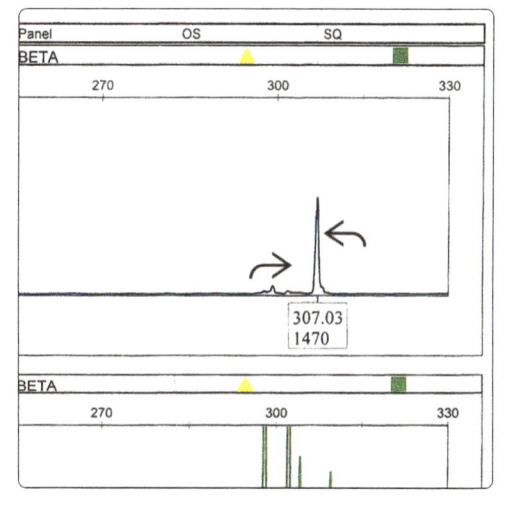

(Left) Wright-Giemsa stain of peripheral blood smear shows 3 lymphocytes, 2 with cytoplasmic, villous projections and 1 with the characteristic "polar" villi ➡. (Right) IGH rearrangement performed by PCR shows a dominant monoclonal peak at position 307 ➡, as expected since SMZL is a B-cell lymphoma.

Molecular Pathology of Lymphoid Neoplasms

331

Hairy Cell Leukemia

KEY FACTS

TERMINOLOGY
- Hairy cell leukemia (HCL): Indolent neoplasm of small mature B cells with abundant cytoplasm and hairy projections
  - Circulating "hairy cells" in peripheral blood
  - Bone marrow involvement with diffuse, interstitial pattern of distribution
  - Extensive splenic involvement, effacement of red pulp

ETIOLOGY/PATHOGENESIS
- *BRAF* V600E mutation
  - Major molecular driver of HCL
  - Highly specific to HCL among small, mature lymphoid neoplasms
- Activated, late clonal B cells
  - Somatic hypermutation of *IGHV* in most cases

CLINICAL ISSUES
- Indolent disease with near-normal life expectancy
- Spleen and bone marrow are major sites of involvement
- Purine nucleoside analogs (pentostatin and cladribine) are most effective therapy but not curative
- 30-40% relapse rate in longitudinal studies
- Durable complete response with BRAF inhibitors (vemurafenib) plus rituximab in relapsed or refractory cases

MOLECULAR
- *BRAF* V600E mutation in virtually all cases
  - Disease-defining genetic event in HCL
  - Constitutively activates MEK/ERK signaling pathway
  - Promotes proliferation and survival

ANCILLARY TESTS
- Bright expression of CD20, CD22, CD11c, CD200, CD25, and CD103 detected on flow cytometry
- Annexin-A1, CD20, CD25, CD103, CD123, cyclin-D1, TRAP, TBX21 (TBET), and *BRAF* V600E mutation-specific antigen detected by IHC

Circulating Hairy Cell

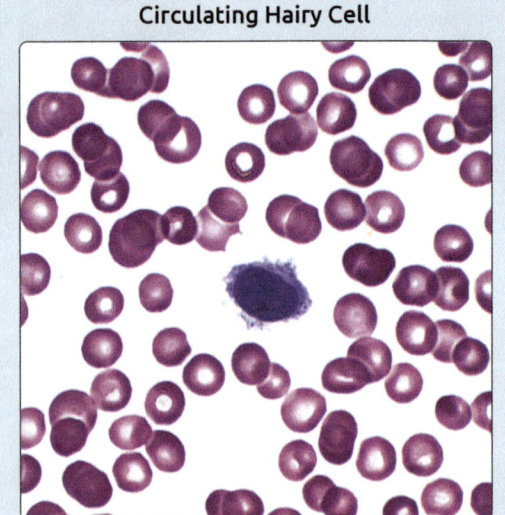

Sanger Sequencing

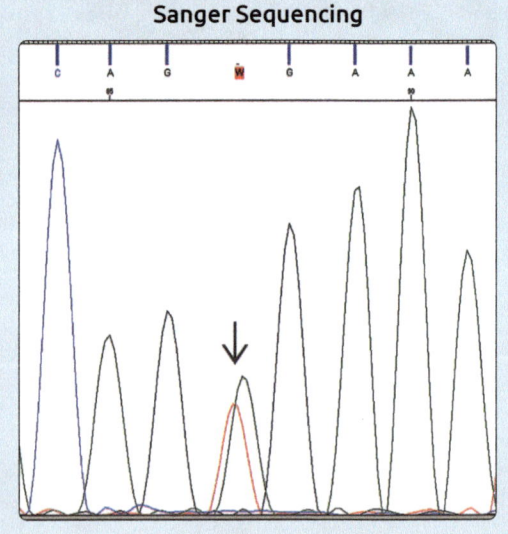

(Left) Wright-stained peripheral blood smear from a 48-year-old man with pancytopenia and profound monocytopenia shows a circulating hairy cell with oval nucleus and cytoplasmic hairy projections. (Right) Sanger sequencing analysis of DNA obtained from circulating hairy cells shows a point mutation in codon 600 of BRAF corresponding to BRAF c.1799T>A (V600E) mutation ➡.

***BRAF* V600E Mutation-Specific IHC**

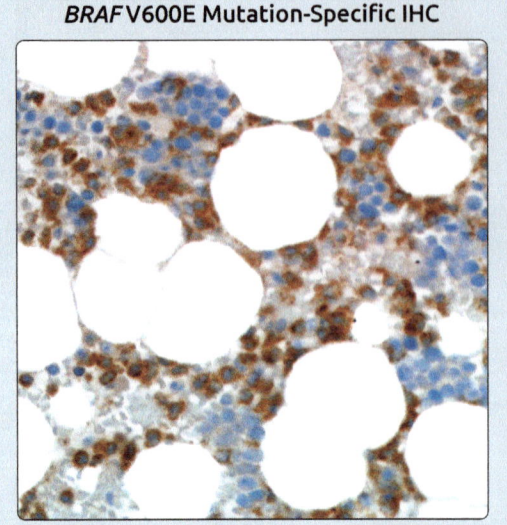

NGS Analysis of Codon 600 of *BRAF*

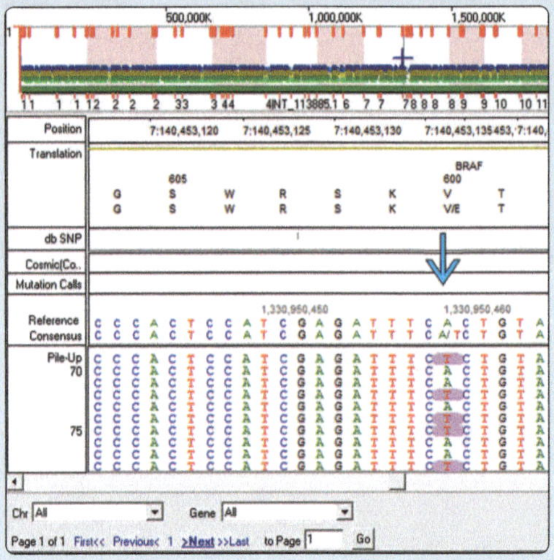

(Left) Bone marrow trephine biopsy using BRAF V600E mutation-specific antibody highlights residual disease in this patient with a recent diagnosis of hairy cell leukemia (HCL). (Right) NGS performed on bone marrow aspirate obtained from a patient with new diagnosis of HCL shows a T > A base substitution ➡ in codon 600 of BRAF corresponding to BRAF V600E mutation. Virtually all HCL cases harbor this mutation.

Hairy Cell Leukemia

TERMINOLOGY

Abbreviations
- Hairy cell leukemia (HCL)

Synonyms
- Leukemic reticuloendotheliosis (old terminology)

Definitions
- Indolent neoplasm of small mature B cells with oval nuclei and abundant cytoplasm
- Usually involves bone marrow, peripheral blood, and spleen
- Occasional circulating "hairy cells" (HCs) in peripheral blood
- Bone marrow involvement with diffuse, interstitial pattern
- Extensive splenic involvement with effacement of red pulp
- *BRAF* V600E somatic mutation in ≥ 95% of cases

ETIOLOGY/PATHOGENESIS

Etiology
- Activated, late clonal B cells
  - Somatic hypermutation of immunoglobulin heavy chain variable region (*IGHV*) in most cases
- Precise nature of HCs and normal counterpart is not entirely clear

Pathogenesis
- *BRAF* c.1799T>A (p.V600E) mutation present in virtually all HCL cases
  - Considered molecular driver of HCL
  - Highly specific to HCL among lymphoid neoplasms
  - Constitutively activates RAF/ERK/MEK signaling pathway
- Production of cytokine and cytokine receptors
  - Tumor necrosis factor alpha (TNF-α) receptors on HCs are involved in their survival
  - IL-6 production induced by TNF
  - Transforming growth factor beta (TGF-β)
    - Linked to suppression of production and normal function of hematopoietic cells
  - Fibroblast growth factor (FGF) and fibronectin synthesis
    - Linked to bone marrow fibrosis
- Expression of adhesion molecules and homing receptors
  - HCs express integrins and CD44
  - Adhesion molecules cooperate with chemokine receptors in tissue homing and retention

CLINICAL ISSUES

Epidemiology
- Incidence
  - ~ 1,000 new cases diagnosed per year in USA
  - Accounts for 2% of all lymphoid leukemias
- Age
  - Middle aged to older patients
  - Median: 52 years
    - Uncommon in young adults
    - Extremely rare in children
- Sex
  - M:F = 5:1

Site
- Spleen and bone marrow are major sites of involvement
- Liver sinusoids and portal tracts may be involved
- Lymph nodes are rarely involved

Presentation
- Weakness and fatigue
- Fever due to neutropenia
- Left upper quadrant pain due to splenomegaly
- Bleeding diathesis due to thrombocytopenia
- Incidental finding at time of routine complete blood count (CBC) in minority of cases

Laboratory Tests
- CBC reveals pancytopenia
  - Anemia in most patients
  - Profound monocytopenia in virtually all cases
  - Neutropenia and thrombocytopenia in ~ 50%
  - Occasional circulating HCs on blood smear review

Natural History
- Indolent disease with near-normal life expectancy with current treatment
- Increased risk of infection due to neutropenia &/or immunosuppressive therapy
- 30-40% relapse rate in longitudinal studies
- Disease-free survival curve does not reach plateau
- Spontaneous splenic rupture may rarely occur

Treatment
- Purine nucleoside analogs (pentostatin and cladribine)
  - Other lymphoid neoplasms mimicking HCL do not respond to purine nucleoside analogs
- ~ 90% morphologic remission with purine nucleoside analog monotherapy
- Poor response to therapy in cases with *IGHV* 4-34 usage or *TP53* mutations
- Rituximab may be useful in eradicating minimal residual disease
- BRAF inhibitors (vemurafenib) plus rituximab
  - Durable complete remission in > 80% of relapsed or refractory HCL

Assessment of Response in Hairy Cell Leukemia
- Complete response (CR)
  - Near normalization of peripheral blood count
    - Hgb > 11g/dL, platelets > 100,000/μL, absolute neutrophils > 1,500/μL
  - No morphologic evidence of HCL in both blood and bone marrow
  - Patients with CR may or may not have MRD on IHC assessment of bone marrow
- Partial response (PR)
  - Near normalization of blood count with minimum of 50% improvement in organomegaly and bone marrow infiltration by HCL
- Progressive disease and relapse
  - 25% increase in organomegaly or 25% decline in hematologic parameters defines progressive disease
  - Reappearance of HCL in blood &/or bone marrow defines morphologic relapse
  - Reappearance of cytopenia below thresholds defined for CR or PR

Hairy Cell Leukemia

BRAF Wildtype Hairy Cell Leukemia
- Clinical and genetic features similar to hairy cell leukemia variant (HCLv)
  - High WBC count similar to HCLv
  - Unmutated immunoglobulin heavy chain variable (IGHV) region or low-level mutated with *IGHV4-34* usage
  - Frequent activating mutations in MAP2K1/MEK1 pathway genes
  - Poor response to purine analogs (e.g., cladribine)

MICROSCOPIC

Blood
- Typically contains rare circulating HCs
  - Small to intermediate in size, oval to indented nuclei with mature chromatin and absent or inconspicuous nucleoli
  - Abundant pale blue cytoplasm with frayed cytoplasmic borders and hairy projections

Bone Marrow Aspirate
- Contains no or only few HCs due to dry tap
- HCs are present on touch imprints of trephine biopsy
  - HC projections are not appreciated on touch preparations

Bone Marrow Trephine Biopsy
- Variable degree of marrow involvement
  - Diffuse interstitial infiltrate throughout marrow space
  - Involvement may appear inconspicuous on H&E
  - Involved marrow may be hypocellular
  - In subset of cases with decreased hematopoiesis, marrow may resemble aplastic anemia
    - CD20 or BRAF V600E antigen essential to highlight subtle HCL infiltrate
  - Neoplastic cells have oval to spindled nuclei with abundant clear cytoplasm
  - Fried egg appearance with distinct cytoplasmic border is typically apparent
- Increased reticulin fibrosis is seen in all cases

Spleen
- HCL infiltrates splenic cords and sinuses of red pulp
- White pulp is often atrophic and effaced
- Red blood cell lakes often seen lined by HCL cells

Liver
- Liver sinusoids may be infiltrated by HCL
- Infiltrate may also extend to portal tracts

Lymph Nodes
- Lymph nodes are usually spared but can be infiltrated in advanced disease
- Involved lymph node demonstrates interfollicular and paracortical pattern of neoplastic distribution with sparing of follicles

ANCILLARY TESTS

Histochemistry
- Reticulin
  - Increased reticulin fibrosis in all HCL cases

Immunohistochemistry
- Expression of pan B-cell antigens CD20, CD22, CD79A, PAX5, and annexin-A1; CD25, CD103, CD123, TRAP, TBX21, BRAF V600E (clone VE1), and cyclin-D1 (weak)
  - Annexin-A1 is specific marker for HCL among other B-cell malignancies
  - Also expressed in granulocytic lineage and T cells
  - Interpretation difficult in low-level involvement by HCL
- CD5 and CD10 are negative in majority of HCL

Flow Cytometry
- Expression of CD20, CD22, CD11c, CD25, CD103, CD123, CD200, and FMC7
- CD10 or CD5 expressed in rare cases

Genetic Testing
- *BRAF* V600E mutation
  - Present in virtually all HCL
  - Disease-defining genetic event in HCL
- Cooccurring mutations
  - *KLF2* and *CDKN1A* (~ 16% each)
- Clonal rearrangement of immunoglobulin heavy chain (*IGH*) gene
- Somatic hypermutation of *IGH* variable region in > 85%
- Chromosomal translocations are uncommon in HCL

DIFFERENTIAL DIAGNOSIS

Hairy Cell Leukemia Variant (ICC)
- Spleen and bone marrow morphology similar to HCL
- More conspicuous nucleoli compared to HCL
- No significant reticulin fibrosis in bone marrow
- Leukocytosis is common with greater degree of circulating neoplastic cells compared to HCL
- In contrast to HCL, monocytes are present in peripheral blood
- CD103 may be expressed, but CD25, annexin-A1, and BRAF V600E are negative
- *BRAF* mutations are not detected in HCLv

Splenic Diffuse Red Pulp Small B-Cell Lymphoma
- Diffuse splenic red pulp involvement is present, as name implies
- Intrasinusoidal pattern of involvement in bone marrow
- Circulating neoplastic cells contain abundant cytoplasm with villous projections
- Annexin-A1, CD25, and CD103 negative

Splenic Marginal Zone Lymphoma
- Splenic involvement is predominantly limited to white pulp
- Bone marrow involvement is predominantly nodular

SELECTED REFERENCES
1. Falini B et al: A comparison of the International Consensus and 5th World Health Organization classifications of mature B-cell lymphomas. Leukemia. 37(1):18-34, 2023
2. Alaggio R et al: The 5th edition of the World Health Organization classification of haematolymphoid tumours: lymphoid neoplasms. Leukemia. 36(7):1720-48, 2022
3. Maitre E et al: Deciphering genetic alterations of hairy cell leukemia and hairy cell leukemia-like disorders in 98 patients. Cancers (Basel). 14(8):1904, 2022
4. Troussard X et al: Hairy cell leukemia 2022: update on diagnosis, risk-stratification, and treatment. Am J Hematol. 97(2):226-36, 2022

Hairy Cell Leukemia

Effacement of Red Pulp

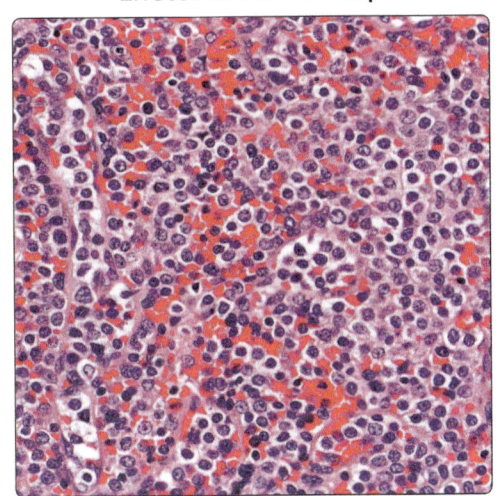

Prominent Interstitial Infiltrate

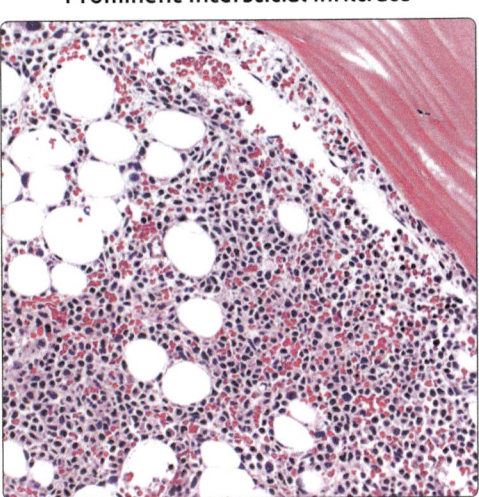

(Left) Massively enlarged spleen shows effacement of red pulp by an infiltrate of hairy cells within splenic cords and sinuses. The neoplastic cells contain oval nuclei with mature chromatin and abundant pale cytoplasm with distinct cytoplasmic borders. (Right) Bone marrow biopsy from the same patient shows a prominent interstitial infiltrate of hairy cells with oval nuclei and abundant clear cytoplasm.

CD20

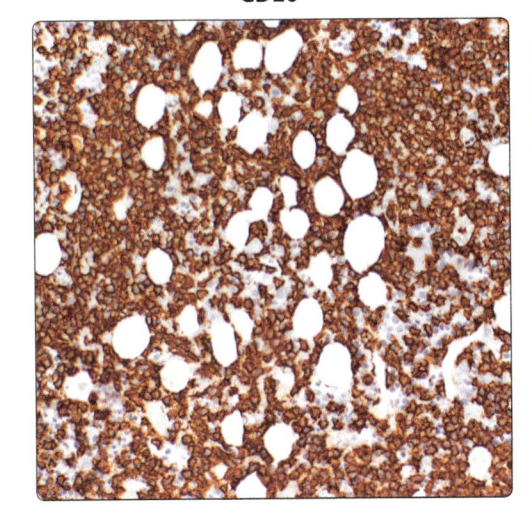

Annexin-A1

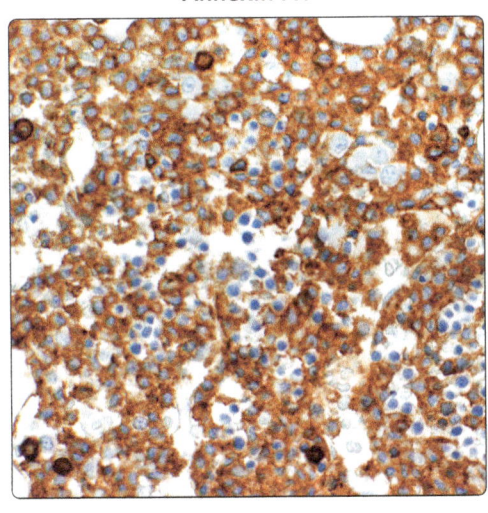

(Left) CD20 of marrow core biopsy highlights an extensive infiltrate of hairy cells. In a subset of cases with hypocellular marrow, the hairy cells can easily be overlooked on morphologic assessment without evaluation of IHC for a B-cell marker. (Right) Annexin-A1 highlights hairy cells with moderate expression of this antigen. The occasional cells with bright expression of annexin-A1 are residual myeloid lineage cells.

Flow Cytometry

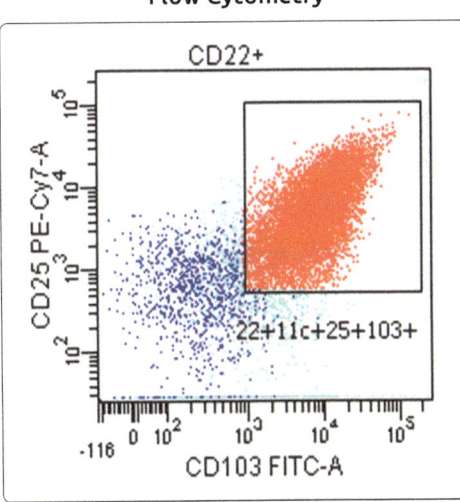

Pyrosequencing

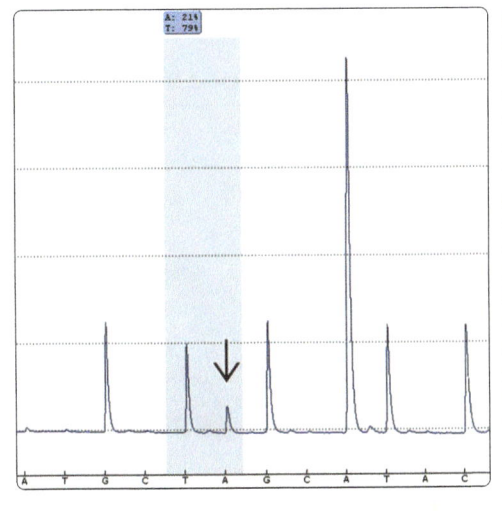

(Left) Flow cytometric analysis with selective gating on bright CD20(+) and λ-light chain-restricted circulating hairy cells shows bright coexpression of CD22, CD11c, CD25, and CD103 (red population). This immunophenotype is virtually diagnostic of HCL. (Right) Pyrosequencing analysis of DNA obtained from bone marrow aspirate shows a BRAF c.1799T>A (V600E) point mutation ➔. The BRAF V600E mutation is present in virtually all HCL cases.

Splenic B-Cell Lymphoma/Leukemia, Unclassifiable

KEY FACTS

TERMINOLOGY
- Splenic B-cell lymphoma/leukemia unclassifiable (SBCLU): Group of mature B-cell lymphomas in ICC classification involving blood, spleen, and bone marrow, which do not fit in other categories of B-cell neoplasm
  - Includes 2 entities: Hairy cell leukemia variant (HCLv) and splenic diffuse red pulp small B-cell lymphoma (SDRPL)
- WHO 5th edition no longer uses term SBCLU but this version includes 2 entities, SDRPL and splenic B-cell lymphoma/leukemia with prominent nucleoli, which is equivalent to HCLv

CLINICAL ISSUES
- Chronic but not curable
- Survival is variable

MACROSCOPIC
- Massive splenomegaly
- Red pulp infiltration

- Sinusoidal distribution in bone marrow

MOLECULAR
- Clonal *IGH* rearrangements
- *BRAF* mutation absent

MICROSCOPIC
- Leukocytosis with lymphocytosis
  - Lymphocytes show abundant cytoplasm
  - Round nuclei with prominent nucleoli in HCLv

ANCILLARY TESTS
- CD20 and other pan B-cell markers (+)
- CD5(-/+), CD10(-/+), CD103(+), TRAP(-/+)
- CD25, annexin A1, and CD123 (-)

TOP DIFFERENTIAL DIAGNOSES
- Classic HCL
- Splenic marginal zone lymphoma

Effaced Architecture

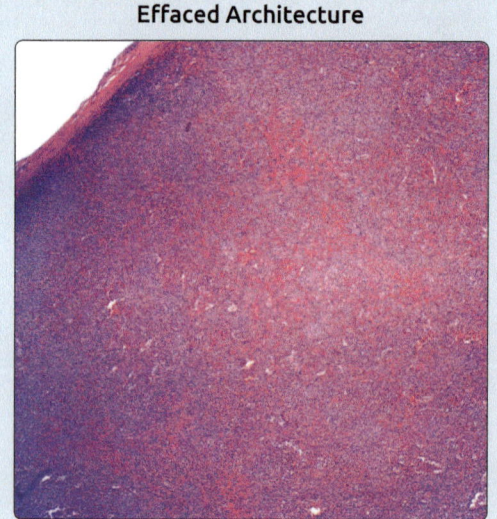

Neoplastic Lymphoid Cells

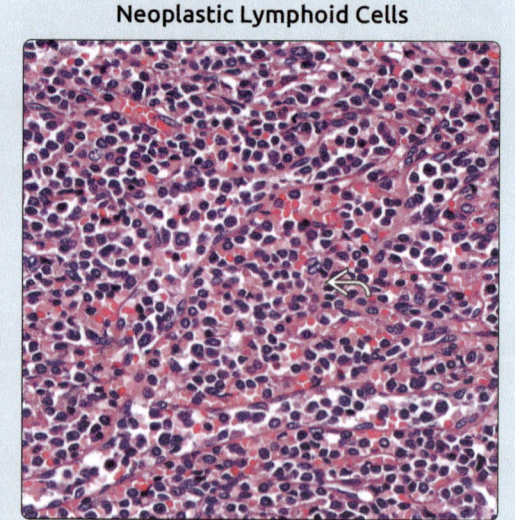

(Left) Low-power view of spleen shows effaced architecture by small lymphocytes involving red pulp and sinuses. (Right) Sinusoidal and red pulp infiltrate with neoplastic lymphoid cells ➡ is shown. This lymphoma did not meet criteria for either hairy cell leukemia variant (HCLv) or splenic diffuse red pulp small B-cell lymphoma (SDRP SBCL). The lymphoma cells expressed CD20, CD11c, BCL2, and DBA44. These were negative for CD5, CD10, CD123, CD103, and BRAF.

Hairy Cell Leukemia Variant

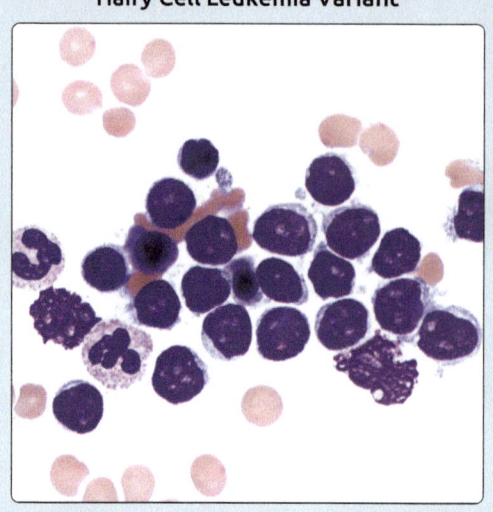

Hairy Cell Leukemia Variant

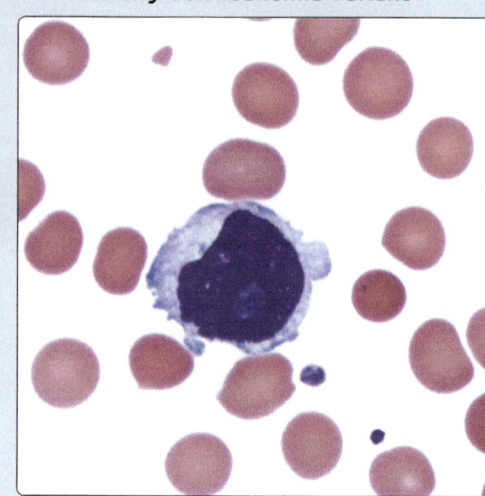

(Left) Bone marrow aspirate smear from a patient with HCLv shows pronounced lymphocytosis. Note central nucleoli. (From DP: Blood & Bone Marrow.) (Right) High-power view of an HCLv cell from an 88-year-old woman with anemia, thrombocytopenia, and normal monocyte count shows prominent nucleolus and partial hairy projections. (From DP: Blood & Bone Marrow.)

Splenic B-Cell Lymphoma/Leukemia, Unclassifiable

TERMINOLOGY

Abbreviations
- Splenic B-cell lymphoma/leukemia unclassifiable (SBCLU), splenic diffuse red pulp small B-cell lymphoma (SDRPL), hairy cell leukemia variant (HCLv)

Synonyms
- Prolymphocytic variant of HCL
- Splenic lymphoma with villous lymphocytes
- Splenic marginal zone lymphoma, diffuse variant
- Splenic B-cell lymphoma/leukemia with prominent nucleoli

Definitions
- SBCLU is group of mature B-cell neoplasms involving blood, spleen, and bone marrow, which do not fit in other categories of B-cell neoplasms
  - International Consensus Classification (ICC) includes 2 entities in SBCLU
    - SDRPL and HCLv
  - WHO 5th edition no longer uses term SBCLU but includes 2 entities
    - SDRPL and splenic B-cell lymphoma/leukemia with prominent nucleoli, which is equivalent to HCLv

ETIOLOGY/PATHOGENESIS

Mature B-Cell Neoplasm
- Etiology uncertain
- Not related to classic HCL or splenic marginal zone B-cell lymphoma
- Uncertain relationship between HCLv and SDRPL

CLINICAL ISSUES

Presentation
- Middle-aged to older patients with male predominance
- Splenomegaly, bone marrow and peripheral blood involvement
- Less often hepatomegaly or lymphadenopathy

Treatment
- Splenectomy if symptomatic
- Older, high-risk patients may benefit from splenic radiation
- HCLv
  - Purine nucleoside analogues with rituximab are 1st line but may not respond
    - Cladribine ± rituximab or pentostatin may be effective
- SDRPL
  - Good response to splenectomy
  - No specific treatment

Prognosis
- Chronic clinical course, but incurable
- HCLv
  - Significantly shorter survival than classic HCL
  - Transformation associated with 17p deletions
- SDRPL
  - Because there are few cases, there is limited information about usual clinical behavior
  - Aggressive behavior associated with *NOTCH1*, *TP53*, or *MAP2K1* mutations

MACROSCOPIC

General Features
- Massively enlarged spleen; hepatomegaly also may occur
- Diffuse involvement of splenic red pulp
- Lack of lymphadenopathy

MOLECULAR

Cytogenetics
- HCLv
  - Complex karyotypes involving 14q32 (*IGH*) and 8q24 (*MYC*), deletion 17p (*TP53*), and trisomy 12 reported
  - Copy number abnormalities most frequent are gains on chromosome 5, losses on 7q and 17p
- SDRPL
  - Complex cytogenetics involving t(9:14)(p13;q32), *PAX5*, and *IGH* reported
  - Copy number abnormalities present in 70% of cases
  - Negative for *CCND1* rearrangements, deletion 7q, trisomy 3 or 18

PCR
- Clonal immunoglobulin heavy chain (*IGH*) rearrangements
  - HCLv
    - Mutated *IGH* variable region in most patients
      - VH4-34 expression associated with symptoms
    - Mutations of *MAP2K1*, *KDM6A*, *CREBBP*, *KMT2C* (MLL3), *TP53*, *U2AF1*, *CCND3*, and *ARID1A*
    - Absence of *BRAF* mutation
  - SDRPL
    - Recurrent *CCND3* mutations and *BCOR* alterations reported
    - Absence of *BRAF* mutation
    - Rare *MYD88*, *NOTCH1*, *NOTCH 2*, *MAPK1*, *SF3B1*, and *TP53* mutations

MICROSCOPIC

Histologic Features
- SBCLU
  - Leukocytosis, varying lymphocytosis often showing villous projections or abundant cytoplasm without monocytopenia
    - HCLv
      - Lymphocytosis with central round nuclei and prominent nucleoli
    - SDRPL
      - Low level of lymphocytosis without prominent nucleoli
  - Involvement of splenic red pulp cords and sinuses often with blood lakes
  - Involvement of bone marrow with intrasinusoidal growth distribution

ANCILLARY TESTS

Immunohistochemistry
- SBCLU
  - Pan B-cell markers positive: CD20(+), CD19(+), CD22(+), CD79a(+), PAX5(+)
  - CD5(-/+), CD10(-/+), CD103(+/-), TRAP(-/+)

Splenic B-Cell Lymphoma/Leukemia, Unclassifiable

- o HCL markers usually negative: CD25(-), annexin A1 (-), CD123(-)
- o HCLv
  - Negative for classic HCL markers: CD25, annexin A1, CD123
  - CD11c, CD103, and FMC7 positive
  - TRAP(-/+); cytochemistry negative or weakly positive
  - BRAF(-)
- o SDRPL
  - Negative with few exceptions for TRAP, CD25, and annexin A1
  - DBA.44 (CD72)(+), IgG(+), frequent IgD(+), CD11c (rare +), CD123 (rare +), CD103 (rare +), cyclin-D3 (+)

DIFFERENTIAL DIAGNOSIS

Classic Hairy Cell Leukemia

- Cytopenias, including monocytopenia
- Leukemic cells may be present in peripheral blood
- Clear fried egg appearance in tissue sections
- CD20(+), CD25(+), CD123(+), TRAP(+), DBA.44(+), annexin A1 (+), BRAF(+)
- *BRAF* 600V mutations by PCR
  - o HCLv does not show monocytopenia, lacks most HCL markers and does not have *BRAF* mutations

Splenic Marginal Zone Lymphoma

- Splenic white pulp expanded with secondary red pulp involvement
  - o Neoplastic B cells have abundant cytoplasm and may appear villous in peripheral blood
    - Polar cytoplasmic projections
- Hilar lymph nodes are often involved
- Associated with hepatitis C
- IgM(+), IgD(+/-), CD11c(+), CD5(-), CD10(-), CD23(-), CD43(-), CD103(-/+), annexin A1 (-)

Chronic Lymphocytic Leukemia/Small Lymphocytic Lymphoma

- Small CD5(+) B-cell lymphoma with lymphocytosis
  - o Small lymphocytes with round nuclei with clumped chromatin and indistinct nucleoli
  - o Prolymphocytes and paraimmunoblasts are evident in tissue and peripheral blood
- Extensive bone marrow involvement; easily aspirated
- Spleen shows white pulp involvement with secondary red pulp nodules
- CD5(+), CD23(+), CD11c(-), IgM(+), IgD(+/-), LEF1(+)

Leukemic Nonnodal Mantle Cell Lymphoma

- Slowly increasing asymptomatic lymphocytosis
- Involves peripheral blood, bone marrow, and spleen
  - o Interstitial or sinusoid growth pattern
- Nodal involvement minimal to absent
- More indolent than classic mantle cell lymphoma
- Cyclin-D1/BCL1(+), CD5(+) variable intensity, CD200(-/+), CD23(-/+), DBA44(+), SOX11(-)
- *CCND1* rearrangement present
- *TP53* aberrations portend more aggressive disease

B-Cell Prolymphocytic Leukemia

- Very rare; many cases reclassified as other small B-cell lymphomas
- Marked lymphocytosis
  - o Small to intermediately sized lymphocytes with prominent nucleoli
  - o Lack cytoplasmic projections
- Marked splenomegaly
- Aggressive disease
- Not diagnosed if previous CLL/SLL
- CD5(+/-), CD10(-), IgM (+), IgD(+/-)

SELECTED REFERENCES

1. Maitre E et al: Novel targeted treatments in hairy cell leukemia and other hairy cell-like disorders. Front Oncol. 12:1068981, 2022
2. Ozkaya N et al: Splenic diffuse red pulp small B-cell lymphoma with cyclin D3 expression. Blood. 140(7):793, 2022
3. Paillassa J et al: Hairy cell leukemia (HCL) and HCL variant: updates and spotlights on therapeutic advances. Curr Oncol Rep. 24(9):1133-43, 2022
4. Paillassa J et al: Updates in hairy cell leukemia (HCL) and variant-type HCL (HCL-V): rationale for targeted treatments with a focus on ibrutinib. Ther Adv Hematol. 13:20406207221090886, 2022
5. Tran J et al: Advances in the treatment of hairy cell leukemia variant. Curr Treat Options Oncol. 23(1):99-116, 2022
6. Zhang XL et al: [Clinical features and prognosis of eight patients with splenic diffuse red pulp small B-cell lymphoma.] Zhonghua Xue Ye Xue Za Zhi. 43(12):1028-33, 2022
7. Liu Q et al: Current and emerging therapeutic options for hairy cell leukemia variant. Onco Targets Ther. 14:1797-805, 2021
8. Matutes E: Diagnostic and therapeutic challenges in hairy cell leukemia-variant: where are we in 2021? Expert Rev Hematol. 14(4):355-63, 2021
9. Schmieg JJ et al: CD5-negative, CD10-negative low-grade B-cell lymphoproliferative disorders of the spleen. Curr Oncol. 28(6):5124-47, 2021
10. Yilmaz E et al: A review on splenic diffuse red pulp small B-cell lymphoma. Curr Oncol. 28(6):5148-54, 2021
11. Suzuki T et al: Clinicopathological analysis of splenic red pulp low-grade B-cell lymphoma. Pathol Int. 70(5):280-6, 2020
12. Andritsos LA et al: Trametinib for the treatment of IGHV4-34, MAP2K1-mutant variant hairy cell leukemia. Leuk Lymphoma. 59(4):1008-11, 2018
13. Angelova EA et al: Clinicopathologic and molecular features in hairy cell leukemia-variant: single institutional experience. Mod Pathol. 31(11):1717-32, 2018
14. Letendre P et al: Novel therapeutics in the treatment of hairy cell leukemia variant. Leuk Res. 75:58-60, 2018
15. Maitre E et al: New generation sequencing of targeted genes in the classical and the variant form of hairy cell leukemia highlights mutations in epigenetic regulation genes. Oncotarget. 9(48):28866-76, 2018
16. Jallades L et al: Exome sequencing identifies recurrent BCOR alterations and the absence of KLF2, TNFAIP3 and MYD88 mutations in splenic diffuse red pulp small B-cell lymphoma. Haematologica. 102(10):1758-66, 2017
17. Mason EF et al: Detection of activating MAP2K1 mutations in atypical hairy cell leukemia and hairy cell leukemia variant. Leuk Lymphoma. 58(1):233-6, 2017
18. Martinez D et al: NOTCH1, TP53, and MAP2K1 mutations in splenic diffuse red pulp small B-cell lymphoma are associated with progressive disease. Am J Surg Pathol. 40(2):192-201, 2016
19. Jain P et al: Relapsed refractory BRAF-negative, IGHV4-34-positive variant of hairy cell leukemia: a distinct entity? J Clin Oncol. 34(7):e57-60, 2016
20. Waterfall JJ et al: High prevalence of MAP2K1 mutations in variant and IGHV4-34-expressing hairy-cell leukemias. Nat Genet. 46(1):8-10, 2014
21. Kreitman RJ et al: Cladribine with immediate rituximab for the treatment of patients with variant hairy cell leukemia. Clin Cancer Res. 19(24):6873-81, 2013
22. Pande P et al: A hairy cell leukaemia variant - a rare case report. J Clin Diagn Res. 7(2):358-60, 2013
23. Shao H et al: Distinguishing hairy cell leukemia variant from hairy cell leukemia: development and validation of diagnostic criteria. Leuk Res. 37(4):401-9, 2013

Splenic B-Cell Lymphoma/Leukemia, Unclassifiable

Hairy Cell Leukemia Variant

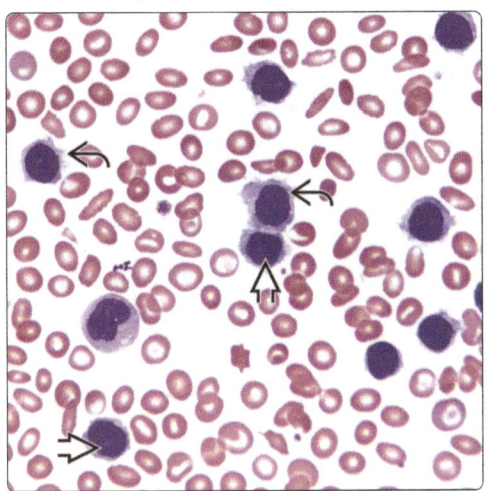

Gross Appearance of Hairy Cell Leukemia Variant

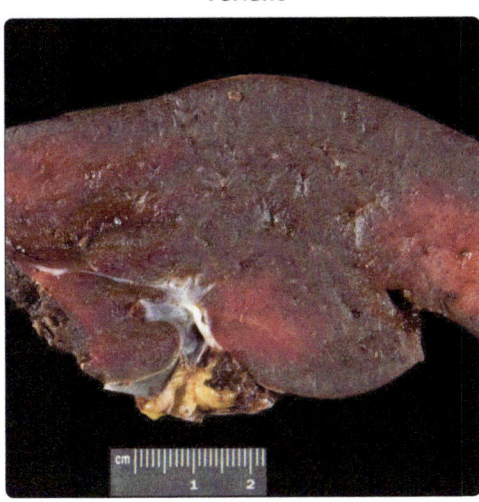

(Left) Peripheral blood smear from a case of HCLv shows the characteristic appearance of neoplastic cells that have lightly basophilic cytoplasm with small villous projections ⇨, oval nuclei with dispersed chromatin, and small nucleoli ⇨. (From DP: Spleen.) **(Right)** Gross photograph of spleen involved by HCLv shows massive enlargement with a diffuse appearance. No nodules are present. (From DP: Spleen.)

Hairy Cell Leukemia Variant

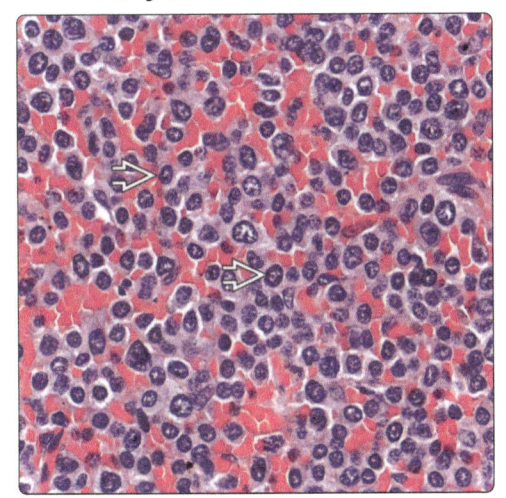

IGH Rearrangement

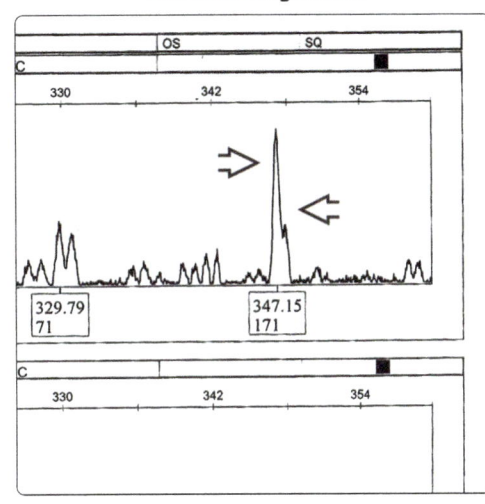

(Left) HCLv shows diffuse red pulp infiltrate of small to intermediate-sized lymphocytes with distinct nucleoli ⇨ and indistinct cytoplasm. Cords and sinuses are inapparent due to lymphocyte density. (From DP: Spleen.) **(Right)** PCR assay or immunoglobulin heavy-chain gene rearrangement shows a single dominant peak ⇨, supportive evidence that this diffuse infiltrate represents B-cell lymphoma.

Hairy Cell Leukemia Variant

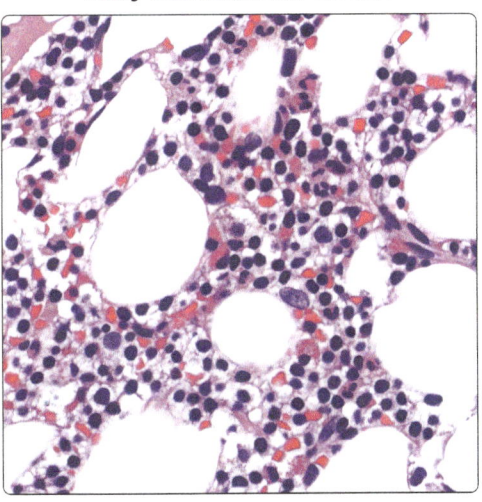

PAX5 Immunohistochemistry

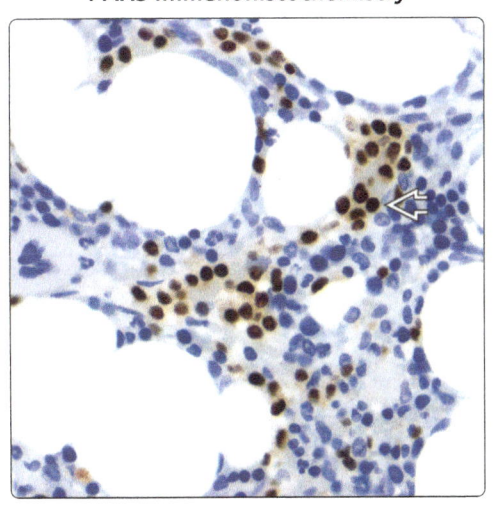

(Left) Bone marrow core biopsy shows a subtle, diffuse interstitial infiltrate of widely spaced mature lymphoid cells mimicking classic HCL. (From DP: Blood & Bone Marrow.) **(Right)** PAX5 of bone marrow involved by HCLv highlights intrasinusoidal distribution of neoplastic cells ⇨. (From DP: Spleen.)

Splenic B-Cell Lymphoma/Leukemia, Unclassifiable

Splenic Diffuse Red Pulp Small B-Cell Lymphoma

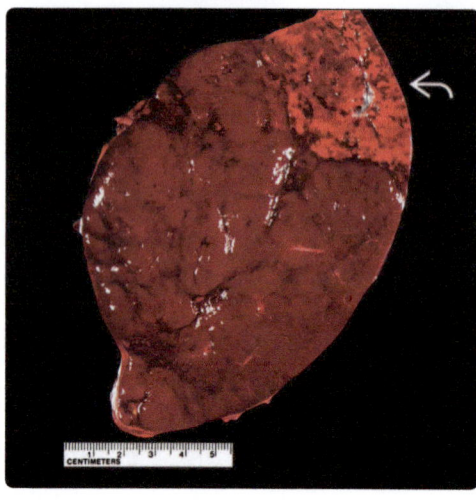

Splenic Diffuse Red Pulp Small B-Cell Lymphoma

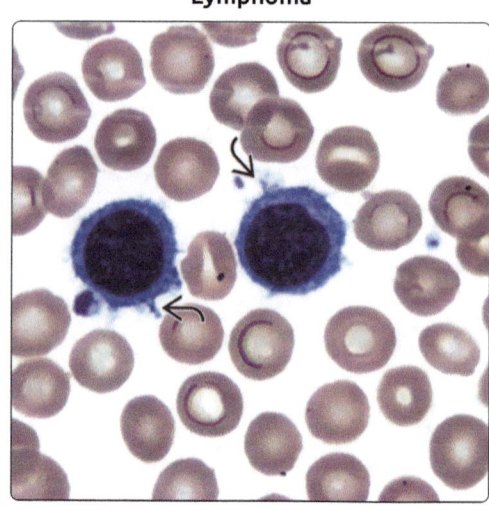

(Left) *Gross photograph of SDRP SBCL shows diffuse enlargement of spleen without nodules. A wedge-shaped infarction ➢ is noted.* (Right) *Wright-Giemsa stain of peripheral blood smear from a patient with SDRP SBCL shows 2 intermediate-sized lymphocytes with small cytoplasmic projections ➢ and condensed chromatin.*

Splenic Diffuse Red Pulp Small B-Cell Lymphoma

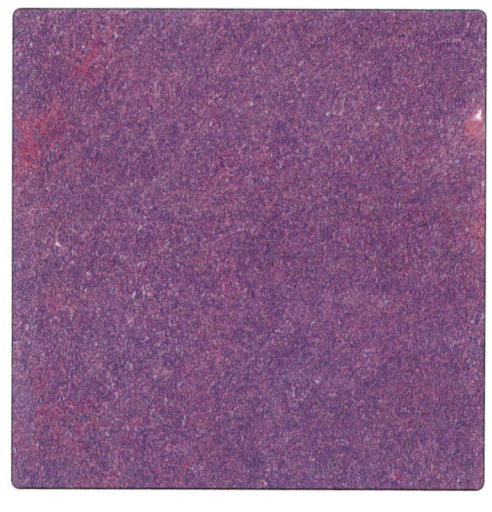

CD20: Splenic Diffuse Red Pulp Small B-Cell Lymphoma

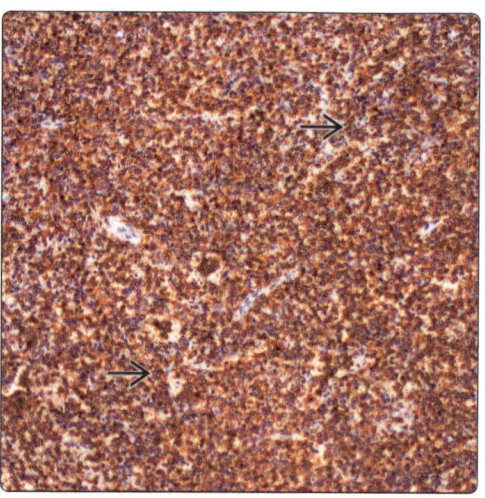

(Left) *Low-power view of spleen involved by SDRP SBCL shows a diffuse pattern of red pulp, along with absence of white pulp nodularity.* (Right) *CD20 shows diffuse replacement by positive lymphocytes ➢ on low-power view of SDRP SBCL. No residual white pulp nodularity is present.*

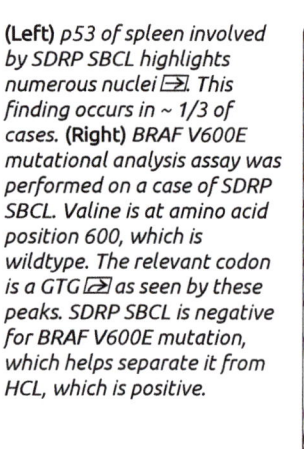

p53: Splenic Diffuse Red Pulp Small B-Cell Lymphoma

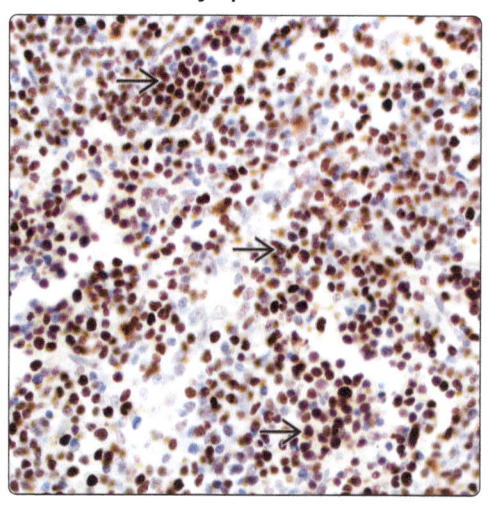

***BRAF* V600E Mutational Analysis Assay**

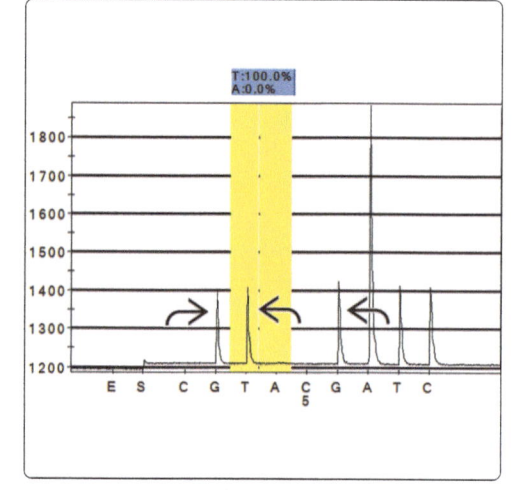

(Left) *p53 of spleen involved by SDRP SBCL highlights numerous nuclei ➢. This finding occurs in ~ 1/3 of cases.* (Right) *BRAF V600E mutational analysis assay was performed on a case of SDRP SBCL. Valine is at amino acid position 600, which is wildtype. The relevant codon is a GTG ➢ as seen by these peaks. SDRP SBCL is negative for BRAF V600E mutation, which helps separate it from HCL, which is positive.*

Splenic B-Cell Lymphoma/Leukemia, Unclassifiable

Gross Appearance of Classic Hairy Cell Leukemia

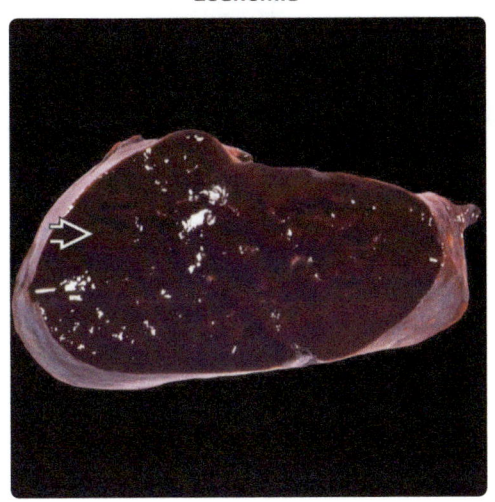

Classic Hairy Cell Leukemia

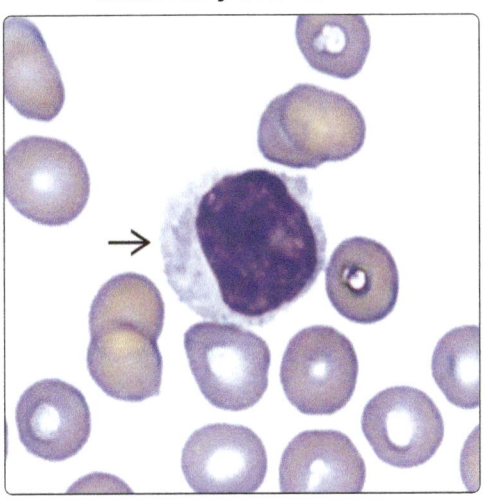

(Left) Spleen involved by classic HCL is shown. There is expansion of the red pulp ⇒, and nodules are not easily discernible. (Right) Characteristic classic hairy cell ⇒ from a patient with HCL is shown. There are cytoplasmic projections and abundant cytoplasm. The nucleoli are indistinct.

Classic Hairy Cell Leukemia

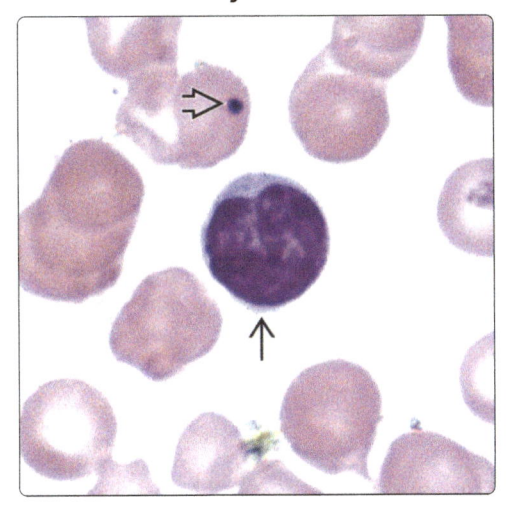

Classic Hairy Cell Leukemia

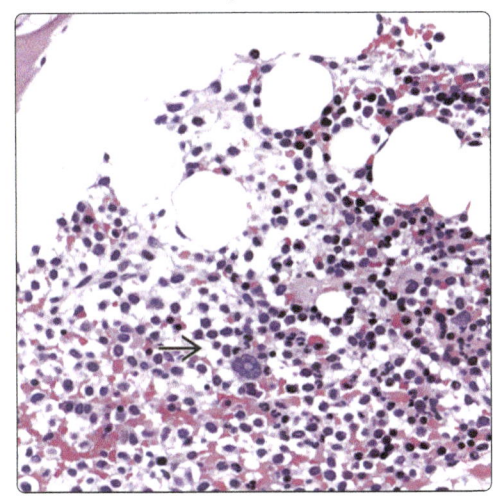

(Left) Peripheral blood smear from a patient with classic HCL shows small projections ⇒ in the cytoplasm, and the nucleus is bilobed. There is a Howell-Jolly body in a red blood cell ⇒, indicating functional asplenia. (Right) Bone marrow core biopsy shows the characteristic fried egg appearance ⇒ of the neoplastic hairy cells. The neoplastic cells contain abundant clear cytoplasm. Reticulin stain shows markedly increased reticulin fibrosis in most cases (not shown).

TRAP Cytochemistry

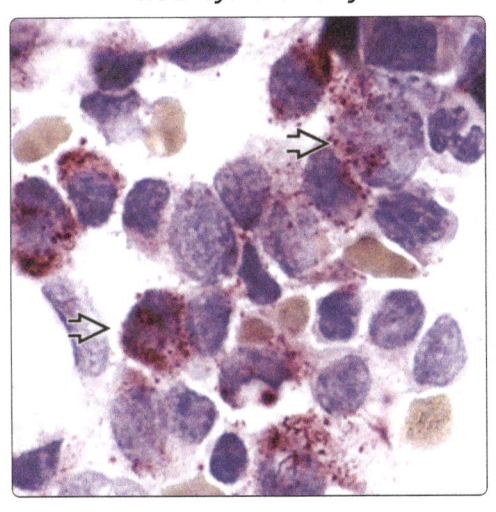

DBA44 Immunohistochemistry

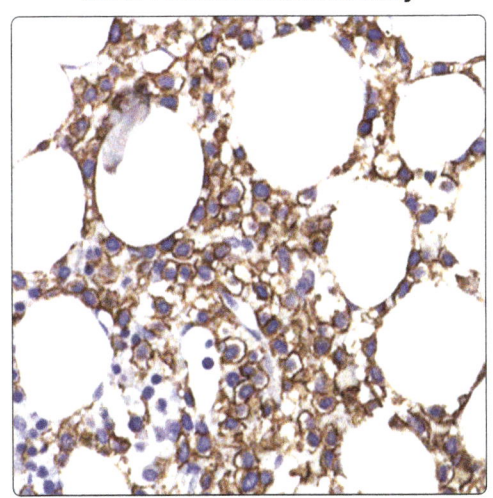

(Left) TRAP of bone marrow aspirate smear shows malignant cells with a granular staining pattern ⇒. TRAP can also be performed on tissue sections with immunohistochemistry, which shows a similar granular appearance. (Right) DBA44 is positive in HCL cells on this bone marrow core biopsy. Other positive markers include TRAP, annexin A1, CD123, and CD25.

Molecular Pathology of Lymphoid Neoplasms

Splenic B-Cell Lymphoma/Leukemia, Unclassifiable

Chronic Lymphocytic Leukemia/Small Lymphocytic Lymphoma

Chronic Lymphocytic Leukemia/Small Lymphocytic Lymphoma

(Left) Peripheral blood smear shows small lymphocytes with clumped chromatin ➡ and scant cytoplasm ➡. The lymphocytes are characteristic of chronic lymphocytic leukemia/small lymphocytic lymphoma (CLL/SLL). No cytoplasmic projections are present. (Right) Gross photograph shows spleen involved by CLL/SLL. There are visible nodules throughout ➡. The white pulp and red pulp are both involved.

Chronic Lymphocytic Leukemia/Small Lymphocytic Lymphoma

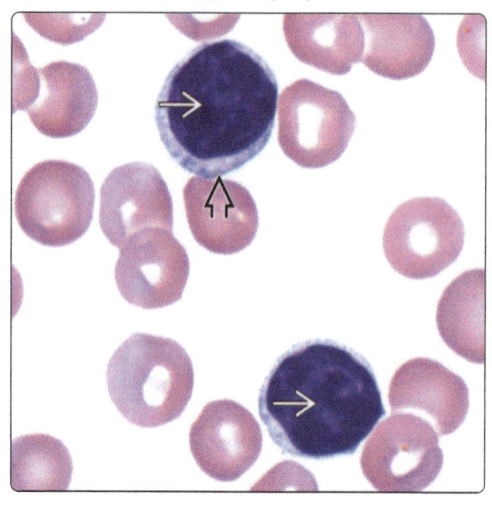

Chronic Lymphocytic Leukemia/Small Lymphocytic Lymphoma

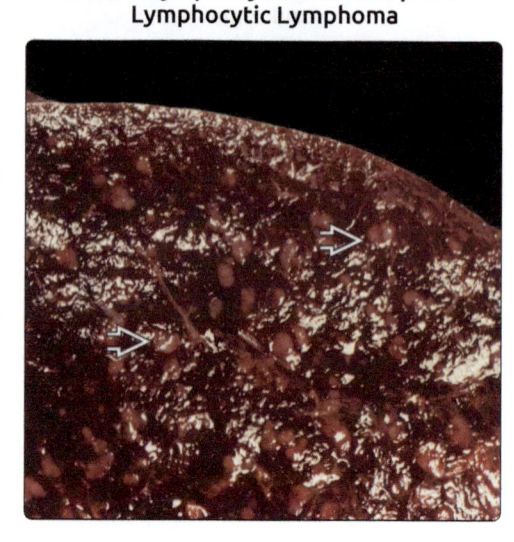

(Left) Paraffin-embedded lymph node shows lighter areas within a background of small lymphocytes, which correspond to proliferation centers ➡. (Right) High-power view shows that the neoplastic cells are predominately round with block-like chromatin ➡. Within the proliferation centers, the larger cells are paraimmunoblasts ➡, and the smaller cells with central nucleoli are prolymphocytes ➡.

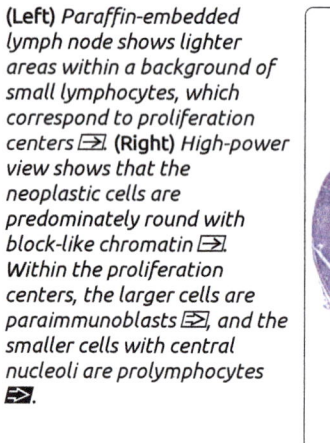

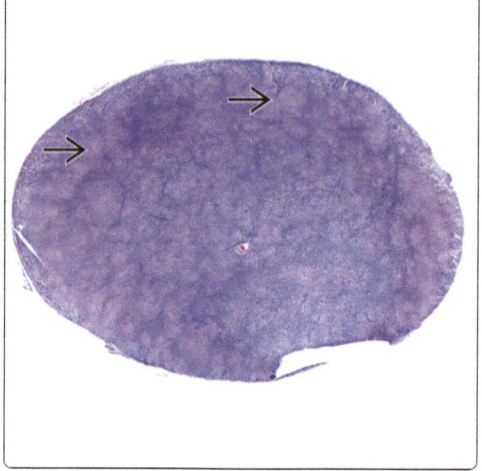

CD5 Immunohistochemistry

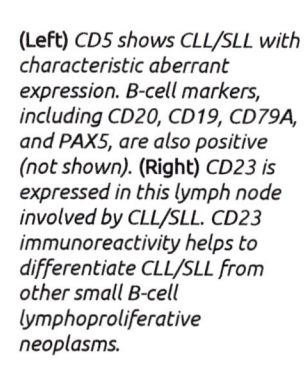

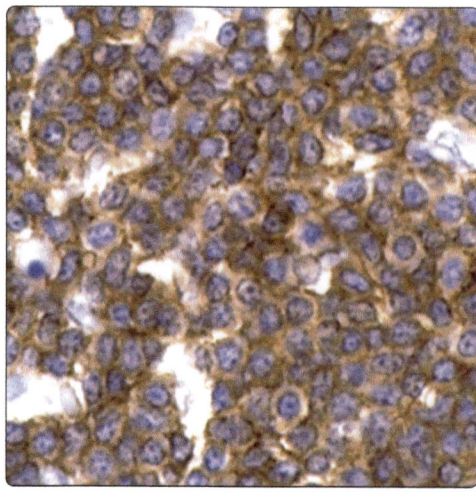

CD23 Immunohistochemistry

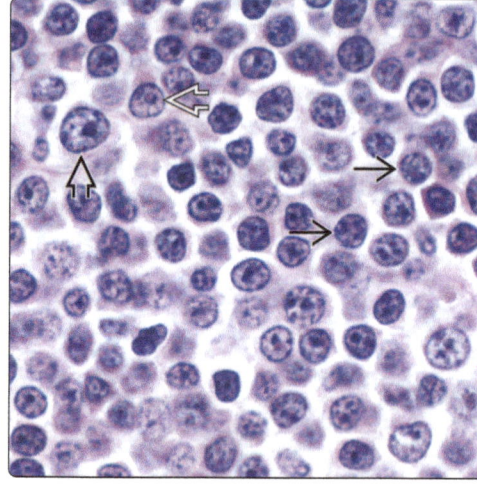

(Left) CD5 shows CLL/SLL with characteristic aberrant expression. B-cell markers, including CD20, CD19, CD79A, and PAX5, are also positive (not shown). (Right) CD23 is expressed in this lymph node involved by CLL/SLL. CD23 immunoreactivity helps to differentiate CLL/SLL from other small B-cell lymphoproliferative neoplasms.

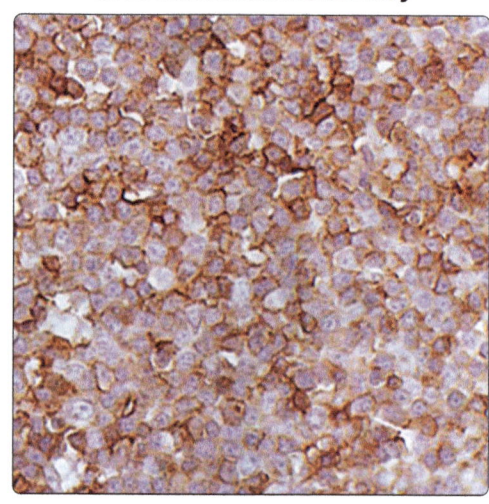

Splenic B-Cell Lymphoma/Leukemia, Unclassifiable

Splenic Marginal Zone Lymphoma

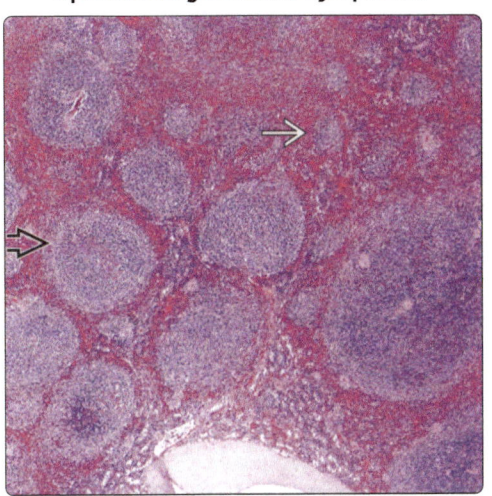

Splenic Marginal Zone Lymphoma

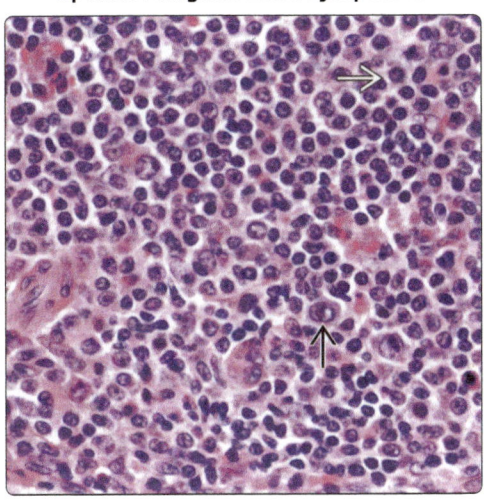

(Left) Splenic marginal zone lymphoma shows multiple lymphoid nodules in the white pulp with secondary involvement of the red pulp ⇒. The nodules show a monocytoid appearance ⇒ at the periphery of the nodules. (Right) Splenic marginal zone lymphoma shows mature lymphocytes with occasional plasmacytoid lymphocytes ⇒. Rare transformed large cells ⇒ are also present.

CD20: Splenic Marginal Zone Lymphoma

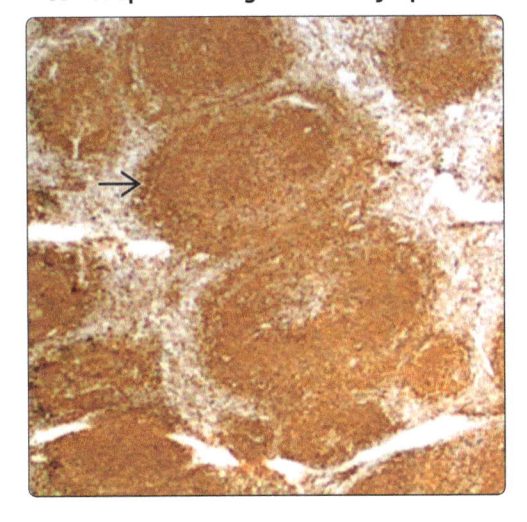

Splenic Marginal Zone Lymphoma

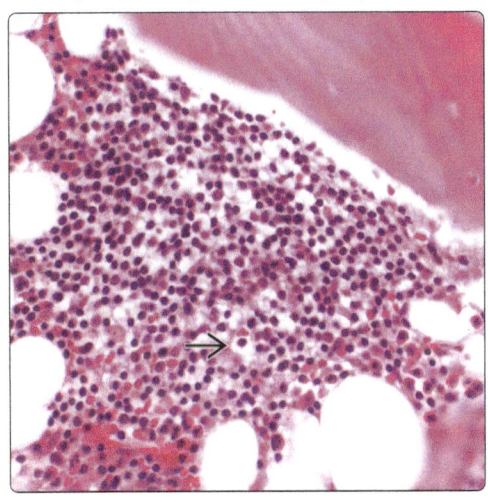

(Left) CD20 of splenic marginal zone lymphoma ⇒ highlights B-cell nodules throughout. The B cells were negative for CD5 and CD10. (Right) Splenic marginal zone lymphoma involving bone marrow shows a lymphoid nodule abutting the bony trabeculae. The cells are monocytoid appearing ⇒ with abundant cytoplasm.

B-Cell Prolymphocytic Leukemia

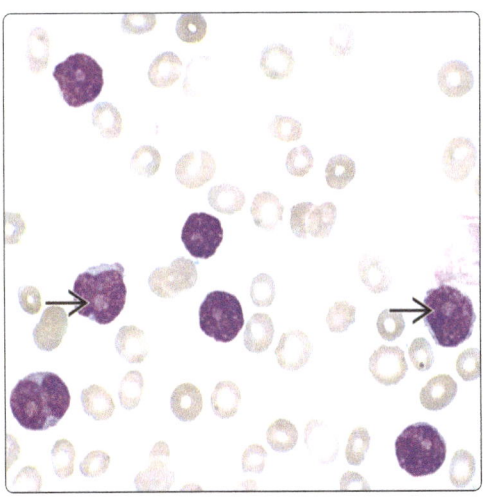

B-Cell Prolymphocytic Leukemia

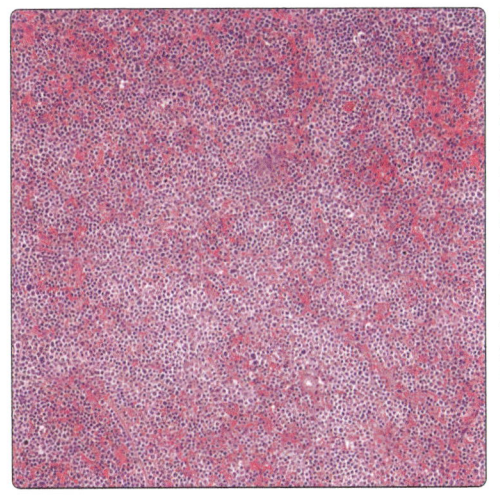

(Left) Peripheral blood smear from a patient with B-cell prolymphocytic leukemia shows neoplastic cells with single "punched-out" nucleoli ⇒ and irregular nuclei. No cytoplasmic projections are seen, as would be expected in HCLv. (Right) Spleen with B-cell prolymphocytic leukemia is shown. The red pulp is diffusely infiltrated with neoplastic cells, and the white pulp architecture is entirely effaced.

Lymphoplasmacytic Lymphoma

KEY FACTS

TERMINOLOGY
- Lymphoplasmacytic lymphoma (LPL)
  - B-cell lymphoma with variable mixture of small B cells, plasmacytoid lymphocytes, and plasma cells
- Waldenström macroglobulinemia (WM)
  - LPL with bone marrow (BM) involvement and IgM monoclonal protein

ETIOLOGY/PATHOGENESIS
- LPL is recognized by both World Health Organization (WHO) 5th edition and International Consensus Classification (ICC) as distinct entity

CLINICAL ISSUES
- Neuropathy, cardiac problems, coagulopathy, &/or gastrointestinal problems in WM
- Usually involves BM, sometimes spleen and lymph node

MOLECULAR
- *MYD88* and *CXCR4* mutational analysis should be performed on most LPL/WM cases
- *MYD88* p.L265P somatic mutation
  - Present in > 90% of LPL but not specific and not required for diagnosis
  - Helps differentiate LPL from other small B-cell lymphomas
- Del (6q23) most common cytogenetic finding

MICROSCOPIC
- Bone marrow infiltration by > 10% small lymphocytes with plasmacytoid &/or plasma cell differentiation

ANCILLARY TESTS
- Monoclonal IgM serum electrophoresis
- Immunohistochemistry or flow cytometry shows 2 monoclonal populations of cells: Mature B cells [CD20(+)] and plasma cells [CD38(+)]

Spectrum of Cell Types

(Left) *Lymphoplasmacytic lymphoma (LPL) shows a spectrum of cell types, including small lymphocytes ➡, plasmacytoid lymphocytes, and plasma cells ➡. (Right) Pyrogram demonstrates MYD88 L265P mutation due to substitution of thymine (T) for cytosine (C) ➡ in codon 265 of the MYD88 gene in a patient with history of LPL.*

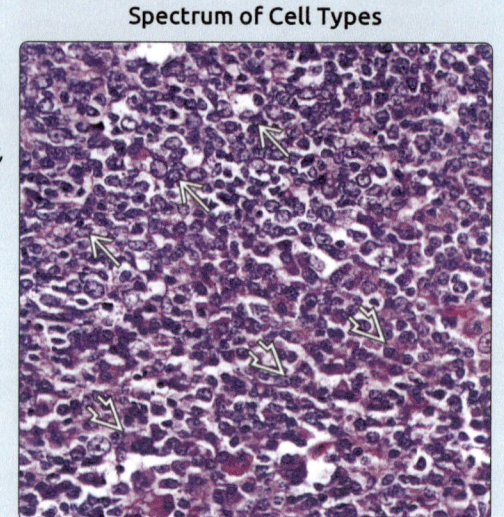

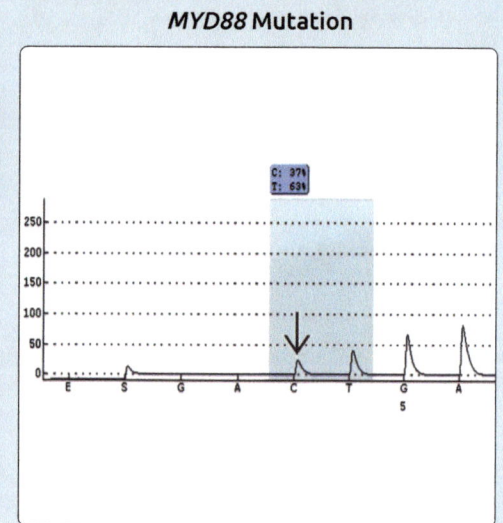

MYD88 Mutation

Clonal IGH Rearrangement

(Left) *Since LPL is a B-cell lymphoma, it typically shows monoclonal IGH rearrangement by PCR testing. In this IGH rearrangement assay, there is a dominant monoclonal peak seen at position 116 ➡. (Right) LPL shows many kappa (+) cells ➡. λ-light chain is negative (not shown).*

κ-Light Chain Restriction

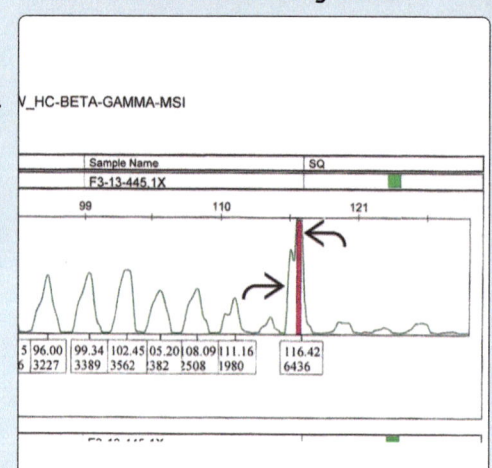

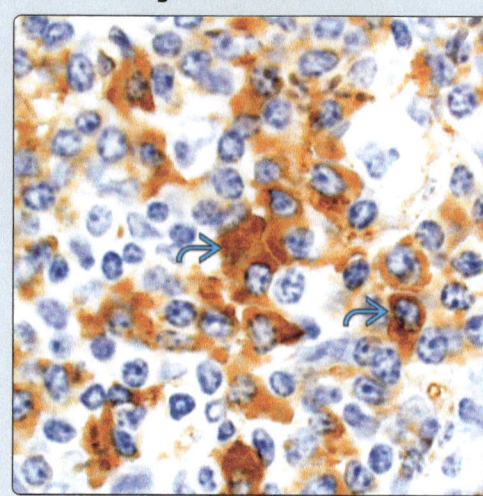

Lymphoplasmacytic Lymphoma

TERMINOLOGY

Abbreviations
- Lymphoplasmacytic lymphoma (LPL)

Synonyms
- Immunocytoma

Definitions
- B-cell lymphoma consisting of variable mixture of small B cells, plasmacytoid lymphocytes, and plasma cells that does not fit criteria for any other B-cell lymphoproliferative disorder
  o Waldenström macroglobulinemia (WM) is LPL with IgM monoclonal protein of any concentration in blood, which is commonly associated with hyperviscosity syndrome
  o MYD88 mutation detected in > 90% of LPL but is not entirely specific for this entity

ETIOLOGY/PATHOGENESIS

Classification of Lymphoplasmacytic Lymphoma
- LPL is recognized by both World Health Organization (WHO) 5th edition and International Consensus Classification (ICC) as distinct entity
  o ICC diagnostic criteria involve identifying abnormal lymphoplasmacytic aggregates in bone marrow (BM) as well as evidence of clonal B cells and plasma cells, even when aggregates are < 10% of marrow cellularity
  o WHO recognizes 2 subtypes of LPL: IgM and non-IgM subtypes
    – Non-WM type LPL
      □ Only 5% of cases of LPL
      □ Have IgG or IgA monoclonal proteins
      □ Includes nonsecretory LPL and IgM LPL without marrow involvement

Etiology
- Unknown
- Risk factors include IgM monoclonal gammopathy of undetermined significance (MGUS)
- Hepatitis has been associated with WM
- Familial cases are seen in up to 20% of WM patients

Cell of Origin
- Memory B cell that has undergone somatic hypermutation
- Lymphoma with plasmacytic differentiation that makes immunoglobulin

CLINICAL ISSUES

Epidemiology
- Incidence
  o ~ 1% of hematopathologic malignancies
- Age
  o Mean at diagnosis: 65 years
- Sex
  o M > F
- Ethnicity
  o White > Asian or Black populations

Site
- BM is usually involved and less often lymph node and spleen
  o Lymphadenopathy in < 25%, but up to 60% at relapse
- Extranodal sites are infrequently involved, including CNS (Bing-Neel syndrome), skin, gastrointestinal tract, and kidney
  o Bing-Neel syndrome is defined as central nervous system involvement with WM

Presentation
- Many symptoms of WM are related to effect of elevated IgM paraprotein
  o Coagulopathy
    – From IgM paraprotein binding to clotting factors, fibrin, or platelets
    – Hyperviscosity with blurred vision and headache
  o Neuropathy with ataxia, gait problems, tremor
  o Cardiac problems
  o Cryoglobulinemia, cold agglutinin hemolysis
  o Gastrointestinal symptoms
    – From IgM depositing in gastrointestinal tract
- Fatigue, shortness of breath, and weakness indicate anemia from BM infiltration
- Bleeding can be seen in thrombocytopenia or from acquired von Willebrand disease
- Hepatosplenomegaly in ~ 15%
- Amyloidosis and light chain deposition disease
- Non-IgM LPL has less hyperviscosity and neuropathy

Laboratory Tests
- Serum/urine protein electrophoresis
  o LPL patients often have serum monoclonal paraprotein
    – IgM is most common
    – IgG and IgA are less common, and each can occur alone or with IgM
    – Not all cases of LPL have monoclonal paraprotein
  o WM **must** show IgM paraprotein
    – IgM paraprotein can be of any concentration
  o IgM paraproteins can occur in other lymphoproliferative disorders and are not specific for LPL or WM
- ↑ erythrocyte sedimentation rate, ↑ LDH, and ↑ β-2-microglobulin can be present
- Cryoglobulin test is sometimes positive

Treatment
- Patients with smoldering WM are often watched and not treated with any specific therapy
  o SWM is defined as having serum monoclonal IgM protein ≥ 3 g/dL &/or ≥ 10% BM lymphoplasmacytic infiltrate but no end organ damage
    – End organ damage includes anemia, constitutional symptoms, hyperviscosity, lymphadenopathy, and hepatosplenomegaly
- Patients with active WM or LPL with end organ damage are treated with therapy, but therapy is not standardized
  o Radiation for local disease
  o Chemotherapy
    – Rituximab + purine analog &/or alkylating agent or bendamustine or bortezomib/dexamethasone are indicated for most patients

Lymphoplasmacytic Lymphoma

- New monoclonal antibodies (ofatumumab), proteasome inhibitors (carfilzomib), rapamycin inhibitors, and Bruton tyrosine kinase inhibitors
- Plasmapheresis reduces circulating IgM
- Splenectomy for chemotherapy-resistant patients
- Autologous or allogeneic stem cell transplant

Prognosis
- Clinical course is indolent
  - Median survival: ~ 5 years
- WM has lower mortality compared to LPL
- WM International Prognostic Scoring System adverse indicators
  - Age > 65 years
  - Hemoglobin < 11.5 g/dL
  - platelets < 100,000
  - β_2 microglobulin > 3 mg/L
  - Serum monoclonal protein > 7 g/dL
- MYD88 wildtype cases have higher risk of diffuse large B-cell lymphoma transformation

MOLECULAR

Gene Alterations
- Molecular studies for MYD88 and CXCR4 mutations are often necessary as ancillary testing for LPL
  - MYD88 alterations can be found in blood, skin, and cerebrospinal fluid
- MYD88 c.794T>C, p.L265P
  - Genomic location: 3: 38141150 (GRCh 38)
  - Considered driver mutation in LPL
  - Positive in > 90% of LPL/WM
    - Helps differentiates LPL from other plasmacytoid small B-cell lymphomas in correct clinical context
      - Negative in most other small B-cell lymphomas and plasma cell myeloma
    - Absence of MYD88 mutation does not exclude diagnosis of LPL
    - Causes gain of function of MYD88 and activates NF-κB pathway and Toll-like receptor (TLR) signaling pathways
  - Other rare non-L265P MYD88 mutations have been reported in 1-2% of LPL
  - MYD88 mutation is not specific or required for LPL diagnosis
    - Also detected in 80% of IgM MGUS, ~ 40% of DLBCL of activated B-cell subtype, DLBCL leg type (~ 70%), central nervous system lymphoma (36%), mucosa-associated lymphoid tissue (MALT) lymphoma (9%), Burkitt lymphoma (4%), small lymphocytic lymphoma/chronic lymphocytic leukemia (3%), and testicular DLBCL
    - Not reported in DLBCL of germinal center B-cell subtype
- CXCR4 mutations
  - Altered in ~ 40% of LPL patients but also in small percentage of other B-cell lymphomas
    - Reported in marginal zone lymphoma and diffuse large B-cell lymphoma of ABC type
    - Not found in IgM MGUS
  - CXCR4 mutations are usually concurrent with MYD88 mutations
  - Nonsense and frameshift mutations affecting C-terminal region
  - Characteristics of LPL with CXCR4 alterations
    - Resistance to Ibrutinib therapy
    - High serum IgM
    - Viscosity
    - Earlier time to treatment
- Other altered genes in LPL/WM
  - TP53, CD79B, KMT2D, MYBBP1A, TAP2, LRP1B, ARID1A, H1-4, and RAPGEF3
- MicroRNA
  - Elevated miR-155, decreased miR-9

Cytogenetics
- Variety of chromosomal aberrations seen
  - 6q21-q25 deletion
    - Most common finding by chromosomal analysis (~ 50% of cases)
      - Increase in number from IgM MGUS to asymptomatic WM to symptomatic WM
      - Implies del6q21-q25 may be associated with progression of disease
    - This finding is not specific for LPL and can also rarely be seen in marginal zone lymphoma (MZL)
  - Trisomy 4, trisomy 18
    - Trisomy 4 and trisomy 18 often occur together
    - Trisomy 4 is not found in other small B-cell lymphomas
  - Trisomy 3, 13q deletions, 17p deletions, 11q deletions
    - Can also be seen in other small B-cell lymphomas, such as small lymphocytic lymphoma/chronic lymphocytic leukemia and MZL
    - del(6q), del(11q), and trisomy 4 are poor prognostic indicators
  - Rare IGH translocations
  - t(9;14)(p13.2;q32.3) (PAX5::IGH) is no longer considered diagnostic of LPL
- No cytogenetic abnormalities are specific for LPL/WM
- No translocations typical of other small B-cell lymphomas, such as t(14;18), t(11;18), or t(11;14) are seen

In Situ Hybridization
- EBER(-)

PCR
- Clonal IGH rearrangement
  - Variable regions of IGH show somatic hypermutation and biased variable gene segments usage
  - VH3-23 overrepresentation and high IGH mutation rate
  - Peripheral blood may show clonal cytotoxic T cells

Chromosomal Microarray
- Losses of 13q14.3, 17p13.3, 11q21-q22, and 7q32.1-q33 are found in LPL but also in MZL

Gene Expression Profiling
- WM, IgM monoclonal gammopathy of undetermined significance and plasma cell myeloma have different gene expression signatures

MICROSCOPIC

Histologic Features
- BM

Lymphoplasmacytic Lymphoma

- o Infiltrated with small B cells, plasmacytoid cells, and plasma cells
  - Lymphoid aggregates with nodular, diffuse, or interstitial growth patterns
    - May be paratrabecular
    - Aggregates can have follicular dendritic cell meshworks
  - Scattered large B cells may represent early transformation to DLBCL
- o Dutcher bodies and Russell bodies are often present
  - Dutcher bodies can also be seen in neoplasms with plasma cell differentiation, including multiple myeloma, MZL, and very rare cases of follicular lymphoma (FL)
- o Mast cells and hemosiderin-laden macrophages may be present
- o Amyloid and crystal-storing histiocytosis sometimes can be seen
- o Residual disease after treatment may show only plasma cells
- Spleen
  - o Infiltrate often involves both white and red pulp
  - o Nodular or diffuse growth patterns
    - Small lymphocytes, plasmacytoid lymphocytes, &/or plasma cells
  - o Neoplastic cells may be focused on mantle zones and marginal zones
- Blood
  - o Absolute lymphocytosis with increased numbers of small lymphocytes, plasmacytoid lymphocytes, and plasma cells
  - o Red blood cell rouleaux formation, especially if elevated IgM paraprotein is present
  - o Rarely cold agglutinin &/or cryoglobulin
- Lymph node
  - o Total or partial effacement of lymph node by malignant cells
  - o Diffuse growth pattern with patent sinuses and preserved follicles
  - o Residual reactive germinal centers are often small &/or atretic
  - o Sometimes plasmacytoid or monocytoid B cells
  - o Often monomorphic predominantly lymphoid infiltrate
  - o Can show follicular colonization and hemosiderin-laden macrophages

Cytologic Features

- Lymphocytes are small in size with coarse chromatin, indistinct nucleoli, and often plasmacytoid features

ANCILLARY TESTS

Immunohistochemistry

- B cells
  - o CD19(+), CD20(+), CD22(+), CD79A(+), and PAX5(+)
  - o CD45RB(+), BCL2(+), CD200(+) (moderate intensity)
  - o Usually CD5, CD10, and CD23 (-)
    - However, expression of CD5, CD23 and CD10 can be seen in some cases and should not be mistaken for different type of small B-cell lymphoma
  - o Cyclin-D1, CD103, and BCL6 (-)
- Plasmacytoid cells
  - o Plasma cell markers CD138, CD38, and MUM1 (+)
  - o CD20 and CD45RB (-)
  - o κ- and λ-light chains show monoclonality in plasma cells
  - o PAX5(+/-)
- Heavy chains
  - o Usually IgM(+)
  - o Sometimes IgA(+) or IgG(+)
  - o IgD(-)
- Congo red will show apple green birefringence if there is amyloid

Flow Cytometry

- Usually 2 separate monoclonal populations
  - o B cells
    - CD19(+), CD20(+), CD45(+), κ- or λ-light chain restricted
    - Usually CD5, CD10, and CD23 (-)
    - Variably reactive for CD25, FMC7, CD43, and CD11c
    - CD103(-)
  - o Plasma cells
    - CD138(+), CD38(+), CD19(+), cytoplasmic κ or λ restriction
    - CD20(-)

DIFFERENTIAL DIAGNOSIS

Nodal Marginal Zone Lymphoma

- Shares many morphologic and phenotypic characteristics with LPL
  - o Both LPL and MZL consist of lymphocytes with plasmacytoid features
  - o Can have IgM paraprotein like LPL
  - o Both MZL and LPL/WM can involve lymph nodes, BM, and spleen
  - o Similar phenotype, positive for B-cell markers and BCL2, but negative for CD5, CD10, and cyclin-D1
- Differences
  - o Most cases lack *MYD88* L265P mutation
  - o More lymphadenopathy, less BM and spleen involvement
  - o Usually no clinical features of WM, including hyperviscosity, visual problems, neurologic changes, and cryoglobulinemia
  - o Areas with monocytoid morphology favor MZL
  - o Cytoplasmic or surface IgM favors LPL
- Sometimes definitive diagnosis may not be possible, and differential must include both MZL and LPL

Extranodal Marginal Zone Lymphoma of Gastrointestinal Tract

- t(11;18)(q21;q21), t(14;18)(q32;q21), and t(1;14)(p22;q32) are detected in MALT lymphoma but not found in LPL/WM
- Only 9% show *MYD88* mutations
  - o *MYD88* p.L265P alterations favors LPL over MZL
- LPL and WM rarely involve extranodal sites
- Associated with *Helicobacter pylori*
- IgM paraprotein is uncommon
- Often shows lymphoepithelial lesions and reactive colonized germinal centers

Lymphoplasmacytic Lymphoma

Incidence of *MYD88* L265P Mutations in 100 Bone Marrow Specimens Involved by Subtypes of Small B-Cell Neoplasms/Multiple Myeloma

Type of Hematopoietic Disorder	Number of Cases With *MYD88* L265P Mutation	Percentage of Cases With *MYD88* L265P Mutation
LPL/WM	30/30	100
CLL/SLL	0/10	0
Follicular lymphoma	0/10	0
HCL	2/10	20
HCL variant	0/10	0
Mantle cell lymphoma	0/10	0
Marginal zone lymphoma	0/10	0, although low % positive in other studies
Plasma cell myeloma	0/10	0

LPL/WM = lymphoplasmacytic lymphoma/Waldenström macroglobulinemia; CLL/SLL = chronic lymphocytic leukemia/small lymphocytic lymphoma; HCL = hairy cell leukemia.

Common Molecular Changes in Mature B-Cell Lymphomas

Type of Lymphoma	Molecular Abnormality
LPL/WM	*MYD88* L265P mutation
Follicular lymphoma	t(14;18)(q32;q21); *IGH::BCL2*
Mantle cell lymphoma	t(11;14)(q31;q32); *CCND1::IGH*
Marginal zone lymphoma	t(11;18)(q22;q21); *BIRC3::MALT1*, lung and gastric, t(14;18)(q32;q21); *IGH::MALT1*, ocular, salivary t(3;14)(p13;q32); *IGH::FOXP1* thyroid, skin, ocular
Splenic marginal zone	del(7)(q22-32)
HCL	*BRAF* mutation
Diffuse large B-cell lymphoma	t(14;18)(q32;q21); *IGH::BCL2*, *BCL6* rearrangements
Burkitt lymphoma	t(8;14); *IGH::MYC*, t(2;8); *IGK::MYC*, t(8;22); *IGL::MYC*

PL/WM = lymphoplasmacytic lymphoma/Waldenström macroglobulinemia; HCL = hairy cell leukemia.

Multiple Myeloma
- Rare cases of IgM(+) multiple myeloma and IgA(+) or IgG(+) LPL
- Has different clinical features, including lytic bone lesions and renal abnormalities
- Usually does not present with clinical features of WM, including hyperviscosity or neurologic problems
- Consists entirely of plasma cells
  - LPL usually has component of monoclonal small B cells
- Usually CD19(-), CD45RB(-), and cyclin-D1 (+/-), unlike LPL/WM
- t(11;14)(q13;q32) in subset of multiple myeloma and not LPL/WM
- No *MYD88* L265P mutation

IgM Monoclonal Gammopathy of Undetermined Significance
- *MYD88* alterations detected in 80%
- IgM protein in serum < 3 g/L
- BM clonal plasma cells < 10%
- No lytic bone lesions
- No evidence of other B-cell hematopoietic disorder
- No myeloma-related organ damage (hypercalcemia, renal insufficiency, anemia, or bone lesions)

Plasmablastic Lymphoma
- Consists of B cells and plasmacytoid cells (like LPL/WM)
- Morphology differs because B cells are large with prominent nucleoli and considerable atypia
- EBER(+)
- Phenotype differs

SELECTED REFERENCES
1. Dogliotti I et al: Diagnostics in Waldenström's macroglobulinemia: a consensus statement of the European Consortium for Waldenström's Macroglobulinemia. Leukemia. 37(2):388-95, 2023
2. Falini B et al: A comparison of the International Consensus and 5th World Health Organization classifications of mature B-cell lymphomas. Leukemia. 37(1):18-34, 2023
3. Gertz MA: Waldenström macroglobulinemia: 2023 update on diagnosis, risk stratification, and management. Am J Hematol. 98(2):348-58, 2023
4. Gustine JN et al: TP53 mutations are associated with mutated MYD88 and CXCR4, and confer an adverse outcome in Waldenström macroglobulinaemia. Br J Haematol. 184(2):242-5, 2019
5. Treon SP et al: Genomic landscape of Waldenström macroglobulinemia. Hematol Oncol Clin North Am. 32(5):745-52, 2018
6. Yu X et al: MYD88 L265P mutation in lymphoid malignancies. Cancer Res. 78(10):2457-62, 2018
7. Patkar N et al: MYD88 mutant lymphoplasmacytic lymphoma/Waldenström macroglobulinemia has distinct clinical and pathological features as compared to its mutation negative counterpart. Leuk Lymphoma. 28(4):564-74, 2015

Lymphoplasmacytic Lymphoma

Plasma Cell Population

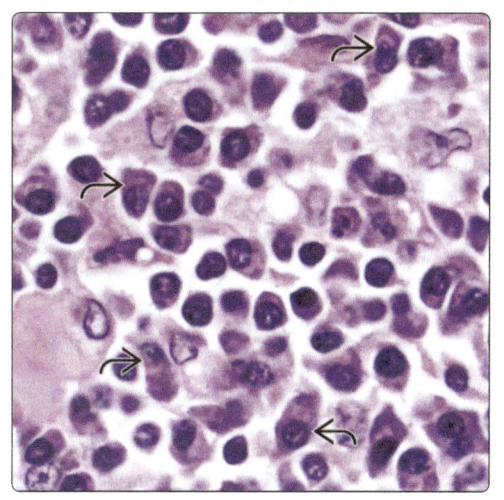

Small B-Cell Population

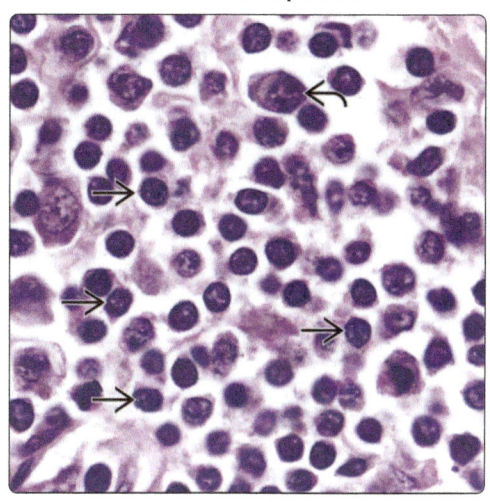

(Left) LPL shows collections of plasma cells ⇨ with eccentrically located nuclei, ample eosinophilic cytoplasm, and perinuclear hofs. (Right) Small B cells are present ⇨ with coarse chromatin, indistinct nuclei, and scant cytoplasm. Only a few plasmacytoid lymphocytes are identified ⇨.

Plasma Cell Population

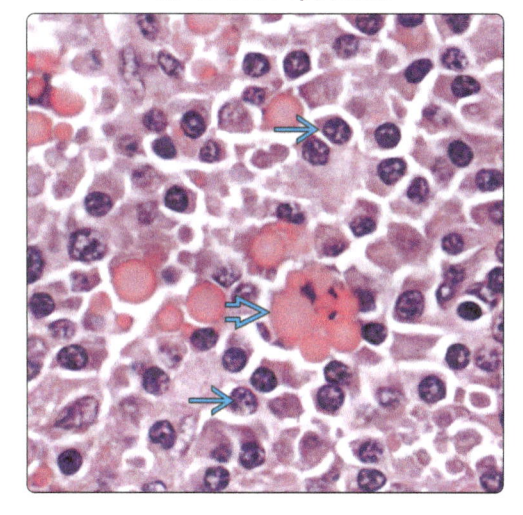

CD38 Immunohistochemistry

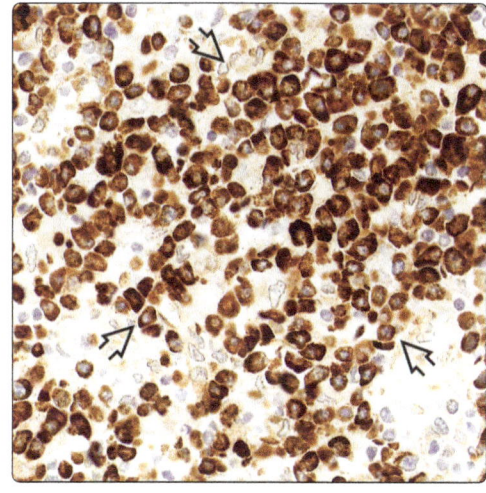

(Left) Plasma cell population ⇨ is shown in this case of LPL. Russell bodies (large, intracytoplasmic, immunoglobulin-containing inclusions) ⇨ are also present. (Right) CD38 highlights clusters of plasma cells ⇨ with a cytoplasmic staining pattern. There were also populations of B cells that expressed CD20, PAX5, and CD22 (not shown).

κ-Light Chain Immunohistochemistry

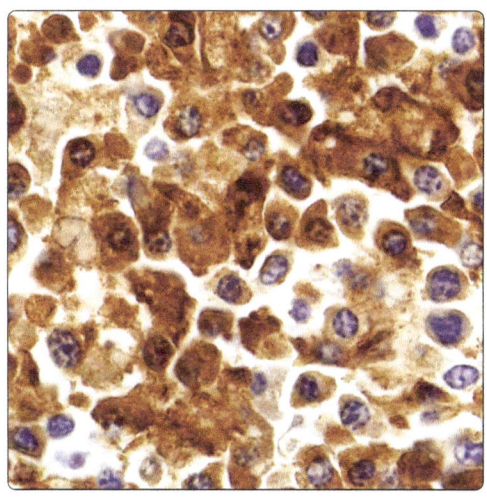

λ-Light Chain Immunohistochemistry

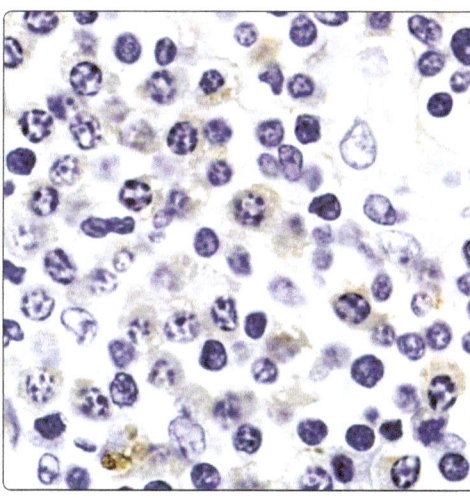

(Left) κ-light chain shows diffuse staining of plasmacytoid cells in LPL. (Right) λ-light chain is negative in plasmacytoid cells. κ and λ stains demonstrate κ restriction and are further proof that this is a clonal proliferation.

Monoclonal Gammopathy of Undetermined Significance

KEY FACTS

TERMINOLOGY
- 2022 ICC and WHO 5th edition for monoclonal gammopathy of undetermined significance (MGUS)
  o Serum monoclonal protein < 3 g/L
  o < 10% clonal plasma cells or B cells in bone marrow
  o Absence of end-organ damage attributable to plasma cell or lymphoplasmacytic disorder
  o No CRAB attributable to plasma cell neoplasm in non-IgM MGUS
  o No evidence of hyperviscosity, lymphadenopathy, amyloidosis
  o No evidence of non-plasma cell B-cell disorder
- 2 types
  o Non-IgM MGUS
    – Progresses to plasma cell neoplasms
    – Heavy chains commonly expressed
    – Light chain MGUS: Abnormal free light chain ratio, no Ig heavy chain
  o IgM MGUS
    – Progresses to lymphoplasmacytic lymphoma

CLINICAL ISSUES
- Absence of specific M protein-related symptoms
- Screening tests for MGUS
  o Serum and urine protein electrophoresis
  o Serum free light chain assay

MICROSCOPIC
- Non-IgM: Bone marrow with < 10% clonal plasma cells
  o Usually mature appearance with mild atypia
  o Scattered interstitial distribution in biopsy sections
- IgM: < 10% clonal lymphoplasmacytic cells

ANCILLARY TESTS
- CD138, CD20, κ and λ immunostains or in situ hybridization
- Flow cytometry to identify monotypic B-cells or plasma cells
- FISH often identifies abnormalities
- NGS may identify *MYD88* or *CXCR4* mutation in IgM MGUS

Non-IgM MGUS Plasma Cell Type

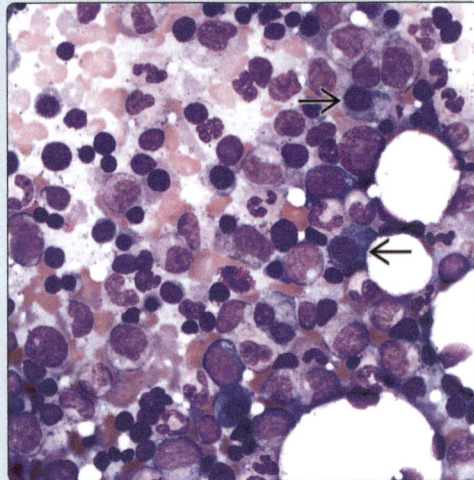

CD138 Immunohistochemistry

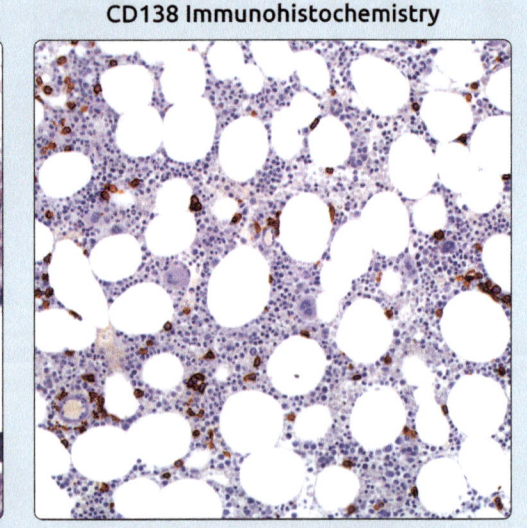

(Left) Mature-appearing plasma cells ➡ are present in marrow aspirate smear with occasional enlarged nuclei and binucleation. Morphologic appearance of plasma cells is not distinguishable from reactive plasma cells. Erythroid and myeloid lineages show appropriate maturation. (Right) CD138 helps to enumerate plasma cells in bone marrow biopsy from a 72-year-old man with monoclonal gammopathy of undetermined significance (MGUS). Plasma cells are interstitial in distribution and comprise < 5% of cellularity.

λ-Light Chain In Situ Hybridization

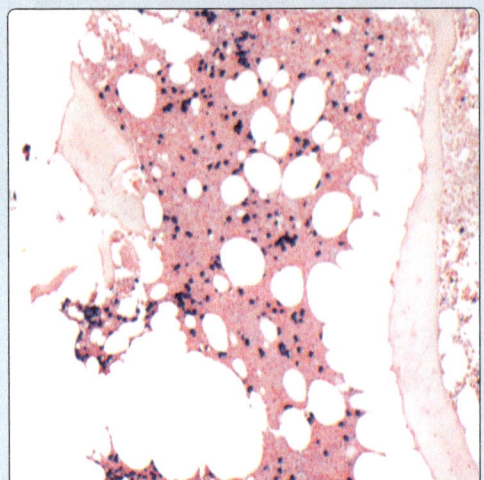

κ-Light Chain In Situ Hybridization

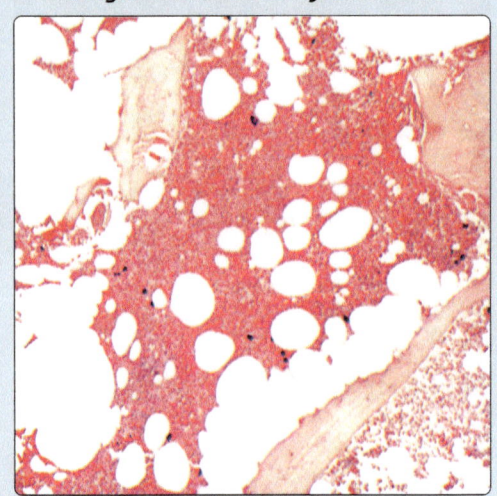

(Left) Bone marrow biopsy from a 76-year-old man with longstanding MGUS is shown. This is a λ in situ hybridization stain showing scattered λ-positive plasma cells. (Right) κ in situ hybridization with only rare positive cells is shown. The patient had both IgG λ monoclonal protein (0.79 g/dL) and free λ-light chains.

Monoclonal Gammopathy of Undetermined Significance

TERMINOLOGY

Abbreviations
- Monoclonal gammopathy of undetermined significance (MGUS)
- Free light chains (FLC)

Synonyms
- Benign monoclonal gammopathy

Definitions
- Asymptomatic disorder in which individual has low-level monoclonal serum immunoglobulin or FLC
  - Serum monoclonal (IgM or non-IgM) protein < 3g/L
  - < 10% clonal or monotypic plasma cells or < 10% clonal or monotypic lymphoplasmacytic cells in bone marrow
  - Absence of end-organ damage attributable to plasma cell neoplasm or lymphoplasmacytic lymphoma (LPL)/Waldenström macroglobulinemia (WM)
    - CRAB: Hyper**c**alcemia, **r**enal insufficiency, **a**nemia, **b**one lesions, and amyloidosis attributable to plasma cell neoplasm (non-IgM MGUS)
    - No evidence of constitutional symptoms, hyperviscosity, lymphadenopathy, hepatosplenomegaly
  - No evidence of a B-cell lymphoproliferative disorder

ETIOLOGY/PATHOGENESIS

Etiology
- Non-IgM: No known cause
- IgM: Possible association with hepatitis C virus

Increased Risk Association
- Non-IgM
  - Familial clustering
    - 3x higher than general population if 1st-degree relative has non-IgM MGUS
    - Higher risk if 1st-degree relative has multiple myeloma/plasma cell myeloma (MM/PCM)
  - Immunosuppression
  - Inflammatory diseases

2022 ICC vs. WHO 5th Edition
- ICC definition of IgM MGUS
  - IgM paraprotein, < 10% bone marrow plasma cells, and lack of lymphoplasmacytic B-cell aggregates
  - Most are precursors of LPL/WM
  - 2 types: IgM MGUS, plasma cell type and IgM MGUS, not otherwise specified (NOS)
    - IgM MGUS plasma cell type: Precursor of IgM multiple myeloma
      - Clonal plasma cells without detectable clonal B-cells and wildtype *MYD88*
      - May show t(11;14)(q13;q32) or other cytogenetic findings seen in MM
    - IgM MGUS, NOS
      - Monoclonal or monotypic B-cells
      - May have *MYD88* or *CXCR4* mutation
  - Non-IgM MGUS
    - Most are precursors of MM
    - Presence of non-IgM serum monoclonal protein < 3g/dL, clonal PC < 10%, and absence of end organ damage that can be attributed to plasma cell disorder (CRAB)
    - Secretes IgG > IgA > IgD > IgE or rarely light chain only
    - No heavy chain is secreted or identified on IFE
    - May be associated with primary amyloidosis
- WHO-HAEM5 definition of IgM MGUS
  - Presence of IgM serum monoclonal proteins < 3g/dL, < 10% bone marrow lymphoplasmacytic cells (clonal B-cells and plasma cells), and no constitutional symptoms attributable to lymphoproliferative disorder
  - Light chain MGUS: FLC ratio < 0.26 or > 1.65
  - In contrast to ICC, no further IgM subclassifications in WHO-HAEM5
- Other conditions associated with clonal Ig secretion in absence of overt malignancy
  - Monoclonal gammopathy of renal significance (MGRS) or clinical significance (MGCS)
    - Represents recognized entity in WHO-HAEM5
    - Do not represent separate disease entities in ICC; instead, can be added descriptively as clinical feature to underlying diagnosis (e.g., MGUS)

CLINICAL ISSUES

Epidemiology
- Incidence
  - Prevalence increases with age for White populations
    - Non-IgM: > 50 years = 3.2%; > 70 years = 5%; > 85 years = 9%
    - IgM: 15% of all MGUS are IgM with prevalence of 0.5% at > 50 years
- Age
  - Median at diagnosis: 70 years for both types
- Sex
  - Slightly more common in men for both types
- Ethnicity
  - Non-IgM MGUS: Black Americans have 2-3x higher risk than White Americans
  - IgM MGUS: More common in White than Black or Asian populations

Presentation
- Often asymptomatic
  - Incidental finding often during routine work-up
  - No M protein-related signs or symptoms
  - Underdiagnosed in general population
- Symptoms associated with MGUS
  - Increased osteoporosis/osteopenia
  - Peripheral neuropathy
  - Thrombotic events, especially deep vein thrombosis

Laboratory Tests
- Screening tests for MGUS
  - Serum protein electrophoresis (SPEP)
    - Perform immunofixation (IFE) to identify immunoglobulin type
  - Urine protein electrophoresis (UPEP) or serum FLC assay
    - If abnormal FLC assay, UPEP is recommended
    - UPEP shows monoclonal light chain in ~ 1/3 of MGUS; requires 24-hour collection

Monoclonal Gammopathy of Undetermined Significance

- Tests to be performed at initial diagnosis
  - Complete blood count and routine chemistry
    - Red cell indices, calcium, and creatinine to evaluate for CRAB
  - Vitamin D levels
  - Bone marrow evaluation
    - Depends on clinical indication; may not be necessary for low-risk MGUS

Treatment
- Drugs
  - Vitamin D and calcium
  - Antiresorptive therapy (bisphosphonates) if osteoporosis or fractures present
  - Corticosteroids or rituximab for peripheral neuropathy

Prognosis
- At present, no reliable biologic markers to predict progression to MM or LPL/WM
- Non-IgM MGUS models for progression
  - Mayo model: Risk based on 3 factors
    - Serum M protein < 1.5 g/dL, IgG subtype, and normal FLC ratio; low risk if all 3 factors within normal
  - Spanish study group model: Risk based on multiparametric flow cytometry techniques to identify abnormal plasma cell populations and DNA ploidy
- IgM MGUS progresses to LPL/WM
  - Progresses to LPL/WM or other B-cell neoplasms or amyloidosis at rate or 1.5% per year
  - MYD88 L265P mutation and higher levels of serum IgM are independent risk factors for progression

MOLECULAR

Cytogenetics
- Non-IgM MGUS
  - Cytogenetic abnormalities in plasma cell type are similar to MM but less frequent
  - Often normal
- IgM MGUS
  - Most common: del 6q, +18q, trisomy 4, 5, 12 and monosomy 8

Fluorescence In Situ Hybridization
- Non-IgM MGUS
  - Similar abnormalities found in MM but less frequent
  - More sensitive than conventional cytogenetic testing
  - Abnormalities detected by FISH
    - Hyperdiploidy in 40-50%
    - Deletion of 13q present in 40-50%
    - Immunoglobulin light chain aberrations
    - High prevalence of immunoglobulin heavy chain translocations (50%)
- IgM MGUS
  - Del 6q, +18q, trisomy 4, 5, 12 and monosomy 8

Array Comparative Genomic Hybridization
- Non-IgM MGUS
  - Show progressive complexities (increased copy number alterations) in MM as compared to MGUS

Other Molecular Alterations
- Non-IgM MGUS
  - Numerous gene mutations, similar to MM
    - 5% of MGUS have activating KRAS and NRAS mutations
  - No specific abnormality distinguishes MGUS from MM
- IgM MGUS
  - Gene expression profile similar to LPL/WM
  - MYD88 L265P can be detected by allele-specific PCR from peripheral blood in 60%
  - CXCR4 S338X mutations in 9-20% and may confer shorter treatment-free interval
  - KMT2D mutations in 5%

MICROSCOPIC

Cytologic Features
- Non-IgM MGUS
  - Peripheral blood
    - May see mild rouleaux formation
  - Bone marrow with < 10% clonal plasma cells
    - Usually mature appearance; rarely mild atypia, including inclusions, enlarged size, and nucleoli
- IgM MGUS
  - Peripheral blood often appears normal
  - Bone marrow
    - < 10% clonal lymphoplasmacytic cells
    - Increased mast cells may be seen

ANCILLARY TESTS

Immunohistochemistry
- Non-IgM MGUS
  - Plasma cells CD138(+), CD19(-), CD56(+/-), CD117(+/-), κ or λ restricted
    - Best way to quantify clonal plasma cells in biopsies
    - κ and λ in situ hybridization is better in determining clonality than immunohistochemical stains
- IgM MGUS
  - Lymphocytes CD20(+), CD138(+), CD56(-), CD5(-/+), CD10(-), κ or λ
  - Light chain restricted PC population may be seen

Flow Cytometry
- Non-IgM MGUS
  - Cytoplasmic light chain restricted plasma cells
    - CD138(+), CD38(+), CD19(-), CD45(+/-), CD56(+/-), CD117(+/-)
    - Analysis underestimates plasma cell percentage
- IgM MGUS
  - CD138(-/+), CD20(+), CD56(-), CD5(-), CD10(-) monotypic B-cells
  - Small monotypic plasma cell population may be present

SELECTED REFERENCES

1. Falini B et al: A comparison of the International Consensus and 5th World Health Organization classifications of mature B-cell lymphomas. Leukemia. 37(1):18-34, 2023
2. Abeykoon JP et al: Monoclonal gammopathy of undetermined significance: evaluation, risk assessment, management, and beyond. Fac Rev. 11:34, 2022
3. Khalili P et al: Evaluation of genes and molecular pathways involved in the progression of monoclonal gammopathy of undetermined significance (MGUS) to multiple myeloma: a systems biology approach. Mol Biotechnol. ePub, 2022

Monoclonal Gammopathy of Undetermined Significance

Slight Increase in Plasma Cells

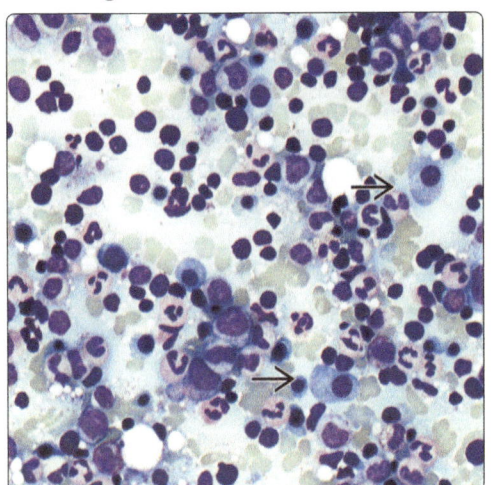

Rare Plasma Cells

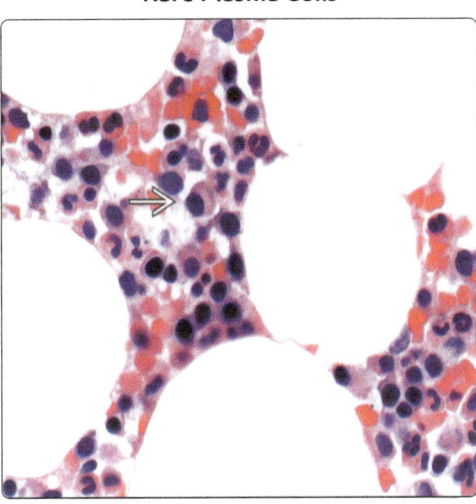

(Left) Bone marrow aspirate smear from an 84-year-old woman with IgG κ MGUS is shown. Plasma cells ➡ represent 8% of the marrow cellularity. The patient had diffuse osteopenia. (Right) Bone marrow biopsy shows single plasma cells ➡ but no sheets or clusters. Trilineage hematopoiesis is seen throughout the marrow. The cellularity was normal for age.

κ-Light Chain In Situ Hybridization

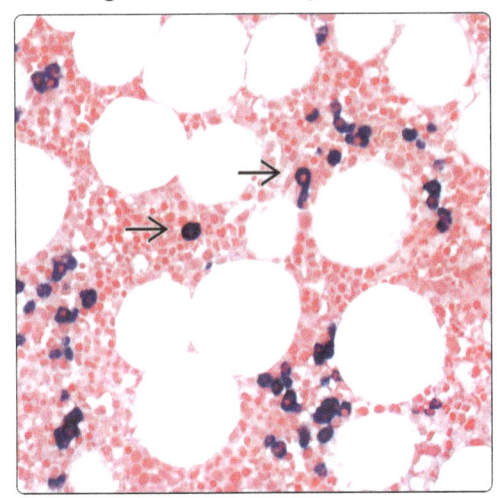

λ-Light Chain In Situ Hybridization

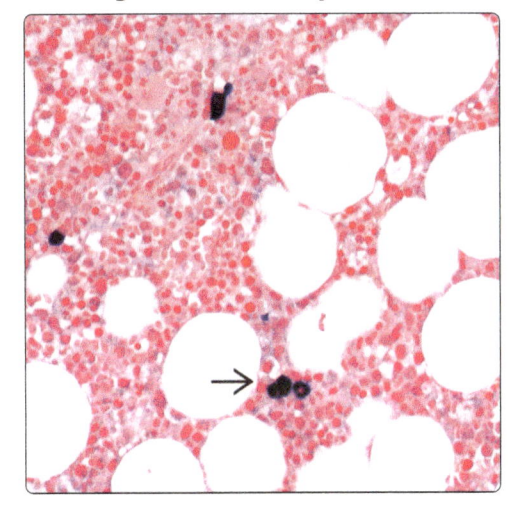

(Left) κ in situ hybridization shows < 10% plasma cells. Positive cells appear blackish-blue in color ➡. In situ hybridization staining often shows less background staining than immunohistochemical staining. (Right) λ in situ hybridization shows rare scattered positive plasma cells ➡. This patient had longstanding MGUS.

CD138 Immunohistochemistry

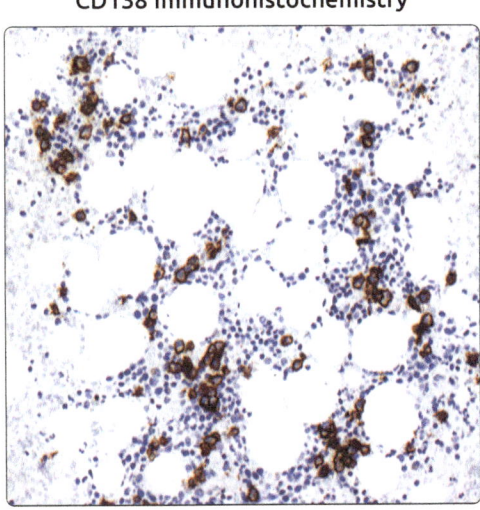

Serum Protein Electrophoresis

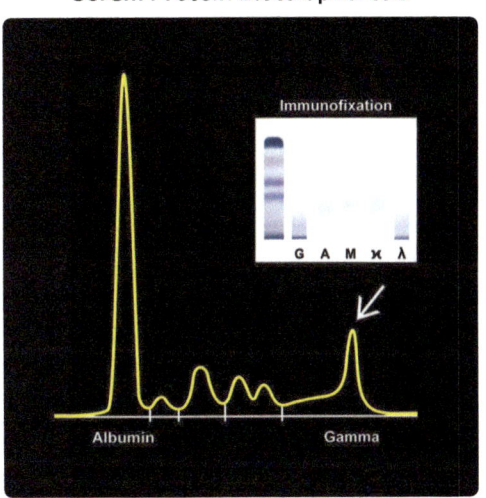

(Left) CD138 shows an increase in plasma cells focally. Overall, the plasma cells were < 10% of the nucleated bone marrow cells. (Right) Serum protein electrophoresis from a patient with MGUS shows a monoclonal component in the γ region ➡ that measures 2.1 g/dL. The associated serum immunofixation has discrete bands in G and λ, identifying the monoclonal component as IgG λ. (From DP: Blood and Bone Marrow.)

Multiple Myeloma (Plasma Cell Myeloma)

KEY FACTS

TERMINOLOGY
- Multiple myeloma (plasma cell myeloma) (MM)
- Diagnosis requires
  - ≥ 10% clonal plasma cells (PCs) in bone marrow (BM) and ≥ 1 myeloma-defining events
    - End-organ damage related to PC disorder or ≥ 1 biomarker of malignancy (≥ 60% PCs, free light chain ratio > 100, or > 1 bone lesion)
- Often preceded by MGUS
- Smoldering MM
  - Requires ≥ 30g/L serum or urinary M protein and clonal BM plasma cells of 10-60%
  - No related end-organ damage, biomarker of malignancy or amyloidosis

CLINICAL ISSUES
- Clinical spectrum spans from asymptomatic to aggressive
- Clinical features: BM plasmacytosis, osteolytic bone lesions, monoclonal gammopathy
- Accounts for 10-15% of hematopoietic malignancies
- Median overall survival
  - ≥ 5 years for standard-risk MM after tandem stem cell transplantation
  - 2-3 years for high-risk disease after therapy
- More favorable prognosis
  - Hyperdiploid (45%) or *CCND* family dysregulation
- More aggressive disease
  - Nonhyperdiploid (40%), especially hypodiploid
  - *NSD2* translocation, *MAF* translocation, *TP53* deletion

MICROSCOPIC
- Peripheral blood: Rouleaux formation
- BM: Clonal PC infiltrate, amyloid, osteoclastic bone lesions

ANCILLARY TESTS
- Cytogenetic/FISH on all newly diagnosed patients
  - Have prognostic and therapeutic implications

Plasma Cell

Plasmacytosis

(Left) Plasma cell (PC) is shown in the peripheral blood of a patient with multiple myeloma (MM), a.k.a. plasma cell myeloma. Circulating PCs are an unfavorable prognostic feature. (Right) Bone marrow aspirate smear shows sheets of PCs, which were light chain restricted by immunohistochemistry. A clonal PC population is necessary for the diagnosis of MM.

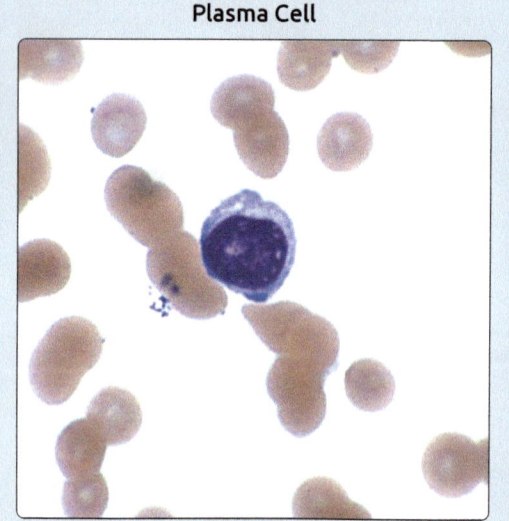

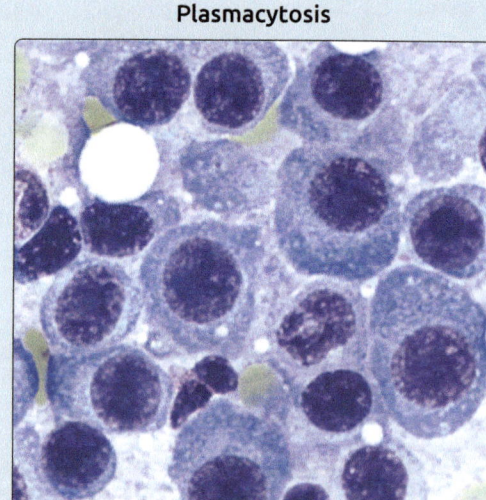

Plasma Cells Mimic Reed-Sternberg Cells

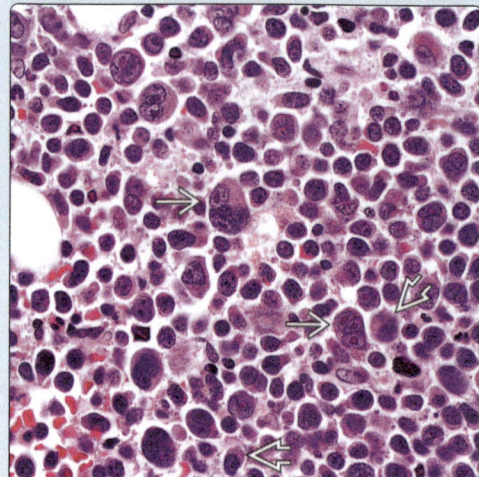

Amyloid Deposition in Vessels and Stroma

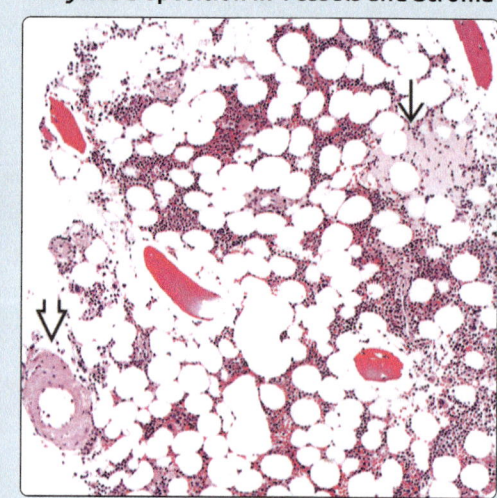

(Left) The polymorphous type of MM has marked cellular pleomorphism and multinucleated cells with prominent nucleoli ➡. Some of the large cells may resemble Reed-Sternberg (RS) cells or anaplastic large cell lymphoma cells. One clue to the diagnosis is the presence of recognizable PCs ➡ in the background infiltrate. (Right) Amyloidosis is a manifestation of end-organ damage (i.e., symptomatic) in MM and is seen in ~ 10% of patients. Focal involvement of stroma ➡ &/or vessel walls ➡ is typical.

Multiple Myeloma (Plasma Cell Myeloma)

TERMINOLOGY

Abbreviations
- Multiple myeloma (MM)

Synonyms
- Plasma cell myeloma (PCM)

Definitions
- Bone marrow (BM)-based plasma cell (PC) neoplasm with clinical spectrum spanning from asymptomatic to aggressive disease
  - Often preceded by monoclonal gammopathy of undetermined significance (MGUS)

CLASSIFICATION

- **ICC vs. WHO-HAEM5**
  - Similar diagnostic criteria in both classifications
    - Demonstration of clonal plasma cells and ≥ 1 myeloma-defining criteria (SLiM-CRAB)
      - MR showing > 1 focal lesions, &/or
      - Serum free light chain ratio > 100, &/or
      - BM plasma cells > 60%, &/or
      - Anemia, &/or
      - Hypercalcemia, &/or
      - Lytic lesions, &/or osteoporosis with compression fractures, &/or
      - Renal impairment
  - In addition, ICC divides MM into 5 subgroups
    - MM with recurrent genetic abnormalities
      - MM with hyperdiploidy
      - MM with *CCND* family translocation
      - MM with *MAF* family translocation
      - MM with *NSD2* translocation
    - MM, not otherwise specified (NOS)

ETIOLOGY/PATHOGENESIS

Environmental Exposure
- Possible link to chemical, toxin, or radiation exposure
- Associated risk factors
  - Increased susceptibility among older individuals; immunosenescence
  - Genetic predisposition
    - Familial clustering
    - Risk 3.7x general population in individuals with 1st-degree relative with MM or MGUS
    - 40% of MM patients have 1st-degree relative with cancer; 10% of these are hematologic neoplasms

Proposed Pathogenesis
- Historic stepwise progression of MGUS to MM has been debated
  - Rate of primary genetic events across MGUS, smoldering MM, and newly diagnosed MM appears to be similar
  - Hyperdiploidy and MM-associated translocations appear to occur early with involvement of almost all tumor cells
    - Include recurrent driver genetic abnormalities that are mostly mutually exclusive
    - Other recurrent genetic abnormalities are acquired later and include
      - 13q, 1q gain
    - Acquired mutational events contributes to acquisition of additional genetic events
      - *KRAS, NRAS, BRAF, FGFR3, ATM, TP53*, and others
  - Disease progression in MGUS and MM is associated with
    - Higher genomic instability, higher tumor mutation burden, novel mutations, biallelic loss of tumor suppressor genes, and complex structural genetic events
  - Some patients with MGUS live for decades without developing MM

CLINICAL ISSUES

Epidemiology
- Incidence
  - ~ 20,000 cases per year in USA and Europe
    - 2nd most common hematologic neoplasm
- Age
  - Peak incidence is 8th decade of life
  - Rarely observed in people < 40 years
  - Incidence increases with age
    - Median at diagnosis: ~ 70 years
- Sex
  - Slight male predominance (M:F = 1.1:1.0)
- Ethnicity
  - Highest incidence in Black populations (~ 9.5/100,000)
  - Lower incidence in White populations (4.1/100,000)
  - Lowest incidence in Asian populations

Presentation
- Clinically defined MM
  - Symptomatic
    - ≥ 10% clonal PCs in BM or plasmacytoma and at least 1 myeloma-defining event (either end-organ damage related to clonal PC or 1 biomarker of malignancy)
      - End-organ damage attributable to PC proliferation [hyper**c**alcemia, **r**enal insufficiency, **a**nemia, and **b**one lesions (CRAB)]
      - Biomarker of malignancy: Clonal PCs ≥ 60%, free light chain (FLC) ratio ≥ 100 or > 1 focal lesion on MR imaging
  - Asymptomatic (smoldering) variant of MM
    - ≥ 30 g/L serum monoclonal (M) protein &/or 10-60% clonal plasma cells in BM
    - No evidence of myeloma-related symptoms or end-organ damage or amyloidosis
    - Differentiated from MGUS due to higher risk of progression and number of PCs
  - Plasma cell leukemia (PCL)
    - Peripheral blood clonal plasma cells ≥ 5% of WBCs
    - Primary PCL
      - Present with renal failure, lymphadenopathy, organomegaly, other extramedullary disease sites, ↑ free light chain, ↓ bone lesions
  - Nonsecretory variant of MM
- Molecularly defined MM
  - MM not otherwise specified
  - MM with recurrent cytogenetic abnormalities
    - *CCND* family translocations, *MAF* family translocations, *NSD2* translocation and hyperdiploidy

Multiple Myeloma (Plasma Cell Myeloma)

Laboratory Tests

- Serum protein electrophoresis (SPEP)
  - Identifies and quantifies monoclonal protein
  - Decrease in uninvolved immunoglobulin classes
- Urine protein electrophoresis (UPEP) or serum free light chain (FLC) assay
  - FLC is best for screening
    - If abnormal, perform UPEP
- Immunofixation electrophoresis
  - To determine immunoglobulin type
- Nephelometric quantitation of immunoglobulins
- Chemistry panel
  - Increased β2-microglobulin (75% at diagnosis)
    - Surrogate marker for tumor burden
  - Lactic acid dehydrogenase and serum albumin
  - Subset of MM patients have
    - Increased uric acid, creatinine, or calcium
    - Decreased albumin

Treatment

- High-dose chemotherapy with autologous stem cell transplant is standard for younger patients
  - Multiple trials using different drugs for pretransplant induction and maintenance therapy
- Bisphosphonates for bone disease
- Anti-MM drugs, including novel agents
  - Immunomodulatory drugs: Thalidomide, lenalidomide, pomalidomide
  - Protease inhibitors: bortezomib, carfilzomib
  - Novel agents used in clinical trials
    - Multikinase inhibitors, MEK inhibitors, farnesyl transferase inhibitors, histone deacetylase inhibitors, heat shock protein 90 inhibitors
    - Elotuzumab (anti-SLAMF7), daratumumab (anti-CD38)
    - Various monoclonal antibodies directed against IL-6 and CS1
    - CAR-T cells

Prognosis

- Overall survival 6 months to 10 years
  - Median survival: ~ 5.5 years
  - Genetic abnormalities are most powerful prognostic factor
    - Genetic findings are highly variable
- Features associated with worse prognosis
  - Increased proliferative rate
  - Increased tumor burden
  - High-risk genetic features
  - Plasmablastic morphology
- International Myeloma Working Group proposed molecular classification
  - 2 major cytogenetic groups
    - Recurrent *IGH* translocations: 40-50%
    - Hyperdiploidy without *IGH* translocations: 55%
  - More favorable prognosis if
    - Hyperdiploid (45%) or cyclin dysregulation
    - *CCND* family translocations (18%): t(11;14)(q13;q32), t(6;14)(p21;q32), t(12;14)(p13;q32)
  - More aggressive disease if
    - Nonhyperdiploid (40%), especially hypodiploid
    - *NSD2* translocation (15%): t(4;14)(p16;q32)
    - *MAF* translocation (~ 8%): t(14;16)(q32;q23), t(14;20)(q32;q11), t(8;14)(q24;q32)
    - *TP53* deletion
- Smoldering MM with > 10% clonal PCs
  - FLC ratio < 0.125 or > 8
    - High risk of progression in first 2 years
- Patient stratification based on pathogenic factors include
  - Age, tumor burden, renal function, comorbidities
  - Serum levels of lactic acid dehydrogenase, β2-microglobulin
  - Albumin, PC labeling index, functional status and cytogenetics

MOLECULAR

Cytogenetics

- Performed on BM specimen at presentation
  - May use IL-6 or IL-4 to stimulate growth due to typically low PC proliferative activity
  - Informative in 30-40% of MM
  - Hyperdiploidy (48-74 chromosomes)
    - Detected in 45% of MM cases
    - Associated with gains of odd-numbered chromosomes, including 5, 9, and 15
    - Better overall survival than nonhyperdiploid
    - Less likely to show del (13q) or -13
  - Nonhyperdiploidy
    - Detected in 40% of MM cases
    - Poor prognostic marker
    - < 48 chromosomes or > 74 chromosomes; includes near-tetraploid karyotypes
    - Associated with *IGH* translocations (70-90%)
    - Hypodiploid (≤ 44 chromosomes)
      - 30% of PCM
      - Associated with *IGH* translocations (88%)
      - ≥ 50% show t(4;14)
    - Pseudodiploid (45-47 chromosomes)
      - 18% of MM
    - Tetraploid (≥ 75 chromosomes)
      - 1-2% of MM
      - Associated with *IGH* translocations (90%)
  - Periodic follow-up to detect clonal evolution or therapy-related myeloid neoplasms recommended
- *IGH* translocations
  - Target *IGH* class switching region in 65% of MM
  - Considered primary "immortalizing" event
  - Associated with dysregulation of *CCND1*, *CCND2*, or *CCND3*

In Situ Hybridization

- FISH detects abnormalities in > 90% of MM
- 54% of cases with normal cytogenetics show abnormalities by FISH
- Interphase fluorescence in situ hybridization (I-FISH)
- Technique of choice for cytogenetic characterization
- Often necessary to perform plasma cell enrichment
  - Enrichment by anti-CD138 microbeads
- Better identification of specific genetic lesions
- Recommended FISH probes for risk stratification
  - 13q14, 17p (TP53)

Multiple Myeloma (Plasma Cell Myeloma)

- t(4;14)(p16;q32) and t(14;16)(q32;q23)
- Ploidy category and t(11;14)(q13;q32)
- Chromosome 1 abnormalities

Chromosomal Microarray

- Identifies discrete minimal common regions of recurrent copy number alterations
  - Deletions of 1p (30%), 6q (33%), 8p (25%), 12p (15%), 13q (59%), 14q (39%), 16q (35%), 17p (7%), 20 (12%), and 22 (18%)
  - Acquired isodisomy or copy number neutral loss of heterozygosity for 1q (8%), 16q (9%), or X (20%)
  - 2 hyperdiploid subgroups: Trisomy 11 ± 1q gain and del(13q)

Molecular Genetics

- Multiple genetic lesions associated with progression
  - Activating mutations
    - MAPK/STAT3 pathway: *NRAS* (20%), *KRAS* (20%), *HRAS*, *FGFR3*, *BRAF* (5-10%)
    - NFκB pathway
  - Inactivating mutations in *RB1*, *TP53*
  - *MYC* dysregulation

Gene Expression Profiling

- Most informative test but limited availability
- 7 distinct gene expression profiles described
  - 2 high-risk disease signatures
    - High proliferation (1q abnormalities)
    - *NSD2* associated
  - 2 moderate-risk disease signatures
    - Hyperdiploid; *MAF/MAFB* gene signature
  - 3 low-risk gene signatures
    - Low bone disease associated
    - *CCND1* or *CCND3* associated

Most Common Cytogenetic Abnormalities

- Abnormal ploidy: Hyperdiploidy; nonhyperdiploidy, including hypodiploidy, pseudodiploidy, and tetraploidy
- Primary *IGH* translocations: t(6;14), t(6;14), t(11;14), t(14;16), t(14;20)
- Common primary or secondary abnormalities: del(1p), gain of 1q21, t(8;14)(q24;q32) or *MYC* variant, del(12p), del (13q) or -13; del (17p)

MICROSCOPIC

Cytologic Features

- Peripheral blood
  - Rouleaux formation
  - Cytopenias
- BM
  - PC infiltrate
    - Multifocal, unevenly distributed plasma cells common
  - Osteoclastic bone lesions; amyloid occasionally

ANCILLARY TESTS

Immunohistochemistry

- CD138, kappa and lambda
  - Helps to establish light chain restriction and quantify PC population in tissue

  - Aberrant CD56 expression (70%), cyclin-D1 (33%), CD117 (35%)

Flow Cytometry

- Routinely underestimates PC percentage
  - Establish clonality in most cases
    - Daratumumab can interfere with light chain interpretation
- MM is CD138(+), CD38(+), CD19(-), CD45(+/-), CD56(+/-)
  - Often weaker CD38, brighter CD138 than normal
  - Aberrant expression of other lineage antigens may be present, including CD20 (15-20%), CD28 (40%), CD33 (15%), CD52 (30%), and CD117 (27%)

DIFFERENTIAL DIAGNOSIS

Reactive Polyclonal Plasmacytosis

- Systemic infections
- Autoimmune disorders
- Unlike MM, plasma cells are polytypic

Monoclonal Gammopathy of Undetermined Significance

- Monoclonal spike on SPEP/UPEP
  - No disease-related end-organ damage or bone lesions
- Small clonal PC population (< 10%), small paraprotein

Lymphoplasmacytic Lymphoma

- Neoplasm with both monoclonal B-cells and monoclonal PCs
  - IgM monoclonal protein
  - Hyperviscosity, often associated with Waldenström macroglobulinemia
  - *MYD88* mutations help to exclude other lymphomas

SELECTED REFERENCES

1. Alaggio R et al: The 5th edition of the World Health Organization classification of haematolymphoid tumours: lymphoid neoplasms. Leukemia. 36(7):1720-48, 2022
2. Campo E et al: The International Consensus Classification of mature lymphoid neoplasms: a report from the Clinical Advisory Committee. Blood. 140(11):1229-53, 2022
3. Hanamura I: Multiple myeloma with high-risk cytogenetics and its treatment approach. Int J Hematol. 115(6):762-77, 2022
4. Gowin K et al: Plasma cell leukemia: a review of the molecular classification, diagnosis, and evidenced-based treatment. Leuk Res. 111:106687, 2021
5. Heider M et al: Multiple myeloma: molecular pathogenesis and disease evolution. Oncol Res Treat. 44(12):672-81, 2021
6. Kleinot W et al: Daratumumab interference in flow cytometry producing a false kappa light chain restriction in plasma cells. Lab Med. 52(4):403-9, 2021
7. Chouman K et al: Characterization of new anti-IL-6 antibodies revealed high potency candidates for intracellular cytokine detection and specific targeting of IL-6 receptor binding sites. Eur Cytokine Netw. 29(2):59-72, 2018
8. Cohen AD: CAR T Cells and other cellular therapies for multiple myeloma: 2018 update. Am Soc Clin Oncol Educ Book. e6-15, 2018
9. Hoang PH et al: Whole-genome sequencing of multiple myeloma reveals oncogenic pathways are targeted somatically through multiple mechanisms. Leukemia. 32(11):2459-70, 2018
10. Merz M et al: Prognostic significance of cytogenetic heterogeneity in patients with newly diagnosed multiple myeloma. Blood Adv. 2(1):1-9, 2018
11. Perrot A et al: Risk stratification and targets in multiple myeloma: from genomics to the bedside. Am Soc Clin Oncol Educ Book. 675-80, 2018
12. Ryland GL et al: Novel genomic findings in multiple myeloma identified through routine diagnostic sequencing. J Clin Pathol. 71(10):895-99, 2018
13. Saxe D et al: Recent advances in cytogenetic characterization of multiple myeloma. Int J Lab Hematol. 41(1):5-14, 2018

Multiple Myeloma (Plasma Cell Myeloma)

ICC and WHO Classifications of Plasma Cell Neoplasms

	Monoclonal Gammopathy of Undetermined Significance (MGUS)	Smoldering Myeloma	Multiple Myeloma
Clonal bone marrow plasma cells	< 10%	10-59%† &/or	≥ 10% or biopsy-proven plasmacytoma < 5% circulating PCs
M protein in serum or urine	Serum non-IgM type < 30 g/L; light chain MGUS: Abnormal serum FLC ratio (< 0.26 or > 1.65) and urine < 500 mg/24 hours	Serum ≥ 30 g/L or urine ≥ 500 mg/24 hours†	Yes; IgG > light chain ≥ IgA > > > IgM, IgD, IgE, biclonal (< 10%) 3% are nonsecretory
Myeloma-defining criteria (SLiM CRAB)	No and no amyloidosis	No and no amyloidosis	Yes; CRAB* &/or ≥ 1 biomarker (SLiM-CRAB): Clonal BM plasma cells ≥ 60%; involved:uninvolved serum FLC ratio ≥ 100**; > 1 focal lesion on MR studies (each ≥ 5 mm in size)

†Must fulfill criteria for clonal BM plasma cells &/or M protein to diagnose smoldering MM. *International Myeloma Working Group diagnostic criteria for CRAB = serum calcium > 0.25 mmol/L (> 1 mg/dL) above upper limit of normal or > 2.75 mmol/L (> 11 mg/dL); renal insufficiency: Creatinine clearance < 40 mL/min or serum creatinine > 177 umol/L (> 2 mg/dL); anemia: Hemoglobin > 2 g/dL below lower limit of normal, or < 10 g/dL; bone lesion. **Involved free light chain level is 100 mg/L or higher.

Genetic Abnormalities in Multiple Myeloma

ICC 2022	% of Cases	Clinical Characteristics*
Hyperdiploid	45	Standard risk, older patients, ↑ IgGκ, ↑ bone disease
MM with CCND family translocation t(11;14) CCND1::IGH t(6;14) CCND3::IGH t(12;14) CCND2::IGH	18-20 16 2-6 < 1	Standard risk; ↑ in nonsecretory MM (83%), ↑ in IgD MM; CCND1::IGH is less responsive to novel therapies compared to many poor risk abnormalities, sensitive to venetoclax due to ↑ BCL2/MCL1
MM with MAF family translocation t(14;16) IGH::MAF t(14;20) IGH::MAFB t(8;14) MAFA::IGH	6-8 3-5 2 1	Poor risk, often ↑ free light chain, 25% present with acute renal failure, aggressive disease; IGH::MAF excluded as high-risk marker in R2-ISSR*, minor impact on progression-free survival
MM with NSD2 translocation t(4;14) NSD2 ± FGFR3::IGH	13-15	Poor risk in 30-40%; depends on NSD2 breakpoint location and other genomic markers (i.e., TP53); bortezomib therapy overcomes poor prognosis
MM, NOS	9-10	More aggressive if hypodiploid (≤ 44 chromosomes)
Other Relevant Genetic Lesions		
1q gain or amplification*	40	High risk if 4+ copies; amplification (≥ 4 copies of 1q21) worse than gain (> 3 copies of 1q21); prognosis related to dosage effect, associated with disease progression, drug resistance; ↑ in smoldering MM before active progression; 70% of relapsing MM; poor response to proteosome inhibitors or venetoclax; bortezomib for consolidation or maintenance therapy
del(17)(p13);TP53 deletion or mutation*	10	Clonal size of PCs with del(17p) important; > 55-60% have worse prognosis; poorest risk if biallelic inactivation of TP53 (4% of cases) by either deletion or mutation; advanced MM stages; aggressive clinical features, 80% of R/R MM and secondary PCL; early BM transplants and bortezomib therapy helpful
Deletion 1p†	5	Poor risk, aggressive clinical presentation, poor response to therapy; biallelic deletion has ultra high risk
MYC translocations	-	Partners include IGH, IGK, IGL, and non-Ig enhancers; contribute to disease progression
Double-hit MM	< 10%	Ultra high risk but different definitions, i.e. ≥ 2 high-risk cytogenetic or molecular abnormalities

*New prognostic factors added to 2nd revision of International Staging System (R2-ISS) and by *† Francophone du Myeloma group. Except for del1p, these alterations are already included in Mayo Clinic mSMART and European Myeloma network prognostic scores.

Multiple Myeloma (Plasma Cell Myeloma)

M-Component on Serum Electrophoresis

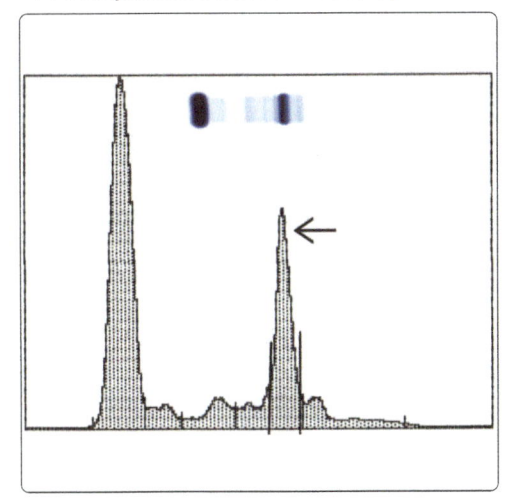

Immunofixation Electrophoresis

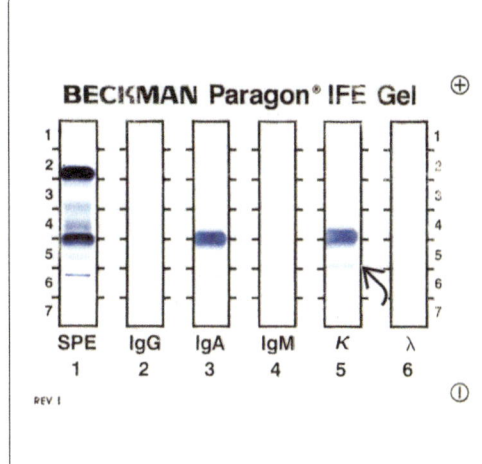

(Left) Serum protein electrophoresis (SPEP) from an older man with lytic bone lesions shows an M-component ➡ in the β2 region measuring 35 g/L. An M-component is found in ~ 97% of MM cases by SPEP or UPEP analysis. (Right) Immunofixation electrophoresis identifies the M-component to be IgAκ with slight free κ light chain ➡. Distribution of M-components in MM includes IgG (~ 50%), IgA (~ 20%), light chain (~ 20%), IgD (~ 2%), biclonal (~ 2%), IgE/IgM (< 1%), and nonsecretory (~ 3%).

Femur With Multiple Lytic Lesions

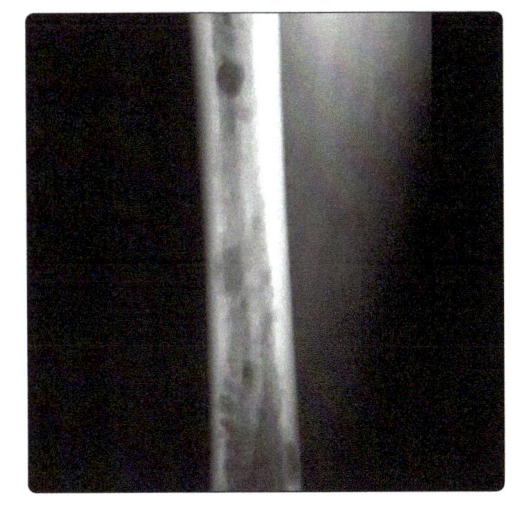

Skull With Multiple Lytic Lesions

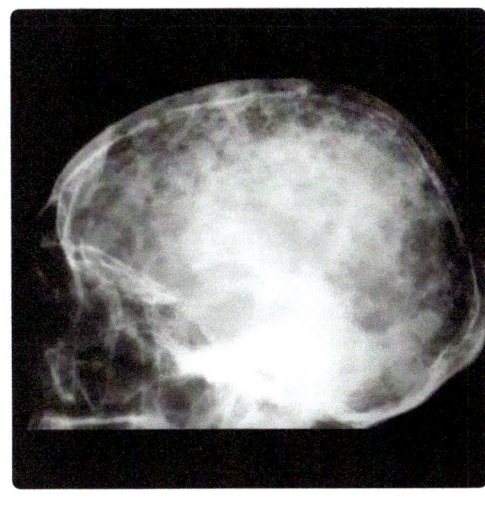

(Left) Lateral radiograph of the femur shows multiple osteolytic lesions with endosteal scalloping of the cortex. Lytic bone lesions or a combination of osteoporosis, osteolysis, or pathologic fractures are found in ~ 75% of MM patients. Biopsies of bone near lytic lesions show prominent osteoclastic activity adjacent to the trabeculae. (Right) Lateral radiograph of the skull shows multiple lytic lesions without surrounding sclerosis involving the calvaria.

Atypical Plasma Cells

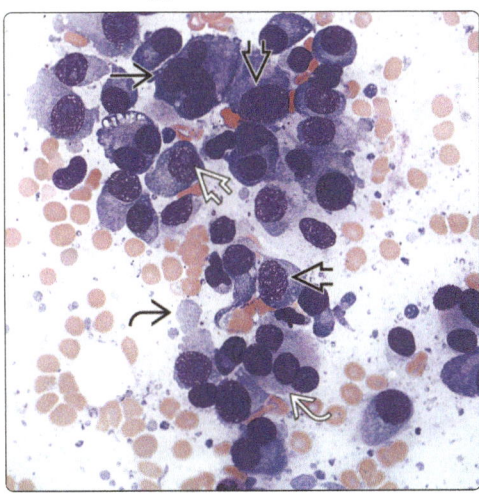

Interphase FISH

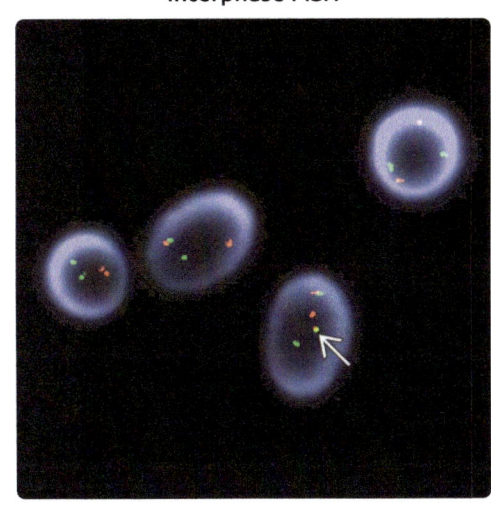

(Left) Features of PC atypia in this bone marrow aspirate smear include pleomorphism ➡, multinucleation ➡, dispersed nuclear chromatin ➡, prominent nucleoli ➡, and cytoplasmic fraying ➡. (Right) Interphase FISH shows FGFR3/IGH fusion ➡ associated with t(4;14). (IGH: Green; NSD2/FGFR3: Red). t(4;14) is linked to high-risk MM when β-2-microglobulin is ≥ 4 mg/L and hemoglobin is ≤ 10 g/dL. del(17)p13 or t(14;16)(q32.3;q23) also indicates high-risk disease.

Molecular Pathology of Lymphoid Neoplasms

Multiple Myeloma (Plasma Cell Myeloma)

CD138 Immunohistochemistry

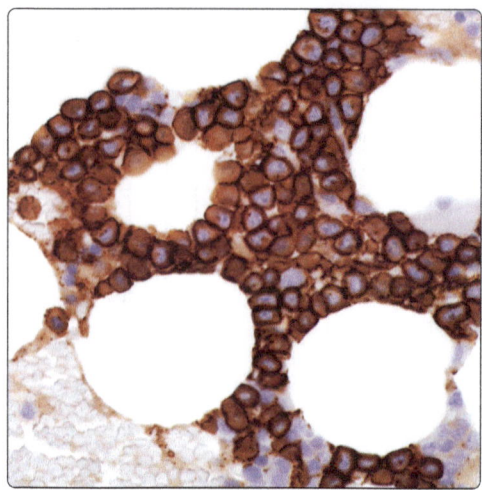

CD56 Immunohistochemistry

(Left) CD138 is the most specific marker for PCs in bone marrow and helps to evaluate for a percentage of PC involvement, particularly when PCs are unevenly distributed in aspirate smears and biopsy sections. (Right) Aberrant immunophenotypes are seen in > 80% of MM cases at diagnosis, including expression of CD56 ➡ in a majority of cases (~ 70%). Lineage infidelity is a feature of PCM with myeloid, T-cell, and B-cell marker expression possible.

κ In Situ Hybridization

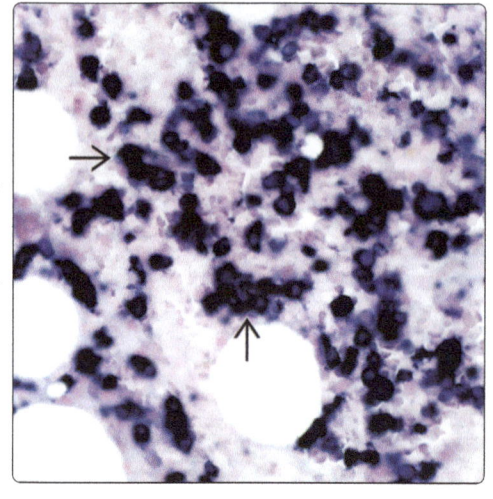

λ In Situ Hybridization

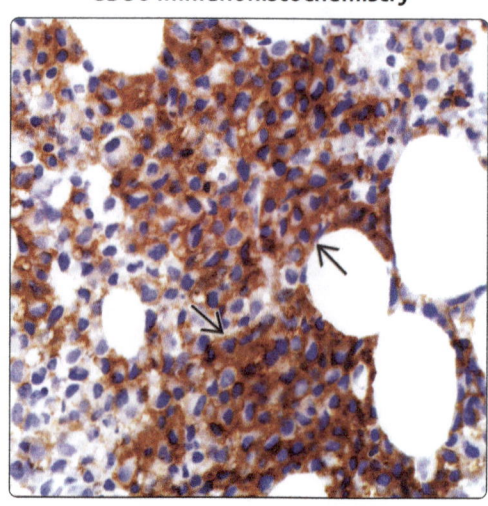

(Left) Clonality in plasma cell neoplasms is best assessed by light chain evaluation. In situ hybridization is often more reliable than immunohistochemistry. PCs are κ positive ➡ in this biopsy. (Right) Only rare λ-positive PCs ➡ are present, confirming clonal PC infiltrate. As CD138 stains a variety of undifferentiated epithelial and mesenchymal neoplasms, light chain expression also confirms plasmacytic process.

Cyclin-D1 Immunohistochemistry

FISH Showing t(11;14)

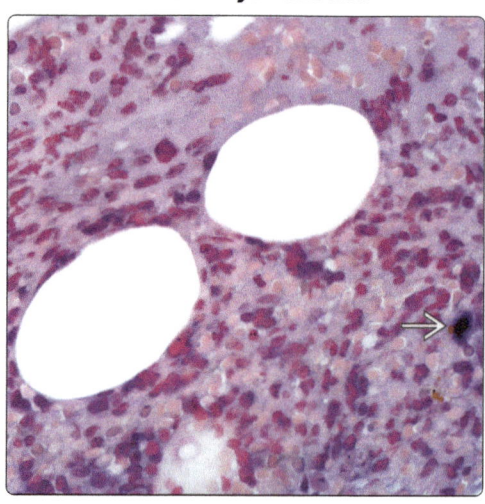

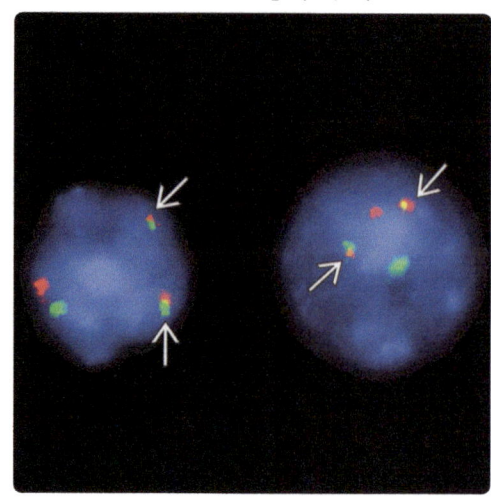

(Left) Cyclin-D1 expression is seen in ~ 1/3 of PCM with only ~ 10% of these having an associated t(11;14)(q13;q32) karyotypic abnormality. The staining pattern is nuclear ➡. (Right) FISH using IGH and CCND1 probes shows IGH::CCND1 fusion signals (orange) ➡ corresponding to t(11;14).

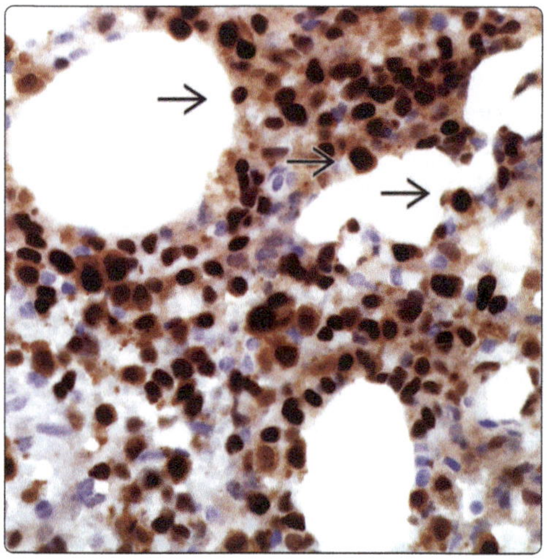

Multiple Myeloma (Plasma Cell Myeloma)

Flow Cytometry for CD138

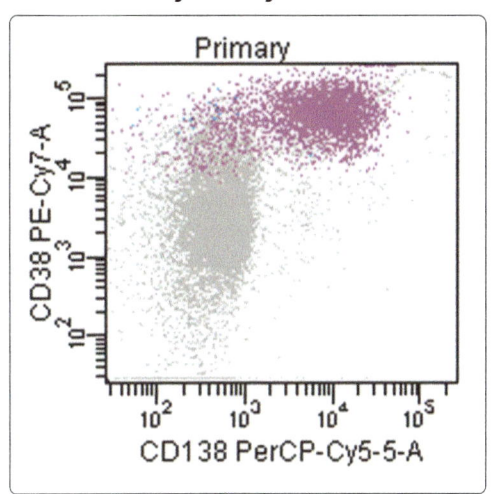

Flow Cytometry for Light Chains

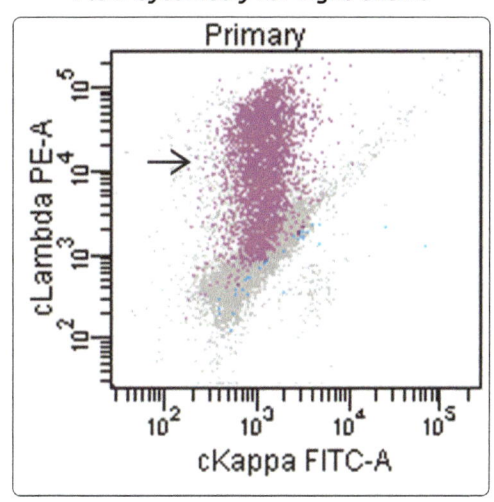

(Left) Flow cytometry identifies the PCs (pink) in this marrow by their bright CD138 and CD38 coexpression. Gating on CD38 alone is problematic, as neoplastic PCs often have dimmer CD38 than normal, and activated/immature T cells, hematogones, and monocytes may be brightly CD38(+). (Right) Evaluation for PC immunoglobulin requires permeabilization of the cell membrane to allow antibodies to enter the cytoplasm. PC clonality is identified by finding cytoplasmic lambda light chain restriction ➡.

Flow Cytometry Showing Plasma Cells With Dim to Negative CD45

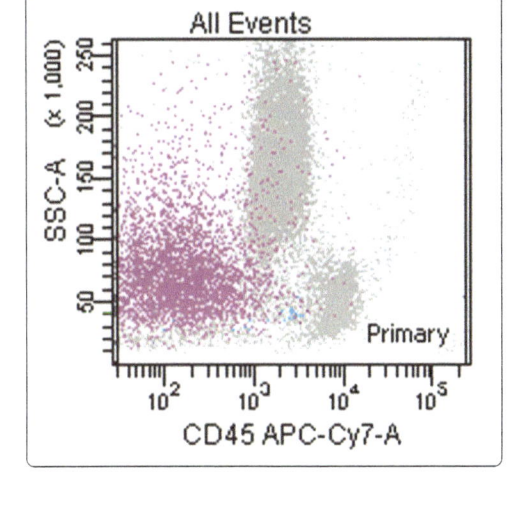

Flow Cytometry Showing Bright CD138 and Aberrant CD56

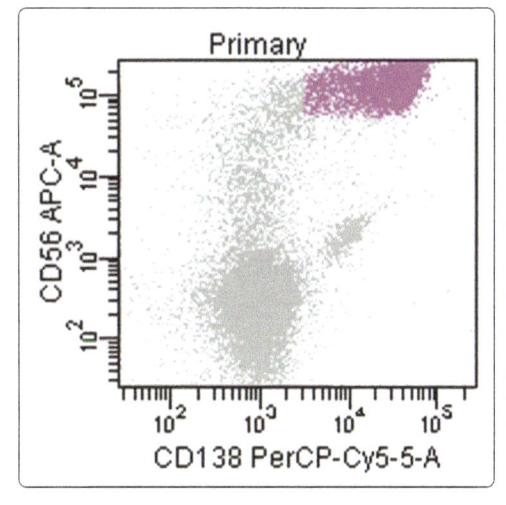

(Left) Compared to normal PCs, which express CD45, neoplastic PCs (pink) variably lose CD45 expression. Normal CD19 expression is also lost in most cases. The neoplastic PCs have no specific forward or side-scatter characteristics. (Right) While aberrant CD56 expression (pink) in PCs supports a clonal process, it does not distinguish between monoclonal gammopathy of undetermined significance and MM. Knowing the pattern of aberrant antigen expression is helpful for monitoring residual disease after therapy.

Plasma Cell Myeloma Karyotype

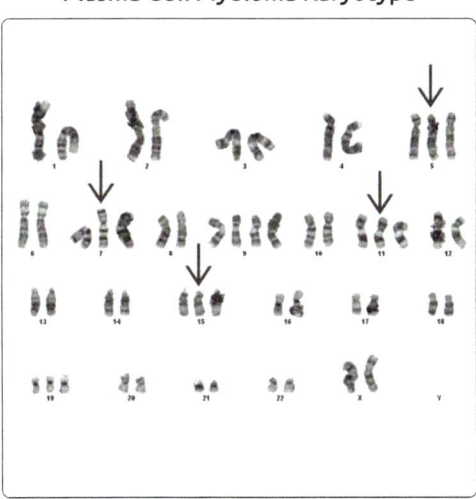

Interphase FISH

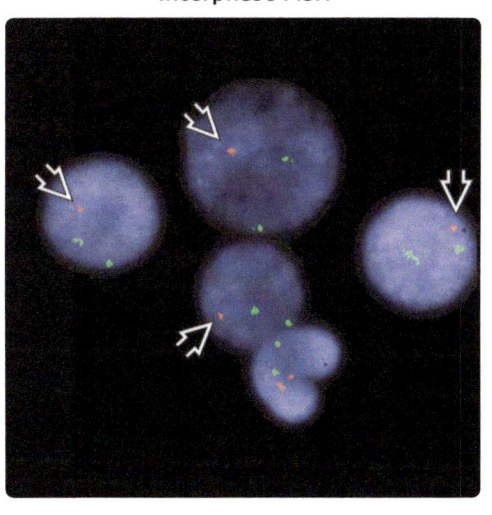

(Left) Karyotype shows 52 ~ 53, XX, +5, +7, +9, +9, +11, +15, +19[cp11]/46, XX. This hyperdiploid karyotype is common for MM and shows multiple trisomies ➡ of the odd-numbered chromosomes. Hyperdiploid MM has a better prognosis than nonhyperdiploid karyotypes unless there are concurrent gains in chromosome 1q. (Right) Interphase FISH analysis shows 2 normal copies of 11q22.3 region (ATM: Green) in all cells and evidence for deletion of 17p13 region (TP53: Red) ➡ in a subset of PCs.

Molecular Pathology of Lymphoid Neoplasms

Follicular Lymphoma

KEY FACTS

TERMINOLOGY
- Follicular lymphoma (FL): B-cell neoplasm composed of germinal center B cells (centrocytes and centroblasts)

ETIOLOGY/PATHOGENESIS
- t(14;18)(q32;q21) juxtaposes *BCL2* at 18q21 adjacent to *IGH* on derivative chromosome 14
  - Found in ~ 90%, is early molecular event causing overexpression of antiapoptotic protein BCL2
  - Subset (~ 10%) of cases will not show t(14;18)(q32;q21)
- t(14;18); *IGH::BCL2* detected in blood of healthy individuals; some later develop FL
- *BCL6* rearrangement in ~ 15%
- Double-hit FL
  - Rare finding in which FL shows both *BCL2* and *MYC* rearrangements
  - Low-grade histology but aggressive clinical behavior

CLINICAL ISSUES
- Indolent clinical course with slow progression but frequent relapses

MOLECULAR
- Monoclonal *IGH* and immunoglobulin light chain gene rearrangements
- Early secondary genetic alterations include *EZH2*, *EPHA7*, *KMT2D*, *TNFRSF14*, *CREBBP*, *EP300*, and *MEF2B*
- Secondary genetic alterations include *MYC* rearrangement, *CDKN2A*, *TP53*, and *BCL6* mutations

MICROSCOPIC
- Neoplastic follicles, fairly uniform in size and shape, containing centrocytes and centroblasts
- Usually loss of tingible body macrophages

ANCILLARY TESTS
- Expresses germinal center makers BCL6, CD10, HGAL, LMO2, and aberrant BCL2

Low-Power Morphology

Classic Cytogenetics

(Left) Low-power view of follicular lymphoma (FL) shows numerous variably shaped follicles in the cortex and medulla. Mantle zones appear attenuated. (Right) Karyotype shows t(14;18)(q32;q21), which is detected in 80-90% of FL cases. The translocation can be revealed by routine cytogenetics or FISH.

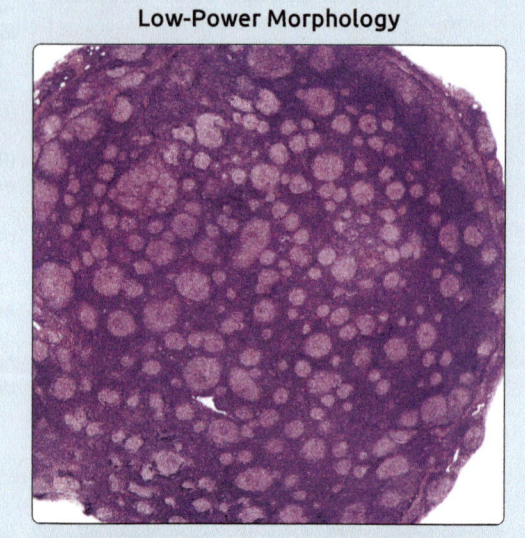

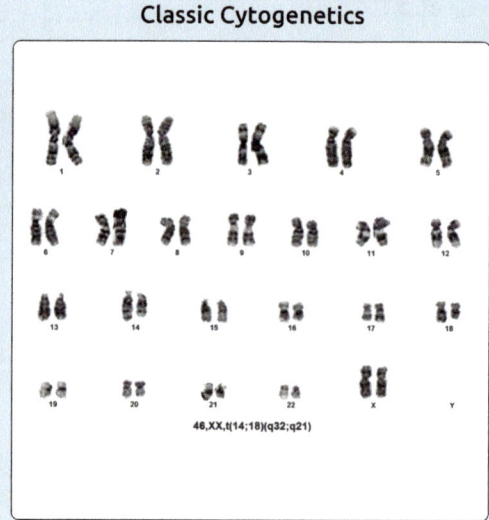

Peripheral Blood Morphology

High-Power Morphology

(Left) Peripheral blood smear from a patient with FL shows leukemic involvement by centrocytes with deeply cleaved nuclei, so-called buttock cells ➡. (Right) Grade 3A FL with follicular pattern is shown. The follicles are composed of many centroblasts, but centrocytes are also present.

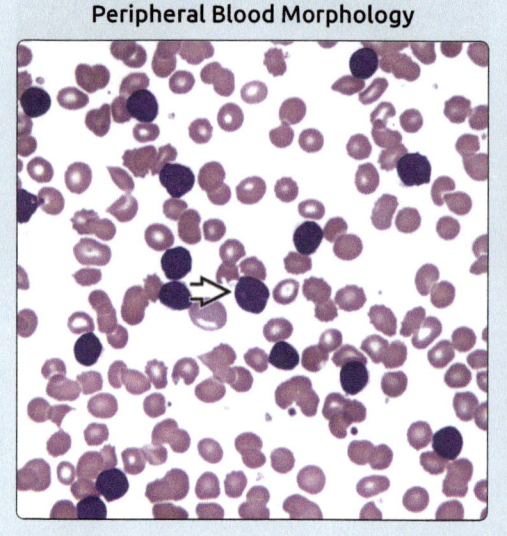

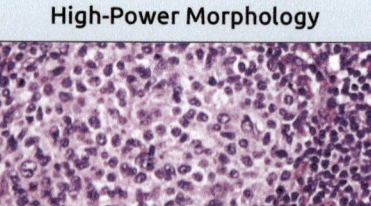

Follicular Lymphoma

TERMINOLOGY

Abbreviations
- Follicular lymphoma (FL)

Definitions
- B-cell neoplasm of germinal center B cells containing centrocytes and centroblasts with follicular, follicular and diffuse, and, rarely, diffuse growth patterns

CLASSIFICATION

WHO-HAEM5
- 3 subtypes of follicular lymphoma
  - Classic follicular lymphoma (cFL)
    - Requires presence of t(14;18)(q32;q21)-IGH::BCL2 rearrangement
    - Grading no longer required
  - Follicular large B-cell lymphoma (FLBCL)
    - New name for high-grade (3B) FL
  - FL with uncommon features
    - Includes diffuse follicular lymphoma variant and FL with "blastoid" or "large centrocyte" cytological features
  - In situ follicular B-cell neoplasm, duodenal-type follicular lymphoma, and testicular follicular lymphoma are considered variants of FL and not distinct entities

ICC
- Morphologic grading of nodal FL (grade 1-2, 3A, and 3B) is retained
- In situ follicular B-cell neoplasia and duodenal-type follicular lymphoma are considered variants of FL
- Pediatric FL remains clearly defined entity
- Testicular follicular lymphoma is considered new distinct entity of FL
- BCL2-rearranged-negative, CD23-positive follicle center lymphoma recognized as specific provisional entity of follicle center lymphoma
  - Frequently but not always diffuse pattern with pelvic/inguinal location and common STAT6 mutations

ETIOLOGY/PATHOGENESIS

t(14;18)(q32;q21); IGH::BCL2
- Juxtaposes BCL2 at 18q21 adjacent to IGH on derivative chromosome 14
- Widely considered initiating molecular event of FL
  - Leads to constitutive expression of BCL2
  - Found in almost 90% of cFL
  - Results in overexpression of BCL2 protein
    - BCL2 is antiapoptotic and confers survival advantage
- Translocation occurs after break at IGH on chromosome 14 due to defective VDJ recombination
  - Rare variants involve IGL instead of IGH
- t(14;18) detected in people without lymphoma
  - Detected in >70% of healthy individuals by sensitive methods, usually in blood, but also in BM, spleen, and lymph nodes
  - Most will never develop FL
  - Usually detected at very low levels
  - Number of t(14;18)+ cells in blood increases with age
  - Healthy individuals with t(14;18) may take up to 15 years to develop FL
  - Higher levels of t(14;18)(+) cells indicate higher risk for FL
  - CREBBP mutations may also be detected
  - Insufficient to induce lymphomagenesis by itself
  - Other molecular changes are necessary for development of lymphoma
- Multiple subclones can be identified in early disease

Other Genes Implicated in Follicular Lymphoma Genesis
- KMT2D and CREBBP early-event gene mutations
  - Induce loss of function of chromatin modifiers
- Gain-of-function mutations include EZH2, ARID1A, MEF2B, and KMT2C
- Loss-of-function mutations and deletion TNFRSF14
- Less frequent mutations of BTK, CARD11, FOXO1, NOTCH1/NOTCH2, RRAGC, STAT6, and TNFAIP3 have been reported
- RRAGC and CTSS do not appear to be mutated in lymphoma other than FL
- CDKN2A, MYC, and TP53 mutations more commonly seen in transformed FL than in cFL

Other Proteins Involved in Apoptosis
- Overexpression of cell death suppressor proteins BCLXL and MCL1
- Decreased expression of cell death promoting proteins BAX (BCL2L4) and BAD
- Overexpression of inhibitors of apoptosis proteins

Germline Susceptibility Factors
- Genotypic analysis has identified susceptibility locus at 6p21.3
  - Contains single gene, chromosome 6 open reading frame 15
- 4x increased lymphoma risk in 1st-degree relatives of patients with FL

Microenvironment
- T cells, macrophages, and follicular dendritic cells all contribute to pathogenesis of FL
  - Follicular dendritic cells prevent apoptosis of FL cells
  - T-follicular helper cells (TFH) and regulatory T cells are increased in FL
    - TFH can stimulate growth of neoplastic B cells
    - CD40L/CD154(+) T cells in secondary follicles inhibit FL cell death
- Endothelial cells and fibroblasts also play role in microenvironment

CLINICAL ISSUES

Epidemiology
- Incidence
  - ~ 20% of non-Hodgkin lymphoma
  - 2nd most common non-Hodgkin lymphoma in Western world
- Age
  - Mostly affects adults
- Sex
  - No sex predilection; only slight male predominance

Follicular Lymphoma

Site
- Lymph nodes most often involved
- Spleen, bone marrow, and peripheral blood also frequently involved
- Can occur at any extranodal site, but gastrointestinal tract, soft tissue, breast, and thoracic vertebrae more commonly affected

Natural History
- Often multifocal lymphadenopathy at diagnosis and often with splenomegaly
- Only ~ 10% are stage I or II at diagnosis
- Indolent clinical course with slow progression but frequent relapses
- 25-60% of cases progress to diffuse large B-cell lymphoma (DLBCL)

Treatment
- "Watch and wait" strategy used in small fraction of patients at initial diagnosis
  - Usually asymptomatic or low-tumor-burden patients
  - Some patients live for decades without treatment
  - Pediatric FL and duodenal-type FL are often indolent and may be treated without chemotherapy
- Radiation can be used for low-stage FL
- Chemotherapy is currently used for patients with higher stage (III-IV) disease
  - Alkylating-based regimens
    - Cyclophosphamide, adriamycin (doxorubicin), vincristine, and prednisone (CHOP) is standard therapy
    - Relapse is universal, and subsequent responses are shorter than initial remission
  - Chimeric monoclonal anti-CD20 antibodies
    - Rituximab widely used, has greatly improved outcomes of FL
    - Rituximab can be single-agent therapy or with other chemotherapy (R-CHOP)
    - Some patients on rituximab develop resistance
    - Newer anti-CD20 antibodies, including obinutuzumab
    - Some newer CD20 antibodies have modified Fc region of antibody
  - Anti-CD22 antibodies (epratuzumab and inotuzumab) are in development
  - Bispecific T-cell engager (blinatumomab) activates T cells exerting cytotoxic activity on B cells
  - More aggressive treatments with high-dose chemotherapy and stem cell transplantation are reserved for resistant disease in patients with good performance status

Prognosis
- Incurable disease
  - Overall 10-year survival: Up to ~ 80%
  - Median overall survival: ~ 14 years
- Adverse prognostic factors in FL International Prognostic Index 2 (FLIPI 2)
  - High serum β2-microglobulin
  - Bulky lymph nodes > 6 cm
  - Bone marrow involvement
  - Hemoglobin < 12 g/dL
  - Age > 60 years
- Pathologic adverse prognostic factors include
  - High histologic grade and diffuse areas > 25% with predominance of large cells
    - These areas are designated as DLBCL
  - High proliferation index
  - Complex karyotype
  - Elevated lactate dehydrogenase
  - Higher number of tumor associated macrophages
  - Presence of *BCL6* rearrangement
  - Elevated serum levels of IL-2R, IL-1RA, and CXCL9
  - Deletion 6q25-27
  - Deletion 1p36.22-p36.33

MICROSCOPIC

Histologic Features
- Lymph node
  - Partial or complete effacement of architecture
  - Follicular (> 70%), follicular and diffuse (25%), and, rarely, diffuse (< 5%) growth patterns
  - Closely packed neoplastic follicles, fairly uniform in size and shape
    - Distributed in cortex, medulla, and perinodal fibroadipose tissue
  - Follicles usually poorly circumscribed with attenuated mantle zones
  - "Cracking" artifact may surround neoplastic follicles
  - Neoplastic follicles are composed of centrocytes and centroblasts
    - Cells randomly distributed throughout individual follicles without polarity
    - Infrequent mitoses and absent or scanty tingible body macrophages
    - Centrocytes: Small to large with angulated, elongated, or twisted nuclei, dark chromatin, and scant cytoplasm
    - Centroblasts: Large cells with oval or multilobated nuclei, vesicular chromatin, 1-3 nucleoli
  - Floral variant
    - Mantle zone lymphocytes penetrate into neoplastic follicles, imparting irregular shapes
    - Better highlighted with follicular dendritic cell markers (e.g., CD21)
    - Often grade 3
- Bone marrow
  - Paratrabecular aggregates of centrocytes and, less frequently, centroblasts
    - Aspirate smears may have scant lymphoma cells or are (-)
  - Interstitial &/or diffuse patterns in advanced disease
- Peripheral blood
  - Marked leukemic involvement in 5-10% of patients
  - Neoplastic cells have highly cleaved nuclei
  - Low-level involvement is detected by molecular methods in ~ 90% of patients

Grading of Follicular Lymphoma
- Grading has prognostic and therapeutic significance
- Most reliably performed on lymph node excisional biopsy specimen
- System is based on mean number of centroblasts per HPF
  - Count at least 10 HPF and divide by 10

Follicular Lymphoma

- Grade 1: 0-5 centroblasts/HPF
- Grade 2: 6-15 centroblasts/HPF
- Grade 3: > 15 centroblasts/HPF
  - Grade 3A: Centrocytes admixed with centroblasts
  - Grade 3B: Sheets of centroblasts with rare or no centrocytes
- 2017 WHO and 2022 ICC recommend lumping cases of FL 1-2 together as low grade
- WHO-HAEM5 classification regards grading of FL as optional
- ICC retains grading of FL
  - Minimal differences in outcome between patients with FL grade 1 vs. 2
  - Any area of DLBCL in FL should be reported as primary and separate diagnosis with estimate of proportion of DLBCL

Reporting Pattern in Follicular Lymphoma
- Most reliably performed on lymph node biopsy specimen
- Follicular: > 75% follicular
- Follicular and diffuse: 25-75% follicular
- Focally follicular: 1-25% follicular
- Diffuse: 0% follicular

Variants of Follicular Lymphoma
- In situ follicular neoplasia, duodenal, testicular, and diffuse

In Situ Follicular Neoplasia
- Considered variant of FL in both WHO-HAEM5 and ICC
- Lymph node with rare, bright BCL2(+) B cells within germinal centers
  - Follicles are CD10(+), BCL6(+), and t(14;18) (+)
  - *EZH2* mutations are identified, so this may be early molecular event

Duodenal Follicular Lymphoma
- FL involving small intestine, usually duodenum
- Considered variant of FL in both WHO-HAEM5 and ICC
- Localized disease; good prognosis, even without treatment
- Follicles are CD10(+), BCL6(+), BCL2(+), and t(14;18) (+)

Testicular Follicular Lymphoma
- Often in children; high-grade morphology, but good prognosis
- Considered new distinct entity of FL in ICC
- No *BCL2* rearrangement

Diffuse Follicular Lymphoma
- Considered variant of FL in WHO-HAEM5 but distinct entity in ICC
  - Designated as *BCL2*-rearranged-negative, CD23-positive follicle center lymphoma in ICC
  - Usually have *STAT6* mutations
  - Coexpression of CD10 and CD23 is characteristic; CD23 expression surrogate to *STAT6* mutations
  - Only microfollicles with weak (+) or (-) BCL2 expression
- Often presents as large mass in inguinal region but does not disseminate in most cases
- By definition, t(14;18)(q32;q21); *IGH::BCL2* is negative
- Del 1p36 (*TNFRSF14*) is often present

DIFFERENTIAL DIAGNOSIS

Reactive Follicular Hyperplasia
- Features that distinguish reactive follicular hyperplasia (RFH) from FL
  - Preserved nodal architecture with follicles located mostly in cortex
  - Variably sized and shaped follicles that are widely spaced
  - Polarization of germinal centers into light and dark zones
  - Presence of tingible body macrophages and mitoses
  - Sharply demarcated mantle zones surround germinal centers
  - BCL2(-) germinal centers
  - No clonal *IGH* rearrangements, no t(14;18)(q32;q21)

Mantle Cell Lymphoma
- Nodular pattern can resemble FL
- Cells are small and uniform with regular or variably irregular nuclear contours; no centroblasts
- Hyalinized blood vessels and scattered histiocytes with pink/eosinophilic cytoplasm
- Immunophenotype
  - CD5(+), CD43(+), cyclin-D1 (+)
- Detection of t(11;14)(q13;q32); *CCND1::IGH* by cytogenetics or FISH
- No t(14;18)(q32;q21); *IGH::BCL2*

Pediatric Follicular Lymphoma
- Considered distinct entity from FL in both ICC and WHO-HAEM5
- Occurs mostly in children and young adults with marked male predominance (M:F = 10:1)
- Typically presents with low-stage disease as isolated neck mass
- Excellent prognosis even without chemotherapy treatment
- Large follicles, high-grade morphology, and high proliferative rate
- CD10(+), BCL6(+), BCL2(-)
- Must lack *BCL2*, *BCL6*, and *MYC* rearrangements

Primary Cutaneous Follicle Center Lymphoma
- Considered distinct entity from FL in both WHO-HAEM5 and ICC
- B-cell lymphoma of follicle center origin that originates in skin, usually on scalp, forehead, or trunk
- Can have follicular, diffuse, and mixed follicular and diffuse growth patterns
- Often appears high-grade with high proliferative rate, but prognosis is excellent, so not graded
- CD10(+/-), BCL6(+), BCL2(-/+), HGAL(+), LMO2(+), CD21(+)/CD35(+) FDC networks
- Usually negative for *BCL2* rearrangement; if positive, should exclude secondary skin involvement by systemic follicular lymphoma

Large B-Cell Lymphoma With *IRF4* Rearrangement
- Considered distinct entity from FL in both WHO-HAEM5 and ICC
- Large B-cell lymphoma defined by *IRF4* rearrangement that encodes MUM1 protein
  - Most commonly t(6;14)(p25;q32); *IRF4::IGH*

Follicular Lymphoma

- Can have follicular, diffuse, and mixed follicular and diffuse growth patterns
- Cases with follicular growth pattern can resemble grade 3B follicular lymphoma/follicular large B-cell lymphoma
- Usually presents as low-stage disease in children and young adults with cervical lymph nodes and Waldeyer ring most common sites of involvement
- Very favorable prognosis status post surgery &/or chemotherapy
- Most commonly CD10(+), BCL6(+), BCL2(+), and MUM1(+) (strong, diffuse staining)
- Must have *IRF4* rearrangement (most commonly *IRF4::IGH*), which can be demonstrated by FISH
- Cannot have *MYC* or *BCL2* rearrangements, but some cases can have *BCL6* rearrangement

MOLECULAR PATHOLOGY

Cytogenetics

- t(14;18)(q32;q21): *IGH::BCL2* in ~ 80-90% of cases
  - Rarely (10%) only karyotypic abnormality
- Cases of FL without t(14;18)(q32;q21)
  - Usually BCL2(-)
  - Show increased *CHEK1* expression and decreased *TCL1A* expression
- Complex karyotype correlates with poorer prognosis
- Chromosome aberrancies
  - Deletions of 1p, 6q, 10q, and 17p
  - Gains of 1q, 2p, 6p, 7, 8, 12, 18q, and X
- On average, FL cases have ~ 6 cytogenetic abnormalities
  - 17p deletions have worse prognosis

In Situ Hybridization

- FISH can detect t(14;18)(q32;q21); *IGH::BCL2* in up to 90% of FL cases
  - Large probes can detect multiple breakpoints

Polymerase Chain Reaction

- Monoclonal *IGH* and immunoglobulin light chain (*IGK* and *IGL*) rearrangements
  - Variable regions of *IGH* undergo extensive and ongoing mutations
  - Mutations can cause false-negative result when using PCR to assess for *IGH* rearrangements
    - Multiple primer sets are therefore required for analysis
- Multiple breakpoints in *BCL2* that must be individually assessed by PCR
  - Major breakpoint cluster region (MBR)
    - ~ 50-60% of FL with t(14;18)
  - Minor breakpoint cluster region (MCR)
    - ~ 5-10% of FL
  - Intermediate cluster region (ICR)
    - ~ 10-15% of FL
  - 5' breakpoint region
    - ~ 5% of FL
- Less *BCL2* rearrangement seen in high-grade FL
- No *BCL2* rearrangement seen in testicular FL

Chromosomal Microarray

- ~ 90% of FL have abnormalities detected by chromosomal microarray (CMA)
  - Gains of 2p15, 7p, 7q, 8q, 12q, 18p, and 18q
  - Losses of 1p36, 3q, 6q, 9p, 11q, 13q, and 17p
- Abnormalities associated with worse prognosis
  - Loss of 6q or 9p21
  - Gain of X
- Abnormalities associated with transformation to DLBCL
  - Gains of 2, 5, and 3q

Molecular Genetics

- Secondary genetic alterations in FL
  - Mutations in *H1-5* (27%), *POU2F2* (8%), *IRF8* (6%), *ARID1A* (11%), *TNFRSF14*, *EPHA7*, *EZH2*, *CREBBP*, *EP300*, *KMT2D*, and *MEF2B*
  - *NOTCH1* and *NOTCH2* mutations uncommon in FL
    - More common in splenic marginal zone lymphoma
    - Patients with mutations have lower frequency of *IGH::BCL2* fusion and more spleen involvement
- Gene alterations associated with transformation to DLBCL
  - *MYC*, *BCL6*
  - *CDKN2A*, *TP53*, or *SUB1*
    - Occurs in FL but is more common at time of transformation to DLBCL
  - *PLA2G6*, *PDGFRB*, and *RAB6A*
  - NFkB pathway genes (*TNFAIP3*, *MYD88*, *BTK*, *IGBP1*, *IRAK1*, *ROCK1*, *TMED7*, *TICAM2*, and *TRIM37*)
- *MYC* rearrangement
  - Uncommon
  - Double-hit FL shows both *BCL2* and *MYC* rearrangement
  - Low-grade histology but aggressive clinical behavior supports double-hit lymphoma
  - Rare finding
- *BCL6* rearrangement
  - Found in any FL type
  - Detected in only 15% of FL with *BCL2* rearrangement
  - More frequently detected in FL without *BCL2* rearrangement (35% of cases)
  - FLBCL has *BCL6* rearrangement in 40% of cases
    - Implies relationship of FLBCL and DLBCL
- Follicular lymphoma without *BCL2* and *BCL6* rearrangements
  - Only ~ 10% of cFL cases
  - More common in FLBCL, diffuse FL, testicular FL and pediatric FL
  - Late germinal center B cell that has not excited germinal center
    - Somatic hypermutation
    - Gene expression profile of late or post germinal center B cell
  - Different genetic pathway
    - *STAT6* > 50% and *KMT2D* < 50%
  - cFL with diffuse growth pattern
    - Usually inguinal lymph nodes and low-stage disease
    - CD23 coexpression common
    - 1p36 deletion and *TNFRSF14* alteration

Gene Expression Profiling

- Genetic signature of FL is similar to that of normal germinal center B cells
- FL has relatively homogeneous gene signature distinct from other small B-cell lymphomas

Follicular Lymphoma

Genetic Abnormalities in Follicular Lymphoma

Gene	Frequency (%)	Effect
BCL2	85	BCL2 overexpression
KMT2D	89	Histone modification
EPHA7	70	Loss of tumor suppressor
BCL6	47	Bystander mutation
TNFRSF14	30	Unknown but found in 1p36 region
CREBBP	30	Histone modification
MEF2B	15	Histone modification
EP300	9	Histone modification
EZH2	7	Oncogenic
TNFAIP3	13	Loss of tumor suppressor
FAS	6	Decrease apoptosis
TP53	< 5	Loss of tumor suppressor

Early and Late Genetic Alterations in Follicular Lymphoma

Early Genetic Alterations	Late Genetic Alterations
t(14;18); IGH::BCL2	MYC
EPHA7, KMT2D	CDKN2A
TNFRSF14, CREBBP, EP300	TP53
MEF2B, EZH2	BCL6

- Grades 1, 2, 3A, and 3B tend to have similar gene expression profiles
  - Even molecular signature of FL grade 3B is closer to lower grade FL than to DLBCL of germinal center type
  - Supportive evidence that FL grade 3B belongs to group of FL and should not be reclassified as DLBCL
  - Grade 3A FL is closer to grades 1-2 than to grade 3B FL
- Nonneoplastic (microenvironment) components of FL are important for disease severity
  - Initial study from Leukemia/Lymphoma Molecular Profiling Project found 2 gene expression profiles: Immune response 1 (IR1) and 2 (IR2)
    - IR1 (good prognosis): Genes related to T cells and macrophages
    - IR2 (poor prognosis): Genes related to monocytes and dendritic cells
- Studies have analyzed t(14;18)(+) FL and t(14;18)(-) FL separately
  - FL with t(14;18)(q32;q21); IGH::BCL2
    - Enriched germinal center B-cell genes
  - FL without t(14;18)(q32;q21); IGH::BCL2
    - Enriched activated B-cell-like, NFκB pathway, and proliferation genes
- Transformed FL has different gene expression than de novo DLBCL
  - Gains of 9p23-24, 6p12, and 17q21.33

MicroRNA

- miR-16, miR-26a, miR-101, miR-29c, and miR138
  - Downregulated in t(14;18)(-) FL

ANCILLARY TESTS

Immunohistochemistry

- Pan B-cell markers (+)
- Germinal center markers (+)
  - BCL6, CD10, HGAL, LMO2
- BCL2(+) in 85-90% of FL grade 1 and grade 2, 50% of FL grade 3
  - BCL2(+) useful to distinguish FL from reactive follicles, which are BCL2(-)
- Follicular dendritic cell meshworks
  - CD21, CD23, and CD35 (+)
- CD23(+/-), IRF4/MUM1(-)
- Usually CD5(-), CD43(-)
  - Small subset (< 5%) can be CD5(+) or CD43(+)
- Grade 3 FL
  - Can be CD10(-), BCL2(-), IRF4/MUM1(+)

SELECTED REFERENCES

1. Amin R et al: The follicular lymphoma epigenome regulates its microenvironment. J Exp Clin Cancer Res. 41(1):21, 2022
2. Campo E et al: The International Consensus Classification of mature lymphoid neoplasms: a report from the Clinical Advisory Committee. Blood. 140(11):1229-53, 2022
3. Khoury JD et al: The 5th edition of the World Health Organization classification of haematolymphoid tumours: myeloid and histiocytic/dendritic neoplasms. Leukemia. 36(7):1703-19, 2022
4. Kumar E et al: Pathogenesis of follicular lymphoma: genetics to the microenvironment to clinical translation. Br J Haematol. 194(5):810-21, 2021
5. Nann D et al: Follicular lymphoma t(14;18)-negative is genetically a heterogeneous disease. Blood Adv. 4(22):5652-65, 2020
6. Xian RR et al: CREBBP and STAT6 co-mutation and 16p13 and 1p36 loss define the t(14;18)-negative diffuse variant of follicular lymphoma. Blood Cancer J. 10(6):69, 2020

Follicular Lymphoma

CD20 Immunohistochemistry

(Left) CD20 highlights neoplastic secondary follicle (germinal center) ⇨ in FL. There are also many B cells ⇨ between the follicles. (Right) BCL6 highlights germinal center B cells within follicles ⇨ as well as within interfollicular B cells ⇨ in this case of FL. The reactivity is stronger in germinal centers than in interfollicular regions. BCL2 is also positive (not shown).

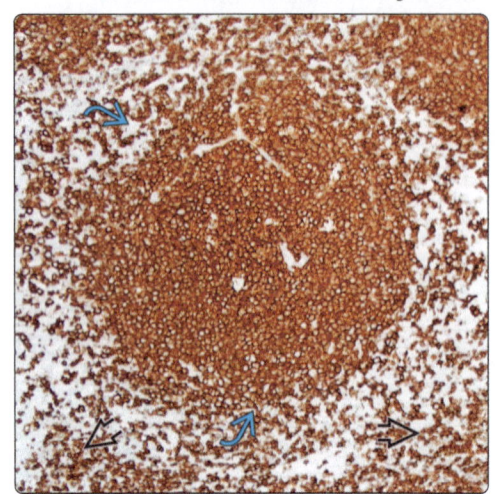

BCL6 Immunohistochemistry

BCL2 Immunohistochemistry

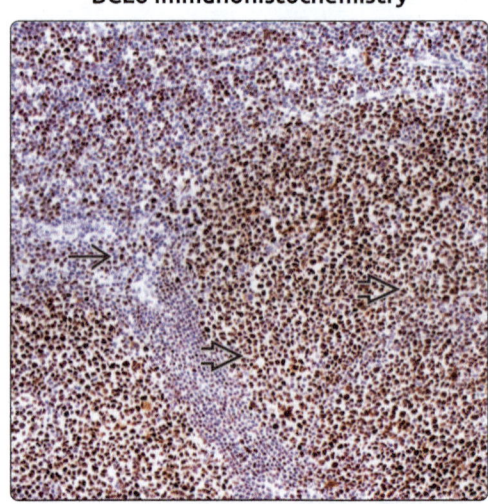

(Left) BCL2 is negative ⇨ in this case of FL. BCL2 is commonly positive in FL but can be negative in a subset of cases. The chance of BCL2 negativity increases in higher grade FL. (Right) FISH performed on lymph node with FL using dual-fusion probes for BCL2 (red ⇨) and IGH (green ⇨) is shown. A yellow fusion signal ⇨ is detected, indicating the presence of t(14;18)(q32;q21)/IGH::BCL2.

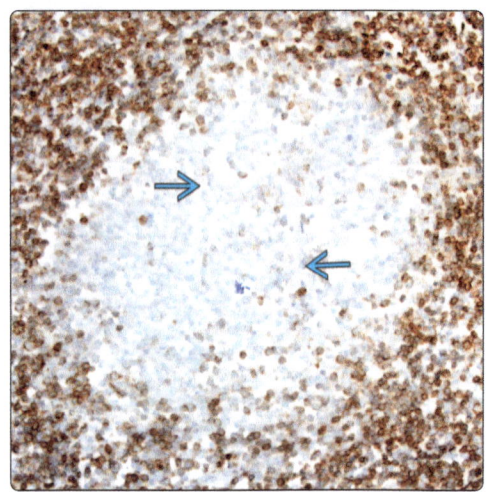

IGH::BCL2 FISH

RT-PCR for IGH::BCL2 Fusion

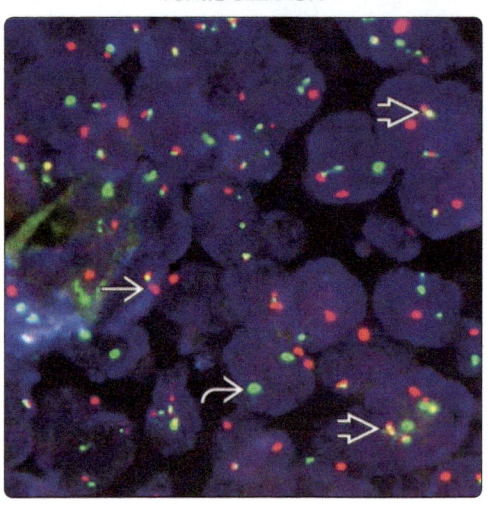

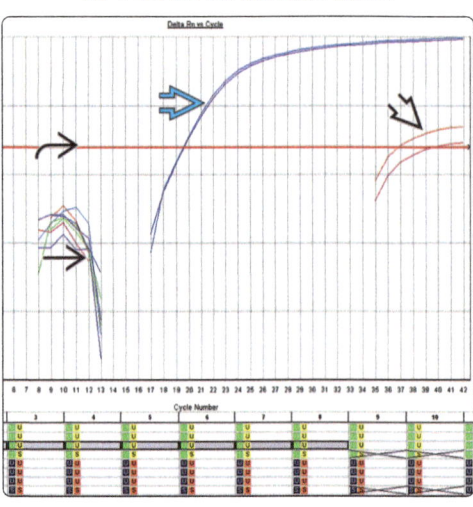

(Left) RT-PCR to assess for IGH::BCL2 fusion involving major breakpoint cluster region is shown. Threshold ⇨, negative control ⇨, high positive control ⇨, and low positive amplification ⇨ are highlighted in a patient sample with FL. (Courtesy S. Chen, MD.) (Right) This case of FL shows a dominant monoclonal peak at position 304 ⇨. FL typically shows monoclonality by PCR, since it is a B-cell lymphoma.

PCR for IGH Rearrangement

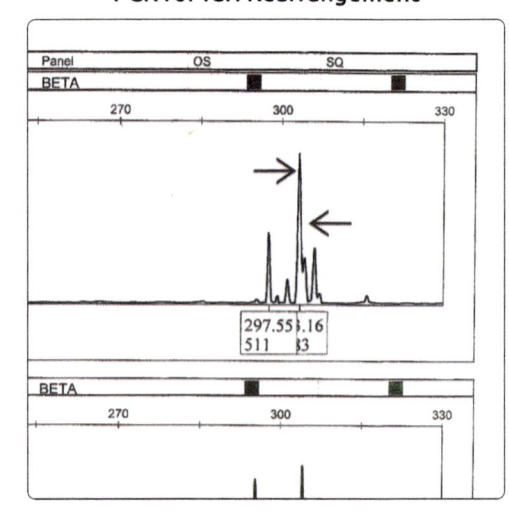

Follicular Lymphoma

Duodenal Follicular Lymphoma

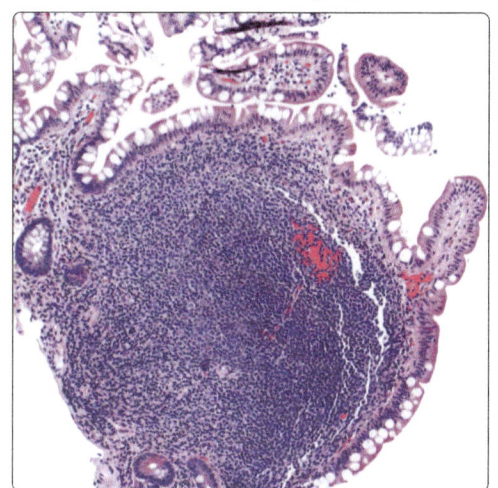

Duodenal Follicular Lymphoma: BCL2

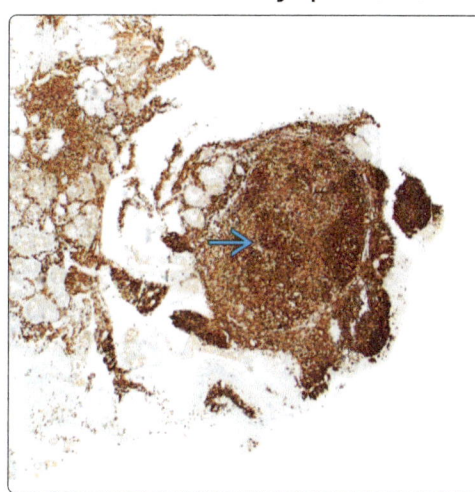

(**Left**) *Duodenal mucosa is involved by an atypical germinal center consisting mostly of small to intermediate-sized centrocytes with only rare centroblasts morphologically indistinguishable from low-grade (WHO grade 1-2) FL.* (**Right**) *Atypical germinal center shows strong, diffuse expression of BCL2 secondary to overexpression ⇨ caused by the presence of t(14;18)(q32;q21); IGH::BCL2.*

Diffuse Follicular Lymphoma

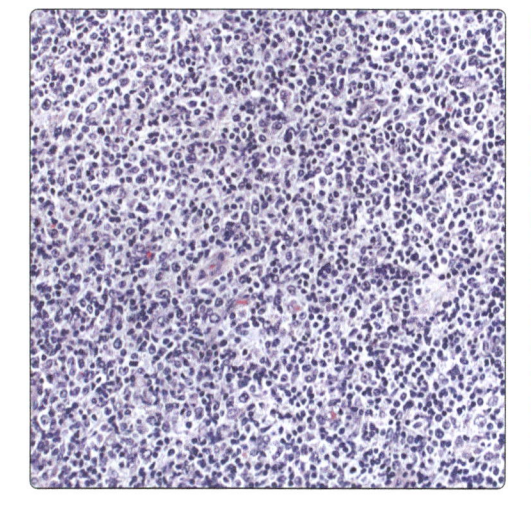

Diffuse Follicular Lymphoma: CD23

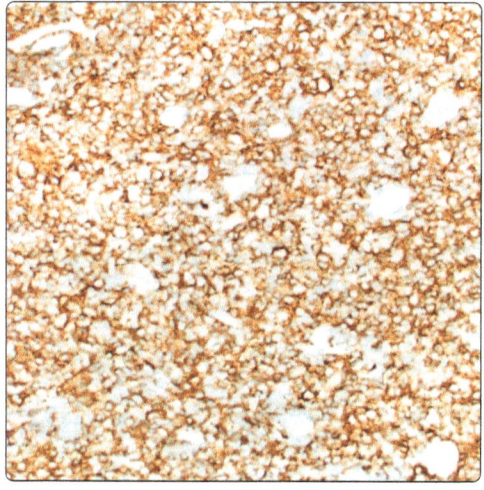

(**Left**) *Diffusely growing proliferation of predominantly small to intermediate-sized centrocytes with occasional scattered centroblasts is shown.* (**Right**) *Lymphoma cells are diffusely positive for CD23, which is a surrogate marker to STAT6 mutations.*

Pediatric Follicular Lymphoma

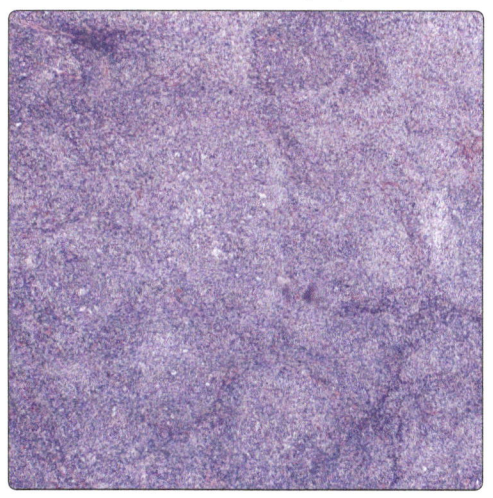

Pediatric Follicular Lymphoma: BCL2

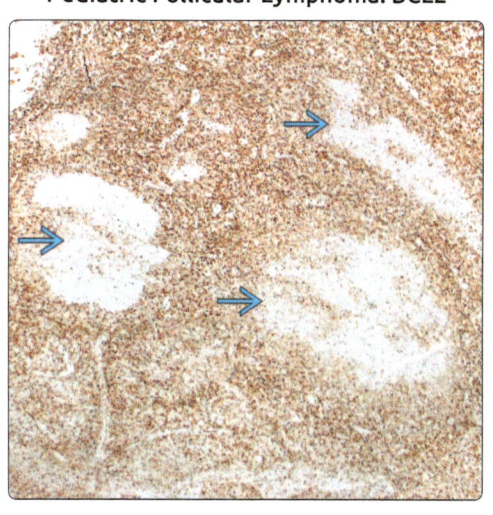

(**Left**) *Lymph node tissue shows architecture effaced by an atypical proliferation of large, irregularly shaped, serpiginous germinal centers lacking well-defined mantle zones and normal polarization.* (**Right**) *Atypical germinal centers are negative for BCL2 ⇨, as pediatric-type follicular lymphoma lacks t(14;18)(q32;q21)/IGH::BCL2.*

Mantle Cell Lymphoma

KEY FACTS

TERMINOLOGY
- B-cell lymphoma characterized by *CCND1::IGH* composed of small to medium-sized lymphocytes with irregular nuclear contours

ETIOLOGY/PATHOGENESIS
- *CCND1::IGH*, t(11;14)(q13;q32) resulting in cyclin-D1 overexpression is considered primary genetic event causing MCL
  o Can be detected by FISH, karyotyping, or PCR

MOLECULAR
- Additional secondary chromosomal aberrations are very common and include loss of 1p, 13q, 17p, gains in 3q
- Other mutated genes often function to regulate cell cycle
  o Cyclin-D1 (-) MCL often shows mutations in other cell cycle regulators (cyclin-D2, cyclin-D3)
- Monoclonal *IGH* and immunoglobulin light chain gene rearrangements

MICROSCOPIC
- Uniform, small to intermediate-sized B cells with irregular nuclear contours
- Pleomorphic, blastoid, prolymphocytoid variants
- In situ MCL
  o Cyclin-D1 (+) B cells in mantle zones of reactive lymphoid tissue with *CCND1* translocations
- Leukemic nonnodal MCL
  o MCL in blood, bone marrow, or spleen without lymphadenopathy

ANCILLARY TESTS
- CD20(+), CD5(+), cyclin-D1 (+), SOX11(+)
- FMC7(+), BCL2(+), CD23(-), CD200(-)

TOP DIFFERENTIAL DIAGNOSES
- Small lymphocytic lymphoma
  o Lacks cyclin-D1 and *CCND1* translocations and is CD23(+)

Diffuse Lymphoid Infiltrate

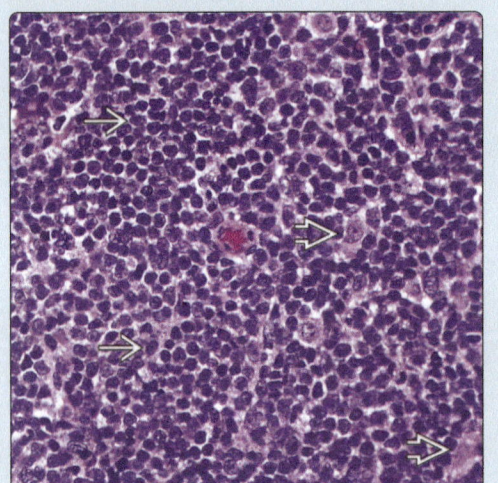

Cyclin-D1 Immunohistochemistry

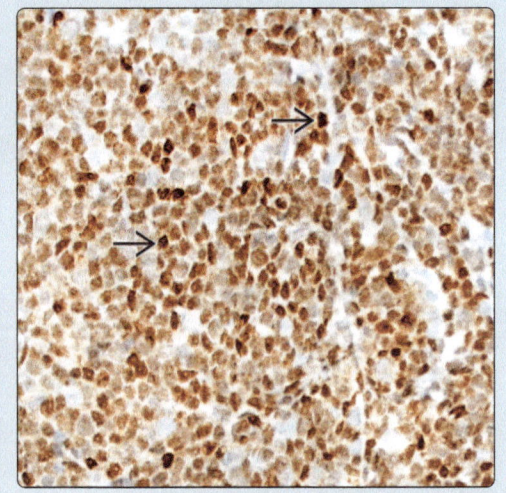

(Left) Mantle cell lymphoma (MCL) shows a diffuse lymphoid infiltrate ➡. There are also scattered histiocytes ➡, a feature typical of MCL. (Right) Cyclin-D1 in MCL shows positive nuclear staining ➡. Most MCL cases are cyclin-D1 (+), although some can be (-). Cytoplasmic staining without nuclear staining is not diagnostic for MCL.

SOX11 Immunohistochemistry

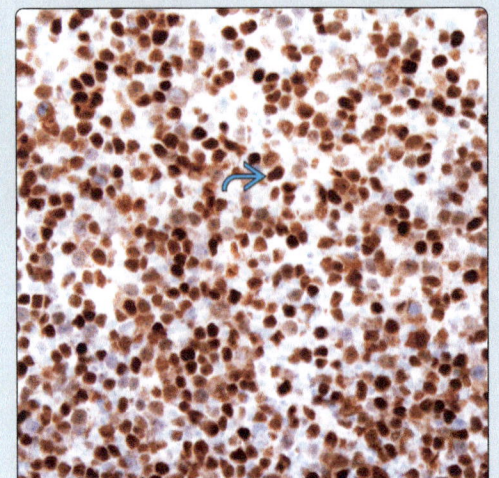

Lymphomatoid Polyposis

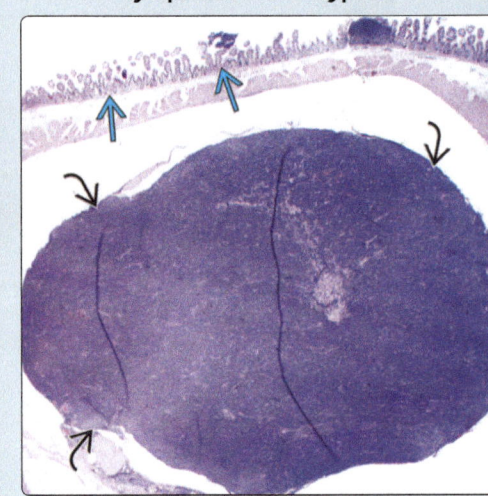

(Left) SOX11 is a newer marker for MCL that shows nuclear positivity ➡ in > 90% of cases. (Right) Lymphomatoid polyposis is the term given to studding of the intestine ➡ with multiple foci of MCL ➡. This example is SOX11(+).

Mantle Cell Lymphoma

TERMINOLOGY

Abbreviations
- Mantle cell lymphoma (MCL)

Definitions
- Mature small B-cell lymphoma comprised of mantle zone B cells, expressing CD5, cyclin-D1 and SOX11, and showing CCND family gene rearrangements most commonly CCND1::IGH
  - Newest WHO divides MCL into
    - Conventional mantle cell lymphoma
    - In situ mantle cell neoplasia
  - International Consensus Classification (ICC) expands definition of MCL to include genetic variants with CCND2 and CCND3 rearrangements with IGH genes in otherwise typical MCL
  - ICC notes that aggressive B-cell lymphomas with secondary CCND1 rearrangements should not be diagnosed as MCL

ETIOLOGY/PATHOGENESIS

CCND1::IGH
- t(11;14)(q13;q32) is primary event in pathogenesis of MCL
  - But is not required since there are CCND1::IGH (-) cases of MCL
- Translocation of CCND1 (cyclin-D1) normally at 11q13 to chromosome to IGH on 14q32
  - Detected in > 95% of cases
  - IGK and IGL are rare alternate translocation partners
  - Overexpression of BCL1 (cyclin-D1), which affects entry into cell cycle
  - Dysregulated cyclin-D1 accelerates transition from G1 to S phase of cell cycle
    - Cyclin-D1 binds CDK4 and CDK6 and activates E2F family of transcription factors by phosphorylating its inhibitor RB1 and p27
    - Overcomes cell cycle suppression of RB1 and p27
    - Which leads to MCL proliferation
- CCND1 rearrangement can be detected in blood of healthy individuals
  - So it may not cause MCL without other gene alterations

Secondary Gene Alterations in MCL
- Found in > 90% of cases
- Copy number changes
  - Gains in 3q, 7p, 8q (MYC), 15q, 18q (BCL2)
  - Losses of 1p, 2q, 6q, 8p, 9p, 10p, 11q (ATM), 13q (RB1), 17p (TP53), 19p
- Tetraploid chromosome clones are more often detected in pleomorphic variant of MCL
- Next-generation sequencing
  - Multiple genes mutated in MCL
  - ATM most common ~ 50% of cases
  - MYC rearrangements and TP53 mutations are commonly seen in aggressive MCL variants
    - Cases with MYC rearrangements should not be considered double hit MCL or high-grade B-cell lymphoma
  - TP53 (~ 25%), CCND1 (25%), KMT2D (20%), NSD2 (12%), SMARCA4 (8%), UBR5 (10%), BIRC3 (8%), NOTCH1 (8%), S1PR1 (10%), and CARD11 (8%)
  - SOX11 is overexpressed with in situ mantle cell neoplasia
    - This suggests it functions in very early MCL pathogenesis
    - It is also implicated in aggressive MCL cases
- MCL without CCND1 rearrangement
  - Some cases have shown cryptic IGK or IGL enhancer rearrangements and strong cyclin-D1 positivity
  - Alternatively CCND2, CCND3, or CCNE1 are alterative rearrangements
    - Also cause cell cycle dysregulation

IGHV Genes
- Most MCL has unmutated or minimally mutated IGVH genes
- Cases of leukemia nonnodal MCL have more somatic hypermutation, indicating that these cells have gone through germinal center
- MCL has preferential usage of IGHV3-21, IGHV4-34, and IGHV1-8 subgroups
- Stereotyped variable heavy chain complementarity-determining region 3 (CDR3) sequences detected in ~ 10% of MCL
  - Indicates there is antigen-driven selection for some MCL

Leukemia Nonnodal Mantle Cell Lymphoma
- Involves blood, bone marrow and spleen, little or no lymphadenopathy
- Show hypermutated immunoglobulin genes (postgerminal center cells)
  - Often uses IGHV1-8 gene, unlike conventional MCL
- Lack expression of SOX11, unlike conventional MCL
- Low Ki-67, often lacks CD5
- CD23 and CD200 positivity
- Indolent but more aggressive if TP53 mutations are acquired or if there is genomic complexity
- Absence of ATM and CCND1 alterations are features

Cell of Origin
- Pregerminal center antigen naive B cell
  - Except leukemic nonnodal mantle cell lymphoma is post germinal center B cell

CLINICAL ISSUES

Epidemiology
- Age
  - Range: 30-78 years (median: 62 years)
- Sex
  - M:F = 2-3:1

Site
- Most cases of MCL involve lymph nodes, but extranodal sites are often involved
  - Common extranodal sites
    - Blood, bone marrow
    - Lymphomatous polyposis is term given to MCL that has multiple polyploid lesions studding gastrointestinal tract
    - Spleen in ~ 40% of patients

Mantle Cell Lymphoma

Presentation
- Widespread lymphadenopathy
- Subset of patients present with lymphocytosis
- Splenomegaly; can be massive
- Leukemic nonnodal MCL occurs with patients with splenic involvement, peripheral blood lymphocytosis, and lacks nodal disease

Laboratory Tests
- Elevated serum β-2-microglobulin or lactate dehydrogenase in 40% of patients
- Flow cytometry will show MCL in blood of most patients
  - Lymphocytosis is usually at low level
    - Can be marked: > 200 x 10⁹/L

Treatment
- Aggressive chemotherapy regimens offer best chance at disease eradication
  - Rituximab plus fractionated cyclophosphamide, vincristine, doxorubicin, and dexamethasone (R-hyper-CVAD)
  - Rituximab plus cyclophosphamide, doxorubicin, vincristine, and prednisone (R-CHOP)
    - For older patients or those with significant morbidity precluding aggressive regimen
- Watch and wait
  - Can be used for patients with low risk
  - In situ MCL and leukemic nonnodal MCL
- Refractory MCL
  - Bortezomib, protease inhibitor
  - Temsirolimus, mTOR pathway inhibitor
  - Ibrutinib is Bruton tyrosine kinase inhibitor
- New therapeutic agents
  - HSP90 inhibitors
  - Histone deacetylase inhibitors
  - Cell cycle regulators

Prognosis
- Currently incurable and usually carries aggressive course
  - Survival has increased to 5-10 years with modern chemotherapy
- Some correlation between morphologic features and prognosis
  - Blastoid and pleomorphic variants are associated with adverse prognosis
- Poor prognostic markers
  - Complex karyotypes, *TP53* alterations, high Ki-67 *CDKN2A* alterations
    - Ki-67 (> 30%) is associated with more aggressive disease
    - p53 expression in > 50% of lymphocytes relates to poor survival
- Leukemic nonnodal mantle cell lymphoma has favorable prognosis

IMAGING

Radiographic Findings
- MCL is usually fluorodeoxyglucose (FDG) PET negative/low

MOLECULAR

Cytogenetics
- Detects *CCND1::IGH* t(11;14)(q13;q32)
  - ~ 70-80% of cases (+) by karyotyping
  - Rare cases may show variant translocations of *CCND1* with immunoglobulin light-chain genes
- Blastoid/pleomorphic variants of MCL
  - High frequency of additional chromosomal abnormalities
  - Tetraploid chromosomes are more frequent
  - Higher frequency of abnormalities of 17p (*TP53*) and 9q (*CDKN2A*)

In Situ Hybridization
- *CCND1* and *IGH* dual fusion probes
  - Most sensitive method for detecting *CCND1::IGH*
  - Can be performed on formalin-fixed tissue sections
  - Typically uses fusion probes
- *IGH* break-apart probes
  - Positive test shows break indicating translocation involving *IGH* on chromosome 14
  - Not specific; will also be seen in other lymphomas involving *IGH*

PCR
- Monoclonal *IGH* and immunoglobulin light-chain gene rearrangements
- *CCND1::IGH* fusion can also be detected by PCR
  - Multiple breakpoints, so less sensitive than FISH or cytogenetics
    - Detected on only 30-40% of cases
  - Often, primers detect only translocation involving major translocation cluster (MTC)

Molecular Genetics
- *CCND1::IGH* (-) MCL
  - May show mutations or translocations in other cell cycle regulators (*CCND2*, *CCND3*)
    - *CCND2* rearrangements are common and can partner with immunoglobulin heavy-chain gene or light-chain genes
    - t(2;12) fuses *CCND2* to *IGK*, t(12;22) fuses *CCND2* to *IGL*
    - t(12;14) fuses *IGH* to *CCND2*
    - *CCND3* translocations have rarely been reported
  - Clinically similar to conventional cyclin-D1 (+) MCL
  - Usually SOX11(+)

Gene Expression Profiling
- Expression of ~ 40 genes can reliably identify MCL cases
- Cases of cyclin-D1 (-) MCL show similar gene expression profile as cyclin-D1 (+) MCL
  - Cyclin-D1 (-) can express other cell cycle regulators (i.e., cyclin-D2)
- Splits MCL patients into different prognostic groups

MICROSCOPIC

Histologic Features
- Lymph node

Mantle Cell Lymphoma

- Architecture effaced by small to medium-sized lymphocytes with diffuse, nodular, or mantle zone growth patterns
- Small lymphocytes with irregular nuclear contours, coarse chromatin, indistinct nucleoli, and scant cytoplasm
- Can show scattered epithelioid histiocytes, hyalinized blood vessels, and small reactive (naked) germinal centers
- Paraimmunoblasts, centroblasts, and proliferation centers are not seen
- Does not transform to diffuse large B-cell lymphoma
  - Instead, cases with larger more atypical lymphocytes are considered blastoid or pleomorphic variants of MCL
- In situ mantle cell neoplasia
  - Cyclin-D1 (+) B cells in mantle zones of reactive lymphoid tissue with *CCND1* translocations
- Morphologic variants of MCL
  - Blastoid: Medium-sized cells with immature chromatin and high mitotic rate (≥ 20/10 HPF)
  - Pleomorphic: Large cells, more prominent nucleoli, and increased mitoses
    - Blastic and pleomorphic variants are more aggressive tumors and have higher Ki-67 index
  - Small cell: Round nuclear contours and low mitotic rate
  - Marginal zone-like: Small cells with abundant pale cytoplasm
    - Can have reactive germinal centers and residual follicular dendritic cell meshworks
  - Prolymphocytoid: Intermediate to large cells with prominent nucleoli

ANCILLARY TESTS

Immunohistochemistry

- Pan B-cell antigens (+), CD5(+)
- Cyclin-D1 (+) with nuclear pattern
  - Negative in ~ 5% of cases
  - Cyclin-D1 (-) cases can have *CCND1* alterations due to mutations in *CCND1* or truncated cyclin-D1 mRNA
- SOX11(+) with nuclear staining
  - Expressed in cyclin-D1 (-) or CD5(-) MCL
  - Not expressed in other small B-cell lymphomas
  - Also (+) in Burkitt lymphoma, B-lymphoblastic lymphoma, and hairy cell leukemia
  - SOX11 is transcription factor involved in neurogenesis
    - Detected in neural tumors, such as astrocytes and small cell lung carcinomas, as well as some soft tissue tumors, including rhabdomyosarcoma
  - Negative in leukemic nonnodal MCL
- IgM/IgD(+) λ-light chains > κ
- BCL2(+), CD43(+/-)
- CD3(-), CD23(-)
  - CD23 can be positive in rare cases
- CD10(-), BCL6(-)
  - Occasional cases express CD10 or BCL6
    - Usually aggressive variants
- LEF1 and CD200 are only rarely (+)
  - These are typically positive in CLL/SLL and negative in MCL
  - More commonly positive in blastoid and pleomorphic variants
  - CD200(+) in leukemic nonnodal MCL
- Proliferation index as determined by Ki-67 is variable and has prognostic significance
  - High index, > 30%, correlates with poorer survival
- p27(+) in cyclin-D1 (-) MCL

Flow Cytometry

- Monotypic surface Ig(+), intermediate to strong
- CD19(+), CD20(+), CD22(+)
- CD79b(+), FMC7(+)
- CD5(+), CD10(-), CD200(-)
  - Occasional cases are CD5(-) and CD10(+)
    - More often in pleomorphic or blastoid variants
- CD23 usually (-) but dimly (+) in ~ 10% of MCL cases
- Cyclin-D1 is technically difficult to assess by flow cytometry
- SOX11(+/-)

DIFFERENTIAL DIAGNOSIS

Chronic Lymphocytic Leukemia/Small Lymphocytic Lymphoma

- Proliferation centers with variable admixture of prolymphocytes
- Usually less irregular nuclear contours than in MCL
- Immunophenotype is very helpful in distinguishing from MCL
  - CD5(+), CD23(+), CD43(+/-)
  - CD200 (bright) with CLL/SLL, and usually dim or (-) in MCL
  - Cyclin-D1 (-), but can be weakly (+) in proliferation centers
- No evidence of *CCND1::IGH*

Plasma Cell Myeloma

- Can express cyclin D1

Diffuse Large B-Cell Lymphoma

- Must be differentiated from MCL pleomorphic and blastoid variants
- Presence of *CCND1::IGH* may be secondary event in progression of some aggressive B-cell lymphomas and should not be diagnosed as MCL
- Lack of CD5 and SOX11 and presence of mutations uncommon in MCL favor diagnosis of DLBCL over MCL

High-Grade B-Cell Lymphoma With *MYC* and *BCL2* Rearrangements

- Double-hit lymphoma
- Can show *CCND1::IGH* but should not be diagnosed as MCL

SELECTED REFERENCES

1. Jain P et al: Mantle cell lymphoma in 2022-A comprehensive update on molecular pathogenesis, risk stratification, clinical approach, and current and novel treatments. Am J Hematol. 97(5):638-56, 2022
2. Obr A et al: TP53 mutation and complex karyotype portends a dismal prognosis in patients with mantle cell lymphoma. Clin Lymphoma Myeloma Leuk. 18(11):762-8, 2018
3. Yang P et al: Genomic landscape and prognostic analysis of mantle cell lymphoma. Cancer Gene Ther. 25(5-6):129-40, 2018

Mantle Cell Lymphoma

Role of Cyclin-D1 on Cell Cycle

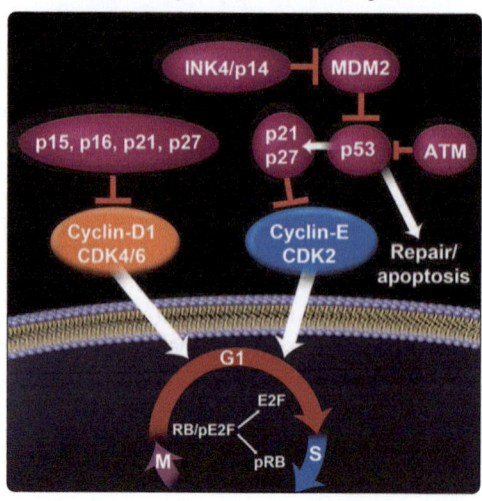

Cytogenetics of t(11;14)(q13;q32)

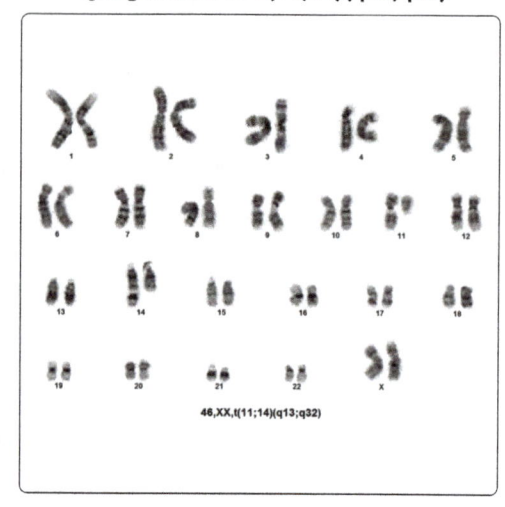

(Left) The role of cyclin-D1 on the cell cycle is shown. Cyclin-D1 cyclin-dependent kinase complexes act on the G1 to S transition. Other genes that are involved in the pathogenesis of MCL are genes that influence the cell cycle. Some of these genes are also depicted. **(Right)** This karyotype shows the t(11;14) translocation involving the IGH gene on chromosome 14 and the CCND1 gene on chromosome 11. (Courtesy T. O'Brien, CG, CM.)

Positive CCND1::IGH by FISH

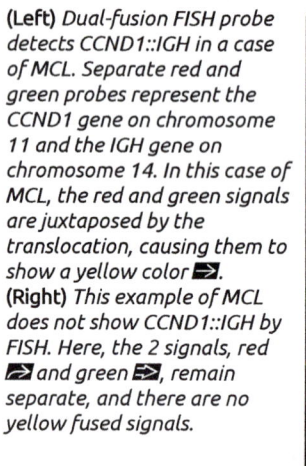

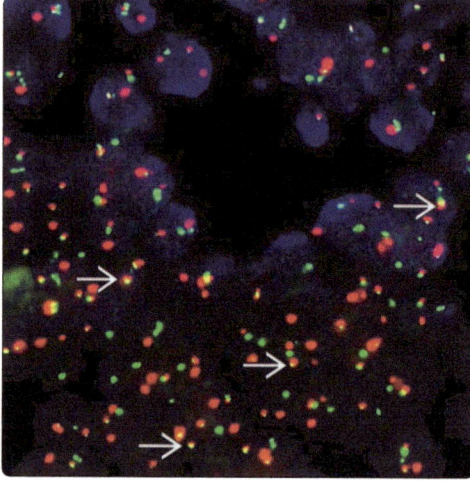

Negative CCND1::IGH by FISH

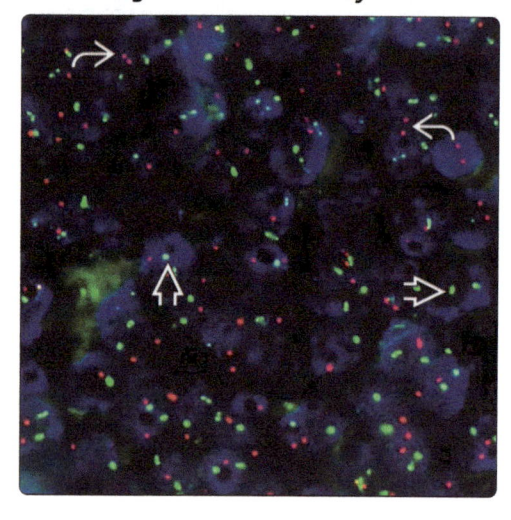

(Left) Dual-fusion FISH probe detects CCND1::IGH in a case of MCL. Separate red and green probes represent the CCND1 gene on chromosome 11 and the IGH gene on chromosome 14. In this case of MCL, the red and green signals are juxtaposed by the translocation, causing them to show a yellow color ➡. **(Right)** This example of MCL does not show CCND1::IGH by FISH. Here, the 2 signals, red ➡ and green ➡, remain separate, and there are no yellow fused signals.

IGH Break-Apart Probe

IGH Gene Rearrangement

(Left) IGH dual-color break-apart probe utilizes a yellow fusion probe in chromosome 14. Note the separated red ➡ and green ➡ signals, which represents a translocation of the IGH gene. **(Right)** This case of MCL shows a dominant monoclonal band by PCR testing for IGH gene rearrangement ➡. IGH monoclonality is typically seen since MCL is a B-cell lymphoma.

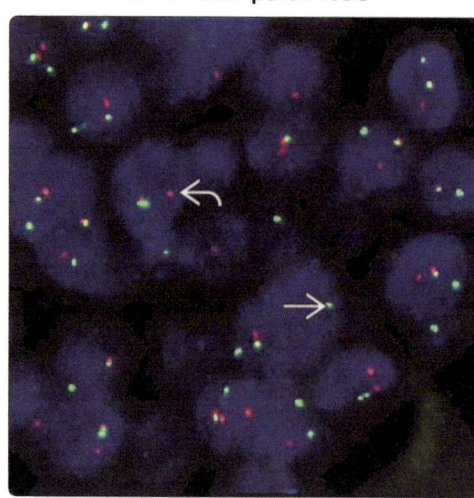

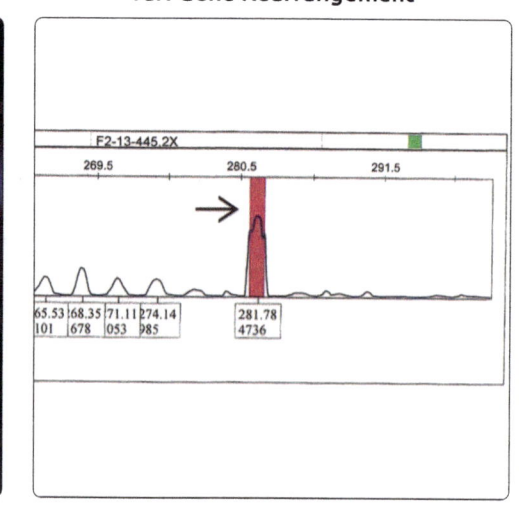

Mantle Cell Lymphoma

Blastoid Mantle Cell Lymphoma

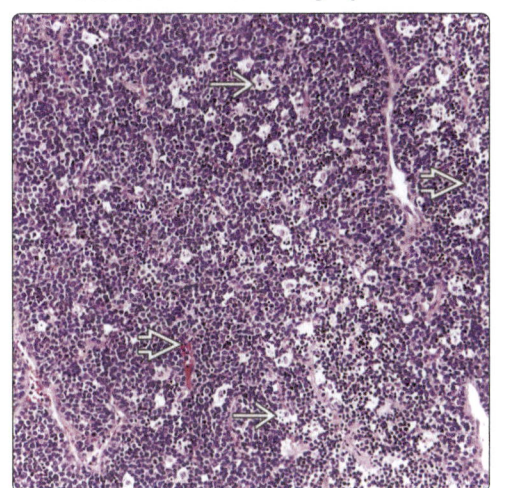

Peripheral Blood

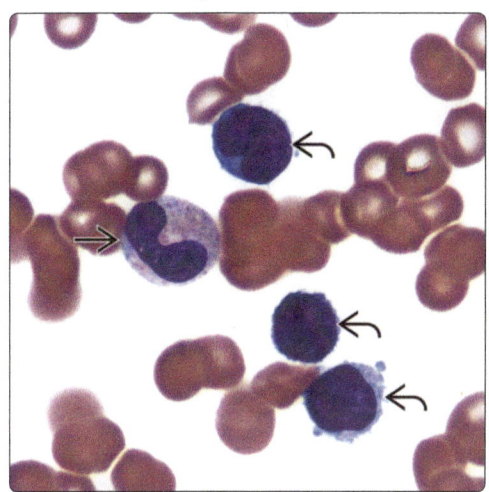

(Left) *Blastoid variant of MCL shows a prominent starry-sky pattern. The "stars" are tingible body macrophages ➡ that appear pale in a "sky" of darker tumor cells ➡.* **(Right)** *Peripheral blood smear shows small lymphocytes with irregular nuclear contours ➡, a common appearance of MCL cells. A band ➡ is shown for comparison. Peripheral blood lymphocytosis occurs in 25% of cases of MCL. Leukemic nonnodal MCL is the term used for MCL in blood, bone marrow, or spleen lacking lymph node adenopathy.*

CD20 Immunohistochemistry

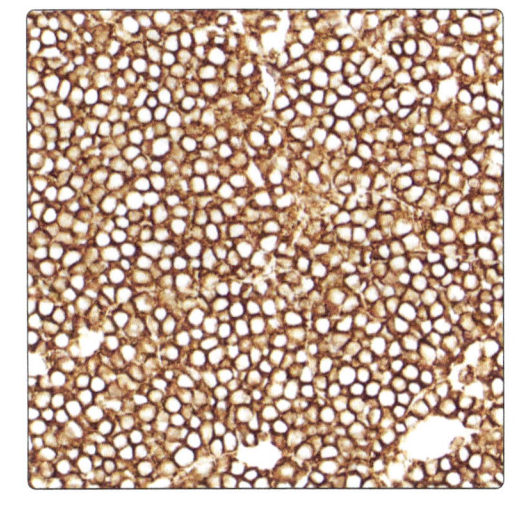

CD5 Immunohistochemistry

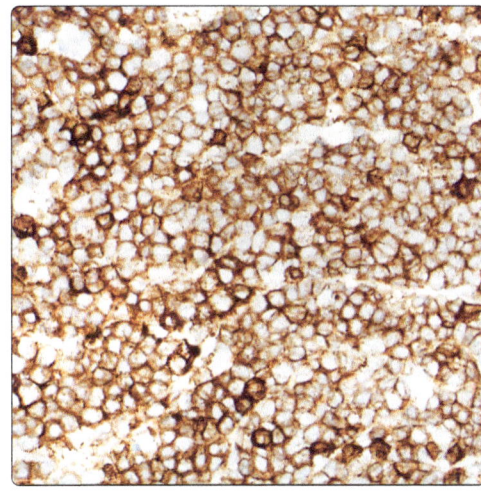

(Left) *CD20 in MCL shows a diffuse infiltrate of B cells. Other B-cell markers, such as PAX5, would also be positive.* **(Right)** *CD5 is strongly coexpressed in the B cells of this case of MCL. CD5 is often positive in MCL and chronic lymphocytic leukemia/small lymphocytic lymphoma but is usually negative in the other small B-cell lymphomas.*

SOX11 Immunohistochemistry

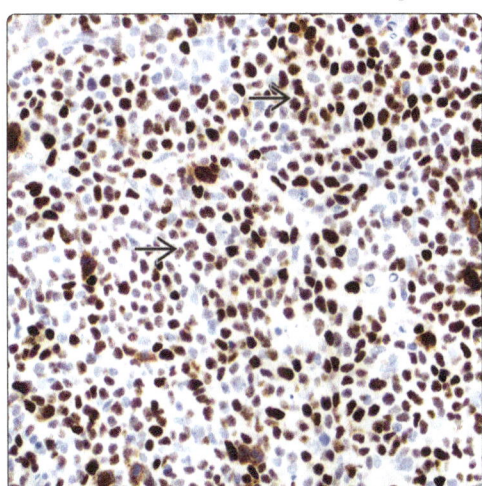

Ki-67 Immunohistochemistry

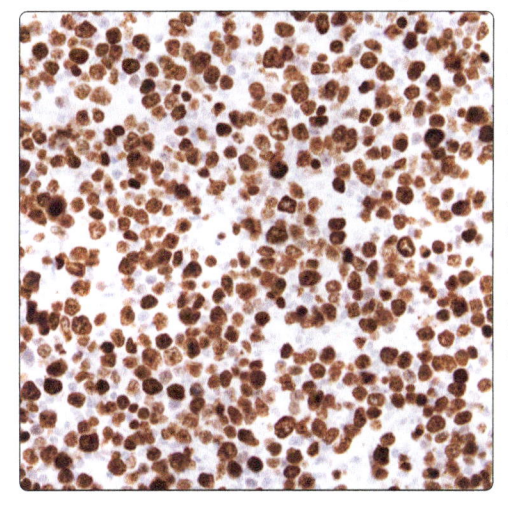

(Left) *SOX11 shows strong reactivity ➡ in most neoplastic nuclei in this case of MCL. SOX11 is highly sensitive for the diagnosis of MCL and can be used to identify cases that are cyclin-D1 (-).* **(Right)** *Ki-67 stain of MCL, pleomorphic variant, shows a very high proliferation rate, where > 90% of tumor cells are positive. A high index correlates with poorer survival.*

Diffuse Large B-Cell Lymphoma

KEY FACTS

TERMINOLOGY
- Diffuse large B-cell lymphoma (DLBCL), not otherwise specified (NOS) (ICC and WHO)
  - Biologically heterogeneous neoplasms composed of large B cells

CLINICAL ISSUES
- Prognosis affected by extent of disease, molecular genetics, and proliferation rate
- DLBCL may result from progression of low-grade B-cell lymphoma or arise de novo

MACROSCOPIC
- Lymphadenopathy
- Mass lesions in extranodal sites

MOLECULAR
- FISH and conventional cytogenetics
  - Stratifies DLBCL, NOS into prognostic groups
  - TP53 mutations may confer worse prognosis
- Molecular subtypes of DLBCL, NOS
  - Germinal center B-cell (GCB) subtype
  - Activated B-cell (ABC) subtype
- No current consensus for mutational subtypes

MICROSCOPIC
- Neoplastic lymphocytes with nuclear size ≥ macrophage nucleus or 2x size of mature normal lymphocyte

ANCILLARY TESTS
- Immunohistochemical features of DLBCL subtypes (Hans scheme most common)
  - GCB subtype: CD10(+), BCL6(+), MUM1(-)
  - Non-GCB (ABC-like) subtype: CD10(-), BCL6(+/-), MUM1(+)
    - GCB has better prognosis that ABC subtype
- Double-expressor DLBCL (poor prognosis)
  - Expresses MYC (≥ 40% of cells) and BCL2 (≥ 50% of cells)
- CD5 expression may portend worse prognosis

Proliferation of Large Lymphoid Cells

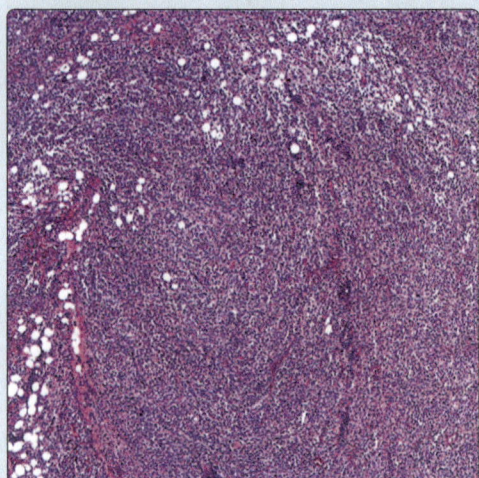

Large B Cells With Plasmacytoid Features

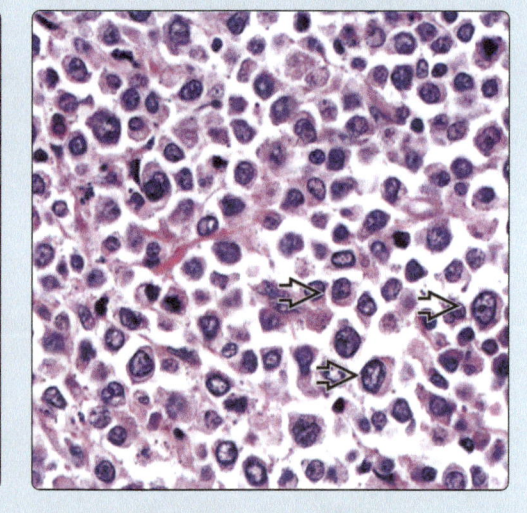

(Left) Low-power view shows diffuse proliferation of large lymphoid cells in soft tissue. The soft tissue is replaced by diffuse sheets of large atypical lymphoid cells. (Right) Diffuse large B-cell lymphoma (DLBCL) shows plasmacytoid features ➡ with abundant eosinophilic cytoplasm.

FISH for Dual-Fusion t(14;18) IGH::BCL2

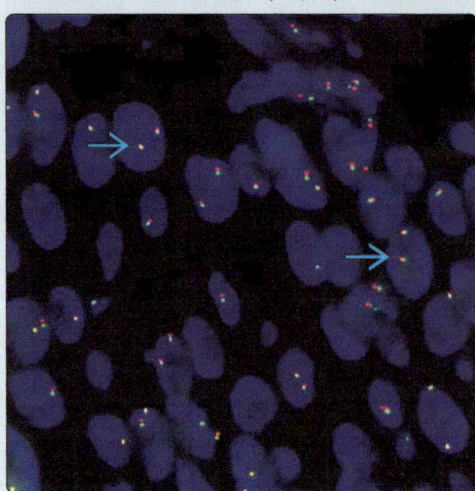

FISH Break-Apart for BCL6

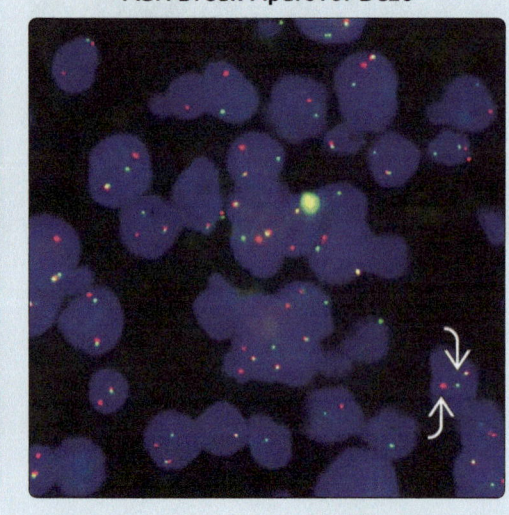

(Left) t(14;18) was detected in this dual-fusion IGH::BCL2 test, as seen by multiple fused (yellow) signals ➡. t(14;18) is frequently seen in DLBCL. (Right) BCL6 rearrangement is detected in this break-apart probe FISH assay, as seen by separate green and yellow signals ➡. BCL6 is among the most common recurring translocations in large B-cell lymphomas.

Diffuse Large B-Cell Lymphoma

TERMINOLOGY

Abbreviations
- Diffuse large B-cell lymphoma (DLBCL), not otherwise specified (NOS)

Definitions
- DLBCL, NOS: Biologically heterogeneous neoplasm composed of large B cells with nuclear size ≥ macrophage nucleus or 2x size of mature small lymphocyte

ETIOLOGY/PATHOGENESIS

Infectious Agents
- No known causative infectious agents, but some cases are associated with Epstein-Barr virus (EBV) and hepatitis C

Immunodeficiency
- Increases incidence of DLBCL
  - Common immune dysfunctions associated with DLBCL includes HIV infection, iatrogenic immunosuppression, congenital immune dysfunction

Classification
- International Consensus Classification (ICC) and World Health Organization (WHO) 5th edition diagnoses are similar
- Divided into morphologic variants, immunophenotypic, and molecular subgroups
  - Morphologic variants
    - Centroblastic
    - Immunoblastic
    - Anaplastic
    - Other rare morphologic variants
  - Cell of origin subtypes by immunophenotyping
    - Germinal center B cell (GCB)-like
    - Non-GCB [activated B cell (ABC)]-like
  - Cell of origin subtypes by gene expression profiling
    - GCB subtype (50-60%)
    - ABC subtype
    - Others (those that do not fit GCB or ABC)
- Other lymphoma of large B cells
  - T-cell/histiocyte-rich large B-cell lymphoma
  - Primary mediastinal (thymic) large B-cell lymphoma
  - Intravascular large B-cell lymphoma
  - DLBCL associated with chronic inflammation
  - Lymphomatoid granulomatosis
  - ALK(+) large B-cell lymphoma
  - Plasmablastic lymphoma
  - HHV8(+) diffuse large B-cell lymphoma
  - Primary effusion lymphoma
  - Primary DLBCL of CNS
  - Primary cutaneous DLBCL, leg type
  - EBV(+) diffuse large B-cell lymphoma, NOS
  - Large B-cell lymphoma with IRF4 rearrangement

CLINICAL ISSUES

Epidemiology
- Age
  - Older adults primarily affected
  - Median: 7th decade, though children and young adults can be affected

Presentation
- Enlarging lymph nodes or extranodal mass
- Frequent B symptoms
- DLBCL may represent transformation from low-grade B-cell lymphoma

Treatment
- Adjuvant therapy
  - Stem cell transplant in cases with certain genetic findings, such as *MYC* translocations
- Drugs
  - R-CHOP (rituximab + cyclophosphamide, doxorubicin, vincristine and prednisone) chemotherapy is primary treatment
  - Less cytotoxic targeted therapies are being developed; bortezomib has efficacy in relapsed DLBCL and ABC subtypes
- Radiation
  - Radiation may be used in limited-stage disease and specific subtypes

Prognosis
- International Prognostic Index (IPI) used for prognostication
  - Clinical variables, including disease stage and patient age, are considered in prognostication
- Morphologic variants have not shown prognostic differences
- Overall 5-year survival ranges from 25-75% depending on prognostic factors
- No single aberrant gene is responsible for diverse nature of DLBCL, NOS
- Unfavorable prognostic factors
  - ABC by gene expression profiling
  - High Ki-67 expression (> 80%)
  - Non-GCB (ABC-like) subtype as determined by immunohistochemistry
  - High expression of MYC may portend poor prognosis, but reports vary
  - Concurrent BCL2 and MYC expression (double expressors) may show poor prognosis
  - *TP53* mutations or loss show worse prognosis
  - *CDKN2A* mutations and trisomy 3 are associated with decreased survival in ABC subtype
  - Decreased CD8(+) tumor-infiltrating T cells or overexpression of PDL1 may confer worse prognosis
- Double-/triple-hit B-cell lymphomas are now classified as separate category of high-grade B-cell lymphoma (HGBCL)
  - HGBCL with rearrangements of *MYC* and *BCL2* (ICC)
  - HGBCL with rearrangement of *MYC* and *BCL6* (ICC)
  - DLBCL/HGBCL with *MYC* and *BCL2* rearrangements (WHO-HAEM5)

MACROSCOPIC

General Features
- Enlarged lymph nodes or extranodal mass lesions

Diffuse Large B-Cell Lymphoma

MOLECULAR

Cytogenetics

- Used for detection of numerical and structural chromosomal abnormalities
  - Identifies common translocation involving *IGH*, *MYC*, and *BCL6*, among others
  - *BCL6* translocations account for most common cytogenetic abnormality in DLBCL
    - Occur most commonly in ABC subtype of DLBCL

Fluorescence In Situ Hybridization

- Routinely performed to detect translocations in DLBCL
  - Commonly used probes include *MYC*, *BCL2*, and *BCL6*
    - Isolated *MYC* rearrangement in 5-15% of DLBCL
    - Molecular studies for mutations common to DLBCL help exclude Burkitt lymphoma (BL)
  - FISH break-apart probe strategy is commonly used
  - FISH targeted probes are used if identification of partner fused gene indicated
- FISH panel that include *MYC*, *BCL2*, and *BCL6* probes helps to separate DLBCL, NOS from so-called double-/triple-hit lymphomas
  - Double-/triple-hit lymphomas are now classified as high-grade B-cell lymphoma with rearrangements of *MYC* and *BCL2* (ICC)
    - Poor prognosis with resistance to therapy
  - DLCBL with *MYC* and *BCL6* rearrangements appear to show clinical behavior between DLBCL and HGBCL but are classified as HGBCL with *MYC* and *BCL6* rearrangements (ICC)
- *IRF4* and *IGH* rearrangements in large B-cell lymphoma
  - Cytogenetically cryptic translocation
  - FISH assay should be done to detect this rearrangement in suspected cases
  - Detected in distinct category of non-Hodgkin lymphoma designated as large B-cell lymphoma with *IRF4* rearrangement
  - Occurs in children and younger age
  - Associated with favorable outcome after treatment

Polymerase Chain Reaction

- Detects clonal *IGH* rearrangement in DLBCL

Molecular Genetics

- Mutated genes implicated in oncogenesis of DLBCL
  - *BCL6*, *MYC*, *PAX5*, *PIM1*, *PIM2*, *SOCS1*, *BACH2*, *CIITA*, and *TCL1A*

Gene Expression Profiling

- Used for prognostication
- Stratifies DLBCL into 3 subtypes
  - GCB subtype: 55%
  - ABC subtype: 35%
  - Other subtype not fitting GCB or ABC: 10%

MicroRNA Expression

- Global microRNA expression profiling
  - Has been used for prognostication
  - Can separate DLBCL of GCB-like from ABC-like subtype

Next-Generation Sequencing

- Confirms distinct genotype in ABC-like, GCB-like, and primary mediastinal LBCL
  - Many mutations discovered have yet to be linked to prognosis
  - No current consensus for classification using mutational subgroups
- Some genetic alterations are shared between GCB and ABC subtypes of DLBCL
- Mutated *TP53* may confer poor prognosis
- Other mutated genes implicated to have adverse prognostic impact
  - *B2M*, *CD58*, *CREBBP*, *EP300*, *KMT2D* (MLL2), *MEF2B*, *FOXO1*, and *BCL6*
- Some mutated gene profile may differ in GCB subtype vs. ABC subtype of DLBCL
  - Mutations in NF-κB and B-cell receptor signaling pathways are more common in ABC-like and include
    - *CD79B*, *CARD11*, *MYD88*, *PRDM1*, *PIM1*, and *TNFAIP3*
  - Mutations in gene involving histone methylation are more common in GCB-like and include
    - *KMT2D* (MLL2), *EZH2*, *CREBBP*, *GNA13*, *MEF2B*, *B2M*, and *TNFRSF14*

MICROSCOPIC

Histologic Features

- Large lymphoid cells with heterogeneous morphology depending on subtype

Cytologic Features

- Large B cells with nuclear size ≥ macrophage nucleus or 2x size of mature normal lymphocyte

ANCILLARY TESTS

Immunohistochemistry

- Positive for pan B-cell markers: CD20, CD19, CD22, CD79A, PAX5
  - Rituximab can greatly reduce expression of CD20, so may require alternate B-cell marker
    - Alternate B-cell marker is required to assess B-cell lineage
- Nonpan B-cell lineage markers typically included in diagnostic work up of DLBCL
  - CD3, CD5, CD10, BCL2, cyclin-D1, BCL6, MUM1, κ, and λ
- Additional helpful diagnostic and prognostic markers recommended to be included in IHC panel
  - Ki-67, MYC, CD138, ALK, HHV8, FOXP1, and CD30
- Germinal center-associated markers
  - CD10, BCL6, LMO2, HGAL, and GCET1
- Several published algorithmic schemes to distinguish GCB- vs. ABC-like DLBCL subtypes and non-GCB type, including
  - Hans, Choi, Visco-Young, Nyman, and Tally
  - Hans algorithm most commonly used
    - GCB subtype CD10(+), BCL6(+/-), and MUM1(-)
    - ABC (non-GCB) subtype CD10(-), MUM1(+), and BCL6(+/-)
- MYC expression
  - Detected in 30-50% of DLBCL
    - Higher than rate of *MYC* rearrangements

Diffuse Large B-Cell Lymphoma

- – May confer worse prognosis but is not useful surrogate for *MYC* rearrangements
- Expression of BCL2 and MYC (so-called "double expressor") worse prognosis
- Expression of CD5 may confer worse prognosis
- Ki-67
  - \> 80% Ki-67 proliferation index may be poor prognostic indicator
    - – Poor prognosis in high Ki-67 proliferation index may only be applicable in DLBCL in older patients and in ABC-like subtypes

Flow Cytometry
- Used for immunophenotyping of lymphoma
  - Commonly used antibody panel for suspected DLBCL cases include CD20, CD19, CD3, CD5, CD10, κ, and λ
  - More specific and prognostic marker are done on paraffin-embedded tissue sections

In Situ Hybridization
- EBER can be (+)
  - Seen most often in immune-suppressed and older individuals
  - May indicate worse prognosis
  - If EBER(+), diagnosis is reclassified as EBV(+) DLBCL except in WHO well-defined lymphoma categories that are EBV associated, including
    - – Lymphomatoid granulomatosis
    - – Plasmablastic lymphoma
    - – DLBCL associated with chronic inflammation
    - – EBV(+) mucocutaneous ulcer

DIFFERENTIAL DIAGNOSIS

Burkitt Lymphoma
- Highly aggressive but curable lymphoma of germinal center-derived B cells
- Monotonous, medium-sized cells with numerous histiocytes and mitoses
- *MYC* rearrangement by FISH or karyotyping is hallmark
- CD20(+), CD10(+), BCL6(+), BCL2(-) or weakly (+)
- Ki-67 shows virtually 100% rate
- EBER(+) in > 90% of endemic BL
- EBER(+) in ~ 20-30% of sporadic BL and in 30-40% of immunodeficiency-associated cases

High-Grade B-Cell Lymphoma
- Heterogeneous group of aggressive lymphomas
  - HGBCL with *MYC* and *BCL2* rearrangements
  - HGBCL with *MYC* and *BCL6* rearrangements
  - LBCL (HGBCL-WHO) with 11q aberrations
  - HGBCL, NOS
    - – DLBCL with blastoid morphology
    - – Excludes lymphoblastic leukemia/lymphoma and blastoid mantle cell lymphoma
- Worse prognosis than DLBCL with resistance to therapy

Mediastinal Gray Zone Lymphoma
- Associated with mediastinal disease, especially primary mediastinal large B-cell lymphoma
- B-cell markers often aberrantly expressed in conjunction with expression of Hodgkin markers

- BOB1/OCT2 can help to differentiate from DLBCL
  - One or other or both should be (-) in classic Hodgkin lymphoma
  - Both typically (+) in DLBCL

Myeloid Sarcoma
- Can be very difficult to differentiate from DLBCL on morphology
- MPO(+), CD34(+/-), CD68(+), CD163(+), CD117(+)
- May be solitary mass but often in bone marrow and peripheral blood

Histiocytic Sarcoma
- Malignant neoplasm composed of neoplastic histiocytes
- Sometimes associated with other lymphomas, including DLBCL
- CD163(+), CD45(+), CD68(+), CD20(-), CD3(-)
- Clonal *IGH* rearrangement may be sometimes detected by PCR in HS

Malignant Melanoma
- Large, malignant-appearing cells
- IHC should differentiate from DLBCL
- Malignant cells in melanoma are S100(+), HMB-45(+), tyrosinase (+), Melan-A (+), SOX10(+)

Poorly Differentiated Epithelioid Neoplasms
- May be difficult to morphologically differentiate from DLBCL on H&E
- Carcinomas are cytokeratin (+), EMA(+), CD45(-)

SELECTED REFERENCES

1. Song JY et al: Diffuse large B-cell lymphomas, not otherwise specified, and emerging entities. Virchows Arch. 482(1):179-92, 2023
2. Alaggio R et al: The 5th edition of the World Health Organization classification of haematolymphoid tumours: lymphoid neoplasms. Leukemia. ePub, 2022
3. Campo E et al: The International Consensus Classification of mature lymphoid neoplasms: a report from the Clinical Advisory Committee. Blood. 140(11):1229-53, 2022
4. Harrington F et al: Genomic characterisation of diffuse large B-cell lymphoma. Pathology. 53(3):367-76, 2021
5. Pileri SA et al: Predictive and prognostic molecular factors in diffuse large B-cell lymphomas. Cells. 10(3), 2021
6. Ennishi D et al: Toward a new molecular taxonomy of diffuse large B-cell lymphoma. Cancer Discov. 10(9):1267-81, 2020
7. Wright GW et al: A probabilistic classification tool for genetic subtypes of diffuse large B cell lymphoma with therapeutic implications. Cancer Cell. 37(4):551-68.e14, 2020
8. Crombie JL et al: Diffuse large B-cell lymphoma and high-grade B-cell lymphoma: genetic classification and Its implications for prognosis and treatment. Hematol Oncol Clin North Am. 33(4):575-85, 2019
9. Chapuy B et al: Molecular subtypes of diffuse large B cell lymphoma are associated with distinct pathogenic mechanisms and outcomes. Nat Med. 24(5):679-90, 2018
10. Ennishi D et al: Double-hit gene expression signature defines a distinct subgroup of germinal center B-cell-like diffuse large B-cell lymphoma. J Clin Oncol. JCO1801583, 2018
11. Guo L et al: Molecular heterogeneity in diffuse large B-cell lymphoma and its implications in clinical diagnosis and treatment. Biochim Biophys Acta Rev Cancer. 1869(2):85-96, 2018
12. Li S et al: Diffuse large B-cell lymphoma. Pathology. 50(1):74-87, 2018
13. Pasqualucci L et al: Genetics of diffuse large B-cell lymphoma. Blood. 131(21):2307-19, 2018
14. Schmitz R et al: Genetics and pathogenesis of diffuse large B-cell lymphoma. N Engl J Med. 378(15):1396-407, 2018
15. Wight JC et al: Prognostication of diffuse large B-cell lymphoma in the molecular era: moving beyond the IPI. Blood Rev. 32(5):400-15, 2018
16. Reddy A et al: Genetic and functional drivers of diffuse large B cell lymphoma. Cell. 171(2):481-94.e15, 2017

Diffuse Large B-Cell Lymphoma

(Left) Low-power view shows lymph node effaced by a diffuse proliferation of lymphocytes extending into soft tissue ⇨. There are no nodular areas in this proliferation. **(Right)** High-power view shows a mixture of small lymphocytes and large cells. The malignant cells are large B cells ⇨. Mitoses ⇨ are noted in the proliferation.

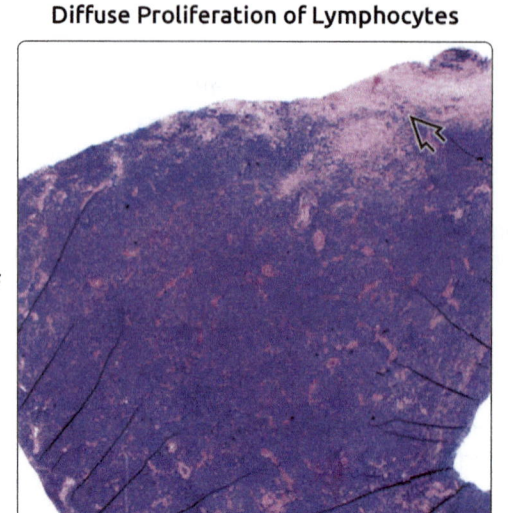

Diffuse Proliferation of Lymphocytes

Large Lymphoid Cells With Interspersed Small Lymphocytes

(Left) DLBCL is a heterogeneous group of B-cell lymphomas that show varying morphologies. This case shows large pleomorphic cells ⇨, some appearing Hodgkin-like. The background shows numerous histiocytes ⇨. **(Right)** DLBCL shows many large cells ⇨ within a background of small, cleaved centrocytes ⇨. There are numerous mitotic figures ⇨.

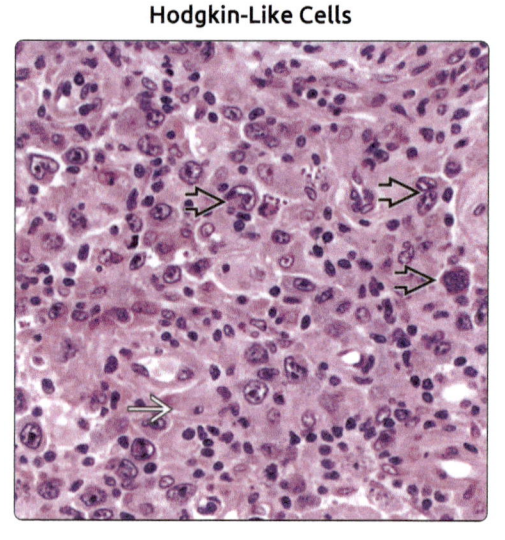

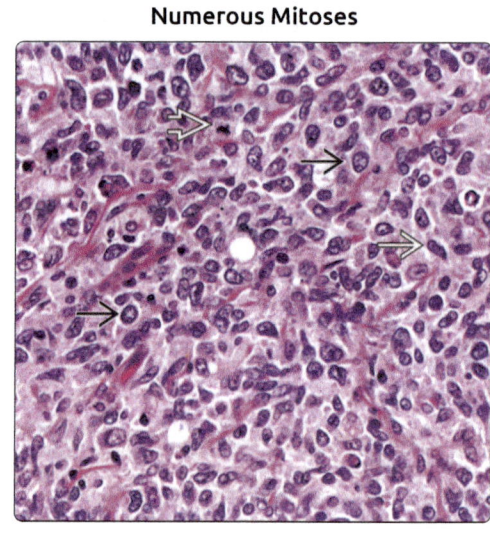

Hodgkin-Like Cells

Numerous Mitoses

(Left) These cells are immunoreactive with CD20, confirming their B-cell lineage. The cells are large and have abundant cytoplasm. **(Right)** CD3 shows numerous small T cells in the background of numerous large B cells. This finding is not unusual in cases of DLBCL.

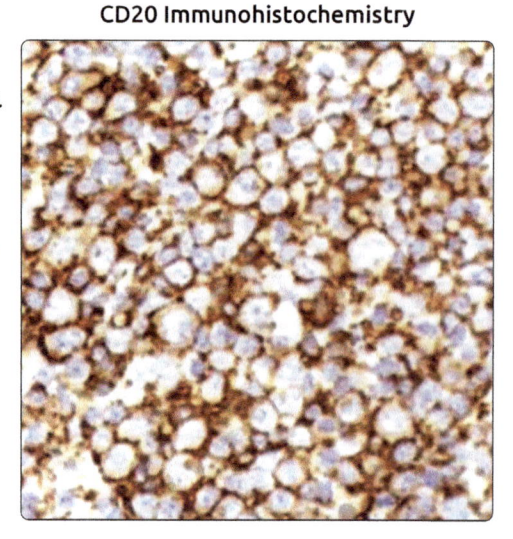

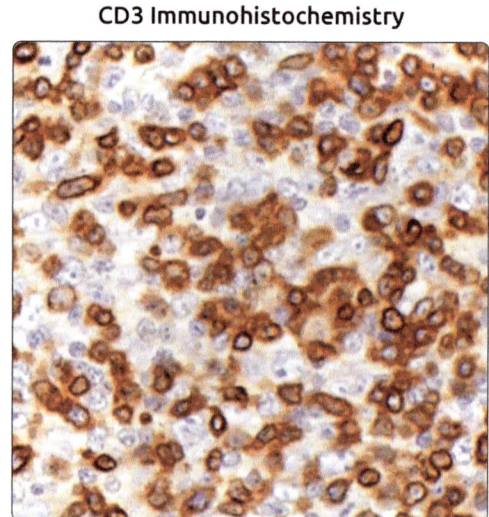

CD20 Immunohistochemistry

CD3 Immunohistochemistry

Diffuse Large B-Cell Lymphoma

Anaplastic Variant

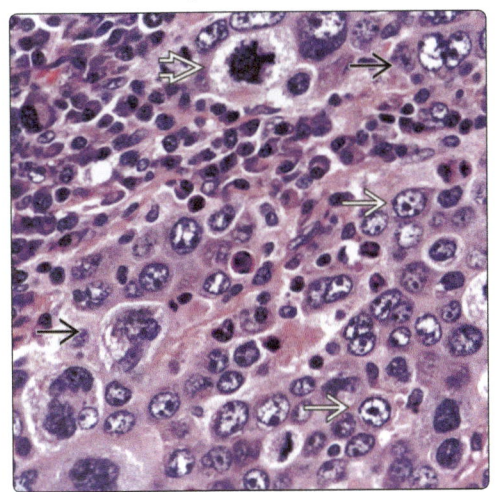

CD20(+) With Sinusoidal Growth Pattern

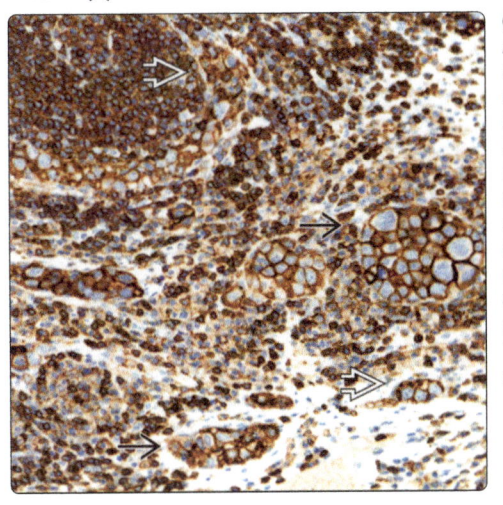

(Left) Anaplastic DLBCL is a morphologic variant. The cells are large and pleomorphic ➡ with bizarre mitoses ➡. There is a range of cell size among the neoplastic cells, including intermediate-sized cells ➡ as well as significantly enlarged cells. (Right) CD20 shows large, anaplastic-appearing B cells ➡. This case also showed CD30 positivity (not shown) in a diffuse membrane pattern. The cells are distributed in a sinusoidal pattern ➡.

Intravascular Large B-Cell Lymphoma

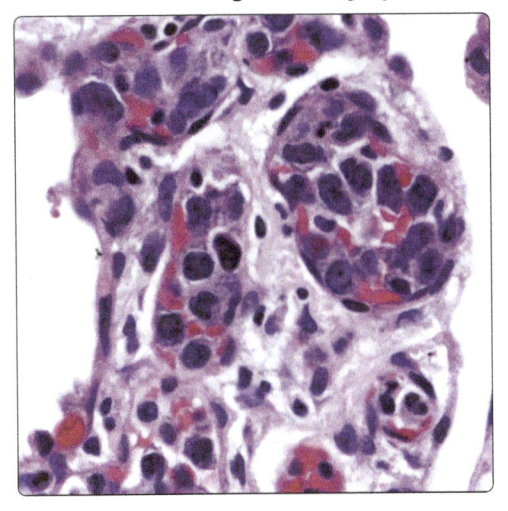

CD20(+) Intravascular Diffuse Large B-Cell Lymphoma

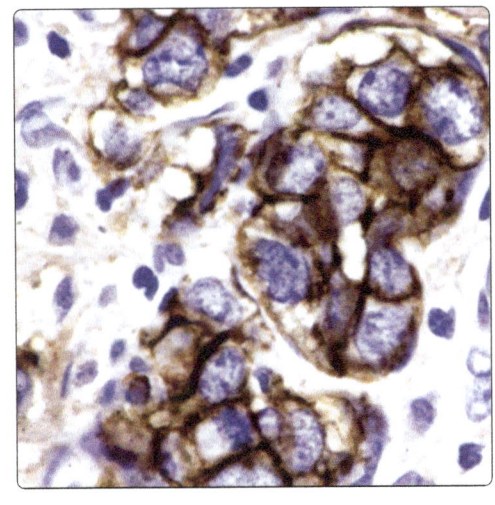

(Left) Intravascular large B-cell lymphoma has a distinct clinicopathologic presentation. Characteristically, there is skin or organ involvement with sparing of the lymph nodes. (Right) CD20 is positive in this case of intravascular large B-cell lymphoma. CD5 or CD10 may be coexpressed in a minority of cases. MUM1 may also be positive.

Primary Mediastinal Large B-Cell Lymphoma

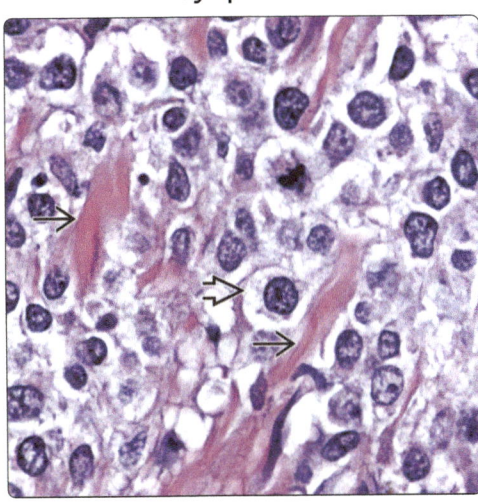

CD79A Immunohistochemistry

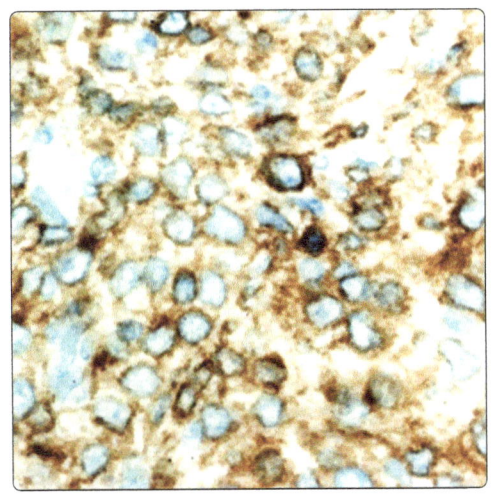

(Left) Primary mediastinal large B-cell lymphoma (PMBL) is shown. This type of large B-cell lymphoma is often localized to the mediastinum and, when disseminated, spares the lymph nodes. PMBL has a unique transcriptional signature, which shares features with classic Hodgkin lymphoma. Sclerosis is often present ➡. Large B cells have abundant cytoplasm ➡. (Right) CD79A shows diffuse staining in PMBL. CD30, MUM1, and CD23 are also expressed in the majority of cases.

Diffuse Large B-Cell Lymphoma

Plasmablastic Lymphoma

EBER In Situ Hybridization

(Left) *Plasmablastic lymphoma (PBL) of the nasopharynx shows CD138 and EBER positivity. CD20 is negative, but CD79A is weakly positive. Ki-67 is near 100%. The cells show plasmacytoid differentiation ➡. PBL is a specific type of DLBCL, but CD56 expression should raise suspicion for plasma cell myeloma rather than PBL.* (Right) *In situ hybridization for EBV (EBER) is positive in this DLBCL with a nuclear pattern of staining ➡.*

Burkitt Lymphoma

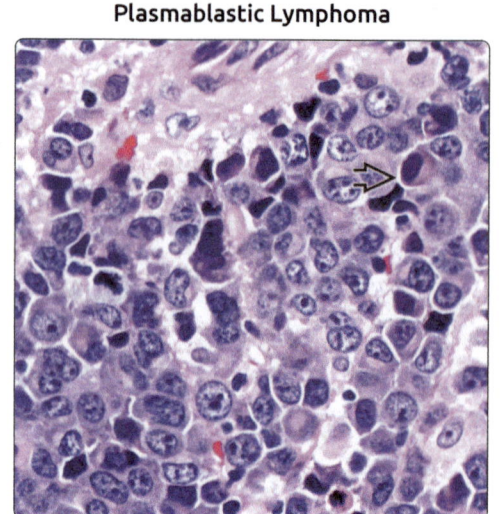

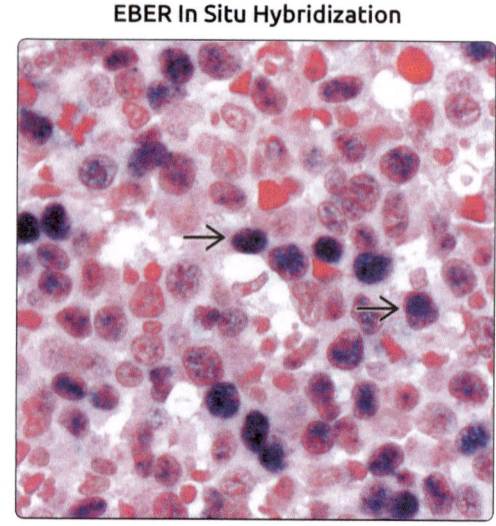

Burkitt Lymphoma

(Left) *Burkitt lymphoma of the nasopharynx shows predominantly intermediate-sized lymphoid cells with relatively fine chromatin ➡. Increased mitotic activity as well as numerous tingible body macrophages are present.* (Right) *High-power view of Burkitt lymphoma shows intermediate-sized cells with apoptosis ➡ and numerous histiocytes ➡ leading to the so-called starry-sky pattern. Mitoses are often numerous.*

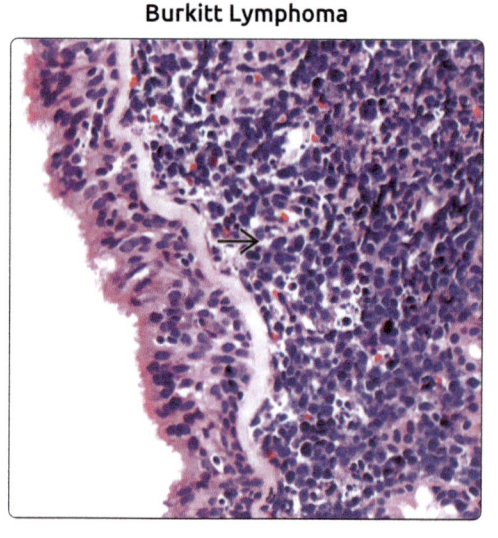

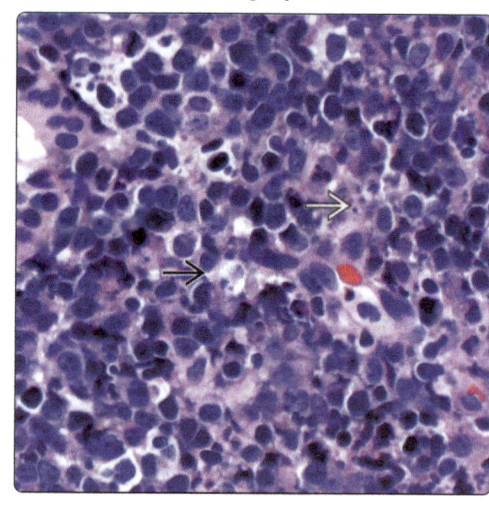

High Proliferation Rate by Ki-67

Burkitt Lymphoma Cytology

(Left) *High Ki-67 staining (virtually 100%) in a case of Burkitt lymphoma is shown.* (Right) *Peripheral blood shows circulating Burkitt lymphoma cells. The cells are large with cytoplasmic and intranuclear vacuoles ➡. Small nucleoli are present ➡. Although these cytologic findings are typically seen in Burkitt lymphoma, they are not pathognomonic and can also be seen in peripheralized DLBCL.*

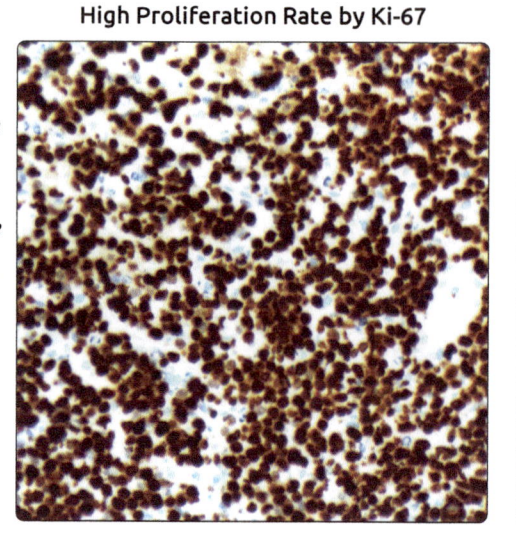

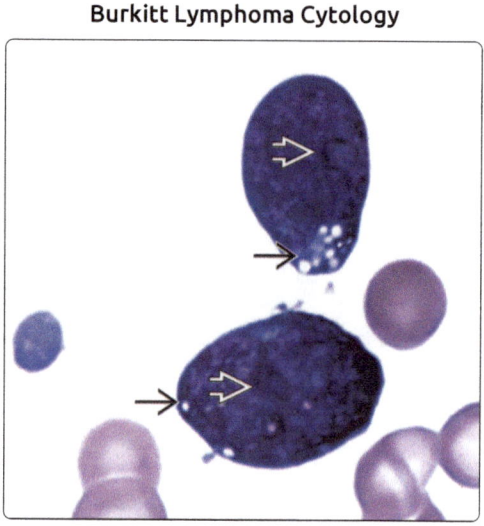

Diffuse Large B-Cell Lymphoma

Epithelioid Angiosarcoma

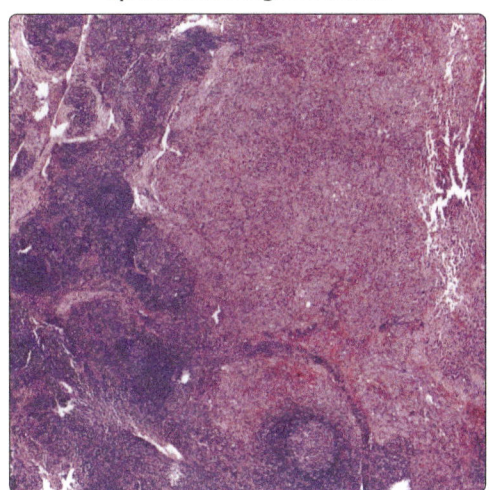

Epithelioid Angiosarcoma

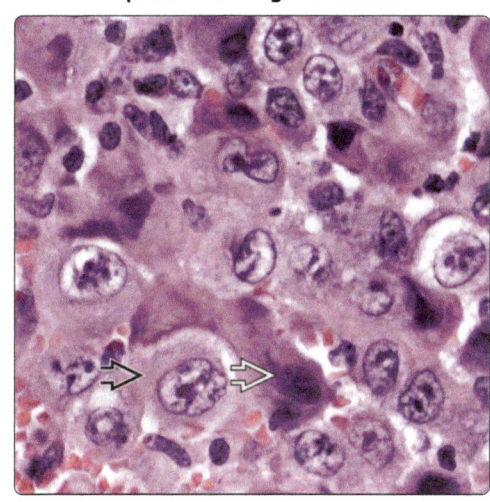

(Left) Low-power view of epithelioid angiosarcoma is shown. The lymph node is subtotally involved by this neoplasm and shows partial retention of the nodal architecture. (Right) High-power view shows large atypical cells, which resemble DLBCL. The cells contain abundant cytoplasm ⇨, and scattered mummified cells are also present ⇨.

CK-PAN Immunohistochemistry

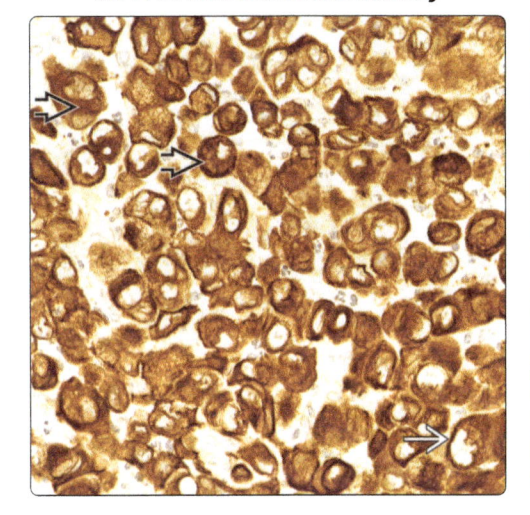

CD31 Immunohistochemistry

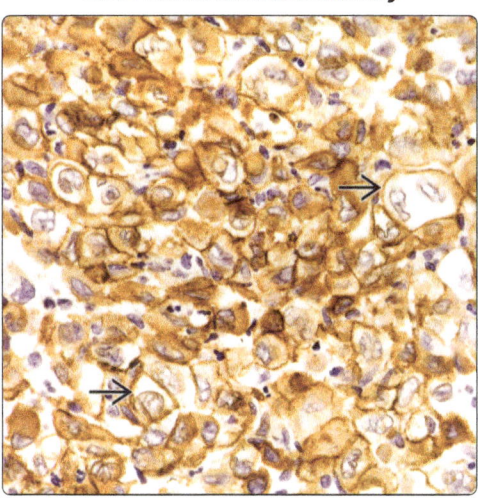

(Left) CK-PAN shows cytoplasmic ⇨ and membrane ⇨ positivity. Epithelioid angiosarcoma shows both epithelial and vascular antigen expression. (Right) Epithelioid angiosarcoma shows expression of CD31, a vascular marker. The membrane pattern of staining is appreciated ⇨.

Malignant Melanoma

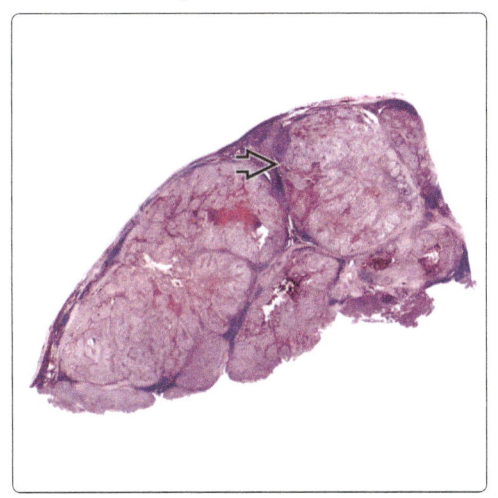

Malignant Melanoma

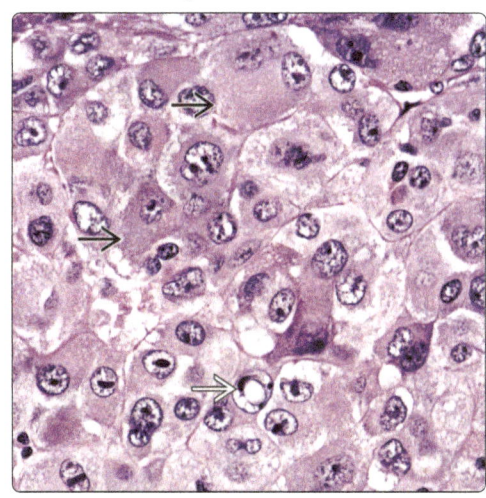

(Left) Low-power view shows spleen effaced by melanoma. Note the vaguely nodular appearance ⇨, but this is likely caused by tissue infiltration rather than true nodularity. (Right) High-power view shows large malignant cells with abundant cytoplasm ⇨ in a case of malignant melanoma. Intranuclear inclusions ⇨ are helpful in differentiating this neoplasm from DLBCL.

Diffuse Large B-Cell Lymphoma

Anaplastic Large Cell Lymphoma

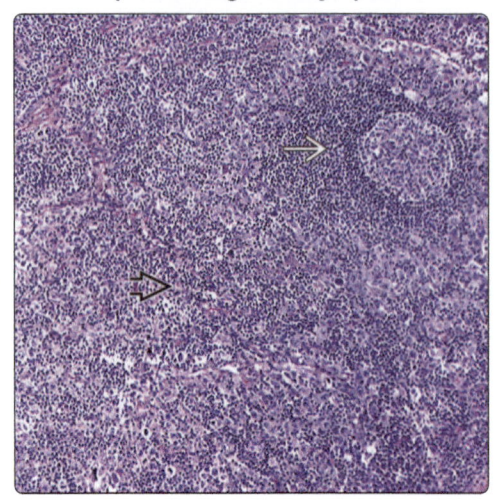

Morphology of Anaplastic Large Cell Lymphoma Cells

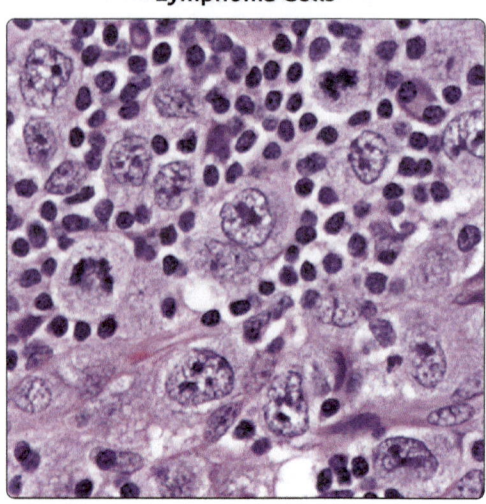

(Left) *Anaplastic large cell lymphoma (ALCL) in a lymph node is shown. The neoplastic cells are in the interfollicular area ⇨ with rare residual lymphoid follicles ➡.* (Right) *ALCL is usually pleomorphic but can appear similar to DLBCL. The cells in this case are somewhat monomorphic but have abundant cytoplasm. There is usually a background of small lymphocytes and eosinophils present.*

CD45 Immunohistochemistry

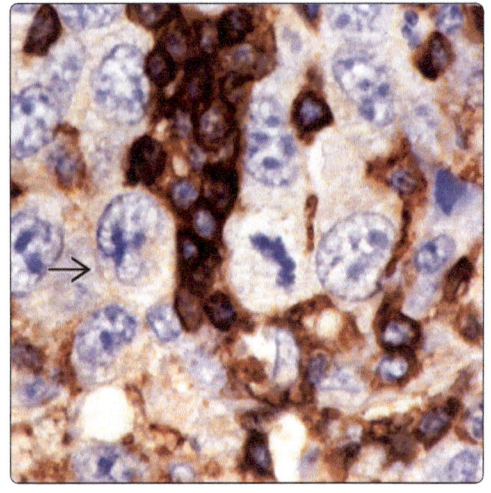

CD30 Immunohistochemistry

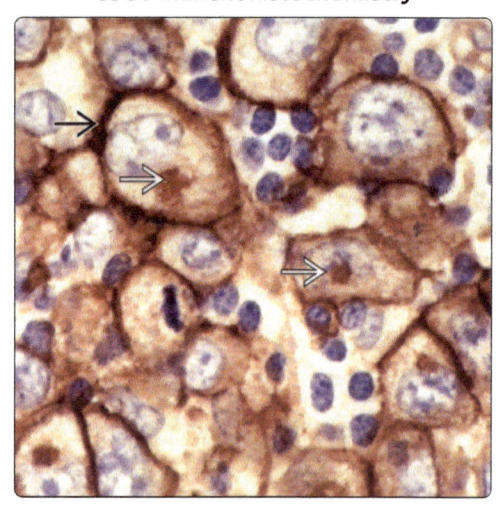

(Left) *CD45 is often variably positive in ALCL. The ALCL cells in this case are negative ⇨.* (Right) *CD30 is uniformly positive in ALCL. In this case, CD30 shows membrane ⇨ and Golgi positivity ➡. T-cell antigens can show variable staining.*

ALK Immunohistochemistry

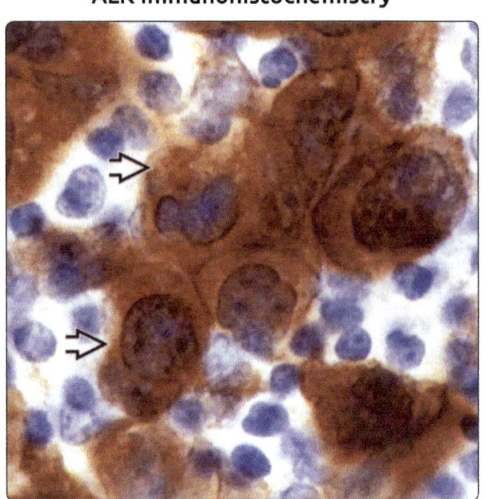

CD43 Immunohistochemistry

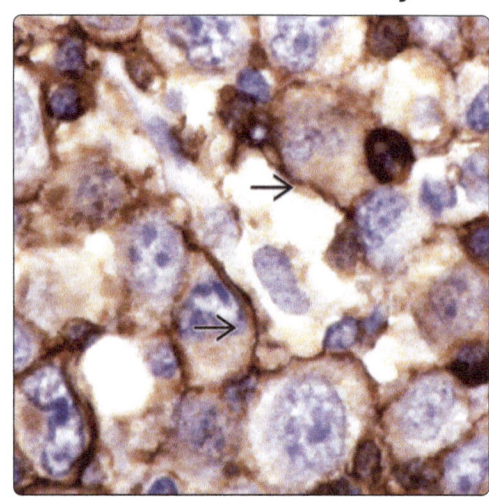

(Left) *ALK expression is nuclear and cytoplasmic in this case of ALK(+) ALCL ⇨, indicating that translocation t(2;5) is likely present. Other patterns of staining can be seen with alternative ALK fusions.* (Right) *T-cell antigens are variable in ALCL. However, CD43 is often positive, even in so-called null phenotype ALCL with a membranous pattern of staining ➡.*

Diffuse Large B-Cell Lymphoma

Histiocytic Sarcoma

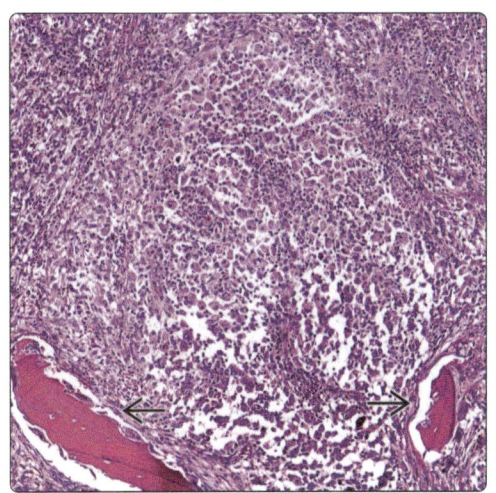

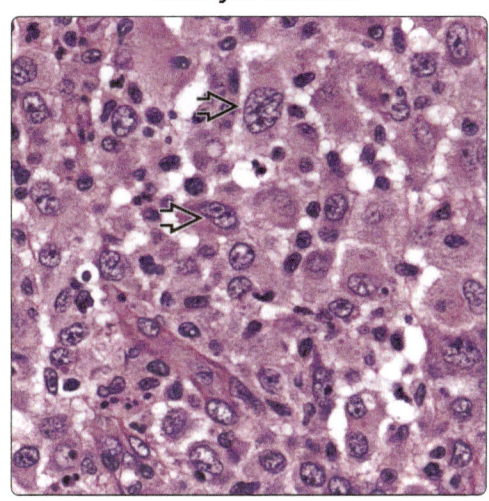

Histiocytic Sarcoma

(Left) Low-power view of histiocytic sarcoma shows malignant cells eroding bone ➔. Sheets and nodular aggregates of neoplastic cells are present. (Right) High-power view of histiocytic sarcoma is shown. The cells are large and appear pleomorphic, similar to DLBCL. There is abundant cytoplasm, and the nuclei are atypical ➔. The behavior of histiocytic sarcoma is variable.

CD163 Immunohistochemistry

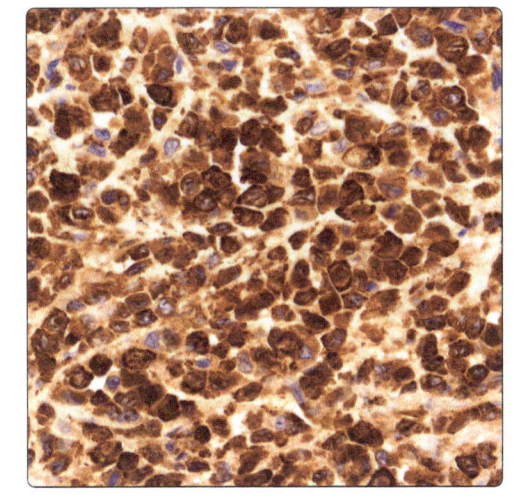

CD68 Immunohistochemistry

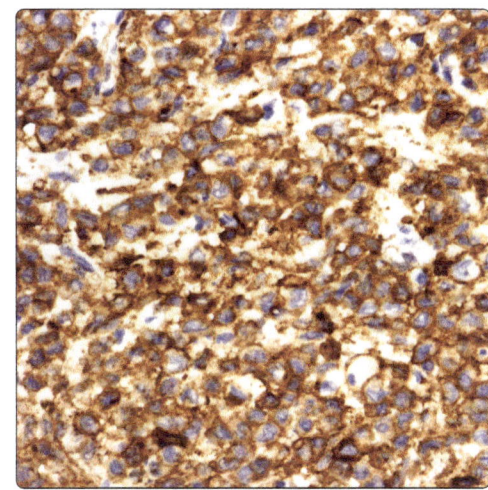

(Left) CD163, a histiocytic marker, stains the neoplastic cells of histiocytic sarcoma. (Right) CD68, another histiocyte marker, also characteristically stains histiocytic sarcoma.

Myeloid Sarcoma

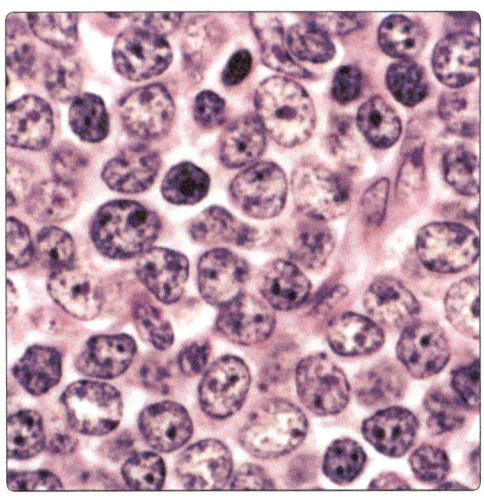

CD34 Immunohistochemistry

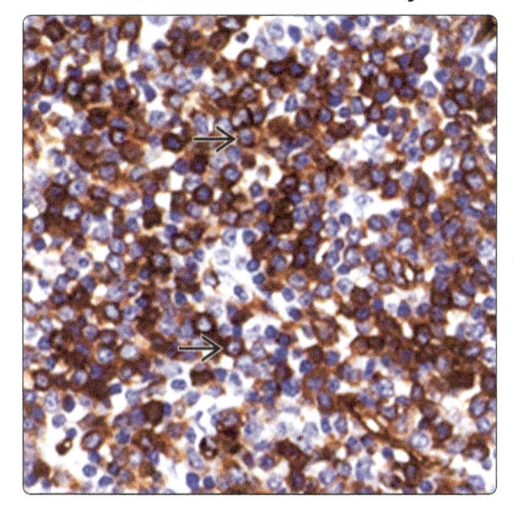

(Left) Large cells with fine chromatin that are fairly uniform in size are shown in this case of myeloid sarcoma, a malignant neoplasm composed of immature myeloid cells. (Right) CD34 highlights neoplastic cells ➔ in this example of myeloid sarcoma. Other immunohistochemical stains that are often positive in myeloid sarcoma include CD117, MPO, and CD68. TdT may rarely be positive.

Burkitt Lymphoma

KEY FACTS

TERMINOLOGY
- Burkitt lymphoma (BL): Highly aggressive lymphoma, often extranodal with high mitotic rate
- Translocation of *MYC* protooncogene to immunoglobulin heavy chain gene, κ-light chain or λ-light chain gene leads to *MYC* activation
  - t(8;14), t(8;22), and t(2;8)

CLINICAL ISSUES
- 3 clinical variants of BL
  - Endemic BL in equatorial Africa and associated with EBV in almost all cases
  - Sporadic BL in West in immunocompetent patients
  - Immunodeficiency-associated BL, more common in HIV

MICROSCOPIC
- B cells with rounded edges (cobblestoning), macrophages with phagocytosed debris (starry-sky pattern)

ANCILLARY TESTS
- Germinal center phenotype: CD10(+), BCL6(+)
- *MYC* translocation is characteristic of BL but can be seen in other non-Hodgkin lymphomas
- BL karyotype is usually simple, unlike other high-grade lymphomas
- Gene expression profiling has distinct profile for BL

TOP DIFFERENTIAL DIAGNOSES
- Diffuse large B-cell lymphoma
  - 15% have *MYC* alterations, but lower proliferative rate, and BCL2 can be strongly (+)
  - *MYC* can have translocations with nonimmunoglobulin genes
- High-grade B-cell lymphoma with *MYC* and *BCL2* rearrangements
  - Worse prognosis
- High-grade B-cell lymphoma with 11q aberration
  - Lacks *MYC* alteration but has 11q aberration

Uniform Lymphoma Cells

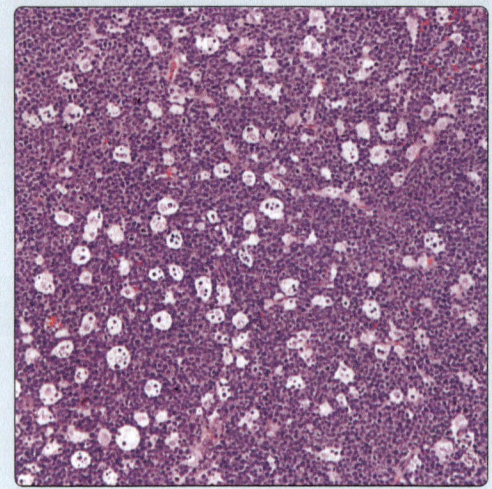

t(8;14) by Cytogenetics

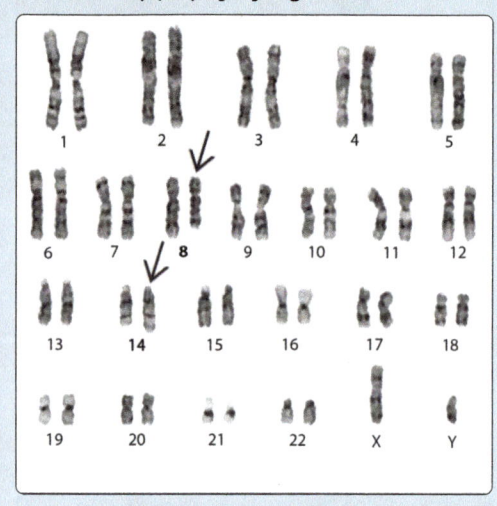

(Left) *H&E of Burkitt lymphoma (BL) shows sheets of uniform lymphoma cells with evenly interspersed, reactive, tingible-body macrophages imparting a characteristic starry-sky pattern.* (Right) *Conventional cytogenetic analysis in a case of BL shows a karyotype with the most common translocation, t(8;14)(q24;q32)➠. (Courtesy L. Abruzzo, MD.)*

Clear Vacuoles

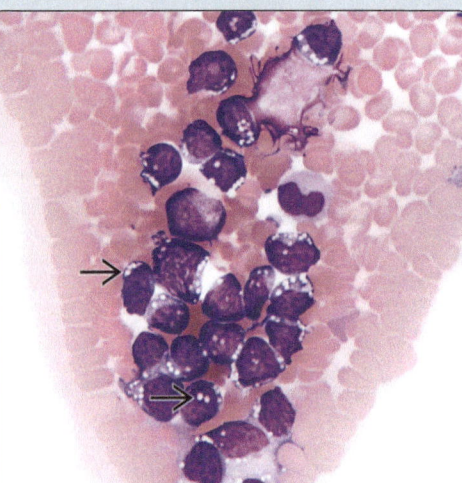

MYC Gene Rearrangement

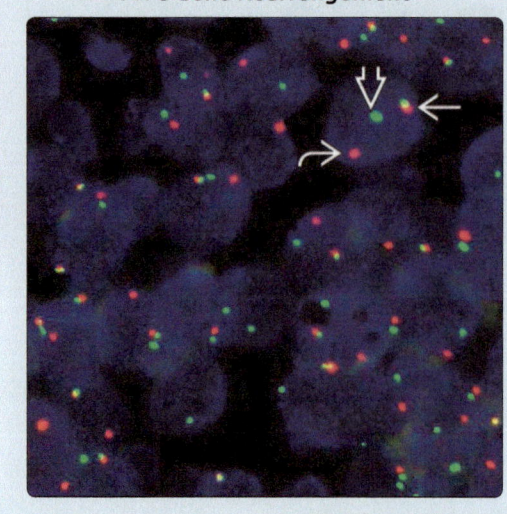

(Left) *Touch imprint of a bone marrow biopsy from a patient with BL is shown. The lymphocytes are often medium-sized with basophilic cytoplasm and numerous clear vacuoles ➠.* (Right) *Break-apart FISH probe looks for MYC rearrangement in a case of BL. MYC rearrangement is identified, as evident by 1 red, ➠ 1 green ➠, and 1 yellow ➠ signal in each cell.*

Burkitt Lymphoma

TERMINOLOGY

Abbreviations
- Burkitt lymphoma (BL)

Synonyms
- Small, noncleaved cell lymphoma, Burkitt type (working formulation)
- Undifferentiated, Burkitt type (Rappaport classification)
- Acute lymphoblastic leukemia, L3 type (French-American-British classification)

Definitions
- Mature aggressive lymphoma of medium-sized B cells with high proliferative index, germinal center phenotype and IG::MYC rearrangement
  - Translocation of MYC protooncogene to immunoglobulin heavy chain gene, κ-light chain gene, or λ-light chain gene leads to MYC overexpression

ETIOLOGY/PATHOGENESIS

Classification
- 3 clinicopathologic variants of BL
  - Endemic
  - Sporadic
  - Immunodeficiency associated
- 2 WHO subtypes
  - Epstein-Barr virus (EBV)-associated BL and EBV(-) BL
  - Some studies indicate that EBV(+) or EBV(-) subtypes correlate better than 3 clinicopathologic variants
  - EBV(+) BL and EBV(-) BL form discrete biologic groups based on their molecular features regardless of epidemiologic content and geographic location
  - EBV(+) BL shows significantly higher somatic mutations compared to EBV(-) cases
  - Distinction of EBV(+) BL vs. EBV(-) BL is recommended by WHO 5th edition

MYC::IG Translocation
- Considered driver mutation of BL
- Juxtapose intact MYC gene to either IGH, IGL or IGK locus resulting in MYC upregulation
  - MYC is involved in many cell pathways: Proliferation, transcription, apoptosis

Infectious Agents
- Evidence that BL is polymicrobial disease
- Association of BL with EBV infection
  - EBV(+) in
    - > 95% of endemic BL cases
    - ~ 30-40% of immunodeficiency-associated BL cases
    - ~ 20% of sporadic BL cases
  - EBV may be early in pathogenesis, so that B cells can avoid apoptosis possibly before MYC translocation
- *Plasmodium falciparum* infection associated with endemic BL
  - Geographic distribution of endemic BL corresponds to distribution of malaria
  - Impact on immunity and viral persistence leading to reactivation of latently infected memory B cells
- Arboviruses associated with endemic BL
  - Mosquitoes carry arboviruses as they carry malaria
    - Arboviruses are RNA viruses, and some have oncogenic properties
- Immunodeficiency
  - HIV can cause chronic antigenic stimulation
  - May exhaust EBV-specific cytotoxic T cells
  - May therefore allow EBV-driven lymphomagenesis
- Some rare inherited disorders have high risk of BL
  - Supports genetic predisposition for BL
  - Includes ataxia telangiectasia, Purtilo/Duncon syndrome/XLP, Williams-Beuren syndrome, and XMEN disease

Dietary Factors
- Diet may be relevant to endemic BL
  - In Africa, link to ingestion of *Euphorbia tirucalli*
    - Plant has phorbol ester-like substance that may act as tumor promoter

CLINICAL ISSUES

Epidemiology
- Incidence
  - Endemic BL
    - Common in equatorial Africa, Northern South America, Papua New Guinea
    - Most common type of lymphoma in equatorial Africa
  - Sporadic BL
    - ~ 1-2% of lymphomas in industrialized nations
- Age
  - Endemic BL
    - Children > 2 years of age and adolescents
    - Median: 8 years
  - Sporadic BL
    - Less common in children
    - ~ 30-50% of childhood lymphomas in USA
  - Immunodeficiency-associated BL
    - Age corresponds to cause of immunodeficiency
    - Most patients HIV positive
- Sex
  - M:F = 3:1

Site
- Most patients with BL present with extranodal disease
- Endemic BL
  - Jaws and other facial bones most often involved
  - Viscera, gonads, gastrointestinal tract
  - Central nervous system involved in up to 20% of patients
- Sporadic BL
  - Abdomen, particularly gastrointestinal tract
  - Orbit, Waldeyer ring, breast, ovaries, and testes
  - Small subset of cases can present in leukemic phase
    - Bone marrow usually extensively involved in these patients
- Immunodeficiency-associated BL (iBL)
  - Lymph nodes preferentially affected
  - Bone marrow and peripheral blood seen in 20% of iBL
- All variants can show CNS involvement

Presentation
- Patients present with rapidly growing mass

Burkitt Lymphoma

- B-type symptoms are common

Laboratory Tests
- Indirect indicators of tumor burden and proliferation
  - High serum β-2-microglobin level
  - High serum lactate dehydrogenase level
- Hyperuricemia can occur due to high tumor cell turnover

Natural History
- Widely disseminated disease
- Rapidly growing progressive masses

Treatment
- Drugs
  - Rapid administration of multiple chemotherapeutic agents with prophylaxis to CNS &/or testes
    - Eliminate disease in privileged or sanctuary sites
  - BL very sensitive to chemotherapy
    - Rapid release of intracellular contents following cell death can result in tumor lysis syndrome

Prognosis
- With highly intensive therapy, most patients with BL have complete response
  - Overall survival rate
    - > 90% for children
    - > 80% for adults
- Worse prognosis in low-/middle-resource settings

IMAGING

CT Findings
- F-18 FDG PET/CT
  - All untreated BL highly FDG avid
  - Extranodal involvement identified in > 50% of BL patients
  - Most patients with sporadic BL have disease localized to abdomen and pelvis
- Conventional cytogenetics may miss some *IG::MYC*
  - Cryptic insertions of *MYC* into *IGH* are reported

MACROSCOPIC

Gross Pathology
- Resection specimens of BL often show large, extranodal mass, often in abdomen
- Fleshy cut surface with areas of necrosis and hemorrhage

MOLECULAR

Cytogenetics
- *MYC* translocations are characteristic
  - Partners are immunoglobulin gene loci: *IGH*, *IGK*, and *IGL*
    - t(8;14)(q24;q32) in ~ 80% of cases
    - t(8;22)(q24;q11) in ~ 15% of cases
    - t(2;8)(p11;q24) in ~ 5% of cases
- Other cytogenetic aberrations common in BL
  - Abnormalities of chromosomes 1 and 13 may be related to poor prognosis
    - Secondary chromosomal abnormalities usually in pediatric BL
  - No evidence of t(14;18); *IGH::BCL2* or *BCL6* translocations
  - Complex karyotype should not be present at time of diagnosis
    - If present, consider other high-grade B-cell lymphoma

In Situ Hybridization
- EBER(+) in > 95% of endemic cases, ~ 30-40% of immunodeficiency-associated cases, and ~ 10-20% of sporadic cases of BL
  - EBNA1 expressed, but EBNA2 and EBNA3 usually absent
  - EBNA2 and EBNA3 are either downregulated in BL or they are not required for neoplastic transformation
- FISH
  - Break-apart probe commonly used to demonstrate *MYC* translocations
    - Does not show which partner gene is involved
  - 90% of cases detect *MYC* rearrangement by FISH
  - 10% of cases do not show *MYC* rearrangement by FISH
    - Other techniques, such as cytogenetics or PCR, may detect *MYC* rearrangement in cases that are negative by FISH

PCR
- *MYC*
  - *MYC* breakpoints
    - Endemic BL has *MYC* breakpoints that can be several hundreds of kilobases upstream of MYC promoter
    - Sporadic BL and iBL have *MYC* breakpoints that are nearby upstream (5') or within 1st exon or intron of *MYC*
    - In *IGK::MYC* and *IGL::MYC*, breakpoints in 8q24 are usually downstream (3') of *MYC*
  - High false-negative rate due to
    - 3 partner genes
    - Extensive breakpoint heterogeneity
- *IGH*
  - Monoclonal *IGH* gene rearrangement
  - False-negative results in subset of cases due to somatic mutations of *IGH* gene
- No evidence of T-cell receptor gene rearrangements

Next-Generation Sequencing
- Detected *TCF3* mutations and its negative regulator *ID3* in BL
  - Activates PI3K pathway, promoting cell survival
  - Activates cell cycle genes, such as *CCND3* activating cell proliferation
  - *TCF3* or *ID3* gene alterations activate BCR signaling
  - Found in EBV(-) and EBV(+) BL
- *TP53* mutations
  - Detected in up to 1/2 of BL cases
  - Common in EBV(-) BL

Chromosomal Microarray
- ~ 65% of BL shows genetic alterations in addition to *MYC* translocations
  - Gains, amplifications, and losses
    - Most frequent gains: 1q, 7/7q, 8q24-qter, 12, amplification of 13q31-32
    - Most frequent loss: 17p12-pter

Gene Expression Profiling
- Shows signatures for BL that are distinct from DLBCL

Burkitt Lymphoma

- High level of expression: *MYC* and target genes
- Low level of expression: NF-κB target genes and major histocompatibility complex class I genes
- Expression of subgroup of germinal center B-cell genes
- No differences exist between pediatric and adult cases of BL
- Although BL subtypes share common gene expression signatures, sporadic BL can be distinguished from endemic and immunodeficiency-associated BL by gene expression profiling
- Some signature differences between endemic BL and sporadic BL
- Double-hit lymphomas can share BL gene expression signature
  - Can show signature intermediate between BL and diffuse large B-cell lymphoma

MYC-Regulated MicroRNAs
- MicroRNAs are small, 20-24 nucleotide, non-protein-coding, single-stranded RNA
  - Inhibit mRNAs from being translated **or** cause them to be degraded
- MicroRNAs that are repressed by MYC
  - miR-15a/16-1, miR-34a, and let-7 family members
  - miR-9 and miR-34b are downregulated on MYC translocation negative BL cases
- MicroRNAs that are activated by MYC
  - miR-17-5p, miR-20a
- EBV miRNAs are beginning to be identified, and their role in BL pathogenesis may soon become apparent

MICROSCOPIC

Histologic Features
- Morphologic features of endemic, sporadic, and immunodeficiency-associated BL are identical
- Diffuse growth pattern
- Starry-sky pattern is prominent due to presence of numerous scattered tingible body macrophages with phagocytosed debris
- Extremely high mitotic rate
- Numerous apoptotic cells and often large areas of necrosis
- Granulomas in BL
  - Often in EBV(+) cases
  - Usually early stage disease, good prognosis
  - Even spontaneous remission

Cytologic Features
- Monomorphic neoplastic cells with respect to nuclear size, shape, and cytoplasm
  - Intermediate cell size with nuclear size ≤ histiocyte nuclei
  - Central nuclei with 2-5 small basophilic nucleoli
  - Some nucleoli are located on nuclear membrane
- Cytoplasm is moderate in amount and highly basophilic
  - Cytoplasm tends to square off with adjacent cells
    - Provides cobblestone or jigsaw puzzle appearance
  - Numerous lipid vacuoles present
    - Cannot appreciate on H&E-stained sections
    - Easily observed on Wright-Giemsa-stained touch imprint
- Rare cases of iBL show plasmacytoid differentiation

- Cases that show more pleomorphic cells are still considered BL, and term "atypical BL" is no longer used

Lymph Nodes
- Diffuse effacement of architecture with prominent starry-sky pattern
- In subset of cases, lymphoid follicles can be colonized, imparting nodular pattern; usually focal

Peripheral Blood and Bone Marrow
- Occasional tumor cells can be found in blood smears of subset of BL patients
  - Careful search may be required to identify neoplastic cells
- Small subset of patients present with overt leukemia
  - High leukocyte count and numerous BL cells in blood smear
  - Bone marrow biopsy specimen is diffusely replaced
    - Starry-sky pattern &/or necrosis can be prominent
  - Blood and bone marrow smears show intermediate-sized cells with numerous cytoplasmic vacuoles

ANCILLARY TESTS

Cytology
- Fine-needle aspiration smears
  - "Dirty" background may be present due to necrosis
  - Numerous mitotic figures and apoptotic cells
  - Nuclei may be round, oval, or clefted
  - Stippled chromatin, 2-5 nucleoli
  - Well-defined rim of basophilic cytoplasm with many vacuoles (Wright-Giemsa)

Histochemistry
- BL is strongly positive for methyl green pyronine stain
  - This is because cells have numerous cytoplasmic polyribosomes
  - Positive in cytoplasmic vacuoles (neutral lipids)
  - Can be shown in frozen sections, touch imprints, or smears

Immunohistochemistry
- Pan B-cell antigens (+), T-cell specific antigens (-)
- Germinal center-associated antigens: CD10, BCL6, HGAL, and MEF2B (+)
  - HGAL variable (+), LMO2(-)
- Aberrant CD43, LEF1, SOX11, and TCL1A can be seen
- MYC expression
- Diffusely (+) in > 80% of cells in almost all cases
- Rare cases MYC(-) despite *MYC* gene rearrangement
- CD45(+), CD43 frequently (+)
- Ki-67 shows very high proliferation rate
  - Usually, virtually every cell is positive with uniform, bright intensity
  - Generally ≥ 95% (100% is not uncommon)
- BCL2(-) or weakly positive
- TdT(-), CD34(-), IRF4(+/-), CD5(-), CD138(-), CD23(-)
- Adipophilin (+) in cytoplasmic lipid vacuoles
- Few reactive T cells admixed within BL
- Monotypic cytoplasmic (c) Ig(+) in subset of cases
  - Plasmacytoid variant of BL is positive for cIg

Burkitt Lymphoma

- Aberrant phenotypes, including CD5(+) and CD10(-), are more often seen in sporadic BL in older patients

Flow Cytometry
- Monotypic surface IgM(+); κ > λ
- CD10(+), CD38(+), CD71(+)
- HLA-DR(+), FMC7(+)
- CD44(+), CD54(+) in most cases; LFA-1(-)

DIFFERENTIAL DIAGNOSIS

Diffuse Large B-Cell Lymphoma
- *MYC* alterations reportedly occur in 10-15%
  - More frequent in highly proliferative cases
  - May have complex karyotype by cytogenetics
- Less often show starry-sky pattern
- Large lymphoma cells with vesicular chromatin
  - Centroblastic and immunoblastic variants
- Subset of cases can have immunophenotype identical to BL
- Proliferation rate usually < 80%

High-Grade B-Cell Lymphoma, NOS
- Some cases are histologically similar to BL, can have *MYC* rearrangement
  - Usually lack CD10 and are strongly BCL2(+)

High Grade B-Cell Lymphoma With *MYC* and *BCL2* Rearrangements
- Previously called double-hit or triple-hit lymphomas
  - t(14;18)(q32;q21); *IGH::BCL2* &/or *BCL6* rearrangements
- May exhibit cytologic spectrum of intermediate- and large-sized cells
- May be BCL2(+) and have variable TDT expression
- Cytogenetic analysis may shows complex karyotype
- Chromosomal microarray may show multiple gains and losses
- Often more aggressive prognosis than DLBCL or BL

High Grade B-Cell Lymphoma With 11q Aberration
- Cases which histologically look like BL with similar phenotype and gene expression profiles but lack *MYC* gene rearrangement
- Chromosome 11q alteration characterized by proximal interstitial gains of 11q23.2-q23.3 and telomeric losses of 11q24.1-qter
- As compared to BL, Burkitt-like lymphoma with 11q aberration is more likely to
  - Occur within lymph nodes
  - Show less MYC protein expression by immunohistochemistry
  - Have more complex karyotypes as seen by classic cytogenetics
  - Display more cytological pleomorphism
  - Sometimes show follicular growth pattern on H&E

B-Lymphoblastic Lymphoma/Leukemia
- Small- to medium-sized blasts with fine chromatin, absent or small inconspicuous nucleoli
- TdT(+), CD34(+), surface Ig(-)
- ~ 3% of cases have t(8;14)(q24;q32)
  - Chromosome breaks are in *IGH* joining regions and many different switch regions

Mantle Cell Lymphoma, Blastoid Variant
- *MYC* translocations have only been rarely reported
  - t(11;14)(q13;q32) typically identified
- Can have prominent starry-sky pattern
- CD5(+), cyclin-D1 (+), unlike BL

Pediatric-Type Follicular Lymphoma
- Intermediate to large blastoid cells
- Usually in follicular pattern
- CD10(+), BCL6(+), BCL2(-)/weak
- Ki-67 > 30%, MYC(-)
- CD21(+) follicular dendritic cell meshworks
- No *MYC*, *BCL2*, *BCL6*, or *IRF4* translocations

DIAGNOSTIC CHECKLIST

Clinically Relevant Pathologic Features
- 3 clinicopathologic variants of BL
  - Endemic, sporadic, and immunodeficiency-associated
    - Endemic BL occurs in equatorial Africa, 100% EBV(+)
- Rapidly growing mass that is frequently extranodal

Pathologic Interpretation Pearls
- *MYC* translocations are characteristic of BL
  - t(8;14)(q24;q32) in ~ 80%
  - Variant translocations, t(2;8)(p12;q24) or t(8;22)(q24;q11) in ~ 20%
- *MYC* translocations can also be found in DLBCL and rarely in B-cell lymphoblastic leukemia/lymphoma and mantle cell lymphoma
- Immunophenotype
  - IgM(+), CD10(+), BCL6(+), Ki-67 high (≥ 95%), BCL2(-)

SELECTED REFERENCES

1. Alaggio R et al: The 5th edition of the World Health Organization Classification of Haematolymphoid Tumours: Lymphoid Neoplasms. Leukemia. 36(7):1720-48, 2022
2. Campo E et al: The International Consensus Classification of Mature Lymphoid Neoplasms: a report from the Clinical Advisory Committee. Blood. 140(11):1229-53, 2022
3. Wilke AC et al: SHMT2 inhibition disrupts the TCF3 transcriptional survival program in Burkitt lymphoma. Blood. 139(4):538-53, 2022
4. Woroniecka R et al: Cryptic MYC insertions in Burkitt lymphoma: new data and a review of the literature. PLoS One. 17(2):e0263980, 2022
5. Ott G et al: [Revised version of the 4th edition of the WHO classification of malignant lymphomas: what is new?.] Pathologe. 40(2):157-68, 2019
6. Swerdlow SH et al: The 2016 revision of the World Health Organization (WHO) classification of lymphoid neoplasms. Blood. 127(20):2375-90, 2016
7. Ferreiro JF et al: Post-transplant molecularly defined Burkitt lymphomas are frequently MYC-negative and characterized by the 11q-gain/loss pattern. Haematologica. 100(7):e275-9, 2015
8. De Souza MT et al: Conventional and molecular cytogenetic characterization of Burkitt lymphoma with bone marrow involvement in Brazilian children and adolescents. Pediatr Blood Cancer. 61(8):1422-6, 2014
9. Greenough A et al: New clues to the molecular pathogenesis of Burkitt lymphoma revealed through next-generation sequencing. Curr Opin Hematol. 21(4):326-32, 2014
10. Said J et al: Burkitt lymphoma and MYC: what else is new? Adv Anat Pathol. 21(3):160-5, 2014
11. Salaverria I et al: A recurrent 11q aberration pattern characterizes a subset of MYC-negative high-grade B-cell lymphomas resembling Burkitt lymphoma. Blood. 123(8):1187-98, 2014
12. Love C et al: The genetic landscape of mutations in Burkitt lymphoma. Nat Genet. 44(12):1321-5, 2012
13. Schmitz R et al: Burkitt lymphoma pathogenesis and therapeutic targets from structural and functional genomics. Nature. 490(7418):116-20, 2012

Burkitt Lymphoma

Molecular Pathology of Lymphoid Neoplasms

FISH *MYC* Break-Apart Probe

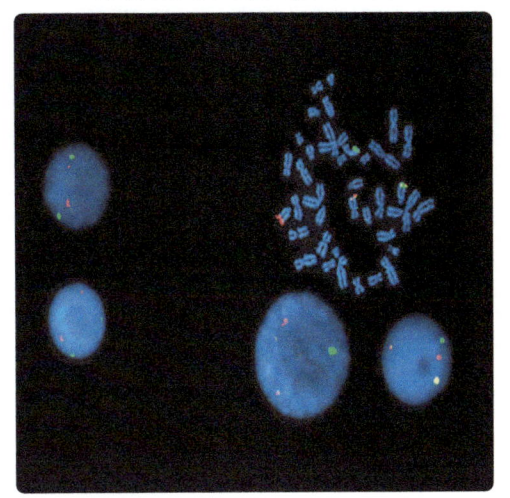

No *MYC* Gene Rearrangement

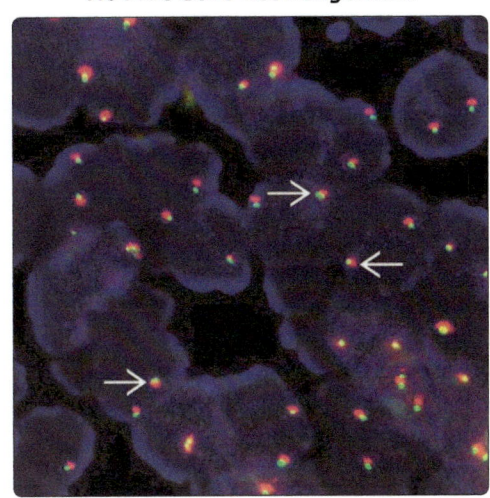

(Left) *In this break-apart FISH probe for MYC, 1 allele shows colocalization of red and green signals (normal), and 1 allele shows segregation of both probes.* **(Right)** *In this break-apart FISH probe for MYC, MYC gene rearrangement is not detected. A normal nucleus produces 2 yellow signals; the red and green signals ➔ remain together. MYC rearrangement is characteristic of BL.*

PCR for *IGH* Gene Rearrangement

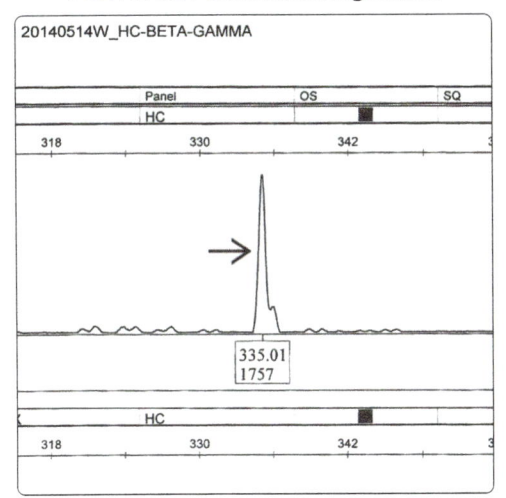

BCL6 Gene Rearrangement

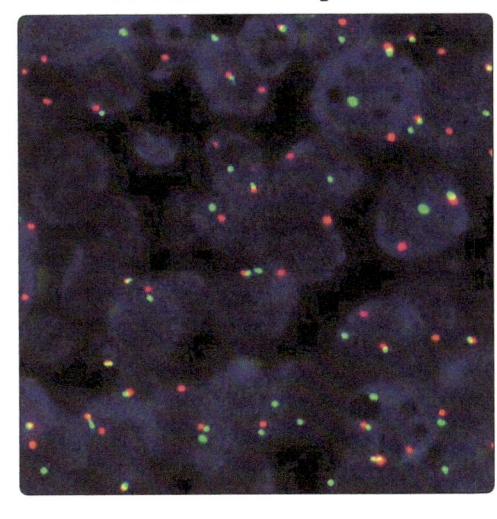

(Left) *This is an example of PCR for immunoglobulin heavy chain gene rearrangement. A dominant monoclonal peak ➔ is observed, indicative of the monoclonality of BL.* **(Right)** *This case, which morphologically looks like BL, shows BCL6 gene rearrangement with separated red and green signals. This case, which also had MYC rearrangement, would now be reclassified as high-grade B-cell lymphoma with MYC and BCL6 rearrangements.*

Classic Cytogenetics

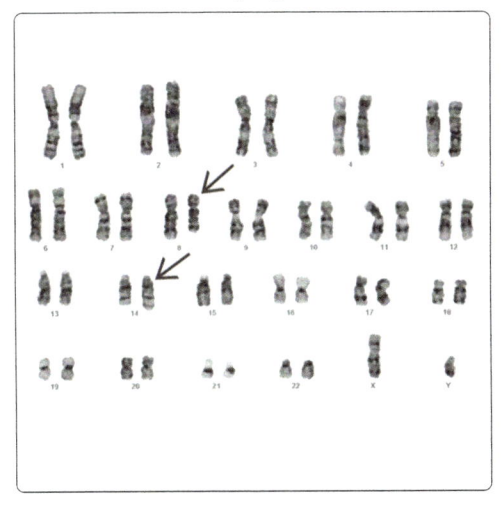

Translocation of *MYC* With *IGL*

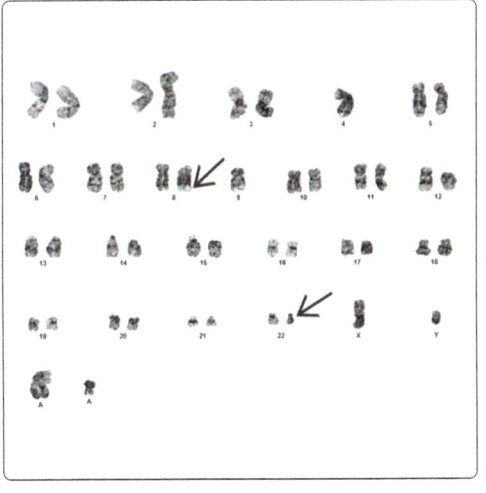

(Left) *Classic cytogenetic karyotyping shows t(8;14)(q24;q32) ➔ in a case of gastric BL. This translocation of the MYC protooncogene to the immunoglobulin heavy chain leads to MYC overexpression. This translocation is detected in ~ 80% of BL cases by cytogenetics.* **(Right)** *This karyotype shows t(8;22)(q24;q11) ➔, which is found in ~ 15% of BL cases. The MYC gene on chromosome 8 translocates with the IGL gene at 22q11.*

Burkitt Lymphoma

(Left) *Graphic shows that breakpoints are different in endemic BL (eBL) and sporadic BL (sBL). In eBL, the breakpoint on IGH occurs usually within the joining region, whereas for sBL, it occurs within the switch regions.* **(Right)** *This case of BL shows medium-sized cells, similar to the size of benign histiocyte nuclei. The lymphoma cells have round nuclear contours, multiple indistinct nucleoli, and basophilic cytoplasm. Macrophages with engulfed pyknotic nuclei are also present.*

Varying Breakpoints in Endemic and Sporadic Subtypes

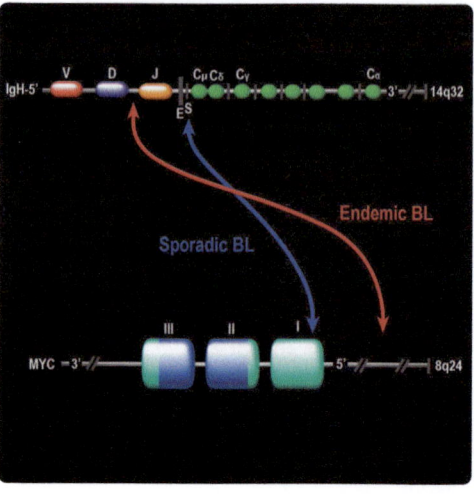

Medium-Sized Cells

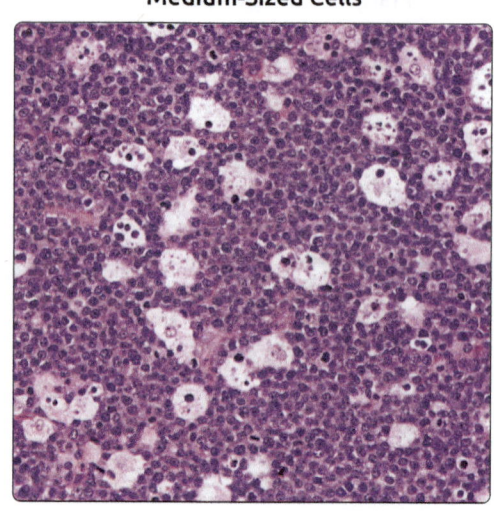

(Left) *CD20 shows that the neoplastic cells are strongly positive ➡. This neoplasm was also positive for CD19, CD38, and CD43 (not shown).* **(Right)** *BL has a germinal center phenotype. CD10 shows that the neoplastic cells are strongly and uniformly positive ➡. Other germinal center markers, such as BCL6, are also typically positive.*

CD20 Immunohistochemistry

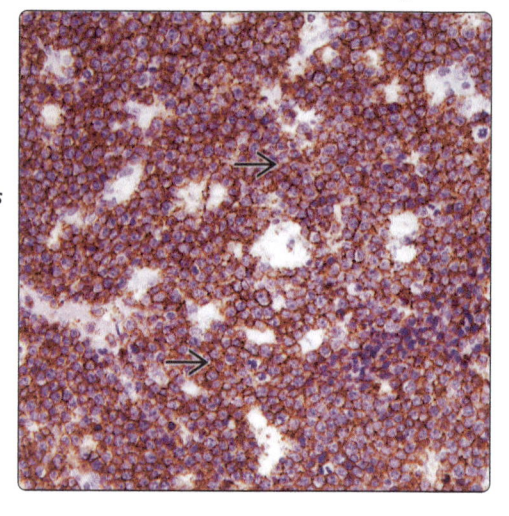

CD10 Immunohistochemistry

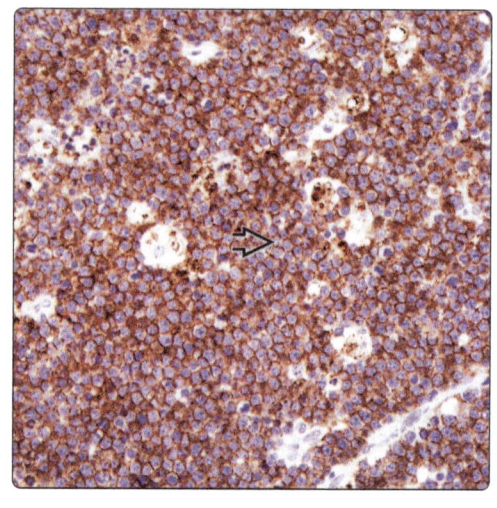

(Left) *In this case of BL, the lymphoma cells are negative for BCL2 ➡. BL is usually BCL2(-), although a subset of cases (~ 20%) may be weakly positive.* **(Right)** *Ki-67 shows that virtually all of the lymphoma cells in BL are strongly positive and therefore proliferating. Typically, BL cases have a very high proliferation rate (> 95%), whereas in cases of diffuse large B-cell lymphoma (DLBCL), Ki-67 proliferation index will not typically exceed 80%.*

BCL2 Immunohistochemistry

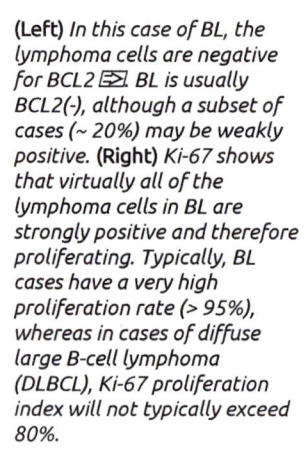

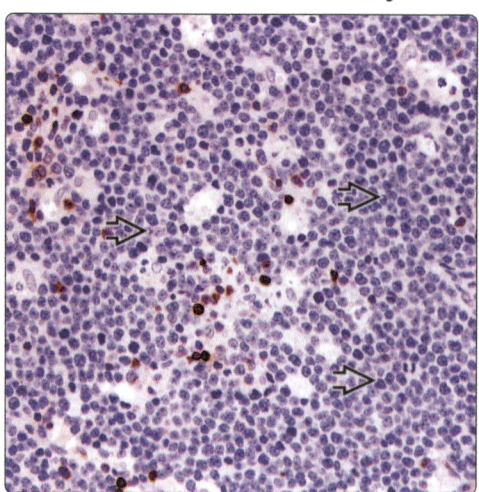

Ki-67 Proliferation Rate

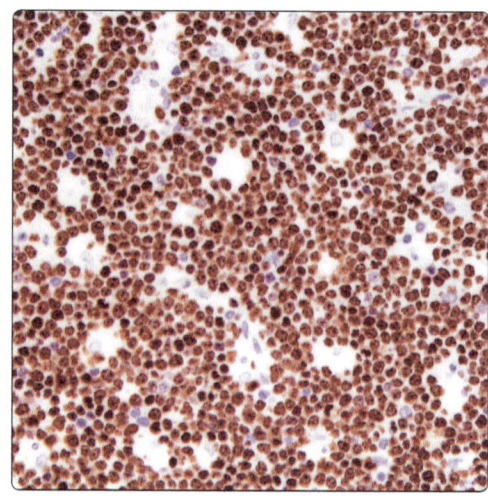

Burkitt Lymphoma

MYC Immunohistochemistry

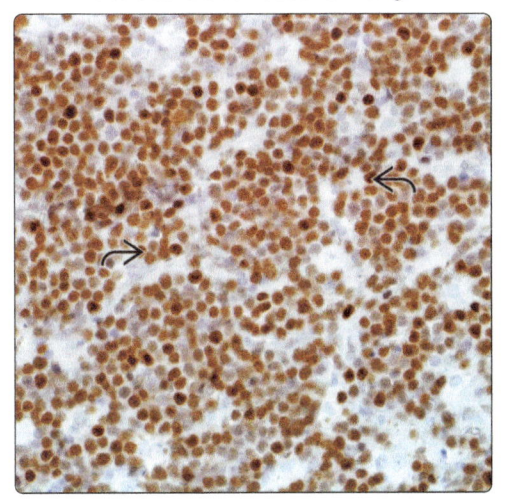

MYC(+) DLBCL

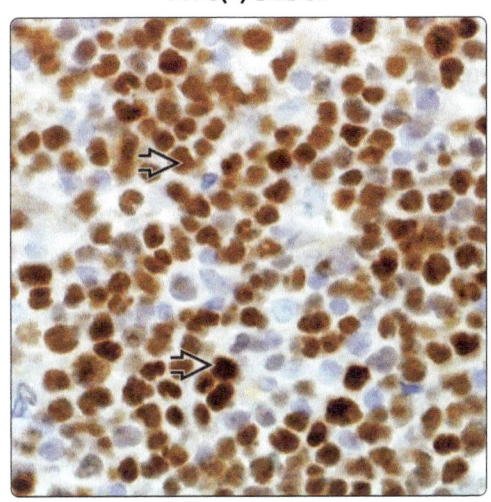

(Left) *MYC shows strong nuclear expression ⇒ in a case of BL. Most BL cases will be positive for MYC.* (Right) *MYC is positive ⇒ in this case of DLBCL. MYC translocations are not specific for BL, but can also be seen in DLBCL and double-hit lymphoma. Therefore, MYC positivity is not specific for BL.*

TCL1 Immunohistochemistry

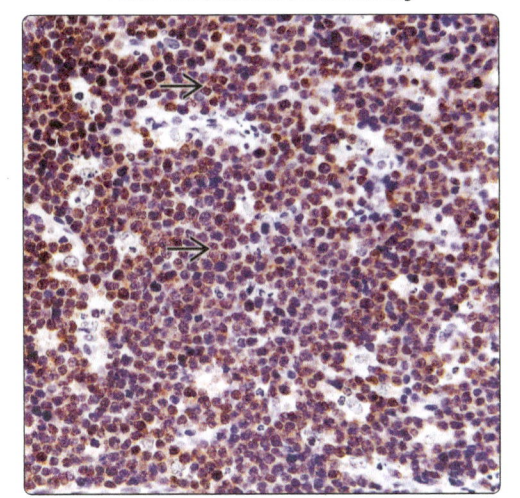

Flow Cytometry: CD19/CD10

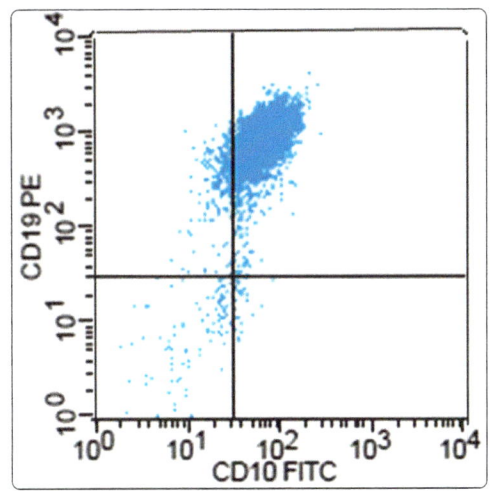

(Left) *TCL1 is expressed in the nuclei of the neoplastic cells ⇒ of BL, which is the only germinal center-derived tumor with uniformly high TCL1 expression.* (Right) *Flow cytometry shows that the BL cells express CD19 and CD10, indicating that they are B cells of germinal center origin.*

Flow Cytometry: κ Restriction

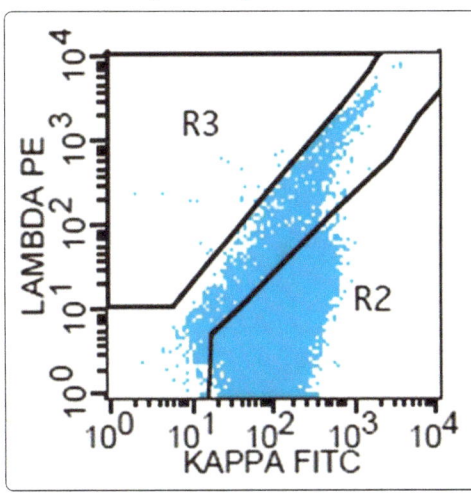

Flow Cytometry: CD10/κ

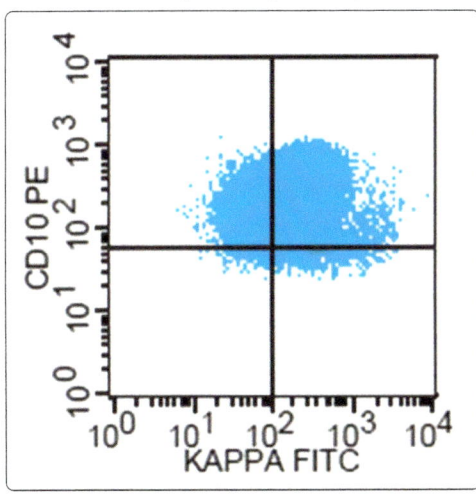

(Left) *Flow cytometry shows that the BL cells have surface immunoglobulin kappa light chain restriction.* (Right) *Flow cytometry shows that the BL cells express CD10 and kappa but were lambda negative (not shown).*

T-Cell Prolymphocytic Leukemia

KEY FACTS

TERMINOLOGY
- T-cell prolymphocytic leukemia (T-PLL) is aggressive mature T-cell neoplasm characterized by small to medium-sized T-cells involving peripheral blood (PB), bone marrow (BM), lymph nodes, and skin
  - Accepted entity both by WHO 5th edition and ICC

CLINICAL ISSUES
- High lymphocyte count
- Hepatosplenomegaly, skin involvement, PB, and BM

CYTOPATHOLOGY
- Atypical small lymphocytes show prominent nucleoli and cytoplasmic blebs
  - Small cell and cerebriform variants
- BM diffusely infiltrated
- Lymph nodes infiltrated by small lymphocytes

MOLECULAR
- Clonal *TRB* or *TRG* by PCR or next-generation sequencing
- Complex cytogenetics common
- Rearrangements involving *TCL1A* (TCL1), *TCL1B* (TML1), or *MTCP1* in 90%
- Most consistent findings inv(14)(q11q32) or t(14;14)(q11;q32) with secondary abnormalities; or t(X;14)(q28;q11)
- *JAK/STAT* signaling abnormalities in up to 75%

ANCILLARY TESTS
- Immunohistochemistry and flow cytometry show pan T-cell markers often without antigen loss
- CD52 &/or TCL1 expression
- CD4(+)/CD8(-) 60%, CD4(+)/CD8(+) 25%, CD4(-)/CD8(+) 15%

TOP DIFFERENTIAL DIAGNOSES
- Adult T-cell leukemia
- T-large granular lymphocyte leukemia

Small to Intermediate-Sized Lymphocytes

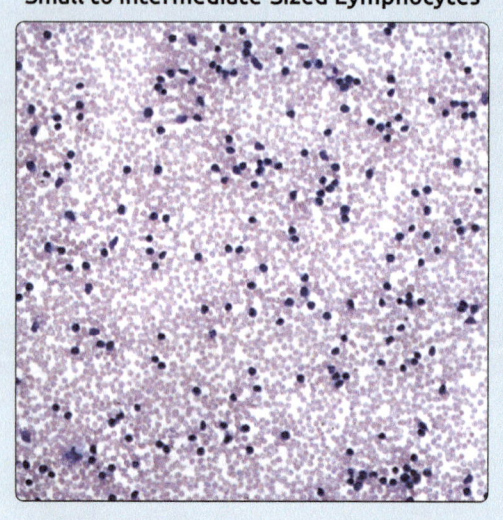

Prominent Nucleoli and Moderate Cytoplasm

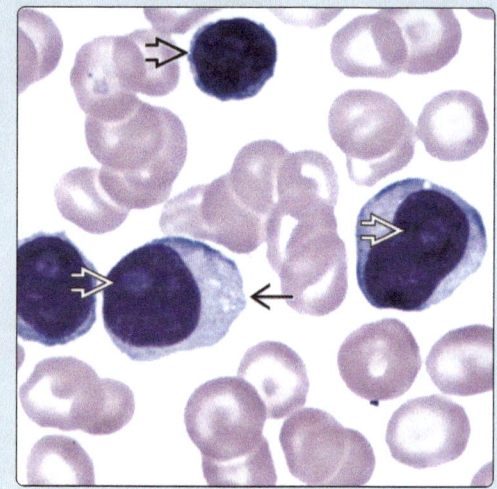

(Left) *An older patient with T-cell prolymphocytic leukemia (T-PLL) presented with a high white count, predominantly composed of small to intermediate-sized lymphocytes.* (Right) *Lymphocytes show prominent nucleoli ➡ and a moderate amount of cytoplasm ➡. The cells are intermediate in size, but larger than a normal, small, mature lymphocyte ➡.*

Moderately Conspicuous Nucleoli

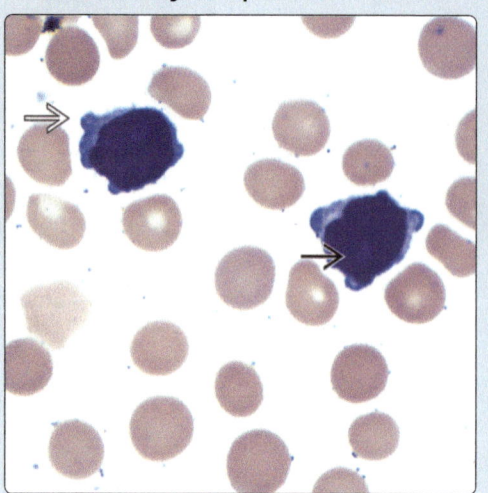

Focal Lymphoid Aggregates

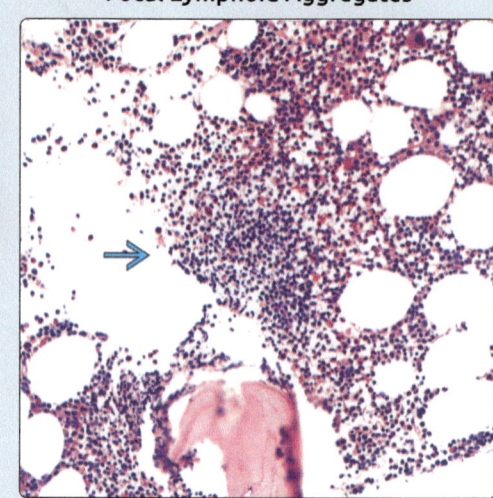

(Left) *Peripheral blood (PB) from a patient with a white count of 23,000 with 67% lymphocytes is shown. The lymphocytes are small, and nucleoli ➡ are moderately conspicuous. Cytoplasmic blebs ➡ are also present.* (Right) *Bone marrow (BM) shows focal lymphoid aggregates ➡, which are composed of T cells expressing TCR α-β, CD3, CD2, CD5, CD7, CD4, and CD52 by flow cytometry. FISH studies showed TCL1 rearrangement.*

T-Cell Prolymphocytic Leukemia

TERMINOLOGY

Abbreviations
- T-cell prolymphocytic leukemia (T-PLL)

Synonyms
- T-chronic lymphocytic leukemia

Definitions
- Aggressive, mature T-cell neoplasm characterized by small- to medium-sized T cells typically involving peripheral blood (PB), bone marrow (BM), lymph nodes, and skin

CLASSIFICATION

T-PLL
- Accepted entity both by WHO 5th edition and ICC

CLINICAL ISSUES

Epidemiology
- Incidence
  - 2% of mature lymphocytic leukemias
  - Median age: 65 years
  - Male predominance (M:F = 3:1)

Presentation
- Very high lymphocyte counts: ≥ 100 x 10⁹/L
- Lymphadenopathy and hepatosplenomegaly
- Skin involvement on 20% of cases
- Subset of patients may have indolent period preceding aggressive progression
- Patients with ataxia-telangiectasia syndrome have increased risk of T-PLL

Treatment
- Induction with alemtuzumab (anti-CD52)
- Followed by hematopoietic stem cell transplant

Prognosis
- Course is aggressive
- 20% overall 5-year survival; commonly < 1 year
- Rare chronic cases reported

MOLECULAR

Cytogenetics
- Complex karyotypes are common with numerical and structural abnormalities at 14q32 locus of *TCL1A*
- Common cytogenetic abnormalities include inv(14), t(14;14), i(8)(q10), monosomy 11 or deletion 11q, monosomy 22, and monosomy 13 as well as various abnormalities of 12p, 5, 7q, 17q, and 17p
- Most consistent findings inv(14)(q11q32) or t(14;14)(q11;q32) (involving *TCL1A* or *TCL1B*) with secondary abnormalities; or t(X;14)(q28;q11) (involving *MTCP1*)

In Situ Hybridization
- Common abnormalities by FISH include *TCL1A* (TCL1), *TCL1B* (TML1), or *MTCP* rearrangement in 90%
- Gains in *MYC* and loss of *ATM* reported

Polymerase Chain Reaction
- T-cell receptor gene rearrangements for *TRB* and *TRG*

Array Comparative Genomic Hybridization
- Multiple chromosomal abnormalities not recognized in conventional karyotyping or FISH
- Gains in chromosome regions include 8q (75%), 5p (62%), 14q (37%), 6p (25%), and 21 (25%)
- Losses in chromosomal regions include 8p (75%), 11q (75%), 13q (37%), and 25% for 6q, 7q, 16q, 17p, and 17q
  - Significance of these losses and gains is uncertain

Molecular Genetics
- Mutations of *JAK1/JAK3*, *IL2RG*, and *STAT5B* lead to STAT5 signaling
- Deletions or missense mutations at ataxia telangiectasia mutated (ATM) locus (11q23) found in 80-90%
- *SAMHD1* mutated in ~ 20%
- Other recurrently mutated genes include *EZH2*, *FBXW10*, *CHEK2*, *HERC1*, *HERC2*, *PRDM2*, *PARP10*, *PTPRC*, and *FOXP1*

Single-Nucleotide Polymorphism-Based Arrays
- Most common gained chromosomal regions were gains in 4q, 5p, 6p, 8q, and 14q
- 250K NspI single-nucleotide polymorphism (SNP) array showed several copy number alterations involving TCL1 oncogene
  - Disruptions in chromosome 14 often unbalanced
  - Chromosomal duplication of 14q32.13-14q32.33 region

MICROSCOPIC

Histologic Features
- PB shows markedly high lymphocyte counts
- BM shows interstitial/diffuse infiltrates
- Lymph nodes show proliferations of small lymphocytes partially effacing architecture
  - Early lesions difficult to distinguish from reactive
- Spleen shows red pulp infiltrates

Cytologic Features
- Lymphocytes are irregular with moderate cytoplasm showing blebs and prominent nucleoli

ANCILLARY TESTS

Immunohistochemistry
- Pan T-cell markers (+); often without loss of antigens
- TCL-1 and CD52 expression

Flow Cytometry
- Pan T-cell markers expressed; often no loss of antigens
- No immature markers, such as CD34, TdT, or CD1a
- CD4(+)/CD8(-) 60%, CD4(+)/CD8(+) coexpression 25-48%, CD8(+)/CD4(-) 15%
- TCL-1 and CD52 are expressed

SELECTED REFERENCES

1. Tian S et al: Epigenetic alteration contributes to the transcriptional reprogramming in T-cell prolymphocytic leukemia. Sci Rep. 11(1):8318, 2021
2. Sun S et al: Current understandings on T-cell prolymphocytic leukemia and its association with TCL1 proto-oncogene. Biomed Pharmacother. 126:110107, 2020

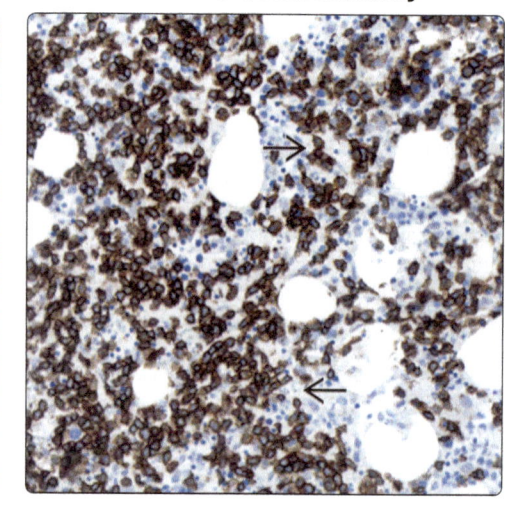

T-Cell Prolymphocytic Leukemia

(Left) Lymph node shows partial effacement ➡ by T-PLL. The immunophenotype of this T-PLL was unusual and showed CD8(+)/CD4(-). There is an infiltrate of small- to medium-sized lymphocytes. There are residual germinal centers ➡, sometimes making differentiation from a reactive process difficult. **(Right)** Malignant lymphocytes ➡ are small and appear mature. There are eosinophils ➡ in the background, but T-PLL does not characteristically show eosinophilia.

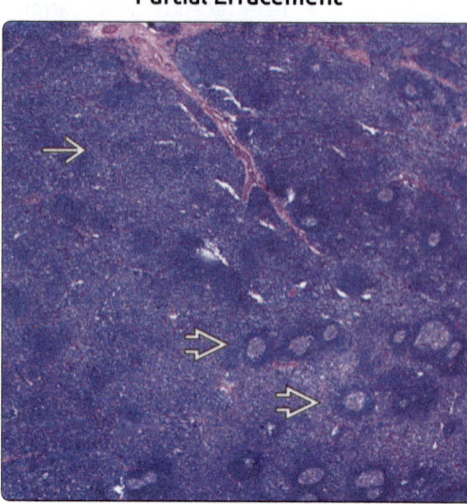

Partial Effacement

Malignant Lymphocytes

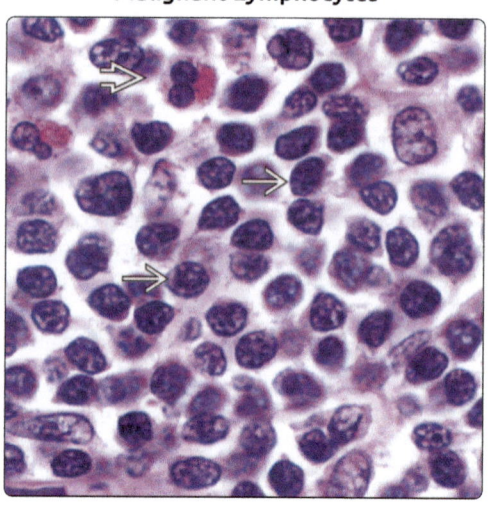

(Left) CD3 shows cytoplasmic positivity. The immunophenotype of T-PLL often does not show loss of T-cell antigens. CD52 is positive. The most common immunophenotype is CD4(+)/CD8(-), but CD4(+)/CD8(+) is present in 25-45% of cases. **(Right)** CD20 is negative in the malignant T-cell population.

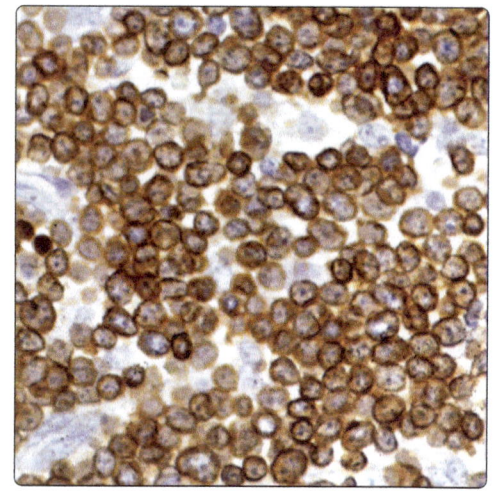

CD3 Immunohistochemistry

CD20 Immunohistochemistry

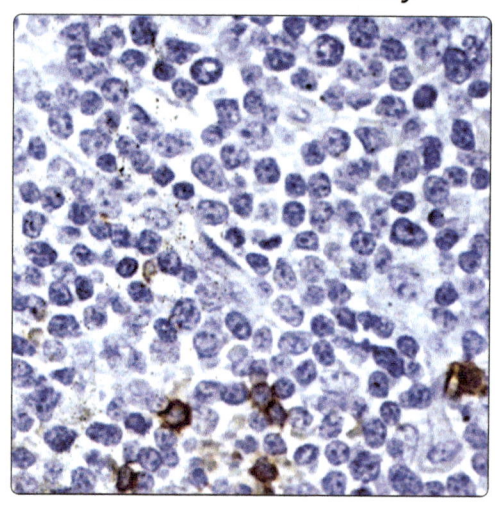

(Left) BM from a patient with T-PLL is hypercellular with extensive involvement by small lymphocytes ➡. **(Right)** CD3 shows numerous positive cells ➡ in this patient with CD8(+)/CD4(-) T-PLL. Often, these patients present with hepatosplenomegaly and very high white counts. The BM is often extensively infiltrated by small T cells.

Hypercellular Bone Marrow

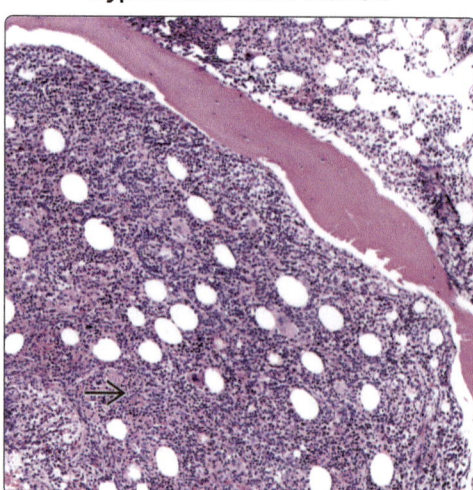

CD3 Immunohistochemistry

T-Cell Prolymphocytic Leukemia

Adult T-Cell Leukemia/Lymphoma

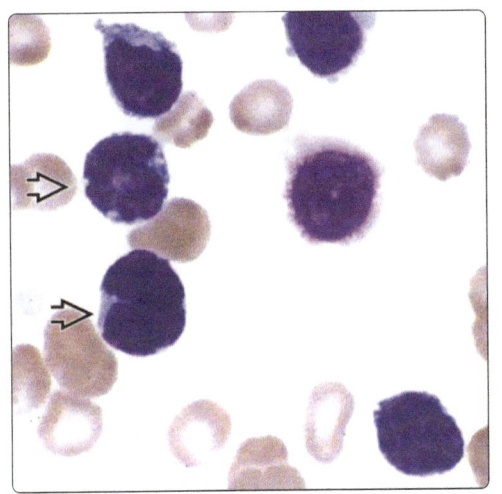

Adult T-Cell Leukemia/Lymphoma

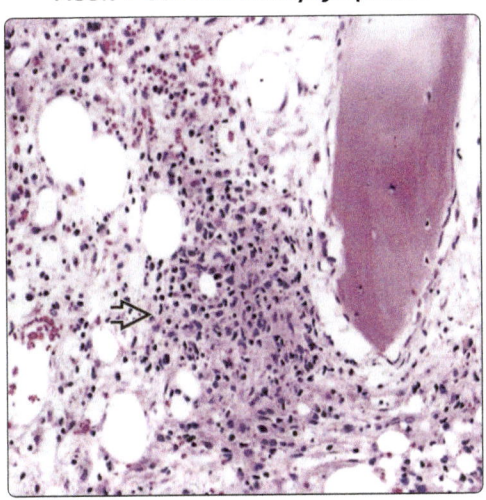

(Left) PB shows characteristic flower-like cells ➡ in adult T-cell leukemia/lymphoma (A-TLL). This leukemia/lymphoma is associated with human T-lymphotropic virus 1 (HTLV-1). The clinical behavior ranges from indolent to aggressive. A-TLL is often in the PB and BM but also infiltrates the lymph nodes. (Right) BM biopsy of ATLL shows a vague lymphoid aggregate ➡. This patient was HTLV-1 positive and progressed to an aggressive T-cell lymphoma in the lymph node.

Sézary Syndrome

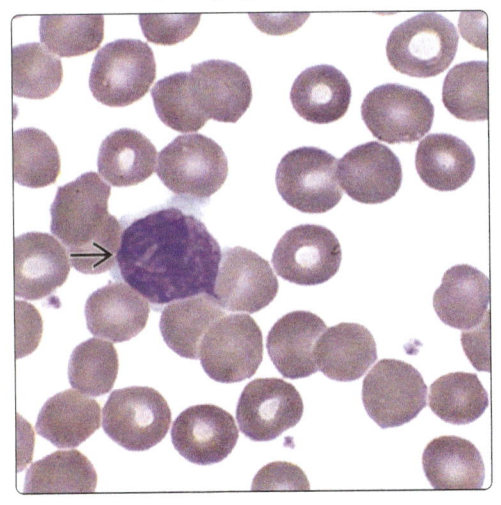

Sézary Syndrome

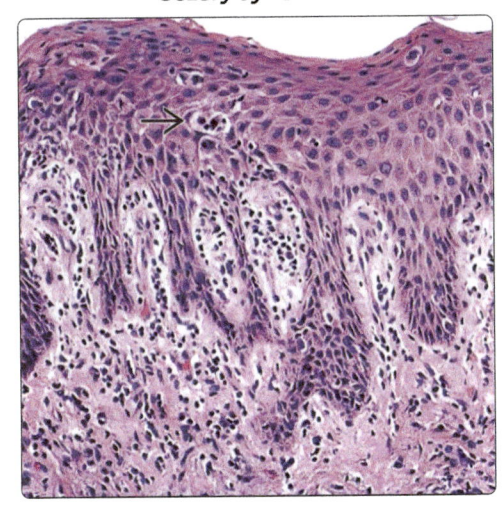

(Left) PB from a patient with Sézary syndrome is shown. The skin was involved diffusely. The lymphocytes show cerebriform nuclei ➡. (Right) Skin biopsy from a patient with Sézary syndrome is shown. The patient had widespread erythroderma. Pautrier microabscesses ➡ are not necessary for the diagnosis of Sézary syndrome but are present here.

Chronic Lymphocytic Leukemia/Small Lymphocytic Lymphoma

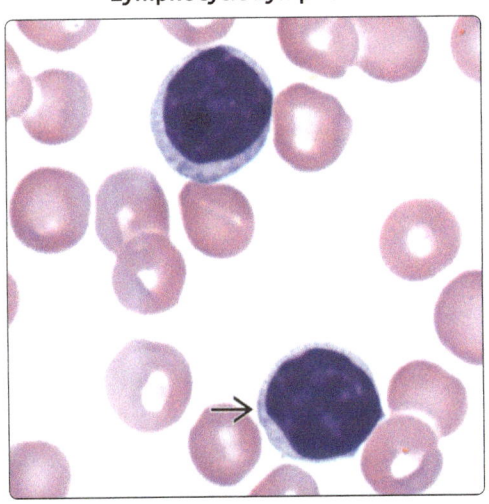

Chronic Lymphocytic Leukemia/Small Lymphocytic Lymphoma

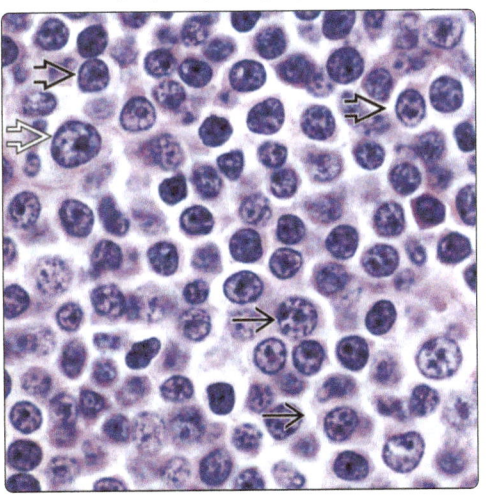

(Left) PB from a patient with chronic lymphocytic leukemia/small lymphocytic lymphoma (CLL/SLL), a B-cell process, is shown. The cells have clumped chromatin with a soccer ball appearance ➡. The absolute lymphocyte count can be very high in CLL/SLL. (Right) Lymph node from a patient with CLL/SLL is shown. The cells have clumped chromatin, similar to the PB lymphocytes ➡. There are also large paraimmunoblasts ➡ and prolymphocytes ➡.

Chronic Lymphoproliferative Disorder of NK Cells

KEY FACTS

TERMINOLOGY
- Chronic lymphoproliferative disorder of NK cells (CLPD-NK)
- Definition: Sustained increase in NK cells (usually ≥ 2 x 10^9/L) without identified cause and chronic indolent clinical course

CLINICAL ISSUES
- Indolent and chronic
- Neutropenia
- May be associated with autoimmune diseases
- Rarely splenomegaly, hepatomegaly, or lymphadenopathy
- May transform to aggressive NK-cell leukemia

MOLECULAR
- Mutations: *STAT3* in SH2 domain detected in 30%; *TET2* ~ 25%; *CCL22* ~ 22%
- *IGH*, *TRG*, and *TRB* are germline (no clonal rearrangement)
- Clonality can be detected by human androgen receptor assay (HUMARA) in female patients

MICROSCOPIC
- Peripheral blood shows mature NK cells
- Moderate cytoplasm with sparse cytoplasmic granules

ANCILLARY TESTS
- Flow cytometry
  - Surface CD3(-), CD3ε(+), CD8(+), CD56(+) but 50% weak to (-), CD2(+/-), CD7 (+/-), CD16(+/-), CD94(+/-)
  - Killer cell immunoglobulin-like inhibitory receptor (KIR)-restricted pattern of expression
- Immunohistochemistry
  - CD3(+), CD56 weak to (-), CD2(-), TIA1(+), granzyme-B (+)

TOP DIFFERENTIAL DIAGNOSES
- Reactive NK-cell proliferation
- T-large granular lymphocytic (T-LGL) leukemia
- Aggressive NK-cell leukemia
- Mycosis fungoides and Sézary syndrome
- Infectious mononucleosis

Large Granular Lymphocytes

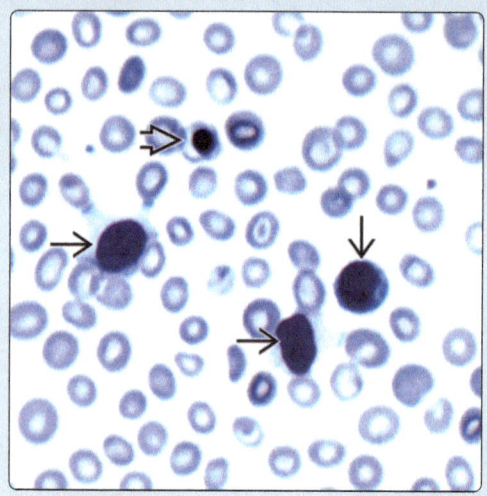

NK Cell in Blood

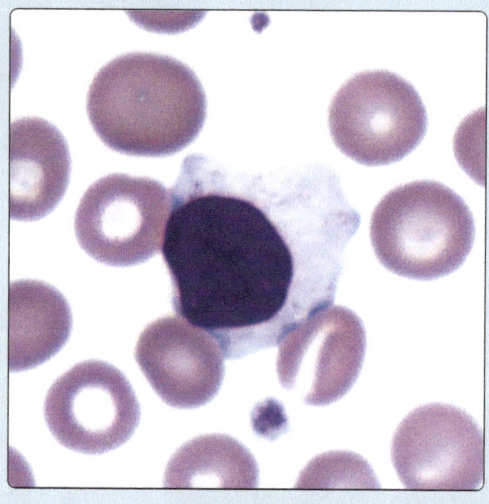

(Left) *Peripheral blood in chronic lymphoproliferative disorder of NK cells (CLPD-NK) shows mature-appearing, large granular lymphocytes ➡ without atypia. Note the nucleated red blood cell ➡. This patient had a chronic clinical course.* (Right) *NK cell shows characteristic appearance of large granular lymphocyte with moderate to abundant cytoplasm and azurophilic granules.*

T-Large Granular Lymphocytic Leukemia in Blood

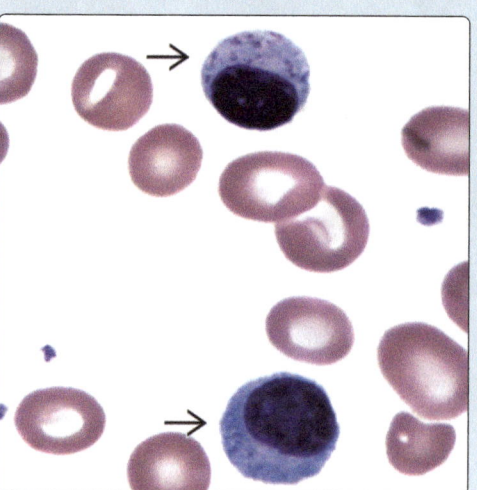

T-Large Granular Lymphocytic Leukemia in Bone Marrow

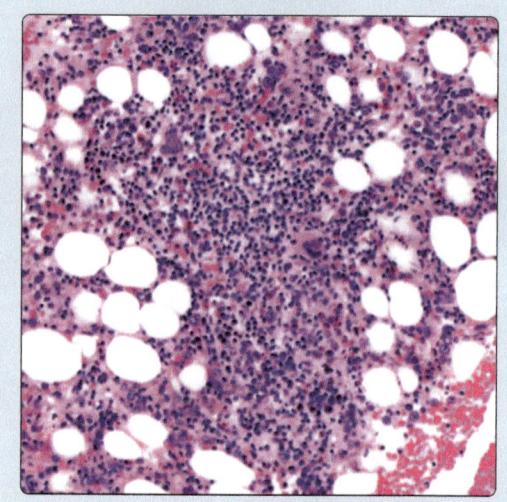

(Left) *Peripheral blood shows T-large granular lymphocytic (T-LGL) leukemia. The cells are characteristic for large granular lymphocytes and cannot be distinguished from benign T large granular lymphocytes or NK cells. Note abundant cytoplasm and small azurophilic granules ➡.* (Right) *Bone marrow shows T-LGL. The aggregates are composed of small lymphocytes. Often, benign aggregates are present, which show central CD20(+) B cells surrounded by small CD3(+) T cells.*

Chronic Lymphoproliferative Disorder of NK Cells

TERMINOLOGY

Abbreviations
- Chronic lymphoproliferative disorder of NK cells (CLPD-NK)
- NK-large granular lymphocytic leukemia (NK-LGLL)

Synonyms
- Chronic NK-cell lymphocytosis
- NK-cell large granular lymphocyte (LGL) lymphocytosis

Definitions
- International Consensus Classification (ICC) vs. WHO 5th edition (WHO-HAEM5)
  - CLPD-NK (ICC)
  - NK-LGLL (WHO-HAEM5)
    - Monoclonal/oligoclonal expansion of NK cells with many similarities with T-large granular lymphocytic (T-LGL) leukemia
- Persistent (> 6 months) increase in peripheral blood NK cells, usually > 2 x 10⁹/L, chronic indolent clinical course, and no clear identifiable cause (prior WHO 4th edition)

ETIOLOGY/PATHOGENESIS

Infectious Agents
- No documented association with infection, including EBV

CLINICAL ISSUES

Presentation
- Predominately adults; median age: 60 years
- Often asymptomatic
- Cytopenias, primarily neutropenia and anemia
- Associated autoimmune diseases
  - Rheumatoid arthritis, vasculitis, polymyositis, Hashimoto thyroiditis
- Often have other neoplasms, both nonhematopoietic and hematopoietic
  - Including plasma cell myeloma, myelodysplastic syndrome, acute myeloid leukemia, chronic myeloid leukemia, and polycythemia vera
- Peripheral blood and bone marrow are involved
  - Intrasinusoidal and interstitial pattern in bone marrow
- Coexisting CLPD-NK and T-LGL leukemia not uncommon

Treatment
- 1st-line options include methotrexate and cyclophosphamide
- STAT3 inhibitors promising

Prognosis
- 5-year overall survival (OS): 94%; 10-year OS: 84%
- OS is similar to T-LGL leukemia
- Patients may die from associated malignancies
- May transform to aggressive NK-cell leukemia (ANKL)

MOLECULAR

Cytogenetics
- Not well studied
- Clonally is difficult to prove in NK cells
- Human androgen receptor assay (HUMARA) can assess clonality in female patients

Polymerase Chain Reaction
- *IGH*, *TRB*, and *TRG* remain in germline status

Molecular Genetics
- Mutations: *STAT3* mutations in SH2 domain present in ~ 30%; *TET2* ~ 25-30%; *TNFAIP3* minority; *JAK3* and *STAT5B* rare
  - Similar mutations also found in T-LGL leukemia and may indicate common pathogenesis
  - p.Y640F and p.D661Y variants account for 80% of somatic *STAT3* mutations
  - Mutation status does not alter prognosis
- Mutations of *CCL22* found in 21.5% of CLPD-NK
  - Mutually exclusive of *STAT3* and *STAT5B* mutations and not found in T-LGL

Gene Expression Profiling
- DNA microarray analysis
  - 15 genes reported to be associated with NK-cell lymphoproliferative diseases
    - Specifically and differentially overexpressed in CLPD-NK/ANKL include *OPTN*, *ZFR*, *BMI1*, *ANXA7*, and *OGT*
    - 10 genes expressed in normal NK cells and CLPD-NK/ANKL, including *TTR*, *ACTN1*, *RNASE6*, *VDR*, and *LILRA4*
  - Neoplastic NK cells are distinct from normal NK cells

MICROSCOPIC

Histologic Features
- Peripheral blood show mature large granular lymphoid cells
  - Uniform-appearing, no immature forms
  - Sparse, coarse cytoplasmic granules
  - Moderate amount of cytoplasm
- Bone marrow may show subtle involvement
  - Interstitial and intrasinusoidal infiltrates
  - Best seen by CD3, TIA1, and CD56

ANCILLARY TESTS

Immunohistochemistry
- Expression of perforin, TIA1, &/or granzyme-B
- Surface CD3(-), CD3ε(+), CD57(+/-), CD2(+/-), CD7(+/-), CD56(+) to dim, CD16(+), CD8 variable, CD5(-)
- EBER in situ hybridization (-)

Flow Cytometry
- Surface CD3(-), CD3ε(+), CD57(+/-), CD2(+/-), CD7(+/-), CD56(+) to dim, CD16(+), CD94(+), CD8 variable, CD5(-)
- Skewed killer cell immunoglobulin-like inhibitory receptor (KIR) repertoire is present
- High frequency of KIR-activating receptor expression compared with healthy individuals

SELECTED REFERENCES

1. Alaggio R et al: The 5th edition of the World Health Organization classification of haematolymphoid tumours: lymphoid neoplasms. Leukemia. 36(7):1720-48, 2022
2. Campo E et al: The International Consensus Classification of mature lymphoid neoplasms: a report from the Clinical Advisory Committee. Blood. 140 (11): 1229-53, 2022, 2022
3. Pastoret C et al: Linking the KIR phenotype with STAT3 and TET2 mutations to identify chronic lymphoproliferative disorders of NK cells. Blood. 137(23):3237-50, 2021

Chronic Lymphoproliferative Disorder of NK Cells

Aggressive NK-Cell Leukemia in Blood

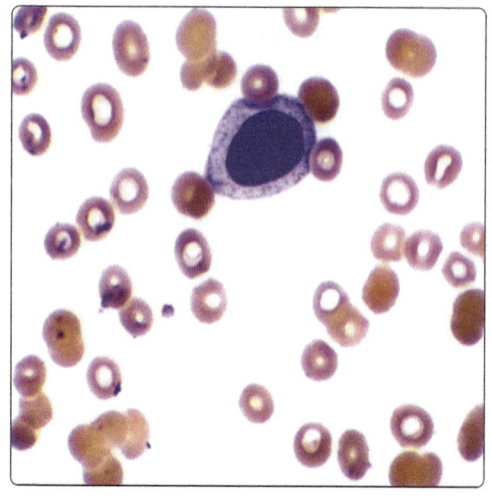

Aggressive NK-Cell Leukemia in Blood

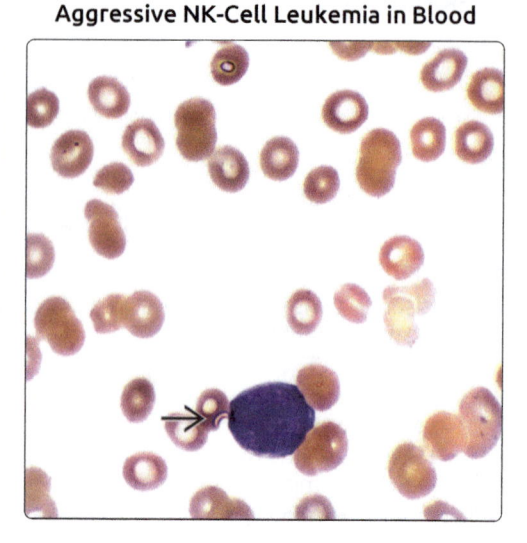

(Left) Aggressive NK-cell leukemia shows the typical appearance of a large granular lymphocyte with moderate cytoplasm and azurophilic granules; however, the nucleus is slightly immature. (Right) In this aggressive NK-cell leukemia, the cell appears immature ⇒, which distinguishes this entity from CLPD-NK. The neoplastic cells can also show atypia, including irregular folding and nucleoli.

Aggressive NK-Cell Leukemia in Bone Marrow

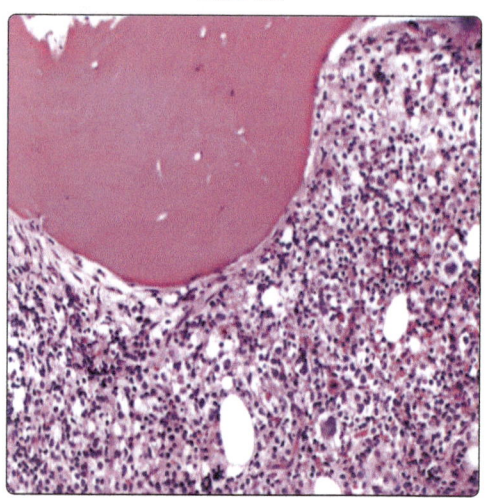

Flow Cytometry of Aggressive NK-Cell Leukemia in Blood

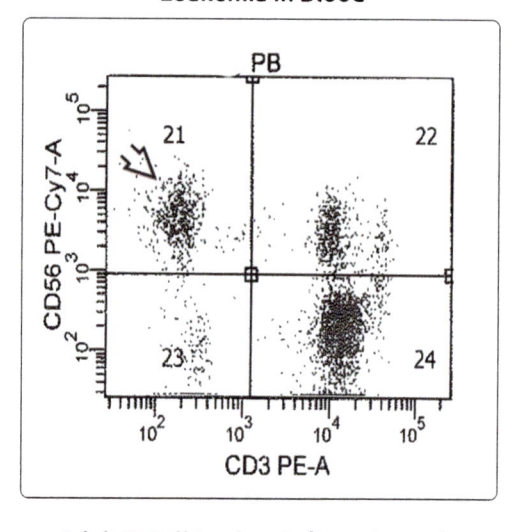

(Left) Bone marrow shows extensive infiltration by neoplastic NK cells in aggressive NK-cell leukemia. The cells have clearing around the nucleus, indicating abundant cytoplasm. (Right) Flow cytometry of aggressive NK-cell leukemia shows an NK-cell immunophenotype with surface CD3(-) and CD56(+) lymphoid population ⇒.

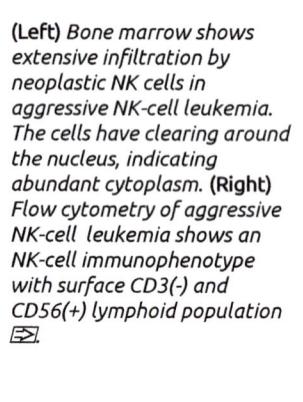

Adult T-Cell Leukemia/Lymphoma in Blood

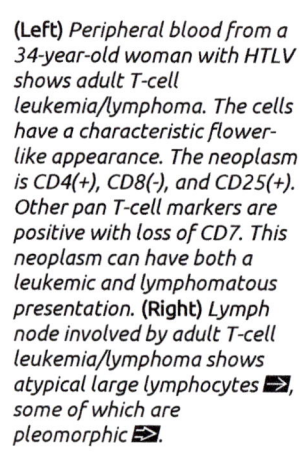

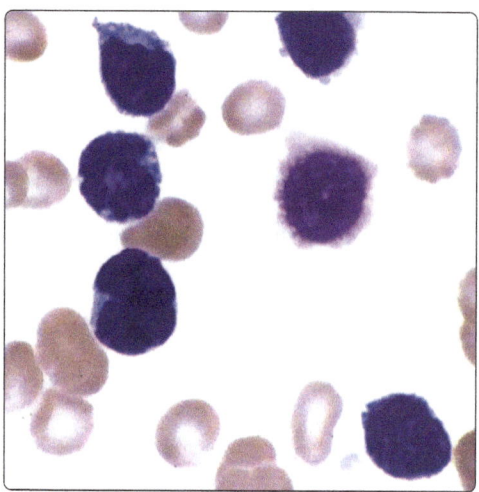

Adult T-Cell Leukemia/Lymphoma in Lymph Node

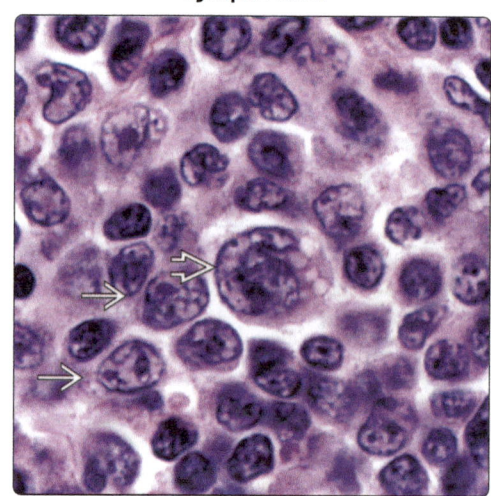

(Left) Peripheral blood from a 34-year-old woman with HTLV shows adult T-cell leukemia/lymphoma. The cells have a characteristic flower-like appearance. The neoplasm is CD4(+), CD8(-), and CD25(+). Other pan T-cell markers are positive with loss of CD7. This neoplasm can have both a leukemic and lymphomatous presentation. (Right) Lymph node involved by adult T-cell leukemia/lymphoma shows atypical large lymphocytes ⇒, some of which are pleomorphic ⇒.

Chronic Lymphoproliferative Disorder of NK Cells

T-Prolymphocytic Leukemia in Blood

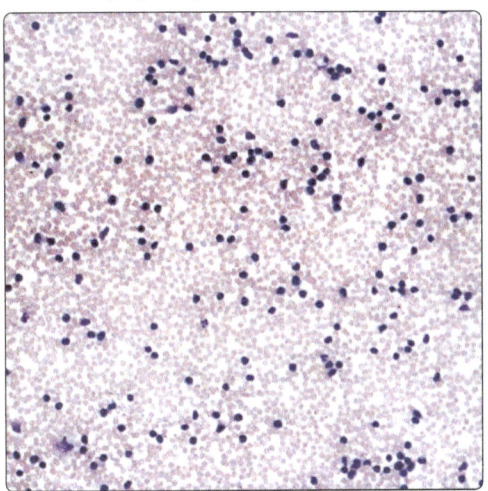

T-Prolymphocytic Leukemia in Blood

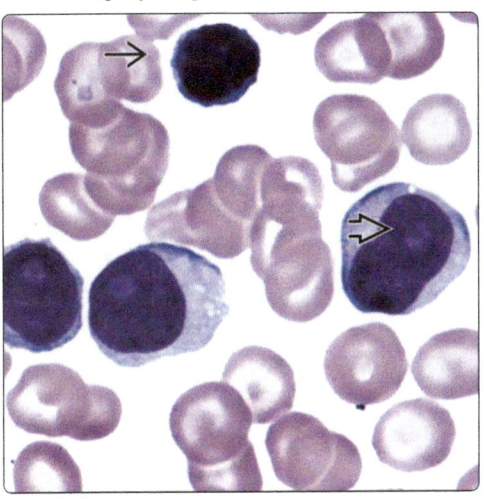

(Left) This older patient presented with significant lymphocytosis and was diagnosed with T-prolymphocytic leukemia (T-PLL). The white count in this neoplasm can often be > 100,000/µL. This T-cell neoplasm has an aggressive course in contrast to CLPD-NK or T-LGLL. (Right) Cells in T-PLL are larger than normal mature lymphocyte ⇥. They are slightly irregular and have prominent nucleoli ⇥. The cells can be CD4(+), CD4 and CD8(+) (double positive), or CD8(+)/CD4(-).

Sézary Cell in Blood

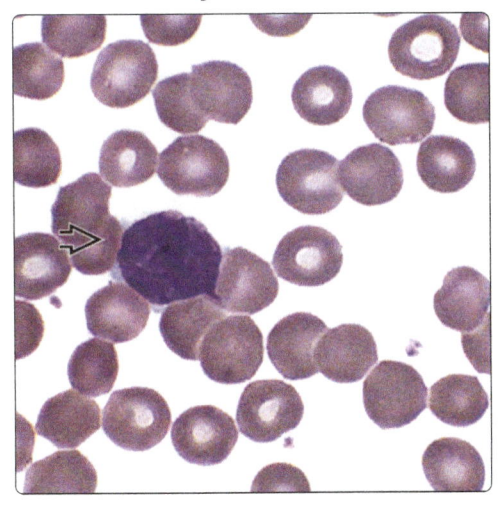

Skin Biopsy of Sézary Syndrome

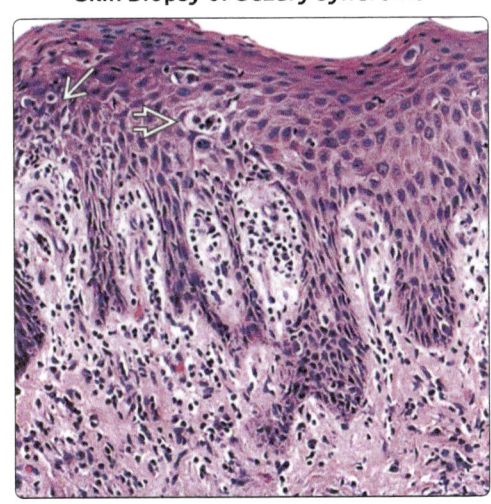

(Left) Neoplastic cell in Sézary syndrome shows irregular nuclei ⇥, which are described as cerebriform. The immunophenotype is CD4(+) with other pan T-cell marker expression. There is often loss of CD7 antigen. (Right) Skin biopsy in Sézary syndrome shows Pautrier microabscesses ⇥ and epidermotropism ⇥ of the small, neoplastic T cells.

Infectious Mononucleosis

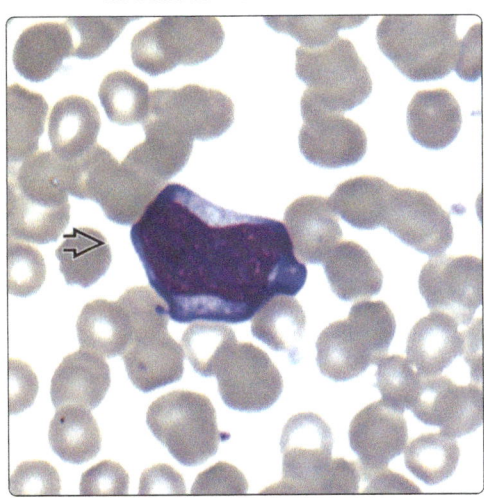

Infectious Mononucleosis

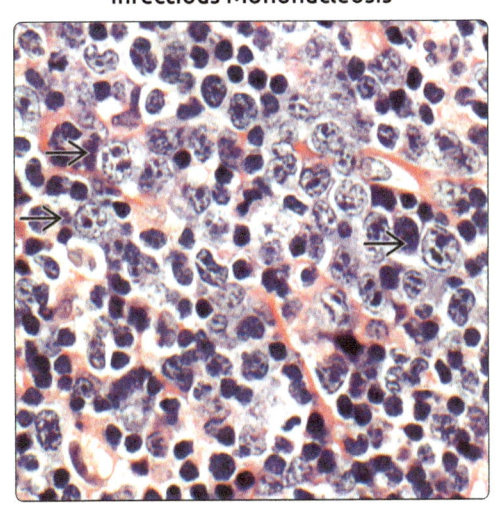

(Left) Atypical lymphocyte ⇥ from a 21-year-old with malaise and sore throat is shown. Monospot test was positive. Deep basophilic cytoplasm is characteristic of infectious mononucleosis but not specific for this entity. (Right) Heterogeneous population of lymphocytes in infectious mononucleosis is shown. Note the numerous immunoblasts ⇥.

Molecular Pathology of Lymphoid Neoplasms

401

Aggressive NK-Cell Leukemia

KEY FACTS

TERMINOLOGY
- Rare systemic neoplastic proliferation of NK cells commonly associated with Epstein-Barr virus (EBV) with aggressive clinical course

ETIOLOGY/PATHOGENESIS
- Associated with EBV, suggesting role in pathogenesis
- Possible leukemic counterpart of extranodal NK-/T-cell lymphoma, nasal type, but genetic differences exist

MOLECULAR
- Chromosomal microarray shows loss of 7p, 17p13.1 and gain of 1q
- Frequent mutations of JAK/STAT pathway; *TP53* mutations
- Germline T-cell receptor gene rearrangements
- Killer lectin-type receptors transcripts absent by RT-PCR

MICROSCOPIC
- Peripheral blood smear shows atypical cells with large, granular, lymphocytic appearance
  - May be pleomorphic or immature in appearance
- Bone marrow may show patchy, interstitial or sinusoidal infiltrates

ANCILLARY TESTS
- Immunohistochemistry
  - CD56(+), CD2(+), CD8(-/+), cCD3ε(+)
  - Surface CD3(-), CD5(-), CD7(-), CD57(-)
  - TIA(+), granzyme-B (+), perforin (+), FASL(+)
- Flow cytometry
  - CD56(+), CD16(-/+), CD2(+), cCD3ε(+)
  - CD8(-/+), surface CD3(-), CD57(-)
  - CD5(-), CD7(-), perforin (+)
- Cytogenetics: Complex karyotype, no specific aberrancies

TOP DIFFERENTIAL DIAGNOSES
- Chronic NK-cell lymphoproliferative disorders
- Extranodal NK-/T-cell lymphoma, nasal type
- T-large granular lymphocytic (T-LGL) leukemia

Circulating ANKL

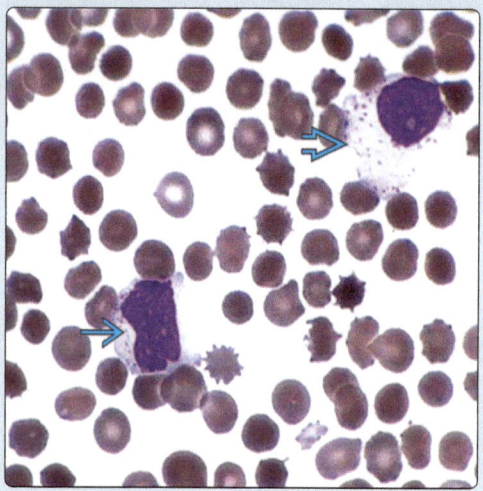

ANKL in Bone Marrow

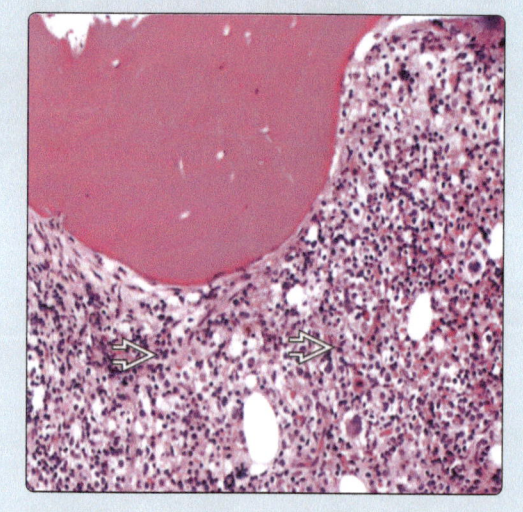

(Left) Wright-stained peripheral blood smear from a patient with aggressive NK-cell leukemia (ANKL) shows circulating neoplastic cells with irregular nuclei ➡ and abundant cytoplasm ➡ with intracytoplasmic granules. (Right) Bone marrow trephine biopsy shows extensive involvement ➡ by ANKL. Involvement of the bone marrow can be variable in ANKL.

ANKL With Blastoid Morphology

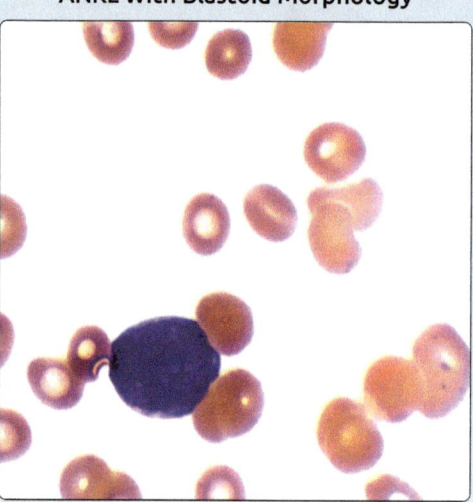

Flow Cytometry

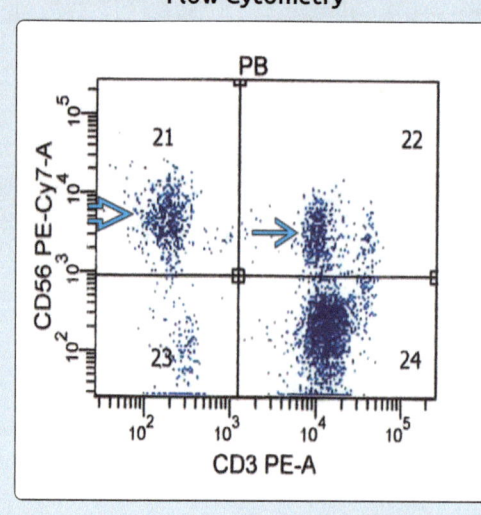

(Left) ANKL shows rare neoplastic blast-like cells in the peripheral blood. Other neoplastic cells showed the characteristic abundant cytoplasm and cytotoxic granules. This cell could be mistaken for a blast. (Right) Flow cytometric analysis shows a population of CD56(+) surface CD3(-) cells ➡, which are the neoplastic NK-cell population. There is also a population of surface CD3(+), CD56(+) cells, which are T-large granular lymphocytes (T-LGL) ➡. The T-LGLs were also CD57(+) and thought to be reactive.

Aggressive NK-Cell Leukemia

TERMINOLOGY

Abbreviations
- Aggressive natural killer (NK)-cell leukemia (ANKL)

Synonyms
- Aggressive NK-cell leukemia/lymphoma

Definitions
- Systemic neoplastic proliferation of NK cells associated with Epstein-Barr virus (EBV) with aggressive clinical course

ETIOLOGY/PATHOGENESIS

Unknown
- EBV is strongly associated with ANKL (85-100% of cases)
  - Suggests role in pathogenesis
  - Rare EBV-negative cases, which are clinicopathologically similar to EBV-positive cases reported
- Possible genetic predisposition
- Common mutations of JAK/STAT and RAS/MAPK pathways
- STAT3 activation and MYC expression are critical to proliferation and survival
- Uncertain relationship to extranodal NK-/T-cell lymphoma
  - Rare cases may evolve from extranodal NK-/T-cell lymphoma or chronic NK-cell leukemia

CLINICAL ISSUES

Epidemiology
- Incidence
  - Rare (< 5% of all lymphoid neoplasms)
- Ethnicity
  - Most frequent in Asia
  - Seen in some indigenous American populations

Presentation
- Most de novo; M = F; median age: 40 years
- Fulminant course with multiorgan failure and disseminated intravascular coagulation
- Hemophagocytic lymphohistiocytosis (HLH) is frequent

Treatment
- Systemic chemotherapy followed by stem cell transplant

Prognosis
- Poor with median survival < 2 months
  - Refractory to available therapies
  - P-glycoprotein, product of multidrug resistance TBC1D9 (a.k.a. MDR1), is expressed on neoplastic cells

MOLECULAR

Cytogenetics
- Often difficult to obtain because of necrosis and lack of adequate viable cells
- Complex karyotypes when cytogenetic analysis is successful
  - Unbalanced translocations often present
    - Most frequent 7p-, 17p-, and 1q+

Chromosomal Microarray
- Loss of 17p13.1 identified in 40%
- Loss of 7p and gain of 1q occur with significant frequency

Molecular Genetics
- T-cell receptor gene rearrangements are in germline status
  - Analysis is not informative in determining clonality in NK neoplasms
  - Southern blot analysis of EBV DNA terminal repeats is informative to assess clonality
- Killer lectin-type receptors (KLR) transcripts not expressed by RT-PCR
- NGS whole-exome sequencing
  - Frequent mutations in JAK/STAT pathway (48%)
  - Commonly mutated genes include TP53 (50%), TET2 (33%), and CREBBP (21%)
  - Other reported mutated genes
    - Mutations in KMT2D and DDX3X
    - Mutations in immune checkpoint genes, including CD274 (a.k.a. PD-L1) and PDCD1LG2 (a.k.a. PD-L2)

MICROSCOPIC

Histologic Features
- Blood
  - ANKL cells are larger than normal large, granular lymphocytes
  - Pale or slightly basophilic cytoplasm with azurophilic granules
  - Slightly immature nuclear chromatin with inconspicuous or distinct nucleoli
- Bone marrow
  - Variable patterns of infiltration; interstitial and sinusoidal; patchy or diffuse
    - Variable cytology ranging from small bland to very pleomorphic cells
  - Necrosis and apoptosis may be prominent
  - Hemophagocytosis is frequently seen
- Tissue biopsy
  - Necrosis, apoptosis, angioinvasion, and angiodestruction are common

ANCILLARY TESTS

Immunohistochemistry
- Neoplastic cells have NK immunophenotype
  - CD56(+), CD16(+), CD2(+), cCD3ε(+), FASL(+), CD94(+)
  - CD57(-), CD8(-/+), sCD3(-), CD5(-), CD7(+/-), CD11b(-/+)
  - TIA(+), granzyme-B (+), and perforin (+)
- Both LMP1 and EBER detected in many cases

Flow Cytometry
- Important for diagnosis
- CD2(+), CD56(+), cCD3ε(+), CD7(+/-), CD57(-), CD8(-) with rare exceptions, CD16(-/+), perforin(+)
- KIR (CD158a-e) is frequently (-)
- Variable expression of killer immunoglobulin-like receptors

SELECTED REFERENCES

1. Quintanilla-Martinez L et al: New concepts in EBV-associated B, T, and NK cell lymphoproliferative disorders. Virchows Arch. 482(1):227-44, 2023
2. Sumbly V et al: Aggressive natural killer cell leukemia: a brief overview of its genomic landscape, histological features, and current management. Cureus. 14(2):e22537, 2022
3. El Hussein S et al: Genomic and immunophenotypic landscape of aggressive NK-cell leukemia. Am J Surg Pathol. 44(9):1235-43, 2020

Aggressive NK-Cell Leukemia

ANKL in Blood

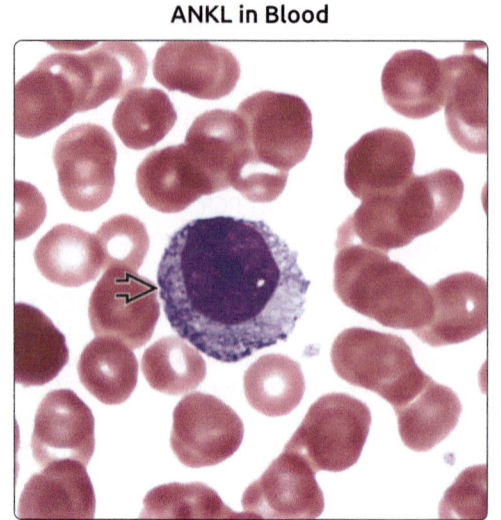

ANKL in Bone Marrow

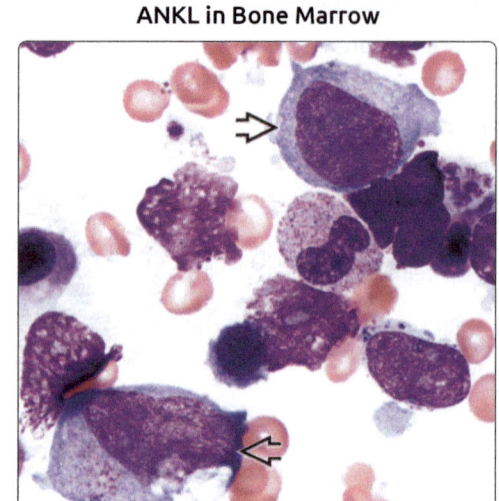

(Left) *Peripheral blood smear from a 17-year-old boy with ANKL shows a rare circulating neoplastic cell. Note the sparse cytoplasmic granules ⇨. Extensive scanning was required to identify neoplastic cells. (From DP: Blood & Bone Marrow.)* (Right) *Bone marrow aspirate smear from a patient with ANKL shows 2 atypical large cells ⇨ with sparse cytoplasmic granules admixed with normal hematopoietic cells. (From DP: Blood & Bone Marrow.)*

ANKL in Bone Marrow

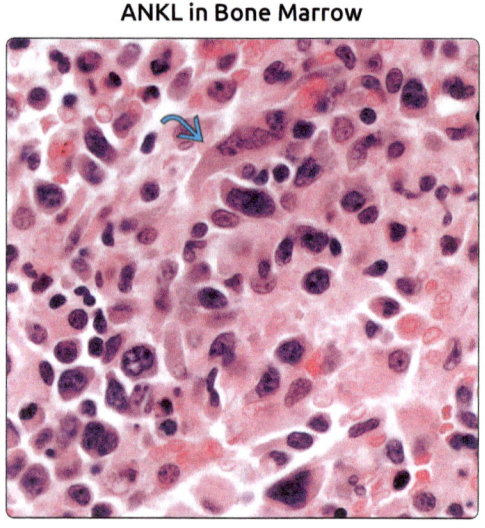

EBER(+) ANKL

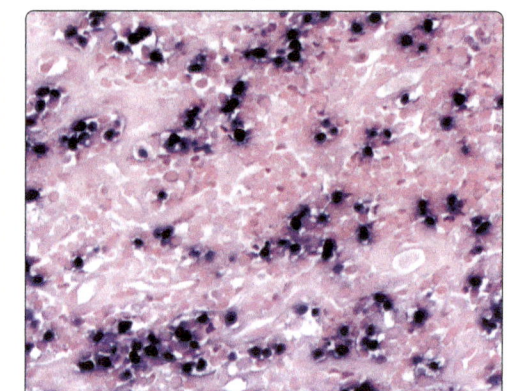

(Left) *Bone marrow core biopsy shows a substantial interstitial infiltrate of variably sized pleomorphic ANKL cells. Note the large, tadpole appearance ⇨ of some neoplastic cells. (From DP: Blood & Bone Marrow.)* (Right) *ISH for EBER shows numerous diffusely infiltrative, positive neoplastic cells in ANKL. EBV positivity is a key diagnostic feature of ANKL. EBV likely plays a key role in pathogenesis of ANKL. (From DP: Blood & Bone Marrow.)*

Hemophagocytic Activity

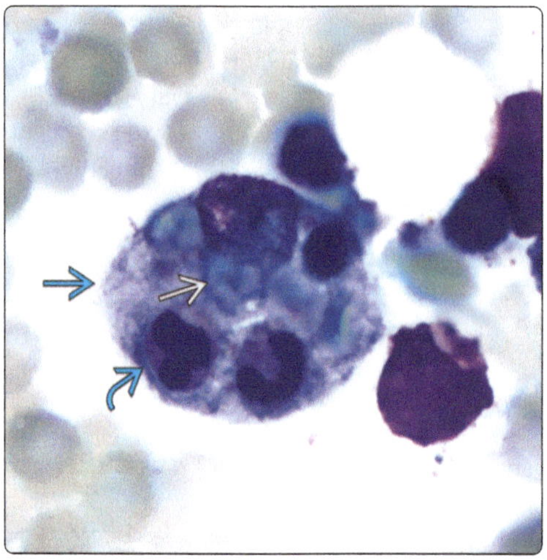

Histiocytes With Erythrophagocytic Activity

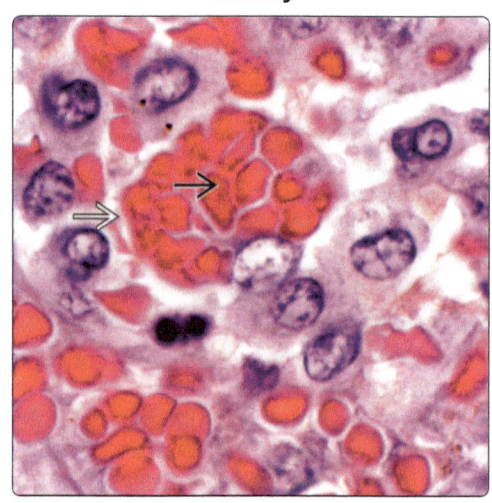

(Left) *Wright-stained bone marrow aspirate smear shows a histiocyte ⇨ with phagocytosed erythroid ⇨ and granulocytic cells ⇨. This patient had familial hemophagocytic syndrome with markedly increased ferritin. Hemophagocytic lymphohistiocytosis is often associated with hematologic malignancy and is not exclusive for ANKL.* (Right) *Bone marrow biopsy shows numerous plump histiocytes ⇨ engorged with red blood cells ⇨.*

Aggressive NK-Cell Leukemia

Extranodal NK-/T-Cell Lymphoma, Nasal Type

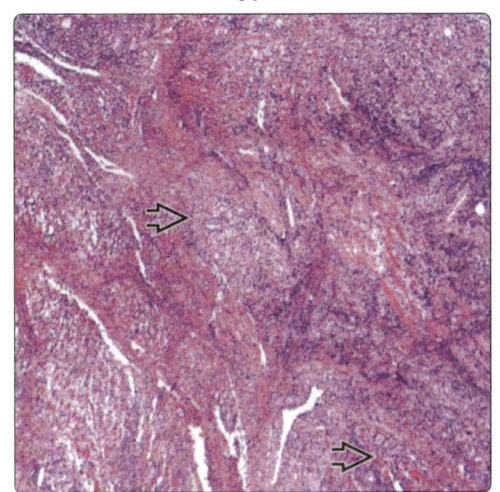

Extranodal NK-/T-Cell Lymphoma, Nasal Type

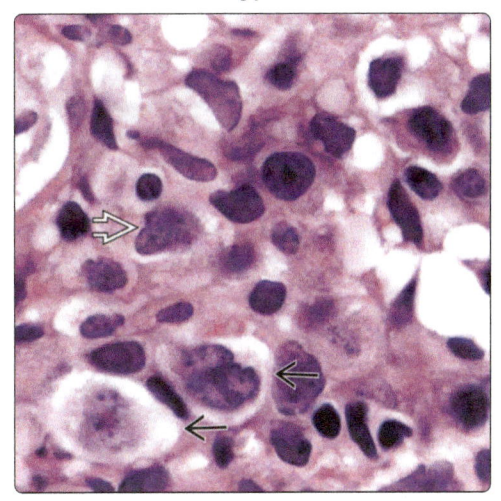

(Left) Nasopharyngeal excisional biopsy of extranodal NK-/T-cell lymphoma (ENKTL) shows extensive infiltration by neoplastic, lymphoid-appearing cells ⇒. (Right) Higher power view shows pleomorphic cells ⇒ with abundant cytoplasm ⇒. There is variation in size and shape. The neoplastic infiltrate is typically angiocentric and angiodestructive. Most ENKTLs show extensive necrosis. The relationship between ENKTL and ANKL is uncertain.

CD56 Immunohistochemistry

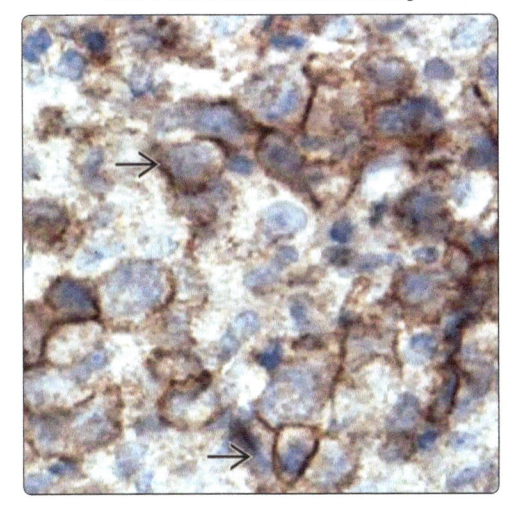

TIA Immunohistochemistry

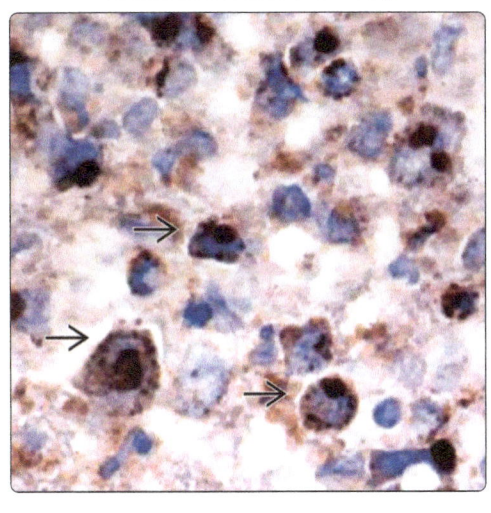

(Left) ENKTL with membrane CD56 positivity ⇒ is shown. This is characteristic for both ANKL and ENKTL. (Right) TIA marks cytoplasmic granules ⇒ characteristic for this stain in ENKTL. Perforin and granzyme-B can also be positive with granular cytoplasmic staining in ENKTL and ANKL by IHC.

Extranodal NK-/T-Cell Lymphoma, Nasal Type

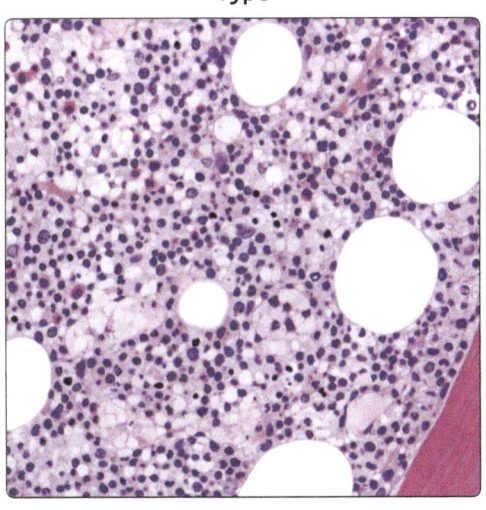

EBER(+) Extranodal NK-/T-Cell Lymphoma

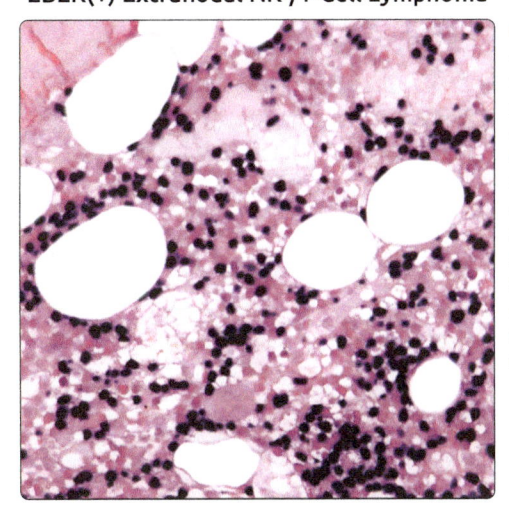

(Left) Bone marrow trephine biopsy shows ENKTL, nasal-type. This patient had disease primarily involving the nasopharynx. (From DP: Lymphomas.) (Right) Bone marrow biopsy shows ENKTL, nasal-type. In situ hybridization for EBER highlights many EBER(+) neoplastic cells present in an interstitial distribution pattern. (From DP: Lymphomas.)

Extranodal NK-/T-Cell Lymphoma

KEY FACTS

TERMINOLOGY
- Predominantly extranodal lymphoma of either NK- or T-cell lineage
- Characterized by EBV infection, necrosis, cytotoxic immunophenotype, and angioinvasion

ETIOLOGY/PATHOGENESIS
- EBV seen in almost all cases, likely involved in pathogenesis
- Rare cases can be (-), and sometimes other T-cell lymphomas can be EBV(+)

CLINICAL ISSUES
- Typically poor outcomes; worst prognosis in extranasal tumors

MOLECULAR
- Monoclonal *TRB* and *TRG* rearrangements detected in T-cell subtype but not NK-cell subtype
- del(6)(q21q25) and i(6)(p10) most common cytogenetic abnormality
  - Isochromosome 7q rarely detected, and trisomy 13 has been reported
- Various gene mutations have been identified, including *FAS*, *TP53*, *CTNNB1*, *KRAS*, and *KIT*
- Gene expression profiling shows activation of JAK/STAT, AKT, and NF-κB pathways may help to develop targeted therapies in future
- Gene expression profiles cluster regardless if NK- or T-cell lineage and are similar to gamma delta T-cell lymphoma

MICROSCOPIC
- Necrosis is seen in majority of cases
- Angiocentricity and angiodestruction

ANCILLARY TESTS
- NK-cell lineage: CD2(+), cytoplasmic CD3-ε(+), CD56(+/-), CD5(-), and CD8(-)
- T-cell lineage: CD2(+), CD3(+), CD5(+), CD8(+/-), and TCRβ(+)

Neoplastic Cells and Mitotic Figures

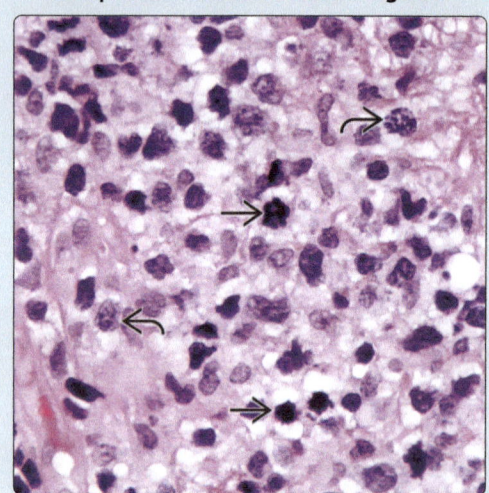

PCR for *TRG* Rearrangement

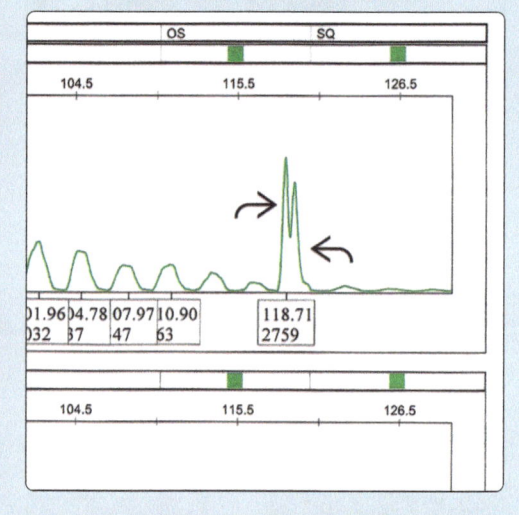

(Left) Extranodal NK-/T-cell lymphoma (ENKTL) shows that the neoplastic cells ➔ are medium sized with irregular nuclear contours and pale cytoplasm. Scattered mitotic figures ➔ are also present. (Right) PCR for T-cell receptor gamma shows a dominant monoclonal peak ➔ in this case of ENKTL. This rearrangement is often seen in ENKTL of T-cell origin but not in those of true NK-cell origin.

Necrosis With Tumor

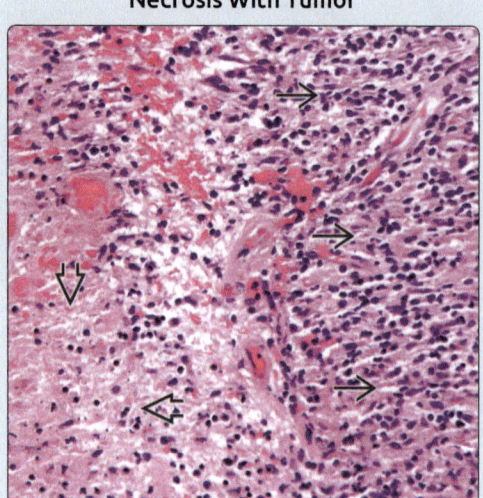

Radiologic Appearance

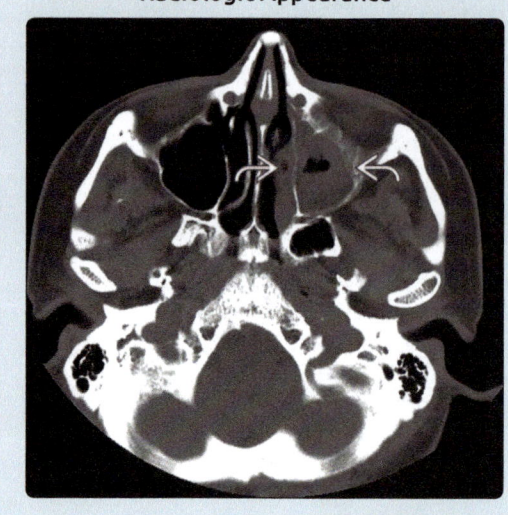

(Left) Biopsy of maxillary sinus from a patient with ENKTL shows extensive coagulative necrosis ➔ and lymphoid infiltrate ➔. ENKTL is commonly associated with coagulative necrosis. (Right) CT in this case of ENKTL shows an opacified maxillary sinus ➔ and thickening of mucosa in the nasopharynx.

Extranodal NK-/T-Cell Lymphoma

TERMINOLOGY

Abbreviations
- Extranodal NK-/T-cell lymphoma (ENKTL)

Synonyms
- Polymorphic reticulosis, malignant midline reticulosis
- Angiocentric T-cell lymphoma type

Definitions
- Predominantly extranodal lymphoma characterized by vascular damage, necrosis, cytotoxic immunophenotype, and associated with EBV
  - Most cases are NK-cell neoplasm, but some are T-cell lineage

Classifications
- ENKTL, nasal type [International Consensus Classification (ICC)]
- ENKTL [WHO 5th edition (WHO-HAEM5)]
  - WHO-HAEM5 dropped qualifier "nasal-type" since disease can present at various extranodal sites

ETIOLOGY/PATHOGENESIS

Infectious Agents
- EBV is consistently present, suggesting its key role in pathogenesis
  - EBV is usually type A
  - Type II latency: EBNA1(+), EBNA2(-), LMP1(+)
  - 30 bp deletion in *LMP1*

Epidemiology
- Common in Asia and in Native Americans of Central and South America
- Rare in USA, but incidence is rising

CLINICAL ISSUES

Epidemiology
- Age
  - Mostly adults
- Sex
  - More common in men

Presentation
- Nasal or extranasal mass
  - Nasal cases usually involve upper aerodigestive tract
    - 80% of cases are nasal subtype
    - Include nasal cavity, nasopharynx, paranasal sinuses, and palate
    - Patients suffer from obstruction, epistaxis, or midline destructive lesion
  - Extranasal cases involve any anatomic site other than nasal/upper aerodigestive tract
    - 20% of cases are extranasal
    - Skin is most common extranasal site
    - Other sites include testis, gastrointestinal tract, kidney, and salivary glands
    - Bone marrow, obtained as part of staging, can be involved

Natural History
- ENKTL, nasal type can disseminate
  - Regional lymph node involvement is not uncommon
  - Bone marrow involvement and leukemic phase occur in subset of cases
  - Can disseminate to virtually any anatomic site

Treatment
- L-asparaginase-based chemotherapy in combination with radiotherapy results in markedly improved outcomes in advanced disease
- Immune checkpoint inhibitor therapy may be beneficial for relapsed/refractory disease
  - Supports finding that immune evasion is important for ENKTL cell survival

Prognosis
- Historically, outcomes were poor with ~ 35% survival rate
  - Recent prognosis is improved with
    - More intense chemotherapy
    - Upfront radiotherapy
- Worst prognosis in extranasal tumors
- Factors associated with poor prognosis
  - High international prognostic index (IPI)
  - Ki-67 proliferation rate > 50%
  - High circulating EBV DNA
  - High-stage disease or age > 60 years

IMAGING

General Features
- Location
  - Typically, imaging studies show mass of upper airways, which may destroy bone, distort midline, or displace adjacent organs

MOLECULAR

In Situ Hybridization
- EBV-encoded early RNA (EBER) is positive in both NK- and T-cell subtypes of ENKTL, nasal type
  - Test is highly sensitive
  - Rare cases can be EBER negative
  - EBER can also rarely be positive in other T-cell lymphomas

PCR
- 10-40% of T-cell tumors carry monoclonal *TRB* and *TRG* rearrangements
- NK-cell tumors do not carry monoclonal T-cell receptor gene rearrangements
  - T-cell receptor genes are germline in true NK-cell neoplasms

Cytogenetics
- Deletion of 6q21-25 is most common cytogenetic abnormality
  - 6q21-25 contains tumor suppressor genes, including *PRDM1*, *HACE1*, and *FOXO3*
- Isochromosome 7q has been detected in rare cases of ENKTL
  - So, isochromosome 7q is **not** specific for hepatosplenic T-cell lymphoma

Extranodal NK-/T-Cell Lymphoma

Molecular Genetics
- Various gene deletions or mutations have been identified
- Alterations have been found in JAK-STAT pathway (*JAK3*, *STAT3*, and *STAT5B*), tumor suppressor genes (*TP53* and *MGA*), and epigenetic regulators (*ARID1A*, *BCOR*, *EP300*, and *KMT2D*)
- *PRDM1* plays role in NK-cell homeostasis
- Promoter hypermethylation of cell cycle regulators (*CDKN2A*, *CDKN2B*, and *CDKN1A*) and tumor suppressor genes (*BCL2L11*, *DAPK1*, and *PTPN6*)
- Overexpression of genes, including *AURKA*, *BIRC5*, *EZH2*, *MYC*, and *PD-L1*, have also been identified
- Increased human trophoblastic cell surface antigen 2 (TROP2) found in ENKTL
  - Increased TROP2 associated with poor prognosis

Gene Expression Profiling
- Profiles cluster regardless if NK-cell or T-cell lineage
- Similar profiles to other gamma delta T-cell lymphomas
  - Other than hepatosplenic T-cell lymphoma
- Platelet-derived growth factor α is overexpressed; *HACE1* is deregulated

Chromosomal Microarray (Array CGH)
- Comparative genomic hybridization (CGH) studies have shown multiple gains and losses
  - Most common site of gain: 2q
  - Common sites of losses: 1p36, 6q16-q27, 4q12, 5q34-q35, 7q21-22, 9p, 11q22-q23, 12p, 12q, and 15q11-q14
- Nasal-type NK-/T-cell lymphoma of skin
  - Gains of 1q, 7q, and loss of 17p

MicroRNA
- Deregulation of miRNAs, including miR-26, miR-101, miR-146a, miR-155, and miR21

MICROSCOPIC

Histologic Features
- Lymphoid infiltrate typically with diffuse pattern
  - Cell size ranges from small to large
  - Mitotic figures commonly and easily seen
  - Coagulative necrosis and apoptotic bodies seen in ~ 90% of cases
  - Mucosal ulceration and inflammation
    - Overlying mucosal epithelium may show pseudoepitheliomatous hyperplasia
  - Angiocentricity and angiodestruction seen in ~ 70% of cases
    - Less commonly recognized in small biopsy specimens
  - Neoplastic cells can have azurophilic cytoplasmic granules on touch imprints
  - Hemophagocytosis can complicate clinical course
- Lymph node
  - Preferentially involves paracortex ± medulla
- Bone marrow
  - ~ 10-20% of staging bone marrows positive for tumor
    - Commonly interstitial infiltrate without discrete aggregates
    - In situ hybridization for EBER can be helpful to detect disease in subtle cases

ANCILLARY TESTS

Immunohistochemistry
- NK-cell lineage in ~ 65-75%
  - CD2(+), CD56(+/-), and CD94(+); cytotoxic markers, including TIA, granzyme B, and perforin (+)
    - Both T and NK cells express epsilon chain of CD3 (CD3-ε)
  - CD4(-), CD5(-), CD8(-), CD16(-), CD57(-), and TCRβ(-)
- T-cell lineage in ~ 25-35%
  - CD2(+), CD3-ε(+), CD5(+), CD8(+/-), TCRβ(+), CD56(-/+); cytotoxic markers (+)
    - T-bet and ETS1 (+); CXCL13 and PD-1 (-/+)
    - CD30(+) in 30%
- EBV latent membrane protein variably expressed
  - Usually fewer cells than EBER in situ hybridization

DIFFERENTIAL DIAGNOSIS

Peripheral T-Cell Lymphoma Involving Upper Aerodigestive Tract
- Histologic features can mimic ENKTL, nasal type
  - Necrosis and involvement of vessels
  - Usually lack CD56 and are negative for EBV
  - Includes cases that are CD3(+), CD56(-), EBV(-), and cytotoxic markers (-)

EBV(+) Nodal T-/NK-Cell Lymphoma
- Disease located primarily in lymph nodes
- Necrosis and angioinvasion not prominent
- Neoplastic cells are often larger
- Mostly have T-cell and not NK-cell phenotype
- Previously classified as peripheral T-cell lymphoma, not otherwise specified
- Different molecular alterations than ENKTL, *TET2* mutations most common

Aggressive NK-Cell Leukemia
- Involves blood and bone marrow
- By definition, always NK-cell lineage

Subcutaneous Panniculitis-Like T-Cell Lymphoma
- Involves subcutis and spares dermis
- CD8(+), CD56(-), and EBV(-)

Infections
- Number of infectious organisms can involve nasal region
- Mixed inflammatory infiltrate with granulocytes
- No evidence of monoclonal gene rearrangements
- EBV(-)

SELECTED REFERENCES

1. Campo E et al: The International Consensus Classification of mature lymphoid neoplasms: a report from the Clinical Advisory Committee. Blood. 140(11):1229-53, 2022
2. Kim H et al: The pathologic and genetic characteristics of extranodal NK/T-cell lymphoma. Life (Basel). 12(1):73, 2022
3. Dong G et al: Genetic manipulation of primary human natural killer cells to investigate the functional and oncogenic roles of PRDM1. Haematologica. 106(9):2427-38, 2021
4. Xiong J et al: Genomic and transcriptomic characterization of natural killer T cell lymphoma. Cancer Cell. 37(3):403-19.e6, 2020

Extranodal NK-/T-Cell Lymphoma

EBER

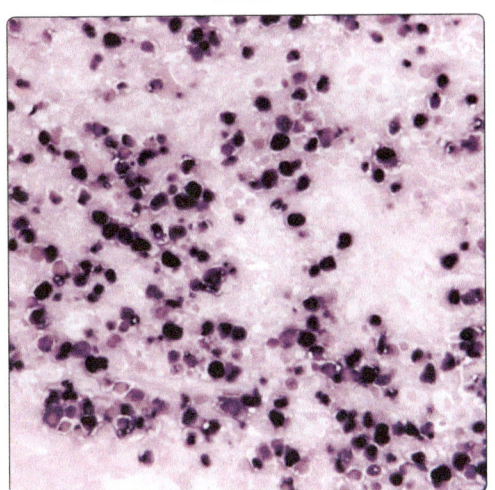

CD3 Immunohistochemistry

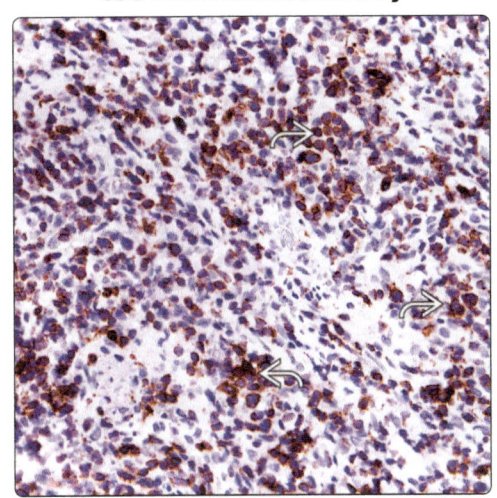

(Left) In situ hybridization for Epstein-Barr virus-encoded small RNA (EBER) is strongly positive. EBV infection is a consistent feature of ENKTL. This test is sensitive and easy to perform. (Right) CD3 shows that the neoplastic cells of ENKTL are immunoreactive ⇒. This antibody detects the epsilon chain of CD3 within the cell cytoplasm. Expression of CD3-ε chain is positive in both T cells and NK cells.

CD56 Immunohistochemistry

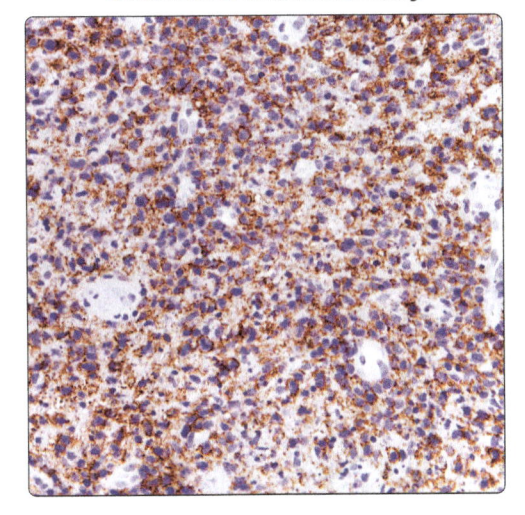

TIA Immunohistochemistry

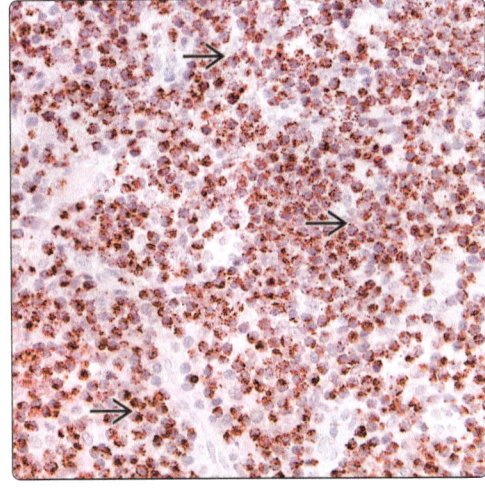

(Left) CD56 is diffusely positive and commonly (but not invariably) expressed in ENKTL of NK-cell lineage. CD56 is highly suggestive of but not entirely specific for NK-cell lineage. (Right) TIA shows many cytotoxic granules ⇒ in this case of ENKTL, nasal type. Other cytotoxic markers, such as GZM-B and perforin (not shown), are also usually immunoreactive in this tumor.

CD8 Immunohistochemistry

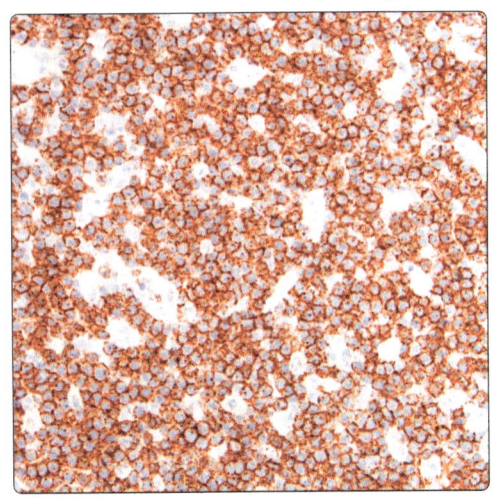

Lymph Node

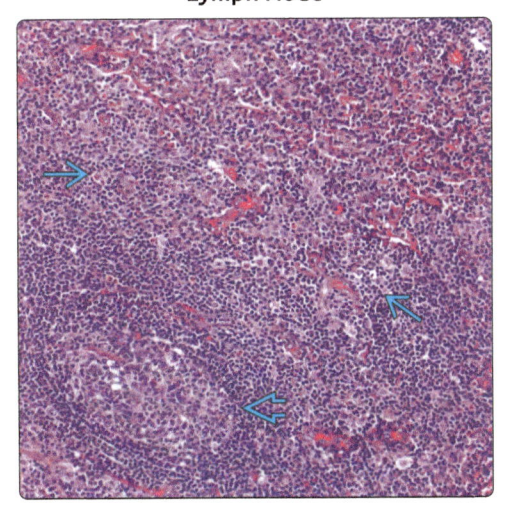

(Left) CD8 shows that the neoplastic cells are positive, supporting T-cell lineage. (Right) In a lymph node, ENKTL is thought to begin in the medullary and paracortical regions ⇒. B-cell regions, such as germinal centers ⇒, in the cortex may be spared.

Adult T-Cell Leukemia/Lymphoma

KEY FACTS

TERMINOLOGY
- Peripheral CD4(+) T-cell neoplasm often disseminated, caused by retrovirus, human T-cell lymphotrophic virus type I (HTLV-I)

ETIOLOGY/PATHOGENESIS
- HTLV-I is causally related to adult T-cell leukemia/lymphoma (ATLL) and necessary for diagnosis
- HTLV-1 encodes HBZ and Tax crucial proteins involved in T-cell proliferation

CLINICAL ISSUES
- 4 clinical subtypes
  - Acute, lymphomatous, chronic, and smoldering
- Presentation depends on subtype
  - Peripheral blood, bone marrow, lymph node, and skin can be involved
  - Hypercalcemia distinguishes aggressive ATLL subtype from other lymphomas

MOLECULAR
- PCR: Used to confirm enzyme immunosorbent assay (EIA) tests for HTLV-I
- Clonal T-cell receptor gene rearrangements by PCR
- Genetically unstable with high number of structural variations, cytogenetics complex, integration of retrovirus in host is random
- Common mutations involve T-cell function or proliferation

MICROSCOPIC
- Peripheral blood shows large flower-like cells
- Bone marrow shows variable lymphoid infiltrates
- Lymph nodes show effacement by atypical pleomorphic cells, Reed-Sternberg-like cells, or bizarre pleomorphic cells

ANCILLARY TESTS
- Immunohistochemistry and flow cytometry
  - CD4(+), CD5(+/-), CD2(+/-), CD7(-), CD25(+)
  - FOXP3 and CCR4 are frequently expressed

Peripheral Blood

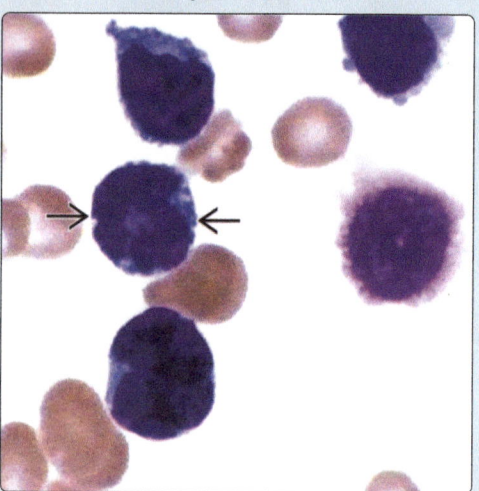

Bone Marrow

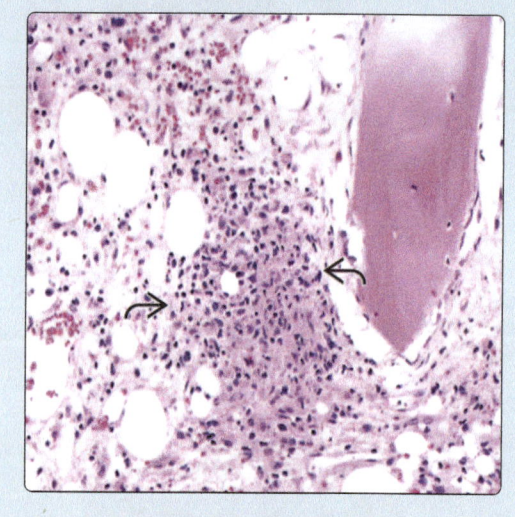

(Left) *Peripheral blood smear shows characteristic flower-like cells in adult T-cell lymphoma/leukemia (ATLL). The nuclei are petal-like ➡ with inconspicuous nucleoli. Peripheral blood abnormalities are commonly present.* (Right) *Bone marrow trephine biopsy from the same patient shows variable involvement with ATLL ➡ and a background that appears hypocellular. This patient had a chronic presentation.*

Cerebrospinal Fluid

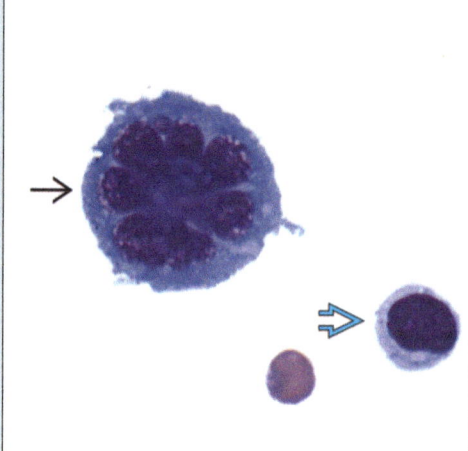

Cerebrospinal Fluid

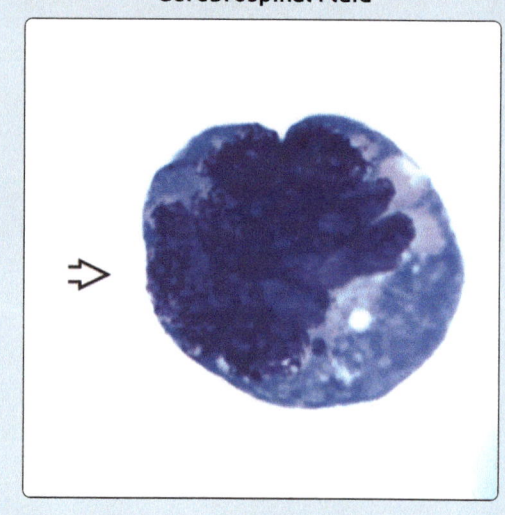

(Left) *Cerebrospinal fluid from a 29-year-old woman with ATLL shows a neoplastic T cell ➡ that is significantly larger than the normal small lymphocyte ➡.* (Right) *Cytospin preparation of cerebrospinal fluid from an HTLV-1 positive patient is shown. Flow cytometry showed the large neoplastic T cells ➡ being positive for CD4, CD3, CD2, and CD30 but negative for CD7. CD25 was also negative in this case, which is unusual.*

Adult T-Cell Leukemia/Lymphoma

TERMINOLOGY

Abbreviations
- Adult T-cell lymphoma/leukemia (ATLL)

Definitions
- Distinct entity recognized by both WHO 5th edition and ICC classifications
- Peripheral CD4(+) T-cell neoplasm often disseminated, caused by retrovirus, human T-cell lymphotrophic virus type I (HTLV-I)

ETIOLOGY/PATHOGENESIS

Environmental Exposure
- Major paths of exposure
  o Breast feeding, blood exposure, sexual transmission

Infectious Agents
- HTLV-I is causally related to ATLL
- ~ 20 million people worldwide infected with HTLV-I
- 1-5% of HTLV-I carriers will develop ATLL
  o Inflammatory diseases related to HTLV-I
    – Tropical spastic paraparesis (TSP), HTLV-I-associated myelopathy (HAM), HTLV-I uveitis and infective dermatitis

Epidemiology
- Endemic in Southern Japan, Africa, Caribbean, Latin America, Australia, and Northeast Iran
- HLA alleles A26, B4002, B4006, and B4801 appear to be predisposed to develop ATLL
- Molecular subtypes are specific to geographic area

Risk Factors
- HTLV-I infection early in life, increased age
- Male sex, family history of ATLL, specific HLA types
- History of infective dermatitis, smoking
- Serum titers against HTLV-I, HTLV-I proviral load

CLINICAL ISSUES

Presentation
- 4 clinical subtypes of ATLL
  o Acute: 60%
    – Most common subtype in children
    – Marked leukocytosis with eosinophilia
    – Hypercalcemia ± osteolytic lesions ± renal dysfunction and neuropsychiatric abnormalities
    – Massive lymphadenopathy, organomegaly, CNS and skin involvement
    – Opportunistic infections
  o Lymphomatous: 20%
    – Lymphadenopathy without peripheral blood involvement
    – ± skin involvement ± hypercalcemia
  o Chronic: 15%
    – Skin involvement, leukocytosis, lymphocytosis, mild lymphadenopathy, and hypercalcemia
  o Smoldering: 5%
    – Normal WBC count with > 5% circulating neoplastic cells, frequent skin or pulmonary lesions but no hypercalcemia

- Most ATLL patients have associated immunodeficiency

Treatment
- Prevention of HTLV-I transmission is key to prevent of ATLL
- Aggressive forms
  o Multidrug chemotherapy and allogenic stem cell transplant
  o Zidovudine and α-interferon ± chemotherapy in Western countries
- Indolent forms
  o No treatment given; watch and wait

Prognosis
- Survival time for acute subtypes: ~ 6 months; lymphomatous: ~ 10 months
- Chronic and smoldering have better survival rate but can progress to acute phase in ~ 25% of patients
- Primary skin disease without systemic involvement has better prognosis than secondary skin involvement
- Poor prognostic indicators
  o > 40 years of age, hypercalcemia, high lactate dehydrogenase (LDH), and high serum CD25
  o Main predictor of disease is proviral load
    – Percentage of HTLV-I-infected peripheral blood mononuclear cells

MACROSCOPIC

General Features
- Nonspecific; organomegaly and skin lesions

MOLECULAR

Cytogenetics
- No consistent cytogenetic abnormalities

Polymerase Chain Reaction
- HTLV-I-integrated site-specific PCR
  o Oligoclonal expansion of HTLV-I infected premalignant cells detected in asymptomatic HTLV-I carriers
  o Used to confirm enzyme immunosorbent assay (EIA) tests for HTLV-I
    – Conventional PCR (tax and pol)
    – Real-time PCR (pol)
- T-cell receptor gene rearrangements
  o Clonal rearrangements of *TRB* &/or *TRG* detected in aggressive disease

Array Comparative Genomic Hybridization
- Paired samples using oligo array CGH using blood and lymph node samples showed that clonal evolution takes place in lymph node
- Numerous TCR subclones exist in lymph node
- Chromosome imbalances were common in lymph node

Molecular Genetics
- HTLV-I genotype is characterized by parallel sequencing technology in asymptomatic carriers, myelopathy/TSP, and ATLL patients
- HTLV-I gene encodes
  o 3 structural proteins: Gag, Pol, and Env
  o 2 crucial regulatory proteins: Tax (p40) and HBZ

Adult T-Cell Leukemia/Lymphoma

- Tax drives viral replication and activates cellular pathways in T-cell proliferation
- HBZ drives cell proliferation
- Both play role in pathogenesis of HTLV-1 and leukemogenesis
- Clonal HTLV-1 integration
  - HTLV-1 integration can be demonstrated on paraffin tissue sections using RNAscope with HTLV-1 HBZ mRNA probes
- Novel fusions and alterations involving genes related to immune function, including
  - *CTLA4::CD28*, *ICOS::CD28* fusions and *REL* C-terminal truncation
  - Recurrent genetic alterations in *HLA-A* and *HLA-B*
  - Structural variants with disruption of 3' UTR of *CD274* (PD-L1)
- *CCR4* mutations in ~ 25% of cases
  - Predicts response to mogamulizumab
- Other reported frequently mutated genes include
  - *PLCG1*, *PRKCB*, *VAV1*, *IRF4*, *FYN*, *CARD11*, *CDKN2A*, *CDKN2B*, and *STAT3*
- Mutations associated with unfavorable prognosis include
  - *TP53* and *PRKCB*; alterations in TCR/NFκB pathway in indolent subtype

MicroRNA (miRNA)
- Dysregulation of miRNA may be involved in pathogenesis of HTLV-I
- ATL patients show polycomb-mediated miR-31 silencing resulting in overexpression of NFκB-inducing kinase following NFκB activation

MICROSCOPIC

Histologic Features
- Peripheral blood
  - Lymphocytosis with large atypical lymphocytes: Flower-like cells
  - Markedly elevated WBC count in acute variant
  - Morphologic involvement of blood may not be detected in lymphomatous or smoldering forms
- Bone marrow
  - Variably involved with subtle or patchy infiltrates
  - Diffuse or interstitial involvement ± fibrosis
  - Increased osteoclasts showing bone resorption
  - > 5% bone marrow involvement is considered prognostically poor
- Lymph node
  - Heterogeneous morphology
  - Diffuse paracortical expansion
  - Least common is angioimmunoblastic T-cell lymphoma-like morphology
- Skin
  - Clinical
    - Patch, plaque, multipapular, tumoral, erythrodermic, and purpuric
  - Histologic findings
    - Perivascular, nodular, and diffuse infiltrate
    - Epidermotropic with microabscesses (Pautrier-like microabscesses)
    - Follicular mucinosis-like in some cases
  - Lymphohistiocytic lesions may be prelude to lymphoma involvement

Cytologic Features
- Cell types
  - Pleomorphic medium and large cells
  - Reed-Sternberg-like cells
  - Anaplastic large cell-like are bizarre large cells with abundant cytoplasm

ANCILLARY TESTS

Immunohistochemistry
- CD4(+), CD5(+/-), CD2(+/-), CD3(+), CD7(-), CD8(-), CD25 strongly (+), CCR4(+), CD30(-/+), FOXP3(+) in ~ 50%, HTLV-1/HTLV-2(+)
- Few are CD4(-), CD8(+) or CD4 and CD8 double (+)

Flow Cytometry
- CD4(+), CD5(+/-), CD2(+/-), CD3(+/-), CD7(-), CD8(-), CD25(+), TCRα/β(+)

Serologic Testing
- EIA tests detect HTLV-I antibody in human serum or plasma in all subtypes
  - Western blot or PCR is used to confirm and separate HTLV-I and HTLV-II
  - PCR is most definitive as western blot is often indeterminate

DIFFERENTIAL DIAGNOSIS

Mycosis Fungoides
- Negative for HTLV-I
- Clinical presentation less acute
- Histologically similar to ATLL
- Similar immunophenotype [CD4(+), CD8(-), CD7(-), CD3(+)]

Peripheral T-Cell Lymphoma
- Negative for HTLV-I
- Serologic testing recommended in endemic areas
- May have same immunophenotype and histology as ATLL

Anaplastic Large Cell Lymphoma
- Negative for HTLV-I
- Bright and uniform expression of CD30

DIAGNOSTIC CHECKLIST

Clinically Relevant Pathologic Features
- HTLV-I positivity is necessary for diagnosis

Pathologic Interpretation Pearls
- Immunophenotype CD4(+), CD8(-), CD25 strongly (+), FOXP3(+) in ~ 50%, TCRα/β(+)
- Clonal T-cell receptor gene rearrangements

SELECTED REFERENCES

1. Alaggio R et al: The 5th edition of the World Health Organization Classification of Haematolymphoid Tumours: Lymphoid Neoplasms. Leukemia. 36(7):1720-48, 2022
2. de Leval L et al: Genomic profiling for clinical decision making in lymphoid neoplasms. Blood. 140(21):2193-227, 2022
3. Kogure Y et al: Whole-genome landscape of adult T-cell leukemia/lymphoma. Blood. 139(7):967-82, 2022

Adult T-Cell Leukemia/Lymphoma

Effaced Lymph Node Architecture

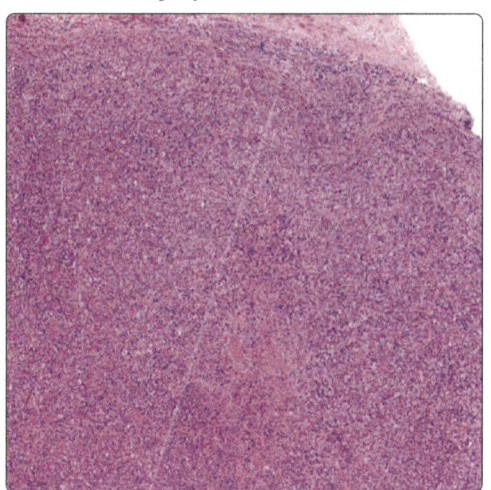

Neoplastic Large T Cells

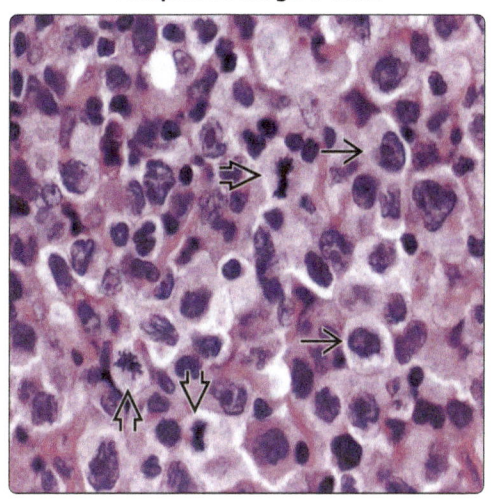

(Left) *Lymph node from a patient with chronic presentation of ATLL in peripheral blood who progressed to lymphomatous clinical picture is shown. The architecture is effaced by a proliferation of large cells with abundant cytoplasm.* (Right) *High-power view of the same lymph node section shows large, pleomorphic cells with abundant cytoplasm ⇨. Numerous mitoses ⇨ are noted. The patient had an aggressive clinical course after transformation to lymphoma.*

CD3 Immunohistochemical Stain

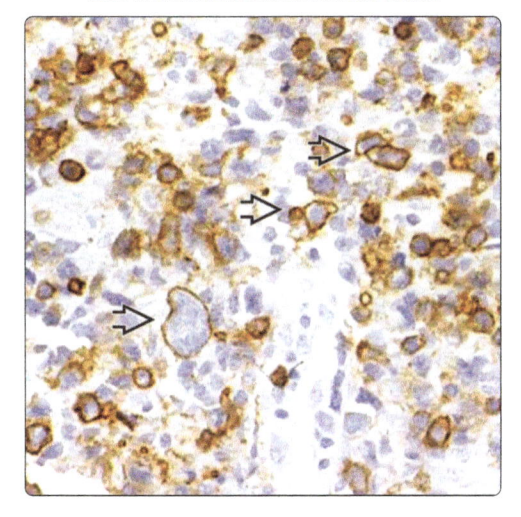

Flow Cytometry

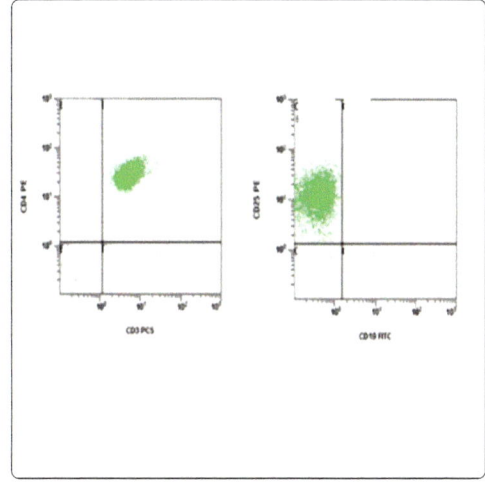

(Left) *ATLL in lymph node shows CD3 positivity ⇨. Neoplastic cells are also CD4 and pan T-cell marker (+) with a loss of CD7 (not shown). ATLL is also commonly positive for CD25.* (Right) *ATLL assessed by flow cytometric immunophenotyping shows a CD3(+), CD4(+), and CD25(+) cell population. The left histogram displays CD4 (y-axis) vs. CD3; the right histogram displays CD25 (y-axis) vs. CD19. (From DP: Lymphomas.)*

Cutaneous Adult T-Cell Leukemia/Lymphoma

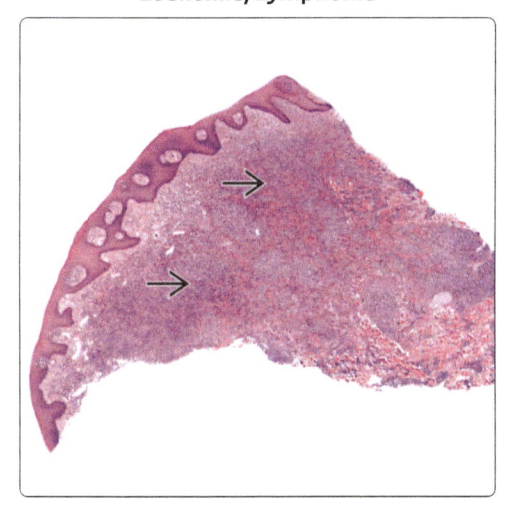

Skin With Pautrier-Like Microabscess

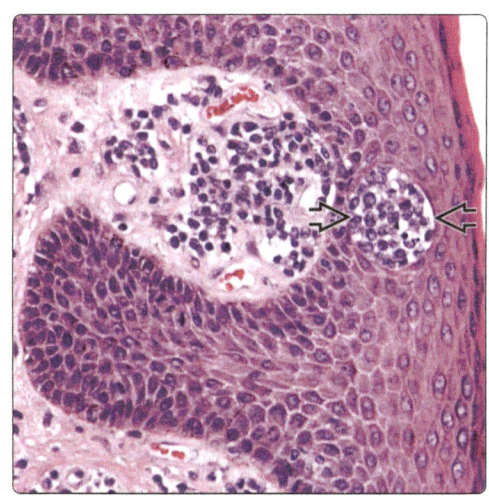

(Left) *Biopsy from a cutaneous nodule in a patient with ATLL shows a dense lymphoid infiltrate ⇨ involving the dermis. (From DP: Lymphomas.)* (Right) *Abundant neoplastic lymphoid cells in the epidermis form a well-circumscribed cluster, giving the appearance of a Pautrier-like microabscess ⇨. Smaller and less cellular intraepidermal aggregates are more characteristic of mycosis fungoides, although sometimes the distinction is not possible. (From DP: Lymphomas.)*

Adult T-Cell Leukemia/Lymphoma

(Left) The majority of the neoplastic cells are pleomorphic and medium to large in size in this high-power image of ATLL involving the skin. (From DP: Lymphomas.) **(Right)** ATLL in the leukemic phase shows neoplastic lymphoid cells with irregular nuclear contours ⇨. Note the intermediate to large size and the flower-like nuclei. (From DP: Lymphomas.)

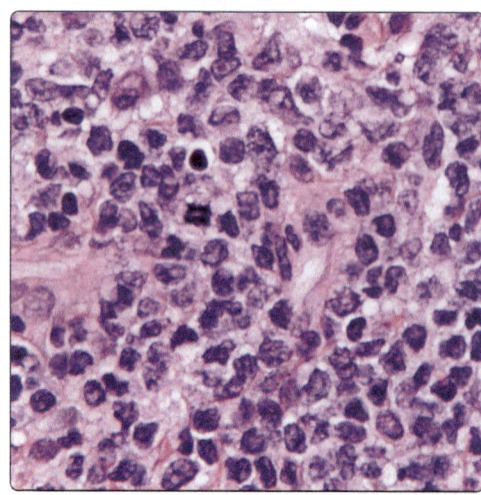

Cutaneous Adult T-Cell Leukemia/Lymphoma

Peripheral Blood

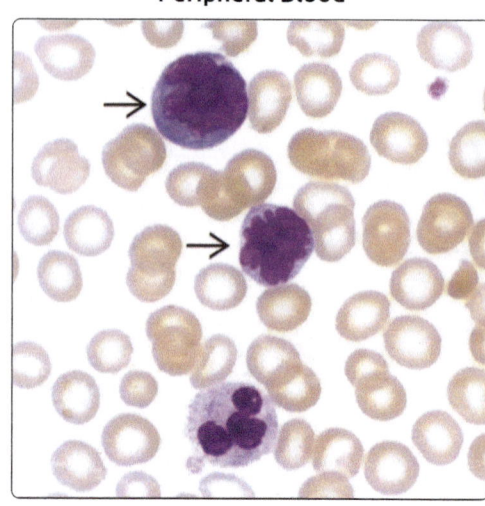

(Left) Bone marrow core biopsy shows ATLL in a 54-year-old African American woman with osteolytic lesions. There is hypercellularity with a polymorphous proliferation of medium to large lymphoma cells ⇨. Numerous osteoclasts ⇨ cause resorption of bone trabeculae. (From DP: Lymphomas.) **(Right)** ATLL involving bone marrow is shown. Increased bone resorption and osteoclasts ⇨ on both sides of the bone trabeculae cause the appearance of an apple core. (From DP: Lymphomas.)

Bony Resorption in Bone Marrow

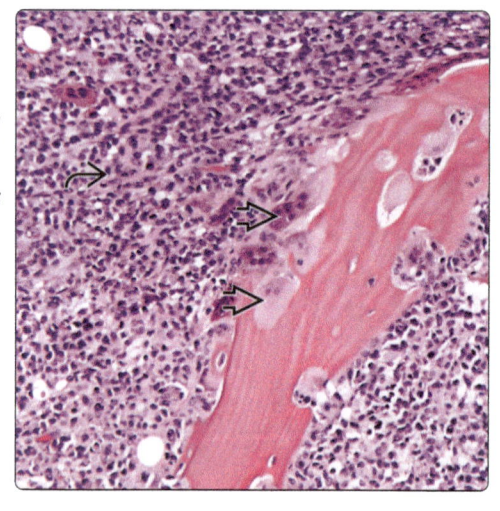

Osteoclastic Activity in Bone Marrow

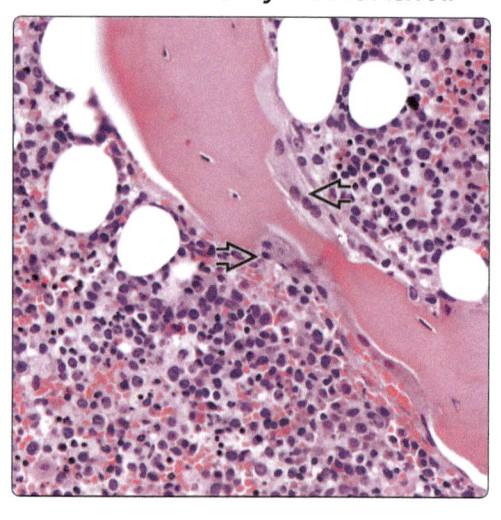

(Left) Lymph node with effacement of the architecture ⇨ is shown. There is no distinction from other lymphomas at this low power. **(Right)** At higher power, the neoplastic cells are irregular with singly distributed large, atypical cells scattered throughout the neoplastic infiltrate. The large cells can resemble Reed-Sternberg cells and may be CD30(+). Integrated human T-cell lymphotrophic virus type I (HTLV-I) into the host genome is necessary for diagnosis. TRG &/or TRB show clonality in most cases.

Effaced Lymph Node

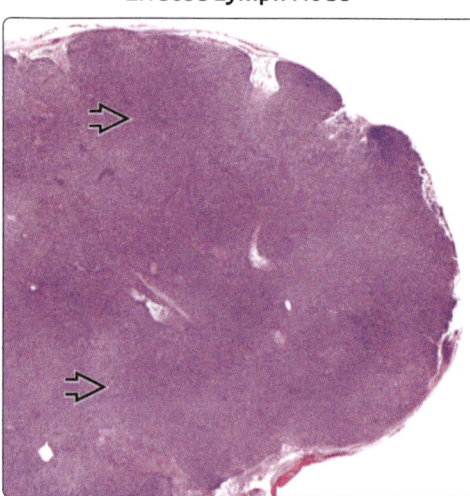

Neoplastic Large T-Cells

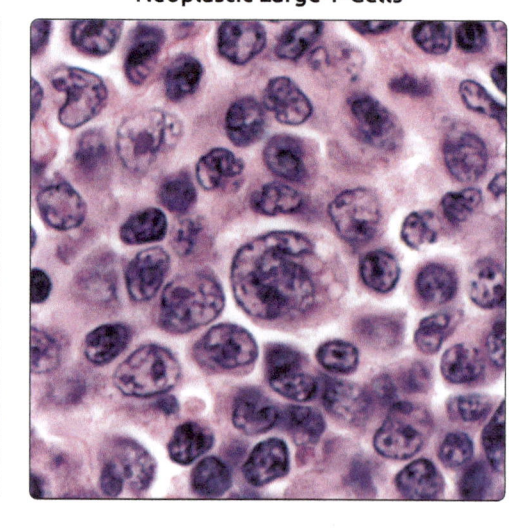

Adult T-Cell Leukemia/Lymphoma

Mycoses Fungoides

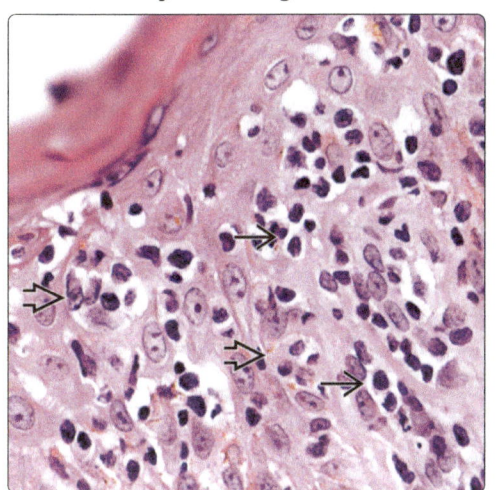

Sézary Syndrome

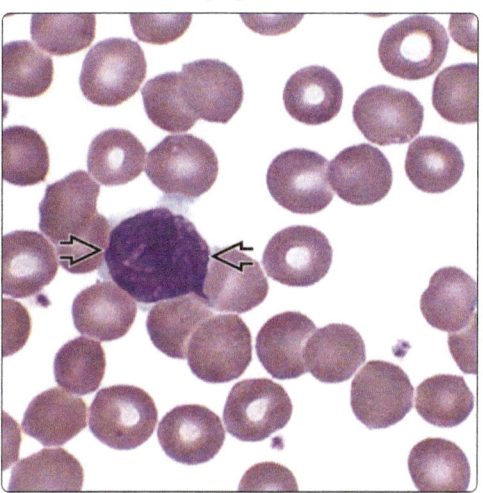

(Left) Skin biopsy from a patient with mycoses fungoides shows similar features to ATLL. Pautrier microabscesses are present ➡ with scattered epidermotropic lymphocytes ➡. (Right) This cell from the peripheral blood of a patient with Sézary syndrome shows a circulating Sézary cell with irregular nuclear contours ➡. The cells are less flower-like than ATLL but are more cerebriform with nuclear irregularities.

Peripheral T-Cell Lymphoma

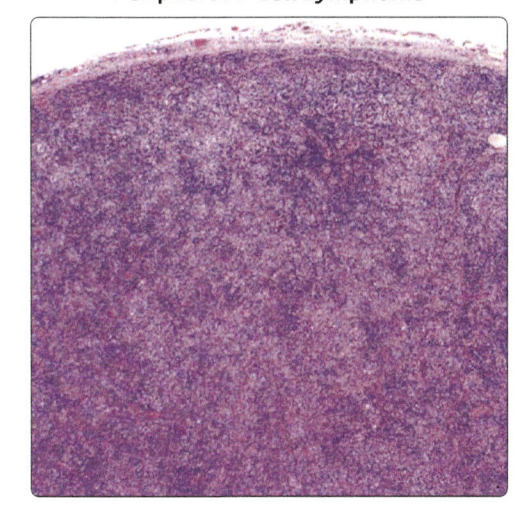

Peripheral T-Cell Lymphoma

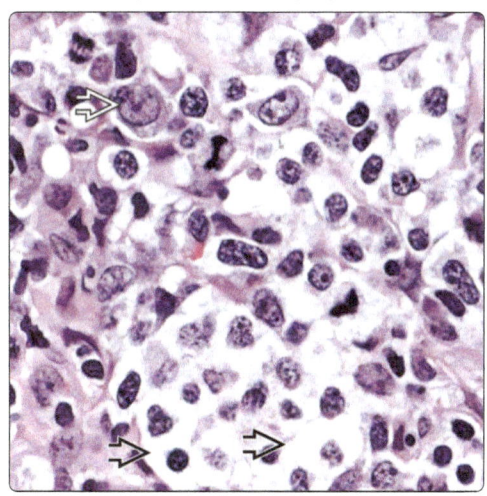

(Left) Lymph node involved by peripheral T-cell lymphoma is shown. There is effacement of the architecture by a proliferation of pale-staining T cells. (Right) The malignant cells in this peripheral T-cell lymphoma have abundant cytoplasm ➡ with some cells showing irregular nuclei ➡. The cells can have a similar immunophenotype to ATLL, but they lack integrated HTLV-I in the host genome.

Anaplastic Large Cell Lymphoma

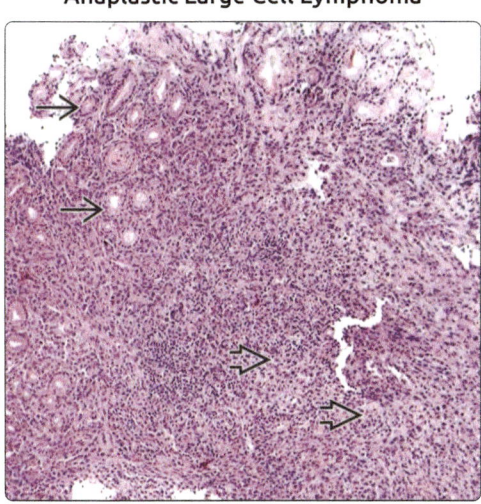

Anaplastic Large Cell Lymphoma

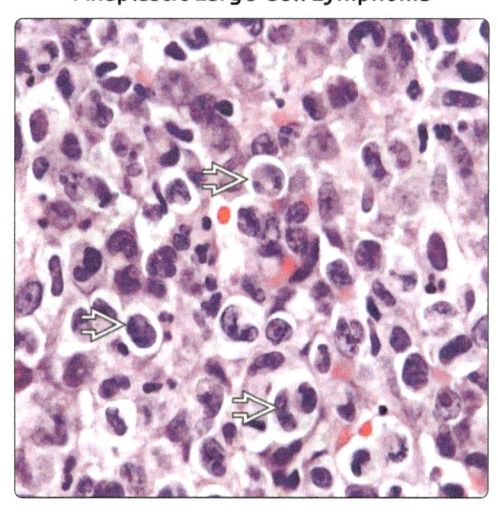

(Left) Section of esophagus and stomach shows an anaplastic large cell lymphoma. There is a dense lymphoid infiltrate ➡. Residual glands are noted ➡. (Right) High-power view shows numerous atypical large cells with pleomorphic nuclei and abundant cytoplasm. This case was CD30(+), which does not distinguish it from ATLL. It also showed variable pan T-cell markers and TIA1 positivity. So-called hallmark cells ➡ are present.

Molecular Pathology of Lymphoid Neoplasms

415

Intestinal T-Cell Lymphoma

KEY FACTS

TERMINOLOGY
- **Abbreviations**
  - World Health Organization, 5th edition (WHO-HAEM5)
  - International Consensus Classification (ICC)

CLASSIFICATION
- Both classifications use same nomenclature for 4 below categories
  - Enteropathy-associated T-cell lymphoma (EATL)
  - Monomorphic epitheliotropic intestinal T-cell lymphoma (MEITL)
  - Indolent NK-cell lymphoproliferative disorder of GI (INKLPD-GIT)
  - Intestinal T-cell lymphoma, not otherwise specified (ITCL, NOS)
- Different designation used in one category by ICC vs. WHO-HAEM5
  - Indolent clonal T-cell LPD of GI tract (ICC)
  - Indolent T-cell lymphoma of GI tract (WHO-HAEM5)
- 1 new distinct category designated as type II refractory celiac disease (RCD-II) (ICC)
  - Not recognized in WHO-HAEM5
  - Previously described as precursor to enteropathy-associated T-cell lymphoma, now defined as distinct entity in ICC

MOLECULAR
- Clonal *TRB* and *TRG* rearrangements in categories in this group except for indolent NK-cell LPD of GI tract
- EBER (-) in all categories in this group
- EATL has *TNFAIP3*, *JAK1*, and *STAT3* alterations
- MEITL has *SETD2*, *STAT5B*, and *MYC* alterations

MICROSCOPIC
- T cells in MEITL are usually more monotonous than EATL

ANCILLARY TESTS
- CD8 and CD56 usually (+) in MEITL, unlike EATL

Enteropathy-Associated T-Cell Lymphoma

(Left) Interface between enteropathy-associated T-cell lymphoma (EATL) ➡ and adjacent residual villi ➡ is shown. Intraepithelial lymphocytes are present within the villi. (Right) PCR for T-cell receptor γ (TRG) shows a dominant monoclonal peak, as is often the case for EATL.

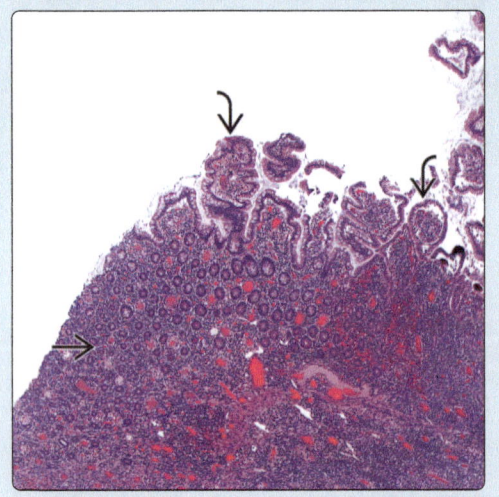

T-Cell Receptor-γ Gene Rearrangement

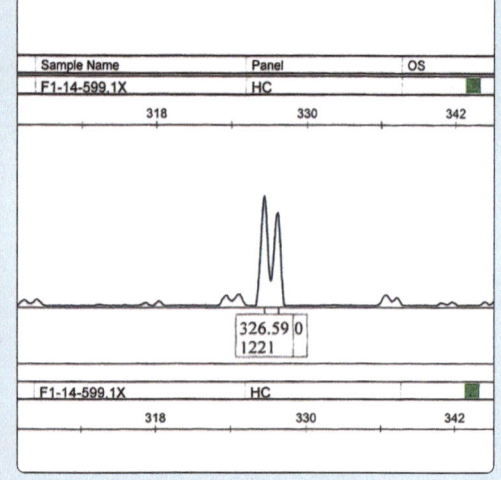

Pleomorphic T Cells

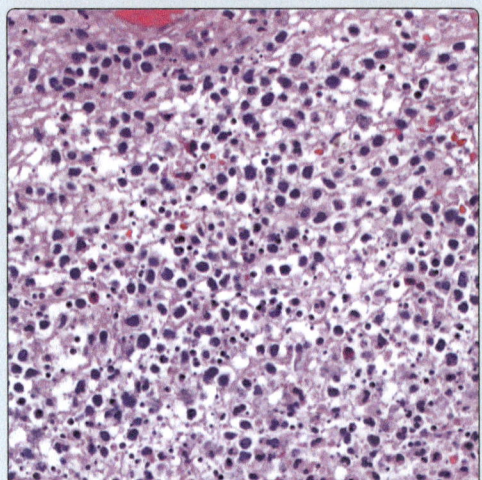

Clear Cytoplasm

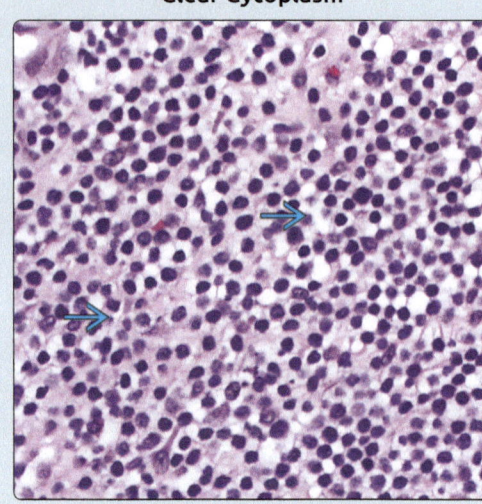

(Left) EATL involving jejunum is shown. Lymphoma cells are large and pleomorphic. Numerous eosinophils and some neutrophils are present in the background. (Right) In this case of monomorphic epitheliotropic intestinal T-cell lymphoma (MEITL), the T-cells have a very homogeneous appearance. The cells often have a clear rim of cytoplasm ➡.

416

Intestinal T-Cell Lymphoma

TERMINOLOGY

Definitions
- Mature T-cell lymphomas, which are primary to GI tract

CLASSIFICATION

ICC and WHO-HAEM5
- Both classifications use same nomenclature for 4 below categories
  - Enteropathy-associated T-cell lymphoma (EATL)
  - Monomorphic epitheliotropic intestinal T-cell lymphoma (MEITL)
  - Indolent NK-cell lymphoproliferative disorder of GI tract (INKLPD-GIT)
  - Intestinal T-cell lymphoma, not otherwise specified (ITCL, NOS)

ICC vs. WHO-HAEM5
- Different designation used in one category by ICC vs. WHO-HAEM5
  - Indolent clonal T-cell LPD of GI tract (ICC)
  - Indolent T-cell lymphoma of GI tract (WHO-HAEM5)
- 1 new distinct category designated as type II refractory celiac disease (RCD-II) (ICC)
  - Not recognized in WHO-HAEM5
  - Previously described as precursor to enteropathy-associated T-cell lymphoma, now defined as distinct entity in ICC

ETIOLOGY/PATHOGENESIS

Enteropathy-Associated T-Cell Lymphoma
- Associated with celiac disease (CD)
  - Serological tests positive; association with HLA-DQ2 or HLA-DQ8, unlike MEITL
  - Pathologic evidence of CD in uninvolved intestinal mucosa
  - Associated clinical findings, such as gluten intolerance, dermatitis herpetiformis, and hyposplenism
  - CD may be diagnosed at time of EATL diagnosis
- Aggressive intestinal T-cell lymphoma of intraepithelial lymphocytes with cellular pleomorphism, often in people with CD
- Poor prognosis with median survival of 7 months
- Present with GI symptoms, often culminating in intestinal perforation and peritonitis
- T-cell type
  - αβ, γδ, or TCR-silent T cells
  - More αβ T-cells than γδ T-cells

Monomorphic Epitheliotropic Intestinal T-Cell Lymphoma
- No association with CD
- No association with HLA-DQ2 or HLA-DQ8
- T-cell type
  - αβ, γδ, or TCR-silent T-cells
  - More γδ T-cells than αβ T-cells

Indolent NK-Cell Lymphoproliferative Disorder of GI Tract
- Could be immune response to GI mucosa antigens
- *Helicobacter pylori*
  - *H. pylori* has been reported at high prevalence in gastric cases of INKLPD-GIT
  - Reported to regress after *H. pylori* treatment
- Previously known as lymphomatoid gastropathy or NK-cell enteropathy and was previously considered reactive
  - However, gene mutations such as *JAK3* have been detected, so it is now considered neoplasm
- Very indolent behavior with spontaneous regression of disease without treatment, rare recurrence often after years
- Superficial mucosal and rarely lymph node infiltrate of atypical cells with NK-cell immunophenotype

Indolent T-Cell Lymphoproliferative Disorder/Lymphoma of GI Tract
- Etiology undetermined; not associated with CD
- Some patients have inflammatory bowel disease or intestine immune disorders, but relationship with indolent T-cell LPD/lymphoma of GI tract is unknown
- No known ethnic predisposition
- Indolent T-cell lymphoma of GI tract (WHO-HAEM5)
  - ICC designates this category as lymphoproliferative disorder similar to terminology used in WHO-HAEM4
    - Changing to "lymphoma" reflects cases of tumor disseminating and morbidity of tumor
  - Term "indolent" is still used to describe protracted clinical course in most cases
  - Clonal T-cell disorder with lamina propria infiltration by small T cells lacking epitheliotropism and with long clinical course

Intestinal T-Cell Lymphoma, Not Otherwise Specified
- Aggressive primary GI T-cell lymphoma that does not fulfill criteria of EATL, MEITL, indolent T-cell lymphoma of GI tract, INKLPD-GIT
  - Often cytotoxic phenotype
  - Often lack epitheliotropism of EATL and MEITL

CLINICAL ISSUES

Epidemiology
- Incidence
  - EATL
    - Most common type of intestinal T-cell lymphoma
    - Greatest frequency in areas with high prevalence of celiac disease, particularly Northern European and United States
    - Accounts for ~ 35% of all small intestinal lymphomas
    - < 5% of all GI tract lymphomas
    - Annual rate of 0.5-1.0 per million people in Western countries
    - Typically occurs ~ 5-10 years after CD diagnosis
      - But can be diseased before or concomitant with CD diagnosis
      - Lymphoma may develop in course of progressive deterioration of RCD
  - MEITL
    - More commonly in Hispanic and Asian populations, unlike EATL
    - Most cases of primary intestinal T-cell lymphoma in Asia but found worldwide

Intestinal T-Cell Lymphoma

- INKLPD-GIT
  - Rare disease that includes cases called NK cell enteropathy or lymphomatoid gastropathy in past
- ITCL, NOS
  - Wide geographic distribution
  - Incidence is low in United States and Europe but high in Asia, involving up to 63% of cases
- Age
  - EATL: Median 60 years
  - MEITL: Median 54-67 years
  - Indolent T-cell LPD/lymphoma of GI tract: Usually in adults and only rarely reported in children
  - INKLPD-GIT: Usually adults from 3rd to 8th decade
  - ITCL, NOS: Median: 49 years; range: 15-78 years
- Sex
  - EATL: M = F
  - MEITL: M:F = 2:1
  - Indolent T-cell LPD/lymphoma of GI tract: M:F = 1.5-2:1
  - IT NOS: M:F = 2:1

Site
- EATL
  - ~ 90% arise in small intestine: Jejunum or ileum
  - Presentation in duodenum, stomach, and colon may occur rarely
    - Lymphomas arising in these sites show genetic alterations similar to classic EATL in jejunum or ileum
    - RCD can involve duodenum, stomach, or colon
  - Patients usually do not have peripheral lymphadenopathy
    - Lymph node may be site of EATL, although it is more commonly extranodal
    - Nodal EATL may potentially represent another type of lymphoma
  - EATL can disseminate to liver, bone marrow, spleen, skin, and other organs
- MEITL
  - Most common in small intestine
    - Jejunum most frequent site
    - ~ 16% involve large intestine
    - ~ 5% involve stomach
    - 20-35% of cases are multifocal GI tumors
  - Mass ± ulceration
  - Can diffusely involve intestinal mucosa
  - Can involve mesenteric lymph nodes
  - Sometimes disseminates to liver, lung, brain, or skin
- INKLPD-GIT
  - Usually involves stomach (70%)
  - Less common in small bowel and large intestine (~ 30%)
  - Similar lesions have been reported in gallbladder and adjacent lymph nodes
- Indolent T-cell LPD/lymphoma of GI tract
  - More commonly in small bowel but can involve other parts of GI tract
  - Including oral cavity and esophagus
  - Involvement of tissue outside of GI tracts
    - Uncommon at time of diagnosis, but can occur with disease progression
    - Includes bone marrow, peripheral blood and tonsil
- ITCL, NOS
  - One or multiple GI sites
  - Colon and small bowel are most common
  - Can disseminate to regional lymph nodes and other GI sites

Presentation
- EATL
  - Clinical history of CD
    - Some cases associated with CD, and some arise de novo
    - Typical symptoms of celiac disease
      - Diarrhea
      - Malabsorption, anemia, weight loss, vitamin deficiencies
      - Dermatitis herpetiformis
    - Most patients have adult-onset CD
      - Rarely, patients have childhood-onset CD
  - Clinical findings of EATL
    - Weight loss, abdominal pain, and diarrhea
    - B symptoms
    - Small bowel obstruction or perforation frequently
- MEITL
  - Abdominal pain, weight loss, obstruction, bleeding or perforation
  - Usually no malabsorption
- INKLPD-GIT
  - Usually asymptomatic or only abdominal pain
  - Lesions seen by endoscopy
  - No history of CD or Crohn disease
  - No systematic lymphadenopathy
- Indolent T-cell LPD/lymphoma of GI tract
  - Abdominal pain, diarrhea, vomiting, and weight loss
  - Mesenteric lymphadenopathy sometimes but no peripheral lymphadenopathy
- ITCL, NOS
  - Symptoms depend on site of involvement
  - Similar presentation to EATL and MEITL, but infrequent malabsorption
  - Gastric cases show epigastric gain and hematemesis
- RCD-II
  - Persistent enteropathy-associated histologic changes on biopsy despite strict gluten-free diet for > 12 months or severe persistent symptoms necessitating clinical intervention independent of duration of gluten-free diet
  - In some cases of RCD-II, intraepithelial lymphocytes show
    - Loss of T-cell antigens, including CD8
    - Monoclonal T-cell receptor gene rearrangement
    - Gain of chromosome 1q
    - Overexpression of interleukin-15, which can be involved in development of T-cell lymphoma

Laboratory Tests
- EATL
  - CD
    - Serology
      - IgA antitissue transglutaminase and IgA endomysial antibody are most sensitive and specific tests
    - HLA typing
      - HLA-DQ2 and HLA-DQ8 typing may be useful in individuals with equivocal findings
  - May have high lactate dehydrogenase levels

Intestinal T-Cell Lymphoma

Treatment
- EATL and MEITL
  - ~ 50% of patients require laparotomy for complications of hemorrhage, perforation, or obstruction
  - Combination chemotherapy is often used
    - Cyclophosphamide, doxorubicin, vincristine, prednisolone (CHOP)
  - Stem cell transplant
- INKLPD-GIT
  - Usually does not show prolonged response to chemotherapy

Prognosis
- EATL
  - Poor
    - Multifocal disease with frequent recurrences
    - Complications include GI bleeding and perforation
    - 5-year survival: 8-20%
    - < 10 months median survival
    - De novo EATL patients have more favorable prognosis than RCD2-related EATL
    - CD30(+) cases of EATL can be treated with CD30 targeted therapy
- MEITL
  - Aggressive intestinal T-cell lymphoma of intraepithelial T lymphocytes, with monomorphic cells, usually in people lacking CD
  - Poor with median survival of 7 months
  - Intestinal perforation, local recurrence, tumor dissemination, and resistance to chemotherapy leads to poor prognosis
- INKLPD-GIT
  - Nonaggressive disease
  - Spontaneous regression of lesions usually after few months
  - Sometimes persistent lesions
  - Gastric cases may have concomitant *H. pylori* infection
  - No dissemination
- Indolent T-cell LPD/lymphoma of GI tract
  - Indolent disease
  - Chronic relapsing course
  - Unfavorable response to chemotherapy
- ITCL, NOS
  - Poor prognosis
  - May be better than EATL or MEITL (some studies)
  - Worse prognostic indicators include high stage of disease and large cell morphology

MACROSCOPIC

General Features
- EATL
  - Tumor can present as ulcers, ulcerated nodules, strictures, and less commonly exophytic mass
    - Mesenteric lymph nodes may be enlarged
  - Remaining small intestinal mucosa may be thin with reduced mucosal folds
- MEITL
  - Large, ulcerated mass with full-thickness infiltration of intestinal wall ± perforation
- INKLPD-GIT
  - Single or multiple superficial elevated lesions
  - Often with erosion, ulcer, or hemorrhage
- Indolent T-cell LPD/lymphoma of GI tract
  - Mucosa thickened with prominent folds, nodules, fissures, polyps, and ulcers
- ITCL, NOS
  - Ulcerated plaques and elevated masses

MOLECULAR

Gene Alterations
- EATL
  - Clonal *TRB* and *TRG* rearrangements
    - Detected in nearly all cases
  - Chromosomal imbalances, including gains of chromosome 7, 1q, and 5q, and losses involving 8p22-23.2, 16q21.1, 11q14.1-q14.2, and 9p21.2-p21.3
  - Mutational landscape overlaps that of RCD-II
    - Except *TNFAIP3* has only been detected in de novo EATL
  - Activating mutations in JAK-STAT pathway
    - Most commonly *JAK1* and *STAT3* and rarely *JAK3*, *STAT5B*, *TYK2*, or *SOCS1*
    - Other reported mutated genes include *TNFAIP3*, *KMT2D*, *BCOR*, *DDX3X*, *KRAS*, *NRAS*, *BRAF*, and *TP53*
- MEITL
  - Clonal rearrangements of *TRB* and *TRG*
  - Copy number alterations
    - Gains of 9q, 1q, and 7q; loss or gain of 8q
  - Genes commonly mutated include
    - *SETD2* (~ 90%), *STAT5B*, *STAT3*, *JAK3*, *BRAF*, *KRAS*, *NRAS*, and *GNA12*
    - *MYC* alterations reported in ~ 20%
    - Both γδ and αβ cases
    - *TP53* alterations also reported
- INKLPD-GIT
  - Negative for clonal rearrangement of *TRB* and *TRG*
  - Reported gene alterations include *JAK3*, *RUNX1T1*, *CIC*, *ERBB4*, and *SETD5*
    - Presence of gene alterations is evidence that INKLPD-GIT is neoplastic
  - JAK3-STAT5 pathway may be activated
    - Since STAT5 IHC is strongly positive
- Indolent T-cell LPD/lymphoma of GI tract
  - Clonal *TRB* and *TRG* rearrangements identified in all cases
  - Recurrent *STAT3::JAK2* fusions identified in subset of CD4(+) cases
  - Cases with *STAT3::JAK2* fusion might be sensitive to JAK inhibitors
  - Other mutated genes include *TET2*, *DNMT3A*, and *KMT2D*
  - *TET2*, *KMT2D* alterations
  - Structural alterations in *IL2* in CD8(+) cases
  - More mutations may be related to presence of disease progression
  - EBER ISH is negative
- ITCL, NOS
  - Genotype is incompletely studied and largely unknown
  - Mutations in genes overlapping with those altered in MEITL and EATL have been reported

Intestinal T-Cell Lymphoma

- Fewer *SETD2*, *STAT5*, and *JAK3* mutations compared to MEITL
- JAK/STAT and MAPK pathway alterations have been found

Array CGH
- Variety of aberrations detected in EATL
  - Some also found in RCD-II
  - Not specific for EATL and also may are seen in other primary intestine T-cell lymphomas
- Chromosomal gain of 9q34
  - Seen in EATL and MEITL
- MEITL
  - Similar to EATL, MEITL shows gains of 9q34.3 and losses at 16q12.1
    - However, alterations of 1q32.2-q41 and 5q34-q35.5 have been reported in MEITL in some studies
    - Gains of 4p15.1, 7q34, 8p11.23, 9q22.31, and 12p13.31 as well as loss of 7p14.1 are thought to be more specific to MEITL

Cytogenetics
- Conventional cytogenetics rarely performed in cases of EATL
- ~ 58-70% show complex chromosomal abnormalities

In Situ Hybridization
- *MYC* break-apart probe can detect gains of *MYC* oncogene (8p24) in MEITL
- EBV-encoded RNA (EBER) negative

PCR
- Monoclonal T-cell receptor γ (*TRG*) and β (*TRB*) rearrangements detectable in all types of intestinal T-cell lymphoma
  - Typically Vδ1 region rearrangements
  - Clonal gene rearrangements found both in tumor and in intraepithelial lymphocytes away from tumor in EATL and MEITL

MICROSCOPIC

Histologic Features
- EATL
  - Tumors vary from scattered or clusters of atypical cells in lamina propria or submucosa to transmural infiltrates of pleomorphic lymphoid cells
  - In most cases, lymphoma cells are medium to large in size and relatively pleomorphic
    - Immunoblast or anaplastic morphology
    - Differs from MEITL, which is monomorphic
    - Round or angulated nuclei, vesicular chromatin, prominent nucleoli, and moderate to abundant pale-staining cytoplasm
  - Inflammatory background
    - Histiocytes, eosinophils, neutrophils, small lymphocytes, and plasma cells
    - May obscure tumor cells
  - Adjacent small intestinal mucosa often shows enteropathy-associated changes
    - Villous atrophy, crypt hyperplasia
    - Increased intraepithelial lymphocytes
    - Increased lamina propria lymphocytes and plasma cells
  - Lymph nodes
    - With EATL can show paracortical or intrasinusoidal involvement by neoplastic T cells
    - May just show necrosis without neoplastic T cells
    - May contain pools of lymphoid fluid called lymph node cavitation
- MEITL
  - Most often monotonous, homogeneous, small to medium-sized lymphocytes within mass
    - Round nuclei, dispersed chromatin, rim of pale cytoplasm, indistinct nucleoli
  - In some cases, neoplastic cells are pleomorphic with open chromatin and distinct nucleoli
  - Less inflammatory background than EATL
  - Less tumor necrosis than EATL
  - Lymphoma invades adjacent mucosa with destruction or expansion of villi and epitheliotropic cells
  - No histological evidence of CD in uninvolved mucosa
- Dense transmural lymphoid infiltrate with ulcer, perforation, and epitheliotropic growth found in both EATL and MEITL
- INKLPD-GIT
  - T cells expanding lamina propria in well-circumscribed infiltrate
  - Medium-sized T cells with fine clumped chromatin, small distinct nucleoli, and moderate pale cytoplasm
  - Paranuclear eosinophilic cytoplasmic granules can be seen
  - Glands can be infiltrated, and there can be epithelial involvement
  - Necrosis seen in occasional cases
  - Mixed inflammation often present
    - Eosinophils, neutrophils and plasma cells
  - Muscularis mucosae should be intact
  - No angioinvasion
  - No villous atrophy or crypt hyperplasia
- Indolent T-cell LPD/lymphoma of GI tract
  - Monotonous small T cells in lamina propria
    - May just be patchy infiltrate
    - T cells have round to ovoid nuclei, fine chromatin, indistinct nucleoli, and moderate cytoplasm
  - May involve submucosa and muscularis mucosae
  - No villous atrophy, but crypt hyperplasia can be present
  - Intraepithelial lymphocytes are usually not increased; however, T cells can infiltrate crypt epithelium or lower parts of villi
  - Rarely shows scattered chronic inflammatory cells
  - Granulomas can be focally identified
- ITCL, NOS
  - T-cell infiltrates of mucosa, which is often transmural and can show ulceration
  - Infiltrate can be patchy or diffuse
  - T cells are medium to large in size; often, vesicular chromatin and prominent nucleoli
  - Epitheliotropism only rarely present

Intestinal T-Cell Lymphoma

ANCILLARY TESTS

Immunohistochemistry

- CD without EATL
  - Intraepithelial lymphocytes often have normal immunophenotype
    - CD3 and CD8 (+); CD5(-)
- EATL
  - CD3, CD2, CD7, CD103, TIA1, granzyme B, &/or perforin (+)
  - CD4, CD5, and CD56 (-)
    - CD30(+) in subset of cases, especially in cases with large-sized neoplastic T cells
    - CD8(+) in ~ 25% of cases and more common in patients without CD
    - αβ > γδ so βF1 more commonly positive than TCR-δ
    - EMA sometimes (+); CD30(+) in most tumors with large cell morphology
    - ALK and EBER ISH (-)
  - Adjacent intraepithelial lymphocytes often show similar aberrant immunophenotype in patients with RCD-II
    - CD3(+); CD5, CD8, and CD4 (-)
    - Often cytotoxic proteins (-)
- MEITL
  - Typically CD8, CD56, CD2, CD3, and CD7 (+)
    - Rarely, either CD8 or CD56 may be (-)
  - TIA1 is expressed in most cases, but granzyme B and perforin expression can be variable
  - CD20 may be aberrantly expressed (~ 20%)
  - CD4, CD5, and CD30 (-)
  - CD103(+)
  - MATK and SYK (spleen tyrosine kinase) are (+), unlike EATL
  - TCR-βF1 and TCR-δ can be (+/-)
  - Adjacent intraepithelial lymphocytes are CD3, CD8, and TIA1 (+) but can be CD56(+/-)
  - γδ > αβ so TCR-δ more commonly (+) than βF1
    - Occasional cases have lack of TCR expression
- INKLPD-GIT
  - cCD3, CD7, CD56, TIA1, and granzyme B (+)
  - Surface CD3, CD4, CD5, TCR-αβ, and EBER ISH (-)
  - CD2(+/-)
  - Ki-67 is low, but can approach 50%
- Indolent T-cell LPD/lymphoma of GI tract
  - CD3(+); downregulation or loss of CD5 or CD7
  - CD4 > CD8 or CD/CD8--
    - CD4(+) cases are FOXP3 and PD1 (-)
    - CD8(+) cases are TIA1(+) but granzyme B (-)
  - βF1(+) αβ T cells in all cases
  - CD56(-/+), CD103(-/+)
  - Ki-67 < 10%
  - CD30(-) except in cases with transformation
- ITCL, NOS
  - CD3(+); most cases aCD4(-)/CD8(-) or CD4(+)
  - Most are TCR-αβ (+) and subset are T-cell receptor silent
  - TIA1 usually (+), but granzyme B and CD30 immunoreactivity variable
  - CD56(-)
  - Ki-67 usually high
  - EBER ISH reported in rare cases

DIFFERENTIAL DIAGNOSIS

Peripheral T-Cell Lymphoma, Not Otherwise Specified

- Uncommonly arises in GI tract
  - Usually involves lymph nodes unless disseminated
- CGH studies of peripheral T-cell lymphoma, not otherwise specified (PTCL-NOS) commonly show
  - Chromosomal gains of 7q, 8q, 17q, and 22q
  - Chromosomal losses of 4q, 5q, 6q, 9p, 10q, 12q, and 13q
- No gain of 9q31.3-qter or deletions of 16q12.1 as seen in EATL
- Histologically similar to EATL and MEITL
- No intraepithelial lymphocytosis or villous blunting
- Often CD4(+) and cytotoxic proteins negative

Extranodal NK-/T-Cell Lymphoma

- Morphologic features overlap with EATL and MEITL
- EBER-positive in virtually all cases, unlike EATL
- No enteropathy-associated changes
- Angiocentric and angiodestructive growth pattern
- Surface CD3(-), cytoplasmic CD3-ε(+)
- CD2(+), CD4(-), CD8(-), CD5(-), CD56(+)
- Cytotoxic proteins positive
- Can involve GI tract, although more common in upper airways and head and neck

DIAGNOSTIC CHECKLIST

Pathologic Interpretation Pearls

- Not all small intestinal T-cell lymphomas are EATL
- Association with CD is proven for EATL but not MEITL
- Most patients with EATL are T-cell receptor (TCR) silent, whereas most patients with MEITL express TCR and derive more frequently from T cells than γδ from αβ T cells
- In difficult cases, *JAK1*, JH1-kinase and *STAT2* SH2 domain alterations favors EATL over MEITL
- *JAK3* and *STAT5* mutations as well as *SETD2* inactivation favors MEITL over EATL
- Lack of malabsorption, negative celiac serologies, usually monomorphic lymphomatous infiltrate with few admixed inflammatory cells, lack of villous atrophy and MATK expression can favor MEITL over EATL
- Absence of epitheliotropism, lack of CD56 expression, and low ki-67 index can favor CD8(+) indolent T-cell LPD/lymphoma of GI tract over MEITL

SELECTED REFERENCES

1. de Leval L et al: Extranodal T- and NK-cell lymphomas. Virchows Arch. 482(1):245-64, 2023
2. Veloza L et al: Monomorphic epitheliotropic intestinal T-cell lymphoma comprises morphologic and genomic heterogeneity impacting outcome. Haematologica. 108(1):181-95, 2023
3. Alaggio R et al: The 5th edition of the World Health Organization classification of haematolymphoid tumours: lymphoid neoplasms. Leukemia. 36(7):1720-48, 2022
4. Campo E et al: The International Consensus Classification of mature lymphoid neoplasms: a report from the Clinical Advisory Committee. Blood. 140(11):1229-53, 2022

Intestinal T-Cell Lymphoma

Pleomorphic T Cells

Monomorphic Epitheliotropic Intestinal T-Cell Lymphoma

(Left) EATL in a patient with a history of celiac disease is shown. The lymphoma cells are large and pleomorphic ➡. There is necrosis and apoptotic debris present. (Right) On the other hand, this example of MEITL (previously called type II EATL) has a different morphology. Instead of being pleomorphic, the neoplasm consists of similar, more monomorphic ➡ T cells. This patient did not have a known history of celiac disease.

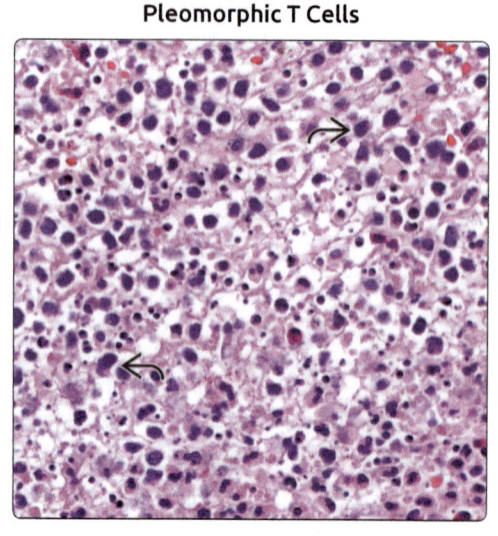

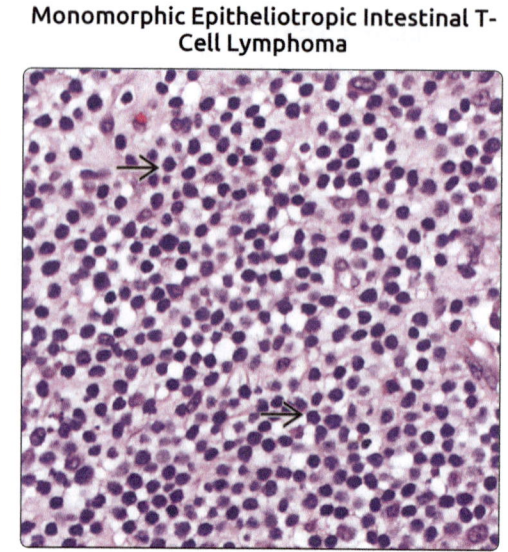

Acute Inflammation

CD3 Immunohistochemistry

(Left) In contrast to MEITL, EATL typically contains marked acute inflammation in the background inflammatory cells as well as necrosis and ulceration. Numerous neutrophils are seen obscuring the malignant tumor infiltrate ➡. (Right) CD3 is diffusely positive ➡ in this case of EATL of the jejunum. Other T-cell markers, such as CD2 and CD5, were negative, an aberrant immunophenotypic feature diagnostic of T-cell lymphoma.

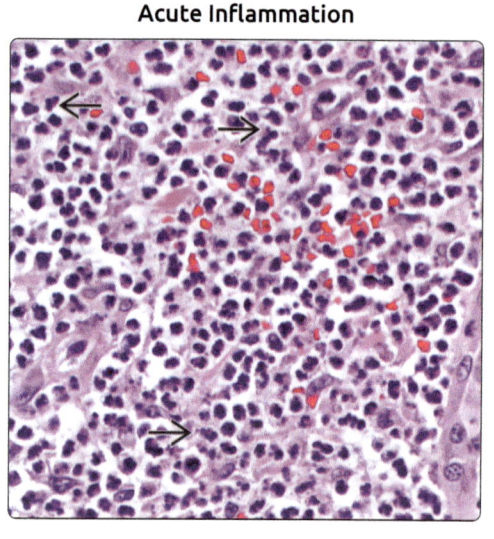

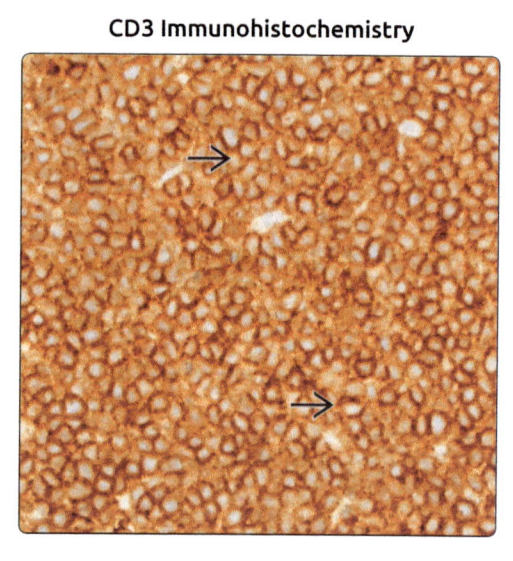

CD56 Immunohistochemistry

CD8 Immunohistochemistry

(Left) CD56 is positive ➡ in this case of MEITL. CD56 is frequently positive in MEITL but negative in EATL, and is thus used to help differentiate these lymphomas. (Right) CD8 is positive in this case of EATL of the ileum. CD8 is more often positive in MEITL than in EATL.

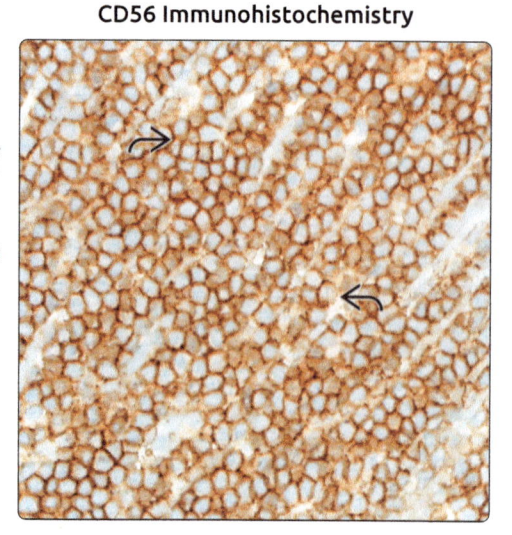

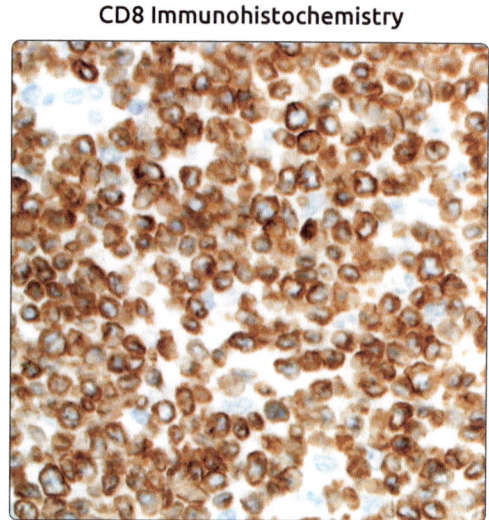

Intestinal T-Cell Lymphoma

Dense Lymphocytic Infiltrate

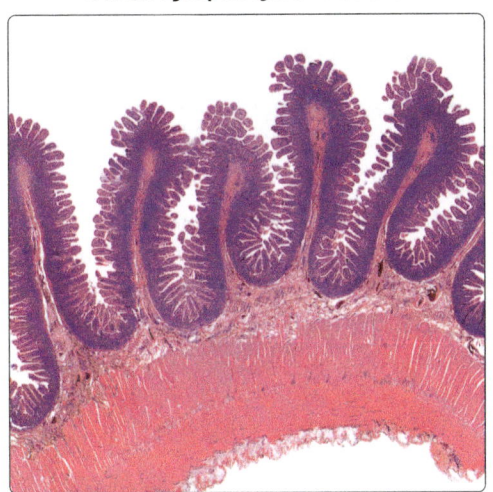

Lamina Propria Involvement

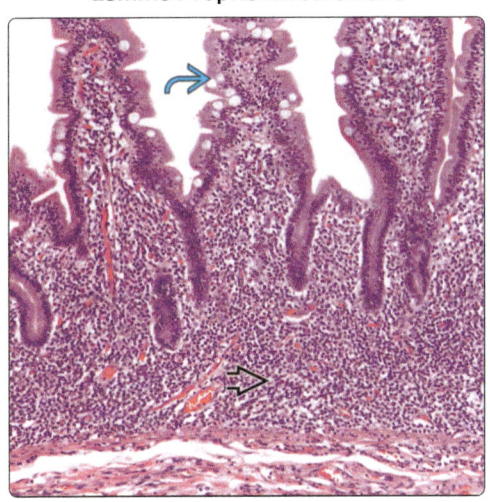

(Left) Indolent T-cell lymphoma of the GI tract shows a dense lymphocytic infiltrate in the lamina propria. Note that the infiltrate does not involve the muscularis mucosae, submucosa, or muscularis propria. (From DP: Lymph Node.) (Right) Indolent T-cell lymphoma of the GI tract shows small intestine involved by a uniform small, lymphocytic infiltrate in the lamina propria ➡. No epitheliotropism is noted ➡.

Small Lymphocytes

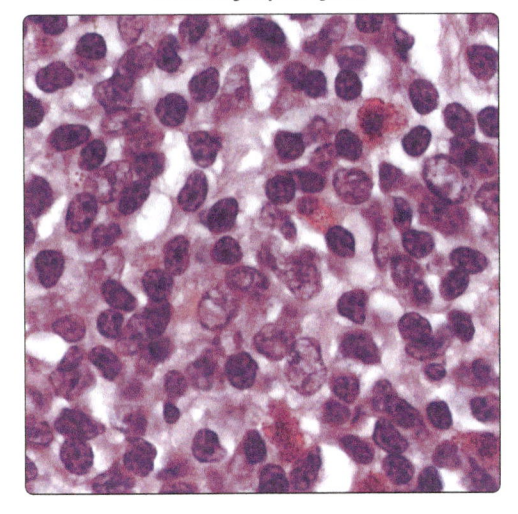

CD8 Immunohistochemistry

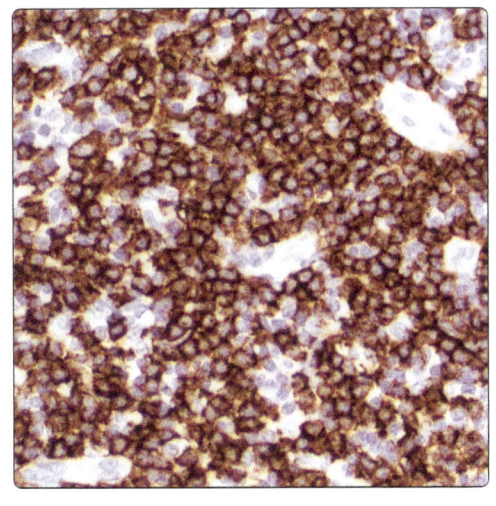

(Left) Small intestine mucosa involved by indolent T-cell lymphoma of the GI tract shows a predominance of small lymphocytes with clumped chromatin. (From DP: Lymph Node.) (Right) CD8 highlights numerous neoplastic small lymphocytes in this case of indolent T-cell lymphoma of the GI tract.

Lymph Node Involvement

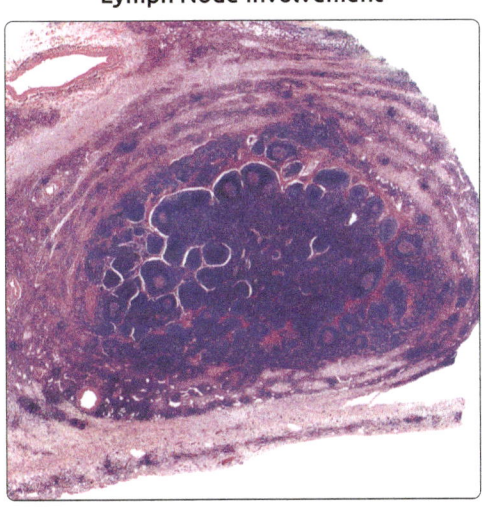

CD8 Immunohistochemistry

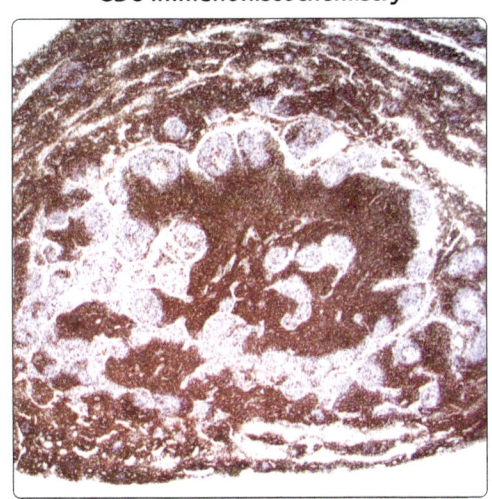

(Left) Mesenteric lymph node involved by indolent T-cell lymphoma of the GI tract shows nodal and perinodal infiltration. The nodal component displays remnants of lymphoid follicles and paracortical areas. (From DP: Lymph Node.) (Right) CD8 highlights most neoplastic small lymphocytes in this case of indolent T-cell lymphoma of the GI tract.

Hepatosplenic T-Cell Lymphoma

KEY FACTS

TERMINOLOGY
- Mature extranodal T-cell lymphoma with poor prognosis
- Cytotoxic lymphocytes usually γδ T cells
- Less commonly αβ T cells
- WHO 5th edition notes that hepatosplenic T-cell lymphoma (HSTCL) is not just disease occurring in young people and that there is dyspoiesis seen in bone marrow of these patients

CLINICAL ISSUES
- Marked splenomegaly, common hepatomegaly
- Minimal or absent lymphadenopathy
- Aggressive disease with poor outcome
- Associated with chronic immunosuppression
  - Can develop after treatment with azathioprine and infliximab for Crohn disease

MOLECULAR
- Isochromosome 7q is primary molecular finding
- Trisomy 8 is less common
- Clonal *TRB* and *TRG* rearrangements detected
- Gene expression profile appears distinct from other T-cell lymphomas
- Cases with αβ T cells and γδ T cells have similar gene expression profiles

MICROSCOPIC
- Spleen, liver, and bone marrow show sinusoidal infiltration
- Occasional cases with blastic cells with prominent nucleoli that mimic acute leukemia

ANCILLARY TESTS
- CD3(+), CD4(-)/CD8(-/+)
  - CD5(-), CD56(+/-), TCR-γδ(+)
  - Nonactivated cytotoxic cells: TIA(+), granzyme B (-)
- Subset of cases express TCR-αβ
  - Similar clinicopathologic and cytogenetic features to TCR-γδ(+) cases

Splenic Involvement

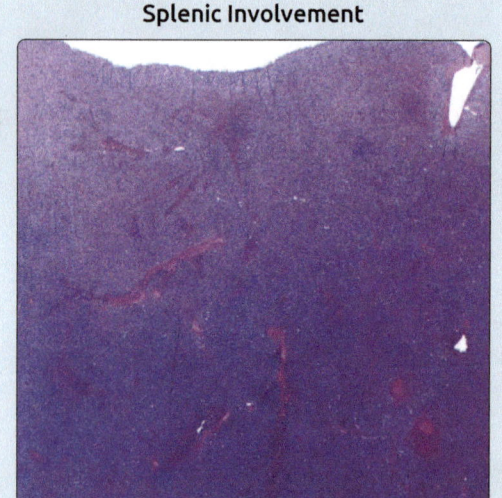

T Cells Infiltrating Red Pulp

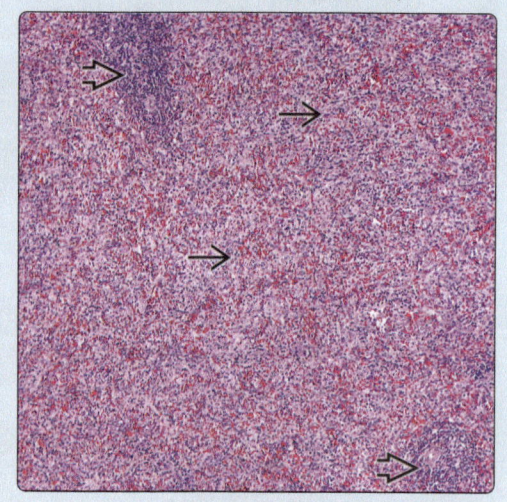

(Left) Hepatosplenic T-cell lymphoma (HSTCL) shows extensive involvement of the spleen. (Right) T cells infiltrate the sinuses of the red pulp ➡. Remnants of white pulp are also seen ➡.

T-Cell Receptor-γ Gene Rearrangement

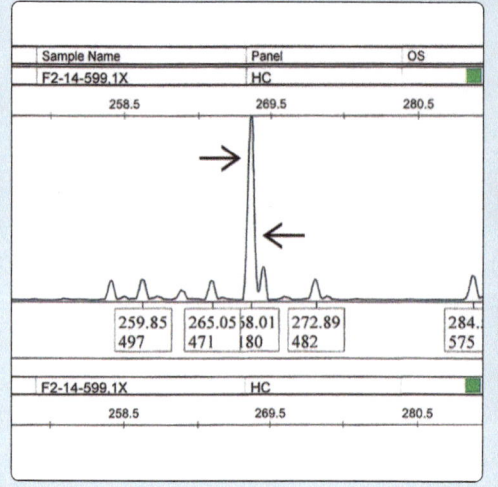

Liver Involvement

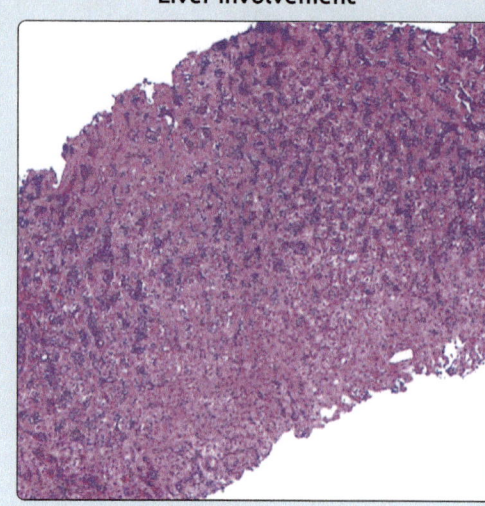

(Left) HSTCL shows a dominant monoclonal peak ➡ on this PCR assay for T-cell receptor-γ gene rearrangement. (Right) HSTCL involving the liver is shown. The sinuses of the liver are filled with the malignant T cells. HSTCL most commonly involves the liver, spleen, and bone marrow.

Hepatosplenic T-Cell Lymphoma

TERMINOLOGY

Abbreviations
- Hepatosplenic T-cell lymphoma (HSTCL)

Synonyms
- Erythrophagocytic T-γ lymphoma

Definitions
- Aggressive systemic mature T-cell lymphoma with cytotoxic T cells and sinusoidal involvement of spleen, liver, and bone marrow
  o Recognized entity by both WHO 5th edition (WHO-HEAM5) and 2022 International Consensus Classification (ICC)
  o Most cases express TCR γδ (~ 75%) followed by TCR αβ (~ 25%), and ~ 5%, are TCR-silent
  o WHO-HAEM5 states that HSTCL is not just disease occurring in young people and notes that bone marrow dyspoiesis is not uncommon in HSTCL

ETIOLOGY/PATHOGENESIS

Association With Chronic Immunosuppression
- 20% of patients
- Solid-organ transplant recipients
- Inflammatory bowel disease patients treated with tumor necrosis factor-α antagonists or thiopurines (infliximab and azathioprine)

CLINICAL ISSUES

Epidemiology
- Incidence
  o < 1% of all non-Hodgkin lymphomas
  o 5% of peripheral T-cell lymphomas
- Age
  o Often in young adults
    – However, 51% of patients are at least 60 years old
- Sex
  o M > F for gamma/delta subtype, W > F for α/β subtype

Presentation
- Systemic (B-type) symptoms
- Splenomegaly
  o Hepatomegaly in ~ 50% of patients
- Minimal or absent lymphadenopathy
  o Peripheral lymph nodes are uncommonly involved
- Cytopenias are common
  o Thrombocytopenia is almost constant
    – Severity correlates with progression
  o Leukemic phase is unlikely at presentation
    – Can occur during course of disease
- High serum lactate dehydrogenase level

Treatment
- Standard anthracycline-containing chemotherapy regimens are not effective
- Platinum-cytarabine regimens and 2'-deoxycoformycin (pentostatin) are often used
- Promise for cure after stem cell transplantation

Prognosis
- Poor
  o Median survival: ~ 12 months
  o No clinical features or biomarkers predict prognosis
  o Patients with T-cell receptor alpha/beta subtype may have poorer prognosis

MACROSCOPIC

General Features
- Spleen
  o Diffuse enlargement; no discrete gross lesions
  o Commonly > 1,000 g
  o Homogeneous and diffusely red-purple parenchyma

MOLECULAR

Cytogenetics
- Isochromosome 7q [i(7)(q10)] is primary finding by karyotyping
  o Found in ~ 70% of cases
  o Though to be early event in HSTCL
  o Common abnormality but not specific for HSTCL
    – Also detected in nasal-type extranodal NK-/T-cell lymphoma and ALK(-) anaplastic large cell lymphoma
  o Ring chromosome 7 has also rarely been reported
  o t(7;15)(p22;q21) reported in single case
- Trisomy 8 is less common than isochromosome 7q
- Loss of Y chromosome in subset of cases

Molecular Alterations
- Isochromosome 7q
  o Common deleted region spans region of 13 Mb continually amplified in HSTCL with ring chromosome 7
  o Mapped common deleted region at 7p22.1p14.1 and common gained region at 7q22.11q31.1
  o Sometimes ring chromosomes can lead to isochromosome 7q
    – TRB and TRG are involved with forming ring 7
  o Loss of 7p22.1p14.1 and gain of 7q22.11q31.1 are associated with overexpression of ABCB1, CHN2, RUNDC3B, and PPP1R9A
- Mutations involving genes in the JAK-STAT pathway and chromatin-modifying genes
  o STAT5B (35% of cases) and STAT3 alterations involve JAK-STAT pathway are detected in HSTCL
  o ARID1B, INO80, (21%) and SETD2 (25%) mutations (chromatin-modifying genes) detected in ~ 60%

In Situ Hybridization
- FISH tests show 2-5 copies of i(7)(q10)
- EBER (-)

Polymerase Chain Reaction
- HSTCL from γδ T-cells show clonal TRG rearrangement
  o Some also show biallelic clonal TRD rearrangement
  o Some γδ cases have shown clonal TRB rearrangement
- HSTCL from αβ T-cells show clonal TRB rearrangement

Gene Expression Profiling
- HSTCL appears to have profile distinct from other T-cell lymphomas

Hepatosplenic T-Cell Lymphoma

- Identified alteration in *CHN2*, *PPP1R9A*, and *ABCB1*, genes on chromosome 7 as part of profile for HSTCL
- Overexpresses genes encoding NK-cell-associated molecules and oncogenes, such as *FOS* and *VAV3*
- Overexpresses *S1PR5* and *ABCB1*
- Hypermethylated genes in HSTCL include
  - *BCL11B*, *CXCR6*, *GIMAP7*, *LTA*
- HSTCL from αβ T-cells have shown similar gene expression profile as compared to HSTCL from γδ T cells

MICROSCOPIC

Histologic Features

- Spleen
  - Red pulp sinuses and cords are infiltrated by T cells
    - White pulp is atrophic
  - Hemophagocytosis can be observed
- Liver
  - Sinusoidal pattern of infiltration
  - Mild portal and periportal infiltrate can be seen
- Bone marrow
  - Hypercellular bone marrow with trilineage hematopoiesis
  - Pattern of infiltration
    - Sinusoidal pattern typically
    - Interstitial or diffuse pattern may occur in advanced disease
    - Pattern can be subtle and difficult to recognize in routine H&E-stained sections
    - Immunohistochemistry for T-cell markers is useful to assess extent and pattern of infiltration
    - Dyspoietic cells often present in bone marrow, although this does not have any clinical impact
    - Erythrophagocytosis can be seen, and hemophagocytic lymphohistiocytosis can rarely develop
- Lymph nodes
  - Enlarged splenic hilar nodes in ~ 10% of cases
  - Neoplastic infiltration usually confined to sinuses

Cytologic Features

- Early-stage disease
  - Relatively monotonous tumor cells small to intermediate in size with irregular nuclear contours
    - Nuclear chromatin loosely condensed with small nucleoli
    - Clear cytoplasm, devoid of azurophilic granules
- Late-stage disease
  - Medium to large cells with prominent nucleoli that resemble blasts
  - Can mimic myelodysplastic syndrome or myeloproliferative neoplasm

ANCILLARY TESTS

Immunohistochemistry

- Immunophenotypic variability from case to case
- In situ hybridization analysis for Epstein-Barr virus encoded RNA (EBER) is negative
- Neoplastic cells are of cytotoxic T-cell lineage
  - CD3(+), CD5(-), CD7(+), CD56(+/-), CD4(-), CD8(-/+)
- TCR-γδ is usually (+), 75% of cases
  - Antibody specific for γδ T cells
  - Loss of TCR-γδ expression (TCR silent) can occur during disease progression
- TCR-βF1 antibody reacting with epitope of framework of α/β TCR is usually (-)
  - Except in αβ-derived HSTCL
  - Clinicopathologic and cytogenetic features similar to TCR-γδ(+) cases
  - More common in female patients
- Cytotoxic phenotype
  - TIA(+), granzyme M (+), granzyme B(-), and perforin (-)
- NK-cell markers CD56 (~ 70%) and CD16 (~ 60%) are often (+)

Flow Cytometry

- Most cases are TCR-γδ(+)
  - TCR-γδ(+) is most reliably determined by flow cytometry
- Few cases express TCR-αβ
- CD2(+), CD3(+), CD7(+), CD16(-/+), CD56(+/-)
- KIR(+), CD94 (dim + or -)
- CD4(-), CD5(-), CD8(-/+), CD57(-)
  - Unusual variations include CD5 expression
- B-cell associated antigens (-), myeloid antigens (-)

DIFFERENTIAL DIAGNOSIS

T-Cell Large Granular Lymphocytic Leukemia

- Older patients with indolent clinical course, unlike HSTCL
- Large, granular lymphocytes in peripheral blood
- Splenic red pulp cords and sinusoids with T-cell infiltrate
- Bone marrow, usually interstitial pattern, but sinusoidal pattern can also seen
- CD8(+), CD57(+), TCR-αβ(+)
  - Activated cytotoxic immunophenotype: TIA(+), granzyme B (+), perforin (+)
  - CD5 (dim +), CD16(+), CD56(-)
- Distinction between HSTCL and T-cell large granular lymphocytic (T-LGL) leukemia can be difficult
  - Neoplastic lymphocytes with azurophilic granules favors T-LGL leukemia
  - TCR-αβ(+), CD8(+), CD57(+), granzyme B (+) favors T-LGL leukemia

T-Cell Prolymphocytic Leukemia

- High white blood cell count, usually > 100 x 10^9/L
- Cytogenetic findings include inv14q or t(14;14)(q11;q32)
- Lymphocytes with prominent nucleoli
- Hepatosplenomegaly; generalized lymphadenopathy in subset
- Splenic red pulp involvement
- T-cell markers (+), CD52 (bright +), TCL1(+/-)

SELECTED REFERENCES

1. Vega F et al: American Registry of Pathology Expert Opinions: recommendations for the diagnostic workup of mature T cell neoplasms. Ann Diagn Pathol. 49:151623, 2020
2. Bergmann AK et al: DNA methylation profiling identifies candidate genes for the pathogenesis of hepatosplenic T-cell lymphoma. Haematologica. 104(3):e104-7, 2018
3. McKinney M et al: The genetic basis of hepatosplenic T cell lymphoma. Cancer Discov. 7(4):369-79, 2017
4. Finalet Ferreiro J et al: Integrative genomic and transcriptomic analysis identified candidate genes implicated in the pathogenesis of hepatosplenic T-cell lymphoma. PLoS One. 9(7):e102977, 2014

Hepatosplenic T-Cell Lymphoma

Liver Involvement

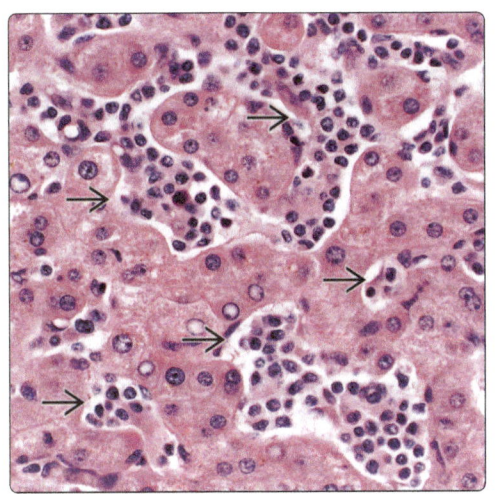

Bone Marrow Involvement

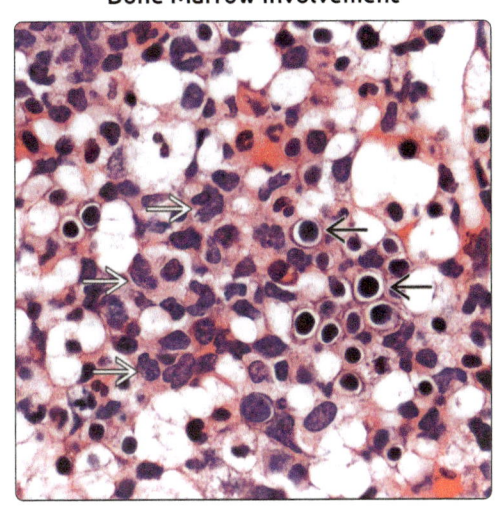

(Left) Numerous neoplastic lymphocytes of HSTCL within liver sinuses ➡ are shown. Subsequent immunohistochemical studies showed that cells were positive for CD3 and CD56 but negative for CD4 and CD8. (Right) Bone marrow involved by HSTCL is shown. Cells suspected to be neoplastic show nuclei with irregular nuclear contours ➡. There are also erythroid precursors ➡ characterized by round nuclei surrounded by a clear halo.

Isochromosome 7q

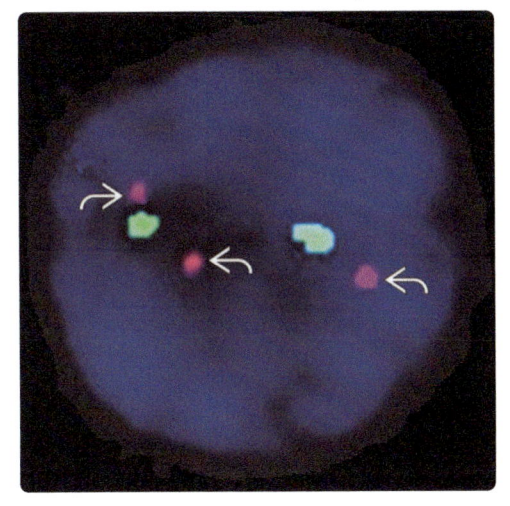

CD3 Immunohistochemistry

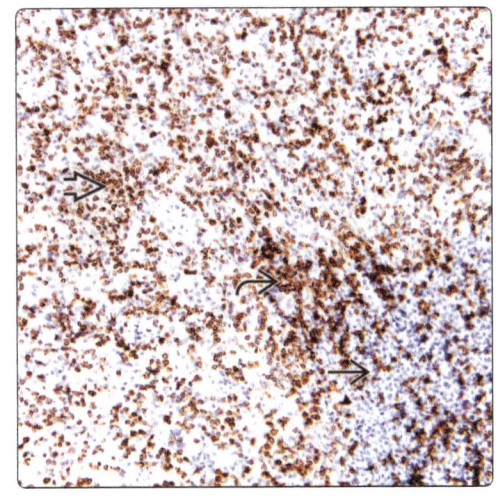

(Left) FISH is positive for the presence of isochromosome 7q, showing an interphase cell with 3 red signals (7q31 regions) ➡ and 2 green signals, indicating the presence of 2 centromeres for chromosome 7. (Right) CD3 highlights T cells of HSTCL distributed mainly in the red pulp of the spleen. Residual attenuated white pulp is noted ➡. CD3 expression is more dim in tumor cells ➡ and stronger in reactive T cells ➡.

CD56 Immunohistochemistry

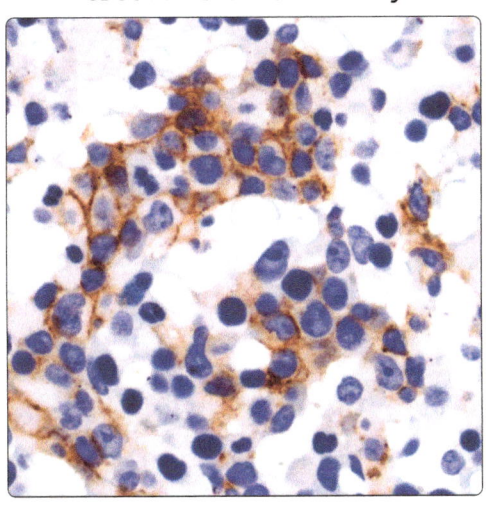

TIA Immunohistochemistry

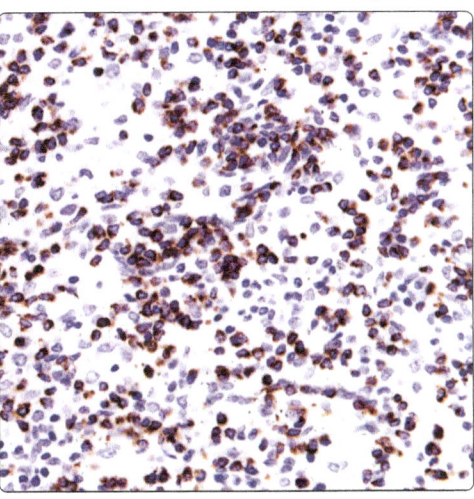

(Left) CD56 highlights the malignant T cells of splenic HSTCL. In contrast, neoplastic lymphocytes of T-cell large granular lymphocytic leukemia are negative for CD56 and positive for CD57. (Right) TIA1 highlights cytoplasmic granules in neoplastic lymphocytes of splenic HSTCL.

Subcutaneous Panniculitis-Like T-Cell Lymphoma

KEY FACTS

TERMINOLOGY
- T-cell lymphoma of CD8(+) αβ cells usually involving subcutaneous tissue with cytotoxic phenotype
- Recognized entity in both WHO 5th edition and ICC 2022

ETIOLOGY/PATHOGENESIS
- Low Tregs, such as CCR4 and FOXP3, may lead to immune activation in SPTCL

CLINICAL ISSUES
- Excellent prognosis
  - Worse if patients has HLH or *HAVCR2* alterations
- Wide age distribution
  - Found in children, adults, and, rarely, infants
- Therapies range from steroids to immunosuppressive drugs (i.e., cyclosporine) to chemotherapy

MOLECULAR
- No specific cytogenetic abnormalities
- Epstein-Barr-encoded RNA (EBER) usually (-)
- Monoclonal T-cell receptor gene rearrangement nearly all cases
- *HAVCR2* germline alterations in 25% act more aggressive
- Multiple gene alterations of epigenetic modifiers, PI3K/AKT/mTOR and JAK-STAT pathways

MICROSCOPIC
- Atypical lobular panniculitic T-cell infiltrate confined to subcutis
- Malignant T cells rim around adipocytes
- Prominent necrosis/apoptosis and angioinvasion

ANCILLARY TESTS
- IHC: TCR-βF1(+), TCR-δ(-), CD8(+), CD4(-), CD56(-), EBER(-)
- Cytotoxic markers (+)

TOP DIFFERENTIAL DIAGNOSES
- γ/δ T-cell lymphoma
- Lupus panniculitis

Typical Appearance

Clonal T-Cell Receptor Gene Rearrangement

(Left) Low-power view of subcutaneous panniculitis-like T-cell lymphoma (SPTCL) shows malignant T cells confined to subcutaneous tissue ➡. The dermis ➡ and epidermis ➡ are both spared and are morphologically unremarkable. (Courtesy M. Tomaszewsky, MD.) (Right) Clonal T-cell receptor gene rearrangement ➡ in a case of SPTCL is shown. The dominant monoclonal peak at ~ 330 base pairs in size is interpreted as a clonal T-cell receptor gene rearrangement.

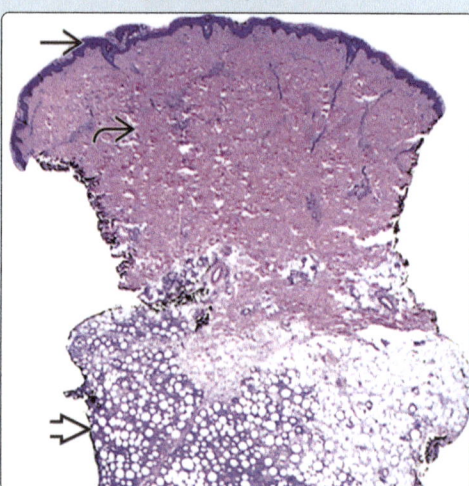

Lobular Pattern

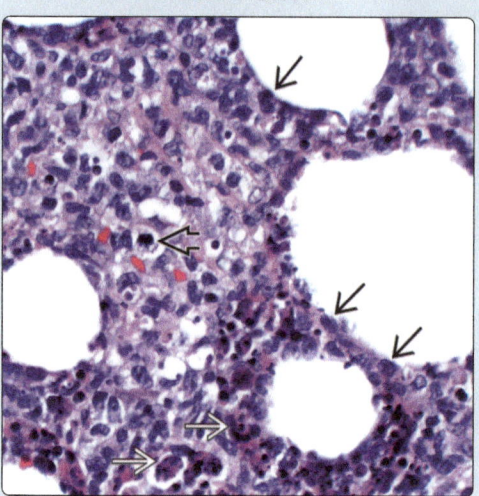

CD3 Immunohistochemistry

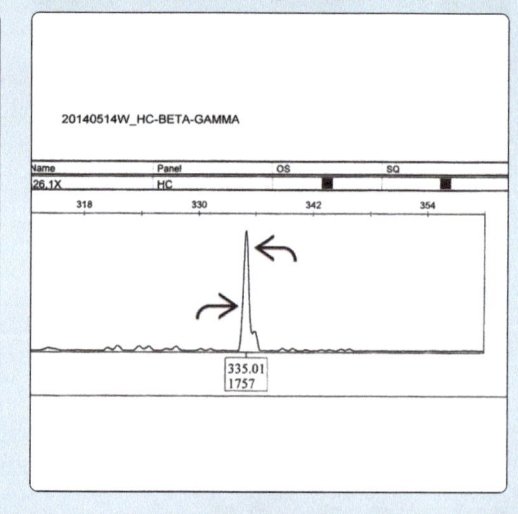

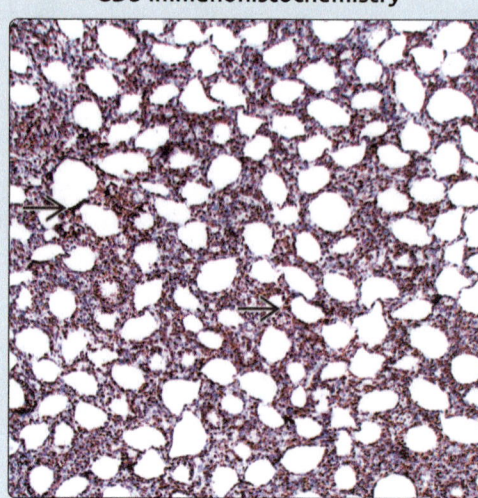

(Left) Lobular pattern of atypical T cells rimming fat cells ➡ is shown. There are also numerous histiocytes containing apoptotic debris ("bean bag cells") ➡ and markedly atypical lymphocytes present between the fat cells with a mitotic figure ➡. (Right) In this case of SPTCL, CD3 strongly highlights the numerous malignant T cells diffusely infiltrating and rimming the fat cells ➡.

Subcutaneous Panniculitis-Like T-Cell Lymphoma

TERMINOLOGY

Abbreviations
- Subcutaneous panniculitis-like T-cell lymphoma (SPTCL)

Definitions
- T-cell lymphoma of CD8(+), αβ (TCR-βF1)(+) cells involving subcutaneous fat, and rarely other sites, with activated cytotoxic phenotype
- Recognized entity in both WHO 5th edition and ICC 2022

ETIOLOGY/PATHOGENESIS

Cell of Origin
- Composed of αβ T-cells
  - Cases of γδ cells are reclassified as cutaneous γ/δ T-cell lymphoma
  - Subcutaneous T-cell lymphomas of γδ type are more aggressive than αβ cases

Autoimmune Disease
- Present in ~ 20% of patients
  - Lupus panniculitis is common
    - Microscopic findings of SPTCL overlap with lupus profundus panniculitis

HAVCR2 Germline Mutations
- HAVCR2 p.T82C reported in 85% of SPTCL patients of East Asian or Polynesian descent
- HAVCR2 p.I97M present in ~ 25% of patients of European descent

Decreased T Regulatory Proteins (Tregs)
- Low Tregs, such as CCR4 and FOXP3, may lead to immune activation in SPTCL

CLINICAL ISSUES

Epidemiology
- Incidence
  - < 1% of all non-Hodgkin lymphoma
    - Presents sporadically without familial involvement
- Age
  - Wide age distribution
    - Found in children and adults
    - Rarely found in infants
    - Affects younger individuals more than other cutaneous T-cell lymphomas
    - Median: ~ 35 years (range: 5 months to 84 years)
- Sex
  - More common in female patients

Site
- Extremities and trunk most common
- Lipophilic involving sites containing fat
  - Usually subcutaneous tissue
  - Rarely mesenteric, perinodal fat or marrow
- Uncommonly disseminates
  - Can involve lymph nodes but not initially

Presentation
- Usually multiple erythematous subcutaneous nodules or plaques
  - Painless mass, rarely ulcerates (unlike cutaneous γ/δ T-cell lymphoma)
  - Symptoms due to mass effects
  - Only rarely single lesion
- B symptoms in up to 50%
- Hemophagocytic lymphohistiocytosis (HLH) in up to 20%
  - Related to release of cytotoxic molecules
  - More often associated with HAVCR2-mutated cases
  - May occur up to 5 years after presenting diagnosis

Treatment
- Therapies range from steroids to immunosuppressive drugs (i.e., cyclosporine) to chemotherapy
  - Chemotherapy may be given after immunomodulary agents fail
  - Chemotherapy and or stem cell transplant can be used for patients with HLH or with HAVCR2 mutations

Prognosis
- Indolent disease
  - 5-year overall survival: ~ 80%
  - Mostly stage I, which is localized to skin
  - Rare systemic spread
    - Including lymph nodes
    - Often years after diagnosis
- HAVCR2-mutated cases have shorter relapse-free survival

MOLECULAR

Cytogenetics
- No specific cytogenetic abnormalities

In Situ Hybridization
- Epstein-Barr-encoded RNA (EBER) typically (-)
  - Rare EBER(+) cases associated with immunocompromised and Asian patients
- Terminal deoxynucleotidyl transferase-mediated dUTP nick-end labeling (TUNEL)
  - May have high apoptotic rate

Polymerase Chain Reaction
- Clonal T-cell receptor gene rearrangement (TRG &/or TRB)
  - Detected in most cases

Molecular Genetics
- HAVCR2 mutations
  - Germline HAVCR2 mutations in a high percentage of patients
    - HAVCR2 p.Y82C variant in ~ 85% of patients of East Asian or Polynesian descent
    - HAVCR2 p.I97M variant in ~ 25% of patients of European descent
  - HAVCR2-mutated cases
    - Tend to be younger (< 30 years) compared to wildtype HAVCR2
    - More often associated with hemophagocytic lymphohistiocytosis
    - Have shorter relapse-free survival
  - Other genes more frequently mutated in HAVCR2-mutated cases
    - UNC13D, PIAS3, KMT2D
- Mutations in immune response-related genes

Subcutaneous Panniculitis-Like T-Cell Lymphoma

- ○ *ASXL1*, *JAK3*, *PIAS3*, and *PLCG2*
- Mutations in epigenetic modifier genes
  - ○ *KMT2D*, *KMT2C*, *BAZ2A*, and *NUP98*

Array Comparative Genomic Hybridization
- Gains of 2q, 4q, 5q, 6q, 13q
- Losses of 1p, 2p, 5p, 7p, 9q, 10q, 11q, 12q, 16, 17p, 19, 20, 22
  - ○ 5q and 13q gains may be more characteristic of SPTCL
    - Not found in other cutaneous T-cell lymphoma

MICROSCOPIC
Histologic Features
- Atypical T-cell infiltrate of subcutaneous fat lobules
  - ○ Lobules involved (lobular panniculitis), septa usually spared
    - Septal pattern rarely seen, which may represent spilling of T cells from lobules
    - No tumor in overlying dermis or epidermis
  - ○ Malignant T-cells rim individual adipocytes
    - Characteristic, but not specific, for SPTCL
  - ○ Neoplastic cells
    - Usually medium in size
    - Mild to marked atypia with irregular nuclear contours
    - Hyperchromatic to vesicular chromatin
    - Pale, clear cytoplasm
  - ○ Initial biopsy commonly shows minimal T-cell atypia
    - Later biopsies show more diagnostic lesion
- Karyorrhexis (apoptosis)
  - ○ Necrosis from released cytotoxic molecules
- Fat necrosis
- Angioinvasion in some cases
  - ○ Poor prognostic indicator
- Reactive inflammatory cells
  - ○ Histiocytes
    - Present with vacuolated, foamy cytoplasm from imbibed material/lipid
    - May show hemophagocytosis
    - Sometimes poorly formed granulomas with multinucleated giant cells
- Usually lacks plasma cells, eosinophils, or neutrophils
  - ○ Plasma cells are only seen in ~ 10% of cases
  - ○ Plasma cells and plasmacytoid dendritic cells favor diagnosis of lobular panniculitis

ANCILLARY TESTS
Immunohistochemistry
- CD3(+), CD8(+), αβ (TCR-βF1)(+), TIA(+), granzyme B (+), and perforin (+)
- Variable loss of CD2, CD5, or CD7
  - ○ CD8(+)/CD4(-) in > 95%
  - ○ CD4(-)/CD8(-) and CD4(+)/CD8(-) rarely
- γδ(-), CD30(-), CD56(-), granzyme M (-), and EBER(-)
- CD123(-), unlike in lobular panniculitis where it highlights plasmacytoid dendritic cells
- Ki-67 proliferative index often high

DIFFERENTIAL DIAGNOSIS
Primary Cutaneous γδ T-Cell Lymphoma
- Panniculitic pattern of tissue involvement, like SPTCL
  - ○ Dermal and epidermal involvement, unlike SPTCL
  - ○ Ulcerated epidermis, contrary to SPTCL
- Immunophenotype
  - ○ TCR-βF1(-), TCR-γδ(+), and CD56(+), unlike SPTCL
  - ○ Usually CD4(-) and CD8(-) (double negative)
- Clinical presentation compared to SPTCL
  - ○ Older median age at diagnosis (~ 60 years)
  - ○ Generalized lesions
  - ○ More B symptoms
  - ○ More often associated with hemophagocytic lymphohistiocytosis
  - ○ Worse prognosis than SPTCL

Reactive Panniculitis
- SLE panniculitis (lobular panniculitis)
  - ○ Difficult to differentiate from SPTCL in some cases
    - Lupus profundus panniculitis and SPTCL can coexist
  - ○ Similarities to SPTCL
    - Inflammation of subcutis in panniculitic pattern
    - No/minimal lymphocyte atypia, like early lesions of SPTCL
    - Self-heal and improve with steroids, like many SPTCL cases
  - ○ Differences from SPTCL
    - CD138 plasma and CD123 plasmacytoid dendritic cells
    - Germinal centers or B-cell aggregates
    - Mixed inflammatory infiltrate with histiocytes, eosinophils, and neutrophils
    - Less T-cell atypia, minimal rimming of fat cells
    - No rimming of CD8(+) T cells
    - Mix of CD4(+) and CD8(+) T cells
    - Cytotoxic markers (-)
    - Vacuolar epidermal change and interstitial mucin
    - Usually polyclonal *TRG* gene rearrangement
    - Rarely oligoclonal T-cell populations are present

SELECTED REFERENCES
1. Goodlad JR et al: Recent advances in cutaneous lymphoma-implications for current and future classifications. Virchows Arch. 482(1):281-98, 2023
2. Koh J et al: Genetic profiles of subcutaneous panniculitis-like T-cell lymphoma and clinicopathological impact of HAVCR2 mutations. Blood Adv. 5(20):3919-30, 2021
3. Geller S et al: C-C chemokine receptor 4 expression in CD8+ cutaneous T-cell lymphomas and lymphoproliferative disorders, and its implications for diagnosis and treatment. Histopathology. 76(2):222-32, 2020
4. Sonigo G et al: HAVCR2 mutations are associated with severe hemophagocytic syndrome in subcutaneous panniculitis-like T-cell lymphoma. Blood. 135(13):1058-61, 2020
5. Fernandez-Pol S et al: High-throughput sequencing of subcutaneous panniculitis-like t-cell lymphoma reveals candidate pathogenic mutations. Appl Immunohistochem Mol Morphol. 27(10):740-8, 2019
6. Polprasert C et al: Frequent germline mutations of HAVCR2 in sporadic subcutaneous panniculitis-like T-cell lymphoma. Blood Adv. 3(4):588-95, 2019
7. Li Z et al: Recurrent mutations in epigenetic modifiers and the PI3K/AKT/mTOR pathway in subcutaneous panniculitis-like T-cell lymphoma. Br J Haematol. 181(3):406-10, 2018
8. Kitayama N et al: CCR4 and CCR5 expression in a case of subcutaneous panniculitis-like T-cell lymphoma. Eur J Dermatol. 27(4):414-5, 2017

Subcutaneous Panniculitis-Like T-Cell Lymphoma

CD4 and CD8 Immunohistochemistry

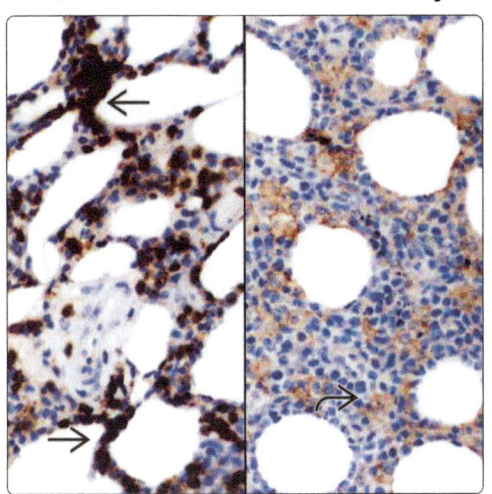

TCR-βF1 Immunohistochemistry

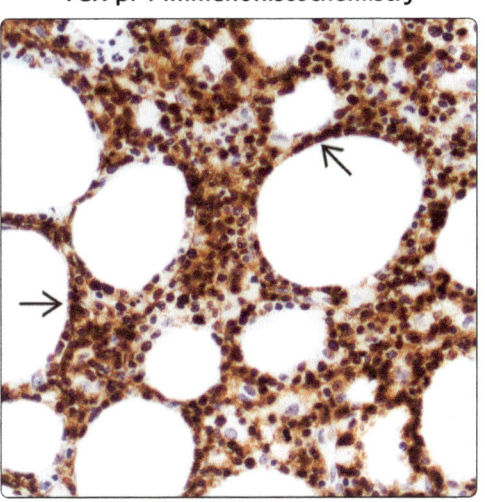

(Left) In this case of subcutaneous panniculitis-like T-cell lymphoma (SPTCL), the malignant T cells strongly express CD8 ⇒ (left) but are nonimmunoreactive for CD4 (right). Only scattered histiocytes ⇒ and reactive T cells are highlighted by CD4. **(Right)** TCR-βF1 is positive in T cells rimming fat ⇒, similar to CD3 and CD8. This is evidence that the cells in SPTCL are αβ cells and not γδ T cells. (Courtesy T. Muzzafar, MD.)

Granzyme B Immunohistochemistry

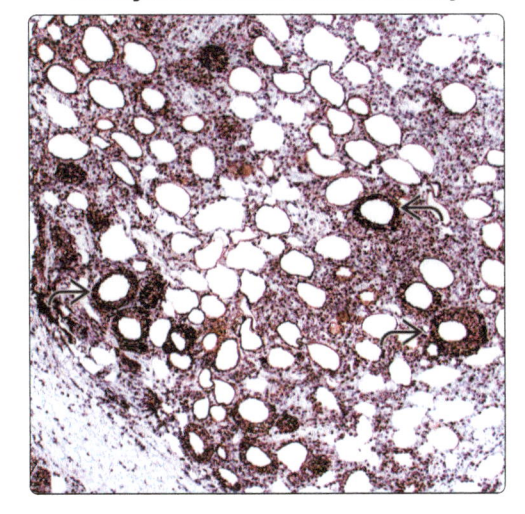

CD56 Immunohistochemistry

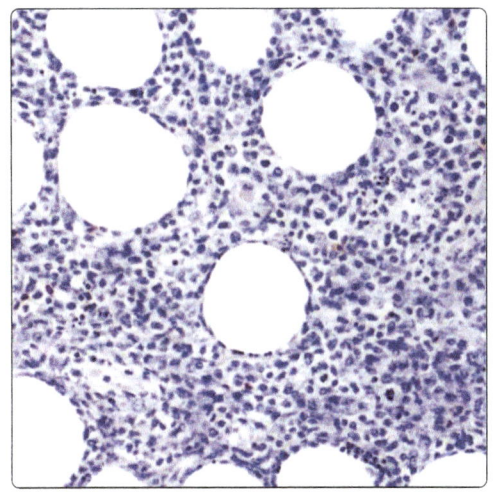

(Left) Granzyme B is a cytotoxic marker that is typically strongly and diffusely positive in SPTCL. Note the staining in areas of fat rimming ⇒. These cells were also positive for other cytotoxic markers, including TIA and perforin (not shown). **(Right)** CD56 is negative in the malignant cells in this case of SPTCL. In cases of cutaneous γ/δ T-cell lymphoma, CD56 is typically positive. Cutaneous γ/δ T-cell lymphoma is more aggressive and is in the differential of SPTCL.

CD123 Immunohistochemistry

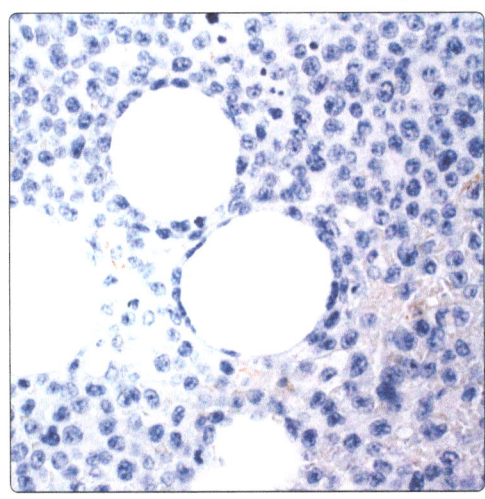

CD68 Immunohistochemistry

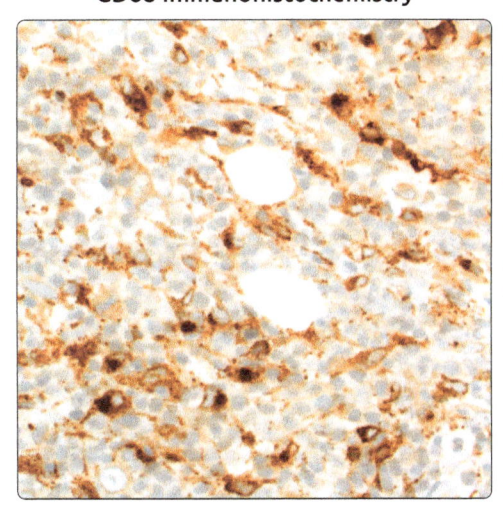

(Left) CD123 is negative in this case of SPTCL. CD123 is often positive in the plasmacytoid dendritic cells of lupus panniculitis and can be used to differentiate these entities. **(Right)** CD68 stains reactive histiocytes in this case of SPTCL. Histiocytes are often prevalent in SPTCL, but plasma cells and eosinophils are usually not common.

Mycosis Fungoides/Sézary Syndrome

KEY FACTS

CLASSIFICATION
- ICC and WHO both recognize mycosis fungoides (MF) and Sézary syndrome (SS) as distinct entities
- MF is primary cutaneous T-cell lymphoma characterized by epidermotropism and clinical course progressing from patches to plaques to tumors
- SS is T-cell proliferation defined by triad of erythroderma, generalized lymphadenopathy, and neoplastic T cells with cerebriform nuclei (Sézary cells) in blood, skin, and lymph nodes

CLINICAL ISSUES
- Overall indolent clinical course
- MF variants include pagetoid reticulosis, folliculotropic MF, syringotropic MF, and granulomatous slack skin

MOLECULAR
- Clonal T-cell receptor gene rearrangements
  - Found in 50% of patch stage, 73% of plaque stage, and 90% of tumor-stage MF
  - Can also be false-negative in early stage and falsely positive in reactive dermatoses
- Deregulation of phosphatidylinositol 3-kinase pathway
- *STAT3* activation and *CDKN2A* inactivation associated with aggressive disease
- Complex karyotypes can be seen

MICROSCOPIC
- Epidermotropism, Pautrier microabscesses
- Cerebriform lymphocytes with halos
- Large cell transformation: Large cells ≥ 25%

ANCILLARY TESTS
- CD3(+), TCR-αβ/βF1(+), CD4(+), CD8(-), CD7(-), and CD26(-)

TOP DIFFERENTIAL DIAGNOSES
- Drug reactions, inflammatory dermatoses

Clinical Appearance

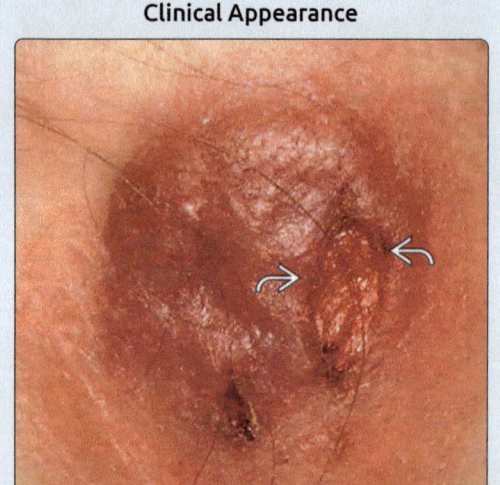

PCR For *TRG* Rearrangement

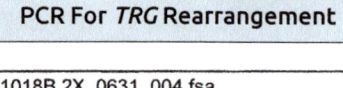

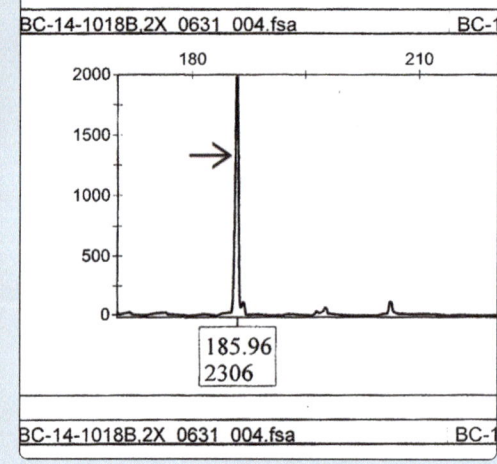

(Left) Clinical photograph of the tumor stage of mycosis fungoides (MF) shows a large and ulcerated lesion ➡. (Right) PCR for TRG rearrangement is performed on skin with MF. The dominant peak ➡ represents a clonal TRG rearrangement, which is expected in this T-cell lymphoma.

Epidermotropism

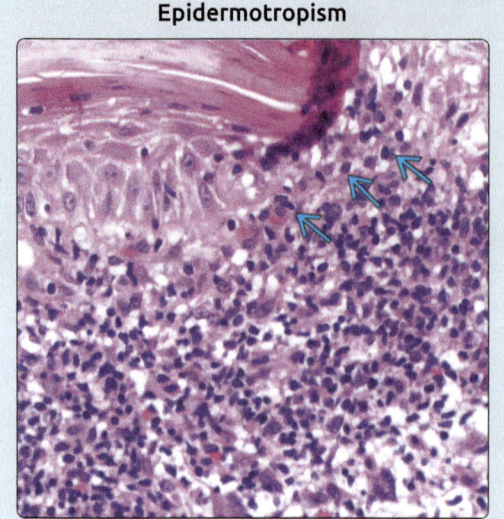

CD3 Immunohistochemistry

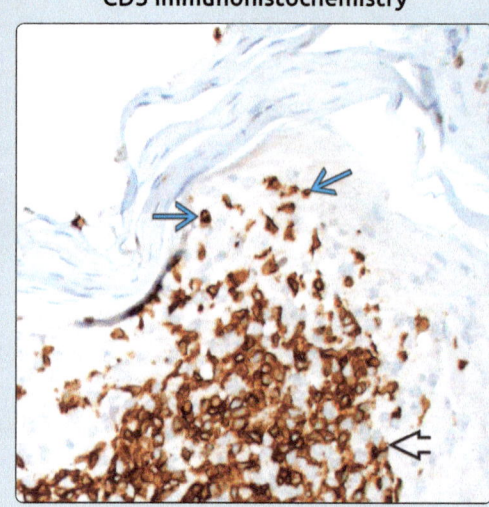

(Left) Epidermotropism with lymphocytes extending into the epidermis is shown. Picket fencing ➡ is seen with lymphocytes lining up along the dermal-epidermal junction. (Right) CD3 shows deep dermal T cells ➡, which also extend upward into the epidermis ➡. This process, known as epidermotropism, is a feature of MF.

Mycosis Fungoides/Sézary Syndrome

TERMINOLOGY

Abbreviations
- Mycosis fungoides (MF)
- Sézary syndrome (SS)

CLASSIFICATION

ICC vs. WHO HAEM5
- ICC and WHO both recognize mycosis fungoides (MF) and Sézary Syndrome (SS) as distinct entities
- MF
  o Primary cutaneous T-cell lymphoma with clinical course progressing from patches to plaques to tumors consisting of clonal T-cells with convoluted nuclear shapes and frequently demonstrating epidermotropism
- SS
  o T-cell proliferation defined by triad of erythroderma, generalized lymphadenopathy, and neoplastic T cells with cerebriform nuclei (Sézary cells) in blood, skin, and lymph nodes
  o Closely related but distinct entity from MF

ETIOLOGY/PATHOGENESIS

Ultraviolet Exposure
- Implicated as causative agent in MF and SS by assessment of genomic signatures

Infection
- Although no clear agent has been identified to cause MF, data shows that antibiotic treatment is related to decrease in percentage of neoplastic T cells, suggesting that microbiome may be factor

CLINICAL ISSUES

Epidemiology
- Incidence
  o MF is most common type of cutaneous T-cell lymphoma
    - > 50% of all cases of primary cutaneous lymphoma
    - 0.6 per 100,000 people per year
  o SS is rare with only 0.36 per 100,000 people per year
- Age
  o Adults (5th-6th decades)
  o Can be seen in patients < 35 years, including children
- Sex
  o M:F = 2:1
- Ethnicity
  o MF has disproportionately higher incidence in Black than in White populations

Presentation
- MF has stepwise evolution of disease from patches to plaques to tumors
  o Patches
    - Mostly on trunk but can arise anywhere on body, including palms and toes
  o Plaques
    - Palpable lesions rise above skin surface
    - Can be associated with patch lesions
  o Tumors
    - Usually manifest as skin nodule(s)
    - Can coexist with patches and plaques
    - Later disease
- MF variants
  o **Pagetoid reticulosis (localized)**
    - a.k.a. Woringer-Kolopp disease
    - Solitary, slow-growing, psoriasiform, crusty or hyperkeratotic patch or plaque
    - Often CD8(+) and CD30(+)
  o **Folliculotropic (pilotropic) MF**
    - MF with involvement of hair follicles and sometimes adnexa
    - Often involves head and neck area
    - Follicular papules (often grouped), alopecia, and acneiform lesions
    - Clinically more aggressive than other MF types; responds less well to skin-directed therapy
    - Morphology shows cystic dilation or cornified plugging
    - T cells involve follicular epithelium and spare interfollicular epidermis
    - Follicular mucinosis and mucinous degeneration of follicular epithelium
    - Should be distinguished as either early stage or advanced stage
      □ Advanced-stage cases have dense dermal interfollicular involvement
      □ For intermediate-stage cases, increased cell size, high Ki-67 proliferative index, and lack of follicular mucinous are features of more advanced disease
  o **Granulomatous slack skin**
    - Pendulous folds of lax skin in axillae and groin, usually in young adults
    - May coexist with classic MF lesions or classic Hodgkin lymphoma
    - T cells with granulomatous infiltrate containing macrophages, multinucleated giant cells, and less elastic fibers
    - Rare disease with indolent course, although some are more aggressive
- SS
  o Leukemic presentation with involvement of skin showing redness over most of body, which is known as erythroderma
  o Lymph node and involvement of other organs in advanced disease
  o Oropharynx, lungs, and CNS are most common
  o Increased secondary cutaneous and systemic malignancies because of immune dysregulation

Laboratory Tests
- Peripheral blood
  o Look for Sézary cells
- Serum lactate dehydrogenase &/or β-2 microglobulin
  o High levels associated with poorer prognosis

Natural History
- Evolution from patches to plaques to tumors over time
- Some patients develop visceral involvement by MF
  o Including lymph nodes, lungs, and spleen

Mycosis Fungoides/Sézary Syndrome

Treatment
- Early-stage MF (stages I and IIA): Direct skin therapy
  - Topical chemotherapy with nitrogen mustard or carmustine
  - Topical corticosteroids and retinoids
  - Phototherapy; local radiation (radiograph or electron beam)
- Advanced-stage MF (stages IIB-IV)
  - Extracorporeal photopheresis
  - Single-agent chemotherapy
    - Methotrexate, pegylated liposomal doxorubicin (Doxil), purine analogs (fludarabine, 2-deoxycoformycin), others
  - Combination chemotherapy: Many regimens have been used
    - Cyclophosphamide, doxorubicin, vincristine, and prednisone (CHOP)
    - Cyclophosphamide, vincristine, and prednisone (CVP)
    - CVP with methotrexate (COMP)
  - Hematopoietic stem cell transplantation

Prognosis
- MF has indolent clinical course with slowly growing lesions, but disease prognosis is based on clinical stage
  - Large cell transformation and blood, lymph node, and visceral organ involvement are associated with poor prognosis
- SS is aggressive disease with 5-year overall survival of 10-30%

MACROSCOPIC

General Features
- Patches
  - Circumscribed lesions with discoloration of variable size, color, and shape
  - Little scaling, not palpable
- Plaques
  - Palpable infiltrate of variable stage (thin and thick)
- Tumors
  - Often exophytic and ulcerated (hence, term fungoides)

MOLECULAR

PCR
- Clonal T-cell receptor (*TRB* and *TRG*) rearrangements
  - Reported in 40-90% of cases of MF
  - Found in 50% of patch stage, 73% of plaque stage, and 90% of tumor-stage MF
  - Early MF can have few epidermotropic T cells, so clonality may be difficult to determine
    - Leading to false-negatives
  - Clonal *TRG* or *TRB* rearrangement also found in ~ 25-65% of benign inflammatory dermatoses
    - Leading to false-positives
    - Identical T-cell clones in > 1 site, such as skin and blood, are more supportive of MF
- Clinical significance of clonal *TRB* and *TRG* rearrangements in MF staging is controversial
  - Clonal gene rearrangement in blood is extremely common in early-stage disease
    - Not synonymous with blood involvement by MF in absence of morphologic or immunophenotypic evidence of disease
  - Clonal gene rearrangement in lymph nodes is common finding

Molecular Genetics
- Tumor suppressor pathways, JAK3/STAT3 and MAPK signal transduction pathways, chromatin modification, T-cell activation pathways, cell cycle regulation, and alterations of NFkB signaling downstream to TCR may all be involved in development of MF/SS
- Complex karyotypes can be seen
- *CDKN2A* inactivation (loss of 9p21) associated with aggressive disease
- *TP53* mutations are frequently identified and are associated with shorter survival
- Deregulation of phosphatidylinositol 3-kinase pathway
  - AKT1 is activated in MF skin lesions
  - Rare *PIK3CA* mutations in exon 9
  - Inactivation of PTEN in subsets of cases
    - *PTEN* mutations in exons 7, 8, and 5
- STAT3 activation
  - Found in tumor-stage MF
  - Possible therapeutic target
- Dysregulated cell cycle
  - Decreased regulatory proteins p14, p15, and p16 induce cell cycle arrest
- *TOX*
  - Transcript levels increased in MF
- *JUNB* amplification
  - Involved in T-cell proliferation and apoptosis
- *FAS* mutation or promoter hypermethylation or nonfunctioning splice variants
  - Leads to decreased or defective FAS activity and dysfunctional apoptosis
- *HNRNPK* and *SOCS1* deletions
  - Reported in tumor-stage of MF
  - Results in activation of JAK-STAT signaling pathway
- SS
  - Has complex numeric alterations similar to MF
  - Gain-of-function mutations in *PLCG1*, *CARD11*, *CD28*, and *CARMIL2* have been identified
    - These involve TCR signaling pathways
    - These increased NFkB activity
  - DNA damage response pathways show genetic alterations in *TP53* and *ATM*
  - JAK-STAT signaling pathways show genetic alterations in *STAT5B* and *JAK3*
  - Chromatin modifiers show genetic alterations, including *ARID1A*, *DNMT3A*, and *TET2*
  - Isochromosome 17q has been identified

Gene Expression Profiling
- Can differentiate MF from adult T-cell leukemia/lymphoma (ATLL)
  - Both diseases show epidermotropism
  - Cutaneous homing genes are different for MF and ATLL

MicroRNA
- May differentiate MF from benign skin disorders

Mycosis Fungoides/Sézary Syndrome

- miR03, miR205, miR326, miR663, and miR711 identify MF with > 90% accuracy

Comparative Genomic Hybridization
- Gains of 1p36, 7, 9q34, 18q24, and 9 with losses of 2q, 9p21, and 17p

MICROSCOPIC
Histologic Features of Skin
- Patch stage
  - Subtle epidermotropic T-cell infiltrates showing hyperconvoluted cerebriform nuclei and clear halos
  - Line up along basal and low layers of epidermis, especially at tips of rete ridges
  - Dermis has band-like lichenoid collection of reactive small lymphocytes and scattered histiocytes
  - In some early lesions, biopsy findings may be nondiagnostic
- Plaque stage
  - T cells colonize upper epidermis, showing pagetoid growth, or may form Pautrier microabscesses, which are intraepidermal clusters of T cells associated with Langerhans cells
    - Characteristic feature, which may only be seen in some cases
    - Confluent Pautrier microabscesses that can result in subcorneal and subepidermal bullae
- Tumor stage
  - Dermal infiltrate becomes more diffuse and prominent
    - Tumor cells range in size from small to large
  - Epidermotropism often lost
  - Large cell transformation
    - Often occurs in tumor stage
    - Large cells comprise ≥ 25% of tumor
    - CD30 can be (+); high Ki-67 proliferation rate
- Folliculotropic or syringotropic MF
  - Involves hair follicles or eccrine ducts/glands
  - Often spares epidermis
  - Sometimes mucinosis of follicles (follicular mucinosis)
- May lose epidermotropism in SS
- Peripheral blood contains Sézary cells in SS
  - Sézary cell count ≥ 1,000/μL
- Lymph nodes
  - Partially or completely effaced by Sézary cells
  - Medium-sized cells with irregular contours
  - Also frequently show dermatopathic lymphadenopathy
  - In early lymph node involvement, MF/Sézary cells may be hard to see and may need flow cytometry to identify
- Bone marrow
  - Can be involved but infiltrate may be interstitial and sparse

Cytologic Features
- Small to medium-sized lymphocytes (unless large-cell transformation)
- "Cerebriform nuclei" have grooved nuclei and nuclear convolutions

ANCILLARY TESTS
Immunohistochemistry
- CD4(+), CD8(-)
  - Rare cases can be CD4(-), CD8(+) or CD4(+), CD8(+)
- CD2(+), CD3(+), CD5(+), βF1(+), and TCR beta+
- Often shows loss of CD2, CD5, CD7 &/or CD26
- CD4:CD8 ratio > 10; CD4(+), CD7(-) cells ≥ 40% or CD4(+), CD26(-) cells ≥ 30% in SS
- CD30(+/-), usually expressed by large cells
- PD1 often (+) but follicular T-helper markers like ICOS often (-)
- CD45(+), CCR4(+), CLA(+), CD52(+), CD25(-/+), STAT3(+)

Flow Cytometry
- Can be performed on skin, peripheral blood, lymph nodes, and other tissue specimens
- CD4:CD8 ratio is often increased
- Typical immunophenotype: CD3(+), CD4(+), CD8(-), CD5(+), TCR-αβ(+), CD7(-), and CD26(-)
- Diminished expression of CD2, CD3, CD4, CD7, or CD5 may be seen

DIFFERENTIAL DIAGNOSIS
Drug Reactions, Inflammatory Dermatoses
- Exocytosis of lymphocytes can simulate MF, but there is often background of spongiosis &/or interface changes
- Often increased numbers of eosinophils in dermis
- Dyskeratotic keratinocytes and parakeratosis may or may not be present
- Usually do not show clonal T-cell receptor gene rearrangement

Cutaneous Anaplastic Large Cell Lymphoma
- Cases of MF with large cell transformation can be uniformly CD30(+), similar to cutaneous anaplastic large cell lymphoma (C-ALCL)
- Clinical findings are different: Usually single nodule in C-ALCL, patches/plaques in MF
- Rarely if ever shows t(2;5) translocation characteristic of systemic ALK(+) ALCL

SELECTED REFERENCES
1. Campo E et al: The International Consensus Classification of mature lymphoid neoplasms: a report from the Clinical Advisory Committee. Blood. 2022;140(11):1229-53. Blood. 141(4):437, 2023
2. Alaggio R et al: The 5th edition of the World Health Organization classification of haematolymphoid tumours: lymphoid neoplasms. Leukemia. 36(7):1720-48, 2022
3. Jones CL et al: Spectrum of mutational signatures in T-cell lymphoma reveals a key role for UV radiation in cutaneous T-cell lymphoma. Sci Rep. 11(1):3962, 2021
4. Bastidas Torres AN et al: Genomic analysis reveals recurrent deletion of JAK-STAT signaling inhibitors HNRNPK and SOCS1 in mycosis fungoides. Genes Chromosomes Cancer. 57(12):653-64, 2018
5. Hashikawa K et al: Microarray analysis of gene expression by microdissected epidermis and dermis in mycosis fungoides and adult T-cell leukemia/lymphoma. Int J Oncol. 45(3):1200-8, 2014
6. Huang Y et al: Evidence of an oncogenic role of aberrant TOX activation in cutaneous T cell lymphoma. Blood. 125(9):1435-43, 2014

Mycosis Fungoides/Sézary Syndrome

(Left) *Patch stage of MF shows an epidermal basal layer infiltrate ➡. The tumor cells are small but have irregular nuclear contours. Epidermotropism can be very subtle in the patch stage.*
(Right) *Plaque stage of MF shows Pautrier microabscesses ➡ in the epidermis, containing small clusters of atypical T cells.*

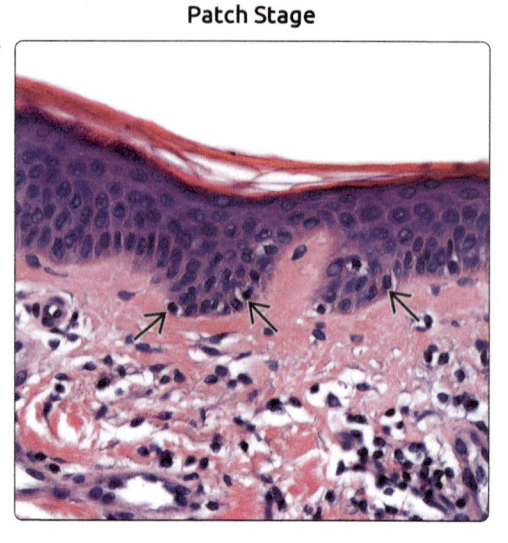

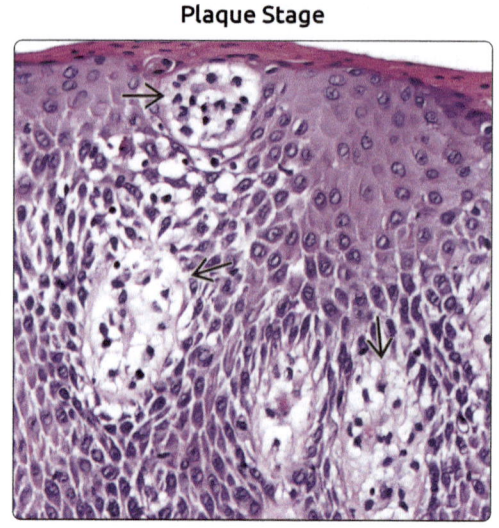

(Left) *Tumor stage of MF does not show epidermotropism. Instead, large tumor cells grow in sheets ➡ in the dermis. Epidermotropism is often lost at the tumor stage.*
(Right) *Peripheral blood smear shows many cerebriform (Sézary) cells ➡, consistent with MF in the leukemic phase [so-called secondary Sézary syndrome (SS)].*

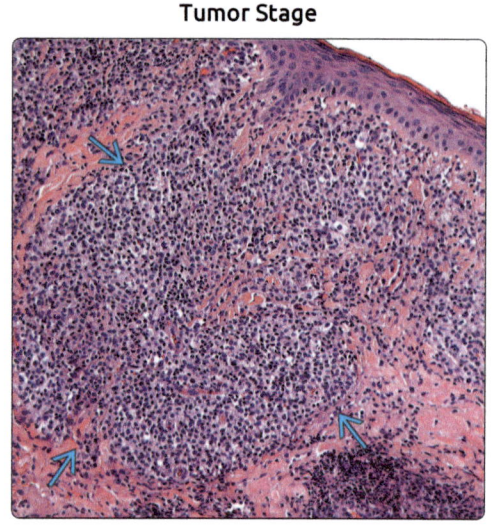

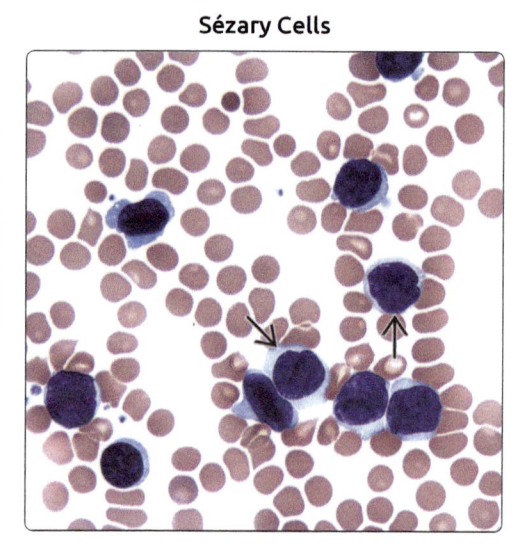

(Left) *IHC for MF usually shows diminished to lost T-cell antigens &/or CD4 restriction. Here, intraepidermal atypical cerebriform lymphocytes within Pautrier microabscesses are CD4(+) ➡.*
(Right) *This case of MF is CD8(+). CD8 highlights the neoplastic intraepidermal T cells ➡ that express CD8 more dimly than reactive CD8(+) T cells in this field. CD8(+) MF is clinically similar to CD4(+) MF.*

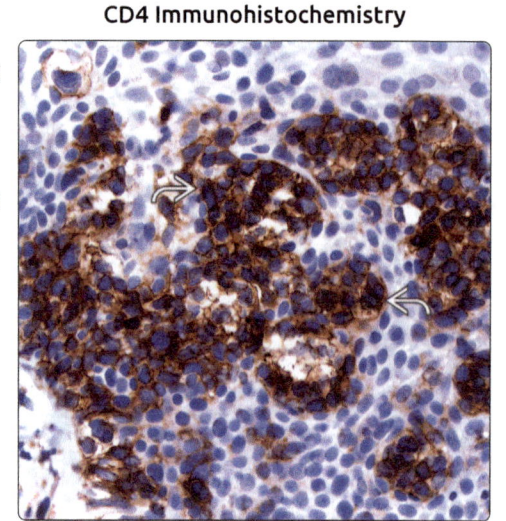

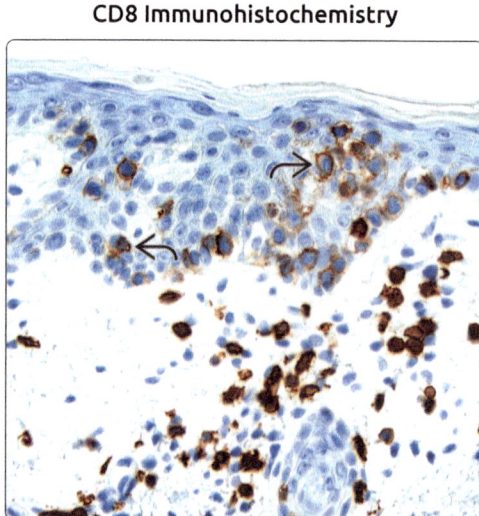

Mycosis Fungoides/Sézary Syndrome

Sézary Cells in Blood

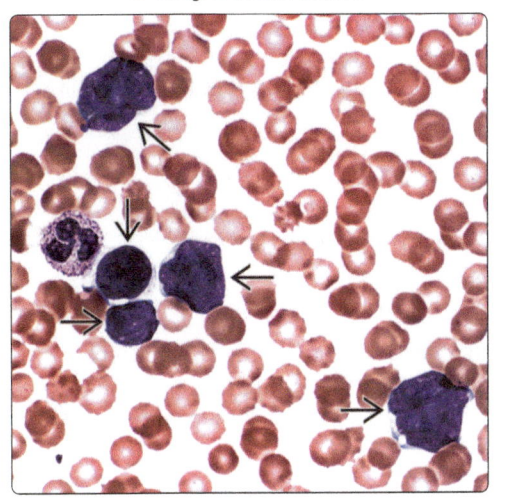

Cerebriform Nuclear Configurations in Sézary Cells

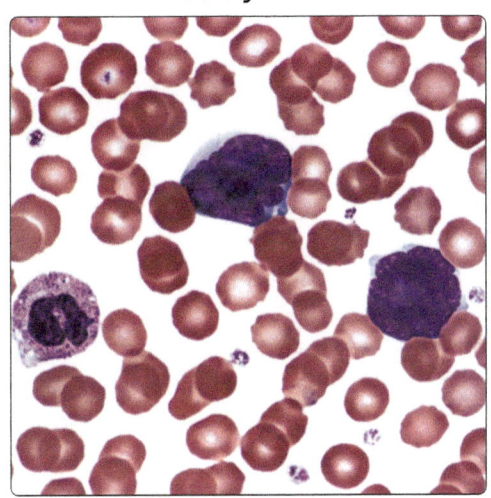

(Left) Peripheral blood smear from an SS patient with significant blood involvement shows the range in size of the circulating Sézary cells ➡. (Courtesy K. Foucar.) (Right) On high magnification, circulating Sézary cells have a distinct cerebriform appearance. Note the prominent, yet subtle, nuclear irregularities.

Small Sézary Cell

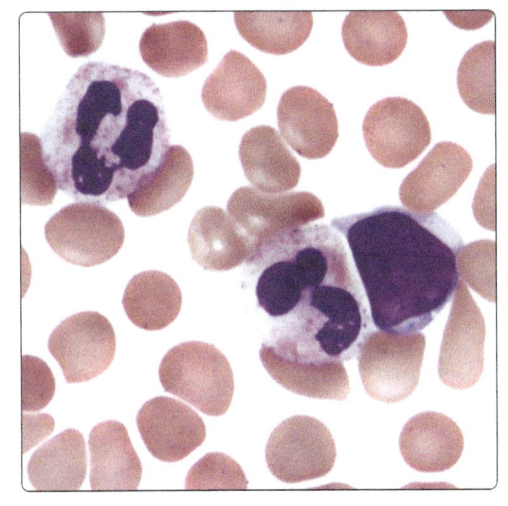

Small Atypical Sézary Cell

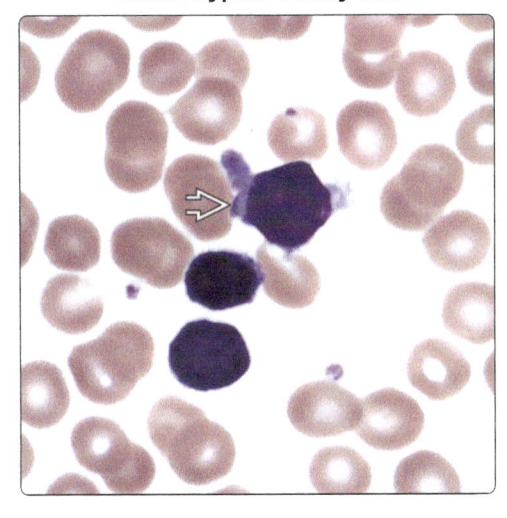

(Left) The spectrum of Sézary cells in the blood often includes smaller, atypical lymphoid cells with condensed chromatin and nucleoli. (Right) Blood smear shows a small, atypical lymphoid cell with subtle nuclear convolutions ➡ as well as 2 more normal-appearing lymphocytes. Without concurrent large, atypical cells and flow cytometry to confirm the Sézary cell phenotype, a diagnosis of SS can be challenging.

Sézary Cells vs. Monocytes

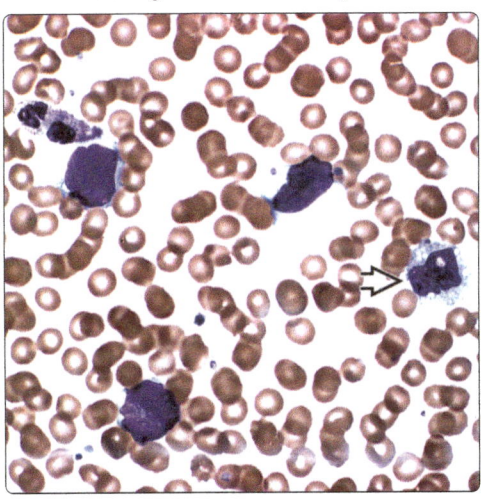

CD3 Immunohistochemistry

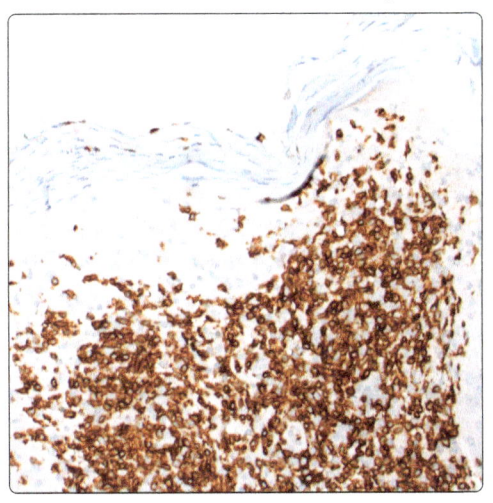

(Left) Peripheral blood smear from an 89-year-old woman with generalized itching is shown. Although the hemoglobin, hematocrit, and platelet counts are preserved, an atypical lymphocytosis is present. Note the comparison to normal monocyte ➡. A diagnosis of SS was made. (Right) CD3 is positive in the neoplastic T cells in the dermis.

Molecular Pathology of Lymphoid Neoplasms

Primary Cutaneous CD30-Positive T-Cell Lymphoproliferative Disorders

KEY FACTS

TERMINOLOGY
- Primary cutaneous anaplastic large cell lymphoma (PC-ALCL): CD30(+) T-cell lymphoproliferative disorders that can contain atypical, usually large cells without evidence of mycosis fungoides
  - Includes lymphomatoid papulosis (LyP) and anaplastic large cell lymphoma (ALCL)
- Primary cutaneous ALCL and LyP recognized by both ICC and WHO and have not undergone significant reclassification in most recent publications

CLINICAL ISSUES
- PC-ALCL shows solitary or localized nodules that can regress but frequently recur and can involve regional lymph nodes
  - Good prognosis (~ 90% 10-year survival)
- LyP shows papules or nodules at various stages of development that can wax and wane

MOLECULAR
- No translocations of *ALK* on chromosome 2p23 in majority cases, unlike systemic ALK(+) ALCL
- *DUSP22* rearrangements and *NPM1::TYK2* fusions, unlike ALK(+) ALCL
  - Common in PC-ALCL
- *TP63* rearrangements only rarely seen
  - More common in systemic, ALK(-) ALCL
- Clonal T-cell receptor gene rearrangements

MICROSCOPIC
- PC-ALCL
  - Polymorphic background infiltrate not prominent
  - Diffuse sheets of large T cells in dermis ± subcutis
  - Hallmark cells with multiple nuclei (horseshoe-shaped) helpful if present
- LyP
  - Different morphology in types A through E

Primary Cutaneous Anaplastic Large Cell Lymphoma

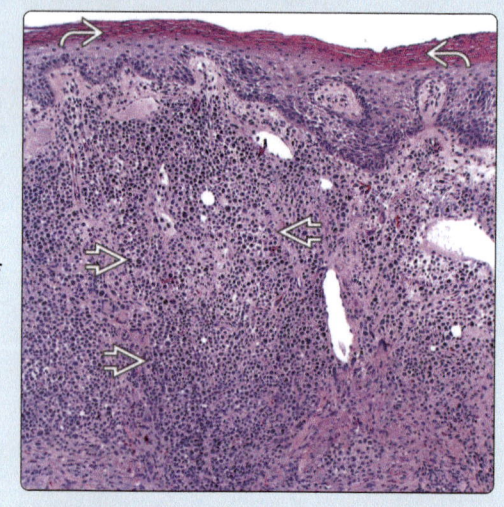

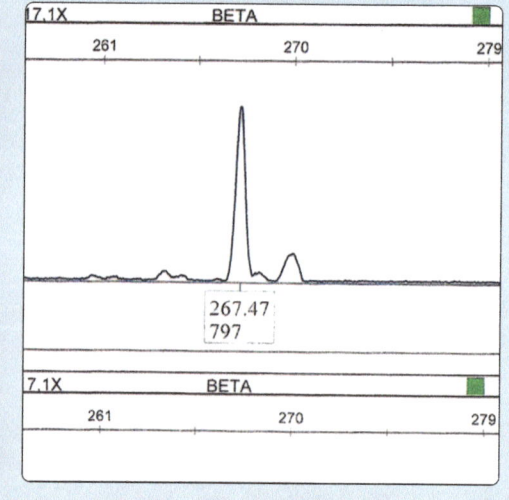

(Left) *Primary cutaneous anaplastic large cell lymphoma (PC-ALCL) shows diffuse, sheet-like proliferation ➔ of numerous large, atypical cells with abundant cytoplasm. The epidermis is not involved ➔.* (Right) *T-cell receptor β gene rearrangement shows a dominant monoclonal peak of 267 bp. TRB and TRG are clonally rearranged in the majority of PC-ALCL.*

Clonal T-Cell Receptor Gene Rearrangement

Lymphomatoid Papulosis, Type B

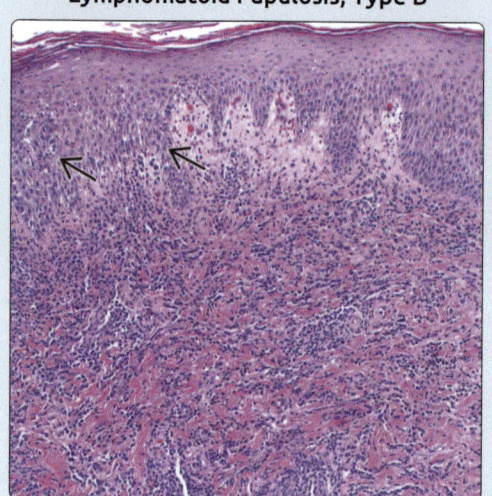

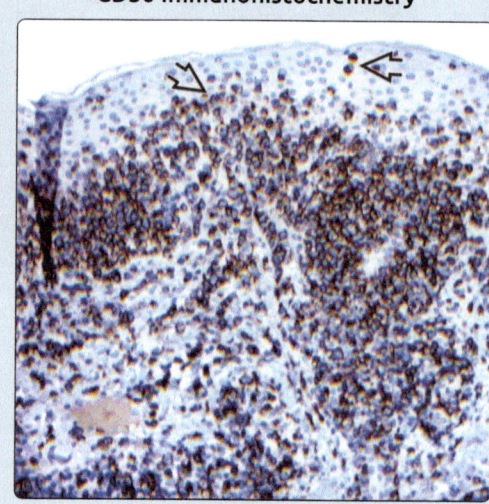

(Left) *Lymphomatoid papulosis (LyP) shows dermal lymphoid infiltrate extending into the epidermis ➔, which is considered to be type B LyP. Because of the epidermotropism, type B LyP can be mistaken for mycosis fungoides.* (Right) *CD30 in the same case shows positive cells in the dermis and within the epidermis ➔. In transformed mycosis fungoides, T cells in the epidermis are typically positive for CD3.*

CD30 Immunohistochemistry

Primary Cutaneous CD30-Positive T-Cell Lymphoproliferative Disorders

TERMINOLOGY

Abbreviations
- Primary cutaneous anaplastic large cell lymphoma (PC-ALCL)
- Lymphomatoid papulosis (LyP)

Synonyms
- Regressing atypical histiocytosis
- Primary cutaneous large cell T-cell lymphoma, CD30(+)

Definitions
- CD30(+) T-cell lymphoproliferative disorder that can contain atypical, usually large cells with spectrum of disease that include
  o Lymphomatoid papulosis (LyP)
  o Primary cutaneous anaplastic large cell lymphoma (PC-ALCL)

CLASSIFICATION

WHO HAEM5 vs. 2022 ICC
- Primary cutaneous CD30(+) T-cell lymphoproliferative disorder
  o Encompass spectrum of disease with overlapping immunophenotype and genetic features
  o Lymphomatoid papulosis (LyP) at one spectrum
  o Primary cutaneous anaplastic large cell lymphoma at other end
- Identical terminology in both 2022 ICC and WHO HAEM5

ETIOLOGY/PATHOGENESIS

Etiology
- Chronic antigen stimulation as well as viral infection and immunosuppression may also play role
- Viral etiology has been proposed but is not proven
- Staphylococcus superantigens have been identified

CLINICAL ISSUES

Epidemiology
- Incidence
  o 2nd most common group of cutaneous T-cell lymphomas after mycosis fungoides
    – 0.1-0.2 per 100,000
    – 20% of systemic ALCL cases involve skin
    – LyP is 1.6 cases per 1 million
- Age
  o Adult/older population; rare in children
- Sex
  o M:F = 2-3:1

Site
- Often trunk, face, and extremities

Presentation
- PC-ALCL presents as solitary or localized nodules, tumors, or papules ± ulceration, and ~ 20% are multifocal
- LyP presents as chronic, recurrent, self-healing lesions at various stages of development
  o May wax and wane
  o Skin lesions in different stages of evolution coexist

Natural History
- PC-ALCL shows partial or complete spontaneous regression (40%) but frequently recurs
  o Extracutaneous dissemination in ~ 10%
    – Usually to regional lymph nodes
- In LyP, skin lesions regress within 3-12 weeks with residual scars or hypo- or hyperpigmentation

Treatment
- PC-ALCL can be treated with radiation for localized nodules, methotrexate for multifocal lesions, and combination chemotherapy for systemic disease

Prognosis
- Primary cutaneous anaplastic large cell lymphomas
  o Better prognosis that most other cutaneous large cell lymphomas
    – ~ 90% 10-year survival
    – Age < 60 years and spontaneous regression are good prognostic indicators
  o Systemic disease is poor prognostic indicator
    – Multifocal skin lesions and local lymph node involvement do not yield worse prognosis
- Lymphomatoid papulosis
  o Excellent prognosis but increased risk for 2nd lymphoma, such as mycosis fungoides and PC-ALCL, in 15-50% of patients
  o Increased risk of squamous cell carcinoma and melanoma

MOLECULAR

Molecular Alterations
- ALK rearrangements
  o PC-ALCL usually do not have ALK rearrangements, unlike systemic ALCL
  o Exceptional PC-ALCL cases with ALK rearrangements have been reported in children and adults
    – Rearrangements can include NPM1 or other fusion partners
  o ALK::NPM1 rearrangement has not been reported in LyP
- DUSP22 rearrangements
  o Located on chromosome 6 at p25.3
  o Reported in 20-25% of PC-ALCL
  o Also reported in small subset of LyP cases
  o Mutually exclusive of ALK rearrangements and not reported in ALK(+) ALCL
  o Can be detected FISH break-apart probes
- TP63 rearrangements
  o Reported in very rare cases of PC-ALCL
  o Typically detected in ~ 38% of systemic ALK(-) ALCL
- NPM1::TYK2 fusion resulting in constitutive activation of STAT3 signaling pathway
  o Found in ~ 15% of PC-ALCL and in small subset of LyP
  o STAT mutations and oncogenic fusion transcripts activating JAK-STAT pathway have been identified
- Signal transduction associated with PI3K, MAPK, and G-protein pathways activated in PC-ALCL
  o Oncogenic fusion transcripts activating JAK-STAT pathway have been identified in LyP
- Genes mutated in PC-ALCL include

Primary Cutaneous CD30-Positive T-Cell Lymphoproliferative Disorders

- *H3K4*, *KMT2D*, *KMT2A*, *SETD2*, *CREBBP*, *STAT3*, and *EOMES*
- SATB1 is expressed in vast majority of LyP cases
- Mutations affecting IL6/JAK1/STAT3 pathways present in ~ 15-30% of PC-ALCL
- No specific findings by cytogenetics

PCR
- Clonal T-cell receptor gene rearrangements, including *TRB* and *TRG*
- In ~ 90% of PC-ALCL and 20-80% of LyP

Chromosomal Microarray
- Imbalances in *CTSB*, *RAF1*, *REL*, and *JUNB*
- Allelic deletions at 9p21-22
- Gains of 7q31 and losses at 6q16-21 and 13q34 in PC-ALCL

Gene Expression Profiling
- *CCR10* and *CCR8* are skin-homing chemokines that are overexpressed
- Leads to skin involvement of PC-ALCL and little extracutaneous spread

MICROSCOPIC

Histologic Features
- PC-ALCL
  - Diffuse sheets of large T cells in dermis ± subcutis
    - Only infrequent epidermotropism ± ulceration
    - Epidermotropism in cases with *DUSP22* rearrangement
    - Usually only found in dermis
    - Can involve lymphatic spaces
  - Tumor cells
    - Large anaplastic, pleomorphic, or immunoblastic appearance
    - Anaplastic cells with roundish shapes ± abundant cytoplasm
      - Small cell and histiocyte-rich variants are rare
    - Mitotic figures
    - Hallmark cells with multiple nuclei (horseshoe-shaped); often not seen but helpful if present
  - Polymorphic background infiltrate (eosinophils and plasma cells) uncommon, unlike LyP
    - Exceptions
      - Ulcerating ALCL has polymorphic infiltrate, fewer CD30(+) cells, and epidermal hyperplasia
      - Neutrophil-rich (pyogenic ALCL) shows clusters of neutrophils with only scattered CD30(+) cells
- LyP
  - Variable histology depending on age of lesion
    - Single LyP lesion may show overlapping features of different subtypes
  - 6 subtypes, including A, B, C, D, E, and LyP with *DUSP22* rearrangements
  - Type A: Scattered large atypical CD30(+) cells with acute inflammatory cells
    - Looks similar to classic Hodgkin lymphoma
  - Type B: Epidermotropic infiltrate of small atypical CD30(+) or CD30(-) cells
    - Looks like early mycosis fungoides
  - Type C: Monotonous or cohesive sheets of CD30(+) cells with few acute inflammatory cells
    - Looks like PC-ALCL
  - Type D: Epidermotropic with small to medium CD8(+) and CD30(+) pleomorphic cells
    - Looks like primary cutaneous aggressive epidermotropic CD8(+) cytotoxic T-cell lymphoma
  - Type E: Angiocentric with small to medium CD8(+) and CD30(+) cells
  - LyP with *DUSP22* rearrangements, biphasic pattern: Epidermotropic with small weak CD30(+) T cells and dense dermal, medium to large, strongly CD30(+) cells
  - Folliculotropic, syringotropic, and granulomatous LyP has been described

ANCILLARY TESTS

Immunohistochemistry
- PC-ALCL
  - CD30(+) in > 75% of tumor cells; CD15(+) in ~ 40% of cases
  - T-cell antigens expressed, including CD2, CD3, CD5, and CD7
    - Can show loss of T-cell antigens
  - CD4(+)/CD8(-)
    - Rarely CD8(+) and CD4(+)/CD8(+)
  - Cytotoxic markers positive
    - Granzyme-B, perforin, TIA
  - EMA(-) and ALK(-) in PC-ALCL
    - Usually EMA(+) and ALK(+) in systemic ALCL
    - ALK(+) skin tumor likely indicates secondary cutaneous ALCL
  - CLA and HOXC5 expressed in PC-ALCL
    - CLA(-) in systemic ALCL
  - Negative for B-cell markers (CD20 and CD79A)
    - Rarely positive for PAX5
- LyP
  - Large atypical cells of type A and type C LyP have same phenotype as PC-ALCL
  - CD4 usually (+) in LyP A, LyP B, and LyP C
  - CD8 usually (+) in LyP D and LyP E
  - Cases with *DUSP22* rearrangement either CD4(-)/CD8(-) or CD8(+)
  - May be TIA1(+); rare CD56; γ/δ TCR, follicular helper T-cell markers (+)

SELECTED REFERENCES

1. Goodlad JR et al: Recent advances in cutaneous lymphoma-implications for current and future classifications. Virchows Arch. 482(1):281-98, 2023
2. Campo E et al: The International Consensus Classification of mature lymphoid neoplasms: a report from the Clinical Advisory Committee. Blood. 40(11):1229-53, 2022
3. Gallardo F et al: Genetics abnormalities with clinical impact in primary cutaneous lymphomas. Cancers (Basel). 14(20):4972, 2022
4. Sundram U: Cutaneous lymphoproliferative disorders: what's new in the revised 4th edition of the World Health Organization (WHO) Classification of Lymphoid Neoplasms. Adv Anat Pathol. 26(2):93-113, 2019

Primary Cutaneous CD30-Positive T-Cell Lymphoproliferative Disorders

CD3 Immunohistochemistry

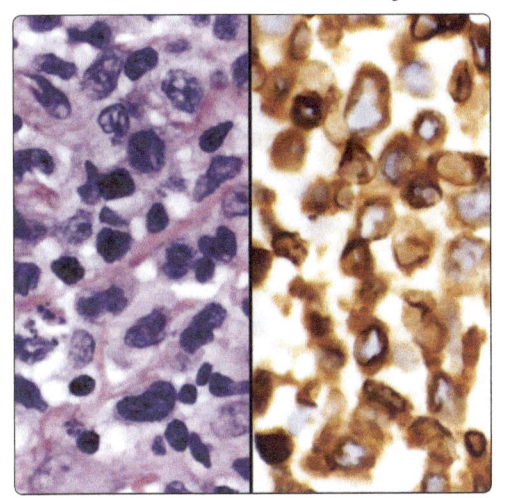

Hallmark Cell

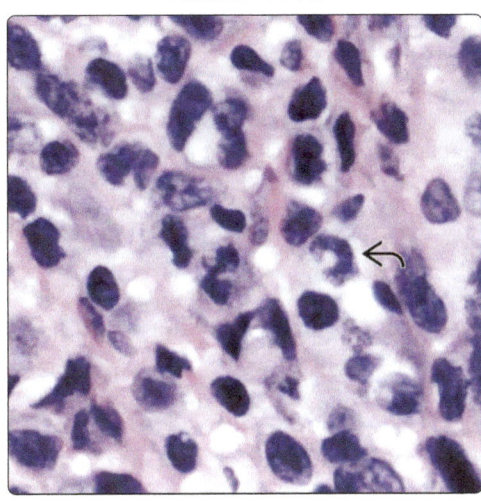

(Left) There are large, anaplastic-appearing malignant cells on H&E (left), which are immunoreactive to CD3 (right), as expected in this case of ALCL. (Right) At high power, rare cells have horseshoe-shaped nuclei of so-called hallmark cells ⇨. These cells are not found in all cases of ALCL.

CD4 Immunohistochemistry

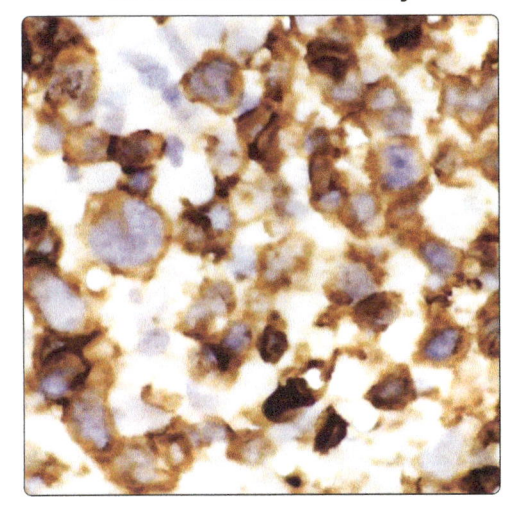

***ALK* Break-Apart Probe**

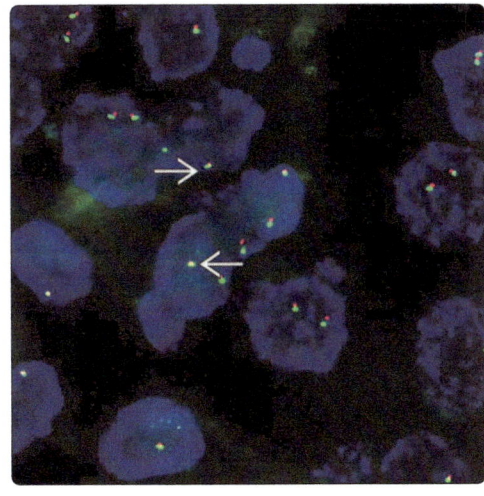

(Left) Tumor cells are CD4(+). CD8 (not shown) was negative. Most cases of ALCL are CD4(+)/CD8(-), and only 5% are CD4(-)/CD8(+). (Right) ALK FISH break-apart probe shows that the signals are fused (yellow) ⇨, indicating that ALK is not rearranged. ALK is rearranged in systemic ALCL but not typically rearranged in PC-ALCL.

ALK Immunohistochemistry

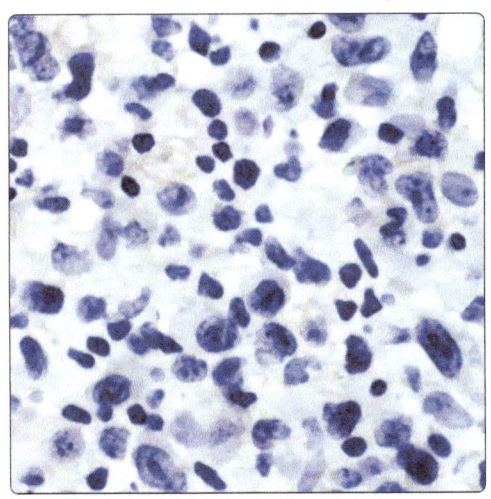

ALK Immunohistochemistry

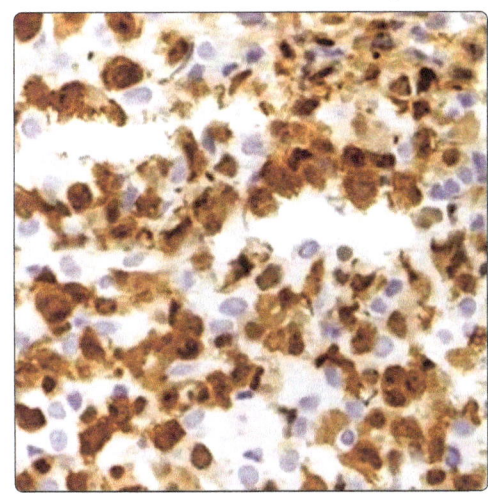

(Left) ALK is negative in this case of PC-ALCL. PC-ALCL is usually ALK(-), differing from systemic ALK(+) ALCL, which is ALK(+) as its name specifies. (Right) ALK(+) systemic ALCL with secondary cutaneous involvement is shown. Currently, systemic ALCL is classified as either ALK(+) or ALK(-), which are considered different diseases.

Peripheral T-Cell Lymphoma, NOS

KEY FACTS

TERMINOLOGY
- Mature T-cell lymphoma encompassing cases not fulfilling criteria of more specific T-cell lymphoma
- Heterogeneous group of tumors
- Both WHO 5th edition and 2022 ICC recognize peripheral T-cell lymphoma, not otherwise specified (PTCL, NOS) as entity
- Nodal T follicular helper (TFH) cell lymphomas and EBV-positive nodal T- and NK-cell lymphomas are excluded from this category

CLINICAL ISSUES
- Sometimes eosinophilia
- Cases with cytotoxic phenotype are more aggressive

MOLECULAR
- Clonal rearrangements of T-cell receptor genes (*TRB* and *TRG*)
- *GATA3* and *TBX21* are distinct molecular subtypes
- Complex karyotypes
- t(5;9); *ITK::SYK*, t(6;14); *IRF4::TRA* (cytotoxic phenotype), t(14;19); *NECTIN2::TRA*

MICROSCOPIC
- Paracortical infiltrate or diffuse effacement of lymph node architecture
- Wide cytological spectrum
- Sometimes increased cells with clear cytoplasm
- Background inflammatory cells often numerous
- ± high rates of proliferation and apoptosis

ANCILLARY TESTS
- Expresses pan T-cell markers
- Loss of ≥ 1 T-cell antigens is aberrant finding
- CD4(+), CD8(-) or CD4(-), CD8(+)
- ± cytotoxic molecules

Increased Cells With Clear Cytoplasm

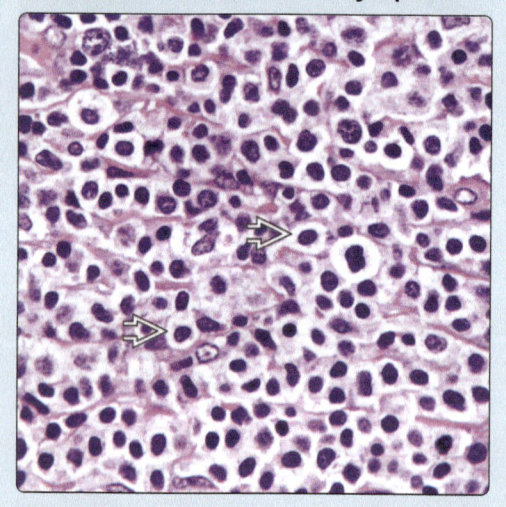

Clonal *TRG* Rearrangement

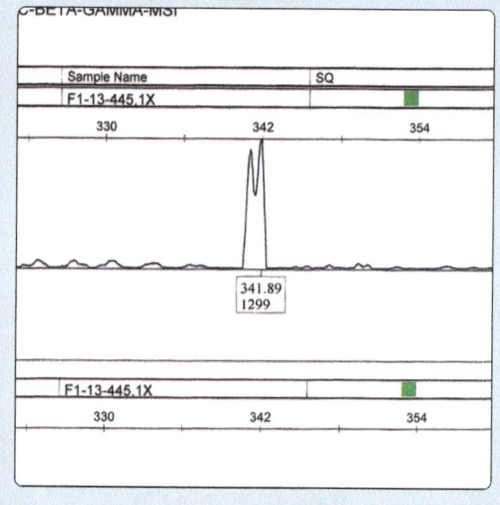

(Left) In this case of peripheral T-cell lymphoma, not otherwise specified (PTCL, NOS) involving a lymph node, the neoplastic cells are monomorphic and show abundant clear cytoplasm ➡. (Right) A dominant monoclonal peak is seen on PCR testing for T-cell receptor γ at position 341, which indicates that this is a monoclonal T-cell process.

T-Zone Pattern

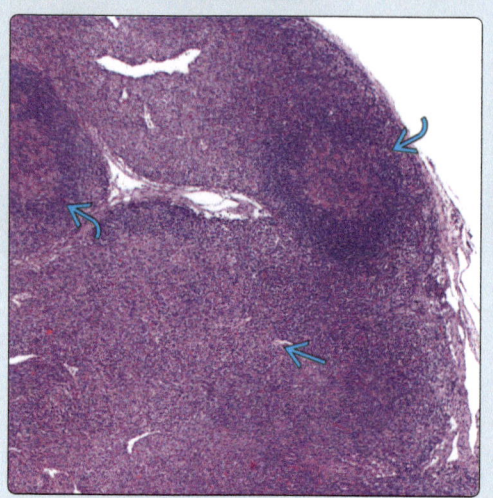

Large Tumor Cells

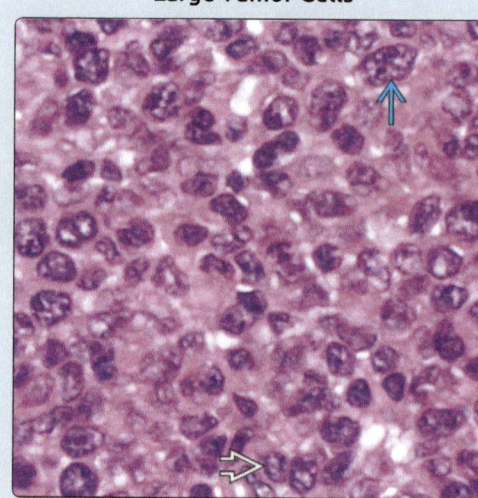

(Left) PTCL, NOS with T-zone pattern is shown. There are malignant T cells ➡, which are surrounding residual reactive germinal centers ➡. (Right) At high power, the tumor cells between the reactive germinal centers are large in size ➡ with atypical nuclear shapes, vesicular chromatin ➡, and pink cytoplasm.

Peripheral T-Cell Lymphoma, NOS

TERMINOLOGY

Abbreviations
- Peripheral T-cell lymphoma, not otherwise specified (PTCL, NOS)

Synonyms
- PTCL, unspecified

Definitions
- Mature T-cell lymphoma encompassing cases not fulfilling criteria of more specific T-cell lymphoma
  o Heterogeneous entity that remains diagnosis of exclusion
  o Both WHO 5th edition (HAEM5) and 2022 International Consensus Classification (ICC) recognize PTCL as entity
  o Nodal T follicular helper (TFH) cell lymphomas and EBV-positive nodal T- and NK-cell lymphomas are excluded from this category

CLINICAL ISSUES

Epidemiology
- Incidence
  o Most common noncutaneous T-cell lymphoma in Western countries
    – ~ 35% of all T-cell neoplasms
    – ~ 6% of all non-Hodgkin lymphomas
- Age
  o Adults (median: ~ 60 years)
- Sex
  o M:F ~ 2:1

Site
- Lymph nodes
  o Most frequently involved
- Bone marrow, spleen, and liver are involved in systemic disease
- Other most common extranodal locations
  o Skin and gastrointestinal tract

Presentation
- Peripheral lymphadenopathy is most common presentation
- B symptoms, particularly with extensive disease
- Usually presents with advanced-stage disease
- Leukemic presentation is uncommon, though blood can be involved
- Cytokine-related paraneoplastic phenomena can occur
  o Pruritus &/or eosinophilia
  o Hemophagocytic syndrome in ~ 3% of case
- Prior to onset of PTCL, immune-mediated disorders can occur, including
  o Hashimoto thyroiditis, rheumatoid arthritis
  o Immune thrombocytopenic purpura

Laboratory Tests
- Serum lactate dehydrogenase (LDH) and β-2 microglobulin can be elevated

Treatment
- Aggressive combination chemotherapy ± consolidation therapy
  o Induction combination chemotherapy regimens combine anthracycline with alkylating agent
  o Consolidation therapy
    – Hematopoietic stem cell transplantation
    – Radiation therapy
- Traditionally treated with B-cell lymphoma chemotherapy regimens
  o Cyclophosphamide, doxorubicin, vincristine, and prednisone (CHOP)
  o Still most commonly used induction therapy
- Treatment for refractory or relapsed PTCL
  o Combination chemotherapy, but there is no consensus on optimal regimen
  o FDA has approved several drugs recently
- Newer treatment options
  o Tyrosine kinase inhibitors
    – Imatinib, dasatinib have been studied
      □ Dasatinib has shown response in PTCL, NOS in phase I/II clinical trials
      □ Imatinib lacks efficacy in relapsed/refractory PTCL, NOS
  o Histone deacetylase inhibitors
    – Romidepsin, belinostat
  o Immune system modulators
    – Brentuximab vedotin, alemtuzumab (anti-CD52 antibody campath), lenalidomide
  o Antifolates
    – Pralatrexate
  o Fusion proteins
    – Denileukin diftitox
  o Nucleoside analogues
    – Pentostatin, gemcitabine
  o Anti-CC chemokine receptor 4 (CCR4) antibody (mogamulizumab)

Prognosis
- Unfavorable
  o Exhibits aggressive clinical behavior
  o Low survival rates
- Poor prognosis has been associated with
  o High stage, age > 60 years, high Ki-67
  o High International Prognostic Index (IPI)
  o GATA3 molecular subtype, cytotoxic phenotype
  o *TP53* and *CDKN2A* alterations
- Better prognosis
  o Small subset of patients with localized disease and low IPI have better outcome

MOLECULAR

Molecular Genetics
- 2 molecular variants have been identified: *TBX21* and *GATA3* mutated
  o This is based on their gene expression profile resembling T helper type 1 (Th1) and Th2 cells, respectively
  o This molecular classification is not routinely used for clinical diagnosis
  o IHC surrogate markers (TBX21, CXCR3, GATA3, CCR4) can separate out these 2 subgroups
  o *TBX21* subtype
    – *TBX21*, a.k.a. T-bet

Peripheral T-Cell Lymphoma, NOS

- Resemble Th1 cells
- Better prognosis
- Fewer copy number alterations
- More mutations in genes that regulate DNA methylation
- May include subgroup with a cytotoxic gene expression program and aggressive behavior
- NFkB pathway is involved
- Mutation in epigenetic regulators (e.g., *TET2*, *DNMT3A*)
  - *GATA3* subgroup
    - Resemble Th2 cells
    - Worse prognosis
    - Greater genomic complexity
    - High *MYC* expression
    - PI3K activation
    - Tumor suppressor genes including *TP53* (17p) deletion, *CDKN2A* (9p) deletion, and *PTEN* (10p) heterozygous deletion
- Other gene alterations
  - Tumor suppressor genes frequently altered
    - *TP63*, *CDKN2A*, *PTEN*, and *TP53*
    - Deletion of *CDKN2A* and *PTEN*, found in 20% of cases, is highly specific finding for PTCL, NOS and rarely found in other mature T-cell neoplasms
  - *PLCG1*, *CD28*, and *VAV1*
    - Fount in PTCL, but also common in other T-cell lymphomas
  - Deregulation of genes involved with apoptosis
    - *MOAP1*, *ING3*, *GADD45A*, *GADD45B*
  - Deregulation of genes involved with chemoresistance
    - *CCN1*, *NNMT*
  - Aberrant tyrosine kinase signaling
    - Overexpress *PDGFRA*

Cytogenetics
- Complex cytogenetic abnormalities
  - Chromosomal gains of 7q and 8q encompassing *CDK6* (7q22) and *CARD11* (7p22.2)
  - 14q11 [T-cell receptor (TCR) loci] are uncommon
- Trisomy 3 is associated with lymphoepithelioid variant of PTCL
- **Recurrent translocations**
  - t(6;14)(p25.3;q11.2); *IRF4::TRA*
    - Translocates *IRF4* oncogene and *TRA* gene
    - Cytotoxic phenotype
  - t(14;19)(q11.2;q13.3); *NECTIN2::TRA* has been identified
    - Results in juxtaposition of *NECTIN2* gene and *TRA* gene
  - t(5;9)(q32;q22); *ITK::SYK*
    - Results in overexpression of SYK

In Situ Hybridization
- EBV-encoded RNA (EBER) (+) in small subset of PTCL
  - More commonly found in background B cells

Polymerase Chain Reaction
- Clonal rearrangements of TCRs (*TRB* and *TRG*) are detected in majority of cases
- *IGH* gene rearrangements in ~ 1/3 of PTCL
  - Regardless of presence of associated B-cell proliferation

Chromosomal Microarray
- Recurrent gains in chromosomes 7q, 8q, 17q, and 22q
- Recurrent losses in chromosomes 4q, 5q, 6q, 9p, 10q, 12q, and 13q

Gene Expression Profiling
- No single shared gene expression signature has been identified for PTCL-NOS
  - Reflects heterogeneity of PTCL, NOS
- Different signatures have been found in PTCL, NOS as compared to AITL, ALK(+) anaplastic large cell lymphoma (ALCL), and ALK(-) ALCL
- NF-κB dysregulation in subset

MICROSCOPIC

Histologic Features
- Variable morphologic features
- Lymph node
  - Paracortical infiltrate or diffuse effacement of architecture
  - Mixed reactive background infiltrate frequently seen
    - Eosinophils, plasma cells, small lymphocytes
    - Clusters of epithelioid histiocytes in lymphoepithelioid variant of PTCL
    - Large B cells can be EBV (+) or (-)
    - Inflammatory background more common in *TBX21* subtype
  - Proliferation of postcapillary venules in interweaving (arborizing) fashion can be seen in some cases
  - Paracortical distribution can mimic benign paracortical hyperplasia
    - Reactive follicles are preserved and can be hyperplastic
    - Small or intermediate-sized neoplastic cells with clear or eosinophilic cytoplasm
    - Commonly associated with vascular proliferation and heterogeneous mixture of reactive cells
  - High rates of proliferation and apoptosis
  - Fibrosis may be identified
    - Fibrous bands can compartmentalize neoplasm, simulating nodular pattern
- Spleen
  - Solitary or multiple fleshy nodules involving white pulp with colonization of periarteriolar sheath
  - Predominant infiltration of red pulp in some cases
- Skin
  - PTCL commonly infiltrates dermis and subcutis
    - Epidermotropism is rare
  - Angiocentricity and adnexal involvement may be seen
  - Necrosis often present

Cytologic Features
- Tumor cells may be small, intermediate, or large in size
  - Most commonly intermediate &/or large cells
- Cytoplasm sparse or abundant
  - Clear, eosinophilic, or basophilic
  - Clear cytoplasm is classic feature
- Nuclei
  - Vesicular, hyperchromatic, or pleomorphic
  - Multinucleated or Reed-Sternberg-like nuclei can occur

Peripheral T-Cell Lymphoma, NOS

Morphologic Variants of Peripheral T-Cell Lymphoma, Not Otherwise Specified

- Lymphoepithelioid (LE-PTCL)
  - a.k.a. Lennert lymphoma
  - Histiocytes numerous and clustered along with T cells
    - T cells less commonly scattered, larger, more atypical cells, including occasional Reed-Sternberg-like B cells [usually EBV(+)]
    - Mimic granulomatous inflammation, often masking neoplastic T cells
    - T cells are usually small and mildly atypical with irregular nuclei and coarse chromatin
    - T cells often CD8(+) but can be CD4(+)
    - Nonactivated cytotoxic phenotype [TIA1(+) and granzyme B (-)]
    - Cases with TFH immunophenotype should be classified as nodal TFH cell lymphoma
    - LE-PTCL has somewhat better prognosis than other forms of PTCL, NOS
- T-zone
  - No longer considered variant of PTCL, NOS
    - Instead, it is considered nonspecific morphologic pattern, which can be seen in PTCL, NOS
- Follicular variant
  - No longer considered variant of PTCL-NOS
  - Reclassified by WHO as AITL and other nodal lymphomas of T follicular helper cell origin

Peripheral T-Cell Lymphoma With Associated B-Cell Proliferation

- ≤ 10% of PTCL cases can be associated with numerous B cells
- B cells are small, mature plasma cells, plasmacytoid large B lymphocytes, or plasmablasts
- B cells are often EBV(+)

ANCILLARY TESTS

Immunohistochemistry

- Mature T-cell immunophenotype
  - Pan T-cell antigens (+)
  - CD4(+)/CD8(-) or CD4(-)/CD8(+)
    - CD4 and CD8 (+) can change over time
    - CD8 is usually (+) in lymphoepithelioid variant
  - TdT(-), CD1A(-), CD99(-)
- Expression patterns of TCR are similar to normal T cells
  - TCR-αβ(+) in 95% of cases
    - β F1 (+) in these cases
  - Small subset are TCR-γδ(+)
    - β F1 (-) in these cases
- Aberrant T-cell immunophenotype
  - Loss of ≥ 1 pan T-cell antigens
    - Frequent absence of CD2, CD3, CD5, CD7, or TCR
  - Coexpression or absence of both CD4 and CD8
  - Rarely, B-cell antigens are aberrantly expressed
    - CD20 most frequent
- Absence of follicular helper T-cell phenotype
  - ≤ 1 TFH marker should be positive
  - CD10, BCL6, ICOS, and CXCL13
- CD30 can be (+), exceptionally with coexpression of CD15
  - CD30 is usually variable (+) in PTCL, but uniformly and brightly (+) in ALCL
  - CD30 (+) cases can be treated with brentuximab
- Cytotoxic molecules can be expressed in ~ 30% of PTCL
  - More common in *TBX21* cases
  - TIA1, granzyme B, and perforin
  - More common in extranodal vs. nodal PTCL
  - Cytotoxic immunophenotype more common in Japan than in United States or Europe
    - These tumors are commonly EBV(+) and could represent T/NK-cell lymphomas
- CD56 can be (+)
- Proliferation rate (Ki-67) of PTCL is highly variable
  - Lower in neoplasms composed of small cells
  - Usually substantial or very high in large-cell neoplasms
- TBX21, GATA3, CXCR3, and CCR4 may be (+)
  - Can be used as surrogate markers to *TBX21* and *GATA3* gene alterations

Flow Cytometry

- Decreased (dim) intensity of antigen expression compared with normal T cells
- Immunophenotype by flow cytometry is same as by immunohistochemistry
- Loss of T-cell markers more reliably assessed by flow cytometry

DIFFERENTIAL DIAGNOSIS

Nodal T Follicular Helper Cell Lymphoma, Angioimmunoblastic Type

- Similar morphology, but prominent high endothelial venules in AITL
- Infiltrate may be more polymorphous than in PTCL, NOS
- EBV(+) B immunoblasts
- Immunophenotype
  - ≥ 2 TFH associated markers (+)
    - BCL6, CXCL13, ICOS, PD1, SAP (+)
  - Follicular dendritic cell (FDC) meshworks hyperplasia
    - CD21(+), CD23(+), &/or CD35(+)
- Unlike PTCL, patients with AITL often also have polyclonal hypergammaglobulinemia
- *RHOA* G17 and *IDH2* R172 mutations
- No deletions of *CDKN2A* and *PTEN*
- *TP53* deletions/mutations rare

Nodal T Follicular Helper Cell Lymphoma, Not Otherwise Specified

- ≥ 2 TFH associated markers (+)
  - BCL6, CXCL13, ICOS, PD1, SAP
- No increase in high endothelial venules
- No FDC meshworks
- *RHOA* G17V mutations detected in some cases
- No deletions of *CDKN2A* and *PTEN*
- *TP53* deletions/mutations rare

ALK(-) Anaplastic Large Cell Lymphoma

- PTCL, NOS can overlap with ALK(-) ALCL histologically
  - Hallmark cells, sinus involvement, and anaplastic cytologic features support ALCL
- *DUSP22* and *TP63* altered in ALK(-) ALCL

Peripheral T-Cell Lymphoma, NOS

Molecular Findings in T-Cell Lymphoma

Type of T-Cell Lymphoma	Molecular Finding	Characteristics
PTCL, NOS	Complex karyotypes, *GATA3* and *TBX21* signatures	
Nodal TFH cell lymphoma, angioimmunoblastic type	*IDH2* mutations, *RHOA* mutations	*IDH2* mutations found in ~ 20% of AITLs
ALK(+) anaplastic large cell lymphoma	t(2;V)(p23;v)	*ALK* fusion proteins, potential therapeutic target
ALK(-) anaplastic large cell lymphoma	*DUSP22* and *TP63* rearrangements	*DUSP22* and *TP63* rearrangements are typically absent in PTCL, NOS
Hepatosplenic T-cell lymphoma	i(7)(q10)	Not entirely specific
Enteropathy-associated T-cell lymphoma	9q gains	Reproducible finding
Enteropathy-associated NK-/T-cell lymphoma	6q deletion and PDGFRA activation	

PTCL, NOS = peripheral T-cell lymphoma, not otherwise specified; AITL = angioimmunoblastic T-cell lymphoma.

- Different gene expression profile than PTCL, NOS
- Strong, uniform CD30(+), EMA(+)
  - CD30 can also be (+) in PTCL, NOS but not uniformly
- *DUSP22* rearrangements
  - Can also occur in PTCL
- JAK1 and STAT3 pathway activation

Adult T-Cell Leukemia/Lymphoma
- Histologically and immunophenotypically, PTCL, NOS and ATLL can be indistinguishable
- Positive serologic studies for human T-cell leukemia virus type 1 (HTLV-1)
- Hypercalcemia
- Leukemic phase is common in ATLL patients
  - Cells in blood smear are multilobated and flower-shaped
- CD4(+), CD25(+), CD30(-/+), CCR4(+), FOXP3(-/+)
- *CCR4* mutations and *IRF4* amplifications

Mycosis Fungoides Involving Lymph Node
- Histologically and immunophenotypically, mycosis fungoides (MF) in lymph node can closely mimic PTCL, NOS
- Clinically, patients with MF involving lymph node have
  - Skin lesions
  - ± Sézary cells in peripheral blood
- MF in lymph node associated with dermatopathic changes

Hepatosplenic T-Cell Lymphoma
- Usually presents differently than PTCL, NOS
  - Marked splenomegaly and hepatomegaly
  - No lymphadenopathy, typically
  - Sinusoidal distribution of tumor cells in liver, spleen, and bone marrow
- Hepatosplenic T-cell lymphoma (HSTCL) cells are monotonous with
  - Medium-sized nuclei and inconspicuous nucleoli
  - Rim of pale cytoplasm
- Immunophenotype
  - CD2(+), surface CD3(+), CD7(+), usually TCR-γ/δ(+)
  - TIA1(+), granzyme M (+), CD4(-), CD5(-), usually CD8(-)
- Isochromosome 7q is present in large subset of cases

Paracortical Hyperplasia
- Increased T cells that have normal phenotype
- Mixed CD4 and CD8 (+) T cells

- Scattered CD30(+) cells
- No monoclonal T-cell receptor gene rearrangement

Classic Hodgkin Lymphoma
- In differential diagnosis of PTCL in cases where Reed-Sternberg-like cells present
- Reed-Sternberg/Hodgkin cells in background of reactive T cells
- T cells have normal phenotype and lack T-cell receptor rearrangements

T-Cell/Histiocyte-Rich Large B-Cell Lymphoma
- In differential diagnosis of PTCL, NOS in cases where scattered large B cells present
- Large atypical B cells in background of small T cells
- T cells have normal phenotype and lack clonal T-cell receptor gene rearrangements

Nodal Marginal Zone Lymphoma
- Neoplastic cells are B cells and can have increased clear cytoplasm similar to PTCL, NOS
- Neoplastic B cells often grown around follicles and colonize them
- Clonal *IGH* rearrangements

SELECTED REFERENCES

1. Feldman AL et al: Classification and diagnostic evaluation of nodal T- and NK-cell lymphomas. Virchows Arch. 482(1):265-79, 2023
2. Weiss J et al: PTCL, NOS: an update on classification, risk-stratification, and treatment. Front Oncol. 13:1101441, 2023
3. Alaggio R et al: The 5th edition of the World Health Organization Classification of Haematolymphoid Tumours: lymphoid neoplasms. Leukemia. 36(7):1720-48, 2022
4. Amador C et al: Gene expression signatures for the accurate diagnosis of peripheral T-cell lymphoma entities in the routine clinical practice. J Clin Oncol. 40(36):4261-75, 2022
5. Maura F et al: CDKN2A deletion is a frequent event associated with poor outcome in patients with peripheral T-cell lymphoma not otherwise specified (PTCL-NOS). Haematologica. 106(11):2918-26, 2021
6. Heavican TB et al: Genetic drivers of oncogenic pathways in molecular subgroups of peripheral T-cell lymphoma. Blood. 133(15):1664-76, 2019
7. Watatani Y et al: Molecular heterogeneity in peripheral T-cell lymphoma, not otherwise specified revealed by comprehensive genetic profiling. Leukemia. 33(12):2867-83, 2019
8. Lone W et al: Molecular insights into pathogenesis of peripheral T cell lymphoma: a review. Curr Hematol Malig Rep. 13(4):318-28, 2018
9. Wang T et al: T-cell receptor signaling activates an ITK/NF-κB/GATA-3 axis in T-cell lymphomas facilitating resistance to chemotherapy. Clin Cancer Res. 23(10):2506-15, 2017

Peripheral T-Cell Lymphoma, NOS

CD3 Immunohistochemistry

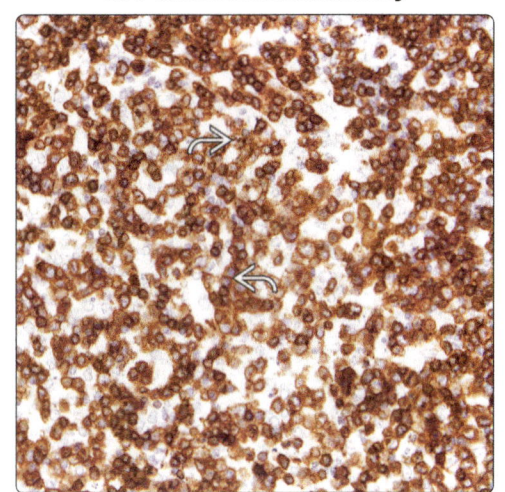

CD5 Immunohistochemistry

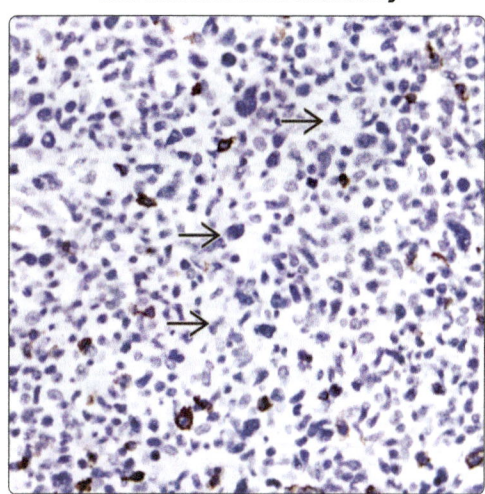

(Left) CD3 is expressed ⇨ in the tumor cells of this case of PTCL, NOS. Most of the lymphoid cells are CD3(+), supporting the T-cell lineage. (Right) CD5(-) neoplastic cells ⇨ are shown. PTCL, NOS often shows an aberrant T-cell immunophenotype with loss of ≥ 1 T-cell markers. Aberrant immunophenotype occurs in ~ 80% of PTCL.

TIA1 Immunohistochemistry

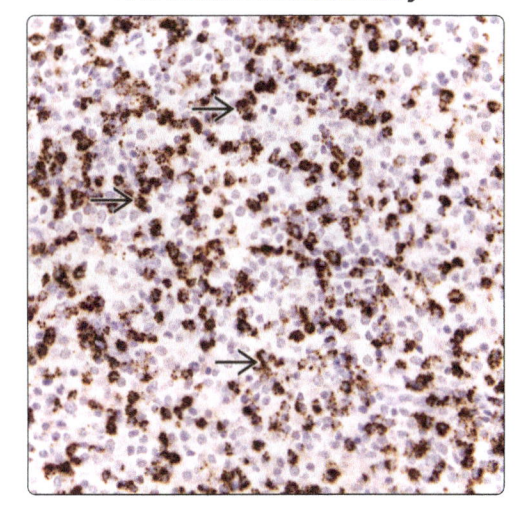

EBER In Situ Hybridization

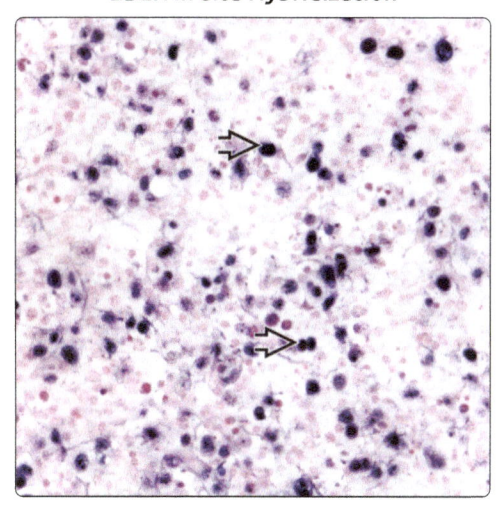

(Left) TIA1 shows increased cytotoxic granules ⇨ in this case of PTCL, NOS. A subset of PTCL, NOS shows cytotoxic immunophenotype. Many of the neoplastic cells are also frequently positive for granzyme B and perforin (not shown). (Right) Epstein-Barr virus-encoded RNA (EBER) ISH shows scattered positive cells ⇨. Both PTCL, NOS and angioimmunoblastic T-cell lymphoma can have scattered EBER(+) B-cells and therefore must be distinguished by other characteristics.

Lymphoepithelioid Variant

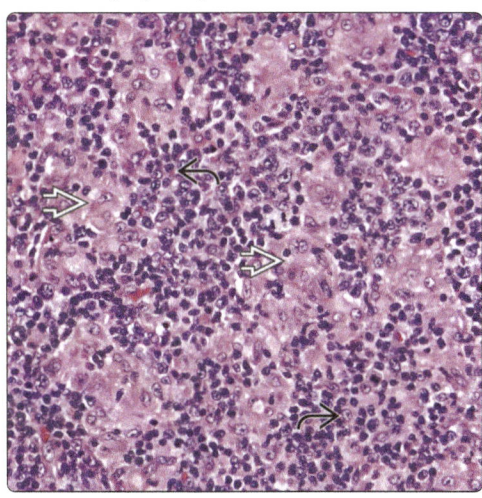

CD3 Immunohistochemistry

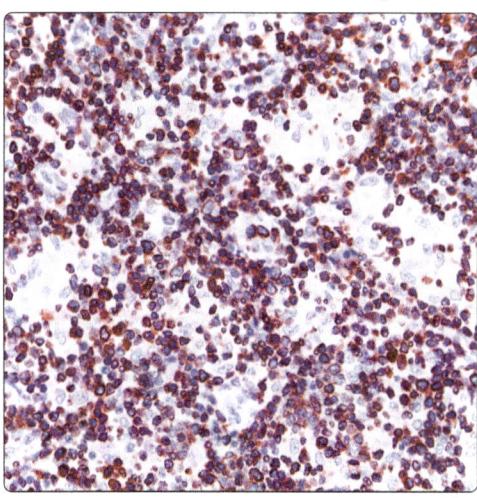

(Left) Lymphoepithelioid variant of PTCL, NOS (a.k.a. Lennert lymphoma) is shown. The neoplastic T cells ⇨ are associated with clusters of epithelioid histiocytes ⇨. (Right) In the same case of Lennert lymphoma, CD3 highlights the neoplastic T cells. Lennert lymphoma can be mistakenly diagnosed as granulomatous inflammation.

Nodal Follicular Helper T-Cell Lymphoma

KEY FACTS

TERMINOLOGY
- Nodal T-follicular helper cell lymphoma (NTFHL): T-cell lymphoma of follicular helper T cells associated with systemic disease, polymorphous infiltrate, and proliferating high endothelial venules
- Both WHO and ICC divide NTFHL into angioimmunoblastic, follicular, and not otherwise specified entities/subtypes

MOLECULAR
- Clonal *TRG* and *TRB* rearrangement, but *IGH* may also be clonal
- *RHOA* G17V mutation
- *IDH2* p.R172 mutation
- *TET2* and *DNMT3A* mutations are early loss-of-function mutations
- EBV-positive B cells present on EBER stain
- Less common mutated genes include *TP53*, *ETV6*, *CCND3*, *EP300*, *JAK2*, and *STAT3*
- T-cell receptor signaling pathway genes *FYN*, *PLCG1*, and *CD28* mutated in ~ 10% of cases
- t(5;9)(q33;q22); *ITK::SYK* more often seen in NTFHL-F

MICROSCOPIC
- Lymph node
  - Tumor cells with clear cytoplasm, arborizing high endothelial vessels, and disrupted follicular dendritic meshworks
  - Germinal centers may be hyperplastic, atretic, or lost
- Skin
  - Dermal lymphocytic infiltrate with eosinophils
  - May be tumor cells in skin or reactive infiltrate

ANCILLARY TESTS
- CD4(+) T cells, CD10(+/-), BCL6(+), CXCL13(+), PD1(+)

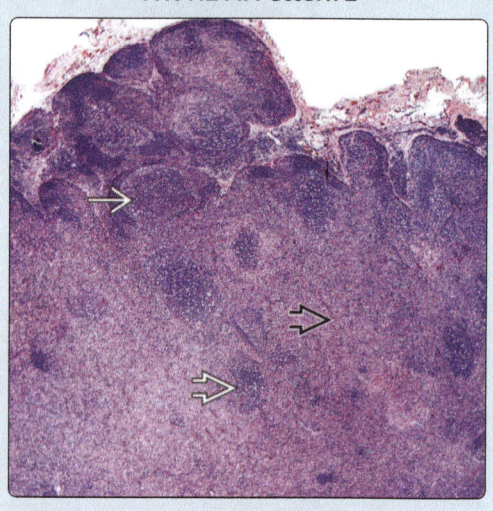

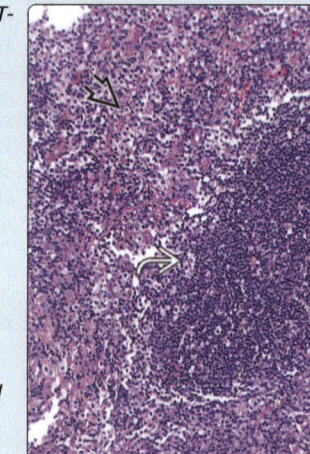

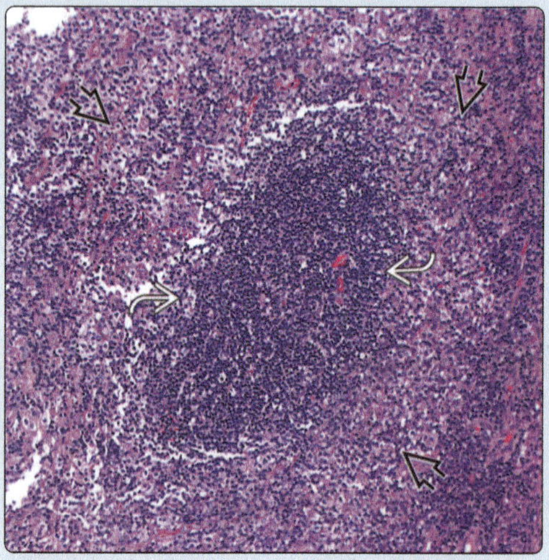

(Left) Nodal follicular helper T-cell lymphoma, angioimmunoblastic type (NTFHL-AI) with pattern 1 morphology is shown. Note the reactive-appearing germinal center ➡ surrounded by neoplastic T cells ➡. (Right) Lymph node involved by NTFHL-AI shows residual small lymphoid follicles ➡, some barely recognizable ➡, and expanded interfollicular ➡ neoplastic T cells. The lymph node is only partially involved by T-cell lymphoma.

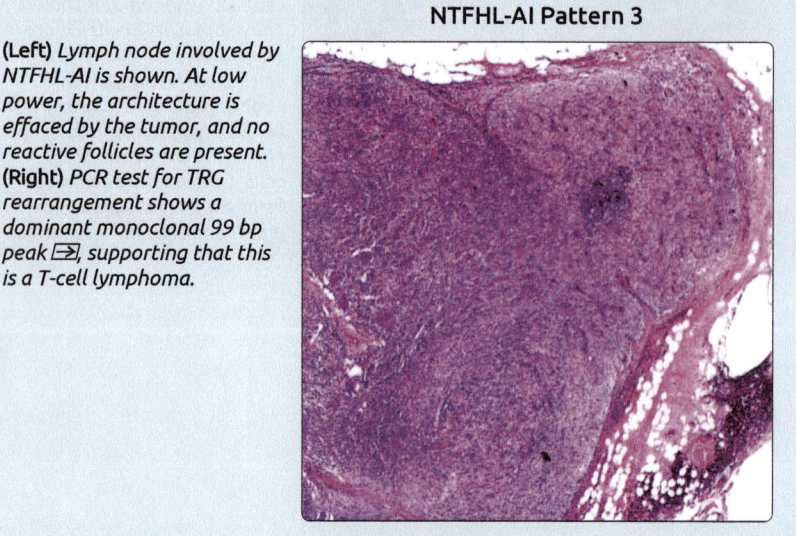

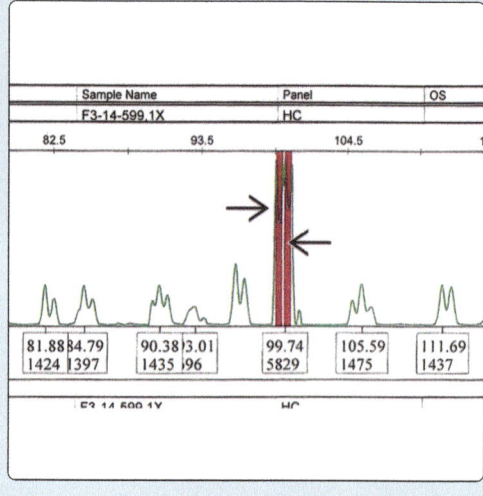

(Left) Lymph node involved by NTFHL-AI is shown. At low power, the architecture is effaced by the tumor, and no reactive follicles are present. (Right) PCR test for TRG rearrangement shows a dominant monoclonal 99 bp peak ➡, supporting that this is a T-cell lymphoma.

Nodal Follicular Helper T-Cell Lymphoma

TERMINOLOGY

Abbreviations
- Nodal T-follicular helper cell lymphoma (NTFHL)

Synonyms
- Angioimmunoblastic lymphadenopathy with dysproteinemia
- Immunoblastic lymphadenopathy
- Immunodysplastic disease (old terminology, not currently used)

Definitions
- NTFHL comprises group of mature T cell neoplasms with phenotypic features of TFH cells
  - All 3 types are T cell lymphomas that express TFH markers and have similar molecular alterations
- NTFHL, angioimmunoblastic type (angioimmunoblastic T-cell lymphoma)
  - Characterized by systemic disease and polymorphous lymphoid infiltrate involving lymph nodes, which show prominent high endothelial venules (HEVs) and follicular dendritic cells (FDCs)
  - Characteristic morphology, phenotype, and genotype better understood than other types
- NTFHL, follicular type displays follicular growth pattern and lacks HEV and extrafollicular FDC proliferation seen in NTFHL, angioimmunoblastic type
- NTFHL-NOS is nodal peripheral T-cell neoplasm with TFH phenotype that does not fulfill criteria for NTFHL, angioimmunoblastic type or NTFHL, follicular type

CLASSIFICATION

WHO 5th Edition (WHO-HAEM5) vs. 2022 International Consensus Classification (ICC)
- Essentially same nomenclature except for 3 categories of NTFHL listed as "subtypes" in ICC designated as "entities" in WHO-HAEM5
- Subtypes/entities of NTFHL include
  - NTFHL, angioimmunoblastic type (NTFHL-AI)
  - NTFHL, follicular type (NTFHL-F)
  - NTFHL, not otherwise specified (NTFHL-NOS)
- In prior WHO 4th edition, NTFHL-AI was called angioimmunoblastic T-cell lymphoma, NTFHL-F was called follicular T-cell lymphoma, and NTFHL-NOS was called nodal peripheral T-cell lymphoma with TFH phenotype

ETIOLOGY/PATHOGENESIS

Follicular Helper T Cell
- CD4(+) T cells that are found within germinal centers of B-cell follicles
- T follicular helper (TFH) cells function in germinal center formation and development of high-affinity antibodies
- Essential in development of high-affinity antibodies
- Produce IL21 and IL4
- Express CD10, PD1, CXCL13, CXCR5, and ICOS

Dysfunction of Immune System
- Patients with NTFHL-AI have hypergammaglobulinemia and other immune dysfunctions
  - Possible mechanism
    - Follicular helper T cells upregulate CXCL13 and CXCR5
    - CXCL13 involved in B-cell recruitment
  - Cytokine dysregulation
    - Patients with NTFHL-AI show abnormal cytokine dysregulation
    - Debated whether skin lesions represent tumor or secondary reaction to cytokines

Drugs
- Implicated as causative agent in some cases

CLINICAL ISSUES

Epidemiology
- Incidence
  - TFH lymphoma comprises 1-2% of all non-Hodgkin lymphoma
  - NTFHL-AI is most common subtype
    - 1,000 new cases per year in USA
    - Comprising 18% of all peripheral T-cell lymphomas
  - NTFHL-F is rare and makes up only 2% of noncutaneous peripheral T-cell lymphoma
  - NTFHL-NOS is rare; incidence unknown
- Age
  - Mostly adults, middle-aged to older
    - Rarely seen in children
  - Median: 63 years
- Sex
  - M > F
- Ethnicity
  - White populations most frequently
  - More common in Europe than in North America

Site
- Lymph node
  - Nearly all cases involve lymph nodes
- Skin
  - Frequent extranodal site
    - ~ 50% of cases have skin lesions
    - Usually secondary to systemic disease
    - Rarely, skin lesion can be 1st manifestation of disease
  - Other organ systems involved
    - Often spleen, liver, and bone marrow
      - No CXCL13 in bone marrow in NTFHL-AI type

Presentation
- Lymph node
  - 1 or more prominent nodes
  - Often generalized lymphadenopathy
- Skin
  - Rash, usually pruritic
    - Maculopapular eruption most common
    - Purpura, erythroderma, papulovesicular lesions, nodules, and urticarial lesions are less common
  - Often generalized lesions
    - Frequently on trunk or extremities
  - Rash can be before, after, or same time as initial diagnosis of NTFHL-AI
- Extracutaneous presentation
  - Hepatomegaly
  - Splenomegaly

Nodal Follicular Helper T-Cell Lymphoma

- B symptoms
- Arthritis/arthralgia
- Ascites
- Leukemic presentation is uncommon, but neoplastic T cells may be detected in blood by flow cytometry

Laboratory Tests
- Complete blood cell count
  - Anemia
    - Autoimmune hemolytic anemia
    - Cryoglobulins/cold agglutinins
    - Sometimes positive Coombs test
  - Lymphocytes
    - Lymphopenia more often
    - Lymphocytosis less often
  - Thrombocytopenia
  - Eosinophilia
- Hyper- or hypogammaglobulinemia
  - Polyclonal
  - Hypoalbuminemia
- ↑ erythrocyte sedimentation rate
- ↑ serum lactate dehydrogenase
- ↑ β-2-microglobulin
- Autoantibodies are sometimes positive
  - Rheumatoid factor
  - Anti-smooth muscle antibody

Natural History
- NTFHL-AI type-related secondary lymphomas
  - Increased risk of developing 2nd lymphoma in patients with NTFHL-AI type
    - Diffuse large B-cell lymphoma is most common 2nd lymphoma
    - Diffuse large B-cell lymphoma usually has positive EBER cells
- Clinical features of NTFHL-F type resemble those of NTFHL-AI type

Treatment
- Combined chemotherapy
  - Treatment strategy in most cases
- Steroids
  - In patients who do not receive chemotherapy
- Autologous stem cell transplant
  - Sometimes follows treatment with chemotherapy
- New therapeutic agents
  - IL21, PD1, CXCL13, and ICOS antibodies are in clinical trials
  - Antiangiogenic therapy is under investigation

Prognosis
- Dismal
  - Median survival: 1-2 years
  - No change in prognosis over past 20 years
- Poor prognostic indicators
  - *TET2*, *DNMT3*, and *IDH2* mutations
  - Males
  - Anemia
  - Mediastinal lymphadenopathy

IMAGING

General Features
- Generalized lymphadenopathy
- Internal organ involvement

MOLECULAR

In Situ Hybridization
- EBV-encoded RNA (EBER)
  - 80-90% of lymph nodes show scattered EBV(+) B cells
    - T cells are EBER(-)
    - Usually negative in skin lesion

PCR
- Clonal T-cell receptor gene rearrangement in 87% lymph nodes with NTFHL-AI
  - Some skin infiltrates show clonal T-cell receptor gene rearrangement
    - Identical clones can be seen in skin and lymph node
  - Clonal *IGH* rearrangement in 25% of lymph nodes with NTFHL-AI type

Gene Alterations
- *RHOA* G17V mutation
  - May be driving molecular event for NTFHL-AI
  - Motility and adhesion gene with loss of GTPase activity
  - G17V variant has dominant-negative effect on RhoA signaling pathway
  - *RHOA* encodes small GTPase, and, when mutated, allows *RHOA* to interact with *VAV1* downstream of T-cell receptor signaling
  - *RHOA* mutation may drive naive CD4(+) T cells to differentiate to TFH cells and facilitate neoplasia
  - Found in ~ 70% of NTFHL-AI but also in NTFHL-NOS and NTFHL-F
  - Also found in 20% of peripheral T-cell lymphoma, not otherwise specified
- *IDH2* R172 mutations
  - *IDH2* alterations are seen in ~ 25% of NTFHL-AI but only rarely in TFHL-F and TFHL-NOS
  - Tumor cells are large in size with clear cell morphology
  - *IDH2* mutations also seen in acute myeloid leukemia and glioblastoma multiforme
  - *IDH2* mutant facilitates production of 2-hydroxyglutarate, which inhibits α-ketoglutarate-dependent dioxygenase
- *TET2* and *DNMT3A*
  - Considered early mutations in TFH cells
  - Loss-of-function mutations in genes that regulate DNA and histone methylation
  - Affects CD4 and CD8 T cells
  - Cause DNA methylation and transcription to be dysregulated
  - NTFHL-AI thought to develop in background of clonal hematopoiesis
  - *TET2* mutations
    - Detected in 80% of cases
    - Also seen in other peripheral T-cell lymphomas with follicular T-helper cell phenotype
    - *TET2* oxidizes 5-methylcytosine successfully to 5-carboxycytosine, promoting cytosine demethylation

Nodal Follicular Helper T-Cell Lymphoma

- o *DNMT3A* mutations
  - *DNMT3A* catalyzes production of 5-methylcytosine in CpG dinucleotides
  - Detected in ~ 35% of cases
- T-cell receptor signaling mutations
  - o *FYN*, *PLCG1*, *CD28*, *ICOS*, and *VAV1* mutations
  - o *CD28* alterations have adverse prognosis
  - o These genes are seen along with *RHOA*, *TET2*, and *DNMT3A* alterations
  - o These genes may also affect other nonneoplastic lymphocytes and may lead to FDC meshwork expansion and high endothelial venules proliferation

Cytogenetics
- No specific chromosomal abnormalities
  - o Trisomy of chromosomes 3, 5, and 21 reported
  - o Loss of 6q, gain of X, or 1p alterations reported
- t(5;9)(q33;q22); *ITK::SYK* fusion
  - o Translocation originally identified in follicular peripheral T-cell lymphoma
  - o Only rarely identified in NTFHL-AL

Chromosomal Microarray
- Recurrent gains of 22q, 19, and 11q13

Gene Expression Profiling
- Has shown differences between NTFHL-AI type and peripheral T-cell lymphoma, not otherwise specified

MICROSCOPIC

Histologic Features
- NTFHL-AI
  - o Lymph node shows effaced architecture, which can be partial or complete
  - o Tumor preferentially involves paracortical areas
    - In early disease, tumor may be only in paracortex
    - Peripheral cortical sinuses of lymph node often patent, unlike in other T-cell lymphomas
  - o Tumor cells
    - Small to medium in size
    - Medium to large clear cells with distinct cell membranes are feature of *IDH2* p.R172 mutant NTFHL-AI
  - o High endothelial venule proliferation
    - ↑ vessels in tumor
    - Usually branching blood vessels
    - Follicular dendritic cells located near blood vessels
    - PAS highlights blood vessels
    - Hyalinized basement membranes and plump endothelial cells
  - o Follicular dendritic cell meshworks
    - Expanded and disrupted in tumor
    - Associated with high endothelial venules
  - o Polymorphic background inflammatory cells
    - Often prominent
    - Eosinophils, reactive small lymphocytes, immunoblasts and histiocytes
    - Epithelioid histiocytes give granulomatous appearance
    - B-cell proliferations may be prominent, consisting of B immunoblasts and plasma cells
    - B immunoblasts can be EBV(+) or EBV(-) and can progress to diffuse large B-cell lymphoma
    - Plasma cells can be polyclonal or monoclonal
  - o Hodgkin/Reed Sternberg (HRS)-like cells may be present
  - o 3 morphologic patterns
    - Pattern 1, hyperplastic follicles
      - □ Large reactive follicles, neoplastic T cells outside of follicles are inconspicuous
      - □ Must distinguish from reactive follicular hyperplasia
      - □ Follicular helper T-cell markers (-) in hyperplasia
    - Pattern 2, atretic follicles
      - □ Prominent perifollicular neoplastic T cells and atretic follicles
      - □ Can be mistaken for Castleman lymphadenopathy
    - Pattern 3, no follicles
      - □ Effaced lymph node
  - o Tumor cell-rich NTFHL-AI
    - Monomorphic appearance with numerous neoplastic T cells and lack of polymorphous inflammatory background infiltrate
    - Can be seen when NTFHL-AI relapses
    - Presence of CD21(+), CD23(+), and CD35(+) expanded FDC meshworks separates tumor cell-rich NTFHL-AI from NTFHL-NOS
- NTFHL-F
  - o Nodular proliferation of monotonous, intermediate-sized lymphoid cells with moderate to abundant clear cytoplasm
  - o 2 reported growth patterns: Follicular lymphoma-like (FL) pattern and progressive transformation of germinal center-like (PTGC) pattern
    - FL-like pattern shows well-defined nodules of T cells, which are surrounded by attenuated mantle zones
    - PTGC-like pattern has large nodules of T cells, and some are disrupted by mantle zone B cells similar to PTGC
  - o Often lacks polymorphous inflammatory background and prominent high endothelial venules seen in NTFHL-AI
  - o May show morphologic overlap with NTFHL-AI type and may not be distinct entity
- NTFHL-NOS
  - o Effacement of lymph node architecture by diffuse infiltrate of medium- to large-sized lymphoid cells
  - o May have T-zone pattern of involving paracortical areas
  - o Unlike NTFHL-AI, typically lacks polymorphous inflammatory background, expanded FDC meshworks, and prominent high endothelial venules
- Skin
  - o Usually nonspecific, variable histologic patterns
  - o Often superficial dermal infiltrates with lymphocytes and eosinophils
  - o Sometimes perivascular lymphocytic infiltrate
  - o Sometimes sheet-like lymphocytic infiltrate
  - o Lymphocytes ± atypia
  - o Hyperplastic capillaries
  - o Usually no epidermotropism present
- Bone marrow
  - o Often involved but may be subtle and difficult to diagnosis
  - o Better to have primary diagnosis from lymph node

Nodal Follicular Helper T-Cell Lymphoma

ANCILLARY TESTS

Immunohistochemistry

- Malignant T cells
  - Positive for T-cell antigens, including CD2, CD3, CD5, and CD7
    - Can aberrantly lose 1 or more T-cell antigens
    - Most commonly lost T-cell antigen is CD7
  - TFH-associated immunophenotypic markers
    - PD1, ICOS, CXCL13, CD10, BCL6, CXCR5, SAP, c-MAF, and CD200
      - PD1, ICOS, CXCL13, CD10, and BCL6 are most commonly used TFH markers
    - Must express 2 or more of these TFH-associated markers
      - None of markers are specific by themselves
      - *RHOA* p.G17V mutant cases usually are immunoreactive for at least 3 TFH markers
      - *IDH2* p.R172 mutant cases are often strongly immunoreactive for CD10, CXCL13, and IDH2
    - PD1 and ICOS are most sensitive
    - CD10 and CXCL13 are most specific
    - CXCL13 usually (+) and CD10 often (-) in cutaneous involvement of TFH lymphoma
    - This phenotype is not seen in reactive paracortex or most other mature T-cell lymphomas
    - NTFHL-NOS type often expresses only PD1 and ICOS (less specific TFH markers)
    - CD10 and BCL6 (+) T cells of NTFHL-F type, and cells can be mistaken for follicular lymphoma
  - Helper T cells [usually CD4(+), CD8(-), and βF1(+)]
  - Follicular dendritic cell (FDC) meshworks
    - CD21, CD23, and CD35, and clusterin (+); FDC meshworks encircle blood vessels
    - FDC meshworks may be subtle in pattern 1 because of expansive follicles
    - In NTFHL-F type, FDC meshworks may be confined to nodules
  - ↑ reactive B immunoblasts
    - Express B-cell markers (CD19, CD20, PAX5, CD79A) and EBER (+/-)
    - Neoplastic T cells EBER(-)
  - HRS-like cells
    - CD30, CD15, and EBER (+/-)
      - CD30 can also be positive in neoplastic T cells
    - May express B-cell markers
    - Often rosetted by malignant TFH cells

Flow Cytometry

- Loss of 1 or more T-cell antigens
  - Surface CD3 may be lost
- CD10 coexpressed on subset of T cells

DIFFERENTIAL DIAGNOSIS

Primary Cutaneous Small/Medium CD4(+) T-Cell Lymphoma

- Also consists of follicular helper cells with same phenotype as NTFHL-AI type and same *RHOA* mutations

Anaplastic Large Cell Lymphoma

- Common in skin
- EBER(-)
- CD30(+); ALK(-), EMA(-)

Follicular Lymphoma and Nodular Lymphocyte-Predominant Hodgkin Lymphoma

- B-cell lymphomas that contain follicular dendritic cells and show some PD1(+) cells
- Cases of NTFHL-F type can be mistaken for follicular lymphoma
- CD10 and BCL6 (+) cells are expressed in B cells in FL and T cells in NTFHL-F

Classic Hodgkin Lymphoma

- Similarities to NTFHL-AI
  - TFHL, angioimmunoblastic type can sometimes have Reed-Sternberg-like cells that look similar to classic Hodgkin lymphoma
  - Both can be EBER(+)
- Differences from NTFHL-AI type
  - No malignant T cells
  - No increased high endothelial venules
  - No increased follicular dendritic cell meshworks
  - No clonal T-cell receptor gene rearrangements
  - Rare in skin
  - CD45(-), CD15(+), and CD30(+)

T-Cell/Histiocyte-Rich Large B-Cell Lymphoma

- Similarities to NTFHL-AI
  - Both tumors have more T cells than B cells
- Differences from NTFHL-AI
  - Large, atypical B cells and small, reactive-appearing T cells
    - Often large, atypical T cells and small B cells in NTFHL-AI
  - Clonal *IGH* rearrangement
  - No increased follicular dendritic cells
  - EBER(-)

EBV(+) Diffuse Large B-Cell Lymphoma

- Both have EBV(+) large cells
- Differences from NTFHL-AI
  - Usually polyclonal T-cell receptor gene rearrangement and clonal *IGH* rearrangement
  - No increased follicular dendritic cells
  - EBV(+) in sheets of large B cells and far fewer in number in NTFHL-AI
  - No aberrant T-cell antigens

Peripheral T-Cell Lymphoma, NOS

- Further studies may determine if current defining criteria of positivity for 2 TFH markers in addition to CD4 are sufficiently robust in excluding peripheral T-cell lymphoma, NOS
- Can express TFH markers
- Often only one TFH marker is positive to differentiate PTCL NOS from NTFHL-AI

Nodal Follicular Helper T-Cell Lymphoma

Clinical and Laboratory Findings

Clinical Finding	Cases (%)	Laboratory Finding	Cases (%)
B symptoms	68-85	Anemia	40-47
Generalized lymphadenopathy	94-97	Other cytopenias	20
Splenomegaly	70-73	Eosinophilia	39
Hepatomegaly	52-72	Hypergammaglobulinemia	50-83
Rash	48-58	Hypogammaglobulinemia	9-27
Arthritis	18	Autoantibodies	66-77
Ascites/effusions	23-37	↑ lactate dehydrogenase	70

NTFHL vs. Peripheral T-Cell Lymphoma, Not Otherwise Specified

Feature	NTFHL, Angioimmunoblastic	PTCL-NOS
High endothelial venules	Increased and arborizing	Normal
Follicular dendritic cells	Increased and disrupted	Normal or decreased
Phenotype	Positive for CD10 and CXCL13	Usually (-) for CD10 and CXCL13
EBV(+) cells	Can be seen in scattered B cells	Variable
RHOA G17V mutation	Found in majority of cases	Found in ~ 20% of cases

Molecular Findings

Molecular Abnormality	Findings
RHOA G17V mutation	May be key molecular abnormality driving pathogenesis
TET2, IDH2, and DNMT3A mutations	Recently described, but not specific for TFH lymphomas
TP53, ETV6, CCND3, and EP300	Loss-of-function mutations
JAK2 and STAT3	Gain-of-function mutations
TRB and TRG rearrangements	Clonal in most cases
IGH rearrangements	Clonal IGH rearrangements well documented, even though this is T-cell lymphoma, not B-cell lymphoma
EBV-encoded RNA (EBER) test	Positive in scattered B cells in lymph node cases; usually negative in skin cases

DIAGNOSTIC CHECKLIST

Clinically Relevant Pathologic Features

- Hypergammaglobulinemia and autoimmune hemolytic anemia

Pathologic Interpretation Pearls

- T-cell lymphoma with arborizing high endothelial venules and increased background inflammatory cells
- CD3(+), PD1(+), EBER(+) B cells, CD10(+), CXCL13(+)

SELECTED REFERENCES

1. Alaggio R et al: The 5th edition of the World Health Organization classification of haematolymphoid tumours: lymphoid neoplasms. Leukemia. 36(7):1720-48, 2022
2. Campo E et al: The International Consensus Classification of mature lymphoid neoplasms: a report from the Clinical Advisory Committee. Blood. 40(11):1229-53, 2022
3. Fujisawa M et al: Activation of RHOA-VAV1 signaling in angioimmunoblastic T-cell lymphoma. Leukemia. 32(3):694-702, 2018
4. Fujisawa M et al: Recent progress in the understanding of angioimmunoblastic T-cell lymphoma. J Clin Exp Hematop. 57(3):109-19, 2017
5. Fukumoto K et al: Review of the biologic and clinical significance of genetic mutations in angioimmunoblastic T-cell lymphoma. Cancer Sci. 109(3):490-6, 2017
6. Leclaire Alirkilicarslan A et al: Expression of TFH markers and detection of RHOA p.G17V and IDH2 p.R172K/S mutations in cutaneous localizations of angioimmunoblastic T-cell lymphomas. Am J Surg Pathol. 41(12):1581-92, 2017
7. Lemonnier F et al: Angioimmunoblastic T-cell lymphoma: more than a disease of T follicular helper cells. J Pathol. 242(4):387-90, 2017
8. Ahearne MJ et al: Follicular helper T-cells: expanding roles in T-cell lymphoma and targets for treatment. Br J Haematol. 166(3):326-35, 2014
9. Hsi ED et al: Diagnostic accuracy of a defined immunophenotypic and molecular genetic approach for peripheral T/NK-cell lymphomas. A North American PTCL study group project. Am J Surg Pathol. 38(6):768-75, 2014
10. Iqbal J et al: Gene expression signatures delineate biological and prognostic subgroups in peripheral T-cell lymphoma. Blood. 123(19):2915-23, 2014
11. Odejide O et al: A targeted mutational landscape of angioimmunoblastic T-cell lymphoma. Blood. 123(9):1293-6, 2014
12. Palomero T et al: Recurrent mutations in epigenetic regulators, RHOA and FYN kinase in peripheral T cell lymphomas. Nat Genet. 46(2):166-70, 2014
13. Piccaluga PP et al: Molecular genetics of peripheral T-cell lymphomas. Int J Hematol. 99(3):219-26, 2014
14. Sakata-Yanagimoto M et al: Disease-specific mutations in mature lymphoid neoplasms: recent advances. Cancer Sci. 105(6):623-9, 2014

Nodal Follicular Helper T-Cell Lymphoma

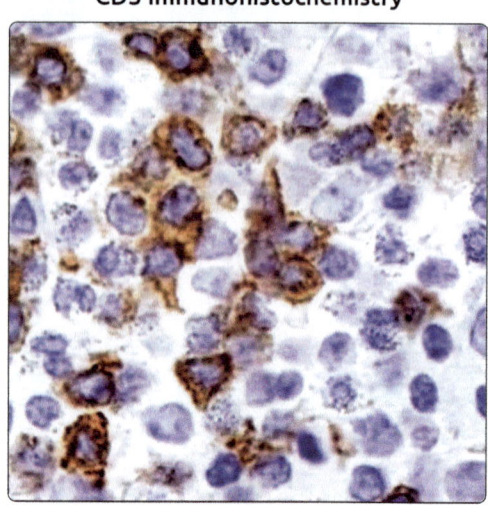

(Left) In NTFHL-AI, the tumor cells are often accompanied by a mixed inflammatory infiltrate. Here, there are scattered eosinophils ⇨ and prominent high endothelial venules ⇨. **(Right)** CD3 is positive in the tumor cells of NTFHL-AI. NTFHL-AI often expresses multiple T-cell antigens but may aberrantly lose 1 or more T-cell markers.

Mixed Infiltrate

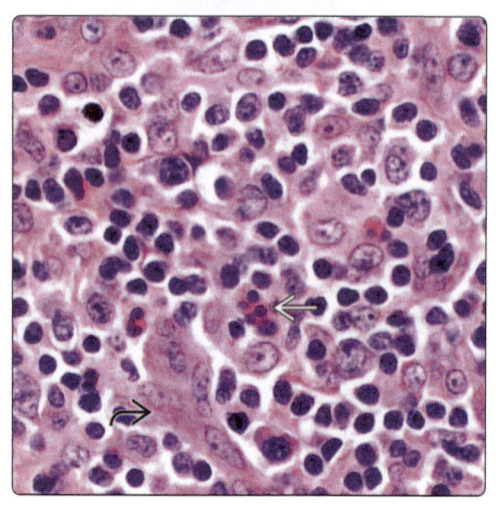

CD3 Immunohistochemistry

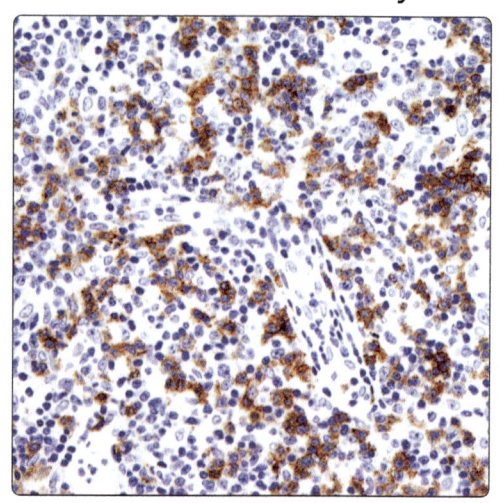

(Left) CD10 is coexpressed in the same T cells. CD10(+) and CD3(+) cells are commonly seen in NTFHL-AI and are considered follicular helper T cells. **(Right)** PD-1 is strongly positive in this case of NTFHL-AI. PD-1 is one of the antigens found in follicular helper T cells that is expressed in NTFHL-AI. (Courtesy S. Wang, MD.)

CD10 Immunohistochemistry

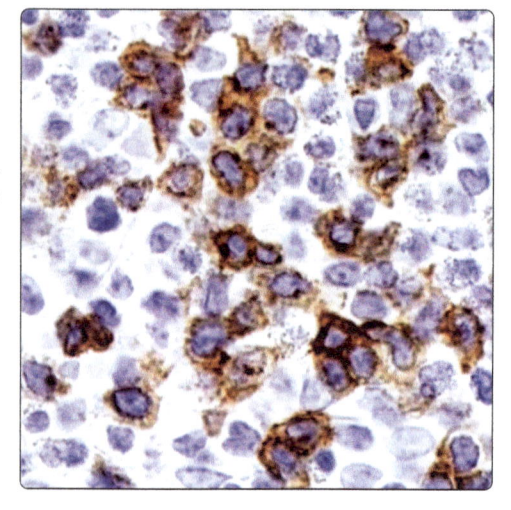

PD-1 Immunohistochemistry

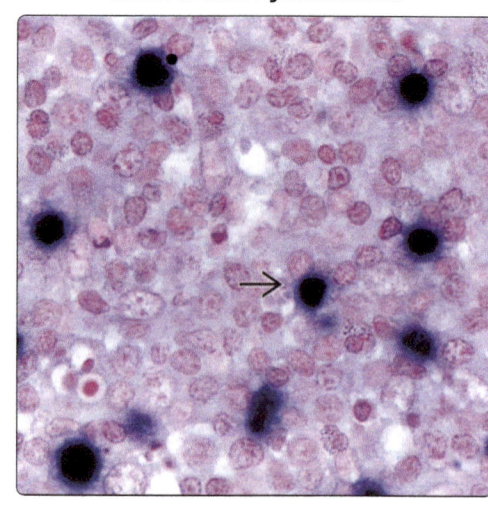

(Left) CD21 shows follicular dendritic cells (FDCs) ⇨ surrounding blood vessels in NTFHL-AI ⇨. Lymph nodes with NTFHL-AI typically show expanded and disrupted FDCs, which are often focused around high endothelial venules. **(Right)** EBER in situ hybridization is positive ⇨ in scattered cells in this case of NTFHL-AI. ~ 80-90% of lymph nodes with NTFHL-AI show EBER(+) cells, but skin lesions are often negative.

CD21 Immunohistochemistry

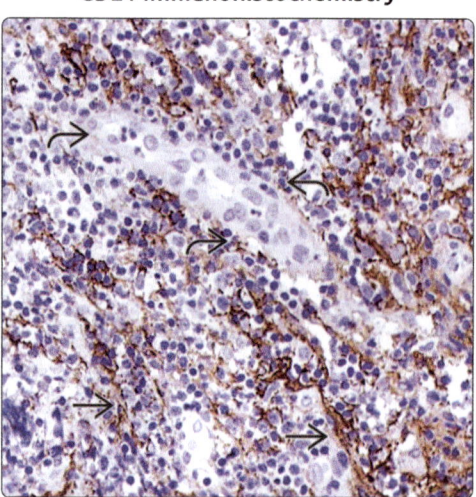

EBER In Situ Hybridization

Nodal Follicular Helper T-Cell Lymphoma

CD4 Immunohistochemistry

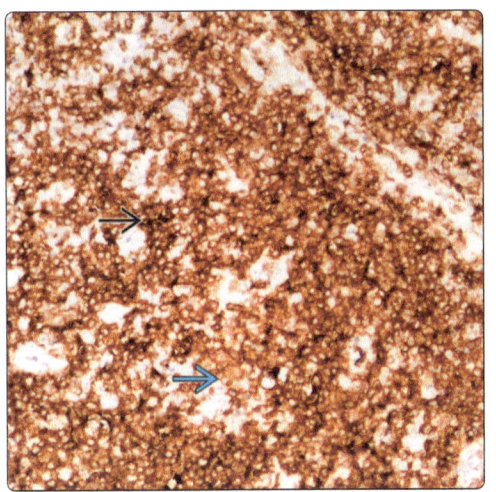

CD20 Immunohistochemistry

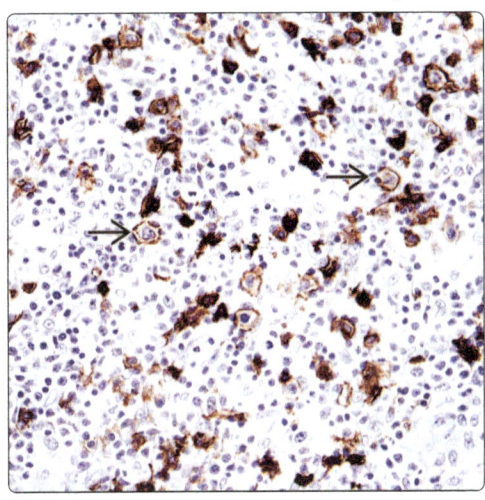

(Left) CD4(+) cells appear to be abundant in both reactive and lymphoma cells. CD4 also reacts with histiocytes, which tend to be large and very faint ➡, compared with the neoplastic CD4(+) T cells, which show dark and diffuse staining ➡. (Right) CD20 highlights scattered B cells in NTFHL-AI, including small B cells as well as B immunoblasts ➡. The number of B cells in NTFHL-AI is highly variable.

NTFHL-AI Involving Bone Marrow: CD3

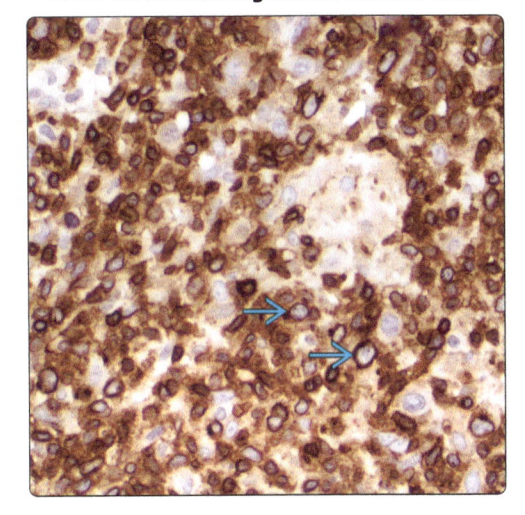

***IGH* Rearrangement**

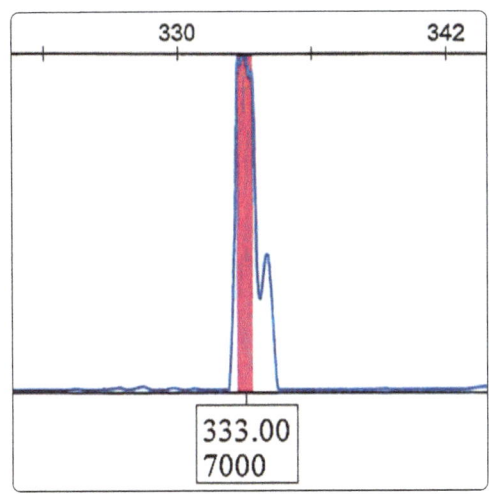

(Left) Most cells in this bone marrow infiltrate of NTFHL-AI are small to intermediate-sized lymphocytes, as highlighted by T-cell marker CD3 ➡. (Right) Dominant monoclonal peak is shown in IGH rearrangement assay by PCR in a patient with NTFHL-AI. Even though NTFHL-AI is a T-cell lymphoma, a subset of cases show clonal IGH rearrangement, which can distinguish NTFHL-AI from most other mature T-cell lymphomas.

NTFHL-AI Involving Bone Marrow

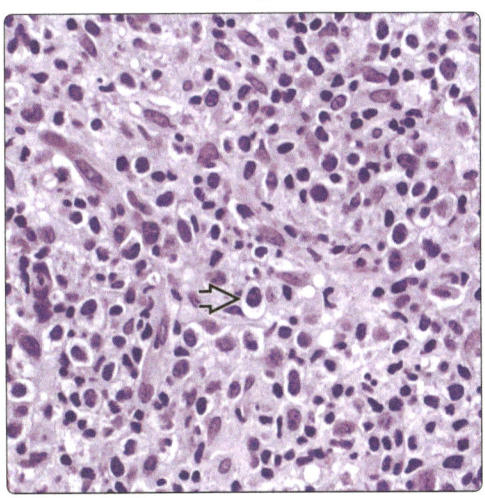

NTFHL-AI Involving Bone Marrow: PD-1

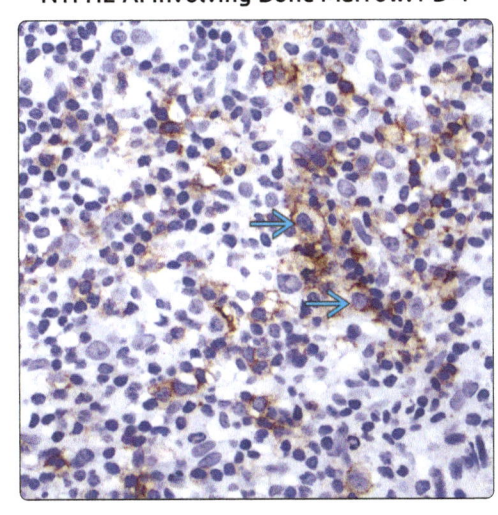

(Left) NTFHL-AI involving bone marrow often presents as a nodular infiltrate, either paratrabecular or nonparatrabecular. The cell infiltrate is polymorphic and can be subtle or show larger cells ➡. (Right) PD-1 highlights scattered intermediate-sized lymphoma cells ➡ of NTFHL-AI.

Anaplastic Large Cell Lymphoma, ALK-Negative

KEY FACTS

TERMINOLOGY
- ALK(-) anaplastic large cell lymphoma (ALCL)
  - T-cell lymphoma with uniform, bright expression of CD30 antigen
    - Morphologically indistinguishable from ALK(+) ALCL
    - Must be distinguished from primary cutaneous ALCL

ETIOLOGY/PATHOGENESIS
- Constitutive activation of JAK-STAT pathway
  - Somatic mutations of *STAT3*, *STAT5B*, and *JAK1*, *JAK3*, and *MSC*
  - Loss-of-function mutations in *SOCS1* and *SOCS2*
  - Fusion of transcription factors with tyrosine kinase genes
    - *NFKB2::ROS1*, *NCOR2::ROS1*, *NFKB2::TYK2*, *PABPC4::TYK2*
    - Leads to concomitant transcriptional and kinase activities
- Mutated genes associated with poor prognosis
  - *TP53*, *STAT3*, *EPHA5*, *JAK1*, *PRDM1*, *LRP1B*, and *KMT2D*
- *DUSP22* rearrangements in ~ 19-30% of cases
  - Defines distinct genetic subtype of ALK(-) ALCL (2022 ICC)
  - *FRA7H* is most common partner gene
- *TP63* rearrangement in ~ 8% of cases
  - *TBL1XR1* is most common partner gene
  - Associated with poor prognosis
- *JAK2* rearrangements reported in ~ 6% of cases
  - Associated with multinucleated Reed-Sternberg-like cells morphology

CLINICAL ISSUES
- Majority of cases present with stage III-IV
- Often with high International Prognostic Index
- Treatment options include
  - Cyclophosphamide, doxorubicin, vincristine, and prednisone (CHOP) is the most commonly used regimen
  - Brentuximab vedotin in relapsed disease

Hallmark Cells

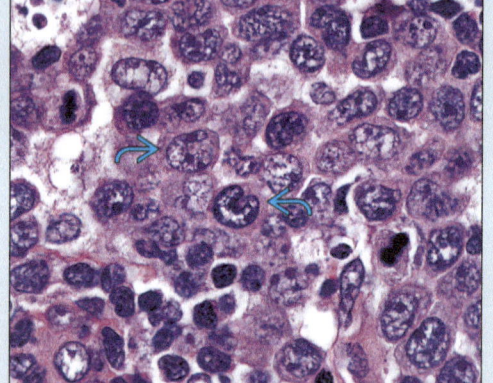

Clonal T-Cell Receptor β Gene Rearrangement

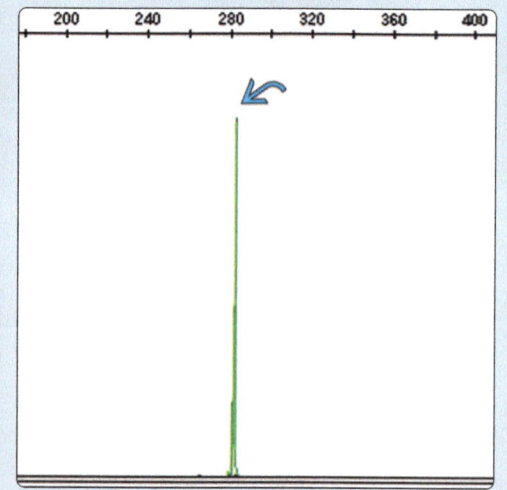

(Left) Lymph node involved by ALK(-) anaplastic large cell lymphoma (ALCL) shows large, neoplastic cells (including hallmark cells ➡) morphologically indistinguishable from ALK(+) ALCL. (Right) Electropherogram of PCR products of T-cell receptor β (TRB) gene shows a prominent peak ➡, consistent with clonal T-cell receptor β gene rearrangement in ALK(-) ALCL.

Scattered ALCL Cells

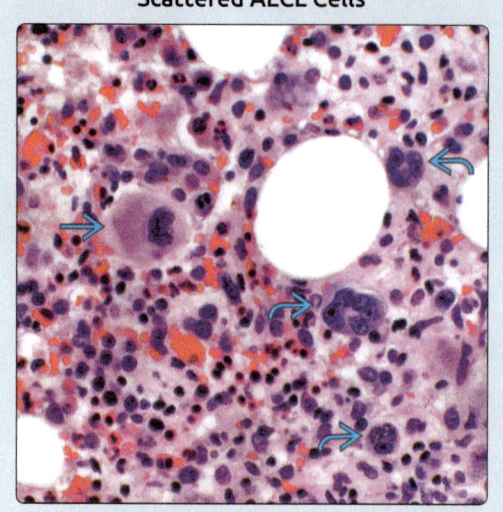

Bright CD30 Expression

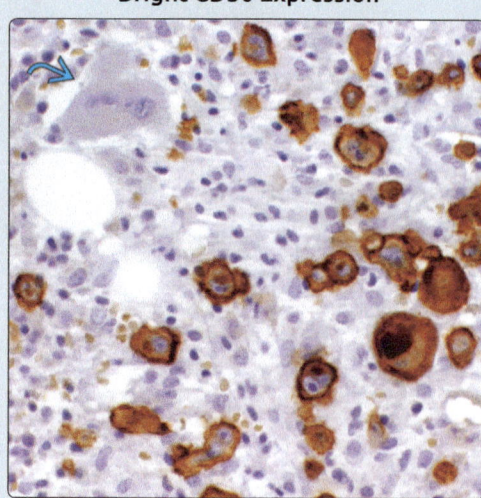

(Left) Bone marrow biopsy shows few scattered ALCL cells ➡ mimicking megakaryocytes ➡ in a patient with history of ALCL. In general, bone marrow involvement in ALCL is uncommon and can be subtle and missed on pure morphologic grounds. (Right) CD30 highlights scattered, brightly positive ALCL cells in this bone marrow core biopsy. An adjacent megakaryocyte ➡ appears negative.

Anaplastic Large Cell Lymphoma, ALK-Negative

TERMINOLOGY

Abbreviations
- Anaplastic large cell lymphoma (ALCL)
- Anaplastic lymphoma kinase (ALK)

Synonyms
- Ki-1 ALCL
  o Initial designation in 1982, not used anymore
- CD30(+) ALCL
  o Outdated terminology, not used anymore

Definitions
- Nodal/systemic ALK(-) ALCL (2022 ICC and 5th WHO classifications)
  o Remains distinct systemic entity of T-cell lymphoma
  o Morphologically indistinguishable from ALK(+) ALCL
  o Strong and uniform expression of CD30
  o By definition, lacks *ALK* rearrangements and ALK protein expression
  o Most cases express cytotoxic granules and T-cell-associated antigens
  o Must be distinguished from primary cutaneous ALCL
  o Genetic subtypes include
    – *DUSP22* rearranged, *TP63* rearranged
    – *JAK2* rearranged in subset of cases with anaplastic and Hodgkin-like morphology

ETIOLOGY/PATHOGENESIS

Molecular Pathogenesis
- Constitutive activation of JAK-STAT pathway
  o Somatic mutations of *STAT3*, *STAT5B*, and *JAK1*, *JAK3*, and *MSC*
  o Loss-of-function mutations in *SOCS1* and *SOCS2*
  o Fusion of transcription factors with tyrosine kinase genes
    – *NFKB2::ROS1*, *NCOR2::ROS1*, *NFKB2::TYK2*, *PABPC4::TYK2*
      □ Leads to concomitant transcriptional and kinase activities
  o Mutated genes associated with poor prognosis
    – *TP53*, *STAT3*, *EPHA5*, *JAK1*, *PRDM1*, *LRP1B*, and *KMT2D*
- *DUSP22* rearrangements in ~ 19-30% of cases
  o Defines distinct genetic subtype of ALK(-) ALCL (2022 ICC)
  o *FRA7H* is most common partner gene
- *TP63* rearrangement in ~ 8% of cases
  o *TBL1XR1* is most common partner gene
  o Associated with poor prognosis
- *JAK2* rearrangements reported in ~ 6% of cases
  o Associated with multinucleated Reed-Sternberg-like cells morphology
- Aberrant expression of ERBB4 truncated transcript
  o Reported in ~ 25% of cases
  o Not reported in ALK(+) ALCL
  o Mutually exclusive of *DUSP22*, *TP63*, *ROS1*, and *TYK2* rearrangements
- *DUSP22* and *TP63* rearrangements have not been reported in ALK(+) ALCL
  o May be seen in other PTCL

CLINICAL ISSUES

Epidemiology
- Incidence
  o Peak incidence in adults with median age ~ 55-60 years
  o Usually older than those with ALK(+) ALCL

Presentation
- Majority of cases present with stage III-IV with B symptoms
- Often with high International Prognostic Index (IPI)
- High lactate dehydrogenase (LDH)
- Lymph node involvement in ~ 50%
- Extranodal involvement in ~ 20%
  o Skin, soft tissue, liver, lung, and bone marrow

Treatment
- Cyclophosphamide, doxorubicin, vincristine, and prednisone (CHOP) is most commonly used regimen
- CHOP induction chemotherapy followed by autologous stem cell transplant
- Addition of other therapeutic agents
  o Addition of anti-CD52 antibody (alemtuzumab) to CHOP
  o Addition of etoposide to CHOP
    – May improve outcome in patients < 60 years of age with normal LDH level
- Investigational agents
  o Pralatrexate and romidepsin approved in relapsed or refractory disease
  o Anti-CD30 antibody (brentuximab vedotin) approved in relapsed ALCL
    – Overall response rate of > 80% in phase II study

Prognosis
- Variable
  o Related to patient's age, IPI score, and underling genetic abnormality
    – 5-year survival ~ 90% in cases with *DUSP22* rearrangements
      □ Older age, extranodal or bone marrow involvement, and high LDH may define clinically high risk in *DUSP22*-rearranged cases
    – 5-year survival ~ 20% in cases with *TP63* rearrangements
    – 5-year survival ~ 40% in cases negative for both *DUSP22* and *TP63* rearrangements
  o In general, prognosis is worse than ALK(+) ALCL

MOLECULAR

Cytogenetics
- t(6;7)(p25.3;q32.3); *DUSP22::FRA7H*
  o Originally reported in 10% of ALK(-) ALCL cases
  o Translocation results in downregulation of *DUSP22* and upregulation of microRNA29
- *TP63* rearrangements in ~ 8% of ALK(-) ALCL cases
  o *DUSP22* and *TP63* rearrangements are mutually exclusive
  o *DUSP22* or *TP63* rearrangements are not reported in ALK(+) ALCL

Anaplastic Large Cell Lymphoma, ALK-Negative

In Situ Hybridization
- FISH break-apart probes are suggested to test for detection of *DUSP22* and *TP63* rearrangements
- FISH for *JAK2* rearrangements might help in classification of cases with anaplastic and Hodgkin-like morphology

PCR
- T-cell receptor gene rearrangements
  - Clonal T-cell receptor gene rearrangements (*TRG* and *TRB*) detected in > 90% of cases

Gene Expression Profiling
- Consistent expression of *TNFSF8*, *BATF3*, and *TMOD1*
  - Gene expression signature appears distinctly different from ALK(+) ALCL and PTCL, NOS

MICROSCOPIC

Histologic Features
- Most common variant
  - Closely mimics classic variant of ALK(+) ALCL
  - Prominent nodal sinus involvement by cohesive, anaplastic-appearing cells
  - May entirely efface nodal architecture
  - Greater degree of anaplasia compared with ALK(+) ALCL in many cases
  - Hallmark cells less prominent than ALK(+) ALCL
- Nonanaplastic variants can be very difficult to recognize
  - Would overlap with CD30 expressing peripheral T-cell lymphoma, NOS
- Histologic recognition of Hodgkin-like variant can be problematic
  - Immunophenotype can overlap with classic Hodgkin lymphoma
  - T-cell antigens expression and clonal T-cell receptor gene rearrangements helpful to distinguish from classic Hodgkin lymphoma

ANCILLARY TESTS

Immunohistochemistry
- Bright and uniform expression of CD30 with membrane and paranuclear patterns
- 1 or more T-cell markers expressed in > 50% of cases
  - Aberrant T-cell antigen expression
  - CD2, CD3, CD4 are often expressed, whereas CD5 may be negative
  - CD3 is negative in many cases
  - CD8 is rarely expressed
- Granzyme-B, TIA1, and perforin expressed in ~ 50%
- CD45 can be negative
- EMA is expressed in subsets of cases
- High proliferation rate on Ki-67 stain
- CD15 can be positive in subsets of cases
- BCL2 is positive in many cases, unlike in ALK(+) ALCL
- LEF1 overexpression in *DUSP22*-rearranged cases
- By definition, ALK protein is consistently negative

DIFFERENTIAL DIAGNOSIS

ALK(+) Anaplastic Large Cell Lymphoma
- Morphologically similar to ALK(-) ALCL
- Shared immunophenotypic features
  - Strong and diffuse expression of CD30 antigen with bright membrane and Golgi pattern
  - Aberrant T-cell antigen loss
  - Expression of cytotoxic granules
- Expression of ALK protein &/or *ALK* rearrangements distinguishes ALK(+) ALCL from ALK(-) ALCL

Cutaneous Anaplastic Large Cell Lymphoma
- Similar to ALK(-) ALCL, cutaneous ALCL is typically negative for ALK expression
  - Rare cases with disease limited to skin have been documented to express ALK protein, particularly in children
- Staging is required to separate primary cutaneous ALCL from secondary involvement by systemic ALK(-) ALCL

Breast Implant-Associated Anaplastic Large Cell Lymphoma
- Definite entity in 2022 updated classifications
- Typically benign clinical course
- Distinct from systemic ALK(-) ALCL
- Presence of mass lesion and lymph node involvement are adverse prognostic features
  - Association with breast implant helps to separate from systemic ALK(-) ALCL

Peripheral T-Cell Lymphoma, Not Otherwise Specified
- Some T-cell lymphomas may express CD30 antigen
  - In contrast to ALK(-) ALCL, expression is weak and often patchy
- Hallmark cells are typically absent in PTCL, NOS

Classic Hodgkin Lymphoma
- Morphologic and immunophenotypic similarities including expression of CD30 and occasionally CD15
- CHL expresses dim PAX5, whereas ALK(-) ALCL is typically negative for PAX5
- Expression of T-cell-associated antigens and clonal T-cell gene rearrangements are helpful in distinguishing ALK(-) ALCL from CHL

Nonhematopoietic Anaplastic Tumors
- CD30 is expressed in embryonal carcinoma
- Immunohistochemistry including cytokeratins can separate metastatic tumors from ALK(-) ALCL

SELECTED REFERENCES

1. Feldman AL et al: Classification and diagnostic evaluation of nodal T- and NK-cell lymphomas. Virchows Arch. 482(1):265-79, 2023
2. Alaggio R et al: The 5th edition of the World Health Organization Classification of Haematolymphoid Tumours: Lymphoid Neoplasms. Leukemia. 36(7):1720-48, 2022
3. Campo E et al: The International Consensus Classification of Mature Lymphoid Neoplasms: a report from the Clinical Advisory Committee. Blood. 140(11):1229-53, 2022
4. Fitzpatrick MJ et al: JAK2 rearrangements are a recurrent alteration in CD30+ systemic T-cell lymphomas with anaplastic morphology. Am J Surg Pathol. 45(7):895-904, 2021
5. Pina-Oviedo S et al: ALK-negative anaplastic large cell lymphoma: current concepts and molecular pathogenesis of a heterogeneous group of large T-cell lymphomas. Cancers (Basel). 13(18):4667, 2021
6. Ravindran A et al: Striking association of lymphoid enhancing factor (LEF1) overexpression and DUSP22 rearrangements in anaplastic large cell lymphoma. Am J Surg Pathol. 45(4):550-7, 2021

Anaplastic Large Cell Lymphoma, ALK-Negative

Hallmark Cells

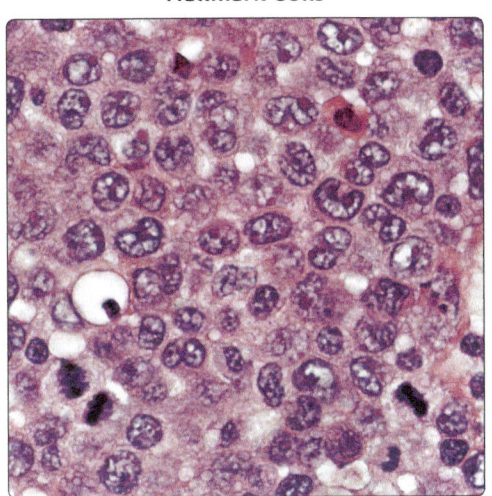

Nodal Intrasinusoidal Distribution

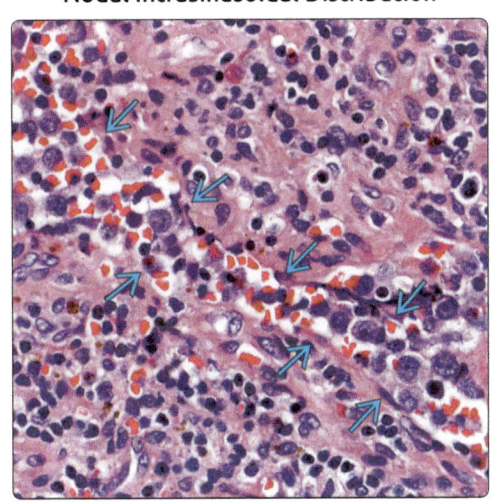

(Left) Numerous hallmark cells are present in this common variant of ALK(-) ALCL with nodal disease. Note the striking morphologic similarity with classic ALK(+) ALCL. (Right) Intrasinusoidal ➡ distribution of neoplastic cells is evident in this lymph node involved by ALK(-) ALCL. In addition to cytomorphologic similarity, the tendency toward nodal sinus distribution of tumor cells is another morphologic feature that overlaps with ALK(+) ALCL.

Bright CD3 Expression

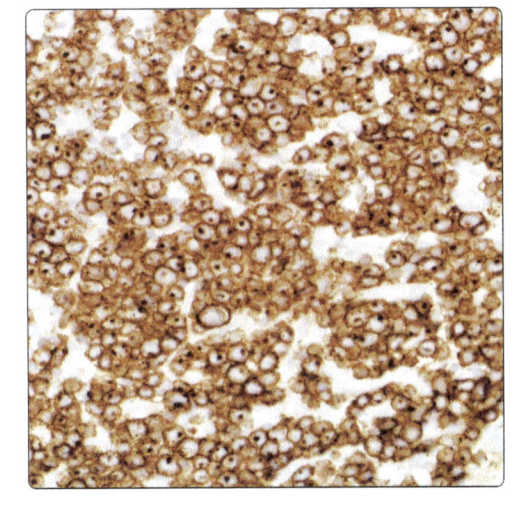

Bright and Uniform CD30 Expression

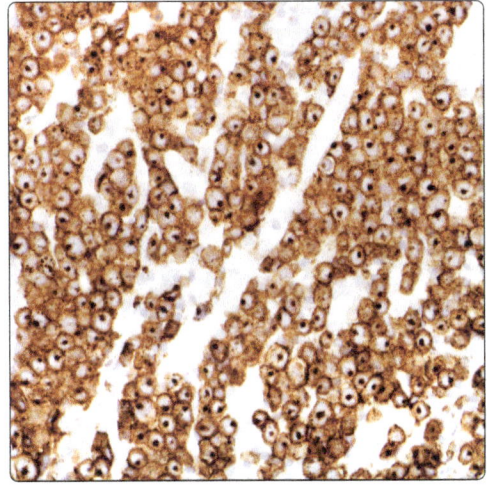

(Left) CD3 shows bright expression by neoplastic cells with prominent membrane and Golgi pattern in this case of nodal ALK(-) ALCL. However, cases often show a null phenotype with lack of CD3 expression. (Right) Bright, uniform expression of CD30 with membrane and prominent Golgi pattern is seen in this case of ALK(-) ALCL. The strong and diffuse expression of CD30 is shared with ALK(+) ALCL.

CD4 Expression

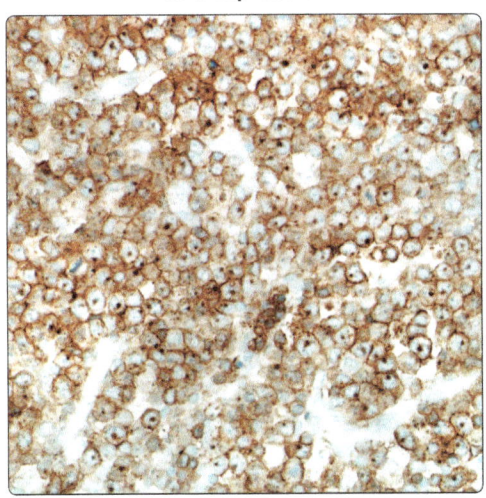

Absence of ALK Expression

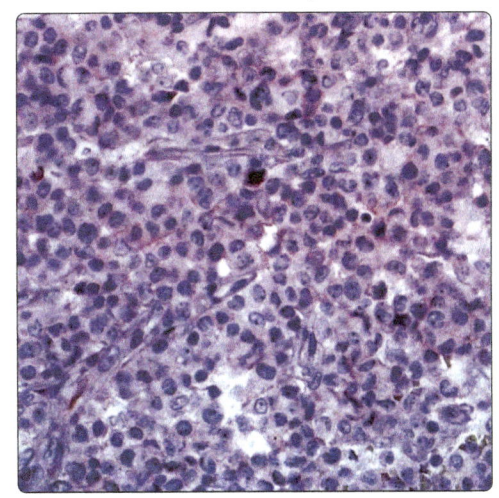

(Left) CD4 shows moderate expression by neoplastic cells in this case of ALK(-) ALCL. The majority of these cases are CD4(+). However, CD8 is also rarely expressed (not shown). (Right) ALK shows absence of expression in this case of nodal ALK(-) ALCL. Inclusion of this antibody is crucial for distinction of ALK(-) ALCL from ALK(+) ALCL.

Anaplastic Large Cell Lymphoma, ALK-Negative

ALK(+) ALCL With Morphologic Features Similar to ALK(-) ALCL

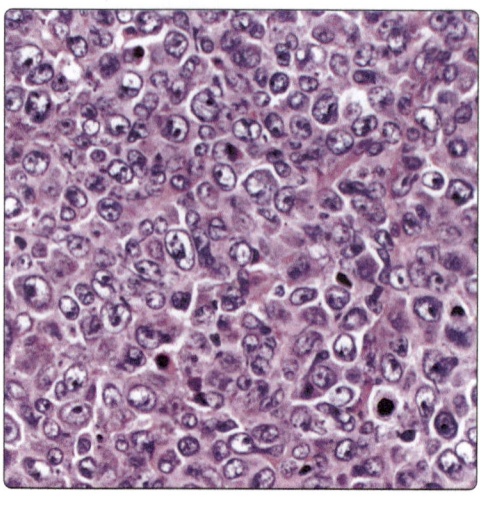

Strong and Uniform CD30 Expression in ALK(+) ALCL

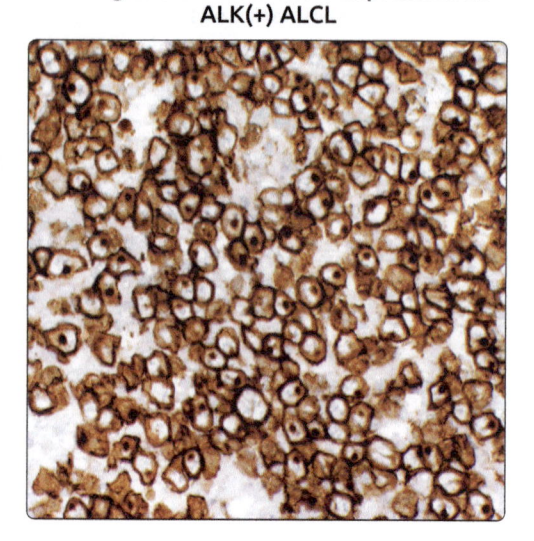

(Left) Common histologic variant of nodal ALK(+) ALCL shows cohesive sheets of anaplastic cells with scattered hallmark cells. Histomorphologic features are similar to ALK(-) ALCL. However, hallmark cells are often more prominent in ALK(+) ALCL. (Right) CD30 shows strong, uniform expression with a membrane and Golgi pattern in this case of ALK(+) ALCL, a feature similar to ALK(-) ALCL.

Subcapsular Sinus Distribution of ALCL Cells in ALK(+) ALCL

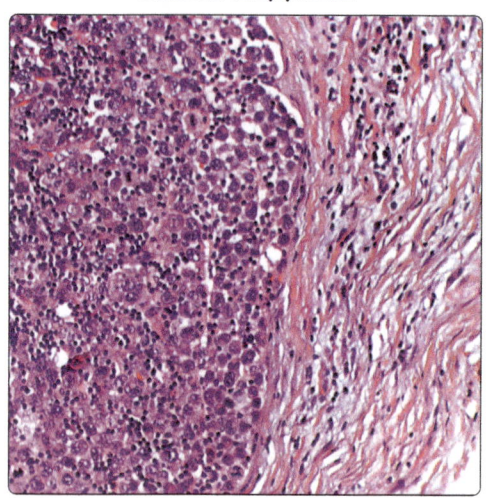

EMA Expression in ALK(+) ALCL

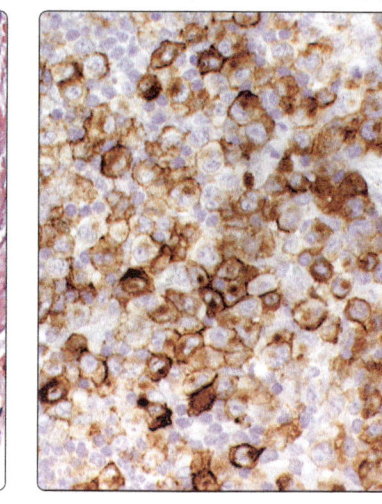

(Left) ALK(+) ALCL shows sheets of anaplastic-appearing cells in the subcapsular sinus. The sinus pattern of involvement is a common feature that is often seen in both ALK(+) and ALK(-) ALCL. (Right) EMA shows variable expression by neoplastic cells in this case of ALK(+) ALCL. Although less frequent, a subset of ALK(-) ALCL also expresses EMA.

ALK Expression in ALK(+) ALCL

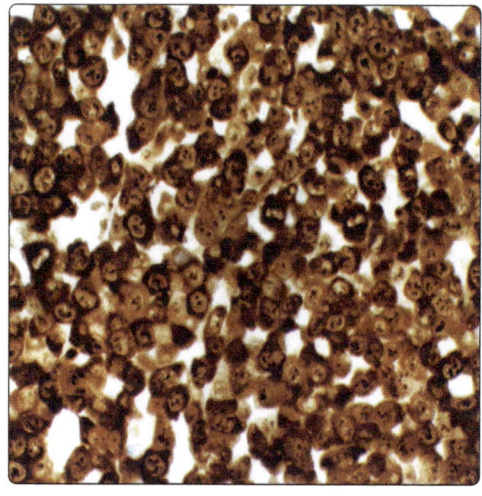

FISH Break-Apart Probe With ALK Rearrangement in ALK(+) ALCL

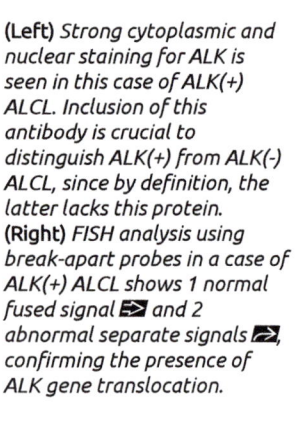

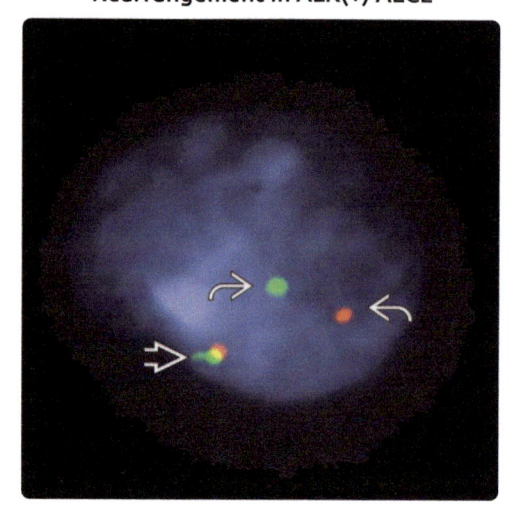

(Left) Strong cytoplasmic and nuclear staining for ALK is seen in this case of ALK(+) ALCL. Inclusion of this antibody is crucial to distinguish ALK(+) from ALK(-) ALCL, since by definition, the latter lacks this protein. (Right) FISH analysis using break-apart probes in a case of ALK(+) ALCL shows 1 normal fused signal ⇨ and 2 abnormal separate signals ⇨, confirming the presence of ALK gene translocation.

Anaplastic Large Cell Lymphoma, ALK-Negative

Classic Hodgkin Lymphoma

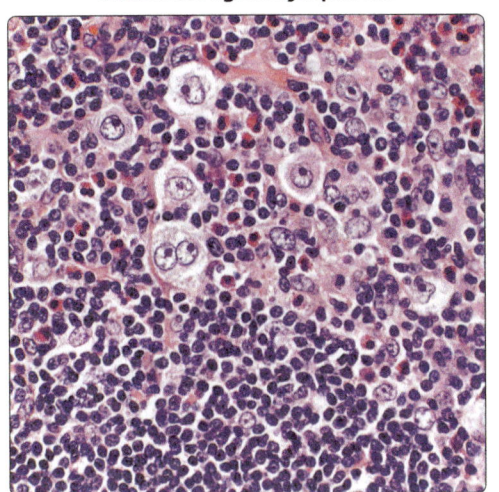

CD45(-) Reed-Sternberg and Hodgkin Cells

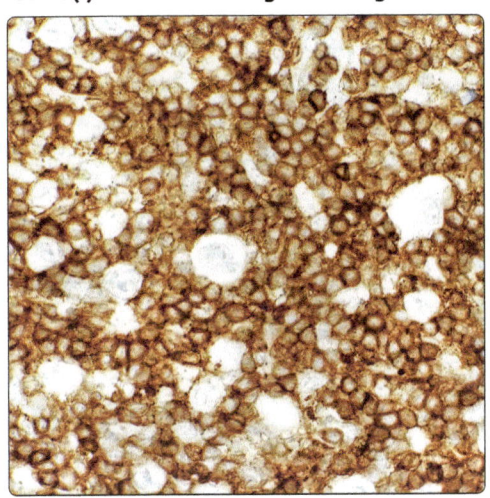

(Left) Classic Hodgkin lymphoma (CHL) shows Reed-Sternberg and Hodgkin cells in an inflammatory background. Rare cases of ALCL, including ALK(-) ones, may contain Hodgkin-like cells and lack cohesive sheets, mimicking CHL. (Right) CD45 highlights small lymphocytes rimming CD45-negative Hodgkin cells in this lymph node involved by CHL. Similarly, some case of ALCL, including ALK(-) ones, may lack CD45.

CD30(+) Reed-Sternberg and Hodgkin Cells

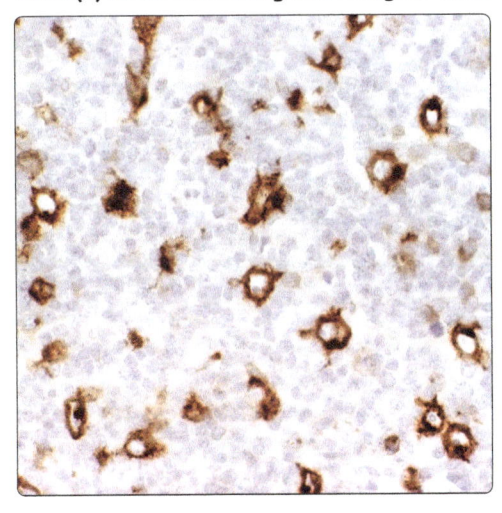

CD15 Expression in Reed-Sternberg and Hodgkin Cells

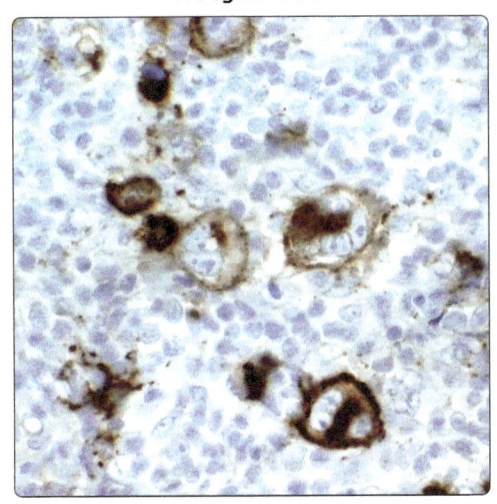

(Left) CD30 highlights Hodgkin cells in this case of nodal CHL. Expression of this antigen is shared with both ALK(+) and ALK(-) ALCL. Therefore, rare morphologic variants of ALCL, such as lymphohistiocytic variant with sparse neoplastic cells, need to be distinguished from CHL. (Right) Expression of CD15 by neoplastic cells is evident in this case of CHL. However, in addition to CHL, CD15 can also be seen in small subsets of both ALK(+) ALCL and ALK(-) ALCL.

CD30(+) and Dim Nuclear PAX5(+) Hodgkin Cells

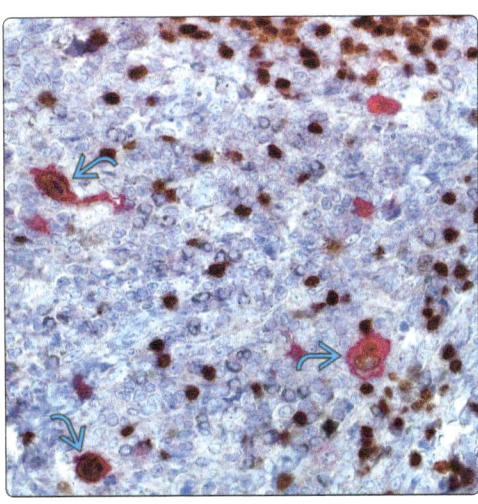

EBER(+) Reed-Sternberg and Hodgkin Cells

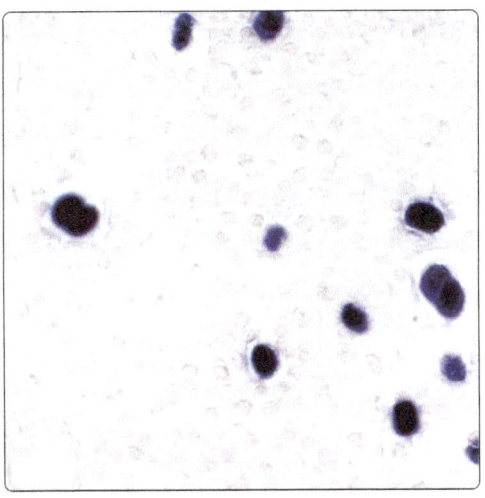

(Left) Lymph node involved by CHL shows bright membrane and paranuclear expression of CD30 (purple) and dim nuclear expression of PAX5 (brown) by Hodgkin cells ⮕. Most CHL expresses dim PAX5, whereas ALK(+) and ALK(-) ALCL are negative. (Right) In situ hybridization for EBV (EBER) highlights EBV-infected neoplastic cells in this case of CHL. ALK(-) ALCL are essentially EBER(-). However, very rare EBER(+) cases have been reported.

Anaplastic Large Cell Lymphoma, ALK-Positive

KEY FACTS

TERMINOLOGY
- ALK-positive anaplastic large cell lymphoma
  - Subtype of T-cell lymphoma composed of large lymphoid cells with kidney-shaped nuclei
  - Uniform and bright expression of CD30
  - Expression of ALK protein

ETIOLOGY/PATHOGENESIS
- Activation of ALK signaling pathway
  - Results from fusion of *ALK* with *NPM1* in majority of cases
  - Less commonly, *ALK* fuses with other partner genes
    - All *ALK* rearrangements upregulate ALK protein

CLINICAL ISSUES
- B symptoms including fever, night sweats, and weight loss
- Majority present at stage III-IV
- Lymph nodes and extranodal sites are commonly involved
  - Common extranodal sites: Skin, soft tissue, bone, lung

- Treatment
  - Anthracycline-based combination chemotherapy
  - Overall 5-year survival: ~ 80%
  - Relapses can be seen in ~ 30% of cases
  - No differences in survival between cases with classic t(2;5) and those with variant translocations

MOLECULAR
- Chromosomal translocations involving *ALK*
  - t(2;5)(p23;q35); *ALK::NPM1* is most common translocation
  - Less common translocations involve *ALK* and other partner genes
- FISH break-apart probes can detect *ALK* rearrangements
- Clonal rearrangements of T-cell receptor genes

MICROSCOPIC
- Heterogeneous with several histologic variants
- All variants contain so-called hallmark cells

Common Variant

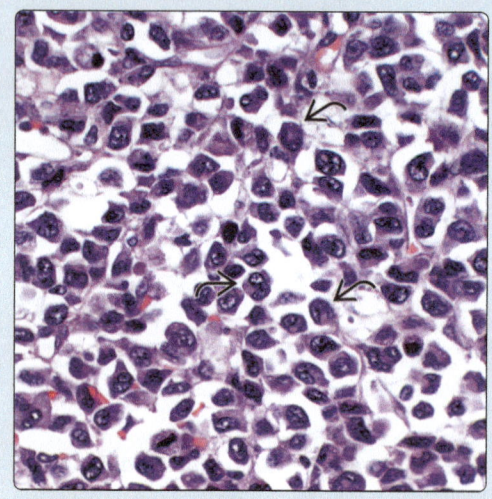

Lymphohistiocytic Variant

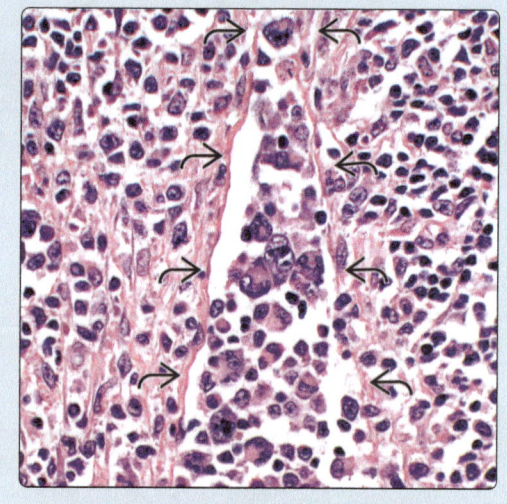

(Left) H&E shows the common variant of anaplastic large cell lymphoma (ALCL). Numerous hallmark cells with horseshoe-like nuclei ➡ are present. Immunohistochemistry showed ALK expression, supporting the diagnosis of ALK(+) ALCL. (Right) H&E shows the lymphohistiocytic variant of ALK(+) ALCL with a subtle population of anaplastic lymphoma cells within nodal sinus ➡. The lymphoma cells can be masked by abundant histiocytes.

ALK Protein Expression

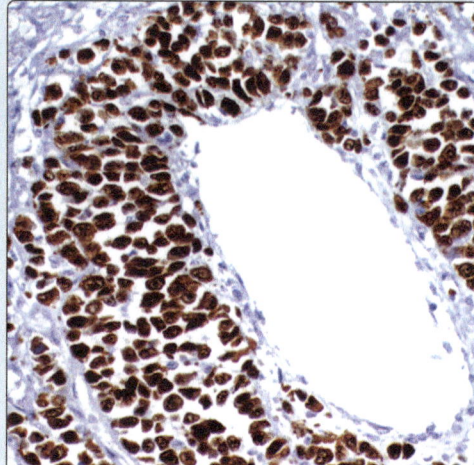

FISH Break-Apart Probe

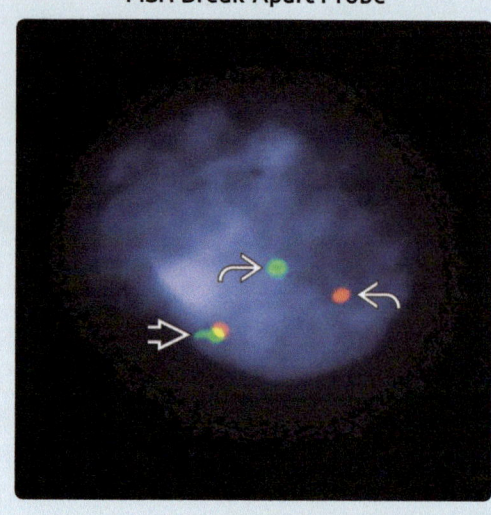

(Left) ALK shows strong nuclear and cytoplasmic expression in this case of ALK(+) ALCL with perivascular accumulation of tumor cells. The staining pattern of ALK suggests ALK::NPM1 rearrangement. (Right) FISH analysis using break-apart probes performed on a lymph node with ALK(+) ALCL reveals 1 normal fused signal ➡ and 2 abnormal separate signals ➡, confirming ALK rearrangement.

Anaplastic Large Cell Lymphoma, ALK-Positive

TERMINOLOGY

Abbreviations
- Anaplastic large cell lymphoma (ALCL)
- Anaplastic lymphoma kinase (ALK)

Synonyms
- Ki-1 ALCL
  - Initial designation in 1982, not used anymore
- CD30(+) ALCL
  - Outdated terminology, not used anymore

Definitions
- Distinct subtype of T-cell lymphoma that has T-cell or null cell phenotype, uniform and bright expression of CD30, and expression of ALK protein

ETIOLOGY/PATHOGENESIS

Molecular Pathogenesis
- Activation of ALK signaling pathway
  - Results from rearrangements of ALK with 1 of several fusion partners
  - ALK::NPM1 in 70-80% of cases
    - ALK fusion with other partner genes in remaining cases
  - All ALK rearrangements upregulate ALK protein
    - ALK protein overexpression results in activation of JAK3/STAT3, PI3K, and RAS/ERK1 signaling pathways
- Distinct molecular signature as determined by gene expression profiling
- Recurrent NOTCH1 mutations, particularly T349P variant

CLINICAL ISSUES

Epidemiology
- Incidence
  - More common in children and adolescents
    - Accounts for 10-15% of childhood lymphomas
    - Accounts for ~ 2% of adult non-Hodgkin lymphomas

Presentation
- B symptoms including fever, night sweats, and weight loss
- Majority of patients present at stage III-IV
  - Peripheral and abdominal lymph nodes involvement
  - Extranodal involvement in 1/3 of cases
    - Includes skin, soft tissue, bone, and lung
  - Blood involvement in subset of small cell variant
  - Bone marrow involvement is uncommon and can be subtle
  - Hemophagocytic lymphohistiocytosis can be seen

Treatment
- Anthracycline-based combination chemotherapy (CHOP) ± etoposide
- Overall response rate ~ 90%
- Relapses can be seen in ~ 30% of cases
  - Usually remains sensitive to chemotherapy
  - Autologous stem cell transplantation
- Treatment of patients with refractory disease
  - Clinical trials using small molecule ALK inhibitors
    - Mutations in ALK kinase domain may emerge that could confer resistance to ALK inhibitor therapy
  - Anti-CD30 (brentuximab vedotin)
  - Allogeneic stem cell transplantation

Prognosis
- Overall 5-year survival: ~ 80%
- No differences in survival between cases with classic t(2;5) and those with variant translocations
- Less favorable prognosis in small cell variant mainly due to disseminated disease at presentation

MOLECULAR

ALK
- Encodes tyrosine kinase receptor that belongs to insulin receptor superfamily
  - Located on short arm of chromosome 2 at p23
  - Originally identified by cloning of ALK::NPM1 fusion gene in case of ALCL

ALK Fusions
- ALK fusions are implicated to be oncogenic
  - NPM1 is most common ALK fusion gene partner in ALK(+) ALCL
- ALK fusion proteins lead to aberrant activation of downstream signaling cascades

Gene Expression Profiling
- Distinct molecular signature as determined by gene expression profiling
  - ALK, BCL6, PTPN12, CEBPB, SERPINA1, and GAS1 significantly overexpressed in ALK(+) ALCL
  - Other reported overexpressed genes
    - TNFRSF8 (CD30), MUC1, GZMB, and PRF1

Cytogenetics
- Chromosomal translocations involving ALK on 2p23
  - t(2;5)(p23;q35); ALK::NPM1 in ~ 75%
  - t(1;2)(q21;p23); TPM3::ALK in ~ 15%
  - t(2;3)(p23;q12); ALK::TFG in ~ 2%
  - t(2;17)(p23;q23); ALK::CLTC in ~ 1%
  - t(2;17)(p23;q25); ALK::RNF213 in ~ 1%
  - t(2;19)(p23;p13); ALK::TPM4 in ~ 1%
  - t(2;22)(p23;q12); ALK::MYH9 in ~ 2%
  - t(x;2)(q12;p23); MSN::ALK in ~ 1%
  - inv(2)(p23q35); ALK::ATIC in ~ 2%
- ALK rearrangements result in upregulation of ALK
  - Constitutive activation of ALK pathway
  - Overexpression of ALK protein

In Situ Hybridization
- FISH using break-apart probes
  - Detects all ALK fusions with various partner genes
  - Cannot determine partner gene fused with ALK
- FISH using targeted probes
  - Targeted probes are used to detect common t(2;5)
  - Not useful for screening of ALK rearrangements

PCR
- Clonal rearrangements of T-cell receptor γ (TRG) and β (TRB) genes detected in > 90% of cases

Anaplastic Large Cell Lymphoma, ALK-Positive

- T-cell receptor clonality is detected in both T-cell and null cell immunophenotype
- RT-PCR for *ALK::NPM1* fusion gene products
  - Can be useful for minimal residual disease detection in cases with *ALK-NPM1* rearrangement
  - Limited clinical utility

Chromosomal Microarray
- Chromosomal imbalances detectable in ~ 60% of cases
  - Gain of 17p that includes gain of *TP53*
  - Gain of 17q24 region to terminal end of long arm (17q24-qter)
  - Loss of 4q13-q21
  - Loss of 11q14 that may include loss of *ATM*

MICROSCOPIC

Histologic Features
- Heterogeneous with several histologic variants
- All variants contain variable numbers of hallmark cells
  - Large cells with kidney-shaped, horseshoe-like, or embryo-shaped nuclei
- Common (classic) variant
  - Accounts for majority of cases
  - Cohesive sheets of large cells with frequent hallmark cells
  - Predominant sinusoidal distribution in lymph nodes with partial involvement
    - Can mimic nonhematopoietic metastatic neoplasms
- Small cell variant
  - Effacement of lymph node architecture
    - Diffuse infiltrate of small, medium, and large cells
    - Low-power appearance of lymph node may resemble reactive or inflammatory process
    - Minor population of hallmark cells can be detected in nodal sinuses and around vessels on careful examination
    - Increased macrophages with erythrophagocytosis
  - Leukemic presentation more common than in other variants
    - Circulating lymphoma cells are typically found at feather edge of blood smear
    - Bone marrow involvement is typically very subtle
  - Cerebrospinal and pleural fluid involvement have been reported
- Lymphohistiocytic variant
  - Neoplastic cells admixed with abundant reactive histiocytes that may mask neoplastic cells
  - Often misdiagnosed as peripheral T-cell lymphoma, NOS
  - Perivascular clusters of hallmark cells are typically present
- Hodgkin-like variant
  - Nodules with sparse or sheets of neoplastic cells separated by thick sclerotic bands
  - Occasional Reed-Sternberg and Hodgkin-like cells
    - Mimics nodular sclerosis classic Hodgkin lymphoma
  - Intrasinusoidal accumulation of neoplastic cells often present
- Sarcomatoid variant
  - Storiform growth pattern with spindled tumor cells
- Monomorphic variant
  - Monomorphous intermediate to large tumor cells
  - Difficult to diagnose in absence of CD30 &/or ALK immunohistochemical stains

ANCILLARY TESTS

Immunohistochemistry
- CD30 strongly and uniformly expressed with membranous and Golgi pattern in all cases
  - Patterns of ALK expression cytoplasmic or membranous in cases with variant translocation
    - Nuclear and cytoplasmic in cases with *ALK::NPM1*
    - Nuclear only in small cell variants; cytoplasmic or membranous in cases with variant translocation
- ≥ 1 T-cell antigens expressed in most cases
  - ~ 70% of cases express CD2, CD4, and CD5
  - Rare cases express CD8
  - TIA1, granzyme B, &/or perforin expressed in most cases
- CD45 variably expressed but can be negative
- CD43 expressed in vast majority of cases
- EMA expressed in most cases
- Rare cases may express CD15
- EBV consistently negative in all cases

DIFFERENTIAL DIAGNOSIS

ALK-Positive Large B-Cell Lymphoma
- Sinusoidal pattern of nodal distribution similar to ALCL
- Strong expression of EMA and CD138
- Lack of CD30 and ALK expression

ALK-Negative ALCL
- Morphologic features similar to ALK(+) ALCL
- Strong expression of CD30 similar to ALK(+) ALCL
- Lack of ALK protein expression

Classic Hodgkin Lymphoma
- Morphologic similarity in particular with Hodgkin-like variant of ALK(+) ALCL
- Expression of CD30 similar to ALK(+) ALCL
- EBV(+) in 40-50% of cases
- Expression of CD15 and dim PAX5 and lack of ALK protein &/or *ALK* rearrangements

Peripheral T-Cell Lymphoma With CD30(+) Cells
- Expression of CD30 is typically variable in PTCL, NOS
- ALK is negative in PTCL, NOS

Primary Cutaneous ALCL
- EMA and ALK are typically negative

Nonhematopoietic Neoplasms
- Immunohistochemistry can easily separate metastatic tumors from ALK(+) ALCL

SELECTED REFERENCES
1. Feldman AL et al: Classification and diagnostic evaluation of nodal T- and NK-cell lymphomas. Virchows Arch. 482(1):265-79, 2023
2. Alaggio R et al: The 5th edition of the World Health Organization Classification of Haematolymphoid Tumours: Lymphoid Neoplasms. Leukemia. 36(7):1720-48, 2022
3. Campo E et al: The International Consensus Classification of Mature Lymphoid Neoplasms: a report from the Clinical Advisory Committee. Blood. 140(11):1229-53, 2022
4. Kaseb H et al: Anaplastic large cell lymphoma. StatPearls, 2022

Anaplastic Large Cell Lymphoma, ALK-Positive

Small Cell Variant

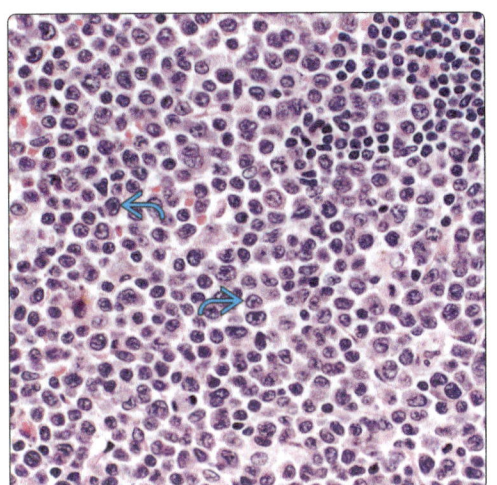

Hodgkin-Like Variant

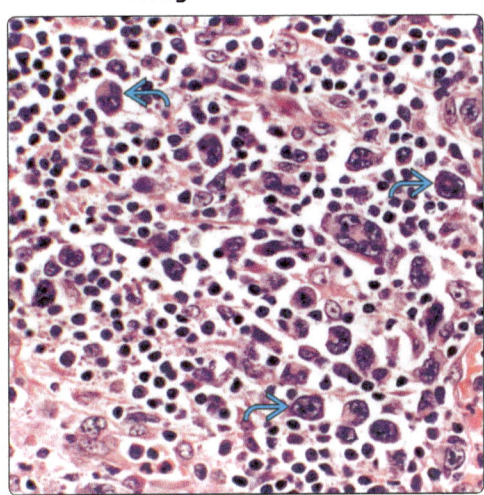

(Left) H&E shows effaced lymph node from a child with disseminated small cell variant of ALK(+) ALCL. There are sheets of relatively uniform and monotonous lymphoma cells. The neoplastic cells are predominantly small to medium-sized with frequent kidney-shaped nuclei ⮕. *(Right)* H&E shows Hodgkin-like variant of ALK(+) ALCL with a highly polymorphous population and occasional hallmark cells ⮕.

Intrasinusoidal ALK(+) ALCL

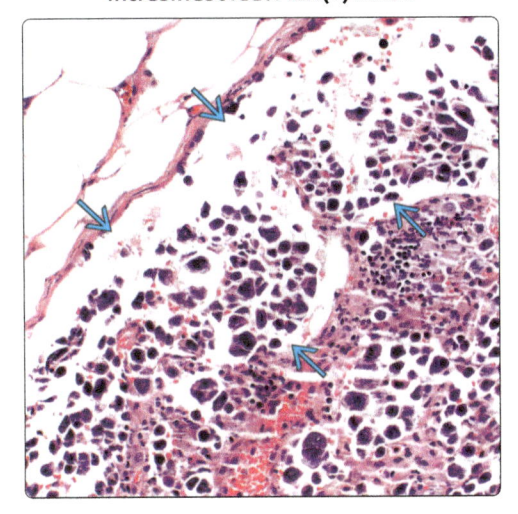

Large Tumor Cells

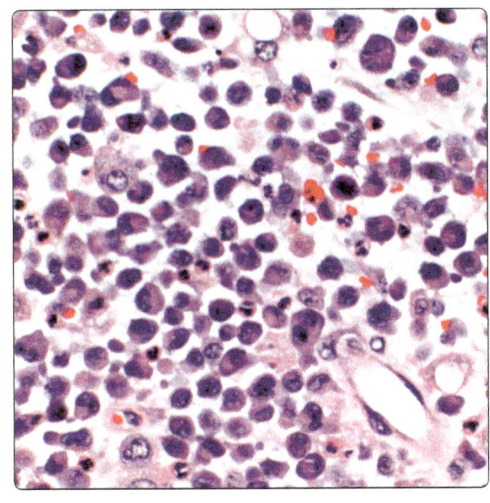

(Left) H&E shows highly polymorphous, anaplastic-appearing large cells with lobulated, hyperchromatic nuclei within subcortical sinuses ⮕, mimicking metastatic tumor of nonhematopoietic origin. The tumor cells strongly expressed CD30 and ALK, confirming the diagnosis of ALK(+) ALCL. *(Right)* H&E shows ALK(+) ALCL with a uniform population of large tumor cells in a loose stroma with scattered background neutrophils.

Circulating Tumor Cells

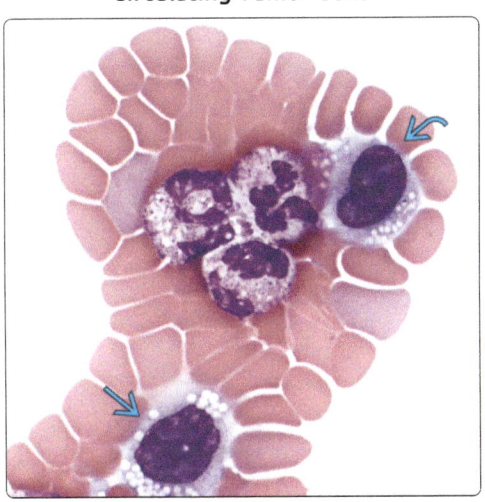

T-Cell Receptor γ Gene Rearrangement

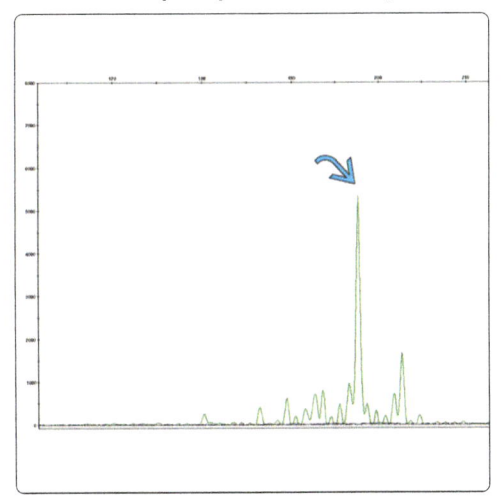

(Left) Peripheral blood smear from a child with disseminated ALK(+) ALCL shows 2 circulating lymphoma cells with kidney-shaped ⮕ and grooved nuclei ⮕ and cytoplasmic vacuoles. *(Right)* Capillary electrophoresis of PCR products of T-cell receptor γ gene performed on DNA extracted from the blood of a patient with circulating ALCL cells shows a prominent peak ⮕ of 198 base-pair in size, confirming the clonal nature of the circulating ALCL cells.

Anaplastic Large Cell Lymphoma, ALK-Positive

Bone Marrow Involvement

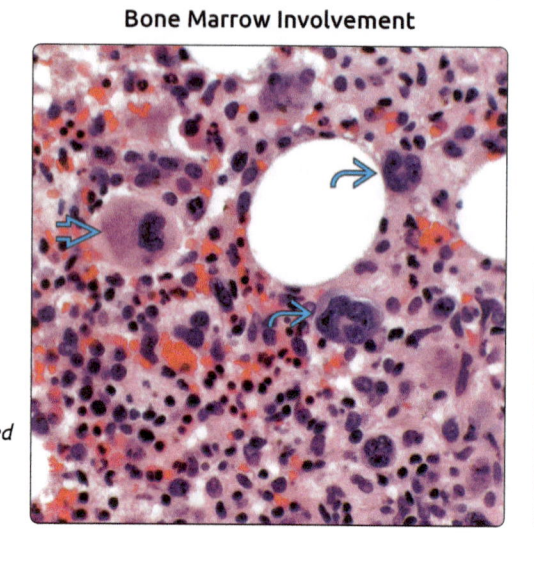

CD3(+) Cells

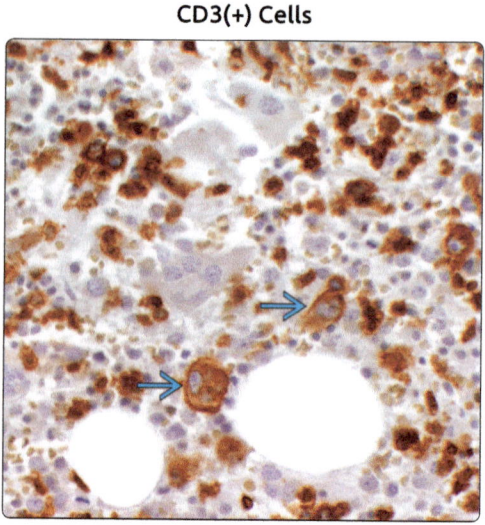

(Left) H&E of bone marrow core biopsy from a patient with systemic ALK(+) ALCL shows a subtle infiltrate of singly distributed, multinucleated lymphoma cells ⇨ that mimic megakaryocytes ➡. (Right) CD3 of bone marrow core biopsy from a patient with systemic ALK(+) ALCL highlights occasional large, multinucleated cells ➡, confirming the T-lineage nature of the cells. The lymphoma cells also expressed ALK protein.

Intrasinusoidal Bright CD30(+) Cells

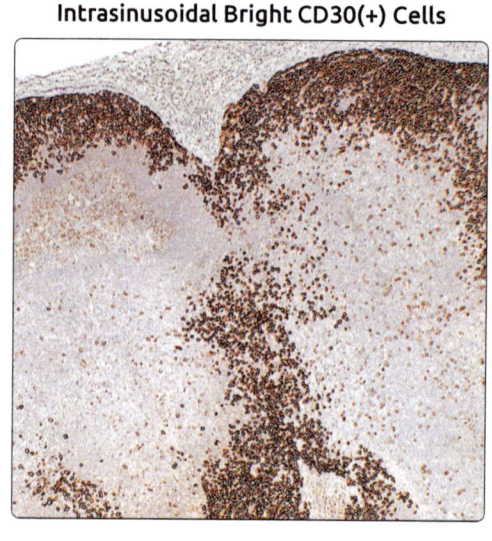

Bright and Uniform CD30(+) With Golgi and Membranous Pattern

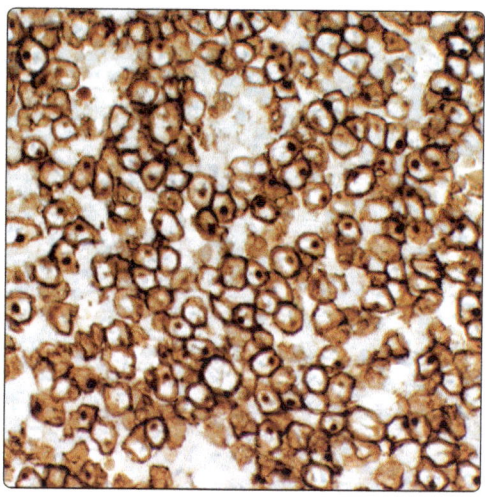

(Left) CD30 highlights numerous positive cells with sinusoidal distribution in this lymph node involved by ALK(+) ALCL. (Right) CD30 shows bright expression by sheets of large lymphoma cells in this lymph node involved by ALK(+) ALCL. Note the bright membranous and Golgi pattern.

CD43(+) Cells

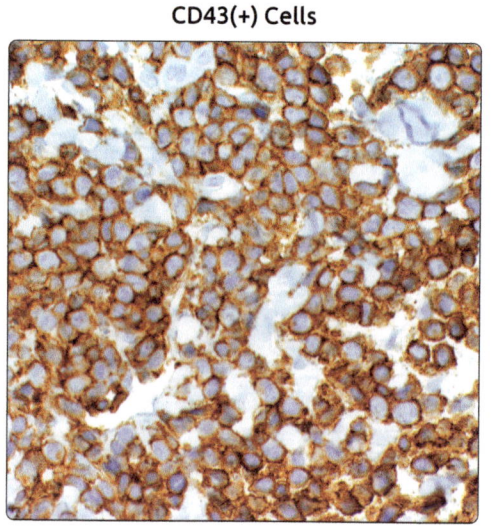

Strong Expression of ALK

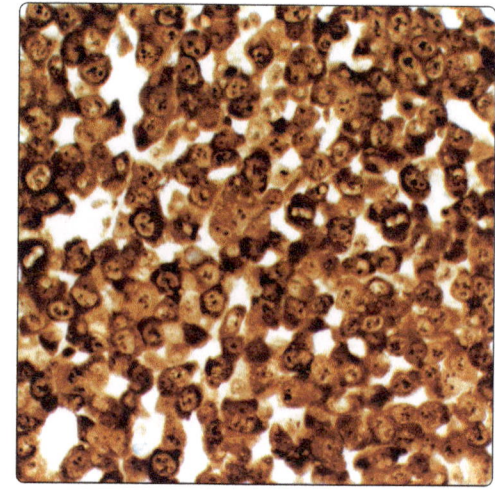

(Left) CD43 of lymph node from a patient with ALK(+) ALCL shows expression of this nonlineage antigen by neoplastic cells. The cells were negative for T-cell associated antigen, consistent with a null cell phenotype, but were positive for clonal T-cell receptor γ gene rearrangement. (Right) ALK shows expression in a membranous and nuclear pattern corresponding to a t(2;5) translocation.

Anaplastic Large Cell Lymphoma, ALK-Positive

Diffuse Large B-Cell Lymphoma With Anaplastic Morphology

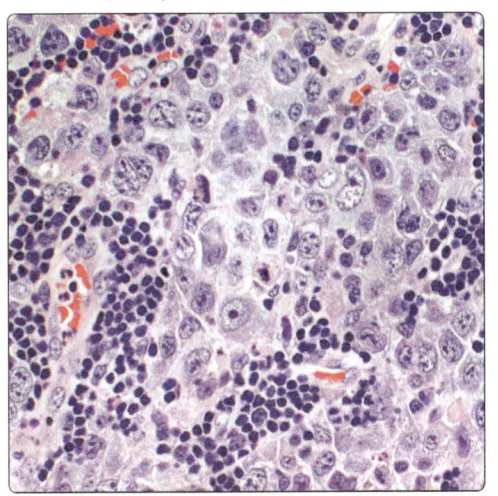

CD30 Expression in Anaplastic Variant of Diffuse Large B-Cell Lymphoma

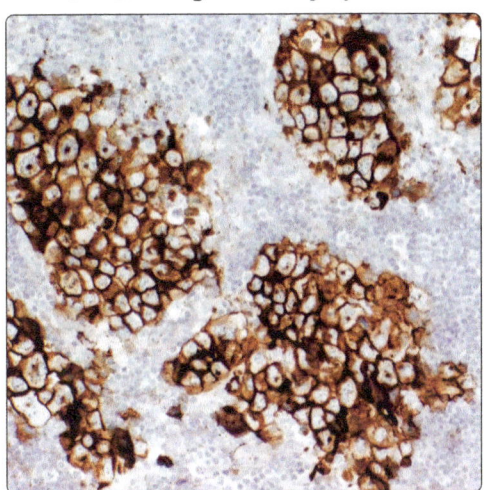

(Left) H&E of lymph node from a patient with anaplastic variant of diffuse large B-cell lymphoma shows cohesive aggregates of anaplastic-appearing large cells in interfollicular regions, mimicking ALCL. *(Right)* CD30 of lymph node from a patient with anaplastic variant of diffuse large B-cell lymphoma shows strong membranous and Golgi patterns of staining of intrasinusoidal anaplastic-appearing large B cells.

Classic Hodgkin Lymphoma

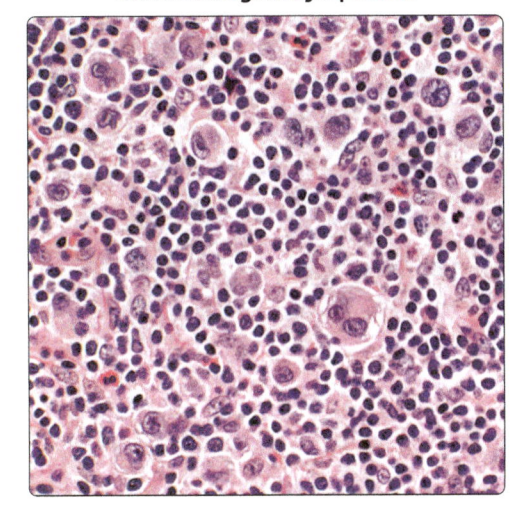

CD45(-) Reed-Sternberg and Hodgkin Cells

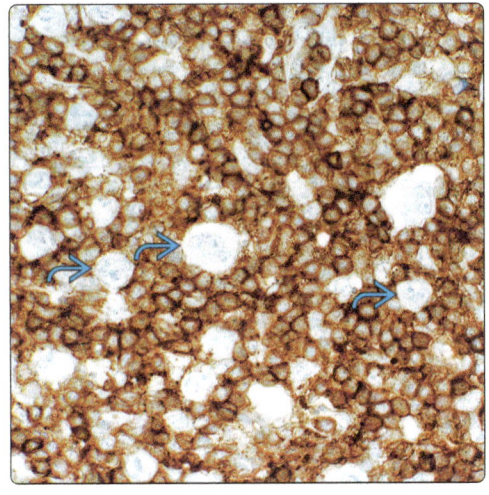

(Left) H&E of lymph node from a young patient with classic Hodgkin lymphoma shows Reed-Sternberg and Hodgkin-like cells as well as occasional hallmark-like cells in an inflammatory background. The cells expressed CD30, CD15, and EBER, confirming the diagnosis. *(Right)* CD45 shows lack of this antigen ➡ on Reed-Sternberg and Hodgkin-like cells. CD45 can also be negative in a subset of ALK(+) ALCL.

CD30(+) Reed-Sternberg and Hodgkin Cells in Classic Hodgkin Lymphoma

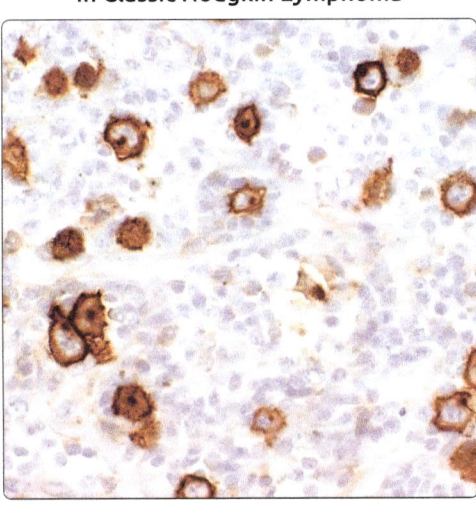

EBER(+) Reed-Sternberg and Hodgkin Cells in Classic Hodgkin Lymphoma

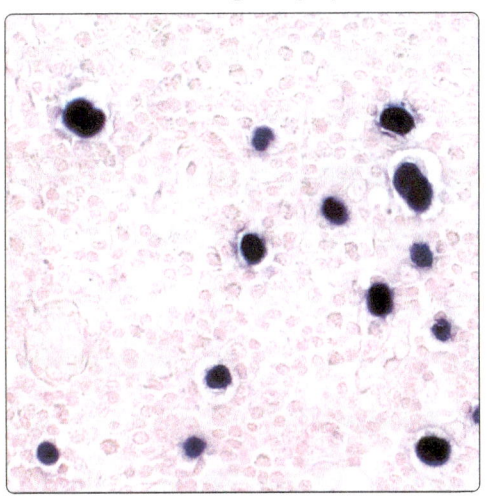

(Left) CD30 highlights bright expression by neoplastic cells in a case of classic Hodgkin lymphoma. The Hodgkin-like cells were also positive for CD15 and negative for CD45. Similar immunophenotypic profile may occasionally be seen in ALCL as well. *(Right)* ISH for EBV shows abundant expression of EBV-encoded mRNA (EBER) by Hodgkin cells in this case of classic Hodgkin lymphoma. EBER is consistently negative in ALCL.

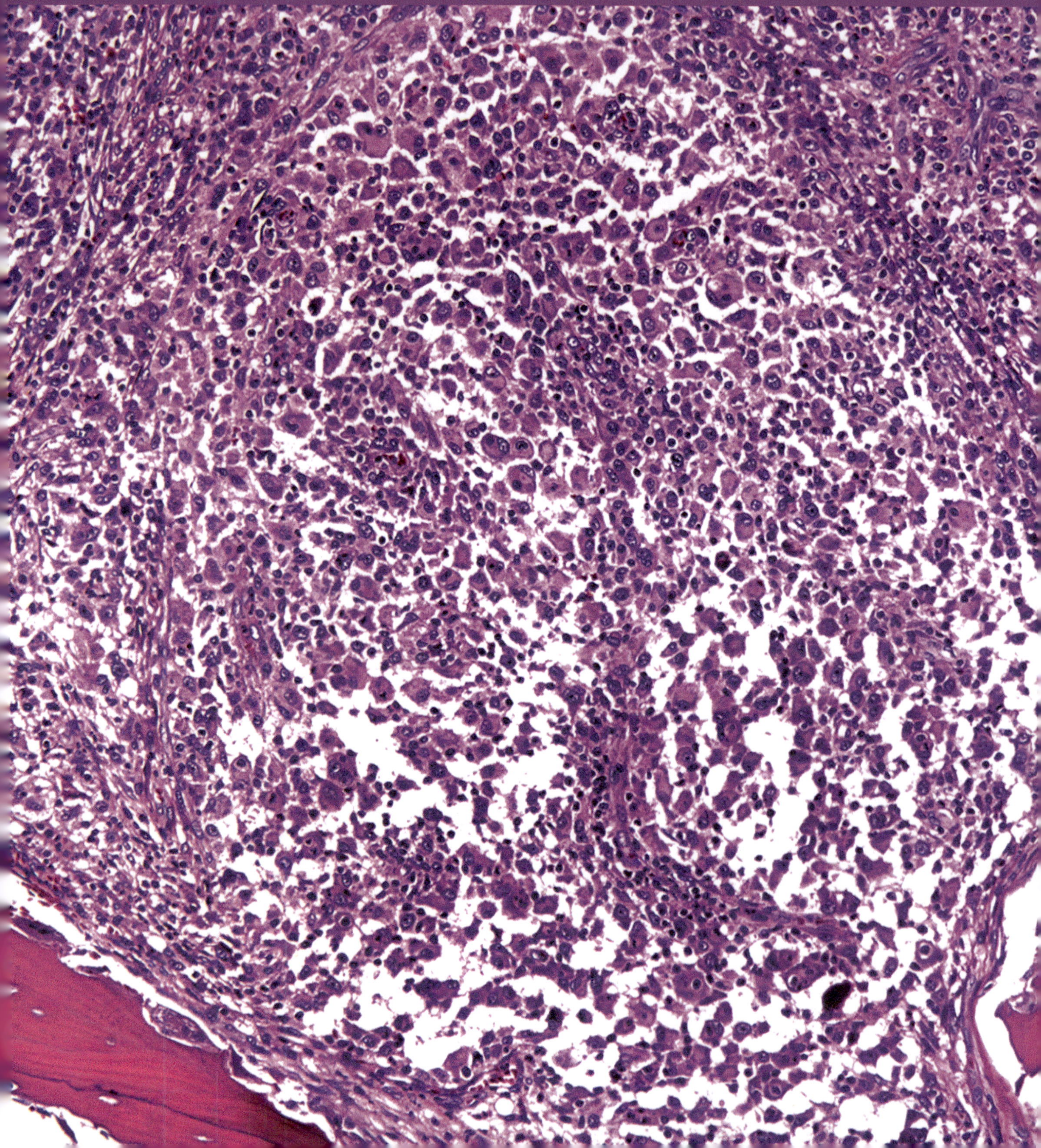

SECTION 7
Molecular Pathology of Dendritic Cell and Histiocytic Neoplasms

Histiocytic Sarcoma	470
Langerhans Cell Histiocytosis	478
Interdigitating Dendritic Cell Sarcoma	484
Follicular Dendritic Cell Sarcoma	488

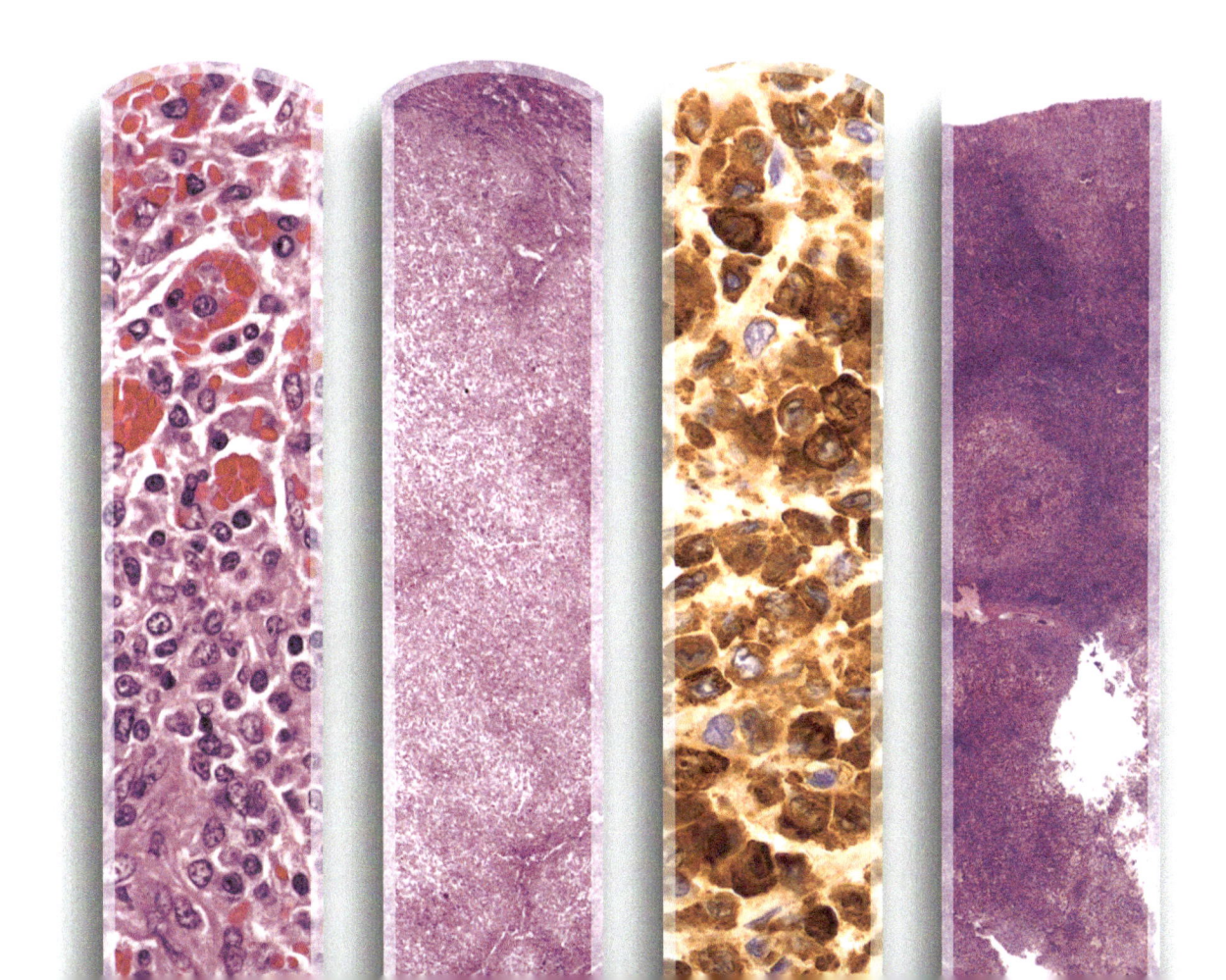

Histiocytic Sarcoma

KEY FACTS

ETIOLOGY/PATHOGENESIS
- Neoplasm consisting of mature malignant histiocytes
- Etiology from pluripotent stem cells and transdifferentiation from prior hematopoietic neoplasm

CLINICAL ISSUES
- Variable presentation, usually extranodal
- Surgical excision can be curable if isolated lesion
- Aggressive if disseminated

MACROSCOPIC
- Mass lesion with variable hemorrhage and necrosis

MOLECULAR
- Recurrent mutations of genes in Ras/Raf/MEK/ERK signaling pathway
  - Mutations in *BRAF* V600E (60% of cases)
- Subset shows mutations in *KMT2D* and *ARID1A*; activating mutations in *CSF1R* and additional receptor tyrosine kinases
- *IGH*, *TRB*, or *TRG* may be clonal with identical clone to one detected in associated lymphoma

MICROSCOPIC
- Spectrum of cytomorphology ranging from bland to overtly malignant cells
- Necrosis and erythrophagocytosis common

ANCILLARY TESTS
- Immunohistochemistry
  - CD45(+/-), CD163(+), CD68(+), CD4(+), lysozyme (+), S100(-/+)
  - CD1a(-), langerin (-), CD21(-), CD35(-)

TOP DIFFERENTIAL DIAGNOSES
- Diffuse large B-cell lymphoma
- Myeloid sarcoma
- Langerhans cell and dendritic cell neoplasms
- Hemophagocytic lymphohistiocytosis
- T-cell lymphoma

Sheets of Large Polygonal Cells

(Left) Histiocytic sarcoma (HS) of the palate shows dyscohesive sheets of large, polygonal cells ➡. The malignant cells are invading bone ➡. (Right) This case of HS is characterized by large, neoplastic cells with foamy cytoplasm and prominent hemophagocytosis ➡. Cells often show atypia ➡ but can also be bland in appearance.

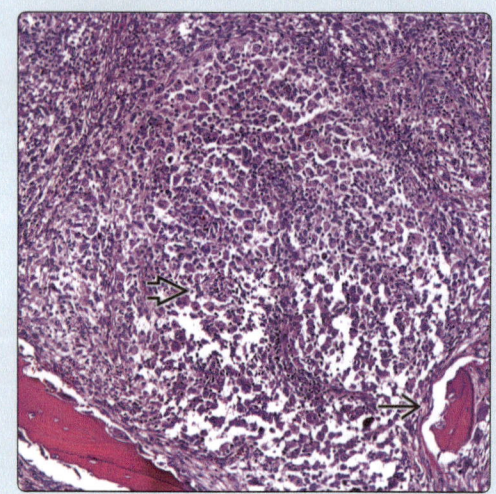

Foamy Cytoplasm and Prominent Hemophagocytosis

Grainy Cytoplasm

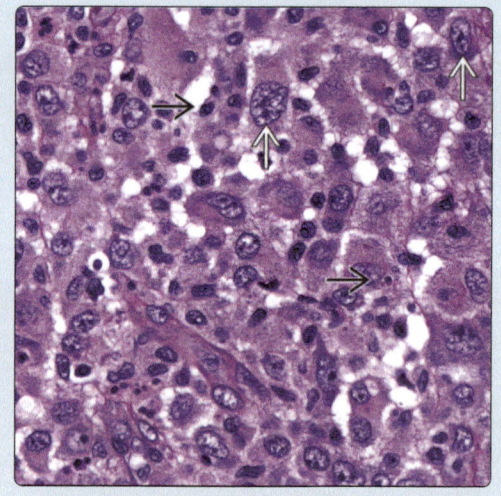

(Left) Lymph node tissue taken at autopsy shows widespread involvement by HS. The cells are relatively bland but have grainy cytoplasm and irregular nuclei ➡. (Right) CD68 shows positive cytoplasmic staining ➡. Other positive markers included CD163, lysozyme, and S100 (not shown).

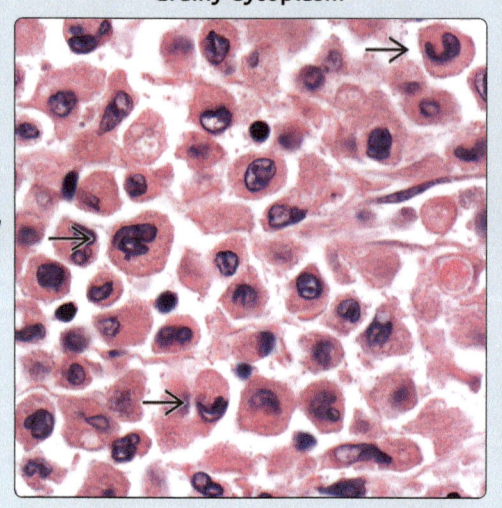

CD68 Immunohistochemistry

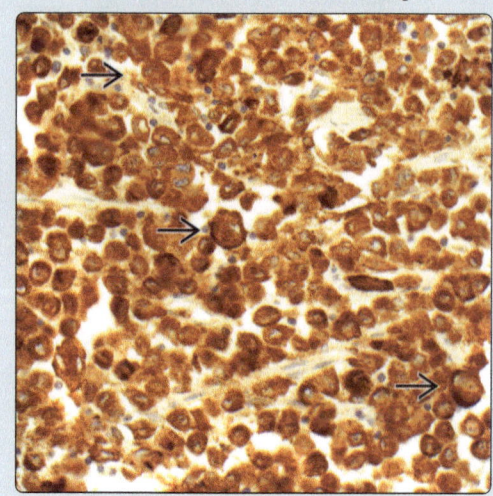

Histiocytic Sarcoma

TERMINOLOGY

Abbreviations
- Histiocytic sarcoma (HS)

Synonyms
- Malignant histiocytosis
- True histiocytic lymphoma

Definitions
- Malignant proliferation of cells with morphologic and immunophenotypic features of mature tissue histiocytes

ETIOLOGY/PATHOGENESIS

Pathogenesis
- De novo HS
  - Derived from hematopoietic stem/progenitor cells
  - Association with mediastinal germ cell tumor suggests common pluripotent germ cell
  - Association with hematopoietic neoplasms suggests common hematopoietic stem cell
- May arise from previous lymphoma, leukemia, or myelodysplasia, and may be clonally related
  - 2 theories: Transdifferentiation and lineage reprogramming
    - Direct transdifferentiation
      - One mature somatic cell transforms into another mature somatic cell without undergoing intermediate pluripotent stage
    - 2-step process-lineage reprogramming
      - Tumor dedifferentiates to early progenitor, then subsequently redifferentiates
    - Evidence that supports transdifferentiation includes patients with both HS and another hematopoietic neoplasm that are clonally related
    - HS generally develops subsequent to hematopoietic neoplasm
  - Rare cases associated with dendritic cell neoplasms

CLINICAL ISSUES

Epidemiology
- Incidence
  - Very rare
    - < 1% of all hematologic malignancies
- Age
  - All ages affected
    - Most common in adults

Site
- Extranodal sites are most common anatomic location, including large bowel, spleen, soft tissue, and skin
  - Lymph node less common primary site
  - Rarely, patients have systemic presentation

Presentation
- Solitary mass
- Systemic symptoms, including fever and weight loss
- Cytopenias common
- Bone marrow involvement is rare
  - Involvement of bone marrow is considered acute monocytic leukemia
- Occasional cases arise from previous lymphoma, leukemia, or myelodysplasia

Treatment
- Surgical excision is curative if low stage
  - Laparoscopic excision is now used in some cases
- Chemotherapy and radiation have varying results
  - Lymphoma-type chemotherapy regiments most commonly used
  - Leukemia-type chemotherapy less common with varying results
  - Rarely, autotransplantation has been used in conjunction with chemotherapy
- *BRAF* inhibitors, such as vemurafenib, are very promising in cases with *BRAF* V600E mutations
- MEK inhibitors, such as trametinib 2, have seen partial response
- Anti-PD1 nivolumab is experimental in PD1/PDL1(+) HS
- Tyrosine kinase inhibitors for HS with *CSF1R* and receptor tyrosine kinase mutations

Prognosis
- Favorable if neoplasm can be completely excised
- High-stage lesions have poor outcomes
- Cases with *BRAF* V600E mutation are not associated with more aggressive disease

MACROSCOPIC

General Features
- Usually solitary mass
- Margins may be infiltrative

Size
- Soft tissue mass may reach up to 12 cm

MOLECULAR

Molecular Genetics
- Recurrent mutations of genes in Ras/Raf/MEK/ERK signaling pathway
  - *BRAF* exon 15 mutational analysis shows *BRAF* V600E mutation in up to 62%
    - Highest frequency of *BRAF* V600E mutation among histiocytic or dendritic cell neoplasms
    - *BRAF* non-V600E, including F595L, G464V, G466R, N581S reported
  - Mutations of *HRAS*, *KRAS*, *PTPN11*, *TP53*, *PTEN*, *PIK3CA*, and *MAP2K1* also reported
- Activating mutations in *CSF1R* and receptor tyrosine kinases
  - *CSF3R*, *KIT*, *ALK*, *MET*, *JAK3*, and *RAF1*; *RET* fusions reported
- Subset shows mutations in *KMT2D* and *ARID1A*

Cytogenetics
- No consistent specific cytogenetic findings
- Early reports of translocation, most likely have associated underlying small B-cell lymphoma

In Situ Hybridization
- Epstein-Barr virus (EBV)-encoded RNA (EBER) (-)

Histiocytic Sarcoma

Polymerase Chain Reaction
- Clonal antigen receptor gene rearrangements for *TRB*, *TRG*, and *IGH* may be seen and do not exclude diagnosis
- When HS is associated with lymphoma, identical clonal gene rearrangements may be present

MICROSCOPIC

Histologic Features
- Neoplastic histiocytic cells are large and dyscohesive
  - Varying morphology from epithelioid to spindle-shaped or pleomorphic
  - Vesicular chromatin, sometimes prominent nucleoli
  - Cytoplasm may be abundant with vacuoles or xanthomatous appearance
- Nodal involvement may show sinusoidal pattern
- Necrosis may be present
- Erythrophagocytosis common systemically or locally

Cytologic Features
- Spectrum of cytomorphology ranges from bland histiocytes to overtly malignant cells

ANCILLARY TESTS

Immunohistochemistry
- At least 2 of following: CD68(+), CD163(+), lysozyme (+), PU.1(+), CD4(+)
- Subset factor XIII(+), CD15(+), CD45(+), S100(+/-)
- Negative for CD1a, CD207 (langerin), CD21, CD35, MPO, CD33, HMB45, SOX10, CD20, CD3, and keratin
- PD1/PDL-1(+) reported

DIFFERENTIAL DIAGNOSIS

Benign Histiocytic Processes
- Infection
  - Special stains often show organisms
- Xanthogranulomatous lesions
- Inflammatory pseudotumor-like lesions
  - Can occur in both soft tissue and lymph node
  - May be mass-like with inflammatory cells
  - Immunohistochemistry may show SMA(+) or EBER(+)
  - In situ hybridization for EBER may be (+) in cases involving spleen or liver

Diffuse Large B-Cell Lymphoma
- Often indistinguishable from HS by morphology
- Large, vesicular nuclei with variable nucleoli
- Immunophenotype
  - B-cell markers (CD20, CD79a, PAX5, and CD22) (+)
- Clonal *IGH* rearrangements present
- t(14;18), *MYC* rearrangements and *BCL6* mutations may be seen

Malignant Melanoma
- Large cells sometimes showing pigment or erythrophagocytosis
- Immunophenotype differentiates from HS
  - S100(+), MART-1/Melan-A (+), HMB-45(+)
  - CD45(-), CD1a(-)
- *BRAF* V600E mutation (+) in 50%

Langerhans Cell Histiocytosis/Langerhans Cell Sarcoma
- Similar in appearance to HS but less atypia unless malignant
- Grooved or twisted nuclei
- Immunophenotype
  - CD163(+), CD1a(+), S100(+), and CD207 (langerin) (+)
  - CD207 (langerin) may be (-) if overtly malignant
- *BRAF* V600E mutation in up to 40%
- Birbeck granules by electron microscopy

Dendritic Cell Neoplasms Other Than Langerhans Cell Histiocytosis/Langerhans Cell Sarcoma
- Includes interdigitating dendritic cell sarcoma, follicular dendritic cell sarcoma, indeterminate dendritic cell tumor, and fibroblastic reticular cell tumor
- Very rare tumors
- Differentiation from HS based on morphology and immunophenotype
- Can be S100(+) &/or CD21(+), depending on type of dendritic cell neoplasm

Hemophagocytic Lymphohistiocytosis
- May be primary or secondary
- Often associated with malignancy (e.g., T-cell lymphoma) or infection (e.g., EBV)
- Phagocytosis is seen in bone marrow, spleen, and liver
- High ferritin levels
- Multiple genes involved, including *PRF1* (perforin), *UNC13D* (Munc 13-4), *STX11* (syntaxin 11), and *STXBP2* (UNC18B)
- Prognosis is poor if not recognized early

Myeloid Sarcoma
- Derived from bone marrow stem cell precursors
- Typical blastic appearance but may look histiocytic
- Bone marrow involvement common
- MPO(+), CD34(+/-), CD117(+/-)

Mature T-Cell Lymphoma
- Most common types that resemble HS: Anaplastic large cell lymphoma and peripheral T-cell lymphoma, not otherwise specified
- Can show erythrophagocytosis
- Immunophenotype shows expression of T-cell-associated antigens
- Clonal *TRB* or *TRG* rearrangements

SELECTED REFERENCES

1. Egan C et al: The mutational landscape of histiocytic sarcoma associated with lymphoid malignancy. Mod Pathol. 34(2):336-47, 2021
2. Egan C et al: Genomic profiling of primary histiocytic sarcoma reveals two molecular subgroups. Haematologica. 105(4):951-60, 2020
3. Hung YP et al: Histiocytic sarcoma. Arch Pathol Lab Med. 144(5):650-4, 2020
4. Said J: Genomic profiling of histiocytic sarcoma: new insights into pathogenesis and subclassification. Haematologica. 105(4):854-5, 2020
5. Durham BH et al: Activating mutations in CSF1R and additional receptor tyrosine kinases in histiocytic neoplasms. Nat Med. 25(12):1839-42, 2019
6. Choi SM et al: KRAS mutation in secondary malignant histiocytosis arising from low grade follicular lymphoma. Diagn Pathol. 13(1):78, 2018
7. Gounder MM et al: Trametinib in histiocytic sarcoma with an activating MAP2K1 (MEK1) mutation. N Engl J Med. 378(20):1945-7, 2018
8. Kumamoto T et al: A case of recurrent histiocytic sarcoma with MAP2K1 pathogenic variant treated with the MEK inhibitor trametinib. Int J Hematol. 109(2):228-32, 2018

Histiocytic Sarcoma

Disseminated Disease

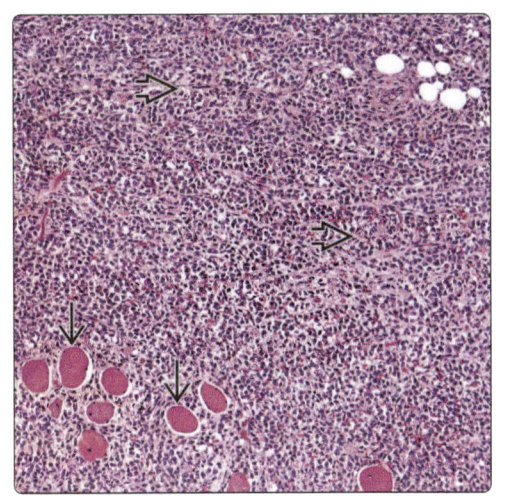

Nuclear Grooves

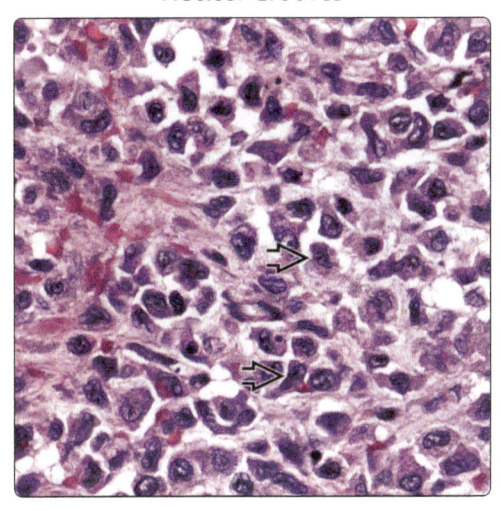

(Left) Malignant histiocytic tumor cells ⇒ infiltrate skeletal muscle ⇒. The tumor presented as a soft tissue mass of the forehead, and it had metastasized from a lymph node. (Right) The tumor cells are large in size, and many have convoluted nuclear grooves ⇒. There is an absence of reactive inflammatory cells.

CD163 Immunohistochemistry

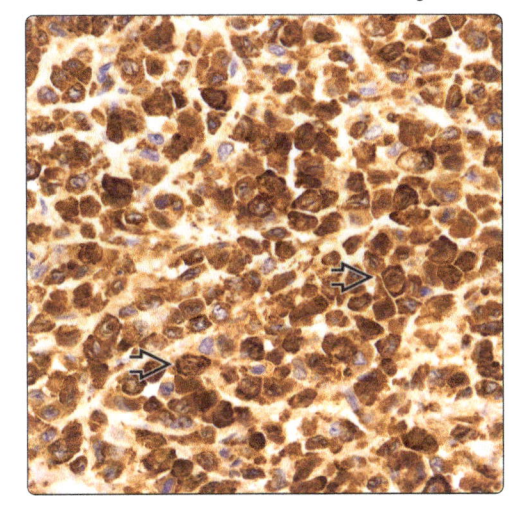

***BRAF* V600E Mutation**

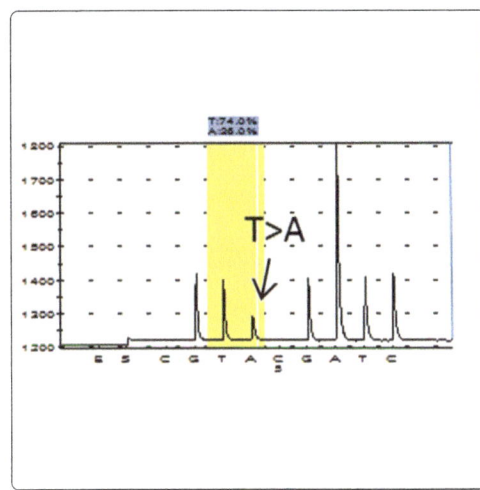

(Left) HS shows both cytoplasmic and membranous staining ⇒ for CD163. The cells were also positive with LCA, other histiocytic markers, and focally for S100 (not shown). (Right) BRAF V600E mutation shows a substitution of nucleotide T for A ⇒. The nucleotide substitution results in an amino acid substitution of valine for glutamic acid. Studies are performed on paraffin-embedded, formalin-fixed tissue.

Effaced Architecture

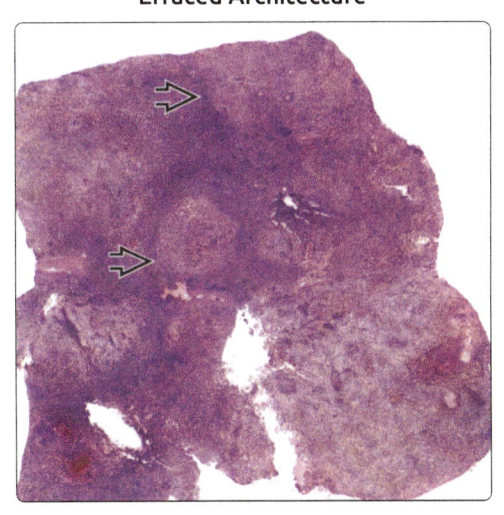

Malignant Histiocytes

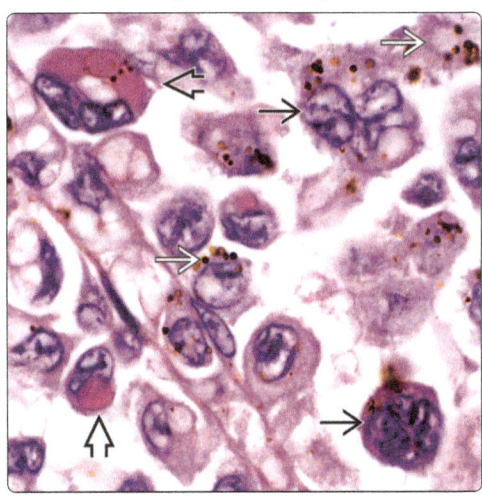

(Left) HS of the spleen shows effaced architecture and numerous vague nodules composed of atypical large malignant histiocytes ⇒. (Right) Malignant histiocytes are dyscohesive, atypical, and pleomorphic ⇒, showing erythrophagocytosis ⇒ and hemosiderin ⇒. Nuclear irregularities are common. The spleen is a common site for HS.

Histiocytic Sarcoma

Langerhans Cell Histiocytosis

(Left) Langerhans cell histiocytosis (LCH) of the spleen shows granuloma-like nodules composed of Langerhans cells ⇨. Other areas are more diffuse ⇨. (Right) LCH is composed of cells that are histocytic with longitudinal nuclear grooves ⇨. Hemophagocytosis (including erythrophagocytosis) can be seen ⇨. Malignant forms of LCH can be very pleomorphic.

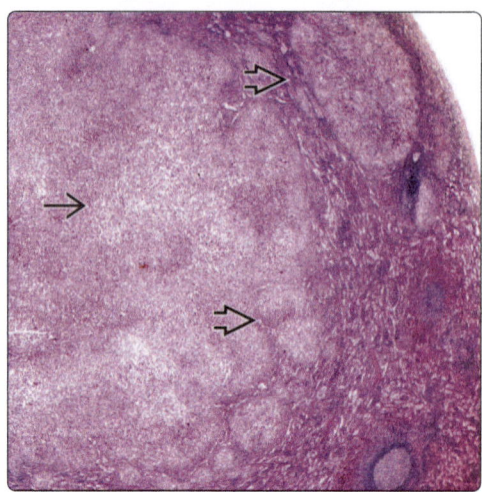

Hemophagocytosis

S100 Immunohistochemistry

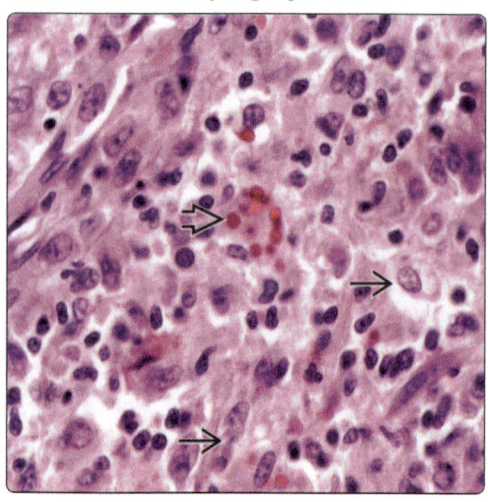

(Left) IHC features distinguishing LCH from HS include uniform positivity for S100. The pattern of staining can be nuclear, cytoplasmic, or membranous. Here, cytoplasmic and membranous staining ⇨ are evident. HS can show patchy S100 positivity. (Right) CD1a shows membranous positivity ⇨ in this case of LCH. Other stains that are positive include CD163, langerin, and sometimes S100. Both LCH and HS can have BRAF mutations.

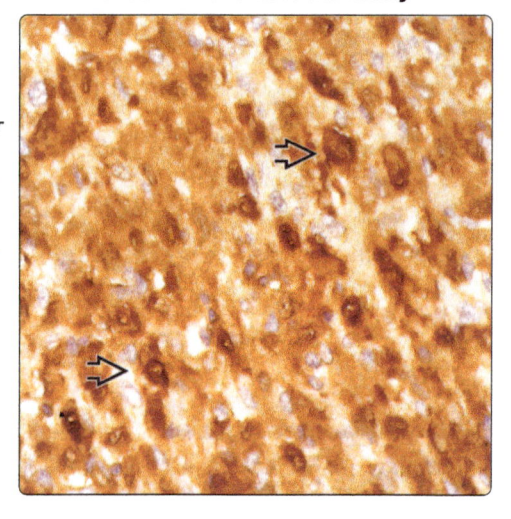

CD1a Immunohistochemistry

Diffuse Large B-Cell Lymphoma

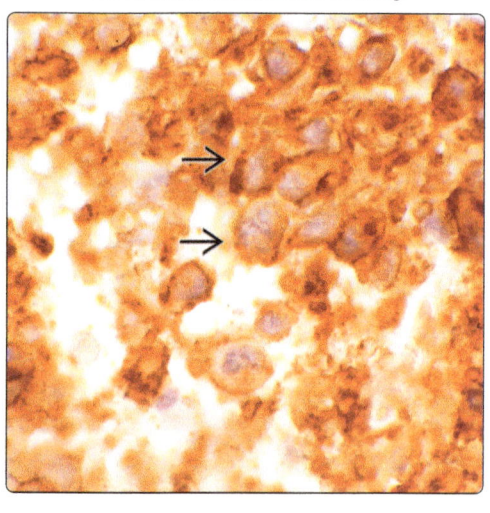

(Left) Diffuse large B-cell lymphoma is shown. The cells are large and pleomorphic with abundant cytoplasm ⇨ and are negative for histiocytic markers but LCA positive (not shown). (Right) Diffuse membranous positivity for CD20 ⇨ helps distinguish diffuse large B-cell lymphoma from HS.

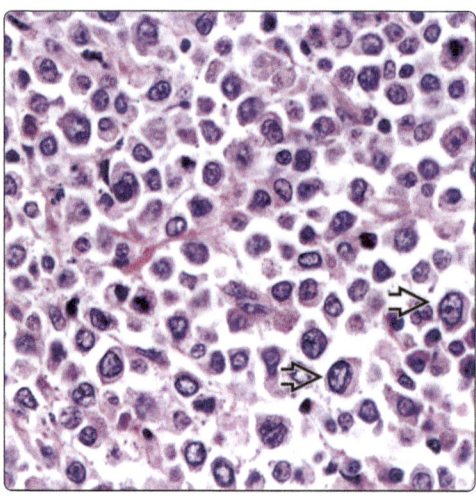

CD20 Immunohistochemistry

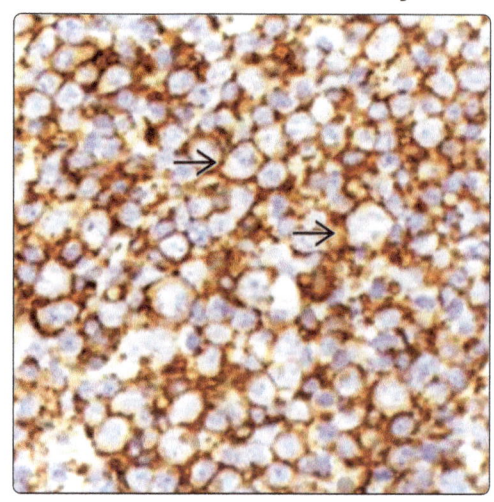

Histiocytic Sarcoma

Malignant Melanoma

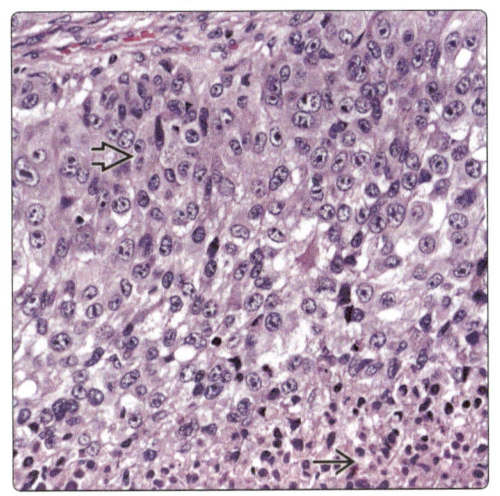

High Power

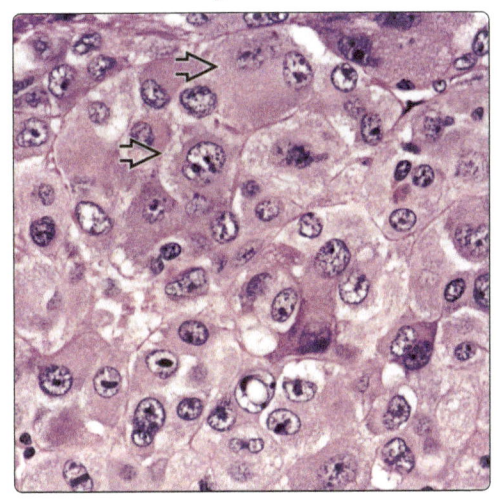

(Left) Malignant melanoma is shown. The cells have a slightly spindled appearance ⇒, which can also be seen in HS. There are areas of apoptosis ⇒, a finding not specific to melanoma. (Right) Malignant melanoma shows large cells with abundant cytoplasm ⇒. Malignant melanoma may show dyscohesive cells, which make it difficult to distinguish from HS without IHC stains.

S100 Immunohistochemistry

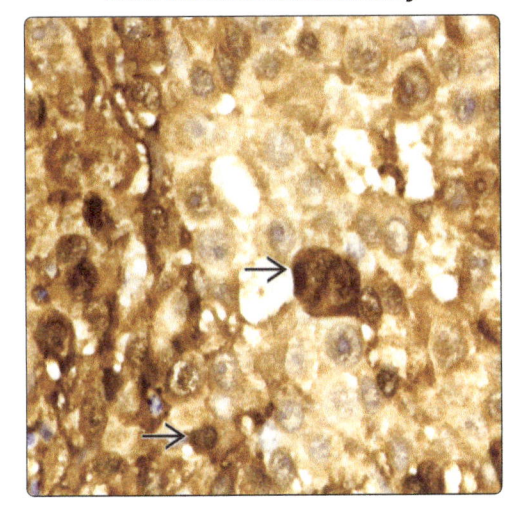

Tyrosinase Immunohistochemistry

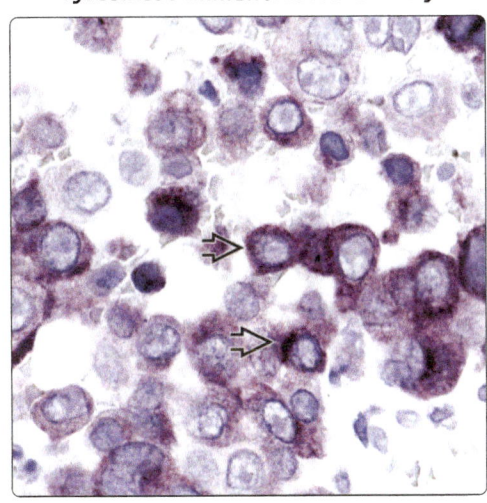

(Left) S100 of malignant melanoma shows both nuclear and cytoplasmic positivity ⇒. Uniform S100 is more characteristic of melanoma than HS, but S100 positivity can also be seen in HS. (Right) Tyrosinase stains positive for malignant melanoma ⇒, a finding which is not seen in HS. HMB-45 is also positive in malignant melanoma, helping to distinguish it from HS.

Myeloid Sarcoma

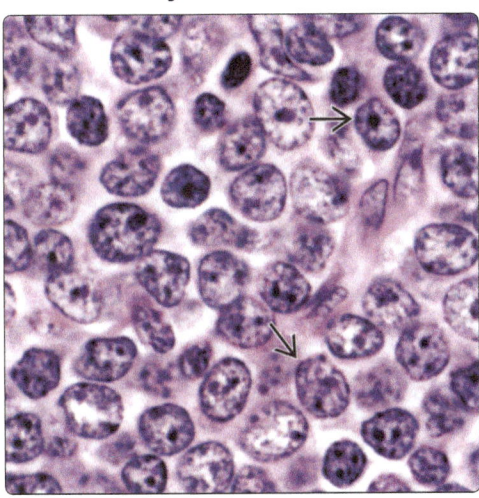

CD34 Immunohistochemistry

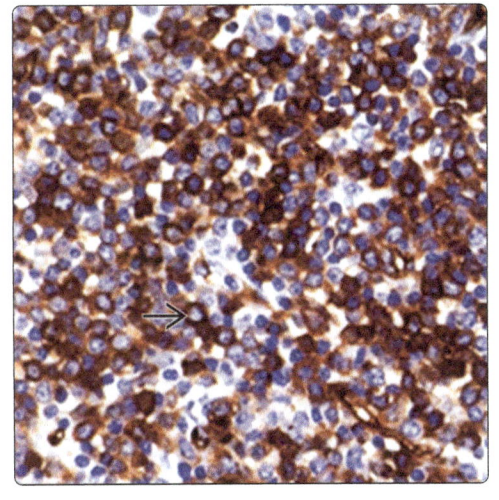

(Left) Myeloid sarcoma shows large, vesicular nuclei, fine chromatin, and moderate cytoplasm ⇒. The blastic appearance of myeloid sarcoma helps distinguish it from HS. (Right) Cells that are positive for CD34 ⇒ are shown. Other markers that are helpful in distinguishing myeloid sarcoma from HS are CD117, MPO, and TdT (rarely positive in myeloid sarcoma). Histiocytic markers do not help, as myeloid sarcoma may be positive.

Histiocytic Sarcoma

(Left) Anaplastic large cell lymphoma (ALCL) is shown. The cells are very pleomorphic and dyscohesive ⇨, similar to HS. **(Right)** CD30 stains almost all of the neoplastic cells in a strong membranous ⇨ and focally Golgi pattern ⇨ in this case of ALCL. This readily available marker helps distinguish ALCL from HS, which is characteristically negative.

Anaplastic Large Cell Lymphoma

CD30 Immunohistochemistry

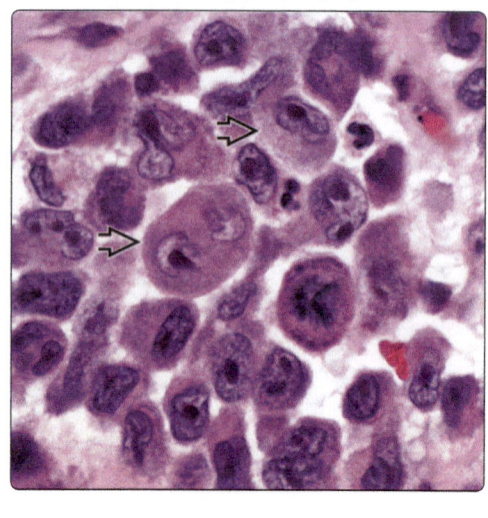

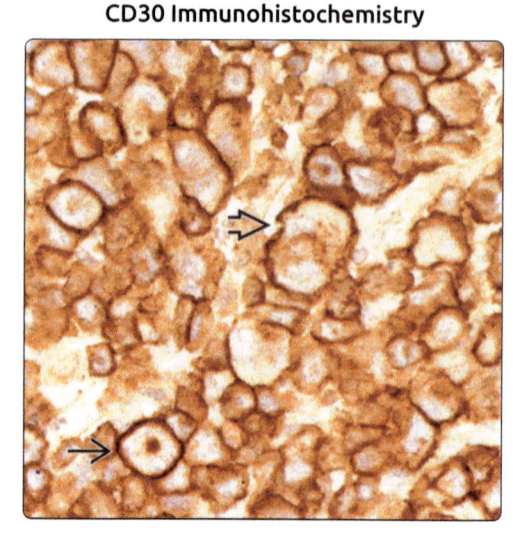

(Left) Familial hemophagocytic lymphohistiocytosis of the spleen shows numerous histiocytes with engulfed red blood cells ⇨. Erythrophagocytosis can also be seen in HS, but clinical presentation is often helpful in diagnosis. **(Right)** Hemophagocytic lymphohistiocytosis shows a histiocyte ⇨ with numerous engulfed red blood cells ⇨. The nuclei ⇨ are bland.

Familial Hemophagocytic Lymphohistiocytosis

Familial Hemophagocytic Lymphohistiocytosis

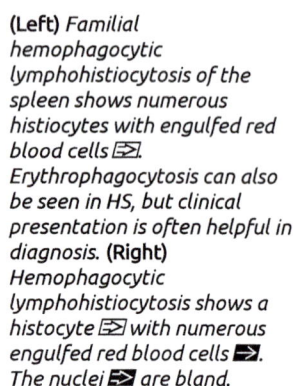

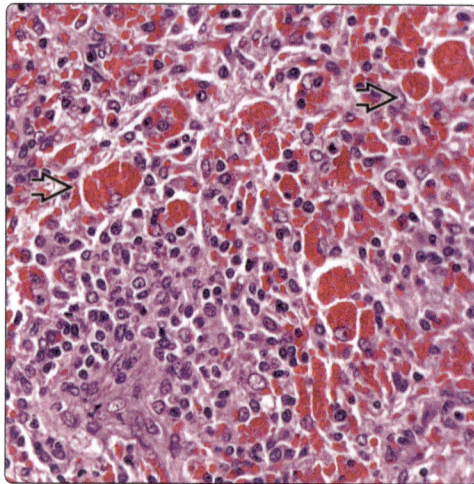

(Left) Lysozyme highlights a histiocyte ⇨ with engulfed red blood cells ⇨. **(Right)** Familial hemophagocytic lymphohistiocytosis shows histiocytes ⇨ with engulfed red blood cells ⇨ and neutrophils ⇨. HS also can show erythrophagocytosis.

Lysozyme Immunohistochemistry

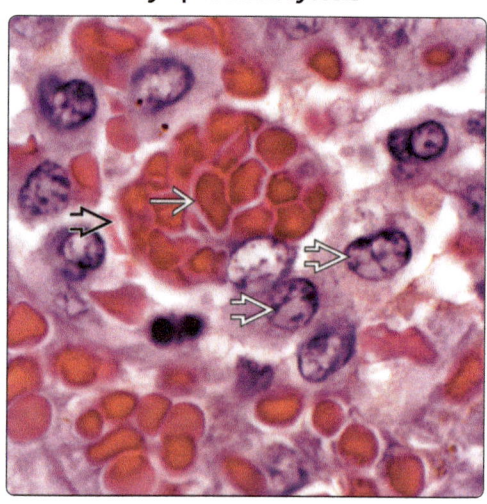

Bone Marrow Aspirate Smear

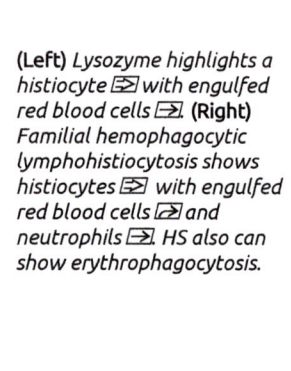

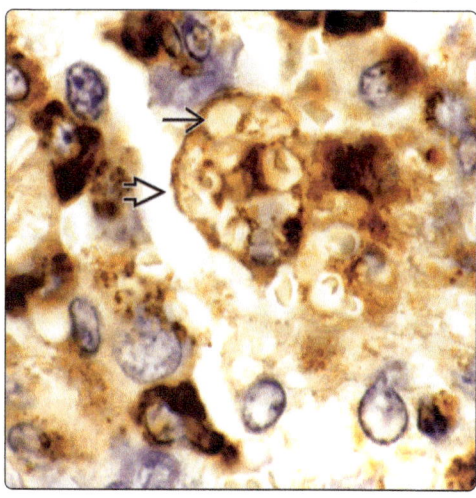

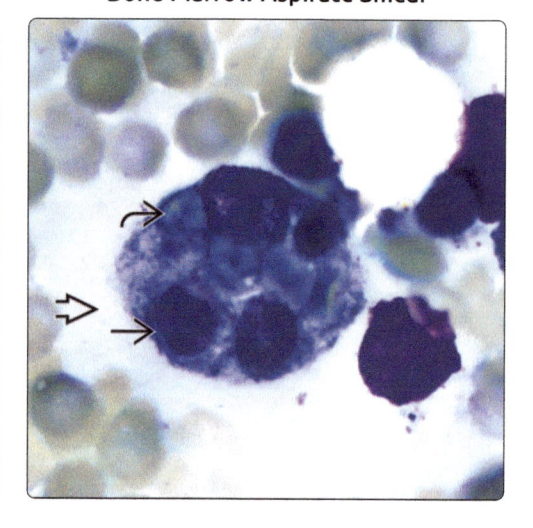

Histiocytic Sarcoma

Peripheral T-Cell Lymphoma, Not Otherwise Specified

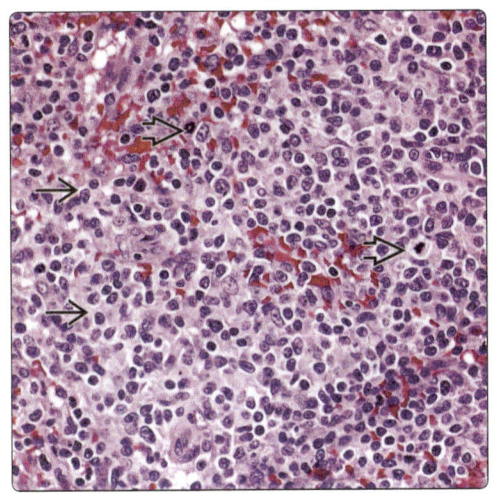

Peripheral T-Cell Lymphoma

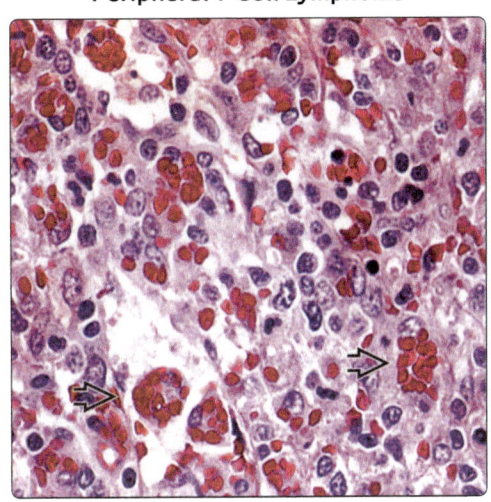

(Left) Peripheral T-cell lymphoma, not otherwise specified shows intermediate-sized lymphocytes ⇨. There are occasional mitoses ⇨. (Right) Numerous histiocytes with erythrophagocytosis ⇨ are shown. Hemophagocytosis is often seen in T-cell lymphomas. The tissues often involved include the bone marrow and spleen.

Interdigitating Dendritic Cell Neoplasm

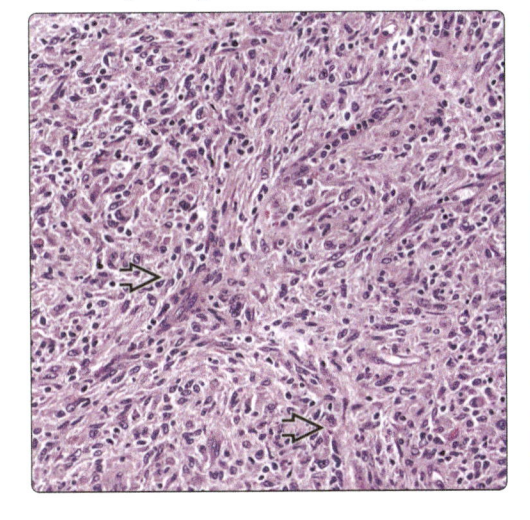

Interdigitating Dendritic Cell Neoplasm

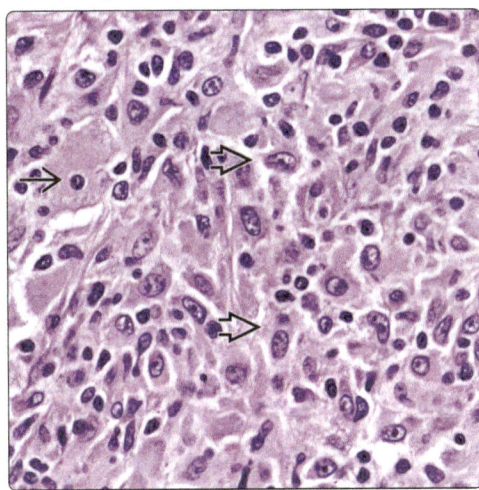

(Left) Interdigitating dendritic cell neoplasm (IDCN) shows a spindled pattern to the cells ⇨, which sometimes helps distinguish it from HS. (Right) The cells are histiocytic in appearance ⇨ with abundant cytoplasm. Rare cells appear to be phagocytizing lymphocytes ⇨.

S100 Immunohistochemistry

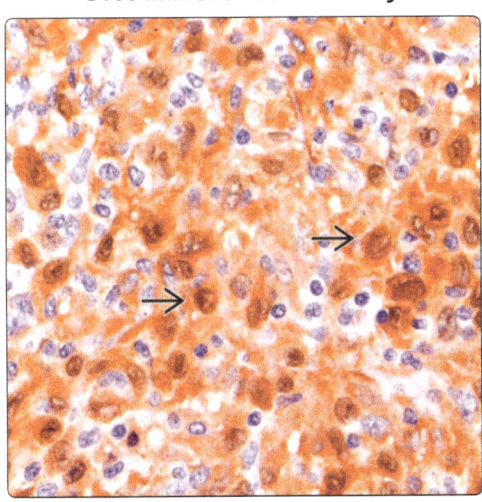

CD68 Immunohistochemistry

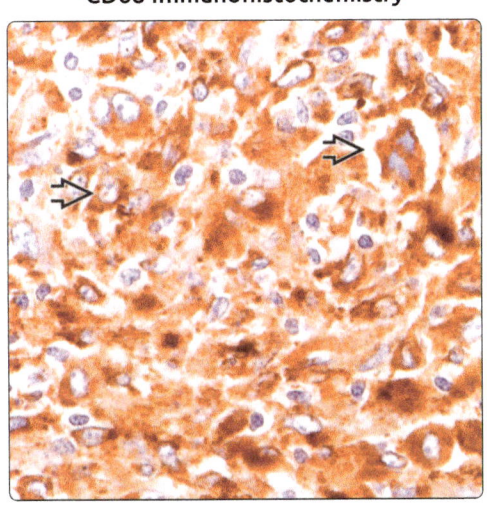

(Left) S100 is positive in IDCN ⇨. CD1a and langerin are negative (not shown). (Right) IDCN is positive for CD68 ⇨. Other markers that are also positive include CD163 and lysozyme.

Langerhans Cell Histiocytosis

KEY FACTS

TERMINOLOGY
- Clonal proliferation of myeloid dendritic cells with expression of CD1a, langerin, and S100
- Recurrent genetic abnormalities involving RAS/RAF/MEK/ERK pathway
  - *BRAF* mutations
  - *MAP2K1* mutations
  - *BRAF* and *MAP2K1* mutations are mutually exclusive in LCH

CLINICAL ISSUES
- 5-10 per 1 million per year in children < 15 years of age
- 1-2 per 1 million per year in adults
- Most cases occur in children; rarely seen in older adults
- M:F = 1.2:1
- Found in any organ but most commonly in bone and skin
- Treatment options are based on disease severity and organ system involvement

MICROSCOPIC
- Morphological features of Langerhans cells
  - Oval-shaped cells ~ 10-15 μm in diameter
  - Coffee bean-shaped, indented, or lobulated nuclei with linear grooves and inconspicuous nucleoli
  - Abundant eosinophilic cytoplasm

ANCILLARY TESTS
- CD1a, langerin, S100, CD68 (weakly), and vimentin (+)
- *BRAF* V600E mutation detection by molecular testing
- NGS testing for *MAPK-ERK* pathway useful for *BRAF* V600E-negative LCH cases

TOP DIFFERENTIAL DIAGNOSES
- Erdheim-Chester disease
- Rosai-Dorfman-Destombes disease
- Langerhans cell sarcoma
- Juvenile xanthogranuloma

Lytic Skull Lesion

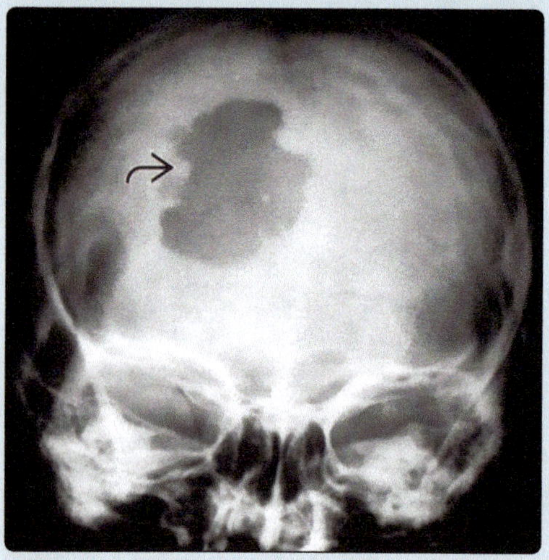

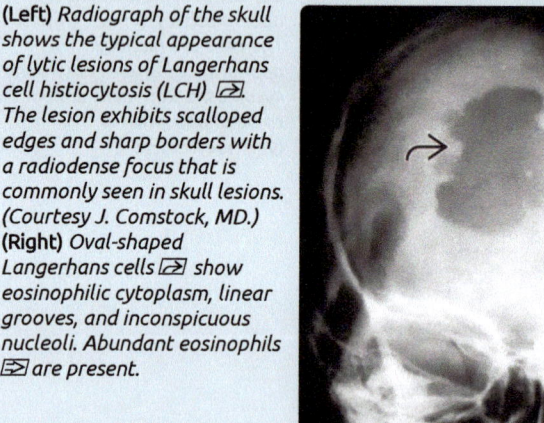

Oval-Shaped Cells

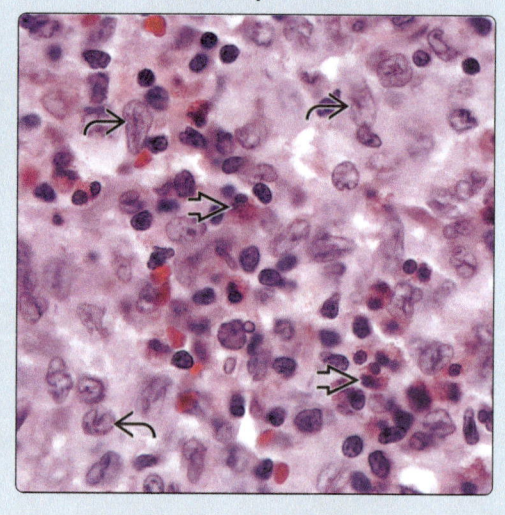

(Left) Radiograph of the skull shows the typical appearance of lytic lesions of Langerhans cell histiocytosis (LCH) ⊿. The lesion exhibits scalloped edges and sharp borders with a radiodense focus that is commonly seen in skull lesions. (Courtesy J. Comstock, MD.) (Right) Oval-shaped Langerhans cells ⊿ show eosinophilic cytoplasm, linear grooves, and inconspicuous nucleoli. Abundant eosinophils ⊿ are present.

BRAF V600E Mutation by Pyrosequencing

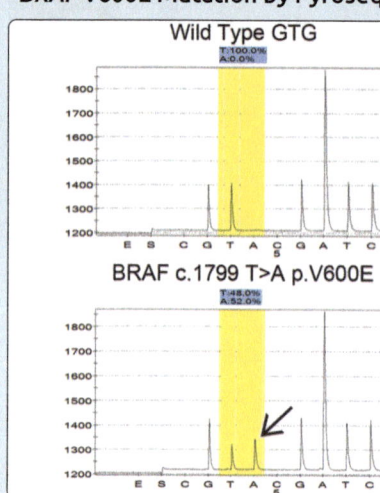

PAS-D Histochemistry

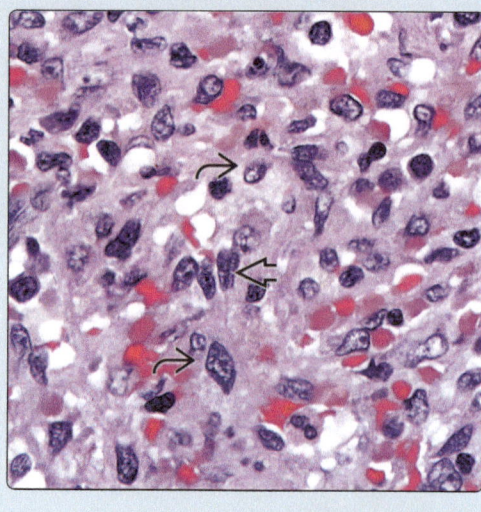

(Left) The top diagram shows wildtype BRAF with GTG detected at the V600 codon of BRAF by pyrosequencing. The bottom diagram shows BRAF c.1799 T>A (p.V600E) mutation ⊿, which occurs due to T>A substitution. (Right) Langerhans cells have linear grooves ⊿. PAS-D is negative for cytoplasmic inclusions ⊿.

Langerhans Cell Histiocytosis

TERMINOLOGY

Abbreviations
- Langerhans cell histiocytosis (LCH)

Synonyms
- Langerhans cell granulomatosis
- Histiocytosis X
- Eosinophilic granuloma (obsolete)
- Hand-Schüller-Christian disease (obsolete)
- Letterer-Siwe disease (obsolete)

Definitions
- Clonal proliferation of myeloid dendritic cells with expression of CD1a, langerin, and S100, Birbeck granules in electronic microscopy, and recurrent genetic abnormalities
- Recurrent genetic abnormalities
  o *BRAF* mutations
  o *MAP2K1* mutations

ETIOLOGY/PATHOGENESIS

Etiology
- LCH originates from misguided differentiation of myeloid dendritic cell precursors
- Clonal X-linked androgen receptor gene assay in female patients proves that LCH is clonal disorder
- Recurrent somatic mutations in *BRAF* and *MAP2K1* occurring in majority of cases support that LCH is neoplastic

CLINICAL ISSUES

Epidemiology
- Incidence
  o 5-10 per 1 million per year in children < 15 years of age; 1-2 per 1 million per year in adults
- Age
  o Most cases occur in children; rarely seen in older adults
- Sex
  o M:F = 1.2:1
- Ethnicity
  o More common among White populations than other ethnic groups

Site
- Virtually in any organs but most commonly in bone and skin
- Other commonly involved sites include pituitary, liver, spleen, hematopoietic system, lungs, lymph nodes, central nervous system, and oral cavity

Presentation
- LCH classification ranges from isolated disease with spontaneous resolution to life-threatening multisystem disease
  o Unifocal (most common)
    – Solitary lesion involving any organs
    – Patients are usually older children or adults
  o Single-system multifocal
    – > 1 lesion involving any organ
    – Patients are usually young children
  o Multisystem
    – ≥ 2 organ/system involvement
    – Patients are usually infants
    – Common presentation includes fever, cytopenia, hepatosplenomegaly, lymphadenopathy, and cutaneous lesions
  o Single-system pulmonary
    – Isolated lung involvement
    – Predominantly smoking related; occurs almost exclusively in smokers or ex-smokers
    – Most patients are young to middle-aged adults
    – Pulmonary LCH with extrapulmonary involvement is classified under multisystem disease
- Mixed histiocytosis
  o LCH cooccurring with Rosai-Dorfman-Destombes disease
  o LCH overlapping with Erdheim-Chester disease (ECD)
  o LCH occur concomitantly with juvenile xanthogranuloma
- LCH concomitantly with hematologic and solid organ neoplasms
  o Myeloid neoplasms and lymphomas
  o Solid organ neoplasms, including lung carcinoma, papillary thyroid carcinoma, and renal cell carcinoma

Treatment
- Options, risks, complications
  o Treatment options depend on extent of organs affected
  o Some cases resolve spontaneously
- Surgical approaches
  o Curettage or excision for solitary bone lesions
- Drugs
  o Topical steroids for localized skin disease
  o Systemic chemotherapy for multisystem involvement
    – Vinblastine and prednisone
- Radiation
  o For inaccessible lesions or vital structures that resection could compromise organ function
  o Adjuvant treatment in cases with incomplete resection
- Treatments designed to inhibit activities of proteins encoded by mutated *BRAF* and *MAP2K1*
  o FDA has granted approval to oral MEK inhibitor cobimetinib (Cotellic) for histiocytic neoplasms
    – LCH, ECD, and Rosai-Dorfman-Destombes disease
  o Vemurafenib, FDA approved for *BRAF* V600E-positive metastatic melanoma
    – Off-label use to treat *BRAF* V600E mutation-positive, refractory, childhood LCH
    – Currently in clinical trials for LCH in adult patients
    – Has shown effectiveness (~ 40% response rate) in adult LCH patients

Prognosis
- Depending on staging of disease
- Favorable if isolated bone lesion or skin lesion with survival rate of ~ 99%
- Poor if multisystem involvement and disseminated with survival rate of ~ 60-70%

IMAGING

Radiographic Findings
- Discrete, punched-out, lytic bone lesions

Langerhans Cell Histiocytosis

MOLECULAR

BRAF Mutations

- BRAF protein is serine/threonine kinase
- Belongs to RAS/RAF/MEK/ERK pathway, plays important role in pathogenesis in LCH
- *BRAF* V600E is most common type of *BRAF* mutation in LCH
  - Found in ~ 60% of LCH patients
  - *BRAF* molecular testing is recommended for diagnosis and targeted therapy
  - Increased risk of initial treatment failure in patients with *BRAF* mutation
  - 2x increased risk for recurrence or relapse in patients with mutation
  - Associates with lower age at diagnosis and higher prevalence of multisystem LCH, high-risk disease, and skin involvement
- Other rare types of *BRAF* alterations
  - *BRAF* exon 12 in-frame deletions
    - May correlate with more lung involvement
  - *MIGA1::BRAF* fusion as alternative genetic mechanism of *BRAF* activation found in LCH patients

MAP2K1 Mutations

- *MAP2K1* encodes protein known as MEK1 protein kinase
  - Functions as downstream effector of *RAF* signaling pathway
    - Enzymatic activities lead to further transduction of signal with *MAPK/ERK* cascade
- ~ 33% of LCH cases harbor somatic *MAP2K1* mutations
  - Most are in-frame deletions, including p.F53_Q58delinsL, p.K57_G61del, p. E102_I103del, p.H100_I103delinsPL, p. E102_I103del, and p. I99_K104del
  - Few are missense mutations, including p.R47Q, p. R49C, p.Q56P, p. C121S, p.G128V, and p. A106T
- *MAP2K1* mutations occur in ~ 50% of *BRAF* wildtype LCH cases
- *MAP2K1* and *BRAF* mutations are mutually exclusive
- *MAP2K1* mutations associated with higher prevalence of single-system (SS)-bone LCH

ARAF Mutations

- Compound mutations *ARAF* Q347_A348del and *ARAF* F351L rarely reported in LCH
- Compound *ARAF* T70M and *BRAF* V600E mutations reported in rare LCH cases

ERBB3 Somatic Mutation

- P921Q detected in 1 *BRAF* wildtype case of LCH

MICROSCOPIC

Histologic Features

- Pathologic features vary depending on anatomic site
  - In general, lesions contain varying numbers (abundant or sparse) of LCH cells accompanied with macrophages, lymphocytes, eosinophils, giant cells, and, less commonly, neutrophils and plasma cells
- Spleen
  - Aggregates of Langerhans cells, mostly in red pulp
  - Secondary white pulp involvement
  - Eosinophils, neutrophils, small lymphocytes, plasma cells, macrophages, and histiocytes are often present
- Lymph node
  - Langerhans cells infiltrate sinus and paracortex
- Liver
  - Langerhans cells infiltrate sinusoidal spaces and intrahepatic biliary system
  - Progressive intrahepatic sclerosing cholangitis can occur
- Lungs
  - Interstitial infiltrate of Langerhans cells with abundant eosinophils, often subpleural in location
- Skin
  - Langerhans cells infiltrate dermis and subcutis tissue and extend to epidermis

Cytologic Features

- Oval cells ~ 10-15 μm in diameter with abundant eosinophilic cytoplasm
- Coffee bean-shaped, indented, or lobulated nuclei with linear grooves and inconspicuous nucleoli

ANCILLARY TESTS

Histochemistry

- PAS-D(-)

Immunohistochemistry

- CD1A (membranous and cytoplasmic) and langerin (CD207) (cytoplasmic granular staining) are specific for Langerhans cells
- S100(+) with both cytoplasmic and nuclear staining in Langerhans cells but not specific
- *BRAF* V600E mutation-specific antibody (VE1) is positive with high concordance with *BRAF* V600E mutation analysis
- Vimentin, CD4, and CD68 (weak) are positive; CD163 is positive in minority of LCH cases (5-10%)
- CD1c, B-cell markers, T-cell markers, CD30, and CD23 are negative

Genetic Testing

- *BRAF* V600E can be tested by variety of molecular platforms to aid in diagnosis and treatment in all LCH patients
  - Digital PCR (dPCR), allele-specific RT-PCR, pyrosequencing, and next-generation sequencing (NGS)
- *BRAF* V600E-negative LCH cases, NGS testing to assess MAPK-ERK pathway mutations
- *IGH*, *IGK*, *TRB*, and *TRG* rearrangement are detected in up to 30% of LCH cases showing monoclonal status

Electron Microscopy

- Birbeck granules
  - Pentalaminar cytoplasmic tennis racket-shaped inclusions
  - Solely found in Langerhans cells
  - Not required for diagnosis

DIFFERENTIAL DIAGNOSIS

Erdheim-Chester Disease

- Rare multisystem non-LCH characterized pathologically by xanthogranulomatous infiltrates and universal long bone involvement

Langerhans Cell Histiocytosis

- Visceral involvement varies; commonly affected organs/sites include central nervous system (cerebellum and brainstem), retroperitoneum, kidney, orbits, skin, pericardium, and lung
- Clusters of macrophages and Touton-type giant cells
- CD163(+); S100, CD1a, and langerin (-)
- Negative for Birbeck granules by electron microscopy
- ~ 50% of ECD patients carry recurrent somatic *BRAF* V600E mutation
- Recurrent somatic mutations in *BRAF* and *PIK3CA* identified in 12-17% of ECD patients

Rosai-Dorfman-Destombes Disease
- a.k.a. sinus histiocytosis with massive lymphadenopathy
- Proliferation of non-Langerhans cell histiocytes
- Patients are often 10-20 years of age
- Commonly presents with enlargement of lymph nodes in neck
- Spleen is usually not involved
- Emperipolesis is hallmark
  - Typically, intact lymphocytes are seen in histiocyte cytoplasm
- S100, CD163, BCL1, and OCT2 (+)
- CD1a and langerin (-)

Langerhans Cell Sarcoma
- High-grade neoplasm of Langerhans cell with overtly malignant cytologic features
- Multiorgan involvement and aggressive clinical course; high mortality rate (> 50%)
- High mitotic activity and fewer eosinophils than LCH
- Same immunophenotype as LCH: CD1a, langerin, and S100 (+)
- Presence of ultrastructural Birbeck granules as seen in LCH
- Skin and soft tissue are most commonly involved
- Rare cases with *BRAF* V600E mutation reported
- Overtly malignant cytologic features as main distinguishing features from LCH

Juvenile Xanthogranuloma
- Benign proliferative disorder of histiocytic cells of dermal dendrocyte phenotype
  - Most common form of non-LCH
- Self-limited dermatologic disorder that is rarely associated with systemic manifestations
- Generally, disease of infancy and early childhood, most in 1st year of life
- Foamy histiocytic dermal infiltrate, often in association with epidermal flattening and ulceration
- Phenotype: CD68 and factor XIIIa (+); CD1a, langerin, CD34, and S100 (-)

Histiocytic Sarcoma
- Malignant histiocytic neoplasm
- Morphology ranges from benign-appearing to overtly malignant
- CD68, CD163, lysozyme, and S100 (+) (variable)
- CD20, CD3, langerin, and CD1a (-)

Interdigitating Dendritic Cell Sarcoma
- Rare neoplasm with splenic red pulp involvement
- Large neoplastic cells forming fascicles or storiform pattern
- S100, vimentin, CD68 (weak), lysozyme, and CD45 (+)
- CD1a and langerin (-)

Familial Hemophagocytic Lymphohistiocytosis
- Infants from birth to 18 months of age
- Overproduction of activated lymphocytes (B and T cells), NK cells, and histiocytes with systemic manifestations, fulminant clinical course, and high mortality rate
- Splenic red pulp with phagocytic histiocytes, which can contain red cells, white blood cells, or platelets
- CD68(+); CD1a, langerin, and S100 (-)
- ~ 40-60% harbor mutations in *PRF1* or *UNC13D*

Lymphoma/Leukemia
- Often has more cytologic atypia than LCH
- Different immunophenotype than LCH
  - Hematopoietic markers (CD45, CD19, CD20, or CD3 based on lineage) (+)
  - Usually CD1a, langerin, and S100 (-)

Granulomatous Disease
- Chronic granulomatous disease and noninfectious granulomas (e.g., sarcoidosis)
  - Splenomegaly and granulomas
- CD1a, langerin, and S100 (-)

Gaucher Disease
- Autosomal recessive inherited lipid storage disease, caused by deficiency of glucocerebrosidase
- Clusters of Gaucher cells may appear similar to Langerhans cells with small nuclei with wrinkled, striated, silk-, or granular-appearing cytoplasm
- Deposition of glucocerebroside in cells of macrophage-monocyte system
- Gaucher cells are PAS(+) and CD1a, langerin, and S100 (-)

DIAGNOSTIC CHECKLIST

Clinically Relevant Pathologic Features
- Combination of lytic bone lesions and skin lesions may point to LCH

Pathologic Interpretation Pearls
- Langerhans cells: Coffee bean-shaped nuclei with linear grooves
- Phenotype: CD1a, langerin, and S100 (+)
- Birbeck granules on electron microscopy
- Positive *BRAF* V600E mutation

SELECTED REFERENCES
1. Kemps PG et al: Clinicogenomic associations in childhood Langerhans cell histiocytosis: an international cohort study. Blood Adv. 7(4):664-79, 2023
2. Goyal G et al: International expert consensus recommendations for the diagnosis and treatment of Langerhans cell histiocytosis in adults. Blood. 139(17):2601-21, 2022
3. FDA: Cobimetinib, FDA-approved drug package insert. Published October 2022. Accessed March, 2023. https://www.accessdata.fda.gov/drugsatfda_docs/label/2022/206192s005lbl.pdf
4. Gulati N et al: Langerhans cell histiocytosis: version 2021. Hematol Oncol. 39 Suppl 1:15-23, 2021
5. Jouenne F et al: Mitogen-activating protein kinase pathway alterations in Langerhans cell histiocytosis. Curr Opin Oncol. 33(2):101-9, 2021
6. Rodriguez-Galindo C et al: Langerhans cell histiocytosis. Blood. 135(16):1319-31, 2020

Langerhans Cell Histiocytosis

CD1a Immunohistochemistry

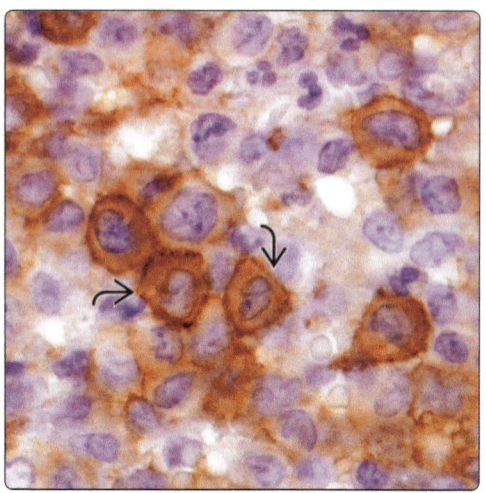

S100 Immunohistochemistry

(Left) *Langerhans cells show positive membranous and cytoplasmic immunoreactivity for CD1a. Grooved nuclei can be seen within the positive-staining cells ⇗. CD1a is specific for Langerhans cells (although not exclusive) and is very useful in cases where the cellularity is low. (Courtesy J. Comstock, MD.)* (Right) *Langerhans cells show positive cytoplasmic and nuclear staining ⇗ for S100. S100 is not specific for LCH; however, cytoplasmic and nuclear positive staining patterns are very helpful for the diagnosis of LCH.*

Langerin Immunohistochemistry

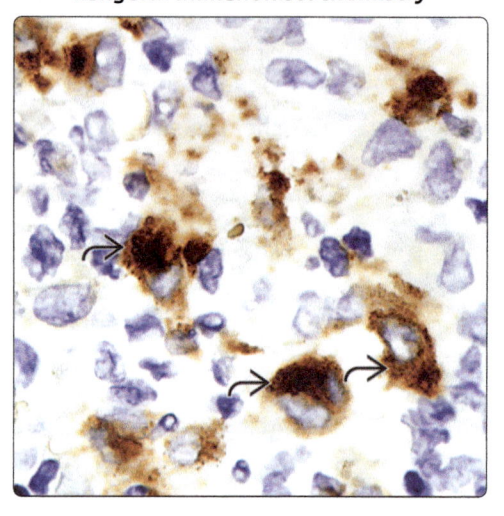

Langerhans Cells

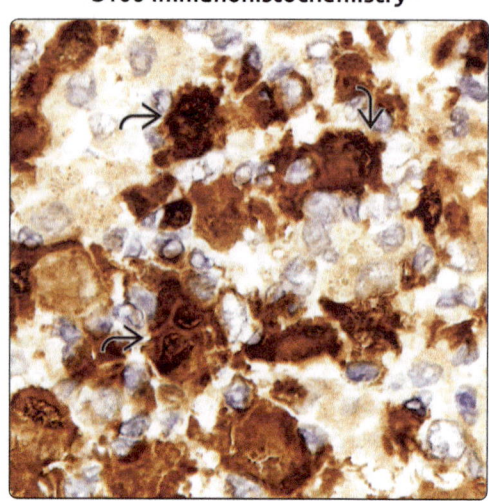

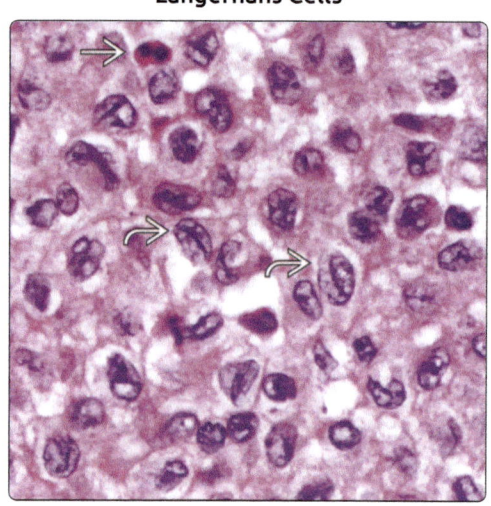

(Left) *Langerhans cells show a cytoplasmic granular staining pattern for langerin ⇗. This is a highly selective marker for Langerhans cells, and it is a relatively specific marker of LCH.* (Right) *High-power view highlights the typical nuclear features of Langerhans cells. The nuclei are folded, show long grooves ⇗, and often resemble coffee beans. An eosinophil ⇗ is seen. (Courtesy J. Comstock, MD.)*

Rosai-Dorfman-Destombes Disease

Histiocytic Sarcoma

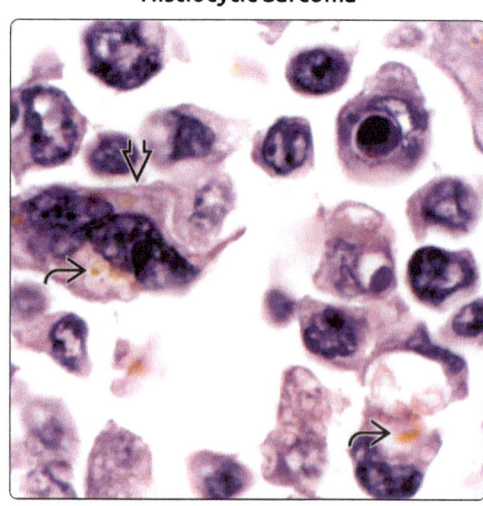

(Left) *Rosai-Dorfman-Destombes disease shows large histiocytes with pale to eosinophilic cytoplasm and centrally located nuclei with vesicular chromatin. Some contain intracytoplasmic lymphocytes and plasma cells (emperipolesis) ⇗.* (Right) *Splenic histiocytic sarcoma shows marked atypia ⇗ and hemosiderin deposits ⇗ from engulfed red blood cells. These cells stain for histiocytic markers CD68 and lysozyme as well as S100. LCH will not show the cellular pleomorphism of histiocytic sarcoma.*

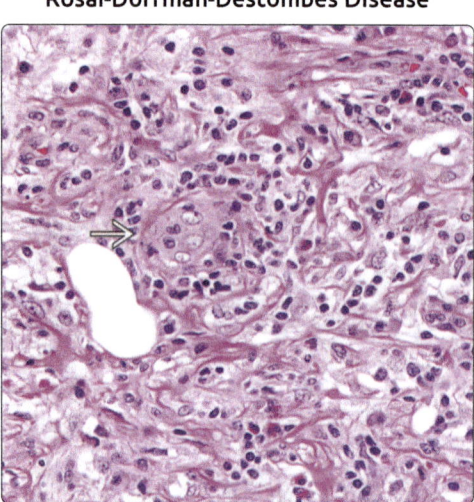

Langerhans Cell Histiocytosis

Familial Hemophagocytic Syndrome

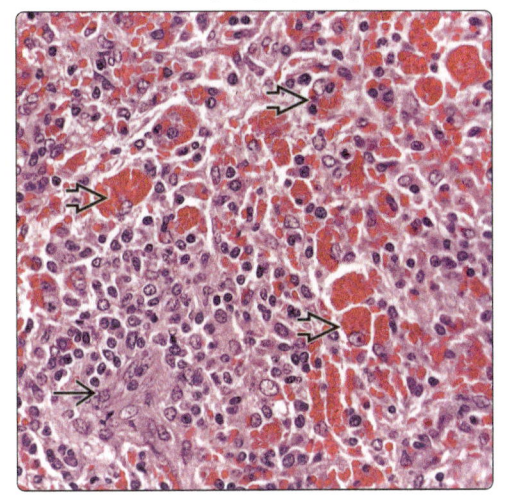

Familial Hemophagocytic Syndrome

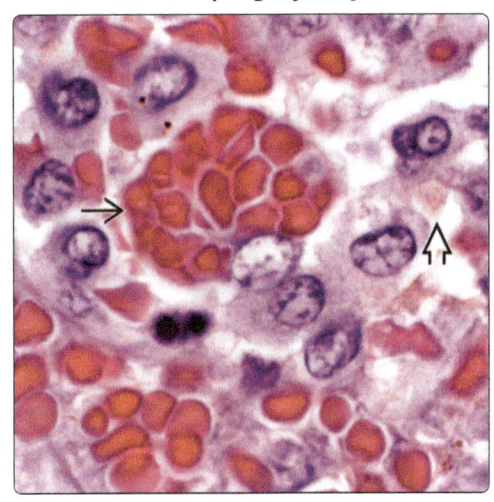

(Left) *Familial hemophagocytic syndrome shows numerous histiocytes with engulfed red blood cells ➡ throughout the spleen. Focal clusters of histiocytes appear granulomatous ➡.* (Right) *Familial hemophagocytic syndrome shows histiocytes with numerous engulfed red blood cells ➡. The histiocytes also contain hemosiderin ➡.*

Noncaseating Granulomas

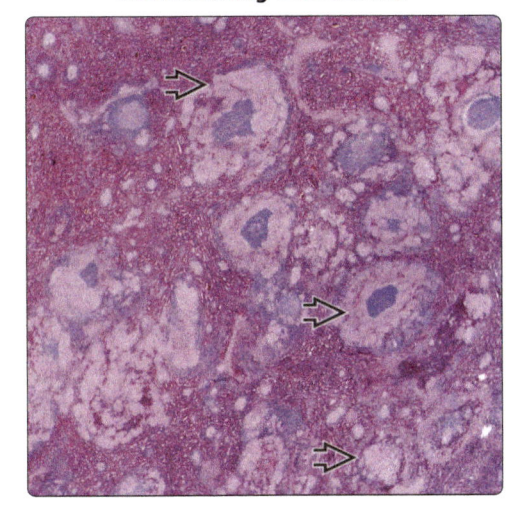

Sarcoidosis

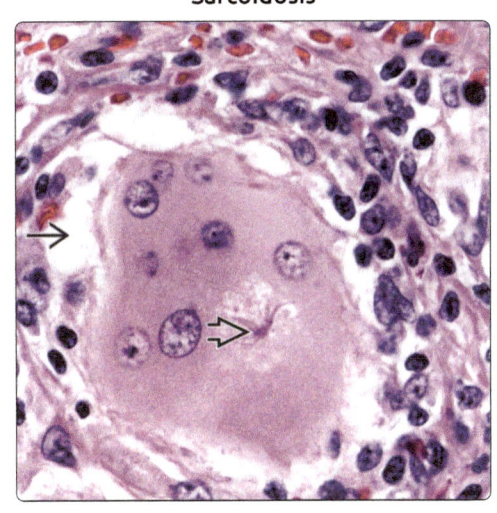

(Left) *Any granulomatous process, both noninfectious and infectious, can appear similar to LCH. This example of sarcoidosis shows well-formed, noncaseating granulomas ➡, better formed than those seen in LCH and hemophagocytosis. Eosinophils are not usually seen in granulomatous inflammation.* (Right) *Giant cell ➡ in a case of sarcoidosis is shown. An asteroid body ➡ is noted in the cell. Giant cells are more common in granulomas.*

Gaucher Disease

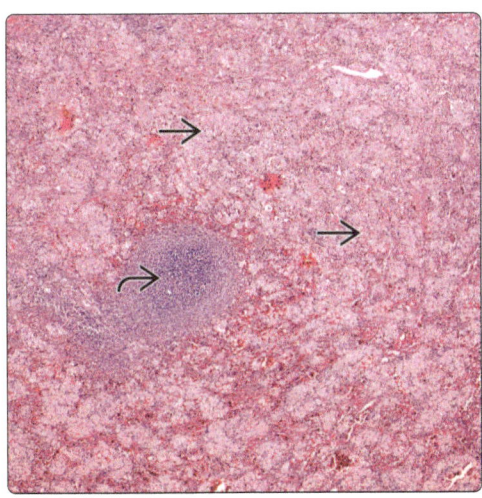

Gaucher Disease

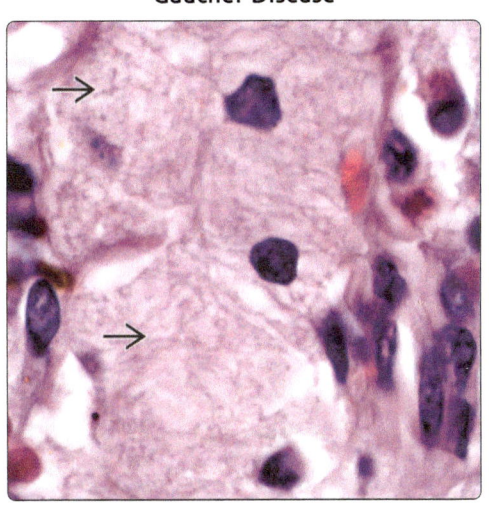

(Left) *Gaucher disease in the spleen shows a granulomatous appearance. There are numerous aggregates composed of engorged histiocytes ➡ filled with glucocerebroside. Focal residual white pulp ➡ is present.* (Right) *Gaucher cells show a wrinkled tissue paper appearance ➡. Glucocerebroside accumulates within the histiocytes due to lack of glucocerebrosidase enzyme.*

Interdigitating Dendritic Cell Sarcoma

KEY FACTS

TERMINOLOGY
- Interdigitating dendritic cell sarcoma (IDCS): Neoplastic proliferation of spindle to epithelioid cells with morphology and phenotype similar to normal IDC

ETIOLOGY/PATHOGENESIS
- Transdifferentiation occurs when histiocytic neoplasm, such as IDCS, develops from B-cell lymphoma

CLINICAL ISSUES
- Single lymph nodes most commonly involved

MOLECULAR
- MAPK pathway alterations, including *BRAF* V600E, *KRAS*, *MAP2K1* mutations, and *CBL::USP2* fusion
  - But similar alterations are seen in other histiocytic/dendritic neoplasms
- No recurrent cytogenetic abnormalities have been reported
- *IGH*, *TRB*, and *TRG* clonal rearrangements usually not detected
  - Except in cases with transdifferentiation with B-cell or T-cell lymphoma
  - *IGH::BCL2* may be detected in both tumors if patient has concurrent IDC sarcoma and follicular lymphoma

MICROSCOPIC
- Spindle-shaped or epithelioid cells
- Sheets, whorls, nests, or fascicles

ANCILLARY TESTS
- Immunohistochemistry
  - S100(+), SOX10(+), CD1a(-), CD68(+/-), CD21(-)
  - Positive for ≥ 1 heme markers
    - CD45/LCA, CD68, CD4, lysozyme

TOP DIFFERENTIAL DIAGNOSES
- Follicular dendritic cell sarcoma
- Melanoma

Nodal Involvement

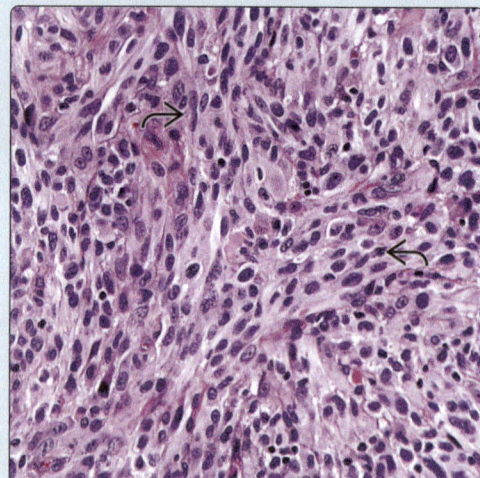

S100 Immunohistochemistry

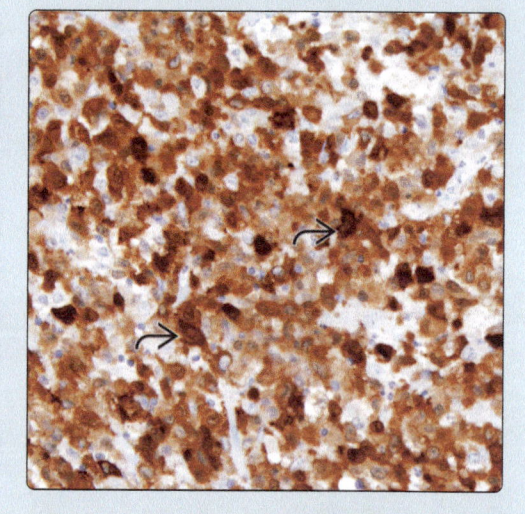

(Left) Interdigitating dendritic cell sarcoma (IDCS) is shown replacing a lymph node. The spindled-shaped neoplastic cells have a loose storiform pattern ⇨. Scattered reactive lymphocytes are present. (Right) S100 is strongly positive ⇨ in IDCS. CD1a was negative (not shown). S100 is the most consistently positive marker in IDCS.

IGH Rearrangement

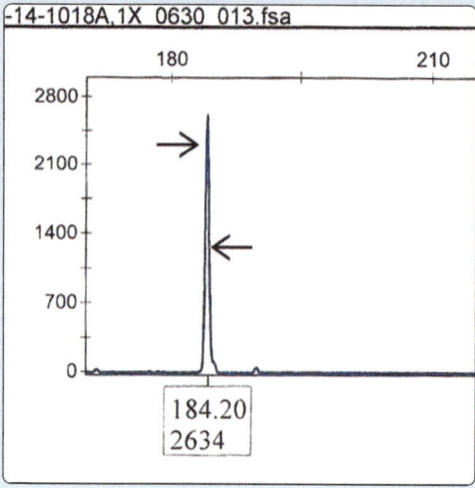

FISH for *IGH::BCL2*

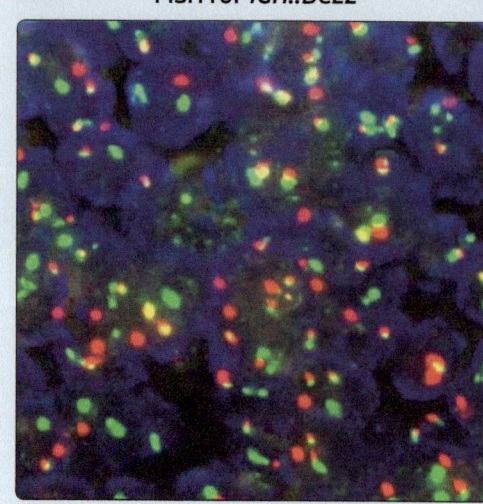

(Left) IGH rearrangement study was performed on a patient with both IDCS and follicular lymphoma (transdifferentiation). The same monoclonal peak ⇨ was identified in both tumors. (Right) FISH dual fusion probe for IGH::BCL2 was performed in the same patient with both IDC sarcoma and follicular lymphoma (transdifferentiation). IGH::BCL2 was identified in both tumors.

Interdigitating Dendritic Cell Sarcoma

TERMINOLOGY

Abbreviations
- Interdigitating dendritic cell sarcoma (IDCS)

Synonyms
- IDC tumor
- Interdigitating dendritic reticulum cell sarcoma

Definitions
- Neoplastic proliferation of spindle to epithelioid cells with morphology and phenotype similar to normal IDC
- IDCS is recognized by both WHO and ICC

ETIOLOGY/PATHOGENESIS

Interdigitating Dendritic Cells
- Stromal antigen presenting cells within lymph nodes
- Normally found in
  - Paracortical areas of lymph node
  - Periarteriolar lymphoid sheaths of spleen
  - T-cell areas of extranodal lymphoid tissue

Transdifferentiation
- Some cases of IDCS are associated with clonally related B-cell lymphomas, and rare cases are associated with T-cell lymphomas
  - Chronic lymphocytic leukemia/small lymphocytic lymphoma is common
  - Usually B-cell lymphoma precedes histiocytic neoplasm
  - IDCS and B-cell lymphomas may share identical clonal *IGH* rearrangements, and both may have *BCL2::IGH* fusion

CLINICAL ISSUES

Epidemiology
- Incidence
  - Exceedingly rare
- Age
  - Wide range
    - Median: 58 years
    - Mostly adults but some in children
- Sex
  - M:F = 1.6:1

Site
- Lymph node
  - Most commonly, single lymph node is involved
  - Cervical, axillary, or inguinal lymph node groups most often affected
- Extranodal sites can be involved
  - Wide variety of extranodal sites
    - Skin and soft tissue most common
    - Liver and spleen
    - Gastrointestinal tract, lung, kidney
  - Bone marrow involved in < 20% of patients

Presentation
- Slow-growing, asymptomatic mass is most common
- Systemic symptoms occur in subset of patients
- Small subset of patients with IDCS also have carcinoma
  - Most common types include breast, stomach, liver, colon carcinomas

Treatment
- Surgical resection and radiation therapy for patients with localized disease
- Currently, there is no established chemotherapy regimen

Prognosis
- Poor clinical course
  - 40-50% of patients develop disseminated disease with poor outcome
    - Median survival with localized disease: ~ 35 months
    - Median survival with disseminated disease: 10 months

MACROSCOPIC

General Features
- Hemorrhage and necrosis can be present

Size
- Variable; 1-6 cm in most studies
- Lobulated mass with firm cut surface

MOLECULAR

Cytogenetics
- No recurrent cytogenetic abnormalities have been reported
  - Lack of information regarding molecular changes due to rarity of tumor

In Situ Hybridization
- *IGH::BCL2* fusion reported in rare cases that developed from follicular lymphoma
  - Identical chromosomal breakpoints in IDCS and follicular lymphoma
- Epstein-Barr virus-encoded RNA (EBER) negative

Polymerase Chain Reaction
- Clonal *IGH*, *TRB*, and *TRG* rearrangements usually not detected
  - Clonal antigen receptor gene rearrangements detected in cases that have undergone transdifferentiation
  - Clonal *IGH* gene rearrangement and trisomy 12 reported in case that developed from chronic lymphocytic leukemia

Molecular Alterations
- Different gene alterations in MAPK pathway
  - *BRAF* V600E, *KRAS*, *MAP2K1*, and *CBL::USP2* alterations have all been identified
  - *BRAF* V600E mutation has been detected in other histiocytic and dendritic neoplasms, including Langerhans cell histiocytosis, histiocytic sarcoma, and FDCS
- Other mutations have been reported
  - *TET2* and *FBXW7*
  - Human androgen receptor assay (HUMARA) has shown clonality in small subset of cases tested

Chromosomal Microarray
- Most cases show identifiable abnormalities
  - Gains include 3q, 13q, trisomy 12
  - Deletions include 7p, 12p, 16p, 18q, 22q

485

Interdigitating Dendritic Cell Sarcoma

- Share some of changes detected in Langerhans cell histiocytosis
- Some cases show no abnormalities

MICROSCOPIC

Histologic Features
- Spindle to epithelioid cell proliferation
  - Typically loose fascicles of spindled cells
  - Can form sheets, whorls, nests or fascicles
  - Cells can show tapered nuclei
  - Vesicular nuclei; grooves; nucleoli can be distinct
  - Abundant eosinophilic cytoplasm with indistinct cell borders
  - Cytologic atypia can be mild or prominent
  - Mitotic rate is usually low
- Partial or complete replacement of lymph node architecture
  - Paracortical or sinusoidal distribution in cases of partial involvement
    - Spares germinal centers
- Inflammatory cells are common in background
  - Small lymphocytes and plasma cells
  - Usually T cells
- Hemophagocytosis is uncommon but has been reported

ANCILLARY TESTS

Immunohistochemistry
- S100 and SOX10 (+) but lacks other specific melanoma markers
- Positive for ≥ 1 heme markers
  - CD45/LCA(+/-), CD68(+/-), CD4(+/-), lysozyme (+/-)
  - CD14(-/+), CD15(-/+), CD33(-/+), CD43(-/+), CD45RO(-/+)
- CD11c(+), HLA-DR(+), fascin (+), β-catenin (+)
- Ki-67 10-70%
- TP53(+), but only several cases have been assessed and reported
- Pan B-cell and pan T-cell antigens (-)
  - PAX5 reported as weakly (+) in IDCS associated with B-cell lymphomas
- EZH2(+) may indicate oncogenesis
  - Also found in histiocytic and dendritic cell neoplasm
  - Including FDC sarcoma, Langerhans cell histiocytosis, and histiocytic sarcoma
  - EZH2(-) in benign histiocytic lesions and normal cells
- Negative markers
  - CD21, CD23, CD35
  - CD1a, langerin, CD163

Electron Microscopy
- Complex interdigitating cell processes and scattered lysozymes
- No Birbeck granules, well-formed desmosomes, or melanosomes

DIFFERENTIAL DIAGNOSIS

Follicular Dendritic Cell Sarcoma
- FDCS may be more spindled than IDCS but can be morphologically indistinguishable
- Features suggestive of FDCS if present
  - Nuclear pseudoinclusions
  - Binucleated, squared off FDCs
  - Reactive small lymphocytes of B-cell lineage
- Immunohistochemistry
  - CD21(+/-), CD23(+/-), CD35(+/-)
  - Clusterin (+), EGFR(+)
  - S100(-), CD68(-/+)
- Electron microscopy shows desmosomes

Melanoma
- Spindle cell melanoma and IDCS have overlapping phenotype and molecular features
  - Both are S100 and SOX10 (+)
  - Both can have *BRAF* mutations
- Dendritic appearance on S100, expression of heme markers, such as CD45, CD4, and CD68, and lack of melanoma specific markers favors diagnosis of IDCS
- Melanoma patients usually have history of melanoma at another anatomic site
- Can only reliably differentiate melanoma from IDCS by electron microscopy
  - Melanosomes by electron microscopy found in melanoma but not in IDCS

Langerhans Cell Sarcoma
- *BRAF* mutations commonly identified (~ 40-50% of cases)
- Usually extranodal sites
  - Most commonly skin and bone
  - Only ~ 20% of patients present with lymph node disease
- Sinusoidal pattern can be present in Langerhans cell sarcoma (LCS)
- Neoplastic IDCs and Langerhans cells are cytologically similar
- Mitotic rate usually high in LCS
  - Often 50 per 10 HPF
- Immunohistochemistry
  - S100(+), CD1a(+), langerin (+)
    - Expression of CD1a and langerin can be focal
    - Langerin and CD1a strong positivity separates LCS from IDC
- Birbeck granules (+/-) by electron microscopy

Histiocytic Sarcoma
- *BRAF* V600E mutations commonly found
- Tumor cells typically have epithelioid appearance without spindling
- Immunohistochemistry
  - CD68(+), CD163(+), lysozyme (+/-), S100(-/+)

SELECTED REFERENCES

1. Jenei A et al: Potential role of MAP2K1 mutation in the trans-differentiation of interdigitating dendritic cell sarcoma: case report and literature review. Front Pediatr. 10:959307, 2022
2. Massoth LR et al: Histiocytic and dendritic cell sarcomas of hematopoietic origin share targetable genomic alterations distinct from follicular dendritic cell sarcoma. Oncologist. 26(7):e1263-72, 2021
3. Tian X et al: Expression of enhancer of zeste homolog 2 (EZH2) protein in histiocytic and dendritic cell neoplasms with evidence for p-ERK1/2-related, but not MYC- or p-STAT3-related cell signaling. Mod Pathol. 31(4):553-61, 2018
4. Xue T et al: Interdigitating dendritic cell sarcoma: clinicopathologic study of 8 cases with review of the literature. Ann Diagn Pathol. 34:155-60, 2018
5. Ninkovic S et al: Interdigitating dendritic cell sarcoma: diagnostic pitfalls, treatment challenges and role of transdifferentiation in pathogenesis. Pathology. 49(6):643-6, 2017

Interdigitating Dendritic Cell Sarcoma

Hemophagocytosis

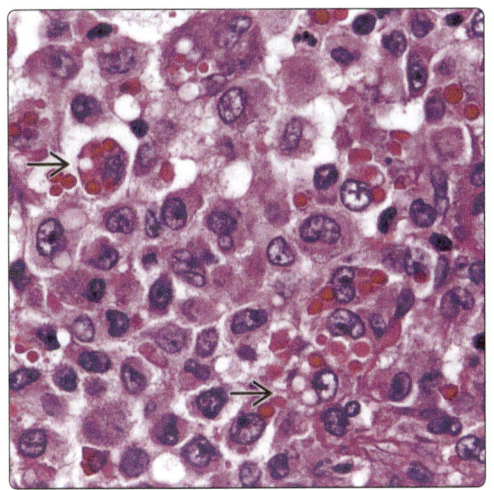

Transdifferentiation

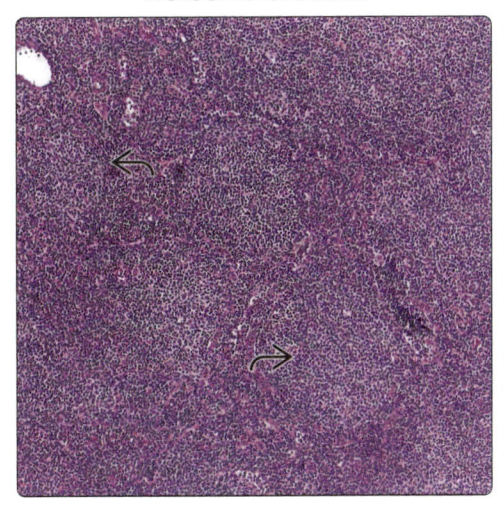

(Left) IDCS shows considerable atypia. The neoplastic cells have abundant eosinophilic cytoplasm and folded nuclei. Hemophagocytosis ➡ was prominent in this neoplasm. (Right) Follicular lymphoma grade 1-2 ➡ is shown. This patient later developed IDCS. Transdifferentiation is the concept in which patients with B-cell lymphoma develop histiocytic or dendritic cell tumors.

Vimentin Immunohistochemistry

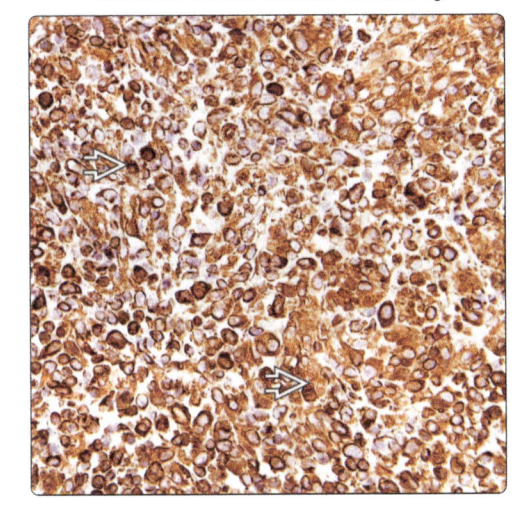

CD68 Immunohistochemistry

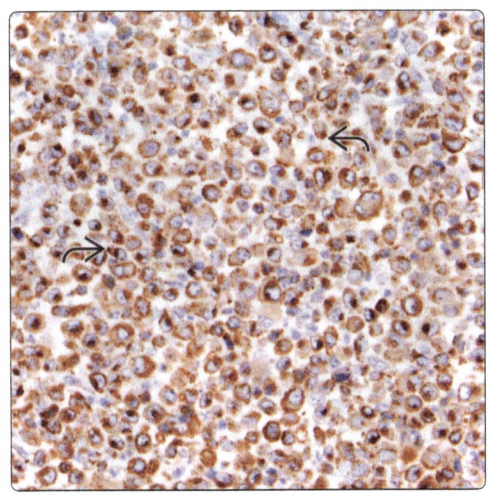

(Left) Vimentin is strongly positive ➡ in the neoplastic cells of this IDCS. The neoplastic cells were also positive for S100 (not shown). (Right) In this example of IDCS involving adipose tissue, the neoplastic cells are positive for CD68 ➡ and were negative for CD163 (not shown).

Fascin Immunohistochemistry

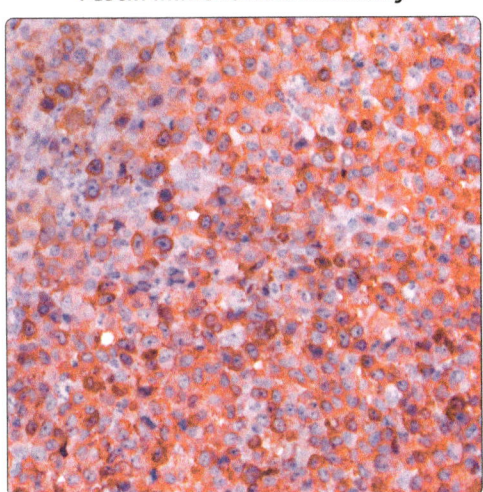

CD43 Immunohistochemistry

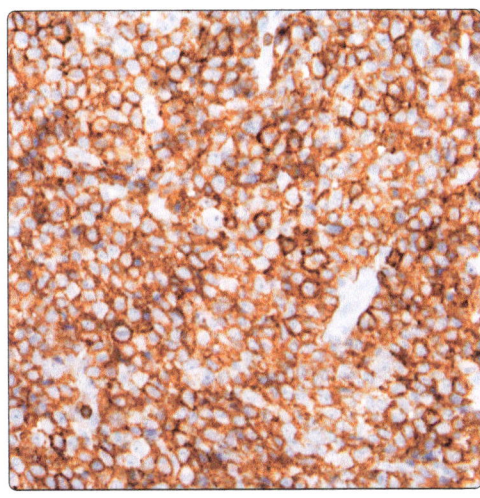

(Left) IDCS involving adipose tissue is shown. The neoplastic cells were positive for fascin and negative for clusterin and CD21 (not shown). (Right) IDCS involving adipose tissue is shown. The neoplastic cells were positive for CD43 and negative for CD3 (not shown).

Follicular Dendritic Cell Sarcoma

KEY FACTS

TERMINOLOGY
- Neoplastic proliferation of follicular dendritic cells (FDCs)
- Recognized sarcoma by WHO and ICC

CLINICAL ISSUES
- Presents as slow-growing, painless mass
- Low- to intermediate-grade soft tissue sarcoma
  - Local excision, frequent recurrence
- Some cases found with hyaline vascular Castleman disease
  - Both have dysplastic follicular dendritic cells

MOLECULAR
- Complex cytogenetics reported
- NFκB pathway alterations, including *BIRC3*, *CYLD*, *NFKBIA*, *SOCS3*, and *TNFAIP2*
- Tumor suppressor genes, such as *CDKN2A*, *RB1*, and *TP53*
- *BRAF* V600E mutations in ~ 18% of cases
- Clonal *IGH* rearrangement in subset of cases

MICROSCOPIC
- Spindled to ovoid cells forming fascicles, storiform arrays, whorls, diffuse sheets, or nodular growth pattern
- Morphologic variants
  - Spindled (typical) or epithelioid
  - Inflammatory pseudotumor-like variant
- High-grade features correlate with aggressive clinical course
- Small lymphocytes interspersed with tumor cells

ANCILLARY TESTS
- Immunophenotype
  - Positive immunostaining for ≥ 2 FDC markers
  - Variable expression of CD21, CD23, CD35, CXCL13, clusterin, and EGFR

TOP DIFFERENTIAL DIAGNOSES
- Interdigitating dendritic cell sarcoma
- Langerhans cell histiocytosis/sarcoma

Spindle Cells

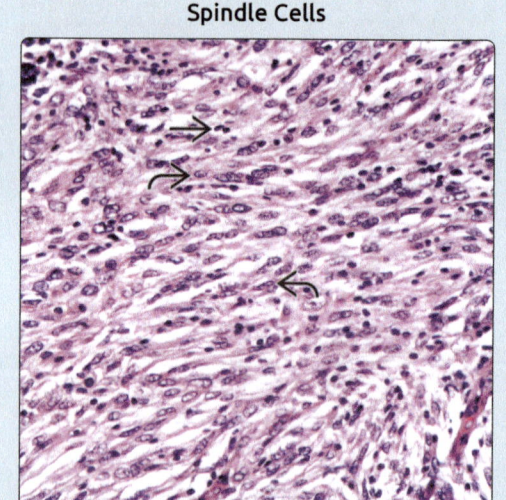

CD21 Immunohistochemistry

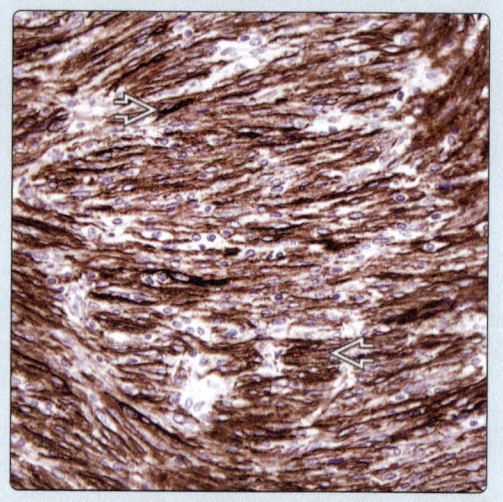

(Left) Lymph node with follicular dendritic cell sarcoma (FDCS) shows spindle cells predominantly arranged in short fascicles. The tumor cells are intimately associated with small lymphocytes. (Right) CD21 is expressed in FDCS involving lymph node. FDC typically expresses CD21.

Complex Karyotype

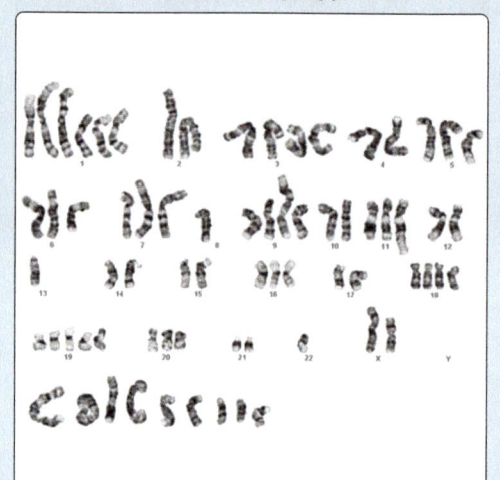

Clonal *IGH* Rearrangement

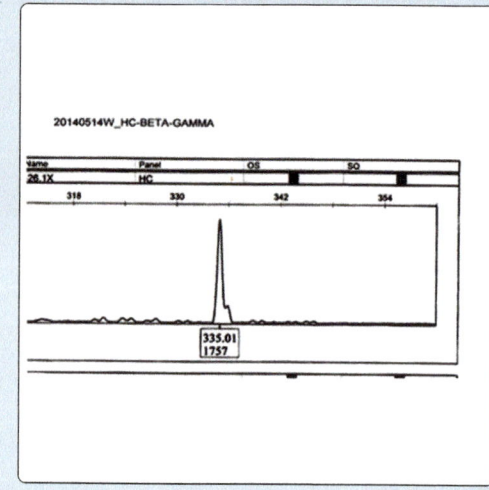

(Left) Complex karyotypes may be seen in FDCS. Chromosome 7 abnormalities have been specifically noted. (Courtesy M. Kempik, MD and D. O'Malley, MD.) (Right) *IGH* rearrangement shows a monoclonal peak. A subset of FDCS can show *IGH* rearrangement.

Follicular Dendritic Cell Sarcoma

TERMINOLOGY

Abbreviations
- Follicular dendritic cell sarcoma (FDCS)

Synonyms
- Dendritic reticulum cell sarcoma

Definitions
- Neoplasm of spindle to ovoid cells consisting of FDCs, expressing FDC markers, usually intermediate in grade
- Recognized sarcoma by the WHO and ICC

ETIOLOGY/PATHOGENESIS

Normal Follicular Dendritic Cells
- Stromal-derived cells localized to B-cell areas in primary and secondary lymphoid follicles
  - Form meshworks via cell-to-cell attachments and desmosomes
- Present antigens to B cells that are involved in B-cell proliferation and differentiation
- Closely related to bone marrow stromal progenitors
  - Have features of myofibroblasts
  - Express antigens related to bone marrow stroma progenitor cells, including CD21, CD23, and CD35

Etiology of Follicular Dendritic Cell Neoplasm
- Hyaline vascular Castleman disease (HVCD) is associated with subset of cases
  - Both HVCD and FDCS have dysplastic FDCs
  - Similar clonal populations have been seen in patient's with both HVCD and FDCS
  - EGFR overexpression has been seen in both FDC sarcomas and dysplastic FDCs of HVCD
- Autoimmune disease also found with some cases
  - Myasthenia gravis and paraneoplastic pemphigus

CLINICAL ISSUES

Epidemiology
- Incidence
  - Rare
- Age
  - Adults
    - Median: 50 years
- Sex
  - No preference
    - Inflammatory pseudotumor-like variant shows female predominance
- Ethnicity
  - More commonly reported in East Asia

Site
- Lymph nodes (~ 30% of cases)
  - Cervical and abdominal lymph nodes most common
- Extranodal sites (~ 70% of cases)
  - Most common in abdomen
  - Can occur in any anatomic site
- Inflammatory pseudotumor-like variant of FDCS
  - Intraabdominal sites, including liver and spleen

Presentation
- Usually slow-growing, painless mass or isolated lymphadenopathy
- Systemic symptoms
  - Common in patients with inflammatory pseudotumor-like variant but otherwise rare in FDCS
  - Fever and weight loss

Treatment
- Complete surgical excision
  - ± adjuvant radiotherapy or chemotherapy

Prognosis
- Most cases behave like low- to intermediate-grade soft tissue sarcoma
  - Local recurrences occur in ~ 40% of patients
  - Metastases in ~ 25% of patients

MOLECULAR

Cytogenetics
- Complex karyotypes can be found
  - Loss of multiple chromosomes
    - Chromosome 7 abnormalities containing *EGFR* locus are reported
  - Cytogenetically diverse findings

Molecular Genetics
- NFkB pathway alterations
  - *BIRC3*, *CYLD*, *NFKBIA*, *SOCS3*, and *TNFAIP2* reported in ~ 50%
- Tumor suppressor genes
  - *CDKN2A*, *RB1*, and *TP53* reported in ~ 25%
- *BRAF* V600E mutations in ~ 18%
- *FDCSP* and *SRGN* expression
- *CD274* (PDL1) and *PDCD1LG2* (PDL2) gains in copy number
- *JAK2* and *BRAF* deletion have been reported
- *HDGFL3::SHC4* fusion in few cases
- Mutations in *KRAS*, *NRAS*, and *PIK3CA* have **not** been reported

In Situ Hybridization
- EBER(-) except in inflammatory pseudotumor-like variant in spleen and liver locations
- *EGFR*
  - Does not show *EGFR* amplification

Polymerase Chain Reaction
- *IGH* rearrangement may be clonal in small subset of cases
  - Presence of *IGH* rearrangement does not exclude diagnosis of FDCS

MICROSCOPIC

Histologic Features
- Spindled to oval neoplastic cells
  - Form fascicles, storiform arrays, whorls, diffuse sheets, or nodular growth patterns
  - Multiple patterns can be seen in same tumor
- Accompanied by reactive inflammatory cells
  - Lymphocytes, plasma cells, and histiocytes
  - Lymphocytes often aggregate around blood vessels or at periphery of tumor

Follicular Dendritic Cell Sarcoma

- FDC neoplasm associated with HVCD
  - HVCD
    - ± regressed (involuted) germinal centers with hyalinization
    - Thick and hyalinized blood vessel walls
    - Vascular proliferation in interfollicular areas
  - Proliferation of FDCs
    - In large sheets, nodular or confluent
    - Often CXCL13(+)

Cytologic Features

- Neoplastic cells with indistinct cell borders and moderate amount of cytoplasm
- Nuclei
  - Oval or elongated with vesicular or granular, finely dispersed chromatin
  - Small but distinct nucleoli
  - Delicate nuclear membranes
  - Nuclear pseudoinclusions are common
  - Binucleated (like normal FDCs) often present
- High-grade FDCS
  - Marked nuclear pleomorphism, cytologic atypia, prominent nucleoli
  - Many mitotic figures

ANCILLARY TESTS

Immunohistochemistry

- 1 or more FDC-associated markers are expressed
  - CD21, CD23, CD35, clusterin, CXCL13, FDCSP, podoplanin (D2-40), SRGN, and SSTR2
  - Reactivity can be patchy and focal
    - Especially in high-grade tumors, epithelioid variant, or inflammatory pseudotumor-like variant
    - CXCL13, CD21, and clusterin are most often positive
    - CD21, CD23, CD35, and clusterin are most specific for FDCS
- Desmoplakin, EGFR, vimentin, fascin, PD-L1 are usually (+)
- Rare cases can be (+) for CD4, CD30, CD31, CD68, CD163, CD45RB, CD20, EMA, keratin, and S100
- Variable Ki-67 proliferative index from 5-75%
- CD1a, langerin, CD123, and CD163 (-)
  - Help exclude Langerhans cell histiocytosis, interdigitating dendritic cell sarcoma (IDCS), blastic plasmacytoid dendritic cell neoplasm, and histiocytic sarcoma
- TDT(+) small cells can be present, indicating indolent T-lymphoblastic proliferation

Electron Microscopy

- Numerous interwoven long villous processes that are connected by desmosomes
- Abundant organelles, including mitochondria and endoplasmic reticulum
- Birbeck granules (-)

DIFFERENTIAL DIAGNOSIS

Interdigitating Dendritic Cell Sarcoma

- Neoplasm most closely related to FDCS
- Physiologic counterpart, IDC, plays important part in antigen presentation, though it appears to be more closely associated to Langerhans cells than FDCs
- Like FDCS, IDCS typically consists of spindle cells arranged in fascicular pattern with bland cytology and admixed lymphocytes
- Unlike FDCS, IDCS is typically CD45(+) and FDC markers (-)
  - CD21, CD23, and CD35 (-)
  - S100(+), vimentin (+)
  - Fascin (+), CD68(+/-), lysozyme (+/-)
  - HMB-45(-), CD1a(-), langerin (-)
- Ultrastructure
  - Complex interdigitating cell processes but no well-formed desmosomes
  - No Birbeck granules
- Appears to be more clinically aggressive than FDC neoplasm

Inflammatory Myofibroblastic Tumor

- Morphologically resembles inflammatory pseudotumor-like variant of FDCS
- Can show proliferations of FDCs
  - Usually seen in liver and spleen
- Spindle cells are myofibroblasts
  - Vimentin (+), actin (+), desmin (+)
  - ALK(+) in ~ 60% of cases
  - FDC-associated markers usually (-), EBER (-)

Langerhans Cell Histiocytosis/Sarcoma

- Mainly intrasinusoidal pattern of distribution in lymph nodes with secondary infiltration of paracortex
- Langerhans cells are oval with grooved, folded, indented, or lobulated nuclei
- Admixed with variable number of eosinophils, histiocytes, neutrophils, and small lymphocytes
- Immunohistochemistry
  - CD1a(+), langerin (+), S100(+)
  - Vimentin (+), CD68(+)
  - FDC-associated markers (-)
- Electron microscopy
  - Birbeck granules (+)
  - No desmosomes/junctional specializations

SELECTED REFERENCES

1. Kafaei L et al: Follicular dendritic cell sarcoma in the setting of Castleman disease. Br J Haematol. 197(5):512, 2022
2. Massoth LR et al: Histiocytic and dendritic cell sarcomas of hematopoietic origin share targetable genomic alterations distinct from follicular dendritic cell sarcoma. Oncologist. 26(7):e1263-72, 2021
3. Nagy A et al: Next-generation sequencing of idiopathic multicentric and unicentric Castleman disease and follicular dendritic cell sarcomas. Blood Adv. 2(5):481-91, 2018
4. Andersen EF et al: Genomic analysis of follicular dendritic cell sarcoma by molecular inversion probe array reveals tumor suppressor-driven biology. Mod Pathol. 0(9):1321-34, 2017
5. Davila JI et al: Comprehensive genomic profiling of a rare thyroid follicular dendritic cell sarcoma. Rare Tumors. 9(2):6834, 2017
6. Facchetti F et al: Histiocytic and dendritic cell neoplasms: what have we learnt by studying 67 cases. Virchows Arch. 471(4):467-89, 2017

Follicular Dendritic Cell Sarcoma

Elongated Neoplastic Cells

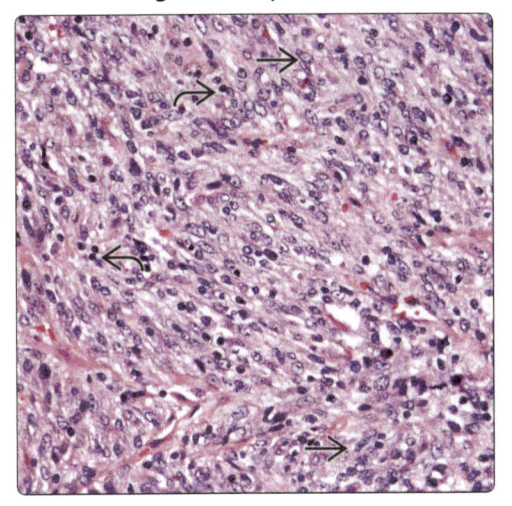

Lymphocytes Associated With Neoplasia

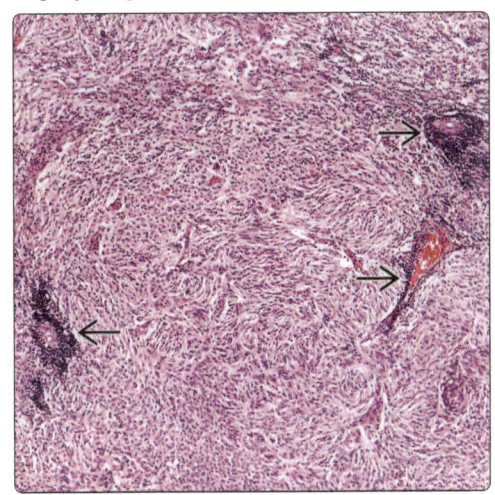

(Left) FDC neoplasm involving a lymph node shows elongated neoplastic cells with low-grade histologic features ➡. The background inflammatory cells can include small lymphocytes ➡, plasma cells, and histiocytes. *(Right)* Neoplastic cells are shown admixed with small lymphocytes. The lymphocytes are often aggregated around the blood vessels ➡.

Vimentin Immunohistochemistry

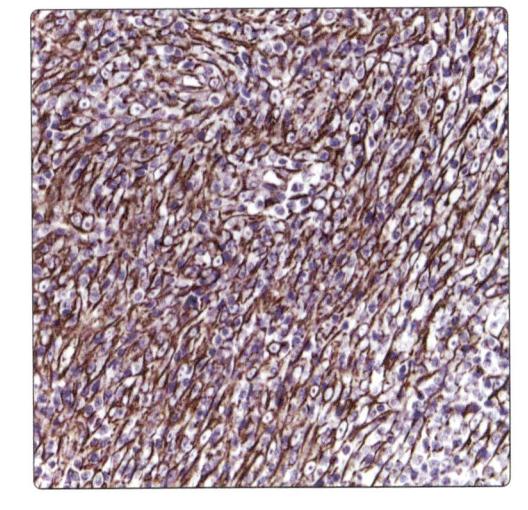

CD35 Immunohistochemistry

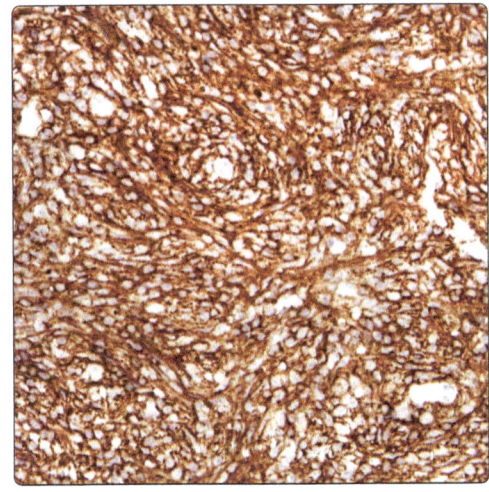

(Left) Vimentin stain of an FDC neoplasm involving lymph node is shown. The neoplastic cells are strongly highlighted by vimentin. *(Right)* The term FDC marker is used for CD21, CD23, and CD35, which are all positive in FDC neoplasms. Here, CD35 strongly and diffusely marks the neoplasm.

CD23 Immunohistochemistry

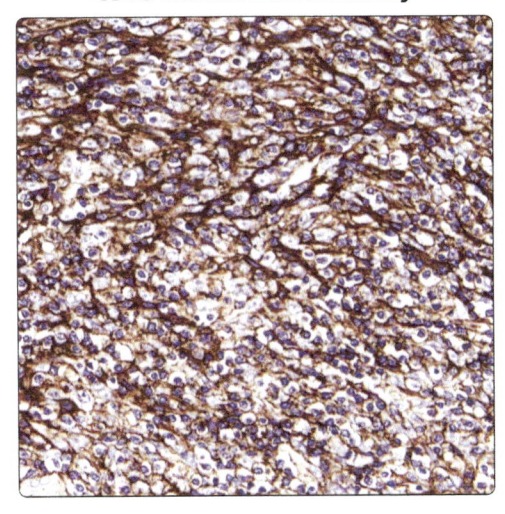

EGFR Immunohistochemistry

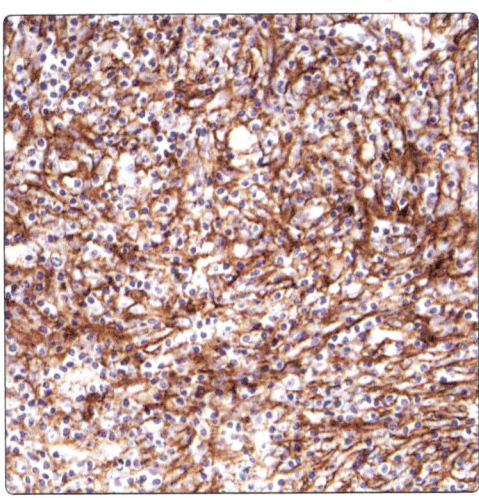

(Left) CD23 stain is strongly positive in this nodal FDC neoplasm. *(Right)* Epidermal growth factor receptor (EGFR) is strongly positive in an FDC neoplasm. FISH for EGFR has not shown amplification of the gene.

SECTION 8
Molecular Pathology of Solid Tumors

Head and Neck, Including Sinonasal Tumors and Salivary Glands

HPV-Associated Head and Neck Carcinomas	494
Head and Neck Mucosal Squamous Cell Carcinoma, Non-HPV Related	500
Important Alterations in Non-HPV-Related Head and Neck Squamous Cell Carcinoma	506
Translocation-Specific Salivary Gland Tumors	508
Translocation-Specific Salivary Gland Tumors (Continued)	518
Nasopharyngeal EBV-Related Squamous Cell Carcinoma	526
Other Head and Neck Tumors	530

Thyroid

Papillary Thyroid Carcinoma	538
Follicular Thyroid Carcinoma	542
Poorly Differentiated Thyroid Carcinoma	546
Anaplastic Thyroid Carcinoma	550
Medullary Thyroid Carcinoma	554

Lung

Adenocarcinoma, Lung	560
Squamous Cell Carcinoma, Lung	568
Small Cell Neuroendocrine Carcinoma	572
Mesothelioma	576

Luminal Gastrointestinal Tract

Gastric Adenocarcinoma	580
Colorectal Adenocarcinoma and Precancerous Lesions	584
Gastrointestinal Stromal Tumor	590

Liver

HNF1A-Inactivated Hepatocellular Adenoma	598
β-Catenin-Activated Hepatocellular Adenoma	602
Inflammatory Hepatocellular Adenoma	606
Hepatocellular Carcinoma	610

Pancreaticobiliary

Pancreatic Ductal Adenocarcinoma	614
Pancreatic Mucinous Cystic Neoplasm	618
Pancreatic Intraductal Papillary Mucinous Neoplasm	620
Cholangiocarcinoma	622

Testis

Testicular Germ Cell Tumors	624

Kidney

Clear Cell Renal Cell Carcinoma	630
Chromophobe Renal Cell Carcinoma	634
Papillary Renal Cell Carcinoma	636
TFE3-Rearranged and TFEB-Altered Renal Cell Carcinomas	638
Wilms Tumor	642
Clear Cell Sarcoma of Kidney	648
Oncocytoma	650
Rhabdoid Tumor of Kidney	652

Bladder

Urothelial Carcinoma	654

Adrenal

Pheochromocytoma/Paraganglioma	660
Adrenal Cortical Carcinoma	666
Neuroblastoma	672
Adrenal Cortical Adenoma	680

Prostate

Prostatic Adenocarcinoma, Acinar Type and High-Grade Prostatic Intraepithelial Neoplasia	684

Breast

ADH and DCIS (Dysplastic, Premalignant)	688
Ductal Carcinomas	694
Lobular Carcinoma	700
Invasive Ductal Carcinoma of No Special Type With Medullary Features	706
Metaplastic Breast Carcinoma	710
Phyllodes Tumors	716
Basal-Like and Triple-Negative Breast Carcinomas	720

Cervix/Vulva/Vagina

Preneoplastic Conditions, Cervix/Vulva/Vagina	730
Squamous Cell Carcinoma, Cervix/Vulva/Vagina	734
Adenocarcinoma, Cervix/Vulva/Vagina	738

Uterus

Endometrial Intraepithelial Neoplasia	742
Uterine Endometrioid Carcinoma	744
Uterine Serous Carcinoma	748
Clear Cell Carcinoma, Uterus	750
Uterine Sarcomas	754

Ovaries/Fallopian Tube

Serous Tumors of Ovary and Fallopian Tube	762
Other Surface Epithelial Tumors of Ovary	768
Sex Cord-Stromal Tumors of Ovary	774
Germ Cell Tumor, Ovary	780

Skin

Premalignant Conditions, Skin	784
Melanoma	788
Squamous Cell Carcinoma, Skin	792
Basal Cell Carcinoma, Skin	796
Sebaceous Tumors	800
Dermatofibroma and Dermatofibrosarcoma Protuberans	802

Bone

Overview of Molecular Pathology of Bone and Soft Tissue Tumors	804
Osteosarcomas	810
Ewing Sarcoma	818
Other Small Round Blue Cell Sarcomas	824
Giant Cell Tumor of Bone	832
Intermediate and Malignant Cartilaginous Tumors of Bone	838

Soft Tissue

Intermediate and Malignant Myofibroblastic/Fibroblastic Tumors	848
Liposarcomas	858
Muscle Sarcomas	868
Intermediate and Malignant Vascular Tumors	878
Malignant Peripheral Nerve Sheath Tumor	886
Representative Genetic Findings in Bone and Soft Tissue Tumors	892

Sarcomas of Uncertain Differentiation

Rare Sarcomas of Uncertain Differentiation With Specific Molecular Alterations	898
Rare Sarcomas of Uncertain Differentiation With Specific Molecular Alterations (Continued)	908

CNS

Glioblastoma, IDH Wildtype	916
Astrocytoma, IDH-Mutant	920
Pilocytic Astrocytoma	924
Oligodendroglioma, IDH Mutant, and 1p/19q Codeleted	928
Ependymal Tumors	932
Medulloblastoma	938
Choroid Plexus Tumors	944
Meningioma	948
Retinoblastoma	952

HPV-Associated Head and Neck Carcinomas

KEY FACTS

ETIOLOGY/PATHOGENESIS
- HPV-16 E6 and E7 oncoproteins disrupt RB1 and TP53 pathways, leading to unchecked cell growth and genetic instability
- HPV-associated head and neck carcinoma patients may also have HPV-negative head and neck mucosal squamous cell carcinoma (HNMSCC) risk factors, such as high alcohol &/or tobacco use

CLINICAL ISSUES
- Most commonly located in oropharynx
  - Oropharyngeal HPV HNMSCC usually has better prognosis than HPV-negative HNMSCC
- HPV+ poorly differentiated neuroendocrine carcinoma (PDNEC) of head and neck is aggressive and appears to behave similarly to HPV-negative high-grade NEC

MICROSCOPIC
- HPV+HNMSCC
  - Nonkeratinizing, immature, basal-like in most cases
  - Unusual histologies include
    - Hybrid: Immature nests with abrupt central keratinization
    - Adenosquamous carcinoma, including some with cilia
    - Undifferentiated carcinoma (lymphoepithelial nasopharyngeal-type morphology) in oropharynx
    - Papillary squamous cell carcinoma
    - Keratinizing squamous cell carcinoma

ANCILLARY TESTS
- All HPV-associated head and neck carcinomas: Overexpression of p16 protein occurs in 95%
  - Diffuse strong expression in tumor cells (> 70%) highly correlates with HPV infection
- Confirmatory high-risk HPV testing required to accurately diagnose morphologically atypical HPV+HNMSCC and HPV-related multiphenotypic sinonasal carcinoma (HMSC)

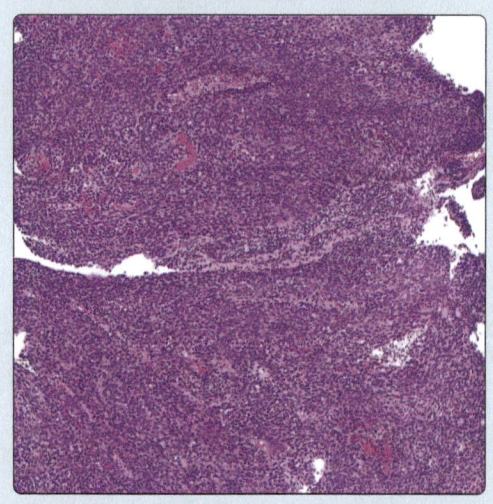

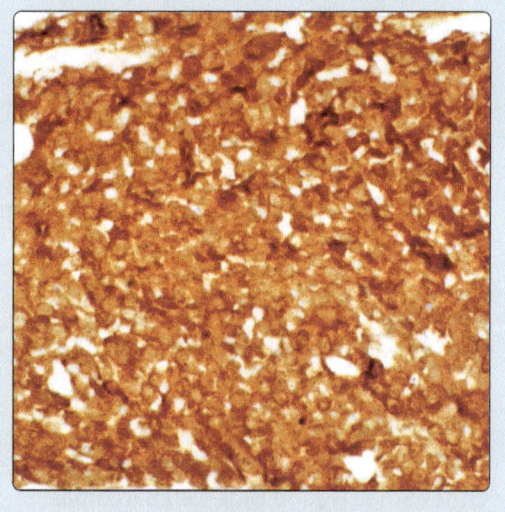

(Left) The most common morphology of human papillomavirus-associated head and neck mucosal squamous cell carcinoma (HPV+HNMSCC) comprises ribbons or nests of basal-like cells that resemble tonsillar crypt nonkeratinizing small squamous cells. **(Right)** About 95% of oropharyngeal HPV+HNMSCC express p16 strongly and diffusely (> 70% cells with nuclear &/or cytoplasmic reactivity).

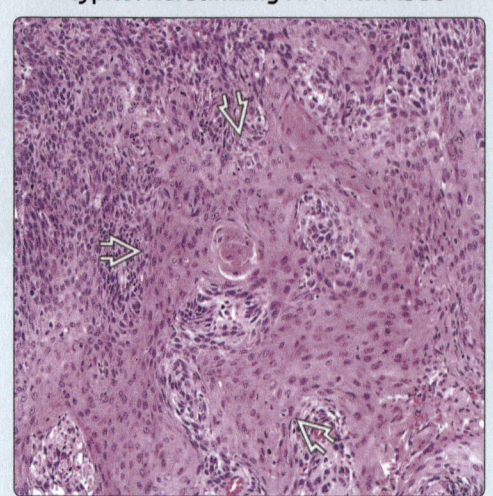

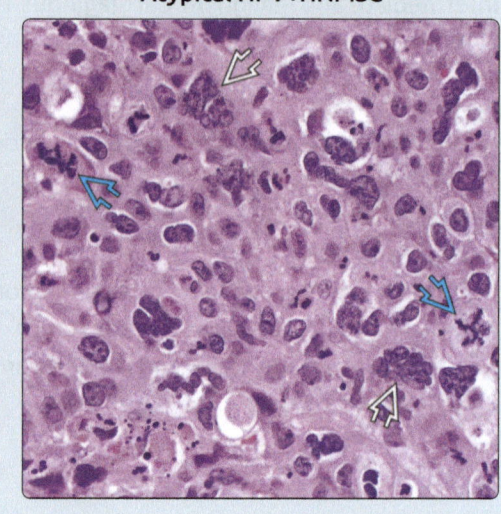

(Left) HPV+HNMSCC from the base of the tongue shows extensive keratinization ➡, an atypical feature. HPV ISH confirmed the presence of the virus. **(Right)** This base of tongue ISH-proven HPV+HNMSCC shows unusual pleomorphism with multinucleation ➡ and atypical mitoses ➡. Because of unconventional histologic features, HPV ISH testing was appropriately performed.

HPV-Associated Head and Neck Carcinomas

TERMINOLOGY

Abbreviations
- Head and neck mucosal squamous cell carcinoma, human papillomavirus associated (HPV+HNMSCC)
- HPV-related multiphenotypic sinonasal carcinoma (HMSC)
- HPV-associated poorly differentiated neuroendocrine carcinoma (HPV+PDNEC)
- Nasopharyngeal carcinoma, HPV-associated (HPV+NPC)

Synonyms
- HPV-related multiphenotypic sinonasal carcinoma was previously called HPV-related carcinoma with adenoid cystic carcinoma-like features

Definitions
- Following 4 entities are head and neck carcinomas associated with HPV
  - HPV+HNMSCC: Invasive, HPV-induced carcinoma of head and neck mucosa composed of malignant squamous cells
  - HMSC: HPV-related sinonasal carcinoma showing salivary tumor-like morphology, positivity for high-risk (HR) HPV, and relatively indolent behavior
  - HPV+PDNEC: High-grade neuroendocrine carcinoma (small cell or large cell morphology) positive for high HR HPV
  - HPV+NPC: Primary carcinoma of nasopharynx positive for HR HPV

ETIOLOGY/PATHOGENESIS

HPV+HNMSCC Infection by HPV Types 16 and 18
- HPV-16 is much more common than HPV-18 (90-95% of all cases)
- Risk factors include
  - High lifetime number of vaginal &/or oral sex partners
  - Seropositivity for HPV viral capsid protein antibodies (15x increased risk)
- Patients may also have non-HPV risk factors, such as high alcohol &/or tobacco use
- Deregulation of cell cycle and apoptosis activation
  - E6 and E7 viral oncoproteins disrupt RB1 (cell cycle) and TP53 (apoptosis) pathways
- Genetic somatic polymorphisms in *TGFB1* and *MDM4* increase risk for developing invasive squamous carcinoma in HPV-infected patients

Other HPV-Associated Head and Neck Carcinomas
- HMSC
  - Most common subtype is HPV-33
- HPV+PDNEC
  - May arise from underlying HPV+HNMSCC

CLINICAL ISSUES

Epidemiology
- Age
  - HPV+HNMSCC: Mostly middle-aged adults
    - On average, 5 years younger than patients with non-HPV HNMSCC
  - Other HPV-associated head and neck carcinomas
    - HMSC: Broad age range from 3rd to 10th decade; average: early 50s
    - HPV+PDNEC: Similar to non-HPV-related PDNEC
    - HPV+NPC: Similar to non-HPV-related NPC
- Sex
  - HPV+HNMSCC: Male predominance
  - HMSC: Slight female predominance

Presentation
- HPV+HNMSCC
  - Mass-like lesion, most commonly in oropharynx
  - Mostly involve palatine tonsils, base of tongue, soft palate
  - Tonsil primary site in ~ 40%
  - May initially present as positive cervical lymph node and occult primary tumor
  - ~ 80% of newly diagnosed oropharynx SCC in USA
    - Most common HNMSCC in nonsmokers and nondrinkers
- HPV+PDNEC: Commonly presents as high-stage oropharyngeal tumor
- HMSC: Commonly presents as large sinonasal mass; usually involves nasal cavity
- HPV+NPC: Can present with positive neck lymph node and occult primary tumor

Treatment
- HPV+HNMSCC
  - Various approaches: Surgical resection with adjuvant chemotherapy or radiation, surgery alone, or radiation alone
    - Deescalation protocol: Less aggressive therapy used in selected patients
      - Reduces iatrogenic morbidity in patients with less aggressive disease
  - Vaccination against HPV high-risk subtypes serves as preventive measure
- Other HPV-associated head and neck carcinomas
  - Too rare to fully determine best treatment protocols
  - HMSC may be treated similar to HPV+HNMSCC
  - HPV+PDNEC is currently treated like small cell carcinoma
  - HPV+NPC may be treated similar to HPV-negative NPC

Prognosis
- Most HPV+HNMSCC have better prognosis than HPV-negative HNMSCC
  - 5-year survival for oropharyngeal HPV+HNMSCC vs. oropharyngeal HPV-negative HNMSCC: ~ 90% vs. ~ 60%, respectively
  - Reasons for improved survival in HPV+HNMSCC incompletely understood
    - Possible factors: Younger age, fewer comorbidities, no alcohol- or tobacco-induced field effect changes, less aggressive genetic alterations in HPV+HNMSCC compared to HPV-negative, more capable immune response, different oral flora, increased radiosensitivity
  - Best predictors of outcome: HPV status and tumor stage
    - Various molecular aberrations cited as prognostic but are not as validated as tumor stage and HPV status

HPV-Associated Head and Neck Carcinomas

- Mutated genes associated with recurrent HPV+HNMSCC or oropharynx: *TSC2, BRIP1, NBN, TACC3, STK11, HRAS, PIK3R1, TP63, FAT1*
  - Behavior of HPV+HNMSCC located at nonoropharyngeal mucosal sites: Not well characterized and likely dissimilar to oropharyngeal HPV-negative HNMSCC
  - Mostly high-stage disease
    – Only 30% of HNMSCC patients (HPV and non-HPV related) are diagnosed at early stage
- Other HPV-associated head and neck carcinomas
  - HMSC: Relatively indolent with few lymph node metastases and no deaths despite T3 or T4 stage
  - HPV+PDNEC: Aggressive tumor with short survival
  - HPV+NPC: May behave similarly to HPV-negative NPC

MOLECULAR

Overview

- HPV+HNMSCC
  - Exhibits marked genetic complexity
  - Some overlap with HPV-negative HNMSCC molecular alterations but also important differences
    – *TP53* mutations and *EGFR* amplification **rare** in HPV+HNMSCC compared to HPV-negative HNMSCC
    – miRNA signature differs
  - Abnormal immune response found in both HPV+HNMSCC and HPV-negative HNMSCC
  - Predisposition to developing invasive carcinoma conferred in part by specific somatic genetic polymorphisms

Cytogenetics

- HPV+HNMSCC more often diploid or near diploid, whereas HPV-negative HNMSCC often complex with tetraploidization

In Situ Hybridization

- All HPV-associated head and neck carcinomas
  - DNA in situ hybridization (ISH) or RNA ISH to detect E6/E7 mRNA
  - ISH results highly concordant with p16 results and qRT-PCR for E6/E7 mRNA
  - Presence of *E6* and *E7* mRNA considered most definitive evidence for **transforming** HPV infection

PCR

- HPV subtypes identified by E6/E7-specific qRT-PCR or multiplex PCR for more high-risk subtypes

Chromosomal Microarray

- HNMSCC-+HPV
  - Copy number gains
    – 3q26-28 (*SOX2/TP63/PIK3CA*) often gained as found also in HPV-negative HNMSCC
    – But *EGFR* and *CCND1* **not** gained as is common in HPV-negative HNMSCC
  - Copy number losses
    – *ATM* commonly lost compared to HPV-negative HNMSCC
    – **No** loss of 3p, *UBR5*, or *CDKN2A* as may be found in HPV-negative HNMSCC

Molecular Genetics of HPV+HNMSCC

- Overexpressed HPV E7 oncoprotein: Inactivates RB1 protein → secondary upregulation of p16 expression by feedback pathways
- Overexpressed HPV E6 oncoprotein: Inactivates p53 protein by ubiquitination
- Altered pathways (protein-protein interaction networks)
  - DNA damage pathway (*BRCA1/BRCA2*, Fanconi anemia genes, *ATM*), FGF pathway, JAK/STAT signaling, immunology-related genes (*HLA-A, HLA-B*) altered more commonly in HPV+HNMSCC
  - PI3K signaling, NOTCH aberrations, SMAD signaling often abnormal in both HPV+HNMSCC and HPV-negative HNMSCC
- HPV+HNMSCC differs from HPV-negative HNMSCC in some specific mutated genes
  - Higher rate of fibroblast growth factor receptor 2/3 (*FGFR2* and *FGFR3*), *DDX3X, KRAS, NF1, FBXW7*, and *BRCA1/BRCA2* mutations than in HPV-negative HNMSCC
- HPV+HNMSCC shares some specific gene alterations with HPV-negative HNMSCC
  - *PIK3CA, KMT2A, NOTCH1* changes
- HPV+HNMSCC patients with smoking history may show tobacco-related mutations, such as in *TP53* and amplification of *EGFR*

Molecular Genetics of Other HPV-Associated Head and Neck Carcinomas

- Too few cases studied to date

MICROSCOPIC

Histologic Features

- HPV+HNMSCC
  - Nonkeratinizing basal-like cells forming nests and ribbons in most cases
    – Cellular, relatively monomorphic tumor cells with hyperchromatic nuclei and high N:C ratio
    – Often have high mitotic rate (high Ki-67 by IHC)
    – Frequent prominent apoptosis and comedonecrosis
  - Hybrid morphology
    – Focal keratinization that is usually abrupt and central in nest of tumor cells
    – Same prognosis as conventional nonkeratinizing type
  - Uncommon HPV-positive histologies include
    – Basaloid SCC, lymphoepithelial carcinoma-like, papillary or nonpapillary keratinizing SCC, adenosquamous carcinoma, including some with cilia
      - Seem to have similar relatively good prognosis as for conventional histology
- HPV-related multiphenotypic sinonasal carcinoma
  - Looks like basaloid or biphasic salivary gland tumor; most commonly adenoid cystic carcinoma but can also be sarcomatoid
    – Usually has solid growth at least focally
  - Overlying mucosa often (70%) shows marked cytologic atypia
- HPV-positive PDNEC
  - Looks like non-HPV associated high-grade NEC, either small cell or large cell type or mixed
- HPV-positive NPC

HPV-Associated Head and Neck Carcinomas

○ Looks like non-HPV-associated NPC; any 1 of 3 histologies; most commonly nonkeratinizing differentiated type

ANCILLARY TESTS

Immunohistochemistry

- Most head and neck HPV-associated carcinomas show marked overexpression of p16 protein
  ○ Surrogate for HPV status when tumor is located in oropharynx or sinonasal region shows appropriate HMSC morphology
  ○ Diffuse strong expression in tumor cells (> 70%) = high correlation with HPV infection
  ○ Rare cases are p16 negative (~ 5%)
  ○ Rare oropharyngeal SCC are diffusely p16 positive but negative for HPV by FISH
    – May behave as well as HPV-positive FISH cases
  ○ Some cases of cutaneous squamous cell carcinoma or HPV-negative HNMSCC are p16 diffusely positive, including those in lymph nodes
    – If there is no oropharyngeal mass, positive node requires HPV testing to confirm or exclude HPV infection
- HPV-related multiphenotypic sinonasal carcinoma
  ○ Commonly shows same cell phenotypes as non-HPV related adenoid cystic carcinoma
    – IHC results are not discriminatory: HMSC is often positive for C-kit, S100, p63 in myoepithelial cells; SOX10, MYB, and p16
  ○ Usually requires HR HPV testing to confirm diagnosis
- HPV-associated PDNEC
  ○ Similar neuroendocrine marker profile as in non-HPV associated NEC
    – Insulinoma-associated protein 1 (INSM1): New marker highly sensitive and specific for neuroendocrine differentiation
  ○ Diffusely p16 positive
- Nasopharyngeal undifferentiated carcinoma, HPV associated
  ○ Diffusely p16 positive
  ○ Similar keratin reactivity pattern as in non-HPV-related NPC

DIFFERENTIAL DIAGNOSIS

DDx for HPV+HNMSCC

- HPV-negative HNMSCC
  ○ More keratinizing and well differentiated than conventional HPV+HNMSCC
  ○ Usually lacks diffuse expression of p16
  ○ Can occur in oropharynx
  ○ Accounts for most squamous cell carcinomas in head and neck mucosal sites outside oropharynx

DDx for HPV-Related Multiphenotypic Sinonasal Carcinoma

- Adenoid cystic carcinoma
  ○ Positive for *MYB* or *MYBL1* fusions
  ○ Negative for HR HPV by DNA or RNA ISH
  ○ Lacks marked atypia of overlying squamous mucosa as seen in ~ 70% of HMSC

- Other salivary gland carcinomas, such as basal cell carcinoma, epithelial-myoepithelial carcinoma, and adenocarcinoma, NOS
  ○ Negative for HR HPV by DNA or RNA ISH

DDx for HPV-Positive Poorly Differentiated Neuroendocrine Carcinomas

- HPV-negative PDNEC
  ○ Often p16 negative
  ○ Negative for HR HPV by DNA or RNA ISH
- Sinonasal undifferentiated carcinoma
  ○ Only focal chromogranin or synaptophysin; few cases tested are negative for INSM1
- HPV+HNMSCC
  ○ Lacks rosettes and distinct cell borders in most cases
  ○ p63 or p40 diffusely positive
  ○ Negative for neuroendocrine markers

DDx for HPV-Positive Nasopharyngeal Carcinoma

- Non-HPV-associated nasopharyngeal undifferentiated carcinoma
  ○ Positive for EBV-encoded RNA (EBER)

DIAGNOSTIC CHECKLIST

Clinically Relevant Pathologic Features

- Age of HPV+HNMSCC patients
  ○ On average, patients are male and 5 years younger than patients with HPV-negative HNMSCC
- HPV+HNMSCC most common in oropharynx (constitutes 60-70% of all squamous cell carcinomas at this site)
  ○ Behavior of HPV-positive HNMSCC outside oropharynx incompletely understood
- HPV+PDNEC head and neck carcinomas are clinically aggressive with poor prognosis similar to HPV-negative high-grade NEC

Pathologic Interpretation Pearls

- Perform p16 immunohistochemistry in all oropharyngeal squamous cell carcinomas regardless of histology
  ○ p16 overexpressing cases: Perform high-risk HPV typing to confirm HPV association in histologically atypical cases

SELECTED REFERENCES

1. de Sousa LG et al: Human papillomavirus status and prognosis of oropharyngeal high-grade neuroendocrine carcinoma. Oral Oncol. 138:106311, 2023
2. Froehlich MH et al: Systematic review of neuroendocrine carcinomas of the oropharynx. Head Neck. 44(7):1725-36, 2022
3. Brennan S et al: The role of human papilloma virus in dictating outcomes in head and neck squamous cell carcinoma. Front Mol Biosci. 8:677900, 2021
4. Shinn JR et al: Oropharyngeal squamous cell carcinoma with discordant p16 and HPV mRNA results: incidence and characterization in a large, contemporary United States cohort. Am J Surg Pathol. 45(7):951-61, 2021
5. Shah AA et al: Consistent LEF-1 and MYB immunohistochemical expression in human Papillomavirus-related multiphenotypic sinonasal carcinoma: A potential diagnostic pitfall. Head Neck Pathol. 13(2):220-4, 2019
6. Hsieh MS et al: Strong SOX10 expression in HPV-related multiphenotypic sinonasal carcinoma: report of six new cases validated by high-risk HPV mRNA in situ hybridization test. Hum Pathol. 82: 264-72, 2018
7. Rooper LM et al: INSM1 is a sensitive and specific marker of neuroendocrine differentiation in head and neck tumors. Am J Surg Pathol. 42(5):665-71, 2018

HPV-Associated Head and Neck Carcinomas

Conventional HPV+HNMSCC

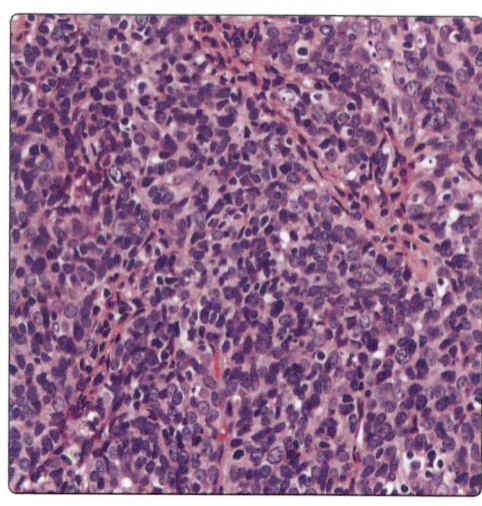

Atypical HPV+HNMSCC: Lymphoepithelial Carcinoma-Like

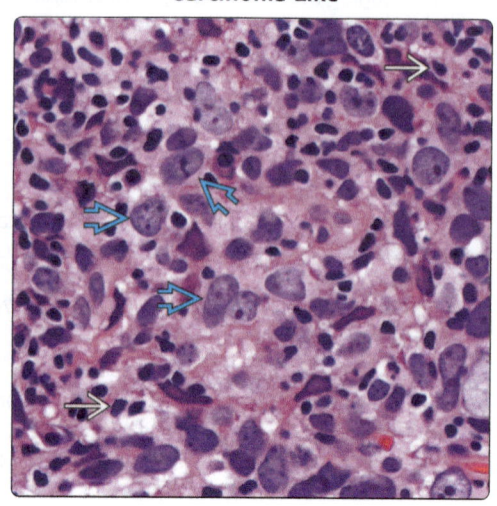

(Left) Classic HPV+HNMSCC morphology consists of loosely cohesive interconnecting nests of nonkeratinizing basal-like squamous cells. (Right) This tumor exhibits a lymphoepithelial architecture with intimately intermixed squamous cells and inflammatory cells ➡. The squamous cells have vesicular nuclei and lack cell borders ➡ with a syncytial growth.

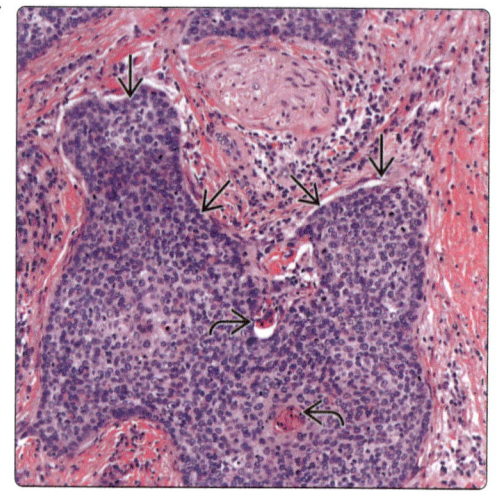

Hybrid HPV+HNMSCC

Hybrid HPV+HNMSCC

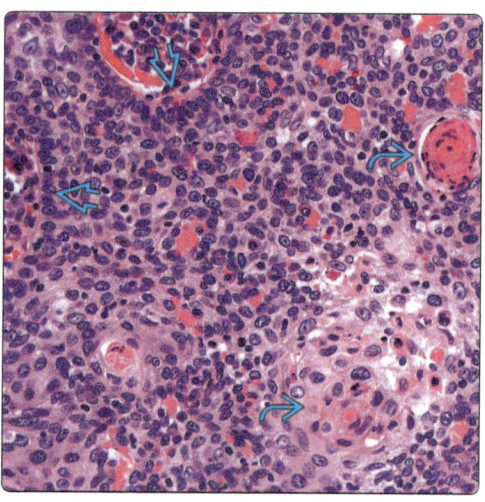

(Left) Hybrid HPV+HNMSCC of the tonsil consists of nests ➡ of basal-like squamous cells with central foci of abrupt keratinization ➡. (Right) Foci of abrupt keratinization ➡ in hybrid HPV+HNMSCC are shown. Note the hint of peripheral palisading ➡ and the predominance of uniform basal-like tumor cells.

Keratinizing HPV+HNMSCC

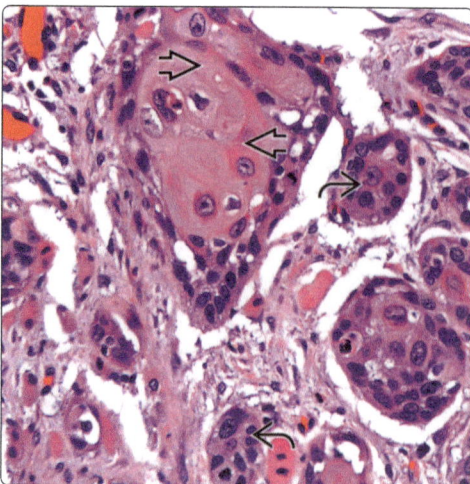

HPV-Positive Chromogenic In Situ Hybridization

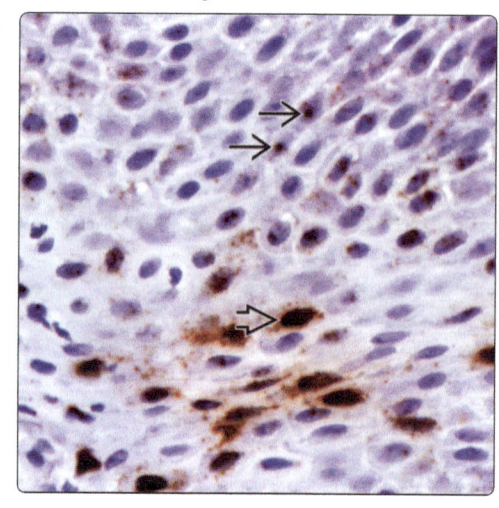

(Left) Keratinizing HPV+HNSCC tonsillar tumor shows an uncommon lower grade morphology ➡ with extensive keratinization ➡. (Right) Pan HPV in situ hybridization shows virally infected cells detectable by these chromogenic labeled probes. Note that the reactivity is nuclear and ranges from punctate ➡ to diffuse ➡ nuclear signal.

HPV-Associated Head and Neck Carcinomas

HPV-Related Multiphenotypic Sinonasal Carcinoma

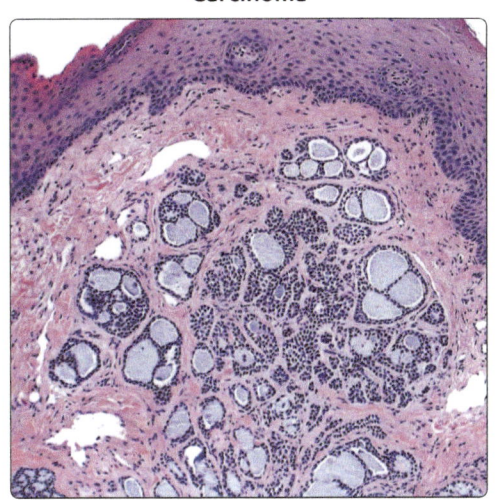

Severe Mucosal Squamous Atypia in HMSC

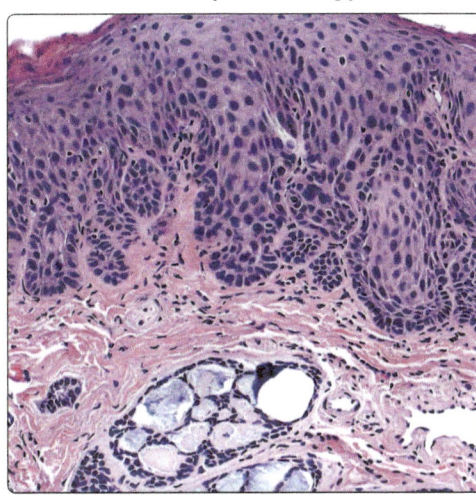

(Left) This case of HPV-related multiphenotypic sinonasal carcinoma (HMSC) mimics the cribriform and basal cell morphology of adenoid cystic carcinoma. (Right) A clue to the diagnosis of HMSC is the presence of severe atypia in the overlying squamous mucosa.

p16 Immunohistochemistry

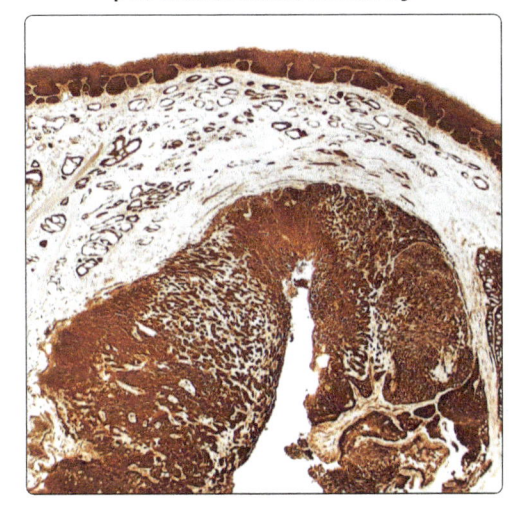

Large Cell Neuroendocrine Carcinoma

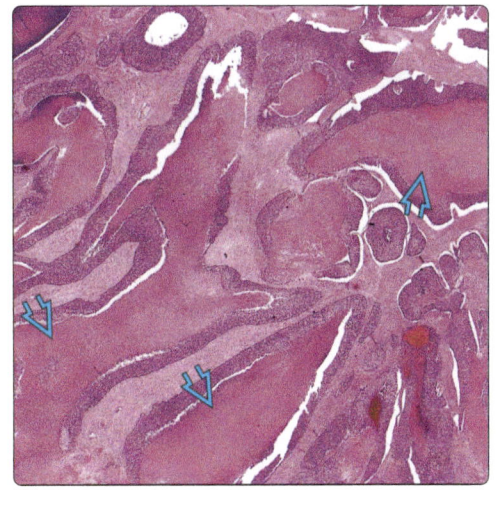

(Left) Note the characteristic diffuse strong reactivity for p16 in this HMSC, including the overlying mucosa. (Right) Laryngeal large cell neuroendocrine carcinoma (NEC) resembles HPV+HNMSCC at low power. Comedonecrosis ➡ is prominent in the irregular, anastomosing nests.

Large Cell Neuroendocrine Carcinoma

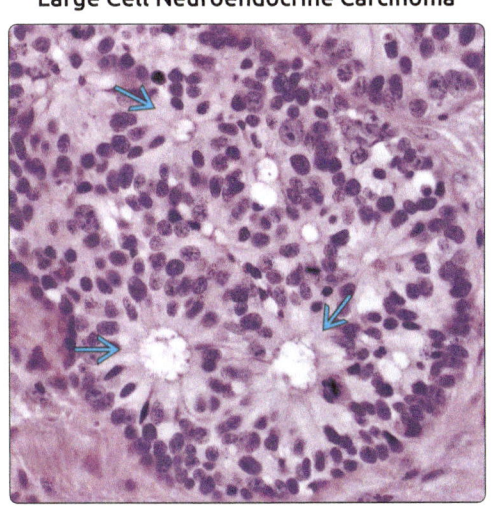

Chromogranin Expression in Large Cell Neuroendocrine Carcinoma

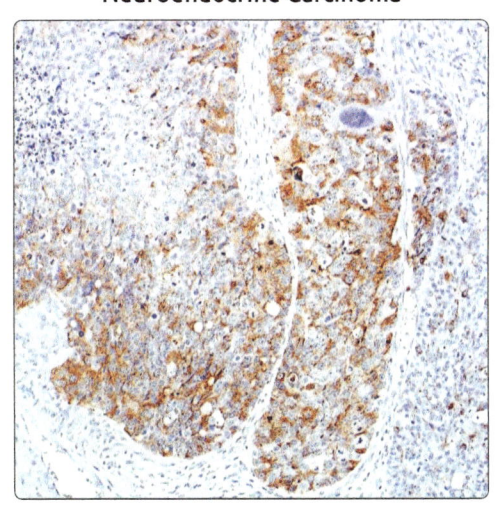

(Left) Large cell NEC shows the same histologic features in the head and neck whether HPV positive or negative. This case from the larynx shows true rosettes ➡ and "salt and pepper" chromatin, clues to the diagnosis. (Right) Laryngeal PDNEC shows patchy chromogranin expression. HPV+PDNEC of the head and neck behaves as aggressively as HPV-negative PDNEC. Accurate diagnosis of head and neck PDNEC is critical because of marked differences in prognosis and treatment compared to HPV+HNMSCC.

Head and Neck Mucosal Squamous Cell Carcinoma, Non-HPV Related

KEY FACTS

ETIOLOGY/PATHOGENESIS
- Tobacco
- Alcohol
- Betel nut quid
- Poor oral hygiene
- Rare inherited germline gene mutations
- Familial genetic risk factors
- Field cancerization effect

CLINICAL ISSUES
- Patients typically male, ≥ 50 years of age
- ~ 66% present with high-stage disease
- Agents targeting multiple pathways may prove most effective, given complexity of head and neck mucosal squamous cell carcinoma, (HNMSCC)-non-HPV pathogenetics
- Best predictors remain clinical/histopathologic and not molecular/genetic

MOLECULAR
- HNMSCC genetic and epigenetic aberrations extremely complex and not entirely understood
  - Genetic complexity complicated by diverse extrinsic factors that affect molecular and epigenetic changes in individual patient's tumor
- Method for selection of best targeted treatment per individual patient not yet determined
- May require multipathway/multiomics approach
- Hundreds of genes reported to be altered
  - Most altered genes function as tumor suppressors
- Recent multiassay analysis of ~ 300 cases of HNMSCC reveals 4 major molecular subtypes [from The Cancer Genome Atlas (TCGA) project]
- New methods to interrogate DNA, RNA, and methylation data from expanded set of TCGA cases reveal new subgroups of squamous cell carcinoma

Representative Gene Alterations in Non-HPV-Associated Mucosal H&N SCC

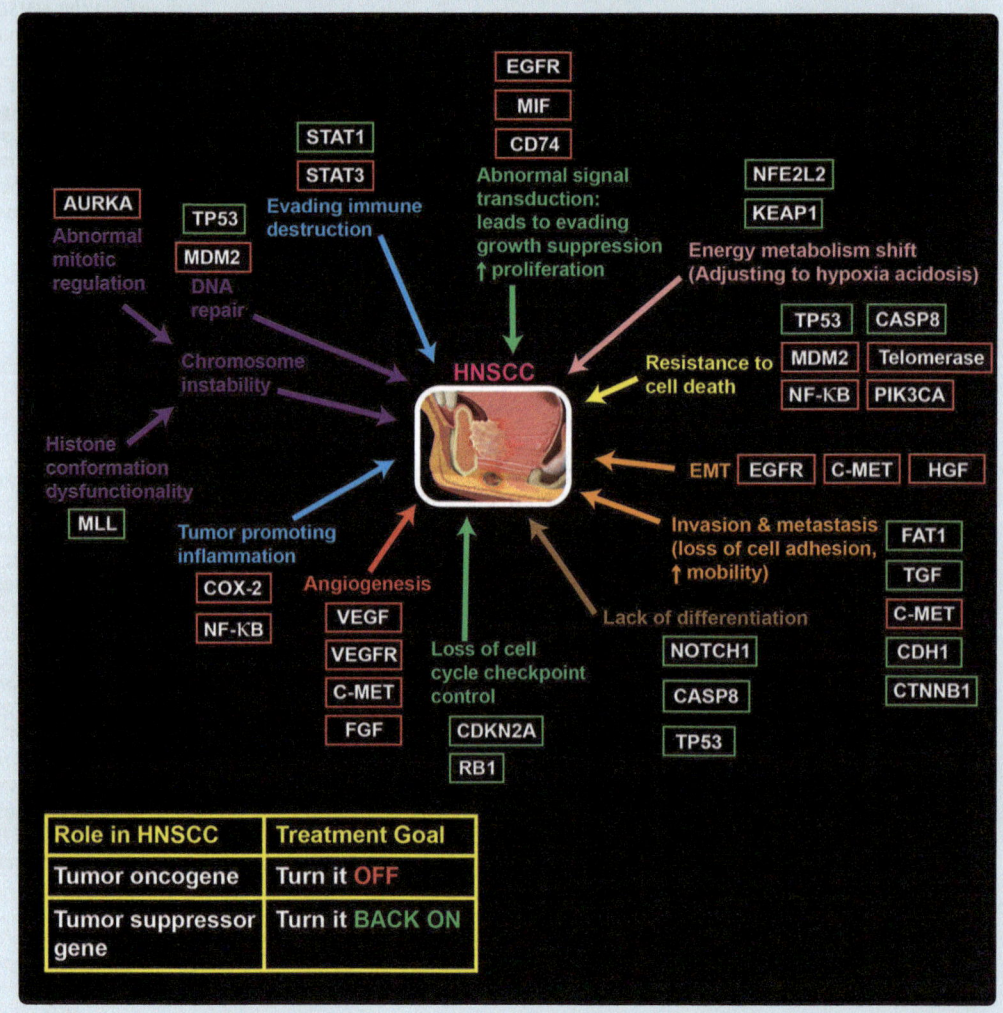

Diagram shows the complex relationship of many molecular genetic and signaling pathway deregulations in head and neck squamous cell carcinoma (SCC).

Head and Neck Mucosal Squamous Cell Carcinoma, Non-HPV Related

TERMINOLOGY

Abbreviations
- Head and neck mucosal squamous cell carcinoma, non-HPV related (HNMSCC-non-HPV)

Definitions
- Invasive squamous cell carcinoma (SCC) of head and neck mucosal sites that is **not** associated with HPV infection

ETIOLOGY/PATHOGENESIS

Environmental Exposure
- Tobacco
  - Smoking associated with 10x higher risk of HNMSCC-non-HPV
  - Activated procarcinogens, including polycyclic aromatic hydrocarbons, react with squamous cells to form DNA adducts
- Alcohol
  - Acetaldehyde reacts with mucosal squamous cells to form DNA adducts
- Betel quid chewing (areca nut)
  - Independently increases risk for oral HNMSCC
- Poor oral hygiene

Genetic Risk Factors
- Rare inherited germline gene mutations
  - Familial atypical multiple mole melanoma syndrome (FAMMMS)
  - *ATR* mutations
  - Fanconi anemia family of gene mutations
- Familial genetic risk factors
  - Combinations of certain single nucleotide polymorphisms increase risk for HNMSCC-non-HPV = high mutagen sensitivity phenotype
  - High risk for forming additional primary tumors in upper aerodigestive tract
  - Certain mitochondrial DNA polymorphisms increase susceptibility
  - Certain miRNA variations increase susceptibility
- Field cancerization effect
  - Mucosa adjacent to carcinoma shares some mutational changes due to widespread toxin exposure

CLINICAL ISSUES

Presentation
- Patients typically male, ≥ 50 year of age
- ~ 66% present with high-stage disease

Treatment
- Standard treatment includes surgical excision ± neck dissection ± radiotherapy
  - High-stage patients may be treated by radiation therapy &/or chemotherapy without surgery
- Immunotherapy effective in some patients and may be combined with other agents
- Molecular targeted therapy
  - Agents targeting multiple pathways may prove most effective given complexity of HNMSCC-non-HPV genetics
  - Many others in clinical trials

Prognosis
- Poor for high-stage disease with overall ~ 60% 5-year survival
- Best predictors remain clinical/histopathologic and not molecular/genetic
  - Histopathological predictors
    - Tumor site in head and neck
    - T stage
    - Tumor volume and thickness
    - Features of leading edge of tumor (invasive front) may also yield prognostic information
    - Presence of perineural invasion
    - Presence, number, and extranodal extent of lymph node metastasis
- Genetic predictors under intense study but not ready for prognosis/prediction per individual patient
  - Proposed molecular/genetic predictors
    - Gene expression signature in primary tumor to predict lymph node metastasis
    - Individual or combined markers to predict outcome
    - Molecular markers to predict response to specific targeted therapies
    - Saliva markers (such as specific miRNAs or proteins) to predict risk for oral SCC
    - Circulating serum/plasma markers for disease monitoring
      - May include specific abnormally elevated miRNAs or lncRNAs
  - Proposed markers not yet validated in large series
  - Prognostic and predictive markers require integration of
    - miRNA signature
    - Gene expression profile
    - Specific gene mutations
    - Genetic intratumoral heterogeneity
    - Methylation signature
    - Proteome signature
    - Immunologic and stromal interactions

MOLECULAR

Overview
- HNMSCC-non-HPV genetic and epigenetic aberrations are complex
  - Driver genes mutated
    - ~ 100 specific genes are consistently found to be mutated: Some are mutated at low frequencies
    - Most function as tumor suppressors: Loss-of-function mutations
  - Alternative splicing of mRNA transcripts is common event
    - Systematically affects ~ 3,500 genes
    - Splicing events lead to multiple isoforms of specific genes, some with pathogenic activity
    - 5 alternately spliced genes independently associated with survival: *C5orf30*, *METTL13*, *RHO11*, *ABCC5*, and *MPZL1*
  - Noncoding RNAs play pathogenic role through aberrant expression
    - MicroRNAs (miRNAs) that normally act as tumor suppressors are downregulated: miR-141, miR-138, miR-145, and others

Head and Neck Mucosal Squamous Cell Carcinoma, Non-HPV Related

- miRNAs that act as oncogenes are upregulated: miR-744-3p, miR-21, and others
- Long noncoding RNAs (lncRNAs) that act as oncogenes are upregulated: HOXA11-AS, RGMB-AS1, XIST, and others
  - Global hypermethylation and hypomethylation are common events
    - Causes include alcohol and tobacco use
- Genetic complexity complicated by diverse extrinsic factors that affect molecular and epigenetic changes in individual patient's tumor
  - Extrinsic factors
    - Sex
    - Ethnicity
    - Type/amount of toxin exposure
    - Tumor site (such as oropharynx, larynx)
    - Immune competence
    - Microbiome of oral cavity
    - Extracellular microenvironmental factors (such as hypoxia, acidosis)
    - Viral infection status
    - Rare inherited disorders
    - Familial predisposition
- Method for selection of best targeted treatment per individual patient not yet determined
  - May require multipathway/multiomics approach

Cytogenetics

- Marked aneuploidy with more karyotype abnormalities more commonly seen in smokers than nonsmokers

Molecular Genetics of Conventional HNMSCC-Non-HPV

- Hundreds of genes are altered (driver and passenger genes)
- Most common altered genes
  - *TP53*: Mutated in 60-80%
    - Mechanism of inactivation: Missense mutations combined with allelic loss
      - Allelic loss occurs rather than copy number loss so that tumors retain 2 copies of mutated *TP53*
  - *CDKN2A*: Frequently lost
  - *CCND1*: Frequently amplified
  - *PIK3CA* (especially in HNMSCC-HPV): Altered in 40%
  - *FAT1*: Altered in 30%
  - *KMT2D/KMT2B*: Altered in 17%
  - *NOTCH1*: Altered in 22%
  - Others include *CASP8, HLA-A, HRAS*, and *TP63*

Gene Expression Profiling of HNMSCC-Non-HPV

- Multiassay analysis of ~ 300 cases of HNSCC reveals 4 major molecular subtypes [from The Cancer Genome Atlas (TCGA) project] and verifies earlier reporting molecular genetic grouping of cases
  - 4 types exhibit reproducible distinct molecular signatures
    - Classic
    - Basal
    - Mesenchymal
    - Atypical
  - Altered gene expression profiles significantly overlap those identified in lung SCC
  - At least 18 targetable molecular alterations
    - Include amplified tyrosine kinases, such as *EGFR, FGFR1, FGFR2, MET*, and *ERBB2*
  - Favorable prognostic group identified by multiple studies, including TCGA
    - Demographically more common in females, nonsmokers, nonalcohol consumers
    - Genes altered
      - *HRAS*: Activating mutation
      - *CASP8* (caspase 8): Inactivating mutation
    - *TP53* is wildtype (unaltered)
    - Low copy number alterations (CNA)
- Pathways typically altered
  - Cell cycle control
    - Aberrant genes (proteins) involved: *TP53* (p53), *CDKN2A* (p16), *CCND1* (cyclin D1)
    - Others include various growth factors, including *EGFR* (EGFR) most commonly
  - Oxidative stress
  - WNT signaling
    - Aberrant genes (proteins) involved: *FAT1, AJUBA*, and *NOTCH1*
      - *FAT1* alterations mutually exclusive with *AJUBA* mutations
  - Cell survival
    - Aberrant genes involved: *PIK3CA* (catalytic p110α subunit of class1 PI3Ks) and *PTEN* (PTEN)
  - Epigenetic regulation
    - Aberrant genes involved: *KMT2D* and *NSD1*
    - Altered miRNAs include decreased miR-let-7c-5p and miRNA-100-5p and increased miR-205-5p and miR-944
      - Affect expression of genes involved in cell cycle control
  - Cross connectivity of altered genes involves multiple additional critical pathways
    - Additional pathways affected include MAPK signaling, Hippo signaling, and others

Molecular Taxonomy of HNMSCC-Non-HPV

- New methods to interrogate DNA, RNA, and methylation data from expanded set of TCGA cases reveal new subgroups of SCC
  - Integrated findings from such studies potentially identify subsets of patients with specific distinct targetable pathways
  - May also potentially identify those patients most likely to respond to immunotherapy
- Assessment of ~ 750-1,400 SCCs from 5 body sites integrated DNA CNA, mutations, methylation, mRNA, miRNA, and protein expression analyses
  - Identified 5 major CNA clusters of SCC
    - Subset of low CNA group significantly correlates with positive HPV status
  - Identified 5 methylation clusters of SCC
  - Identified 6 mRNA clusters of SCC
  - Identified 6 protein expression clusters of SCC
  - Identified 5 miRNA clusters of SCC
- *DEF::AFF2* fusion carcinoma: Rare, nonkeratinizing SCC of sinonasal region

Head and Neck Mucosal Squamous Cell Carcinoma, Non-HPV Related

- Recently identified as a specific fusion-driven type of head and neck SCC
- Histology: Papillary and ribbon-like growth of uniform nonkeratinizing cells often eliciting neutrophilic inflammation
- Behavior: Locally aggressive and can metastasize

MICROSCOPIC

Histologic Features

- Squamous differentiation and invasion through basement membrane required for diagnosis
- 3 grades
  - Well differentiated (resembles normal squamous epithelium)
  - Moderately differentiated (more nuclear atypia with increased mitoses, some atypical)
  - Poorly differentiated (immature cells, absent to sparse keratinization, high mitotic rate)
- Characteristics of invasive front may better predict behavior than overall grade
  - Expansive
    – Rounded nodules of tumor with pushing smooth margins
    – Less aggressive
  - Infiltrative
    – Cords, single cells irregularly invading stroma
    – More aggressive
- Keratinization in form of squamous pearls may be seen in all grades
- Most HNMSCC-non-HPV are moderately differentiated

DIFFERENTIAL DIAGNOSIS

HNMSCC-HPV

- Location
  - Oropharynx (Waldeyer ring) mucosa most commonly
- Differentiation
  - Most poorly differentiated
  - Keratinization absent or sparse
- Most cases express p16 IHC diffusely and strongly, in contrast to most cases of HNMSCC-non-HPV
  - Rare HNMSCC-non-HPV also overexpress p16
    – May require HPV FISH to rule out HNMSCC-HPV

Sinonasal Undifferentiated Carcinoma

- Location
  - Nasal cavity, sinuses
- Differentiation
  - Nests, sheets of undifferentiated cells
  - No keratinization
  - Prominent necrosis &/or apoptosis
  - Vesicular nuclei, high N:C ratio
  - High mitotic rate
- IHC
  - Positive: Keratins 7, 8, 19
  - Negative: Keratins 5, 6

NUT Midline Carcinoma

- Location
  - Midline structures of head and neck
- Differentiation
  - Poorly differentiated
  - Foci of abrupt keratinization common
  - Cells often show cytoplasmic clearing with monotonous round nuclei
- IHC
  - NUT
    – Positive in 100%
    – Speckled nuclear reactivity
- Molecular tests
  - FISH or PCR can be done but unnecessary for diagnosis due to high sensitivity/specificity of NUT antibody

Undifferentiated EBV-Related Nasopharyngeal Carcinoma

- Location
  - Nasopharynx in most cases
- Differentiation
  - Poorly differentiated
    – Round to plump spindly cells
    – Nuclei usually vesicular with macronucleoli
  - Keratinization usually absent to uncommonly sparse
- Tumor stroma
  - Rich in infiltrating lymphocytes &/or plasma cells in most cases
  - Desmoplasia usually absent
- In situ hybridization
  - Positive for nuclear EBV-encoded RNA (EBER)

DIAGNOSTIC CHECKLIST

Clinically Relevant Pathologic Features

- Most patients older than patients with HPV-related SCC
- Most patients have ↑ tobacco use ± ↑ EtOH use compared to patients with HPV-related SCC
- Most tumors occur away from Waldeyer ring (site of most HPV-related SCC)

Pathologic Interpretation Pearls

- Grade of many tumors is moderate compared to poorly differentiated squamous cell carcinoma of HPV, NUT, and EBV-related head and neck SCC
- Treatment decisions based on expression of targetable proteins and other molecular genetic and epigenetic factors

SELECTED REFERENCES

1. Ruangritchankul K et al: DEK::AFF2 fusion carcinomas of head and neck. Adv Anat Pathol. 30(2):86-94, 2023
2. Falco M et al: Overview on molecular biomarkers for laryngeal cancer: looking for new answers to an old problem. Cancers (Basel). 14(7), 2022
3. Dlamini Z et al: Genetic drivers of head and neck squamous cell carcinoma: aberrant splicing events, mutational burden, HPV infection and future targets. Genes (Basel). 12(3), 2021
4. Xing L et al: Systematic profile analysis of prognostic alternative messenger RNA splicing signatures and splicing factors in head and neck squamous cell carcinoma. DNA Cell Biol. 38(7):627-38, 2019
5. Leemans CR et al: The molecular landscape of head and neck cancer. Nat Rev Cancer. 18(5):269-82, 2018

Head and Neck Mucosal Squamous Cell Carcinoma, Non-HPV Related

Well-Differentiated Keratinizing SCC

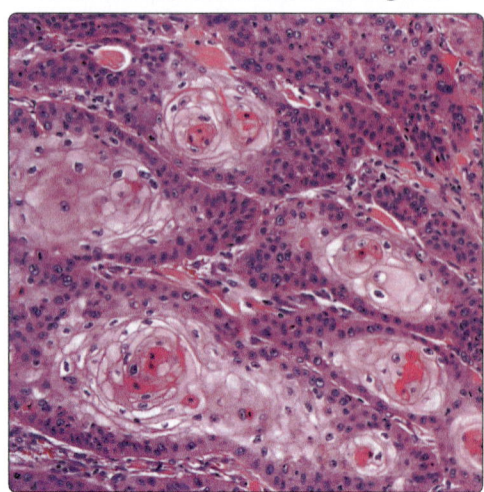

Well-Differentiated Keratinizing SCC

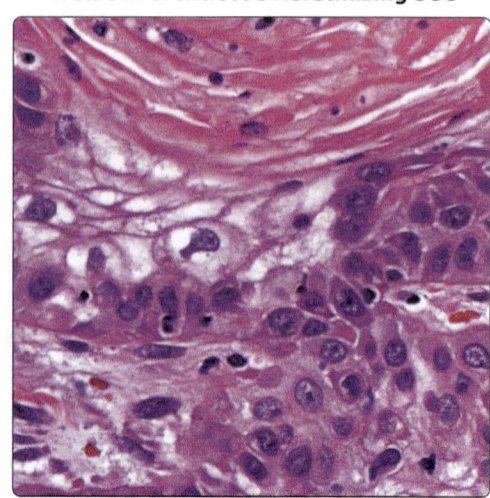

(Left) Well-differentiated SCC is shown growing as interconnecting nests. (Right) High-power view of the same case shows characteristic abrupt keratinization, generally mild nuclear atypia, and intercellular bridges (tonofilaments).

Moderately Differentiated SCC

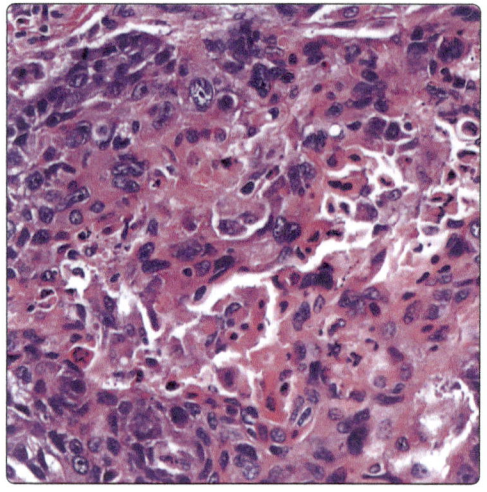

Moderately Differentiated SCC

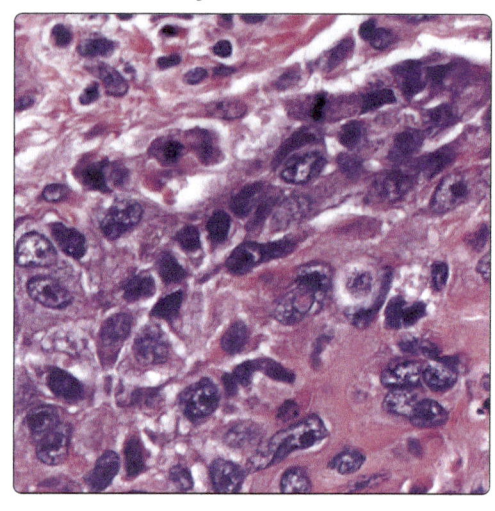

(Left) Moderately differentiated head and neck SCC is characterized by increased nuclear atypia and mitotic activity but often retains some keratinization, as seen here. (Right) High-power view of the same case shows more range in nuclear size and shape but with retention of defined cell borders and intercellular bridges.

Poorly Differentiated SCC

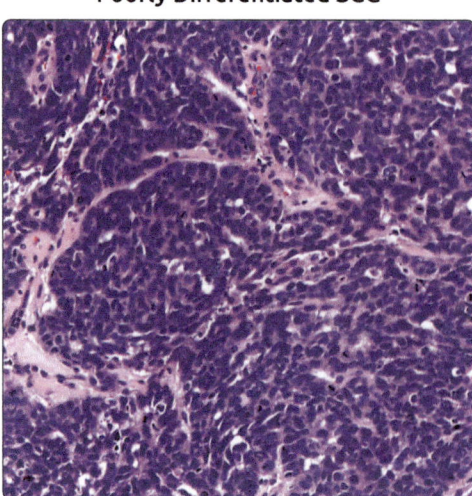

Poorly Differentiated SCC

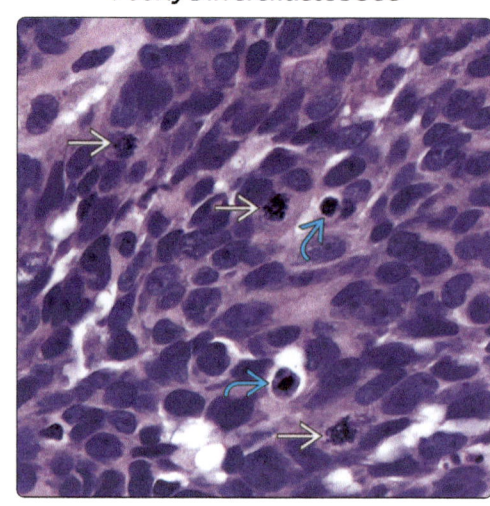

(Left) This example of poorly differentiated head and neck SCC is basaloid, but it lacks some of the features commonly seen in basaloid SCC, such as central comedo-type necrosis, perinodular clefting, hyaline matrix, and myxoid stroma. (Right) At high power, this basaloid head and neck SCC-non-HPV is composed of cells resembling basal cell carcinoma with a high mitotic rate ➡ and apoptosis ➡. This tumor was p16 negative and located on the lateral aspect of the tongue.

Head and Neck Mucosal Squamous Cell Carcinoma, Non-HPV Related

Well-Differentiated SCC

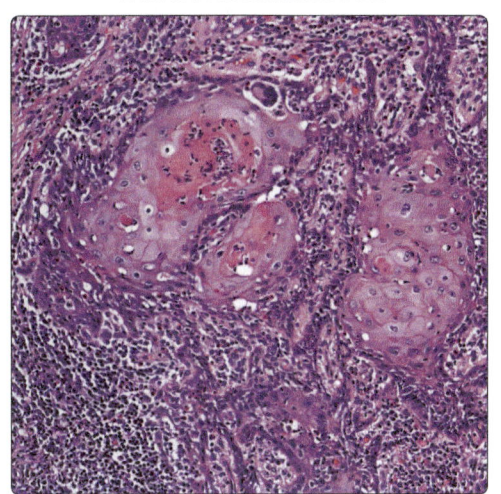

Intense Inflammation

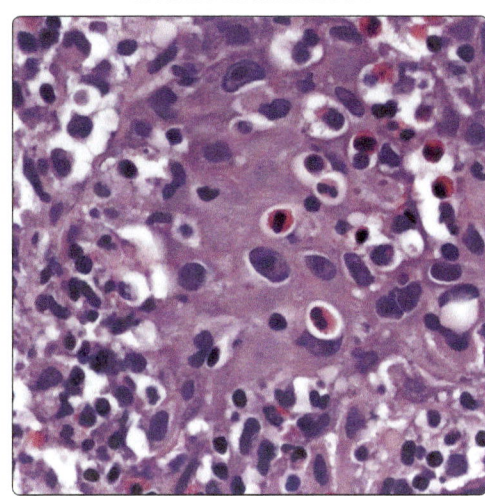

(Left) This well-differentiated head and neck SCC is 1 of 2 tumors found in the oral cavity of an 82-year-old woman with a heavy smoking history. (Right) Higher power view of the base of the same patient's anterior oral tumor reveals a marked inflammatory cell reaction. The degree of inflammation varies in SCC and may play a role in tumor progression.

Second Primary SCC

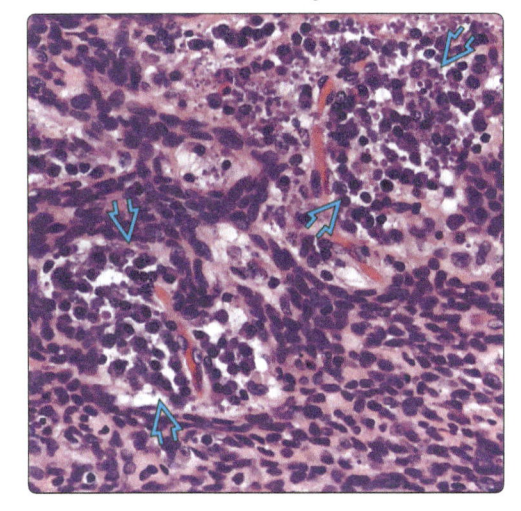

Aggressive Invasive Front

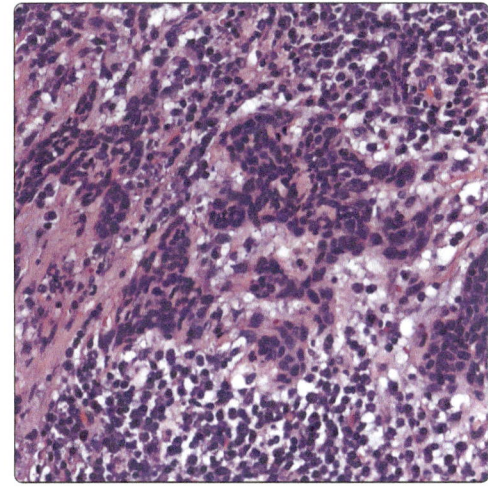

(Left) The 2nd head and neck SCC in the same patient shows less keratinization but is still markedly inflamed, containing plasma cells ⇨. Field cancerization accounts for the development of multiple independent primaries in patients with a heavy smoking &/or alcohol history. (Right) The base of the 2nd tumor in the same patient is composed of irregular strands of malignant cells trailing off into the inflamed stroma. This type of jagged invasive front is associated with a more aggressive course.

Focal Sarcomatoid Appearance in SCC

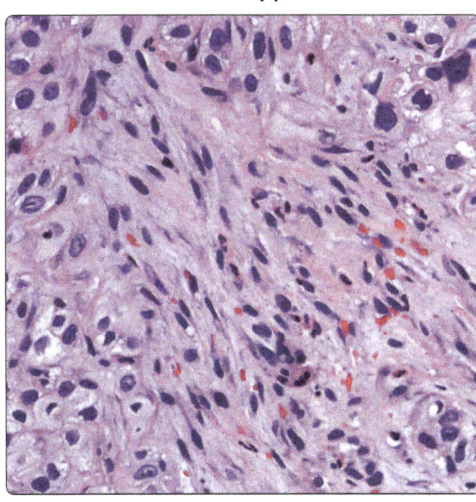

Cytologically Low-Grade Sarcomatoid SCC

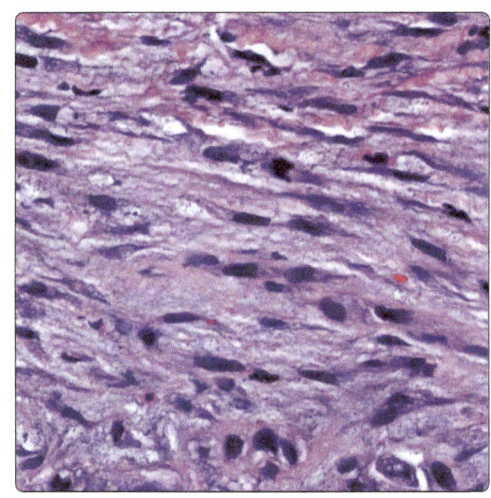

(Left) This head and neck SCC-non-HPV tumor is focally sarcomatoid and contains spindle-shaped tumor cells. (Right) In this sarcomatoid head and neck SCC-non-HPV, the spindle tumor cells assume a relatively bland appearance. Most sarcomatoid SCC contain conventional areas and are more cytologically atypical than this example.

Important Alterations in Non-HPV-Related Head and Neck Squamous Cell Carcinoma

Important Genetic and Epigenetic Alterations in Non-HPV Head and Neck Mucosal Squamous Cell Carcinoma

Site of Alteration (Chromosome Location)	Normal Function	Pathophysiology	Percent, Alteration, and Tumor
TP53 (17p)	Functions as TS by causing cell cycle arrest, apoptosis, repair of damaged DNA	Mutation, inhibition (by other altered gene products), or deletion; cells with damaged DNA continue to divide, leading to additional mutations; diffuse IHC expression most common in high-grade tumors; TP53 mutations associated with poor outcome and poor response to radiation or chemotherapy	40-62% mutated; can also be inactivated, altered in ~ 80% of HNSCC
EGFR (7p)	GFR (receptor tyrosine kinase): Activates MAPK, AKT1, ERK, and JAK/STAT pathways	High gene copy numbers and O/E leads to uncontrolled proliferation; lack of apoptosis, angiogenesis, invasion, and metastasis	80-90% O/E, but only 1-7% have activating mutations; 10% altered in nonoropharyngeal SCC of keratinizing and nonkeratinizing histology
CDKN2A (9p)	p16 protein product functions as TS by regulating cell cycle via interactions with RB1	Loss of cell cycle regulation; some are hypermethylated; there is loss of p16 expression by IHC in most non-HPV-related HNMSCC; however, p16 is expressed in most HPV-associated HNMSCC	30% have copy number variation; 9-12% mutated
CCND1 (11q)	Forms complex that regulates CDK4 involved in G1/S transition of cell cycle and also interacts with RB1	Amplification-O/E helps drive abnormal DNA replication	25% CNA (increased); 0.6% mutated
NOTCH1 (9p)	Cell differentiation, lineage commitment	LOF mutation causes loss of TS function	15% mutated
MET (7q)	TK that functions as oncogene	Activating mutations promote EMT and angiogenesis; may confer chemotherapy resistance	14% mutated
FAT1 (4q)	Functions as TS by maintaining cell adhesion	LOF mutations facilitate tumor cell migration and invasion	12-80% mutated; may be most common in oral HNSCC,-non-HPV
NFKB1 (4q), NFKB2 (10q)	Transcription factor mediating inflammation and immune function	Upregulated	Increasing upregulation in advanced-stage tumors
PTEN (10q)	Functions as TS by inhibiting PI3K pathway	PI3K/AKT abnormally activated promoting cell growth, survival, transformation, and drug resistance	7-10% mutated; IHC may show loss of PTEN protein
HRAS (11p)	GTPase that functions as oncogene	O/E or mutation increases proliferation, survival; oncogenic activation confers resistance to cetuximab therapy	4-9% mutated (higher rates may occur in Indian and East Asian patients)
CASP8 (2q)	Involved in programmed cell death	Mutated cells avoid destruction	10% mutated
KMT2D (MLL2) (12q)	Codes for histone methyltransferase and acts as TS	May be mutated or O/E, and helps regulate transcription estrogen receptor gene	10-20% mutated
KEAP1 (19p)	Works with NFE2L2 (NRF2) in antioxidant pathway (oxidative stress response)	Mutated KEAP1 reduces activity of PI3K/AKT pathway inhibitors	Unknown
NFE2L2 (2q)	Transcription factor involved in response to inflammation and injury through regulation of genes with ARE	Abnormalities of NFE2L2 lead to loss of cell homeostasis and increased susceptibility to various carcinogens	Unknown
B2M (15q)	Codes for serum protein associated with MHC class I antigens	Mutation reduces immunogenicity of tumor	Unknown

Important Alterations in Non-HPV-Related Head and Neck Squamous Cell Carcinoma

Important Genetic and Epigenetic Alterations in Non-HPV Head and Neck Mucosal Squamous Cell Carcinoma (Continued)

Site of Alteration (Chromosome Location)	Normal Function	Pathophysiology	Percent, Alteration, and Tumor
RAC1 (7p)	Codes for Ras GTPase involved in cell growth, cytoskeleton, and other functions	O/E leads to radioresistance and loss of sensitivity to cisplatin chemotherapy	Unknown
FBXW7 (4q)	Member of ubiquitin ligase complex, which functions as tumor suppressor	LOF leads to lack of NOTCH1, cyclin-E1, and MYC protein degradation; LOF reduces efficacy of MTOR inhibitors	5-11% mutated
PIK3CA (3q)	Component of PI3K that functions as oncogene	Increases cell growth, survival, and alters cytoskeleton	21% CNA; 5-20% mutated; more common in HNSCC-HPV tumors [30% of HPV(+) tumors]
RB1 (13q)	Acts as tumor suppressor and cell cycle regulator	LOF mutation enables evasion of growth suppressors	3-20% mutated
TGFB1 (19q)	Multiple functions, including modulating AKT1 and epithelial mesenchymal transition	LOF mutation enables evasion of growth suppressors; increased expression suppresses cell-mediated toxicity, including activated T cells	Unknown percentage of LOF or increased expression
MDM2 (12q)	Controls p53 protein levels	O/E suppresses normal p53 activity and leads to chromosomal instability; certain SNPs of MDM2 lead to increased risk and earlier onset of nonoropharyngeal, non-HPV HNMSCC	Unknown
VEGFB (11q), VEGFA (6p), PDGFB (22q), FGF1 (5q), CXCL8 (4q)	Angiogenesis and control of interferon production	O/E promotes angiogenesis and negatively alters immune response	Unknown
CDH1 (16q), CTNNA1 (5q), CTNNB1 (3p)	Cell adhesion and growth control	Downregulation leads to loss of cohesion and proliferation	Unknown
SPARC (5q)	Tissue invasion	O/E leads to invasion and metastasis	Unknown
PTGS2 (1q)	Involved in inflammation	O/E leads to tumor promoting inflammation	Unknown
MIF (22q)	Interacts with CD74	O/E leads to inhibition of p53 and activation of ERK, MAPK, and P13K/AKT pathways	Unknown
CD74 (5q)	Cell surface receptor	O/E has same effects as MIF O/E	Unknown
ATM (11q), CDKN2B (9p), TIMP3 (22q), MGMT (10q), RARB (3p), DAPK1 (9q), CCNA1 (13q), RASSF1 (3p), DCC (18q)	TS genes	Hypermethylation causes lack of transcription, leading to loss of tumor suppression	Unknown
AURKA (20q), AURKB (17p)	Cell cycle regulators	O/E leads to genomic instability and aneuploidy	Unknown, but most tumors with O/E are poorly differentiated
TERT (5p)	Controls cell senescence	O/E causes replicative immortality	Unknown
HLA-A (6p), TAP1 (6p), TAP2 (6p), TAPBP (6p)	Promote immune surveillance and tumor cell destruction	Downregulation protects tumor cells from immune destruction	Unknown
miRNAs (> 30)	MicroRNAs functioning predominantly as TS	Abnormal regulation of various microRNAs promotes tumor cell proliferation, antiapoptosis, angiogenesis, migration, invasion, and metastasis	High percentage microRNA signature in sputum may predict risk of oral SCC
Long noncoding RNAs (lncRNAs)	Regulate gene expression through multiple mechanisms, including sponging microRNAs	Abnormal differential expression can be pro-oncogenic, such as facilitating EMT, invasion and metastasis	Common in HNMSCC-non-HPV and includes: MALAT1, HOTAIR, UCA1, CCAT1, ZFAS1, and many others

ARE = antioxidant response elements; EMT = epithelial to mesenchymal transition; HNMSCC = head and neck mucosal squamous cell carcinoma; IHC = immunohistochemistry; LOF = loss of function; mAB = monoclonal antibody; O/E = overexpression; TK = tyrosine kinase; TKI = tyrosine kinase inhibitor; TLRs = toll-like receptors; TS = tumor suppressor; SNP= single nucleotide polymorphism. (Note that this table is not a complete list, as many other genes are involved in the pathogenesis of HNMSCC-non-HPV.)

Translocation-Specific Salivary Gland Tumors

KEY FACTS

TERMINOLOGY

- Primary salivary gland tumors that have specific gene alterations
  - Pleomorphic adenoma (PA), mucoepidermoid carcinoma (MEC), adenoid cystic carcinoma (ADCC), acinic cell carcinoma (AcC), polymorphous adenocarcinoma (PMC) and related cribriform carcinoma (CribC), secretory carcinoma (SC)
  - Range from benign to high-grade malignant

CLINICAL ISSUES

- Targeted therapy potentially effective in aggressive high-grade salivary gland tumors
  - TRK inhibitors may be option in SC that is uncommonly high stage or aggressive and exhibits *NTRK3* fusion partner
- Targeted therapies continue to develop
  - May require use of several agents to target multiple dysregulated pathways

MOLECULAR

- Expression profiling may identify targetable pathways
  - EGFR antibodies, mTOR inhibitors, PI3K, and RET inhibitors may be beneficial in particular patients
  - Activating, targetable mutations individually rare and not generally restricted to specific salivary gland subtypes
    - e.g., mutations of PIK3 pathway genes present in ~ 20% of high-grade MEC, salivary duct carcinoma, ADCC

DIAGNOSTIC CHECKLIST

- Specific salivary gland tumor genetic alterations have diagnostic utility, especially in clinically or histologically atypical cases
- Some tumors show overexpression of corresponding gene fusion protein, such as PLAG1, MYB, NR4A3, or pan-TRK, facilitating diagnosis by IHC

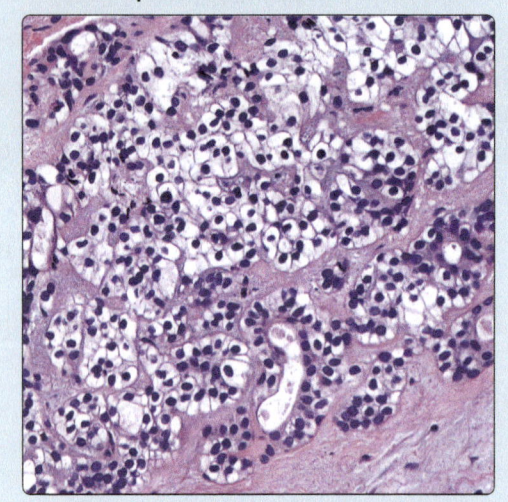

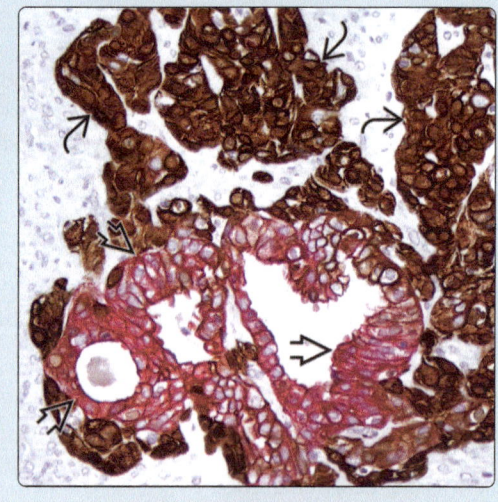

(Left) *Pleomorphic adenoma shows clusters of clear myoepithelial cells, one of many morphological variants found in this tumor.* **(Right)** *CK-PAN highlights mucinous cell differentiation ⇨ and intermediate cell differentiation ⇨ in this mucoepidermoid carcinoma.*

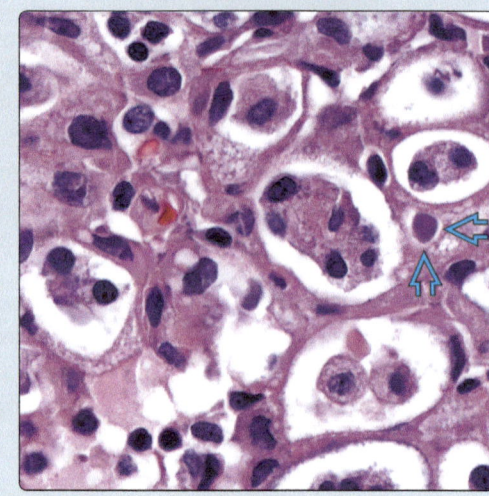

(Left) *Secretory carcinoma shows pseudopapillary ⇨, microcystic ⇨, and solid areas. Mixed architectural patterns are commonly seen in these tumors.* **(Right)** *Tumor cells are relatively large and resemble zymogen-poor acinar cells. Nuclear atypia is mild in this case and in most cases. Note the microcyst with eosiniophilic secretion ⇨.*

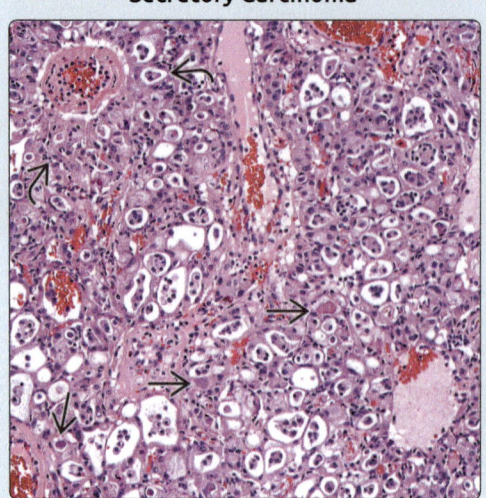

Translocation-Specific Salivary Gland Tumors

TERMINOLOGY

Definitions

- Primary salivary gland tumors with specific gene alterations
  - Pleomorphic adenoma (PA)
  - Mucoepidermoid carcinoma (MEC)
  - Adenoid cystic carcinoma (ADCC)
  - Acinic cell carcinoma (AcC)
  - Polymorphous adenocarcinoma and cribriform adenocarcinoma (PMC; CribC)
  - Secretory carcinoma (SC) (previously termed mammary analog secretory carcinoma)

ETIOLOGY/PATHOGENESIS

PA

- Most show overexpression of PLAG1 protein
- Some have *HMGA2* amplification or rearrangement
- Some show neither PLAG1 overexpression nor *HMGA2* alterations

MEC

- *CRTC1*::*MAML2* or *CRTC3*::*MAML2*

ADCC

- *MYB*::*NFIB* upregulates MYB protein expression
- *MYBL1*::*NFIB* uncommon alternate fusion
- c-kit overexpressed
- NOTCH genes commonly altered
- Rare cases do not rely on MYB overexpression for tumorigenesis

AcC

- *SCPP*::*NR4A3*/*NOR-1* rearrangement in majority of cases
- *HTN3*::*MSANTD3* in ~ 4% of cases

PMC AND CribC

- PMC: *PRKD1* hotspot activating mutations
- CribC: *PRKD1*/*PRKD2*/*PRKD3* rearrangements

SC

- *ETV6*::*NTRK3*
  - *ETV6*: Transcriptional regulator
  - *NTRK3*: Membrane receptor kinase
- Other *ETV6* fusions less common and very rare non-ETV6 fusions

CLINICAL ISSUES

Epidemiology

- Incidence
  - PA: Most common benign salivary gland tumor
  - MEC: Most common malignant salivary gland tumor; also occurs in children
  - ADCC: 2nd most common malignant salivary gland tumor
  - AcC: 3rd most common malignant salivary gland tumor; also occurs in children
  - PMC and CribC: Relatively common malignant minor salivary gland carcinomas
  - SC: Rare salivary gland tumor that may be underdiagnosed due to histologic similarities with other tumor types

Site

- **PA and MEC**
  - Majority occur in major salivary glands, especially parotid
- **MEC**
  - Palate most frequent minor salivary gland location
    - Other rare sites: Lacrimal glands, intraosseous in gnathic bones, lungs, others
- **ADCC**
  - Major salivary glands most common; accounts for 30% of epithelial tumors in minor salivary glands
  - Other rare sites: Lacrimal glands, lungs, uterine cervix, breast, others
- **AcC**
  - Major salivary glands with parotid gland involved in ~ 90-95%
  - Rarely occurs in minor salivary glands or sinonasal region
- **PMC and CribC**
  - Minor salivary glands in almost all cases
- **SC**
  - Fairly common in minor salivary glands as well as major glands
  - May be misdiagnosed in minor salivary glands as AcC
  - May rarely occur in thyroid gland and sinonasal region

Prognosis

- **PA**
  - Conventional PA: Local recurrence rate ~ 2% with complete excision
    - Recurrences often multifocal and difficult to resect
    - Recurrences occur 5-10 years or later after initial excision
  - **Metastasizing PA (a.k.a. benign metastasizing PA)**
    - 25% death due to disease
  - **Carcinoma ex pleomorphic adenoma (Ca ex PA)**
    - Prognosis depends on degree of extension beyond periphery of parent PA
    - Non- or minimally invasive (< 1.5 mm beyond capsule of PA): Excellent prognosis similar to conventional PA
    - Early invasion up to 6 mm still confers good prognosis
    - Widely invasive Ca ex PA: Invasive **tumor type, size, and grade** affect prognosis, but tumor is generally aggressive
- **MEC**
  - Overall relatively favorable prognosis with ~ 8% death rate
  - High-grade tumors behave worse
  - Tumors with Ki-67 proliferation index > 10% behave worse
- **ADCC**
  - High 5-year survival, but most patients eventually die of disease
  - Solid and anaplastic variants pursue more rapid course
  - Low rate of regional lymph node metastasis, but confers worse prognosis if present
- **AcC**
  - High 5-year and 10-year survival
  - Distant metastases (~ 20% of cases) worsens survival
  - High-grade transformation associated with poor 5-year survival
- **PMC and CribC**

Translocation-Specific Salivary Gland Tumors

- PMC: Up to 33% local recurrence and ~ 15% local lymph node involvement; distant metastases rare
- CribC: Generally indolent but with higher rate of regional lymph node metastases
- SC
  - Low local recurrence rate (10-15%) and low regional lymph node metastasis rate with only rare distant metastases
  - Rare anaplastic/transformed variant behaves more aggressively

MOLECULAR

In Situ Hybridization

- PA
  - *PLAG1* and *HMGA2* fusions common (found in 66% by FISH)
    - Histology and prognosis: Same for both *PLAG1* and *HMGA2* fusions
    - Most common fusion partner for *PLAG1* is *CTNNB1* in t(3;8)
    - Salivary duct carcinoma: Some cases show rearrangement of *PLAG1* or *HMGA2*, consistent with origin in prior PA with subsequent tumor transformation
    - *PLAG1* rearrangements also seen in some myoepithelial tumors of skin/soft tissue
- MEC
  - t(11;19); *CRTC1::MAML2*
    - May be present in higher percentage (~ 80%) of low-grade MEC than high-grade MEC (~ 50%)
    - High-grade MEC lacking t(11;19) may represent different tumor
  - Other rare fusion reported: t(11;15); *CRTC3::MAML2* (~ 5%)
- ADCC
  - t(6;9); *MYB::NFIB* most common
    - Present in ~ 90% of cases by FISH and RT-PCR
  - t(8;9); *MYBL1::NFIB*
  - Other rare fusion reported: *NFIB::AIG1*
- AcC
  - t(4;9)(q13;q31); *SCPP::NR4A3/NOR-1* rearrangement in most cases
  - Other rare fusion reported: *NR4A2* (~ 2%)
  - NR4A3 and NR4A2 fusions increase expression of NR4A proteins
    - High expression of MYB protein may cooccur; associated with high-grade transformation and short survival
- PMC and CribC
  - PMC: *PRKD1* mutations
  - CribC: *PRKD1*, *PRKD2*, or *PRKD3* fusions
- SC
  - *ETV6::NTRK3*; t(12;15)(p13;q25) most common fusion
  - *ETV6* break-apart probe can confirm diagnosis in appropriate clinical and histologic context
    - FISH may not be required for diagnosis in cases with typical histologic and IHC findings
  - Other tumors with *ETV6::NTRK3* fusions include congenital fibrosarcoma, congenital mesoblastic nephroma, acute myeloid leukemia, primary thyroid SC, ALK-negative inflammatory myofibroblastic tumor, some GIST, and some radiation-induced papillary thyroid carcinoma
  - Other fusions recently reported
    - t(12;10); *ETV6::RET*
    - t(12;7); *ETV6::MET*

Molecular Genetics

- General comments
  - Most salivary gland tumors show low tumor mutation burden (low TMB)
    - High-grade adenocarcinoma NOS: Highest rare of TMB > 10 mut/Mb ~ 20%
    - May explain relatively low overall response rate to current immune checkpoint inhibitors (ICPI)
      - Typically, cut-off of 20 mutations/Mb tends to predict response to ICPI
  - More fusion partners and entire new fusions are likely to be found as increasing numbers of cases are tested by RNASeq and other methods
  - Molecular testing may be required to determine optimal targeted therapy
    - SC with *ETV6::NTRK3* fusions would likely benefit from TRK inhibitors
      - However, rare SC with *ETV6::RET* fusion will not benefit from TRK inhibitors but may benefit from RET inhibitors
  - Salivary gland tumors generally have low rate of currently actionable alterations
    - *TP53* most frequently mutated gene; ranges from 14-60% of cases depending on tumor type
    - PIK3 pathway genes (*PIK3CA*, *PTEN*, *RICTOR*, *TSC2*, *NF1*); altered in 0-27% of cases depending on tumor type
      - PIK3 pathway inhibitors available
    - *BRAF* activating mutations rare (5% of cases)
- PA
  - Fusions and amplifications of *PLAG1* and *HMGA2* found in most cases
  - Ca ex PA has same genetic alterations as PA but with additional carcinogenic genetic changes
    - *CDKN2A* loss occurs in ~ 50% of Ca ex PA but is absent in PA
    - MicroRNAs: 13 significantly up- or downregulated in Ca ex PA compared to PA
      - Most differentially regulated microRNAs interact with *TP53*
- MEC
  - *CRTC1/CRTC3::MAML2*
    - Disrupt NOTCH signaling pathway
    - Upregulate *EGFR* ligand, amphiregulin → ↑ cell growth and survival
  - *CDKN2A*: Hypermethylated in 35%
- ADCC
  - Low TMB but high diversity of mutations
  - Cell cycle regulatory genes: *TP53* (especially in high-grade ADCC), *CDKN2A* (also suppressed by hypermethylation) mutated

Translocation-Specific Salivary Gland Tumors

- Other pathways or cell functions mutated
  - Chromatin remodeling genes, such as SMARC histones and histone modifiers (35%)
  - FGF/IGF/PI3K pathway (30%; solid histology only)
  - Cell adhesion molecules (30%), NOTCH signaling pathway (13%)
    - NOTCH pathway mutations confer worse prognosis
    - IHC expression of NOTCH1 protein identifies more aggressive tumors
- AcC
  - Enhancer portion of secretory calcium-binding phosphoprotein (*SCPP*) is rearranged upstream of *NR4A3/NOR-1* → ↑ NR4A3 expression
    - NR4A3/NOR-1 protein: Transcriptional activator
      - *NR4A3::NOR-1* fusion also found in extraskeletal myxoid chondrosarcoma; other partners involved than in AcC
  - *NR4A2* fusions also rarely occur; result in same histology; driven by effects of elevated NR4A2 transcriptional activity
- PMC and CribC
  - *PRKD1-3* activating mutations and fusions
    - Encode kinase involved in protein kinase C (PKC) and diacylglycerol (DAG) pathways
    - Fusion partners *ARID1A* and *DDX3X* involved in DNA repair and chromatin remodeling
- SC
  - *ETV6::NTRK3*: Chimeric protein tyrosine kinase
    - Activates RAS/MAPK pathway and PI3K/AKT pathway
  - *ETV6::RET*

Gene Expression Profiling

- ADCC
  - *MYB* overexpressed in 100% of cases
    - Fusion gene product: ↑ MYB transcriptional regulatory activity
    - *MYB* has at least 80 known target genes involved in cell cycle control, cell survival, proliferation, apoptosis, and hemostasis
  - Other overexpressed oncogenes: *KIT, SNAI2, EGFR, VEGFA, BDNF, NGF*
  - Underexpressed genes: *HOXC5, ACVRL1, AQP5, DUSP6, CDH1*
    - *CDH1* hypermethylated in 50%

ANCILLARY TESTS

PA

- IHC
  - Classic PA: Not usually performed but positive for myoepithelial markers (SMA, S100, GFAP, p63, calponin) and ductal epithelial markers (CK7, etc.)
    - PLAG1 often positive; may be helpful in sparse samples, such as FNA
  - Ca ex PA: Higher Ki-67 proliferation rate (~ 35%) compared to PA; p53 often overexpressed; ERBB2 (HER2) ± overexpressed
    - Salivary duct carcinoma Ca ex PA expresses AR (androgen receptor)
- In situ hybridization not usually performed

MEC

- IHC not usually performed in low-grade tumors
  - CK7 and p63 positive
  - p27 (KIP1) expression associated with improved disease-free and overall survival
- In situ hybridization
  - t(11;19); *CRTC1::MAML2*
    - *MAML2* FISH break-apart probe commercially available

ADCC

- IHC not usually performed in low-grade tumors
  - Myoepithelial and ductal epithelial markers positive
  - C-kit: Diffuse strong expression in most cases
    - Mutations of *KIT* rare in ADCC
  - MYB: Diffuse, strong expression relatively specific
  - Loss of E-cadherin expression correlates with poorer clinical outcome
  - NOTCH protein overexpression correlates with worse prognosis
- In situ hybridization
  - t(6;9); *MYB::NFIB*
    - Present in 90% of well-preserved samples
  - *NFIB::AIG1*: Other rare translocation

AcC

- IHC
  - NR4A3/NOR-1 protein: Diffuse nuclear expression in ~ 98% of cases; sensitive and specific
  - Other proteins expressed: DOG1, SOX10
- In situ hybridization or NGS demonstrate *SCPP::NR4A3/NOR-1* rearrangement in most cases

PMC and CribC

- IHC
  - Positive for S100 (typically diffusely); CK7 and p63 positive, but p40 is typically negative; usually patchy for C-kit
  - Variably positive (commonly negative) for myoepithelial markers (SMA, calponin, GFAP)
- Genetic testing
  - Not usually performed for diagnosis or prognosis
    - *PRKD1* mutation in exon 15 present in ~ 75%
    - *PRKD1-3* rearrangements predominantly in cribriform carcinoma

SC

- IHC
  - Positive for pan-TRK antibody, keratins, S100, vimentin, MUC4, mammaglobin, and GATA3
  - Distinctive histologic features combined with characteristic IHC reactivity allows diagnosis without recourse to FISH
- In situ hybridization
  - t(12;15); *ETV6::NTRK3*; rarely other *ETV6* partners
    - *ETV6* break-apart probe commercially available
    - For selection of targeted therapy in rare aggressive case, may require fusion partner information (e.g., *NTRK3*, *RET*, or *MET*)

Translocation-Specific Salivary Gland Tumors

DIFFERENTIAL DIAGNOSIS

DDx for Pleomorphic Adenoma
- Myoepithelioma/myoepithelial carcinoma
  - Lacks chondroid matrix and ductal differentiation of PA
- Ca ex PA
  - More pleomorphic than PA, often with increased mitoses and necrosis
  - Specific subtypes of salivary carcinoma can also form malignant component

DDx for Mucoepidermoid Carcinoma
- Necrotizing sialometaplasia
  - Retains lobular configuration, lacks mucous cells, shows inflamed desmoplastic stroma
  - Squamous pearls common and absent in nearly all MEC
- Adenosquamous carcinoma
  - Controversial entity: May represent high-grade MEC
- Salivary duct carcinoma
  - Can have mucous cells like MEC but also commonly resembles comedo-type DCIS of breast
  - Typically tumors cells more pleomorphic than MEC cells
  - Ancillary studies, such as IHC [positive AR, often positive ERBB2 (HER2) in salivary duct carcinoma] and negative FISH for t(11;19); *CRTC1::MAML2*
- Metastatic squamous cell carcinoma
  - Usually much more cytologic atypia than in MEC
  - Tends to be CK7(-)/p63(+) compared to MEC [diffusely CK7(+)/p63(+)]
  - FISH for t(11;19) negative in metastatic squamous cell carcinoma

DDx for Adenoid Cystic Carcinoma
- Polymorphous low-grade adenocarcinoma (PLGA)
  - Haphazard array of patterns, including targetoid, sheets, tubules, and cribriform
  - Pale vesicular nuclei compared to more hyperchromatic nuclei of ACC
  - FISH for t(6;9); *MYB::NFIB* negative in PLGA
  - IHC
    - Positive: S100 more diffusely, strongly positive in most cases compared to weak and patchy in ADCC; C-kit patchier than in most cases of ADCC; diffuse strong MYB expression in some ADCC and absent in PLGA
- Basal cell adenoma/adenocarcinoma
  - FISH for t(6;9); *MYB::NFIB* is negative in basal cell adenoma/adenocarcinoma
  - Lacks cribriform pattern found in many ADCC
- Adenocarcinoma, not otherwise specified (NOS) for high-grade ADCC
  - Lacks cribriform pattern found focally in some high-grade ADCC
  - FISH for t(6;9); *MYB::NFIB* negative in adenocarcinoma, NOS of salivary gland

DDx for Acinic Cell Carcinoma
- SC
  - Morphologic overlap can be considerable; zymogen granules less pronounced in SC
  - IHC
    - Positive: pan-TRK, S100
    - Negative: NR4A3
  - FISH or sequencing positive for *ETV6* rearrangement

DDx for Polymorphous Carcinoma and Cribriform Adenocarcinoma
- ADCC, adenocarcinoma NOS, PA (unencapsulated in minor salivary glands)

DDx for Secretory Carcinoma
- AcC
  - FISH negative for t(12;15); *ETV6::NTRK3*
    - *ETV6* break-apart probe commercially available
  - Basophilic cytoplasm due to ↑ number of zymogen granules
  - Immunohistochemistry
    - Negative: pan-TRK, S100, mammaglobin, MUC4 as in SC
    - Positive: NR4A3/NOR-1 in ~ 98% of cases
- Intraductal carcinoma (nonapocrine, nononcocytic type)
  - Can mimic SC by histology and IHC
  - FISH is negative for *ETV6* break-apart probe in intraductal carcinoma
  - FISH is positive for *NCOA4::RET*, *STRN::ALK*, *TUT1::ETV5*, or *KIAA217::RET* in most cases of typical intraductal carcinoma

SELECTED REFERENCES

1. Klubíčková N et al: A minority of cases of acinic cell carcinoma of the salivary glands are driven by an NR4A2 rearrangement: the diagnostic utility of the assessment of NR4A2 and NR4A3 alterations in salivary gland tumors. Virchows Arch. 482(2):339-45, 2023
2. Nishida H et al: Histopathological aspects of the prognostic factors for salivary gland cancers. Cancers (Basel). 15(4), 2023
3. Sharma P et al: Diagnostic accuracy of pan-TRK immunohistochemistry in differentiating secretory carcinoma from acinic cell carcinoma of salivary gland-a systematic review. J Oral Pathol Med. 52(3):255-62, 2023
4. Kim H et al: Identification of differentially expressed microRNAs as potential biomarkers for carcinoma ex pleomorphic adenoma. Sci Rep. 12(1):13383, 2022
5. Lassche G et al: Identification of fusion genes and targets for genetically matched therapies in a large cohort of salivary gland cancer patients. Cancers (Basel). 14(17), 2022
6. Skálová A et al: Update from the 5th edition of the World Health Organization classification of head and neck tumors: salivary glands. Head Neck Pathol. 16(1):40-53, 2022
7. Lee DY et al: Oncogenic orphan nuclear receptor NR4A3 interacts and cooperates with MYB in acinic cell carcinoma. Cancers (Basel). 12(9), 2020
8. Wong KS et al: NR4A3 immunohistochemistry reliably discriminates acinic cell carcinoma from mimics. Head Neck Pathol. ePub, 2020
9. Xu B et al: Histologic classification and molecular signature of polymorphous adenocarcinoma (PAC) and cribriform adenocarcinoma of salivary gland (CASG): an international interobserver study. Am J Surg Pathol. 44(4):545-52,, 2020
10. Xu B et al: Misinterpreted myoepithelial carcinoma of salivary gland: a challenging and potentially significant pitfall. Am J Surg Pathol. 43(5):601-9, 2019
11. Katabi N et al: PLAG1 immunohistochemistry is a sensitive marker for pleomorphic adenoma: a comparative study with PLAG1 genetic abnormalities. Histopathology. 72(2):285-93, 2018
12. Rito M et al: Salivary gland neoplasms: does morphological diversity reflect tumor heterogeneity. Pathobiology. 85(1-2):85-95, 2018
13. Skálová A et al: The role of molecular testing in the differential diagnosis of salivary gland carcinomas. Am J Surg Pathol. 42(2):e11-27, 2018

Translocation-Specific Salivary Gland Tumors

Molecular Alterations of More Common Salivary Gland Tumors (7 Tumors)

Tumor	Major Gene Alteration(s)	Chromosome Site/Abnormality	Prevalence
Pleomorphic adenoma	PLAG1 rearrangements HMGA2 rearrangements	8q12 12q14	25-30% 10-15%
Mucoepidermoid carcinoma	CRTC1::MAML2 CRTC3::MAML2	t(11;19) t(11;15)	40-80% 5%
Adenoid cystic carcinoma	MYB::NFIB MYBL1::NFIB	t(6;9) t(8;9)	25-50% Rare
Acinic cell carcinoma	NR4A3::NOR-1 fusion/activation NR4A2 fusion MSANTD3 fusion/amplification	9q31 (NR4A3::NOR-1) 2q22.23 (NR4A2) 19q31 (MSANTD3)	85-90% 1% 4%
Polymorphous adenocarcinoma	PRKD1 mutations	14q12	~75%
Cribriform adenocarcinoma	ARID1A::PRKD1 DDX3X::PRKD1 PRKD2 rearrangement PRKD3 rearrangement	t(1;14) t(X;14) 19q13 2p22	~40% for PRKD1 fusions ~15% ~20%
Secretory carcinoma	ETV6::NTRK3 ETV6::RET ETV6::MET ETV6::Other partners VIM::RET	t(12;15) t(12;10) t(12;7) Unknown t(10;10)	Majority Rare Rare Rare Exceptionally rare

Clinicopathologic Features of More Common Salivary Tumors (7 Tumors)

Tumor	Age Range	Most Common Site	Most Common Histologic Features	Typical IHC Reactivity
Pleomorphic adenoma	A > C MA	Major >> minor SG	Diverse patterns Ductal and myoepithelial cells Myxochondroid matrix	PLAG1(+) (C) MyoEp markers (+) Ductal markers (+)
Mucoepidermoid carcinoma	A > C MA & O	Major > minor SG	Patterns range by grade Intermediate cells, epidermoid cells and mucocytes; ± clear cells	p63, p40, CK5/6 (+) in epidermoid cells MyoEp markers (-)
Adenoid cystic carcinoma	MA & O	Major = minor SG	Cribriform, tubular solid, mixed 2 cell types: Ductal and myoepithelial	MYB(+) (C) Ductal markers (+) MyoEp markers (+) C-kit diffuse (+) (U)
Acinic cell carcinoma	A > C MA	Major >> minor SG	Diverse patterns: Solid, microcystic, trabecular, papillary-cystic Typically 2 cell types: Serous acinar and intercalated duct cells	NR4A3/NOR-1(+) in ~98% DOG1(+) SOX10(+)
Secretory carcinoma	MA & O	Major > minor SG	Diverse patterns, including microcystic with secretions Intercalated duct cell	Pan-TRK(+) Mammaglobin (+) GATA3(+) S100(+) (U)
Polymorphous adenocarcinoma and cribriform adenocarcinoma	MA & O	Minor SG	PMC: Diverse patterns even in one case; uniform terminal ductal cells with open chromatin CribC: Multinodular, solid, microcystic, and cribriform most commonly; cells usually bland with pale nuclei ± grooves	PMC & CriBC: p63(+) CK5/6(+), CK7(+) S100 diffuse (U) C-kit patchy (U) p40(-)

A > C = adults more than children, MA = middle-aged; MA & O = middle-aged adults and older; major SG = major salivary glands; minor SG = minor salivary glands; IHC = immunohistochemical; ductal markers: Keratin 7, pankeratin (AE1/AE3), EMA; MyoEp markers: SMA, calponin, GFAP, p63, S100; (U) = usually, (C) = commonly.

Translocation-Specific Salivary Gland Tumors

Pleomorphic Adenoma

(Left) *Pleomorphic adenoma is characterized by a haphazard mix of matrix material that ranges from myxoid ⇨ to myxochondroid with interspersed clusters or streams of myoepithelial cells and small ducts or nests formed by epithelial cells.* (Right) *In this pleomorphic adenoma, ductal epithelial cells ⇨ form tight clusters of eosinophilic cells and are surrounded by pale myoepithelial cells ⇨. These 2 cell types may sometimes be difficult to distinguish from each other.*

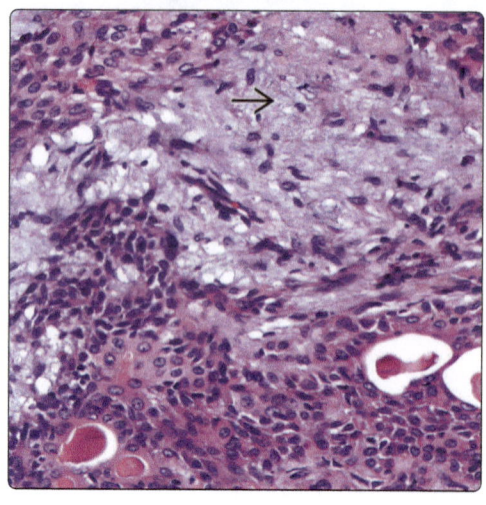

2 Main Cell Types of Pleomorphic Adenoma

Pleomorphic Adenoma With Squamous Metaplasia

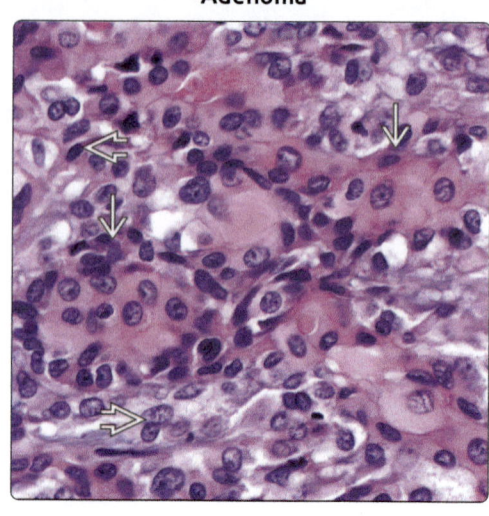

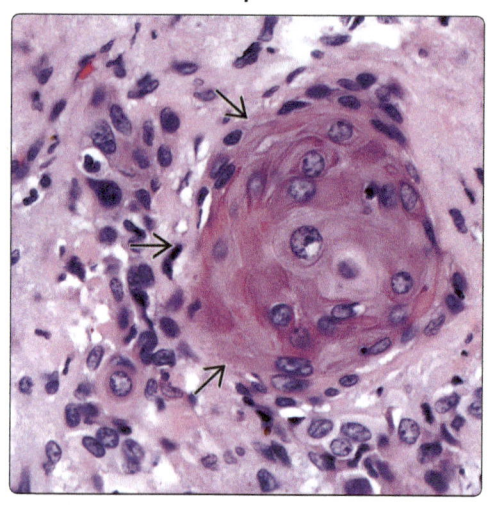

(Left) *Squamous metaplasia ⇨ is a common occurrence in pleomorphic adenoma and can cause potential diagnostic confusion, especially in an FNA specimen.* (Right) *Rarely, the stroma of pleomorphic adenoma may be almost entirely composed of myxochondroid matrix ⇨. These stroma-rich tumors may have a higher rate of local recurrence.*

Stroma-Rich Pleomorphic Adenoma

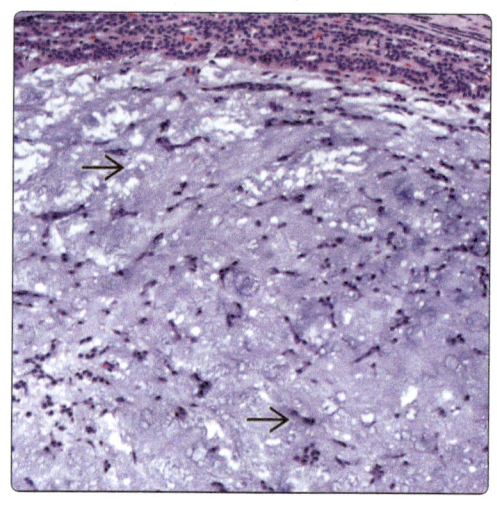

Carcinoma Ex Pleomorphic Adenoma

(Left) *Typical myxochondroid matrix ⇨ and low-grade histology ⇨ abut carcinoma ⇨ characterized by solid growth, increased pleomorphism and mitotic activity.* (Right) *Markedly pleomorphic tumor cells with abundant apocrine-like cytoplasm form a focus of salivary duct carcinoma arising in longstanding pleomorphic adenoma. The malignant cells expressed AR (not shown).*

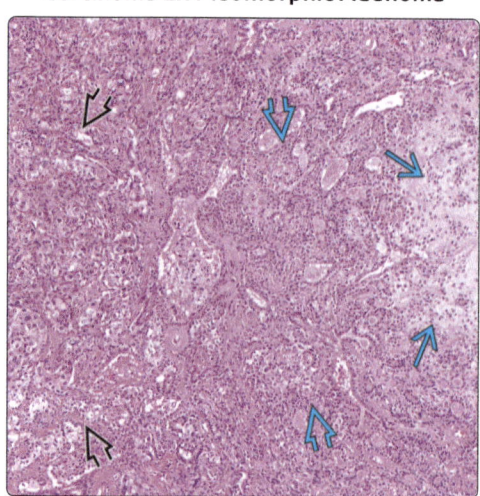

Salivary Duct Carcinoma Arising in Carcinoma Ex Pleomorphic Adenoma

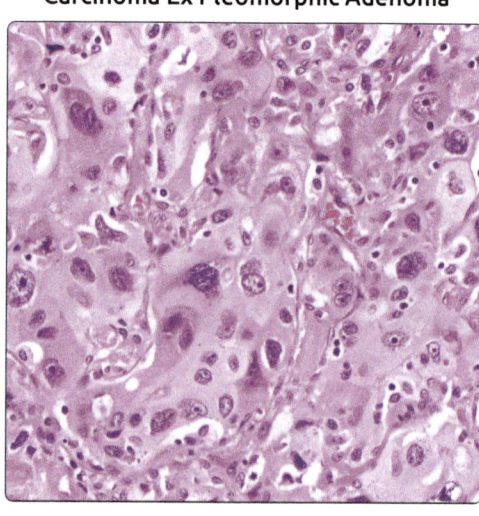

Translocation-Specific Salivary Gland Tumors

Low-Grade Mucoepidermoid Carcinoma

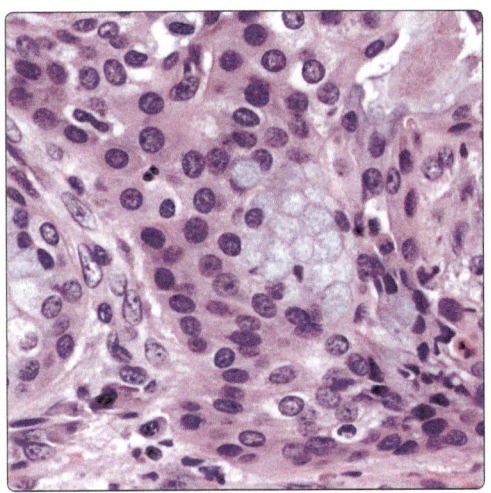

Intermediate Cells of Mucoepidermoid Carcinoma With Atypia

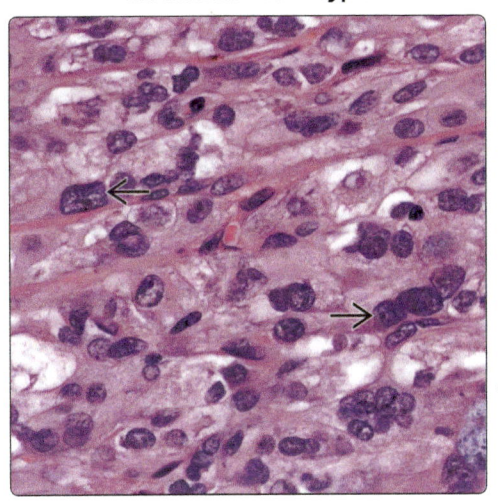

(Left) Epidermoid and mucous cells show minimal nuclear atypia characteristic of grade 1 tumors. Overt keratinization is rare in mucoepidermoid carcinoma, and, if prominent, should prompt strong consideration of another diagnosis. The epidermoid component tends to predominate in high-grade cases. (Right) Intermediate cells exhibit increasing nuclear atypia ⇒. Nuclear atypia is just one component evaluated in mucoepidermoid carcinoma grading systems.

Clear Cells

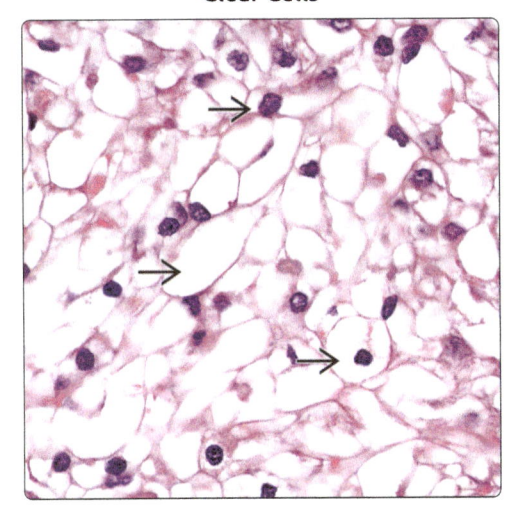

Intermediate-Grade Mucoepidermoid Carcinoma

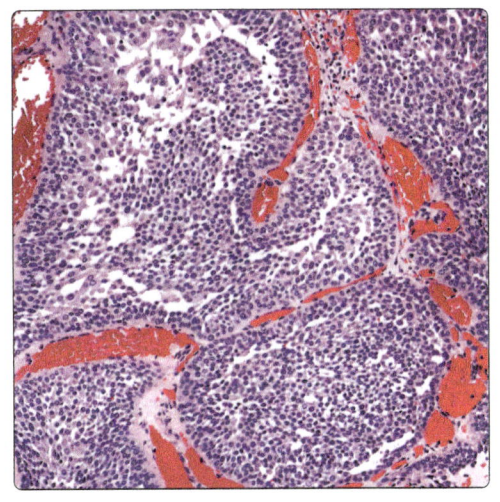

(Left) Mucoepidermoid carcinoma shows clear cells ⇒ common in mucoepidermoid carcinoma containing abundant glycogen. (Right) Intermediate-grade mucoepidermoid carcinoma contains only rare scattered mucous cells and few cysts, features consistent with higher grade tumor. However, the mitotic rate is low, and marked nuclear atypia is absent. Tallied together, these features are consistent with intermediate grade.

Oncocytic Variant of Mucoepidermoid Carcinoma

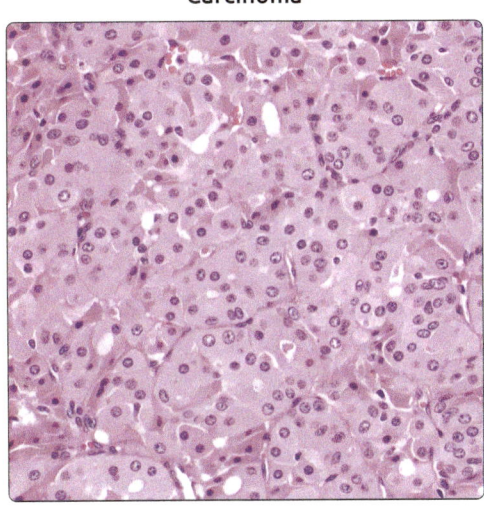

Oncocytic Variant of Mucoepidermoid Carcinoma

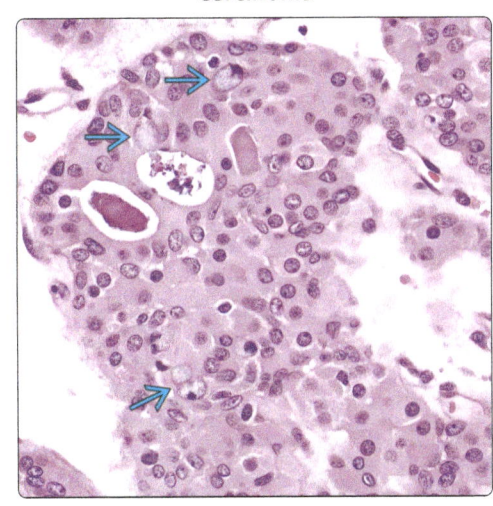

(Left) Oncocytic variant can mimic other oncocytic salivary gland tumors. Most cases will show the CRTC1/CRTC3::MAML2 fusion on ancillary testing. Some tumors also contain a clear cell component not seen in this case. (Right) Goblet cells ⇒ are scattered among oncocytic tumor cells.

Translocation-Specific Salivary Gland Tumors

Adenoid Cystic Carcinoma, Cribriform Pattern

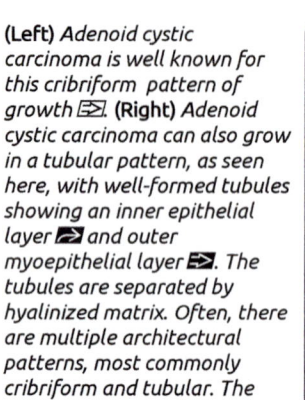

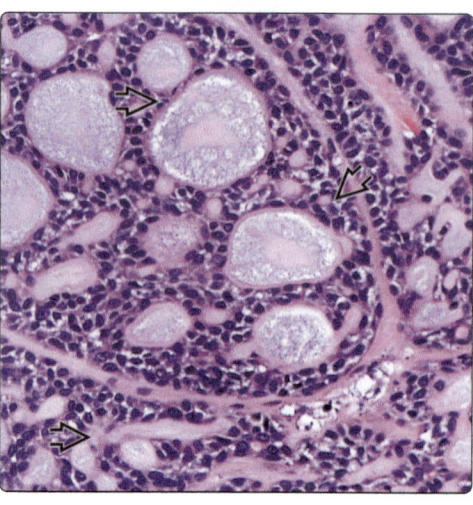

Adenoid Cystic Carcinoma, Tubular Pattern

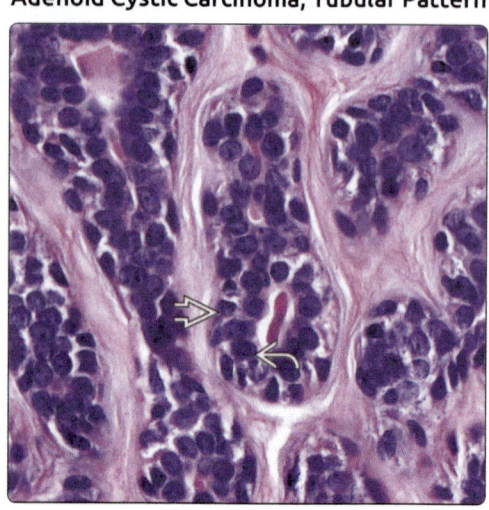

(Left) *Adenoid cystic carcinoma is well known for this cribriform pattern of growth ⇨.* (Right) *Adenoid cystic carcinoma can also grow in a tubular pattern, as seen here, with well-formed tubules showing an inner epithelial layer ⇨ and outer myoepithelial layer ⇨. The tubules are separated by hyalinized matrix. Often, there are multiple architectural patterns, most commonly cribriform and tubular. The solid pattern usually signals a more aggressive course.*

Polymorphous Carcinoma

Polymorphous Adenocarcinoma

(Left) *True to its name, polymorphous carcinoma usually features a number of architectural patterns in a single tumor. Note infiltration of normal mucinous acini ⇨.* (Right) *Polymorphous adenocarcinoma shows a vague cribriform pattern that at low power could suggest adenoid cystic carcinoma.*

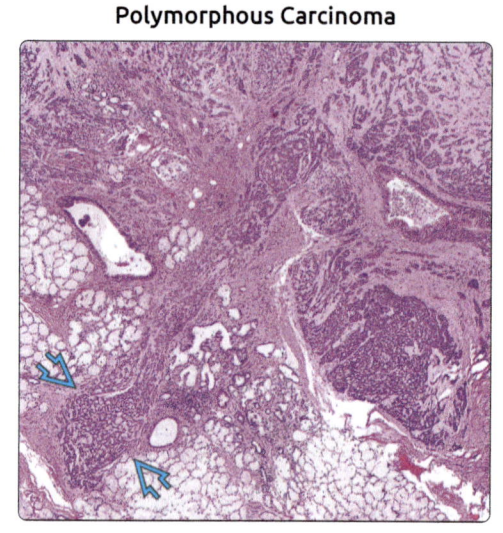

Cribriform Adenocarcinoma

Cribriform Adenocarcinoma

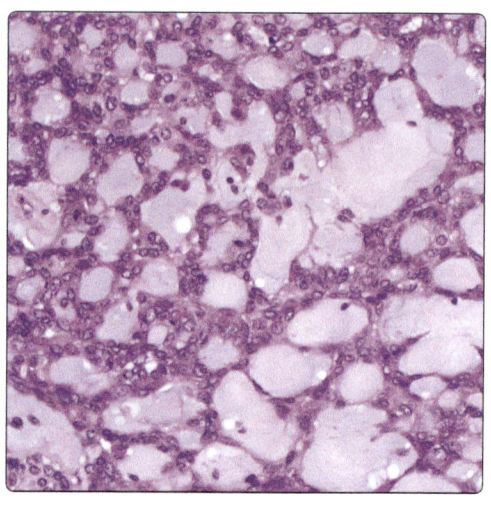

(Left) *This patient's cribriform adenocarcinoma occurred in the tongue base, a common location.* (Right) *Tumor nuclei are characteristically vesicular to clear with accentuated chromatinic rims ⇨. Nuclear grooves may also be identified ⇨, reminiscent of papillary thyroid carcinoma.*

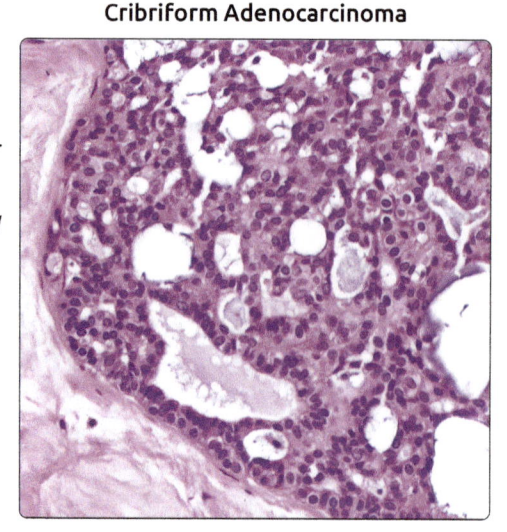

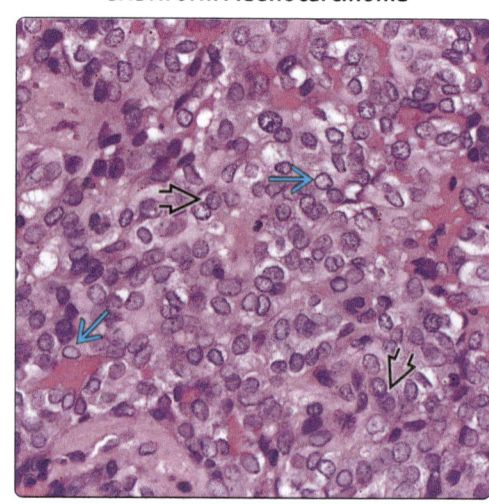

Translocation-Specific Salivary Gland Tumors

p63 Immunohistochemistry in CribC

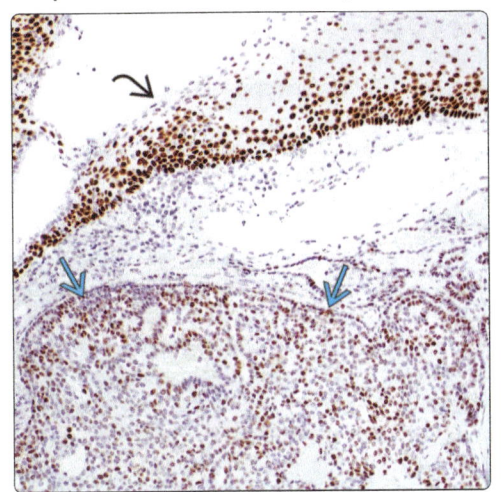

p40 Immunohistochemistry in CribC

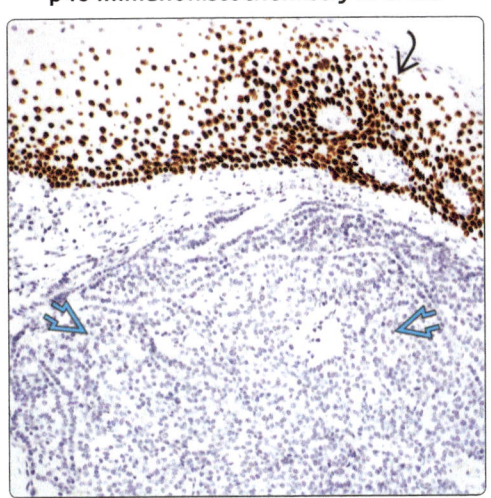

(Left) Cribriform adenocarcinoma usually expresses p63 ➡. Note the p63-positive overlying squamous mucosa ➡. (Right) In contrast to strong reactivity for p63, cribriform adenocarcinoma typically lacks reactivity for p40 ➡. Note the p40 internal positive control comprising normal tongue mucosa ➡.

Acinic Cell Carcinoma

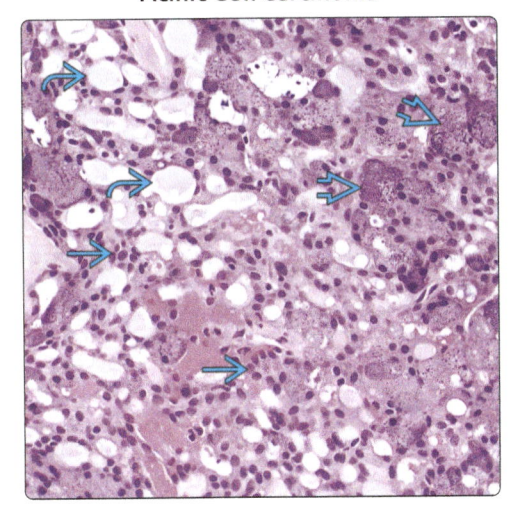

DOG1 Immunohistochemistry in Acinic Cell Carcinoma

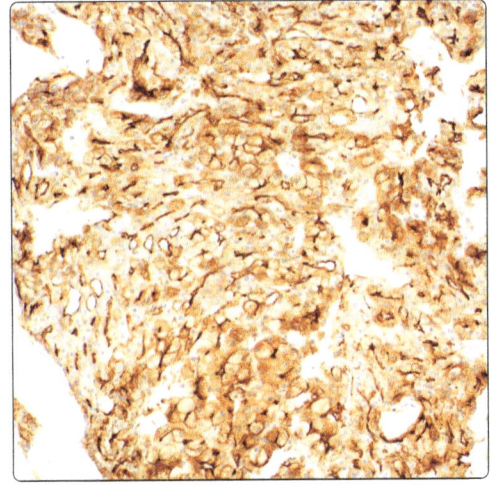

(Left) A common architectural pattern in acinic cell carcinoma comprises sheets of mixed intercalated duct cells ➡ and serous acinar cells ➡ punctuated by microcysts ➡. However, acinic cell carcinoma can show a diversity of architectures, including cystic-papillary, solid, and trabecular. (Right) DOG1 is usually diffusely expressed in acinic cell carcinoma. Expression can be luminal and cytoplasmic, as in this case. A more specific antibody that is diffusely positive in ~ 98% of acinic cell carcinoma is NR4A3.

Acinic Cell Carcinoma With High-Grade Transformation

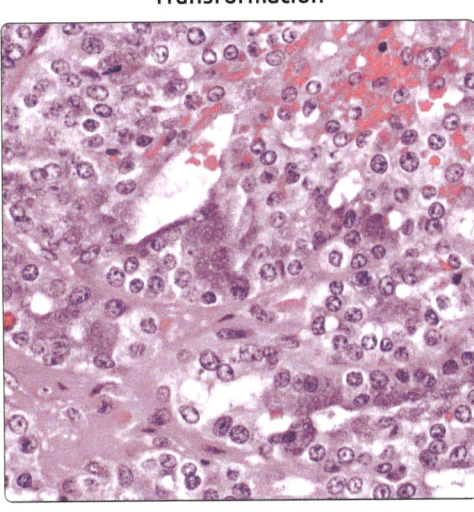

Acinic Cell Carcinoma With High-Grade Transformation

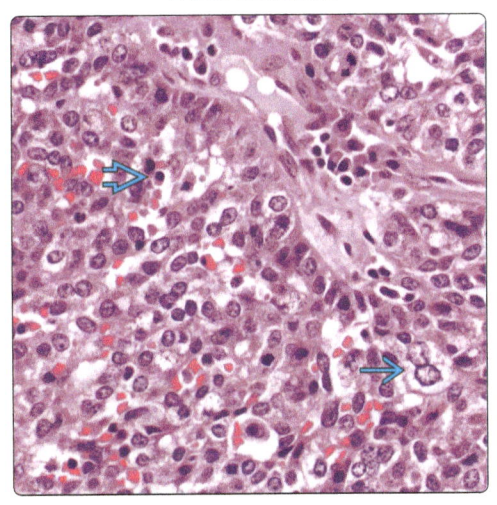

(Left) Lower grade area of acinic cell carcinoma with high-grade transformation shows neoplastic serous acinar cells with variable amounts of zymogen granules and mild nuclear atypia. (Right) High-grade transformed area shows increased cytologic atypia ➡ and individual cell necrosis ➡. Increased mitotic activity, high Ki-67 proliferation index, and foci of geographic necrosis were additional features found in high-grade areas.

Translocation-Specific Salivary Gland Tumors (Continued)

KEY FACTS

TERMINOLOGY

- 7 primary salivary gland (SG) tumors with gene fusions
  - Hyalinizing clear cell carcinoma (HCCC)
  - Epithelial myoepithelial carcinoma (E-MC)
  - Myoepithelial carcinoma (MyoEpC)
  - Basal cell adenoma/carcinoma (BCA/BCC)
  - Intraductal carcinoma (IntDC)
  - Salivary duct carcinoma (SDC)
  - Microsecretory adenocarcinoma (MS-AdCa)

CLINICAL ISSUES

- Targeted therapy is potentially effective in aggressive, high-grade SG tumors
- Targeted therapies continue to develop
  - May require use of several agents to target multiple dysregulated pathways

MOLECULAR

- Expression profiling per patient's high-grade tumor may identify targetable pathways
  - EGFR antibodies, mTOR inhibitors, PI3K, and RET inhibitors may be beneficial
  - Activating, targetable mutations rare per individual case and not generally restricted to specific SG subtypes

DIAGNOSTIC CHECKLIST

- SG tumors are rare and can show morphologic overlap
- E-MC, MyoEpC, and SDC may arise in setting of preexisting pleomorphic adenoma
- Presence of specific SG tumor gene alterations has diagnostic utility, especially in clinically or histologically atypical cases
- High-quality biospecimens preferred to optimize detection of translocations with techniques such as RNAseq or NanoString

Intraductal Carcinoma

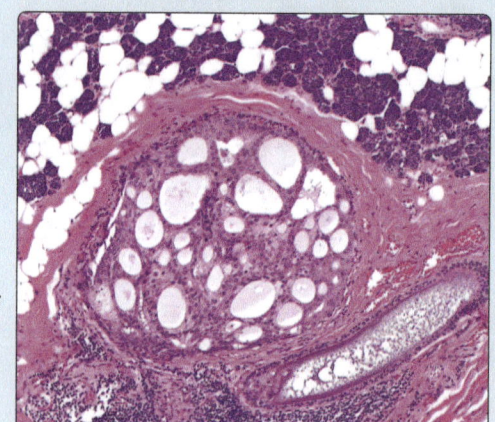

AR Expression in Intraductal Carcinoma

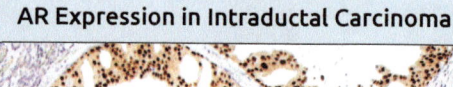

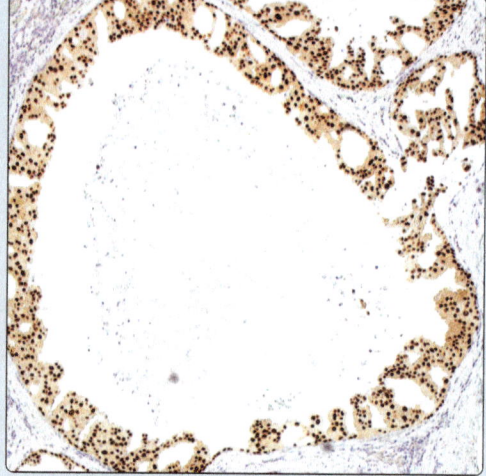

(Left) Histologically, intraductal carcinoma (IDC) can mimic ductal carcinoma in situ (DCIS) of any nuclear grade. Previous terms for IDC were "low-grade cribriform cystadenocarcinoma" or "low-grade salivary duct carcinoma," but the lesion can appear low grade or high grade. (Right) This case of IDC strongly expresses AR, which is usually positive in cases with apocrine features.

Hyalinizing Clear Cell Carcinoma

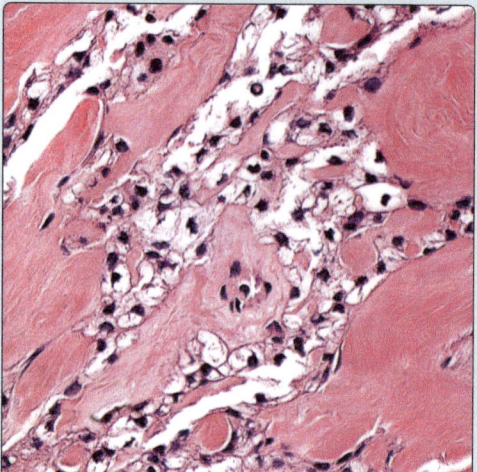

Hyalinizing Clear Cell Carcinoma

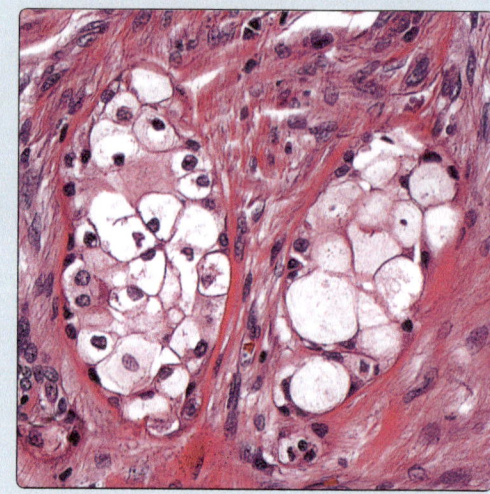

(Left) High-power view of clear cell carcinoma displays cords and trabeculae of epithelial cells with variably clear cytoplasm set within a densely collagenized, acellular stroma. (From DP: Head & Neck.) (Right) The epithelial cells are round to polygonal with well-defined cytoplasmic borders. Intracytoplasmic glycogen accumulation accounts for cell expansion and clear presentation. (From DP: Head & Neck.)

Translocation-Specific Salivary Gland Tumors (Continued)

TERMINOLOGY

Definitions

- 7 primary salivary gland (SG) tumors with specific gene alterations
  - Hyalinizing clear cell carcinoma (HCCC)
  - Epithelial-myoepithelial carcinoma (E-MC)
  - Myoepithelial carcinoma (MyoEpC)
  - Basal cell adenoma/carcinoma (BCA/BCC)
  - Intraductal carcinoma (IntDC)
  - Salivary duct carcinoma (SDC)
  - Microsecretory adenocarcinoma (MSAdCa)

CLINICAL ISSUES

Epidemiology

- Incidence
  - E-MC, MyoEpC, and HCCC: Rare SG tumors that may be underdiagnosed due to histologic similarities with other tumor types
  - BCA/BCC: Uncommon as benign; rare as malignant
  - IntDC: Rare
  - SDC: May arise from preceding pleomorphic adenoma
  - MS-AdCa: Rare (< 100 cases reported)

Site

- HCCC: Minor SGs of oral cavity most commonly involved
- E-MC: Parotid > submandibular > other sites
- MyoEpC: Parotid > minor SG of palate > submandibular SG
- IntDC: Parotid most commonly
- SDC: Parotid most commonly
- BCA/BCC: Parotid most commonly
- MS-AdCA: Minor SGs of oral cavity; rarely in parotid

Presentation

- HCCC: Slow-growing, painless mass
- E-MC: Slow-growing, painless mass in most cases
- MyoEpC: Painless to rapidly growing, painful mass or with other facial nerve symptoms
- BCA/BCC: Usually painless mass; few BCAs associated with dermal eccrine tumors
- IntDC: Asymptomatic mass or swelling
- SDC: Rapidly growing mass, usually painful and often with lymphadenopathy of cervical chain
- MS-AdCa: Slow-growing, painless mass

Treatment

- Complete surgical excision required for all of these tumor types
  - HCCC with rare anaplastic or transformed variant may require radical excision and adjuvant therapy

Prognosis

- HCCC
  - Low local recurrence rate (15-20%) and low regional lymph node metastasis rate with only rare distant metastases
  - Very rare anaplastic/transformed variant behaves more aggressively
- E-MC
  - Typical case can locally recur; rare lymph node and distant metastases
- MyoEpC
  - Some cases metastasize, usually to lungs
  - Some cases cured by resection alone
- BCA/BCC
  - BCA: Membranous variant has 25% local recurrence rate; other types < 10%
  - BCC: Local recurrence rate of ~ 33%; local and distant metastases and death due to tumor are rare
- IntDC
  - Cured by complete excision
- SDC
  - Aggressive with local recurrences, lymph node and distant metastases; ~ 50% 5-year survival
- MS-AdCa
  - Indolent in almost all cases out of < 100 cases reported; single case of metastasis and single case of high-grade transformation

MOLECULAR

In Situ Hybridization

- HCCC
  - t(12;22); *EWSR1*::*ATF1* present in ~ 95% of cases
    - Fuses *EWSR1* to *ATF1*
    - Other tumors with *EWSR1*::*ATF1* fusions include clear cell sarcoma, angiomatoid fibrous histiocytomas, and clear cell sarcoma of GI tract
    - Clear cell odontogenic carcinoma has *EWSR1*::*ATF1* fusion; intraosseous variant of HCCC
- IntDC
  - Intercalated type: t(10;10); *NCOA4*::*RET*
  - Apocrine type: t(6;10); *TRIM27*::*RET*
- MyoEpC
  - *EWSR1* rearrangements with unknown partner
    - *EWSR1* fusions occur predominantly in clear cell variant
  - *PLAG1* fusions occur in cases presumably arising from pleomorphic adenoma (n = 40 cases studied)
    - t(8;8); *FGFR1*::*PLAG1*
    - t(1;8); *TGFBR3*::*PLAG1*
    - *MT-ND4*::*PLAG1*; translocation between mitochondrial-encoded *ND4* and nuclear *PLAG1*

Molecular Genetics

- General comments
  - Most SG tumors show low tumor mutation burden (low TMB)
    - High-grade adenocarcinoma NOS: Highest rare of TMB > 10 mut/Mb ~ 20%
      - Data derive from 623 SG tumors assessed for up to 315 genes (Foundation One assay platform)
    - May explain relatively low overall response rate to current immune checkpoint inhibitors (ICPI)
      - Typically, cut-off of 20 mutations/Mb tends to predict response to ICPI
  - More fusion partners and entire new fusions are likely to be found as increasing numbers of cases are tested by RNASeq and other methods
  - Molecular testing may be required to determine optimal targeted therapy

Translocation-Specific Salivary Gland Tumors (Continued)

- ○ SG tumors generally have low rate of currently actionable alterations
  - – *TP53* most frequently mutated gene; ranges from 14-60% of cases depending on tumor type
  - – PIK3 pathway genes (*PIK3CA, PTEN, RICTOR, TSC2, NF1*): Altered in 0-27% of cases depending on tumor type
    - □ PIK3 pathway inhibitors available
  - – *BRAF*-activating mutations rare (5% of cases)
- HCCC
  - ○ EWSR1::ATF1 fusion protein: Constitutive transcription activator
    - – May suppress *TP53*
    - – May decrease expression of *SH3RF1*
  - ○ EWSR1::CREM fusion protein: Constitutive transcription activator
    - – *ATF1* and *CREM* in CREB family of transcription factors
- E-MC
  - ○ *HRAS* mutations present in ~ 33%
    - – Predominantly found in cases with intact *PLAG1* and *HMGA2*
  - ○ Cases with presumed preceding PA (up to ~ 80% of cases)
    - – *PLAG1* rearrangements ± hyperploidy
    - – *HMGA2* rearrangements ± hyperploidy or hyperploidy alone
  - ○ High-grade E-MC
    - – Additional alterations variably involving tumor suppressor genes, such as *TP53, SMARCB1*
- MyoEpC
  - ○ *PLAG1* rearrangements found in 70% (n = 40 cases)
  - ○ Higher number copy number alterations independently predict risk of recurrence (n = 40 tumors)
  - ○ *EWSR1* rearrangements with unknown partner(s): Few cases
    - – *EWSR1* rearrangements also found in some myoepitheliomas of SG
  - ○ Low TMB: 0.5 mutations/Mb (megabase)
  - ○ Intratumoral heterogeneity present despite low TMB
- BCA/BCC
  - ○ *CTNNB1* (β-catenin) mutations: 50% of BCA but rare or absent in BCC
  - ○ *CYLD* LOH: present in cases with familial dermal cylindromatosis and sporadically
    - – Membranous variant of basal cell adenoma affected
    - – Rare basal adenocarcinomas also positive for *CYLD* loss of heterozygosity (LOH)
  - ○ Basal cell adenocarcinoma: Lack molecular genetic data
- IntDC
  - ○ Intercalated duct type: *NCOA4*::*RET* and *TRIM27*::*RET* mutations
  - ○ Apocrine type: *PIK3CA* and *HRAS* hotspot mutations
- SDC
  - ○ *ERBB2* amplification: ~ 35%
    - – *TP53* mutated in ~ 85% of cases with *ERBB2* amplification (Foundation One data)
      - □ *TP53* mutated overall in ~ 55%
  - ○ *PIK3CA* mutations: > 20%
    - – Also found at > 20% frequency in MEC, ADCC, and adenocarcinoma, NOS
  - ○ *HRAS/NRAS* mutations: ~ 30%
  - ○ Androgen receptor: Mutations, extra gene copies (altered in at least 80%)
  - ○ *FOXO1*: Mutated in some cases
    - – Plays role in androgen receptor signaling
  - ○ *PLAG1* and *HMGA2* rearrangements found in cases arising from pleomorphic adenoma
- MS-AdCA
  - ○ MEF2C::SS18 fusion protein is oncogenic

Gene Expression Profiling

- SDC
  - ○ Expression profile remarkably similar to apocrine carcinoma of breast
  - ○ *EGFR* commonly overexpressed

ANCILLARY TESTS

Hyalinizing Clear Cell Carcinoma

- IHC
  - ○ Positive for keratins, including CK5/6 and p63 if squamous differentiation present
  - ○ Negative for myoepithelial markers (S100, SMA, calponin) in most cases
- In situ hybridization
  - ○ t(12;22); *EWSR1*::*ATF1* and uncommon t(10;22); *EWSR1*::*CREM*

Epithelial-Myoepithelial Carcinoma

- IHC: EMA and C-kit stain ductal cells; S100, actin, calponin, p63, and p40 stain myoepithelial cells
- Genetic testing: Not usually performed currently

Myoepithelial Carcinoma

- IHC: Must react for at least 2 myoepithelial markers, such as p63, p40, S100, actin, calponin, and GFAP
- Genetic testing: Rare cases may show *EWSR1* rearrangement by ISH

Basal Cell Adenoma/Adenocarcinoma

- IHC: Tubular/trabecular cases usually express nuclear β-catenin and LEF1, myoepithelial markers and C-kit; membranous variant also expresses myoepithelial markers and C-kit
- Genetic testing: Germline testing in familial cases for *CYLD* alterations; otherwise not usually performed currently

Intraductal Carcinoma

- IHC: Often AR positive; S100, mammaglobin, and GATA3 with preserved peripheral myoepithelial rim expressing p63, S100, and actin
- Genetic testing: Not usually performed currently

Salivary Duct Carcinoma

- IHC: AR positivity almost requirement; HER2, GATA3, GCDFP, and mammaglobin often positive; negative to only focally positive for p40, p63, and CK5/6
- Genetic testing: Not usually performed currently

Microsecretory Adenocarcinoma

- IHC: Nonspecific but positive for S100, SOX10, and p63; negative for p40
- FISH or sequencing: Shows *SS18* (18q11.2) rearrangement or fusion with *MEF2C* (5q14)

Translocation-Specific Salivary Gland Tumors (Continued)

DIFFERENTIAL DIAGNOSIS

DDx for Hyalinizing Clear Cell Carcinoma
- Clear cell-containing SG tumors
  - May be positive for myoepithelial markers, which are absent in CCC
- Mucoepidermoid carcinoma
  - Usually lacks prominent hyalinized stroma
  - FISH for *EWSR1* break-apart probe is positive in CCC
  - FISH for t(11;19); *CRTC1::MAML2* fusion is positive in MEC
- Metastatic clear cell renal cell carcinoma (RCC)
  - Lacks distinctive architectural patterns found in most cases of CCC
  - Lacks squamous and mucinous cells that are fairly common in CCC
  - IHC
    - Positive: RCC, vimentin, and PAX8 in many cases; negative in CCC
  - FISH for *EWSR1* break-apart probe is positive in CCC and negative in metastatic clear cell RCC

DDx for Polymorphous Carcinoma
- Adenoid cystic carcinoma
  - Biphasic with distinct myoepithelial cells and ductal luminal cells
  - Positive for MYB by IHC in most cases
- Adenocarcinoma, NOS
  - Usually higher grade nuclear features
- Pleomorphic adenoma (unencapsulated in minor SGs)
  - Biphasic with distinct myoepithelial cells and ductal luminal cells

DDx for Basal Cell Adenoma/Adenocarcinoma
- Pleomorphic adenoma
  - Myxochondroid matrix
  - More heterogeneous appearance in most cases
- Canalicular adenoma
  - One cell type without ducts
  - Hypocellular stroma
  - S100 diffusely positive

DDx for Epithelial-Myoepithelial Carcinoma
- Pleomorphic adenoma
  - Myxochondroid matrix
  - Noninfiltrative into surrounding gland
- BCC

DDx for Myoepithelial Carcinoma
- Myoepithelioma
  - Noninvasive
- CCC for cases with clear myoepithelial cells
- Various spindle cell tumors for cases composed of spindle cells

DDx for Intraductal Carcinoma
- Sclerosing polycystic adenosis
  - Resembles proliferative fibrocystic change of breast with interspersed fibrosis
  - Contains intermixed acinar cells and myoepithelial cells
  - Lacks malignant nuclear features
- Secretory carcinoma
  - Lacks peripheral rim of p63-expressing myoepithelial cells as seen in nests of intraductal carcinoma

DDx for Salivary Duct Carcinoma
- Salivary adenocarcinoma NOS
- High-grade mucoepidermoid carcinoma
  - Lacks expression of AR
  - Some cases positive for *MAML2* fusion
- Metastatic adenocarcinoma

DDx for Microsecretory Adenocarcinoma
- Secretory carcinoma: Expresses mammaglobin; positive for *ETV6* fusion
- Adenoid cystic carcinoma: Has myoepithelial AND ductal cells; positive for *MYB*, *MYB1*, &/or *NFIB* rearrangements
- Sclerosing microcystic adenocarcinoma: Sparse cellularity with more prominent stroma; 2 cell population

DIAGNOSTIC CHECKLIST

Pathologic Interpretation Pearls
- Specific SG tumor mutations have diagnostic utility, especially in clinically or histologically atypical cases
- High-quality biospecimens required to optimize detection of translocations
- Additional translocations likely to be found in other SG tumors

SELECTED REFERENCES

1. Bishop JA et al: Microsecretory adenocarcinoma of salivary glands. Adv Anat Pathol. 30(2):130-5, 2023
2. Weinreb I et al: Microcribriform adenocarcinoma of salivary glands: a unique tumor entity characterized by an SS18::ZBTB7A fusion. Am J Surg Pathol. 47(2):194-201, 2023
3. Bishop JA: Proceedings of the North American Society of Head and Neck Pathology, Los Angeles, CA, March 20, 2022: Emerging entities in salivary gland tumor pathology. Head Neck Pathol. 16(1):179-89, 2022
4. Skalova A et al: Clear cell neoplasms of salivary glands: a diagnostic challenge. Adv Anat Pathol. 29(4):217-26, 2022
5. Skálová A et al: Update from the 5th edition of the World Health Organization classification of head and neck tumors: salivary glands. Head Neck Pathol. 16(1):40-53, 2022
6. Bishop JA et al: Microsecretory adenocarcinoma: a novel salivary gland tumor characterized by a recurrent MEF2C-SS18 fusion. Am J Surg Pathol. 43(8):1023-32, 2019
7. El Hallani S et al: Epithelial-myoepithelial carcinoma: frequent morphologic and molecular evidence of preexisting pleomorphic adenoma, common HRAS mutations in PLAG1-intact and HMGA2-intact cases, and occasional TP53, FBXW7, and SMARCB1 alterations in high-grade cases. Am J Surg Pathol. 42(1):18-27, 2018
8. Rito M et al: Salivary gland neoplasms: does morphological diversity reflect tumor heterogeneity. Pathobiology. 85(1-2):85-95, 2018
9. Skálová A et al: The role of molecular testing in the differential diagnosis of salivary gland carcinomas. Am J Surg Pathol. 42(2):e11-27, 2018
10. Skálová A et al: Molecular profiling of salivary gland intraductal carcinoma revealed a subset of tumors harboring NCOA4-RET and novel TRIM27-RET fusions: a report of 17 cases. Am J Surg Pathol. 42(11):1445-55, 2018
11. Weinreb I et al: Recurrent RET gene rearrangements in intraductal carcinomas of salivary gland. Am J Surg Pathol. 42(4):442-52, 2018
12. Dalin MG et al: Multi-dimensional genomic analysis of myoepithelial carcinoma identifies prevalent oncogenic gene fusions. Nat Commun. 8(1):1197, 2017
13. Ni H et al: EWSR1 rearrangement is present in a subset of myoepithelial tumors of salivary glands with variable morphology and does not correlate with clinical behavior. Ann Diagn Pathol. 28:19-23, 2017
14. Patel KR et al: Mammaglobin and S-100 immunoreactivity in salivary gland carcinomas other than mammary analogue secretory carcinoma. Hum Pathol. 44(11):2501-8, 2013
15. Simpson RH: Salivary duct carcinoma: new developments--morphological variants including pure in situ high grade lesions; proposed molecular classification. Head Neck Pathol. 7 Suppl 1:S48-58, 2013

Translocation-Specific Salivary Gland Tumors (Continued)

Molecular Alterations of 7 Salivary Gland Tumors

Tumor	Major Gene Alteration(s)	Chromosome Site/Abnormality	Prevalence
Hyalinizing clear cell carcinoma	EWSR1::ATF1 EWSR1::CREM	t(12;22) t(10;22)	80-90% Rare
Epithelial-myoepithelial carcinoma	HRAS PLAG1, HMGA2 rearrangements	11p15 8q12; 12q14	33% Up to 80%
Myoepithelial carcinoma	EWSR1 rearrangements PLAG1 rearrangements	22q12 8q12	Minority Up to 70%
Basal cell adenoma/carcinoma	CTNNB1 mutation CYLD LOH or mutation	3p22 16q12	~70% tubulotrabecular BCA/BCC ~80% membranous BCA/BCC
Intraductal carcinoma - Intercalated duct type - Apocrine duct type	RET rearrangements Similar to salivary duct carcinoma	10q11 See below	~50% >50%
Salivary duct carcinoma	ERBB2 (HER2) amplification PIK3CA mutation HRAS mutation	17q12 3q26 11p15	~40% ~20%
Microsecretory adenocarcinoma	MEF2C::SS18	t(5;18)	~100%

Clinicopathologic Features of 7 Salivary Tumors

Tumor	Age Range	Most Common Site	Most Common Histologic Features	Typical IHC Reactivity
Hyalinizing clear cell carcinoma	MA&O	Minor > major SG	Sheets, nests Often hyalinized stroma Clear and eosinophilic cells ± mucocytes and squamous cells	Pankeratins (+) p63(+/-) S100(-)
Epithelial-myoepithelial carcinoma	MA&O	Major > minor SG	Tight bilayered tubules of outer, often clear MyoEp and inner ductal cells ± MyoEp overgrowth	PanK: Ductal cells only MyoEp markers in MyoEp cells
Myoepithelial carcinoma	MA&O	Most in parotid	Sheets and nests of MyoEp cells with spindled, round epithelioid, clear ± plasmacytoid features	PanK(+) S100 usually diffuse Other MyoEp markers (+)
Intraductal carcinoma	MA&O	Most in parotid	Intraductal proliferation of varying patterns resembling breast DCIS Low- to rarely high-grade nuclei	Ductal cell markers in luminal cells Outer cells (+) for MyoEp markers
Basal cell adenoma and adenocarcinoma	MA&O	Most in parotid	Solid, tubular, membranous 2 main cell types: Basal-like outer cells and inner pale large cells Stroma often cellular Ducts often present, scattered	Ductal and MyoEp markers (+)
Salivary duct carcinoma	MA&O	Most in parotid	Nodules of high-grade cells often with some comedonecrosis Apocrine in majority of cases Other morphologies include mucin-rich, sarcomatoid, and micropapillary	AR: Diffuse (+) GATA3, PanK (+) HER2(+) in 50%
Microsecretory adenocarcinoma	MA&O	Oral cavity; rare cases in skin or external auditory canal	Microtubules containing bluish secretions is the predominant architecture Background fibromyxoid stroma Cell type: Intercalated duct-like cell forming microcysts; often flattened; no significant cytologic atypia	SOX10(+) S100(+) p63(+) p40, mammaglobin, calponin (-)

MA&O = middle-aged adults and older; major SG = major salivary glands; minor SG = minor salivary glands; ductal markers = keratin 7, pankeratin (like AE1/AE3), EMA; MyoEp markers = SMA, calponin, GFAP, p63, S100.

Translocation-Specific Salivary Gland Tumors (Continued)

Basal Cell Adenoma

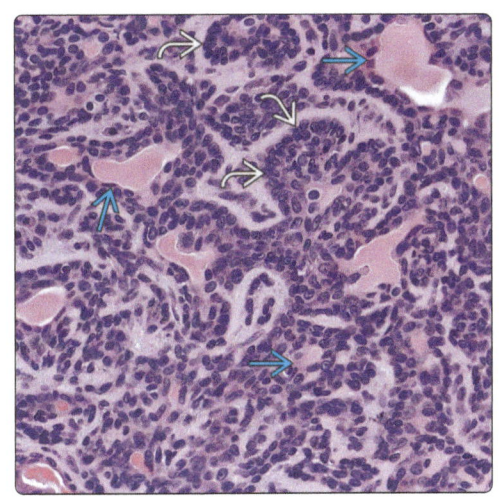

Basal Cell Adenoma

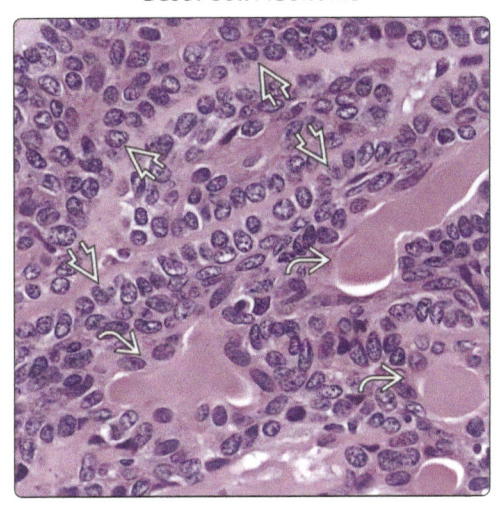

(Left) Tubular variant of basal cell adenoma (BCA) shows numerous duct lumina ⇨ and peripheral palisading of basal cells ⇨ surrounding central paler cells. Note the somewhat cellular stroma. (Right) Tumor cells are uniform and comprise an outer layer of basaloid cells with myoepithelial features ⇨ and an inner layer of larger, paler cells. Ducts may be present ⇨. Squamous metaplasia can also occur (not shown).

Epithelial-Myoepithelial Carcinoma

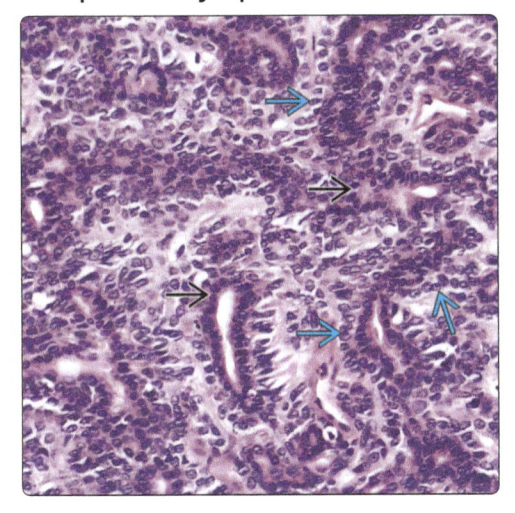

Epithelial-Myoepithelial Carcinoma With Loss of Typical Linked Structures

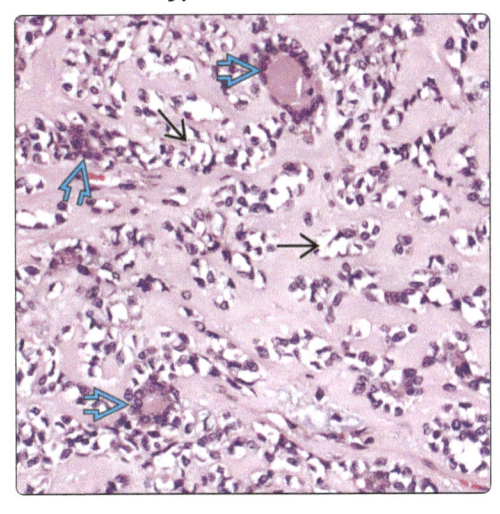

(Left) Back-to-back, serpentine ribbons of tightly associated outer (often clear) myoepithelial cells ⇨ and inner ductal cells ⇨ comprise the classic growth pattern of epithelial-myoepithelial carcinoma (E-MC). (Right) Some cases of E-MC contain areas of tumor with overgrowth of myoepithelial cells (clear cytoplasm ⇨) compared to ductal cells ⇨.

CAM5.2 Expression in Epithelial-Myoepithelial Carcinoma

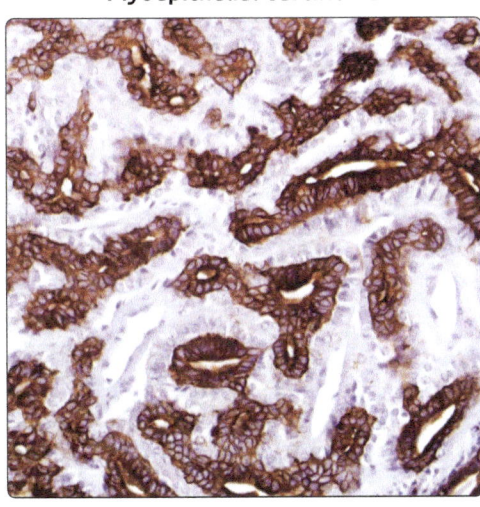

p63 Expression in Epithelial-Myoepithelial Carcinoma

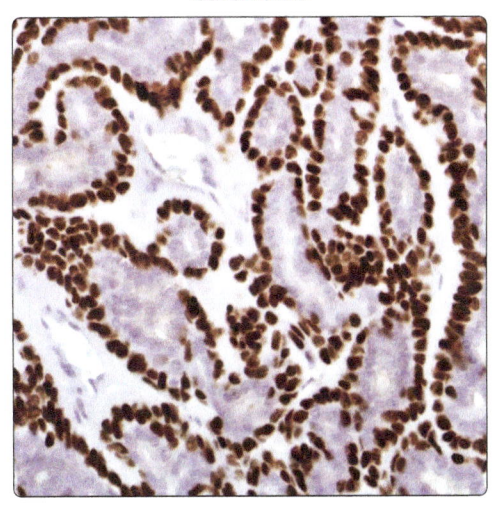

(Left) CAM5.2 is strongly expressed in the inner ductal cell layer. (Right) By contrast, p63 is strongly and diffusely expressed in the outer myoepithelial cells with no reactivity in the inner ductal cells.

Translocation-Specific Salivary Gland Tumors (Continued)

Salivary Duct Carcinoma

Salivary Duct Carcinoma: Comedonecrosis

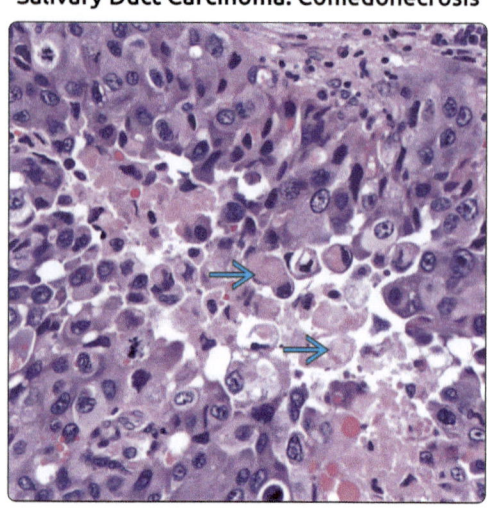

(Left) *Salivary duct carcinoma (SDC) commonly grows as irregular, solid nests of central necrosis.* (Right) *True comedonecrosis is typical with central accumulation of nonviable cells in various stages of dissolution ➡.*

GCDFP-15 Expression in Salivary Duct Carcinoma

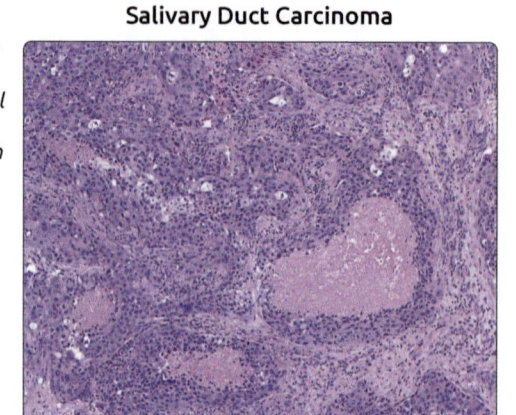

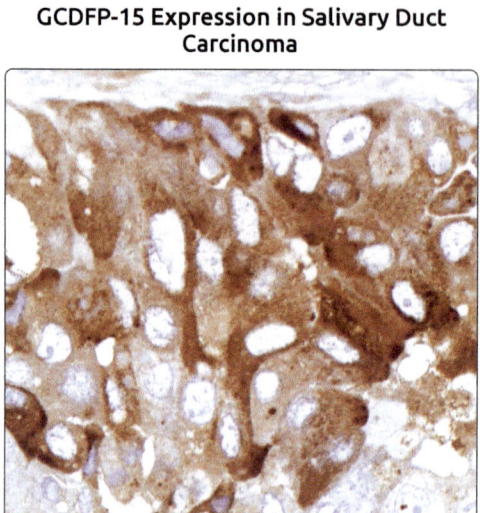

HER2 Expression in Salivary Duct Carcinoma

(Left) *GCDFP-15 is commonly expressed in SDC. Mammaglobin and GATA3 also may be expressed in SDC as well as AR (seen in nearly all cases).* (Right) *This case of SDC shows strong, diffuse, circumferential HER2 expression.*

Salivary Duct Carcinoma

Salivary Duct Carcinoma: Apocrine Cells

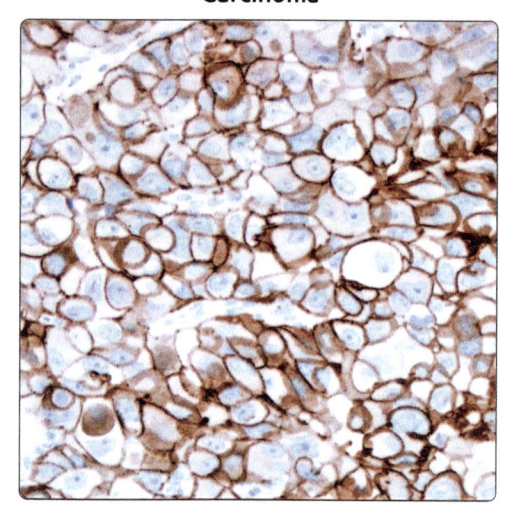

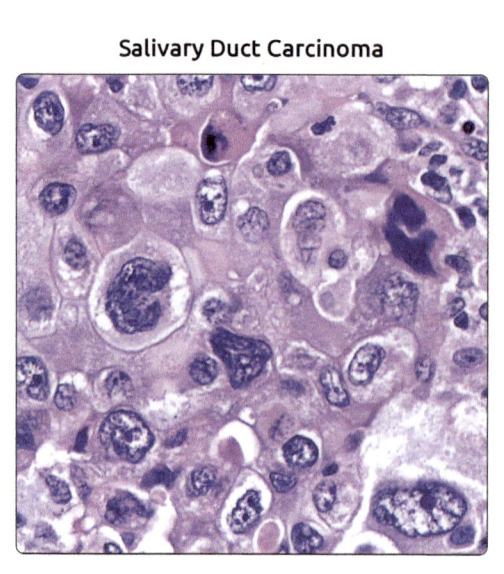

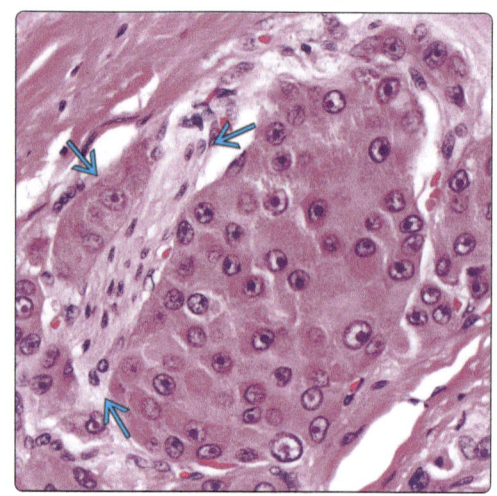

(Left) *Pleomorphism is often marked in SDC.* (Right) *SDC mimics breast carcinoma with apocrine differentiation, which is striking in this example. Note the perineural invasion ➡.*

Translocation-Specific Salivary Gland Tumors (Continued)

Myoepithelial Carcinoma

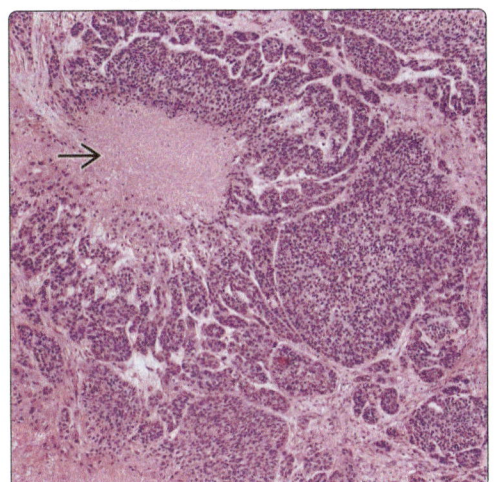

Myoepithelial Carcinoma

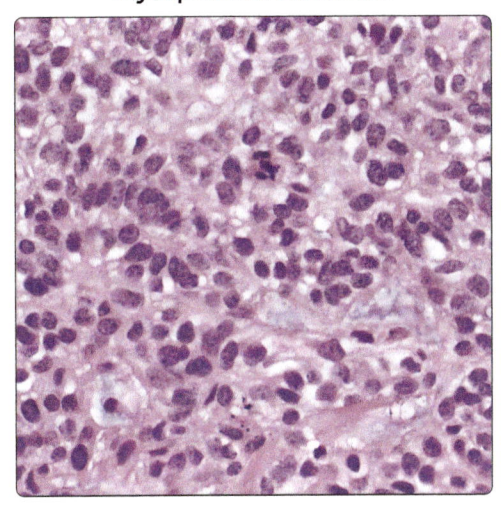

(Left) Myoepithelial carcinoma often consists of merging nodules of tumor. Central necrosis ➡ may mimic SDC at low power. (Right) Myoepithelial cells range in cytologic appearance from spindled to epithelioid or plasmacytoid. Here, the tumor cells are epithelioid with pale pink to clear cytoplasm, indistinct borders, and ovoid, relatively uniform nuclei.

p40 Expression in Myoepithelial Carcinoma

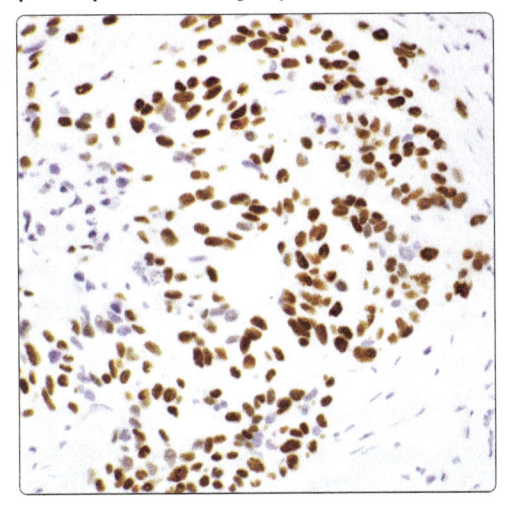

S100 Expression in Myoepithelial Carcinoma

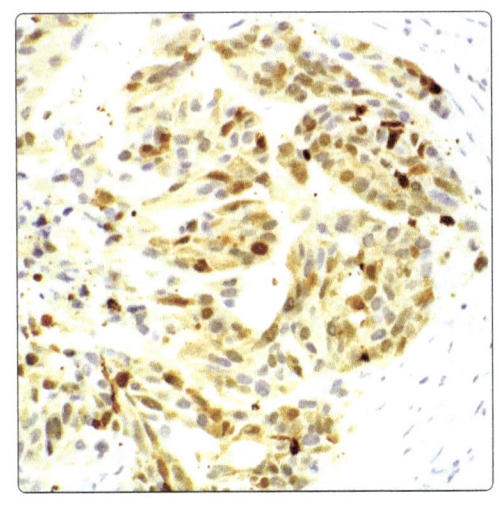

(Left) Characteristically, myoepithelial tumors express a mix of antigens. Tumor cells often express p63 or p40, as in this case. (Right) In the same same case, some tumor cells also express S100.

SMA Expression in Myoepithelial Carcinoma

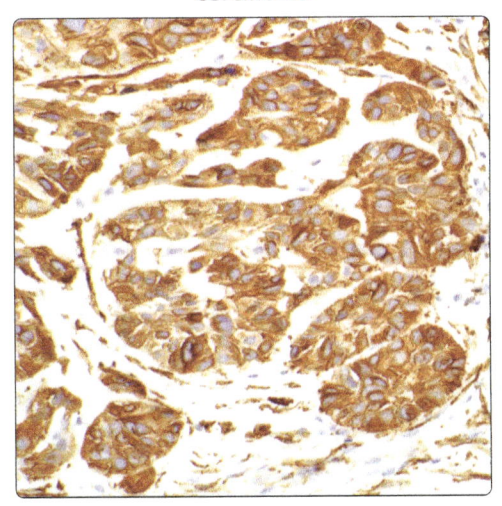

Myoepithelial Carcinoma

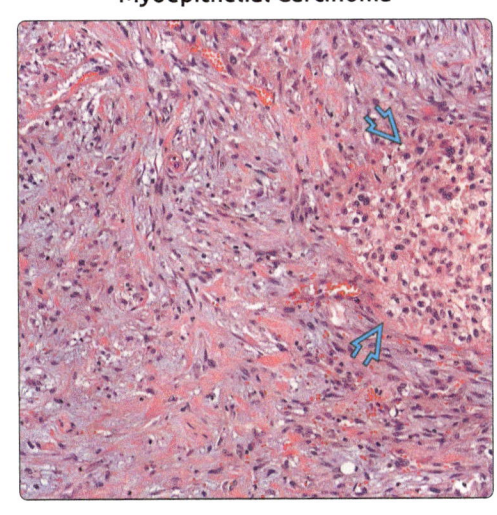

(Left) Consistent with myoepithelial differentiation, tumor cells also express SMA in the same case. (Right) This case of myoepithelial carcinoma consists predominantly of spindled tumor cells set in a fibrous to myxoid background. Clear epithelioid myoepithelial cells are also present ➡.

525

Nasopharyngeal EBV-Related Squamous Cell Carcinoma

KEY FACTS

TERMINOLOGY
- Squamous cell carcinomas of nasopharynx associated with Epstein-Barr virus (EBV) infection

ETIOLOGY/PATHOGENESIS
- EBV infection: Double-stranded DNA virus of human herpesvirus family
- Infection alone insufficient for inducing cancer
- Specific HLA types increase risk: HLA-A2, HLA-B17, HLA-Bw46, HLA-Bw58, HLA-DRB1, HLA-DQB1
- Certain populations at increased risk: Han Chinese, some Native American groups, Africans from Northern and Central regions

CLINICAL ISSUES
- Most common presentation: Cervical neck mass without other symptoms
- Others symptoms: Epistaxis, nasal stuffiness/obstruction, nasal discharge, headache, serous otitis media, pain

MOLECULAR
- Mutations less common than gains, losses and hypermethylation
- Tumorigenic pathways upregulated include EGFR, WNT, PI3K/AKT, MAPK, NF-κB, NOTCH3, mTOR, JNK, and retinoid signaling pathways
- EBER ISH performed on formalin-fixed, paraffin-embedded tissue sections
- 3p deletion and 12p gain: Early events (according to metaanalysis of multiple CGH studies)
- Polymorphisms of viral oncogenes may influence infection efficiency and transforming potential
- Host cell miRNAs abnormally differentially expressed
- Significance of specific miRNAs varies across studies, but recurring findings include downregulation of specific tumor suppressor miRNAs
- Host long noncoding RNAs also deregulated

Nasopharynx

(Left) The nasopharynx (purple and superior blue area) comprises the posterior nasal cavity extending inferiorly to the soft palate. It contains the eustachian tube orifice and fossa of Rosenmüller. (Right) Epstein-Barr encoded RNA (EBER) ISH is invaluable in confirming the diagnosis of nasopharyngeal carcinoma, Epstein-Barr virus related (EBV+NPC). Here, almost all tumor nuclei are positive for EBER.

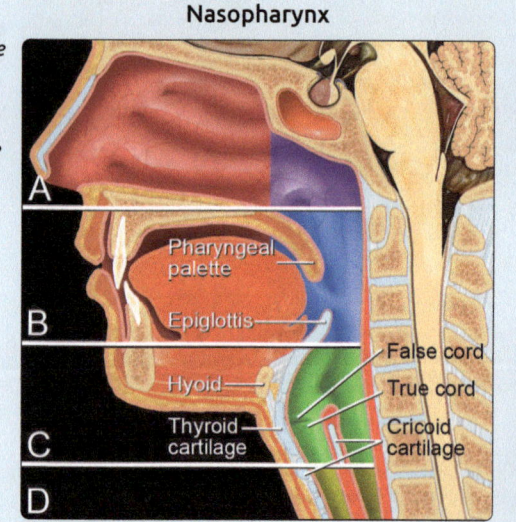

EBER ISH

Latent Membrane Protein 1: Selected Extracellular Effects

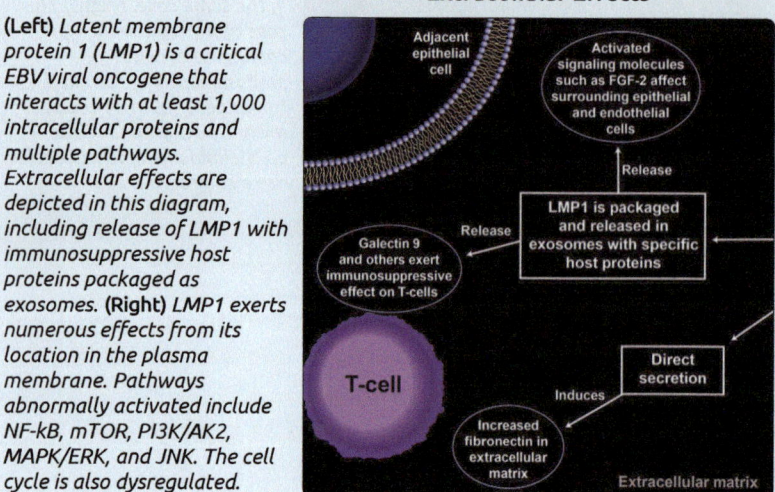

Latent Membrane Protein 1: Selected Intracellular Effects

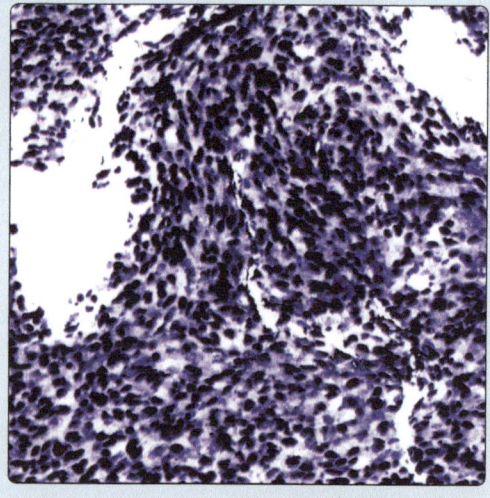

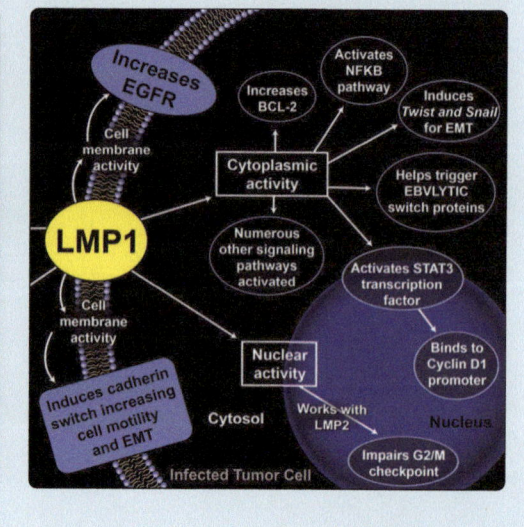

(Left) Latent membrane protein 1 (LMP1) is a critical EBV viral oncogene that interacts with at least 1,000 intracellular proteins and multiple pathways. Extracellular effects are depicted in this diagram, including release of LMP1 with immunosuppressive host proteins packaged as exosomes. (Right) LMP1 exerts numerous effects from its location in the plasma membrane. Pathways abnormally activated include NF-kB, mTOR, PI3K/AK2, MAPK/ERK, and JNK. The cell cycle is also dysregulated.

Nasopharyngeal EBV-Related Squamous Cell Carcinoma

TERMINOLOGY

Abbreviations
- Epstein-Barr virus-positive nasopharyngeal carcinoma (EBV+NPC)

Definitions
- Carcinoma with squamous differentiation within nasopharynx associated with EBV infection

ETIOLOGY/PATHOGENESIS

Environmental Exposure
- Factors that influence development of NPC
  - Poor hygiene, diet high in nitrosamines (such as salted fish, especially early in life), inhaled smoke of various types, including tobacco

Infectious Agents
- EBV infection
  - Double-stranded DNA virus of human herpesvirus family
  - Infection alone insufficient for inducing cancer

Genetic Factors
- Specific HLA types increase risk
  - HLA-A2, HLA-B17, HLA-Bw46, HLA-Bw58, HLA-DRB1, HLA-DQB1
- Geographic/ethnic predilection: Primarily Han Chinese

CLINICAL ISSUES

Presentation
- Symptoms often nonspecific
  - Asymptomatic cervical neck mass most common
- M:F ~ 2-3:1

Prognosis
- Stage
  - Best predictor: Most patients present at high stage
  - Overall 5-year survival rate: ~ 70%
  - 95% survival for patients with low-stage disease using radiotherapy alone
- Other prognostic factors: Older age, male sex, certain HLA types (HLA-Aw33-C3-B58/DR3 haplotype worse prognosis), cervical node metastasis
- Molecular prognostic factors: Many altered genes are proposed to be prognostic, but most are from single studies

MOLECULAR

Complex Molecular Genetic Alterations
- Include deregulated pathways, repressed tumor suppressor genes, viral protein oncogenic effects, and activated oncogenes
- Mutations less common than gains, losses, and hypermethylation
  - Copy number variations (CNVs): More frequent than in other head and neck squamous cell carcinomas
  - Somatic mutations occur in genes that normally stabilize genome
  - DNA mismatch repair genes: At least 1 of 4 genes is lost in ~ 50% of NPC
- Role of viral microRNAs
  - EBV BART microRNAs inhibit key tumor suppressor genes, cell adhesion genes, such as *CDH1* (E-cadherin), immune response genes, and cytokine/chemokine receptors
  - May serve as early serum markers of EBV+NPC
- Field cancerization occurs in nasopharynx mucosa
  - Inactivation of *RASSF1A* and *CDKN2A* found in normal mucosa adjacent to in situ and invasive tumor
  - Telomerase is activated and BCL2 protein is overexpressed in precursor (dysplastic) lesions and invasive tumors
  - EBV latent infection is found in high-grade dysplasia
    – Facilitates transformation to invasive tumor by abnormally activating specific signaling pathways, enhancing genetic instability, suppressing effective immune response, and inducing epigenetic changes

In Situ Hybridization
- Epstein-Barr-encoded RNA (EBER)
  - Identifies small nuclear viral RNAs present in tumor cell nuclei (~ 100,000 per infected cell)
  - Found in ~ 100% of EBV+NPC
  - EBER ISH: Gold standard for diagnosis of EBV+NPC
    – Performed on formalin-fixed, paraffin-embedded tissue sections

Molecular Genetics
- **Tumor suppressor genes lost or downregulated**
  - *DLC1, RASSF1A, DLEC1, PTPRG, CDKN2A, CHFR, MGMT, DAPK1, OPCML, CRYAB, NFKBIA, THY1*
- **Oncogenes mutated &/or upregulated**
  - *LTBR, CCND1, PIK3CA, NOTCH3, BMI1*
- **Gene fusions and rearrangements**
  - Uncommon
  - e.g., *UBR5::ZNF423, RARS::MAD1L1*, others; appear to be pathogenic
- **Viral oncogenic proteins**
  - Polymorphisms of viral oncogenes may influence infection efficiency and transforming potential
  - Latent membrane protein 1 (LMP1)
    – Expressed in tumor cell membrane
    – Mimics constitutively activated tumor necrosis factor
    – Induces expression of EGFR
    – Inhibits TP53-mediated apoptosis
    – Activates NF-κB → ↑ cell proliferation, inhibits antitumor inflammation
    – LMP1 forces infected epithelial cells to produce abnormal exosomes that directly affect NPC microenvironment
      □ Other proteins in abnormal exosomes repress T lymphocytes and induce procarcinogenic cytokine release
      □ LMP1-loaded exosomes circulate systemically and are protected from enzymatic degradation
    – Release of LMP1 by infected tumor cell causes "cadherin switch"
      □ Cadherin switch = upregulation of N-cadherin and downregulation of E-cadherin
      □ Enhances epithelial to mesenchymal transition (EMT) and tumor cell migration

Nasopharyngeal EBV-Related Squamous Cell Carcinoma

- o EBV nuclear antigen-1 (EBNA-1)
  - Impairs CD8-positive T-cell response
- o LMP2
  - Role in tumor growth
  - Other roles to be determined
- o BART1 latent protein encoded by BART1 EBV gene homologous to human protooncogene *CSF1R*
- Ephrin A2: Primary EBV receptor on epithelial cells
- Molecular alterations vary across individual tumors
  - o However, NF-kB signaling is commonly affected
  - o Additional mutations appear to be required for intraepithelial-latent EBV infection to cause NPC
    - Hot spot mutations that enable carcinogenesis include alterations that cause loss of p16 protein

Gene Expression Profiling

- Upregulated pathways include
  - o EGFR, Wnt, PI3K/AKT, MAPK, NF-κB, NOTCH3, mTOR, JNK, and retinoid signaling pathways

Epigenetic Findings

- Host cell miRNAs abnormally differentially expressed
  - o Significance of specific miRNAs varies across studies, but recurring findings include downregulation of specific tumor suppressor miRNAs
    - miR-29a and miR-29b significantly downregulated according to several studies
    - miR-142 and miR-141 expression negatively correlated with survival in several studies
    - let-7 downregulated according to several studies
- Host long noncoding RNAs (lncRNAs) also deregulated
  - o Small nucleolar RNA host gene-1 (*SNHG1*) lncRNA: Upregulated in NPC and other carcinomas
    - Promotes expression of *NAUK1*: Facilitates EMT

MICROSCOPIC

Histologic Features

- **Nasopharyngeal nonkeratinizing undifferentiated carcinoma**
  - o 3 architectural patterns
    - Discrete nests of tumor embedded in lymphoplasmacytic inflammation (Regaud pattern)
    - Dispersed tumor cells intermingled with lymphocytes/plasma cells (Schmincke pattern)
    - Sheets of tumor cells with absent or acute inflammation
  - o Syncytial growth occurs with all 3 architectural patterns
  - o Large, round to spindled tumor cells; indistinct borders; high nuclear:cytoplasmic ratio; vesicular nuclei often with prominent nucleoli
  - o High mitotic and apoptotic rates
  - o Desmoplastic reaction often absent
- **Nasopharyngeal nonkeratinizing differentiated carcinoma**
  - o Architecture mimics high-grade transitional cell carcinoma with anastomosing stratified ribbons of tumor ± prominent cyst formation and pavementing
  - o Discrete tumor cell borders, moderate to high nuclear:cytoplasmic ratio, often marked nuclear pleomorphism
  - o High mitotic rate and apoptotic rates with areas of geographic necrosis common
- Some tumors combine features of both differentiated and undifferentiated types
- No significance to histologic subtype of differentiated or undifferentiated

ANCILLARY TESTS

Immunohistochemistry

- Positive: AE1/AE3, p63, CK5/6
  - o Undifferentiated variant shows interlacing or meshwork of positive tumor cells with interspersed lymphocytes
- Negative: CK7, CK20, neuroendocrine markers, NUT antibody, melanocytic markers; SMARCB1 expression intact

In Situ Hybridization

- EBER ISH almost always performed

Serologic Testing

- IgA against viral capsid antigen (VCA): ~ 70-90% sensitivity
- IgG against early EBV antigens: ~ 70-90% sensitivity

DIFFERENTIAL DIAGNOSIS

HPV-Negative Head and Neck Mucosal Squamous Cell Carcinoma

- Often keratinizing and of lower grade than EBV+NPC
- Usually elicits desmoplastic reaction in surrounding stroma
- EBER ISH negative or at most few cells positive

HPV-Positive Head and Neck Mucosal Squamous Cell Carcinoma

- Usually nonkeratinizing and high-grade-like EBV+NPC
- Diffusely positive for p16
- Positive for HPV by ISH or PCR; negative for EBER ISH or at most only few cells positive

Lymphomas

- May require IHC to distinguish EBV+NPC Schmincke pattern from high-grade lymphoma

Melanoma

- May show prominent cytoplasmic ± extracellular melanin pigment, multinucleated tumor giant cells, mixed spindle and epithelioid morphology with discrete cell borders, nuclear pseudoinclusions
- Some cases may exhibit syncytial undifferentiated histopathology and require IHC to distinguish from EBV+NPC
  - o S100, HMB-45, melanocyte antigen, SOX10 or combination expressed in great majority of cases
  - o Rare cases negative for all melanocytic markers

SELECTED REFERENCES

1. Liu X et al: Nasopharyngeal carcinoma progression: accumulating genomic instability and persistent Epstein-Barr virus infection. Curr Oncol. 29(9):6035-52, 2022
2. Chen FM et al: The prognostic value of deficient mismatch repair in stage II-IVa nasopharyngeal carcinoma in the era of IMRT. Sci Rep. 10(1):9690, 2020
3. Rider MA et al: The interactome of EBV LMP1 evaluated by proximity-based BioID approach. Virology. 516:55-70, 2018

Nasopharyngeal EBV-Related Squamous Cell Carcinoma

Loose Sheets of Tumor Cells

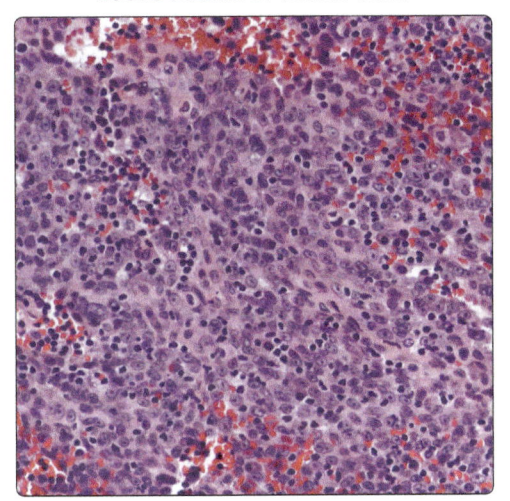

Lymphoepithelial Pattern

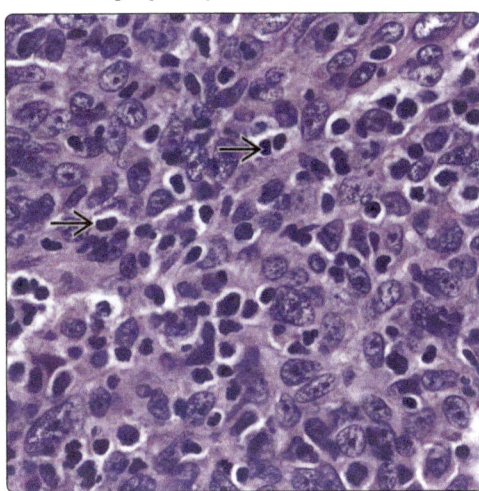

(Left) EBV+NPC shows loose sheets of tumor cells with scant intermingled lymphocytes. (Right) EBV+NPC most often exhibits a lymphoepithelial pattern of intimately intermixed tumor cells and inflammatory cells. In such cases, large cell lymphoma enters the histologic differential. The lymphocytes ➡ are small in size with coarse chromatin and indistinct nucleoli.

Differentiated Nonkeratinizing Histology

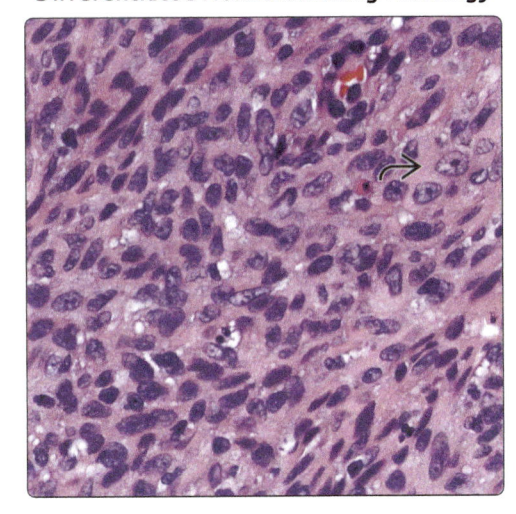

Diffuse p63 Expression

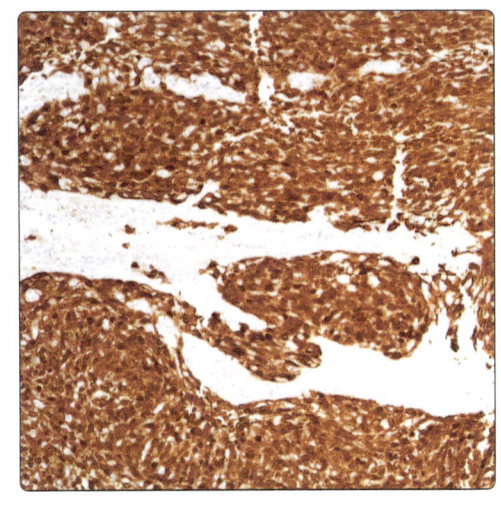

(Left) In this case of NPC, tumor cells contain a moderate amount of eosinophilic cytoplasm ➡, but keratin foci and intercellular bridges are absent. (Right) p63 is positive in this case of EBV+NPC. Most EBV+NPC diffusely express CK5 and p63.

Spindled Tumor Cells

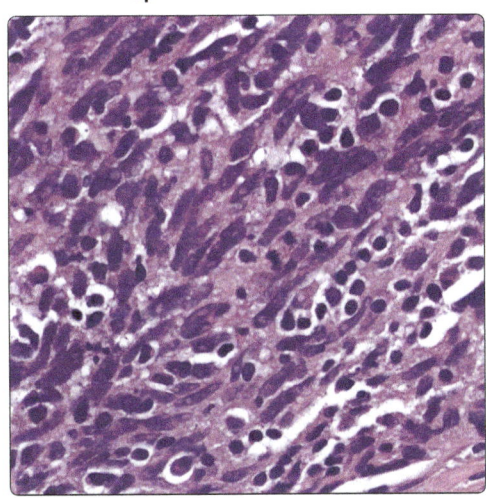

EBER Expression in NPC With Lymphoepithelial-Like Histology

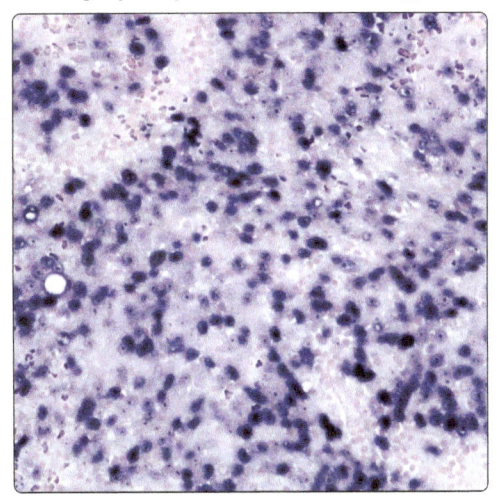

(Left) Spindled tumor cells can occur in NPC, as in this example. (Right) Consistent with dispersed (lymphoepithelial) cell pattern on H&E, EBER ISH highlights scattered tumor nuclei filled with abundant viral RNA. Nearly all tumor nuclei are reactive.

Other Head and Neck Tumors

KEY FACTS

TERMINOLOGY
- 10 malignant neoplasms of sinonasal region
- NUT carcinoma, SMARCB1- and SMARCA4-deficient carcinomas also occur outside head and neck

ETIOLOGY/PATHOGENESIS
- Intestinal-type sinonasal adenocarcinoma: Long-term exposure to wood and leather dust, possibly other inhaled substances
- No known risk factors for nonintestinal type sinonasal adenocarcinoma, NMC, ONB, and SMM

MOLECULAR
- Sinonasal undifferentiated carcinoma: *IDH2* or *IDH1* mutations present in ~ 50% and may represent distinct subset
- SMARCB1-deficient sinonasal carcinoma and other SMARC-protein deficient sinonasal tumors: Loss of *SMARCB1* or *SMARCA4* is defining feature
- NMC: All *NUT* fusions lead to novel protein that deregulates MYC protein
- Olfactory neuroblastoma: *TP53* mutation, p53 wildtype overexpression, and *MYC*, *KDR*, *TAOK2*, *MAP4K2*, and *SIN3B* mutations found in varying percentages
- Sinonasal mucosal melanoma: Incidence of various genetic changes may be related to anatomic location (e.g., sinus vs. nasal cavity), patient population, and possibly specific risk factors

TOP DIFFERENTIAL DIAGNOSES
- Poorly differentiated head and neck squamous cell carcinoma
- Small round blue cell tumors, including some lymphomas, melanomas, and sarcomas
- Metastatic adenocarcinomas or primary salivary carcinomas enter differential for sinonasal adenocarcinomas and SMARCB1-deficient sinonasal adenocarcinoma

Sinonasal Region / **Sinonasal Undifferentiated Carcinoma**

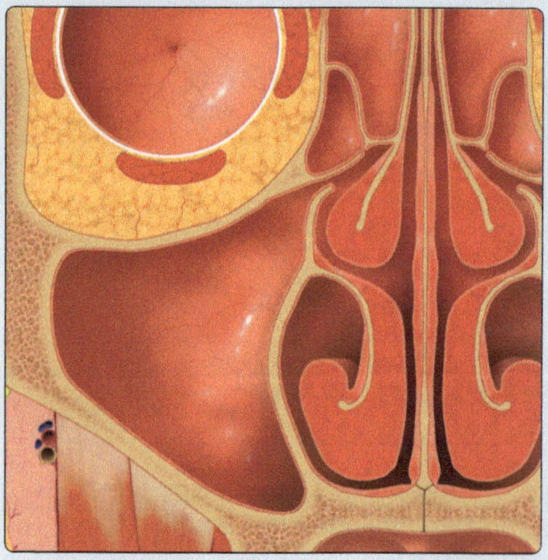

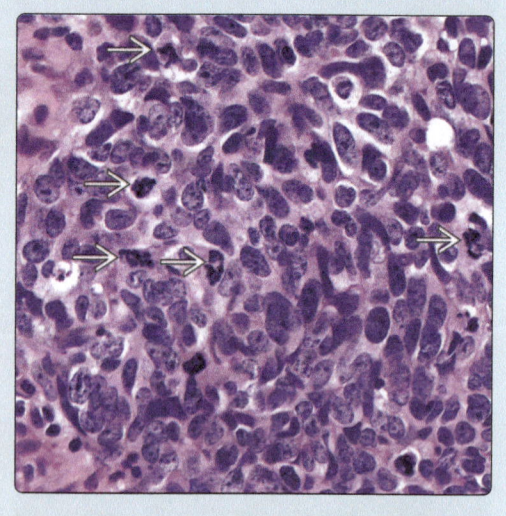

(Left) Coronal graphic through the mid portion of the sinonasal cavity shows the most common locations for these tumors. (Right) Sinonasal undifferentiated carcinoma (SNUC) is highly proliferative. Note the mitotic figures ➡, a characteristic feature of this rapidly growing, locally aggressive carcinoma.

BAF Complex / **Tumors With Abnormalities of BAF Complex**

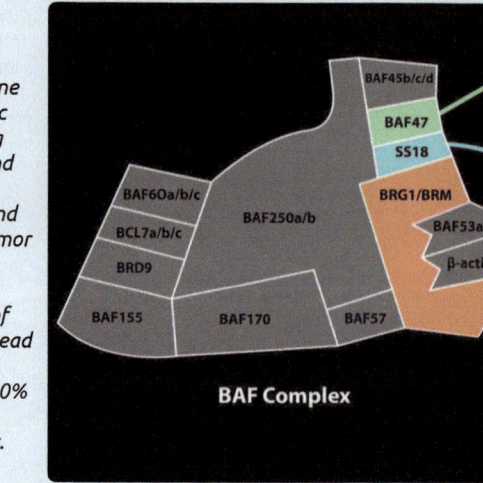

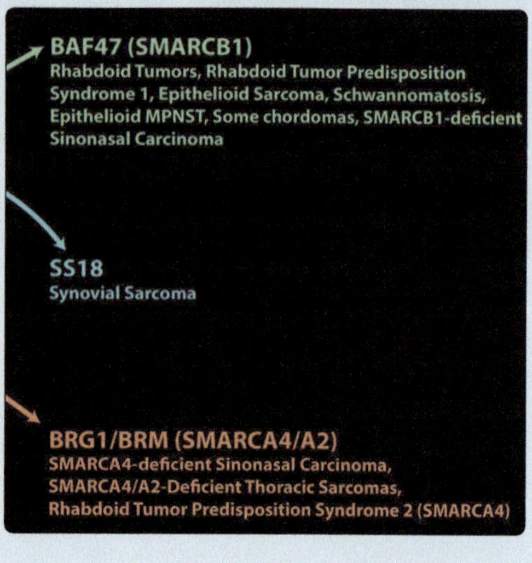

(Left) The BAF complex of proteins (a.k.a. SWI/SNF nucleosome remodeling complex) helps regulate gene expression at the epigenetic level by specifically altering chromatin configuration and consequently gene access. (Right) Numerous benign and malignant tumors and 3 tumor syndromes are driven by genetic alterations of BAF complex proteins. Several of these tumors occur in the head and neck, including the sinonasal region. Overall, 20% of malignant tumors show BAF complex abnormalities.

BAF47 (SMARCB1)
Rhabdoid Tumors, Rhabdoid Tumor Predisposition Syndrome 1, Epithelioid Sarcoma, Schwannomatosis, Epithelioid MPNST, Some chordomas, SMARCB1-deficient Sinonasal Carcinoma

SS18
Synovial Sarcoma

BRG1/BRM (SMARCA4/A2)
SMARCA4-deficient Sinonasal Carcinoma, SMARCA4/A2-Deficient Thoracic Sarcomas, Rhabdoid Tumor Predisposition Syndrome 2 (SMARCA4)

Other Head and Neck Tumors

TERMINOLOGY

Abbreviations
- Sinonasal undifferentiated carcinoma (SNUC)
- SMARCB1-deficient sinonasal carcinoma (SMARCB1-defSNC), SMARCB1-deficient adenocarcinoma (SMARCB1-defSNAdeno), teratocarcinosarcoma, SMARCA4-deficient sinonasal carcinoma (SMARCA4-defSNC)
- NUT (midline) carcinoma (NMC)
- Sinonasal adenocarcinoma (SNAC)
- Olfactory neuroblastoma (ONB)
- Sinonasal mucosal melanoma (SMM)
- Biphenotypic sinonasal sarcoma (BSS)

Definitions
- Malignant neoplasms of sinonasal region of varying cell types and differentiation
  - All except NUT carcinoma occur exclusively in head and neck (SMARCB1-deficient carcinomas of other cell types occur elsewhere)

ETIOLOGY/PATHOGENESIS

Environmental Exposure
- SNUC
  - Prior radiation therapy may be risk factor
- SNAC, intestinal type
  - Long-term exposure to wood and leather dust, and possibly other inhaled substances
  - Chronic inflammation proposed as mechanism for metaplasia that could transform to neoplasia
    - Release of cytokines (TNF, IL-1β) upregulates NFκB pathway and expression of COX2
    - Release of reactive oxygen and reactive nitrogen species may generate mutagenic DNA adducts
    - Mutations in *TP53* and *KRAS*
- SMARCB1-defSNC and other SMARC protein-deficient sinonasal tumors
  - Unknown whether some tumors may be caused by rhabdoid tumor predisposition syndrome (RTPS) = germline *SMARCB1* or SMARCA4 alterations
  - SMARCB1-deficient tumors
    - SMARCB1-deficient sinonasal carcinoma: ~ 150 cases reported
    - SMARCB1-deficient sinonasal adenocarcinoma: ~ 25 cases reported
  - SMARCA4-deficient tumors
    - SMARCA4-deficient sinonasal carcinoma
    - Teratocarcinosarcoma may also show partial loss of SMARCA2

Pathogenesis
- SNUC
  - *IDH2/IDH1* mutations found in ~ 50%: Block cellular differentiation
- SMARCB1-defSNC and other SMARC protein-deficient sinonasal tumors
  - Loss of SMARCB1 or SMARCA4 → widespread deregulated gene expression
- NUT (midline) carcinoma
  - NUT fusion protein blocks cellular differentiation and deregulates cell cycle
- BSS
  - PAX3 fusion protein dysregulates genes involved in nerve and muscle differentiation

CLINICAL ISSUES

Presentation
- SNUC
  - Acute onset (weeks to few months) of rapidly growing sinonasal mass with erosion of surrounding tissues including bone
  - M > F (2-3:1)
  - Can occur at any age, but 50-60s most common
- SMARCB1-defSNC and other SMARC protein-deficient sinonasal tumors
  - SMARCB1-defSNC and SMARCB1-deficient sinonasal adenocarcinoma: Broad age range; mean: 52 years
  - SMARCA4-deficient sinonasal carcinoma: Most common in men in 4th and 5th decade
  - Teratocarcinosarcoma: Broad age range from children to older adults
- NUT (midline) carcinoma
  - Broad age range described; first in children and young adults
  - M = F in head and neck; slight female predominance overall in other sites
  - Most patients symptomatic due to rapidly growing midline mass
  - No association with smoking
- SNAC
  - Usually middle-aged and older adults
  - Intestinal type: Symptoms of ethmoid sinus or nasal vault obstruction
    - M > F (6:1)
- ONB
  - All ages (median: 50 years); bimodal distribution in adolescents and older adults
  - F slightly > M
  - May present with symptoms of nasal obstruction
- SMM
  - Wide age range but 50-70 years most common
  - M > F
  - May present with symptoms of nasal obstruction
- BSS
  - Broad age range (mean: ~ 50 years)
  - F > M (relatively low number of cases reported thus far)
  - Presents with nonspecific sinus or sinonasal symptoms

Prognosis
- SNUC
  - Rapidly fatal in most cases; median survival: ~ 18 months
- SMARCB1-defSNC and other SMARC protein-deficient sinonasal tumors
  - Aggressive; Many patients dead of disease at 2 years
- NUT (midline) carcinoma
  - Rapidly fatal; median survival: ~ 7-9 months
    - Patients with fusion partner other than *BRD4* may do better
  - Targeted therapy with TBX21 (BET) inhibitors
- SNAC
  - Intestinal type: 60% 5-year overall survival

Other Head and Neck Tumors

- Low-grade nonintestinal type: ~ 90% 5-year survival
- High-grade nonintestinal type: ~ 15% 5-year survival
- ONB
  - ~ 80% 5-year overall survival and ~ 70% overall 10-year survival
  - Metastases and recurrences may occur many years after initial diagnosis
- SMM
  - ~ 30% overall 5-year survival
- BSS
  - Locally invasive with ~ 40% risk of local recurrence but no reported metastases or deaths

MOLECULAR

General Comments
- Low case numbers of newly recognized tumor types means molecular genetic data incomplete

Cytogenetics
- NUT (midline) carcinoma differs from other high-grade head and neck squamous cell carcinoma by having simple karyotype

In Situ Hybridization
- NUT (midline) carcinoma
  - *BRD4::NUTM1*; t(15;19)(q14,p13.1)
    - 70% of cases
  - *BRD3::NUTM1*; t(9;15)(q34.2;q14)
  - Fusion of *NUTM1* to *BRD4*, *BRD3* causes lack of differentiation in association with high proliferative rate
  - *NSD3::NUTM1*; t(8;15)(p12;q15): 3rd, rare *NUTM1* translocation partner
  - *NUTM1::variant* = *NUTM1* fused with genes other than *BRD4*, *BRD3*, and *NSD3*
    - 15% of cases
- SNAC, nonintestinal type
  - Subset of low-grade tumors shows t(12;15)(p13;q25); *ETV6::NTRK3* and *ETV6::RET* fusions similar to secretory carcinoma of salivary gland
- BSS
  - Rearrangements of *PAX3* account for majority of cases
    - t(2;4)(q35;q31.1); *PAX3::MAML3* most common (90%)
    - Other PAX3 fusions include *PAX3::FOXO1*, *PAX3::NCOA1/NCOA2*, and *PAX3::WWTR1*

Molecular Genetics
- SNUC
  - *IDH2* or *IDH1* single nucleotide variants: Present in ~ 50% of SNUC
    - May represent distinct subset
    - Most common mutation is *IDH2* R172X
  - *TP53* mutations common, including in *IDH1/IDH2*-mutated cases
  - c-KIT protein often overexpressed (80%) and may be mutated
  - *SOX2* amplification and increased protein expression reported in ~ 35% of cases
  - Other findings in *IDH2/IDH1* wildtype SNUC: *NOTCH1* gain-of-function and *TET2* loss-of-function mutations
- SMARCB1-defSNC and other SMARC protein-deficient sinonasal tumors
  - Very few studies to date; only ~ 25 cases of SMARCB1-deficient sinonasal adenocarcinoma reported
  - SMARCA4-defSNC
    - Additional mutations include inactivating *APC* or activating *CTNNB1* mutations (n=2 cases)
- NUT (midline) carcinoma
  - All translocations lead to novel protein that deregulates *MYC* directly or indirectly
- SNAC
  - Intestinal type
    - Overexpression: *EGFR* (20-33%), *PTGS2* (40-60%), *TP53* (~ 70%)
    - Mutated: *KRAS* (15-40%), *TP53* (up to ~ 85%)
    - LOH at 9p21 (*CDKN2A*) (45%) or epigenetic silencing (~ 66%)
  - Nonintestinal, poorly differentiated sinonasal adenocarcinoma
    - *IDH1/IDH2* mutations: Present in ~ 30-40%
- ONB
  - *TP53* mutation, TP53 wildtype overexpression, and *MYC*, *KDR*, *TAOK2*, *MAP4K2*, and *SIN3B* mutations described in few cases
- SMM
  - Incidence of various genetic changes may be related to location (sinus versus nasal cavity), patient population, and possibly specific risk factors
  - *NRAS* mutations, when present, occur in codons G12 and G13, and infrequently in codon Q61 as in cutaneous melanoma
    - Agents inhibiting or silencing RAS effectors, such as BRAF, CRAF, and PIK3CA inhibitors, may prove to be effective multitargeted therapy
  - *KIT* mutations, when present, do not correlate with KIT protein overexpression by IHC
  - *CCND1* amplification does not correlate with cyclin-D1 expression
  - Tumor suppressor genes lost: *PTEN* (~ 50%), *CDKN2A* (~ 55%)
    - Loss of PTEN and presence of pAkt proteins may indicate possible responsiveness to PI3K-Akt-mTOR inhibitors
  - *PIK3CA* activating mutation
- BSS
  - *PAX3* fusion alters expression of genes involved in neural crest, muscle development, and embryonic development
    - *NTRK3*, *ALX1*, *ALX3*, *ALX4*, *DBX1*, *GREM1*, *MYOCD*, *MYOD1*, *BMP5*, *FGFR2*, and others

Gene Expression Profiling or Affected Pathways
- SNUC
  - *IDH2/IDH1*-mutated cases show *TP53* (~ 50%), activating *KIT* (~ 45%), or activating PI3K pathway member (~ 35%) mutations
- SNAC
  - Intestinal type: *LGALS4* (galectin 4) upregulated and *CLU* (clusterin) downregulated (9 cases studied)
- SMM
  - Diffuse activation of PI3K/Akt and RAS-MAPK pathways
  - *NRAS* mutations (14-60%), *BRAF* mutations (0-6%), *KIT* mutations (0-40%), *CCND1* amplifications (0-29%)

Other Head and Neck Tumors

Epigenetic Findings
- **SNUC**
  - Hypermethylated phenotype may possibly associate with *IDH2/IDH1*-mutated cases (as occurs in other *IDH2/IDH1*-mutated tumors)
- **SMARCB1-defSNC and other SMARC protein-deficient sinonasal tumors**
  - SMARCB1 and SMARCA4 are part of SWI/SNF (**swi**tch **s**ucrose **n**on**f**ermentable) complex that epigenetically regulates chromatin remodeling
    - SMARCB1 or SMARCA4 loss adversely affects SWI/SNF complex, disrupting gene expression, cell proliferation, and differentiation
- **SNAC, intestinal type**
  - Promoter methylation of multiple genes, including *CDKN2A*, *CDH13*, *ESR1*, and *APC*

MICROSCOPIC

Histologic Features
- **SNUC**
  - Low power
    - Hypercellular sheets, nests ± cords, often with geographic necrosis; no glands
    - *IDH2/IDH2* cases uncommonly show glandular or tubular type structures
  - High power
    - Cells lack keratinization and intercellular bridges; N:C ratio usually ↑
    - Mitotic rate and apoptotic rate usually ↑
- **SMARCB1-defSNC and other SMARC protein-deficient sinonasal tumors**
  - SMARCB1-defSNC
    - Basaloid type: Negative for overt squamous differentiation; basaloid tumor cells often with desmoplastic stroma
    - Eosinophilic type: Nests/sheets of pink cells often with rhabdoid &/or plasmacytoid cells
    - Other rare histologies include sarcomatoid (spindle cells) or basaloid type with glands
  - SMARCB1-defSNAdeno
    - Glands must be present; can appear yolk-sac-like
  - SMARCA4-defSNC
    - Resembles high-grade neuroendocrine carcinomas or SNUC
  - Teratocarcinosarcoma
    - Mix of neuroepithelial, epithelial, and mesenchymal elements in varying proportions
- **NUT (midline) carcinoma**
  - Range of appearances that can mimic SNUC, NPC-EBV, and conventional high-grade SCC when NMC contains foci of keratinization
  - Nonspecific poorly differentiated appearance of NMC most likely leads to underdiagnosis and misdiagnosis as SNUC, HNSCC, or small cell undifferentiated carcinoma
  - All patients with poorly differentiated carcinomas in head and neck that are negative for HPV or EBV should be tested with NUT antibody to exclude NUT midline carcinoma
- **SNAC**
  - Intestinal type
    - 4 subtypes: Colonic (40%), mucinous (~ 20%), solid (~ 20%), and papillary (~ 20%)
    - Graded from well to poorly differentiated
  - Nonintestinal type
    - Variable architecture, including glands, papillae, back-to-back acini, solid (in high-grade tumors) and mixed pattern
    - Cells range from cuboidal to columnar ± pseudostratification
    - Mild to moderate nuclear atypia and low mitotic activity in low-grade tumors
    - High mitotic activity, ↑ nuclear atypia in high-grade tumors
- **ONB**
  - Morphology varies by grade
  - Low grade (Hyams I-II)
    - Lobular architecture with neurofibrillary matrix and mild to moderate cellular atypia ± Homer Wright and Flexner rosettes
  - High grade (Hyams III-IV)
    - Less prominent lobular architecture, little to no neurofibrillary matrix, more prominent nuclear atypia, pleomorphism, often necrosis
- **SMM**
  - Low power: Variety of architectures, from sheets to trabeculae
  - High power: Variety of cell shapes, including spindled, small round blue cell, epithelioid, and multinucleated
  - Tumors commonly show high mitotic rates, necrosis
  - Melanin pigment present in some cases
- **BSS**
  - Low power: Fascicles and herringbone pattern most common surrounding variably hyperplastic normal glands and mucosa
  - High power: Tumor cells are uniform, spindled with variably slender, buckled nuclei; negative for pleomorphism and necrosis

ANCILLARY TESTS

Immunohistochemistry
- **SNUC**
  - Positive: Pankeratins (diffuse), p63 and p40 (absent to focal), EMA (usually positive), IDH1/IDH2 positive in *IDH1/IDH2*-mutated cases
  - Variable: S100, neuroendocrine markers, p16 (may be diffusely positive), membranous C-kit
- **SMARCB1-defSNC and other SMARC protein-deficient sinonasal tumors**
  - SMARCB1-defSNC: Positive: Pankeratins, claudin 4 (in 80% at > 5% reactivity; recently reported); p63, keratin 5, and keratin 7 (each ~ 50%); Negative: Loss of SMARCB1 is defining feature; also negative for HR HPV, EBER, and NUT
  - SMARCB1-defSNAdeno: Loss of SMARCB1; often positive for CK7, glypican-3; ± SALL4, HepPAR
  - SMARCA4-defSNC: Loss of SMARCA4; positive for pan-keratin, synaptophysin; ± chromogranin, CD56
  - Teratocarcinosarcoma: Loss of SMARCA4 (diffuse or patchy); positive for other markers consistent with differentiation
- **NUT (midline) carcinoma**

- Positive
  - NUT-specific antibody (except in keratinized foci), pankeratins
- Variable
  - p63, S100, neuroendocrine markers, CD34
- SNAC
  - Intestinal type
    - Positive for keratin 20, villin, CDX2
    - Variably positive for keratin 7; abnormal nuclear expression of β-catenin (30-50%)
  - Nonintestinal type
    - Positive for keratin 7; negative for villin, CDX2, and SATB2
- ONB
  - Positive
    - NSE, S100 protein in sustentacular pattern
  - Negative (or at most, focal)
    - Epithelial markers
  - Variable
    - Chromogranin, synaptophysin
- SMM
  - Positive
    - Melanocytic markers (S100, SOX10, HMB-45, melan-A, tyrosinase)
  - Negative
    - Keratins, chromogranin, synaptophysin
- BSS
  - Positive
    - S100 and SMA are both reactive but may be diffuse, patchy or only few cells positive; PAX3 positive (PAX3 may also be positive in RMS), desmin (~ 60%), myogenin (~ 20%); TLE1 may be positive (also positive in synovial sarcoma); MYOD1 is more sensitive than myogenin for skeletal muscle differentiation
  - Negative
    - SOX10

DIFFERENTIAL DIAGNOSIS

DDx for SNUC

- Other high-grade tumors, including NPC-EBV, SMM, high-grade ONB, small cell neuroendocrine carcinoma, poorly differentiated conventional SCC, SMARCB1-defSNC, high-grade lymphoma, and small round blue cell sarcomas
  - IHC may be required to confirm diagnosis

DDx for SMARCB1-defSNC and Other SMARC Protein-Deficient Sinonasal Tumors

- SMARCB1-defSNC: SNUC, epithelioid sarcoma, basaloid squamous cell carcinoma, high-grade tumors with eosinophilic cells, including adenocarcinomas
- SMARCA4-defSNC: Neuroendocrine carcinoma, SNUC, olfactory neuroblastoma
- SMARCB1-defSNAdeno: SNAC, metastatic adenocarcinoma, germ cell tumors, salivary gland tumors
- Teratocarcinosarcoma: Broad, especially in small biopsies when only one component is sampled

DDx for NUT (Midline) Carcinoma

- Same differential as for SNUC

- IHC required for diagnosis: Speckled nuclear expression of NUT-specific antibody ~ 90% sensitive and 100% specific at this site
  - May diffusely express p16, raising possibility of HNSCC-HPV
    - NMC negative for HPV by ISH compared to HNSCC-HPV

DDx for SNAC

- Some salivary gland tumors, metastatic adenocarcinoma, respiratory epithelial adenomatoid hamartoma (REAH)

DDx for ONB

- Neuroendocrine carcinomas
  - IHC usually required to make correct diagnosis
- Ewing family of tumors when patient is adolescent/young adult
- Lymphoma (for high-grade ONB)
- High-grade squamous cell carcinoma (for high-grade ONB)
- Melanoma (for high-grade ONB)

DDx for SMM

- Other high-grade malignant tumors of head and neck and metastatic melanoma

DDx for BSS

- Cellular schwannoma, malignant peripheral nerve sheath tumor, monophasic synovial sarcoma, leiomyosarcoma, spindle cell RMS

DIAGNOSTIC CHECKLIST

Pathologic Interpretation Pearls

- Precursor lesion absent to rarely found in these tumors
- IHC almost always required to exclude mimics

SELECTED REFERENCES

1. Agaimy A: Proceedings of the North American Society of Head and Neck Pathology, Los Angeles, CA, March 20, 2022: SWI/SNF-deficient sinonasal neoplasms: an overview. Head Neck Pathol. 16(1):168-78, 2022
2. Taverna C et al: Towards a molecular classification of sinonasal carcinomas: clinical implications and opportunities. Cancers (Basel). 14(6), 2022
3. Le Loarer F et al: Clinicopathologic and molecular features of a series of 41 biphenotypic sinonasal sarcomas expanding their molecular spectrum. Am J Surg Pathol. 43(6):747-54, 2019
4. Agaimy A et al: Hereditary SWI/SNF complex deficiency syndromes. Semin Diagn Pathol. 35(3):193-8, 2018
5. Andreasen S et al: Biphenotypic sinonasal sarcoma: demographics, clinicopathological characteristics, molecular features, and prognosis of a recently described entity. Virchows Arch. 473(5):615-26, 2018
6. Arnaud O et al: BAFfling pathologies: alterations of BAF complexes in cancer. Cancer Lett. 419:266-79, 2018
7. Jo VY et al: Expression of PAX3 distinguishes biphenotypic sinonasal sarcoma from histologic mimics. Am J Surg Pathol. 42(10):1275-85, 2018
8. Mito JK et al: Immunohistochemical detection and molecular characterization of IDH-mutant sinonasal undifferentiated carcinomas. Am J Surg Pathol. 42(8):1067-75, 2018
9. Rooper LM et al: INSM1 is a sensitive and specific marker of neuroendocrine differentiation in head and neck tumors. Am J Surg Pathol. 42(5):665-71, 2018
10. Savas S et al: The SWI/SNF complex subunit genes: their functions, variations, and links to risk and survival outcomes in human cancers. Crit Rev Oncol Hematol. 123:114-31, 2018
11. Shair KHY et al: New insights from elucidating the role of LMP1 in nasopharyngeal carcinoma. Cancers (Basel). 10(4), 2018
12. Siegfried A et al: RREB1-MKL2 fusion in biphenotypic "oropharyngeal" sarcoma: new entity or part of the spectrum of biphenotypic sinonasal sarcomas? Genes Chromosomes Cancer. 57(4):203-10, 2018

Other Head and Neck Tumors

Sinonasal Undifferentiated Carcinoma

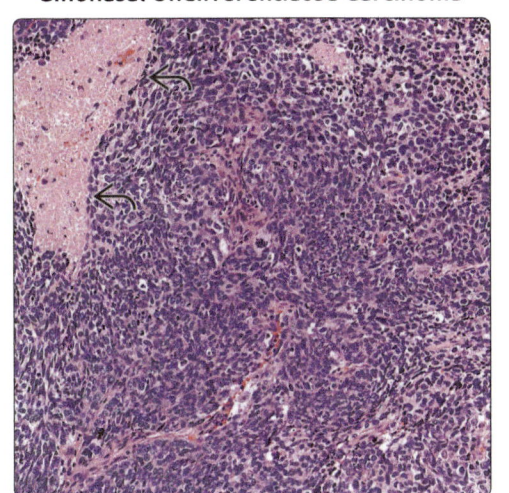

Sinonasal Undifferentiated Carcinoma

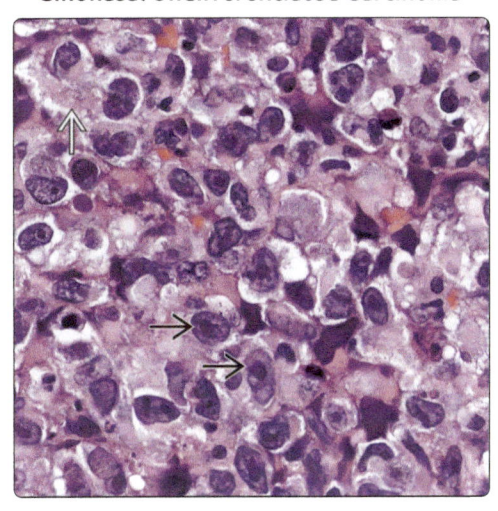

(Left) *SNUC often contains foci of geographic necrosis ⇨ and, by definition, lacks overt squamous or glandular differentiation.* (Right) *SNUC shows sheets of mononuclear cells with prominent nucleoli ⇨ and pale eosinophilic cytoplasm ➡. Macronucleoli are common in SNUC tumor cells.*

EMA Expression in Sinonasal Undifferentiated Carcinoma

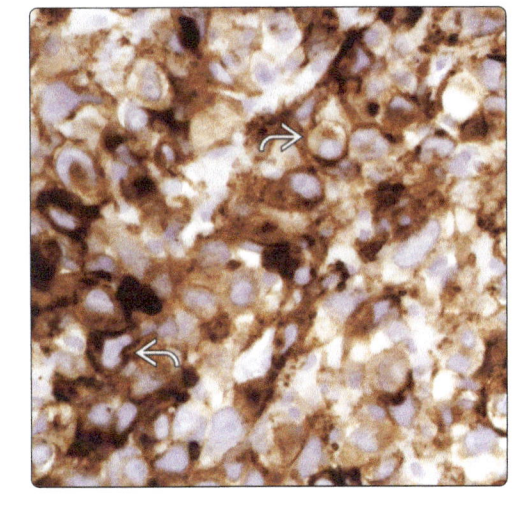

Diffuse p16 Expression in Sinonasal Undifferentiated Carcinoma

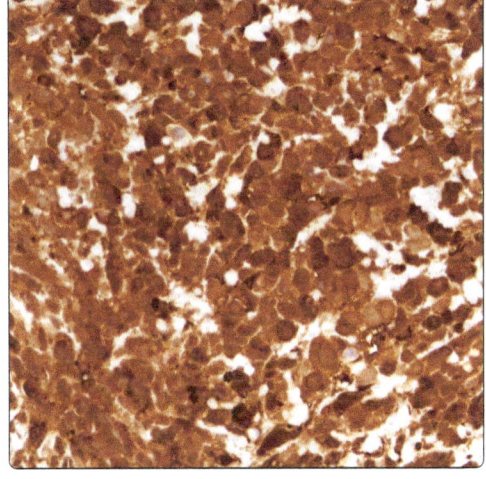

(Left) *EMA is diffusely expressed ⇨ in this case of SNUC and is generally found in up to 40% of cases.* (Right) *SNUC shows strong, diffuse expression of p16. This antibody shows both nuclear and cytoplasmic staining. Such reactivity should not be mistaken for an etiologic association with human papillomavirus.*

Sinonasal Melanoma

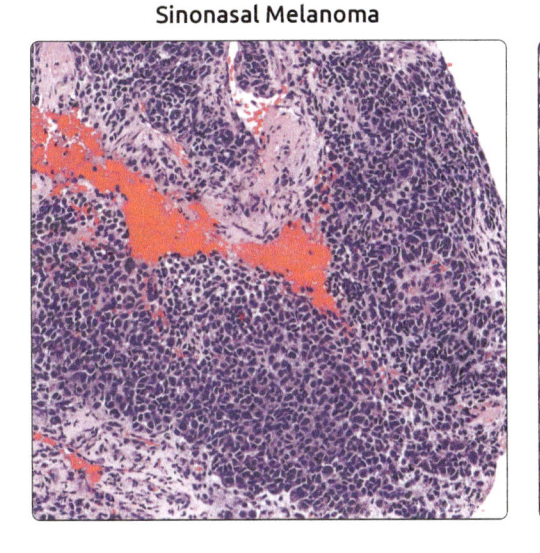

Sinonasal Melanoma

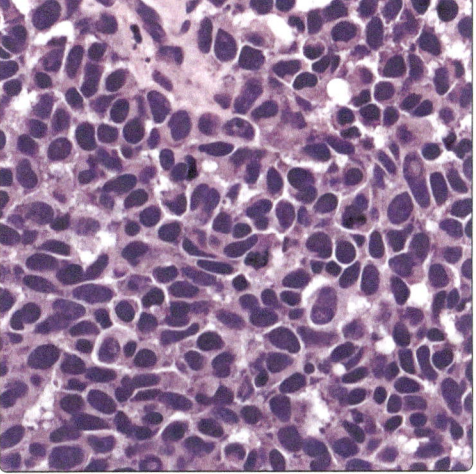

(Left) *Melanoma of the nasal cavity is shown. At this magnification, it easily resembles sinonasal undifferentiated carcinoma, poorly differentiated squamous carcinoma, and high-grade neuroendocrine carcinoma.* (Right) *Sinonasal melanoma shows slightly dyscohesive, round, epithelioid tumor cells, some of which contain single macronucleoli. Strong diffuse expression of S100 and HMB-45 (not shown) confirmed the diagnosis.*

Other Head and Neck Tumors

Olfactory Neuroblastoma

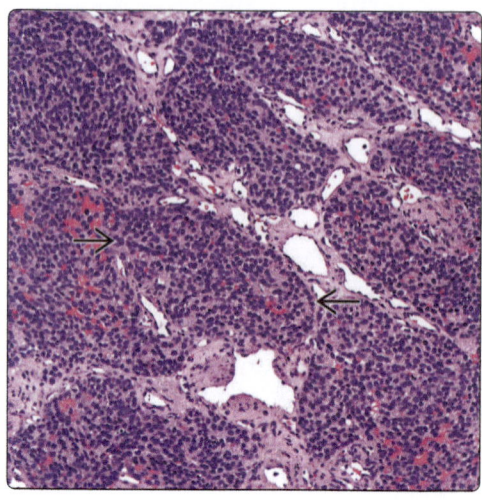

High-Grade Olfactory Neuroblastoma

(Left) Olfactory neuroblastoma grows as circumscribed lobules ➡ surrounded by a fibrotic, highly vascular stroma. This is the most common low-power morphology of olfactory neuroblastoma. (Right) Some higher grade olfactory neuroblastomas show more of a small round blue cell appearance, as in this example. In these cases, IHC is often required to make the diagnosis.

NUT (Midline) Carcinoma

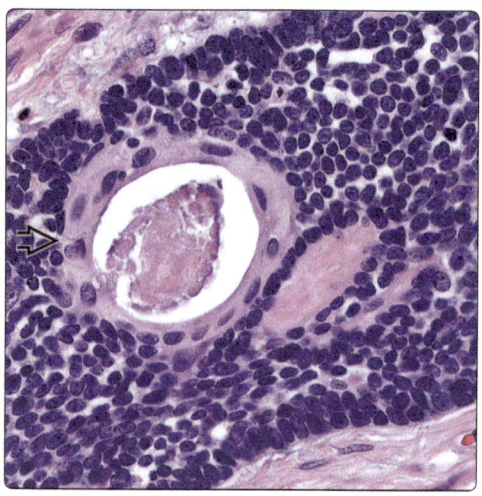

NUT (Midline) Carcinoma: Atypical Morphology

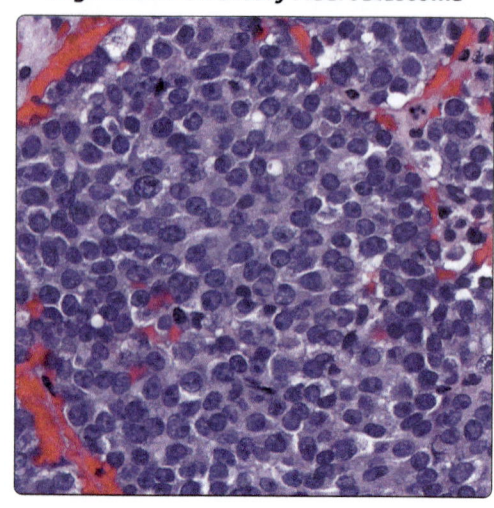

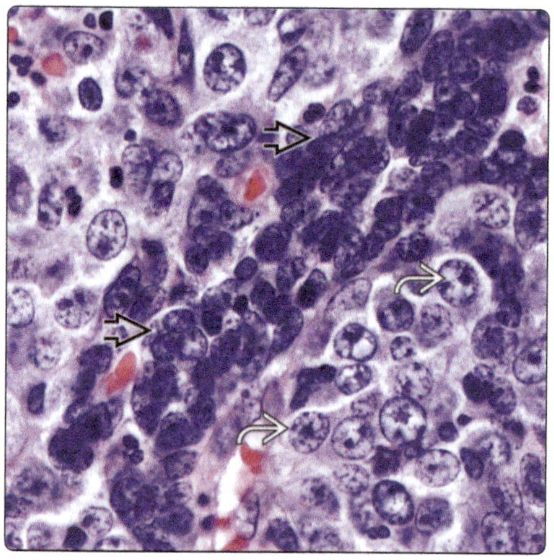

(Left) Abrupt keratinization ➡ is a classic feature of NUT (midline) carcinoma. (Right) NUT (midline) carcinoma (confirmed by FISH for NUT rearrangement) shows an unusual dual-cell morphology: Small round blue cells ➡ and larger cells with vesicular nuclei ➡ and pale amphophilic cytoplasm. NUT IHC should be strongly considered for any high-grade epithelial malignancy in the midline head and neck.

Sinonasal Adenocarcinoma, Intestinal Type

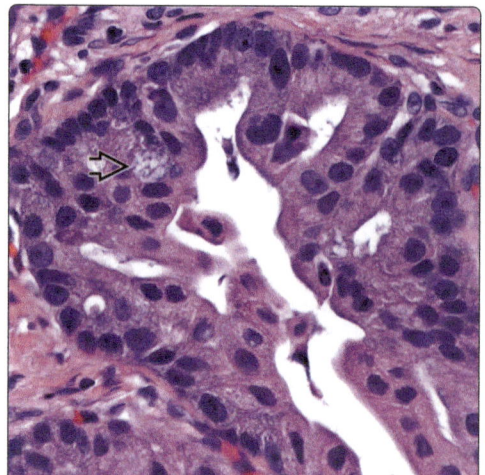

High-Grade Sinonasal Adenocarcinoma, Nonintestinal Type

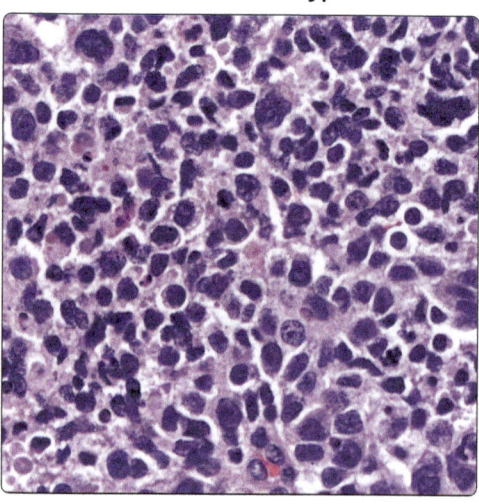

(Left) Low-grade intestinal-type sinonasal adenocarcinoma shows a mucous cell ➡. Strong reactivity for CDX2 and CK7 (not shown) would be expected. (Right) High-grade nonintestinal-type sinonasal adenocarcinoma often consists predominantly of solid sheets of cells. IHC is required to make the diagnosis.

Other Head and Neck Tumors

SMARCB1-Deficient Sinonasal Carcinoma

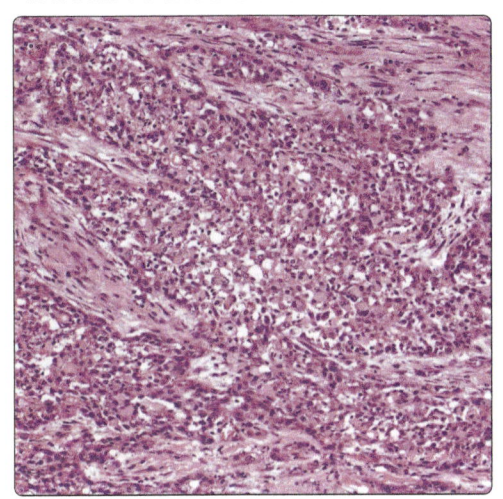

SMARCB1-Deficient Sinonasal Carcinoma With Prominent Rhabdoid Cells

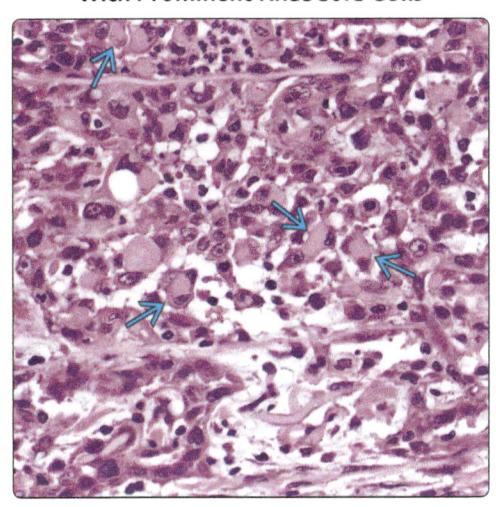

(Left) SMARCB1-deficient sinonasal carcinoma may histologically mimic SNUC, a basaloid carcinoma, or an eosinophilic malignancy. (Right) SMARCB1-deficient sinonasal carcinoma contains abundant rhabdoid cells ➡. Some cases have very few or no rhabdoid/plasmacytoid cells. This case expressed p40 and CK7 and showed loss of SMARCB1 by IHC.

Biphenotypic Sinonasal Sarcoma

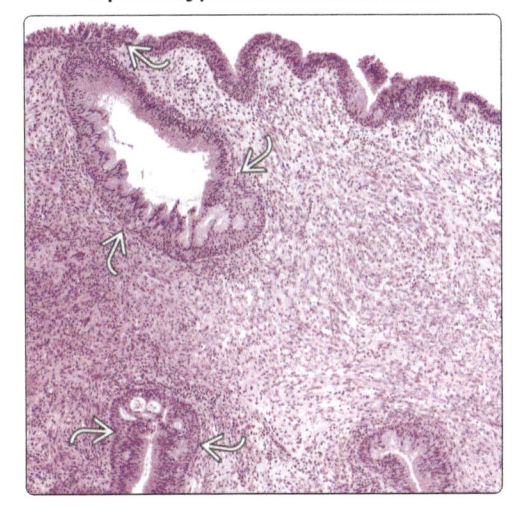

Biphenotypic Sinonasal Sarcoma

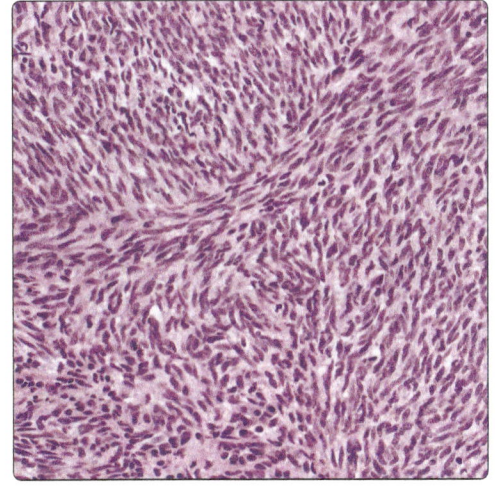

(Left) A characteristic feature of biphenotypic sinonasal sarcoma (BSS) is the reactive hyperplasia that occurs in the sinonasal mucosa and seromucinous glands ➡. Such hyperplasia is a diagnostic clue and should not be interpreted as biphasic tumor. (Right) BSS most commonly mimics a cellular schwannoma, malignant peripheral nerve sheath tumor, or synovial sarcoma. Note the intersecting fascicles of uniform spindled cells with slightly buckled, slender nuclei. Necrosis and pleomorphic cells are absent.

SMA Expression in Biphenotypic Sinonasal Sarcoma

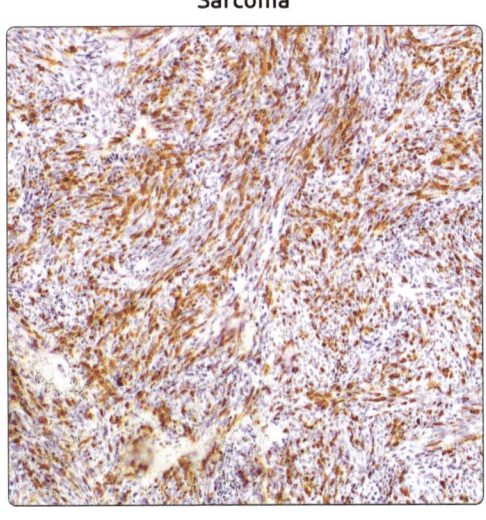

S100 Expression in Biphenotypic Sinonasal Sarcoma

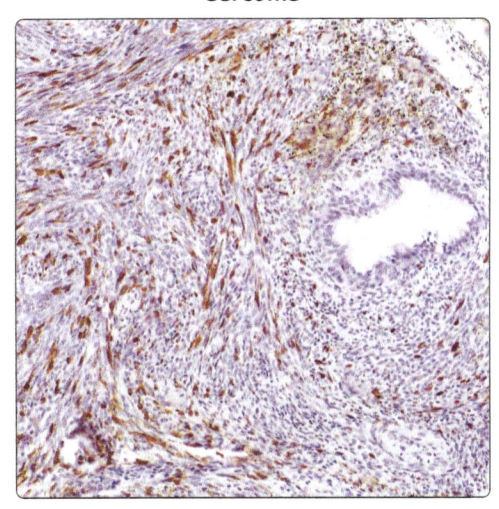

(Left) Similar to expression of S100 in BSS, SMA reactivity can be very focal and patchy (as in this case) or diffuse by IHC. (Right) BSS shows expression of S100. Expression may be very focal, patchy as in this case, or diffuse.

Papillary Thyroid Carcinoma

KEY FACTS

TERMINOLOGY
- Papillary thyroid carcinoma (PTC)

CLINICAL ISSUES
- Most common subtype of thyroid cancer (85-90%)
- Female predominance
- Strong association with radiation exposure
- Most cases present as nodule
- Frequent metastasis to cervical lymph nodes

MOLECULAR
- Gene mutations
  - *BRAF* mutations
    - 60-80% of classic PTC
    - > 90% of tall cell variant
    - p.V600E most common variant
  - RAS mutations
    - < 10% in classic PTC
  - *TERT* promoter mutations in 5-15%
- Gene rearrangements
  - *RET* in up to 25%
  - *PAX8::PPARG* fusion in up to 10% in follicular variants
  - *NTRK1* and *NTRK3* in < 5%
  - *ALK* in < 5%
- miRNA dysregulation
  - miR-146b, miR-221, and miR-222

MICROSCOPIC
- Papillary growth
- Characteristic nuclear features
  - Ground-glass nuclei
  - Nuclear pseudoinclusions
  - Nuclear grooves
- Psammoma bodies
- Several histologic subtypes

Gross Appearance

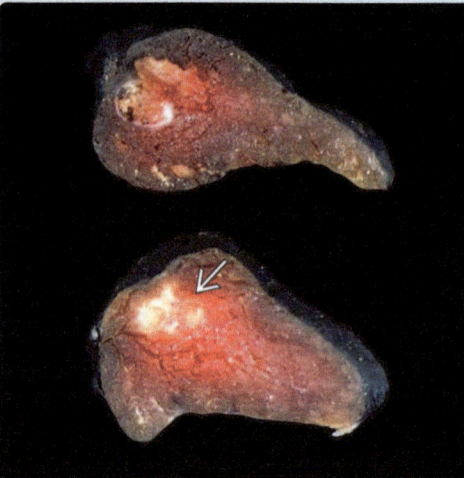

Classic Papillary Growth

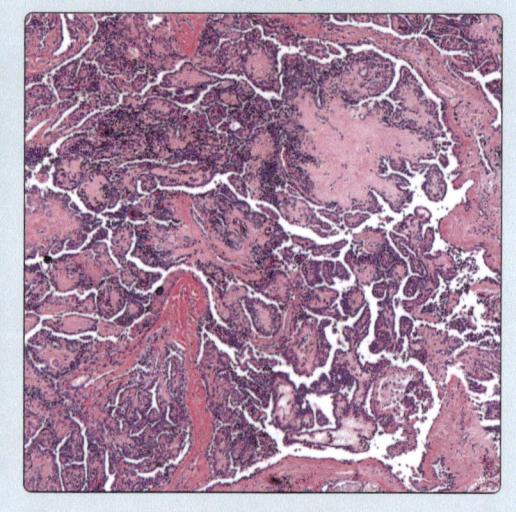

(Left) Gross photograph shows a nodule of papillary thyroid carcinoma (PTC) ➡ with an ill-defined border and infiltrative appearance. It is pale tan to whitish in color. The tumor is easily discernible from the adjacent normal thyroid parenchyma. (From DP: Endocrine.) (Right) Conventional PTC shows classic papillary growth with true fibrovascular cores, which are typically seen in this entity.

Classic Papillary Architecture

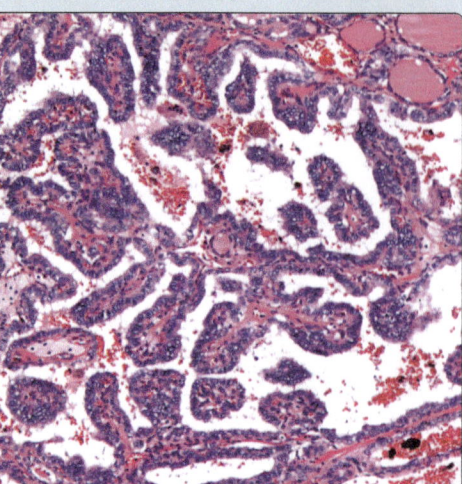

Allele-Specific PCR

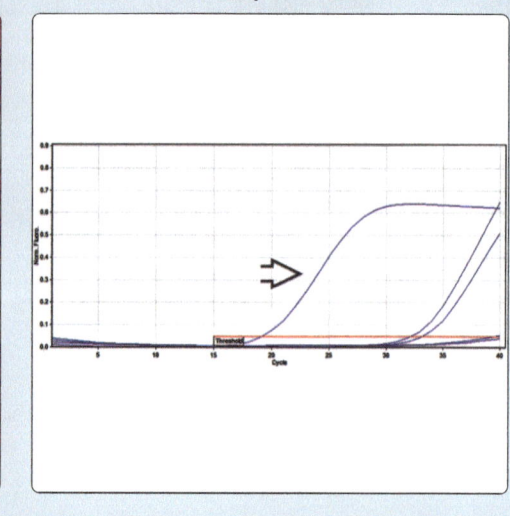

(Left) This patient presented with a thyroid nodule, and FNA cytology was highly suggestive of PTC. Excision shows the classic papillary architecture seen in the majority of conventional PTC. (Right) Allele-specific PCR was performed to detect the BRAF V600E mutation in a patient with PTC with atypical morphology. Here, there is amplification of the BRAF-mutated allele ➡.

Papillary Thyroid Carcinoma

TERMINOLOGY

Abbreviations
- Papillary thyroid carcinoma (PTC)

Definitions
- Most common type of thyroid carcinoma, typically characterized by papillary architecture and well-defined cytological features, including
  o Characteristic empty-appearing nuclei
  o Longitudinal nuclear grooves
  o Psammoma bodies in some cases

ETIOLOGY/PATHOGENESIS

Environmental Exposure
- Strong association with radiation exposure

Cell of Origin
- Follicular cells of thyroid gland

CLINICAL ISSUES

Epidemiology
- Incidence
  o Most common type of thyroid cancer (~ 85-90%)
- Sex
  o F:M = 4:1

Presentation
- Most cases present as thyroid nodule
- Worrisome symptoms and signs at presentation
  o Rapid increase in size
  o Dyspnea, dysphagia, or hoarseness
  o Firmness, lack of mobility, or large size
  o Presence of lymphadenopathy
- May also be found incidentally in thyroid tissue removed for other conditions
- Regional lymph node metastasis usually presents at diagnosis in ~ 50% of PTC
- Distant metastases are uncommon
  o Lung is most common site of metastasis

Treatment
- Surgery
  o Complete or partial thyroidectomy ± neck dissection
- Radioiodine therapy
- Targeted therapies
  o Tyrosine kinase inhibitors
    – Targeting *BRAF* &/or *RET* signaling pathways
    – Mainly considered in patients with aggressive disease or with distant metastasis and for tumors refractory to conventional therapies

Prognosis
- In general, well-differentiated tumors have very good prognosis
  o 90-95% overall survival
- Males and patients > 45 years of age tend to have more aggressive disease
- Regional lymph node metastasis has no significant impact on long-term prognosis
- Distant metastasis is predictor of poor outcome
- Prognostic impacts of *BRAF* or other gene mutations are controversial

MACROSCOPIC

General Features
- Most tumors are solid, whitish, firm, and clearly invasive
- < 10% are encapsulated
- Cystic changes seen in ~ 10% of PTC
- Calcifications may be present

MOLECULAR

Cytogenetics
- Diploid or near-diploid chromosomal DNA content
  o Aneuploidy or complex karyotypes usually associated with high-grade features
- Low rate of loss of heterozygosity

MAPK-Related Gene Alterations
- *BRAF* mutations
  o *BRAF* V600E mutation has been strongly associated with papillary phenotype
    – Seen in ~ 60-80% of classic variant
    – Seen in > 90% of tall cell variant
  o c.1799T>A results in valine to glutamate substitution in codon 600 (p.V600E)
    – Accounts for 98% of *BRAF* mutations
  o *BRAF* mutation has been associated with aggressive behavior and poor outcome in some studies
- *KRAS*, *NRAS*, and *HRAS* mutations
  o Strong association with invasive encapsulated follicular variant of PTC (25-45%)
  o < 10% in classic PTC
  o Mutations in *BRAF*, *NRAS*, *HRAS*, and *KRAS* are essentially mutually exclusive

Other Gene Mutations
- *TERT* promoter mutations
  o Present in 5-15% in most series
  o p.C228T is most common mutation
  o Can coexist with *BRAF* V600E mutations
  o Associated with poor prognosis
- Low-frequency gene mutations
  o Other low-frequency (< 5%) somatic mutations include
    – *HRAS*, *KRAS*, *MEK1*, *EIF1AX*, *PPM1D*, *CHEK2*, *MED12*, and *RBM10*

Gene Fusions
- *RET* rearrangements
  o 16 different partner genes are reported
  o Fusion of tyrosine kinase domain of *RET* oncogene (10q11.21) to 5' portion of partner genes
  o Present in 5-25% of PTC
    – Strong association with radiation-related PTC
    – Common in tumors from children and young adults
  o *RET::CCDC6* fusion (~ 60%)
    – *CCDC6* at 10q21.2
    – Can be detected by cytogenetics
    – Associated with typical papillary growth and microcarcinomas
    – Tend to have more benign clinical course

Papillary Thyroid Carcinoma

- *RET::NCOA4* fusion (~ 30%)
  - *NCOA4* at 10q11.22
  - Not detected by conventional cytogenetics
  - Often correlate with solid variant of PTC and with more aggressive clinical behavior
- *RET::PRKAR1A* fusion (~ 5%)
  - *PRKAR1A* at 17q24.2
- *BRAF* rearrangements
  - Present in ~ 2-3% of PTC
  - Diverse gene partners, including *AKAP9* and *AGK*
- *PAX8::PPARG* rearrangement
  - More common in EFV-PTC (~ 10%)
  - *PAX8* at 2q13 fused with *PPARG* at 3p25
- *NTRK1* and *NTRK3* rearrangements
  - Present in < 5% of PTC
  - Common fusion partners of *NTRK1* include *TPM3*, *TPR*, and *TFG*
  - Common fusion partner of *NTRK3* is *ETV6*
    - Common in radiation-associated PTC
  - Associated with aggressive features
- *ALK* rearrangements
  - Reported in ~ 1-5% of PTC
  - Rearrangements include *STRN::ALK* and *EML4::ALK*
  - Predominantly follicular infiltrative pattern and solid growth
  - May respond to ALK inhibitors (e.g., crizotinib)
- MicroRNA dysregulation
  - High levels of miR-146b, miR-221, and miR-222

MICROSCOPIC

Histologic Features

- Classic subtype shows characteristic papillary growth
- Papillae are usually complex, branching with central fibrovascular core, and randomly oriented
- Lined by neoplastic cells with
  - Ground-glass or optically clear nuclei (in formalin-fixed tissue only)
  - Nuclear pseudoinclusion
  - Nuclear grooves (usually parallel to long axis)
- Mitotic activity is rarely increased
- Psammoma bodies may be present in ~ 50% of PTC
- Lymphatic invasion is commonly present
- Extrathyroidal extension found in ~ 25% of PTC
- Involvement of cervical lymph nodes is very common (> 80%)
- Vascular (blood vessel) invasion is rare (up to 7%)

Histologic Subtypes

- Infiltrative follicular variant (IFVPTC)
  - Infiltrative growth pattern of classic PTC
  - Predominant follicular architecture with nuclear atypia
  - Common molecular alterations
    - *BRAF* mutations
    - *RET* translocations, *NTRK* and *ALK* fusions
- Encapsulated
  - Classic PTC enveloped by thick, fibrous capsule
  - Capsule may be intact or infiltrated by tumor
- Tall cell and columnar cell variant
  - Tall cells
    - Basal nuclei with abundant eosinophilic cytoplasm
    - Tumor cell height at least 3x width
    - Tall cells at least 30% of tumor
    - Strongest association with *BRAF* mutations (up to 80%)
    - *TERT* promoter mutations frequently found
  - Columnar cells
    - Lacks conventional nuclear features of PTC
- Diffuse sclerosing variant
  - Diffuse lobular involvement, dense sclerosis, squamous metaplasia, and dense lymphocytic infiltrate
  - Psammoma bodies are abundant
  - Solid or papillary growth with extensive lymphovascular invasion
    - Common nodal and distant metastasis
  - *RET* rearrangements common
  - *BRAF* V600E mutations (20%)
  - Disease-free survival rate lower than conventional PTC
- Other variants
  - Hobnail, solid/trabecular, oncocytic, spindle cell, clear cell, Warthin-like

ANCILLARY TESTS

Immunohistochemistry

- Positive for pancytokeratin, CK19, PAX8, thyroglobulin, and TTF-1
- S100, vimentin, EMA, CA125, HBME-1, galectin-3 variably positive
- Galectin-3 and HBME-1 show higher specificity for PTC cells
- BRAF pV600 (VE1 clone) highly sensitive and specific for detection of mutation

DIFFERENTIAL DIAGNOSIS

Papillary Hyperplasia in Graves Disease and Adenomatous Goiter

- Lacks characteristic nuclear features of PTC

Follicular Adenoma and Carcinoma

- Frequently microfollicular pattern with thick, fibrous capsule
- Lacks characteristic nuclear features of PTC
- *RAS*-like molecular signature

Medullary Carcinoma

- May have papillary growth pattern
- Positive for calcitonin and neuroendocrine markers
- Amyloid deposits frequently present

SELECTED REFERENCES

1. Baloch ZW et al: Overview of the 2022 WHO Classification of thyroid neoplasms. Endocr Pathol. 33(1):27-63, 2022
2. Prete A et al: Update on fundamental mechanisms of thyroid cancer. Front Endocrinol (Lausanne). 11:102, 2020
3. Haroon Al Rasheed MR et al: Molecular alterations in thyroid carcinoma. Surg Pathol Clin. 12(4):921-30, 2019
4. Acquaviva G et al: Molecular pathology of thyroid tumours of follicular cells: a review of genetic alterations and their clinicopathological relevance. Histopathology. 72(1):6-31, 2018
5. Giordano TJ: Follicular cell thyroid neoplasia: insights from genomics and The Cancer Genome Atlas research network. Curr Opin Oncol. 28(1):1-4, 2016
6. Cancer Genome Atlas Research Network: integrated genomic characterization of papillary thyroid carcinoma. Cell. 159(3):676-90, 2014

Papillary Thyroid Carcinoma

True Papillae

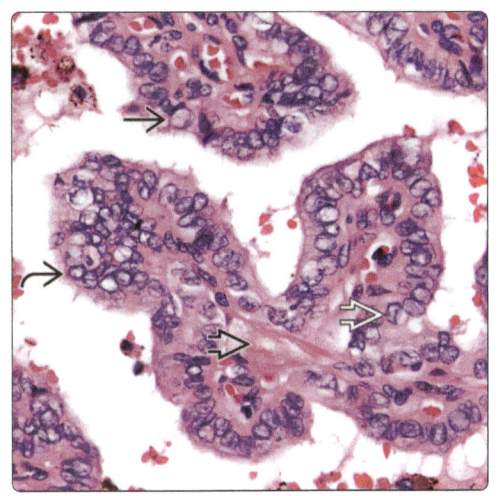

Nuclear Pseudoinclusions

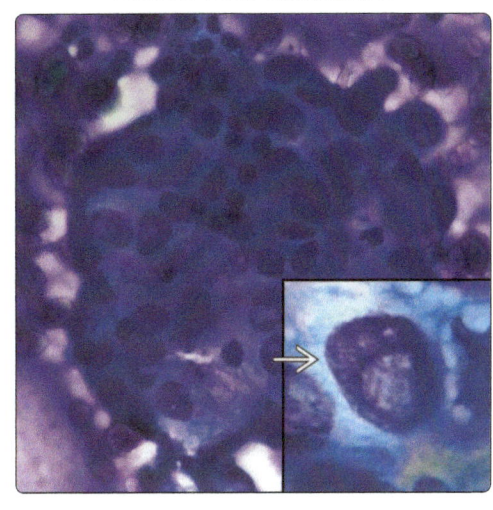

(Left) *True papillae show a central fibrovascular core ⇨ lined by a single layer of neoplastic cells with distinctive morphologic features, including elongated, clear (ground-glass) nuclei ⇨, nuclear pseudoinclusions ⇨, and nuclear grooves ⇨.* (Right) *FNA of thyroid nodule shows a papillary structure composed of cells with fine chromatin and distinctive nuclear pseudoinclusions ⇨.*

Nuclear Pseudoinclusions

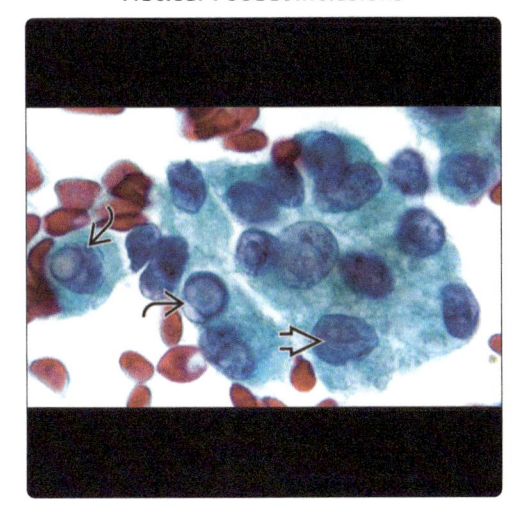

HBME-1 Immunohistochemistry

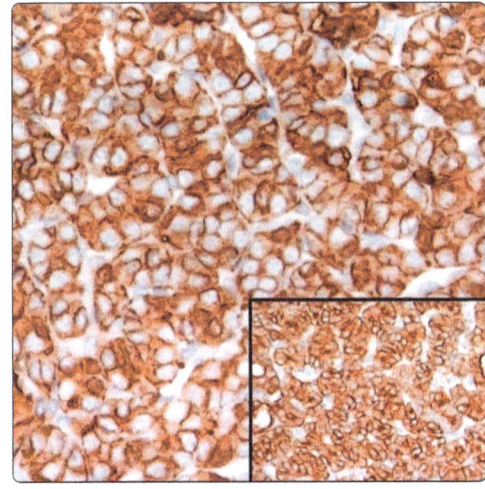

(Left) *Papanicolaou stain of FNA shows the characteristic nuclear features of PTC, including nuclear pseudoinclusions ⇨ and nuclear grooves ⇨ (parallel to long axis).* (Right) *IHC can be helpful when difficult morphologic cases are encountered. This is a follicular variant of PTC with predominance of microfollicles and rare PTC-type nuclei. Cells demonstrate strong positivity for HBME-1 and CK19 (inset).*

CK19 Immunohistochemistry

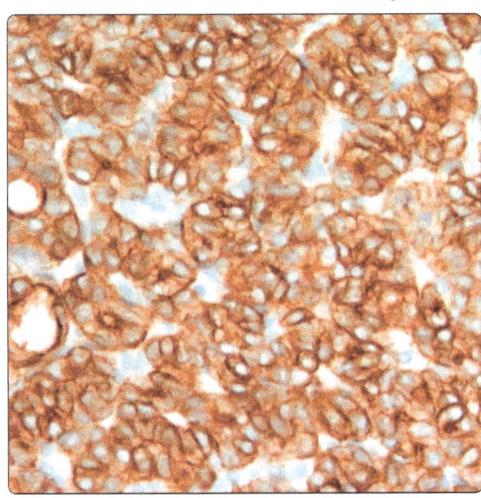

FISH Using Break-Apart *RET* Probes

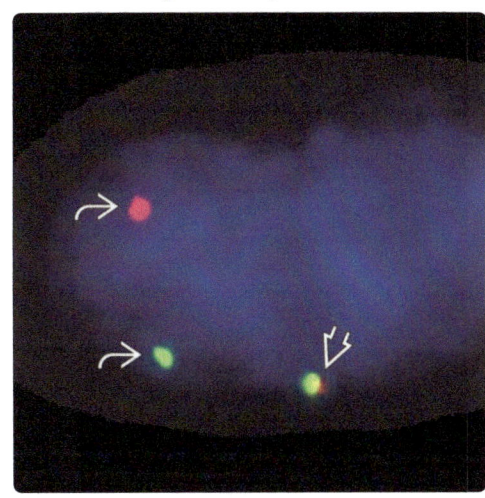

(Left) *CK19 is diffusely and strongly expressed within PTC and its variants; however, it is normally absent or focally expressed in other thyroid lesions.* (Right) *FISH using break-apart probes for RET rearrangements at 10q11.21 is shown. Yellow fusion signal ⇨ is normal, and separated green and red signals ⇨ are abnormal and indicative of RET rearrangement.*

Molecular Pathology of Solid Tumors

541

Follicular Thyroid Carcinoma

KEY FACTS

TERMINOLOGY
- Follicular thyroid carcinoma (FTC)
  - Malignant thyroid tumor with follicular cell differentiation
  - Lacks features of other distinctive thyroid malignancies

CLASSIFICATION
- WHO 5 edition histologic subtypes
  - Minimally invasive (capsular invasion only)
  - Encapsulated angioinvasive
  - Widely invasive

ETIOLOGY/PATHOGENESIS
- Inherited syndromes associated with increased risk for FTC
  - *PTEN* hamartoma tumor syndrome (PHTS)
  - Carney complex
  - Werner syndrome
  - McCune-Albright syndrome
  - Li-Fraumeni syndrome

CLINICAL ISSUES
- 5-10% of all thyroid malignancies
- Female predilection
- Usually single "cold" nodule but in inherited cases can be multifocal and bilateral

MOLECULAR
- RAS family mutations present in 30-50%
- *PPARG* rearrangement seen in up to 10-40%
- PI3K-PTEN-AKT signaling pathway
  - *PTEN* and *PIK3CA* mutations in < 10%
- *TERT* promoter mutation in 10-35%
- None of these mutations are exclusive and diagnostic of FTC, as they can be seen in other thyroid carcinomas and follicular thyroid adenoma

MICROSCOPIC
- Capsular &/or vascular invasion are required for diagnosis

Fibrous Capsule and Adjacent Thyroid | **Capsular Invasion**

(Left) Low-power microphotograph of follicular carcinoma shows a well-encapsulated tumor surrounded by a thick, irregular fibrous capsule ⇨. Adjacent thyroid demonstrates normal histology ⇨. (Right) Capsular invasion is diagnostic of follicular carcinoma. Tumor cells are seen ⇨ invading across the entire thickness of the fibrous capsule ⇨ (classic mushroom sign).

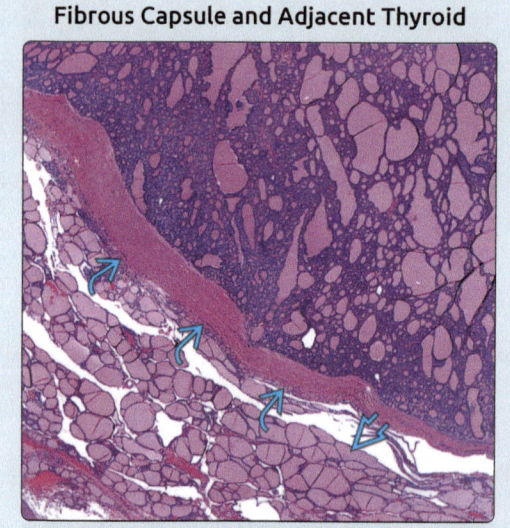

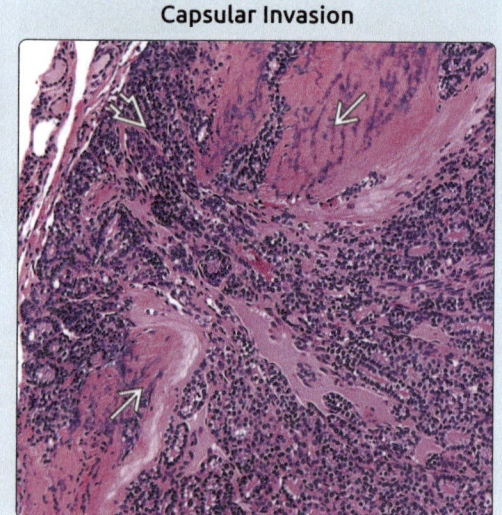

FISH | ***NRAS* Pyrosequencing**

(Left) Dual-fusion interphase FISH can be used to identify the t(2;3)(q14.1;p25.2) translocation associated with the PAX8::PPARG rearrangement ⇨ seen in up to 50% of follicular thyroid carcinoma (FTC) (PAX8 = red signal; PPARG = green signal). (Right) Pyrogram shows DNA sequence of codon 61 within exon 3 of the NRAS gene. Top image shows wildtype sequence (CAA). Bottom image shows c.182A>G (CGA) mutation ⇨. This p.Q61R mutation is the most common NRAS mutation found in FTC.

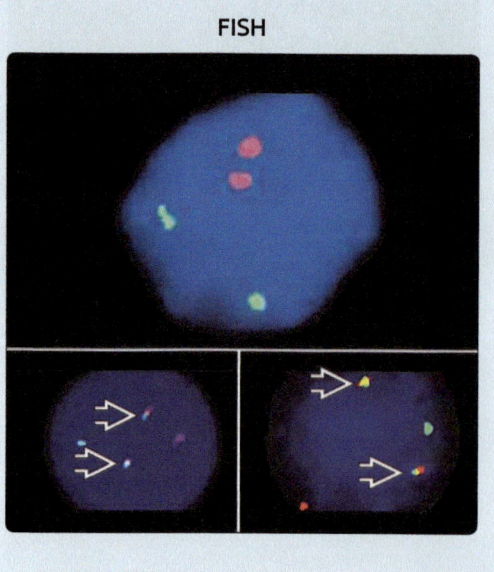

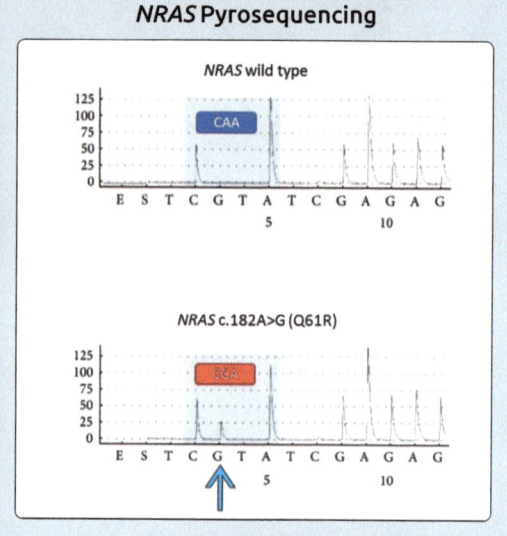

Follicular Thyroid Carcinoma

TERMINOLOGY

Abbreviations
- Follicular thyroid carcinoma (FTC)

Definitions
- Malignant thyroid tumor with follicular cell differentiation

CLASSIFICATION

WHO 5th Edition
- Minimally invasive FTC (capsular invasion only)
- Encapsulated angioinvasive FTC
- Widely invasive FTC

ETIOLOGY/PATHOGENESIS

Sporadic FTC
- Accounts for majority of cases

Hereditary FTC
- Accounts for 10% of cases

Associated Inherited Syndromes
- *PTEN* hamartoma tumor syndrome (PHTS)
  o Characterized by benign hamartomatous and malignant tumors and germline *PTEN* pathogenic variants
  o Includes Cowden syndrome (CS), Bannayan-Riley-Ruvalcaba syndrome (BRRS), *PTEN*-related Proteus syndrome (PS), and Proteus-like syndrome
  o Inherited in autosomal dominant manner
  o Particularly increased risk for epithelial tumors in CS
    - Breast cancer lifetime risk: 85%
    - Thyroid cancer (usually follicular, rarely papillary, never medullary) lifetime risk: 35%
    - Endometrial cancer lifetime risk: 28%
  o Thyroid tumors are often multiple and bilateral
  o Epithelial thyroid cancer (especially FTC) is major diagnostic criteria for PHTS
- Carney complex
  o Autosomal dominant, caused by *PRKAR1A* mutations
  o Characterized by skin pigmentary abnormalities, myxomas, endocrine tumors or overactivity, and schwannomas
    - Up to 75% have multiple thyroid nodules, most being nonfunctioning adenomas
    - ~ 5% can develop thyroid carcinomas (papillary or follicular)
- Werner syndrome
  o Autosomal recessive disorder caused by *WRN* mutations
  o Characterized by premature aging and increased cancer predisposition
    - Most common tumors are soft tissue sarcomas, osteosarcomas, melanomas, and thyroid carcinomas (usually FTC)
- Other familial syndromes associated with FTC include DICER1, McCune-Albright, and Li-Fraumeni
  o Li-Fraumeni syndrome often associated with aggressive behavior

Preexisting Thyroid Disease
- Follicular adenomas more common than FTC (~ 5:1)
- May be precursor lesions, as both can harbor similar molecular alterations

CLINICAL ISSUES

Epidemiology
- Incidence
  o Constitutes ~ 5-10% of all thyroid malignancies
  o Increased prevalence in iodine-deficient areas (25-40%)
- Age
  o Sporadic cases usually in 5th-6th decades
  o Hereditary cases affect patients at earlier age
- Sex
  o Female predilection

Presentation
- Solitary painless nodule
- Slow growing, may develop local symptoms with larger size
- Patients usually euthyroid

Treatment
- Total thyroidectomy ± adjuvant radioactive iodine or external beam radiation therapy are available options, depending on tumor stage

Prognosis
- Metastases are usually blood borne rather than nodal
  o Lungs and bone are most common sites
- Prognosis is directly related to degree of encapsulation and vascular invasion
- Hereditary tumors are usually more aggressive

IMAGING

Ultrasonographic Findings
- Usually shows well-circumscribed nodule
- Cannot distinguish adenoma from FTC

Scintigraphy
- "Cold" nodule on isotopic scan

MACROSCOPIC

General Features
- Solid, encapsulated, round tumors with light tan cut surface
- Minimally invasive tumors often show fibrous, thicker capsule (similar to follicular adenomas)
- Widely invasive tumors show extensive permeation of capsule
- Hereditary tumors may be multifocal and bilateral

MOLECULAR

Cytogenetics
- Complex karyotypes, hyperdiploidy, extra copies of chromosome 7, and chromosomal losses are common
- Aneuploidies can be identified in both FTC and adenomas
  o Loss of heterozygosity (LOH), ~ 20% per chromosome arm
- Chromosomal translocations
  o t(2;3); *PAX8::PPARG* in 10-40% of cases
    - Associated with more overt invasion
  o t(3;7); *PPARG::CREB3L2* reported rarely

Follicular Thyroid Carcinoma

In Situ Hybridization
- Dual-color FISH can be used to identify *PAX8::PARG* fusion

Molecular Genetics
- RAS-type family mutations
  - Family of genes that include protooncogenes *NRAS*, *HRAS*, and *KRAS*
    - GTPases fundamental in transduction of intracellular signals from cell membrane
  - Constitutive activation observed in tumors originating from follicular cells
  - Most common mutations are codon 61 of *NRAS* and *HRAS*
    - Associated with more aggressive behavior and less favorable prognosis
    - Present in 30-50% of FTC and 20-40% of follicular thyroid adenomas (FTA)
- PI3K-PTEN-AKT pathway
  - *PTEN*
    - Negatively regulates *AKT1* and is key regulator of PI3K/PTEN/AKT signaling pathway
    - Inactivating mutations identified in up to 10% of sporadic FTC
  - *PIK3CA*
    - Mutations in exons 9 and 20 reported in up to 10% of sporadic FTC
    - Amplifications also detected
- *TERT*
  - Hotspot mutations in promoter region (C228T and C250T)
  - Present in 10-35% of FTC
  - Associated with aggressive clinical behavior and poor prognosis
- *DICER1* somatic mutation
  - Associated with macrofollicular architecture
- *TSHR* mutations (rarely reported)

MicroRNA
- Global microRNA expression in FTC and adenomas has demonstrated significant dysregulation
  - Upregulation of miR-181 and miR200; downregulation of miR-199
  - miR-7-5p and miR206 proposed as FTC markers with differential expression as compared with FTA

Molecular Panels
- Potentially useful when trying to differentiate benign from malignant nodules
- Numerous commercially available tests (Affirma, ThyroSeq, ThyGenX/ThyraMIR, and Rosetta GX)

MICROSCOPIC

Histologic Features
- Cells often show round or oval nuclei
- Various architectural patterns, including solid, trabecular, microfollicular, and macrofollicular
- WHO 5th edition classifies as minimally invasive, encapsulated, angioinvasive, and widely invasive carcinomas
- Criteria for capsular invasion
  - Tumor extension through entire thickness of capsule
  - Tumor bud still covered by thin capsule; however, it extends beyond outer capsular surface
  - Presence of satellite nodule with cytoarchitectural features similar to main tumor
    - Caution with fine-needle aspiration rupture artifact
- Criteria for vascular invasion
  - Vessel should be of venous caliber
  - Located in or immediately outside capsule (rather than within tumor)
  - Contains 1 or more clusters of tumor cells attached to wall and protruding into lumen

ANCILLARY TESTS

Immunohistochemistry
- Reactive for thyroglobulin, TTF-1, PAX8, and low-molecular-weight keratins
- No definitive marker to differentiate adenoma from carcinoma is available

DIFFERENTIAL DIAGNOSIS

Follicular Thyroid Adenoma
- Main differential diagnosis
- Similar cellular morphology
- Thin, fibrous capsule without evidence of capsular or vascular invasion

Atypical Adenoma or Follicular Lesion of Uncertain Malignant Potential
- Cellular follicular lesion with thickened capsule
- Partial capsular invasion may be present
- Vascular invasion should be absent

Follicular Variant of Papillary Thyroid Carcinoma
- Nuclear features (i.e., nuclear grooves, pseudonuclear inclusions, nuclear clearing, and overlapping nuclei) help to separate from FTC

Follicular Variant of Medullary Carcinoma
- Cells usually show abundant eosinophilic cytoplasm and coarsely clumped chromatin, often with plasmacytoid appearance
- Positive for calcitonin

SELECTED REFERENCES

1. Basolo F et al: The 5(th) edition of WHO classification of tumors of endocrine organs: changes in the diagnosis of follicular-derived thyroid carcinoma. Endocrine. 80(3):470-6, 2023
2. WHO Classification of Tumours Editorial Board: Endocrine and Neuroendocrine Tumours. 5th ed. IARC, 2022
3. Baloch ZW et al: Overview of the 2022 WHO classification of thyroid neoplasms. Endocr Pathol. 33(1):27-63, 2022
4. Acquaviva G et al: Molecular pathology of thyroid tumours of follicular cells: a review of genetic alterations and their clinicopathological relevance. Histopathology. 72(1):6-31, 2018

Follicular Thyroid Carcinoma

Capsular and Angioinvasion

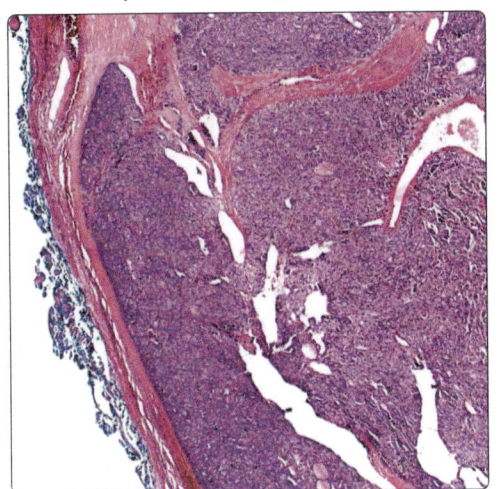

Vascular Invasion

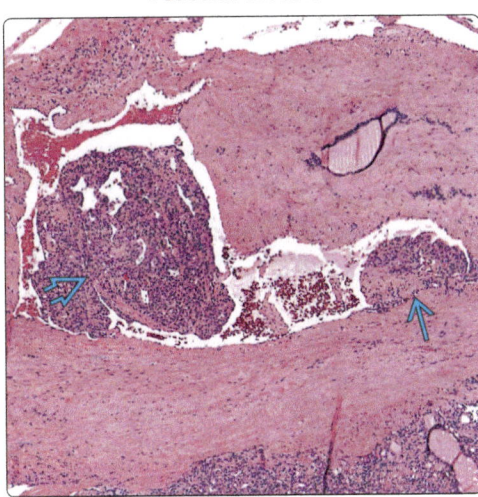

(Left) FTC shows extensive capsular and angioinvasion. *(Right)* Vascular invasion is one of the required histologic features for the diagnosis of FTC. Tumor cells are present within the lumen ⇨ of a large-caliber vessel and are focally attached to the vascular wall ⇨.

Marked Cellularity

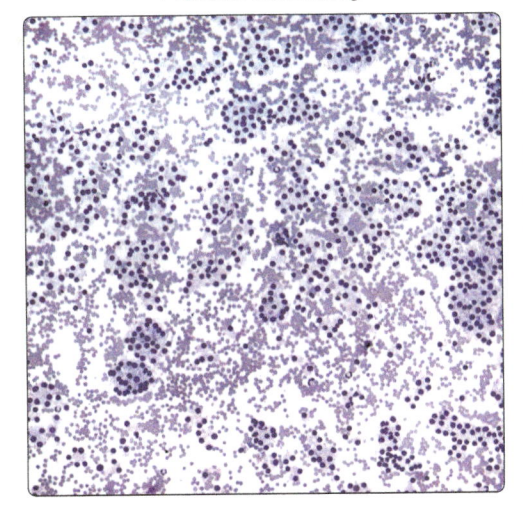

Microfollicles

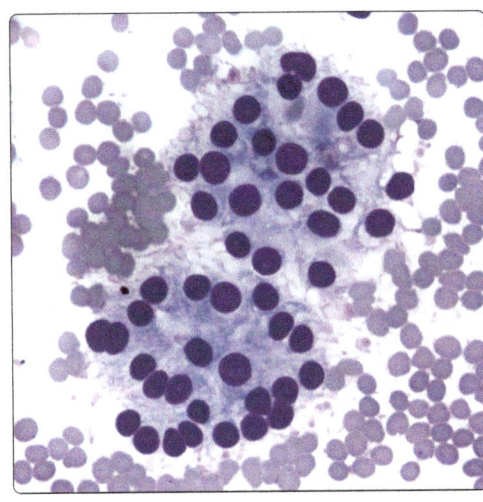

(Left) FNA of a solitary large thyroid nodule shows marked cellularity with predominance of microfollicles, enlarged follicular cells, and near absence of colloid. Subsequent partial thyroidectomy showed FTC. *(Right)* On high power, the microfollicles are better appreciated. For follicular lesions, FNA is a screening procedure, as the diagnosis of FTC relies entirely on histologic features.

Thyroglobulin

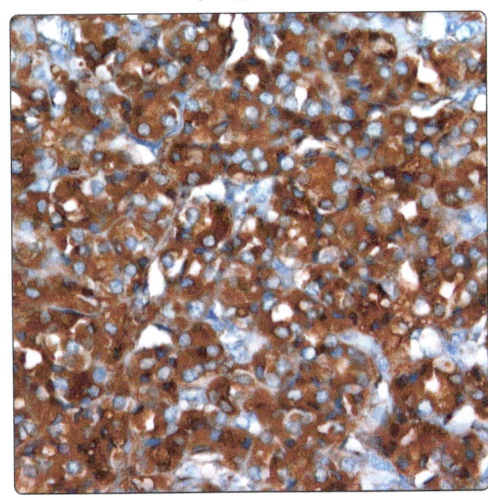

TTF-1

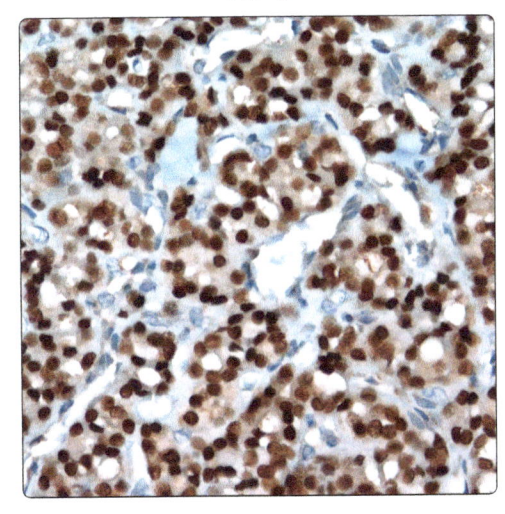

(Left) Thyroglobulin is positive in this case of FTC. Follicular carcinomas are usually positive for thyroglobulin and TTF-1. *(Right)* TTF-1 shows nuclear positivity in this case of FTC. Unfortunately, no reliable immunohistochemical markers are available to differentiate FTC from follicular adenomas, other benign lesions, and other thyroid carcinomas.

Poorly Differentiated Thyroid Carcinoma

KEY FACTS

TERMINOLOGY
- Poorly differentiated thyroid carcinomas (PDTC): Malignant thyroid follicular neoplasm with intermediate morphological and biologic attributes between well-differentiated and undifferentiated thyroid carcinoma
- Subtype of high-grade, follicular, cell-derived, nonanaplastic thyroid carcinoma

CLINICAL ISSUES
- Usually ≥ 6th decade of life
- More common in women than in men
- Frequently present with nodal metastases and extrathyroidal extension
- Death from disease is common

MACROSCOPIC
- Foci of necrosis common
- Infiltrative margins

MOLECULAR
- *NRAS* mutations common
- *BRAF* somatic point mutations reported in ~ 10%
- *TERT* promoter mutations represent most common alteration in PDTC (40%) and are associated with high risk of distant metastasis
- *TP53* somatic mutations in ~ 20-30%
- *CTNNB1* mutations in up to 25%

MICROSCOPIC
- Histological features
  - Insular, trabecular, and solid growth patterns frequently seen
  - Neoplastic cells are usually small and monotonous with high N:C ratio
- Cytological features
  - Microfollicles can be identified
  - Focal atypia and increased mitoses

Insular Growth Pattern

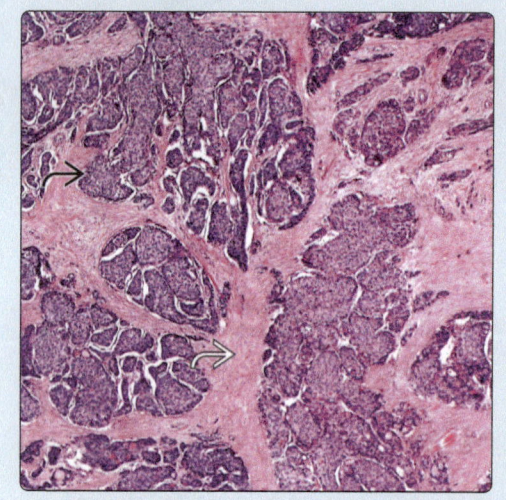

Mitoses

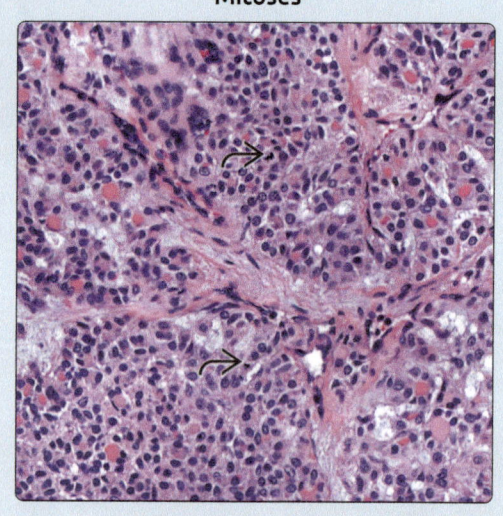

(Left) Poorly differentiated thyroid carcinoma (PDTC) shows an insular growth pattern ➡ defined by well-defined cell nests surrounded by fibrous septa ➡. (Right) PDTC shows increased mitotic activity ➡. PDTC typically shows ≥ 3 mitoses per 10 HPF.

Aspirate Smear

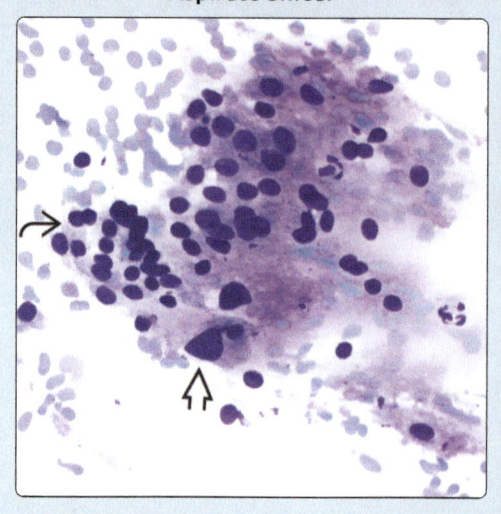

Atypical Morphologic Features

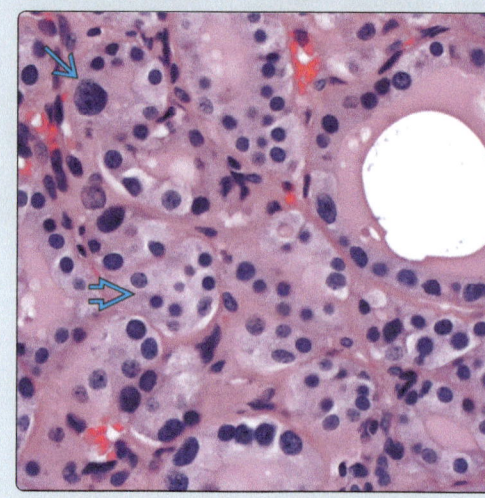

(Left) Aspirate of PDTC shows tumor cells small to intermediate in size with occasional pleomorphism ➡. Microfollicles are present ➡. (Right) Corresponding histology shows scattered nucleomegaly ➡ and microfollicles ➡.

Poorly Differentiated Thyroid Carcinoma

TERMINOLOGY

Abbreviations
- Poorly differentiated thyroid carcinoma (PDTC)

Synonyms
- Insular carcinoma

Definitions
- Malignant thyroid follicular neoplasm with intermediate morphological and biologic attributes between well-differentiated and undifferentiated thyroid carcinoma
- Subtype of high-grade, follicular, cell-derived, nonanaplastic thyroid carcinoma

ETIOLOGY/PATHOGENESIS

Preexisting Conditions
- Genetic and environmental factors (iodide deficiency) may play role
- Can develop in setting of longstanding goiter
- Usually arise de novo

CLINICAL ISSUES

Epidemiology
- Incidence
  o Vary in different geographic regions
  o Accounts for ~ 2% of all thyroid carcinomas in North America
- Age
  o Usually ≥ 6th decade of life
- Sex
  o More common in women than in men

Presentation
- Rapidly growing solitary neck (thyroid) mass
- Frequently present with nodal metastases and extrathyroidal extension
- Pulmonary and bone metastases also common at time of diagnosis

Treatment
- Similar to what is used for undifferentiated carcinomas
  o Surgical resection
  o Radiation and chemotherapy
  o Radioiodine therapy
- Often resistant to conventional therapies

Prognosis
- Intermediate behavior between well-differentiated and undifferentiated thyroid carcinomas
- 5-year survival rates approach 50%
- Death from disease is common

MACROSCOPIC

General Features
- Tend to be solid and gray-white
- Foci of necrosis common
- Infiltrative margins

Size
- Range: 2-13 cm
  o Mean: ~ 6 cm

MOLECULAR

Molecular Alterations
- Overview
  o Genetic mutations unique for PDTC have not been identified
  o PDTC harbors molecular alterations seen in both well-differentiated and undifferentiated carcinomas
  o *BRAF* V600E or RAS mutations (27% and 24% of cases, respectively) are mutually exclusive main drivers in PDTC
  o *TERT* promoter mutations represent most common alteration in PDTC (40%) and are associated with high risk of distant metastasis
- *HRAS*, *KRAS*, and *NRAS*
  o Encodes proteins involved in activation of PI3K/AKT/mTOR signaling pathways
    – Regulator of cell division, cell differentiation, and apoptosis
  o *NRAS* mutations are most common
    – Ranges from 20-55% of PDTC
    – Most common mutations involve codon 61
    – Result in constitutive activation of downstream signaling pathways
    – Lead to uncontrolled growth and cell division
    – Possible association with aggressive tumor behavior and poor prognosis
- *BRAF*
  o Encodes BRAF protein
    – Serine-threonine tyrosine kinase
    – Regulator of cell division, differentiation, cell migration, and apoptosis
  o *BRAF* mutations
    – Somatic point mutations reported in ~ 10% of PDTC
    – Described in PDTC with PTC-like nuclei
    – Also occur in cases with coexisting foci of PTC
    – *BRAF* V600E (c.1799T>A; p.V600E) accounts for majority of *BRAF* mutations
    – *BRAF* V600E is likely early event
    – Results in constitutive activation of MAPK signaling pathway
    – *BRAF* mutations are linked with silencing of iodine transporting genes
    – Targeting BRAF may facilitate iodine uptake ability of thyroid cancer cells
- *TERT* gene
  o Encodes telomerase reverse transcriptase
    – Limitless self-renewal is attained by telomere maintenance, essentially through telomerase *TERT* activation
    – Mutations of TERT promoter lead to TERT-protein overexpression
    – Mutations generate de novo binding elements for ETS-family transcription factors activated by MAPK signaling, such as GABPA
  o Clinical significance
    – TERT-based immunotherapy: TERT-protein overexpression could increase TERT-antigen presentation by cancer cells and increase susceptibility to T-cell recognition and attack

Poorly Differentiated Thyroid Carcinoma

- *TP53*
  - Encodes TP53 protein
  - Tumor suppressor gene and regulator of cell division
  - Somatic mutations (exons 5-9) reported in ~ 20-30% of PDTC
    - Codon 273 most often affected
    - Extremely rare event in well-differentiated carcinomas
- *CTNNB1*
  - Encodes β-catenin
    - Critical for establishment and maintenance of epithelial layers
    - Transmission of contact inhibition signal
    - Involved in WNT signaling pathway
  - Mutations reported in up to 25% of PDTC
    - Activating mutations cluster in exon 3
    - Leading to WNT pathway activation

MICROSCOPIC

Histologic Features

- Insular, trabecular, and solid growth patterns are common
- Neoplastic cells are usually small and monotonous with high N:C ratio
- Round, hyperchromatic to vesicular nuclei
- Increased mitotic activity ≥ 3/10 HPF
- Atypical mitoses in ~ 20% of cases
- Necrosis common
- Invasive growth common, including
  - Extrathyroidal extension
- Extensive vascular invasion in ~ 60-70% of cases
- Minor component of differentiated thyroid carcinomas may be found

Cytologic Features

- Hypercellular aspirate
- Microfollicles can be identified
- Colloid fragments are usually scant but can be seen
- Neoplastic cells present singly, in trabeculae, or in solid spheres
- Monomorphous, small to intermediate-sized cells with round, hyperchromatic nuclei
- Increased mitoses and necrosis
- Commonly show nuclear features of papillary or follicular carcinoma

ANCILLARY TESTS

Immunohistochemistry

- Positive
  - TTF-1
  - PAX8
  - Cytokeratins
  - Focal p53
  - BCL2
- Ki-67 highlights proliferative index of 10-30%

DIFFERENTIAL DIAGNOSIS

Undifferentiated Thyroid Carcinoma

- Most often arise from preexisting tumor
- Nuclear pleomorphism more prominent
- Often with spindle-shaped and epithelioid cells admixed with pleomorphic or osteoclast-type giant cells
- Usually negative for thyroglobulin and TTF-1
- Ki-67 shows high proliferation index, often > 30%

Papillary Carcinoma, Solid Variant

- Show nuclear features characteristics of PTC, including
  - Nuclear enlargement and irregularities
  - Nuclear grooves and inclusions
  - Nuclear crowding and overlapping
- Ki-67 highlights proliferative index of < 10%

Medullary Thyroid Carcinoma

- Can be associated with syndromes
  - Multiple endocrine neoplasia 2
  - Hereditary medullary thyroid cancer
- Classic neuroendocrine nuclear chromatin pattern
  - Coarsely granular, salt and pepper texture
  - Inconspicuous nucleoli
- Calcitonin, chromogranin, synaptophysin, and CD56 (+)
- Thyroglobulin negative

Carcinoma Showing Thymus-Like Differentiation

- Moderate nuclear pleomorphism
- Presence of Hassall corpuscles
- CD5 and p63 (+)
- TTF-1 (-)
- Thyroglobulin (-)

SELECTED REFERENCES

1. Alwelaie Y et al: Revisiting the cytomorphological features of poorly differentiated thyroid carcinoma: a comparative analysis with indeterminate thyroid fine-needle aspiration samples. J Am Soc Cytopathol. S2213-945(23)00044-3, 2023
2. Ibrahimpasic T et al: Poorly differentiated carcinoma of the thyroid gland: current status and future prospects. Thyroid. 29(3):311-21, 2019
3. Acquaviva G et al: Molecular pathology of thyroid tumours of follicular cells: a review of genetic alterations and their clinicopathological relevance. Histopathology. 72(1):6-31, 2018
4. Manzella L et al: New insights in thyroid cancer and p53 family proteins. Int J Mol Sci. 18(6), 2017
5. Liu R et al: TERT promoter mutations in thyroid cancer. Endocr Relat Cancer. 23(3):R143-55, 2016
6. Penna GC et al: Molecular markers involved in tumorigenesis of thyroid carcinoma: focus on aggressive histotypes. Cytogenet Genome Res. 150(3-4):194-207, 2016
7. Omur O et al: An update on molecular biology of thyroid cancers. Crit Rev Oncol Hematol. 90(3):233-52, 2014
8. Patel KN et al: Poorly differentiated thyroid cancer. Curr Opin Otolaryngol Head Neck Surg. 22(2):121-6, 2014
9. Bell JL et al: Insulin-like growth factor 2 mRNA-binding proteins (IGF2BPs): post-transcriptional drivers of cancer progression? Cell Mol Life Sci. 70(15):2657-75, 2013
10. Hannallah J et al: Comprehensive literature review: recent advances in diagnosing and managing patients with poorly differentiated thyroid carcinoma. Int J Endocrinol. 2013:317487, 2013
11. Huang C et al: Carcinoma showing thymus-like differentiation of the thyroid (CASTLE). Pathol Res Pract. 209(10):662-5, 2013
12. Soares P et al: Genetic alterations in poorly differentiated and undifferentiated thyroid carcinomas. Curr Genomics. 12(8):609-17, 2011
13. Asioli S et al: Poorly differentiated carcinoma of the thyroid: validation of the Turin proposal and analysis of IMP3 expression. Mod Pathol. 23(9):1269-78, 2010

Poorly Differentiated Thyroid Carcinoma

High N:C Ratio

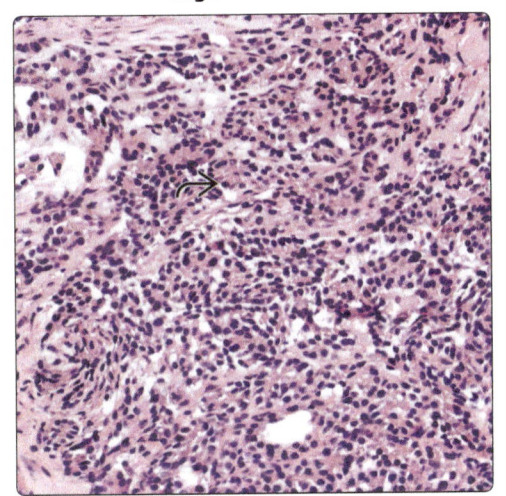

Follicular Variant Transformation

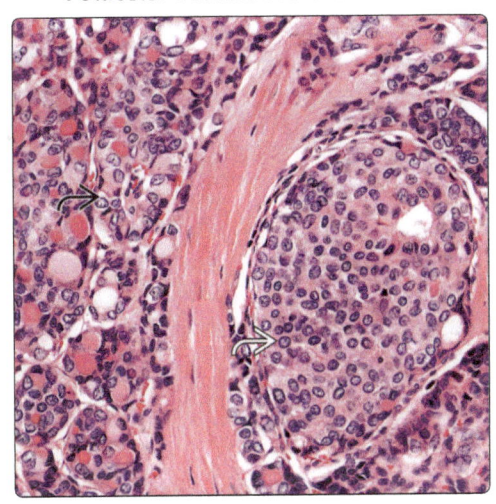

(Left) Neoplastic cells in this case of PDTC are small and monotonous with round nuclei ⇨ and high N:C ratio. (Right) This case of PDTC is raised in the background follicular variant of papillary thyroid carcinoma ⇨. The nuclei in the PDTC show nuclear features characteristic of papillary thyroid carcinoma ⇨.

Vascular Invasion

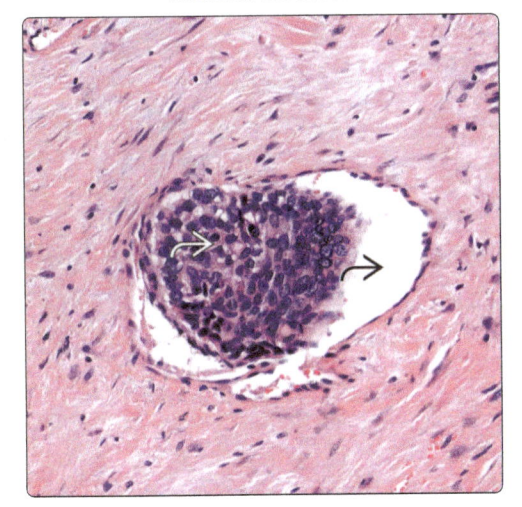

Scant Colloid

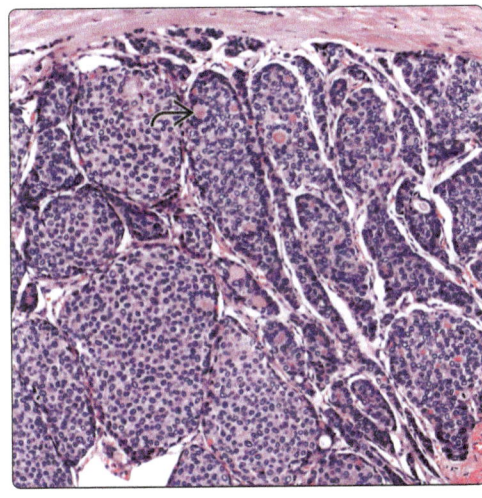

(Left) Cluster of PDTC ⇨ within a vascular space ⇨ is shown. Extensive vascular invasion is typically seen in the majority of PDTC. (Right) PDTC shows scattered microfollicle containing small deposits of colloid ⇨. Scant colloid deposits may be seen in PDTC.

Trabecular Growth Pattern

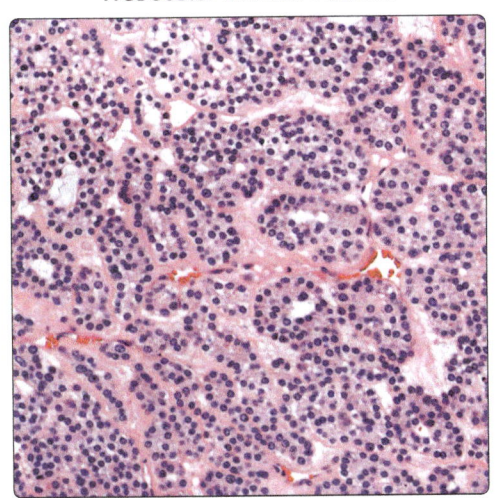

Ki-67 Immunohistochemistry

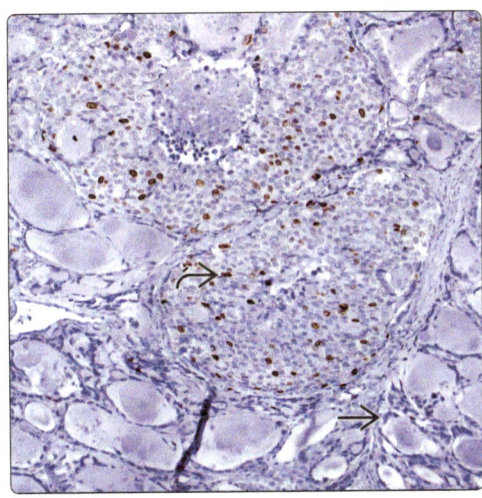

(Left) PDTC shows a trabecular growth pattern, which is defined by cells arranged in cords and small ribbons. (Right) Ki-67 shows a relatively high proliferation index among the neoplastic cells of PDTC ⇨. Notice the absence of Ki-67 expression among background nonneoplastic thyroid follicles ⇨.

Molecular Pathology of Solid Tumors

Anaplastic Thyroid Carcinoma

KEY FACTS

ETIOLOGY/PATHOGENESIS
- History of radiotherapy (external and radioactive iodine)
- Can arise from follicular-derived thyroid neoplasms
  - Papillary carcinoma and variants
  - Follicular carcinoma and variants
  - Poorly differentiated carcinoma

CLINICAL ISSUES
- Rapidly enlarging, hard neck or thyroid mass (weeks to months)
- Accounts for > 60% of thyroid cancer mortality
- More frequent in endemic goiter regions (iodine deficiency)
- Frequent metastases at presentation
- Mortality rate > 90%

MOLECULAR
- *TP53* mutated in up to 80%
- *CTNNB1* mutated in up to 65%
- *NRAS*, *HRAS*, and *KRAS* mutated in up to 60%
- *BRAF* V600E mutation is detected in ~ 40%
- *PIK3CA* alterations in up to 40%
- *TERT* promoter mutations detected in up to 50%

MICROSCOPIC
- Multiple variants: Spindle cell, pleomorphic giant cell, squamoid, osteoclastic, angiomatoid, carcinosarcoma, paucicellular, and rhabdoid

ANCILLARY TESTS
- Usually negative for TTF-1 and thyroglobulin
- Cytokeratin reactivity in majority of cases (up to 80%)
- Positivity for PAX8 also seen in up to 50% of cases
- Strong expression of p53 often present (> 50%)

Pleomorphic/Bizarre Cells

Osteoclast Giant Cells

(Left) Proliferation of malignant cells in anaplastic thyroid carcinoma (ATC) is shown. Note the profoundly pleomorphic/bizarre cells ⇨. (Right) Osteoclastic variant of ATC contains osteoclastic giant cells with bland aggregated nuclei ⇨. These cells are CD68(+) histiocytes.

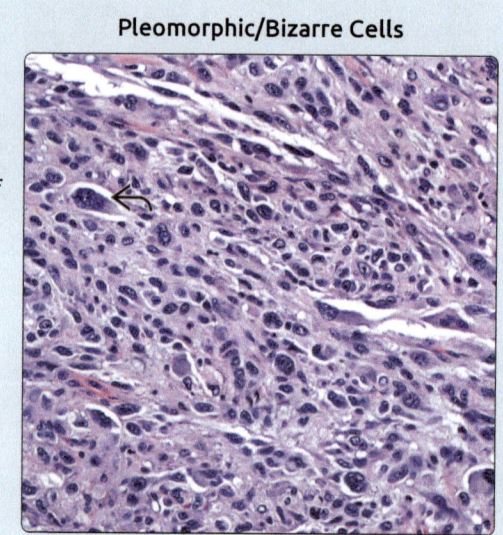

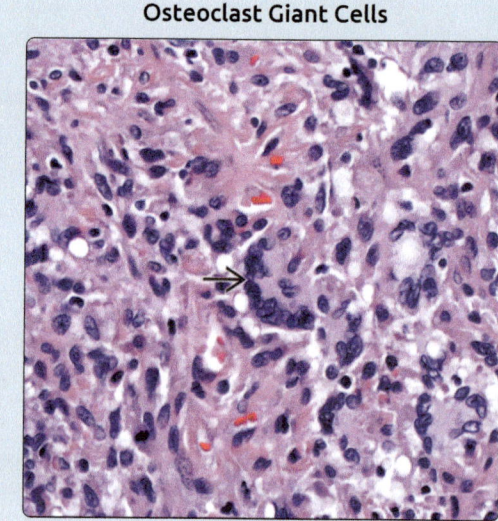

Epithelioid Cells

Squamoid Features

(Left) Aspirate of ATC can be very cellular with numerous large fragments and sheets ⇨ of epithelioid cells. (Right) Tumor cells are largely epithelioid in this case with squamoid features ⇨. Nuclei are hyperchromatic and vary in size and shape ⇨.

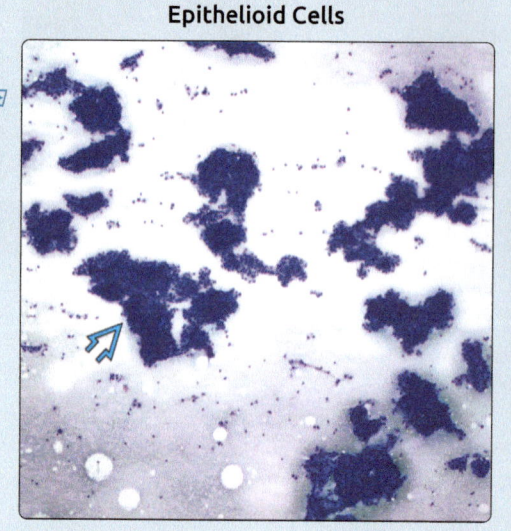

Anaplastic Thyroid Carcinoma

TERMINOLOGY

Abbreviations
- Anaplastic thyroid carcinoma (ATC)

Definitions
- Highly aggressive malignant thyroid follicular cell-derived neoplasm with potential focal features of thyroid follicular differentiation

ETIOLOGY/PATHOGENESIS

Environmental Exposure
- History of radiotherapy (external and radioactive iodine)

Preexisting Conditions
- Follicular cell-derived thyroid neoplasms
  - Papillary carcinoma and variants
  - Follicular carcinoma and variants
  - Poorly differentiated carcinoma

CLINICAL ISSUES

Epidemiology
- Incidence
  - Represents < 5% of all thyroid gland malignancies
  - Accounts for > 60% of thyroid cancer mortality
- Age
  - Majority of patients > 65 years at diagnosis and rarely < 50 years of age
- Sex
  - F:M = 1.5:1

Presentation
- Rapidly enlarging, hard neck or thyroid mass (weeks to months)
- Often with history of prior thyroid disease (benign or malignant)

Treatment
- Conventional therapies
  - Surgical resection, radiation, chemotherapy, and radioiodine
  - Multimodality therapy required

Prognosis
- Rapidly progressive local disease
- Frequent metastases at presentation
- Mortality rate: > 90%

MACROSCOPIC

General Features
- Large (> 5 cm) with normal thyroid tissue effacement and marked extrathyroidal invasion

MOLECULAR

Molecular Alterations
- Overview
  - Early driver events: *RAS* and *BRAF* p.V600E mutations
  - Late driver events: *TP53* and *TERT* promoter mutations
  - ATC gains additional mutations, such as frequent alterations in PIK3CA-PTEN-AKT-mTOR pathway, SWI-SNF complex, histomethyltransferases, and mismatch repair genes
- *BRAF*
  - Encodes BRAF protein
    - Serine-threonine tyrosine kinase
    - Regulator of cell division, differentiation, cell migration, and apoptosis
  - Somatic point mutations reported in ~ 30% of ATC
  - *BRAF* V600E (c.1799T>A; p.V600E) accounts for majority of *BRAF* mutations
    - Results in constitutive activation of MAPK signaling pathway
  - Clinical relevance
    - *BRAF* V600E mutation appears to predict sensitivity to BRAF inhibitors
    - BRAF inhibitors should be considered in *BRAF*-mutated ATC cases
    - Dramatic response to BRAF inhibitor reported in case of ATC with complete resolution of lung metastases
- *HRAS*, *KRAS*, and *NRAS*
  - Encode proteins involved in activation of PI3K/AKT/mTOR signaling pathways
    - Regulator of cell division, cell differentiation, and apoptosis
  - Mutations in *HRAS*, *KRAS*, and *NRAS*
    - Detected in ~ 30% of ATC
    - Most frequent mutations in *HRAS* and *NRAS* involve codon 61 and include *NRAS* Q61R mutation
    - Leads to uncontrolled growth and cell division
  - Clinical relevance
    - Positive predictive value for malignancy if detected in FNA biopsy samples from thyroid nodules
- *TP53*
  - Tumor suppressor gene and regulator of cell division
  - Somatic mutations reported in ~ 50% of ATC
    - Inactivating mutations
- *TERT*
  - Encodes protein component with reverse transcriptase activity
    - Maintains telomere end by addition of telomere repeat TTAGGG
  - *TERT* mutations
    - Promoter mutations including C228T and C250T
    - Present in ~ 50% of ATC
    - Abnormally active telomerase results in immortalization of cells
- *CTNNB1*
  - Encodes β-catenin
    - Critical for establishment and maintenance of epithelial layers
    - Involved in WNT signaling pathway
  - Point mutations in exon 3 reported in up to 65% of ATC
    - Gain-of-function mutations
    - Leads to constitutive activation of β-catenin
    - Excess β-catenin promotes unchecked growth and division of cells
- *PIK3CA*

Anaplastic Thyroid Carcinoma

- o Encodes p110 kDa catalytic subunit of phosphatidylinositol 3-kinase (PI3K)
  - – Activates PI3K/AKT/mTOR pathway to regulate cell cycle progression, adhesion, and migration
- o *PIK3CA* mutations
  - – Somatic mutations occur in ~ 10-20% of ATC
- o *PIK3CA* copy gain/amplification
  - – Amplification of *PIK3CA* genomic locus is found in ~ 40% of ATC
  - – Gain-of-function mutations leads to increased activity in *PIK3CA*
- o Clinical relevance
  - – Multiple PIK3CA inhibitors available and have shown response in clinical trials
- *PTEN* promoter region methylation
  - o Commonly associated with ATC
  - o Silence *PTEN* normal activity
    - – Results in activation of PI3K/AKT loop
  - o Frequently associated with mutations in *BRAF* and *PIK3CA* in thyroid tumors
- Deregulation of microRNAs in ATC
  - o Upregulated expression of several microRNAs (miRs) reported in ATC cell lines and tumors, including
    - – miR-17-3p, miR-17-5p, miR18a, miR19a, miR19b, miR20a, and miR92-1
  - o Downregulated expression of several miRNAs in ATC, including
    - – MiR-26a, miR30d, miR125b
  - o miRNA testing may prove useful for early detection or prognostic biomarkers

MICROSCOPIC

Histologic Features

- Multiple histologic variants: Spindle cell, pleomorphic giant cell, squamoid, osteoclastic, angiomatoid, carcinosarcoma, paucicellular, and rhabdoid
- Pure squamous cell carcinoma in thyroid, without histomorphologic and immunophenotypic expression of thyroid follicle cells, is considered ATC with squamous cell carcinoma phenotype
- Extensive invasive growth with desmoplastic (reactive) stroma
- Significant necrosis, hemorrhage, and degeneration
- Marked pleomorphism
- Variety of patterns: Sheet-like, storiform, fascicular, angiomatoid, and meningothelial
- Increased mitotic activity, including atypical forms

Cytologic Features

- Hypercellular aspirate of single cells, clusters, &/or sheets
- Necrotic background with acute inflammatory infiltrate
- Marked nuclear pleomorphism with bizarre nuclei
- Malignant squamous cells
- Spindle cells frequently present

ANCILLARY TESTS

Immunohistochemistry

- Cytokeratin reactivity in majority of cases (up to 80%)
- Positivity for PAX8 also seen in ~ 50% of cases
- Usually negative for TTF-1 and thyroglobulin
- Strong expression of p53 is often present (> 50%)

Flow Cytometry

- Nearly 100% are aneuploid

DIFFERENTIAL DIAGNOSIS

Metastases

- Clinical and radiographic impression critical in evaluation and separation from primary tumor
- Pertinent IHC panel can be useful

Primary Sarcomas

- Growth pattern may overlap with ATC
- Pertinent immunohistochemical panel be helpful (e.g., desmin, CD34, S100)

Melanoma

- Immunoreactivity to S100, HMB-45, and MART-1 is useful

Diffuse Large B-Cell Lymphoma

- Immunoreactivity to hematopoietic markers (e.g., CD20, CD45)

Other Thyroid Carcinomas

- Poorly differentiated carcinoma
  - o No pronounced pleomorphism
  - o Preserved TTF-1 expression
- Medullary thyroid carcinoma
  - o Immunoreactive to calcitonin, CEA, and neuroendocrine markers
- Spindle epithelial tumor with thymus-like elements (SETTLE)
  - o Predominantly bland-appearing spindle cells in lobules separated by thin, fibrous septa
  - o Most cases tend to be biphasic with glandular/acinar formation
- Intrathyroid thymic carcinoma
  - o No significant atypia with squamoid appearance
  - o Neoplastic cells CD5 and CD117 (+)

SELECTED REFERENCES

1. Deeken-Draisey A et al: Anaplastic thyroid carcinoma: an epidemiologic, histologic, immunohistochemical and molecular single institution study. Hum Pathol. 82:140-8, 2018
2. Giordano TJ: Genomic hallmarks of thyroid neoplasia. Annu Rev Pathol. 13:141-62, 2018
3. Ahn S et al: Comprehensive screening for PD-L1 expression in thyroid cancer. Endocr Relat Cancer. 24(2):97-106, 2017
4. Bonhomme B et al: Molecular pathology of anaplastic thyroid carcinomas: a retrospective study of 144 cases. Thyroid. 27(5):682-92, 2017
5. Chintakuntlawar AV et al: Expression of PD-1 and PD-L1 in anaplastic thyroid cancer patients treated with multimodal therapy: results from a retrospective study. J Clin Endocrinol Metab. 102(6):1943-50, 2017
6. Oishi N et al: Molecular alterations of coexisting thyroid papillary carcinoma and anaplastic carcinoma: identification of TERT mutation as an independent risk factor for transformation. Mod Pathol. 30(11):1527-37, 2017
7. Xu B et al: Genomic landscape of poorly differentiated and anaplastic thyroid carcinoma. Endocr Pathol. 27(3):205-12, 2016

Anaplastic Thyroid Carcinoma

Spindle Cell Variant

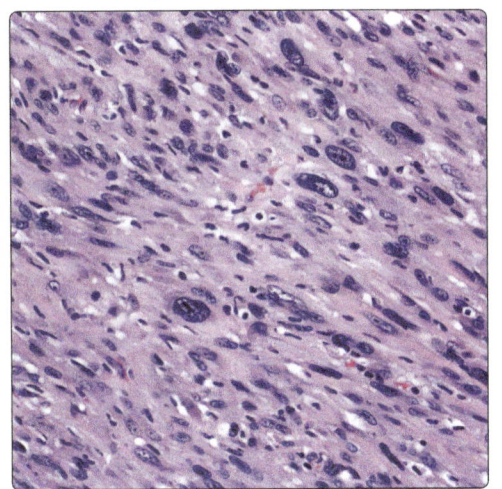

Squamous Cell Carcinoma Variant

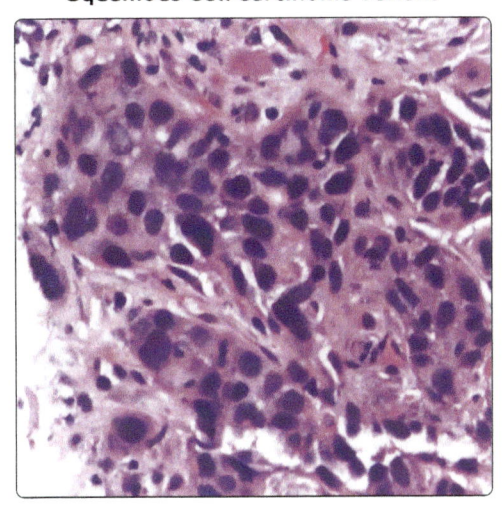

(Left) Spindle cell variant is the most common variant of ATC. Pleomorphic malignant cells are present in fascicles in this subtype of ATC resembling high-grade sarcoma. (Right) ATC shows a squamous cell carcinoma phenotype. The neoplastic cells are positive for p40 but negative for TTF-1 and PAX8. However, this must be differentiated from secondary involvement by squamous cell carcinoma from another site.

ATC Arising From Papillary Thyroid Carcinoma

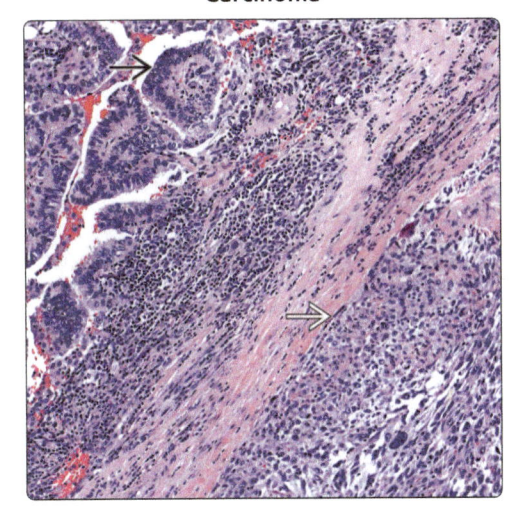

Osteoclastic Variant

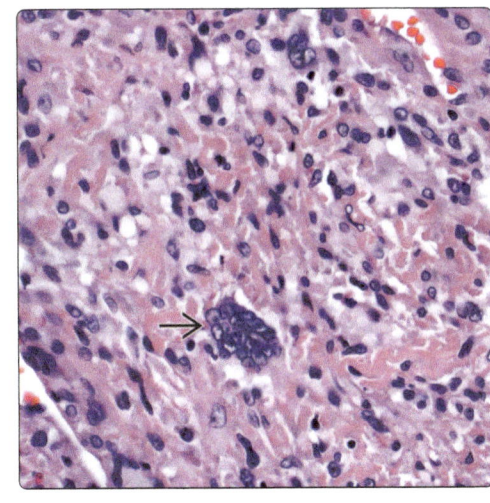

(Left) ATC ➡ arising from an adjacent, preexisting papillary thyroid carcinoma ➡ is shown. (Right) Osteoclastic variant of ATC is shown. The multinucleated cells ➡ are CD68(+), whereas the malignant cells are CD68(-).

Pleomorphic Giant Cell Variant

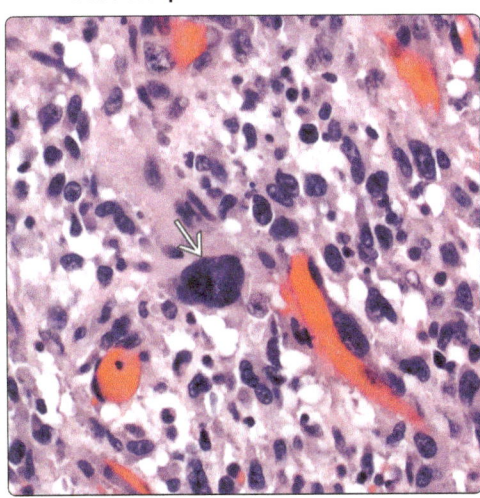

Rhabdoid Variant

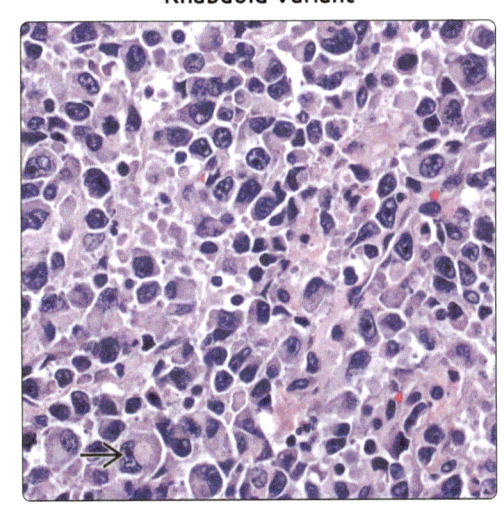

(Left) Pleomorphic giant cell variant is the 2nd most common variant of ATC. Numerous pleomorphic/bizarre and multinucleated cells ➡ are shown. In contrast to the osteoclastic variant, the multinucleated cells are negative for CD68. (Right) Rhabdoid variant of ATC is shown. The malignant cells have dense hyaline-type cytoplasm and eccentric nuclei ➡.

Medullary Thyroid Carcinoma

KEY FACTS

TERMINOLOGY
- Malignant thyroid tumor composed of parafollicular neural crest-derived C cells

ETIOLOGY/PATHOGENESIS
- ~ 20-30% of medullary thyroid carcinoma (MTC) cases are hereditary and associated with *RET* mutations
- Associated with MEN2 syndromes
- Neoplastic C-cell hyperplasia is precursor lesion in hereditary MTC

CLINICAL ISSUES
- 5-10% of all thyroid malignancies; most cases sporadic (70-80%)
- Often single "cold" thyroid nodule
- Increased serum calcitonin and CEA levels
- Germline *RET* mutation analysis indicated in all MTC patients, C-cell hyperplasia, clinical features of MEN2 syndrome, or 1st-degree relative with MEN2

MOLECULAR
- Hereditary MTC
  - Exclusive association with *RET* mutations
  - In MEN type 2A, mutations most commonly seen in exons 10 and 11
  - In MEN type 2B, mutation in exon 16 (M918T) is most common
- Sporadic MTC
  - Somatic *RET* mutations present in ~ 50% of cases
  - *HRAS* and *KRAS* mutations may also be present
  - *RAS* mutations are mutually exclusive with *RET*

MICROSCOPIC
- Eccentric nuclei with finely granular chromatin
- Stromal amyloid can be seen in up to 80% of cases

ANCILLARY TESTS
- Positive for calcitonin and CEA

Gross Appearance

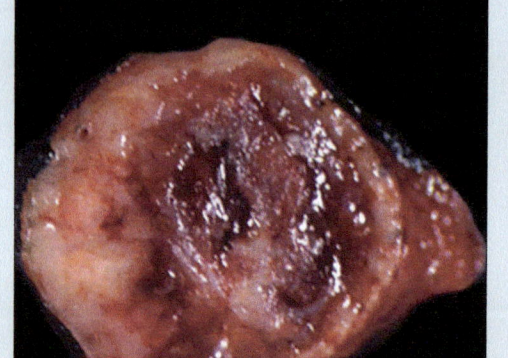

Trabecular Growth Pattern

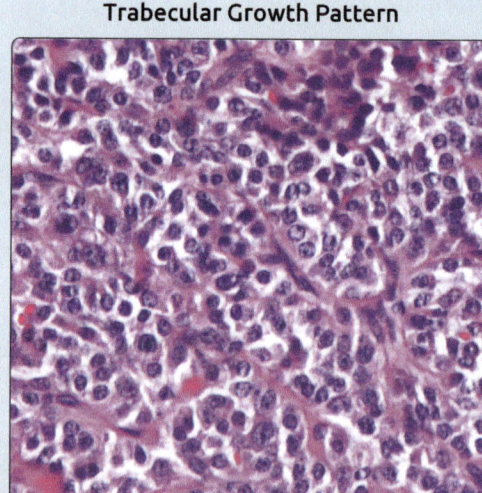

(Left) *Gross cut surface of thyroid lobe shows a well-circumscribed, white-gray-yellow thyroid tumor. Medullary thyroid carcinoma (MTC) is usually firm and gritty. Areas of hemorrhage are present. (From DP: Endocrine.)* (Right) *MTC shows a trabecular growth pattern. Individual cells are relatively round with coarsely clumped chromatin nuclear pattern and small nucleoli. Mitotic activity is low.*

Solid Growth Pattern

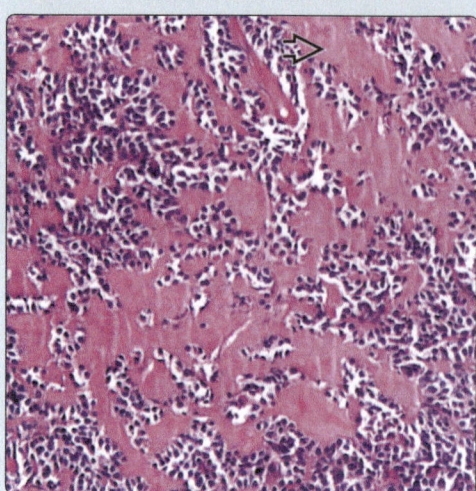

RET M918T Mutation

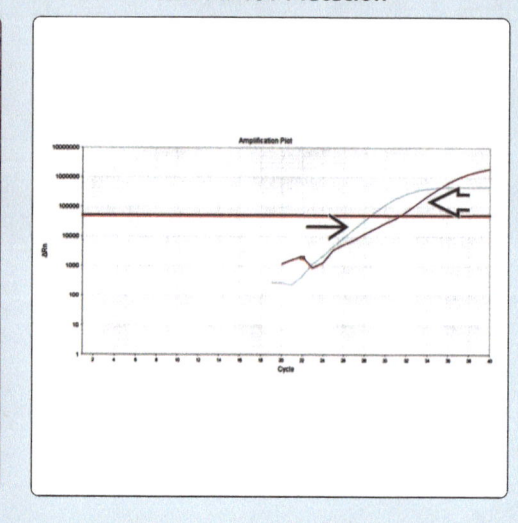

(Left) *MTC from a patient who presented with bilateral thyroid nodules is shown. A solid growth pattern with a nest of neuroendocrine cells and associated dense, amorphous stroma compatible with amyloid ⇨ is present.* (Right) *Real-time PCR shows an M918T mutation ⇨ in the RET gene, confirming the diagnosis of multiple endocrine neoplasia (MEN) type 2B (MEN2b) syndrome. Blue color amplification curve represents positive control ⇨. (Courtesy G. Potikyan, PhD.)*

Medullary Thyroid Carcinoma

TERMINOLOGY

Abbreviations
- Medullary thyroid carcinoma (MTC)

Definitions
- Malignant neoplasm of thyroid composed of neural crest-derived parafollicular C cells

ETIOLOGY/PATHOGENESIS

Syndromic Association
- ~ 20-30% of MTC cases are hereditary
- Exclusively associated with germline *RET* mutations
- Clinical syndromes
  - Multiple endocrine neoplasia (MEN) type 2A (MEN2a)
    - 95% of cases of MEN2
    - 4 variants
      - Classic MEN2a
      - MEN2a with cutaneous lichen amyloidosis (CLA)
      - MEN2a with Hirschsprung disease (HD)
      - Hereditary isolated MTC (former familial MTC)
    - Classic form associated with MTC (95%), pheochromocytoma (50%), and parathyroid disease (20-30%)
    - MTC usually presents at early age (20-30 years)
  - MEN type 2B (MEN2b)
    - ~ 5% of cases of MEN2
    - All patients with MEN2b develop aggressive form of MTC at very young age (< 10 years)
    - Pheochromocytomas occur in ~ 50% of cases, often bilateral
    - Additionally, mucosal neuromas, gastrointestinal ganglioneuromatosis (40%), and marfanoid habitus (75%) can also be seen
- Hereditary forms are autosomal dominant with high penetrance
- Neoplastic C-cell hyperplasia
  - Precursor lesion in hereditary MTC cases
  - Well-defined clusters of cells (usually > 50) with atypia
  - Almost always found in vicinity of MTC

Sporadic Medullary Thyroid Carcinoma
- Somatic *RET* mutations in ~ 25-60% of cases
- Usually occur in 5th-6th decades
- Lack other associated MEN features and family history
- Mainly unifocal presentation without coexisting C-cell hyperplasia

CLINICAL ISSUES

Epidemiology
- Relatively rare; accounts for 2% of thyroid malignancies
- Most common in female patients
- Can be hereditary (25%) or sporadic (75%)
- Affects mainly adults
  - Mean age: ~ 45 years (sporadic) and ~ 35 years (hereditary)
  - MTC in MEN2b usually develops at very early age (< 5 years)

Presentation
- Often presents as painless, "cold" thyroid nodule
- Symptoms of carcinoid &/or Cushing syndromes may be present
- Nonthyroid findings
  - Mucosal neuromas, parathyroid tumors, hypertension
- Regional and distant metastasis can be seen at diagnosis
  - Up to 50% have nodal metastasis
  - Up to 20% present with distant metastasis
  - More common with sporadic cases and those associated with MEN2b

Laboratory Tests
- Screening for calcitonin and CEA levels are recommended for known familial cases
- Germline *RET* mutation analysis indicated in all individuals with
  - Diagnosis of MTC or primary C-cell hyperplasia
  - Clinical features of MEN2
  - Family history of MEN2/FMTC in 1st-degree relative
    - De novo mutations common in MEN2b
    - 5-10% of MEN2a/FMTC present with new mutations

Treatment
- Surgery is primary treatment
  - Total thyroidectomy and lymph node dissection
- Poor response to chemotherapy, radioactive iodine, and external radiation therapy
- Targeted tyrosine kinase inhibitors (TKIs) have been approved for advanced disease
  - Vandetanib and cabozantinib used in numerous clinical trials
- Prophylactic surgery
  - Age at prophylactic surgery depends on mutation risk level

Prognosis
- Considerable variability
- Long-term survival: ~ 90% for patients with localized disease, 70-80% with regional metastasis, and 40-50% with distant metastasis
- Important prognostic factors include tumor stage and age at presentation

MACROSCOPIC

General Features
- Often relatively well circumscribed
- Usually solid, firm, and nonencapsulated
- Majority arise in midportion or upper 1/2 of gland
  - Greater concentration of C cells
- Sporadic cases tend to present as solitary thyroid mass
- Hereditary cases often have multicentric and bilateral disease

MOLECULAR

Molecular Genetics
- *RET*
  - *RET* protooncogene located at 10q11.21; composed of 21 exons
  - Encodes transmembrane receptor tyrosine kinase

Medullary Thyroid Carcinoma

- o Important role in development of parathyroids, urogenital system, and neural crest
- RET protein structure
  - o Extracellular domain
  - o Transmembrane domain
  - o Intracellular domain (2 tyrosine kinase domains: TK1 and TK2)
  - o Involved in activation of multiple signaling pathways, including RAS/RAF/MAP kinase, PI3K/AKT, and STAT3
- Germline mutations in *RET*
  - o Mutations lead to constitutive activation of kinase signaling pathway
  - o Important genotype-phenotype correlations based on location of mutation
  - o *RET* mutations in MEN2a commonly occur in extracellular domain, particularly in codons 609, 611, 618, and 620 of exon 10 and codon 634 of exon 11
    - Codon 634 mutations most commonly seen in MEN2a
    - Associated with earliest onset of MTC and highest risk of pheochromocytoma and hyperparathyroidism
    - CLA almost exclusively seen with codon 634 mutations
  - o *RET* mutations in MEN2b consist of single point mutation in exon 16 (M918T) in ~ 95% of cases
    - Results in constitutive activation of TK2 domain
    - Often associated with very early onset of disease (< 1 year) and aggressive tumors
    - ~ 2-3% of cases harbor mutation in exon 15 (A883F), often associated with older age and less aggressive tumors
  - o *RET* mutations in hereditary isolated MTC
    - ~ 40 mutations have been described, mainly in exons 5, 8, 10, 11, and 13-16, corresponding to cysteine-rich domain and TK1
    - Mutations outside cysteine-rich domain (exons 13-16) are associated with latest onset of disease
- Gene mutations in sporadic MTC
  - o *RET* mutations
    - Somatic mutations are detected in ~ 50% of cases
    - Most common mutation is in exon 16 (M918T)
    - Present in ~ 75-95% of cases and associated with more aggressive disease
    - Additional mutations in exons 10, 11, 15, and 16 have been reported
  - o *KRAS*, *HRAS*, and *NRAS* mutations
    - Mutations in exons 2-4 involving *HRAS* and *KRAS* have been identified in 10-45% of *RET* wildtype cases
    - *NRAS* mutations are very rare
    - *RET* and *HRAS*/*KRAS* mutations appear to be mutually exclusive

Recommended Testing Strategies

- Most laboratories perform selective exon sequencing
- American Thyroid Association recommendations
  - o Mutational analysis of MEN2-specific *RET* exons either in single or multitiered approach
    - Recommended testing for exon 10 (codons 609, 611, 618, and 620), exon 11 (codons 630 and 634), and exons 8, 13, 14, 15, and 16
    - If negative or when clinical criteria for MEN2 is met, sequencing of entire coding region of *RET* is recommended
  - o For MEN2b, analysis should include mutational analysis of exons 15 (A883F) and 16 (M918T) of *RET*
    - If negative, sequencing of entire coding region of *RET* is recommended

MICROSCOPIC

Histologic Features

- Tumor cells are round to polygonal with medium-sized nucleus and ample amphophilic cytoplasm
- Nuclear chromatin is finely granular and disperse (salt and pepper chromatin)
- Stromal amyloid can be seen in 50-90% of cases
- Coarse calcifications and rare psammoma bodies may be present
- Numerous histologic variants have been described
  - o Spindle cell, papillary, follicular, clear cell, oncocytic, paraganglioma-like, melanotic, and squamous
- Grading system (WHO 2022, 5th edition)
  - o High-grade (at least 1 of 3)
    - Mitotic count ≥ 5 per 2 mm²
    - Ki-67 proliferation index ≥ 5%
    - Tumor necrosis

Cytologic Features

- Singly dispersed or loosely cohesive cells with eccentric nuclei ("plasmacytoid")
- Nuclear grooves and cytoplasmic pseudoinclusions can be seen
- Binucleated or multinucleated cells may be present
- Amyloid material can be identified

Primary C-Cell Hyperplasia

- Considered neoplastic process and precursor lesion for MTC
- Nodular aggregates with > 50 C cells/LPF (100x) with atypia
- Commonly associated with hereditary tumors but can be seen in sporadic cases as well

ANCILLARY TESTS

Histochemistry

- Congo red
  - o Reactivity: Positive
  - o Staining pattern: Amyloid shows light green birefringence with polarization

Immunohistochemistry

- Usually positive for calcitonin, calcitonin gene-related peptide (CGRP), chromogranin, synaptophysin, CEA, and TTF-1
- Thyroglobulin is usually negative

DIFFERENTIAL DIAGNOSIS

Follicular Carcinoma

- Lacks amyloid deposits
- Thyroglobulin positive
- Calcitonin negative

Medullary Thyroid Carcinoma

Genotype-Phenotype Correlation and ATA Risk Levels for Aggressive Medullary Thyroid Carcinoma

ATA Risk Level (MTC Aggressiveness)	RET Mutations	Associated Syndrome
Moderate risk (MOD)	Mutations other than M918T, C634, and A883F (continually updated list at www.arup.utah.edu/database/MEN2/MEN2_welcome.php)	MEN2a/FMTC
High risk (H)	**Exon 11**: C634R/G/F/S/W/Y; **exon 15**: A883F	MEN2a/FMTC
Highest risk (HST)	**Exon 16**: M918T	MEN2b

ATA = American Thyroid Association; MTC = medullary thyroid carcinoma; FMTC = familial MTC; MEN2a = multiple endocrine neoplasia type 2A; MEN2b = multiple endocrine neoplasia type 2B.

ATA Recommendations For Management Based on Risk Categories

ATA Risk Level	Recommendation
Moderate risk (MOD)	Physical examination, US of neck, and measurement of serum Ctn levels beginning ~ 5 years of age; long-term screening at every 6-month or annual evaluations
High risk (H)	Thyroidectomy performed at ≤ 5 years of age based on elevated Ctn levels
Highest risk (HST)	Thyroidectomy within 1st year of life

ASAP = as soon as possible; ATA = American Thyroid Association; Ctn = calcitonin.

Distinguishing Features Between Hereditary and Sporadic Medullary Thyroid Carcinoma

Features	Hereditary Medullary Thyroid Carcinoma	Sporadic Medullary Thyroid Carcinoma
Age at presentation	MEN2a: ~ 20-30 years (variable based on RET mutation); FMTC: ~ 50 years (variable based on RET mutation); MEN2b: < 1 year	Usually 50-60 years
Tumor characteristics	Multicentric and bilateral	Solitary mass, unilateral
C-cell hyperplasia	Neoplastic type; frequent (~ 90%)	Reactive; variable (10-40%)
Lymph node metastasis	May be present at diagnosis (variable based of RET mutation)	Usually present at diagnosis
Most common molecular alterations	Germline RET mutations: MEN2a: Exon 11 (codon 634); MEN2b: Exon 16 (M918T); FMTC: Exons 10, 11, 13-16	Somatic RET mutations (~ 50%): M918T (75-95%); HRAS and KRAS mutations (10-45%) in RET wildtype cases

FMTC = familial medullary thyroid carcinoma; MEN2a = multiple endocrine neoplasia type 2A; MEN2b = multiple endocrine neoplasia type 2B.

Papillary Carcinoma
- Nuclear features, including longitudinal nuclear grooves, are characteristic but can also be seen in MTC
- Thyroglobulin positive
- Calcitonin negative
- BRAF V600E mutation detected in ~ 45% of cases

Paraganglioma
- Rare in thyroid
- Negative for calcitonin; zellballen structures with S100(+) sustentacular cells

Extraosseous Plasmacytoma
- Distinct immunohistochemical profile, including CD138 expression and κ- or λ-light chain restriction

Metastatic Neuroendocrine Tumors
- Salt and pepper chromatin pattern
- Can be positive for calcitonin and CEA in rare cases

Amyloid Goiter
- Involves thyroid gland diffusely
- May infiltrate fat
- Congo red stain is positive; calcitonin negative

SELECTED REFERENCES
1. Xu B et al: International medullary thyroid carcinoma grading system: a validated grading system for medullary thyroid carcinoma. J Clin Oncol. 40(1):96-104, 2022
2. Barletta JA et al: Genomics and epigenomics of medullary thyroid carcinoma: from sporadic disease to familial manifestations. Endocr Pathol. 32(1):35-43, 2021
3. Accardo G et al: Genetics of medullary thyroid cancer: an overview. Int J Surg. 41 Suppl 1:S2-6, 2017
4. Chernock RD et al: Molecular pathology of hereditary and sporadic medullary thyroid carcinomas. Am J Clin Pathol. 143(6):768-77, 2015
5. Wells SA Jr et al: Revised American Thyroid Association guidelines for the management of medullary thyroid carcinoma. Thyroid. 25(6):567-610, 2015

Medullary Thyroid Carcinoma

Bilateral Tumor Nodules

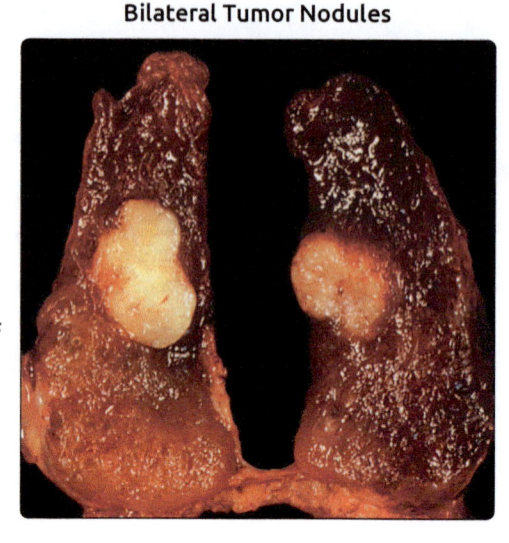

Encapsulated Nodule

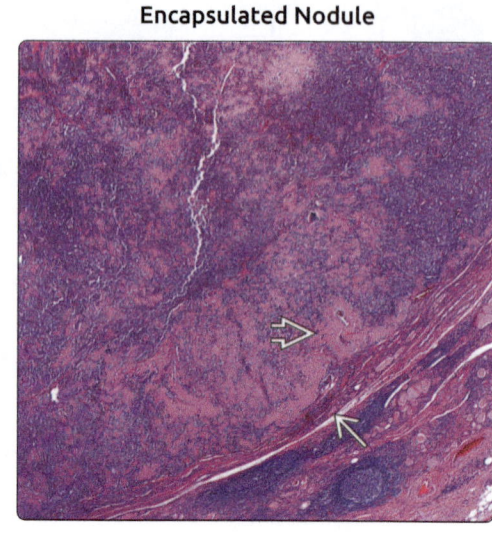

(Left) *Gross photograph of bilateral MTC from a patient with MEN type 2A (MEN2a) shows the characteristic well-circumscribed tumor nodules. MEN-associated tumors are usually bilateral and multifocal. (From DP: Familial Cancer Syndromes.)* (Right) *MTC shows a well-circumscribed, encapsulated nodule ⇨ composed of sheets of medium-sized monotonous cells and associated amyloid deposits ⇨.*

Amyloid Spheres

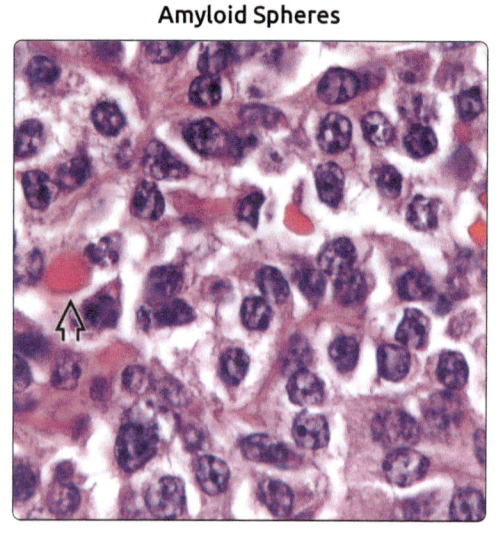

Calcitonin Immunohistochemistry

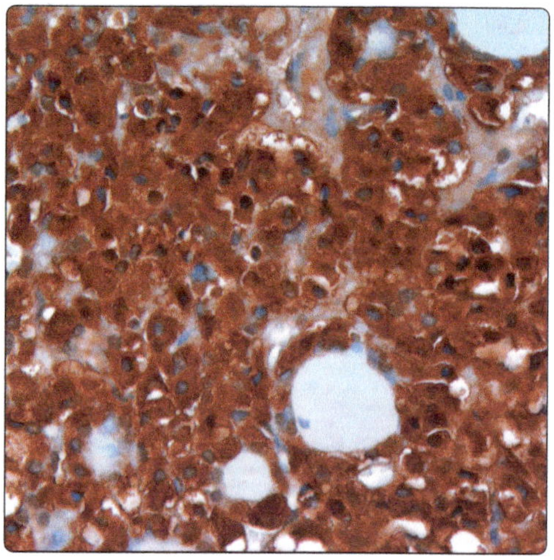

(Left) *MTC shows a solid proliferation of predominantly round cells with granular amphophilic cytoplasm and mid-sized nuclei. Amyloid spheres are also appreciated ⇨.* (Right) *Calcitonin shows strong cytoplasmic expression by neoplastic cells, characteristic of MTC.*

Amyloid Deposits

Congo Red Stain

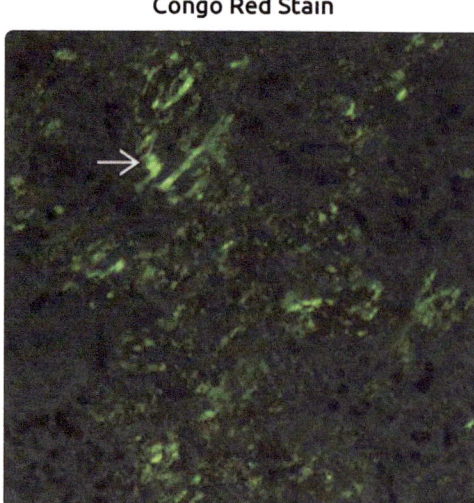

(Left) *Extensive deposition of dense amorphous material is suggestive of amyloid. Although not essential for the diagnosis of MTC, variable amounts of amyloid deposits are commonly seen in MTC.* (Right) *Congo red-stained section under polarized light shows characteristic apple green birefringence ⇨, confirming amyloid deposition.*

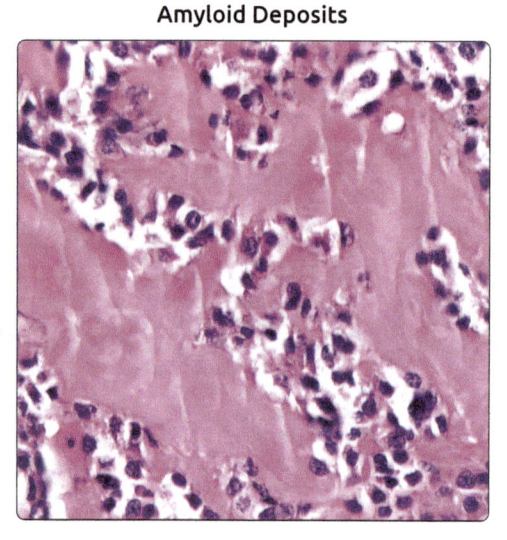

Medullary Thyroid Carcinoma

Absent Colloid

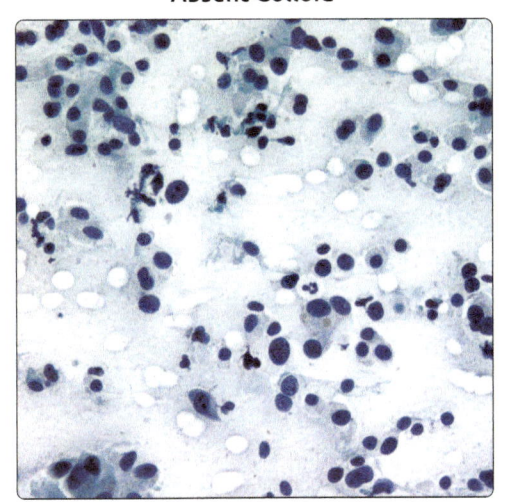

Classic Cytology

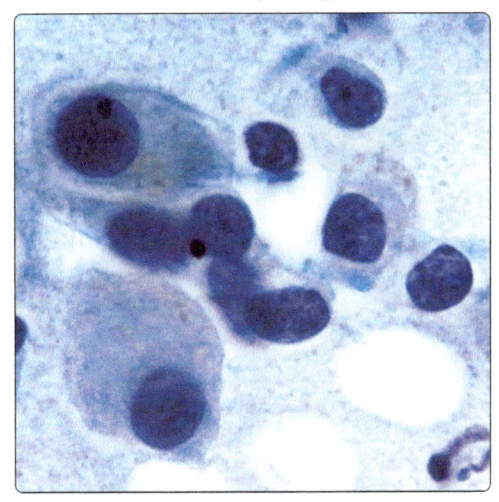

(Left) *FNA shows a characteristic cellular specimen with clusters of loosely cohesive, round to oval cells of variable sizes with eccentrically located nuclei of MTC cells. Colloid is absent.* (Right) *Classic cytology of MTC shows eccentric, round nuclei resembling "plasmacytoid cells" and ample granular cytoplasm. The chromatin has a salt and pepper appearance, and nucleoli are inconspicuous.*

Amyloid Deposits

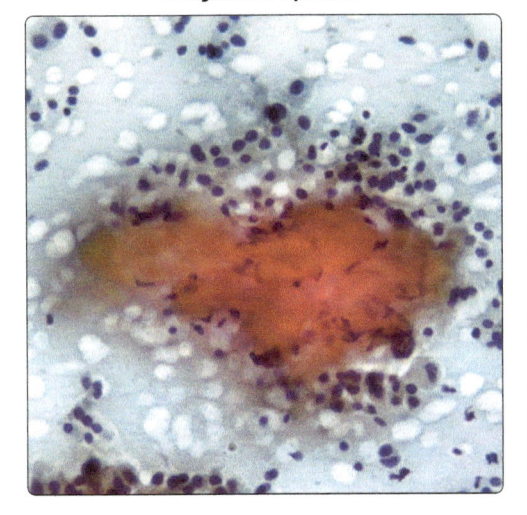

Calcitonin Immunohistochemistry

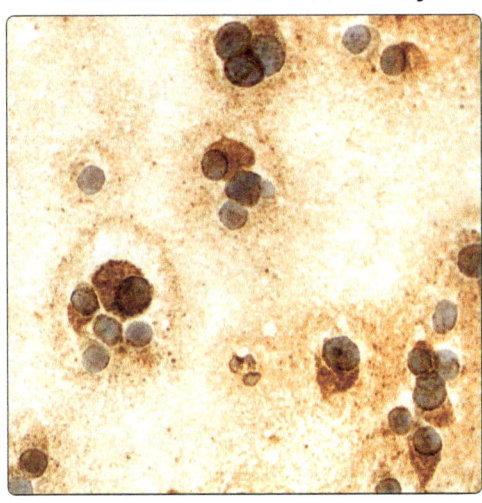

(Left) *FNA shows deposits of amorphous material most consistent with amyloid in a patient with MTC. The background is cellular and loosely cohesive.* (Right) *Calcitonin shows coarse granular cytoplasmic staining of FNA. The MTC cells show the characteristic salt and pepper, neuroendocrine-type nuclear chromatin. (From DP: Familial Cancer Syndromes.)*

C-Cell Hyperplasia

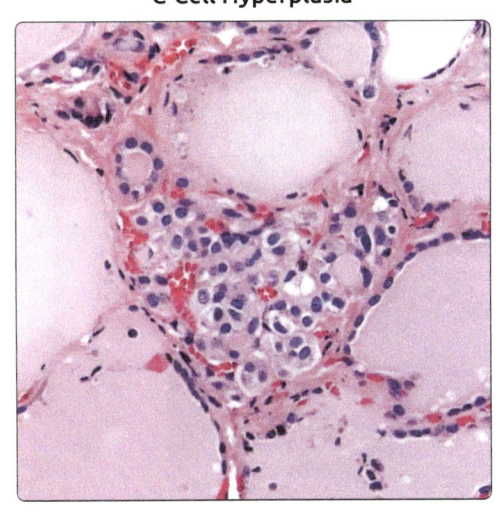

C-Cell Hyperplasia

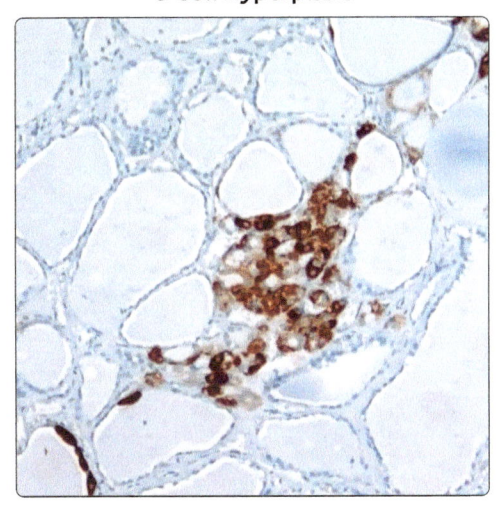

(Left) *As opposed to sporadic cases, hereditary MTC is frequently accompanied by C-cell hyperplasia. In many cases, the C-cell hyperplasia can be easily identified on H&E-stained sections.* (Right) *Calcitonin highlights collections of C cells. In MEN2 patients, foci of C-cell hyperplasia are typically present in the vicinity of the main tumor as well as in the contralateral thyroid lobe.*

Molecular Pathology of Solid Tumors

559

Adenocarcinoma, Lung

KEY FACTS

TERMINOLOGY
- Malignant epithelial neoplasm with glandular differentiation

MACROSCOPIC
- Peripheral or central tumors (0.6 cm to > 10 cm)

MOLECULAR
- *KRAS* mutations (prevalence: 25-35%)
- *EGFR* mutations (prevalence: 10-35%)
- *ALK* rearrangements (prevalence: 4-7%)
- *ROS1* fusions (prevalence: 1-2%)
- *BRAF* mutations (prevalence: 1-4%)
- High tumor mutation burden and PD-L1 expression predict response to immune checkpoint inhibitor (ICI) therapy

MICROSCOPIC
- Acinar, solid, and papillary growth patterns

ANCILLARY TESTS
- Immunohistochemistry
  - TTF-1 and napsin (+); p63 and p40 (-)
- Molecular/biomarkers
  - NCCN guidelines version 5.2022
    - Molecular and biomarker targets for analysis
      - *EGFR*, *ALK*, *ROS1*, *BRAF*, *KRAS*, *MET*, *RET*, *NTRK1/NTRK2/NTRK3*
      - PD-L1 by immunohistochemistry
  - CAP/IASLC/AMP 2017 guideline statement
    - Must test for *EGFR*, *ALK*, and *ROS1* in all cases
    - Consider testing for *BRAF*, *KRAS*, *ERBB2* (HER2), *MET*, and *RET*

TOP DIFFERENTIAL DIAGNOSES
- Adenocarcinoma from extrathoracic origin
- Atypical adenomatous hyperplasia
- Adenoid cystic carcinoma
- Papillary carcinoma of thyroid origin

Signaling Pathways in Lung Adenocarcinoma

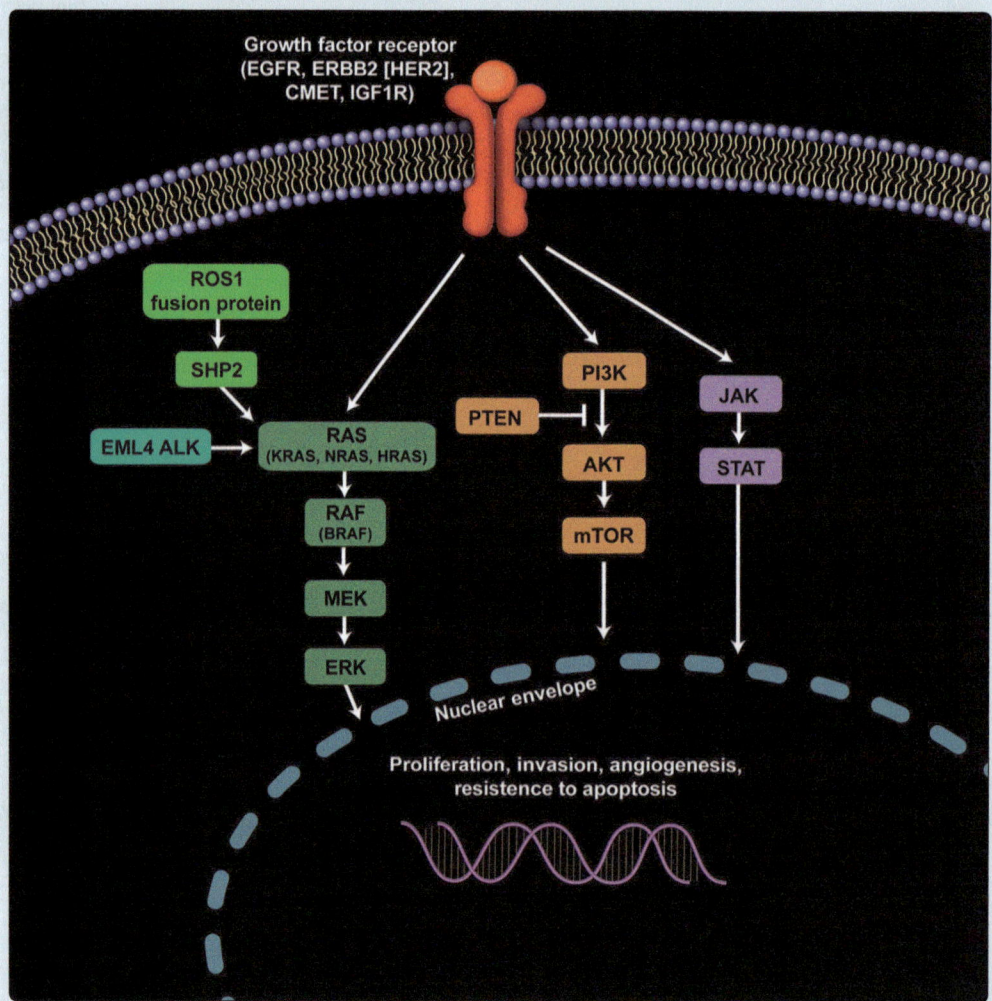

Some of the common growth factor receptors and downstream signaling pathways that become dysregulated in lung adenocarcinoma are illustrated in this simplified graphic. Gene amplification &/or mutation events often lead to increased signaling activity and activation of downstream effectors, resulting in uncontrolled cell proliferation, tumor invasion, angiogenesis, and resistance to normal apoptotic signals. Gene mutations are largely mutually exclusive events, though it is not uncommon for tumors to acquire additional gene mutations &/or gene amplifications in response to the evolutionary pressure exerted while undergoing single-agent targeted therapy.

Adenocarcinoma, Lung

TERMINOLOGY

Definitions
- Malignant epithelial neoplasm with glandular differentiation

ETIOLOGY/PATHOGENESIS

Environmental Exposure
- Close association with tobacco use

Etiology
- Likely originates from endobronchial glands

CLINICAL ISSUES

Epidemiology
- Incidence
  - Adenocarcinomas have become more prevalent than any other non-small cell lung carcinoma (NSCLC)
    - Most common NSCLC
- Age
  - More common in adults
    - 6th and 7th decades of life
    - May also occur in younger individuals

Presentation
- Cough, weight loss, difficulty breathing, chest pain, Cushing syndrome, superior vena cava syndrome, Pancoast syndrome, and hemoptysis

Treatment
- Surgical approaches
  - Segmentectomy, lobectomy, pneumonectomy
- Adjuvant therapy
  - Chemotherapy &/or radiation therapy
  - Targeted therapy for cases with certain gene mutations, amplifications or rearrangements (e.g., EGFR, ALK, ROS1)

Prognosis
- Depends on stage at time of diagnosis
- Presence of certain gene mutation(s) &/or gene rearrangement(s) may have better prognosis
- Tumors with better differentiated histology may have more favorable outcome
- Pulmonary function and other medical conditions may affect prognosis
- Advanced NSCLC generally carries poor prognosis
  - Overall survival of 10-12 months within U.S. population
  - Responsible for most cancer-related deaths worldwide

MACROSCOPIC

General Features
- Peripheral or central tumors
  - Tumors may show necrosis &/or hemorrhage
  - Homogeneous tan cut surface
  - Well circumscribed but not encapsulated

Size
- Varies from 0.6 cm to > 10 cm

Sections to Be Submitted
- Tumor in relation to pleural surface
  - Pleural involvement crucial for staging tumors < 3 cm in size

MOLECULAR

Molecular Genetics
- *KRAS* mutations
  - Prevalence: 25-35% in lung adenocarcinoma (5% in lung squamous cell carcinoma)
    - More common in mucinous adenocarcinomas, non-Asians, and smokers
    - Concurrent *EGFR* and *KRAS* mutations in < 1% of tumors
  - Well-described mutation in NSCLC subtypes
  - Transmits growth signals from variety of tyrosine kinase receptors
    - Most commonly involved in RAF/MEK/ERK signal transduction pathway
  - Mutations have mostly been used as prognostic markers and have not influenced treatment decisions
    - Exception is *KRAS* p.G12C, which has been shown to respond to sotorasib
  - Activating mutations most common in codons 12 and 13 but can also occur in codon 61
    - Activating mutations may portend worse prognosis
    - Predictor of resistance to targeted therapy with EGFR-specific tyrosine kinase inhibitors (TKIs)
  - Detection methods
    - Multiplex PCR, next-generation sequencing, and pyrosequencing methods all provide acceptable performance characteristics
    - Expanded *KRAS* mutation testing may be best performed by multiplex PCR &/or next-generation sequencing
- *EGFR* mutations
  - Prevalence: 10-35% of lung adenocarcinoma in Western populations (3% in lung squamous cell carcinoma)
  - Certain mutations predict response to *EGFR*-specific TKIs (e.g., gefitinib, erlotinib)
    - Acquired resistance inevitably develops ~ 10 months from initiation of treatment
      - *EGFR* T790M is secondary resistance-associated kinase domain mutation; accounts for 50% of all acquired resistance mutations; confers increased sensitivity to 3rd-generation TKI (osimertinib)
      - *EGFR* C797S is resistance-associated mutation that occurs during osimertinib treatment for T790M-positive disease in 10-20% of cases
      - Other more rare *EGFR* resistance mutations include L792H, G796R, L718Q, M766Q, and G724S
      - *MET* amplification also observed in 5-20% of patients who develop EGFR-TKI resistance; confers increased sensitivity to *MET* TKIs
      - *EGFR* D761Y and exon 20 insertions are less common resistance-associated mutations
      - *PIK3CA* mutations
  - Mutations more frequent in Asian ethnicity (as high as 50%), F > M, adenocarcinoma (nonmucinous) histology, and never-smokers
  - Majority of mutations found in exons 18-21 of tyrosine kinase domain

Adenocarcinoma, Lung

- Most common sensitizing *EGFR* mutations include exon 19 deletions and exon 21 L858R substitution mutation
  - Account for 85-90% of mutations
  - Enhance EGFR kinase activity
- Consider germline testing to exclude familial lung cancer syndrome if *EGFR* T790M mutation detected in treatment-naive patient
- Detection methods
  - PCR-based methods (e.g., multiplex PCR, next-generation sequencing) are essential for mutation analysis of exons 18, 19, 20, and 21
  - Immunohistochemistry using EGFR exon 19 E746-A750 deletion and exon 21 L858R mutation-specific antibodies have limited value
    - Not recommended
  - EGFR amplification status as evaluated by FISH or CISH
    - Should not be used to predict *EGFR* mutation status &/or response to anti-EGFR therapy
    - Not recommended

- *ALK* rearrangements
  - Prevalence of 4-7% in lung adenocarcinomas
    - Enriched in younger and never-smoker cohorts
  - Primarily occurs as paracentric inversion with *EML4* (echinoderm microtubule-like protein 4)
    - Other rare fusion partners include *KIF5B*, *TFG*, *KLC1*, and *HIP1*
  - *ALK* activation leads to downstream activation of canonical PI3K/AKT, MAPK, ERK1/2, and STAT pathways
  - Primarily seen in lung adenocarcinomas, young patients, and light or nonsmokers
  - Most commonly occur independent of *KRAS* and *EGFR* mutations
    - Not absolutely mutually exclusive
    - Rare dual oncogenic driver mutations reported
  - Most patients develop resistance to therapy via *ALK* kinase domain mutations (e.g., G1202R, L1196M, F1174L, C1156Y)
    - Usually develops 12 months from initiation of therapy
  - Detection methods
    - FISH analysis is considered gold standard for *ALK* NSCLC mutation testing
      - Abbot Vysis *ALK* break-apart FISH probe kit FDA approved in 2011
    - IHC stains using certain *ALK* clones (i.e., D5F3 and 5A4) may also be used to detect *ALK* rearrangements without FISH confirmation
      - ALK D5F3 (Cell Signaling Technology), ALK 5A4 (Novocastra)
    - RT-PCR and NGS can detect *EML4::ALK* fusions if designed appropriately

- *ROS1* fusions
  - Receptor tyrosine kinase of insulin receptor family
  - Prevalence: 1-2%
  - *ROS1* fusions coexisting with *EGFR* mutations are rare
  - Transforming event is gene fusion involving *ROS1*
    - Fusion partners *CD74*, *SDC4*, *SLC34A2*, *LRIG7*, *EZR*, *TPM3*, and *DEPP1* have been reported
    - Fusions result in chimeric protein with oncogenic activity
  - Resistance mutations have been described (e.g., G2032R, D2033N, S1986F)
  - Detection methods
    - FISH analysis is considered current gold standard for detection
    - IHC may be used as initial screening method; cases with indeterminate &/or positive staining should be confirmed by FISH
      - Recommended IHC antibody clone: ROS1 D4D6 (Cell Signaling Technology)
      - Cases with indeterminate &/or positive staining should be confirmed by FISH

- *ERBB2* (HER2) overexpression/amplification and mutations
  - Prevalence of ERBB2 overexpression by IHC (3+) and amplification by FISH: 7-35%
  - Prevalence of *ERBB2* mutations: 2-4% in lung adenocarcinoma
  - Signal transduction proceeds via PI3K/AKT/mTOR pathway
  - Activating mutations occur in exons 18-21 of tyrosine kinase domain
    - More common in females, Asians, never smokers, or light smokers
  - Detection methods
    - IHC and FISH are commonly employed methods to detect overexpression and amplification
    - NGS methods can provide information regarding both gene amplification and mutation status

- *BRAF* mutations
  - Prevalence: 1-4% in lung adenocarcinomas (< 1% in lung squamous cell carcinomas)
  - Member of RAF kinase family
    - Located downstream from MAPK pathway
    - Involved in RAS/RAF/MEK/ERK signaling pathway
  - *BRAF* V600E mutations account for ~ 50% of *BRAF* mutations
    - Non-V600 mutations tend to occur in exons 11 and 15
      - *BRAF* G469A and D594G reported
  - Detection methods
    - NGS, PCR, and pyrosequencing-based methods are most commonly employed

- *RET* fusions
  - Prevalence: 1-2%
    - As high as 15% when enriched for patients without *EGFR*, *ALK*, *ROS1*, or *KRAS* mutations
  - Oncogenic *KIF5B::RET* fusions occur via paracentric inversion on chromosome 10q11.2
    - Accounts for 90% of fusions
  - Less common fusion partners include *CCDC6*, *TRIM33*, and *NCOA4*
  - More commonly seen in light/never-smokers, younger cohorts, and poorly differentiated histology
  - Detection methods usually involve FISH break-apart probes, PCR, or NGS-based methods
    - NGS technologies may be used to detect *RET* fusions
    - FISH may also be employed
    - RT-PCR may not detect new partners or isoforms
    - IHC has shown low sensitivity and specificity for detection of *RET* rearrangements
      - Not recommended

- *MET* amplification and mutations
  - Pathologic activation via mutations, gene amplification, and protein overexpression

Adenocarcinoma, Lung

- *MET* amplification
  - Prevalence of 4% (1% in lung squamous cell carcinomas)
  - Rare de novo event but common mechanism of EGFR-TKI-induced resistance
  - Observed in 5-20% of patients who developed resistance to anti-EGFR therapy
- *MET* exon 14-skipping mutations
  - Prevalence of 3-4%
  - Results in deletion of juxtamembrane domain
  - Leads to enhanced *MET* receptor signaling
- Encodes for hepatocyte growth factor tyrosine kinase receptor
- Initiates downstream signaling via PI3K pathway
- Detection methods
  - NGS technologies preferred
- *PIK3CA* mutations or amplification
  - Prevalence
    - 1-3% in lung adenocarcinoma
    - 6% in lung squamous cell carcinoma
  - Role of mutations and amplification in oncogenesis is unclear
    - Mutations frequently occur concurrently with known activating mutations in genes such as *EGFR* and *KRAS*
  - Response to *PIK3CA* inhibitors is unknown
- *NTRK1/NTRK2/NTRK3* fusions
  - Prevalence: 3%
  - Transmembrane kinase receptor
    - Signal propagation via RAS/RAF/MAPK pathway
  - Novel gene fusions include
    - *MPRIP::NTRK1* and *CD74::NTRK1*
- *DDR2* mutations
  - Prevalence
    - 2-3% in lung adenocarcinoma
    - 3-4% in lung squamous cell carcinoma
- *FGFR1*, *FGFR2*, and *FGFR3*
  - Gene amplifications, mutations, and translocations are most frequent mechanisms of activation
    - Often occur with *TP53* and *PIK3CA* mutations and *PDGFRA* amplification
  - *FGFR1* amplification is rare in adenocarcinoma (1-3%)
    - More commonly observed in squamous cell carcinoma (~ 20%)
  - Transmembrane tyrosine kinase
    - Induces signal cascades via RAS/RAF/MAPK and PI3K/AKT pathways
  - *FGFR2* and *FGFR3* activating mutations have been described in lung squamous cell carcinoma
  - Detection methods include FISH (amplifications and translocations) and NGS technologies (amplifications, mutations, and translocations)
- *IGF1R*
  - Transmembrane tyrosine kinase
    - Mediates cell proliferation through RAS/RAF/MAPK and PI3K/AKT pathways
  - Frequency of *IGF1R* deregulation in NSCLC has not been well defined
- *MAP2K1*
  - Enriched in smokers
  - Prevalence of ~ 1% in NSCLC
- *NRAS*
  - Prevalence of ~ 1% in NSCLC
  - High prevalence of codon 61 mutations
  - Enriched in smokers
- *NRG1/NRG2*
  - Typically occur as oncogenic fusions with number of genes
  - Account for < 1% of NSCLC
  - Often lead to activation of ErbB-mediated downstream signaling
- Targeted therapies available for some alterations
  - *EGFR*, *ALK*, *ROS1*, *BRAF*, *MET*, *RET*, *KRAS*, *ERBB2*, *PI3K*, *NTRK1/NTRK2/NTRK3*, *PD1*, *IDH1/IDH2*, and *FGFR*
- High tumor mutation burden (TMB)
  - Benefit from immune checkpoint inhibitor (ICI) therapy
  - Higher cut offs for TMB high (i.e., > 19 mutations per megabase) is better predictor for response to ICI therapy

Samples Suitable for Molecular Characterization

- Paraffin-embedded tissue derived from biopsy or resection specimens remain gold standard
  - Tumor enrichment with macrodissection is often required
    - Helps reduce false-negatives related to contamination of nontumor (wildtype) DNA
- Cytology samples (e.g., FNA) may also be suitable
- Liquid samples
  - Analysis of DNA extracted from circulating tumor cells or cell-free DNA in plasma/serum
  - Often used to detect or monitor for known mutations or emerging resistance-associated mutations (i.e., *EGFR* T790M)
  - May be prone to false-negative results

MICROSCOPIC

Histologic Features

- Consist of mixture of architectural patterns (lepidic, acinar, papillary, micropapillary, solid)
- Classified according to predominant architectural pattern
  - **Lepidic**
    - Bland pneumocytic cells growing along surface of alveolar walls
    - Invasive (nonlepidic) component > 5 mm should be present
  - **Acinar**
    - Round to oval neoplastic glands
    - ± mucin
  - **Papillary**
    - Glandular tumor cells growing along fibrovascular cores
  - **Micropapillary**
    - Glandular tumor cells forming papillary tufts and florets
    - Lack fibrovascular cores
  - **Solid**
    - Polygonal tumor cells arranged in sheets
    - Lacking lepidic, papillary, micropapillary, and acinar growth patterns
- Clear cell and signet-ring features
  - Can be seen in variety of growth patterns

Adenocarcinoma, Lung

- o Not considered distinct architectural pattern
- Invasion
  - o Nonlepidic pattern with myofibroblastic stroma containing invasive tumor
  - o Vascular or pleural involvement
  - o Spread through airspace

ANCILLARY TESTS

Immunohistochemistry

- Tumor cells commonly express TTF-1 and CK7
  - o TTF-1 and p63 or p40 may serve as initial focused panel to help differentiate adenocarcinoma from squamous cell carcinoma
    - TTF-1 diffuse positivity and p63/p40 negativity support diagnosis of lung adenocarcinoma
    - TTF-1 negativity and p63/p40 positivity support diagnosis of squamous cell carcinoma
    - CK5/6 (positive in lung squamous cell carcinoma) and napsin (positive in lung adenocarcinoma) may serve as additional markers
- PD-L1
  - o Used to help predict tumor response to immunotherapy
  - o Multiple PD-L1 clones exist (i.e., 22C3, 28-8, SP142, SP263, E1L3N)
    - Selection of clone dependent on type of therapy being considered (e.g., pembrolizumab, nivolumab)
    - Several are components of FDA-approved companion diagnostics

Recommendations for Molecular Testing in NSCLC

- College of American Pathologists (CAP), International Association for the Study of Lung Cancer (IASLC), and Association for Molecular Pathology (AMP)
  - o Revised guidelines updated in 2018
  - o Establishes standards for *EGFR*, *ALK*, and *ROS1* testing to help guide targeted therapies
  - o Evaluation may also include *KRAS*, *MET*, *RET*, *BRAF*, and *ERBB2* (HER2) if panel-based approach is employed
  - o Multiplexed genetic sequencing panels are preferred over multiple single-gene tests
- National Comprehensive Cancer Network (NCCN) version 5.2022
  - o Recommend using broad panel-based approach with DNA and RNA sequencing
  - o Molecular targets for analysis should include *EGFR*, *ALK*, *ROS1*, *BRAF*, *KRAS*, *MET*, *RET*, and *NTRK1/NTRK2/NTRK3*
  - o PD-L1 testing by IHC
  - o Emerging markers may be included as part of larger pan-cancer panel
  - o Plasma cell-free DNA testing
    - May be considered in certain clinical scenarios
      □ Patient unfit for invasive tissue sampling
      □ Limited initial diagnostic panel
      □ Insufficient tissue for molecular analysis
    - High specificity but compromised sensitivity
      □ Up to 30% false-negative rate

DIFFERENTIAL DIAGNOSIS

Adenocarcinoma from Extrathoracic Origin

- Immunohistochemistry positive for TTF-1 and CK7 would favor lung origin in vast majority of cases

Atypical Adenomatous Hyperplasia

- Lesion ≤ 0.5 cm in diameter
- Shares similar histological features with bronchioloalveolar carcinoma

Adenoid Cystic Carcinoma

- Shows characteristic double layer-forming glands
- Immunohistochemical studies show myoepithelial differentiation

Papillary Carcinoma of Thyroid Origin

- Tumors with papillary pattern may show similar histological features
- Positive TTF-1 and negative staining for thyroglobulin favor primary lung cancer

Mesothelioma

- Immunohistochemistry positive for WT-1, calretinin, CK5/6, and D2-40

DIAGNOSTIC CHECKLIST

Pathologic Interpretation Pearls

- Size of lesion will separate carcinoma from atypical adenomatous hyperplasia (AAH)
- Cases designated as AAH are < 0.5 cm in diameter

SELECTED REFERENCES

1. National Comprehensive Cancer Network: NCCN guidelines for NSCLC, version 5.2022 https://www.nccn.org/professionals/physician_gls/pdf/nscl.pdf. Reviewed December 29, 2022. Accessed December 29, 2022
2. Ricciuti B et al: Association of high tumor mutation burden in non-small cell lung cancers with increased immune infiltration and improved clinical outcomes of PD-L1 blockade across PD-L1 expression levels. JAMA Oncol. 8(8):1160-8, 2022
3. Dehem A et al: 1341P NRAS mutated non-small cell lung cancer (NSCLC) patients: characteristics and outcomes. https://doi.org/10.1016/j.annonc.2021.08.1942. Reviewed September 2021. Accessed February 2023
4. Rosas D et al: Neuregulin 1 gene (NRG1). A potentially new targetable alteration for the treatment of lung cancer. Cancers (Basel). 13(20):5038, 2021
5. Skoulidis F et al: Sotorasib for lung cancers with KRAS p.G12C mutation. N Engl J Med. 384(25):2371-81, 2021
6. Meador CB et al: Acquired resistance to targeted therapies in NSCLC: updates and evolving insights. Pharmacol Ther. 210:107522, 2020
7. International Association for the Study of Lung Cancer: CAP/IASLC/AMP molecular guidelines for NSCLC. https://www.iaslc.org/articles/capiaslcamp-molecular-testing-guideline-open-comment-period. Reviewed April 24, 2019. Accessed April 24, 2019
8. Vestergaard HH et al: A systematic review of targeted agents for non-small cell lung cancer. Acta Oncol. 57(2):176-86, 2018
9. Ruiz-Ceja KA et al: Current FDA-approved treatments for non-small cell lung cancer and potential biomarkers for its detection. Biomed Pharmacother. 90:24-37, 2017
10. Minguet J et al: Targeted therapies for treatment of non-small cell lung cancer–recent advances and future perspectives. Int J Cancer. 138(11):2549-61, 2016
11. Berge EM et al: Targeted therapies in non-small cell lung cancer: emerging oncogene targets following the success of epidermal growth factor receptor. Semin Oncol. 41(1):110-25, 2014
12. Shaw AT et al: Crizotinib in ROS1-rearranged non-small-cell lung cancer. N Engl J Med. 371(21):1963-71, 2014

Adenocarcinoma, Lung

Gross Appearance

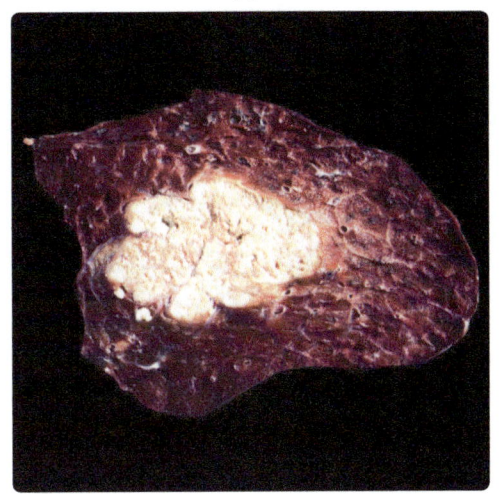

Acinar Pattern

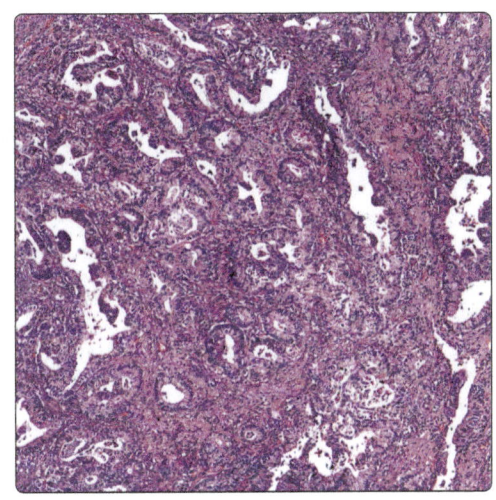

(Left) Gross photograph shows a peripherally located lung adenocarcinoma. The mass is relatively well demarcated but not encapsulated. It is tan and nodular. (Right) Lung adenocarcinoma with an acinar pattern of growth is shown. The neoplastic glandular proliferation is composed of glands of different sizes in a back-to-back arrangement.

Combined Mucinous and Nonmucinous Components

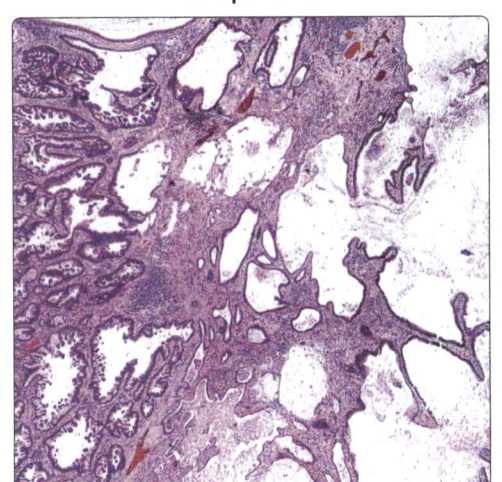

Well-Differentiated Tumor

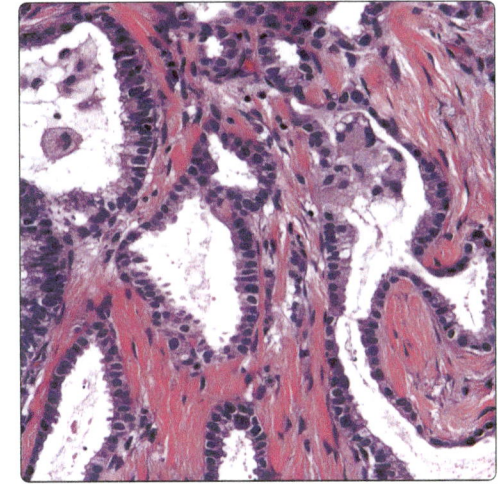

(Left) In this adenocarcinoma, a nonmucinous component merges with a mucinous component showing cystic changes, while the nonmucinous component shows a more acinar component. (Right) High-power view shows well-differentiated adenocarcinoma composed of malignant glands with low cuboidal epithelium.

Multinucleated Giant Cells

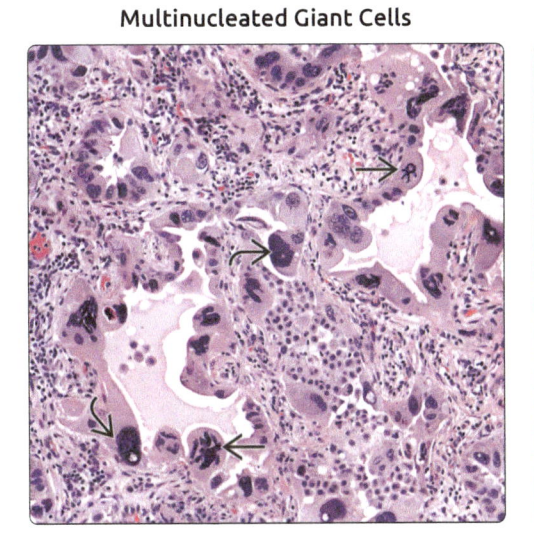

Acinar Pattern With Necrosis

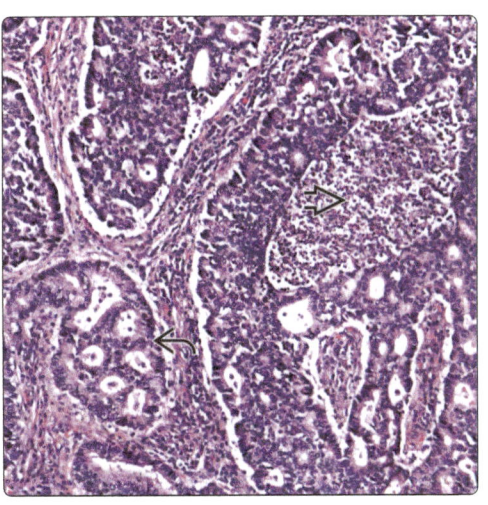

(Left) Lung adenocarcinoma with numerous multinucleated giant cells ⇨ is shown. Note the presence of atypical bizarre mitotic figures ⇨. (Right) Lung adenocarcinoma with comedo-like necrosis ⇨ and acinar pattern ⇨ is shown. The pattern has a vague neuroendocrine morphology, while in some areas it shows conventional glandular differentiation.

Adenocarcinoma, Lung

Papillary Carcinoma

Micropapillary Adenocarcinoma

(Left) High-power view shows true papillary carcinoma of the lung. Note the presence of true papillae. The nuclear characteristics of this tumor may mimic those seen in thyroid carcinomas. (Right) High-power view shows micropapillary adenocarcinoma of the lung. Note that the micropapillae filling the alveolar spaces are devoid of fibrovascular core, contrary to true papillae.

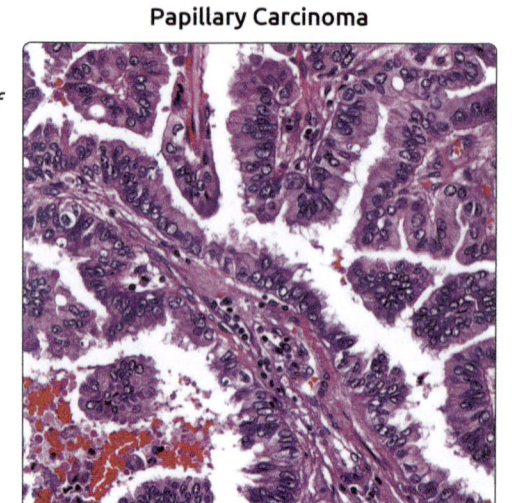

Adenomatoid-Like Adenocarcinoma

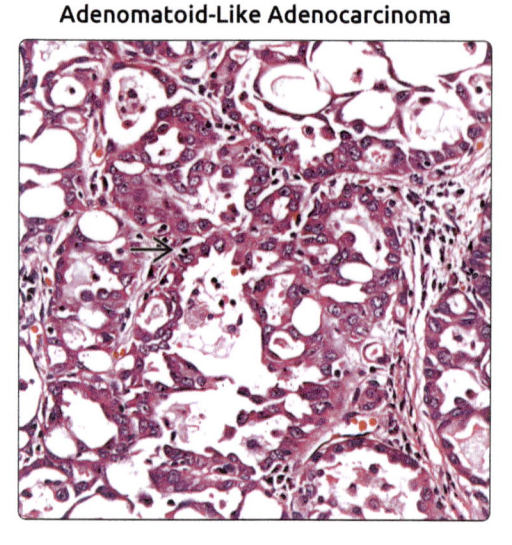

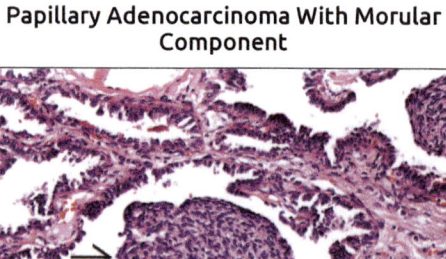

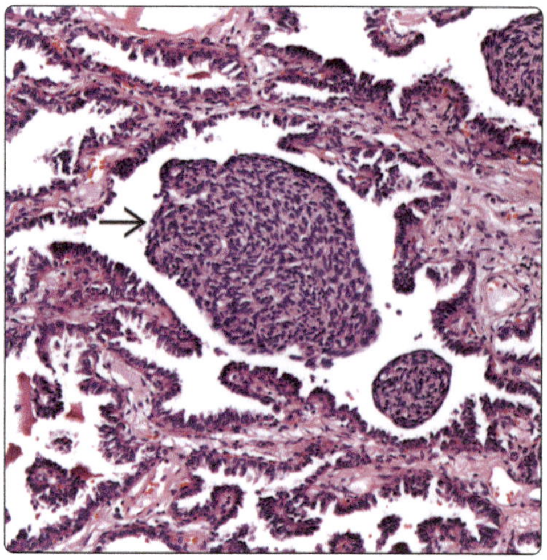

Hepatoid Pattern

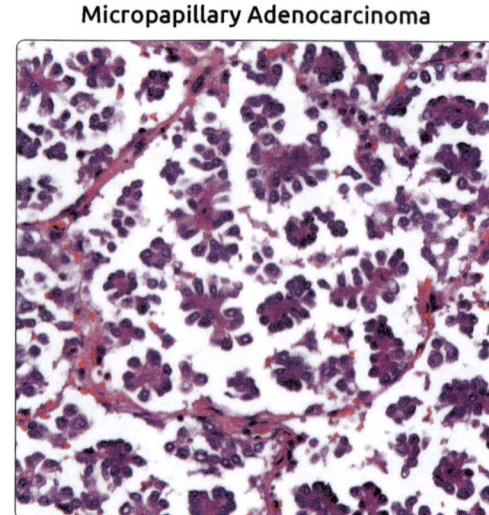

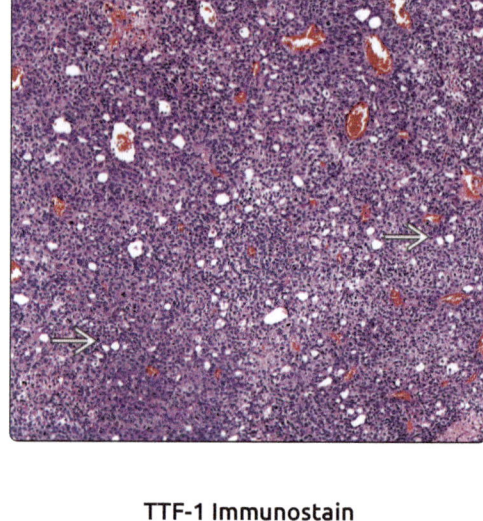

(Left) High-power view shows an adenomatoid tumor-like adenocarcinoma. Note the presence of a more glandular component, nuclear atypia, and rare mitotic figures ➡. These areas are more in keeping with "garden variety" adenocarcinoma. (Right) Medium-power view shows a hepatoid adenocarcinoma of the lung. The sheets of neoplastic cells admixed with fat droplet-like areas ➡ impart a hepatic-like look to this neoplasm.

Papillary Adenocarcinoma With Morular Component

TTF-1 Immunostain

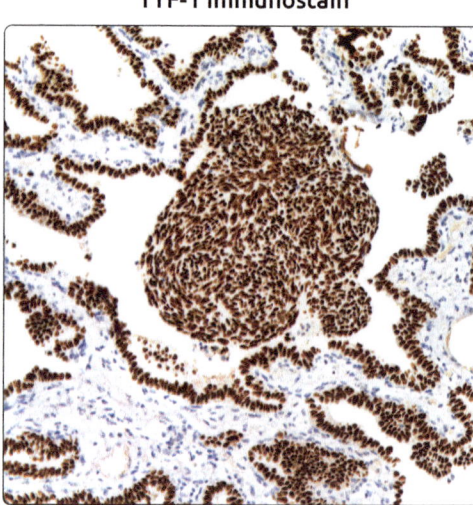

(Left) High-power view shows a papillary adenocarcinoma with morular component. Note the presence of "morules" ➡ within the alveolar spaces, in contrast to those seen in monophasic blastomas, which are in the interstitium at the bases of the glands. (Right) TTF-1 shows strong nuclear staining in the morular component of the tumor. Note that adjacent neoplastic glands are also positive.

Adenocarcinoma, Lung

Next-Generation Sequencing Pileup Diagram

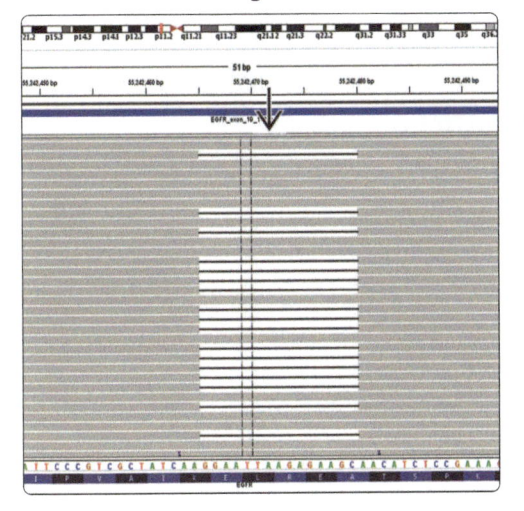

EGFR by FISH

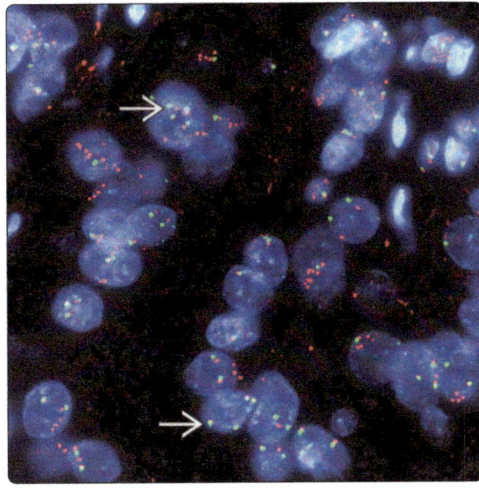

(Left) Next-generation sequencing (massive parallel sequencing) pileup of PCR-amplified products of exon 19 of EGFR gene shows a 15 bp deletion ⇒ involving codons 746-750. EGFR exon 19 deletions typically confer enhanced sensitivity to EGFR small molecule inhibitors. **(Right)** FISH shows EGFR gene amplification ⇒. Although amplification may occur with EGFR mutations, it is nonspecific and should not be used as a surrogate marker for EGFR mutation status.

ALK Break-Apart FISH

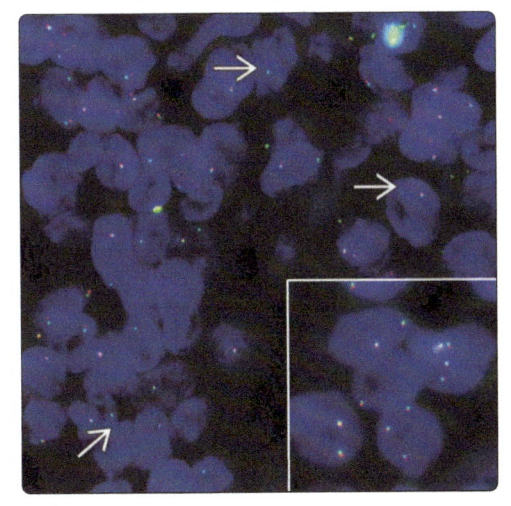

ALK Immunohistochemistry

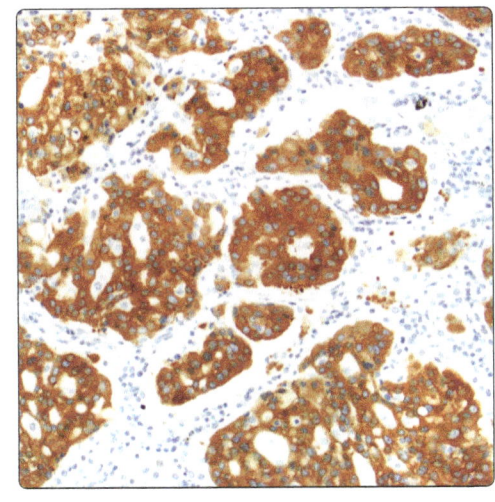

(Left) FISH for ALK in non-small cell lung carcinoma (NSCLC) using the Abbot Vysis ALK break-apart probe shows many separated green and red signals (break-apart) ⇒, consistent with ALK rearrangement. Normal FISH study is shown in the inset. Note the predominance of the yellow signals (green + red), consistent with intact ALK. **(Right)** ALK using D5F3 clone shows diffuse positive cytoplasmic reactivity that is characteristic of ALK-rearranged NSCLC.

ROS1(+) Pattern by FISH

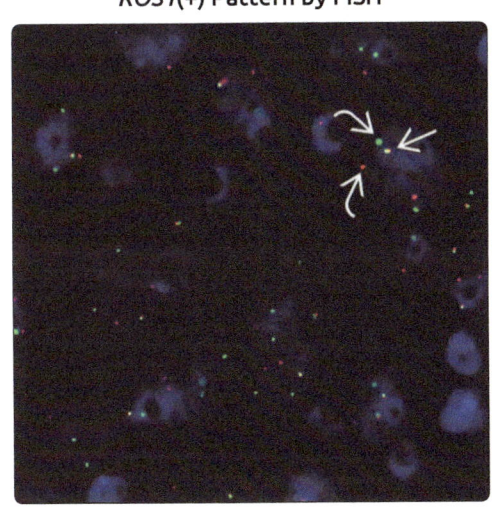

ROS1 Immunohistochemistry

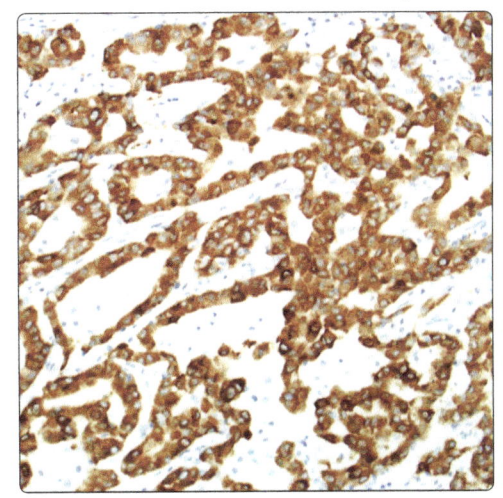

(Left) FISH assay using a dual-color, break-apart probe designed for the detection of ROS1 rearrangements shows the typical ROS1-positive pattern with both fused (native ROS1) ⇒ and split red and green signals ⇒ indicative of ROS1 rearrangement. **(Right)** ROS1 (D4D6 clone) shows diffuse cytoplasmic reactivity with some focal membranous accentuation. This pattern of staining is typical of ROS1-rearranged NSCLC. FISH should be used to confirm the IHC findings.

Squamous Cell Carcinoma, Lung

KEY FACTS

TERMINOLOGY
- Malignant epithelial neoplasm with squamous (epidermoid) differentiation

MACROSCOPIC
- Central or peripheral tumors
- White or light brown in color with homogeneous cut surface

MOLECULAR
- Lung squamous cell carcinoma (SCC) is characterized by complex genomic alterations
- Most lung SCC contain somatic mutations of *TP53*
- Unknown genetic alterations in 21-39%

MICROSCOPIC
- Solid, cystic, or spindled

ANCILLARY TESTS
- Limited IHC panel recommended (TTF-1, p63/p40)
- Broad panel-based approach recommended by NCCN
  - *EGFR, ALK, ROS1, BRAF, KRAS, MET, RET, ERBB2, NTRK1/2/3*
- PD-L1 testing by immunohistochemistry

TOP DIFFERENTIAL DIAGNOSES
- Small cell carcinoma
  - In cases of small cell variant of SCC, may be able to identify in situ squamous component
  - Chromatin pattern of small cell carcinoma (salt and pepper) not present in small cell variant of SCC
- Sarcoma
  - In spindle cell variant of SCC, may identify residual focal areas of squamous differentiation
- Large cell neuroendocrine carcinoma
  - In cases of basaloid SCC, large cell neuroendocrine carcinoma may enter differential diagnosis

Disrupted Signaling Pathways in Squamous Cell Carcinoma

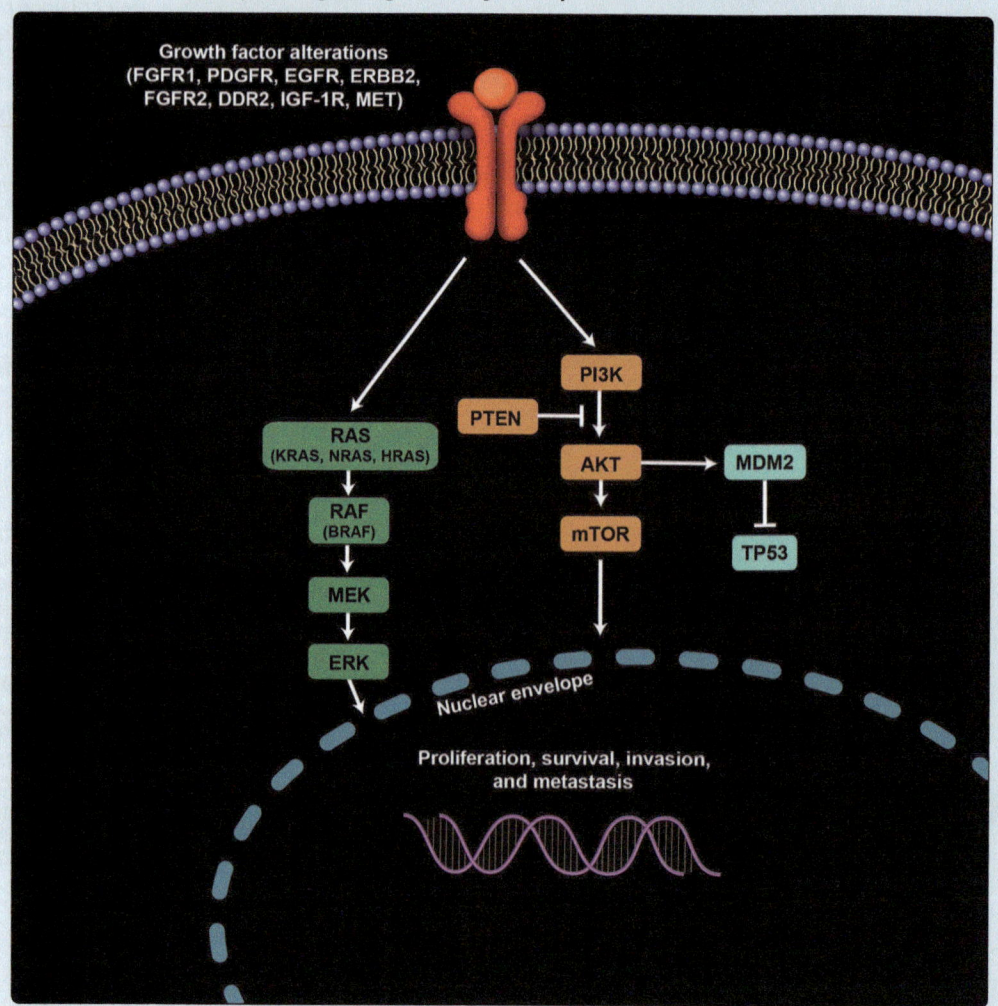

Important signaling pathways involved in the development of lung SCC are shown. Important growth factor receptors, which may either be mutated (i.e., DDR2, PDGFR, EGFR, FGFR1/2) &/or amplified (i.e., EGFR, ERBB2, FGFR1, PDGFRA, IGF1R, MET), result in aberrant signaling and oncogenesis. In the RAS/RAF signaling cascade, mutations have been described in KRAS, HRAS, NRAS, and BRAF. In the PI3K/AKT signaling cascade, mutations have been described in PIK3CA and AKT1. PTEN, a negative regulator in this pathway, is mutated in 10% of lung SCC, while MDM2, a negative regulator of TP53, is amplified in 10%. TP53 mutations occur in 65-81% of lung SCC.

Squamous Cell Carcinoma, Lung

TERMINOLOGY

Abbreviations
- Squamous cell carcinoma (SCC)

Definitions
- Malignant epithelial neoplasm with squamous (epidermoid) differentiation
- Accounts for 30% of non-small cell lung cancers (NSCLC)
  o NSCLC comprises ~ 85% of newly diagnosed lung cancers

ETIOLOGY/PATHOGENESIS

Environmental Exposure
- Strongly associated with tobacco smoke

CLINICAL ISSUES

Epidemiology
- Lung cancer is leading cause of cancer-related deaths worldwide
  o 1.5 million deaths per year

Presentation
- Cough
- Shortness of breath
- Hemoptysis
- Chest pain

Treatment
- Options, risks, complications
  o Surgical approaches
    – Wedge resection
    – Lobectomy
    – Pneumonectomy
  o Radiation therapy &/or platinum-based chemotherapy
  o Targeted therapy
    – PI3K/AKT/mTOR pathway and receptor tyrosine kinase (RTK) signaling
      □ EGFR amplification
      □ BRAF mutation
      □ FGFR1 amplification or mutation
    – Potential driver mutations include
      □ PIK3CA mutations
      □ PTEN mutations/deletion
      □ FGFR1 amplifications
      □ PDGFRA amplification/mutation
      □ BRAF mutation
      □ DDR2 mutations
      □ ERBB family mutations
    – Anti-EGFR therapy
      □ Necitumumab, afatinib, and erlotinib
    – Anti-VEGF therapy
      □ Ramucirumab
    – CDK4/6 pathway
  o Immune checkpoint inhibitors
    – Anti-CTLA4, anti-PD-L1, and anti-PD1 agents
      □ Nivolumab, pembrolizumab, atezolizumab, durvalumab, avelumab, ipilimumab

Prognosis
- Depends on stage at time of diagnosis

MACROSCOPIC

General Features
- Central or peripheral tumors
- White or light brown in color with homogeneous cut surface
- Cut surface may show areas of hemorrhage &/or necrosis
- Tumors may be predominantly cystic
- Tumor size may vary from 2 cm to > 10 cm in diameter

MOLECULAR

Molecular Genetics
- Lung SCC is characterized by complex genomic alterations
  o Somatic mutation rates are higher in lung cancers than in other solid tumors (mean of 11.6 mutations/Mb in lung SCC)
  o Important to distinguish driver mutations (potential therapeutic targets) from passenger mutations
- Statistically significant recurrent mutations
  o TP53 (65-83%), KMT2D (10-40%), SOX2 (18%), KMT2C (8-16%), PIK3CA (4-16%), CCND1 (16%), CDKN2A (7-42%), NFE2L2 (10-20%), PTEN (5-15%), FAT1 (6-20%), LRP1B (15-48%), KEAP1 (12%), NOTCH1 (4-10%), STK11 (5%), EGFR variant III (vIII) mutation (5%), AKT1 (5%), DDR2 (4%), BRAF (4%), FGFR2 (3%), KRAS (3-5%), HRAS (3%), and FGFR1 (14%)
- Other less frequently described mutations
  o ADGRB3, ERBB4, RUNX1T1, FBXW7, NRAS, GRM8, RB1, and HLA-A
- EGFR mutations described in lung adenocarcinoma (deletions and mutations in exons 18-21) are rare in lung SCC
  o Presence may suggest unsampled adenosquamous component
  o EGFR vIII mutations may be observed
    – vIII mutations refer to inframe deletions of exons 2-7 in EGFR
    – May respond to irreversible EGFR inhibitors
- Gene amplification
  o FGFR1 (15-20%), SOX2 (20%), PIK3CA (20%), MDM2 (10%), PDGFRA (9%), EGFR (9%), EPHA2 (7%), MET (6%), ERBB2 (4%), TP63, and IGF1R
- Unknown genetic alterations observed in 21-39% of cases

Next-Generation Sequencing
- Application of next-generation sequencing (NGS) has allowed for comprehensive profiling of genetic alterations
  o Genetic alterations include single nucleotide variations, insertions and deletions, copy number alterations, and chromosomal rearrangements
  o Allows for better and more comprehensive characterization of cancer genomes

Chromosomal Microarray
- Useful in identification of expression level changes (overexpression and underexpression)
  o Often correspond to copy number alterations
  o Recurring copy number alterations frequently involve

Squamous Cell Carcinoma, Lung

- Gains in 1q31, 3q25-27, 5p13-14, 8p12, 8q23-24
- Losses in 3p21, 8p22, 9p21-22, 13q22, 17p12-13
○ Changes may signal oncogenic or tumor suppressor candidate genes

MICROSCOPIC

Histologic Features
- Keratinization, keratin pearls, and intercellular bridges

Predominant Pattern
- Cystic, spindled, and solid

ANCILLARY TESTS

Immunohistochemistry
- Limited panel recommended to preserve tissue
  ○ TTF-1 and p63/p40 to help differentiate adenocarcinoma from SCC
    - TTF-1(-) and p63/p40(+) support diagnosis of SCC
    - TTF-1(+) and p63/p40(-) support diagnosis of lung adenocarcinoma
    - CK5/6 may serve as additional marker (positive in SCC)
  ○ PD-L1 by immunohistochemistry
    - Multiple clones available (e.g., 22C3, 28-8, SP263, SP142, E1L3N)
    - Several have similar staining characteristics

NCCN Guidelines Version 1.2023
- Testing recommendations
  ○ Broad panel-based approach by NGS is recommended
  ○ Recommended targets for analysis
    - EGFR, ALK, ROS1, BRAF, KRAS, MET, RET, ERBB2, NTRK1/NTRK2/NTRK3
  ○ PD-L1 testing by immunohistochemistry

CAP/AMP/IASLC Revised Guidelines Updated in 2017
- Although recommendations are specific to lung adenocarcinoma, testing justified in small biopsies where adenosquamous component cannot be excluded
- Establishes standards for EGFR, ALK, and ROS1 testing to help guide targeted therapies
- Evaluation may also include KRAS, MET, RET, BRAF, and ERBB2 (HER2) if panel-based approach is employed
- Multiplexed genetic sequencing panels are preferred over multiple single-gene tests

DIFFERENTIAL DIAGNOSIS

Small Cell Carcinoma
- In cases of small cell variant of SCC, presence of in situ squamous component will be helpful for diagnosis
- Chromatin pattern of small cell carcinoma (salt and pepper) not present in small cell variant of SCC
- May show positive staining for neuroendocrine markers and TTF-1

Sarcoma
- May identify residual focal areas of squamous differentiation in spindle cell variant of SCC
- Immunohistochemical markers for mesenchymal origin may prove useful

Large Cell Neuroendocrine Carcinoma
- In cases of basaloid SCC, large cell neuroendocrine carcinoma may enter differential diagnosis
- Basaloid SCC is negative for neuroendocrine markers
- Immunomarkers for neuroendocrine origin will show positive staining

DIAGNOSTIC CHECKLIST

Pathologic Interpretation Pearls
- Presence of keratinization, keratin pearls, &/or intercellular bridges

GRADING

In Situ Squamous Cell Carcinoma
- Tumor is limited to bronchial mucosa, full thickness

Well-Differentiated Squamous Cell Carcinoma
- Tumor shows obvious keratinization, and, at high-power view, intercellular bridges are apparent

Moderately Differentiated Squamous Cell Carcinoma
- Tumors show more cellular and nuclear atypia
  ○ Keratinization is not obvious

Poorly Differentiated Squamous Cell Carcinoma
- Sheets of tumor cells with only focal keratinization, high mitotic activity, and prominent cellular and nuclear atypia

SELECTED REFERENCES

1. NCCN Guidelines Version 1.2023 Non-Small Cell Lung Cancer. Published 2023. Accessed 2023. https://www.nccn.org/professionals/physician_gls/pdf/nscl.pdf
2. Catalog of Somatic Mutations in Cancer (COSMIC). Published 2023. Accessed 2023. https://cancer.sanger.ac.uk/cosmic
3. Niu Z et al: Signaling pathways and targeted therapies in lung squamous cell carcinoma: mechanisms and clinical trials. Signal Transduct Target Ther. 7(1):353, 2022
4. Joshi A et al: Molecular characterization of lung squamous cell carcinoma tumors reveals therapeutically relevant alterations. Oncotarget. 12(6):578-88, 2021
5. Ding Y et al: Comparative study on the mutational profile of adenocarcinoma and squamous cell carcinoma predominant histologic subtypes in Chinese non-small cell lung cancer patients. Thorac Cancer. 11(1):103-12, 2020
6. Friedlaender A et al: Next generation sequencing and genetic alterations in squamous cell lung carcinoma: where are we today? Front Oncol. 9:166, 2019
7. Lindeman NI et al: Updated molecular testing guideline for the selection of lung cancer patients for treatment with targeted tyrosine kinase inhibitors: guideline from the College of American Pathologists, the International Association for the Study of Lung Cancer, and the Association for Molecular Pathology. J Mol Diagn. 20(2):129-59, 2018
8. Tsironis G et al: Breakthroughs in the treatment of advanced squamous-cell NSCLC: not the neglected sibling anymore? Ann Transl Med. 6(8):143, 2018
9. Hirsh V: New developments in the treatment of advanced squamous cell lung cancer: focus on afatinib. Onco Targets Ther. 10:2513-26, 2017
10. Soldera SV et al: Update on the treatment of metastatic squamous non-small cell lung cancer in new era of personalized medicine. Front Oncol. 7:50, 2017
11. Langer CJ et al: Incremental innovation and progress in advanced squamous cell lung cancer: current status and future impact of treatment. J Thorac Oncol. 11(12):2066-81, 2016
12. Kenmotsu H et al: Prospective genetic profiling of squamous cell lung cancer and adenosquamous carcinoma in Japanese patients by multitarget assays. BMC Cancer. 14:786, 2014
13. Cancer Genome Atlas Research Network: Comprehensive genomic characterization of squamous cell lung cancers. Nature. 489(7417):519-25, 2012. Erratum in: Nature. 491(7423):288, 2012

Squamous Cell Carcinoma, Lung

EGFR Amplification

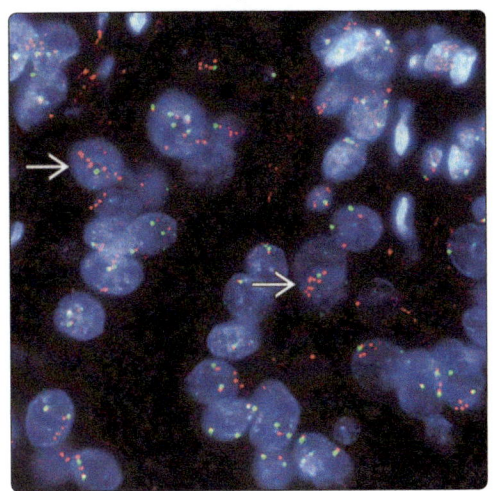

PIK3CA Mutation: IGV

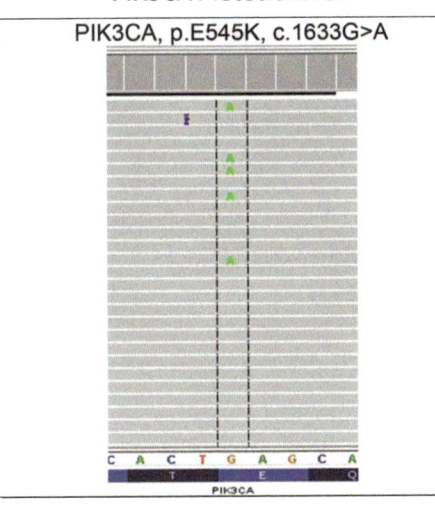

(Left) FISH shows EGFR gene amplification ➡. Amplification of EGFR occurs in ~ 9% of lung SCC, while mutations in EGFR are commonly seen as in-frame deletions of exons 2-7 (e.g., EGFR variant III mutations). (Right) Next-generation sequencing shows a G > A mutation at codon 1633 of PIK3CA. The reference sequence is listed along the bottom. PIK3CA mutations are observed in ~ 16% of lung SCC.

In Situ Squamous Cell Carcinoma

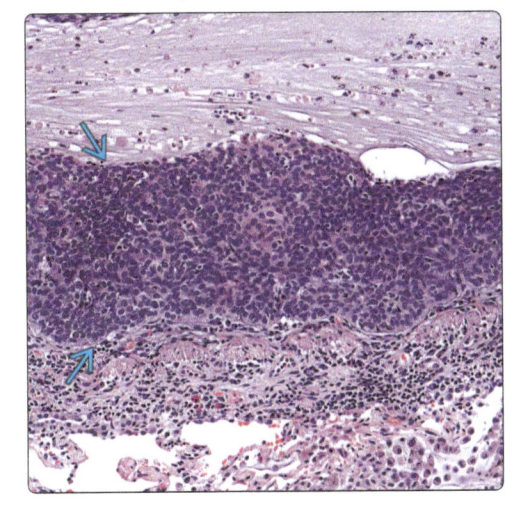

Invasive Squamous Cell Carcinoma

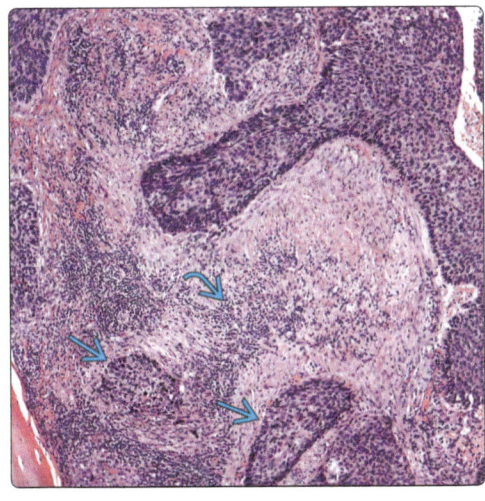

(Left) The bronchial mucosa is replaced by a full-thickness neoplastic cellular proliferation ➡, characteristic of in situ SCC. Note the mild inflammatory reaction adjacent to the neoplastic cells. (Right) Predominantly in situ SCC with focal areas of minimally invasive tumor is shown. Tumor islands of SCC ➡ are admixed with an inflammatory reaction ➡.

Squamous Cell Carcinoma

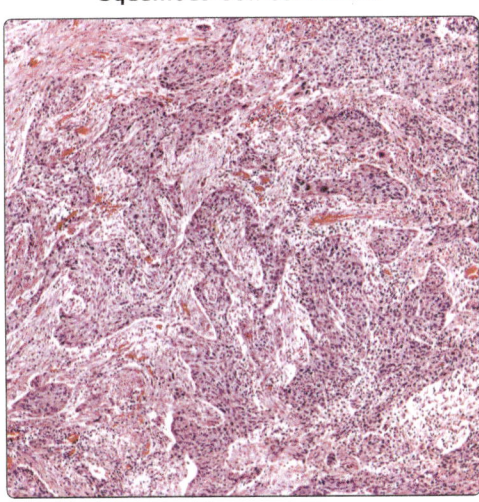

Poorly Differentiated Squamous Cell Carcinoma

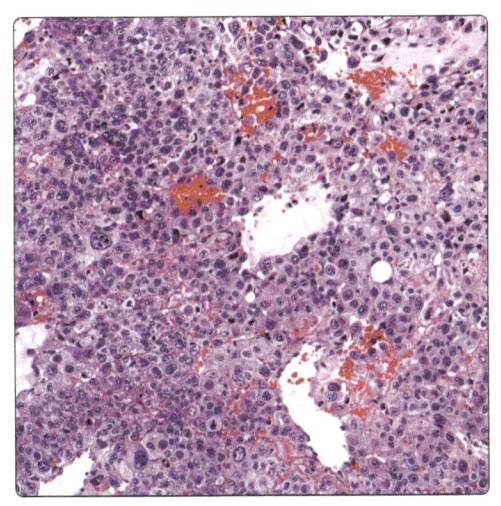

(Left) Moderately differentiated SCC does not show marked keratinization, but the growth pattern and cytologic atypia are typical of SCC. (Right) Sheets of neoplastic cells with focal perivascular arrangement are seen in this example of poorly differentiated SCC. The tumor shows only focal single-cell keratinization.

Small Cell Neuroendocrine Carcinoma

KEY FACTS

CLINICAL ISSUES
- Currently accounts for ~ 15% of all primary lung carcinomas
- Cough, hemoptysis, weight loss, chest pain, dyspnea; paraneoplastic syndromes can occur
- Usually presents as late-stage disease; 2- and 5-year survival rates of ~ 8% and 2%, respectively

MOLECULAR
- Currently no known actionable mutations
  - So-called small cell transformation of *EGFR*-mutant lung adenocarcinomas developing tyrosine kinase inhibitor resistance reported
- Frequent aneuploidy and chromosomal alterations > 10 Mb, most frequent of which are deletions of 3p, 13q, and 17p
- *TP53* mutations in ~ 90%, *RB1* mutations in ~ 80-100%, and *PTEN* mutations in ~ 15-20%
- *MYC* family member amplification, downregulation of *CDH1* (E-cadherin), alteration of intrinsic apoptotic pathway, and mutations in genes that encode histone modifiers are also seen

MICROSCOPIC
- Tumor cells are generally small with scant cytoplasm, salt and pepper chromatin, nuclear molding, and frequent mitotic/apoptotic figures

ANCILLARY TESTS
- Positive for keratins, neuroendocrine markers, and TTF-1

TOP DIFFERENTIAL DIAGNOSES
- Basaloid variant of squamous cell carcinoma
- Poorly differentiated adenocarcinoma
- Large cell neuroendocrine carcinoma
- Lymphoma

Gross Features

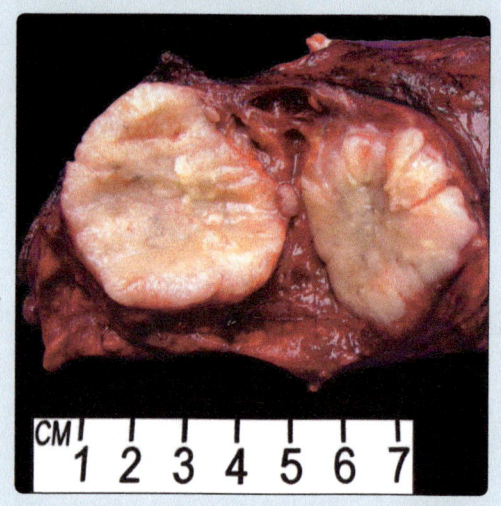

Microscopic Features

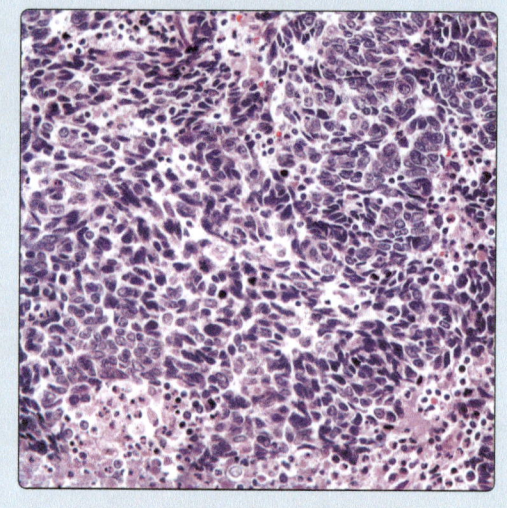

(Left) The cut surface of small cell neuroendocrine carcinoma (SCNEC) shows a uniform, pale-tan to yellow, fish flesh appearance, more closely resembling lymphoma than other types of carcinoma. (Right) Several classic features of SCNEC are seen here, including frequent mitoses, hyperchromasia, nuclear molding, absent/inconspicuous nucleoli, stippled chromatin, and necrosis. (From DP: Thoracic.)

Cytologic Features

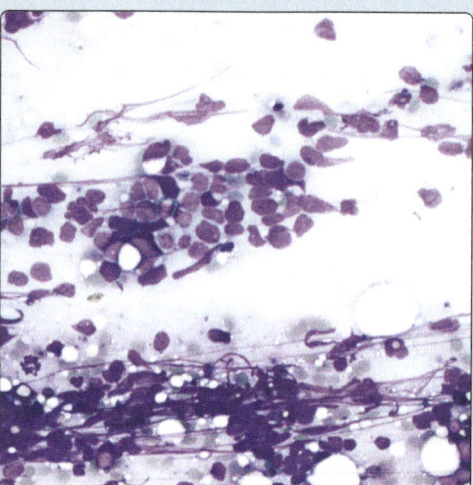

Chromogranin Immunohistochemistry

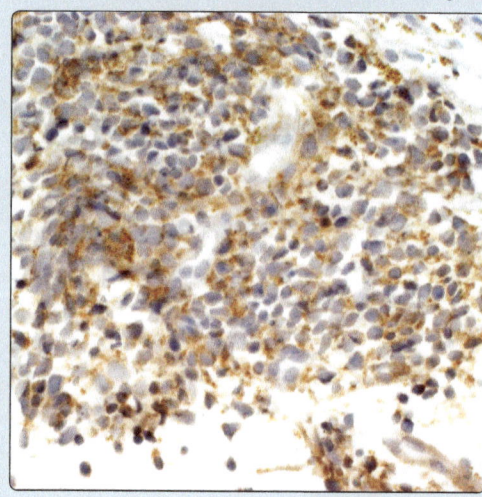

(Left) Scant cytoplasm gives a small round blue cell tumor appearance to cytologic preparations. Classic characteristics, including nuclear molding, mitotic activity, and crush artifact can all be seen in this image. (Right) Generic neuroendocrine markers (chromogranin shown here) stain cytoplasmic neurosecretory granules, albeit at a lesser intensity than in well-differentiated neuroendocrine tumors (carcinoids).

Small Cell Neuroendocrine Carcinoma

TERMINOLOGY

Abbreviations
- Small cell neuroendocrine carcinoma (SCNEC)

Synonyms
- Small cell lung carcinoma (SCLC)
- Small cell undifferentiated carcinoma
- High-grade neuroendocrine carcinoma, small cell type

Definitions
- High-grade epithelial primary lung carcinoma with morphologic &/or immunohistochemical evidence of neuroendocrine differentiation

ETIOLOGY/PATHOGENESIS

Environmental Exposure
- Strongly associated with cigarette smoking
- Tumor mutational profiling shows clear smoking signature demonstrating link to tobacco carcinogens

Pathogenesis
- Mechanism of tumorigenesis is not completely understood
- Tumor suppressor (TS) inactivation or loss may play crucial role in tumorigenesis
  - *TP53* and *RB1* mutations in virtually all cases
  - Functional inactivation of *TP53* and *RB1*
  - Cell cycle and transcription dysregulation
- Other tumor suppressor genes affected
  - *PTEN*, *MLL*, *NOTCH1*, *CREBBP*
  - Putative TS genes *ROBO1*, *FHIT*
- Changes in lung stroma and immune microenvironment may contribute
- Precursor cell has not been identified
  - Possible cells of origin include neuroendocrine cell or pluripotent stem cell capable of differentiation

CLINICAL ISSUES

Epidemiology
- Incidence
  - Accounts for ~ 15% of all primary lung carcinomas
  - 250,000 new cases and > 200,000 deaths globally per year (~ 30,000 cases per year in USA)
  - Reported incidence is decreasing in correlation with decreasing prevalence of cigarette smoking

Presentation
- Generally presents as late-stage disease
  - SCNEC is only rarely incidental finding (< 5% of cases)
- Nonspecific signs and symptoms similar to non-SCLC include cough, hemoptysis, weight loss, chest pain, and dyspnea
- Paraneoplastic syndromes: Ectopic production of antidiuretic hormone (hyponatremia), parathyroid hormone-like peptides (hypercalcemia), ACTH (Cushing syndrome)
  - Rarely, Eaton-Lambert syndrome (pseudomyasthenia)
- Compression of superior vena cava, esophagus, or recurrent laryngeal nerve

Treatment
- Stage-based treatment algorithm
  - TNM stage I early-stage tumors may be treated with surgery with adjuvant chemotherapy or radiotherapy
  - TNM stage I-III locally advanced tumors treated with concomitant chemoradiotherapy ± prophylactic cranial irradiation
  - TNM stage IV metastatic disease treated with chemotherapy ± PDL1 inhibitor
- SCNEC is highly responsive to initial chemotherapy
  - ~ 70% of cases have rapid clinical response, followed by recurrence and systemic spread within 1-2 years

Prognosis
- SCNEC is most aggressive primary lung carcinoma featuring early metastases and poor prognosis
  - Nonmetastatic disease 5-year survival rate of ~ 30% and median survival of 25-30 months
  - Metastatic disease 2- and 5-year survival rates of ~ 8% and 2%, respectively

IMAGING

General Features
- Tumors usually large, centrally located, and at advanced stage at presentation
  - ~ 90% located at lobar or main bronchus
- Mediastinal lymphadenopathy concurrently detected in majority of cases
- Narrowing &/or displacement of vasculature or bronchi and pleural or pericardial effusions common findings

MACROSCOPIC

General Features
- Grossly, resembles lymphoma rather than other carcinomas
  - Composed of soft and friable irregular masses
  - Cut surfaces show uniform, pale-tan to yellow, fish flesh appearance with necrotic areas

MOLECULAR

Cytogenetics
- Characterized by frequent aneuploidy and chromosomal alterations > 10 Mb; may be caused by carcinogens in tobacco smoke
  - Deletion of 17p
    - Results in loss of TS gene *TP53*
  - Deletion of 13q
    - Results in loss of multiple TS genes, most important of which is *RB1*, which normally inhibits cell cycle progression; others include *BRCA2* and *ING1*
  - Deletion of 3p
    - Early event in pathogenesis of both SCNEC and non-SCLC
    - Highly related to cigarette smoking
    - Putative TS genes located on 3p include *ROBO1*, *FHIT*, *BAP1*, *CTNNB1*, *TUSC2*, *HYAL2*, *MLH1*, *SEMA3B*, and *VHL*
- Other chromosomal alterations include losses of 1p, 4p, 4q, 5q, 8p, 10q, and 11q and gains of 3q, 5p, 8q, and 18q

Small Cell Neuroendocrine Carcinoma

Molecular Genetics

- Genomic alterations
  - Loss of *TP53* and *RB1* TS genes occurs frequently in SCLC
    - *TP53* mutations in ~ 90% of cases
    - *RB1* mutations in ~ 80-100% of cases
  - Amplification of MYC family genes (*MYC, MYCL,* and *MYCN*) in subset of SCLC tumors
    - To date, these mutations have been mutually exclusive, suggesting genetic epistasis
  - Amplification of *FGFR1, IARS1,* and *GNAS*
  - Loss-of-function events in
    - RB family member genes *RBL1* and *RBL2*
    - TS *PTEN* gene mutations in ~ 15-20% of cases
    - NOTCH receptors (tumor suppressor role in SCLC)
    - Recurrent mutations seen in *CREBBP, EP300,* and *KMT2A* (MLL) genes that encode histone modifiers
    - WNT signaling pathway alterations may play role in chemoresistant SCLC
  - Downregulation of *CDH1* (E-cadherin) and associated epithelial to mesenchymal transition facilitating tumor invasion
  - Upregulation of *BCL2* and downregulation of *BAX*, resulting in inverted *BAX:BCL2* ratio favoring antiapoptosis

Gene Expression Profiling

- Only limited number of studies currently describe genome-wide expression profiling in SCNEC
  - Initial studies have shown high-level expression of *INSM1, ASCL1, CHGA, NRXN1,* and *NCAM1*

MICROSCOPIC

Histologic Features

- Typically diffuse, patternless growth pattern; however, vague neuroendocrine architecture (rosettes, organoid growth, peripheral palisading) occasionally observed
- Most SCNEC show prominent areas of necrosis and nuclear crush artifact
- Some SCNEC demonstrate Azzopardi phenomenon
  - Accumulation of densely basophilic nucleic acid material around intratumoral vasculature
- Combined SCNEC contain non-small cell carcinoma (NSCC) component
  - NSCC components include adenocarcinoma, squamous cell carcinoma (SCC), and large cell carcinoma (LCC)
  - To establish diagnosis of combined SCNEC and LCC, large cells must comprise ≥ 10% of tumor
  - Giant cell carcinoma and spindle cell carcinoma components also seen, but rare

Cytologic Features

- Tumor cells small, ~ 2-3x size of mature lymphocyte
  - Can be round, oval, fusiform, or spindled
- Chromatin coarsely granular and stippled
- Nuclear molding prominent
- Nucleoli generally absent to inconspicuous
- Mitoses and apoptoses frequent (often > 50 mitoses per 10 HPF, Ki-67 index > 65%)

ANCILLARY TESTS

Immunohistochemistry

- Keratins
  - Positive for LMW keratins (in particular CK8, CK18, and CK19), CAM5.2, and AE1/AE3
    - Punctate or dot-like perinuclear zone of positivity
  - Negative for HMW keratins
  - Positive for CK7 in < 50% of cases and negative for CK20
- Neuroendocrine markers: Chromogranin-A, synaptophysin, CD56 (NCAM), CD57 (Leu7), and NSE
  - \> 90% of all SCNEC positive for at least 1 neuroendocrine marker
  - NSIM1 emerging biomarker positive in some cases
- TTF-1 positive in 90-95% of cases
  - Not specific for pulmonary origin; extrapulmonary SCNEC frequently positive for TTF-1 as well
- Negative for Napsin A, CD45, p40, and p63
  - Rarely, p40 and p63 may be focally positive

Genetic Testing

- Molecular testing not routinely performed in diagnosis or treatment of SCLC
- Currently no known targetable mutations
- Molecular testing should be performed only in following settings
  - Newly diagnosed SCLC in never-smoker to clarify diagnosis or identify targetable mutation
  - Combined SCLC with adenocarcinoma component
- ~ 14% of *EGFR*-mutated NSCLC acquire SCLC morphology and express neuroendocrine markers as manifestation of EGFR-inhibitor resistance

DIFFERENTIAL DIAGNOSIS

Basaloid/Small Cell Variant of Squamous Cell Carcinoma

- Positive for high-molecular-weight keratins, p63, and p40
- Negative for TTF-1, neuroendocrine markers, and CK7

Poorly Differentiated Adenocarcinoma

- Usually negative for neuroendocrine markers and shows at least focal glandular architecture

Large Cell Neuroendocrine Carcinoma

- Increased cell size, decreased N:C ratio
- Often show prominent nucleoli; typically occur in peripheral lung (vs. central with SCNEC)

Lymphoma

- Positive for CD45, lymphoid markers
- Negative for keratins, neuroendocrine markers, and TTF-1

Merkel Cell Carcinoma

- CK20 positive, CK7 usually negative

SELECTED REFERENCES

1. Beasley MB et al: Small cell lung carcinoma. In: WHO Classification of Tumours: Thoracic Tumours, 5th ed. IARC, 2021
2. Rudin CM et al: Small-cell lung cancer. Nat Rev Dis Primers. 7(1):3, 2021
3. Semenova EA et al: Origins, genetic landscape, and emerging therapies of small cell lung cancer. Genes Dev. 29(14):1447-62, 2015

Small Cell Neuroendocrine Carcinoma

Neuroendocrine Features

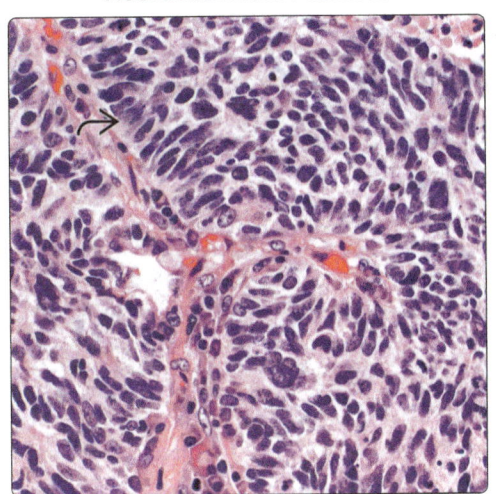

Atypical Mitoses

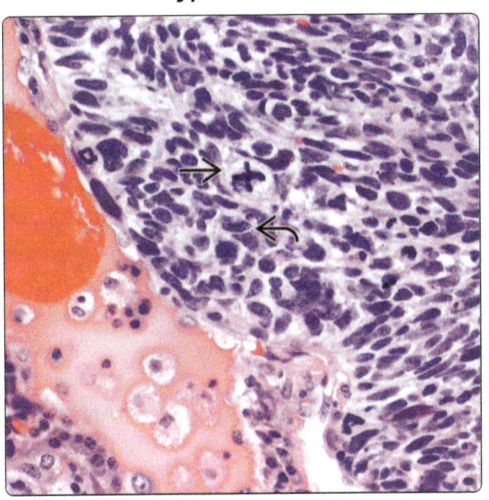

(Left) *A vaguely organoid architecture and a suggestion of peripheral palisading ⇨ are shown. The nuclei demonstrate neuroendocrine-type chromatin (salt and pepper), nuclear molding, inconspicuous nucleoli, and significant anisonucleosis.* (Right) *SCNEC shows overtly malignant cells with high nuclear:cytoplasmic ratios, nuclear molding ⇨, and numerous mitoses, including a highly atypical tetraploid mitotic figure ⇨.*

Cytologic Features

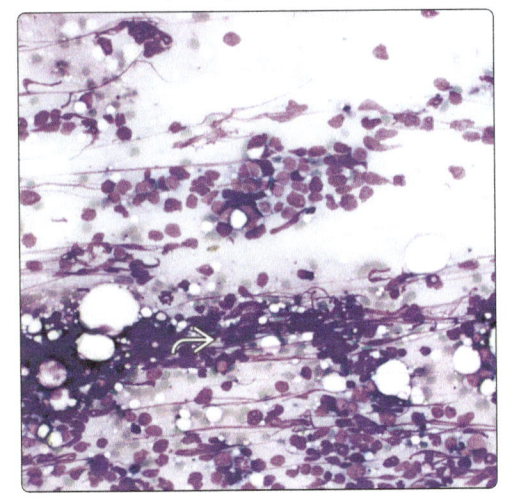

Soft Tissue Invasion

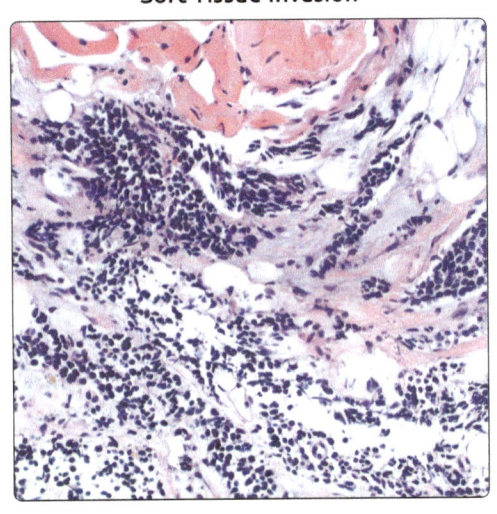

(Left) *Smear of an involved mediastinal node shows a slightly dyscohesive population of SCNEC cells with prominent crush artifact ⇨, a feature frequently seen in cytologic and histologic preparations. High-grade lymphoma could not be completely excluded on the basis of this image.* (Right) *SCNEC metastasis to the chest wall shows malignant cells infiltrating through adipose tissue and skeletal muscle. SCNEC frequently presents with metastases.*

Chromogranin Immunohistochemistry

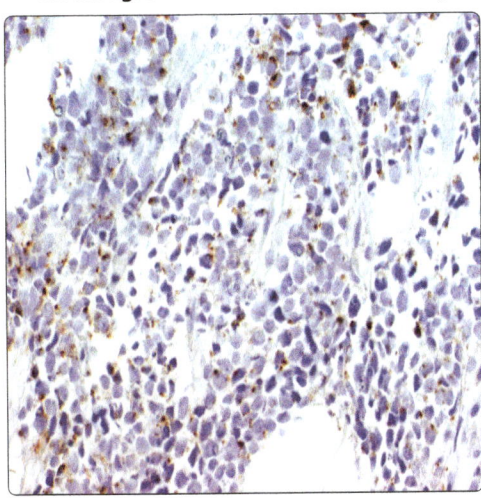

TTF-1 Immunohistochemistry

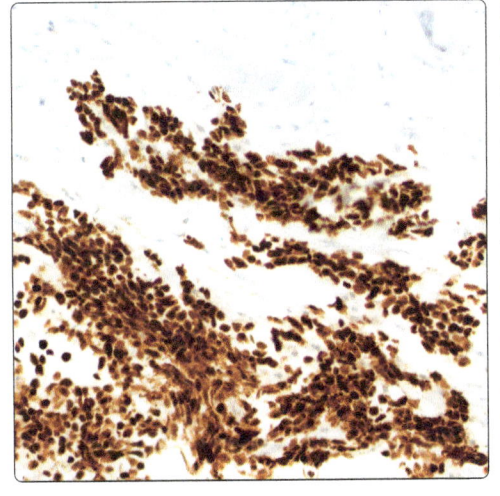

(Left) *Although of only weak to moderate intensity, cytoplasmic staining can be seen for chromogranin here. Chromogranin stains the neurosecretory granules and can demonstrate weaker (or even negative) staining in poorly differentiated tumors such as SCNEC as compared to well-differentiated neuroendocrine tumors (e.g., carcinoids).* (Right) *Nuclear TTF-1 positivity is seen in 85-90% of pulmonary SCNEC, but TTF-1 can also be positive in extrapulmonary high-grade neuroendocrine carcinomas.*

Mesothelioma

KEY FACTS

TERMINOLOGY
- Definition: Tumor of malignant mesothelial cells

CLASSIFICATION
- Benign and preinvasive mesothelial tumors
  - Adenomatoid tumors of pleura
  - Well-differentiated papillary mesothelial tumor
  - Mesothelioma in situ
- Malignant pleural mesothelial tumors
  - Localized pleural mesothelioma
    - Circumscribed mass without diffuse serosal spread
    - Carries BAP1 and TRAF7 mutations
  - Diffuse pleural mesothelioma
  - 3 histologic subtypes
    - Epithelioid, sarcomatous, and biphasic

ETIOLOGY/PATHOGENESIS
- Majority caused by occupational exposure to asbestos
  - Typically develops 20-40 years after exposure
- Other established causes
  - Therapeutic and occupational radiation exposure
  - BAP1 tumor predisposition syndrome
    - Family members with BAP1 tumor predisposition syndrome may be at high risk of developing mesothelioma with small amounts of asbestos exposure

MOLECULAR
- Frequently mutated genes include BAP1, NF2, TP53, SETD2, DDX3X, ULK2, RYR2, CFAP45, SETDB1, and DDX51
  - BAP1 somatic mutations present in ~ 20% of cases
  - Loss of BAP1 may serve as predictive biomarker for immunotherapy in peritoneal mesothelioma

ANCILLARY TESTS
- Positive for calretinin, WT1, CK5/6, D2-40, mesothelin, and GATA3
- Loss of BAP1 &/or CDKN2A &/or MTAP

Asbestos Body

Epithelioid Mesothelioma

(Left) Iron-stained histologic section of lung from a patient with known history of asbestos inhalation shows a ferruginous body consistent with an iron-coated asbestos fiber. (Right) Well-differentiated epithelioid mesothelioma is shown. Neoplastic cells are generally cuboidal and have relatively uniform nucleoli. Tubulopapillary formation may be seen.

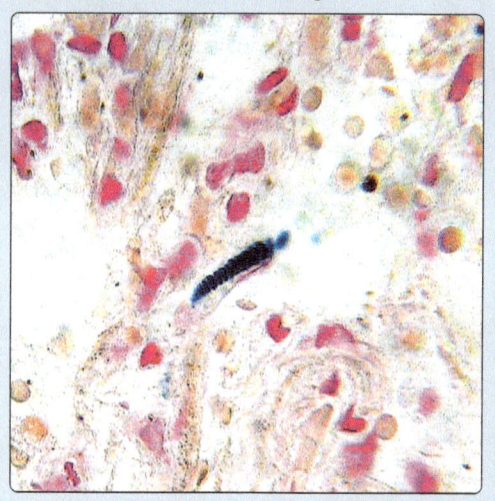

Sarcomatous Mesothelioma

CDKN2A Mutation

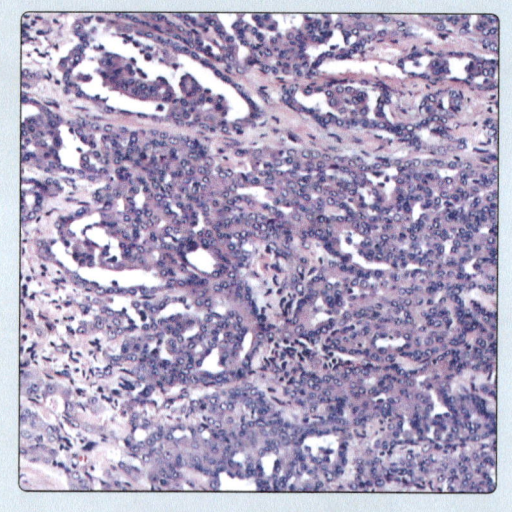

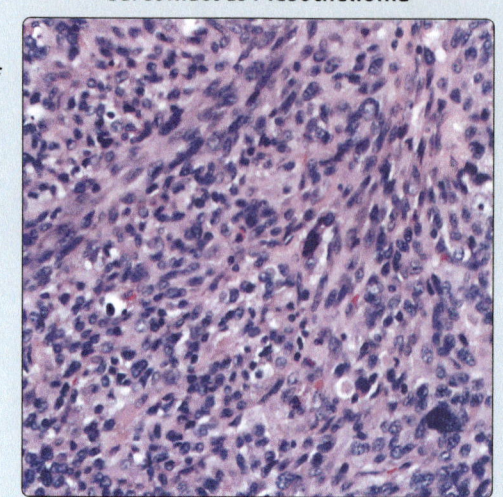

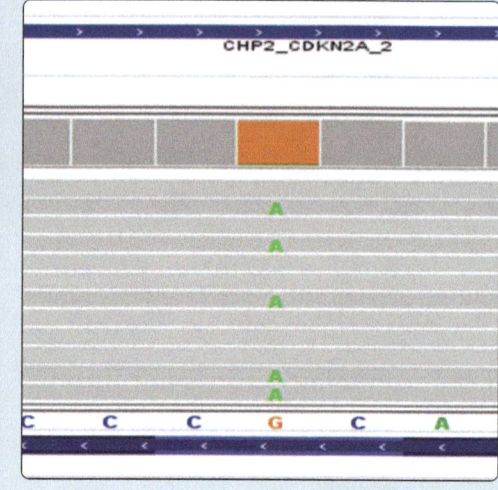

(Left) Sarcomatous mesothelioma is the least common histologic subtype of mesothelioma. It is characterized by highly pleomorphic spindle cell proliferation with nuclear pleomorphism. (Right) NGS pileup of CDNK2 gene performed on DNA extracted from pleural mesothelioma reveals c.401C>T base substitution corresponding to p.A134V missense mutation.

Mesothelioma

TERMINOLOGY

Abbreviations
- Benign mesothelial tumors (BMT)
- Preinvasive mesothelial tumors (PMT)
- Localized pleural mesothelioma (LPM)
- Diffuse pleural mesothelioma (DPM)

Definitions
- Tumor of malignant mesothelial cells

CLASSIFICATION

World Health Organization (WHO) 5th Edition Classification of Mesothelial Tumors
- Benign and preinvasive mesothelial tumors
  o Adenomatoid tumors of pleura
  o Well-differentiated papillary mesothelial tumor
  o Mesothelioma in situ
- Malignant pleural mesothelial tumors
  o Localized pleural mesothelioma
    – Present as circumscribed mass without diffuse serosal spread
    – Carries *BAP1* and *TRAF7* mutations
  o Diffuse pleural mesothelioma
    – 3 histologic subtypes
      □ Epithelioid
      □ Sarcomatous
      □ Biphasic

ETIOLOGY/PATHOGENESIS

Environmental Exposure
- Majority of mesotheliomas caused by occupational exposure to asbestos
  o Mesothelioma typically develops 20-40 years after exposure
  o ~ 10% lifetime risk of malignant mesothelioma in asbestos workers
  o Amosite and crocidolite fibers more carcinogenic than serpentine asbestos
  o Serpentine fibers account for 90% of asbestos types in USA
  o Family members of asbestos workers are also at risk via exposure to asbestos fibers brought home on clothing
  o Inhaled asbestos fibers initiate inflammatory response in lung
    – Phagocytosed asbestos fibers by mesothelial cells may initiate oncogenic cascade
  o High incidence of mesothelioma with exposure to erionite (asbestos-like) fiber in Cappadocia, Turkey
- Other established causes
  o Radiation exposure
    – Therapeutic and occupational radiation without documented asbestos exposure
  o *BAP1* tumor predisposition syndrome
    – Family members with *BAP1* tumor predisposition syndrome may be at risk of developing mesothelioma
    – Small amounts of asbestos exposure in patients with germline mutations reported to increase risk of mesothelioma
    □ Remains controversial; further studies may be indicated
- Other factors involved in pathogenesis of mesothelioma
  o Genomic alterations
    – Copy number losses and some gains
    – Somatic mutations in multiple genes, including *BAP1*

CLINICAL ISSUES

Epidemiology
- Incidence
  o ~ 3,300 new yearly cases in USA per SEAR data
  o Peak incidence in 5th and 6th decades of life

Site
- Pleural mesothelioma accounts for most cases
- Less common sites include mesothelial-lined tissue in peritoneum, pericardium, and tunica vaginalis

Presentation
- Up to 40 years latency period after asbestos exposure
- Nonspecific symptoms and signs
  o Cough, dyspnea, focal chest pain, and pleural effusion
  o Pleural plaques are common
- Paraneoplastic syndromes
  o Hypercalcemia, hypoglycemia, and hypercoagulability can be seen

Treatment
- Surgical approaches
  o Complete removal of tumor impossible in most cases
  o May offer survival advantage
- Adjuvant therapy
  o Cisplatinum and pemetrexed combination therapy
    – ~ 3-month survival benefit over cisplatinum alone in phase III clinical trial
- Radiation
  o Used for either palliative intent or to control residual microscopic tumor post surgery
- Multimodality therapy
  o Surgical resection, chemotherapy, and radiation
    – May improve survival
- Targeted therapies
  o Chimeric antigen receptor (CAR) T-cell therapy
    – Patient's T cells engineered to target cancer cell antigens
  o Antimesothelin antibody
    – Being evaluated in ongoing clinical trials
  o Anti-VEGF antibody (bevacizumab)
    – Cisplatin-pemetrexed-bevacizumab combination is now accepted standard therapy in France

Prognosis
- Most patients die of disease within 2 years of diagnosis
- Median survival ranges from 9-18 months

IMAGING

MR Findings
- Can detect invasion into diaphragm or mediastinum

CT Findings
- May show pleural nodularity

Mesothelioma

MOLECULAR

Cytogenetics

- Nonspecific structural and numerical chromosomal abnormalities can be detected
  - Frequent recurring focal or arm-level deletions, including
    - Losses involving 1p, 3p, 4q, 6q, 9p, 13q, 14q, and 22q
  - Gains involve 1q, 5p, 7p, 8q, and 17q
  - Homozygous deletion of *CDKN2A* in 67-83% in epithelioid and biphasic mesotheliomas and in up to 100% in the sarcomatoid mesotheliomas
    - Loss of *CDKN2A* is strongly associated with shorter overall survival
  - *CDKN2A* is frequently codeleted with *MTAP*
    - *MTAP*-deficient tumors may show increased sensitivity to PRMT inhibitors
- Fusion genes
  - Recurrent fusions involving *NF2*, *BAP1*, *SETD2*, *PBRM1*, and *PTEN* have been reported
  - *ALK* fusions reported in rare cases of peritoneal mesothelioma in children and young adults
  - *EWSR1* fusions have been reported in rare cases of epithelioid pleural and peritoneal mesotheliomas in younger patients without history of asbestos exposure
  - No gene fusions were identified in TCGA cohort of 73 pleural mesotheliomas

FISH

- Can detect deletion of *CDKN2A*

Molecular Genetics

- Activating mutations in oncogenes are rare
- Recurrently mutated genes detected by targeted next-generation sequencing (NGS)
- Frequently mutated genes include *BAP1*, *NF2*, *TP53*, *SETD2*, *DDX3X*, *ULK2*, *RYR2*, *CFAP45*, *SETDB1*, and *DDX51*
  - *BAP1* somatic mutations present in ~ 20% of cases
    - *BAP1*-altered pleural mesotheliomas demonstrate mRNA signature of activated dendritic cells and with higher expression of PDL1 per The Cancer Genome Atlas (TCGA) data in pleural mesothelioma
    - Loss of *BAP1* may serve as predictive biomarker for immunotherapy in peritoneal mesothelioma
    - Sarcomatoid mesotheliomas are also positive for PDL1 (CD274) per one recent study
  - *TP53* somatic mutations detected in ~ 8% of mesotheliomas, associated with aggressive clinical behavior
  - *TP53* and *SETDB1* comutations associated with genome-wide loss of heterozygosity per TCGA data
    - Affects > 80% of genome ("genomic near-haploidization"), mostly in young female patients
- *YAP1* amplification in subsets of cases

MICROSCOPIC

Histologic Features

- Epithelioid type: Tubulopapillary, glandular, and solid patterns resembling adenocarcinomas
  - Less differentiated tumors may show sheets of polygonal cells
- Sarcomatous type: Spindled cell proliferation that resembles sarcoma
  - No epithelial component
- Biphasic (mixed) type: Contains both epithelioid and sarcomatoid elements

ANCILLARY TESTS

Immunohistochemistry

- Positive for calretinin, WT1, CK5/6, D2-40, mesothelin, and GATA3
  - Essential for diagnosis and in differential diagnosis
- Negative for TTF-1, Napsin A, CEA, CD15, BEREP4, and MOC31
- Loss of BAP1, MTAP, Merlin, &/or CDKN2A
  - Triple loss of BAP1, MTAP, and Merlin expression reported to be 90% sensitive for mesothelioma

Molecular Testing

- Blood-based biomarkers, such as calretinin and others, are under evaluation but currently not recommended for clinical use
- *BAP1* or *CDKN2A* loss testing by FISH or NGS desirable

DIFFERENTIAL DIAGNOSIS

Lung Carcinomas Including Adenocarcinoma

- Lack expression of mesothelial-associated antigens
- Expression of pulmonary adenocarcinoma markers, including TTF-1 and Napsin A

Metastatic Tumors

- Clinical history
- Lack mesothelial-associated markers
- Expression of tumor-specific markers would help to distinguish from mesothelioma

Other Rare Tumors

- Sarcomas, including synovial sarcoma

SELECTED REFERENCES

1. Kwon J et al: BAP1 as a guardian of genome stability: implications in human cancer. Exp Mol Med. 55(4):745-54, 2023
2. Calvet L et al: YAP1 is essential for malignant mesothelioma tumor maintenance. BMC Cancer. 22(1):639, 2022
3. Carbone M et al: Medical and surgical care of patients with mesothelioma and their relatives carrying germline BAP1 mutations. J Thorac Oncol. 17(7):873-89, 2022
4. Chapel DB et al: Clinical and molecular validation of BAP1, MTAP, P53, and Merlin immunohistochemistry in diagnosis of pleural mesothelioma. Mod Pathol. 35(10):1383-97, 2022
5. Churg A et al: Well differentiated papillary mesothelial tumor: a new name and new problems. Mod Pathol. 35(10):1327-33, 2022
6. Davis A et al: An update on emerging therapeutic options for malignant pleural mesothelioma. Lung Cancer (Auckl). 13:1-12, 2022
7. Hiltbrunner S et al: Genomic landscape of pleural and peritoneal mesothelioma tumours. Br J Cancer. 127(11):1997-2005, 2022
8. IARC: WHO Classification of Tumours: Thoracic Tumours, 5th ed. IARC, 2021
9. Kiesgen S et al: Chimeric antigen receptor (CAR) T-cell therapy for thoracic malignancies. J Thorac Oncol. 13(1):16-26, 2018
10. Brosseau S et al: A review of bevacizumab in the treatment of malignant pleural mesothelioma. Future Oncol. 13(28):2537-46, 2017
11. Disselhorst MMJ et al: Optimal therapy of advanced stage mesothelioma. Curr Treat Options Oncol. 18(8):48, 2017
12. Galetta D et al: Primary thoracic synovial sarcoma: factors affecting long-term survival. J Thorac Cardiovasc Surg. 134(3):808-9, 2007

Mesothelioma

Epithelioid Mesothelioma

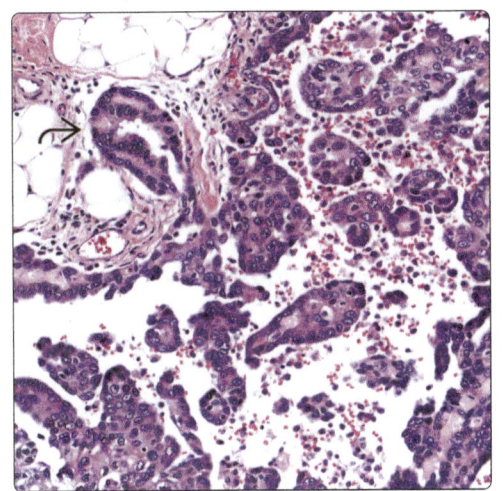

Calretinin Immunohistochemistry

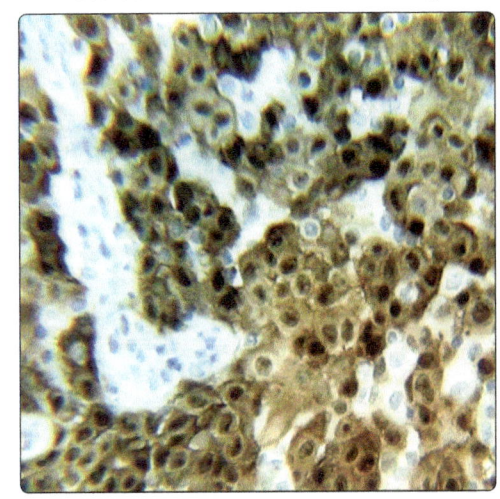

(Left) Epithelioid mesothelioma with tubulopapillary differentiation is shown. Invasion into adjacent fibroadipose tissue ⇲ is present. (Right) Calretinin of well-differentiated pleural mesothelioma is shown. Neoplastic cells show prominent nuclear and cytoplasmic staining, which is characteristic of epithelioid mesothelioma.

WT1 Immunohistochemistry

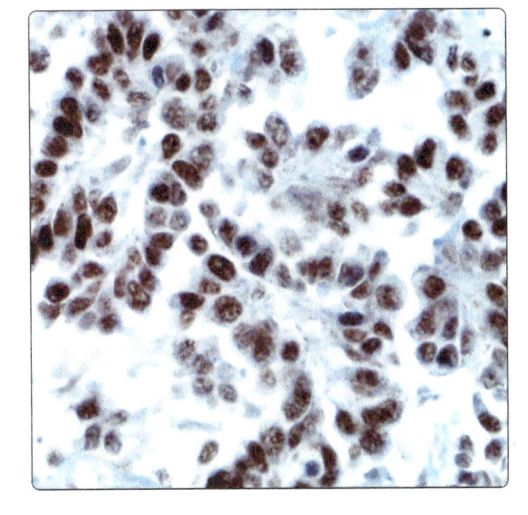

D2-40 Immunohistochemistry

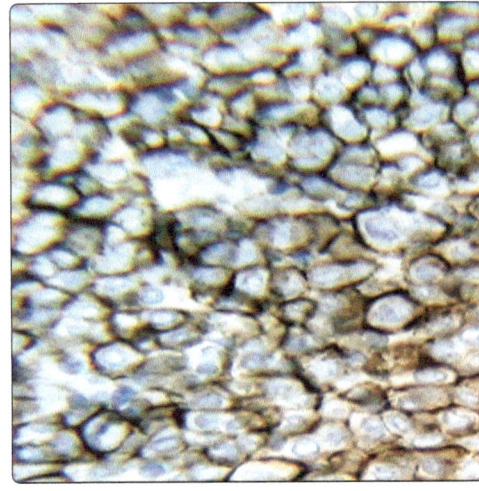

(Left) WT1 of epithelioid pleural mesothelioma shows strong and uniform nuclear positivity among neoplastic cells with no cytoplasmic staining. (Right) D2-40 of epithelioid mesothelioma is shown. Notice that the neoplastic cells show strong and thick cytoplasmic membrane staining.

CK5/6 Immunohistochemistry

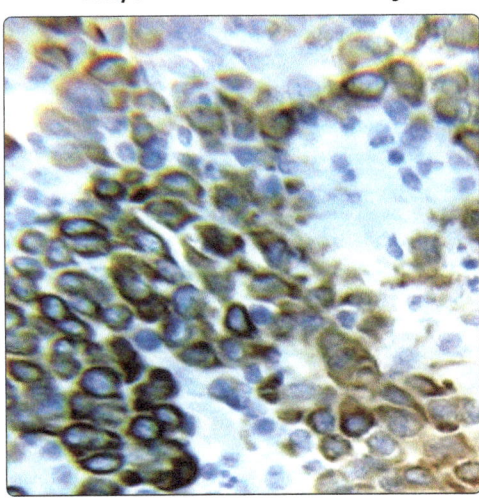

BAP1 Immunohistochemistry

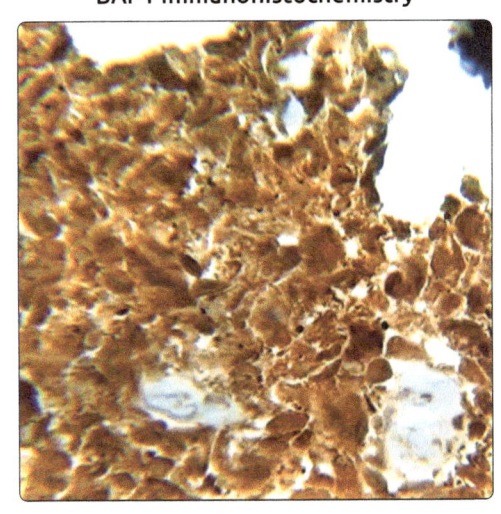

(Left) CK5/6 of well-differentiated epithelioid mesothelioma is shown. The neoplastic cells exhibit strong cytoplasmic positivity with no nuclear staining. (Right) BAP1 of sarcomatous mesothelioma shows strong nuclear expression by neoplastic cells. Diagnosis of sarcomatous mesothelioma can be challenging. A broad panel of antibodies that include mesothelial-associated markers could prove helpful to establish the correct diagnosis.

Gastric Adenocarcinoma

KEY FACTS

TERMINOLOGY
- Gastric adenocarcinoma (GA)
  - Malignant epithelial neoplasm of stomach
  - Comprises > 95% of all stomach cancers

ETIOLOGY/PATHOGENESIS
- Multifactorial disease, including genetic alterations and environmental factors
  - *Helicobacter pylori* responsible for 75-95% of all GA cases
  - Epstein-Barr virus association in ~ 10% of all GA cases
  - > 10% of cases are genetic or hereditary associated

CLINICAL ISSUES
- Most common in Eastern Asia, Eastern Europe, and South America
- Lowest rates in North America and Africa
- Stage is strongest prognosticator
- FDA-approved targeted therapeutic agents
  - HER2 inhibitor for GA with ERBB2 (HER2) overexpression
  - Immune checkpoint inhibitors for cases with MSI-H, PD-L1(+), or TMB-H
  - TRK inhibitors for GA with *NTRK1/NTRK2/NTRK3* fusions
  - RET inhibitor for GA with *RET* fusions
  - BRAF inhibitors for GA with *BRAF* V600E mutation

ANCILLARY TESTS
- *ERBB2* (HER2) testing
  - Overexpression defined as IHC 3(+) or IHC 2(+) and FISH (+)
    - FISH: *ERBB2*:*CEP17* ratio ≥ 2 defines *ERBB2* amplification
- MSI or MMR
  - Universal microsatellite instability by PCR or MMR deficiency (dMMR) by IHC is recommended for all patients with newly diagnosed GA
  - Genetics referral required for all LS-related dMMR
- *NTRK1/NTRK2/NTRK3*, *RET*, *BRAF* analysis by NGS panel

ERBB2 (HER2) Signaling Pathway

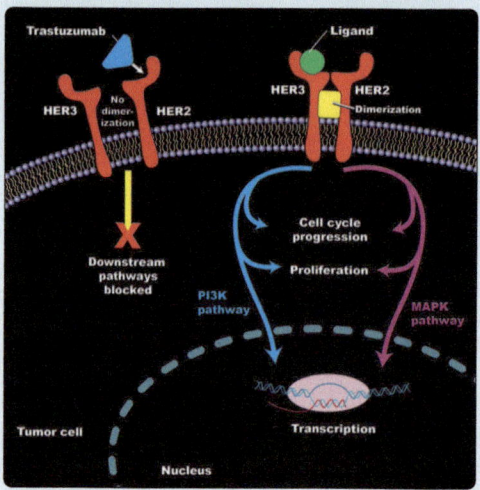

(Left) *Graphic shows the trastuzumab blockade mechanism. Trastuzumab binds to the ERBB2 (HER2) receptor, preventing dimerization and subsequently blocking downstream signal transduction pathways.*

Gross Appearance

(Right) *Gross photograph shows gastric adenocarcinoma forming a well-delineated mass with heaped-up borders and a large central crater.*

Signet-Ring Cell Adenocarcinoma

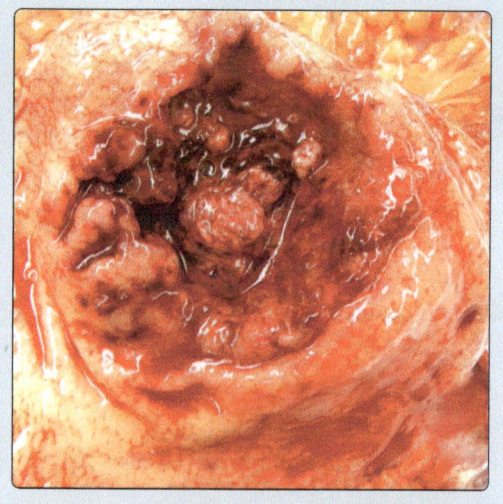

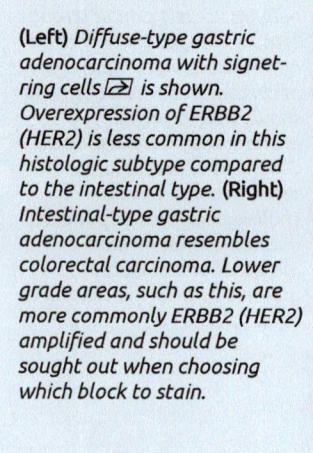

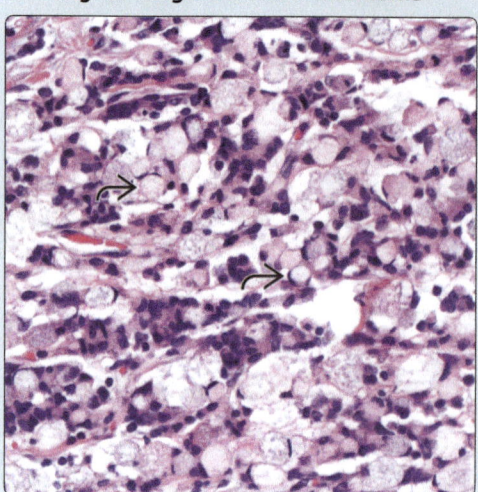

(Left) *Diffuse-type gastric adenocarcinoma with signet-ring cells ⇨ is shown. Overexpression of ERBB2 (HER2) is less common in this histologic subtype compared to the intestinal type.*

Intestinal-Type Adenocarcinoma

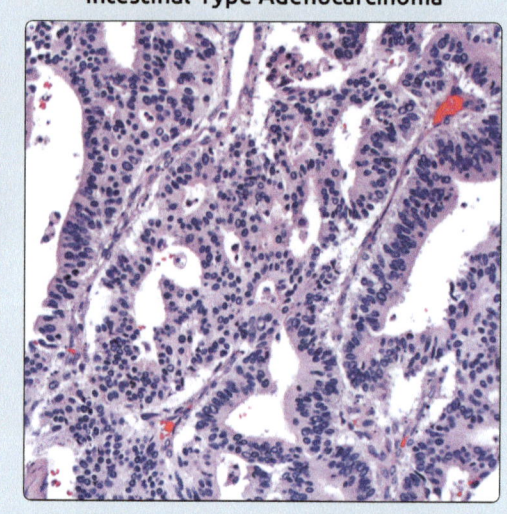

(Right) *Intestinal-type gastric adenocarcinoma resembles colorectal carcinoma. Lower grade areas, such as this, are more commonly ERBB2 (HER2) amplified and should be sought out when choosing which block to stain.*

Gastric Adenocarcinoma

TERMINOLOGY

Abbreviations
- Gastric adenocarcinoma (GA)

Definitions
- Malignant epithelial neoplasm of stomach
  - Comprises > 95% of all stomach cancers

ETIOLOGY/PATHOGENESIS

Underlying Causes
- Multifactorial disease
- Arises from sequential genetic alterations
- Risk involves environmental and genetic factors

Environmental Factors
- Infectious agents
  - *Helicobacter pylori*
    - Responsible for 75-95% of all cases
    - 3x increase in lifetime odds of developing GA
  - Epstein-Barr virus (EBV)
    - ~ 10% of GA worldwide are EBV-associated
      - Proximal stomach, diffuse type histology and early onset
- Autoimmune gastritis associated chronic inflammation
- Smoking, heavy alcohol use, diet high in salt and nitrite

Genetic Factors and Hereditary GA
- Responsible for minority of gastric cancers (< 10%)
- Hereditary diffuse gastric cancer (HDGC)
  - Autosomal dominant (AD) with germline mutations in *CDH1* in ~ 50%
    - Non-*CDH1*-mutated HDGC harbors germline mutations in *PALB2, CTNNA1, MSH2, RECQL5, ATM*, or *BRCA2*
  - 67-83% lifetime risk of developing GA
  - Most common form of hereditary GA
  - Associated with early-onset GA
    - Prophylactic gastrectomy at 18-40 years of age or
    - Screening endoscopy every 6-12 months
- Juvenile polyposis
  - AD with germline mutations in *SMAD4* or *BMPR1A*
  - ~ 9-50% lifetime risk of developing GA
- Peutz-Jeghers syndrome
  - AD disorder with germline mutations in *STK11*
  - ~ 29% risk of developing GA
- Lynch syndrome (LS)
  - AD, germline mutation in mismatch repair (MMR) genes
    - 2nd-hit mutation leads to MMR deficiency (dMMR)
  - 1-13% lifetime risk of developing GA
  - GA is 2nd most common cancer in LS
- Gastric adenocarcinoma and proximal polyposis of stomach (GAPPS)
  - Germline mutation in *APC*
  - Typically arises in fundic gland polyps
- Other hereditary cancer syndromes
  - Li-Fraumeni, Bloom, ataxia telangiectasia, Cowden, hereditary breast and ovarian cancer syndrome, and xeroderma pigmentosum

CLINICAL ISSUES

Epidemiology
- Incidence
  - > 1 million new cases and > 768,000 deaths per year worldwide
  - > 26,000 patients diagnosed annually in United States
  - 5th most common cancer and 3rd most common cause of cancer death worldwide
- Age
  - Most common in 5th decade and older
  - Younger presentation in hereditary syndromes
    - Average age at cancer diagnosis in HDGC is 37 years
  - Early-onset cases (patients < 50 years of age) increasing in USA
- Sex
  - M:F = 2:1
- Geographical distribution
  - 1/2 of worldwide cases of GA occur in Eastern Asia
  - Other high incidence areas include Eastern Europe and South and Central America
  - Lowest rates seen in North America and parts of Africa
  - Incidence has decreased substantially in United States and Western Europe over past several decades

Presentation
- Early cancer may be asymptomatic
- Advanced cancer may show nonspecific symptoms
  - Iron deficiency anemia, weight loss, abdominal pain, early satiety, dysphagia, indigestion, and vomiting

Endoscopic Findings
- Early cancers may be subtle
  - Thickened mucosal fold, plaque or focal erosion
- Advanced cancers
  - Ulcer or mass
  - Diffuse gastric wall thickening (linitis plastica)

Treatment
- Endoscopic mucosal resection
  - Option for treatment of cancers confined to mucosa or submucosa (early gastric cancer)
  - Combined with endoscopic US for staging
  - FNA of suspicious lymph nodes
- Total or subtotal gastrectomy with lymph node dissection
  - For advanced GA invading beyond submucosa
  - Neoadjuvant and adjuvant chemoradiation may be used
- FDA-approved targeted therapeutic agents
  - *ERBB2* (HER2) inhibitors (e.g., trastuzumab)
    - For GA with ERBB2 protein overexpression &/or *ERBB2* amplification
  - Immune checkpoint inhibitors
    - Pembrolizumab/nivolumab
    - For GA with MSI-H, PD-L1(+), or high tumor mutational burden (TMB-H)
  - TRK inhibitors: Entrectinib/larotrectinib
    - For GA with *NTRK1/NTRK2/NTRK3* fusions
  - RET inhibitor: Selpercatinib
    - For GA with *RET* fusions
  - BRAF inhibitors: Dabrafenib/tametinib
    - For GA with *BRAF* V600E mutation

Gastric Adenocarcinoma

Prognosis
- Stage at diagnosis is strongest prognosticator
- 5-year survival rates per tumor (T) stage
  - T1a: > 90%; T1b: 80%; T2: 60-80%; T3: 35-44%; T4: 16%

MACROSCOPIC

General Features
- Predominantly in antrum, often in lesser curvature
- Polypoid, fungating, ulcerated, or diffusely infiltrative

Size
- Ranges from microscopic to large and bulky

MOLECULAR

Gene Mutations
- *ERBB2* (HER2)
  - *ERBB2* amplification or ERBB2 protein overexpression results in constitutive activation of ERBB2 signaling pathway
    - ERBB2 overexpression is reported in 5-30% of cases
    - Independent predictor of poor prognosis

Proposed Molecular Classifications
- The Cancer Genome Atlas Project (TCGA)
  - 4 subtypes: EBV, microsatellite instability, genomically stable, and chromosomal instability

MICROSCOPIC

Major Histologic Subtypes (Lauren Classification)
- Intestinal
  - Gland-forming tumor with columnar to cuboidal cells
  - May also form papillary structures
  - Seen in *H. pylori*-associated GA
- Diffuse
  - Poorly cohesive cells that are isolated or arranged in small aggregates
  - Variably with signet-ring, plasmacytoid, anaplastic, and histiocytic features
  - Seen in EBV- and hereditary-associated GA
- Indeterminate
  - Mixed intestinal and diffuse types

WHO Classification
- Tubular and papillary (corresponds to Lauren intestinal type)
- Mucinous and poorly cohesive, including those with signet-ring cells (corresponds to Lauren diffuse type)
- Mixed (corresponds to Lauren indeterminate type)

ANCILLARY TESTS

Immunohistochemistry
- Positive for CK7, CK20, and CDX2
- Diffuse subtype is negative for E-cadherin
- EBER positive in EBV-associated cases
- ERBB2
  - Positive IHC is defined as IHC 3(+) or IHC 2(+) and FISH (+)
  - IHC interpretation criteria differ from those used in breast cancer
- MMR
  - MMR proficient (pMMR) tumor
    - Intact nuclear expression of MLH1, PMS2, MSH2, and MSH6 protein
  - MMR deficient (dMMR) tumor
    - Negative staining with positive internal control (mononuclear and stomal cells)
    - Lack of MSH2/MSH6, PMS2, or MSH6 expression is associated with LS
    - Lack of MLH1/PMS2 expression may be sporadic or LS associated
      - *MLH1* promoter gene methylation is typical present in sporadic tumors
      - Lack of *MLH1* promoter gene methylation may support LS but requires direct sequencing of MMR genes for confirmation
      - Genetic counseling referral required for all LS-related dMMR proteins
- Programmed death ligand-1 (PD-L1)
  - Combined positive score ≥ 1 indicates PD-L1 expression

Genetic Testing
- *ERBB2* (HER2) ISH
  - Perform if ERBB2 IHC score is (2+)
  - Targeted *ERBB2* centromeric *CEP17* probes used
  - *ERBB2:CEP17* ratio ≥ 2 defines *ERBB2* amplification
- Gene mutation testing
  - Comprehensive genomic profiling for tissue-limited case
    - *NTRK1/NTRK2/NTRK3*, RET, BRAF, ERBB2, MSI, and TMB by NGS
- MSI
  - MSS: No changes in any of 5 NCI-designated or mononucleotide microsatellite markers
  - MSI-high (MSI-H): Changes in ≥ 2 microsatellite markers
- TMB
  - TMB-high (TMB-H): Defined as ≥ 10 mutations/megabase of DNA

DIFFERENTIAL DIAGNOSIS

Lymphoma
- Diffuse large B-cell lymphoma may mimic diffuse-type GA
- Cytokeratin (-), CD45(+), CD20(+)

Metastatic Carcinoma
- Lobular breast carcinoma may mimic signet-ring cell GA
- ER(+), PR(+), GATA3(+), mammaglobin (+), GCDFP-15(+)

Dense Histiocyte Infiltration
- Seen in gastric xanthoma and Whipple disease
- CD68(+), CD163(+), cytokeratin (-)

SELECTED REFERENCES

1. National Comprehensive Cancer Network: NCCN clinical practice guidelines in oncology. Accessed on April 7, 2023. https://www.nccn.org/professionals/physician_gls/pdf/gastric.pdf
2. Lordick F et al: Gastric cancer: ESMO clinical practice guideline for diagnosis, treatment and follow-up. Ann Oncol. 33(10):1005-20, 2022
3. Bartley AN et al: HER2 testing and clinical decision making in gastroesophageal adenocarcinoma: guideline from the College of American Pathologists, American Society for Clinical Pathology, and American Society of Clinical Oncology. Arch Pathol Lab Med. 140(12):1345-63, 2016
4. Correa P et al: The gastric precancerous cascade. J Dig Dis. 13(1):2-9, 2012

Gastric Adenocarcinoma

ERBB2 (HER2)-Nonamplified FISH

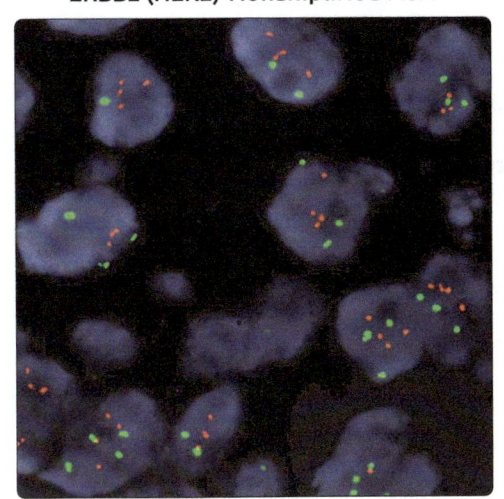

ERBB2 (HER2)-Amplified FISH

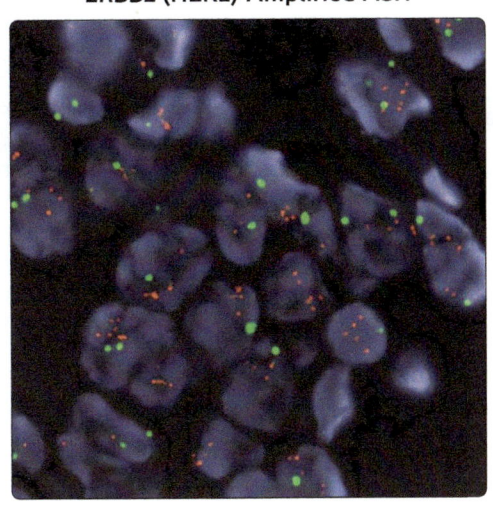

(Left) *FISH shows a nearly equal number of ERBB2 (HER2) and chromosome 17 centromeric signals (orange and green, respectively) yielding an ERBB2:CEP17 ratio of 1.2. A ratio of ≥ 2 is necessary to consider a tumor amplified for ERBB2 (HER2).* (Right) *FISH shows an increase in ERBB2 (HER2) signals (orange) compared to CEP17 signals (green). The ERBB2:CEP17 ratio is 3.8, indicating ERBB2 amplification.*

HER2 Positive With Score of 3(+)

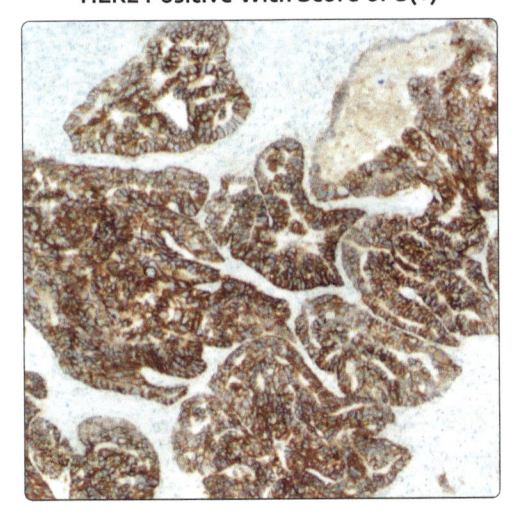

HER2 Equivocal With Score of 2(+)

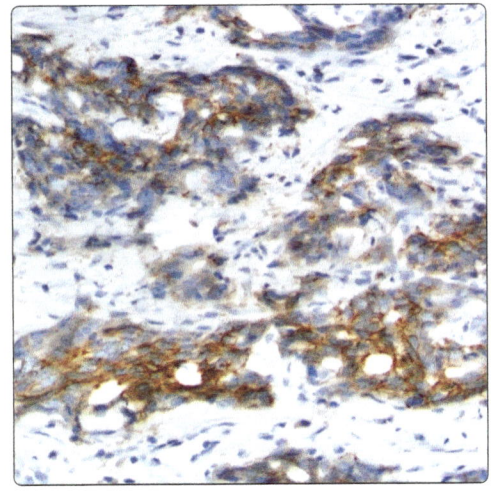

(Left) *Intestinal-type adenocarcinoma shows 3(+) positivity on HER2 stain. Strong, membranous reactivity is evident at low power.* (Right) *In contrast, evaluation at higher power was required to resolve the HER2 positivity in this adenocarcinoma. This is a resection specimen, so at least 10% of the tumor cells must be positive to render a score of 2(+). Notice many cells show incomplete lateral and basolateral staining.*

HER2 With Score of 1(+)

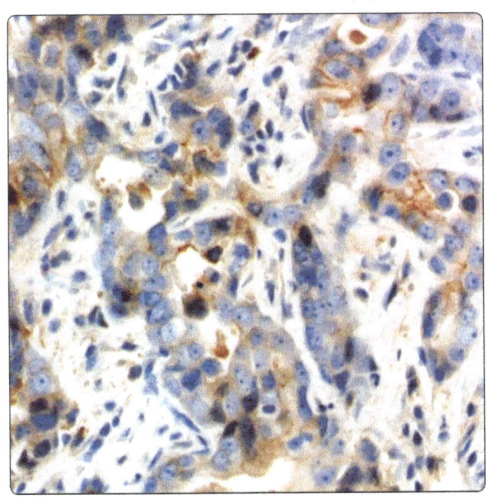

Heterogeneous HER2 Staining

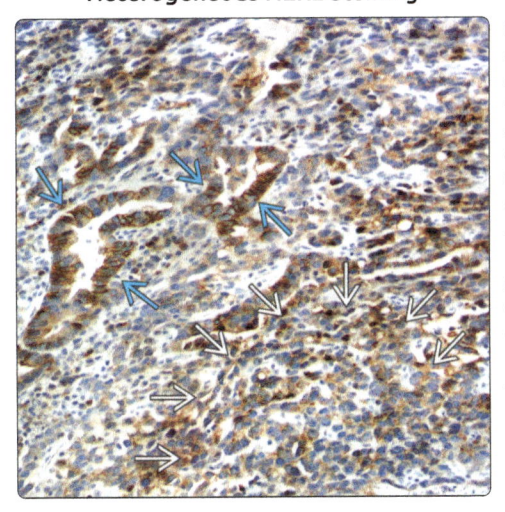

(Left) *HER2 shows faint, barely perceptible membranous reactivity in this adenocarcinoma, which was scored 1(+). Weak staining is only seen at high power.* (Right) *It is not uncommon for adenocarcinomas to show heterogeneous HER2 staining. This stain reveals 2(+) positivity in the well-differentiated component of this gastric adenocarcinoma (upper left) ➡ and 0-1(+) staining in the poorly differentiated component (lower right) ➡.*

Colorectal Adenocarcinoma and Precancerous Lesions

KEY FACTS

TERMINOLOGY
- Colorectal adenocarcinoma (CRC) is malignant epithelial neoplasm of colon
- Colorectal precancerous lesions are dysplastic epithelial neoplasms that typically present as adenomatous polyps or flat dysplastic lesions

ETIOLOGY/PATHOGENESIS
- CRC arises from sequential genetic alterations through various carcinogenic pathways
- Risk involves environmental and genetic factors

CLINICAL ISSUES
- Molecular subtyping of CRC helps refine patient prognosis
  - Sporadic MSI-H CRC shows most favorable outcome, especially with *BRAF* wildtype
  - MSS, *BRAF*-mutated CRC shows worst prognosis
- Effectiveness of EGFR inhibition for advanced-stage disease depends on downstream mutations
  - *KRAS*, *BRAF*, and *NRAS* mutations confer resistance to anti-EGFR therapy

ANCILLARY TESTS
- *KRAS*, *NRAS*, *BRAF* gene mutation testing
- NGS panel may detect other clinically actionable mutations
- LS screen testing
  - Universal LS screening recommended in all patients with newly diagnosed CRC
  - MSI by PCR, MMR by IHC or both
  - Reflex *BRAF* V600 testing
    – Perform if MSI-H &/or lacks MMR IHC expression (dMMR)
    – Reflex *MLH1* promoter methylation
      □ Perform if MSI-H &/or lacks MLH1 IHC expression
  - LS positive screen
    – MSI-H, dMMR IHC, *BRAF* wt, *MLH1* promoter nonmethylated
    – Genetics referral required for all LS positive screens

Colonic Adenocarcinoma With MSI-H

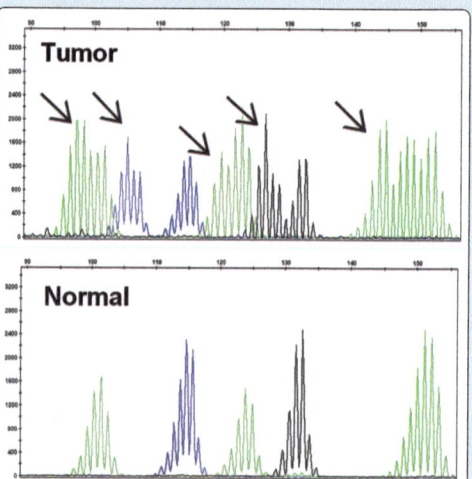

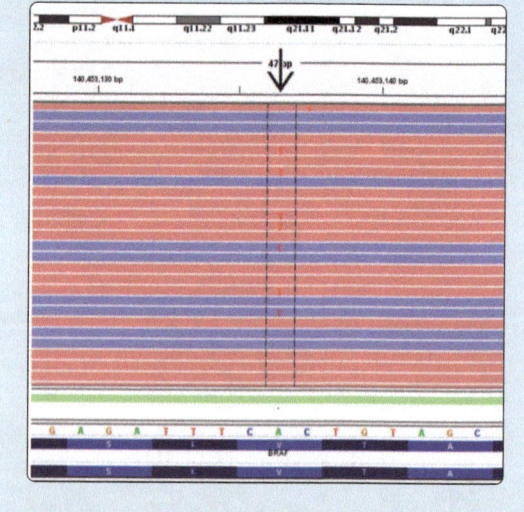

(Left) PCR analysis of paired tumor and normal DNA in colorectal adenocarcinoma (CRC) using 5 mononucleotide markers shows microsatellite instability in all 5 loci ➔, consistent with high degree of microsatellite instability (MSI-H). (Right) NGS of MSI-H CRC shows T to A ➔ base substitution in codon 600 of BRAF, diagnostic of BRAF V600E mutation. Presence of BRAF mutation supports sporadic CRC and virtually excludes Lynch syndrome (LS).

BRAF Mutation

EGFR Signaling Pathway

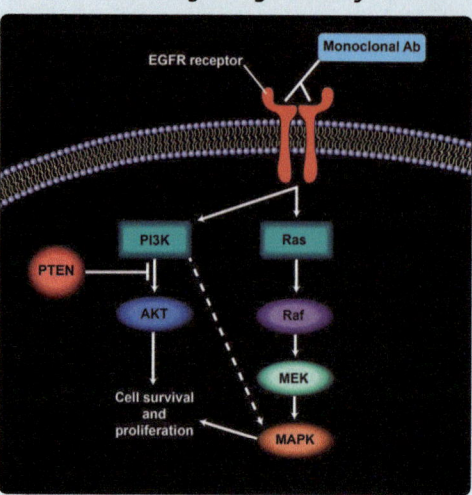

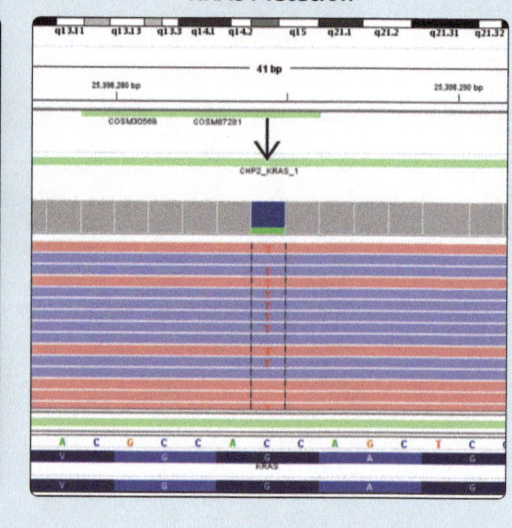

(Left) Monoclonal antibodies block ligand binding in the extracellular domain of the EGFR receptor, which inhibits activation of downstream oncogenes. However, mutation in KRAS results in constitutive activation of the EGFR signaling pathway. KRAS mutations confer resistance to anti-EGFR therapy. (Right) NGS of CRC shows a 35G>A (G12D) ➔ mutation in exon 2 of KRAS. The presence of an activating KRAS mutation confers resistance to anti-EGFR therapy.

KRAS Mutation

Colorectal Adenocarcinoma and Precancerous Lesions

TERMINOLOGY

Abbreviations
- Colorectal adenocarcinoma (CRC)

Definitions
- Malignant epithelial neoplasm of colon
- Colorectal precancerous lesions are epithelial-derived dysplastic epithelial changes that typically present as adenomatous polyps or flat dysplastic lesions
  o Some precancerous lesions progress to CRC

ETIOLOGY/PATHOGENESIS

Underlying Cause
- CRC arises from sequential genetic alterations through various carcinogenic pathways
- Risk involves environmental and genetic factors

Environmental Factors
- Western diet with high calorie and animal fat content
- Alcohol, smoking, sedentary lifestyle
- Chronic inflammation: Increased incidence in inflammatory bowel disease
- Protective factors: Diet high in vegetables, fiber, whole grains, exercise, and prolonged NSAID use

Carcinogenic Pathways of CRC and Precancerous Lesions
- **Chromosomal instability (CIN) pathway**
  o Sporadic and hereditary
  o Adenoma-carcinoma sequence
    – Accounts for ~ 60-70% of sporadic CRC
    – Inactivation of *APC* is initial mutation, present in 80% of adenomas and CRC
    – Activating mutations in *KRAS* (early event)
    – 18q loss of heterozygosity: Loss of *DCC/SMAD4*
    – Inactivation of *TP53* tumor suppressor gene
  o Sequential accumulation of mutations in *KRAS*, *DCC*, *SMAD4*, and *TP53* drives progression to CRC
- **Serrated adenoma/CpG island methylator phenotype (CIMP) pathway**
  o Sporadic and hereditary
  o MSI-high (MSI-H) or MSI-low (MSI-L)
    – MSI-H tumors account for ~ 15% of all sporadic CRC
  o *BRAF* V600E mutation
  o CIMP-high (CIMP-H)
    – Hypermethylation of promoter *MLH1*
      □ Loss of MLH1 leads to defective mismatch repair
  o Sessile serrated adenomas are precursors that progress to CRC
- **Mismatch repair (MMR) pathway**
  o Hereditary Lynch syndrome (LS) tumors, 2-4% of all CRC
  o MSI-H
  o *BRAF* wildtype (wt) in almost all cases
  o *MLH1* promoter methylation test more sensitive to separate hereditary from sporadic MSI-H cases
    – *MLH1* promoter hypermethylated in sporadic cases and only rarely in LS
  o MMR mutation results in defective DNA MMR proteins
    – Resulting accumulation of other mutations drives progression to CRC
- Other pathway classification systems
  o Cancer Genome Atlas Project
    – 3 groups: Chromosomal instability, hypermutated, and ultramutated
  o Consensus Molecular Subtypes Consortium
    – 5 groups: MSI, canonical, metabolic, mesenchymal, and mixed features

Precancerous Lesions
- **Tubular/tubulovillous adenoma (TA/TVA)**
  o Precursor polyps to conventional CRC
  o Inactivating *APC* mutation
    – Leads to development of dysplasia in aberrant crypt foci and early adenomas
  o Subsequent CIN pathway mutations drives progression to CRC
- **Sessile serrated lesion (SSL)**
  o Precursor polyp to CIMP-H, MSI-H CRC
  o Initiating *BRAF* mutation
  o Progressive CpG island hypermethylation
  o *MLH1* promoter hypermethylation commonly seen with progression to cytologic dysplasia
- **Traditional serrated adenoma**
  o Poorly characterized compared to TA and SSL
  o Molecularly diverse
    – May harbor *KRAS* or *BRAF* mutations as early events
    – May show low or high CIMP, or non-CIMP
  o Associated with *MGMT* promoter methylation
  o Typically do not show *MLH1* promoter hypermethylation or loss of MLH1 protein expression, and not associated with MSI-H CRC
  o WNT pathway activating mutations (*CTNNB1*, *APC*, *RNF43*) can occur but appear to be late events
  o May give rise to *BRAF*- or *KRAS*-mutated MSS CRC
- **Microvesicular hyperplastic polyp**
  o *BRAF* mutations present in ~ 70%
  o ~ 47-73% are CIMP positive
  o Speculation that these may be precursors to SSL
- **Goblet cell-rich hyperplastic polyp**
  o *KRAS* mutations in ~ 50%

Genetic Factors and Hereditary CRC
- **Lynch syndrome**
  o Autosomal dominant (AD) with germline mutation in MMR genes: *MSH2* (50%), *MLH1* (30-40%), *MSH6* (~ 7-10%), *PMS2* (< 5%)
    – 2nd-hit somatic mutation leads to MMR deficiency (dMMR)
  o 70% lifetime risk of developing CRC
  o Most common form of hereditary CRC
  o Associated with early-onset CRC
- **Serrated polyposis syndrome**
  o Genetic alterations similar to serrated pathway CRC
  o ~ 25-40% risk of of developing CRC
- **Familial adenomatous polyposis (FAP)**
  o Germline *APC* mutation with 2nd-hit somatic mutation
  o ~ 90-100% risk of developing CRC
  o Often thousands of colonic tubular adenomas
  o Attenuated FAP has < 100 adenomas with ~ 70% risk for development of CRC
- **MUTYH-associated polyposis**

Colorectal Adenocarcinoma and Precancerous Lesions

- o *MUTYH* mutations result in heritable predisposition to colon and gastric cancer
- o Biallelic mutations in *MUTYH* with 35-53% risk of CRC in adulthood
- Juvenile polyposis
  - o Germline mutations in *SMAD4* or *BMPR1A* with autosomal dominant pattern
  - o Polyps appear benign, but patient has ~ 40% risk of developing CRC
- Peutz-Jeghers syndrome
  - o AD disorder with germline mutations in *STK11*
  - o ~ 40% risk of developing CRC
- PTEN hamartoma tumor syndromes
  - o Germline mutations in *PTEN* associated with variety of syndromes, including Cowden, Bannayan-Riley-Ruvalcaba, and others
  - o ~ 13-16% risk of developing CRC

CLINICAL ISSUES

Epidemiology
- Incidence
  - o ~ 1.9 million new cases per year worldwide and 150,000 new cases per year in United States
  - o 3rd most common cancer worldwide
- Age
  - o Median at diagnosis was 72 years in 2000, now is 66 years
  - o Early-onset cases (< 50 year) have steadily increased in past few decades and are projected to continue increasing

Presentation
- Often asymptomatic, identified on screening
- Change in bowel habits
- Iron-deficiency anemia (right sided tumors)
- Hematochezia (left-sided tumors)
- Tenesmus (rectal tumors)

Treatment
- Surgical resection for stage I tumors
- Adjuvant chemotherapy after surgical resection for stage III CRC and high-risk stage II tumors
- Patients with stage II MSI-H CRC may not benefit from adjuvant 5-fluorouracil (5-FU)-based chemotherapy
- Targeted EGFR antibodies in advanced-stage disease with wildtype *KRAS*, *BRAF*, and *NRAS*
- Immune checkpoint inhibitors are FDA approved for advanced dMMR/MSI-H tumors
- TRK inhibitors are a treatment option for *NTRK* fusion positive metastatic CRC
- Selpercatinib RET inhibitor is treatment option for *RET* fusion positive metastatic CRC
- Tucatinib and trastuzumab combination is now FDA approved for *ERBB2* (HER2)-amplified CRC for some patients with advanced disease

Prognosis
- Association of molecular subtypes and patient survival
  - o MSI-H CRC shows most favorable outcome, especially with wildtype *BRAF*
  - o MSS, *BRAF*-mutated CRC shows worst prognosis

MACROSCOPIC

General Features
- Exophytic, fungating mass
- Annular mass with circumferential mural growth (apple core lesion)
- MSI-H and MSS/CIMP-H tumors are frequently located in right colon
- MSS/CIMP-negative tumors are frequently located in left colon

MOLECULAR

Gene Mutations
- *KRAS* and *NRAS*
  - o *RAS* mutation testing mandatory for all patients who are candidates for anti-EGFR therapy
  - o Activating mutations in 40%-50% (*KRAS*) and 1-6% (*NRAS*) of CRC respectively
    - Presence of mutation precludes treatment with anti-EGFR monoclonal antibodies (cetuximab and panitumumab)
      □ Significantly reduced response to EGFR blockade
- *BRAF* V600E
  - o Mutually exclusive of *KRAS* mutation in most cases
  - o Associated with reduced response to anti-EGFR targeted therapy in advanced CRC unless given with BRAF inhibitor
    - Insufficient evidence to recommend *BRAF* mutational status as predictive test for EGFR blockade
  - o Indicates poor prognosis in MSS or MSI-L CRC
    - *BRAF* mutation analysis should be performed in select patients for prognostic stratification
- *ERBB2* (HER2) amplification
  - o Detected in ~ 3% of CRC
  - o Appears to exclusively occur in MSS, *RAS/BRAF* wt CRC
  - o Appears to correlate with resistance to EGFR blockade, but currently not recommended for determining patient eligibility for EGFR blockade
  - o Combination of tucatinib and trastuzumab is now FDA-approved for some patients with *ERBB2* (HER2)-amplified tumors and advanced disease
- *PIK3CA*
  - o Activating mutations in 10-30% of all CRC
  - o Unclear whether mutations are of prognostic significance, though poor survival inconsistently reported in resectable stage I-III CRC
  - o Clinical effect of *PIK3CA* mutations on response to anti-EGFR therapy has shown conflicting results
    - Insufficient evidence to recommend *PIK3CA* mutational status for therapy selections outside of clinical trial
- MMR genes
  - o *MLH1*, *MSH2*, *MSH6*, and *PMS2*
    - Code for mismatch repair proteins responsible for DNA repair
  - o Inactivated through germline mutations or methylation
  - o *EPCAM*
    - Deletions of 3' end of *EPCAM* in 1-3% of LS
    - Mutations result in epigenetic silencing of *MSH2* and subsequent loss of MSH2/MSH6 protein expression

Colorectal Adenocarcinoma and Precancerous Lesions

- Germline *MSH2* mutation analysis usually includes testing for *EPCAM* deletions

MICROSCOPIC

Histologic Features
- Conventional CRC
  - Most are well- to moderately differentiated
  - ~ 15% are poorly differentiated with solid growth
- Microscopic features characteristic of MSI-H CRC
  - Mucinous, medullary, poorly differentiated, and signet ring cell phenotypes
  - Abundant tumor-infiltrating lymphocytes
  - Crohn-like peritumoral lymphoid aggregates

ANCILLARY TESTS

Genetic Testing
- **Gene mutation testing**
  - *KRAS*, *NRAS*, *BRAF* mutation by single gene or NGS panel
  - NGS panel may detect other clinically actionable mutations
  - *ERBB2* (HER2) amplification by IHC, FISH, or NGS in *RAS*/*BRAF* wildtype cases
- **Lynch syndrome screen testing**
  - Universal LS screening is recommended for all patients with newly diagnosed CRC
  - MMR by IHC or MSI by PCR or both for sensitivity near 100%
    - MMR IHC/MSI discordance rate: ~ 2%
      - Discordant show normal MMR IHC/MSI-H, as some dMMR mutations do not result in loss of immunoreactivity or MSI-H
  - Microsatellite instability (MSI)
    - 80-90% sensitivity for identifying LS
    - Test by PCR or NGS
    - MSI-H: Changes in ≥ 40% or ≥ 2 of 5 National Cancer Institute (NCI)-designated or mononucleotide microsatellite markers
    - Microsatellite stable (MSS): No changes in microsatellite markers
  - MMR IHC
    - 85% sensitivity for identifying LS
    - Shows MLH1, PMS2, MSH2, and MSH6 protein expression or loss
- **MMR IHC interpretation**
  - MMR proficient (pMMR) tumor
    - Intact nuclear expression of MLH1, PMS2, MSH2, and MSH6 protein
    - Associated with sporadic tumors
  - Uninterpretable IHC
    - Negative staining with negative internal control
    - Requires repeat IHC
  - MMR-deficient (dMMR) tumor
    - Negative staining of tumor with positive internal control (nonneoplastic mononuclear and stromal cells)
    - Lack of MSH2/MSH6, PMS2 or MSH6 expression
    - Mutated *MSH2* leads to loss of MSH2 and MSH6 expression but not vice versa for mutated *MSH6*
    - Mutated *PMS2* leads to loss of PMS2 expression
    - Mutated *MSH6* leads to loss of MSH6 expression
    - Seen in LS-associated CRC
    - Reflex to *BRAF* V600E and MSI testing
    - Lack of MLH1/PMS2 expression
      - Mutated or methylated *MLH1* leads to loss of MLH1 and PMS2 expression, but not vice versa for mutated *PMS2*
      - Seen in sporadic or LS-associated CRC
      - Reflex to *MLH1* promoter methylation testing &/or *BRAF* V600E mutation testing
  - Caveats
    - ~ 30-60% of patients with loss of MSH2 expression may have biallelic somatic mutations (not LS)
    - False-positive loss of MSH6 expression can occur in neoadjuvant-treated CRC
      - Repeat IHC on pretreatment diagnostic biopsy
    - MSI-H may not occur in CRC with germline *MSH6* mutation
  - Reflex BRAF V600E testing
    - Perform if MSI-H &/or lacks MMR IHC expression (dMMR)
      - *BRAF* mutation is associated with sporadic CRC
      - *BRAF* wildtype is associated with LS
  - Reflex MLH1 promoter methylation testing
    - Perform if MSI-H &/or lacks MLH1 IHC expression
    - Presence of *MLH1* promoter hypermethylation indicates *MLH1* silencing
      - Typically seen in MSI-H sporadic CRC and only rarely in LS
    - Lack of significant promoter methylation suggests germline mutations in the MMR gene *MLH1*
      - Typically seen in LS
  - Lynch syndrome positive screen
    - MSI-H, dMMR IHC, *MLH1* promoter nonmethylated
- **Germline testing**
  - Genetics referral required for all LS-positive screens for further evaluation
    - Evaluation may include germline MMR gene mutation testing and genetic counseling if indicated

DIFFERENTIAL DIAGNOSIS

Metastatic Carcinomas
- Lack or only weakly express CRC markers, such as CK20, CDX2, and SATB2

SELECTED REFERENCES

1. National Comprehensive Cancer Network (NCCN). NCCN clinical practice guidelines in oncology. Accessed April, 2023. https://www.nccn.org/professionals/physician_gls/pdf/colon.pdf
2. Bartley AN et al: Mismatch repair and microsatellite instability testing for immune checkpoint inhibitor therapy: guideline from the College of American Pathologists in Collaboration with the Association for Molecular Pathology and Fight Colorectal Cancer. Arch Pathol Lab Med. 146(10):1194-210, 2022
3. Sepulveda AR et al: Molecular biomarkers for the evaluation of colorectal cancer: guideline from the American Society for Clinical Pathology, College of American Pathologists, Association for Molecular Pathology, and the American Society of Clinical Oncology. J Clin Oncol. 35(13):1453-86, 2017
4. Müller MF et al: Molecular pathological classification of colorectal cancer. Virchows Arch. 469(2):125-34, 2016

Colorectal Adenocarcinoma and Precancerous Lesions

MMR-Deficient Adenoma

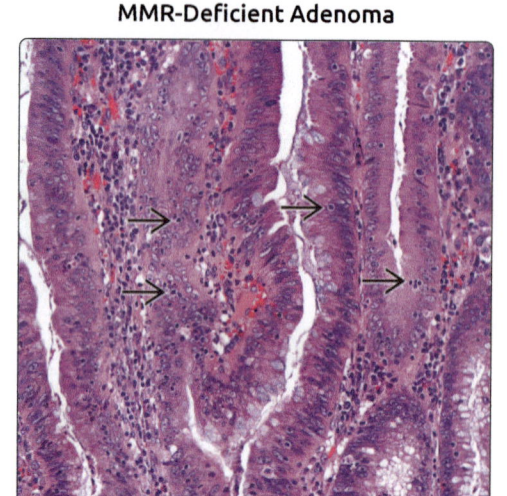

MSH2 Immunohistochemistry

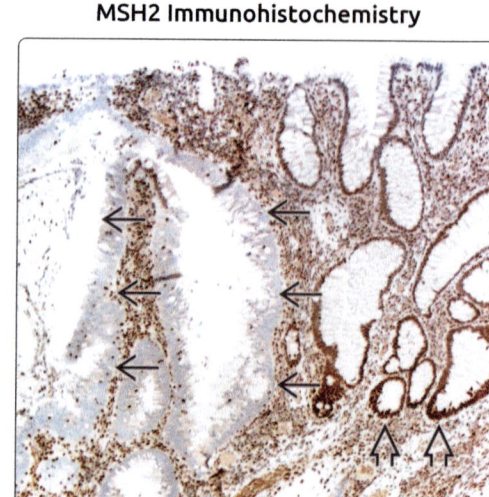

(Left) *Adenoma shows numerous tumor-infiltrating lymphocytes ⇒. MMR IHC is not routinely done on adenomas due to lack of sensitivity in preinvasive lesions, but this unusual finding prompted the stain.* (Right) *MSH2 shows loss of nuclear staining in the adenoma ⇒ and intact staining in the normal crypts ⇒ as well as in the stromal cells and lymphocytes that serve as internal controls.*

Medullary Carcinoma

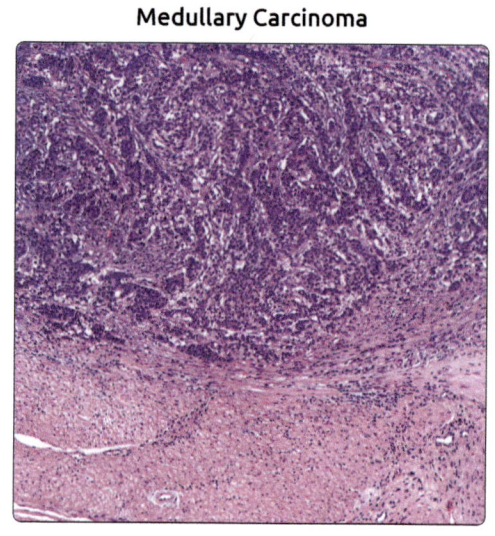

Signet-Ring Cell Carcinoma

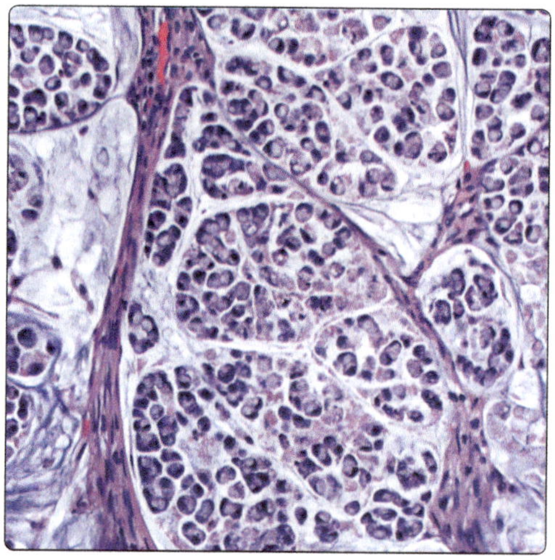

(Left) *MSI-H carcinoma shows a medullary phenotype characterized by tumor growth in solid sheets with no gland formation and a pushing, expansive border. Close examination reveals abundant tumor-infiltrating lymphocytes.* (Right) *MSI-H carcinoma shows a signet-ring cell phenotype.*

Mucinous Carcinoma

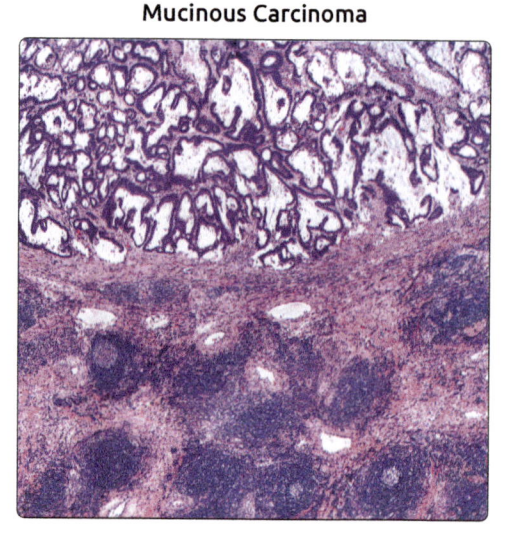

Conventional Adenocarcinoma

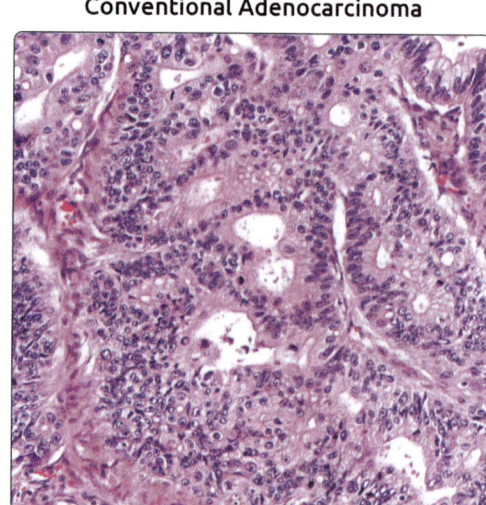

(Left) *Mucinous histology is also often seen in MSI-H colorectal carcinomas. This tumor additionally shows a Crohn-like peritumoral lymphocytic response, evident by prominent lymphoid aggregates at the invasive edge.* (Right) *Conventional colorectal adenocarcinoma arising from the chromosomal instability pathway (APC gene mutation, etc.) shows obvious gland formation and cribriform architecture.*

Colorectal Adenocarcinoma and Precancerous Lesions

Traditional Serrated Adenoma

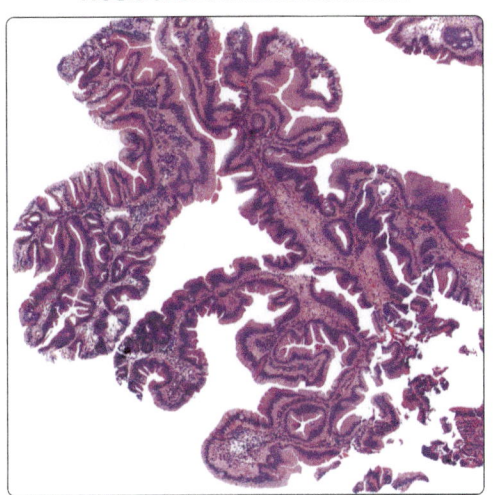

Ectopic Crypts

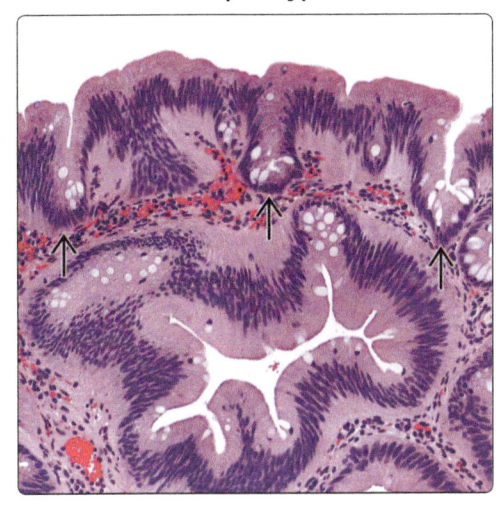

(Left) *Traditional serrated adenomas are uncommon but histologically distinct polyps. At low power, they have a villiform configuration and appear brightly eosinophilic due to their characteristic pink cytoplasm. These polyps may have admixed areas of conventional adenoma and sessile serrated adenoma.* **(Right)** *Small abortive crypts that fail to reach the muscularis mucosa (termed "ectopic crypts")* ➔ *can be found in the majority of traditional serrated adenomas.*

Microvesicular Hyperplastic Polyp

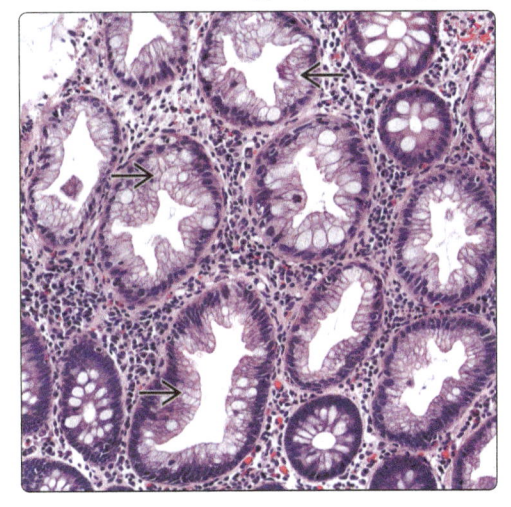

Goblet Cell-Rich Hyperplastic Polyp

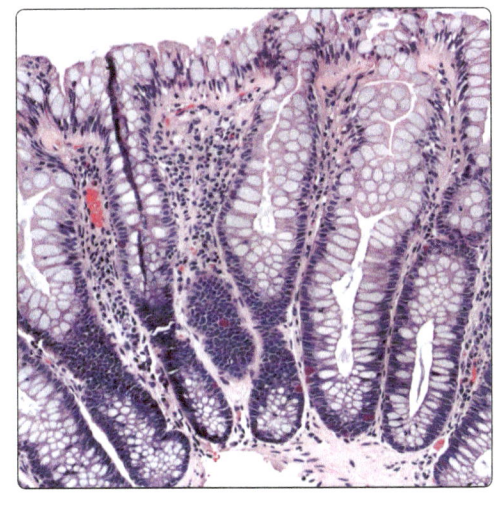

(Left) *Microvesicular hyperplastic polyps have obvious serrations that are present near the surface of the polyp. Their mucin is contained in goblet cells and in small microvesicles* ➔. *These polyps often have BRAF mutations and show a propensity toward hypermethylation.* **(Right)** *Goblet cell-rich hyperplastic polyps often lack prominent serrations, and their mucin is confined to goblet cells. KRAS mutations are more common in these polyps.*

Sessile Serrated Adenoma

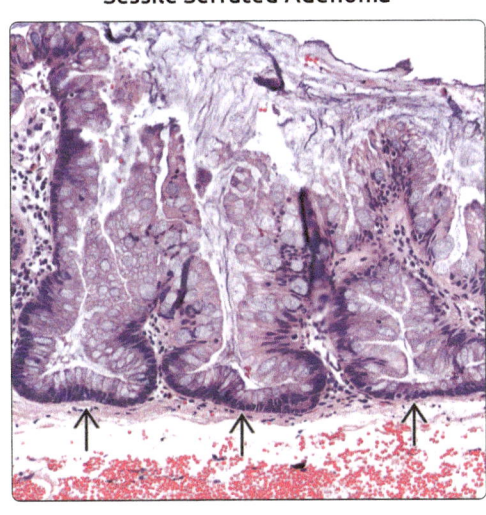

Juvenile Polyp

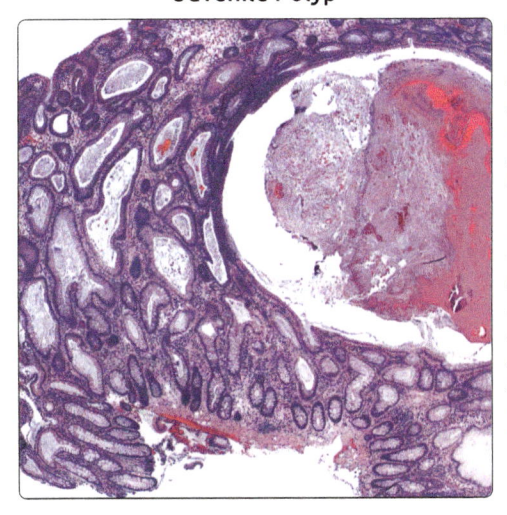

(Left) *Sessile serrated adenomas resemble microvesicular hyperplastic polyps in that they have obvious serrations and mucin present in small microvesicles. However, the serrations extend deep to the bases of the crypts, which are dilated and distorted* ➔. **(Right)** *Hamartomatous juvenile polyp in a patient with a SMAD4 mutation is shown. These polyps resemble inflammatory polyps but have markedly dilated glands containing abundant inspissated mucin.*

Gastrointestinal Stromal Tumor

KEY FACTS

TERMINOLOGY
- Mural-based mesenchymal tumor of gastrointestinal (GI) tract with differentiation toward interstitial cells of Cajal and characteristic histologic, immunohistochemical, and molecular features

ETIOLOGY/PATHOGENESIS
- Acquired mutually exclusive *KIT* or *PDGFRA* mutations in most cases
  - *KIT* somatic mutation in 75% of cases
  - *PDGFRA* somatic mutation in 10% of cases
  - Promotes ligand-independent cell proliferation
- *KIT* and *PDGFRA* wildtype GIST
  - Most demonstrate lack of function of succinate dehydrogenase (SDH) complex (SDH-deficient GIST)
    – Comprise 8% of all gastric GIST
  - *BRAF* mutation
    – Activation of RAS/RAF/MEK pathway
- Genetic factors and syndrome associations
  - Neurofibromatosis type 1 (NF1)
  - Familial GIST syndrome
  - Carney-Stratakis dyad
  - Carney triad

CLINICAL ISSUES
- Most common GI mesenchymal neoplasm
- Nonspecific symptoms at presentation
- Tumor behavior is primarily determined by location, size, mitotic rate, and mutation status
- Specific mutations render important information regarding treatment options
- Primary treatment consists of surgery and tyrosine kinase inhibitors (TKIs)
- Imatinib TKI
  - Tumor response depends on specific mutation
  - Acquired resistance may occur due to secondary resistance-associated mutations
- 2nd generation TKIs
  - Multikinase inhibitors, which act on other tyrosine kinases, such as VEGFR in addition to PDGFRA and KIT
  - Used to overcome imatinib TKI resistance
- TRK inhibitors: Entrectinib/larotrectinib
  - For GIST with *NTRK1/NTRK2/NTRK3* fusions
- BRAF inhibitors: Dabrafenib/trametinib
  - For GIST with *BRAF* V600E mutation

MOLECULAR
- Morphologic-molecular associations
  - Spindle cell GIST is typically *KIT* mutated
  - Adult gastric epithelioid GIST: *PDGFRA* mutated
  - Pediatric gastric epithelioid GIST: SDH deficient

ANCILLARY TESTS
- **Immunohistochemistry**
  - CD117
    – Positive in > 90% of GIST, including nearly all *KIT*-mutated tumors
    – Positive in SDH-deficient and *BRAF*-mutated GIST
  - DOG1
    – Usually captures CD117-negative GIST
  - PDGFRA
    – Expressed in GIST of any type
  - SDHB
    – Best stain for identifying SDH-deficient GIST
  - SDHA
    – Loss of expression reliably predicts tumor and subsequent germline *SDHA* mutation
- **Gene mutation testing**
  - *KIT, PDGFRA, BRAF, NF1, NTRK1/NTRK2/NTRK3*, and *FGFR* analysis by NGS panel
  - Genetics referral required for the following
    – *KIT, PDGFRA*, and SDHB IHC negative tumors
    – *NF1* mutation-positive tumors
    – Evaluation may include germline mutation analysis

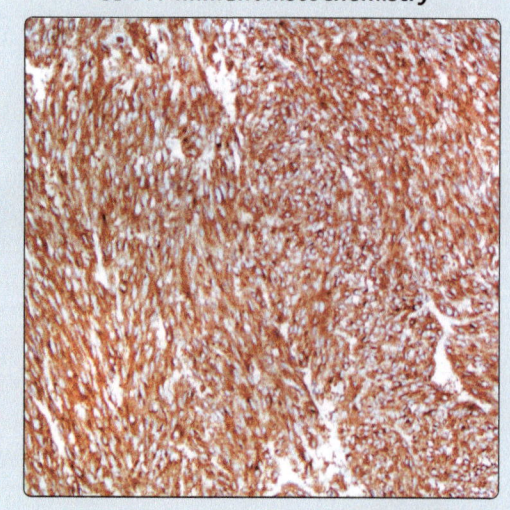

(Left) Sequence analysis using massive parallel sequencing (next-generation sequencing) on DNA extracted from a gastrointestinal stromal tumor (GIST) shows 6 bp (TGGAAG) deletion ➡ in exon 11 of the *KIT* gene. (Right) CD117 shows strong and diffuse cytoplasmic positivity in this GIST. Expression of CD117 is characteristic of most GIST.

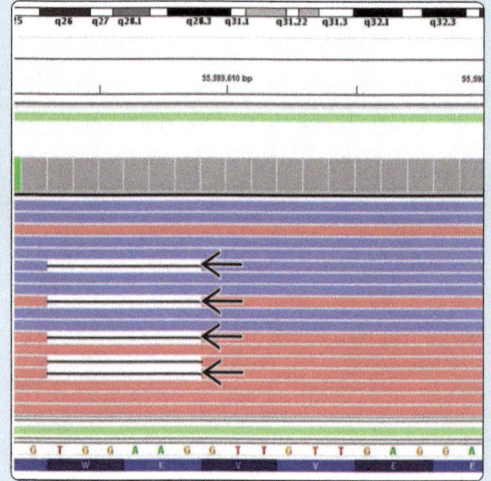

Gastrointestinal Stromal Tumor

TERMINOLOGY

Abbreviations
- Gastrointestinal stromal tumor (GIST)

Definitions
- Mural-based mesenchymal tumor of gastrointestinal (GI) tract with differentiation toward interstitial cells of Cajal and characteristic histologic, immunohistochemical, and molecular features
  - Composed of spindled &/or epithelioid cells
  - CD117 &/or DOG1 immunohistochemical positivity

ETIOLOGY/PATHOGENESIS

Underlying Cause of GIST
- Acquired mutually exclusive *KIT* or *PDGFRA* mutations in most cases
  - *KIT* somatic mutation in 75% of cases
  - *PDGFRA* somatic mutation in 10% of cases
  - Promotes ligand-independent cell proliferation
- *KIT* and *PDGFRA* wildtype GIST
  - Most show lack of function of succinate dehydrogenase (SDH) complex (SDH-deficient GIST)
    - SDH subunit gene mutation in ~ 60% of cases
    - *SDHC* gene promoter hypermethylation in ~ 40% of cases
    - Comprise 8% of all gastric GIST
  - *BRAF/KRAS* mutations
    - Activation of RAS/RAF/MEK pathway
    - Comprise 7-13% of all wildtype GIST in stomach and small intestine
- Genetic factors and syndrome associations
  - Neurofibromatosis type 1 (NF1)
    - Inactivating germline mutations in *NF1*
    - Constitutes 1-2% of all GIST
    - Multifocal, most commonly involves small bowel
  - Familial GIST syndrome
    - Germline mutations in *KIT* or *PDGFRA*
    - Multiple GIST along GI tract
    - Associated with aggressive behavior
  - Carney-Stratakis dyad
    - AD disorder with germline mutations in *SDH*
    - GIST in pediatric, adolescent, and young adult patients
    - GIST and paragangliomas
  - Carney triad
    - SDH-deficiency by *SDHC* gene promoter hypermethylation
    - Predominantly affects young women
    - GIST, pulmonary chondroma, and paraganglioma

CLINICAL ISSUES

Epidemiology
- Incidence
  - Most common GI mesenchymal neoplasm
  - 10-20 per million annually
  - Subclinical GIST more common
    - Up to 25% incidence of small incidental gastric GIST seen at autopsy
- Age
  - Older adults in *KIT* and *PDGFRA*-mutated GIST (median: 60-65 years)
  - Young adults and children in SDH-deficient GIST
    - Nearly all gastric GIST in patients < 21 years of age SDH deficient

Site
- Stomach: ~ 60%
- Jejunum/ileum: ~ 30%
- Duodenum: ~ 5%
- Rectum: < 5%
- Very rare in esophagus and appendix

Presentation
- Nonspecific symptoms
  - Gastric discomfort
  - GI obstruction
  - GI bleeding
  - Asymptomatic abdominal mass

Endoscopic Findings
- Round, mural, nonmucosal-based mass
- Small GIST usually found incidentally

Treatment
- Options, risks, complications
  - Primary treatment consists of surgery and tyrosine kinase inhibitors (TKIs)
- Surgical approaches
  - Wedge resection for single gastric GIST < 5 cm
  - Distal gastrectomy for large GIST involving pylorus or lesser curvature
  - Total gastrectomy for large, multiple, or recurrent GIST
  - Segmental resection for intestinal GIST
- Drugs
  - Imatinib (Gleevec) TKI
    - Inhibits receptor tyrosine kinases, including KIT
    - Tumor response depends on specific mutation
    - Neoadjuvant therapy to shrink GIST before surgery
    - 1st-line drug of choice to prevent recurrence in high-risk resected tumors
    - Acquired resistance may occur due to secondary resistance-associated mutations
  - 2nd-generation TKIs
    - Multikinase inhibitors, which act on other tyrosine kinases, such as VEGFR in addition to PDGFRA and KIT
    - Used to overcome imatinib resistance
    - Avapritinib
      □ FDA-approved for GIST with *PDGFRA* exon 18 or D842V mutation
    - Sunitinib, regorafenib, and pazopanib
      □ For unresectable SDH-deficient GIST
    - Ripretinib for patients already treated with ≥ 3 TKIs
  - TRK inhibitors: Entrectinib/larotrectinib
    - For GIST with *NTRK1/NTRK2/NTRK3* fusions
    - NCCN recommends as preferred 1st-line treatment
  - BRAF inhibitors: Dabrafenib/trametinib
    - For GIST with *BRAF* V600E mutation

Prognosis
- Risk stratification

Gastrointestinal Stromal Tumor

- Malignant potential determined by anatomic site, tumor size, and mitotic rate per 50 HPF for *KIT*- and *PDGFRA*-mutated GIST
- Mutation status
  - *KIT*-mutated GIST more aggressive than *PDGFRA*-mutated or triple-negative (KIT/PDGFRA/BRAF) GIST
  - *PDGFRA* exon 12, *BRAF*, and *KIT* exon 11 mutations associated with most favorable outcome
  - *KIT* exon 9 and *PDGFRA* exon 18 (non-D842V) mutations have worst outcome
- Less aggressive behavior seen in
  - Gastric GIST
  - *PDGFRA*-mutated GIST
- Intestinal and SDH-deficient GIST much less predictable than *KIT*-/*PDGFRA*-mutated GIST with same prognostic factors
  - Lifelong follow-up required due to 20-25% risk of liver metastases and risk of developing other syndrome-related tumors
  - Longer survival with metastatic disease compared to *KIT*-mutated GIST
  - More prone to recurrence compared to *KIT*- and *PDGFRA*-mutated GIST

IMAGING

CT Findings
- Peripheral contrast enhancement most common

Endoscopic Ultrasound
- Muscularis propria-based tumor
- Homogeneous, hypoechoic, round lesion with smooth margins
- Features more common in aggressive tumors
  - Heterogeneous, cystic, irregular borders, and size > 3 cm

MACROSCOPIC

General Features
- Well-defined, round to oval tumor in muscularis propria
- Firm to fleshy or gelatinous cut surface
- Hemorrhage and cystic degeneration in large tumors
- Tumor necrosis uncommon (poor prognostic factor)

Size
- Range from submillimeter to > 20 cm

MOLECULAR

KIT Mutations
- Relative frequency: 75-80%
- Exon 11
  - Highest imatinib response rate
  - Found in 70% of GIST
    - Common in gastric GIST
  - Mutations include deletions, insertions, and substitutions
  - Isolated inframe deletions most common and usually involve 5' end between codons 550-560
    - 557 and 558 deletions associated with aggressive behavior compared to other exon 11 mutations in gastric GIST
  - Point mutations usually associated with benign behavior
  - Probability of primary resistance (defined as tumor progression within first 6 months) to imatinib is ~ 5%
- Exon 9
  - Found in 10-15% of GIST, more common in jejunum/ileum
  - 6 bp insertion/duplication of AY residues encoded by codons 502-503 (most common)
  - Probability of primary resistance: ~ 16%
  - Shorter progression-free and overall survival compared to imatinib-treated exon 11-mutated GIST
  - More responsive to treatment with sunitinib
- Exon 13 and 17
  - Each found in ~ 1-2% of GIST
  - Point mutations most common
    - K642E in exon 13
    - N822K in exon 17
  - Exon 13 mutations may indicate poor prognosis in gastric GIST
  - No prognostic significance for exon 17 mutations
  - Variably sensitive to imatinib

PDGFRA Mutations
- Relative frequency: ~ 10%
- Lower malignant potential than *KIT*-mutated GIST
- Exon 18
  - D842V most common *PDGFRA* mutation
  - Found in 5% of GIST
  - Strongly resistant to imatinib
  - Responds to avapritinib
- Other exon 18 mutations (deletions and substitutions) uncommon
  - Found in 1% of GIST
  - Variable mutation-specific response to imatinib
- Exon 12
  - V561D common, followed by insertions and deletions
  - Found in 1% of GIST
  - Most respond to imatinib

SDH Deficiency
- Relative frequency: ~ 8%
- SDH-deficient GIST has lack of function of SDH complex
  - Complex consists of 4 subunits encoded by similarly named genes (*SDHA*, *SDHB*, *SDHC*, and *SDHD*)
- Inactivated by *SDHC* gene promoter hypermethylation or SDH subunit mutations
  - Mutations include substitutions (majority), deletions, splice-site, frameshift, and duplications
- *SDHA* is most commonly mutated gene (~ 35% frequency)
  - Usually germline mutations with low disease penetrance
  - So far not associated with familial tumor syndromes
  - Occurs in older patients (median age: 34 years)
- *SDHB*, *SDHC*, and *SDHD* mutations (~ 20-30% frequency)
  - Usually germline mutations
- 10-20% SDH-deficient GIST associated with Carney triad or Carney-Stratakis syndrome
- Resistant to imatinib

BRAF V600E Mutation
- Prognostic significance still unclear
- Candidate for therapy with *BRAF*-targeted drugs
- Show predilection for small bowel location

Gastrointestinal Stromal Tumor

Secondary Mutations
- Lead to development of imatinib resistance (secondary resistance-associated mutations)
- Secondary resistance defined as tumor progression 12-36 months following period of good response or stable disease
- Seen in 44-83% of GIST that progress after imatinib treatment
- *KIT* exons 13, 14, 17, and 18 are common targets
  - Sunitinib effective against secondary exon 13 and 14 mutations
  - Regorafenib effective 3rd-line therapy for exon 17 and 18 mutations
- Secondary *PDGFRA* mutations less frequent
  - Usually in exons 14 and 18

MICROSCOPIC

Histologic Features Indicating Aggressive Behavior for all GIST
- High mitotic rate
- Tumor necrosis
- Hypercellularity and sarcomatous appearance
  - Epithelioid sarcomatous tumors have slightly better prognosis than spindle cell counterparts
- Tumor extension into mucosa

KIT-Mutated GIST
- Spindle cell type most common; epithelioid and mixed types also occur
- Spindle cells arranged in fascicles or nodules
- Eosinophilic cytoplasm
- Elongated nuclei with vesicular chromatin and inconspicuous nucleoli
- Paranuclear vacuoles (artifact of fixation)
- Nuclear palisades in gastric tumors
- Skeinoid fibers in benign small intestinal tumors

PDGFRA-Mutated GIST
- Commonly epithelioid type
- Round to polygonal cells with distinct cell borders or with syncytial appearance
- Eosinophilic to pale or clear cytoplasm
- May have stromal sclerosis, myxoid change, or scant interstitial matrix
- Rhabdoid and plasmacytoid forms, binucleate and multinucleated giant cells

SDH-Deficient GIST
- Usually pure epithelioid type, less commonly mixed spindle/epithelioid
- Often multinodular or plexiform growth pattern
  - Most characteristic feature
- Hypercellularity is common
- Pleomorphism and tumor necrosis are rare
- Lymphovascular invasion seen in up to 50% of cases

BRAF V600E-Mutated GIST
- No known distinguishing histologic features

Features Described Following Imatinib Treatment
- Hypocellularity
- Stromal hyalinization, fibrosis, &/or myxoid change
- Necrosis
- Rhabdomyoblastic differentiation

ANCILLARY TESTS

Immunohistochemistry
- CD117
  - Positive in > 90% of GIST, including nearly all *KIT*-mutated tumors
  - Usually diffuse cytoplasmic positivity but may show membranous and perinuclear dot-like positivity
  - Staining patterns and extent of staining do not correlate with type of *KIT* mutation or response to imatinib
  - CD117 negative or only weakly positive GIST are usually epithelioid with *PDGFRA* mutations
  - Positive in SDH-deficient and *BRAF*-mutated GIST
- DOG1
  - Highly sensitive and specific marker for GIST
  - Positive in > 95% of tumors
  - Usually captures CD117-negative GIST
  - Small bowel tumors are negative, usually CD117 positive
- PDGFRA
  - Expressed in GIST of any type
    - Not surrogate marker for *PDGFRA* mutation
    - Also expressed in other tumors
- SDHB
  - Expression lost in **all** SDH-deficient GIST regardless of specific subunit alteration
    - Best stain for identifying SDH-deficient GIST
    - No genotype/phenotype correlation
- SDHA
  - Loss of expression reliably predicts tumor and subsequent germline *SDHA* mutation
    - Good genotype/phenotype correlation
- CD34
  - Positive in 70% of all GIST, but not specific
    - Consistently expressed in gastric spindle cell GIST
    - Negative in non-SDH-deficient gastric epithelioid GIST
- SMA
  - Negative or only focally positive in ~ 19-30% of GIST
  - Almost never expressed in SDH-deficient GIST
- Desmin
  - Usually negative
  - Focally expressed in 5% of epithelioid type tumors
  - Expressed in imatinib-treated tumors with rhabdomyoblastic differentiation
- S100
  - Usually negative
  - Focally expressed in < 1% of epithelioid-type tumors

Genetic Testing
- **Gene mutation testing**
  - *KIT*, *PDGFRA*, *BRAF*, *NF1*, and *FGFR* mutations and *NTRK1*/*NTRK2*/*NTRK3* fusions by NGS panel
  - Genetics referral required for the following
    - *KIT*, *PDGFRA*, and SDHB IHC-negative tumors
    - *NF1* mutation-positive tumors
    - Evaluation may include germline mutation analysis

Gastrointestinal Stromal Tumor

Clinical Prognostication of GIST From Largest Series (Untreated With Imatinib)

Size	Mitoses per 50 HPF	Metastases	Risk
Gastric Gastrointestinal Stromal Tumors			
≤ 2 cm	≤ 5	None	None to negligible
> 2 and ≤ 5 cm	≤ 5	2%	Low
> 5 and ≤ 10 cm	≤ 5	4%	Low
> 10 cm	≤ 5	12%	Intermediate
≤ 2 cm	> 5	None	Low
> 2 and ≤ 5 cm	> 5	16%	Intermediate
> 5 and ≤ 10 cm	> 5	55%	High
> 10 cm	> 5	88%	High
Small Bowel Gastrointestinal Stromal Tumors			
≤ 2 cm	≤ 5	None	None to negligible
> 2 and ≤ 5 cm	≤ 5	4%	Low
> 5 and ≤ 10 cm	≤ 5	24%	Intermediate
> 10 cm	≤ 5	52%	High
≤ 2 cm	> 5	50%	High
> 2 and ≤ 5 cm	> 5	85%	High
> 10 cm	> 5	90%	High

DIFFERENTIAL DIAGNOSIS

Leiomyoma
- Intersecting fascicles of brightly eosinophilic spindle cells
- Nuclei with blunted ends
- SMA(+), desmin (+), CD117(-), and DOG1(-)
  - Potential pitfall: CD117 and DOG1 may stain colonizing Cajal cells interspersed among smooth muscle bundles

Schwannoma
- Prominent lymphoid cuff
- Gastric schwannomas lack features of soft tissue counterparts
  - Verocay bodies, hyalinized vessels, and encapsulation
- S100(+), CD117(-), and DOG1(-)

Fibromatosis
- Arises in mesentery and extends into muscularis propria
- Poorly circumscribed with infiltrative growth pattern
- Nuclear β-catenin (+), CD34(-), DOG1(-), and CD117 usually negative

Glomus Tumor
- Rare in GI tract
- May mimic epithelioid GIST
- Positive for smooth muscle markers (SMA, H-caldesmon, and calponin), but desmin (-), CD117(-), and DOG1(-)

Clear Cell Sarcoma-Like Tumor of GI Tract
- Sheet-like or nested epithelioid or spindle cells with eosinophilic to clear cytoplasm
- Eccentric nuclei may impart plasmacytoid appearance
- S100(+), CD56(+/-), synaptophysin (+/-), CD117(-), DOG1(-), and CD34(-)
- *EWSR1::ATF1* or *EWSR1::CREB1* fusions

DIAGNOSTIC CHECKLIST

Clinically Relevant Pathologic Features
- *KIT*- and *PDGFRA*-mutated GIST
  - Tumor behavior determined by location, size, and mitotic rate
  - Specific mutations render important information regarding treatment options and response to imatinib

Pathologic Interpretation Pearls
- General morphologic-molecular associations
  - Spindle cell GIST typically *KIT* mutated
  - Gastric epithelioid GIST
    - In adult patient, typically *PDGFRA* mutated
    - In pediatric patient, typically SDH deficient

SELECTED REFERENCES

1. National Comprehensive Cancer Network: NCCN clinical practice guidelines in oncology. Accessed on April 18, 2023. http://chrome-extension://efaidnbmnnnibpcajpcglclefindmkaj/https://www.nccn.org/professionals/physician_gls/pdf/gist.pdf
2. Cao Z et al: GISTs with NTRK gene fusions: a clinicopathological, immunophenotypic, and molecular study. Cancers (Basel). 15(1), 2022
3. Recht HS et al: Carney-Stratakis syndrome: a dyad of familial paraganglioma and gastrointestinal stromal tumor. Radiol Case Rep. 15(11):2071-5, 2020
4. Paolo Dei Tos A et al: Gastrointestinal stromal tumour. In: WHO Classification of Tumours Editorial Board. Digestive system tumours. IARC, 2019
5. Sanchez-Hidalgo JM et al: Gastrointestinal stromal tumors: a multidisciplinary challenge. World J Gastroenterol. 24(18):1925-41, 2018
6. Schaefer IM et al: What is new in gastrointestinal stromal tumor? Adv Anat Pathol. 24(5):259-67, 2017
7. Miettinen M et al: Gastrointestinal stromal tumors. Gastroenterol Clin North Am. 42(2):399-415, 2013
8. Miettinen M et al: Succinate dehydrogenase-deficient GISTs: a clinicopathologic, immunohistochemical, and molecular genetic study of 66 gastric GISTs with predilection to young age. Am J Surg Pathol. 35(11):1712-21, 2011

Gastrointestinal Stromal Tumor

Paranuclear Vacuoles

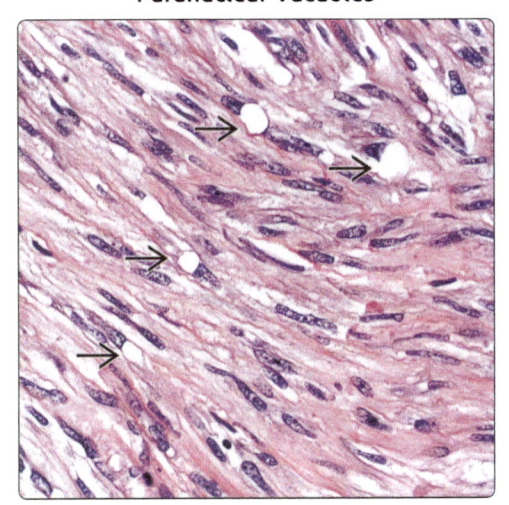

Epithelioid GIST

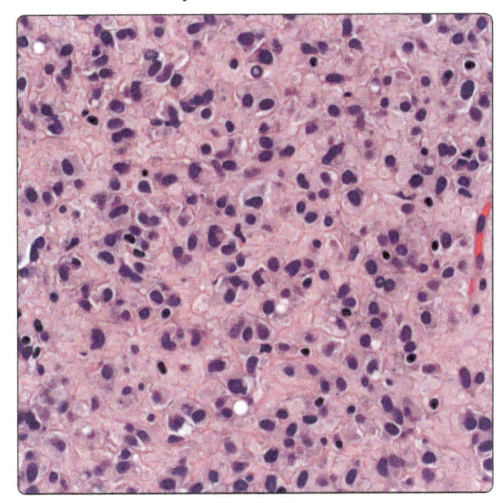

(Left) Typical low-risk spindle cell gastric GIST is shown. The cytoplasm is eosinophilic and fibrillary but not as brightly eosinophilic as what is seen in smooth muscle tumors. Paranuclear vacuoles ⇒ are evident and are a relatively common finding in low-risk GIST. (Right) This small intestinal GIST has an epithelioid phenotype and harbored a KIT exon 11 deletion. The epithelioid cells are polygonal with well-defined borders and round, uniform nuclei.

Low-Grade GIST

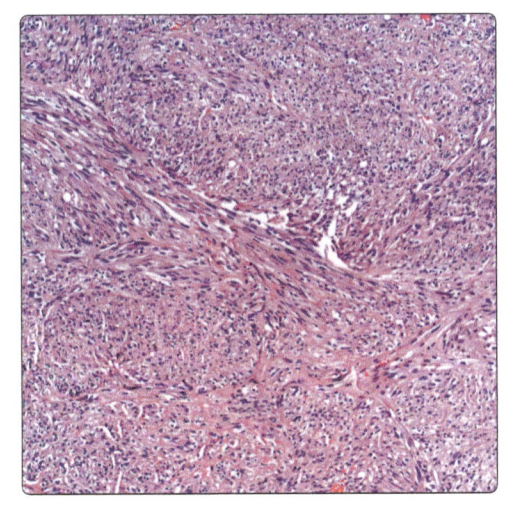

High-Grade GIST: Increased Cellularity

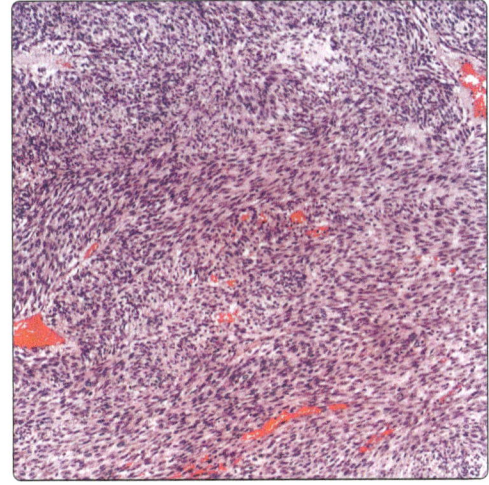

(Left) GIST with low cellularity is indicative of low-grade tumor. In addition to low cellularity, low-grade GIST lacks necrosis, lacks marked cytologic atypia, and has a low mitotic index. (Right) Increased cellularity is readily evident in this high-risk GIST. An accurate mitotic count is essential to ensure proper risk assessment in all GIST.

High-Grade GIST: Necrosis

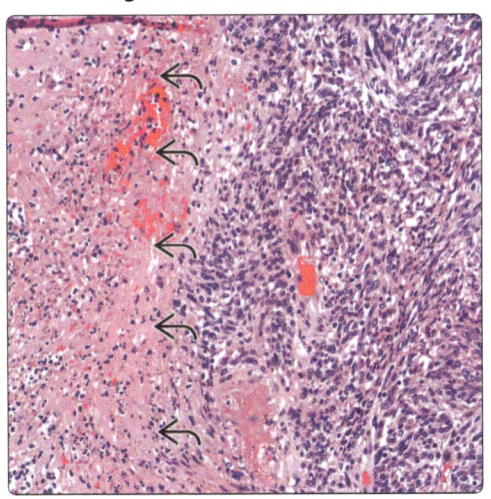

High-Grade GIST: Mitoses

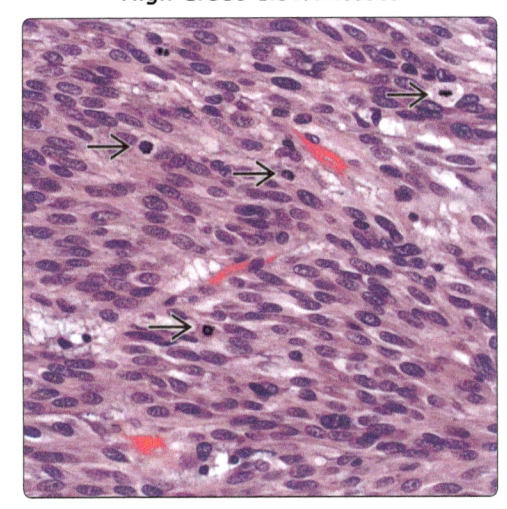

(Left) Area of necrosis ⇒ in high-risk GIST is shown. As in most soft tissue tumors, necrosis is a histologic indicator of aggressive behavior. (Right) High-risk GIST shows abundant mitoses ⇒ (~ 90 per 50 HPF). The high mitotic index in combination with the tumor size (11 cm in this case) and gastric location imparts an 88% risk of metastasis.

Gastrointestinal Stromal Tumor

Epithelioid GIST With Giant Cells

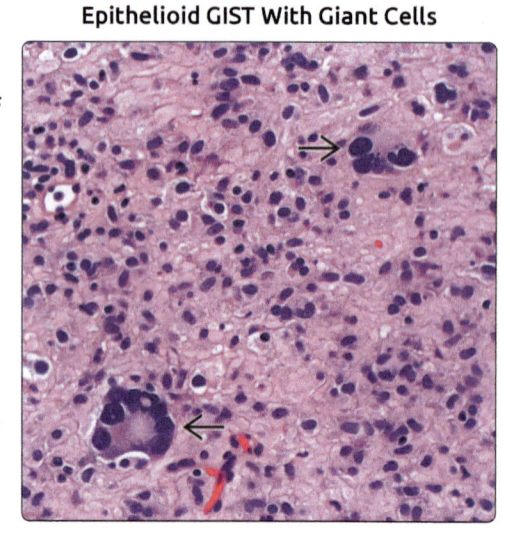

Plasmacytoid Cells

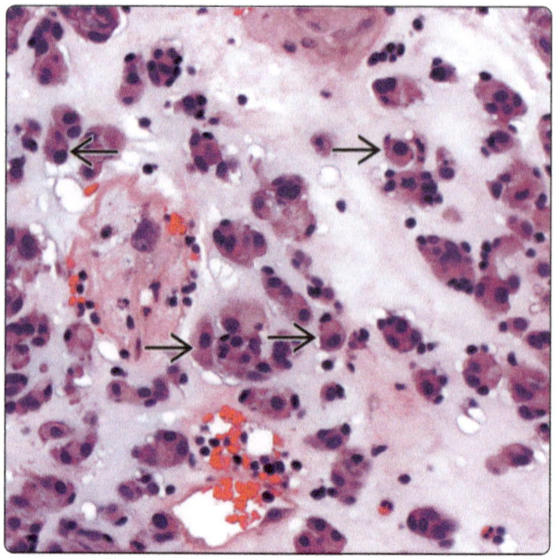

(Left) Variant microscopic features include tumor giant cells ⇒, which are seen in this epithelioid GIST. **(Right)** Another variant feature, plasmacytoid morphology ⇒, is shown. This GIST has cells with round, uniform nuclei that are eccentrically located within abundant pink cytoplasm. The stroma has a chondromyxoid appearance. CD117 or DOG1 are recommended in the work-up of any unusual, mural-based, gastrointestinal mesenchymal tumor to exclude the possibility of GIST.

Imatinib-Treated GIST

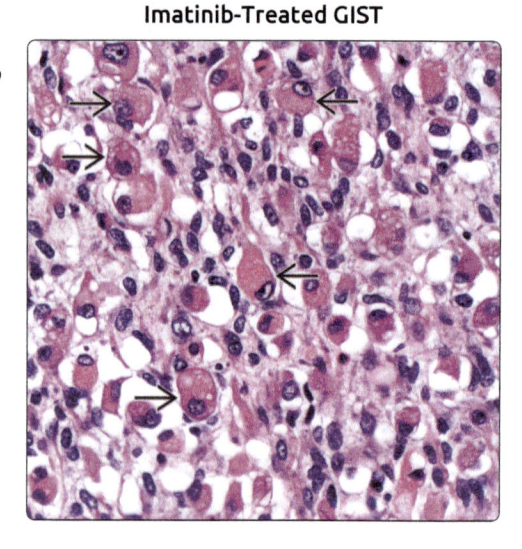

Desmin in Treated GIST

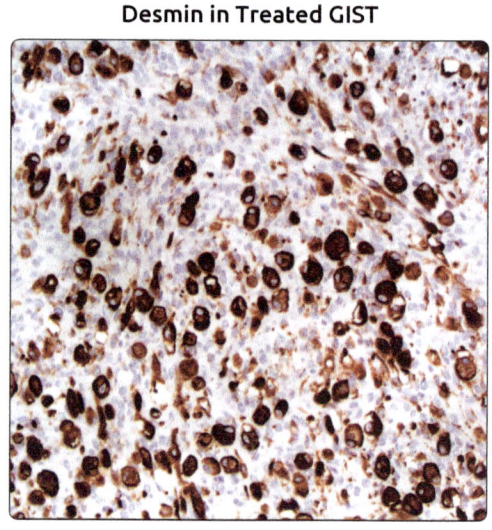

(Left) Gastric GIST resected after treatment with imatinib is shown. There is prominent rhabdomyoblastic differentiation as evident by large, polygonal cells with eccentrically placed vesicular nuclei harboring prominent nucleoli and brightly eosinophilic cytoplasm reminiscent of rhabdomyosarcoma ⇒. **(Right)** Desmin is strongly positive in neoplastic cells.

Myogenin in Treated GIST

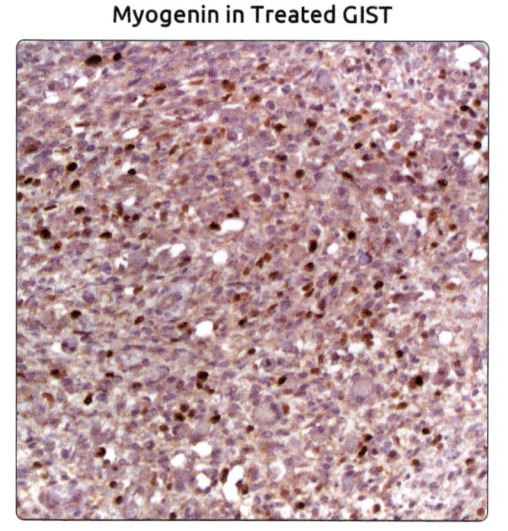

CD117 in Treated GIST

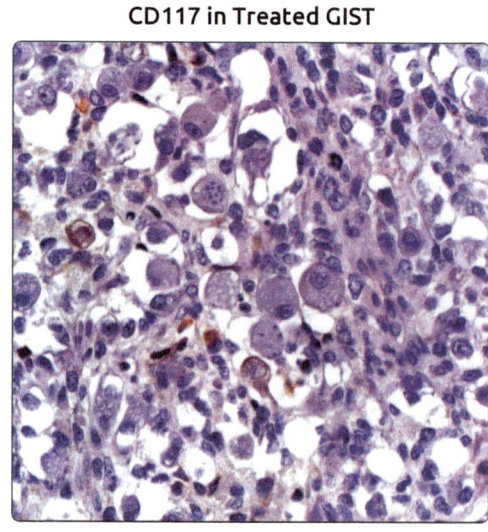

(Left) Myogenin shows patchy but obvious positivity, consistent with skeletal muscle differentiation. **(Right)** CD117 is negative in rhabdomyoblastic cells. This is a known phenomenon that may occur in previously treated tumors. Knowing the treatment history of this GIST was essential in arriving at the correct diagnosis, as the morphologic appearance and staining pattern were atypical.

Gastrointestinal Stromal Tumor

Gastric Leiomyoma

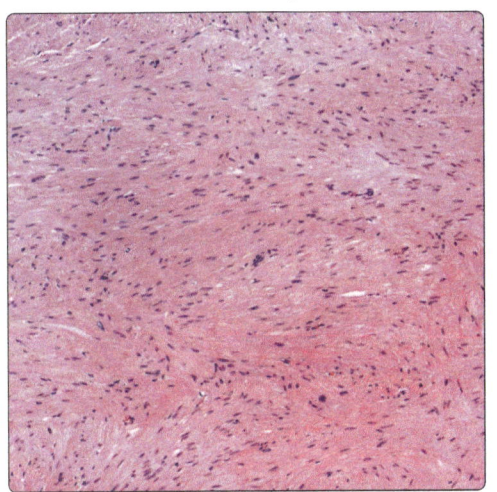

Desmin in Leiomyoma

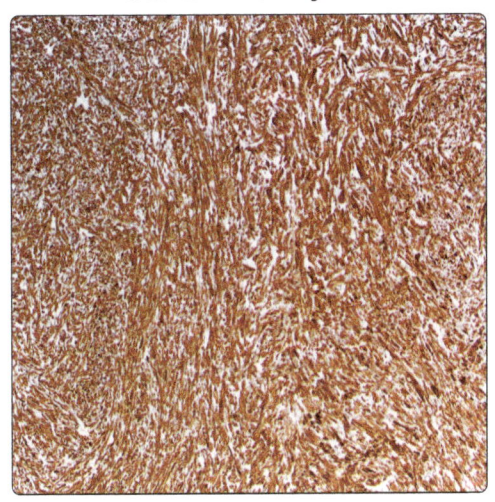

(Left) Gastric leiomyoma is composed of spindle cells with more brightly eosinophilic cytoplasm compared to GIST and is less cellular, though it shares the fascicular growth pattern seen in many spindle cell GIST. Leiomyoma commonly arises in muscularis mucosa, whereas GIST arises in muscularis propria. (Right) Desmin stain in the same case shows strong positivity. GIST are generally negative for this marker.

CD117 in Interstitial Cells Of Cajal

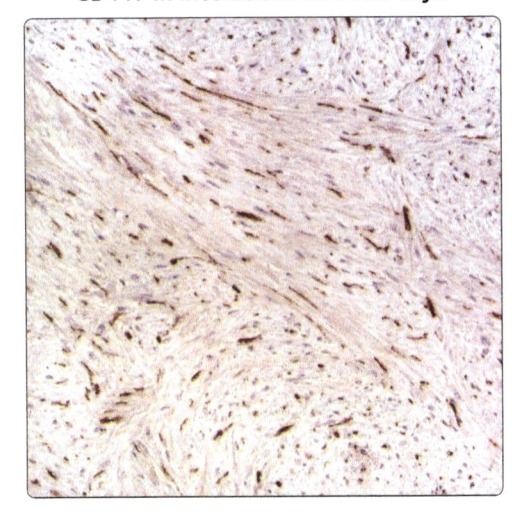

Clear Cell Sarcoma-Like Tumor

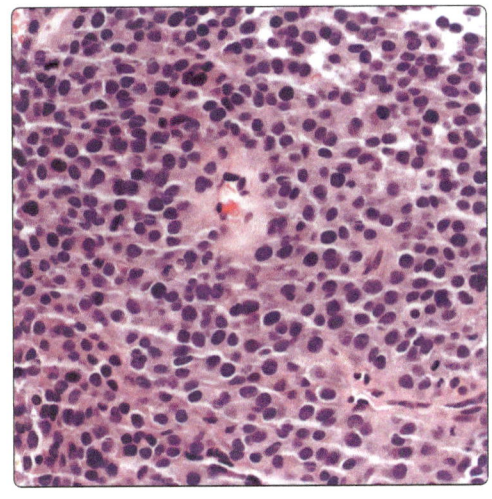

(Left) CD117 stain in the same case shows patchy positivity in some spindle cells, indicating colonizing interstitial cells of Cajal. This pattern should not be confused with the diffuse positivity seen in GIST. (Right) Clear cell sarcoma-like tumor of the gastrointestinal tract was initially suspected to be epithelioid GIST. However, it was CD117 and DOG1 negative and had a t(12;22)(q13;q12)/EWSR1::ATF1 fusion.

Gastric Schwannoma

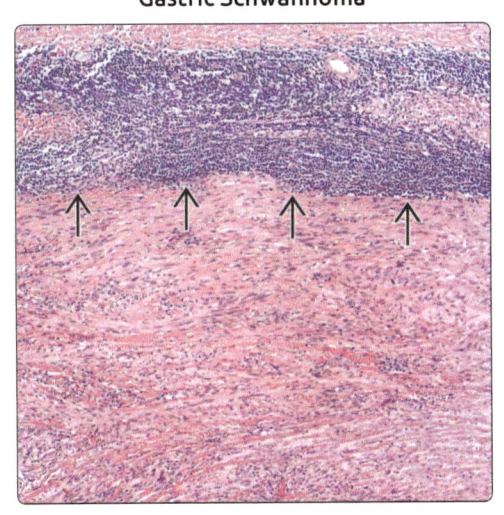

S100 Immunohistochemistry

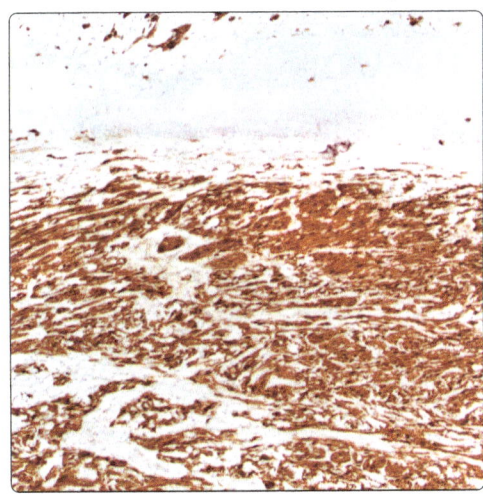

(Left) Gastric schwannoma shows the hallmark finding of a prominent peripheral lymphoid cuff ➡. This feature is important to recognize, as gastric schwannomas often lack the typical features of their soft tissue counterparts, such as Antoni A/B areas, Verocay bodies, and hyalinized vessels. (Right) S100 is strongly positive in schwannoma. One would not expect this degree of positivity in GIST.

HNF1A-Inactivated Hepatocellular Adenoma

KEY FACTS

TERMINOLOGY
- HNF1A-inactivated hepatocellular adenoma (H-HCA)
- Benign liver neoplasm composed of hepatocytes with inactivating mutation of HNF1A

ETIOLOGY/PATHOGENESIS
- Associated with oral contraceptives
- Associated with MODY3 and familial hepatic adenomatosis

CLINICAL ISSUES
- Minimal risk of malignant transformation
- Almost exclusively seen in women
- Asymptomatic incidental finding
- Solitary or multiple

IMAGING
- MR shows diffuse signal dropout with use of chemical shift sequence
  - Indicates marked fatty change

MACROSCOPIC
- Yellow/pale cut surface due to diffuse fatty change
- Typically lacks hemorrhage and peliosis

MOLECULAR
- Biallelic inactivating HNF1A mutations
  - Leads to steatosis and downregulation of L-FABP
- 90% somatic mutations
- 10% germline mutation with 2nd-hit somatic mutation

MICROSCOPIC
- Diffuse marked steatosis
- No cytoarchitectural atypia
- Lack of prominent sinusoidal dilatation and peliosis
- No inflammatory infiltrates or ductular reaction

ANCILLARY TESTS
- Negative L-FABP IHC staining

(Left) Transition of normal liver to HNF1A-inactivated hepatocellular adenoma (H-HCA) is shown. Diffuse steatosis, the hallmark feature, is readily apparent. (Right) L-FABP is negative in HNF1A-inactivated H-HCA and positive in background liver.

Diffuse Steatosis

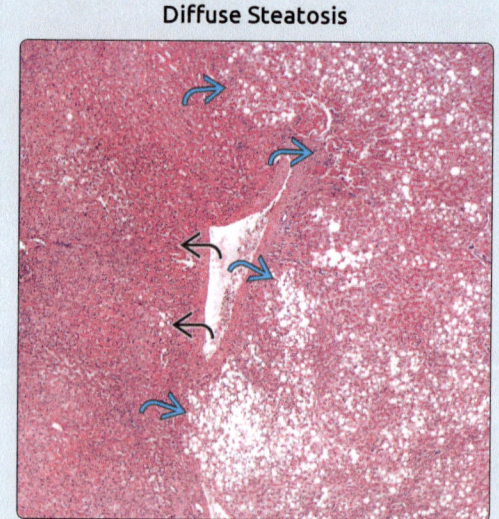

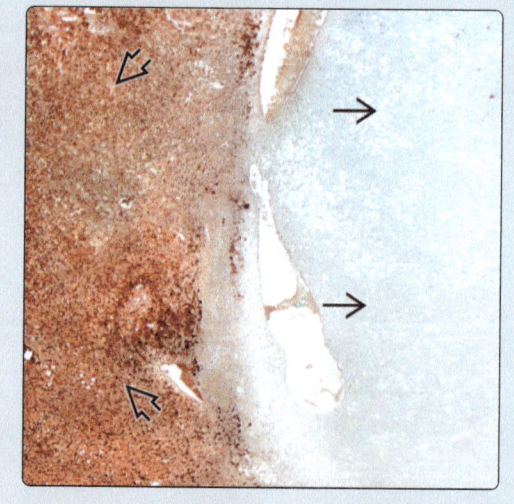

L-FABP Immunohistochemistry

(Left) H-HCA shows groups of nonsteatotic hepatocytes insinuating themselves among steatotic islands, creating a lobular appearance at low power. (Right) As with any HCA, unpaired parenchymal arteries are ubiquitous, though these lack the supportive fibrous connective tissue and inflammation seen in inflammatory HCA (I-HCA) and are not present within bridging fibrous septa as seen in focal nodular hyperplasia.

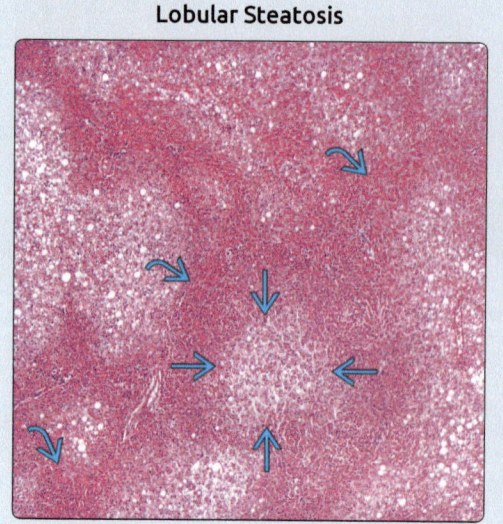

Lobular Steatosis

Unpaired Arteries

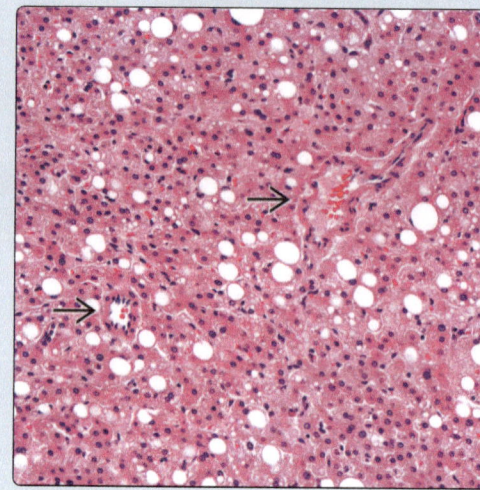

HNF1A-Inactivated Hepatocellular Adenoma

TERMINOLOGY

Abbreviations
- *HNF1A*-inactivated hepatocellular adenoma (H-HCA)

Synonyms
- Liver fatty acid binding protein (L-FABP)-negative hepatic adenoma

Definitions
- Benign liver neoplasm composed of hepatocytes with inactivating mutation of *HNF1A*
  - *HNF1A* controls hepatocyte differentiation in addition to glucose and lipid metabolism

ETIOLOGY/PATHOGENESIS

Definite Mechanisms Unclear
- Associated with oral contraceptives containing estrogen
- Associated with familial hepatic adenomatosis and maturity-onset diabetes of young, type 3 (MODY3)
- 90% biallelic somatic mutations in *HNF1A*
- 10% arise from heterozygous germline mutation in *HNF1A* with 2nd-hit somatic mutation (MODY3-related cases)
- Germline *CYP1B1* mutations also predispose to tumor development

CLINICAL ISSUES

Epidemiology
- Incidence
  - Constitutes 30-35% of all HCA
- Sex
  - Vast majority occur in women of childbearing age
  - Constitutional mutations affect both sexes

Presentation
- Commonly asymptomatic, incidental finding
- Solitary mass or multiple lesions
- May present as adenomatosis
  - Defined as ≥ 10 HCA
- H-HCA arising from germline mutation more common in
  - Younger patients (mean age: 23)
  - Patients not using oral contraceptives
  - Patients with MODY3
  - Patients with familial hepatic adenomatosis

Treatment
- Cessation of exogenous hormones
- Surgical resection for tumors > 5 cm
- Embolization
- Radiofrequency ablation for tumors < 4 cm
- Liver transplant may be necessary in cases of extreme adenomatosis with unresectable tumors
- Genetic counseling regarding family history of hepatic adenomas and MODY3 in selected cases

Prognosis
- Favorable; minimal risk of transformation to hepatocellular carcinoma

IMAGING

General Features
- Round, well-marginated mass with high fat content
- Best evaluated with MR

MR Findings
- T1-weighted gradient-echo images
  - Diffuse and homogeneous signal dropout
    - Indicates abundant intracellular steatosis
- T2-weighted images
  - Isointense to slightly hyperintense
- Gadolinium-enhanced T1-weighted images
  - Moderate arterial-phase enhancement with no persistent portal venous and delayed-phase enhancement

MACROSCOPIC

General Features
- Round, well-defined mass with little or no fibrous capsule
- Yellow/pale cut surface due to diffuse fatty change
- Typically lacks hemorrhage and peliosis
- Noncirrhotic background liver sometimes with steatosis

MOLECULAR

Diagnostically Relevant Molecular Alterations
- Biallelic mutations in *HNF1A* tumor suppressor gene
  - 50% are nonsense, frameshift, or splicing alterations
  - 35% are gene deletions
  - 15% are substitutions
  - Hotspot mutations at codons 291 and 206
    - Codon 291 mutations most frequently found in MODY3 patients
    - Codon 206 mutations specific to adenomas
- *HNF1A* encodes transcription regulator hepatocyte nuclear factor 1 α (HNF1A)
- HNF1A plays role in cell differentiation and metabolic regulation
  - Loss of function promotes lipogenesis leading to tumoral steatosis
  - Loss of function also associated with development of fatty liver in mice
- *FABP1* encodes L-FABP and is positively regulated by *HNF1A*
  - *HNF1A* inactivation downregulates *FABP1*, leading to diminished L-FABP expression
    - Can be detected by loss of L-FABP by IHC

MICROSCOPIC

Histologic Features
- Background of noncirrhotic liver
- Marked diffuse steatosis
  - Mild/focal steatosis is rare but may occur
- Steatotic hepatocytes intermingled with clear hepatocytes
- Lobular appearance at low power due to strands of normal-appearing hepatocytes penetrating tumor
- No cytologic atypia and few if any pseudoglandular structures
- No inflammatory infiltrates

HNF1A-Inactivated Hepatocellular Adenoma

- No ductular reaction
- No to mild sinusoidal dilatation
- Has other typical features of HCA, not otherwise specified (NOS)
  - Hepatocytes arranged in plates of 1-2 cells thick
    - Not always reliably evaluated with reticulin stain due to steatosis
  - Lack of portal tracts
  - Parenchymal unpaired arteries

ANCILLARY TESTS

Immunohistochemistry

- L-FABP
  - Negative
    - Surrogate marker for HNF1A inactivation
  - Normal liver and other HCA subtypes show intact L-FABP expression corresponding to proper upregulation by HNF1A
- Glutamine synthetase
  - Negative or focal physiologic-type staining (positivity isolated to 1-2 hepatocytes surrounding venular structures)
- β-catenin
  - Normal membranous staining
- Serum amyloid associated protein (SAA) and C-reactive protein (CRP)
  - Usually negative
  - May show focal patchy cytoplasmic positivity
    - In these cases, best to compare with background liver if available
    - Can be interpreted as consistent with H-HCA in setting of negative L-FABP staining

DIFFERENTIAL DIAGNOSIS

Other HCA Subtypes

- Inflammatory HCA
  - May show focal to moderate steatosis but usually not as diffuse as H-HCA
  - Inflammatory infiltrates grouped around vessels
  - Moderate to marked sinusoidal dilatation
  - Peliosis
  - Bile ductular reaction
  - SAA and CRP positivity with increased expression compared to nonneoplastic liver
  - L-FABP positive
  - Genotype includes frequent mutations in *IL6T* and occasional *CTNNB1* comutation
- β-catenin-activated HCA
  - Cytoarchitectural atypia
  - Lack of diffuse steatosis
  - Glutamine synthetase diffusely positive
  - β-catenin with nuclear and cytoplasmic positivity
  - L-FABP positive
- HCA unclassifiable
  - L-FABP positive
  - Lacks immunomorphologic features of other defined HCA subtypes

Well-Differentiated Hepatocellular Carcinoma

- Most problematic distinguishing H-HCA from WD-HCC with marked steatosis
  - Background cirrhosis indicates hepatocellular carcinoma
- Liver cell plates ≥ 3 cells thick
  - May be difficult to interpret in steatotic lesions
    - Best interpreted in nonsteatotic areas if present in tumor
  - Loss of reticulin staining is confounding in steatosis and may not be helpful
- Trabecular pattern &/or pseudoglandular architecture typically seen
- Endothelial wrapping
- Hepatocytes with high N:C ratio
- Mitoses
- Other IHC stains
  - Glypican-3 positive
  - Heat shock protein 70 (HSP70) positive
    - Negative staining for these 2 markers is not uncommon in WD-HCC and therefore only positive staining is helpful
  - Glutamine synthetase diffusely positive

Focal Nodular Hyperplasia

- Fibrous septa form obvious nodules
- Central scar
- Fibrous tissue with thick-walled, unpaired arteries
- Peripheral ductular reaction
- Glutamine synthetase expression with geographic or map-like positivity
- L-FABP positive

DIAGNOSTIC CHECKLIST

Clinically Relevant Pathologic Features

- HCA subtype with minimal risk of malignant transformation
- Consider patient demographics and family history
  - Associated with MODY3 and familial hepatic adenomatosis

Pathologic Interpretation Pearls

- Benign-appearing hepatocellular neoplasm in noncirrhotic liver with diffuse steatosis
- Lacks inflammatory infiltrates and ductular reaction
- L-FABP negative
- Glutamine synthetase, SAA, and CRP are all usually negative
- Membranous β-catenin staining

SELECTED REFERENCES

1. Hytiroglou P et al: Etiology, pathogenesis, diagnosis, and practical implications of hepatocellular neoplasms. Cancers (Basel). 14(15), 2022
2. Kim H et al: Hepatocellular adenomas: recent updates. J Pathol Transl Med. 55(3):171-80, 2021
3. WHO Classification of Tumours Editorial Board: Digestive system tumours. IARC, 2019.
4. Védie AL et al: Molecular classification of hepatocellular adenomas: impact on clinical practice. Hepat Oncol. 5(1):HEP04, 2018
5. Nault JC et al: Molecular classification of hepatocellular adenoma associates with risk factors, bleeding, and malignant transformation. Gastroenterology. 152(4):880-94.e6, 2017

HNF1A-Inactivated Hepatocellular Adenoma

Neoplastic Hepatocyte Cords

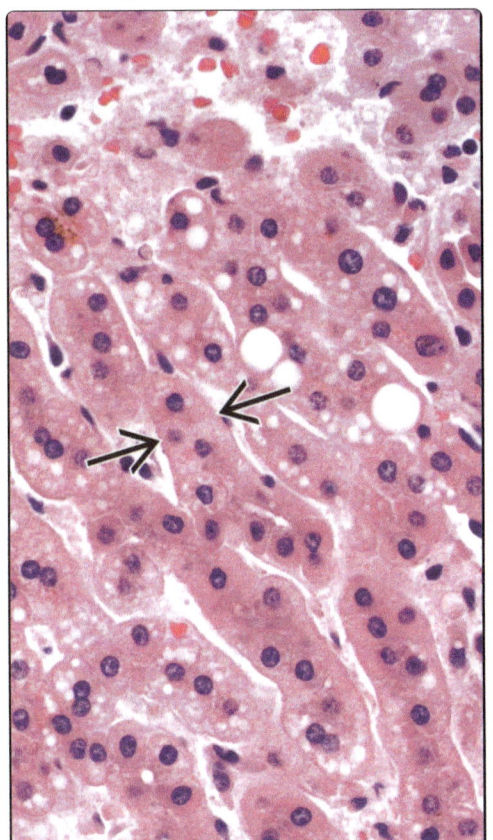

Diffuse Steatosis

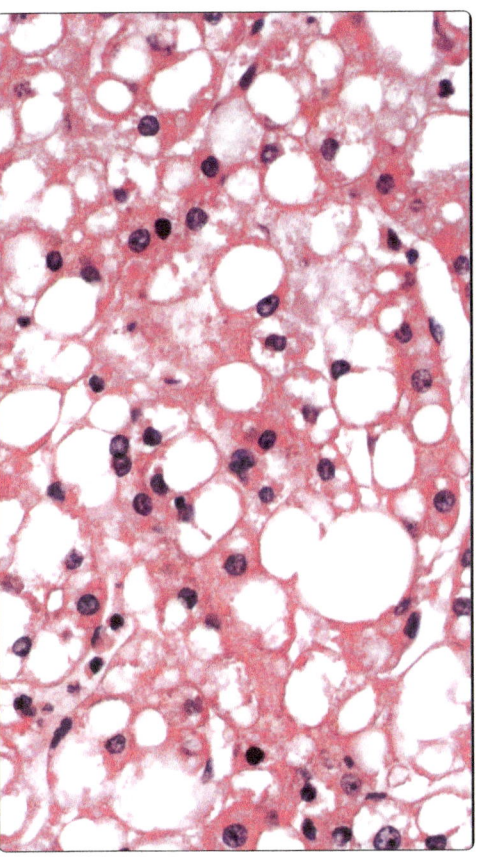

(Left) Neoplastic hepatocytes are arranged in cords of 1-2 cells thick ➡. This is best appreciated in minimally steatotic areas of the lesion, as seen here. (Right) Interpreting hepatocyte plate thickness on H&E is often very difficult in fatty areas, as seen here. This can be a challenging exercise if one is dealing with small biopsy specimens. Reticulin stain may not be useful either, as reticulin loss commonly occurs in steatotic areas.

Mixed-Morphology Hepatic Adenoma

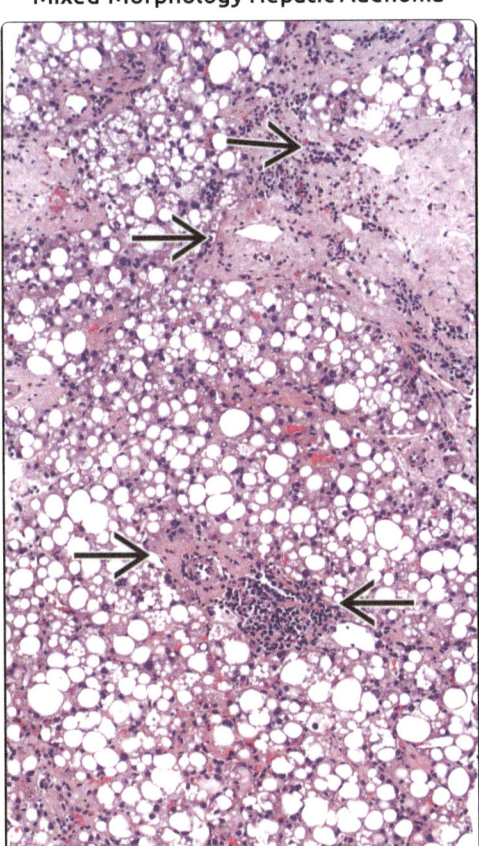

CRP Immunohistochemistry

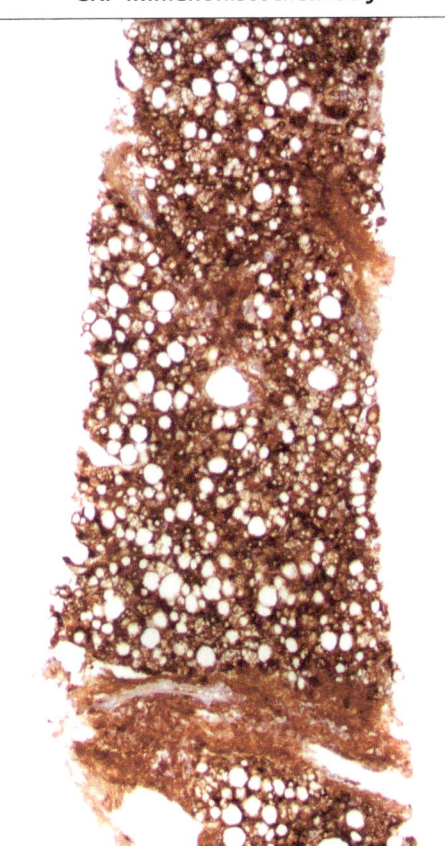

(Left) Biopsy shows features of both H-HCA and I-HCA. The former is suggested by the obvious diffuse steatosis, while the latter is suggested by the unpaired arteries embedded in fibrous connective tissue with associated inflammation ➡. (Right) Fortunately, IHC helped to solve the morphologic dilemma. L-FABP was positive and CRP (pictured) was diffusely positive, consistent with I-HCA.

β-Catenin-Activated Hepatocellular Adenoma

KEY FACTS

ETIOLOGY/PATHOGENESIS
- Associated with
  - Activating β-catenin mutation
  - Administration of androgenic steroids
  - Glycogen storage disease

CLINICAL ISSUES
- Overrepresented in male patients
- Higher risk of malignant transformation compared to other HCA subtypes

MOLECULAR
- Activating *CTNNB1* mutation, which encodes β-catenin
  - Nuclear and cytoplasmic stabilization of β-catenin
  - Glutamine synthetase (GS) overexpression
- *TERT* promoter mutations facilitates telomerase reactivation and promotes malignant transformation

MICROSCOPIC
- Tendency toward cytoarchitectural atypia compared to other HCA subtypes
  - Pseudoglandular structures prominent
  - Cytologic atypia, primarily nuclear hyperchromasia and high N:C ratio
- Lack of atypia does not exclude diagnosis

ANCILLARY TESTS
- Nuclear and cytoplasmic β-catenin immunohistochemical expression
- Glutamine synthetase (GS) immunohistochemistry
  - Surrogate marker for β-catenin activation
    - Exon 3 (other than S45): Diffuse, homogeneous staining
    - Exon 3 S45: Diffuse, heterogeneous staining (starry-sky pattern)
    - Exon 7/8: Faint staining ± some perivascular staining

Pseudoglandular Change

Cytologic Atypia

(Left) β-catenin-activated hepatocellular adenoma (b-HCA) shows abundant pseudoglandular change ➡, evident by neoplastic hepatocytes forming small rosettes with obvious lumina. (Right) Other areas of the same b-HCA show notable cytologic atypia ➡. This tumor was identified in a teenage football player who was suspected of taking steroids. The frank cytoarchitectural atypia was considered sufficient evidence for malignant transformation.

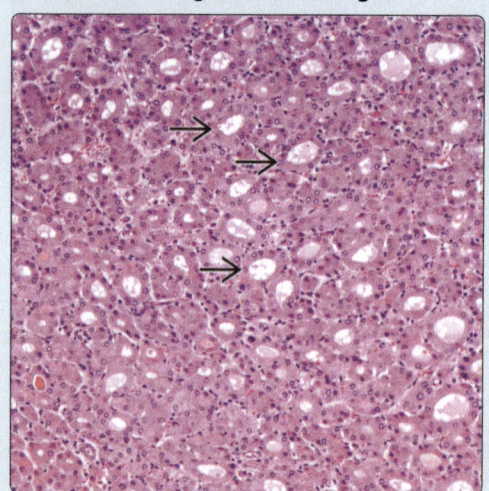

β-Catenin: Aberrant Nuclear Expression

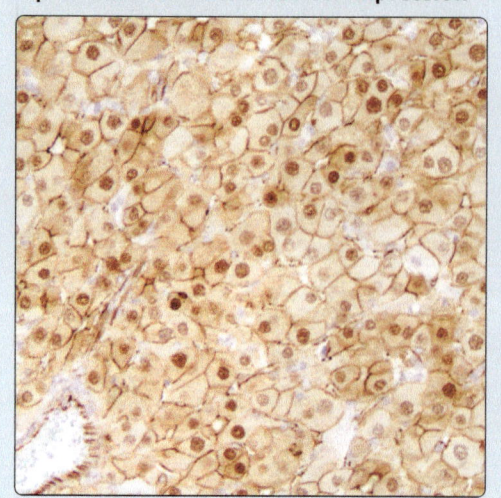

b-HCA Without Atypia

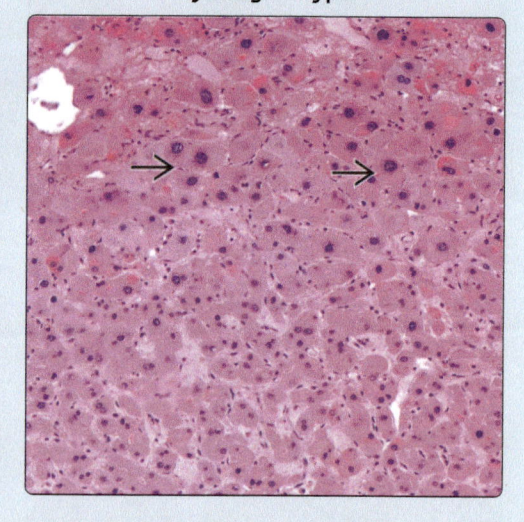

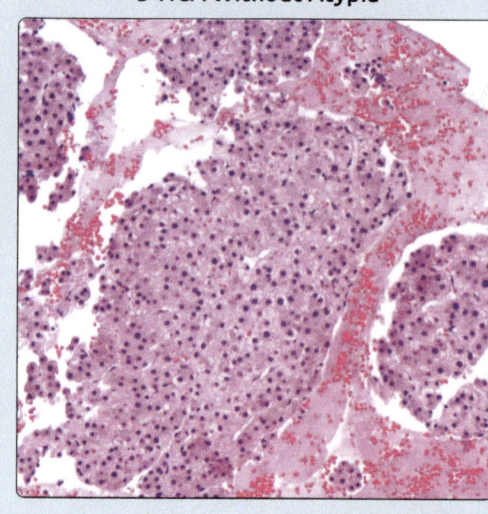

(Left) β-catenin shows patchy nuclear expression in b-HCA. (Right) Cell block preparation from FNA of b-HCA in a patient with glycogen storage disease shows no cytoarchitectural atypia, indicating that one cannot solely rely on morphology to identify these tumors.

β-Catenin-Activated Hepatocellular Adenoma

TERMINOLOGY

Abbreviations
- β-catenin-activated hepatocellular adenoma (b-HCA)

Synonyms
- β-catenin-mutated hepatic adenoma

Definitions
- Benign liver neoplasm composed of hepatocytes
- Increased risk of malignant transformation compared to other HCA subtypes

ETIOLOGY/PATHOGENESIS

Definite Mechanisms Unclear
- Activating β-catenin mutation
- Associated with
  o Administration of androgenic steroids
  o Glycogen storage disease

CLINICAL ISSUES

Epidemiology
- Incidence
  o Comprises ~ 10% of all HCA
- Sex
  o More common in male patients compared to other HCA subtypes

Presentation
- Liver mass
  o Usually solitary
  o Rarely multiple, except if associated with glycogenosis
  o Arises in noncirrhotic liver
- Symptoms
  o Nonspecific
    – Abdominal pain
    – Asymptomatic (incidental finding)

Treatment
- Cessation of exogenous steroids
- Surgical resection favored
- Embolization
- Radiofrequency ablation for tumors < 4 cm

Prognosis
- Complete surgical resection is curative
- Highest risk of malignant transformation of all HCA subtypes
  o Up to 46% of b-HCA associated with hepatocellular carcinoma (HCC) or borderline tumors in one study

IMAGING

MR Findings
- T1-weighted gradient-echo images
  o Hyper- or isointense
  o Absence or only focal signal dropout on chemical shift sequence due to lack of fatty component
    – May help differentiate from HNF1-α-inactivated HCA
- T2-weighted images
  o Hyper- or isointense
- Gadolinium-enhanced T1-weighted images
  o Strong arterial-phase enhancement with persistent enhancement during portal venous and delayed phase
  o Some cases with portal venous washout mimicking hepatocellular carcinoma

MACROSCOPIC

General Features
- Gross features cannot be used to reliably differentiate b-HCA
- Noncirrhotic background liver
- Round, well-defined mass with little to no fibrous capsule
- Tan to brown uniform parenchyma
- May have areas of hemorrhage or degenerative change, especially in large lesions
- Mild patchy to no steatosis
  o May help differentiate from *HNF1A*-inactivated HCA

MOLECULAR

Diagnostically Relevant Molecular Alterations
- *CTNNB1* mutation activates β-catenin within WNT signaling pathway
  o Large deletions and most hotspot mutation involve exon 3
    – Frequently involve the β-Trcp consensus site (codons D32-S37, "exon 3 hotspot")
    – High levels of β-catenin activation
    – High risk of HCC transformation
  o Non-β-Trcp consensus site exon 3 mutations
    – T41 and S45 codons are the most frequently mutated
    – Moderate to weak levels of β-catenin activation
  o Rare mutations involving other exons
    – Exon 7 (K335) and 8 (W383, R386 and N387) most common
    – Weak β-catenin activation
  o *CTNNB1* mutations also present in 10-15% of inflammatory hepatocellular adenomas (b-IHCA)
- Most mutations adversely affect glycogen synthase kinase 3-beta (GSK3B) phosphorylation site of β-catenin
  o Results in abnormal cytoplasmic and nuclear stabilization of β-catenin
    – Can be detected by immunohistochemistry
  o β-catenin transcriptionally activates genes responsible for cell proliferation and differentiation
    – Includes downstream upregulation of glutamine synthetase, which is detected by immunohistochemistry
- Telomerase reactivation through *TERT* promoter mutations promotes malignant transformation
- β-catenin mutations also found in 20-34% of hepatocellular carcinoma
  o These are predominantly missense mutations and are rarely deletions, which contrasts with b-HCA

MICROSCOPIC

Histologic Features
- Background of noncirrhotic liver
- Steatosis is unusual
- No portal tracts in lesional tissue

β-Catenin-Activated Hepatocellular Adenoma

- Benign hepatocytes arranged in plates of 1-2 cells thick
  - Best seen with reticulin stain
- Parenchymal unpaired arteries
- Atypical features more common than in other HCA subtypes
  - Pseudoglandular architecture
  - Cytologic atypia, primarily nuclear hyperchromasia and high N:C ratio
- Few have features of inflammatory HCA
  - These appear to lack cytoarchitectural atypia

ANCILLARY TESTS

Immunohistochemistry

- **Glutamine synthetase (GS)**
  - Diffuse increased expression
  - Surrogate marker for β-catenin activation (based on type of *CTNNB1* mutation)
    - Exon 3 (other than S45): Diffuse, homogeneous staining
    - Exon 3 S45: Diffuse, heterogeneous staining (starry-sky pattern)
    - Exon 7/8: Faint staining ± some perivascular staining
  - More sensitive but less specific than β-catenin IHC
- **β-catenin**
  - Aberrant nuclear and cytoplasmic expression
  - May be very focal and observed only in isolated hepatocytes within entire lesion
    - Lack of aberrant staining on biopsy samples does not exclude b-HCA
  - Some β-catenin mutations may not result in aberrant expression of β-catenin
    - Exon 3 (other than S45): Nuclear staining
    - Exon 3 S45: Weak or no nuclear staining
    - Exon 7/8: No nuclear staining
- **Serum amyloid-associated protein (SAA) and C-reactive protein (CRP)**
  - Usually negative
  - Cytoplasmic expression seen in small subset with features of inflammatory HCA
- **Liver fatty acid binding protein (L-FABP)**
  - Positive staining

Molecular Testing

- Not routinely used for diagnosis
- May be necessary for accurate diagnosis if β-catenin stain is negative and glutamine synthetase is patchy but abnormal

DIFFERENTIAL DIAGNOSIS

Other HCA Subtypes

- **HNF1A-inactivated HCA**
  - Marked diffuse steatosis
  - No cytoarchitectural atypia
  - Immunohistochemical stain for L-FABP is negative
  - Membranous β-catenin staining
  - Glutamine synthetase is negative or shows physiologic-type staining around venular structures
- **Inflammatory HCA**
  - Inflammatory infiltrates commonly grouped around vessels
  - Variable sinusoidal dilatation and peliosis
  - Bile ductular reaction present within small amount of connective tissue
  - Immunohistochemical stains for SAA and CRP are positive
  - Most are negative for glutamine synthetase and show membranous β-catenin staining
    - ~ 10% have β-catenin mutation resulting in diffuse glutamine synthetase positivity and N:C β-catenin staining
- **HCA, unclassifiable**
  - HCA with typical morphology lacking any of above described immunohistochemical profiles

Well-Differentiated Hepatocellular Carcinoma

- Background cirrhotic liver
- Liver cell plates ≥ 3 cells thick
- Prominent pseudogland formation or trabecular pattern
- Endothelial wrapping
- Hepatocytes with high N:C ratio
- Mitotic activity

Focal Nodular Hyperplasia

- Fibrous septa within lesion form obvious nodules
- Central scar
- Scar and septa contain large, thick-walled, unpaired arteries and harbor peripheral ductular reaction at junction with parenchyma
- No cytoarchitectural atypia
- Glutamine synthetase stain shows geographic or map-like positivity

DIAGNOSTIC CHECKLIST

Clinically Relevant Pathologic Features

- Well-differentiated hepatocellular neoplasm in male patients without cirrhosis should raise suspicion of b-HCA if features do not meet criteria for HCC
- b-HCA can also arise in typical clinical setting of female patient on oral contraceptives
- IHC work-up to exclude this potentially aggressive lesion is indicated in majority of cases

Pathologic Interpretation Pearls

- Cytoarchitectural atypia in HCA is suggestive of b-HCA, but lack of atypical features does not exclude this diagnosis
- Nuclear β-catenin positivity may be patchy within any given lesion, so lack of staining on biopsy does not exclude b-HCA
- Diffuse positive glutamine synthetase staining is sensitive surrogate marker for β-catenin activation

SELECTED REFERENCES

1. Hytiroglou P et al: Etiology, pathogenesis, diagnosis, and practical implications of hepatocellular neoplasms. Cancers (Basel). 14(15), 2022
2. Kim H et al: Hepatocellular adenomas: recent updates. J Pathol Transl Med. 55(3):171-80, 2021
3. WHO Classification of Tumours Editorial Board: Digestive system tumours. IARC, 2019
4. Bioulac-Sage P et al: Hepatocellular adenoma: classification, variants and clinical relevance. Semin Diagn Pathol. 34(2):112-25, 2017

β-Catenin-Activated Hepatocellular Adenoma

b-HCA With Peliosis

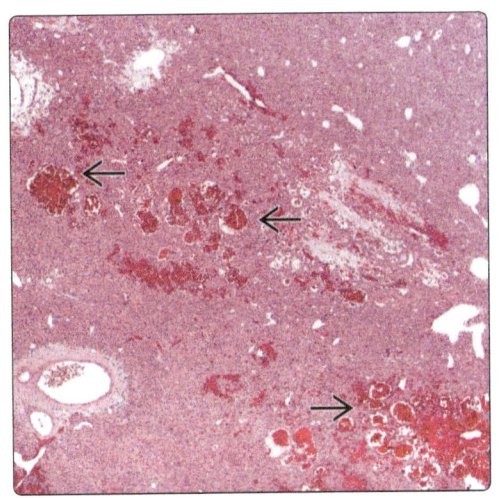

Unpaired Arteries

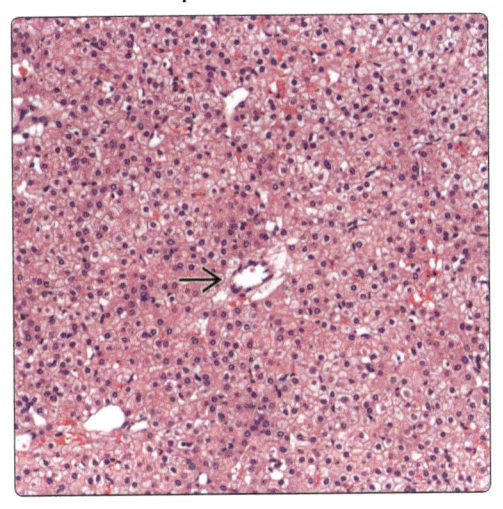

(Left) This case of b-HCA arose in a woman on oral contraceptives. At low power, it resembles most hepatocellular adenomas, as it is composed of sheets of benign-appearing hepatocytes and lacks portal tracts. Areas of peliosis ⇒ are scattered throughout. (Right) Unpaired arteries ⇒ are present and there is no cytoarchitectural atypia. IHC stains were needed to determine that this was, in fact, a β-catenin-activated tumor.

Reticulin

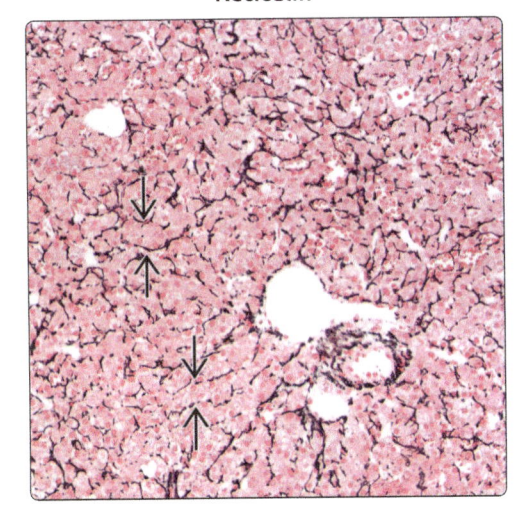

β-Catenin: Normal Membranous Expression

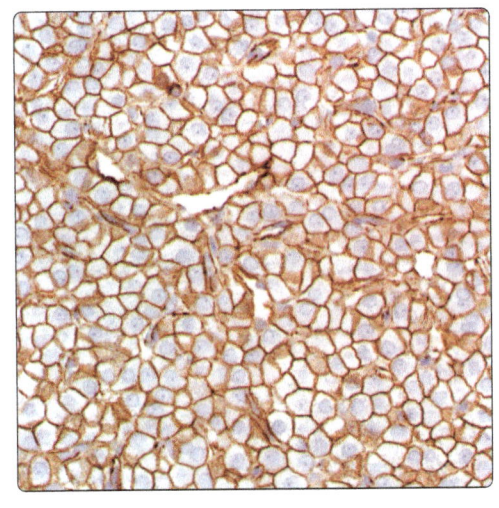

(Left) Reticulin highlights an intact network with liver cell plates 1-2 cells thick ⇒. (Right) β-catenin shows normal membranous positivity without nuclear or cytoplasmic labeling. This staining pattern was seen in many sections taken from this tumor and enforces the fact that negative nuclear β-catenin does not exclude the possibility of β-catenin-activated adenoma.

Positive Glutamine Synthetase

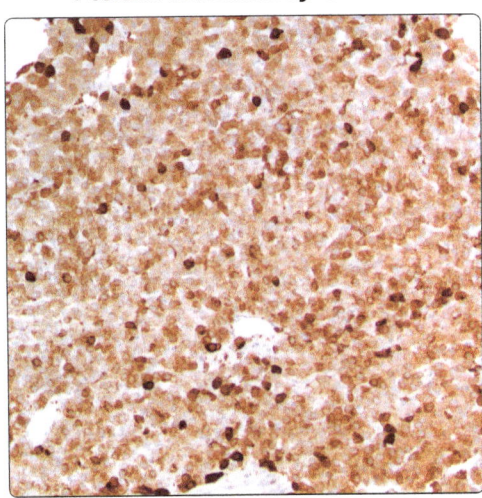

Physiologic Glutamine Synthetase

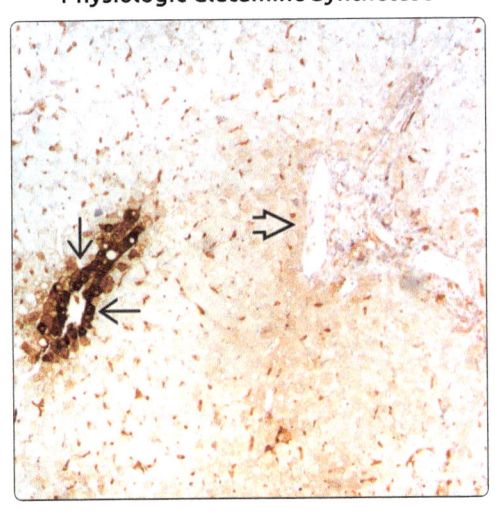

(Left) Glutamine synthetase shows diffuse positivity. Subsequent molecular testing identified a CTNNB1 exon 3/codon 45 missense substitution, which we now know does not often show nuclear β-catenin expression by IHC. (Right) For comparison, the staining pattern of glutamine synthetase in normal liver is shown. Glutamine synthetase normally highlights a 1-2 hepatocyte cell layer rim surrounding central veins ⇒. Notice that periportal and zone 2 hepatocytes closer to portal tract ⇒ lack positivity.

Inflammatory Hepatocellular Adenoma

KEY FACTS

TERMINOLOGY
- Inflammatory hepatocellular adenoma (I-HCA)

ETIOLOGY/PATHOGENESIS
- Associated with obesity and high alcohol intake

CLINICAL ISSUES
- Propensity for multifocal lesions
- May be associated with symptoms of systemic inflammatory syndrome
- Very little risk of malignant transformation in absence of β-catenin mutation

MOLECULAR
- Activating *IL6ST* mutation causing upregulation of gp130
- Sustained activation of IL-6/JAK/STAT signaling pathway
- Upregulation of C-reactive protein (CRP) and serum amyloid-associated protein (SAA), which can be detected by immunohistochemistry
- 10% also harbor coexisting β-catenin mutations

MICROSCOPIC
- Unpaired arteries embedded in fibrous tissue
- Ductular reaction
- Inflammatory infiltrates
- Sinusoidal dilatation and peliosis

ANCILLARY TESTS
- Immunohistochemical positivity for SAA and CRP

TOP DIFFERENTIAL DIAGNOSES
- Focal nodular hyperplasia
  - Geographic glutamine synthetase positivity
  - CRP and SAA are usually negative
  - Nodular architecture and central scar
- β-catenin-activated I-HCA
  - Diffuse glutamine synthetase positivity ± nuclear/cytoplasmic β-catenin expression

Typical Appearance | **Dilated Sinusoids**

(Left) Inflammatory hepatocellular adenoma (I-HCA) is characterized by inflammatory infiltrates grouped around vessels ➡ and prominent sinusoidal dilatation ➡. (Right) I-HCA shows the markedly dilated sinusoids ➡. Note the absence of portal tracts. (From DP: Hepatobiliary & Pancreatic.)

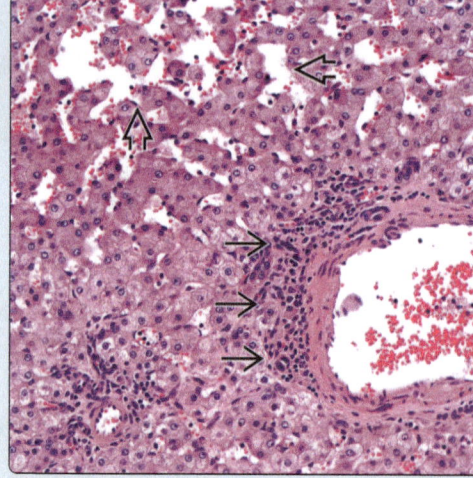

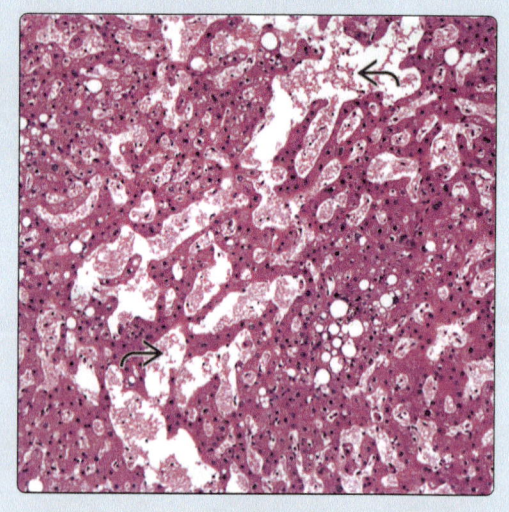

Abortive Portal Tracts: Low Power | **Abortive Portal Tract: High Power**

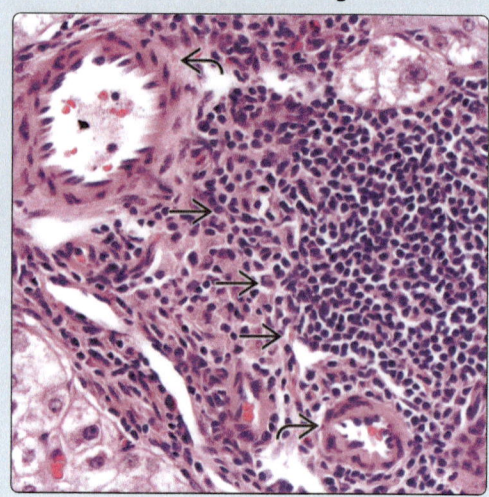

(Left) I-HCA shows randomly dispersed foci of fibrous connective tissue harboring vascular structures, patchy inflammatory infiltrates, and no bile ducts, termed "abortive portal tracts" ➡. Note the lack of nodularity despite the presence of the fibrotic foci. (Right) Inflammatory infiltrates ➡ consist predominantly of lymphocytes and plasma cells. Neutrophils, when present, are usually associated with reactive ductules. Notice the absence of similar caliber bile ducts paired with the arteries ➡.

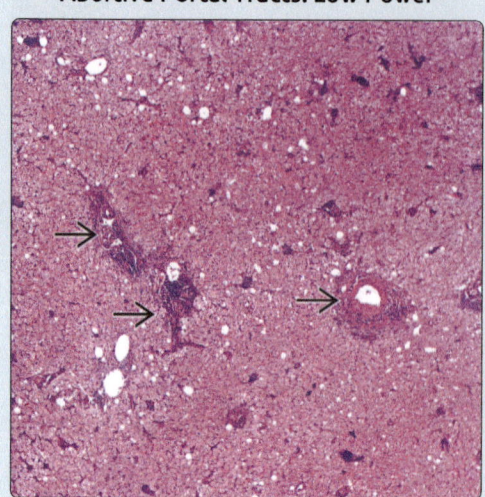

Inflammatory Hepatocellular Adenoma

TERMINOLOGY

Abbreviations
- Inflammatory hepatocellular adenoma (I-HCA)

Synonyms
- Telangiectatic hepatic adenoma
- Telangiectatic focal nodular hyperplasia (T-FNH)
  - Term no longer used

Definitions
- Benign hepatocellular neoplasm with overexpression of acute-phase inflammatory response proteins
  - C-reactive protein (CRP)
  - Serum amyloid-associated protein (SAA)

ETIOLOGY/PATHOGENESIS

Definite Mechanisms Unclear
- Contributing factors
  - Alcohol intake
  - Obesity
  - Oral contraceptives containing estrogen
  - Associated with glycogen storage disease
- Some cases arise in patients with systemic inflammatory syndrome, which may regress after hepatectomy
- 60% arise from somatic activating mutations in *IL6ST*, which encodes glycoprotein 130 (gp130)
- 10% have coexisting β-catenin mutations

CLINICAL ISSUES

Epidemiology
- Incidence
  - Comprises 35-40% of all HCA
- Sex
  - Predominantly occurs in women

Presentation
- Asymptomatic incidental finding
- Symptoms related to mass effect or tumor rupture and hemorrhage
- Masses may be solitary or multiple
  - Multifocality may be more common than in other HCA subtypes
- Occasionally symptoms of systemic inflammatory syndrome &/or chronic anemia
  - Fever and leukocytosis
- May have elevated systemic CRP and ESR levels in up to 50% of cases
- More common in obese patients and those with excessive alcohol consumption

Treatment
- Surgical resection for tumors > 5 cm
- Radiofrequency ablation for tumors < 4 cm
- Embolization

Prognosis
- Favorable
  - Vast majority of cases will not progress to hepatocellular carcinoma
- Increased risk of malignant transformation if associated with β-catenin mutation

MACROSCOPIC

General Features
- Round, well-defined mass with little or no fibrous capsule
- Heterogeneous with areas of congestion and hemorrhage
  - May correspond to areas of microscopic peliosis
- Noncirrhotic background liver

MOLECULAR

Diagnostically Relevant Molecular Alterations
- Majority (60%) of I-HCA have somatic monoallelic activating mutations of *IL6ST*, which encodes gp130 in interleukin 6 (IL-6) signaling pathway
  - Most are inframe deletions
- Gp130 is cell surface signaling receptor that binds IL-6
- Gain-of-function mutations specifically target residues responsible for gp130-IL-6 interface
- Results in constitutively active gp130 in absence of IL-6
  - Sustained activation of IL-6/JAK/STAT transcription pathway
    - Subsequent upregulation of acute-phase reactants CRP and SAA, which can be detected with immunohistochemistry
    - Induction of hepatocellular proliferation
- 10% of I-HCA also harbor coexisting β-catenin mutations
  - Suggests cooperative effect of these signaling pathways in malignant transformation
- Less common genes mutated in JAK/STAT pathway include *FRK* (10%), *STAT3* (5%), *GNAS* (5%), and *JAK1* (3%)
  - These are usually mutually exclusive

MICROSCOPIC

Histologic Features
- Outside of tumor, liver is noncirrhotic
- Intratumoral inflammatory infiltrates commonly grouped around vessels
  - Predominantly lymphocytes and plasma cells
  - Few neutrophils and histiocytes
    - Neutrophils usually associated with bile ductular reaction
- Thick-walled unpaired arteries lying in fibrous connective tissue
  - Termed "abortive portal tracts"
- Usually no bridging fibrous septa
- Bile ductular reaction present in fibrotic foci
  - Mimics focal nodular hyperplasia (FNH)
- Prominent sinusoidal dilatation
- Peliosis
- Steatosis in nontumoral liver is more common in this subtype
  - Most cases lack diffuse intratumoral steatosis
  - Steatosis, if present, is heterogeneously distributed within neoplasm
- Lack of cytoarchitectural atypia
  - Even in cases with coexisting β-catenin mutations
- Other typical features of HCA not otherwise specified
  - Hepatocytes arranged in plates of 1-2 cells thick

Inflammatory Hepatocellular Adenoma

- Lack of portal tracts
- Presence of parenchymal unpaired arteries

ANCILLARY TESTS

Immunohistochemistry

- SAA and CRP
  - Commonly diffuse cytoplasmic positivity restricted to tumoral hepatocytes
  - Patchy positivity can be seen
    - Intensity of expression is greater than in background liver if available for comparison
- Glutamine synthetase
  - Negative or focal physiologic staining around venular structures
  - Diffuse positivity seen in I-HCA with associated β-catenin mutation
- β-catenin
  - Membranous staining
  - Nuclear staining seen in I-HCA with associated β-catenin mutation
- Liver fatty acid binding protein (L-FABP)
  - Positive

Molecular Testing

- May be necessary to evaluate for β-catenin mutation if immunohistochemistry is equivocal in select cases

DIFFERENTIAL DIAGNOSIS

Other HCA Subtypes

- β-catenin-activated HCA
  - Difficult differential diagnosis as 10% of I-HCA also harbors β-catenin mutation
  - No reliable morphologic features to differentiate I-HCA with β-catenin mutation from typical I-HCA
  - Negative glutamine synthetase and membranous β-catenin staining in typical I-HCA
  - Diffuse glutamine synthetase ± nuclear/cytoplasmic β-catenin staining in I-HCA with β-catenin mutation
  - SAA and CRP positivity in all I-HCA cases regardless of β-catenin status
  - β-catenin mutation trumps inflammatory subtype
    - Classify I-HCA with β-catenin mutation as β-catenin-activated I-HCA
- HNF1A-inactivated HCA
  - Diffuse steatosis
  - Lack of inflammatory infiltrates, peliosis, sinusoidal dilatation, and ductular reaction
  - L-FABP negative
  - SAA and CRP negative
- HCA unclassifiable
  - SAA and CRP negative
  - Lacks immunomorphologic features of other defined HCA subtypes

Well-Differentiated Hepatocellular Carcinoma

- Background of cirrhosis
- Liver cell plates ≥ 3 cells thick
- Trabecular &/or pseudoacinar architecture
- Endothelial wrapping
- Hepatocytes with low N:C ratio
- Presence of mitoses

Focal Nodular Hyperplasia

- Difficult differential diagnosis, especially on core biopsy
- FNH has dystrophic, thick-walled arteries embedded in fibrous tissue with ductular reaction and inflammation similar to I-HCA
- FNH usually lacks
  - Parenchymal unpaired arteries
  - Prominent sinusoidal dilatation
- FNH usually shows thick bridging fibrous bands creating nodular architecture
  - Rare I-HCA can be nodular
- Glutamine synthetase
  - Geographic or map-like staining pattern in FNH
- SAA and CRP
  - Usually negative
  - Patchy positivity can be seen in FNH and is more common with CRP
  - Patchy SAA &/or CRP positivity in face of geographic glutamine synthetase in tumor with typical features of FNH should be considered FNH
- Neoplasms previously classified as telangiectatic FNH are now all considered I-HCA

DIAGNOSTIC CHECKLIST

Clinically Relevant Pathologic Features

- 10% of I-HCA have β-catenin mutations, and these have increased risk of malignant transformation
- No histologic features to differentiate β-catenin-activated I-HCA from typical I-HCA
  - Immunohistochemistry is needed to make this distinction
- β-catenin gene (CTNNB1) mutation trumps inflammatory subtype
  - Classify I-HCA with β-catenin mutation as β-catenin-activated I-HCA

Pathologic Interpretation Pearls

- Benign-appearing hepatocellular neoplasm in noncirrhotic liver with
  - Sinusoidal dilatation
  - Inflammatory infiltrates
  - Fibrotic foci harboring thick-walled arteries and ductular reaction
  - Expression of SAA and CRP by immunohistochemistry

SELECTED REFERENCES

1. Hytiroglou P et al: Etiology, pathogenesis, diagnosis, and practical implications of hepatocellular neoplasms. Cancers (Basel). 14(15), 2022
2. Kim H et al: Hepatocellular adenomas: recent updates. J Pathol Transl Med. 55(3):171-80, 2021
3. WHO Classification of Tumours Editorial Board. Digestive system tumours. IARC, 2019
4. Bioulac-Sage P et al: Hepatocellular adenoma: classification, variants and clinical relevance. Semin Diagn Pathol. 34(2):112-25, 2017
5. Joseph NM et al: Diagnostic utility and limitations of glutamine synthetase and serum amyloid-associated protein immunohistochemistry in the distinction of focal nodular hyperplasia and inflammatory hepatocellular adenoma. Mod Pathol. 27(1):62-72, 2014
6. Katabathina VS et al: Genetics and imaging of hepatocellular adenomas: 2011 update. Radiographics. 31(6):1529-43, 2011

Inflammatory Hepatocellular Adenoma

Thick-Walled Arteries

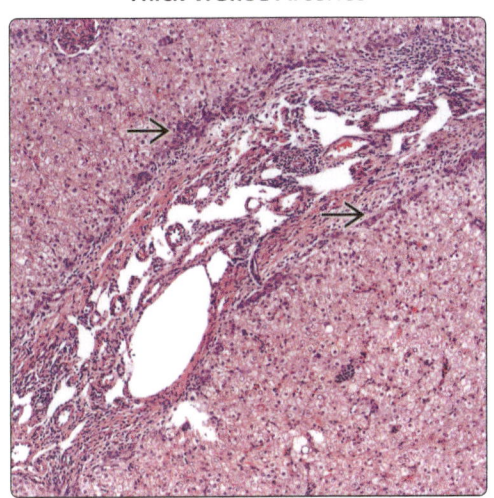

Ductular Reaction

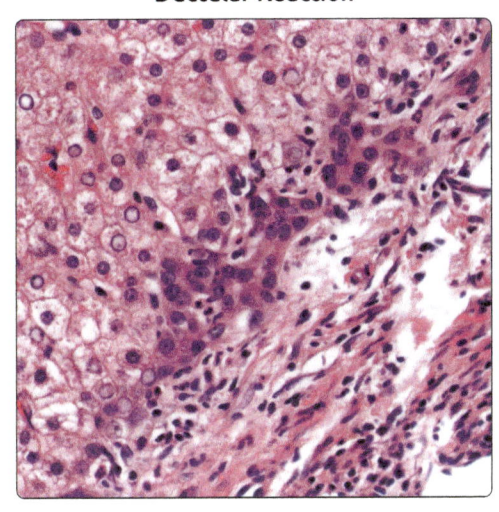

(Left) I-HCA shows many thick-walled, unpaired arteries with a notable peripheral ductular reaction ⇨ at the interface with the neoplastic hepatocytes. Similar features are also seen in focal nodular hyperplasia, in which these arteries are termed "dysplastic arteries." (Right) Reactive ductules differ from their native counterparts in that they are peripherally located, maintain slit-like lumina, and nearly always harbor an accompanying infiltrate of neutrophils.

CRP Immunohistochemistry

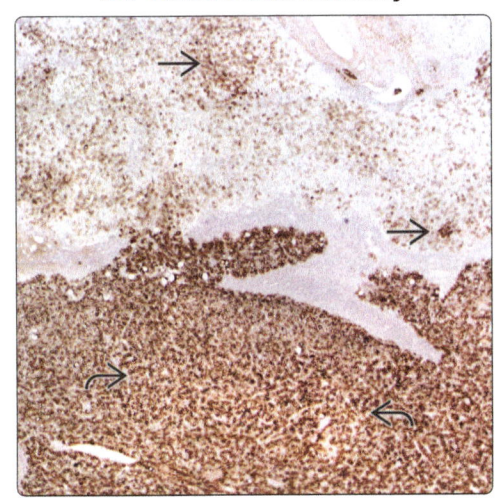

Focal Nodular Hyperplasia

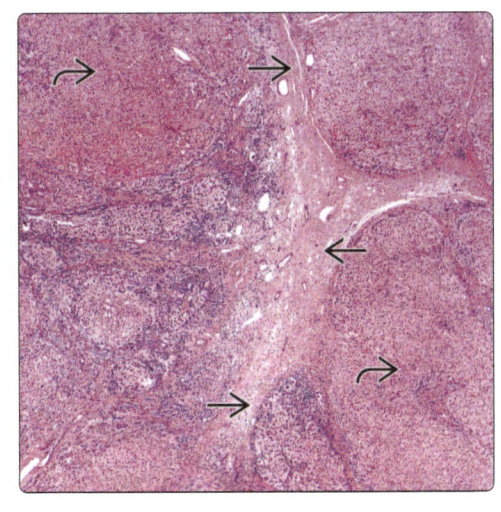

(Left) CRP shows diffuse, strong expression in neoplastic cells ⇨. Note the background nonneoplastic liver ⇨, which only shows patchy staining. (Right) Focal nodular hyperplasia represents the most difficult differential diagnosis. A prominent central scar ⇨ and nodular architecture ⇨ allow for proper identification.

Glutamine Synthetase Stain in Focal Nodular Hyperplasia

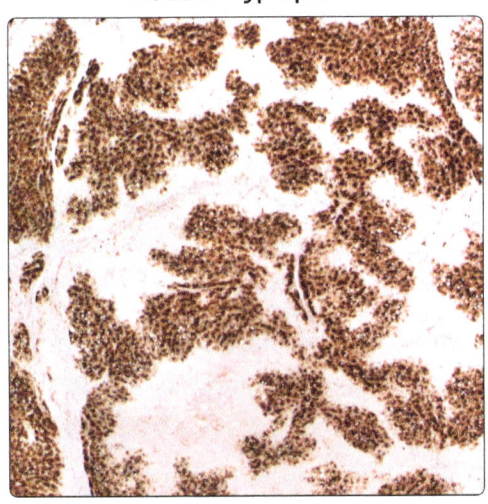

Glutamine Synthetase Stain in I-HCA

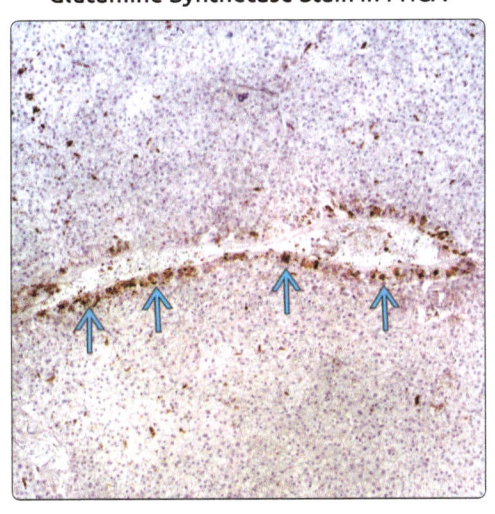

(Left) Glutamine synthetase shows geographic or map-like positivity in focal nodular hyperplasia (FNH). This staining pattern is best appreciated at low power and is not seen I-HCA. (Right) In contrast to FNH, glutamine synthetase is predominantly negative in I-HCA, though focal physiologic staining in 1-2 hepatocytes surrounding intratumoral venules can be seen ⇨. Diffuse, strong positivity would indicate the possibility of β-catenin mutation.

Hepatocellular Carcinoma

KEY FACTS

ETIOLOGY/PATHOGENESIS

- Cirrhosis is major risk factor for hepatocellular carcinoma (HCC)
  - Alcohol-induced cirrhosis is most common risk factor for HCC in USA and in Western countries
  - Alcohol acts synergistically with other risk factors, such as HBV, HCV, diabetics, obesity, and smoking
  - Some inherited disorders are associated with cirrhosis
    - Hemochromatosis, hereditary tyrosinemia, Wilson disease, α-1-antitrypsin deficiency
  - Metabolic syndrome is increasingly important risk factor
- Hepatitis B is leading cause of HCC globally
- Nonalcoholic fatty liver disease (NAFLD) and NASH are emerging risk factors of HCC in Western countries
- HCV infection
- Primary mechanism for HCC may be due to inflammatory hepatocyte damage due to oxidative stress
- Diabetes, obesity, hypertension, and dyslipidemia are associated with elevated risk of HCC
- Males have elevated risk for HCC compared to females

CLINICAL ISSUES

- Tumor size, number of lesions, vascular invasion, and tumor spread determine prognosis
- Surgery is primary treatment for resectable HCC
- Orthotopic liver transplantation is potentially curative treatment for early-stage HCC
- Sorafenib may improve survival in advanced HCC
- Newer therapies include regorafenib
- Immune based treatments like nivolumab are undergoing evaluation for HCC treatment

MOLECULAR

- HCC tumors are commonly aneuploid
- Chromosomal losses include 1p, 4q, 5q, 6q, 8p, 9p, 13q, 16p, 16q, and 17p
- Chromosomal gains include 1q, 6p, 8q, and 17q
- *DNAJB1::PRKACA* fusion reported as specific recurrent abnormality in fibrolamellar subtype of HCC
- The most commonly mutated genes include *TP53*, *CTNNB1*, *AXIN1*, and *RB1*
- Common gene amplifications include *MYC*, *MET*, *TERT*, and *CCND1*
- Common gene deletions include *CDKN2A* and *PTEN*
- Epigenetic alterations in HCC
  - Most common hypermethylated genes include *BMP4*, *CDKN2A*, *GSTP1*, and *NFATC1*
  - Common hypermethylated genes in HBV-positive HCC include *DAB2IP*, *BMP4*, *ZFP41*, *SPDYA*, and *CDKN2A*
- Major signaling pathways implicated in hepatic carcinogenesis include Wnt-β catenin, Ras signaling, PI3K/Akt/mTOR, Rb and DLC1/Rho/ROCK pathways
- Molecular alterations are not currently in routine use in clinical practice for diagnostic purposes

MICROSCOPIC

- Tumor cells of well-differentiated HCC resemble normal liver cells
- Mallory-Denk bodies are identified in 20% of tumors
- Desmoplastic stroma is commonly sparse or absent
- Subset of HCC contains abundant eosinophilic cytoplasm with desmoplastic stroma, which is known as fibrolamellar variant of HCC

ANCILLARY TESTS

- Hep-Par1, pCEA, Glypican-3, Arg-1, glutamine synthetase staining by IHC

TOP DIFFERENTIAL DIAGNOSES

- Metastatic tumors from distant organ sites (e.g., colorectal)
- Hepatocellular adenomas
- Intra- and extrahepatic cholangiocarcinoma
- Focal nodular hyperplasia
- Gallbladder adenocarcinoma

Trabecular Pattern

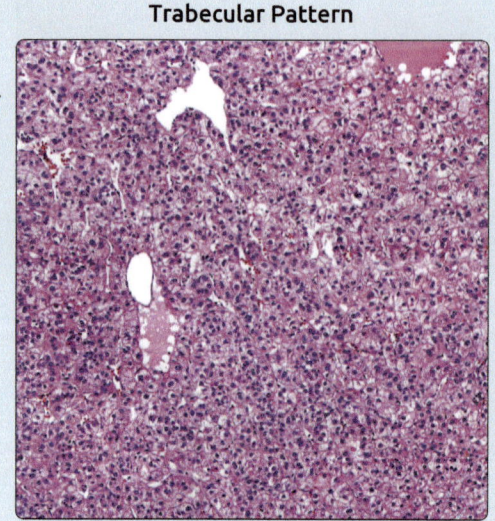

Pseudoacinar Pattern

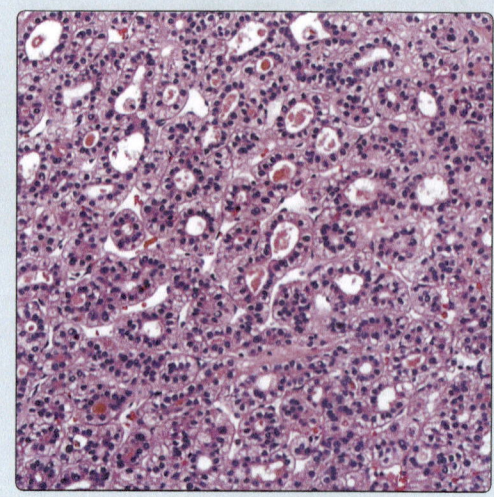

(Left) *Hepatocellular carcinoma (HCC) can form trabecular, solid, pseudoacinar (a.k.a. pseudoglandular) and macrotrabecular growth patterns. This field shows the trabecular pattern of HCC with cord-like proliferation of neoplastic cells with ≥ 3 nuclei in a single cord.* (Right) *HCC shows the presence of pseudoacinar formation.*

Hepatocellular Carcinoma

TERMINOLOGY

Abbreviations
- Hepatocellular carcinoma (HCC)

Definitions
- Primary hepatocyte-derived malignant neoplasm of liver

ETIOLOGY/PATHOGENESIS

Cirrhosis
- Major risk factor for HCC, some inherited disorders associated with cirrhosis
  - e.g., hemochromatosis, hereditary tyrosinemia, Wilson disease, α-1-antitrypsin deficiency

Viral Hepatitis
- Chronic hepatitis B virus (HBV) infection
  - Leading cause of HCC in Asia and Africa
  - ~ 56% of HCC cases globally are due to HBV infections
  - Seropositive HBV patients (HBsAg positive) have 98x increased risk of HCC
  - HBx protein derived from HBV is key mediator of hepatic carcinogenesis through inactivation of TP53 pathway
- Hepatitis C virus (HCV) infection
  - Major cause of HCC in Western hemisphere
  - ~ 17x increased risk of HCC among chronic HCV carriers
  - Primary mechanism for HCC may be due to inflammatory hepatocyte damage secondary to oxidative stress

Alcohol-Related Liver Disease
- Alcohol-induced cirrhosis is common risk factor in USA and in Western countries
- Alcohol acts synergistically with other preexisting risk factors, such as HBV, HCV, diabetics, obesity, and smoking
- Heavy alcohol consumption → 6x increased risk for HCC in cirrhotic patients
- P450 enzyme encoded by *CYP2E1* metabolizes endogenous and exogenous substrates, resulting in production of reactive oxygen species and DNA damage

Environmental Factors
- Aflatoxin (fungal mycotoxin) may play direct causative role in HCC worldwide including sub-Saharan Africa
  - Present in contaminated foodstuffs, e.g., rice and peanuts
  - Converted by cytochrome P450 system into reactive epoxide intermediate which binds to DNA; uniquely causes DNA damage in *TP53* at codon 249
  - Acts synergistically with coexisting HBV and HCV infections to triple risk of HCC

Diabetes and Metabolic Factors
- Diabetes, obesity, hypertension, and dyslipidemia are associated with elevated risk of HCC
  - 2-3x increased risk of HCC in diabetic patients
  - Increased lipid peroxidation and free reactive oxygen species (ROS) generation is implicated in genotoxic damage
  - Obese patients (BMI > 30) have 2-4x increased risk
  - Obesity leads to chronic hyperinsulinemia, which elevates insulin growth factor 1 (IGF1) and promotes cellular proliferation and resistance to apoptosis
  - Both obesity and diabetes are also associated with nonalcoholic steatohepatitis (NASH), which can cause cirrhosis
  - Diabetes, NAFLD, and obesity are important, emerging drivers of HCC worldwide

CLINICAL ISSUES

Epidemiology
- Incidence
  - In 2020, ~ 905,700 HCC cases were diagnosed with 830,200 deaths globally
  - 5th most common malignancy in men and 8th most common malignancy in women worldwide
    - 3rd leading cause of death in cancer patients worldwide
  - East Asia (China and Japan): As high as 35.5 cases per 100,000 in some geographical areas
  - North America: ~ 4 cases per 100,000
    - Incidence doubled from 1975 to 1998 in USA
- Geographically dependent
  - 7th decade in USA
  - Peak is 5th decade in China
    - Mainly due to the high prevalence of hepatitis B in China

Presentation
- Initial symptoms may include right upper quadrant abdominal pain
- Anorexia or early satiety is 2nd most common symptom
- Late-stage symptoms include jaundice, fever, bone pain due to metastatic lesions, complications of portal venous hypertension including esophagogastric varices, ascites, thrombocytopenia, and coagulopathy
- Hepatomegaly is seen in 90% of patients
- 50% of patients may show hepatic bruit and splenomegaly

Treatment
- Surgery is primary treatment for resectable tumors
- Orthotopic liver transplantation is potentially curative treatment for early-stage HCC
- Highest survival seen in patients with single lesion < 5 cm with no evidence of gross vascular invasion
- Tumor ablation may improve local tumor control and overall survival
- Sorafenib may improve survival in advanced HCC

Prognosis
- Tumor size, number of lesions, vascular invasion, and tumor spread determine prognosis
- Only 10-23% of HCC patients are eligible for curative resection
- Patients with early HCC undergoing liver transplant have 5-year overall survival (OS) of 44-78%

MACROSCOPIC

General Features
- Single or multiple masses may be seen
- Numerous cirrhotic-appearing nodules may be present in background
- Tumor may be encapsulated or diffusely infiltrative
  - Encapsulated HCC often arises in background of cirrhosis

Hepatocellular Carcinoma

- Tumor is often soft and varies in color from tan to grayish-white; green if bile production present
- May involve portal vein of liver, depending on size

MOLECULAR

Cytogenetics
- HCC tumors are commonly aneuploid
- Chromosomal losses include
  - 1p, 4q, 5q, 6q, 8p, 9p, 13q, 16p, 16q, and 17p
- Chromosomal gains include
  - 1q, 6p, 8q, and 17q
- DNAJB1::PRKACA fusion reported as specific recurrent abnormality in fibrolamellar subtype

Molecular Genetics
- Molecular alterations are complex and occur in multistep progression
- Most commonly mutated genes include
  - TP53, CTNNB1, AXIN1, and RB1
- Epigenetic alterations in HCC
  - Most common hypermethylated genes include BMP4, CDKN2A, GSTP1, and NFATC1
  - Common hypermethylated genes in HBV-positive HCC include DAB2IP, BMP4, ZFP41, SPDYA, and CDKN2A
  - Other reported promoter hypermethylation genes include CDH1, SLC7A10, DLC1, PTEN, and SFRP1
- Major signaling pathways implicated in hepatic carcinogenesis
  - Wnt-β catenin, Ras signaling, PI3K/Akt/mTOR, Rb and DLC1/Rho/ROCK pathways
- Molecular alterations are not currently in routine use in clinical practice for diagnostic purposes

MICROSCOPIC

Histologic Features
- Tumor cells of well-differentiated HCC resemble normal liver cells
- Prominent nuclei and nucleoli are seen with high N:C ratio and eosinophilic, finely granular cytoplasm
- Bile canaliculi are commonly identified in between neoplastic hepatocytes
  - Mallory-Denk bodies are identified in 20% of tumors
- Trabecular pattern is often present microscopically, with thickened cords of tumor cells and sinuses with dilated canaliculus leading to pseudoglandular pattern formation
- Desmoplastic stroma is commonly sparse or absent
- Occasionally, abundant stroma is present, leading to scirrhous pattern
- Subset of HCC contains abundant eosinophilic cytoplasm with desmoplastic stroma, which is known as fibrolamellar variant of HCC
- Some variants of HCC may include abundant clear cells (clear cell carcinoma)
- Other patterns include tumors with osteoclast-like giant cells, tumors with spindle cell metaplasia, and tumors with sarcomatoid patterns

ANCILLARY TESTS

Immunohistochemistry
- Commonly used immunostains in HCC diagnosis
  - Polyclonal carcinoembryonic antigen (pCEA) and CD10 highlight very distinctive canalicular pattern
  - Hep Par-1(+) in ~ 90% of HCC vs. < 4% in other tumors
  - Glypican-3 (GPC-3) expressed in ~ 80%
  - Arg-1 expressed in both normal hepatocytes and ~ 90% of HCC
  - Glutamine synthetase (GS) is diffusely expressed with cytoplasmic pattern in up to 70% of HCC
    - GS is also expressed in β-catenin-activated hepatic adenomas
  - α-fetoprotein is expressed in 50% of HCC tumors
  - CD34 sinusoidal expression is typically increased in HCC but is not always reliable marker
  - Other immunostains commonly used include HSP70, annexin-A2, CK7, and MOC-31

DIFFERENTIAL DIAGNOSIS

Metastatic Tumor
- Typically lack distinct canalicular pattern with polyclonal CEA and CD10
- Arg-1 is expressed in carcinomas with hepatocellular differentiation and is typically absent in carcinomas of metastatic origin
- Nonhepatocellular tumor-specific markers can also prove useful

Hepatocellular Adenoma
- Mostly in women of childbearing age; strong association with use of contraceptive pills
- Intact reticulin pattern of staining in adenoma but decreased and disorganized in HCC
- Glypican-3 typically absent
- Glutamine synthetase not helpful in separating HCC from β-catenin pathway hepatocellular adenoma (expressed in both diseases)

Cholangiocarcinoma
- Markers specific for HCC, including Hep-Par1 and glutamine synthetase, can prove helpful

Focal Nodular Hyperplasia
- May be confused with HCC in small biopsies
- Glypican-3 absent

SELECTED REFERENCES

1. Llovet JM et al: Molecular pathogenesis and systemic therapies for hepatocellular carcinoma. Nat Cancer. 3(4):386-401, 2022
2. Rumgay H et al: Global burden of primary liver cancer in 2020 and predictions to 2040. J Hepatol. 77(6):1598-606, 2022
3. Pittman ME et al: Anatomic pathology of hepatocellular carcinoma: histopathology using classic and new diagnostic tools. Clin Liver Dis. 19(2):239-59, 2015
4. Swanson BJ et al: A triple stain of reticulin, glypican-3, and glutamine synthetase: a useful aid in the diagnosis of liver lesions. Arch Pathol Lab Med. 139(4):537-42, 2015
5. Ma L et al: Epigenetics in hepatocellular carcinoma: an update and future therapy perspectives. World J Gastroenterol. 20(2):333-45, 2014
6. El-Serag HB: Epidemiology of viral hepatitis and hepatocellular carcinoma. Gastroenterology. 142(6):1264-73, 2012
7. Guichard C et al: Integrated analysis of somatic mutations and focal copy-number changes identifies key genes and pathways in hepatocellular carcinoma. Nat Genet. 44(6):694-8, 2012
8. White DL et al: Association between nonalcoholic fatty liver disease and risk for hepatocellular cancer, based on systematic review. Clin Gastroenterol Hepatol. 10(12):1342-59, 2012

Hepatocellular Carcinoma

Moderately Differentiated HCC

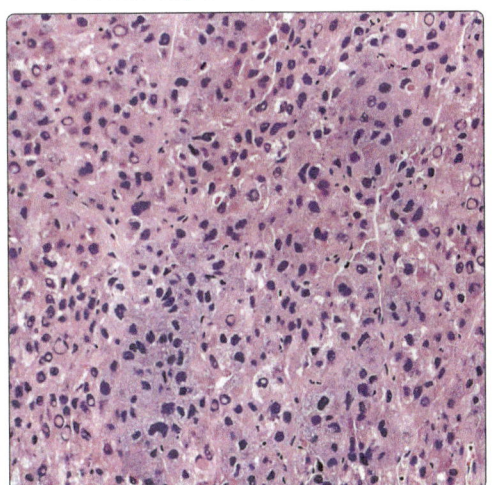

2 Different Patterns of Differentiation

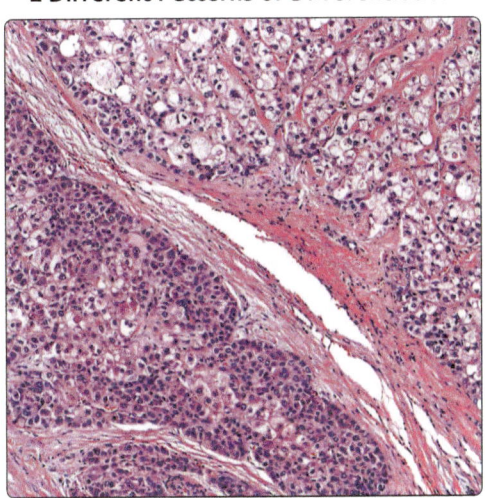

(Left) *Moderately differentiated HCC is shown. The neoplastic cells have variably enlarged, pleomorphic nuclei with irregular nuclear contours.* (Right) *2 different histologic patterns of HCC are shown, including clear cell and sheet-like foci.*

Clear Cell Pattern

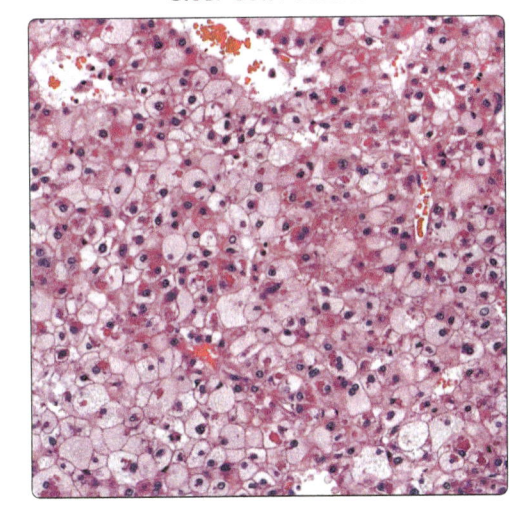

HSP70 Expression

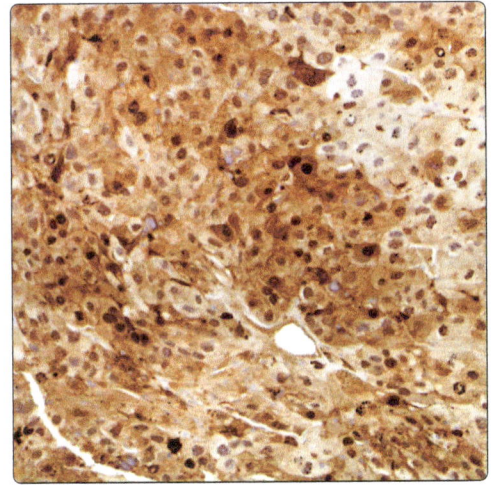

(Left) *Predominance of clear cells with a sheet-like pattern is shown in this case of HCC.* (Right) *HSP70 highlights neoplastic cells of HCC. HSP70 expression is also seen in other neoplasms, including carcinoma of the breast, and lung, and prostate and squamous cell carcinoma.*

Glutamine Synthetase Expression

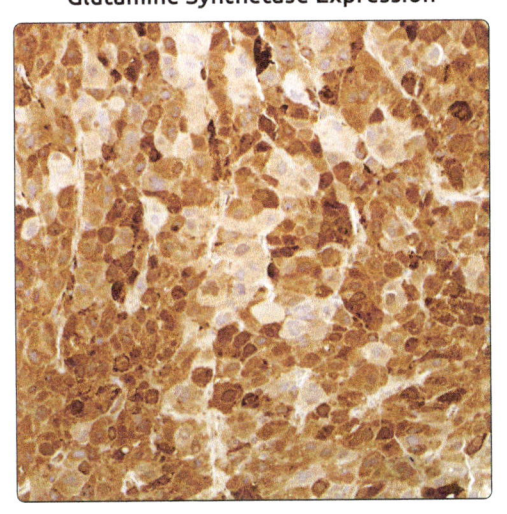

Hep-Par1 Expression

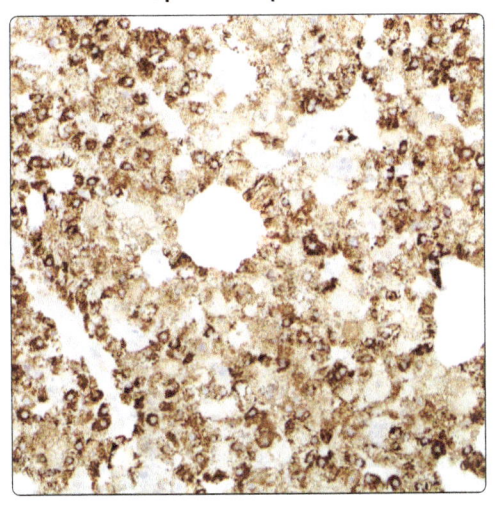

(Left) *Glutamine synthetase shows cytoplasmic and nuclear staining of neoplastic cells with variable staining pattern in this case of HCC. Glutamine synthetase is also expressed in β catenin pathway hepatocellular adenoma.* (Right) *Hep-Par1 shows bright cytoplasmic expression by neoplastic cells in this case of HCC.*

Pancreatic Ductal Adenocarcinoma

KEY FACTS

ETIOLOGY/PATHOGENESIS
- Multifactorial (environmental, preexisting medical, and hereditary factors)
- Precursor lesions
  - Pancreatic intraepithelial neoplasia
  - Intraductal papillary mucinous neoplasm
  - Mucinous cystic neoplasm

CLINICAL ISSUES
- Often nonspecific symptoms, such as epigastric pain and weight loss
- Painless jaundice and pruritus if common bile duct is obstructed
- 5-year survival < 5%

MACROSCOPIC
- Solid and firm mass with ill-defined borders
- Common bile duct and duodenum invasion are common

MOLECULAR
- Genetic alterations associated with carcinogenesis of PDA are generally secondary to
  - *KRAS* activating mutation
  - *TP53* inactivation
  - *SMAD4* inactivation
  - *CDKN2A* inactivation

MICROSCOPIC
- Proliferation of haphazardly arranged, small, tubular structures lined by mucinous cells
- Perineural invasion and vascular invasion
- Glands adjacent to muscular blood vessels
- Variation in nuclear shape and size

TOP DIFFERENTIAL DIAGNOSES
- Chronic pancreatitis
- Neuroendocrine neoplasm

Nuclear Pleomorphism

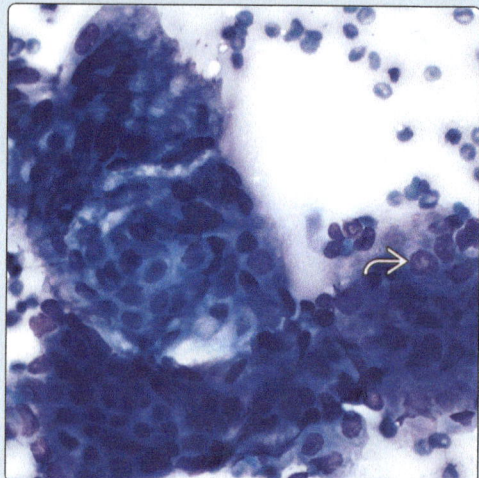

Perineural Invasion

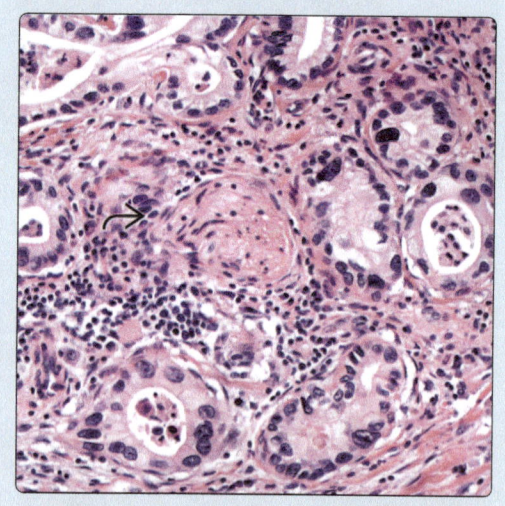

(Left) Diff-Quik preparation of FNA of pancreatic ductal adenocarcinoma shows sheets of atypical ductal cells. The ductal cells are disorganized with nuclear pleomorphism ⊃. (Right) Pancreatic duct adenocarcinoma shows perineural invasion ⊃. This feature is very common in pancreatic ductal adenocarcinoma.

Mild Nuclear Atypia

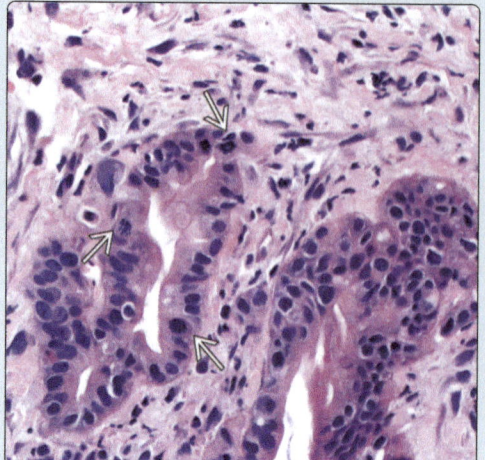

Marked Pleomorphic Nuclei

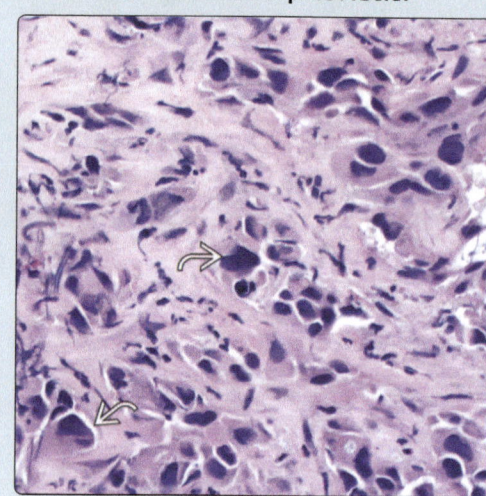

(Left) In well-differentiated ductal adenocarcinoma, the growth pattern and cytologic appearance closely resemble nonneoplastic ductules with mild nuclear variation. Here, mitotic figures are easily identified ⊃. (Right) In poorly differentiated ductal adenocarcinoma, the neoplastic cells may not form glands. Here, they are dyscohesive with marked pleomorphic nuclei ⊃.

Pancreatic Ductal Adenocarcinoma

TERMINOLOGY

Abbreviations
- Pancreatic ductal adenocarcinoma (PDA)

Synonyms
- Pancreatic adenocarcinoma
- Pancreatic tubular adenocarcinoma
- Pancreatic infiltrating ductal carcinoma

Definitions
- Infiltrating epithelial neoplasm of pancreatic ductal origin
  - > 90% of pancreatic neoplasms have ductal origin

ETIOLOGY/PATHOGENESIS

Overview
- Multifactorial

Environmental Risk Factors
- Tobacco smoking
  - 2-3x greater risk than nonsmokers
- Diet high in saturated fats and low in vegetables/fruits
- Heavy consumption of alcohol

Medical Risk Factors
- Chronic pancreatitis
- Obesity
- Diabetes mellitus
- Previous cholecystectomy or partial gastrectomy

Hereditary Risk Factors
- Family history of pancreatic cancer
- Hereditary pancreatitis
  - Mutations in *PRSS1*
- Hereditary breast cancer syndrome
  - Mostly due to *BRCA2* mutations
- Familial atypical multiple mole-melanoma syndrome
  - Mutations in *CDKN2A*
- Peutz-Jeghers syndrome
  - Mutations in *STK11*
- Hereditary nonpolyposis colorectal cancer syndrome (Lynch syndrome)
  - Mutations in DNA mismatch repair genes
- Fanconi anemia
  - Mutations in *FANCC* and *FANCG*

Precursor Lesions
- Pancreatic intraepithelial neoplasia
- Intraductal papillary mucinous neoplasm
- Mucinous cystic neoplasm

CLINICAL ISSUES

Epidemiology
- Incidence
  - 10-12 cases per 100,000
  - 4th leading cause of death from cancer in United States
- Age
  - Usually between 60-80 years at diagnosis
- Sex
  - Slight male predominance
- Ethnicity
  - Higher rates seen in Black populations than in White populations in United States

Presentation
- Painless jaundice and pruritus if common bile duct is obstructed
- Often nonspecific symptoms, such as epigastric pain and weight loss

Treatment
- Surgical resection if resectable at presentation
  - ~ 20% of patients have resectable tumor
- Neoadjuvant therapy prior to resection may be used

Prognosis
- 5-year survival: < 5%

MACROSCOPIC

General Features
- Solid and firm mass with ill-defined borders
- Adjacent areas of fibrosis secondary to chronic pancreatitis
- Common bile duct and duodenum invasion are common
- Focal narrowing of pancreatic and common bile ducts with proximal dilation

MOLECULAR

Cytogenetics
- Common chromosomal deletions
  - 18q21, 17p13, 9p21, 8p22, 1p36
- Common chromosomal gains
  - 8q24, 20q13, 1q25

Molecular Genetics
- *KRAS*
  - Functions as oncogene
  - Somatic point mutation in ~ 70% of cases
    - Mutations likely play early role in oncogenesis
    - Results in constitutive activation of RAS/MAPK signaling pathway
  - Clinical relevance
    - Mutations are associated with altered sensitivity to trametinib, bleomycin, selumetinib, refametinib, and gefitinib
- *TP53*
  - Functions as tumor suppressor gene
  - Prevents cells with mutated or damaged DNA from dividing
  - Regulates cell division and growth
  - Inactivating mutations in ~ 40% of cases
    - Prevents tumor cells from apoptosis
  - Clinical relevance
    - Mutations are associated with altered sensitivity to 5-fluorouracil, rucaparib, CX-5461, bleomycin, and dabrafenib
- *SMAD4*
  - Involved in signal transduction via TGF-β signaling pathway
  - Loss-of-function mutations in ~ 10%
    - Results in deregulation of TGF-β signaling pathway
    - Promotes tumor growth
  - Clinical relevance

Pancreatic Ductal Adenocarcinoma

- Inactivation is likely associated with increase metastatic potential and treatment failure
- Molecular heterogeneity is common
- Worse outcomes are associated with alterations of 3 of 4 main driver genes
  - Patients whose tumors lacked CDKN2A expression have worse disease-free survival (DFS)
  - *KRAS* mutant tumors have worse DFS
  - *TP53* status is associated with shorter DFS
  - *SMAD4* status is not associated with pattern of disease recurrence
  - Patients have worse DFS and overall survival with greater number of altered driver genes
- Other mutated genes
  - Genes mutated with 5% or less frequency in COSMIC data
    - *CDKN2A*
    - *LRP1B*
    - *KMT2C* (MLL3)
    - *ARID1A*
    - *RNF43*
    - *KMT2D*
    - *ATM*
    - *GNAS*
    - *TGFRB2*
    - *MAP2K4*
    - *NF1*
    - *RBM10*

MICROSCOPIC

Histologic Features

- Conventional type
  - Proliferation of haphazardly arranged, small, tubular structures lined by mucinous cells
  - Perineural invasion and vascular invasion are typical
  - Glands adjacent to muscular blood vessels
  - Neoplastic cells with generous cytoplasm containing mucin or with clear cell change
  - Variation in nuclear shape and size
- Histologic variants and patterns
  - Foamy gland pattern
    - Well-differentiated ductal carcinoma
    - Foamy, microvesicular cytoplasm
  - Large duct pattern
    - Infiltrating microcystic (dilated) glands in clusters
    - Malignant ducts with irregular contours
    - Intraluminal necrotic debris with neutrophils
  - Vacuolated pattern
    - Cribriform nests of neoplastic cells
    - Signet ring-like appearance
  - Lobular carcinoma-like pattern
    - Reminiscent of lobular breast carcinoma
    - Conventional tubular-type often present
  - Solid nested pattern (clear cell carcinoma)
    - Morphologic features of neuroendocrine neoplasm
    - Prominent gland formation
  - Micropapillary pattern
    - Neoplastic cells in micropapillary pattern
    - Clusters of tumor cells in lacunar spaces
  - Mucinous (colloid) carcinoma
    - Neoplastic cells floating in pools of mucin
  - Medullary carcinoma
    - Neoplastic cells in syncytial pattern
    - Lack of desmoplasia
    - Associated with inflammatory infiltrate
  - Adenosquamous carcinoma
    - Malignant glands and squamous cells
  - Hepatoid carcinoma
    - Neoplastic cells in nests or trabeculae
    - Hepatocellular differentiation
  - Undifferentiated carcinoma
    - Minimal features of epithelial differentiation
    - Osteoclast-like giant cells can be seen

Cytologic Features

- Hypercellular aspirate of ductal cells
- Uneven distribution of ductal cells within sheet
- Isolated malignant ductal cells
- Enlarged nuclei with irregular nuclear contours
- Anisonucleosis (> 4:1 variation in size)

ANCILLARY TESTS

Immunohistochemistry

- Positive for CK7, CK8, CK18, CK19, EMA, CEA, CA19-9, CA125, and B72.3
- Loss of expression of SMAD4 (55%)
- Overexpression of p53 (50-75%)
- CK20 and MUC2 positive in mucinous (colloid) carcinoma

DIFFERENTIAL DIAGNOSIS

Chronic Pancreatitis

- Ductules retain normal lobular configuration
- No significant nuclear abnormalities
- Clinical history can also prove helpful

Ampullary/Periampullary Carcinomas

- Presence of precursor in situ ampullary lesions

Acinic Cell Carcinoma

- Neoplastic cells in acinar, trabecular, and solid patterns
- Positive for trypsin and chymotrypsin
- Negative for CK7

Neuroendocrine Neoplasms

- Nuclear features with "salt and pepper" chromatin
- Positive for chromogranin and synaptophysin

SELECTED REFERENCES

1. COSMIC: Catalogue of Somatic Mutations In Cancer. v98. Published March 2019. Updated May 23, 2023. Accessed July 17, 2023. https://cancer.sanger.ac.uk/cosmic.
2. Kimura H et al: CKAP4, a DKK1 receptor, is a biomarker in exosomes derived from pancreatic cancer and a molecular target for therapy. Clin Cancer Res. 25(6):1936-47, 2019
3. Qian ZR et al: Association of alterations in main driver genes with outcomes of patients with resected pancreatic ductal adenocarcinoma. JAMA Oncol. 4(3):e173420, 2018
4. Zhao L et al: Gene expression profiling of 1200 pancreatic ductal adenocarcinoma reveals novel subtypes. BMC Cancer. 18(1):603, 2018
5. Martinez-Useros J et al: UNR/CDSE1 expression as prognosis biomarker in resectable pancreatic ductal adenocarcinoma patients: a proof-of-concept. PLoS One. 12(8):e0182044, 2017

Pancreatic Ductal Adenocarcinoma

Increased Nuclear:Cytoplasmic Ratio

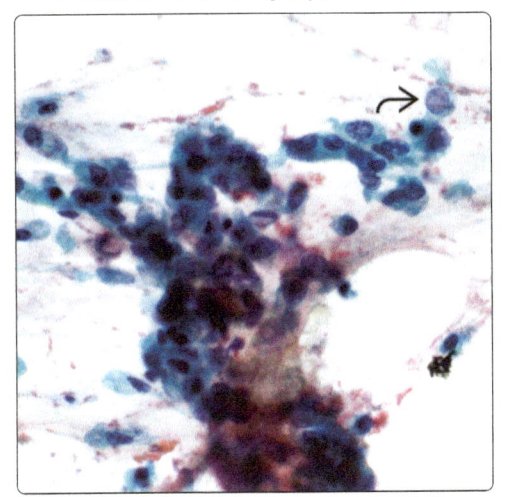

Thick-Walled Vessel

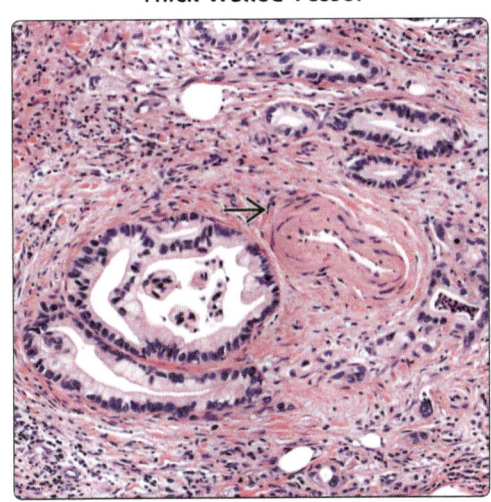

(Left) Pap-stained FNA of pancreatic duct adenocarcinoma shows single neoplastic cells with nuclear enlargement and increased nuclear:cytoplasmic ratio ➡. (Right) Pancreatic duct adenocarcinoma shows distribution of neoplastic glands in close proximity to a thick-walled vessel ➡. This is a common feature in pancreatic carcinomas.

Colloid (Mucinous) Variant

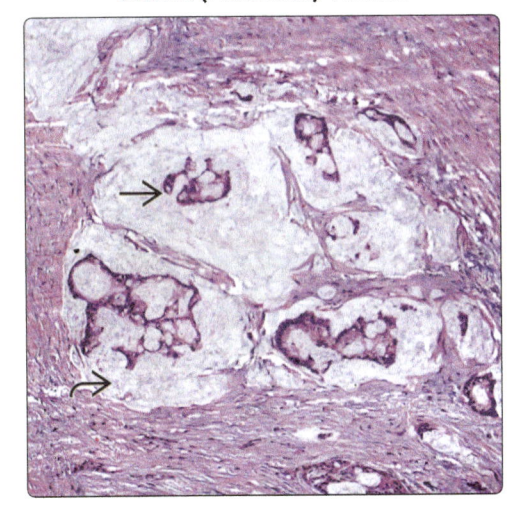

Foamy Gland Pattern

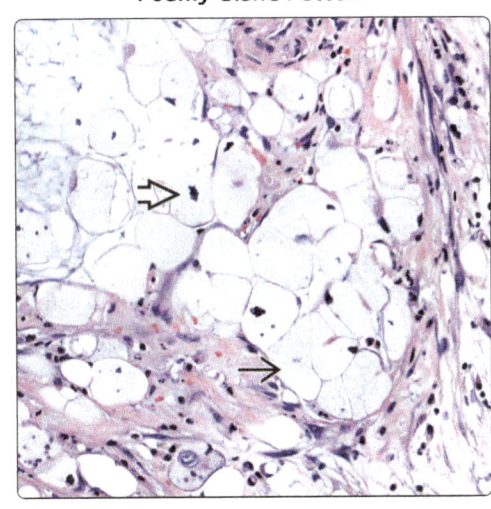

(Left) Colloid (mucinous) variant of pancreatic duct adenocarcinoma shows neoplastic glands ➡ floating in large pools of mucin ➡. (Right) Foamy gland pattern of pancreatic duct adenocarcinoma shows neoplastic cells with microvesicular cytoplasm ➡ and raisinoid nuclei ➡.

Perineural Invasion

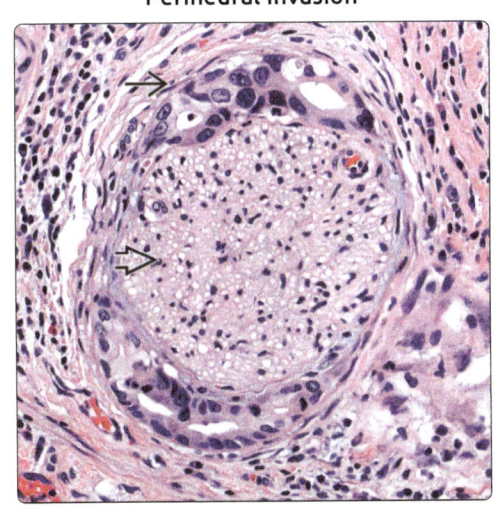

Lymph Node Metastasis

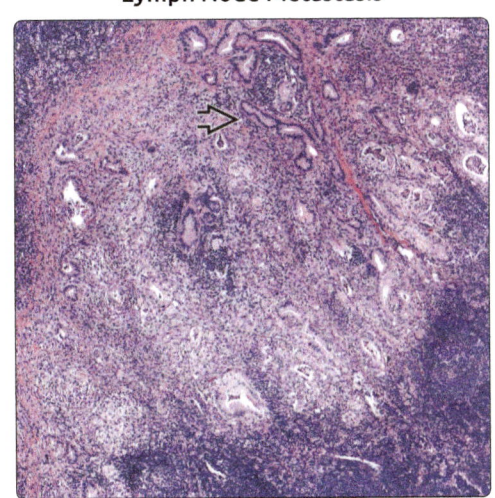

(Left) Pancreatic duct adenocarcinoma with perineural invasion is shown. The neoplastic glands ➡ are surrounding the nerve ➡. (Right) Pancreatic ductal adenocarcinoma ➡ shows extensive involvement of the excised lymph node.

Pancreatic Mucinous Cystic Neoplasm

KEY FACTS

TERMINOLOGY
- Neoplasm composed of mucin-producing epithelial cells with ovarian-type stroma lacking connection with ducts

CLINICAL ISSUES
- Occurs virtually only in women
- Slow growing and asymptomatic in most cases
  - Larger tumors may be symptomatic
- 5-year survival rate
  - > 95% in cases without invasive carcinoma
  - 20-60% in cases with invasive carcinoma
- Mostly in body and tail of pancreas

MACROSCOPIC
- Typically single, multilocular cysts surrounded by thick, fibrotic capsule filled with thick mucin
- No connection to pancreatic ducts and their branches

MOLECULAR
- *KRAS* mutations
  - Detectable in PMCN with even low-grade dysplasia
- *TP53* and *SMAD4* mutations are late events
  - Associated with invasive carcinoma component

MICROSCOPIC
- Histologic features
  - Mucinous epithelium with varying degree of dysplasia
  - Ovarian-type stroma in cyst wall
- Cytologic features
  - Epithelial cells with varying degree of dysplasia
  - Thick, colloid-like mucin

TOP DIFFERENTIAL DIAGNOSES
- Intraductal papillary mucinous neoplasm
- Serous cystadenoma

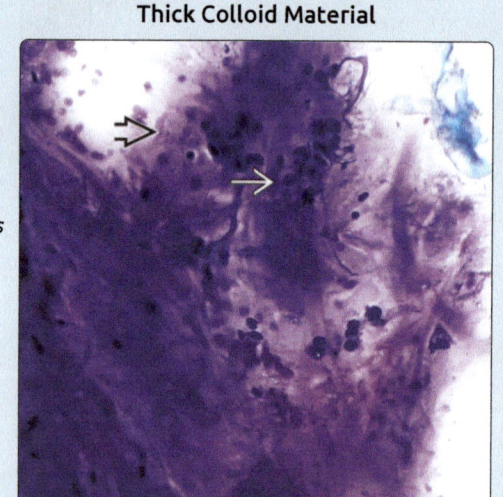

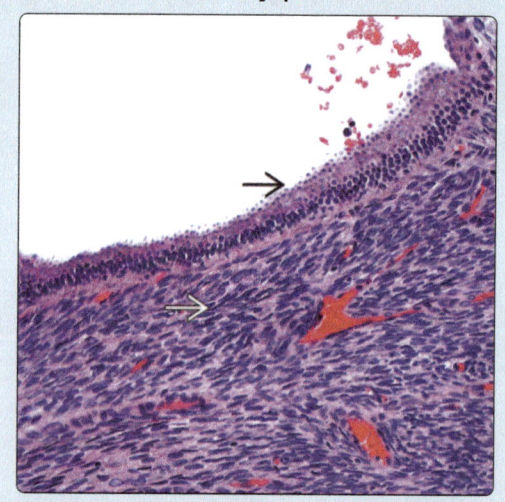

(Left) Aspirate smear of pancreatic mucinous cystic neoplasm (PMCN) shows predominantly thick colloid material ⇨. Note the inflammatory and epithelial cells embedded in the pool of mucin ⇨. (Right) PMCN shows tall, columnar, mucin-producing epithelium ⇨ with low-grade dysplasia and a distinctive underlying ovarian-type stroma ⇨ required for the diagnosis.

Thick Colloid Material

Mucin-Producing Epithelium With Low-Grade Dysplasia

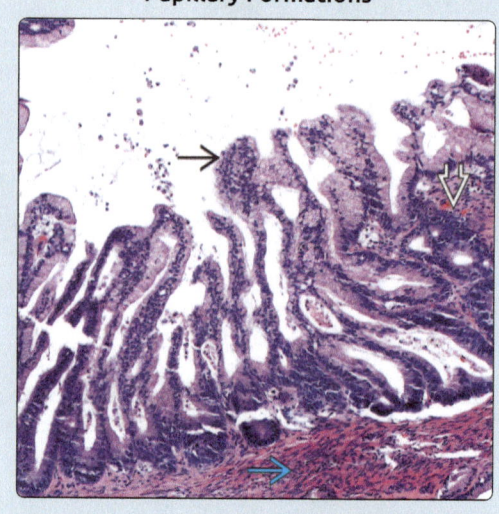

(Left) Pap-stained cytologic smear of PMCN shows malignant epithelial cells with high nuclear:cytoplasmic ratio ⇨, consistent with an associated concurrent pancreatic adenocarcinoma. (Right) PMCN shows abundant papillary formations ⇨ with pseudostratified, hyperchromatic nuclei and some cribriform architecture ⇨. An ovarian stroma is present ⇨.

Pancreatic Mucinous Cystic Neoplasm With Pancreatic Adenocarcinoma

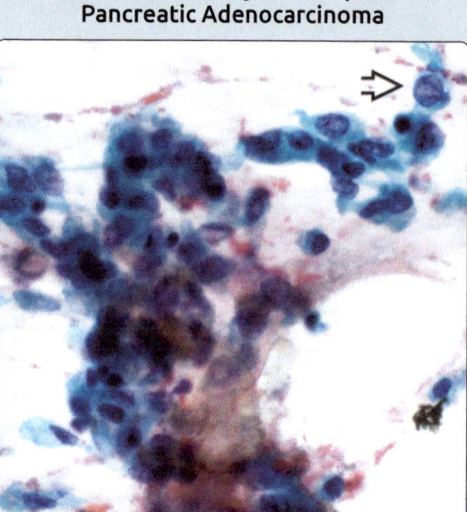

Papillary Formations

Pancreatic Mucinous Cystic Neoplasm

TERMINOLOGY

Abbreviations
- Pancreatic mucinous cystic neoplasm (PMCN)

Synonyms
- Mucinous cystic neoplasm of pancreas

Definitions
- Neoplasm composed of mucin-producing epithelial cells with ovarian-type stroma lacking connection with ducts

CLASSIFICATION

Mucinous Cystic Neoplasm
- Mucinous cystic neoplasm with low-grade dysplasia
- Mucinous cystic neoplasm with high-grade dysplasia
- Mucinous cystic neoplasm with associated invasive carcinoma

CLINICAL ISSUES

Epidemiology
- Age
  - Mean at diagnosis: 40-50 years
- Sex
  - Virtually cases all in women (F:M = 20:1)

Site
- Vast majority in body and tail of pancreas

Presentation
- Slow growing and asymptomatic in majority of cases
- Larger tumors can be symptomatic

Treatment
- Surgical resection is treatment of choice

Prognosis
- Considered precursor lesion for pancreatic cancer
- Prognosis is variable
  - 5-year survival rate
    - > 95% in cases without invasive carcinoma
    - 20-60% in cases with invasive carcinoma

MACROSCOPIC

General Features
- Typically single, multilocular cysts surrounded by thick, fibrotic capsule filled with thick mucin
- No connection to pancreatic ducts and their branches

MOLECULAR

Molecular Alterations
- *KRAS* mutations
  - Seen in 50-60% of PMCN
  - Mutations appear to be early event
    - Detectable with even low-grade dysplasia
  - Present in ~ 80% of PMCN with high-grade dysplasia and those associated with adenocarcinoma
  - Mutations are activating somatic mutations mainly involving codon 12 of exon 2 of *KRAS*
  - Can serve as diagnostic biomarker, especially in fine-needle aspiration cytology specimens
- *RNF43* mutations
  - Inactivating somatic mutations seen in up to 38%
  - Mainly associated with high-grade PMCN
  - Testing may prove useful as diagnostic marker in pancreatic cyst fluid
- *TP53* mutations
  - Inactivating mutations similar to other cancers
  - Reported in overall 41% of PMCN
  - *TP53* mutations are late events with invasive carcinoma
- *SMAD4* mutations
  - Inactivating somatic mutations
  - Late events and mostly observed in PMCN associated with infiltrating carcinoma
- *CDKN2A* mutations
  - Inactivating somatic mutations reported in up to 43% of cases
- *PIK3CA* mutations
  - Reported with low frequency of ~ 75 in PMCN
    - Associated with high-grade dysplastic epithelium

MICROSCOPIC

Histologic Features
- Mucinous epithelial lining with varying degree of dysplasia
- Ovarian type stroma in cyst wall

Cytologic Features
- Thick, colloid-like mucin
- Epithelial cells with varying degree of dysplasia

ANCILLARY TESTS

Immunohistochemistry
- Ovarian-type stroma of PMCN expresses ER, PR, calretinin, &/or inhibin

DIFFERENTIAL DIAGNOSIS

Intraductal Papillary Mucinous Neoplasm
- Connected to pancreatic ducts &/or its branches
- No ovarian stroma

Pancreatic Pseudocyst
- Cyst not lined by epithelium
- No mucin production

Serous Cystadenoma
- Lined by glycogen-rich cuboidal cells
- No mucin production

Solid Pseudopapillary Neoplasm
- Usually in young women
- No mucin production

SELECTED REFERENCES

1. Sawai H et al: Invasive ductal carcinoma arising in mucinous cystic neoplasm of pancreas: a case report. Am J Case Rep. 20:242-7, 2019
2. Cowan RW et al: Genetic progression of pancreatic cancer. Cancer J. 20(1):80-4, 2014
3. Fukushima N et al: Mucinous cystic neoplasms of the pancreas: update on the surgical pathology and molecular genetics. Semin Diagn Pathol. 31(6):467-74, 2014

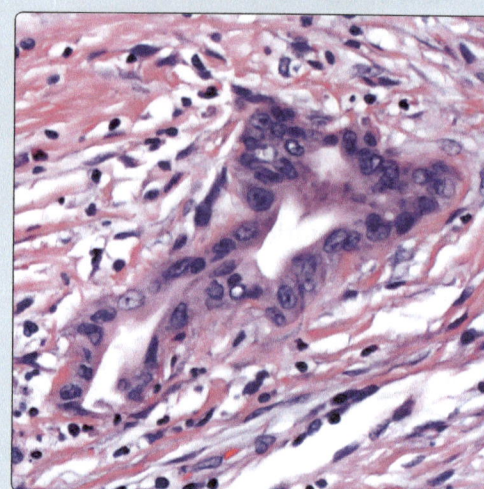

Pancreatic Intraductal Papillary Mucinous Neoplasm

KEY FACTS

TERMINOLOGY
- Pancreatic cystic neoplasm composed of mucin-producing epithelial cells with papillary formations connected to main pancreatic duct &/or its branches

CLINICAL ISSUES
- Accounts for 20-50% of resected pancreatic cystic tumors
- Commonly in pancreatic head
- Invasive adenocarcinoma can arise within intraductal papillary mucinous neoplasm (IPMN)
- Excellent prognosis for completely resected tumors with low- or even high-grade dysplasia
- 5-year survival: ~ 40% in IPMN with associated invasive carcinoma

MACROSCOPIC
- Dilated main duct filled with mucin and lined by small papillary formations
- Multilocular (grape-like) cystic lesions in branch duct type

MOLECULAR
- Genes commonly mutated in IPMN
  - *GNAS*
  - *KRAS*
  - *RNF43*
  - *TP53*

MICROSCOPIC
- Histologic features
  - Mucinous neoplastic epithelium in papillae
  - Types: Gastric, biliary, or intestinal
- Cytologic features
  - Dysplasia: Low or high grade
  - Thick, colloid-like mucin

TOP DIFFERENTIAL DIAGNOSES
- Pancreatic mucinous cystic neoplasm
- Serous cystadenoma

Thick Mucin

Gastric and Intestinal Epithelium

(Left) Diff-Quik-stained cytologic preparation of intraductal papillary mucinous neoplasm (IPMN) shows thick mucin with only rare inflammatory-type-appearing cells. **(Right)** IPMN shows papillary formations lined by gastric ➡ and intestinal ➡ epithelium with low-grade dysplasia.

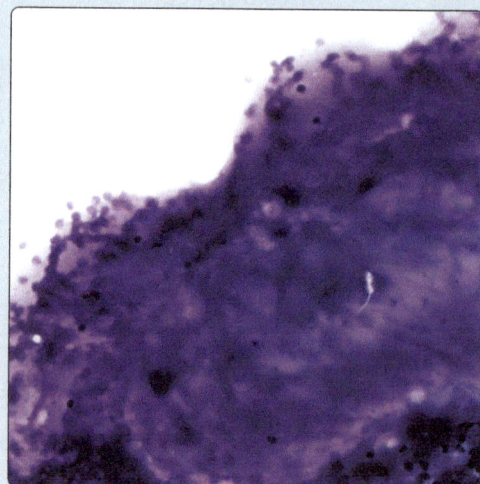

High-Grade Dysplasia

Associated Invasive Carcinoma

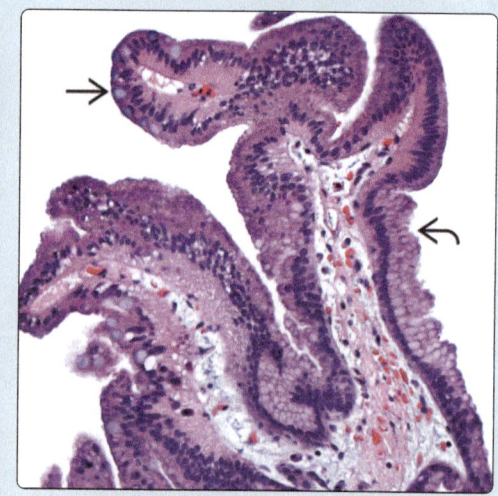

(Left) IPMN shows papillary formations lined with high-grade dysplasia. The epithelial lining shows architectural complexity with micropapillae ➡. The nuclei are round with loss of polarity ➡. **(Right)** Invasive carcinoma associated with IPMN is shown.

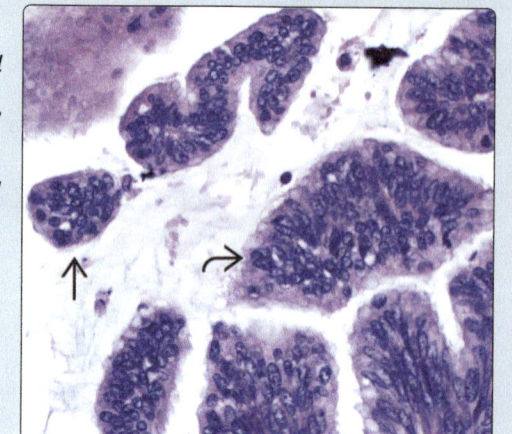

Pancreatic Intraductal Papillary Mucinous Neoplasm

TERMINOLOGY

Abbreviations
- Intraductal papillary mucinous neoplasm (IPMN)

Definitions
- Pancreatic cystic neoplasm composed of mucin-producing epithelial cells with papillary formations connected to main pancreatic duct &/or its branches
- Can be low-grade, high-grade or associated with invasive carcinoma

CLASSIFICATION

Subtypes
- Gastric, intestinal, or pancreatobiliary

CLINICAL ISSUES

Site
- Commonly in pancreatic head

Presentation
- Accounts for 20-50% of resected pancreatic cystic tumors
- Branch duct-type often detected incidentally
- Majority are asymptomatic
- Increase risk of other synchronous or metachronous malignancies (e.g., gastric or colon cancer)

Treatment
- Surgical resection for main duct type
  - Relatively high incidence of associated invasive carcinoma

Prognosis
- Excellent prognosis for completely resected tumors with low- or even high-grade dysplasia
  - Recurrence or metastatic lesions may occur in small subset of cases several years post complete resection
- 5-year survival: ~ 40% in IPMN associated invasive carcinoma

MACROSCOPIC

General Features
- Dilated main duct filled with mucin and lined by small papillary formations
- Multilocular (grape-like) cystic lesions in branch duct type

MOLECULAR

Molecular Alterations
- Mutations detected by targeted next-generation sequencing (NGS) panel
  - *GNAS* mutations
    - Activating somatic mutations present in 50-70% of IPMN
    - Mutation at codon 201 found exclusively in IPMN
      - Common mutations include R201H and R201C
    - Concurrent *KRAS* mutations detected in ~ 37% of cases
    - *GNAS* mutation testing can serve as diagnostic molecular biomarker
    - *GNAS* mutations absent in pancreatic mucinous neoplasm
    - *GNAS* mutation may play role in transformation of IPMN
    - *GNAS* mutations associated with
      - Intestinal subtype of IPMN
      - MUC2 expression
      - Pancreatic ductal adenocarcinoma and IPMN
  - *KRAS* mutations
    - Activating somatic mutations, typically in codon 12 of exon 2
    - Seen in 60-80% of cases
    - *KRAS* mutations are early events associated with dysplastic epithelium
    - Diagnostic molecular biomarker but is not specific for IPMN
  - *RNF43* mutations
    - Somatic mutations in ~ 50% of IPMN
    - Associated with *GNAS* &/or *KRAS* mutations in virtually all cases
  - *TP53* mutations
    - Mutations reported in ~ 10% of IPMN
    - Mutations are associated with high-grade dysplasia and invasive cancer
  - *BRAF* mutations
    - Detected in ~ 6% of cases
  - Other gene mutations detected with low frequency (< 5%)
    - *CDKN2A, CTNNB1, IDH1, STK11, PTEN*

MICROSCOPIC

Histologic Features
- Mucinous neoplastic epithelium in papillae
  - Subtypes: Gastric, biliary, or intestinal
  - Dysplasia: Low or high grade

Cytologic Features
- Thick, colloid-like mucin
- Epithelial cells with varying degree of dysplasia

DIFFERENTIAL DIAGNOSIS

Pancreatic Mucinous Cystic Neoplasm
- Multiloculated cysts with thick walls
- No connection to pancreatic ducts &/or branches
- Distinct ovarian-type stroma

Pancreatic Pseudocyst
- Associated with history of pancreatitis
- Cyst not lined by epithelium
- No mucin production

Serous Cystadenoma
- Cyst with central stellate scar
- Lined by glycogen-rich cuboidal cells
- No mucin production

SELECTED REFERENCES

1. Ohtsuka T et al: Clinical assessment of the GNAS mutation status in patients with intraductal papillary mucinous neoplasm of the pancreas. Surg Today. 49(11):887-93, 2019

Cholangiocarcinoma

KEY FACTS

ETIOLOGY/PATHOGENESIS
- Parasitic infestations of *Clonorchis sinensis* (Chinese liver fluke) and *Opisthorchis viverrini* (Southeast Asian liver fluke) common in Southeast Asia
- Hepatocholelithiasis (stones in liver and biliary tract)
- Chronic inflammation plays key role in pathogenesis of cholangiocarcinoma

CLINICAL ISSUES
- Incidence of idiopathic cholangiocarcinoma (ICC) is increasing in Western world, including North America, Europe, Japan, and Australia
- Regional hotspots of CC (northeast Thailand) due to factors such as fluke infestation

MOLECULAR
- *FGFR2* fusion genes identified in 7-14% of cases
- Targeted therapies (e.g., TAS-120) available for patients with *FGFR2* fusion changes
- *IDH1*, *IDH2*, *HER2*, *NTRK*, and *RET* mutational changes are treatment targets in CC

MICROSCOPIC
- Neoplastic cells in CC are arranged in tubules and glands, forming cribriform pattern, and can also form solid cords, nests, or papillary structures
- Uncommon histologic variants include mucinous, adenosquamous, clear cell, spindle cell, and sarcomatoid

ANCILLARY TESTS
- Specific molecular markers for ICC and ECC are currently unavailable
- ICC is strongly positive for CK7 and CK19; ECC is more often positive for CK20

TOP DIFFERENTIAL DIAGNOSES
- Metastatic adenocarcinoma
- Hepatocellular carcinoma

Desmoplastic Stromal Response

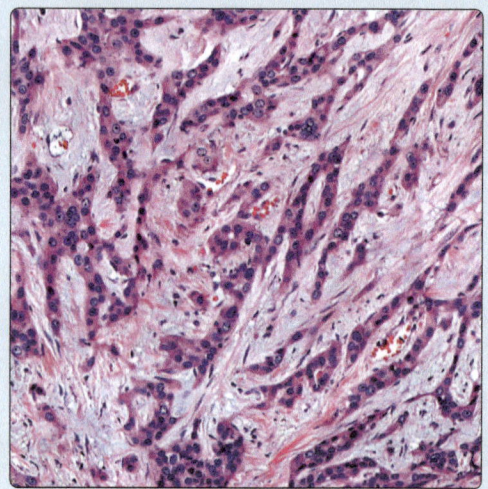

Perineural Invasion

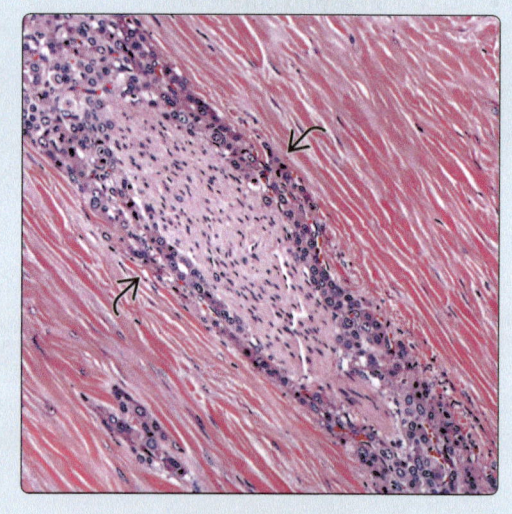

(Left) Cholangiocarcinoma with infiltrating cords of neoplastic cells associated with desmoplastic stromal response is shown. The tumor cells are moderately differentiated. (Right) Infiltrating neoplastic cells in markedly fibrotic stroma are shown in this case of cholangiocarcinoma. Perineural invasion is present ⇗.

Glandular Proliferation

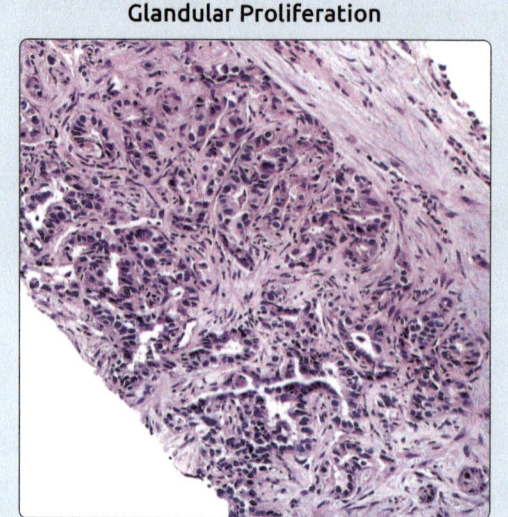

CK19 Immunohistochemistry

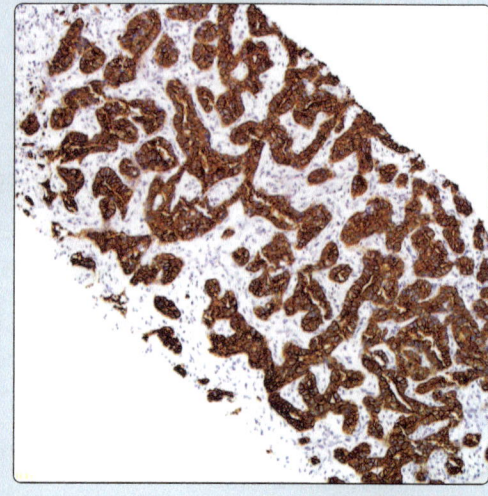

(Left) Core needle biopsy of cholangiocarcinoma shows a well- to moderately differentiated glandular proliferation within a desmoplastic stroma. (Right) CK19 shows bright expression in cholangiocarcinoma.

Cholangiocarcinoma

TERMINOLOGY

Abbreviations
- Cholangiocarcinoma (CC)
  - Intrahepatic cholangiocarcinoma (ICC)
  - Extrahepatic cholangiocarcinoma (ECC)

Definitions
- Malignant neoplasm arising from bile ducts
  - ICC arises in liver
  - ECC arises outside liver (hilum to ampulla of Vater)
  - Hilar CC (a.k.a. Klatskin tumor) arises in hilum of right and left hepatic ducts

ETIOLOGY/PATHOGENESIS

Risk Factors
- Primary sclerosing cholangitis, inflammatory disease of bile ducts in Western world
- Parasitic infestations, including *Clonorchis sinensis* and *Opisthorchis viverrini* in China and Thailand, respectively
- Congenital liver disease, such as Caroli disease
- Choledochal cysts
- Hepatocholelithiasis
- Other risk factors
  - Chronic liver disease (hepatitis B or C)
  - Alcoholic liver disease

Other Less-Defined Associations
- HIV infection
- Diabetes
- Obesity
- Thorotrast administration

CLINICAL ISSUES

Epidemiology
- Incidence of ICC is increasing in Western world, including North America, Europe, Japan, and Australia
- Accurate reclassification of metastatic adenocarcinoma as CC may be reason for apparent increase in incidence
- ICC accounts for 15-20% of all primary liver cancers
- Regional hotspots of CC (northeast Thailand) have incidence of 96/100,000 due to factors such as fluke infestation
- Median age of presentation: ~ 50 years worldwide; > 65 years in Western world
- Slight male predominance

Presentation
- Anorexia and early satiety may be present
- Right upper abdominal quadrant pain and hepatomegaly in ICC
- Rapid onset of painless, deep jaundice in hilar and ECC

Treatment
- Combination of surgery, radiation, and chemotherapy
- Liver transplantation is option with localized ICC

Prognosis
- Overall poor survival
- TNM staging at diagnosis determines outcomes for CC
- 5-year survival in localized stage I ICC: ~ 15%; decreases to 2% with distant metastasis

MACROSCOPIC

General Features
- ICC typically large in size at diagnosis
- Hilar CC and ECC are small and cause obstruction early on
- CC is grossly firm and white to tan in color

MOLECULAR

Molecular Genetics
- *IDH1* and *IDH2* mutations reported in up to 13% in ICC
- *KRAS* and *BRAF* mutations reported in ~ 45% and 22% of CC, respectively
- Newly identified targets include *BAP1* (9-12%) and *ARID1A* (15-36%)
- *FGFR2* fusion genes identified in 7-14% of cases
- *HER2* copy number changes are commonly seen in ECC
- 3 most altered genes in liver fluke-associated CC include *TP53* (~ 44%), *KRAS* and *SMAD4* (each ~ 17%)
- Rare genomic changes in CC include *NTRK* and *RET* fusions (< 0.2%)

MICROSCOPIC

Histologic Features
- Neoplastic cells are arranged in tubules and glands, forming cribriform pattern
- Can form solid cords, nests, or papillary structures
- Desmoplastic reaction is often identified in CC and plays key role in therapeutic nonresponse
- Tumor immune microenvironment plays key role in response to therapy

ANCILLARY TESTS

Immunohistochemistry
- No specific IHC marker available currently
- Diagnosis is typically made by exclusion of metastatic adenocarcinoma using tumor-specific IHC markers
  - Site-specific markers, such as CDX2 for colon, TTF-1 for lung, and PSA for prostate cancer, may be used to separate metastatic diseases from primary CC
- ICC is strongly positive for CK7 and CK19; ECC is more often positive for CK20
- p53 is positive in 20-80% cases of CC but is not specific

DIFFERENTIAL DIAGNOSIS

Metastatic Adenocarcinoma
- Tumor-specific IHC can help to separate from CC

Hepatocellular Carcinoma
- IHC markers specific for HCC, including AFP, Hep-Par1, and glutamine synthetase can prove helpful

SELECTED REFERENCES
1. Ilyas SI et al: Cholangiocarcinoma - novel biological insights and therapeutic strategies. Nat Rev Clin Oncol. 20(7):470-86, 2023
2. Sumbly V et al: Ivosidenib for IDH1 mutant cholangiocarcinoma: a narrative review. Cureus. 14(1):e21018, 2022

Testicular Germ Cell Tumors

TERMINOLOGY

Abbreviations
- Testicular germ cell tumor (TGCT)

Synonyms
- Term germ cell neoplasia in situ (GCNIS) replaced old term intratubular germ cell neoplasia unclassified (IGCNU)
- Term spermatocytic tumor replaced old term spermatocytic seminoma

ETIOLOGY/PATHOGENESIS

Pathogenetic Factors
- GCNIS
  - Noninvasive precursor lesion to seminomas and adult nonseminomatous germ cell tumor (NSGCT)
  - Typically seen in seminiferous tubules adjacent to invasive germ cell tumors
- Invasive TGCTs
  - Likely originate from primordial germ cells (early fetal developing germ cells) via common precursor GCNIS
- GCNIS and seminoma share many phenotypic characteristics with primordial germs cells and gonocytes, consistent with premeiotic origin
  - Express many transcription factors associated with pluripotency, including POU5F1 and NANOG
- Gains of short arm of chromosome 12
  - Likely key transformational event that drives invasive phenotype
  - Most commonly isochromosome 12p
  - Present in invasive TGCTs
  - Pure GCNIS lacks these alterations
- TP53 protein is consistently expressed in GCNIS and invasive TGCTs but not mutated
- Loss of PTEN protein expression is common event in progression from GCNIS to invasive TGCT
- Loss of CDKN2C and p21 expression and gain of MDM2 expression is associated with invasive growth
- Postpubertal teratoma
  - Thought to arise from GCNIS through intermediary of malignant nonteratomatous germ cell tumor
  - This intermediary can give rise to metastasis
- Spermatocytic tumor
  - Biologically different from other adult TGCTs
  - Thought to arise from premeiotic germ cell that lacks residual embryonic traits
  - Progenitor cell thought to be either mature spermatogonia or primary spermatocyte
  - Lacks chromosome 12p abnormality

TESTICULAR GERM CELL TUMORS IN PREPUBERTAL MALES

Yolk Sac Tumor, Prepubertal Type
- Most common TGCT in children
- Occurs from birth to 9 years of age
  - Median age: 18 months
- Presents as painless testicular mass
- Often diagnosed at low stage confined to testis
  - Excellent prognosis
    - 5-year survival of > 90%
- Metastasis rare at presentation
- Consistently lack association with GCNIS
- Histologically almost always pure yolk sac tumor
- Prepubertal yolk sac tumors are aneuploid
- Consistently lacks chromosome 12p abnormality

Teratoma, Prepubertal Type
- 2nd most common TGCT in children
- Median age: 13 months
- Biologically different from postpubertal teratoma
  - Not associated with GCNIS
  - Benign, does not have metastatic potential
  - Includes dermoid cyst and epidermoid cyst
- Histologically more organoid appearance and lack of cytologic atypia
- Normal karyotype

Seminoma

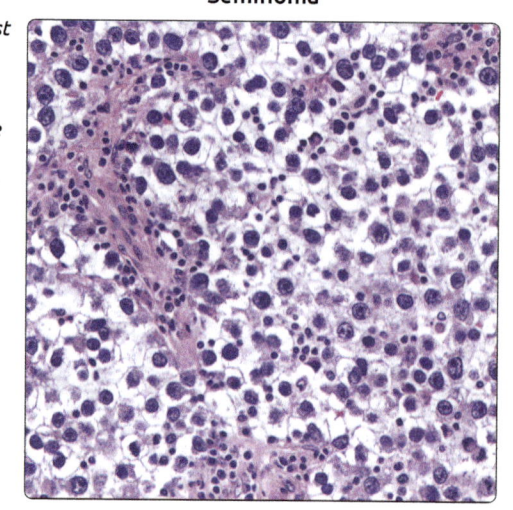

CD117 Immunohistochemistry in Seminoma

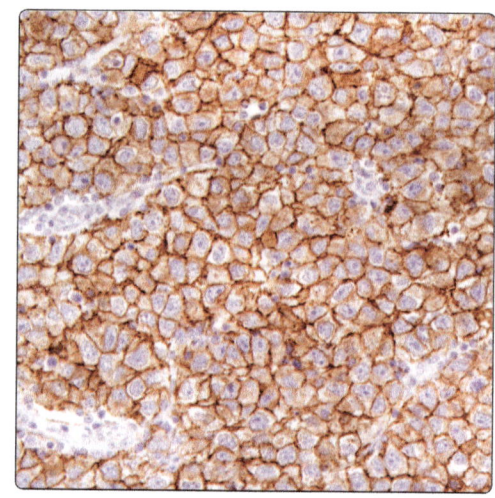

(Left) Seminomas are the most common type of adult testicular germ cell tumors (TGCTs). Tumor cells grow in sheets surrounded by delicate fibrous septa with scattered lymphocytes. Cells have well-defined borders, clear cytoplasm, large nuclei, and prominent nucleoli. (Right) Seminomas typically show strong immunohistochemical staining for CD117 in a membranous pattern. This marker can help with the differential diagnosis from nonseminomatous germ cell tumors (NSGCTs), especially embryonal carcinoma.

Testicular Germ Cell Tumors

TESTICULAR GERM CELL TUMORS IN POSTPUBERTAL MALES

Classification
- Pure seminoma
- Mixed malignant germ cell tumors
- NSGCTs
  o Includes mixed germ cell tumors
- Teratoma, postpubertal type (mature or immature)
- Dermoid cyst and epidermoid cyst
- Spermatocytic tumor

CLINICAL ISSUES

Epidemiology
- Malignant germ cell tumors comprise ~ 1% of all malignancies in males
- Most common malignancy in male patients 15-35 years of age
- Seminoma age range: 35-45 years
- Nonseminoma age range: 25-35 years
- More frequent in White populations and in Northern European countries
- Incidence increasing, thought in part to be due to environmental factors
- ~ 5% are bilateral
- ~ 50% of malignant TGCTs are pure seminomas
- ~ 1/3 of malignant TGCTs are mixed with varying proportions of seminoma, embryonal carcinoma, yolk sac tumor, choriocarcinoma, postpubertal teratoma
- **Spermatocytic tumor**
  o Most patients > 50 years (mean age: 55 years)

Risk Factors
- Positive family history
- Inherited genetic factors dominate risk of TGCTs and are highly polygenic in nature
- Cryptorchidism, prior TGCT, infertility, microlithiasis
- Hypospadias, other genital malformations, disorders of sex development (gonadal dysgenesis, androgen insensitivity syndrome)
- Patients with GCNIS on testicular biopsy have 50% risk of progression to invasive TGCT within 5 years
- Patients with gonadal dysgenesis in presence of Y chromosome (46,XY or 45,X/46,XY) at risk for TGCTs
  o Gonadal dysgenesis with presence of gonadoblastoma locus on Y chromosome (GBY locus) has 25% lifetime risk for TGCT
  o *TSPY1* (Yp11.2) gene mapped to GBY locus may act as oncogene in gonadal dysgenesis
  o Gonadoblastoma is precursor lesion for invasive TGCTs in patients with gonadal dysgenesis
- Environmental risk factors
  o Dietary factors, increased intrauterine exposure to estrogens and antiandrogens
  o Synthetic hormones, pesticides, herbicides, other chemicals, thought to be due to antiandrogen properties (endocrine disruptors)
- Risk likely related to combination of genetic and environmental factors

Treatment and Prognosis
- **Pure seminoma**
  o Orchiectomy for clinical stage I
    – Postoperative surveillance preferred over adjuvant chemotherapy or radiation
  o Postsurgical management of metastases depends on stage and medical center, includes radiation to lymph nodes &/or chemotherapy
  o Retroperitoneal lymph node dissection considered in some cases after primary chemotherapy
  o Seminomas are sensitive to cisplatin-based chemotherapy and to radiation therapy
  o Cure rate for clinical stage I and II seminomas is > 95%
- **Malignant NSGCTs**
  o Orchiectomy for stage I
    – Postoperative surveillance or lymph node dissection or chemotherapy
  o Postsurgical management of metastases depends on stage and medical center, includes lymph node dissection, or chemotherapy or surveillance
  o Most NSGCTs, except teratomas, are sensitive to cisplatin-based chemotherapy
  o Cure rate for patients with clinical stage II and nonbulky retroperitoneal involvement > 95%
  o Survival rate with bulky clinical stage II disease is 70-80%
  o 10-20% of patients with metastatic TGCTs develop treatment resistance
- **Yolk sac tumor**
  o Metastases are more resistant to chemotherapy than other NSGCT components
  o Prognosis is worse than other NSGCT components
- **Choriocarcinoma**
  o Most patients present with metastases, often to lung, liver, or brain
  o Prognosis is worse than other malignant TGCTs
- **Teratoma, postpubertal type**
  o Postpubertal teratomas are malignant with substantial risk of metastasis
    – Mature histology does **not** equal benign clinical behavior
  o Presence of immature elements in teratoma has no known prognostic significance and should not be mentioned in diagnosis
  o Resistant to chemotherapy and radiation
- Pure dermoid cysts and epidermoid cysts are benign
- Very rare subtype of postpubertal teratoma is benign
- **Spermatocytic tumor**
  o Vast majority of cases are clinically benign
  o Metastases are rare and typically associated with sarcomatoid transformation

Laboratory Tests
- 3 serum markers used for staging and follow-up
  o Elevated AFP is marker for yolk sac tumor component
  o Elevated β HCG is marker for choriocarcinoma component, may be elevated in seminomas containing syncytiotrophoblastic cells
  o Elevated LDH is nonspecific marker

Testicular Germ Cell Tumors

MOLECULAR PATHOLOGY

Cytogenetics

- Gains of excess material of chromosome 12p are genetic hallmark of adult malignant TGCTs
  - Vast majority of seminomas and NSGCTs have isochromosome 12p (i12p)
  - Remainder have excess 12p material in derivative chromosome
  - Occurs in adult TGCTs of all histologic types (seminoma, embryonal carcinoma, yolk sac tumor, choriocarcinoma, postpubertal teratoma, but not spermatocytic tumor)
  - Detected in most somatic malignancies arising in adult malignant TGCTs
- Amplification and overexpression of genes in 12p11.2-12.1 region in ~ 10% of TGCTs
- Premalignant GCNIS without associated invasive TGCT lacks gain of chromosome 12p
- Recurrent small scale focal gain at 2q32.1 encompassing gene *FSIP2* in 15-20% of malignant TGCTs
- Median DNA content
  - Hypertriploid in seminomas
  - Hypotriploid in malignant NSGCTs
- Other recurrent chromosomal abnormalities in TGCTs include
  - Gains of chromosomes 7, 8, 17, 21, 22, X, and chromosomal material from 12p
  - Losses of chromosomes 4, 11, 13, 18, Y
- Most postpubertal teratomas are aneuploid, presence of cytologic atypia correlates with aneuploidy, i(12p) can be found

Molecular Genetics

- Mean mutation rate in malignant TGCTs low at 0.5 somatic mutations per megabase of DNA
  - Mutations reported in subset of seminomas most often affect *KIT*, *CDC27*
- Significant somatic mutations in seminomas in *KIT*, *KRAS*, *NRAS*, *PIK3CA*
- *KIT* is most frequently mutated driver gene in seminomas
  - Activating mutations in 25-35% of seminomas
  - Mutation most common in exon 17
  - Most frequent mutations are D816V and D816H
- KIT-KITLG signaling is major pathway implicated in tumorigenesis as predisposing risk factor and as somatic driver event
- Subset of pure seminomas defined by *KIT* mutations, globally demethylated DNA, and decreased *KRAS* copy number
- *KRAS* mutations in 5-25%
- *TP53* mutations generally absent
- High rates of alterations in *TP53-MDM2* axis identified in cisplatin-resistant cases
- Genome-wide association studies identified multiple single nucleotide polymorphisms (SNPs) associated with susceptibility to TGCTs
  - Many genes associated with these SNPs are related to KIT-KITL receptor tyrosine kinase signaling, telomere maintenance, and cell-cycle control

Chromosomal Microarray

- Confirms excess of 12p genetic material in adult TGCTs
- Some studies identified chromosomal aberrations associated with cisplatin resistance

Gene Expression Profiling

- Distinct gene expression signatures reported for seminoma, embryonal carcinoma, yolk sac tumor, choriocarcinoma, and teratoma
- Gene expression patterns of GCNIS, seminoma, and embryonal carcinoma overlap with early fetal germ cells
- Genes overexpressed in seminoma include *KIT*, *POU5F1*, *NANOG*, *POU2AF1*, *PROM1*, *CLEC11A*, and *MCFD2*
- Genes overexpressed with progression from GCNIS to invasive TGCTs include *POU5F1*, *NANOG*, *DPPA3*, and *GDF3*
  - These genes are located at 12p13, which is characteristically amplified in invasive TGCTs

Epigenetics

- Epigenetic changes are necessary for development and maturation of normal germ cells
  - DNA of fetal germ cells generally hypomethylated
  - After birth DNA becomes hypermethylated
- Epigenetic changes also present in malignant TGCTs
  - GCNIS and seminomas have low levels of DNA methylation
  - Embryonal carcinomas show intermediate to high degree of DNA methylation
  - More differentiated TGCTs (yolk sac tumor, choriocarcinoma, and postpubertal teratoma) show higher degree of DNA methylation
- Most seminomas are hypomethylated and sensitive to chemotherapy
- GCNIS, seminoma, and embryonal carcinoma have patterns of genomic imprinting similar to early fetal germ cells
- Methylation is absent in subgroup of seminomas with *KIT* or *KRAS* mutation
- Epigenetic silencing of tumor suppressor genes *BRCA1*, *MGMT*, *RASSF1A*, and *RAD51C* in NSGCTs

MicroRNAs

- miR371a-3p overexpressed in seminomas, embryonal carcinomas, and mixed NSGCTs
- Serum levels of miRNA 371/372/373/367 elevated in patients with seminoma, embryonal carcinoma, and yolk sac tumor

Spermatocytic Tumor

- DNA content ranges from diploid to hypertetraploid
- Gains of chromosome 9 are consistent finding
- Amplification of *DMRT1* locus on chromosome 9 may be involved in pathogenesis
- Mutations in *HRAS* or *FGFR3* genes in ~ 25% of cases
- Many genes overexpressed by gene expression profiling, including *SSX2*, *SSX4*, *PRSS50*, *CTCFL*, and *DMRT1*

MICROSCOPIC PATHOLOGY

Germ Cell Neoplasia In Situ

- Neoplastic cells located along thickened basement membranes of seminiferous tubules
- Cytologically most often resemble seminoma cells

Testicular Germ Cell Tumors

Seminoma
- Sheets of neoplastic cells with intervening delicate fibrous septa
- Septa have associated chronic inflammation, mostly lymphocytes; may be granulomatous
- Well-defined cell borders and clear cytoplasm
- Large hyperchromatic nuclei, prominent nucleoli
- Occasional syncytiotrophoblastic cells present in 10-20% of cases

Embryonal Carcinoma
- 3 major architectural patterns are solid, tubular or glandular, and papillary
- Large tumor cells with amphophilic cytoplasm and ill-defined cell borders
- Crowded large vesicular or smudged nuclei with nuclear overlap, prominent nucleoli, frequent mitoses
- Common as component of mixed malignant TGCT, rare in pure form

Yolk Sac Tumor, Postpubertal Type
- Numerous different histologic patterns
- Microcystic/reticular pattern most common
  - Cells with cytoplasmic vacuoles often resemble lipoblasts
  - Cells may also be arranged in reticular pattern
- Endodermal sinus pattern
  - Schiller-Duval bodies (glomeruloid bodies) have central blood vessel surrounded by fibrous rim and neoplastic cells
- Other patterns are papillary, solid, glandular/alveolar, macrocystic, polyvesicular vitelline, myxoid, sarcomatoid/spindle cell, hepatoid, parietal
- Intracellular round hyaline globules characteristic
- Deposits of extracellular basement membrane material common, called parietal differentiation

Trophoblastic Tumors
- Most commonly choriocarcinoma
  - Mixture of mononuclear trophoblastic cells and multinucleated syncytiotrophoblastic cells
  - Usually extensive hemorrhage and necrosis
  - Rare in pure form
- Placental site trophoblastic tumor (PSTT), epithelioid trophoblastic tumor (ETT), and cystic trophoblastic tumor (CTT) extremely rare

Teratoma, Postpubertal Type
- Pure teratoma typically associated with
  - GCNIS in adjacent seminiferous tubules
  - Tubular atrophy, sclerosis, and hypospermatogenesis
- Variable combinations of somatic-type tissue components, often in organoid arrangements
  - Endodermal: Enteric-type glands, respiratory epithelium, seromucous glands
  - Mesodermal: Cartilage, smooth muscle, skeletal muscle, and bone
  - Ectodermal: Squamous epithelial nests and cysts, neuronal tissue, pigmented choroidal epithelium
- > 50% of mixed malignant TGCTs have teratomatous component
- Presence of immature elements with cytologic atypia has no known prognostic significance
  - Primitive cellular stroma with mitotic activity forming cuffs around glands is common
  - Immature elements include neuroectoderm, blastema, embryonic tubules
- Secondary malignant components in teratomas have histology of overt sarcoma or carcinoma
  - More common in metastatic sites after chemotherapy
- Pure dermoid cysts and epidermoid cysts are benign
  - Not associated with GCNIS
  - Dermoid cysts have hair and skin adnexal structures
  - Lack other histologic components of teratoma

Spermatocytic Tumor
- Grow in sheets and cords with 3 major cell types
  - Small cells with smudgy chromatin, similar in size to lymphocytes
  - Intermediate-sized cells with granular chromatin
  - Large cells with nuclei up to 100 μm diameter; chromatin has filamentous appearance

ANCILLARY TESTS

Immunohistochemistry
- GCNIS
  - Positive for OCT3/4, CD117, NANOG, SALL4, podoplanin (D2-40), PLAP, and SOX17
- Seminoma
  - Positive for OCT3/4, CD117, NANOG, SALL4, podoplanin (D2-40), PLAP, and SOX17
- Embryonal carcinoma
  - Positive for OCT3/4, CD30, NANOG, SALL4, pancytokeratin, PLAP (patchy and weak), and SOX2
- Yolk sac tumor
  - Positive for AFP, glypican-3, pancytokeratin, HNF1 β, and SALL4
- Choriocarcinoma
  - Syncytiotrophoblasts positive for β HCG, GATA3, glypican-3, and pancytokeratin
  - Cytotrophoblasts positive for SALL4, GDF3, p63, GATA3
- Spermatocytic tumor
  - Often positive for CD117, SALL4, DMRT1, SSX2, and MAGE-A4

SELECTED REFERENCES

1. Hwang MJ et al: Somatic-type malignancies in testicular germ cell tumors: a clinicopathologic study of 63 cases. Am J Surg Pathol. 46(1):11-7, 2022
2. Al-Obaidy KI et al: Testicular tumors: a contemporary update on morphologic, immunohistochemical and molecular features. Adv Anat Pathol. 28(4):258-75, 2021
3. Al-Obaidy KI et al: Molecular characteristics of testicular germ cell tumors: pathogenesis and mechanisms of therapy resistance. Expert Rev Anticancer Ther. 20(2):75-9, 2020
4. Looijenga LHJ et al: Report from the International Society of Urological Pathology (ISUP) Consultation Conference on Molecular Pathology of Urogenital Cancers: IV: Current and Future Utilization of Molecular-Genetic Tests for Testicular Germ Cell Tumors. Am J Surg Pathol. 44(7):e66-79, 2020
5. Hu R et al: Spermatocytic seminoma: a report of 85 cases emphasizing its morphologic spectrum including some aspects not widely known. Am J Surg Pathol. 43(1):1-11, 2019
6. Lafin JT et al: New insights into germ cell tumor genomics. Andrology. 7(4):507-15, 2019
7. Shen H et al: Integrated molecular characterization of testicular germ cell tumors. Cell Rep. 23(11):3392-406, 2018
8. Litchfield K et al: The genomic landscape of testicular germ cell tumours: from susceptibility to treatment. Nat Rev Urol. 13(7):409-19, 2016

Testicular Germ Cell Tumors

(Left) The neoplastic cells of germ cell neoplasia in situ (GCNIS) ➡ are located in seminiferous tubules on the luminal side of the thickened basement membrane. They have clear cytoplasm, well-defined cell borders, large hyperchromatic nuclei, and prominent nucleoli. **(Right)** Immunohistochemical stain for OCT3/4 highlights nuclei of GCNIS cells. No staining is seen in adjacent uninvolved tubules in the right lower corner.

Germ Cell Neoplasia In Situ

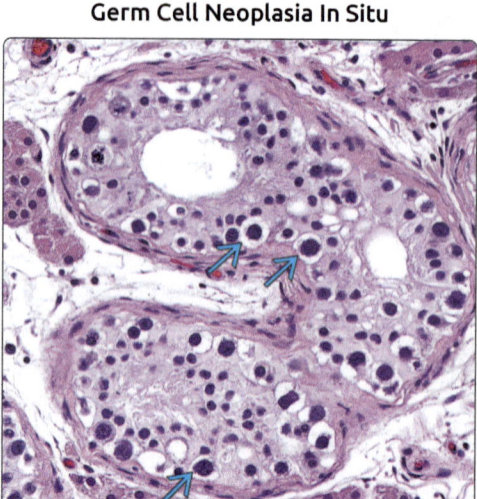

GCNIS Nuclei Positive for OCT3/4

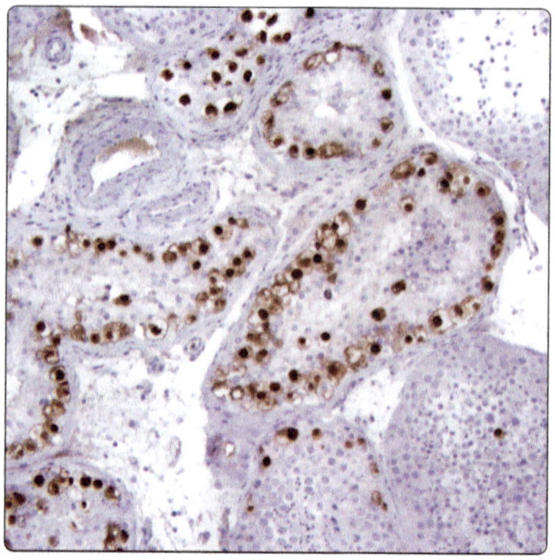

(Left) Embryonal carcinoma is a common component of adult mixed TGCTs. Tumor cells have indistinct cell borders with large pleomorphic nuclei, nuclear overlap, and coarse chromatin. Mitoses are common. **(Right)** Embryonal carcinomas are typically positive for CD30 by immunohistochemistry with a membranous staining pattern. This finding can help with the differential diagnosis from seminomas and other components of NSGCTs.

Embryonal Carcinoma

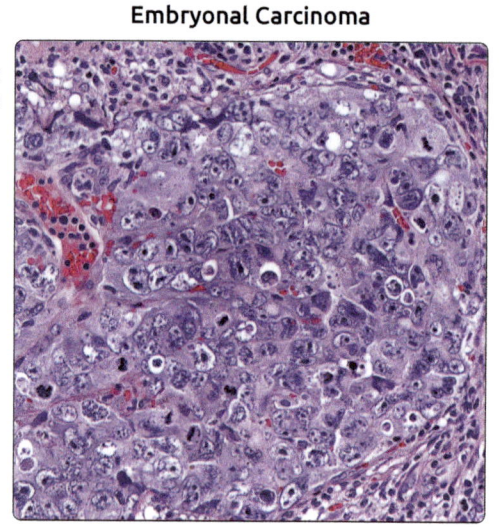

CD30 Immunohistochemistry in Embryonal Carcinoma

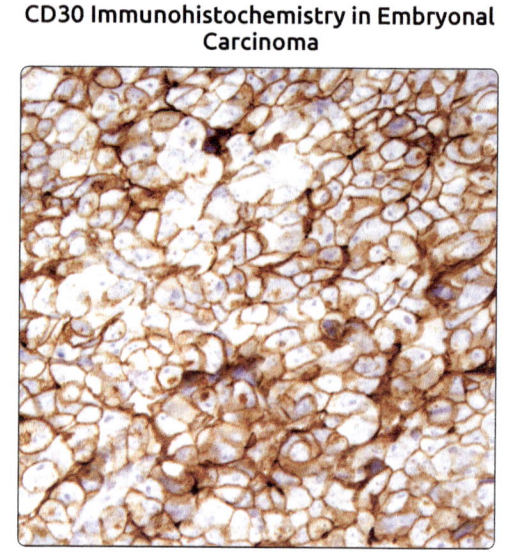

(Left) The most common histologic pattern in yolk sac tumors is the microcystic pattern. Tumor cells show prominent cytoplasmic vacuoles, which may mimic lipoblasts. Hyaline globules are also common in yolk sac tumors ➡. **(Right)** Schiller-Duval bodies (glomeruloid bodies) are a characteristic finding in the endodermal sinus pattern of a yolk sac tumor. They are composed of a central blood vessel surrounded by a thin fibrous rim and a layer of neoplastic cells ➡.

Microcystic Pattern of Yolk Sac Tumor

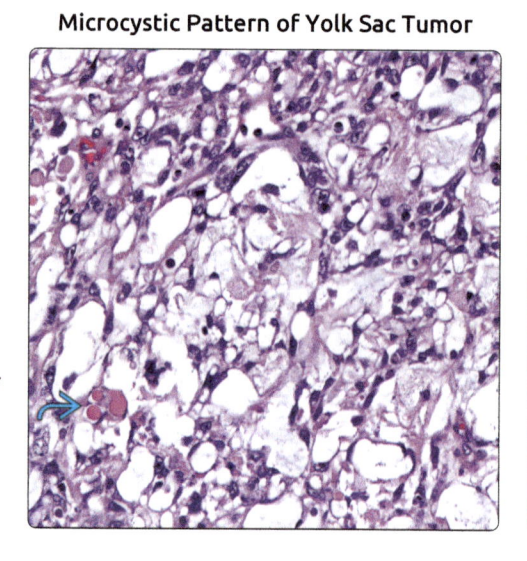

Schiller-Duval Body in Yolk Sac Tumor

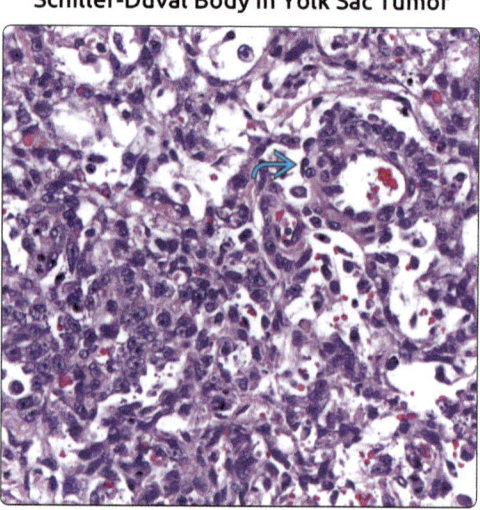

Testicular Germ Cell Tumors

Mature Teratoma

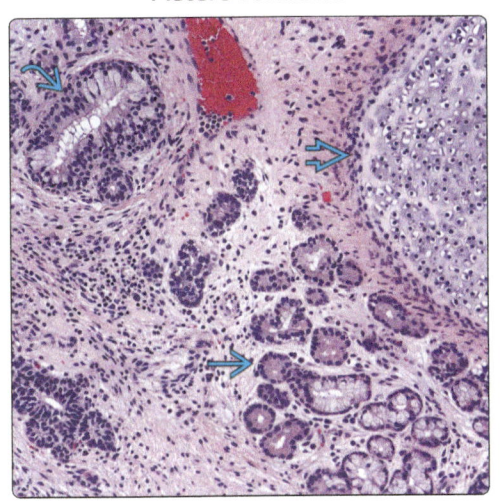

Immature Elements in Teratoma

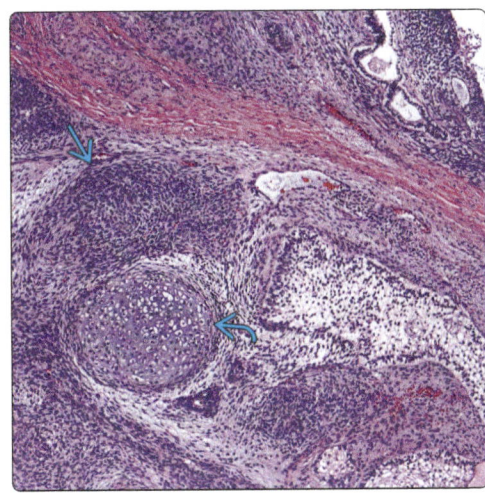

(Left) This mature teratoma shows an island of hyaline cartilage ⇒, seromucous glands, ⇒ and respiratory-type epithelium ⇒. (Right) The presence of immature elements and cytologic atypia in postpubertal-type testicular teratomas have no known prognostic significance. Nests of blastema ⇒ are collections of small immature cells with ovoid hyperchromatic nuclei and scant cytoplasm. Cytologic atypia is seen in the hyaline cartilage ⇒.

Immature Neuroectodermal Elements in Teratoma

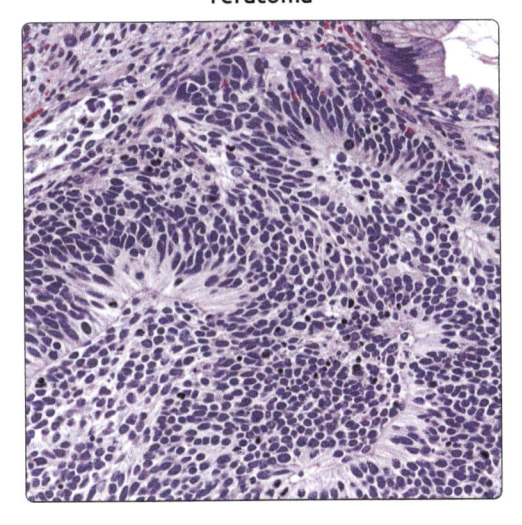

Choriocarcinoma

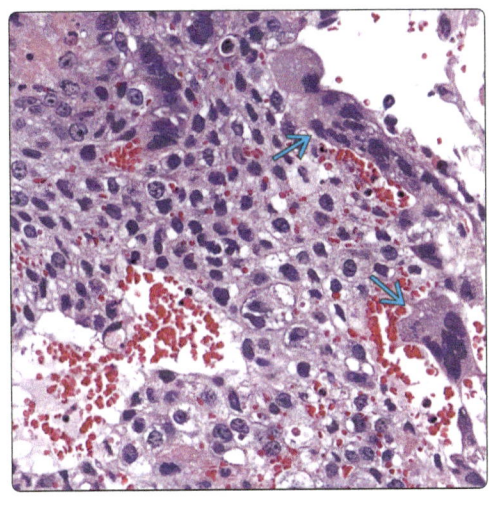

(Left) Highly immature neuroectoderm in teratomas is composed of small cells with hyperchromatic nuclei. These cells are arranged in tubules and pseudorosettes to form neuroepithelium. (Right) Choriocarcinomas are composed of a mixture of mononuclear trophoblastic cells, often with clear cytoplasm, and multinucleated syncytiotrophoblast cells with eosinophilic cytoplasm ⇒. Hemorrhage and necrosis are typically abundant.

HCG-β Immunohistochemistry in Choriocarcinoma

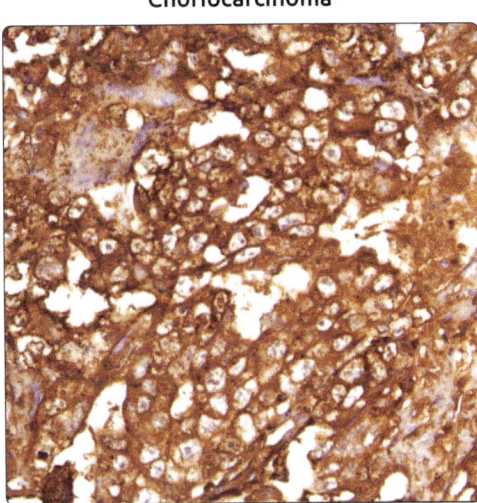

Spermatocytic Tumor

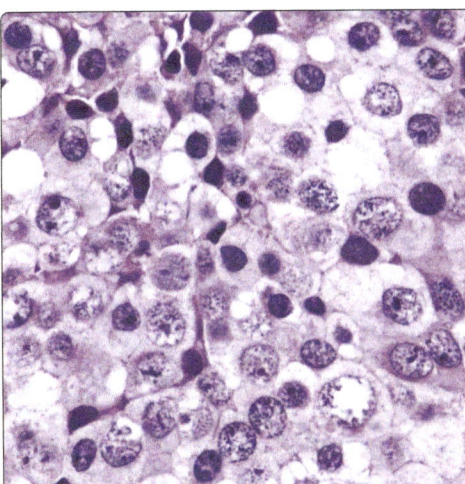

(Left) Immunohistochemical stain using HCG-β antibody reveals strong expression of this antigen in a case of testicular choriocarcinoma. (Right) Spermatocytic tumors are composed of 3 major cell types that grow in nests and sheets. There are small cells similar in size to lymphocytes, intermediate-sized cells, and large cells with nuclei up to 100 μm in diameter.

Clear Cell Renal Cell Carcinoma

KEY FACTS

TERMINOLOGY
- Malignant epithelial tumor thought to arise from epithelial cells of proximal nephron

ETIOLOGY/PATHOGENESIS
- Biallelic *VHL* alteration leads to loss of VHL protein (pVHL) function
  - Results in constitutive stabilization and increased levels of HIF-α transcription factors
  - Increased HIF-α levels induce expression of many downstream genes
  - Downstream genes are involved in regulation of angiogenesis, cell proliferation, energy metabolism, and tumor progression
- ~ 40% of pVHL wildtype cases harbor biallelic inactivation of *ELOC* at 8q21

CLINICAL ISSUES
- Sporadic in 95% of cases
- ~ 5% of cases occur in familial setting of autosomal dominant von Hippel-Lindau (VHL) syndrome

MOLECULAR
- *VHL* tumor suppressor gene located at 3p25 and inactivated by mutation, deletion, or abnormal promoter methylation
- Tumor suppressor genes *PBRM1*, *BAP1*, and *SETD2* located at 3p21 and mutated in some cases
  - *BAP1*-mutated tumors associated with poor prognosis
- Mutations in genes encoding signaling proteins of PI3K-AKT-mTOR pathway in 20-30% of cases
- Genetic alterations in cell cycle components common

MICROSCOPIC
- Grows in sheets, nests, microcysts, and macrocysts
- Tumor nests surrounded by delicate vascular network
- WHO/ISUP grading system based on nucleolar grade

Karyotype With 3p Deletion

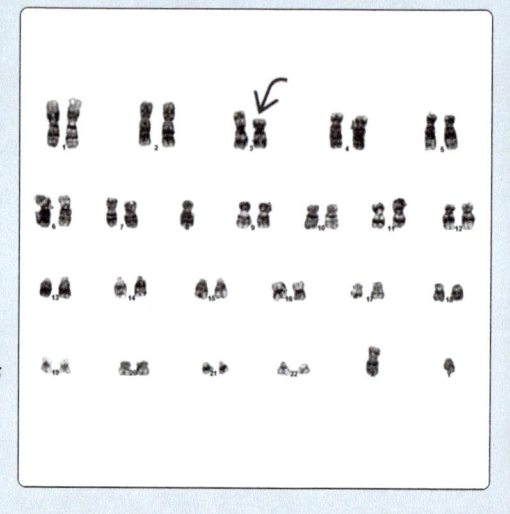

Gross Appearance

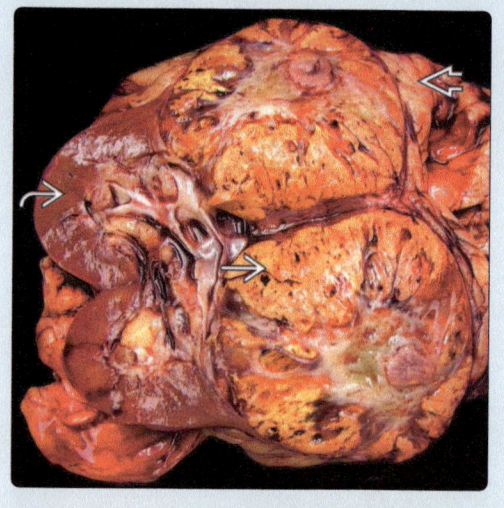

(Left) Karyotype of clear cell renal cell carcinoma (CC-RCC) shows deletion of 3p ➢, which harbors the VHL gene. Loss of the 3p chromosomal region is the cytogenetic hallmark of this tumor. Monosomy 8 is also present in this case. (Right) Gross photograph shows characteristic features of CC-RCC with golden-yellow cut surface ➢. The tumor bulges into perinephric adipose tissue ➢ and replaces large portions of the normal kidney parenchyma ➢.

Characteristic Histology

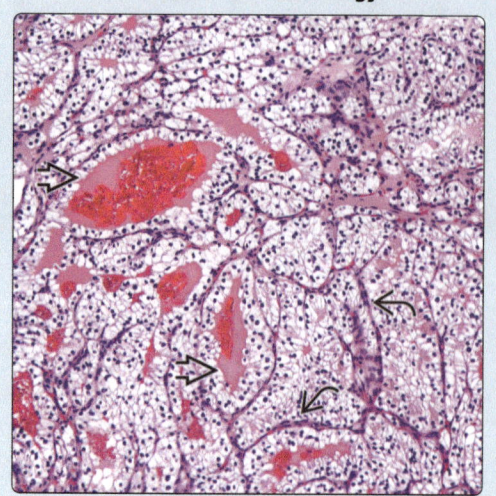

CAIX

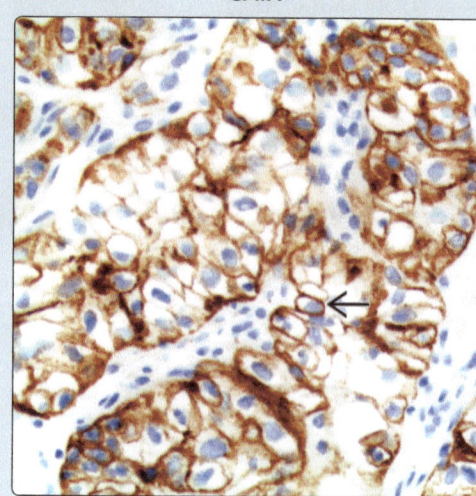

(Left) CC-RCC shows tumor cell nests surrounded by a delicate vascular network ➢. Microcysts lined by tumor cells are characteristic of this tumor ➢ and are filled with proteinaceous fluid &/or blood. (Right) CAIX is a useful marker for CC-RCC, staining tumor cell membranes in a circumferential (box-shaped ➢) pattern. It is often positive in higher grade and sarcomatoid tumors.

Clear Cell Renal Cell Carcinoma

TERMINOLOGY

Abbreviations
- Clear cell renal cell carcinoma (CC-RCC)

Definitions
- Malignant epithelial tumor thought to arise from epithelial cells of proximal nephron

ETIOLOGY/PATHOGENESIS

Molecular Pathogenesis
- Impaired degradation of HIF-α represents common pathogenetic mechanism in *VHL*-mutated and *VHL* wildtype tumors
- In normal cells, wildtype VHL protein (pVHL) binds to E3 ubiquitin ligase complex
  o Leads to proteolytic degradation of HIF-α transcription factors
- In CC-RCC, biallelic *VHL* alteration leads to loss of pVHL function
  o Results in reduced proteolytic degradation, constitutive stabilization, and increased levels of HIF-α transcription factors
  o Increased HIF-α levels induce expression of many downstream genes
    – Downstream genes are involved in regulation of angiogenesis, cell proliferation, energy metabolism, and tumor progression
    – Genes include *VEGFA*, *PDGFB*, *TGFA*, *EGFR*, *IGFBP2*, *SLC2A1*, *EPO*, and *CXCR4*
  o Dysregulated pVHL-mediated HIF-α degradation results in pseudohypoxia
    – HIF-α activation drives switch from normoxic mitochondrial respiration to glycolysis as main source of energy (Warburg effect)
- Sporadic CC-RCC
  o 2 consecutive steps lead to inactivation of both *VHL* alleles
  o *VHL* inactivated by mutation, deletion, or abnormal promoter methylation
- von Hippel-Lindau (VHL) disease
  o Heterozygous inheritance of single deleted or inactivated germline *VHL* allele
  o Loss or inactivation of 2nd *VHL* allele results in clinical disease expression
- *VHL* wildtype CC-RCC
  o ~ 40% of *VHL* wildtype cases harbor biallelic inactivation of *ELOC*
    – *ELOC* mutations functionally impair degradation of HIF-α, leading to constitutive HIF1-α activity
    – *ELOC* mutations are always mutually exclusive with *VHL* mutations

Risk Factors
- Tobacco smoking, obesity, hypertension
- Acquired cystic kidney disease requiring dialysis

CLINICAL ISSUES

Epidemiology
- CC-RCC accounts for 60-70% of all RCC
- Most patients > 40 years of age

Presentation
- Sporadic in 95% of cases
- ~ 5% of cases occur in familial setting of VHL syndrome
  o Cancer syndrome with autosomal dominant inheritance
  o Occurs in 1 out of 36,000 live births
  o Patients develop CC-RCC, often multiple and bilateral
  o Other associated tumors
    – Capillary hemangioblastomas of CNS and retina
    – Pheochromocytoma
    – Pancreatic and inner ear tumors
    – Often numerous small foci of clear cell tumors and cysts

Treatment
- Partial nephrectomy (nephron-sparing surgery) or radical nephrectomy
- Ablative techniques for nonsurgical candidates include radiofrequency ablation or cryoablation
- Systemic therapies for stage IV disease include
  o Axitinib and pembrolizumab, cabozantinib and nivolumab, or lenvatinib and pembrolizumab
  o Tyrosine kinase inhibitors, including pazopanib, sunitinib, or tivozanib
  o Cytokine (cytotoxic) therapy with interferon-α or high-dose interleukin-2
  o mTOR inhibitors everolimus or temsirolimus
  o Therapeutic efficacy rather modest
  o Recent studies explored therapeutic efficacy of monoclonal antibodies against immune checkpoint inhibitors CTLA-4, PD-1, and PD-L1
  o Currently no predictive markers available in clinical practice

Prognosis
- Depends on pathologic stage, grade, and presence or absence of sarcomatoid features

MOLECULAR

Molecular Genetics
- Alterations of *VHL* gene at 3p locus
  o *VHL* is tumor suppressor gene located on 3p25.3
  o Biallelic *VHL* alteration in > 90% of sporadic CC-RCC
  o *VHL* alteration occurs through
    – Loss of 1 copy of 3p
    – 2nd hit by inactivating mutations or promoter hypermethylation of remaining allele
    – *VHL* is epigenetically silenced by promoter methylation in up to 20% of cases
- Alterations of other genes at 3p locus
  o Copy number loss of 3p found in > 90% of cases
  o Other tumor suppressor genes located at 3p include *PBRM1*, *BAP1*, and *SETD2*
  o *PBRM1* mutated in ~ 40% of cases
    – 2nd most commonly mutated gene in CC-RCC
  o *BAP1* loss-of-function mutations in ~ 10% of cases
    – *BAP1*-mutated tumors are typically high grade with poor prognosis
  o *PBRM1* and *BAP1* mutations largely (not entirely) mutually exclusive

Clear Cell Renal Cell Carcinoma

- o *SETD2* mutated in ~ 13% of cases
- o *PBRM1*, *BAP1*, and *SETD2* involved in chromatin remodeling
- Alterations at other chromosomal loci
  - o Gains of 5q, 7q; losses of 8p ± loss of 8q
  - o Loss of heterozygosity at 9p, 14q, 18q
  - o Losses of 14q, 4p, and 9p have been associated with poor prognosis
    - – *HIF1A* likely target of 14q deletions
  - o Copy number gains of 5q in up to 70% of cases
    - – Often leads to *SQSTM1* upregulation
- Genetic alterations affecting signaling pathways
  - o Mutations in genes that encode signaling proteins of PI3K/AKT/mTOR pathway
    - – Found in 20-30% of cases
    - – Typically in mutually exclusive manner
    - – Mutated genes include *PTEN*, *TSC1* or *TSC2*, *PIK3CA*, *PIK3CB*, *PIK3CG*, *AKT1*, *AKT2*, *AKT3*, *RHEB*, and *MTOR*
  - o Genetic alterations in components of cell cycle and senescence regulation
    - – Found in ~ 40% of sporadic cases
    - – Typically in mutually exclusive manner
    - – Include mutations or deletions of *CDKN2A*, *TP53*, *RB1*, *ATM*, *CHEK2*, or *MDM2*
    - – *CDKN2A* alterations (mutations, hypermethylation, deletions) in 16%, associated with poor prognosis
    - – Gains of chromosomal regions harboring *MYC* or *MDM4*
- Ultradeep sequencing shows intratumoral heterogeneity
  - o ~ 75% of driver mutations are subclonal
- Epigenetic changes
  - o *RASSF1* tumor suppressor gene on 3p21 methylated in 30-50% of sporadic cases
    - – Suggests that *RASSF1* inactivation typically results from combination of allelic loss and methylation
  - o Numerous genes have mean combined methylation-mutation rate of > 20%
    - – Include *FAM107A* in ~ 40% and *DLEC1* in ~ 30% of cases, both located on 3p
  - o Epigenetically silenced *FHIT* in ~ 50% of cases
    - – Several Wnt pathway inhibitors inactivated by methylation, including *SFRP1*, *SFRP4*, *SFRP5*, *DKK1*, *DKK2*, and *DKK3*
- Gene expression profiling
  - o Profiles of mRNA expression and protein expression identified molecular subclasses of CC-RCC
  - o 4 different microRNA expression profiles identified that predict survival
- Aberrant DNA methylation and histone protein modification are frequent in CC-RCC
  - o Represent potentially reversible mechanisms of tumor suppressor gene inactivation

MICROSCOPIC

Histologic Features

- Tumor cells grow in sheets, nests, microcysts and macrocysts
  - o Surrounded by abundant thin blood vessels forming delicate vascular network
  - o Microcysts contain eosinophilic fluid &/or red blood cells
- Tumor cells have clear cytoplasm and distinct cell membranes
  - o Cytoplasmic lipids and glycogen dissolved during tissue processing
- Cells with granular eosinophilic cytoplasm more often seen in higher grade tumors
- Presence of coagulative tumor necrosis has adverse prognostic significance and should be reported
- Nuclei vary from small and round to pleomorphic with bizarre shapes
- Nucleoli vary from inconspicuous to prominent
- Tumors with sarcomatoid or rhabdoid morphology are high grade by definition
- International Society of Urologic Pathology grading system
  - o Grade 1: Absent or inconspicuous nucleoli at 400x
  - o Grade 2: Nucleoli conspicuous at 400x but inconspicuous at 100x
  - o Grade 3: Nucleoli conspicuous at 100x
  - o Grade 4: Extreme nuclear pleomorphism ± multinucleated tumor giant cells or sarcomatoid or rhabdoid morphology

ANCILLARY TESTS

Immunohistochemistry

- Positive for pancytokeratin, EMA, vimentin, carbonic anhydrase IX (CAIX), PAX2, PAX8, RCCma, and CD10

DIFFERENTIAL DIAGNOSIS

Chromophobe Renal Cell Carcinoma

- Positive for CK7 and CD117
- Negative for CAIX

Clear Cell Papillary Renal Cell Tumor

- Tumor cells have apical alignment of low-grade nuclei
- Positive for CK7, cup-like staining for CAIX

SELECTED REFERENCES

1. Jonasch E et al: Clear cell renal cell carcinoma ontogeny and mechanisms of lethality. Nat Rev Nephrol. 17(4):245-61, 2021
2. Trpkov K et al: New developments in existing WHO entities and evolving molecular concepts: the Genitourinary Pathology Society (GUPS) update on renal neoplasia. Mod Pathol. 34(7):1392-424, 2021
3. D'Avella C et al: Mutations in renal cell carcinoma. Urol Oncol. 38(10):763-73, 2020
4. Williamson SR et al: Report from the International Society of Urological Pathology (ISUP) Consultation Conference on Molecular Pathology of Urogenital Cancers: III: Molecular Pathology of Kidney Cancer. Am J Surg Pathol. 44(7):e47-65, 2020
5. Ricketts CJ et al: The cancer genome atlas comprehensive molecular characterization of renal cell carcinoma. Cell Rep. 23(1):313-26.e5, 2018
6. Turajlic S et al: Deterministic evolutionary trajectories influence primary tumor growth: TRACERx Renal. Cell. 173(3):595-610.e11, 2018
7. Chen F et al: Multilevel genomics-based taxonomy of renal cell carcinoma. Cell Rep. 14(10):2476-89, 2016
8. Frew IJ et al: A clearer view of the molecular complexity of clear cell renal cell carcinoma. Annu Rev Pathol. 10:263-89, 2015
9. Su D et al: Molecular pathways in renal cell carcinoma: recent advances in genetics and molecular biology. Curr Opin Oncol. 27(3):217-23, 2015
10. Brugarolas J: Molecular genetics of clear-cell renal cell carcinoma. J Clin Oncol. 32(18):1968-76, 2014
11. Gerlinger M et al: Genomic architecture and evolution of clear cell renal cell carcinomas defined by multiregion sequencing. Nat Genet. 46(3):225-33, 2014
12. Sato Y et al: Integrated molecular analysis of clear-cell renal cell carcinoma. Nat Genet. 45(8):860-7, 2013

Clear Cell Renal Cell Carcinoma

Characteristic Microcysts

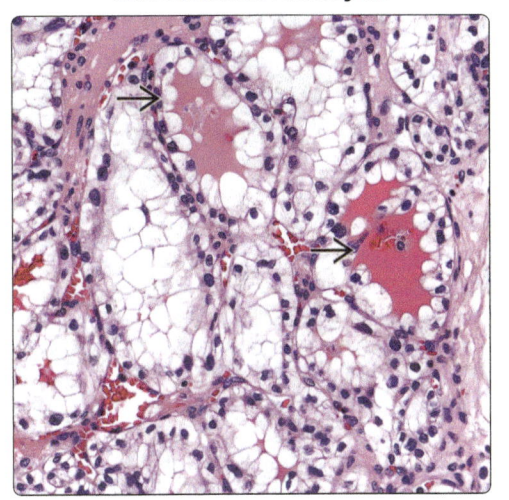

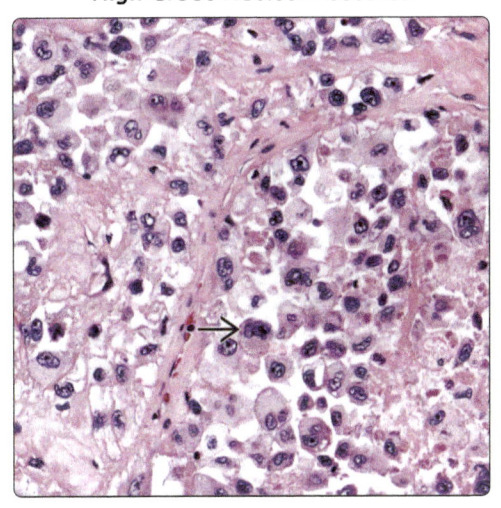

High-Grade Nuclear Features

(Left) Nested growth pattern and microcysts ➡ characteristic of CC-RCC are shown. Tumor cells have well-defined borders. Their cytoplasm appears clear, as cytoplasmic lipids and glycogen are dissolved during tissue processing. (Right) Tumor cells with eosinophilic cytoplasm and high-grade nuclear features are present in this case of CC-RCC. Large nuclei with bizarre nuclear shapes ➡ and prominent nucleoli are seen.

Spindle-Shaped Tumor Cells in Sarcomatoid CC-RCC

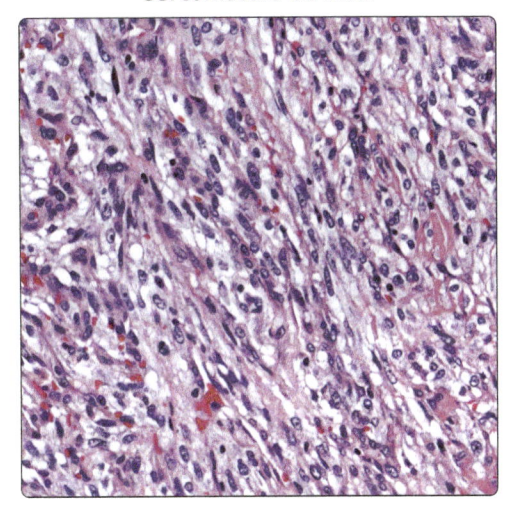

RCCma Immunohistochemistry

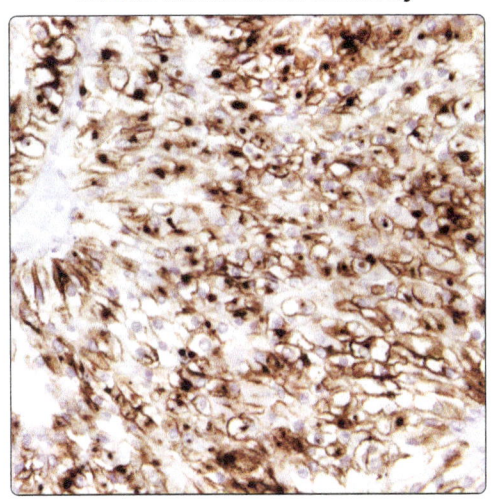

(Left) CC-RCC shows sarcomatoid differentiation characterized by the presence of malignant spindle cells. Tumors with sarcomatoid differentiation are high-grade by definition and are associated with a poor prognosis. (Right) CC-RCC shows immunoreactivity for RCCma in a membranous distribution. RCCma is specific for RCC and can help in the work-up of metastatic carcinomas of unknown primary origin.

PAX8 Immunohistochemistry

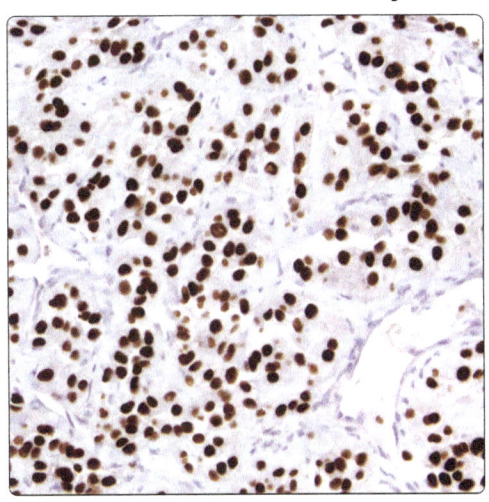

CD10 Immunohistochemistry

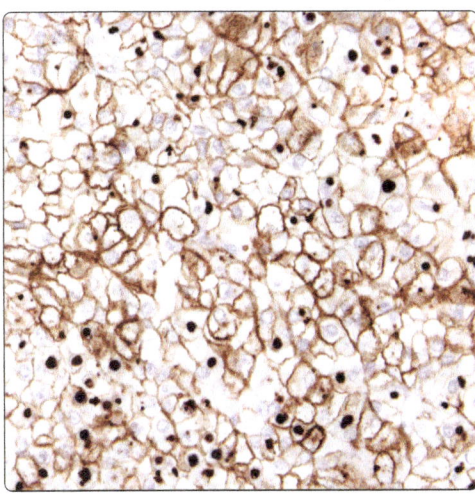

(Left) Nuclear labeling for PAX8 in CC-RCC is shown. PAX8 is a sensitive marker for RCC of various histologic types but also labels tumors from other primary sites, including thyroid or gynecologic origin. (Right) CD10 shows predominantly membranous reactivity in this case of CC-RCC. CD10 is typically positive in CC-RCC, but it is not specific for renal tumors.

Chromophobe Renal Cell Carcinoma

KEY FACTS

ETIOLOGY/PATHOGENESIS
- Chromophobe renal cell carcinoma (ChRCC)
  - Malignant epithelial neoplasm arising from cells of distal nephron

CLINICAL ISSUES
- Comprises ~ 5% of all renal cell carcinomas
- Mean age: 5th decade
- 5-year survival: ~ 90% after surgery; mortality rate: ~ 10%
- Incidence of metastatic disease: 5-10%
- No established treatment for systemic disease
- Familial cases associated with autosomal dominant Birt-Hogg-Dubé syndrome

MOLECULAR
- Hypodiploid DNA content
- Loss of chromosomes 1, 2, 6, 10, 13, 17, 21
- Commonly mutated genes: *TP53* (20-30%), *PTEN* (6-9%)
- Mutations in PI3K/AKT/mTOR pathway in ~ 15%
- Mutations in mitochondrial DNA in ~ 20%
- Rearrangement in *TERT* promoter region in ~ 10%
- Expression of *FOXI1* and *RHCG* enriched in CH-RCC

MICROSCOPIC
- Variable admixture of larger pale cells and smaller cells with perinuclear halos
- Larger cells with transparent flocculent cytoplasm
- Smaller cells with granular, eosinophilic cytoplasm and perinuclear halos
- Nuclei are hyperchromatic with irregular, wrinkled contours; binucleation common
- Eosinophilic variant of ChRCC almost entirely composed of intensely eosinophilic cells
- Coagulative tumor necrosis associated with worse prognosis
- Sarcomatoid transformation associated with more aggressive clinical course

Binucleated Cells

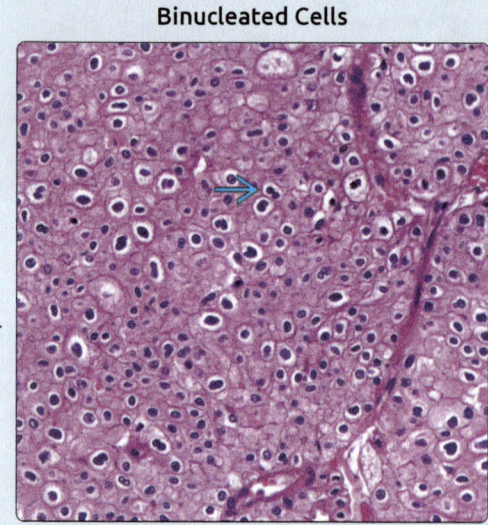

Large and Small Tumor Cells

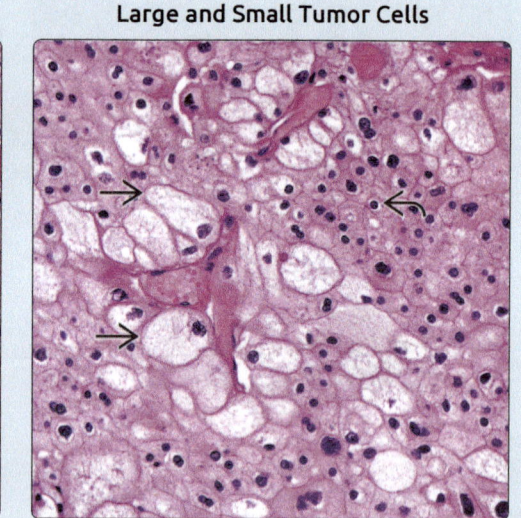

(Left) *This case of chromophobe renal cell carcinoma (ChRCC) is composed of sheets of tumor cells with granular eosinophilic cytoplasm, perinuclear halos, and well-defined cell membranes. Multiple binucleated cells are present ➡.* (Right) *Larger tumor cells ➡ in ChRCC have transparent, slightly flocculent cytoplasm and prominent, plant-like cell membranes. Smaller cells have less abundant granular cytoplasm and occasional perinuclear halos ➡.*

Eosinophilic Variant

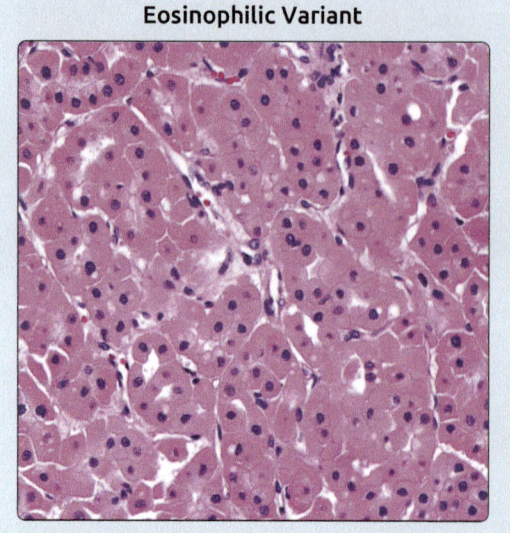

CD117 Immunohistochemistry

(Left) *Eosinophilic variant of ChRCC has a nested growth pattern and cells with granular eosinophilic cytoplasm, histologic features that overlap with renal oncocytoma. This case was diffusely positive for CK7 by immunohistochemistry, confirming the diagnosis.* (Right) *Membranous immunostaining for CD117 is typical for ChRCC but is also seen in renal oncocytomas.*

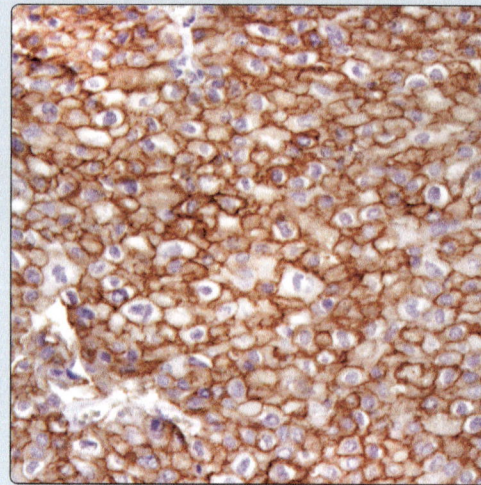

Chromophobe Renal Cell Carcinoma

TERMINOLOGY

Abbreviations
- Chromophobe renal cell carcinoma (ChRCC)

Definitions
- Malignant epithelial neoplasm of kidney

ETIOLOGY/PATHOGENESIS

Pathogenesis
- Thought to arise from cells of distal nephron

CLINICAL ISSUES

Epidemiology
- Comprises ~ 5% of all renal cell carcinomas
- Mean age: 5th decade; age range: 27-86 years

Presentation
- May present with hematuria, pain, flank mass
- Most cases discovered incidentally on imaging
- Most cases present at stage 1 or 2 at diagnosis
- Incidence of metastatic disease: 5-10%
- Sporadic cases
  - Accounts for majority of cases
  - Not associated with *FLCN* mutations
- Familial cases
  - Associated with Birt-Hogg-Dubé (BHD) syndrome
    - Autosomal dominant inheritance
    - Caused by mutations of *FLCN*, which encodes folliculin
    - Characterized by cutaneous fibrofolliculomas, pulmonary cysts that predispose to spontaneous pneumothorax, bilateral multifocal renal tumors
  - Other renal tumors in BHD syndrome include hybrid oncocytic chromophobe tumor (HOCT) and oncocytoma

Treatment
- Partial or radical nephrectomy
- Ablative techniques, including radiofrequency ablation or cryoablation for nonsurgical candidates
- Sunitinib and everolimus have low response rate
- Immune checkpoint inhibitors have limited antitumor effect

Prognosis
- 5-year survival: ~ 90% after surgery; mortality rate: ~ 10%
- Metastatic ChRCC has poor prognosis

MACROSCOPIC

General Features
- Typically circumscribed mass, not encapsulated
- Cut surface typically homogeneous beige or tan
- Some cases have hemorrhage and necrosis

MOLECULAR

Molecular Genetics
- Hypodiploid DNA content
- Nonrandom losses of chromosomes 1, 2, 6, 10, 13, 17, 21
- Less frequent loss of chromosomes 3, 5, 8, 9, 11, 18, Y
- Most commonly mutated genes include *TP53* (20-30%) and *PTEN* (6-9%)
  - *TP53* and *PTEN* mutations and imbalanced chromosome duplication enriched in metastatic ChRCC
- Mutations in PI3K/AKT/mTOR pathway in ~ 15%
- Genes upregulated include *ADAP1*, *SDCBP2*, *HOOK2*, *BAIAP3*, and *SPINT1*
- Mutations in mitochondrial DNA in ~ 20%
- Rearrangement in *TERT* promoter region in ~ 10%
- Genes mutated in < 5%: *FAAH2*, *PDHB*, *PDXDC1*, and *ZNF765*
- Expression of *FOXI1* and *RHCG* enriched in oncocytic neoplasms, including ChRCC

MICROSCOPIC

Histologic Features
- Sheets and nests of tumor cells surrounded by delicate fibrous septa containing blood vessels
- Variable admixture of larger pale cells and smaller cells with perinuclear halos
  - Larger cells have transparent, slightly flocculent cytoplasm and prominent plant-like cell membranes
  - Smaller cells have less abundant granular and eosinophilic cytoplasm and perinuclear halos
- Hyperchromatic nuclei with irregular wrinkled contours; binucleation common
- Eosinophilic variant of ChRCC almost entirely composed of intensely eosinophilic cells
- ChRCC not graded according to WHO and ISUP
- Coagulative tumor necrosis associated with worse prognosis
- Sarcomatoid transformation associated with aggressive clinical course

ANCILLARY TESTS

Histochemistry
- Hale colloidal iron stain positive in most cases

Immunohistochemistry
- Positive for pan-CK, EMA, PAX8, CK7, CD117, Ksp-cadherin, EPCAM (Ber-EP4), and claudin-7

DIFFERENTIAL DIAGNOSIS

Renal Oncocytoma
- Round, vesicular nuclei without perinuclear halo
- CK7 negative or only focally positive

SELECTED REFERENCES

1. Moch H et al: Chromophobe renal cell carcinoma: current and controversial issues. Pathology. 53(1):101-8, 2021
2. Trpkov K et al: New developments in existing WHO entities and evolving molecular concepts: the Genitourinary Pathology Society (GUPS) update on renal neoplasia. Mod Pathol. 34(7):1392-424, 2021
3. Skala SL et al: Next-generation RNA sequencing-based biomarker characterization of chromophobe renal cell carcinoma and related oncocytic neoplasms. Eur Urol. 78(1):63-74, 2020
4. Williamson SR et al: Report from the International Society of Urological Pathology (ISUP) Consultation Conference on Molecular Pathology of Urogenital Cancers: III: molecular pathology of kidney cancer. Am J Surg Pathol. 44(7):e47-65, 2020
5. Ricketts CJ et al: The Cancer Genome Atlas comprehensive molecular characterization of renal cell carcinoma. Cell Rep. 23(1):313-26.e5, 2018

Papillary Renal Cell Carcinoma

KEY FACTS

CLINICAL ISSUES
- Most cases are sporadic
- Familial cases in hereditary papillary renal cell carcinoma (PRCC) syndrome
- Subclassification into type 1 and type 2 tumors no longer recommended, according to WHO 5th edition

MOLECULAR
- Sporadic cases commonly have trisomy 7, trisomy 17, loss of Y chromosome
- Significantly mutated genes include MET, CDKN2A, SETD2, NF2, KDM6A, SMARCB1, FAT1, BAP1, PBRM1, STAG2, NFE2L2, and TP53
- Formerly type 1 tumors typically have altered MET status (~ 80%) by mutation, splice variant, or fusion
- Formerly type 2 tumors are genetically heterogeneous
- Altered cancer-associated pathways include chromatin remodeling and Hippo signaling pathways
- Mutations or promoter hypermethylation of CDKN2A associated with poor prognosis
- Activation of or mutations in NRF2-ARE pathway genes
- High-grade tumors have alterations in TERT promoter and ARID1A mutations
- Distinct subgroup has CpG island methylator phenotype (CIMP) that is associated with poor survival

MICROSCOPIC
- Papillary architecture with fibrovascular cores
  - Typically lined by single layer of tumor cells
- Graded according to WHO/International Society of Urological Pathology (ISUP) grading system based on nucleolar prominence
- Sarcomatoid change present in ~ 5% of cases

ANCILLARY TESTS
- Positive for pancytokeratin, EMA, cytokeratin 7, CD10, AMACR (P504S), PAX2, PAX8, and RCCma

Low-Grade PRCC

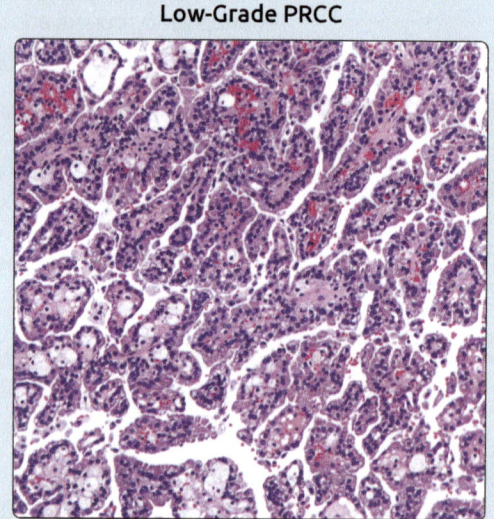

Low-Grade PRCC

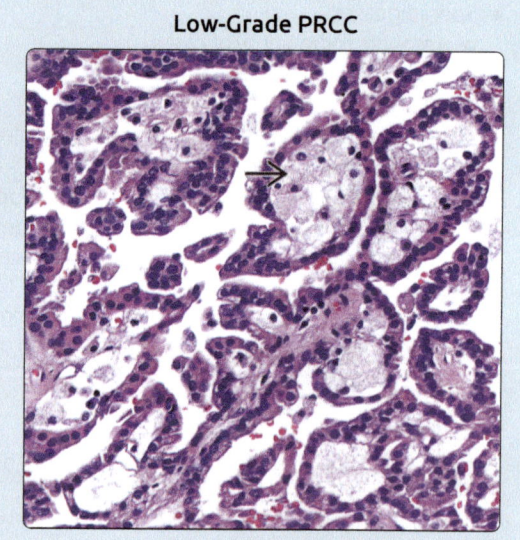

(Left) Papillary renal cell carcinoma (PRCC) is composed of papillary fronds lined by a single layer of small tumor cells with round to ovoid nuclei and modest to relatively scant cytoplasm. (Right) The fibrovascular cores of PRCC often contain collections of foamy macrophages ➔. Tumor cells are small with modest to scant amphophilic cytoplasm and small, monotonous nuclei. This tumor was formerly classified as type 1 PRCC.

High-Grade PRCC

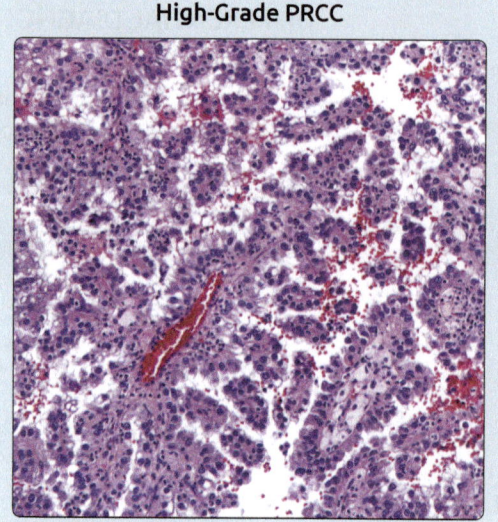

High-Grade PRCC

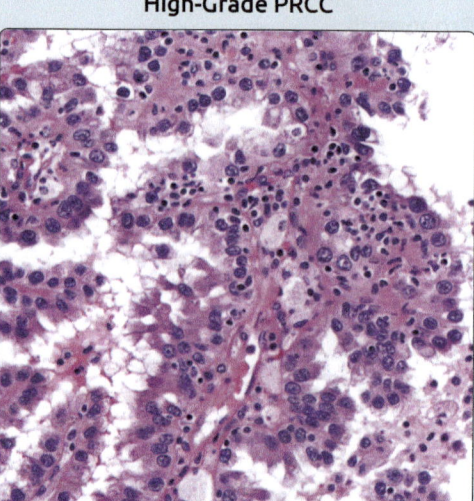

(Left) PRCC shows papillary fronds with fibrovascular cores lined by tumor cells with more abundant eosinophilic cytoplasm. (Right) Neoplastic cells of the same tumor show abundant eosinophilic cytoplasm, large nuclei, and prominent nucleoli. This tumor was formerly classified as type 2 PRCC.

Papillary Renal Cell Carcinoma

TERMINOLOGY

Abbreviations
- Papillary renal cell carcinoma (PRCC)

Definitions
- Malignant epithelial neoplasm of kidney with papillary architecture thought to arise from proximal nephron

CLINICAL ISSUES

Epidemiology
- Accounts for 10-15% of renal cell carcinomas
- 2nd most common type of renal cell carcinoma
- Subclassification into type 1 and type 2 tumors no longer recommended according to WHO 5th edition

Presentation
- Most cases are sporadic
- Mean age: 52-66 years
- Familial cases
  - Hereditary PRCC
    - Autosomal dominant inheritance
    - Tumors are typically multiple and bilateral
    - Caused by activating germline mutations in tyrosine kinase domain of *MET* oncogene located at 7q31

Treatment
- Partial nephrectomy (nephron-sparing surgery) or radical nephrectomy
- Ablative techniques, including radiofrequency ablation or cryoablation for nonsurgical candidates
- For systemic disease
  - Tyrosine kinase inhibitors
  - mTOR inhibitors
  - Monoclonal antibodies against immune checkpoint inhibitors PD-1, PD-L1, CTLA-4

Prognosis
- Depends on grade, stage, and presence or absence of sarcomatoid change

MOLECULAR

Molecular Genetics
- Heterogeneous molecular alterations
- Sporadic cases commonly have trisomy 7, trisomy 17, loss of Y chromosome
- Often gains of chromosomes 3, 8, 12, 16, and 20
- Losses of chromosomes 1p, 4q, 6q, 9p, 11p, 13q, 14q, 18, 21q, and X
- Significantly mutated genes identified by whole-genome sequencing
  - *MET*, *CDKN2A*, *SETD2*, *NF2*, *KDM6A*, *SMARCB1*, *FAT1*, *BAP1*, *PBRM1*, *STAG2*, *NFE2L2*, *TP53*
  - *TFE3* and *TFEB* fusions in ~ 10% of cases
- Formerly type 1 tumors
  - ~ 80% have altered *MET* status, either by mutation (~ 15%), splice variant, or fusion
- Formerly type 2 tumors are genetically heterogeneous
- Altered cancer-associated pathways include chromatin remodeling and Hippo signaling pathways
- Mutations in *SETD2*, *BAP1*, *PBRM1* located on chromosome 3p
- Mutations or promoter hypermethylation of *CDKN2A* associated with poor prognosis
- Activation of or mutations in NRF2-ARE pathway genes (*NFE2L2*, *CUL3*, *KEAP1*, *SIRT1*) in aggressive tumors
  - Mutations in key genes of this pathway lead to constitutive activation of NRF2 transcription factor responsible for cell proliferation under oxidative stress
- High-grade tumors have alterations in *TERT* promoter and *ARID1A* mutations
- *TP53* mutations associated with poor survival
- Distinct subgroup has CpG island methylator phenotype (CIMP) that is associated with poor survival
  - Some of these cases also have *FH* mutation

MICROSCOPIC

Histologic Features
- Papillary architecture with fibrovascular cores
  - Typically lined by single layer of tumor cells
- Tubular, solid, and glomeruloid areas may be seen
- Fibrovascular cores often contain collections of foamy macrophages
- Necrosis may be present
- Sarcomatoid change present in ~ 5% of cases
- Graded according to WHO/International Society of Urological Pathology (ISUP) grading system based on nucleolar prominence
  - Type 1 PRCC
  - Type 2 PRCC

ANCILLARY TESTS

Immunohistochemistry
- Positive for pancytokeratin, EMA, cytokeratin 7, CD10, AMACR (P504S), PAX2, PAX8, and RCCma

DIFFERENTIAL DIAGNOSIS

Clear Cell Papillary Renal Cell Carcinoma
- Tumor cells have clear cytoplasm with apical alignment of low-grade nuclei
- Negative for AMACR and CD10

SELECTED REFERENCES

1. Angori S et al: Papillary renal cell carcinoma: current and controversial issues. Curr Opin Urol. 32(4):344-51, 2022
2. Mendhiratta N et al: Papillary renal cell carcinoma: Review. Urol Oncol. 39(6):327-37, 2021
3. Trpkov K et al: New developments in existing WHO entities and evolving molecular concepts: The Genitourinary Pathology Society (GUPS) update on renal neoplasia. Mod Pathol. 34(7):1392-424, 2021
4. D'Avella C et al: Mutations in renal cell carcinoma. Urol Oncol. 38(10):763-73, 2020
5. Williamson SR et al: Report from the International Society of Urological Pathology (ISUP) Consultation Conference on Molecular Pathology of Urogenital Cancers: III: Molecular Pathology of Kidney Cancer. Am J Surg Pathol. 44(7):e47-65, 2020
6. Ricketts CJ et al: The cancer genome atlas comprehensive molecular characterization of renal cell carcinoma. Cell Rep. 23(1):313-26.e5, 2018
7. Cancer Genome Atlas Research Network et al: comprehensive molecular characterization of papillary renal-cell carcinoma. N Engl J Med. 374(2):135-45, 2016
8. Durinck S et al: Spectrum of diverse genomic alterations define non-clear cell renal carcinoma subtypes. Nat Genet. 47(1):13-21, 2015

TFE3-Rearranged and TFEB-Altered Renal Cell Carcinomas

TERMINOLOGY

Abbreviations
- Microphthalmia-associated transcription factor (MiT)-family translocation renal cell carcinoma (RCC)

Synonyms
- MiT family translocation RCC
- Translocation-associated RCC

Definitions
- RCC harboring translocation involving member of MITF transcription factor gene family
  o Most commonly TFE3
  o Less commonly TFEB
- Established category of RCC since 2016 WHO classification

TRANSLOCATION-ASSOCIATED RCC GROUPS

TFE3-Rearranged Renal Cell Carcinoma
- Defined by translocations involving TFE3 fusion
- TFE3 located at Xp11.23
  o Fused with 1 of several partner genes via chromosomal translocations
    - Partner genes include ASPSCR1, PRCC, SFPQ, NONO, CLTC, RBM10, MED15, PARP14, LUC7L3, KHSRP, DVL2, and EWSR1
- Most common translocations
  o t(X;17)(p11.23;q25.3); ASPSCR1::TFE3 fusion
    - Identical to translocation detected in alveolar soft part sarcomas
  o t(X;1) with PRCC::TFE3 fusion
- Less common translocations
  o t(X;1) with SFPQ::TFE3 fusion
  o inv(X); NONO::TFE3 fusion
  o t(X;17); CLTC::TFE3 fusion
- RNA sequencing identified cases with MED15::TFE3 and other novel gene fusions
- Normal functions of TFE3
  o Encodes TFE3 protein
    - Basic helix-loop-helix/leucine zipper transcription factor
    - Homodimerize or heterodimerize to bind consensus hexanucleotide E-box DNA sequence
    - Regulates differentiation of melanocytes, hematopoietic cells, and osteoclasts

Melanotic Xp11 Translocation Carcinoma
- Extremely rare melanotic epithelioid renal neoplasm bearing TFE3 fusion
  o Some cases harbor t(X;1); SFPQ::TFE3 fusion
  o Pathologic features overlap with TFE3-rearranged RCC, melanoma, and perivascular epithelioid neoplasm (PEComa)

TFEB-Altered Renal Cell Carcinoma
- Includes TFEB-rearranged RCC, also designated t(6;11) RCC, and TFEB-amplified RCC
- TFEB-rearranged RCC initially defined by t(6;11)
  o Results in TFEB::MALAT1 fusion and overexpression of TFEB protein
  o Other gene fusion partners described
- TFEB-amplified RCCs extremely rare

ETIOLOGY/PATHOGENESIS

TFE3-Rearranged Renal Cell Carcinoma
- Chimeric mRNA transcripts encode N-terminal portion of fusion partner linked to C terminus of TFE3
- TFE3 fusion partners have constitutively active promoters
  o Most TFE3 fusion partners likely play regulatory role in mRNA splicing or mitosis
- TFE3 protein is involved in regulation of several signaling pathways that may contribute to carcinogenesis
  o TGFB1 and ETS transcription factors, E-cadherin expression, CD40L-dependent lymphocyte activation, mTOR signaling, folliculin signaling, and cell cycle regulation

TFEB-Rearranged Renal Cell Carcinoma
- t(6;11)(p21.1;q13.1) translocation results in TFEB::MALAT1 fusion

Papillary Architecture

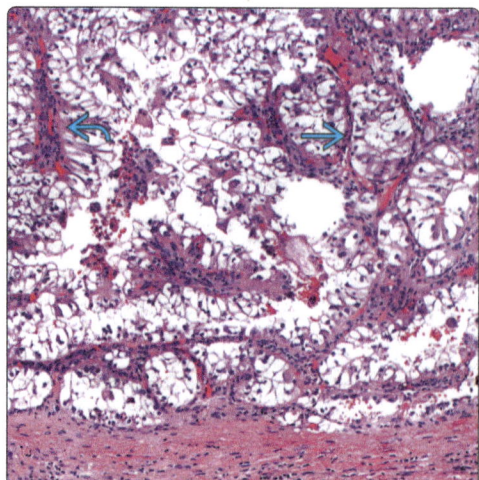

Tumor Cells With Voluminous Clear Cytoplasm

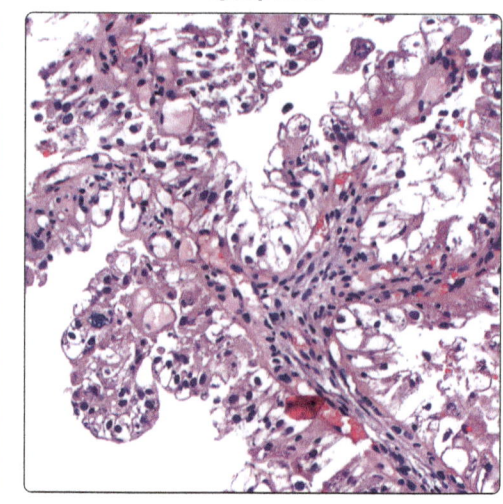

(Left) TFE3-rearranged renal cell carcinoma (RCC) in a 5-year-old girl shows a papillary growth pattern with delicate fibrovascular cores ➡, as well as nested areas ➡. IHC for TFE3 showed characteristic strong diffuse nuclear staining. (Right) Papillary area of the same tumor shows tumor cells with large, voluminous, and clear cytoplasm. Cell borders are well defined, and nuclei vary in size and shape.

TFE3-Rearranged and TFEB-Altered Renal Cell Carcinomas

- o Leads to upregulation of *TFEB*
- *TFEB* encodes helix-loop-helix transcription factor
  - o TFEB protein is regulator of metabolic pathways and mTOR pathways that may contribute to carcinogenesis
  - o TFEB fusion protein may contribute to carcinogenesis via activation of these pathways

CLINICAL ISSUES

TFE3-Rearranged Renal Cell Carcinoma

- **Epidemiology**
  - o Rare: Most cases reported in children and young adults
    - Overall, most patients < 50 years of age; rare cases reported in older populations
  - o M ~ F
  - o To date, most molecularly confirmed cases have *ASPSCR1*::*TFE3* fusion or *PRCC*::*TFE3* fusion
  - o Xp11 translocation carcinomas account for ~ 50% of all pediatric RCC
  - o Overall incidence of RCC is much higher in adults than in pediatric age group
    - 1-4% of adult RCC Xp11 translocation carcinomas
      - □ Therefore, adult cases of Xp11 translocation carcinomas likely outnumber pediatric cases
  - o Up to 15% of pediatric cases have history of prior chemotherapy
- **Clinical presentation**
  - o ~ 50% of cases present with abdominal pain, flank pain, or hematuria
  - o Adults often present with advanced disease and distant metastasis
  - o Some present as palpable mass
  - o Some discovered incidentally
  - o *ASPSCR1*::*TFE3* carcinomas tend to present at more advanced stage than *PRCC*::*TFE3* carcinomas
    - *ASPSCR1*::*TFE3* carcinomas have greater likelihood of positive lymph nodes and distant metastasis
- **Treatment and prognosis**
  - o Nephrectomy with extended lymphadenectomy
  - o No established systemic therapy for metastatic disease
    - Limited experience with mTOR inhibitors, tyrosine kinase inhibitors, and immune checkpoint inhibitors
  - o Overall outcome similar to clear cell RCC
  - o Older age and advanced stage are poor prognostic factors
  - o Outcome data limited because tumors are rare and natural history is highly variable
  - o On short-term follow-up, children with regional lymph node metastases tend to have favorable prognosis
    - Long-term follow up data is necessary before favorable outcome can be confirmed
  - o Adults appear to have worse prognosis and do poorly when presenting with systemic disease
  - o Systemic metastases portend grim prognosis
  - o Multivariate analysis of all molecularly confirmed cases found that
    - Older age and advanced stage are independent predictors of death
    - *ASPSCR1*::*TFE3* tumors appear to be most aggressive with worse prognosis, tends to present at more advanced stage

Melanotic Xp11 Translocation Carcinoma

- Extremely rare; few cases with limited reported follow-up
- Melanotic Xp11 translocation carcinomas and PEComa harboring *TFE3* fusions may represent distinct entities
  - o Pathologic features may overlap with Xp11 translocation RCC

TFEB-Rearranged Renal Cell Carcinoma

- Rare; ~ 100 cases reported to date
- Age range: 3-77 years
  - o Majority of cases in young adults (mean: 28.5; median: 25 years)
- ~ 50% of cases present with abdominal pain or hematuria
- Less aggressive than Xp11 translocation carcinomas on limited reported cases
  - o Aggressive in ~ 17% of cases
- Aggressive tumors occur in older patients and tend to be larger in size

MOLECULAR PATHOLOGY

TFE3-Rearranged Renal Cell Carcinoma

- **Cytogenetics**
  - o Xp11 translocations detected by cytogenetics
    - t(X;17)
    - t(X;1)
    - inv(X)
- **In situ hybridization**
  - o FISH assay with *TFE3* break-apart probe
    - Can confirm presence of Xp11 translocation in formalin-fixed, paraffin-embedded archival tissue blocks
    - Probes bind to centromeric and telomeric portions of *TFE3*
      - □ Show fusion signals in normal tissue
      - □ Show split signals in *TFE3* rearranged translocation carcinomas
- **Other molecular genetic abnormalities**
  - o *TFE3* fusions activate MET signaling
  - o Frequent mutations in chromatin remodeling genes
  - o Xp11 carcinomas differentially express multiple microRNAs associated with cell signaling

Melanotic Xp11 Translocation Carcinoma

- Carry translocations involving *TFE3*
  - o Some cases have *SFPQ*::*TFE3* fusion

TFEB-Rearranged Renal Cell Carcinoma

- **Cytogenetics**
  - o t(6;11) detected by cytogenetics
    - Results in fusion of *MALAT1* with *TFEB*
- **In situ hybridization**
  - o FISH assay can confirm diagnosis in paraffin-embedded tissue

MACROSCOPIC PATHOLOGY

TFE3-Rearranged Renal Cell Carcinoma

- Mostly circumscribed ± pseudocapsule
- *PRCC*::*TFE3* tumors may have calcified pseudocapsule
- Cut surface yellow-tan to gray; hemorrhage and necrosis common

TFE3-Rearranged and TFEB-Altered Renal Cell Carcinomas

- Some cases have infiltrative edges

TFEB-Rearranged Renal Cell Carcinoma
- Typically intact pseudocapsule, 2-12 cm diameter
- Solid, focal cysts; homogeneous tan-yellow cut surface

MICROSCOPIC PATHOLOGY

TFE3-Rearranged Renal Cell Carcinoma
- Broad spectrum of architectural and cytologic features
- Some histologic features are characteristic of tumors with specific translocations, but considerable overlap exists
- Characteristic histologic features
  - Papillary, pseudopapillary, solid, and alveolar architecture
  - Large cells with voluminous clear cytoplasm, distinct cell borders
  - Common in ASPSCR1::TFE3 carcinomas; high nuclear grade, psammomatous calcifications, and dyscohesive tumor cells
- PRCC::TFE3 carcinomas
  - Typically more nested architecture; either demarcated or merging papillary areas; lower grade nuclei
- NONO::TFE3 carcinomas
  - Often glandular, tubular, or papillary architecture
  - Apical nuclei with subnuclear vacuoles reminiscent of secretory endometrium
  - Other features include eosinophilic or granular cytoplasm, oncocytoma-like features, spindle cells
- MED15::TFE3 carcinomas
  - Cystic architecture; papillary and solid areas; uniform round nuclei

Melanotic Xp11 Translocation Carcinoma
- Overlapping histologic features with Xp11 translocation carcinoma, melanoma, and PEComa
- Composed of solid sheets and nests of polygonal epithelioid cells
- Clear or finely granular cytoplasm containing variable amounts of finely granular melanin pigment

TFEB-Rearranged Renal Cell Carcinoma
- Broad range of growth patterns, including solid and nested
- 2 distinct cell populations of larger and smaller cells
  - Larger epithelioid cells predominate with
    - Well-defined cell borders; abundant clear, finely granular, or eosinophilic cytoplasm
    - Round and uniform or vesicular nuclei with prominent nucleoli
  - Smaller cells comprise 2nd cell population
    - Clustered around nodules of basement membrane material
    - Smaller nuclei with dense chromatin
    - Cases without small cell component have been reported
    - Areas resembling epithelioid angiomyolipoma, clear cell RCC with cystic change, or chromophobe RCC may be seen
    - Papillary, tubulocystic, or oncocytoma-like features may be seen

ANCILLARY TESTS

TFE3-Rearranged Renal Cell Carcinoma
- Immunohistochemistry
  - Positive for TFE3 with antibody against C-terminal portion of fusion protein
    - Stain is highly fixation dependent in archival material
    - TFE3 also stains alveolar soft part sarcoma
  - Positive for CD10, RCCma, and AMACR; most cases positive for PAX2 and PAX8; ~ 60% positive for cathepsin K
    - Other common subtype of RCC negative for cathepsin K
    - ASPSCR1::TFE3 carcinoma negative for cathepsin K
  - Some cases positive for Melan-A, HMB-45
    - SFPQ::TFE3 and CLTC::TFE3 translocation carcinomas rarely stain with Melan-A or HMB-45
  - Underexpress vimentin, cytokeratins, EMA
  - Most cases negative for MITF

Melanotic Xp11 Translocation Carcinoma
- Immunohistochemistry
  - Positive for TFE3; patchy positivity for Melan-A and HMB-45
  - Negative for CD10, PAX2, PAX8 (in contrast to typical TFE3-rearranged RCC), and MITF (in contrast to melanoma)

TFEB-Rearranged Renal Cell Carcinoma
- Immunohistochemistry
  - TFEB positive, sensitive and specific for t(6;11) RCC
    - Stain is highly fixation dependent in archival material
  - Positive for Melan-A, HMB-45, PAX8, cathepsin K, AMACR, and CD68 (KP1 clone)
    - Cathepsin K positive in almost all t(6;11) RCC
  - Negative or only focally positive for cytokeratins

SELECTED REFERENCES

1. Wei S et al: A review of neoplasms with MITF/MiT family translocations. Histol Histopathol. 37(4):311-21, 2022
2. Argani P: Translocation carcinomas of the kidney. Genes Chromosomes Cancer. 61(5):219-27, 2022
3. Xia QY et al: Clinicopathologic and molecular analysis of the TFEB fusion variant reveals new members of TFEB translocation renal cell carcinomas (RCCs): expanding the genomic spectrum. Am J Surg Pathol. 44(4):477-89, 2020
4. Caliò A et al: t(6;11) renal cell carcinoma: a study of seven cases including two with aggressive behavior, and utility of CD68 (PG-M1) in the differential diagnosis with pure epithelioid PEComa/epithelioid angiomyolipoma. Mod Pathol. 31(3):474-87, 2018
5. Wang XT et al: RNA sequencing of Xp11 translocation-associated cancers reveals novel gene fusions and distinctive clinicopathologic correlations. Mod Pathol. 31(9):1346-60, 2018
6. Argani P et al: RBM10-TFE3 renal cell carcinoma: a potential diagnostic pitfall due to cryptic intrachromosomal Xp11.2 inversion resulting in false-negative TFE3 FISH. Am J Surg Pathol. 41(5):655-62, 2017
7. Classe M et al: Incidence, clinicopathological features and fusion transcript landscape of translocation renal cell carcinomas. Histopathology. 70(7):1089-97, 2017
8. Marchionni L et al: MicroRNA expression profiling of Xp11 renal cell carcinoma. Hum Pathol. 67:18-29, 2017
9. Saleeb RM et al: Melanotic MiT family translocation neoplasms: expanding the clinical and molecular spectrum of this unique entity of tumors. Pathol Res Pract. 213(11):1412-8, 2017
10. Xia QY et al: Xp11 translocation renal cell carcinomas (RCCs) with RBM10-TFE3 gene fusion demonstrating melanotic features and overlapping morphology with t(6;11) RCC: interest and diagnostic pitfall in detecting a paracentric inversion of TFE3. Am J Surg Pathol. 41(5):663-76, 2017

TFE3-Rearranged and TFEB-Altered Renal Cell Carcinomas

Solid and Papillary Growth Patterns

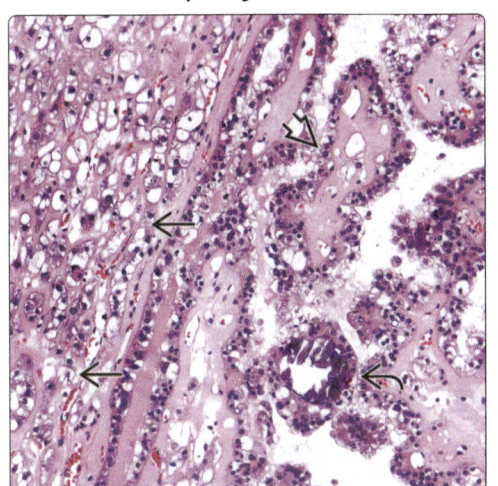

Polygonal Cells With Clear Cytoplasm

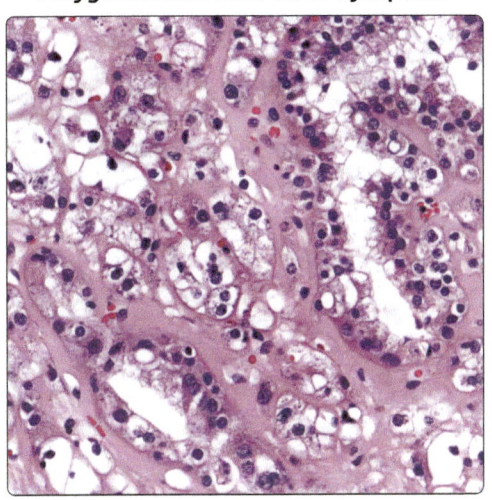

(Left) *TFE3-rearranged RCC in a 30-year-old woman is shown. Areas of solid growth ⇨ are sharply demarcated from papillary areas ⇨ with broad, hyalinized fibrovascular cores. A psammoma body is present ⇨. Strong, diffuse nuclear staining characteristic of TFE3 was present.* (Right) *Higher power view of the same tumor shows polygonal cells with clear to granular cytoplasm and well-defined cell borders. Nuclei are mostly round.*

Solid Alveolar Growth Pattern

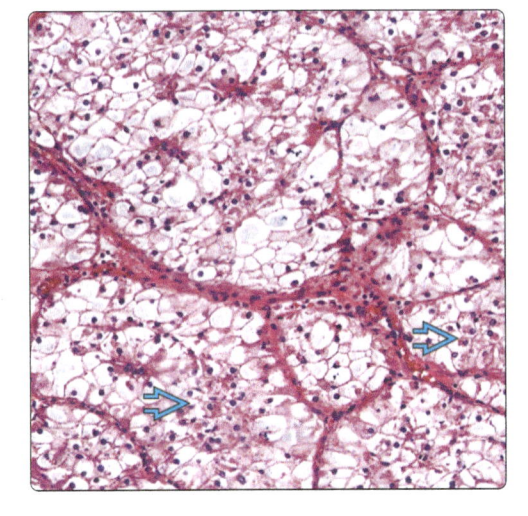

TFE3 Immunohistochemistry

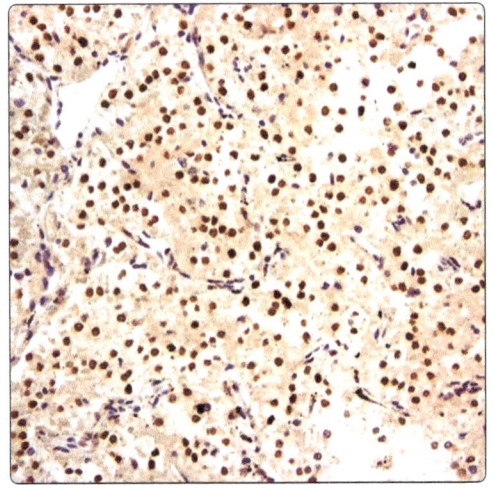

(Left) *Solid alveolar growth pattern is not uncommon in TFE3-rearranged RCC. Solid alveoli may show central cell dyscohesion ⇨, and morphologically may mimic alveolar soft part sarcoma. This pattern is commonly associated with ASPSCR1::TFE3 fusion. (From DP: Genitourinary.)* (Right) *TFE3 shows strong nuclear staining in ASPSCR1::TFE3 carcinoma. This finding is characteristic of TFE3-rearranged RCC irrespective of fusion partner. (From DP: Genitourinary.)*

Biphasic Growth Pattern

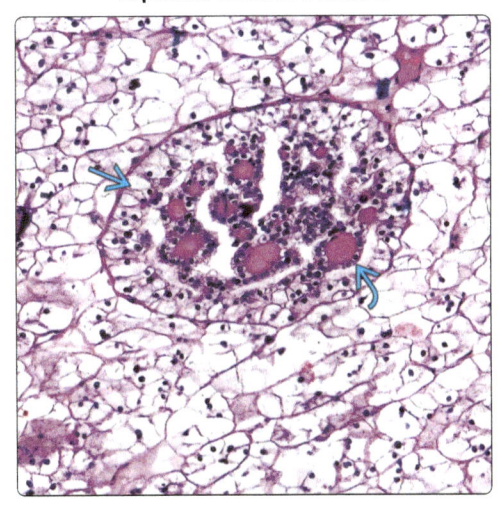

TFEB Immunohistochemistry

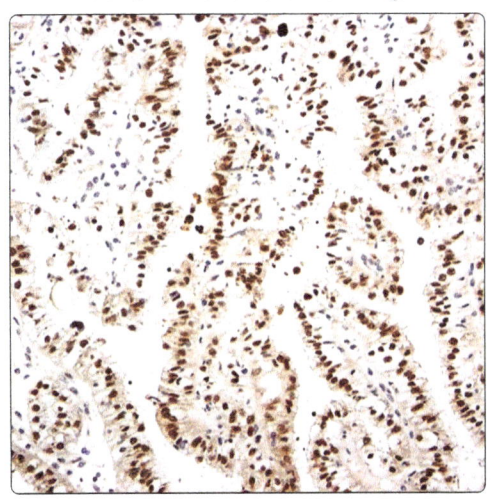

(Left) *Biphasic growth pattern characteristic of t(6;11) translocation carcinoma shows smaller cells located within a tubular structure ⇨. These cells are arranged around hyaline nodules ⇨ composed of basement membrane material. (From DP: Genitourinary.)* (Right) *Strong, diffuse staining for TFEB is highly specific for t(6;11) translocation carcinomas but may focally stain some lymphocytes. (From DP: Genitourinary.)*

Wilms Tumor

KEY FACTS

TERMINOLOGY
- Wilms tumor (WT): Malignant nephroblastic tumor, often with multiphasic differentiation

ETIOLOGY/PATHOGENESIS
- Syndromic associations in 10%
  - **W**T, **a**niridia, **g**enitourinary abnormalities, mental **r**estriction (WAGR) syndrome, sporadic aniridia
  - Denys-Drash and Frasier syndromes
  - Beckwith-Wiedemann syndrome
  - Familial nephroblastoma
  - Other syndromes include Bloom, Perlman, Li-Fraumeni, Sotos, Simpson-Golabi-Behmel, trisomy 18, CLOVES

CLINICAL ISSUES
- Most common pediatric renal tumor
- 5-10% have bilateral or multicentric tumors
- ~ 75% of cases < 5 years of age

MOLECULAR
- *WT1* deletions or mutations
  - Germline: WAGR syndrome, sporadic aniridia, Denys-Drash syndrome, sporadic tumors
  - Somatic mutations occur in 12% of tumors
- *WT2* locus alterations
  - Germline alterations in Beckwith-Wiedemann syndrome
  - Somatic loss of heterozygosity (LOH) and loss of imprinting (LOI) at 11p15 in 70% of tumors
- Other mutated genes include *CTNNB1*, *AMER1*, *TP53*, and microRNA processing genes
- Gain of 1q: Strongest predictor of adverse outcome
- If 1q normal, LOH at 1p and 16q predicts relapse in favorable histology WT
- *WT1* mutation and LOH/LOI at 11p15
  - Predict recurrence in very low-risk WT with surgery only
- *TP53* mutations or loss at 17p13 associated with anaplasia and worse prognosis

Gross Appearance

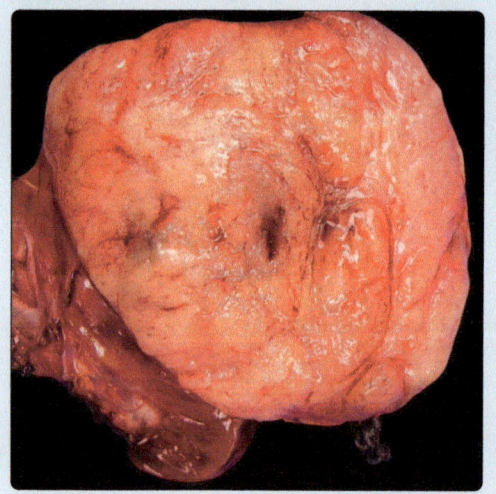

Triphasic Morphology

(Left) Gross photograph of a large, well-circumscribed Wilms tumor (WT) shows its tan-white, bulging cut surface. The tumor is separated from nonneoplastic kidney by a thin, fibrous pseudocapsule (not shown). (Right) Typical histologic appearance of WT is shown. Note the triphasic morphology with epithelial ➡, blastemal ➡, and stromal ➡ components. However, some tumors may be biphasic or monophasic.

Anaplastic Change With Nuclear Enlargement and Abnormal Mitosis

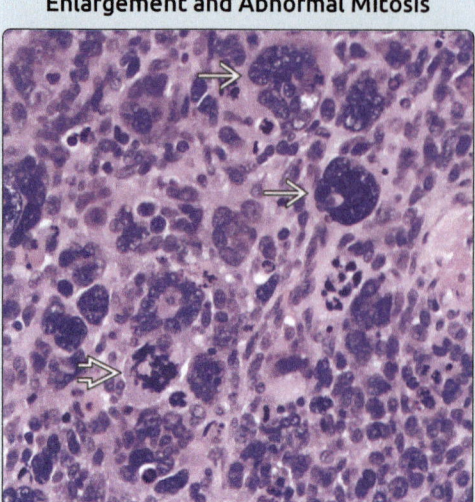

Nuclear Staining for WT1

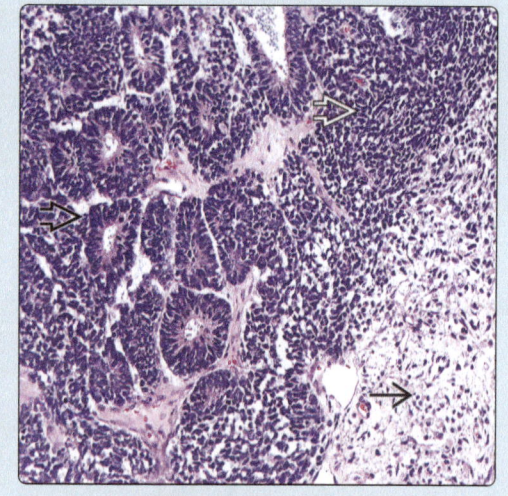

(Left) This area of blastema shows anaplastic change, the definition of which includes presence of definite large, hyperchromatic cells (3x size of typical blastemal cells in 2 axes) ➡ and large, abnormal multipolar mitoses ➡. Anaplasia is a very important indicator of aggressive behavior in WT. (Right) WT shows diffuse strong nuclear staining for WT1 in blastemal and epithelial areas.

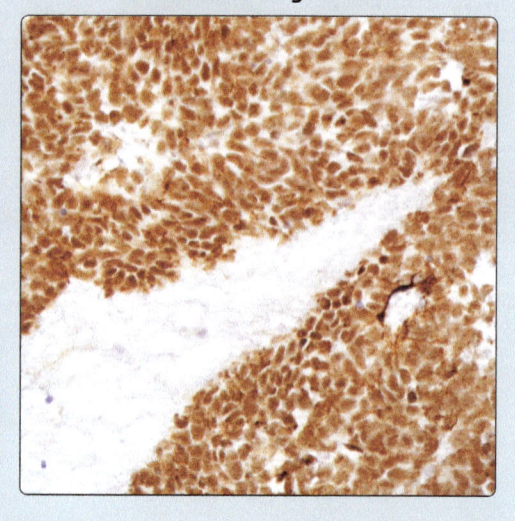

Wilms Tumor

TERMINOLOGY

Abbreviations
- Wilms tumor (WT)

Synonyms
- Nephroblastoma

Definitions
- Malignant renal tumor from nephrogenic blastema, typically with multiphasic differentiation

ETIOLOGY/PATHOGENESIS

Developmental Anomaly
- WT: Syndromic/congenital anomaly associations in 10-15%
  o Can be grouped into nonovergrowth and overgrowth phenotypes based on absence or presence of overgrowth of somatic tissues
  o Renal ultrasound surveillance recommended every 3 months from birth/diagnosis until at least age 8 years in predisposing syndromes
- Nonovergrowth phenotype syndromes with *WT1* inactivation mutations
  o **W**ilms tumor, **a**niridia, **g**enitourinary anomalies, developmental delay (**r**estriction) (WAGR) syndrome
    – Deletions of several contiguous genes, including *PAX6* in addition to *WT1*
  o Denys-Drash syndrome, Frasier syndrome, isolated genitourinary abnormalities, and sporadic aniridia
    – All associated with *WT1* mutations and predisposition to WT development
    – Sporadic aniridia associated with WT; precise mapping of breakpoint needed to determine if *WT1* is involved
  o Other syndromes associated with predisposition for WT development
    – Li-Fraumeni syndrome, Bloom syndrome, Fanconi anemia with biallelic mutations in *BRCA2* or *PALB2*, trisomy 18 (Edwards syndrome)
- Overgrowth phenotype syndromes with predisposition to WT development
  o Beckwith-Wiedemann syndrome (BWS)
    – *WT2* mutations linked to predisposition to WT
  o Perlman syndrome with *DIS3L2* mutations
    – Associated with high risk of WT development
  o 9q22.3 microdeletion syndrome
    – Deletion invariably encompasses *PTCH1*
  o Isolated hemihypertrophy
  o Congenital lipomatous overgrowth, epidermal nevi, scoliosis and spinal deformities (CLOVES) syndrome with somatic *PIK3CA* mutations
  o Other syndromes with predisposition to WT include Sotos syndrome and Simpson-Golabi-Behmel syndrome
- Familial WT
  o 1-2% of patients with WT have 1 or more relatives with isolated WT
  o Familial cases show higher rate of bilateral tumors and earlier age of diagnosis
  o Genetic linkage has identified several candidate genes/loci, including loci at 17q12-q21 and 19q13.4
  o Rare mutations in *WT1*, *BRCA2*, and *CTR9* in familial WT

Nephrogenic Rests
- Abnormal clusters of embryonic kidney cells that persist into postnatal life
  o Thought to be WT precursors
- Perilobular nephrogenic rests (PLNR)
  o Located at periphery of renal lobule; may be multifocal
  o *IGF2* dysregulated WT often associated with PLNR (including with hemihypertrophy and overgrowth syndromes)
  o Well-circumscribed, blastemal-predominant histology
- Intralobular nephrogenic rests (ILNR)
  o Located within renal lobule, usually isolated lesions
  o *WT1* mutated WT often associated with ILNR PLNR (including with WAGR and Denys-Drash syndromes)
  o Irregular, stromal-predominant histology

Pathogenesis
- Pathways involved in development of WT include *IGF2* overexpression (70%, including alterations at *WT2* locus), abnormalities in *WNT* signaling (30%, including mutations in *WT1*, *CTNNB1*, and *AMER1*), and abnormalities in microRNA processing (20%)
- Later events: 1p/16q loss, 1q gain, *TP53* mutations
- > 40 genes somatically mutated in WT

CLINICAL ISSUES

Epidemiology
- Most common pediatric renal tumor
  o > 95% of pediatric renal tumors
  o ~ 7 cases per million < 15 years of age
- 5-10% have bilateral or multicentric tumors
- Average age at presentation
  o 42-47 months for unilateral tumors
  o 30-33 months for bilateral tumors
- ~ 75% of cases present in patients < 5 years of age; 98% in patients < 10 years of age; peak incidence at 2-3 years of age
- Rare cases may occur in adults

Presentation
- Usually abdominal mass noted by parent
- Pain, malaise, hematuria, hypertension (20-30%)

Treatment
- Multimodal therapy, including surgery, chemotherapy, and radiotherapy
- Differences between treatment protocols in North America vs. Europe, but both have excellent results
- Surgery
  o Children's Oncology Group (COG) in North America recommends nephrectomy at time of diagnosis, followed by chemotherapy and radiotherapy in some patients
  o International Society of Pediatric Oncology (SIOP) in Europe advocates preoperative chemotherapy prior to nephrectomy
  o Nephron-sparing surgery considered for bilateral tumors
  o Surgery only may be considered in very low-risk WT
- Chemotherapy following nephrectomy at diagnosis (COG protocols in North America)

Wilms Tumor

- Depends on factors, such as stage, tumor weight, and presence of anaplasia
- WT with unfavorable histology (diffuse anaplasia) treated more aggressively
- Favorable histology WT (FHWT) with combined loss of heterozygosity (LOH) of 1p and 16q may be treated more aggressively
- Stage III/IV tumors with LOH of 1p and 16q may be treated more aggressively
- Other markers that may allow risk stratification of otherwise very low-risk WT include 11p15 methylation status, *WT1* mutations, LOH at 11p15
- Radiation therapy
  - Used postoperatively in high-stage tumors and tumors with anaplasia

Prognosis

- Overall survival: > 90%
- Unfavorable factors include high stage, unfavorable histology (diffuse anaplasia)
- Stage at diagnosis, tumor weight, patient age, and histology used to stratify patients into risk groups
  - Very low risk, low risk, standard risk, favorable histology, and high risk
- Molecular alterations help further risk stratifications
  - Gain of 1q is strongest predictor of poorer survival in unilateral FHWT
  - If 1q is normal, 1p/16q LOH may predict worse outcome
  - 11p15 LOH and methylation status predict recurrence in very low-risk WT treated by surgery alone
  - *TP53* mutations or loss at 17p13 associated with anaplasia and worse prognosis
  - LOH at 4q, 14q, 11q associated with anaplasia and worse prognosis
  - *MYCN* amplification and *MYCN* P44L mutation associated with poor prognosis

COG Staging (Conceptual Summary)

- Stage I: Tumor limited to kidney and completely resected
- Stage II: Tumor with regional extension but completely resected
- Stage III: Residual tumor after surgery but confined to abdomen
- Stage IV: Hematogenous metastases, positive lymph nodes beyond abdomen/pelvis
- Stage V: Bilateral kidney tumors at time of diagnosis

MACROSCOPIC

General Features

- Minority of tumors are multicentric or bilateral
- Clearly demarcated, often encapsulated
- May have hemorrhage and necrosis

MOLECULAR

Cytogenetics

- Partial gains of 1q
- Partial losses of 1p, 1q, 4q, 11q, 14q, 16q, and 22q
- Complete loss of chromosomes 22, 16, 11, and 12
- Trisomy of chromosomes 12, 18, 13, and 8
- Rearrangements and deletions of 11p13 may occur

Molecular Genetics

- *WT1* mutations
  - Both somatic and germline *WT1* mutations occur in WT
  - Somatic *WT1* inactivating mutations or deletions in 12%
  - Germline *WT1* mutations occur in association with syndromes and with sporadic WT
  - Mutations in WAGR syndrome
    - Contiguous gene deletion syndrome involving multiple genes, including *WT1* and *PAX6*
    - ~ 50% of patients with WAGR syndrome develop WT
  - Sporadic aniridia
    - Results from deletion that involves *PAX6* and may include part or all of *WT1*
    - Risk of WT is 40-50% if deletion involves *WT1*
  - WT and isolated genitourinary anomalies
    - *WT1* deletions, frameshift and nonsense mutations
  - Denys-Drash syndrome
    - Most have germline missense mutations in exon 8 or 9 of *WT1*
    - Risk for WT: > 90%
  - Frasier syndrome
    - Point mutation in *WT1* intron 9 donor splice site
    - Rare cases with WT
  - Isolated WT without syndromic findings
    - Germline *WT1* mutations can be found in 2% of cases
  - Tumors with *WT1* mutations usually have stromal-predominant histology and muscle differentiation
  - Tumors with *WT1* mutations are often associated with mutations in *CTNNB1*
- *WT2* alterations
  - *WT2* locus maps to 11p15.5 and includes
    - *H19-ICR* (imprinting control region) with *IGF2* and *H19*, and *CDKN1C* and *KCNQ1OT1*
    - *IGF2* codes for growth factor; *H19* produces noncoding RNA tumor suppressor
    - Normally, in *H19-ICR*, both *IGF2* and *H19* are imprinted with paternal allele-only *IGF2* expression and maternal allele-only expression of *H19*
    - Loss of imprinting (LOI) as result of hypermethylation of *H19-ICR* results in aberrant biallelic expression of *IGF2* and decreased expression of *H19* from maternal allele
  - Other functional abnormalities at *WT2* locus seen in WT and BWS include LOH, mutations, paternal uniparental disomy (UPD), microdeletions, microduplications, and microinsertions
  - Both somatic and germline alterations in *WT2* occur in WT
    - Alterations in *WT2*, including LOH and LOI, occur as somatic change in 70%
    - Germline alterations in *WT2* occur in BWS and in sporadic tumors
  - Beckwith-Wiedemann syndrome is associated with several abnormalities at *WT2* locus, including
    - Microdeletions, hypermethylation at *H19-ICR*
    - Mutation of *CDKN1C*, microduplication at imprinting center 2
    - Paternal UPD of 11p15
  - Sporadic tumors without syndromic findings may show constitutional alterations at *WT2* locus, including

Wilms Tumor

- Hypermethylation at *H19-ICR*
- Paternal UPD of 11p15
- Microdeletion and microinsertion
    - Tumors with LOI are usually stroma poor
- *AMER1* mutations
    - Somatic mutations in ~ 15-20% of WT
    - Germline mutations do not predispose to WT
    - Associated with epigenetic abnormalities at 11p15
- *CTNNB1* mutations
    - Somatic mutations in ~ 15% of WT
    - Almost always seen in association with mutations in either *WT1*, or *AMER1*, or *MLLT1*
    - Late event (not seen in nephrogenic rests)
- *TP53* mutation
    - Strongly associated with unfavorable histology
        - Up to 75% of anaplastic WT harbor *TP53* mutations
- *MYCN* alterations
    - Copy number gain and high expression seen in WT and associated with diffuse anaplasia
- Mutations in miRNA processing genes
    - Seen in ~ 20% of WT, generally mutually exclusive
    - Germline mutations in *DICER1* (DICER1 syndrome) and *DIS3L2* (Perlman syndrome) predispose to WT
    - Sporadic mutations in WT include *DROSHA*, *DICER1*, *DIS3L2*, *XPO5*, *DGCR8*, and *TARBP2*
- *FBXW7* mutations
    - Somatic deletions or mutations found in 4% of WT
- *CTR9* mutations
    - Germline inactivating mutations predispose to WT
- *PTCH1* alterations
    - Virtually all 9q22.3 microdeletion syndrome cases have deletion of 1 copy of *PTCH1*
    - Associated with increased risk for WT development
- *MLLT1* mutations
    - Seen in 4% of WT; associated with *CTNNB1* mutations
- *REST* mutations
    - Germline and sporadic mutations described
- *SIX1* and *SIX2* mutations
    - Sporadic mutations seen; associated with microRNA processing gene mutations
- *BRAF* p.V600E mutation
    - Subset of epithelial-predominant WT in adults and children
    - Morphologic overlap with metanephric adenoma
    - May respond to BRAF targeted therapy
- *TRIM28* mutations
    - Germline or somatic mutations associated with WT with monomorphic epithelial histology
    - Seen in young children, very good prognosis

MICROSCOPIC

Histologic Features

- WT typically shows triphasic appearance with mixture of blastema, epithelial, and stromal elements
- Only 1 or 2 components may be present in some cases
- Blastema
    - Densely packed small round cells with little cytoplasm, darkly staining nuclei, and inconspicuous nucleoli
    - Usually numerous mitoses
    - Diffuse, nodular, and serpiginous growth patterns
- Epithelial components
    - Typically tubules, cysts, or glomeruloid structures lined by cuboidal or columnar cells
    - May see squamous, mucinous, or other epithelial differentiation
    - Poorly formed rosette structures may be seen
- Stromal components
    - Usually fibroblastic or myxoid spindle cells
    - Heterologous differentiation may be present: Skeletal and smooth muscle, fat, bone, cartilage, neural elements
- Anaplasia
    - Areas of tumor with definitely hyperchromatic large cells (3x diameter of blastemal cells in 2 axes) and large multipolar mitoses
    - "Focal anaplasia" includes being confined to 1 or few discrete loci within primary tumor with no anaplasia or marked nuclear atypia elsewhere
    - "Diffuse anaplasia" includes more extensive anaplasia, anaplastic tumor at margin, intravascular anaplastic tumor, or anaplastic tumor at extrarenal site
    - Diffuse anaplasia in WT is unfavorable histology

ANCILLARY TESTS

Immunohistochemistry

- WT1 expressed in blastemal and epithelial components

Genetic Testing

- Germline testing
    - May be indicated depending on clinical findings

DIFFERENTIAL DIAGNOSIS

Clear Cell Sarcoma

- Delicate fibrovascular septa
- WT1 negative, cyclin-D1 positive

Rhabdoid Tumor

- SMARCB1 (INI1) negative, WT1 negative

Other Small Round Blue Cell Tumors

- Neuroblastoma
    - Neuroendocrine markers positive, WT1 negative
- Ewing sarcoma
    - CD99 and NKX2.2 positive, WT1 negative

Metanephric Adenoma

- CD57 positive, WT1 negative or weak

Papillary Renal Cell Carcinoma

- CK7 and AMACR positive, WT1 negative

SELECTED REFERENCES

1. NIH: Wilms tumor and other childhood kidney tumors treatment (PDQ). Updated May 2023. https://www.cancer.gov/types/kidney/hp/wilms-treatment-pdq
2. WHO Classification of Tumours Editorial Board: Urinary and male genital tumours. IARC, 2022
3. Gadd S et al: Genetic changes associated with relapse in favorable histology Wilms tumor: a Children's Oncology Group AREN03B2 study. Cell Rep Med. 3(6):100644, 2022
4. Phelps HM et al: Biological drivers of Wilms tumor prognosis and treatment. Children (Basel). 5(11), 2018

Wilms Tumor

Nephrogenic Rest

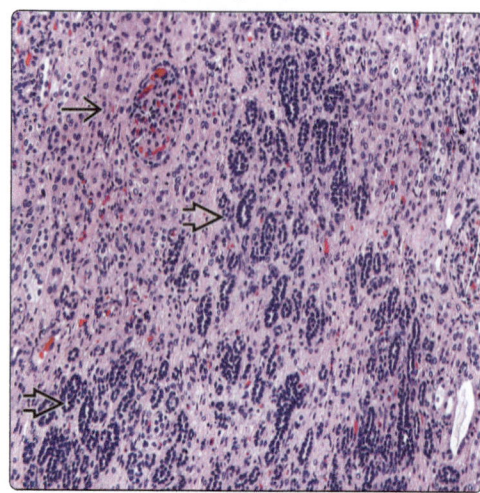

Nuclear Staining for WT1

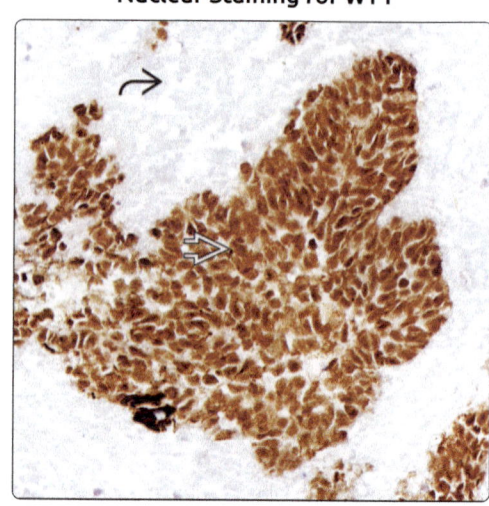

(Left) Nephrogenic rests are believed to be the precursor lesions for WT. This intralobular rest is composed mainly of small tubules ⇨, interdigitating between areas of normal nonneoplastic kidney parenchyma ⇨. Usually, intralobular nests have more stroma. **(Right)** WT1 shows diffuse nuclear staining in areas of blastema ⇨ in this case of WT. Note that the stromal compartment ⇨ is generally negative for WT1.

Epithelial Component With Glands

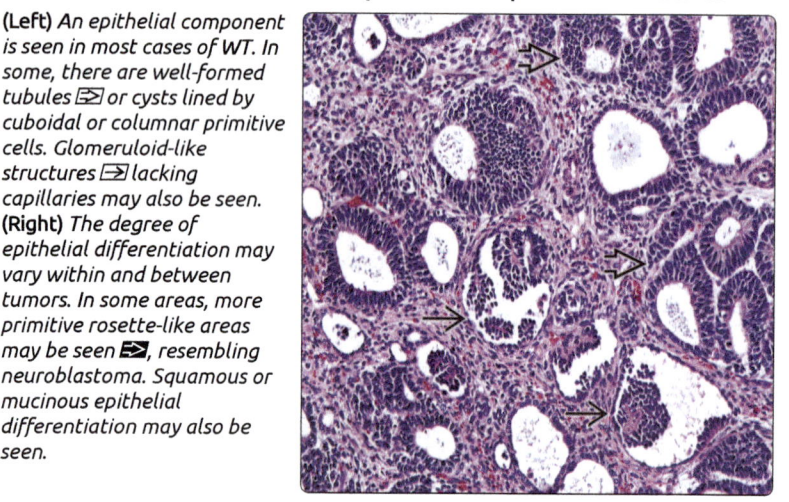

Less Well-Formed Glands (Rosette-Like)

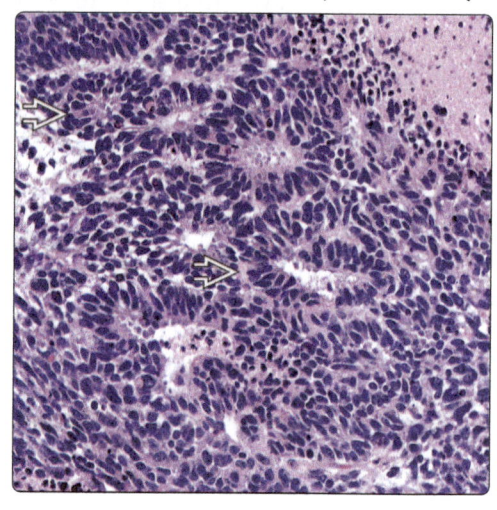

(Left) An epithelial component is seen in most cases of WT. In some, there are well-formed tubules ⇨ or cysts lined by cuboidal or columnar primitive cells. Glomeruloid-like structures ⇨ lacking capillaries may also be seen. **(Right)** The degree of epithelial differentiation may vary within and between tumors. In some areas, more primitive rosette-like areas may be seen ⇨, resembling neuroblastoma. Squamous or mucinous epithelial differentiation may also be seen.

Fibromyxoid Stromal Component

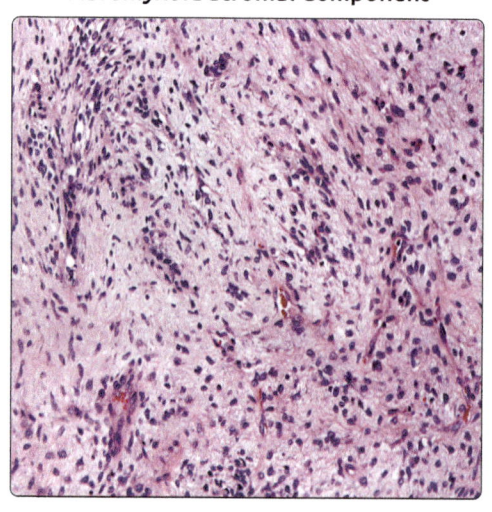

Smooth Muscle Stromal Component

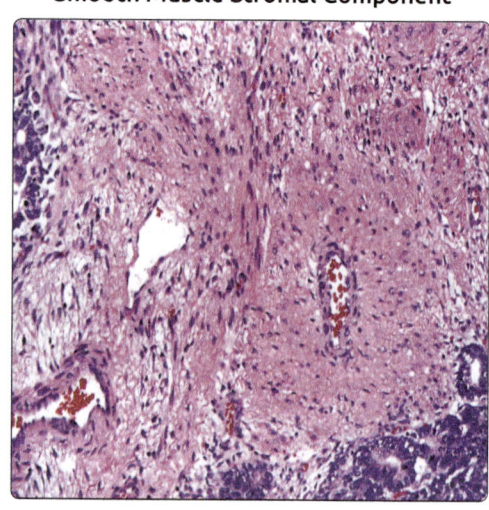

(Left) The stromal component of WT is most commonly composed of fibromyxoid loose spindle cells, as seen here. However, great variability in the stroma may be seen with many different lines of differentiation. **(Right)** Stroma in WT may be more fibrous or show differentiation toward smooth muscle, as seen here. Other heterologous lines of differentiation include differentiation toward skeletal muscle, cartilage, fat, neural tissue, or bone.

Wilms Tumor

Blastemal and Stromal Components

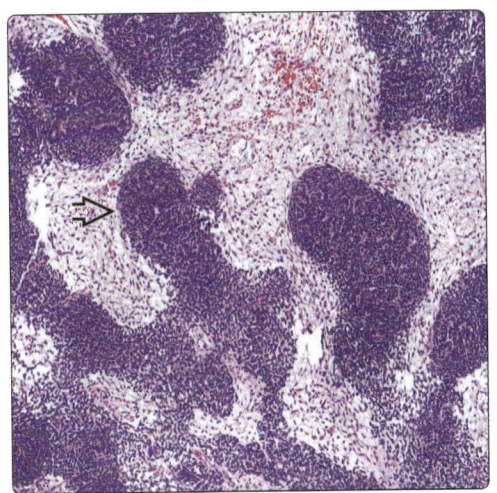

Diffuse Pattern of Blastema

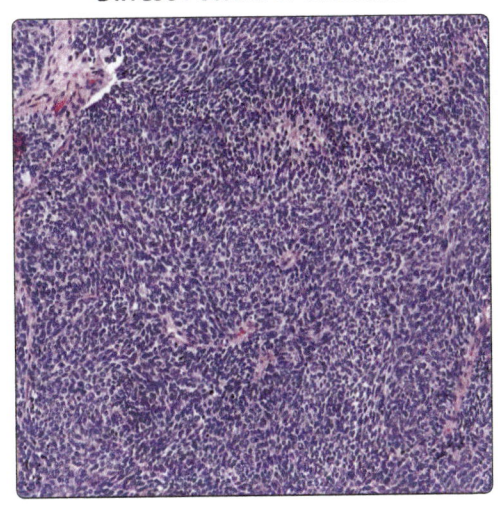

(Left) The blastemal component of WT is composed of areas of densely packed primitive cells with little evidence for cytologic differentiation. Blastema may show serpiginous (as seen here), nodular, or diffuse patterns. Here, there are well-defined anastomosing regions of blastema ⇒, sharply delimited from surrounding stroma. *(Right)* The diffuse pattern of blastema may be associated with an infiltrative tumor margin with invasion of tissues surrounding the kidney.

Blastema With Densely Packed Small Cells

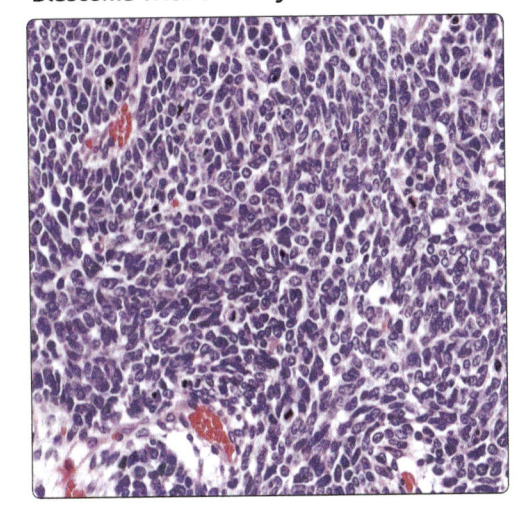

Anaplastic Change

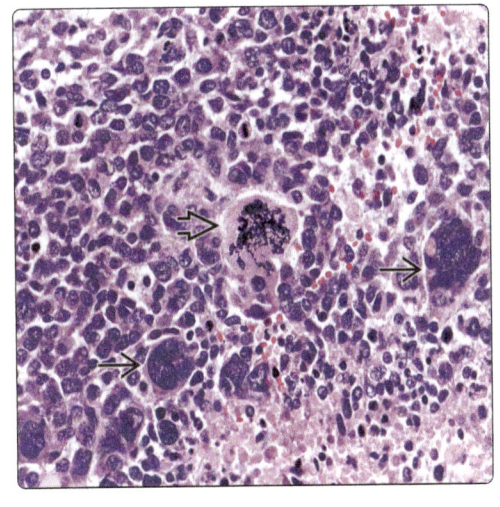

(Left) The blastemal cells are small, densely packed, and overlapping, with little cytoplasm, and are mitotically active. *(Right)* Anaplasia is a very important poor prognostic feature in WT. The definition includes presence of definitely hyperchromatic, large cells (3x size of normal blastemal cells in 2 axes) ⇒ and large, abnormal, multipolar mitoses ⇒. Without the large, abnormal mitoses, the histologic finding would be termed "nuclear unrest."

Rhabdomyoblastic Differentiation

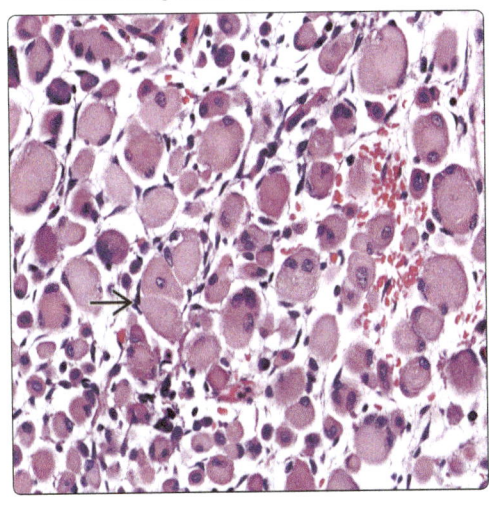

Extensive Necrosis and Macrophages Post Chemotherapy

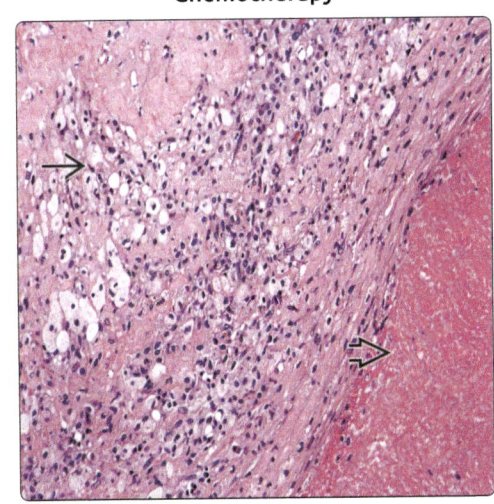

(Left) WT shows diffuse, predominantly (> 50%) skeletal muscle/rhabdomyoblastic stromal differentiation ⇒, termed "fetal rhabdomyomatous nephroblastoma." The tumor has a good prognosis despite chemoresistance. *(Right)* If chemotherapy is given before surgery, the tumor may show necrosis ⇒, and there may be foamy macrophages ⇒. Residual diffuse anaplasia or extensive blastema are poor prognostic features.

Clear Cell Sarcoma of Kidney

KEY FACTS

TERMINOLOGY
- Clear cell sarcoma of kidney (CCSK): Rare, aggressive pediatric sarcoma of kidney composed of variably pale cells and branching fibrovascular septa with molecular findings of BCOR mutations or YWHAE::NUTM2 fusion

ETIOLOGY/PATHOGENESIS
- Biology poorly understood, cell of origin unclear
- No familial or syndromic association
- No known associated germline genetic mutations

MOLECULAR
- Internal tandem duplication (ITD) in exon 15 of BCOR is present in majority of cases
- Rearrangement of YWHAE with NUTM2B or NUTM2E due to t(10;17)(q22;p13) translocation seen in minority of cases
- BCOR::CCNB3 fusion seen in rare cases
- BCOR ITD, YWHAE::NUTM2 fusion, and BCOR::CCNB3 fusion are all mutually exclusive and associated with BCOR overexpression
- No clinicopathologic distinguishing features between tumors with BCOR ITD and tumors with YWHAE::NUTM2 fusion; BCOR::CCNB3 fusion seen in slightly older population
- CCSK thought to be part of family of tumors sharing BCOR ITD and morphologic features, including infantile undifferentiated round cell sarcoma, primitive myxoid mesenchymal tumor of infancy, CNS high-grade neuroepithelial tumor with BCOR ITD, and high-grade endometrial stromal sarcoma with BCOR ITD

TOP DIFFERENTIAL DIAGNOSES
- Blastema-predominant Wilms tumor
- Primitive neuroectodermal tumor
- Cellular congenital mesoblastic nephroma
- Rhabdoid tumor of kidney

Nests and Cords of Tumor Cells With Branching Small Septal Vessels

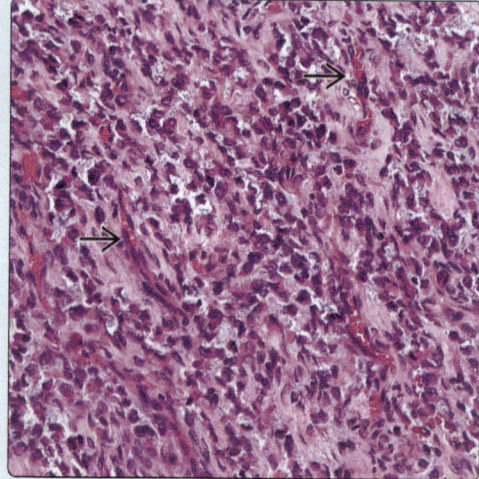

Pale Cytoplasm With Indistinct Cell Borders and Fine Nuclear Chromatin

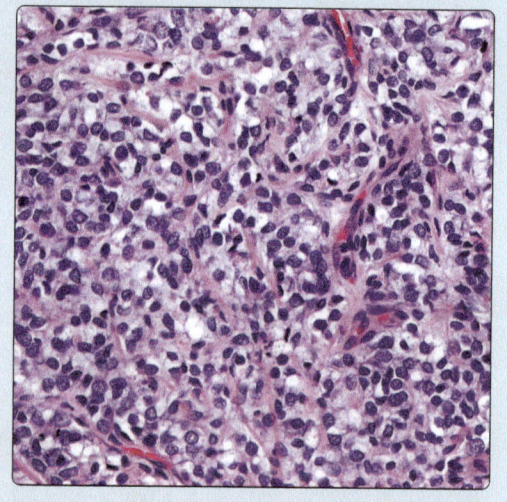

(Left) Clear cell sarcoma of the kidney (CCSK) shows classic histologic pattern with nests and cords of tumor cells separated by delicate, branching, fibrovascular septa ➡. (From DP: Pediatric Neoplasms.) (Right) CCSK shows predominance of round/oval cells with pale cytoplasm, indistinct cell borders, fine nuclear chromatin, and inconspicuous nucleoli. (From DP: Pediatric Neoplasms.)

Myxoid Variant

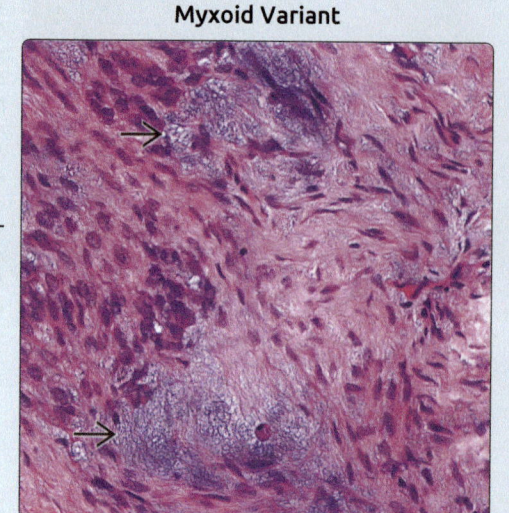

Sclerosing Variant

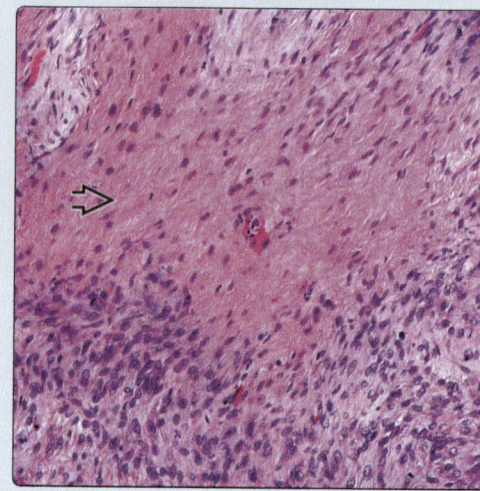

(Left) Myxoid variant of CCSK shows amphophilic myxoid material ➡ separating cords of tumor cells. (From DP: Pediatric Neoplasms.) (Right) Sclerosing variant of CCSK shows tumor cells separated by acellular hyaline or osteoid-like material ➡. (From DP: Pediatric Neoplasms.)

Clear Cell Sarcoma of Kidney

TERMINOLOGY

Abbreviations
- Clear cell sarcoma of kidney (CCSK)

Definitions
- Rare, aggressive pediatric sarcoma of kidney composed of variably pale cells and branching fibrovascular septa with molecular findings of *BCOR* mutations or *YWHAE::NUTM2* fusion

ETIOLOGY/PATHOGENESIS

Developmental Anomaly
- No familial or syndromic association
  - Cell of origin unclear, biology poorly understood
  - No known associated germline genetic mutations

CLINICAL ISSUES

Epidemiology
- 3-5% of pediatric renal malignancies
- 50% diagnosed by age 12-36 months
  - Mean age: 3 years; highest incidence in children 2-3 years; very rare in adults

Presentation
- Abdominal mass, pain, hematuria, fever
- 5% have metastasis at presentation: Lymph nodes, bone, lung, abdomen, retroperitoneum, brain, liver

Treatment
- Radical nephrectomy, postoperative radiotherapy, chemotherapy

Prognosis
- Overall long-term survival: ~ 69%; stage I: ~ 98%
- Late relapses (> 3 years) uncommon
- Doxorubicin has improved survival
- Adverse: Age < 2 years or > 4 years, high stage
- Not related to histologic variants or mutation type

MACROSCOPIC

General Features
- Unilateral, unicentric, well demarcated, 2.3-24 cm in size
- Heterogeneous solid appearance; may be cystic
- 5% show extension into renal vein

MOLECULAR

Cytogenetics
- t(10;17)(q22;p13); *YWHAE::NUTM2E* in minority of cases

Molecular Genetics
- Internal tandem duplication (ITD) in exon 15 of *BCOR* seen in majority of cases
- Rearrangement of *YWHAE* with *NUTM2B* or *NUTM2E* due to t(10;17)(q22;p13) translocation seen in minority of cases
- *BCOR::CCNB3* fusion seen in rare cases
- *BCOR* ITD, *YWHAE::NUTM2* fusion, and *BCOR::CCNB3* fusion are all mutually exclusive and result in upregulation of BCOR mRNA and protein
- CCSK thought to be part of family of tumors sharing *BCOR* ITD and morphologic features, including infantile undifferentiated round cell sarcoma, primitive myxoid mesenchymal tumor of infancy, CNS high-grade neuroepithelial tumor with *BCOR* ITD, and high-grade endometrial stromal sarcomas with *BCOR* ITD
- No clinicopathologic distinguishing features between CCSKs with *BCOR* ITD and CCSK with *YWHAE::NUTM2* fusion; CCSK with *BCOR::CCNB3* fusion seen in slightly older population
- *BCOR* ITD can be detected by DNA and RNA-based NGS methods, but data analysis may need additional bioinformatic steps
- Rare molecular findings
  - *IRX2::TERT* fusion
  - *EGFR* amplification, point mutation, or ITD
  - *PTEN* mutations

MICROSCOPIC

Histologic Features
- Classic: Nests and cords of cells with pale cytoplasm, fine nuclear chromatin, indistinct nucleoli, and septal branching small blood vessels; seen at least focally in > 90% of cases
- Variants: Myxoid, sclerosing, cellular, epithelioid, palisading, storiform, spindle, and anaplastic

ANCILLARY TESTS

Immunohistochemistry
- Positive: BCOR, cyclin-D1, TLE1, SATB2, BCL2, and CD10
- BCOR positivity not completely sensitive or specific for CCSK, also may be seen in synovial sarcoma and renal malignant solitary fibrous tumor
- Cyclin-D1 positivity: Sensitive for CCSK, but may also be seen in Ewing sarcoma, neuroblastoma, and other round cell sarcomas
- Cyclin-B3 may be positive in tumors with *BCOR::CCNB3* fusion
- Negative: Epithelial markers, vascular markers, neural markers, muscle markers, CD99, and WT1

DIFFERENTIAL DIAGNOSIS

Blastema-Predominant Wilms tumor
- Bilateral, multicentric, nephrogenic rests
- WT1 positive, BCOR and cyclin-D1 negative

Primitive Neuroectodermal Tumor
- Translocation involving *EWSR1*
- CD99 positive

Rhabdoid Tumor of Kidney
- Prominent nucleoli
- Loss of SMARCB1, BCOR and cyclin-D1 negative

Cellular Congenital Mesoblastic Nephroma
- *ETV6::NTRK3* fusion

SELECTED REFERENCES

1. Al-Ibraheemi A et al: Assessment of BCOR internal tandem duplications in pediatric cancers by targeted RNA sequencing. J Mol Diagn. 23(10):1269-78, 2021

Oncocytoma

KEY FACTS

TERMINOLOGY
- Benign renal epithelial neoplasm with eosinophilic cytoplasm due to numerous mitochondria

ETIOLOGY/PATHOGENESIS
- **Cell of origin**
  - Believed to arise from intercalated cells of renal collecting tubules

CLINICAL ISSUES
- Benign neoplasm
  - Does not metastasize
- Treatment includes surgical resection or surveillance

MOLECULAR
- Many oncocytomas have no detectable clonal cytogenetic abnormalities
- May have losses of chromosomes 1, 14, 21, X, Y
- Subset have structural rearrangements of involving 11q13 chromosomal region
- *CCND1* is located at 11q13, correlating with overexpression of cyclin-D1 protein
- 11q13 locus is also at proximity of genes encoding mitochondrial proteins, including *NDUFC2*, *SDHD*, *UCP2*, and *UCP3*
- Somatic loss-of-function mitochondrial DNA (mtDNA) mutations involving genes of mitochondrial complex I
- May be seen in Birt-Hogg-Dubé syndrome with germline *FLCN* mutations
- Metabolomics profiling show adaptive upregulation of glutathione biosynthesis

TOP DIFFERENTIAL DIAGNOSES
- Chromophobe renal cell carcinoma, eosinophilic-type
- Clear cell renal cell carcinoma, eosinophilic-type
- SDH-deficient renal cell carcinoma
- Other oncocytic tumors
- Oncocytoma-like epithelioid angiomyolipoma

Gross Appearance

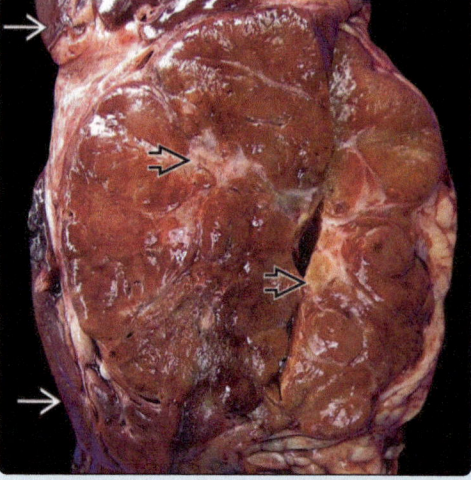

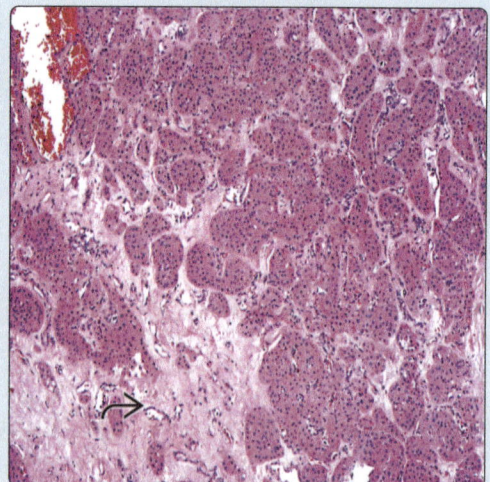

(Left) Gross photograph of renal oncocytoma shows a well-circumscribed, brown mass with areas of stellate scarring present centrally. Residual normal kidney is present but not grossly invaded by tumor. (Right) Microscopically, renal oncocytoma typically shows solid nests of oncocytic cells with granular, eosinophilic cytoplasm and often areas of hypocellular, myxoid to fibrous edematous stroma.

Nests of Oncocytic (Eosinophilic) Cells and Edematous Stroma

Abundant Eosinophilic Cytoplasm and Round Uniform Nuclei

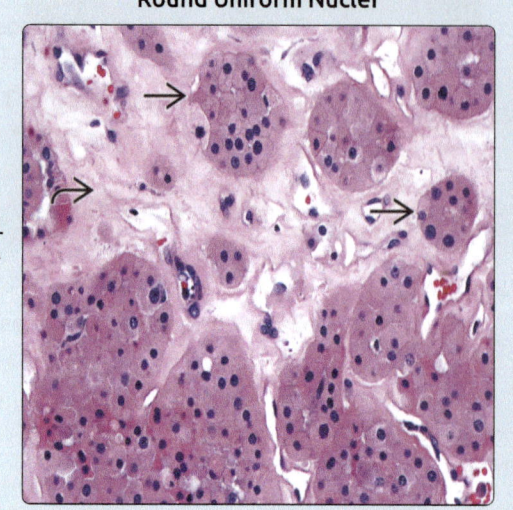

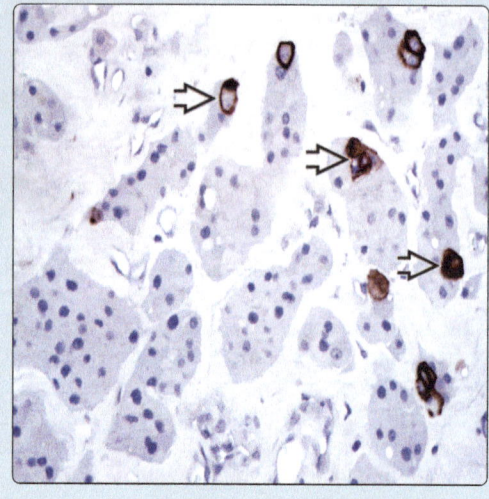

(Left) Renal oncocytoma shows cells with abundant granular, eosinophilic cytoplasm, round, uniform nuclei, and nucleoli, which may be prominent. A characteristic edematous matrix is present. (Right) CK7 usually shows negative or very focal staining of single or small groups of cells.

Focal Staining for CK7 in Oncocytic Cells

Oncocytoma

TERMINOLOGY

Definitions
- Benign renal epithelial neoplasm with eosinophilic cytoplasm due to numerous mitochondria

ETIOLOGY/PATHOGENESIS

Cell of Origin
- Believed to arise from intercalated cells of renal distal tubules

CLINICAL ISSUES

Presentation
- 6-9% of renal epithelial tumors
- Age range: 2nd-10th decades; peak incidence in 7th decade
- 75-80% are asymptomatic, discovered incidentally
- Some cases present with hematuria, abdominal mass, flank pain, hypertension, erythrocytosis
- Rare hereditary cases, many of which represent Birt-Hogg-Dubé (BHD) syndrome
- Multiple oncocytomas may be seen in renal oncocytosis, most of which are thought to be due to BHD

Treatment
- Surgical resection
- May consider surveillance if biopsy findings are very convincing for oncocytoma

Prognosis
- Benign neoplasm, does not metastasize

MACROSCOPIC

General Features
- Well circumscribed, nonencapsulated
- Classically mahogany brown, may be tan
- Central stellate scar in ~ 1/3 of tumors
- Necrosis is not typical

MOLECULAR

Cytogenetics
- Many oncocytomas have no detectable clonal cytogenetic abnormalities
- May have losses of chromosomes 1, 14, 21, X, Y
- Translocations involving *CCND1* at 11q13
  - t(5,11)(q35;q13) and t(9,11)(p23,q13)
  - Other chromosomal partners of 11q13 locus include 1, 6, 7, 8
- Oncocytomas may also show cytogenetic mosaicism
- Unlike chromophobe carcinoma, oncocytoma does not typically show losses of chromosomes 2, 6, 10, 17

Molecular Genetics
- 11q13 breakpoints have been found near *CCND1*, correlating with overexpression of cyclin-D1
- 11q13 locus located in proximity of genes encoding mitochondrial proteins, including *NDUFC2*, *SDHD*, *UCP2*, and *UCP3*
- Somatic loss-of-function mitochondrial DNA (mtDNA) mutations, especially involving subunits of mitochondrial complex I
- Some tumors may show microsatellite instability
- May be seen in BHD syndrome with germline *FLCN* mutations

MICROSCOPIC

Histologic Features
- Usually solid nests, cysts, and tubules may be seen
- Often areas of hypocellular myxoid edematous stroma
- Cells with granular eosinophilic cytoplasm due to accumulation of mitochondria
- Uniform round nuclei; may have prominent nucleoli
- Degenerative atypia may be seen
- Generally should not see necrosis, well-formed papillae, mitoses, raisinoid nuclei, or perinuclear halos

ANCILLARY TESTS

Immunohistochemistry
- Positive for CD117
- CK7 negative or only focal scattered positive cells

DIFFERENTIAL DIAGNOSIS

Chromophobe Carcinoma, Eosinophilic Subtype
- Irregular raisinoid nuclei, perinuclear halos
- Often diffuse staining for cytokeratin 7
- Frequent losses of chromosomes 2, 6, 10, 17

Clear Cell Carcinoma, Eosinophilic Subtype
- Fine capillary vasculature, nuclear irregularities
- CA9 positive, CD117 negative

Succinate Dehydrogenase-Deficient Renal Cell Carcinoma
- Nuclear pleomorphism and cytoplasmic inclusions
- Negative for SDHB and CD117

Other Oncocytic Tumors
- Heterogeneous group of low-grade tumors, including emerging entities eosinophilic vacuolated tumor and low-grade oncocytic tumor, and BHC-associated hybrid oncocytic chromophobe tumor

Other Entities With Eosinophilic Cytoplasm
- Includes low-grade fumarate hydratase-deficient RCC, MiT family translocation RCC, and eosinophilic solid and cystic RCC

DIAGNOSTIC CHECKLIST

Pathologic Interpretation Pearls
- Currently, differentiation of oncocytoma from mimics is primarily on morphology and immunohistochemistry

SELECTED REFERENCES

1. Oszwald A et al: Update on classification of oncocytic neoplasms of the kidney. Curr Opin Urol. 33(3):239-44, 2023
2. Amin MB et al: Low grade oncocytic tumors of the kidney: a clinically relevant approach for the workup and accurate diagnosis. Mod Pathol. 35(10):1306-16, 2022

Rhabdoid Tumor of Kidney

KEY FACTS

TERMINOLOGY
- Highly aggressive pediatric sarcoma of kidney with poor prognosis, characteristically showing loss of function of SMARCB1 in most cases

CLINICAL ISSUES
- Very uncommon after 3 years of age
- ~ 67% of patients present at advanced stage
- Prognosis very poor; 5-year survival: < 15% to 25%

MOLECULAR
- Most rhabdoid tumors of kidney (RTK): Biallelic loss of function of SMARCB1 located at 22q11
  - Germline mutations or deletions in ~ 35%: Mostly de novo
  - Inherited inactivation of SMARCB1 allele: Rhabdoid tumor predisposition syndrome 1
  - 2 somatic events may be seen in ~ 65%
  - Abnormalities include mutations, deletions, and duplications
- Rare RTK: Loss of function of SMARCA4
  - Inherited inactivation of SMARCA4 allele: Rhabdoid tumor predisposition syndrome 2
- Very low mutation rate except at SMARCB1 locus

ANCILLARY TESTS
- Immunohistochemistry for SMARCB1 (INI1) is negative in at least 98% of RTK
- SMARCA4 (BRG1) is negative in rare tumors

TOP DIFFERENTIAL DIAGNOSES
- Renal medullary carcinoma and epithelioid sarcoma
- Other histologic mimics retain SMARCB1 expression
- Renal cell carcinomas may show rhabdoid change

DIAGNOSTIC CHECKLIST
- Germline mutational testing and genetic counseling should be considered for all patients with rhabdoid tumors

---

Sheets of Tumor Cells With Eosinophilic Cytoplasm and Eccentrically Placed Nuclei

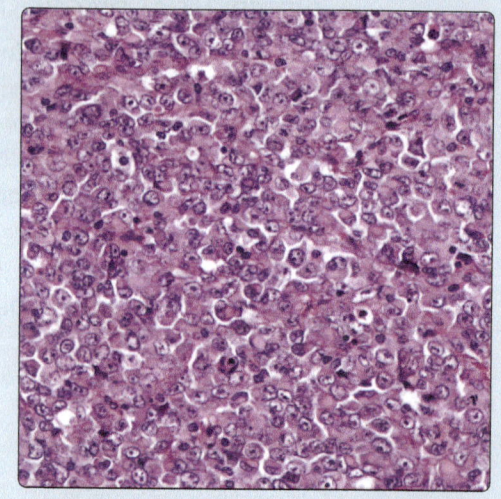

Vesicular Round Nuclei With Prominent Nucleoli and Thick Nuclear Membranes

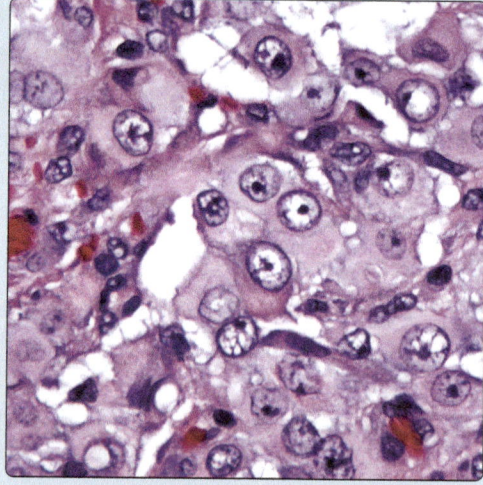

(Left) Classic histology of rhabdoid tumor of the kidney (RTK) includes monotonous sheets of loosely cohesive tumor cells with abundant eosinophilic cytoplasm and eccentric nuclei with prominent nucleoli. (From DP: Genitourinary.) (Right) RTK shows vesicular, round nuclei with thick nuclear membranes and prominent nucleoli. (From DP: Pediatric Neoplasms.)

Abundant Eosinophilic Cytoplasm With Eosinophilic Cytoplasmic Inclusions

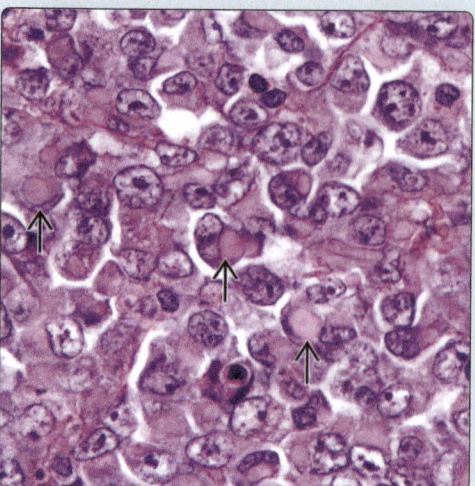

Loss of SMARCB1 in Tumor Cells and Preservation in Benign Cells

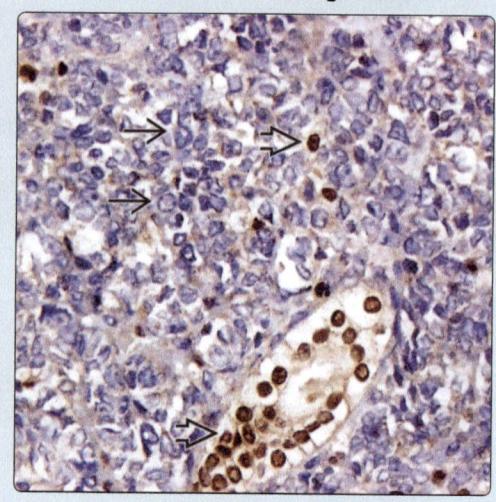

(Left) Classic histology of RTK includes abundant eosinophilic cytoplasm and cytoplasmic inclusions ➔, which represent intermediate filaments. (From DP: Genitourinary.) (Right) Characteristic loss of nuclear SMARCB1 in tumor cells ➔ is seen in at least 98% of rhabdoid tumors. Expression is preserved in nonneoplastic cells ➔. (From DP: Genitourinary.)

Rhabdoid Tumor of Kidney

TERMINOLOGY

Abbreviations
- Rhabdoid tumor of kidney (RTK)

Definitions
- Highly aggressive pediatric sarcoma of kidney with pleomorphic cells, prominent nucleoli, and cytoplasmic inclusions, characteristically showing loss of SMARCB1 IHC and loss of function of *SMARCB1* in most cases

ETIOLOGY/PATHOGENESIS

SMARCB1
- Normal function
  o Tumor suppressor gene
  o Part of SWI/SNF chromatin remodeling complex
- Biallelic loss of function of *SMARCB1*
  o Seen in > 98% of cases
  o Mutations include germline or somatically acquired
- Familial rhabdoid tumors
  o Rhabdoid tumor predisposition syndrome 1
    – Inherited inactivation of 1 allele of *SMARCB1*
    – Multifocal tumors and schwannomatosis in adults
  o Rhabdoid tumor predisposition syndrome 2
    – Inherited inactivation of 1 allele of *SMARCA4*

CLINICAL ISSUES

Presentation
- 1.5-3% of pediatric renal malignancies
- Median age at diagnosis: 11-13 months; M:F = 1.4:1
- ~ 67% of patients present at advanced stage
- 10-15% are associated with brain tumors (either RTK metastasis or atypical teratoid/rhabdoid tumors of brain)

Treatment
- Surgery, radiotherapy, multiagent chemotherapy, autologous stem cell transplantation

Prognosis
- Very poor; 5-year survival from < 15% to 25%
  o Worse if age < 6 months, high stage, presence of AT/RT

MOLECULAR

Cytogenetics
- May show monosomy of chromosome 22

Molecular Genetics
- Characteristic loss of function of *SMARCB1*
  o Germline mutations or deletions in ~ 35%
    – Point or frameshift mutations in 40%
    – Heterozygous loss in 26%
    – Deletion of 1 or more exons in 23%
    – Duplications in 9%
    – Most of germline mutations are de novo (not inherited)
    – In minority, parent is carrier of germline abnormality, giving rise to rhabdoid tumor predisposition syndrome 1; gonadal mosaicism may also occur
  o Somatically acquired abnormalities
    – Deletion in 46%, copy-neutral loss of heterozygosity (LOH) in 29%, and frameshift mutation in 23%
  o 2 somatic events may be seen in ~ 65%
    – Homozygous deletion (most common)
    – Deletion, intragenic deletion, or frameshift or point mutation
- Loss of function of *SMARCA4*
  o Rarely described in familial and sporadic cases of RTK and atypical teratoid/rhabdoid tumor
  o Tumors retain SMARCB1 protein expression
  o May result in rhabdoid tumor predisposition syndrome 2
- Whole-exome sequencing
  o Very low mutation rate except at *SMARCB1* locus
    – Suggests tumorigenesis is driven by epigenetic changes
- Germline mutational testing and genetic counseling should be considered for all patients with rhabdoid tumors
- NGS detects *SMARCB1* and *SMARCA4* alterations
- NGS should be used with other testing, such as SNP arrays, to show loss of the other allele

MICROSCOPIC

Histologic Features
- Classic histology
  o Sheets of large cells with eosinophilic cytoplasm
  o Vesicular nuclei with prominent nucleoli
  o Perinuclear eosinophilic cytoplasmic inclusions
    – Represent aggregates of intermediate filaments
    – May be difficult to detect in some cases
- Histologic variants
  o Sclerosing, epithelioid, spindle cell, lymphomatoid, vascular, pseudopapillary, myxoid, and cystic
    – Classic areas are usually also present

ANCILLARY TESTS

Immunohistochemistry
- SMARCB1 (INI1) is negative in at least 98% of RTK
- SMARCA4 (BRG1) is negative in rare tumors
- Can express neuroepithelial, epithelial, and mesenchymal markers; CD99(+) in > 50%

DIFFERENTIAL DIAGNOSIS

Renal Medullary Carcinoma and Epithelioid Sarcoma
- Show *SMARCB1* loss similar to RTK
- Tend to occur in older patients

Other Histologic Mimics, Including Clear Cell Sarcoma and Congenital Mesoblastic Nephroma
- Typically retain SMARCB1 expression by IHC

Renal Cell Carcinomas (Nonmedullary)
- May have rhabdoid areas; SMARCB1 generally retained

SELECTED REFERENCES
1. Sirohi D MD et al: SWI/SNF-deficient neoplasms of the genitourinary tract. Semin Diagn Pathol. 38(3):212-21, 2021
2. Pawel BR: SMARCB1-deficient tumors of childhood: a practical guide. Pediatr Dev Pathol. 21(1):6-28, 2018

Urothelial Carcinoma

KEY FACTS

TERMINOLOGY
- Malignant neoplasm derived from urothelium

MOLECULAR
- 2 important clinicopathologic categories of urothelial carcinoma
  - Nonmuscle invasive bladder cancer
    - Tends to recur rather than progress
    - Typically associated with low-grade papillary histology
    - Associated with *FGFR3*, *HRAS*, and *PIK3CA* mutations, and chromosome 9 losses
  - Muscle invasive bladder cancer (MIBC)
    - Tends to progress and metastasize
    - Usually high-grade histology
    - High rate of mutations and genomic amplifications
- Comprehensive genomic analysis of MIBC has shown dysregulation of several pathways
  - p53/cell cycle regulation (89% of tumors), including alterations in *TP53*, *CDKN2A*, *RB1*, *CDKN1A*, and *MDM2*
  - RTK/RAS/PI(3)K (71% of tumors), including mutations in *FGFR3*, *EGFR*, *ERBB2*, *ERBB3*, *PIK3CA*, and *PTEN*
  - Chromatin modification pathways: Histone-modifying genes (52% of tumors), SWI/SNF complex (26%), including mutations in *ARID1A*, *KMT2D*, *KMT2C*, *KDM6A*, *EP300*, and *CREBBP*
  - DNA repair pathway (16% of tumors), including alterations in *ATM*, *ERCC2*, and *RAD51B*
- Mutational signature
  - MIBC has high somatic mutation rate, driven mainly by APOBEC-mediated mutagenesis
  - Tumors with profile of high APOBEC-signature mutagenesis, high mutational burden, and predicted high neoantigen load have 75% 5-year survival
- International Consensus Molecular Classification combines expression profiling studies of MIBC to show 6 subtypes with biologic relevance: Luminal-papillary, luminal nonspecified, luminal-unstable, stroma-rich, basal/squamous, and neuroendocrine-like

Gross Appearance

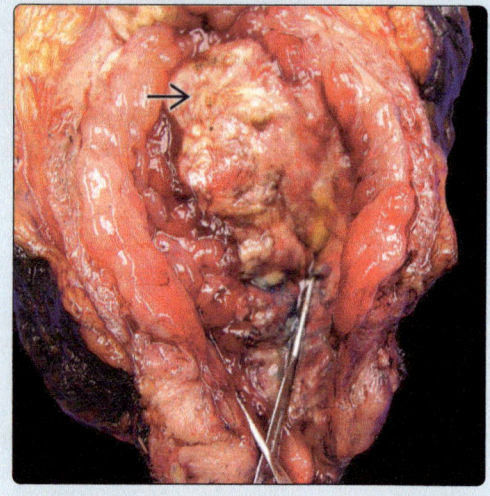

Papillary Urothelial Carcinoma, Low Grade

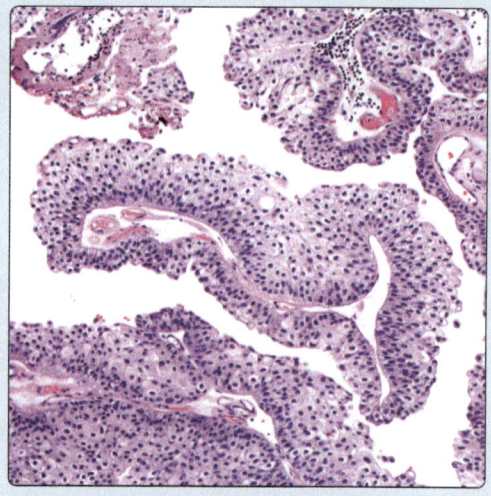

(Left) Opened cystectomy specimen shows urothelial carcinoma presenting as an ulcerated, irregular, exophytic mass ➡. Cystectomy is typically performed for muscle-invasive localized (T2/T3) tumors. *(Right)* Frond-like proliferation composed of fibrovascular cores lined by neoplastic urothelial cells with low-grade cytologic atypia is shown. There is no invasion of subepithelial connective tissue (lamina propria). This is a Ta stage tumor.

Urothelial Carcinoma In Situ

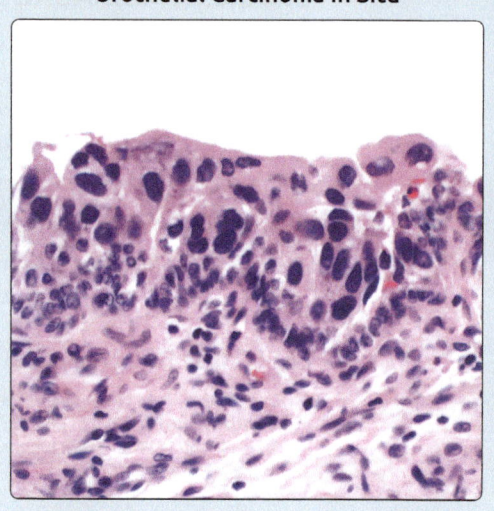

Invasion of Muscularis Propria

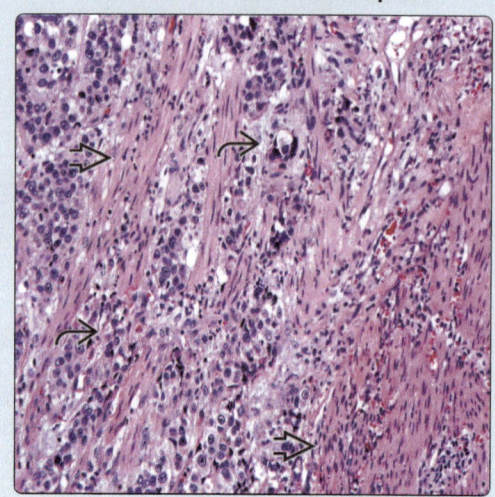

(Left) Urothelial carcinoma in situ shows a flat surface proliferation of neoplastic urothelial cells with high-grade cytologic atypia (enlarged, irregular, hyperchromatic cells). There is no lamina propria invasion. This is a Tis stage tumor. *(Right)* Nests of urothelial carcinoma cells ➡ infiltrating between muscle bundles ➡ of the muscularis propria are shown. Muscle invasion (stage T2) is a key finding for prognosis and therapy.

Urothelial Carcinoma

TERMINOLOGY

Synonyms
- Transitional cell carcinoma

Definitions
- Malignant neoplasm derived from urothelium
  - 2 important clinicopathological phenotypes of urothelial carcinoma
    - Superficial nonmuscle invasive bladder cancer (NMIBC)
    - Muscle invasive bladder cancer (MIBC)

ETIOLOGY/PATHOGENESIS

Environmental Exposure
- Tobacco smoke
  - Carcinogens, such as 4-aminophenol
  - Smokers have 2-5x increased risk
  - Estimated to give rise to 30-50% of bladder cancers
- Occupational carcinogen exposure
  - Especially in rubber and dye industries with exposure to aniline dyes, β-naphthylamine, and benzidine
- Drugs
  - Cyclophosphamide, phenacetin
- Arsenic in drinking water
- Pelvic radiation

Infectious Agents
- Viruses
  - May contribute to development of small percentage of bladder tumors
    - Viral DNA and RNA transcripts described in 4-6% of cases
    - Viruses, including CMV, BK polyomavirus, and HPV-16
- *Schistosoma haematobium*
  - Particularly associated with bladder squamous cell carcinoma

Tumorigenic Pathways
- Papillary pathway
- Flat, carcinoma in situ (CIS) pathway
- Invasive carcinoma can arise from both

Pathogenic Role of APOBEC-Mediated Mutagenesis
- High mutational load is driven mainly by APOBEC-signature mutagenesis
- Major driver of mutagenesis in both NMIBC and MIBC

Hereditary Factors
- In general, not major contributor
- Polymorphisms in *NAT2* and *GSTM1* (carcinogen detoxifying genes) genes may confer some increased risk
- Lynch syndrome associated with increased risk of urothelial cancer of ureter and renal pelvis (upper urinary tract)

CLINICAL ISSUES

Epidemiology
- Incidence
  - 10th most common cancer worldwide
  - 200,000-220,000 deaths worldwide per year
- Age
  - Most diagnosed in 6th decade or older
- Sex
  - 4x more common in men
- Geographic variability
  - Highest incidence in Southern Europe and Egypt
  - Lowest incidence in Far East

Presentation
- Painless gross or microscopic hematuria
- Bladder irritative symptoms including urinary frequency, urgency, dysuria
- Mass or obstructive symptoms

Treatment
- Surgical approaches
  - Transurethral resection
    - Noninvasive papillary tumors (Ta), T1 tumors
  - Cystectomy
    - T2/T3 tumors, sometimes for T1/Ta tumors
- Intravesical therapy
  - Chemotherapy (e.g., mitomycin C)
    - Low- to intermediate-risk Ta papillary tumors
  - Bacillus Calmette-Guérin (BCG) therapy
    - Intermediate- to high-risk Ta tumors, T1 tumors, CIS
- Systemic chemotherapy
  - Cisplatin-based protocols
    - Metastatic disease
    - Neoadjuvant therapy prior to cystectomy
- Immunotherapy with immune checkpoint inhibitors
  - Metastatic disease; possibly also in neoadjuvant setting

Prognosis
- MIBC
  - Overall 5-year cancer-specific survival rate: < 50%
  - Stage is most important prognostic factor
    - Prognosis worsens with increase in stage
    - 5-year survival with tumor spread to regional lymph nodes: ~ 34%
    - 5-year survival with distant metastasis: ~ 6%
  - Certain histological subtypes have poorer outcome, including small cell, micropapillary, and sarcomatoid
  - Grade is not as important prognostic factor after muscle invasion has occurred
- NMIBC
  - 5-year survival: ~ 90%
  - Risk of recurrence: Up to 75%; progression: ~ 10-15%
  - Risk increases with tumor size, number of tumors, grade, prior recurrence, presence of lamina propria invasion, and additional presence of CIS

MOLECULAR

Cytogenetics
- NMIBC
  - Chromosome 9 deletion in > 50%
    - Appears to be early event in carcinogenesis
  - Gains of 3q, 7p, and 17q can be seen
    - Testing (UroVysion) for these may provide diagnostic and prognostic information
  - Other early events include 9q, 9p, 11p deletions

Urothelial Carcinoma

- Other later events include 8p, 17p, 11q deletions and gain of 20q
- Few genomic rearrangements and near diploid karyotype compared to MIBC
- MIBC
  - Frequently aneuploid with multiple alterations

Molecular Genetics

- **NMIBC**
  - *FGFR3*-activating point mutations
    - Up to 80% of Ta tumors, 10-30% of T1 tumors
  - *HRAS* or *KRAS*
    - 10-15% of NMIBC
    - Mutually exclusive with *FGFR3* mutations
  - *PIK3CA*-inactivating point mutations
    - 40-50% of Ta tumors, 6-20% of T1 tumors
    - Frequently co-occur with *FGFR3*, *HRAS*, or *KRAS* mutations
  - *TERT* promoter mutations
    - Most common alteration in urothelial carcinoma, seen across grades, stages, and subtypes
    - 70-80% of Ta/T1 tumors, 65% of CIS
    - Early event in tumorigenesis
    - Not seen in benign entities
    - Seen in majority of tumors with *FGFR3* mutations
    - Can be detected in urine samples
  - *CCND1* amplification
    - Detected in ~ 20%
  - *STAG2*-inactivating mutations
    - Ta tumors: 32-36%; T1 tumors: 18-27%
  - Chromatin modifier genes
    - Majority of tumors have inactivating (indel, nonsense, splice site) mutations in at least one of these genes
      - *KDM6A, KMT2A, KMT2C, KMT2D, ARID1A, EP300, CREBBP*
  - DNA damage repair genes
    - Seen more commonly in high-grade Ta and T1 tumors
    - *ERCC2, ATR, ATM, FANCA, BRCA1, BRCA2, POLE*
  - Other mutated genes: *TSC1, RHOB*
- **MIBC**
  - The Cancer Genome Atlas (TCGA) 2017 project has shown deregulation of several pathways
    - TP53/cell cycle pathway in 89%
    - RTK/RAS/PI(3)K pathway in 71%
    - Chromatin modification pathways: Histone modifiers (52%), SWI/SNF complex (26%)
    - DNA repair pathway (16%)
  - High level of genomic amplifications and deletions
    - 34 significantly amplified and 32 significantly deleted recurrent focal somatic copy number alterations (CNAs) in TCGA study
    - *CDKN2A* deletion in 22%
    - Other likely targeted deleted genes include *RB1, KDM6A, CREBBP, ARID1A, RAD51B, PTEN, PTPRB, NCOR1,* and *CDKN2B*
    - Amplified genes include *AHR, EGFR, GATA3, CCND1, PPARG, MDM2, E2F3, SOX4, ERBB2, YWHAZ, MYC, CCNE1, FGFR3, MYCL, ZNF703, BCL2L1, KRAS,* and *TERT*
  - Gene fusions include
    - *FGFR3::TACC3, TSEN2::PPARG,* and *MKRN2::PPARG*
  - Mutation signatures
    - MIBC has high somatic mutation rate, driven mainly by APOBEC-mediated mutagenesis
    - Tumors with profile of high APOBEC-signature mutagenesis, high mutational burden, and predicted high neoantigen load have 75% 5-year survival
    - > 50% of APOBEC-signature mutations are clonal, suggesting that they are generated early in tumorigenesis
    - Mutations include
      - *TP53* (48%), *KMT2D* (28%), *KDM6A* (26%), *ARID1A* (25%), *PIK3CA* (22%), *KMT2C* (18%), *RB1* (17%), *EP300* (15%), *STAG2* (14%), *FGFR3* (14%), *ATM* (14%), *CREBBP* (12%), *ELF3* (12%), *FAT1* (12%), *SPTAN1* (12%), *ERBB2* (12%), *KMT2A* (11%), and *ERBB3* (10%)
      - *TERT* promoter mutations most common alteration in urothelial carcinoma (70-80%)
  - Mutually exclusive mutations include
    - *CDKN2A* and *TP53*; *CDKN2A* and *RB1*; *TP53* and *MDM2*; *FGFR3* and *TP53*
  - Co-occurring mutations include
    - *TP53* and *RB1*; *TP53* and *E2F3*; *FGFR3* and *CDKN2A*; *FGFR3* and *STAG2*
- Alterations associated with histological subtypes
  - Plasmacytoid subtype
    - Somatic *CDH1*-truncating mutations (84%) or promoter hypermethylation: Loss of E-cadherin expression
    - *CDH1* germline alterations not described
  - Micropapillary subtype
    - *ERBB2* amplification
  - Small cell/neuroendocrine carcinoma subtype
    - Loss of function of *TP53* (90%) and *RB1* (87%)
  - Nested subtype
    - High rates of *TERT* promoter mutations; may have mutations in *TP53, JAK3,* and *CTNNB1*
    - Large nested subtype: Large majority have *FGFR3* alterations
  - Sarcomatoid subtype
    - Enriched in *TP53, RB1,* and *PIK3CA* mutations
    - Expression features of basal molecular group
  - Squamous differentiation
    - Clusters with basal/squamous molecular group
  - Glandular differentiation
    - High rates of *TERT* promoter and chromatin remodeling gene alterations, similar to usual urothelial carcinoma
- Potentially predictive alterations
  - Alterations in *ERCC2* and other DNA damage repair genes may predict better response to cisplatin-based regimens, immune checkpoint inhibitors, and radiation therapy
  - Tumors with *FGFR3* alterations may respond to anti-FGFR agents
  - Tumor mutation burden, mismatch repair deficiency, and PD-L1 expression in tumor/immune cells help predict response to immune checkpoint inhibitor therapy

Urothelial Carcinoma

Gene Expression Profiling

- Classification of MIBC based on mRNA expression clustering
  - May have predictive/prognostic and therapeutic implications
- International Consensus Molecular Classification (Kamoun 2020): 6 consensus molecular classes
  - Effort by Bladder Cancer Molecular Taxonomy Group to unify multiple existing classifications
  - Resulted in 6 consensus molecular classes, showing differences in oncogenic mechanism, histology, tumor microenvironment, and prognosis (worse survival: Neuroendocrine-like, basal/squamous, luminal unstable)
- Luminal-papillary (24% of cases)
  - Enriched in papillary histology (59%); younger patients, lower stage, better prognosis
  - Enriched in *FGFR3* (55%) and *KDM6A* (38%) alterations, and *CDKN2A* deletions (33%)
- Luminal nonspecified (8%)
  - Enriched in micropapillary subtype (36%); commonly associated with CIS, older patients
  - Associated with fibroblastic, and B- and T-cell signatures
- Luminal-unstable (15%)
  - Higher cell cycle activity, most genomic alterations (highest somatic mutation load, most CNAs)
  - Associated with *PPARG* alterations (89%), *TP53* (76%) and *ERCC2* (22%) mutations, amplifications of 6p22.3 region (76%) and *ERBB2* (22%)
- Stroma-rich (15%)
  - Characterized by stromal (smooth muscle, endothelial, fibroblastic, and myofibroblastic) and immune (B- and T-cell) signatures
- Basal/squamous (35%)
  - Enriched in *TP53* (58%) and *RB1* (20%) mutations (coexist in 14%), genomic deletion at 13p14.2 (49%)
  - Associated with CD8 T- and NK-cell signatures
  - Enriched in squamous histology (42%), more common in women, higher stage, poorer prognosis
- Neuroendocrine-like (3%)
  - *TP53* and *RB1* in 90%
  - Neuroendocrine histology in 72%
  - Poor prognosis

MICROSCOPIC

Histologic Features

- Papillary lesions
  - Papilloma and papillary urothelial neoplasm of low malignant potential (PUNLMP)
    - Hyperplastic and neoplastic urothelium thrown into papillary structures with central thin, fibrovascular core
    - Urothelium appears normal and hyperplastic, respectively
  - Low-grade urothelial carcinoma
    - Low-grade cytologic atypia; branching and fusion of papillae
  - High-grade urothelial carcinoma
    - High-grade cytologic atypia, more branching and fusion of papillae, may have associated invasion
- Flat lesions
  - CIS
    - Noninvasive, usually multifocal
    - Disordered, mitotically active, cytologically high grade
    - Subepithelial proliferation of small capillaries common
- Invasive carcinoma
  - Tumor invades through basement membrane into lamina propria (T1) or muscularis propria (T2)
  - Most are high grade, and most arise from dysplasia or CIS, or from high-grade papillary tumors
  - Histological subtypes include nested, micropapillary, plasmacytoid, small cell, and sarcomatoid
  - Aberrant differentiation, including squamous, glandular, trophoblastic, and müllerian, can occur

ANCILLARY TESTS

Immunohistochemistry

- CIS (flat)
  - Full-thickness staining for CK20; p53 nuclear staining
- Urothelial carcinoma
  - Frequently positive for CK7 and CK20
  - Positive for high-molecular-weight cytokeratins, p63, and GATA3
  - PD-L1 expression in tumor and immune cells helps predict response to immune checkpoint inhibitor therapy

In Situ Hybridization

- UroVysion
  - Interphase FISH-based assay testing for aneuploidy of chromosomes 3, 7, and 17, and for loss of 9q21 in urothelial cells in urine
  - FDA approved for surveillance of recurrence in patients with previously diagnosed urothelial carcinoma
  - Also approved for screening of high-risk patients (smokers) with hematuria
  - Improves sensitivity of urine cytology for detection of urothelial carcinoma
  - Reported sensitivity: 69-87%; specificity: 89-96%
  - May provide prognostic information for NMIBC recurrence
  - When performed after BCG therapy, may provide predictive information for therapy failure

DIFFERENTIAL DIAGNOSIS

Papillary/Polypoid Cystitis

- Commonly associated with indwelling catheters
- No significant cytologic atypia

Pseudocarcinomatous Hyperplasia

- Benign reactive epithelial proliferation
- Usually in setting of prior radiation or chemotherapy

SELECTED REFERENCES

1. WHO Classification of Tumours Editorial Board: Urinary and male genital tumours. IARC, 2022
2. Kamoun A et al: A consensus molecular classification of muscle-invasive bladder cancer. Eur Urol. 77(4):420-33, 2020
3. Robertson AG et al: Comprehensive molecular characterization of muscle-invasive bladder cancer. Cell. 171(3):540-56.e25, 2017

Urothelial Carcinoma

(Left) Flat carcinoma in situ shows a disordered proliferation of large, high-grade urothelial cells. Mitoses ⇒ and capillary neovascularization ⇒ are present. **(Right)** p53 shows full-thickness staining of carcinoma in situ. This may be a useful adjunct to morphological assessment; in contrast to what is found in carcinoma in situ, nuclear p53 staining is absent or only focal in normal urothelium.

Urothelial Carcinoma In Situ

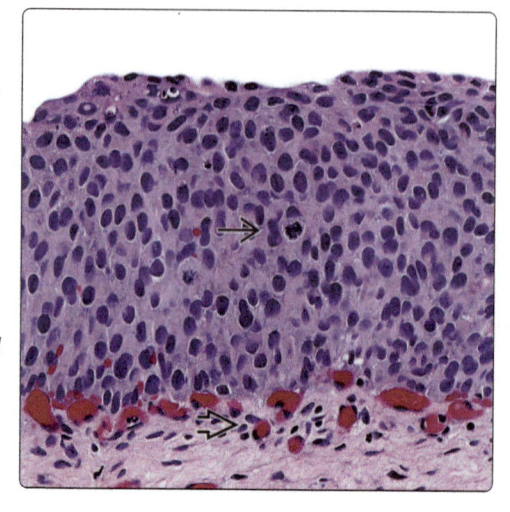

Carcinoma In Situ: p53

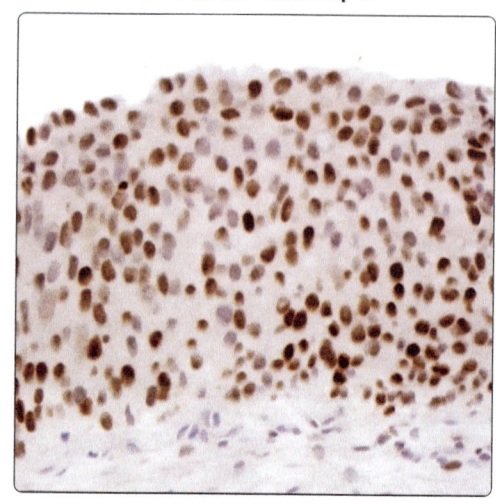

(Left) CK20 shows diffuse, full-thickness cytoplasmic staining of carcinoma in situ. Normal urothelium typically shows staining of the surface umbrella cell layer only. **(Right)** Low-grade papillary urothelial carcinoma shows a papillary proliferation of urothelial cells on fine fibrovascular cores ⇒. There is some fusion ⇒ of papillae, but cellular polarization and maturation is orderly, and high-grade cytology is not seen.

Carcinoma In Situ: CK20

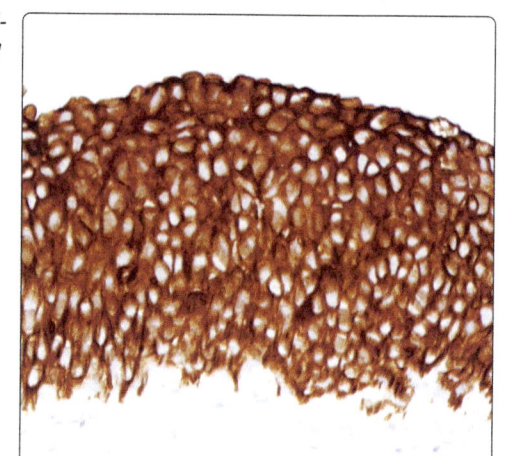

Low-Grade Papillary Urothelial Carcinoma

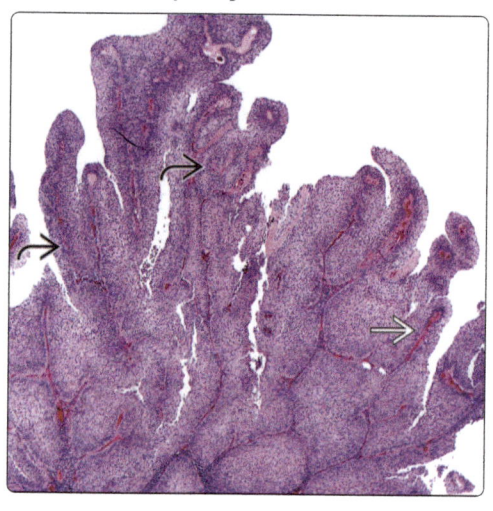

(Left) High-power view shows low-grade papillary urothelial carcinoma with relative preservation of polarization. While there may be occasional hyperchromatic nuclei, the overall cytology of the urothelial cells is low grade. **(Right)** High-grade papillary urothelial carcinoma shows focal visible fibrovascular cores ⇒, but the papillae are ill-formed, fused, or anastomosed, and the urothelium appears disordered with markedly atypical cells.

Preservation of Cell Polarization

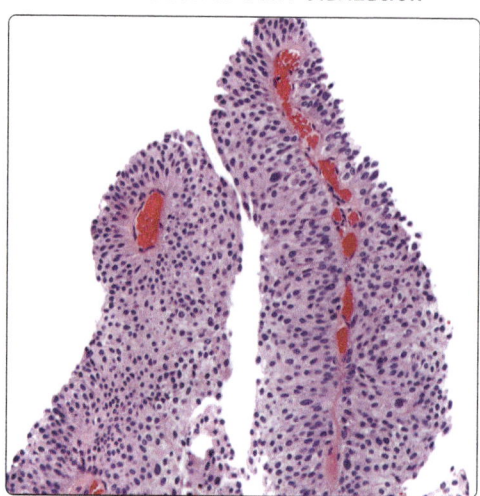

High-Grade Papillary Urothelial Carcinoma

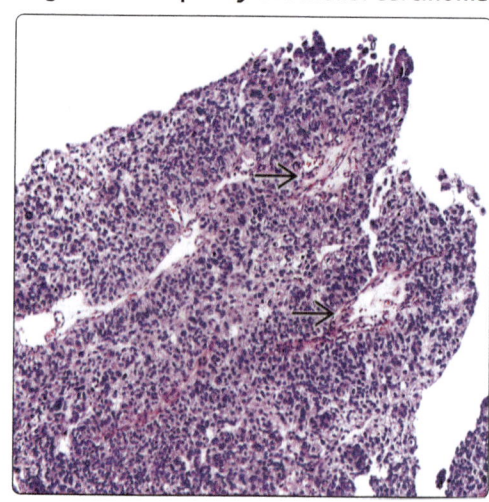

Urothelial Carcinoma

Atypia and Loss of Polarization

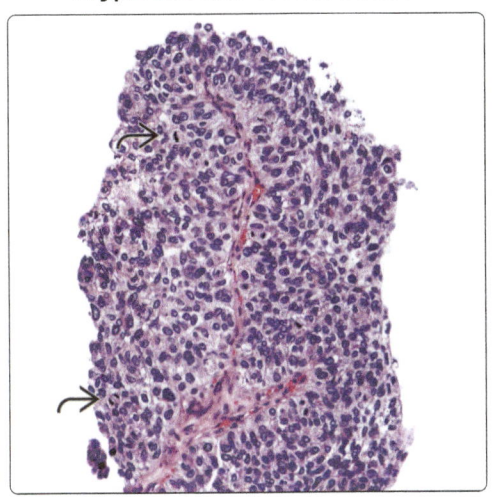

Invasion of Lamina Propria

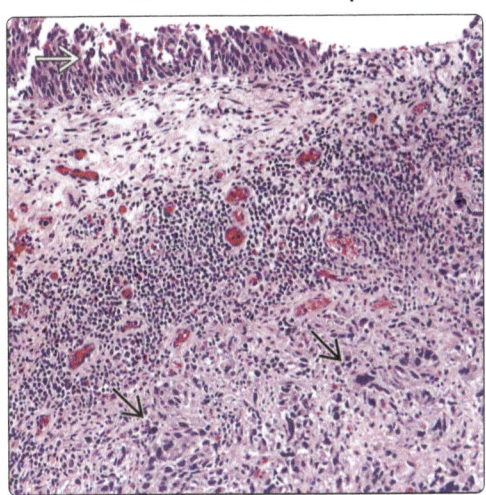

(Left) *High-grade papillary urothelial carcinoma is shown. The papillary urothelium is disordered, and normal polarization is lost. There is high-grade cytologic atypia, and multiple mitotic figures ⇨ are present.* (Right) *Urothelial carcinoma with invasion of lamina propria ⇨ is shown. Normal surface urothelium ⇨ is present. This tumor shows high-grade cytology and is infiltrating as small nests and sheets.*

Squamous Differentiation

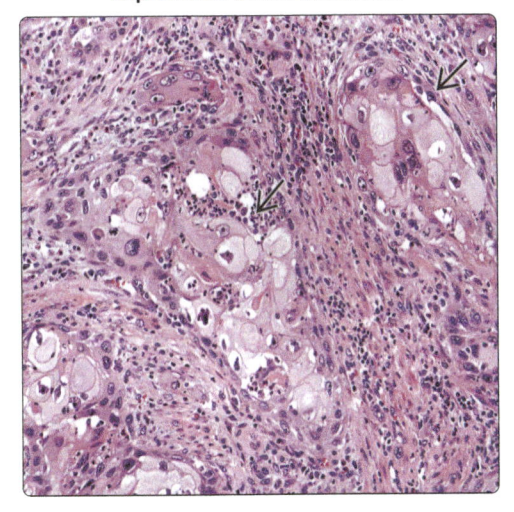

Normal Urothelial Cell

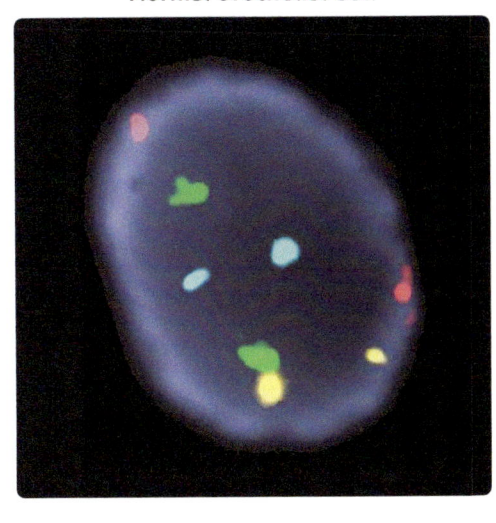

(Left) *Invasive urothelial carcinoma with aberrant squamous differentiation ⇨ is shown. Urothelial carcinoma can be phenotypically quite plastic, and aberrant differentiation is not uncommon.* (Right) *Normal urothelial cell from urine tested by FISH using UroVysion Vysis probe sets for chromosomes 3q (red), 7p (green), 17q (aqua), and 9p21 region (gold) is shown. There are 2 intact signals visible for each of the probes.*

Deletion of 9p21 Region

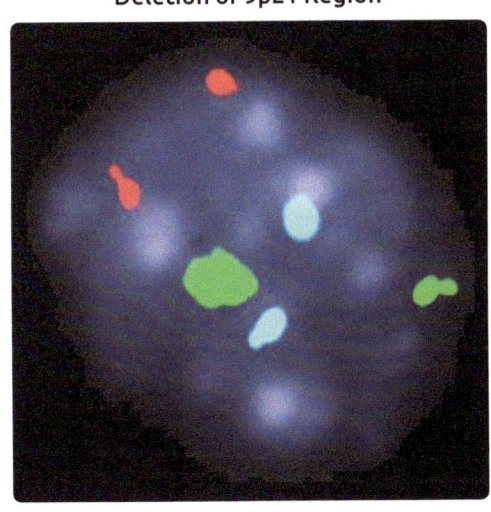

Chromosomal Aneuploidy

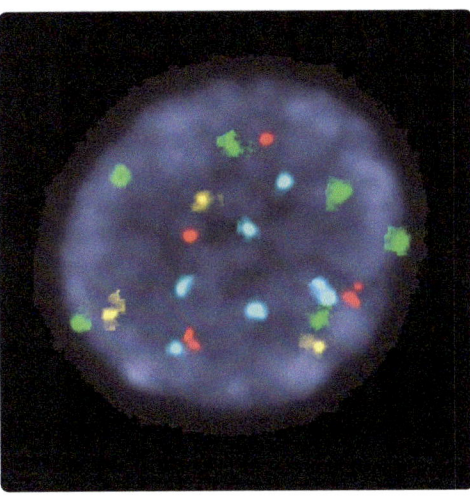

(Left) *Urothelial cell shows homozygous deletion for the 9p21 chromosomal region (loss of both of the gold signals), consistent with positive UroVysion test. Note that 2 normal signals are present for the probes for chromosomal regions 3q, 7p, and 17q.* (Right) *Urothelial cell shows abnormal numbers for each probe set (> 2 green, red, aqua, and gold signals), indicating chromosomal aneuploidy. This constitutes a positive result for this test.*

659

Pheochromocytoma/Paraganglioma

KEY FACTS

CLINICAL ISSUES
- Identification of patients with hereditary pheochromocytoma involves clinical assessment, biochemical testing, and pathology leading to directed genetic testing

MOLECULAR
- Majority of pheochromocytomas appear to arise sporadically
  - Many sporadic tumors have no known somatic driver mutation
  - *NF1* inactivation somatic mutation is most common mutation, found in > 25% of sporadic cases
  - Up to 1/3 of sporadic cases have no known genetic driver mutation
- > 40% of PPGL hereditary; at least 10 known susceptibility genes
  - *RET, VHL, NF1, SDHA, SDHB, SDHC, SDHD, SDHAF2, KIF1B, TMEM127,* and *MAX*
- *SDHB* mutation associated with extraabdominal location, high probability of metastasis, and poor prognosis

MICROSCOPIC
- Classic pattern is small nests (zellballen) of neuroendocrine cells with interspersed small blood vessels
- Numerous variant and combined patterns exist, including diffuse growth, large zellballen, spindle cells, cell cords
- Sustentacular cells variably present, best seen with IHC

ANCILLARY TESTS
- IHC for SDHB and SDHA can triage patients for appropriate genetic testing
- Positive for TYH, DBH, GATA3, INSM1, chromogranin A, and synaptophysin
- Sustentacular cells stain for S100 and SOX10

Gross Appearance

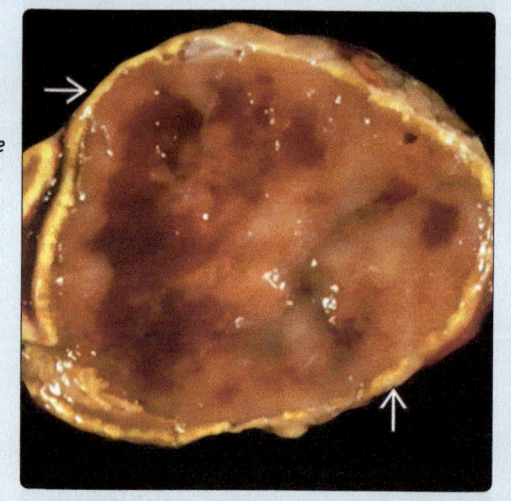

Radiologic Appearance

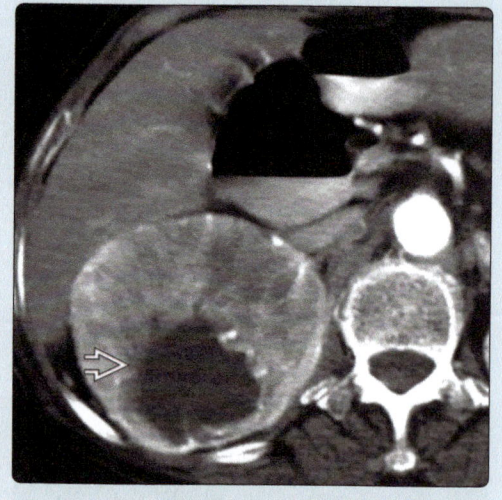

(Left) *Typical gross appearance of a pheochromocytoma (PCC) shows a gray-pink cut surface with areas of hemorrhage, which distinguishes it from the yellow-brown of adrenal cortex ➡.* (Right) *Axial CECT shows a large, well-circumscribed, moderately enhancing right adrenal PCC with a hypodense area of necrosis ➡.*

Thin Fibrovascular Septa

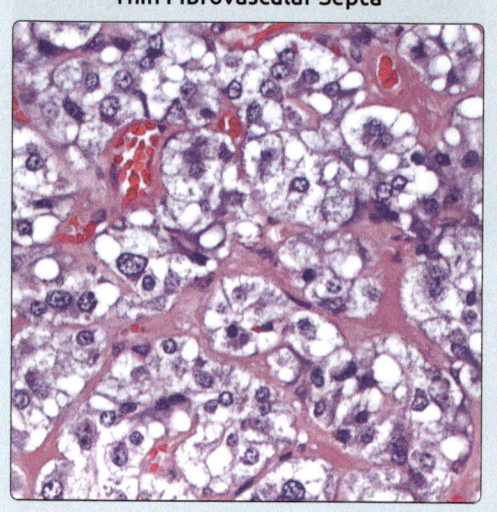

Hyaline Globules

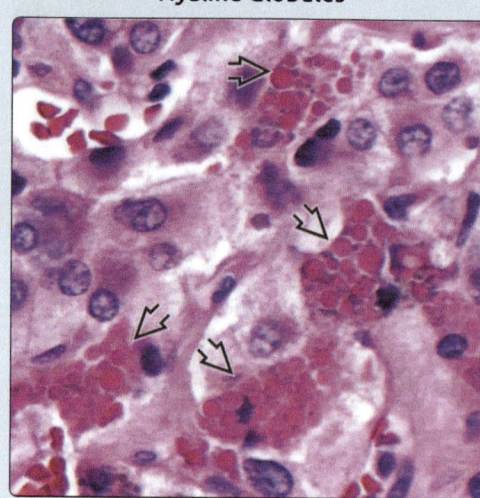

(Left) *The usual pattern of PCC is small groups of cells surrounded by thin fibrovascular septa (zellballen). The cells have abundant eosinophilic or amphophilic cytoplasm.* (Right) *PCC in patients with multiple endocrine neoplasia type 2 (MEN2) syndrome may have numerous hyaline globules ➡ that are particularly conspicuous.*

Pheochromocytoma/Paraganglioma

TERMINOLOGY

Abbreviations
- Pheochromocytoma (PCC)
- Paraganglioma (PGL)
- Pheochromocytoma/paraganglioma (PPGL)

Synonyms
- Intraadrenal PGL
- Adrenal sympathetic PGL

Definitions
- PCC: Neuroendocrine neoplasm derived from neural crest cells that arises from adrenal medulla chromaffin cells
- PGL: Neuroendocrine neoplasm derived from neural crest progenitor cells that arises from extraadrenal sympathetic or parasympathetic paraganglia
  - Sympathetic (sympathoadrenal) PGL arises in vicinity of sympathetic chains and along sympathetic nerve branches in pelvic organs and retroperitoneum
  - Parasympathetic PGL [head and neck PGL (HNP)] arises mainly from branches of vagus and glossopharyngeal nerves in head and neck, sometimes mediastinum
  - PCC is intraadrenal sympathetic PGL

ETIOLOGY/PATHOGENESIS

Developmental Anomaly
- Normal paraganglia, from which PPGL arise, consist of neural crest-derived neuroendocrine cells associated with sympathetic and parasympathetic nerves
  - Adrenal medulla and organ of Zuckerkandl are major sympathetic paraganglia; others are microscopic
  - Carotid bodies are major parasympathetic paraganglia; others are microscopic

Environmental Influences
- High-altitude PGL in people living in some mountainous areas
  - Mostly carotid PGL

Hereditary Influences
- > 40% of adults and up to 80% of children with PPGL have hereditary susceptibility gene germline mutation
- Highest inheritable proportion of any known human tumor
  - At least 18 known susceptibility genes, including
    - *RET*, *SDHA*, *SDHB*, *SDHC*, *SDHD*, *SDHAF2*, *NF1*, *VHL*, and *TMEM127*
  - Hereditary PPGL often found after other stigmata point to hereditary tumor syndrome (usually MEN2, VHL, NF1)
  - Variants of some hereditary syndromes can cause only PPGL (VHL type 2C)
  - Mutations of some genes (e.g., *TMEM127*) cause hereditary but nonsyndromic PPGL
  - Multiple tumors or tumors presenting in children suggest hereditary disease
  - Tumors with *RET* or *NF1* mutations almost always intraadrenal
  - *SDHD*- and *SDHAF2*-related PGL show parent of origin-dependent expression
    - Tumor development only with paternal inheritance

CLINICAL ISSUES

Epidemiology
- Incidence is ~ 0.6 cases per 100,000 person-years
- Age at diagnosis: 50-60 years in most cases; ~ 20% occur in children

Site
- ~ 98% of sympathetic PGL located in abdomen or pelvis; 90% are intraadrenal (PCC)
- Most parasympathetic PGL are carotid, jugulotympanic, or vagal

Presentation
- < 25% present with classic triad of headache, palpitations, and diaphoresis
- Many are discovered incidentally on imaging for other work-up or surveillance of germline mutation positive patients
- Sympathoadrenal PPGLs may show signs and symptoms of catecholamine excess
  - Tumors with *SDHB* mutation are more likely than other sympathoadrenal PPGL to be clinically silent
- Parasympathetic PGL are usually clinically silent mass lesions
- Sporadic tumors typically solitary, usually in adults

Laboratory Tests
- Plasma metanephrine, normetanephrine, and 3-methoxytyramine more sensitive than corresponding catecholamines for tumor detection
- Succinatemutaion analysis
- PCC can be adrenergic or noradrenergic; extraadrenal PGL is almost always noradrenergic; HNP can lack ability for catecholamine biosynthesis
- Genotype affects biochemical function
  - Noradrenergic PCC raises suspicion of von Hippel-Lindau (VHL) syndrome

Treatment
- Complete surgical excision with adrenergic blockade
- Metastatic disease treatment includes surgery, ablation, chemotherapy, and radionuclide therapy
- Molecular targeted therapy undergoing clinical trials
  - Tyrosine kinase inhibitors
  - HIFA2 inhibitors
  - Checkpoint inhibitor immunotherapy

Prognosis
- Overall survival for patients with PPGL is 63% at 5 years
- Most patients with metastases die from complications of excess catecholamines or destructive local growth

Malignancy
- WHO 2017 states that all PPGL should be considered malignant
- Metastatic disease
  - Risk of metastasis and prognosis vary with tumor location and genotype
    - ~ 10% metastasis for PCC; > 20% for PGL
    - Best predictor of metastasis is presence of *SDHB* mutation (43%)

Pheochromocytoma/Paraganglioma

- Metastatic tumors with *SDHB* mutation have worst prognosis
  - Must be to sites where normal paraganglia are not present to avoid confusion with new primary tumor
  - Currently, no established histologic criteria to predict whether primary PPGL will metastasize
    - Most accepted adverse histologic findings include high proliferative rate, comedonecrosis and diffuse growth pattern
  - Metastases can develop years or decades after resection of primary tumor
- All patients must receive lifelong follow-up

MACROSCOPIC

General Features

- Circumscribed, unencapsulated; ~ 3-5 cm, can be > 10 cm
- Cut surface usually pink-gray to tan
  - Distinguishes PCC from yellow-gold color of most adrenal cortical tumors
- Cystic degeneration and necrosis sometimes present
- Sample for micronodules in uninvolved adrenal tissue
  - May represent synchronous microPCC associated with hereditary disease

MOLECULAR

Sporadic PPGL

- Majority of PCC appear to arise sporadically
- Up to 1/3 of sporadic cases have no known genetic driver mutation
- *NF1* inactivation mutation is most common somatic mutation seen in > 25% of sporadic tumors
- Germline mutations in known susceptibility genes may be seen in up to 16% of sporadic-appearing cases
  - Changes in copy number of hereditary susceptibility genes may be present

Hereditary PPGL

- Identification of multiple susceptibility genes demonstrated extensive tumor genetic heterogeneity
- Most striking feature is genetic diversity
  - ≥ 10 susceptibility genes now established
- Most attributable to mutations in *RET, VHL, NF1, SDHA, SDHB, SDHC, SDHD, SDHAF2, KIF1B, TMEM127,* and *MAX*
  - Occult germline mutations of susceptibility genes common in patients with apparently sporadic tumors
- Mutations in SDH family of genes account for up to 80% of familial PPGL aggregations
  - ~ 30% of pediatric tumors
  - > 40% of malignant tumors
- Multiple endocrine neoplasia type 2 (MEN2)
  - Autosomal dominant syndrome caused by mutation in *RET* protooncogene
  - Activating *RET* mutations predispose to PCC
    - Often recurrent and bilateral in 50-80% of cases
- Familial PPGL syndromes
  - PGL syndromes encompass group of inherited syndromes that involve mutations in genes that encode components of succinate dehydrogenase (SDH) mitochondrial enzyme complex 2
    - SDH is composed of 4 subunits: A, B, C, and D
  - Germline mutations in SDH family of genes give rise to familial PPGL syndrome, sometimes only referred to as familial PGL
    - PGL1, PGL2, PGL3, and PGL4 caused by mutations in *SDHD, SDHAF2, SDHC,* and *SDHB*, respectively
    - Head and neck PGL common
    - *SDHA*-related PGL rare and caused by loss-of-function mutation in *SDHA*
- Carney triad
  - Mean age of presentation of PPGL is 28 years
    - Only 16% present with PCC
- VHL syndrome
  - Autosomal dominant, caused by mutation of *VHL*
  - ~ 10-26% of VHL patients develop PPGL, but risk varies between different families
  - Mean age of onset of PCC in VHL is ~ 30 years
- Neurofibromatosis type 1 (NF1)
  - Autosomal dominant, caused by *NF1* mutation
  - PCC occur in 20-50% of individuals with NF1 and hypertension
  - NF1-associated PPGL typically has characteristics similar to those of sporadic tumors with relatively late mean age of onset and ~ 10% risk of malignancy
  - Gangliocytic duodenal PGL may also occur
  - ~ 84% of PCC are unilateral
- Carney-Stratakis dyad
  - Inherited predisposition to gastrointestinal stromal tumor (GIST) and PGL caused by inactivating germline mutations in *SDHB, SDHC,* or *SDHD*
  - Only rare cases reported to be associated with PCC
- Recently identified hereditary forms of PPGL involve transmembrane-encoding gene, *TMEM127*, and *MAX*
  - No specific syndrome has been described for *TMEM127*
  - *MAX* mutations occur in families with PCC, but no specific syndrome has been described yet

Gene Expression Profiling

- The Cancer Genome Atlas has classified PPGL into 3 molecular clusters
- Cluster I: Mutations disrupt hypoxia-signaling pathways
  - Krebs cycle/VHL/EPAS1-related
  - Genes include *VHL*, SDHx, and *FH*
- Cluster II: Mutations disrupt kinase-signaling pathways
  - Genes include *RET, NF1, TMEM127,* and *MAX*
- Cluster III: Mutations affect WNT-signaling pathway
  - *MAML3* oncogene fusions and *CSDE1* mutations in sporadic adult PCC

MICROSCOPIC

Histologic Features

- Wide architectural and cytologic variation
- Classic pattern is small nests (zellballen) of neuroendocrine cells (chief cells) with interspersed small blood vessels
- Numerous variant and combined patterns exist, including diffuse growth, large zellballen, spindle cells, cell cords
- Sustentacular cells variably present, best seen with IHC
  - Possibly nonneoplastic cell type induced or attracted by tumor-derived factors
- Cavernous blood vessels sometimes prominent, especially in HNP

Pheochromocytoma/Paraganglioma

Tumor Distributions in Major Familial Paraganglioma Syndromes

Syndrome	Gene	Adrenal	Other Sympathetic	Head & Neck	Other Tumors
MEN2A and MEN2B	RET	+++	+/-	+/-	**Medullary thyroid carcinoma**, parathyroid adenoma (MEN2A only)
VHL	VHL	+++	++	+/-	**RCC, hemangioblastoma**, endolymphatic sac tumor, neuroendocrine tumor (carcinoid), pancreatic endocrine tumor
NF1	NF1	+++	+/-	+/-	**Neurofibroma**, GIST, neuroendocrine tumor (carcinoid)
PGL1	SDHD	++	++	++	
PGL2	SDHAF2		+/-		
PGL3	SDHC	+/-	+/-	+++	GIST
PGL4	SDHB	++	+++	+	RCC, GIST
SDHA-related	SDHA		+		GIST
Carney-Stratakis dyad	SDHB, SDHC, or SDHD	++	+	+	GIST
Familial pheochromocytoma	TMEM127	+	+/-	+/-	
MAX related	MAX	+			

GIST = gastrointestinal stromal tumor; MEN2 = multiple endocrine neoplasia type 2; VHL = von Hippel-Lindau; RCC = renal cell carcinoma.

Cytologic Features

- Tumor cells resemble normal chromaffin cells, vesicular nuclei, inconspicuous or large nucleoli
- Nuclear pseudoinclusions, embracing cells, extracellular hyaline globules variably present
- Basophilic, amphophilic, or clear cytoplasm

ANCILLARY TESTS

Immunohistochemistry

- Positive for TYH, DBH, GATA3, INSM1, chromogranin A and synaptophysin
  - TYH expression correlates with catecholamine synthesis; can be negative, especially in parasympathetic PGL
    - Elevated metanephrine after resection of TYH(-) PGL suggests 2nd primary, not metastasis
- Sustentacular cells positive for S100 and SOX10
- Ki-67 proliferative index essential reporting criteria
  - Established risk factor for development of metastases
  - Reported as % positive tumor cells in 10 HPF within hotspot area
- Molecular markers for germline mutation screening
  - SDHB, SDHA for SDHx mutations
    - SDHB protein lost in PPGL with SDHA, SDHB, SDHC, or SDHD mutations
    - SDHA protein lost only when SDHA is mutated
  - FH for fumarate hydratase mutations

Genetic Testing

- Germline testing with genetics consultation in appropriate clinical context

DIFFERENTIAL DIAGNOSIS

Adrenal Cortical Carcinoma

- Positive for Melan A, SF1
- Negative for chromogranin, TYH, GATA3
- Synaptophysin and inhibin positive in both cortical and medullary tumors; do not use in this differential diagnosis

Other Neuroendocrine Tumors

- Neuroendocrine carcinomas and carcinoids, pancreatic endocrine tumors, medullary thyroid carcinoma
- Keratins are usually positive

Hepatocellular Carcinomas

- Absence of neuroendocrine markers, presence of keratins &/or tissue-specific markers

Renal Cell Carcinoma

- Absence of neuroendocrine markers, presence of keratins &/or CD10, RCC, and other tissue-specific markers

Alveolar Soft Part Sarcomas

- Absence of neuroendocrine markers, presence of soft tissue-specific marker TFE3

Glomus Tumors and Glomangiomas

- Location: Outside adrenal
- Presence of neuroendocrine markers, S100, GFAP

SELECTED REFERENCES

1. de Krijger RR et al: Phaeochromocytoma; sympathetic paraganglioma; parasympathetic paraganglioma. In: WHO Classification of Tumours Editorial Board. Endocrine and neuroendocrine tumours. IARC, 2022
2. Neumann HPH et al: Pheochromocytoma and paraganglioma. N Engl J Med. 381(6):552-65, 2019

Pheochromocytoma/Paraganglioma

Zellballen Arrangement

Cellular Atypia

(Left) The classic histologic pattern of PCC is a small zellballen cellular arrangement. The groups of cells are surrounded by thin, fibrovascular cores. The cells have eosinophilic and pale cytoplasm. (Right) The growth of this PCC is patternless with thin, fibrous septa but lacking the zellballen cellular arrangement. There is marked variability in cell size, with scattered pleomorphic cells surrounded by tumor cells with clear cytoplasm.

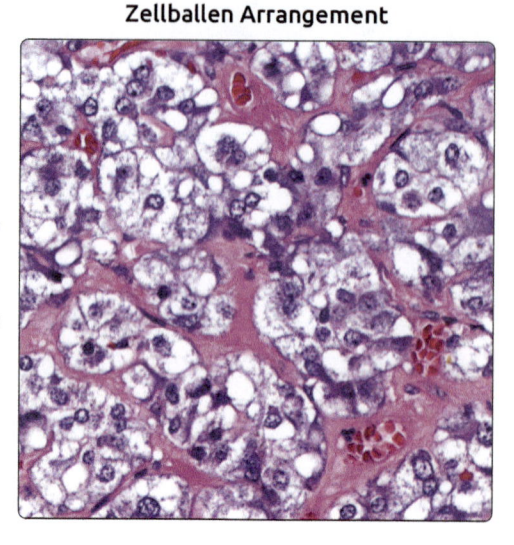

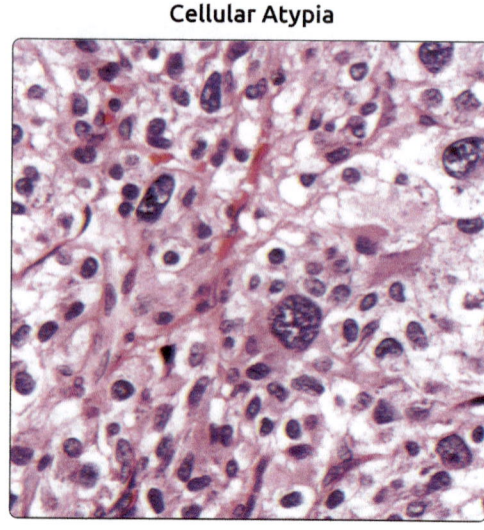

Hyaline Globules

Cytoplasmic Variation

(Left) Hyaline globules ⇨ are present in some PCC/paragangliomas (PGL) but also may be seen in some adrenal cortical neoplasms. They tend to be particularly conspicuous in PCC of patients with MEN2. (Right) PCC may contain cells with ample basophilic, amphophilic, or clear cytoplasm. Here, the characteristic basophilic granular cytoplasm of these tumors is shown.

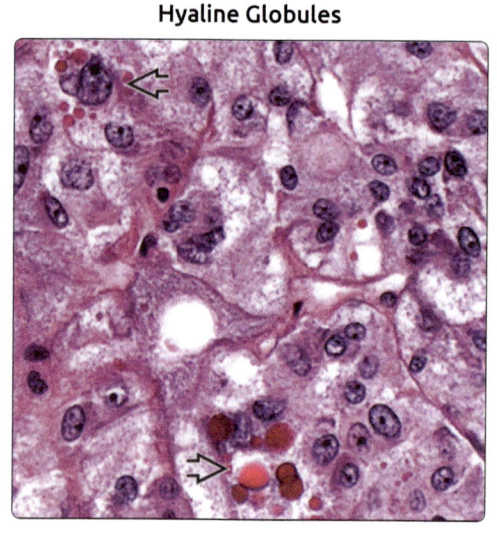

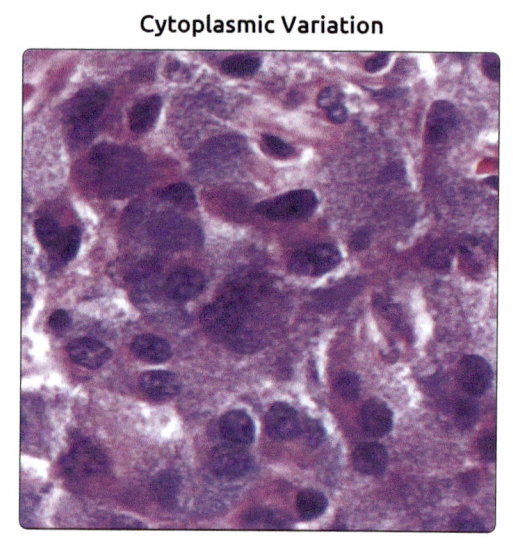

Mitotic Activity

Architectural Variation

(Left) A mitotic figure ⇨ is present in this malignant PCC with a diffuse pattern, lacking the classic zellballen pattern. This tumor is composed of compact eosinophilic cells, which may be associated with more aggressive behavior. (Right) Although the classic histologic pattern of PCC is a zellballen pattern, numerous variants and combined patterns exist, including diffuse growth, large zellballen, spindle cells, and cell cords. Mitotic figure ⇨ is shown.

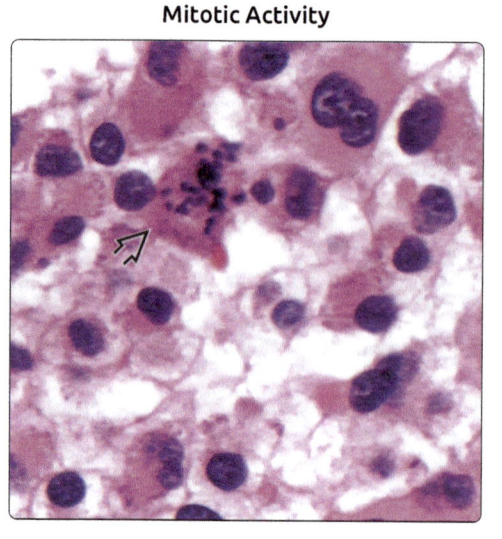

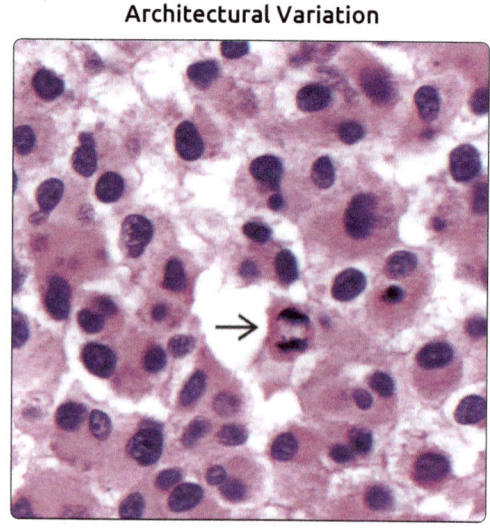

Pheochromocytoma/Paraganglioma

Chromogranin-A

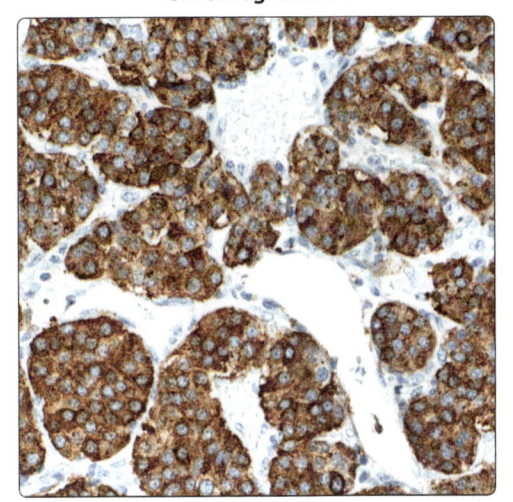

Synaptophysin

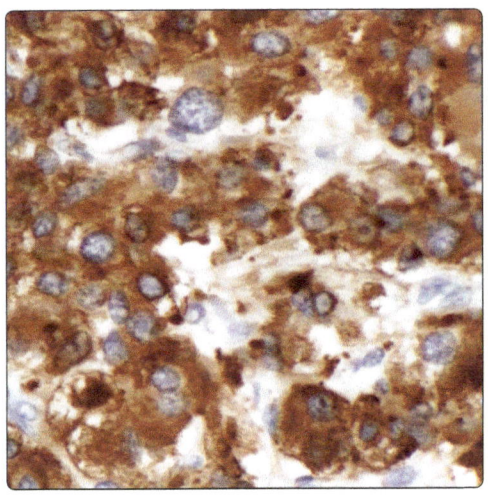

(Left) Chromogranin-A shows granular immunoreactivity in the neuroendocrine cell nests between cavernous blood vessels in a carotid PGL. Note the negativity of the endothelial cells for this marker. (From DP: Endocrine.) (Right) Synaptophysin shows granular immunoreactivity in the nests of neuroendocrine cells of PCC in a patient with MEN2A. Neuroendocrine immunostains may show significant variability of staining in PCC.

SDHA

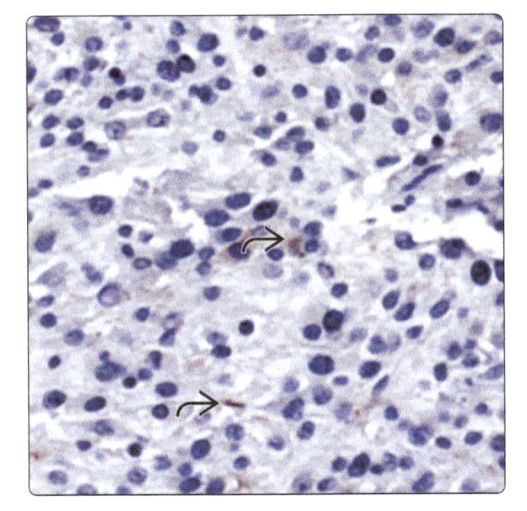

SDHB

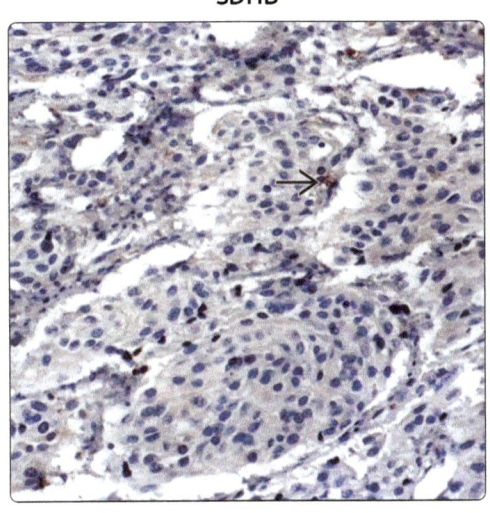

(Left) Tumor cells in PCC with mutations of the SDHA gene are negative for SDHA protein. The sustentacular cells and endothelial cells ⊠ serve as intrinsic positive controls. (Right) Tumor cells in PCC with mutations of the SDHA, SDHB, SDHC, or SDHD genes are negative for SDHB protein, whereas sustentacular cells ⊠ and endothelial cells serve as intrinsic positive controls.

S100

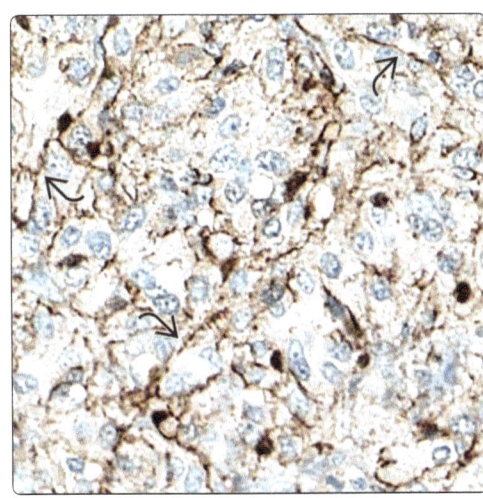

Proliferative Index by Ki-67

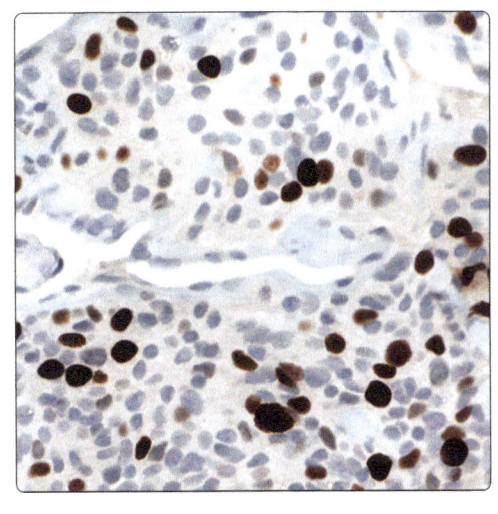

(Left) S100 in PGL shows nuclear and cytoplasmic staining of sustentacular cells, which sometimes have conspicuous cytoplasmic processes ⊠. The chief cells are usually negative for this marker but sometimes show weak staining. (Right) High Ki-67 labeling index is unusual in PCC/PGL and, when present, may be associated with aggressive tumor behavior. This carotid PGL showed angioinvasion and soft tissue infiltration. (From DP: Endocrine.)

Adrenal Cortical Carcinoma

KEY FACTS

TERMINOLOGY
- Adrenal cortical carcinoma (ACC): Malignant epithelial neoplasm derived from cells of adrenal cortex

ETIOLOGY/PATHOGENESIS
- Pathogenesis not fully understood
- Acquisition of somatic driver mutations in most cases
- 90% of ACC sporadic
  - Genetic predisposition in 10%

CLINICAL ISSUES
- Functional tumors often present with features related to excess hormone production
- Complete, radical surgery followed by mitotane, combination chemotherapy and pembrolizumab
- Currently no targetable molecular alterations in ACC
- Prognosis closely related to pathologic stage and feasibility of complete resection
- Local recurrence and metastatic disease common
- Overall 5-year survival: 37-47%

MOLECULAR
- Complex molecular landscape includes driver gene mutations, LOH, and whole-genome doubling
  - Cause cell cycle activation, Wnt pathway activation, and epigenetic modification

MICROSCOPIC
- No single feature diagnostic of malignancy
- Multiple systems for diagnosis (Hough, van Slooten, Weiss)

ANCILLARY TESTS
- Positive for vimentin, inhibin, SF1, melan-A, synaptophysin, calretinin, and IGF2
- MSI or MMR recommended for all patients with newly diagnosed ACC
- Tumor mutational burden
- Germline testing with genetics consultation in appropriate clinical context

---

Gross Appearance

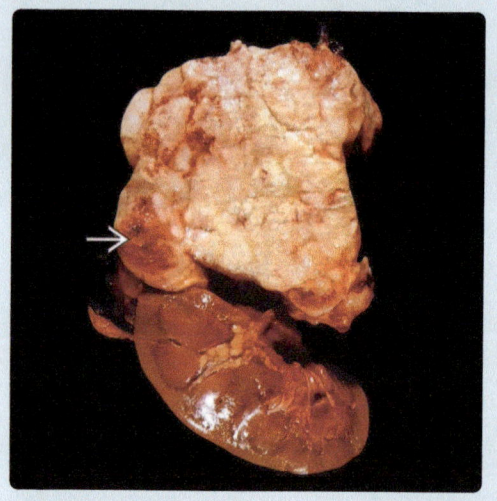

Radiologic Features

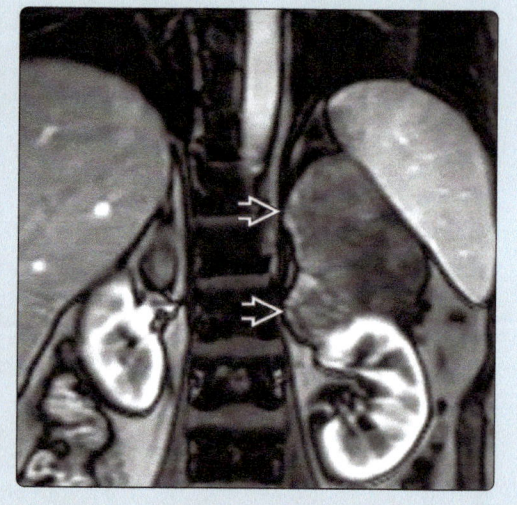

(Left) Adrenal cortical carcinoma (ACC) tends to appear grossly as large, solid masses in the suprarenal region, typically measuring > 5 cm. Focal areas of necrosis and hemorrhage ➡ are usually present. (From DP: Endocrine.) (Right) Radiologic image shows a large left adrenal gland mass ➡ pushing the kidney down and compressing the adjacent spleen. The interior is mottled and shows mixed intensity. (From DP: Endocrine.)

Microscopic Features

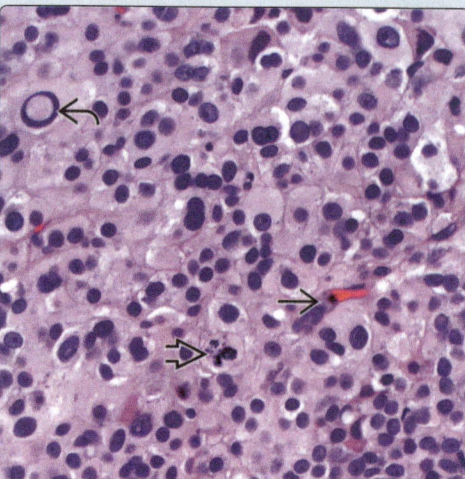

Clear and Eosinophilic Cytoplasm

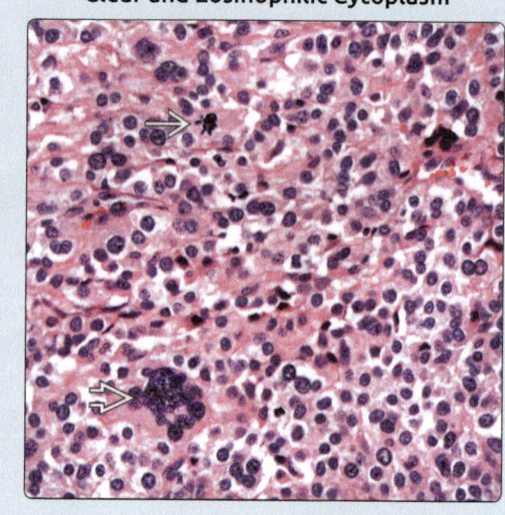

(Left) Tumor cells are separated by inconspicuous fibrovascular septa ➡. Nuclear pleomorphism, atypical mitotic figures ➡, and intranuclear pseudoinclusions ➡ are common. (Right) ACC shows tumor composed by slightly pleomorphic round cells with both clear and eosinophilic cytoplasm. An atypical mitotic figure ➡ and a multinucleated giant cell ➡ are indicated. (From DP: Endocrine.)

Adrenal Cortical Carcinoma

TERMINOLOGY

Abbreviations
- Adrenal cortical carcinoma (ACC)

Synonyms
- Adrenocortical carcinoma

Definitions
- Malignant epithelial neoplasm derived from cells of adrenal cortex

ETIOLOGY/PATHOGENESIS

Possible Multistep Process
- Acquisition of somatic driver mutations in most cases
- Adrenal cortical hyperplasia and adenoma share subset of molecular alterations with ACC and may represent precursor lesions
- 90% of ACC sporadic
- Genetic predisposition in 10%

Hereditary Tumor Syndrome Associations
- Li-Fraumeni syndrome (LFS)
  o 50-80% of children and 5.8% of adults with ACC have LFS
  o Inactivating mutations in *TP53* tumor suppressor gene
  o *CHEK2* mutation affects production of cell cycle regulator and tumor suppressor protein
- Lynch syndrome (LS)
  o ~ 3% of adults with ACC have LS
  o Inactivating mutations in mismatch repair genes
- Multiple endocrine neoplasia 1 (MEN1)
  o ~ 2% of adults with ACC have MEN1
  o *MEN1* mutation affects production of menin tumor suppressor protein
- Familial adenomatous polyposis (FAP)
  o Seen in < 1% of adults with ACC
  o Germline mutation in *APC* tumor suppressor gene
- Beckwith-Wiedemann syndrome
  o Mutations in *IGF2*, *CDKN1C*, and *H19*

CLINICAL ISSUES

Epidemiology
- 1-2 cases per million in USA
- ~ 3% of endocrine neoplasms and 0.2% of all malignancies
- Bimodal age distribution: 1st decade of life and 50-60 years
- F:M = 1.5-2.5:1

Presentation
- Can be separated on basis of hormone production
  o Nonfunctional tumors have no measurable hormone production
    – Sometimes detected incidentally
  o Functional tumors produce hormones, often leading to clinical signs/symptoms
- > 50% of ACC presents with symptoms of hormonal dysfunction
- Presentation depends on specific hormone excess (glucocorticoid > androgen > mineralocorticoid > > estrogen)
  o Glucocorticoids
    – Cushing syndrome
    – Protein wasting, striae, skin thinning, diabetes, hypertension, gonadal dysfunction, muscle atrophy, osteoporosis, central obesity, moon facies, and psychiatric disorders
  o Androgens
    – Virilization in women
    – Excess testosterone in men
    – Precocious puberty in children
    – Adrenal virilization-feminization syndrome due to adrenal mass is considered sign of malignancy in adults
  o Mineralocorticoids
    – Typically deoxycorticosterone (DOC); hyperaldosteronism almost never seen
    – Hypertension and hypokalemia
  o Estrogens
    – Gynecomastia and testicular atrophy in men
    – Menstrual irregularities, endometrial hyperplasia
    – Precocious puberty in children
- Highly necrotic tumors of either type can present with fever, potentially mimicking infectious process

Treatment
- Surgical approaches
  o Complete surgical excision provides optimal therapy
- Drugs
  o Mitotane
    – May help prolong disease-free survival following surgical therapy
    – Can also be used following incomplete resection, for metastatic disease, or for nonresectable tumors
  o Multiagent chemotherapy
    – Combinations of mitotane, etoposide, doxorubicin, cisplatin, and streptozocin
    – Failure is common, may be due to increased expression of multidrug resistance protein 1 (MDR1)
  o Pembrolizumab
    – Alone or in combination with mitotane
    – 3 phase II studies showed 14-23% overall response rate, 54% clinical benefit in one, and 52% disease control in another
- Radiation
  o Radiotherapy may help control residual disease
- Targeted therapy undergoing clinical trials
  o Tyrosine kinase inhibitors
  o Checkpoint inhibitor immunotherapy
  o Radioimmunotherapy
  o Cancer peptide therapeutic vaccine

Prognosis
- Overall 5-year survival: 37-47%
- Better prognosis for stage I/II tumors
- Feasibility of complete resection is most significant prognostic factor
- Local recurrence is common
- ~ 40% of patients present with metastases
  o Common sites include lung, liver, lymph nodes, and bone

Adrenal Cortical Carcinoma

IMAGING

General Features
- Large, heterogeneous suprarenal masses with frequent hemorrhage and calcifications
- Irregular borders, often with displacement or invasion of adjacent structures
- PET scan useful for detecting distant metastases

MACROSCOPIC

General Features
- Typically large, bulky, lobulated tumors
- 3-40 cm (median: 8-10 cm) and usually > 100 g (up to 5 kg)
- Depending on lipid content, cut surfaces are red-brown to yellow-orange
- Frequent degenerative changes, including hemorrhage, necrosis, fibrosis, cystic change, and calcifications

AJCC/UICC Staging System
- Stage I: Confined to gland, ≤ 5 cm
- Stage II: Confined to gland, ≥ 5 cm
- Stage III: Extends beyond gland, but no invasion of adjacent organs
- Stage IV: Distant metastases or adjacent organ involvement

MOLECULAR

General Statements
- Molecular pathogenesis of ACC is uncertain
- Currently no known targetable molecular alterations in ACC
- ACC and adrenal cortical adenoma (ACA) share subset of known molecular alterations

Cytogenetics
- Frequent chromosomal aberrations
  o Duplications, numerical alterations and rearrangements
    – Gains in chromosomes, 4, 5, 12, and 19
    – Losses in 1, 2, 3, 4, 6, 9, 11, 13, 15, 17, 18, 22, and X
  o Aneuploid DNA pattern has frequently been reported with these chromosomal imbalances

Chromosomal Microarray
- Copy number alterations
  o Allelic losses in chromosomes 1, 2q, 3, 6p, 7p, 8p, 9, 10, 11, 13q, 14q, 15q, 16, 17, 19q, and 22q
  o Increased copy number in 5, 6q, 7, 8q, 12, 16q, and 20
  o Gains in 6q, 7q, and 12q and losses in 3, 8, 10p, 16q, 17q, and 19q associated with decreased overall survival
- Early studies show strong relationship between tumor size and number of genetic aberrations detected using chromosomal microarray

Molecular Genetics
- Rearrangements, loss of heterozygosity (LOH), and abnormal imprinting of 11p15.5 locus
  o Lead to downregulation of CDKN1C and H19 and upregulation of IGF2
    – Overexpression of IGF2 seen in sporadic ACC cases
    – Associated with more malignant phenotype and higher risk of ACC recurrence
- Mutations of TP53
  o Tumor suppressor gene involved in cell proliferation
  o Somatic TP53 mutations occur in 20-35% of adult cases
  o Germline mutations in 50-80% of children with ACC
    – Indicates presence of LFS
  o Inactivation of TP53 is associated with aggressive phenotype and poor clinical outcome
  o LOH has also been seen in 80-85% of ACC
    – Does not always correlate with TP53 mutation
- Mutations of CTNNB1 and ZNRF3 deletions
  o Seen in ~ 31% of cases
    – Associated with decreased overall survival
  o Constitutive activation of Wnt/β-catenin pathway
    – Promotes cell proliferation, motility, epithelial to mesenchymal transition, and resistance to apoptosis
    – Seen in both ACA and ACC
- Somatic mutation in MEN1
  o Tumor suppressor gene
    – LOH of MEN1 locus at 11q13 in ~ 85% of cases
- Inactivating germline mutations of PDE11A
- Mutation in PRKAR1A gene locus 17q24
  o PRKAR1A encodes component of cAMP signaling pathway implicated in endocrine tumorigenesis
  o Mutations associated with Carney complex syndrome
- TERT, CDK4, ZNRF3, and RB1 are altered in > 30% of cases
  o Affect cell cycle regulation and chromosome maintenance
- Homologous recombination deficiency (HRD)
  o HRD-associated mutation signatures have been identified in subset of ACC

Gene Expression Profiling
- Upregulation of IGF2
  o Differences in expression of DLGAP5 and PINK1 may allow for discrimination between benign and malignant adrenocortical tumors
- High expression of BUB1 and low expression of PINK1
  o May allow for selection of tumors with poor prognosis

Epigenomics
- Hypermethylation of tumor suppressor genes and regulators of cell cycle, including CDKN2A, GATA4, DLEC1, HDAC10, PYCARD, and SCGB3A1
  o Methylation levels inversely correlated to mRNA expression levels
- MicroRNA expression
  o Upregulation of miR-503 and miR-483
  o Downregulation of miR-335 and miR-195
- SWI/SNF complex (ARID1B, SMARCA4, SMARCC2) mutations
  o Involved in chromatin remodeling
- KMT2C, KMT2A, and ATRX mutations
  o Involved in histone modification
- KDM5A copy gain
  o Increased expression antagonizes MEN1 histone methyltransferase activity

Genomic Characterization
- The Cancer Genome Atlas Project on ACC (ACC-TCGA)
  o 3 molecular subtypes with distinct clinical outcomes and therapeutic targets
  o CoC1: Good prognosis
    – Lower frequency of somatic alterations, genomically quiet

Adrenal Cortical Carcinoma

- Steroid low/immune-high, and CIMP-low
  - **CoC2**: Intermediate prognosis
    - Somatic alterations activating the Wnt pathway
    - ± whole-genome doubling (WGD)
    - Steroid-high and CIMP-intermediate
  - **CoC3**: Poor prognosis
    - Higher frequency of somatic alterations leading to cell cycle and Wnt pathway activation
    - Genomically noisy, proliferative, WGD
    - Steroid-high and CIMP-high
- Confirmation of known alterations: *CTNNB1*, *TP53*, *CDKN2A*, *RB1*, and *MEN1*
- New driver genes: *PRKAR1A*, *RPL22*, *TERF2*, *CCNE1*, and *NF1*
- Somatic alterations: 45%, 40%, and 20% involved cell cycle activation, Wnt pathway activation, and epigenetic modification, respectively
- WGD associated with aggressive clinical course

MICROSCOPIC

Histologic Features

- ACC demonstrates morphologic spectrum from overtly malignant appearing to normal adrenal appearing
  - Inter- and intratumoral heterogeneity
- Distinction between ACC and ACA can be challenging
- Multiple architectural patterns, including patternless sheets, trabeculae, and nests
- Necrosis may be present and is suggestive of malignancy
- Fibrous connective tissue bands
- Loss of reticulin network

Cytologic Features

- Increased N:C ratio
- Bland to markedly pleomorphic nuclei, multinucleation common, nuclear hyperchromatism, vesicular chromatin, and prominent nucleoli
- Intranuclear pseudoinclusions
- Frequently increased mitotic activity; may see atypical mitotic figures
- Clear to eosinophilic cytoplasm
- Cytologic distinction of benign vs. malignant adrenocortical tumors is difficult
  - Marked pleomorphism, nuclear membrane irregularities, and macronucleoli favor carcinoma
- FNA helpful in identification of metastases

ANCILLARY TESTS

Immunohistochemistry

- Positive for vimentin, inhibin, melan-A, SF1, and calretinin
- Positive for synaptophysin, but usually negative for chromogranin
- Focal, weak positivity for cytokeratins can be seen
- Ki-67 proliferative index > 5%
- 2022 WHO classification ancillary tools to consider
  - IGF2
    - Highlights juxtanuclear granular expression in 80% of ACC in adults
    - Shown to be best diagnostic ancillary tool
  - Gordon-Sweet silver
    - Highlights altered reticulin framework
- DAXX &/or ATRX
  - Global loss of expression correlates with poorer clinical outcome
- p53
  - Abnormal expression (overexpression or global loss) seen in adverse molecular clusters
    - Seen in LFS-associated ACC
- β-catenin
  - Nuclear expression seen in adverse molecular clusters
    - May be seen in FAP-associated ACC
- Mismatch repair (MMR)
  - MMR deficiency (dMMR): Lack of MMR protein expression with positive internal control
    - dMMR proteins can be seen in subset of sporadic tumors and in LS

Genetic Testing

- Microsatellite instability (MSI)
  - Testing available by PCR or NGS
  - Microsatellite stable (MSS): No changes in any of 5 NCI-designated or mononucleotide microsatellite markers
  - MSI-high (MSI-H): Changes in ≥ 2 microsatellite markers
    - Associated with both sporadic MSI-H pathway tumors and LS
- Tumor mutational burden (TMB)
  - FDA-approved test is recommended by NCCN
  - TMB-high is defined as ≥ 10 mutations/megabase
- Germline testing with genetics consultation in appropriate clinical context

DIFFERENTIAL DIAGNOSIS

Adrenal Cortical Adenoma

- Multiple systems used to distinguish benign from malignant adrenocortical tumors
  - Hough, Weiss, van Slooten
- Histologic features suggestive of malignancy
  - High-grade cytology, increased mitotic activity (> 5/50 HPF), atypical mitoses, confluent tumor necrosis, lymphovascular and capsular invasion, and diffuse architecture (> 1/3 of tumor)

Renal Cell Carcinoma

- Positive for EMA and CD10; strong keratin reactivity

Hepatocellular Carcinoma

- Positive for Hep-Par1, CEA, AFP, and keratins

Pheochromocytoma

- Positive for chromogranin and INSM1
- S100-positive sustentacular cells highlight zellballen pattern

SELECTED REFERENCES

1. Mete O et al: Adrenal cortical carcinoma. In: WHO Classification of Tumours Editorial Board. Endocrine and neuroendocrine tumours. IARC, 2022. https://tumourclassification.iarc.who.int/chapters/53
2. Lavoie JM et al: Whole-genome and transcriptome analysis of advanced adrenocortical cancer highlights multiple alterations affecting epigenome and DNA repair pathways. Cold Spring Harb Mol Case Stud. 8(3), 2022
3. Mete O et al: Overview of the 2022 WHO classification of adrenal cortical tumors. Endocr Pathol. 33(1):155-96, 2022
4. National Comprehensive Cancer Network: NCCN clinical practice guidelines in oncology. Accessed June 30, 2023. https://www.nccn.org/professionals/physician_gls/pdf/neuroendocrine.pdf

Adrenal Cortical Carcinoma

Gross Appearance

Cut Section

(Left) This small (5-cm) ACC was detected incidentally. Its lobulated cut surface shows a clear demarcation between homogeneous, adenoma-like periphery ⇨ and clearly malignant central lobule with hemorrhage and necrosis ⇨. Normal adrenal parenchyma is also present ⇨. (Right) Encroachment of this ACC into periadrenal soft tissue ⇨ supports diagnosis of malignancy. Hemorrhage and necrosis are also seen ⇨.

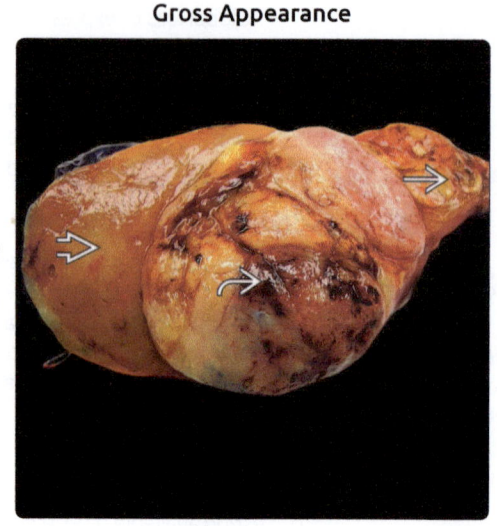

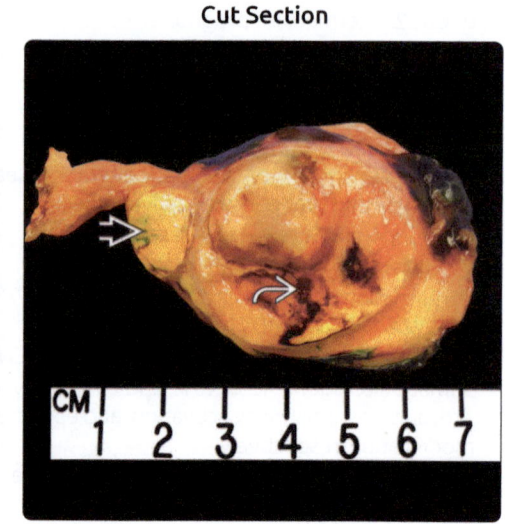

Vascular Invasion

Cytologic Features

(Left) Juxtaposition between ACC composed of small uniform cells ⇨ and residual normal adrenal tissue ⇨ is shown. Tumor invasion of a large intraparenchymal vessel ⇨ is noted. (From DP: Endocrine.) (Right) Cytologic diagnosis of ACC can be challenging, although marked nuclear pleomorphism and membrane irregularity ⇨ favors carcinoma. Caution is advised, however, as patchy "endocrine atypia" can be seen in adenoma.

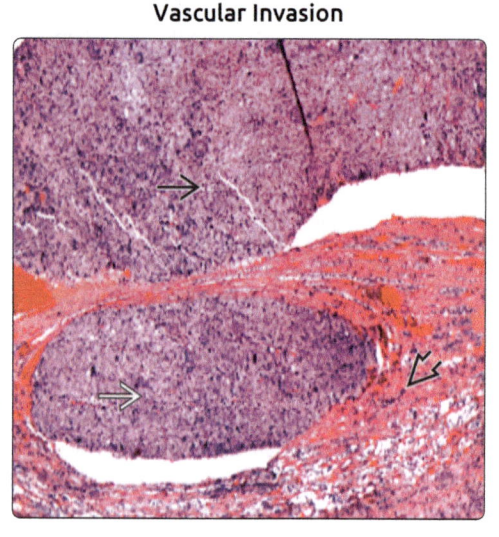

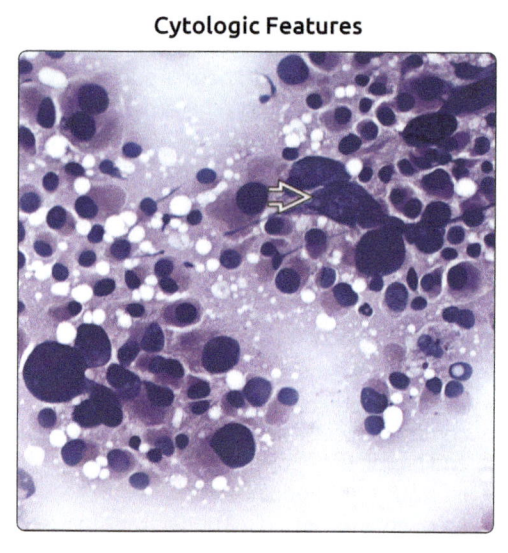

Vascular Invasion

Cytologic and Mitotic Atypia

(Left) This tumor invades a vessel wall ⇨ and is composed of small, uniform cells with clear cytoplasm. Atypical large, multinucleated cells ⇨ are also shown. (From DP: Endocrine.) (Right) ACC composed of small, compact eosinophilic cells, some with prominent nucleoli intermixed with scattered, bizarre multinucleated cells ⇨ is shown. Several mitotic figures, including atypical mitoses ⇨, are present. (From DP: Endocrine.)

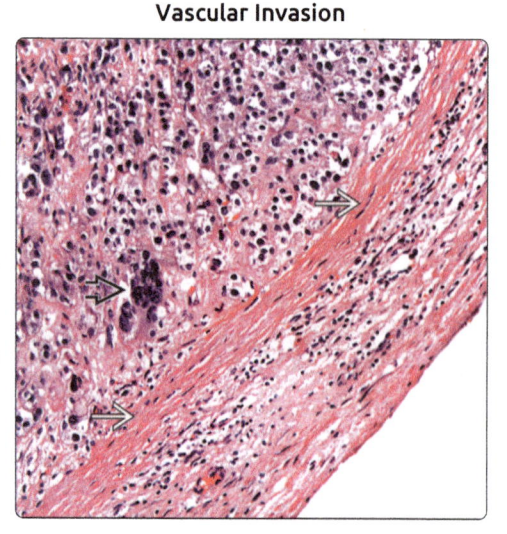

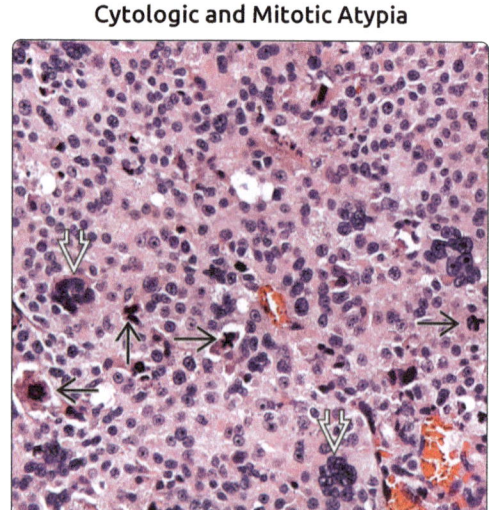

Adrenal Cortical Carcinoma

Nuclear Features

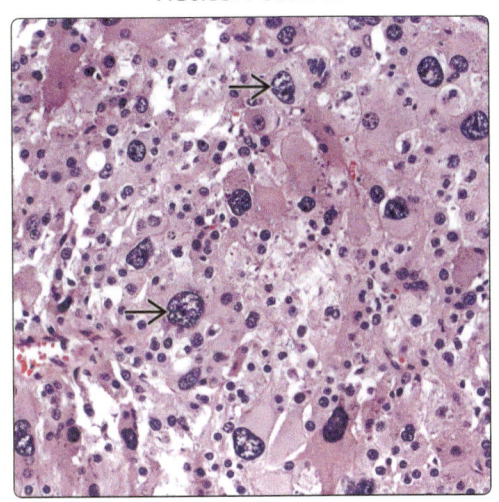

Inhibin Immunohistochemistry

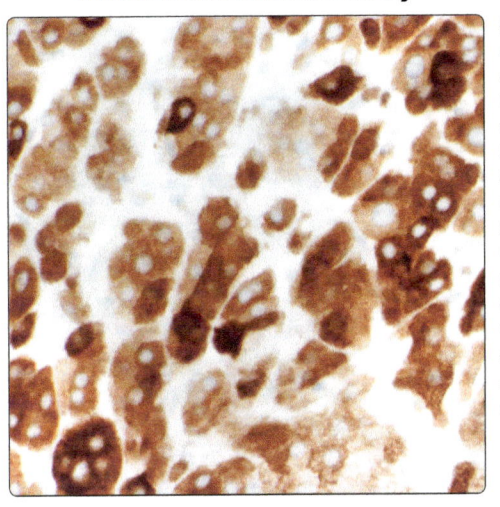

(Left) ACC shows an admixture of cells with varying levels of atypia. Highly atypical cells with large nuclei, coarse chromatin, and irregular nuclear membranes ➡ are seen intercalating between comparatively bland cells with small, compact nuclei. (Right) Cytoplasmic inhibin staining is characteristic. IHC helps differentiate ACC from other diagnostic considerations, such as renal cell carcinoma, pheochromocytoma, and hepatocellular carcinoma.

Tumor Necrosis

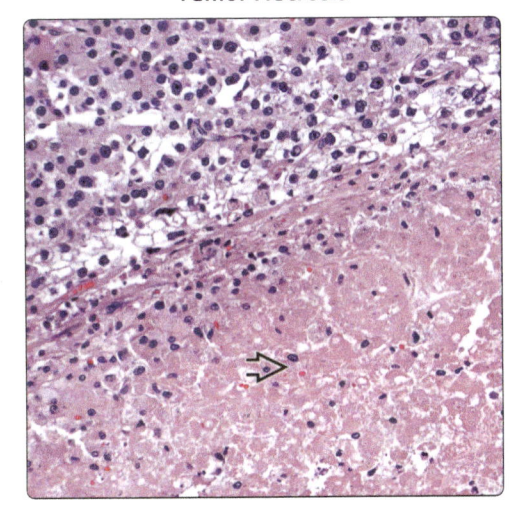

Soft Tissue Invasion

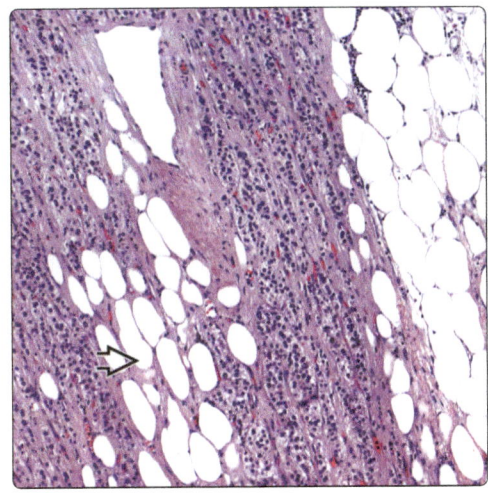

(Left) Tumor necrosis ➡, while occasionally seen in adenoma, is suggestive of malignancy and is a histologic criterion in all schemata used to separate benign from malignant cortical tumors. (Right) ACC invading periadrenal fat ➡ is shown. Although this is a feature of malignancy, caution is advised in making this interpretation, as some adenomas can show lipomatous metaplasia, mimicking extraadrenal extension.

Pulmonary Metastasis

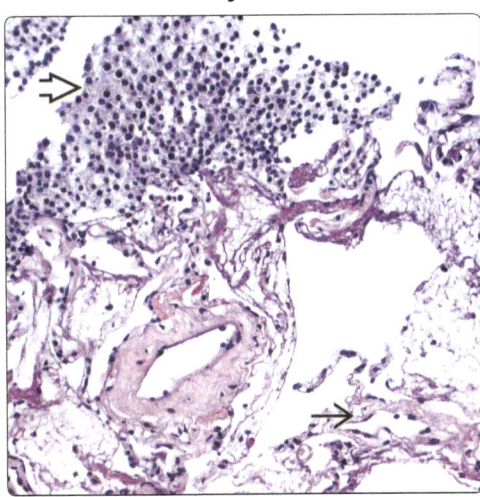

Melan-A Immunohistochemistry

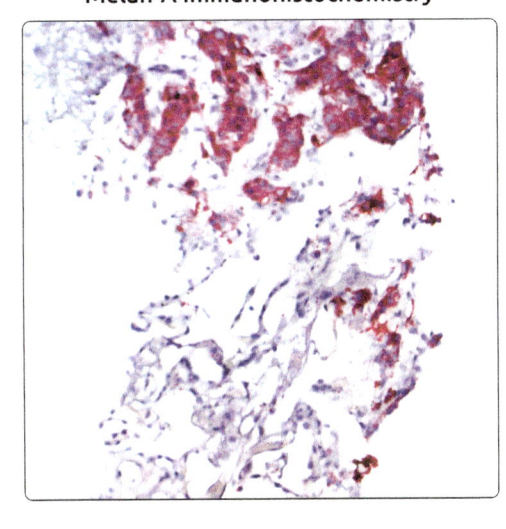

(Left) Lung biopsy shows a focus of metastatic ACC ➡. The tumor nodule is composed of compact, relatively bland cells with clear to eosinophilic cytoplasm. Adjacent lung parenchyma ➡ is seen. (Right) Melan-A highlights neoplastic cells within lung parenchyma. Other diagnostic considerations for tumors with this immunomorphology would include pulmonary clear cell tumor ("sugar tumor") and metastatic melanoma.

Neuroblastoma

KEY FACTS

TERMINOLOGY
- Neuroblastoma (NB): Malignant pediatric neoplasm derived from embryonic neural crest cells

CLINICAL ISSUES
- 85% of patients < 5 years of age
- Tumors arise along sympathetic chain
- ~ 67% have metastases on presentation

MOLECULAR
- Worse prognosis
  - *MYCN* amplification
  - *TERT* rearrangements
  - *ATRX* mutations
  - Deletion of 11q and 1p, gain of 17q
  - Diploid/near-diploid or tetraploid DNA index

MICROSCOPIC
- INPC classification
  - Undifferentiated NB
  - Poorly differentiated NB
  - Differentiating NB
  - Nodular ganglioneuroblastoma
  - Intermixed ganglioneuroblastoma
- Combination of histologic subclassification, mitotic-karyorrhectic index, and age at diagnosis used to determine favorable vs. unfavorable histology

ANCILLARY TESTS
- NB84, protein gene product 9.5 (PGP9.5), PHOX2B, and neuroendocrine markers
- Liquid biopsy (circulating tumor nucleic acid) may become standard of care especially for evaluating response to therapy

TOP DIFFERENTIAL DIAGNOSES
- Other small round blue cell tumors
- Ganglioneuroma

Sympathetic Chain

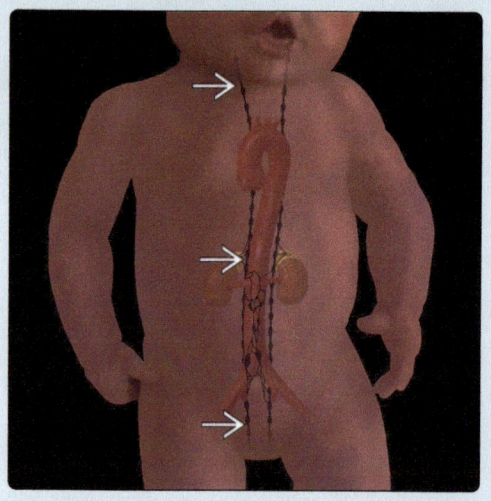

Adrenal Neuroblastoma

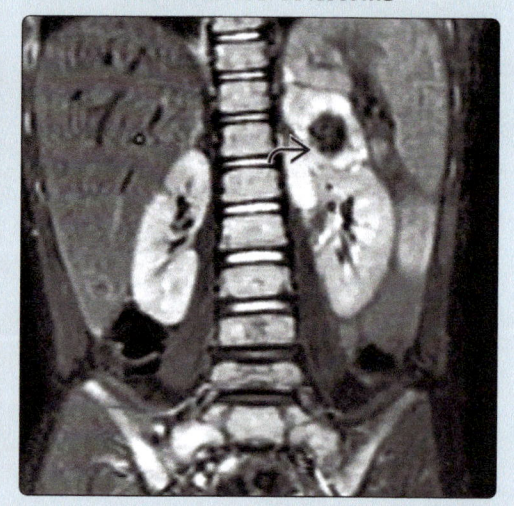

(Left) *Migration of primordial neural crest cells results in formation of the sympathetic chain ➡, which includes the adrenal medulla. Neuroblastoma (NB) can occur anywhere along this axis.* (Right) *T2 MR shows adrenal neuroblastoma with central necrosis ➡. NB can occur anywhere along the sympathetic chain, but the adrenals are the most common site. (From DP: Endocrine.)*

Metastatic Neuroblastoma

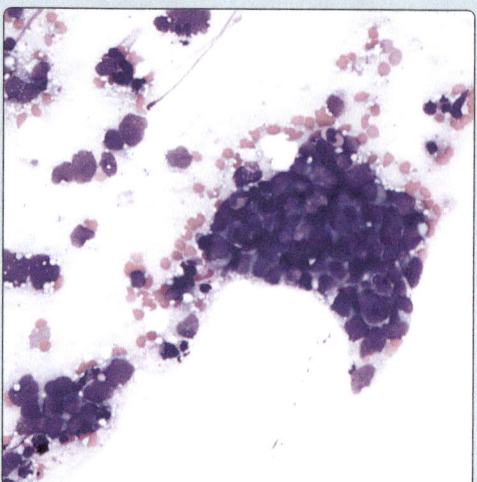

Metastatic Neuroblastoma

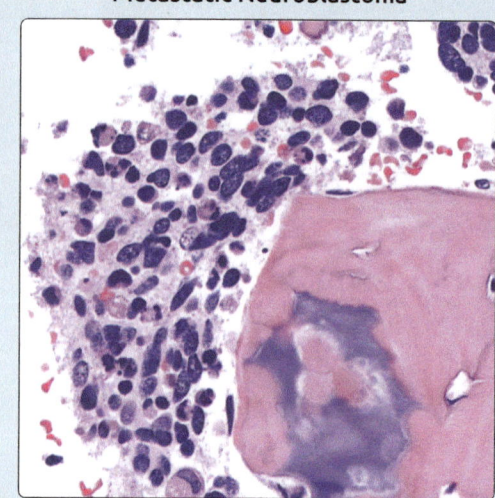

(Left) *Touch prep of positive bone marrow shows clusters of neuroblasts. The tumor cells are larger than surrounding lymphocytes with a high N:C ratio and hints of nuclear molding.* (Right) *Core biopsy of positive bone marrow shows paratrabecular location of clusters of tumor cells exhibiting "salt and pepper" type chromatin and individual cell necrosis.*

Neuroblastoma

TERMINOLOGY

Abbreviations
- Neuroblastoma (NB)
- Ganglioneuroblastoma (GNB)

Synonyms
- Schwannian stroma-poor neuroblastic tumor
- Peripheral neuroblastic tumor

Definitions
- Malignant pediatric neoplasm arising from sympathoadrenal lineage of neural crest during development
  o NB is undifferentiated/poorly differentiated
  o GNB is moderately differentiated, showing variable tumor cell differentiation into mature ganglion cells

ETIOLOGY/PATHOGENESIS

Developmental Anomaly
- Derived from embryonic neural crest cells
  o Primordial, multipotent cell population giving rise to sympathetic ganglia and adrenal medulla
  o Neuroblastoma can therefore arise anywhere along sympathetic chain
    – Cervical, thoracic, abdominal, pelvic

CLINICAL ISSUES

Epidemiology
- Incidence
  o 4th most common malignant tumor in children; 1 in 7,000 live births
  o Most common congenital neoplasm
    – ~ 20-30% of cases are congenital
  o Majority are sporadic
    – 2-3% are autosomal dominant familial cases
- Age
  o 50% of patients diagnosed by age 2
  o 85% of patients < 5 years of age
  o Most familial cases present before 1 year of age

Site
- Majority of NB intraabdominal (65%)
  o Adrenal (40%)
  o Extraadrenal (25%)
- Incidence of extraabdominal NB matches relative distribution of extraabdominal sympathetic ganglia
  o Thorax (20%)
  o Neck (5%)
  o Pelvis (5%)
  o Other (16%)

Laboratory Tests
- Urine catecholamine metabolites and dopamine have been used for screening
  o Vanillylmandelic acid (VMA)
  o Homovanillic acid (HVA)
- Lactate dehydrogenase (LDH)
  o > 1,500 IU/L associated with worse prognosis
- Ferritin
  o > 142 ng/mL associated with worse prognosis
- Neuron-specific enolase (NSE)
  o > 100 ng/mL associated with worse prognosis

Natural History
- Some cases undergo spontaneous regression/maturation, including stage IV with disseminated disease limited to liver, skin, or bone marrow (IV-S)
  o Most commonly in infants < 1 year of age
  o Causative factor(s) unknown
- Incidentally discovered ganglioneuromas in distribution of sympathetic chain often assumed to be spontaneously regressed NB

Treatment
- Highly standardized and based on low-/intermediate-/high-risk stratification
- Combinations of surgery, chemotherapy, and radiotherapy
- Stem cell transplantation is considered in high-risk group

Prognosis
- 5-year survival by International Neuroblastoma Staging System (INSS) stage at diagnosis
  o Stage 1: > 90%
  o Stage 2: 70-80%
  o Stage 3: 40-70%
  o Stage 4
    – < 1 year of age: > 60%
    – 1-2 years of age: 20%
    – > 2 years of age: 10%
  o Stage 4-S: > 80%
- International Neuroblastoma Risk Group (INRG) staging system
  o Pretreatment (presurgical) risk stratification system
  o Based on specific clinical criteria and image-defined risk factors (IDRFs)
  o Allows comparison of clinical trials conducted by different cooperative groups
- Adverse prognostic factors
  o MYCN oncogene amplification
  o TERT rearrangements
    – Mutually exclusive from MYCN amplification and ATRX mutations
  o ATRX mutations
    – Mutually exclusive from MCYN amplification and TERT rearrangements
  o Diploid/near-diploid or tetraploid DNA index
  o Deletion of 11q and 1p
  o Gain of 17q
  o Older age at time of diagnosis
  o Histologic subtype
    – Undifferentiated NB and nodular GNB at any age
    – Poorly differentiated NB > 1.5 years
    – Differentiating NB > 5 years
  o High mitotic-karyorrhectic index (MKI)
  o Increased levels of ferritin, NSE, LDH, creatine kinase BB, and chromogranin-A
  o Pattern of urinary catecholamine excretion
  o Lack of high-affinity nerve growth factor receptors
  o Many other specific gene and epigenetic aberrations reported to be predictive

Neuroblastoma

- Require independent, prospective validation

IMAGING

General Features
- Extensive radiographic evaluation is required to determine extent of disease and identify metastatic foci
- Meta-iodobenzylguanidine (MIBG) scintigraphy scans are widely used for initial staging
  - High sensitivity/specificity due to radiolabeled MIBG incorporation into catecholamine-secreting tumor cells
  - ~ 10% of patients will have MIBG-negative disease

MACROSCOPIC

General Features
- Typically solitary mass up to 10 cm (average 6-8 cm)
- Variably firm, gray to white cut surfaces, depending on amount of stroma present
- Hemorrhage, cystic degeneration, and calcifications can be seen, particularly in postchemotherapy specimens
- Cases with nodular appearance warrant additional sampling to exclude nodular GNB (worse prognosis)

MOLECULAR

General Statements
- Relative paucity of recurrent somatic mutations
- Very few recurrent genetic aberrations in druggable pathways

Cytogenetics
- In general, low-/intermediate-risk NB has numerical chromosomal gains, while high-risk NB has intrachromosomal rearrangements and segmental alterations
  - In recent series of 493 NB cases, tumors with only whole-chromosome copy number variations showed no disease-related deaths
- Large segmental chromosomal aberrations may confer poor prognosis
  - Deletion of 11q23
    - Included as prognostic factor in INRG classification system
    - Inversely associated with MYCN amplification
    - Associated with older age at diagnosis
  - Deletion of 1p and gain of 17q are also well-established markers of poor prognosis
  - Other chromosomal losses and gains include deletions of 3p, 4p, 9p, and 14q, and gains of 1q, 2p, 7q, and 11p
- Tumor cell ploidy/DNA index
  - Near-diploidy or tetraploidy is associated with worse prognosis
    - More common in advanced-stage tumors
  - Hyperdiploidy is associated with better prognosis
    - Seen in majority of NB

Molecular Genetics
- MYC family oncogene (MYCN and MYC) overexpression
  - MYCN (2p24.3) transcription factor that regulates growth, differentiation, proliferation, and survival of developing neural crest cells
  - Expression is regulated by several signaling pathways, including hedgehog and Wnt
  - Amplification of MYCN is most common genetic abnormality in sporadic NB
    - Defined as ≥ 10 copies for diploid genome or > 4x signal relative to chromosome 2
    - Majority of MYCN-amplified tumors overexpress MYCN protein
  - Amplification is seen in 20-25% of all NB cases, but in 30-40% of high-risk patients
  - Associated with poor outcomes, including advanced-stage disease, aggressive behavior, and high risk of relapse
  - MYCN amplification is inversely associated with 11q deletion
  - By contrast, MYCN gain is associated with 11q aberration
    - MYCN gain = 2-4x increase in signal relative to centromeric reference probe
    - MYCN gain confers increased risk for death in certain patient subgroups, including patients with non-high-risk disease
  - Subset of NB shows overexpression of MYC protein, independent of genomic amplification
    - Associated with aggressive clinical behavior
- Telomere abnormalities
  - Telomere reverse transcriptase (TERT) overexpression
    - Direct transcriptional overexpression of TERT in MYC-driven cases
    - Genomic rearrangements of TERT in non-MYC-drive cases
  - Alternative lengthening of telomeres (ALT) phenotype
    - ATRX mutations
  - Significant association between ATRX mutations and age at diagnosis
    - Seen in 17% of children between 18 months and 12 years of age with stage 4 disease
    - Seen in 44% of patients > 12 years of age
    - No ATRX mutations have been found in children < 18 months of age with stage 4 disease
  - No ATRX mutations have been identified in patients with MYCN amplification
- Somatic ALK activating mutations and amplifications
  - Mutations seen in ~ 10% of sporadic NB
  - High-level amplification present in ~ 3-4% of NB
  - Activating ALK mutations or amplifications are associated with poor prognosis
  - Potential target for molecular therapy
- Whole-genome sequencing has identified recurrent genetic mutations in ARID1A and ARID1B
- NTRK1 protein overexpression
  - Associated with better prognosis

Familial Neuroblastoma
- Accounts for ~ 2-3% of all NB
- Heterogeneous etiology, thought to involve mutations in important signaling pathways responsible for development of sympathoadrenal lineage
  - Heterozygous mutations in PHOX2B (4p12)
    - Encodes paired homeodomain transcription factor promoting cell cycle exit and neuronal differentiation
  - ALK mutations

Neuroblastoma

- Expressed in developing sympathoadrenal lineage of neural crest
- Thought to regulate balance between differentiation and proliferation
- Likely pathways include MAPK and Ras-related protein 1 (RAP1)
- Evidence suggests PHOX2B protein can directly regulate *ALK* expression
- 20% risk of developing bilateral adrenal and multifocal primary tumors
- Autosomal dominant
- Potential susceptibility loci at 16p12-p31, 4p16, 2p21-p25.1, 12p12.1-p13.33
  - Suggests possible oligogenic model in which 2 loci have synergistic effect on NB
- Genome-wide association studies have identified predisposing single nucleotide polymorphisms (SNPs)
  - *CASC15*, *NBAT1*, *BARD1*, *LMO1*, *DUSP12*, *HSD17B12*, *DDX4*, *IL31RA*, *HACE1*, and *LIN28B*

MICROSCOPIC

Histologic Features

- Histologic evaluation begins with assessment/quantification of tumor cell differentiation
  - Neuroblasts
    - Undifferentiated component
    - Small round blue cells
    - Very scant cytoplasm
  - Ganglion cells/ganglionic differentiation
    - Represents differentiation/maturation of tumor cells
    - Cell size increases
    - Increased amounts of eosinophilic or amphophilic cytoplasm
    - Cytoplasm can contain Nissl substance (basophilic granules composed of endoplasmic reticulum)
    - Chromatin becomes vesicular
- Background stroma also shows different levels of differentiation
  - Neuropil
    - Eosinophilic, fibrillary extracellular material
  - Schwannian stroma
    - Resembles collagen
- Homer Wright pseudorosettes
  - Circular aggregates of neuroblasts surrounding central core of cytoplasmic processes (not true lumen)
  - Can be helpful in distinguishing NB from other small round cell tumors but only seen in minority of cases
- Mitotic-karyorrhectic index (MKI)
  - Applied to stroma-poor tumors (undifferentiated, poorly differentiated, differentiating NB subtypes)
  - MKI index is combined with tumor subtype and patient age to determine favorable vs. unfavorable histology status
  - Quantification of mitotic and karyorrhectic cells (per 5,000 tumor cells)
    - Low: < 100
    - Intermediate: 100-200
    - High: > 200

International Neuroblastoma Pathology Committee Classification

- a.k.a. Shimada classification
- **Undifferentiated NB**
  - No ganglionic differentiation
  - No or minimal neuropil
  - No or minimal Schwannian stroma
  - Confirmatory immunohistochemical testing is required to exclude other small round cell tumors
- **Poorly differentiated NB**
  - < 5% of tumor cells show ganglionic differentiation
  - Undifferentiated neuroblasts are primary cell type
  - Neuropil can be present
  - No or minimal Schwannian stroma
- **Differentiating NB**
  - > 5% of tumor cells show ganglionic differentiation
  - More abundant neuropil
  - More prominent schwannian stroma
    - Must be < 50%
- **Intermixed GNB**
  - Microscopic nests of neuroblastoma within schwannian stroma
  - > 50% schwannian stroma
- **Nodular GNB**
  - Grossly identifiable nodules, which microscopically will represent undifferentiated NB component
  - Abrupt demarcation between stroma-poor neuroblastoma and stroma-rich component
  - Fibrous pseudocapsule often seen surrounding NB component
  - > 50% schwannian stroma
- Posttreatment resection specimens are not histologically classified
  - "Neuroblastoma with treatment effect" is sufficient
- Histologic classification using metastatic tissue is permitted if specimen is pretreatment

ANCILLARY TESTS

Immunohistochemistry

- NB84
  - Highly sensitive for neuroblastoma
  - Decreased specificity; can be positive in other small round cell tumors
    - Ewing sarcoma/PNET, medulloblastoma, desmoplastic small round cell tumor
- NSE
  - Most sensitive but least specific
  - Found at least focally even in undifferentiated NB
- S100
  - Positive in schwannian stroma
- Additional positive immunohistochemical stains
  - Chromogranin
  - Synaptophysin
  - CD56
  - Protein gene product 9.5 (PGP9.5)
  - PHOX2B

Neuroblastoma

Favorable vs. Unfavorable Histology in Neuroblastic Tumors

Classification	MKI	Age at Diagnosis	Histologic Category
Neuroblastoma, undifferentiated	Any	Any	Unfavorable
Neuroblastoma, poorly differentiated	High	Any	Unfavorable
	Low to intermediate	> 1.5 years	Unfavorable
	Low to intermediate	< 1.5 years	Favorable
Neuroblastoma, differentiating	High	Any	Unfavorable
	Intermediate	> 1.5 years	Unfavorable
	Intermediate	< 1.5 years	Favorable
	Low	> 5 years	Unfavorable
	Low	< 5 years	Favorable
Nodular ganglioneuroblastoma	*	*	Unfavorable or favorable

*The determination of favorable vs. unfavorable histology in nodular ganglioneuroblastoma is based on the neuroblastoma component. MKI = mitosis-karyorrhexis index.

Neuroblastoma Staging System

Stage	Definition
1	Localized confined tumor; complete gross excision; contralateral nodes negative
2A	Unilateral tumor; incomplete gross excision; identifiable ipsilateral and contralateral nodes negative
2B	Unilateral tumor ± complete gross excision; identifiable ipsilateral nodes positive; identifiable ipsilateral and contralateral nodes negative
3	Tumor infiltrating across midline without positive nodes or unilateral tumor with positive contralateral nodes
4	Distant metastases to nodes, bone, liver, skin, &/or bone marrow
4-S	Patient < 1 year of age; localized tumor (stage 1 or 2); distant metastases confined to skin, liver, &/or bone marrow

DIFFERENTIAL DIAGNOSIS

Ganglioneuroma/Maturing Ganglioneuroma
- Schwannian stroma with admixed single cells (vs. nests of cells seen in GNB)

Non-Hodgkin Lymphoma
- Positive for CD45 and B- or T-cell associated antigens
- Negative for NB84, neuroendocrine markers

Ewing Sarcoma/Primitive Neuroectodermal Tumor
- Usually occurs in older patients
- Strong CD99 membranous positivity and usually FLI-1 positive
- 20% show low-molecular-weight keratin positivity
- Specific gene fusions, most commonly *EWSR1::FLI1*

Wilms Tumor
- Classically shows triphasic or biphasic morphology
- WT-1 immunoreactivity
- Negative for neuroendocrine markers

Alveolar Rhabdomyosarcoma
- Usually occurs in older patients
- Often shows classic alveolar pattern (tumor cells clinging to central fibrovascular cores)
- Cells generally have higher degree of anisonucleosis and more abundant cytoplasm
- Immunoreactivity for muscle markers (MYOD1, desmin, myogenin)
- t(1;13); *PAX7::FOXO1* or t(2;13); *PAX3::FOXO1*

Desmoplastic Small Round Cell Tumor
- Primarily affects young adults
- Classic desmoplastic stroma
- Polyphenotypic by IHC
  - Combined desmin and WT1 positivity with cytokeratins &/or EMA immunoreactivity in most cases

SELECTED REFERENCES

1. Mete O et al: Overview of the 2022 WHO classification of paragangliomas and pheochromocytomas. Endocr Pathol. 33(1):90-114, 2022
2. Salemi F et al: Neuroblastoma: essential genetic pathways and current therapeutic options. Eur J Pharmacol. 926:175030, 2022
3. Shimada H et al: Neuroblastoma. In: WHO Classification of Tumours Editorial Board. Paediatric tumours. IARC, 2022
4. Sokol E et al: The evolution of risk classification for neuroblastoma. Children (Basel). 6(2), 2019
5. Schulte M et al: Cancer evolution, mutations, and clonal selection in relapse neuroblastoma. Cell Tissue Res. 372(2):263-8, 2018
6. Ahmed AA et al: Neuroblastoma in children: update on clinicopathologic and genetic prognostic factors. Pediatr Hematol Oncol. 34(3):165-85, 2017
7. Campbell K et al: Association of MYCN copy number with clinical features, tumor biology, and outcomes in neuroblastoma: a report from the Children's Oncology Group. Cancer. 123(21):4224-35, 2017
8. Cheung NK et al: Neuroblastoma: developmental biology, cancer genomics and immunotherapy. Nat Rev Cancer. 13(6):397-411, 2013
9. Suganuma R et al: Peripheral neuroblastic tumors with genotype-phenotype discordance: a report from the Children's Oncology Group and the International Neuroblastoma Pathology Committee. Pediatr Blood Cancer. 60(3):363-70, 2013

Neuroblastoma

Undifferentiated/Poorly Differentiated Neuroblastoma

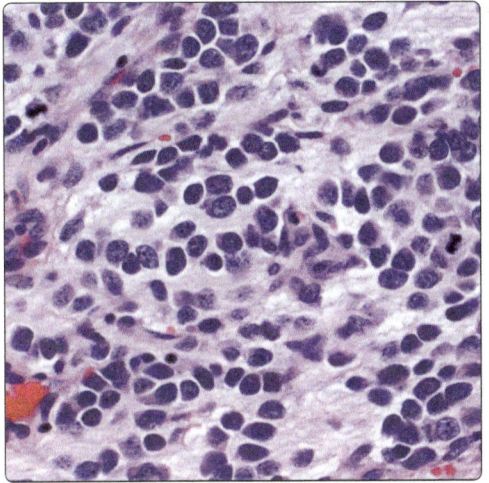

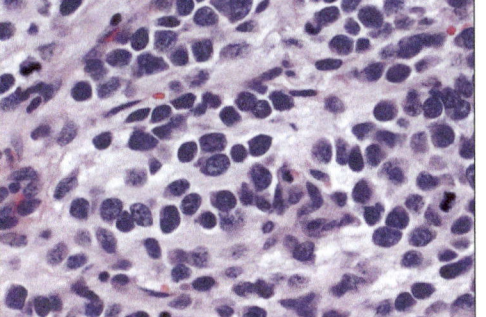

Undifferentiated/Poorly Differentiated Neuroblastoma

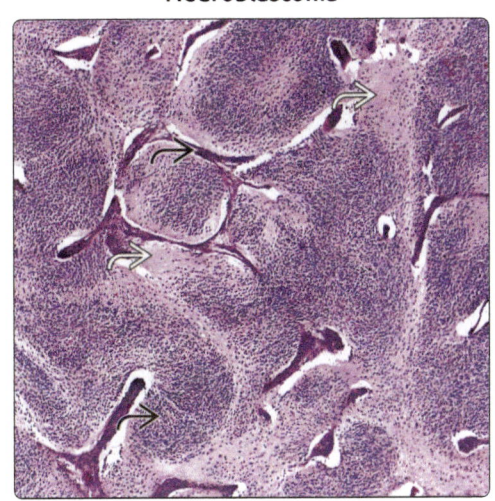

(Left) Undifferentiated/poorly differentiated NB appear histologically similar to other high-grade small round cell tumors. Clinical/laboratory findings may favor NB, but immunohistochemistry is ultimately required for diagnosis. (Right) Poorly differentiated NB shows thin septa composed of schwannian stroma ➡. Pale, eosinophilic neuropil ➡ is seen in places between the nodules or nests of NB cells. (From DP: Endocrine.)

Undifferentiated/Poorly Differentiated Neuroblastoma

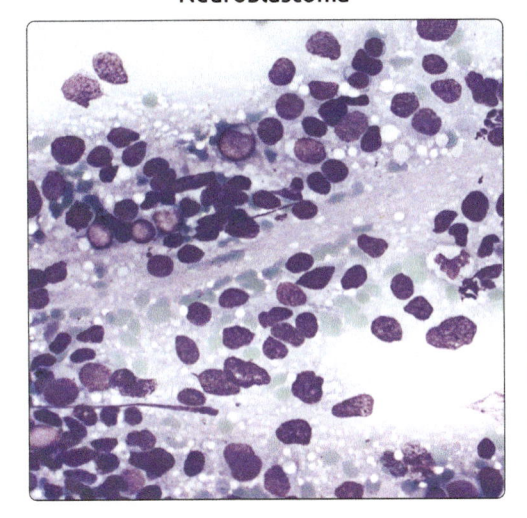

Homer Wright Rosettes

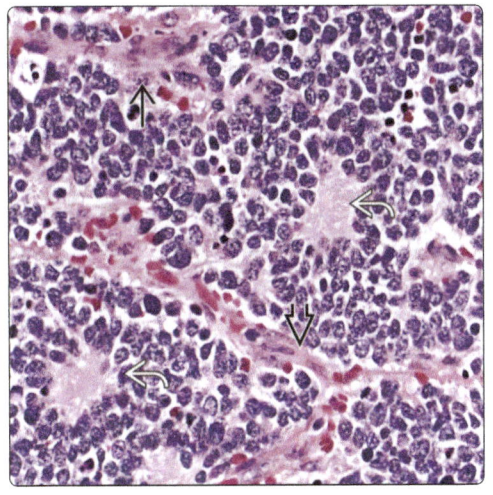

(Left) The cytologic features of this undifferentiated NB are those of other small round blue cell tumors. Fine-need aspiration is useful for confirming metastases. (Right) Homer Wright rosettes ➡ are composed of neuroblasts surrounding a central core of neurites without a central lumen. These can be found in varying numbers in poorly differentiated NB but are not specific. Small foci of schwannian stroma ➡ are also seen, which may form thin bands ➡. (From DP: Endocrine.)

Acellular Components

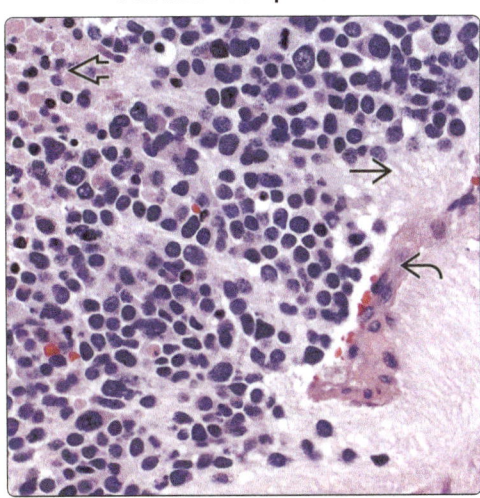

Liver Metastasis

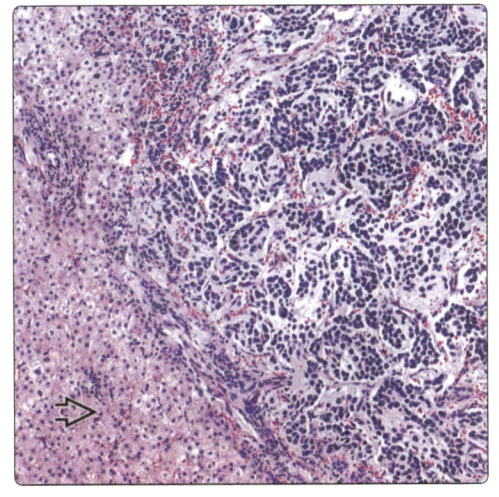

(Left) Distinction between fibrillary neuropil ➡ and collagen-like schwannian stroma ➡ may require higher magnification. Further distinction between stromal elements and necrotic foci is made easier by nonviable tumor "ghost cells" ➡. (Right) Liver metastases are common in NB, as shown in this poorly differentiated NB involving hepatic parenchyma ➡. Cases in which metastases are limited to the liver, skin, &/or bone marrow have a significantly better prognosis.

Neuroblastoma

Differentiating Neuroblastoma

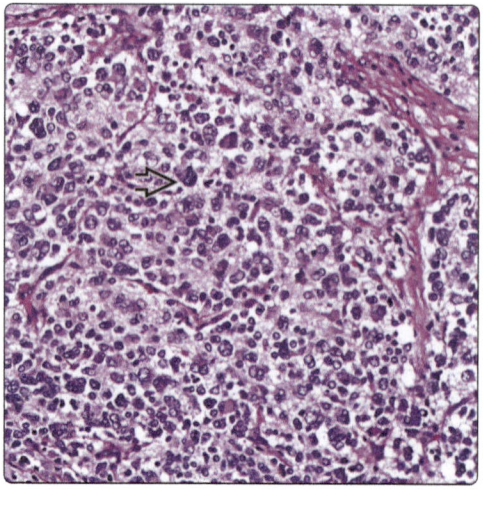

Intermixed Ganglioneuroblastoma

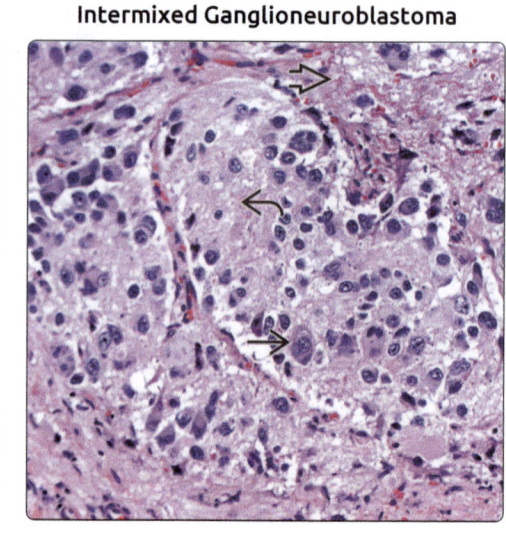

(Left) In this example of differentiating neuroblastoma, > 5% of the neuroblasts show differentiation with increased cytoplasm and vesicular nuclei ➡. (From DP: Endocrine.)
(Right) Intermixed ganglioneuroblastoma (GNB) shows maturing ganglion cells ➡ surrounded by schwannian stroma ➡ and neuropil ➡. Neuropil has a fibrillary appearance because it is composed of tangles of eosinophilic neuritic processes.

Schwannian Stroma and Mature Ganglion Cells

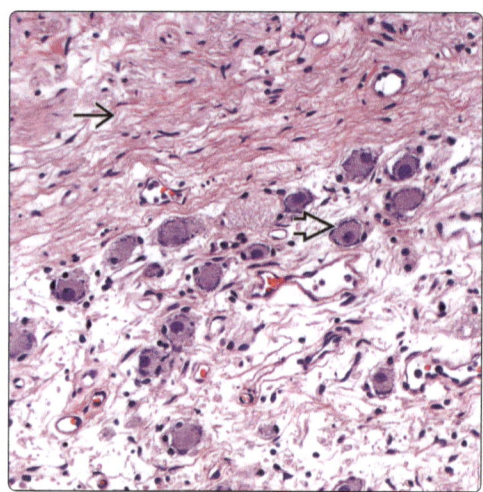

Degenerative Changes

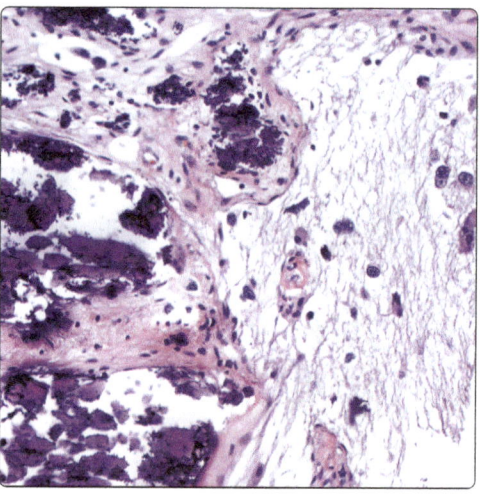

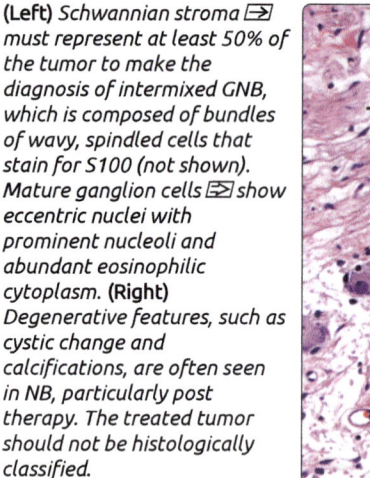

(Left) Schwannian stroma ➡ must represent at least 50% of the tumor to make the diagnosis of intermixed GNB, which is composed of bundles of wavy, spindled cells that stain for S100 (not shown). Mature ganglion cells ➡ show eccentric nuclei with prominent nucleoli and abundant eosinophilic cytoplasm. (Right) Degenerative features, such as cystic change and calcifications, are often seen in NB, particularly post therapy. The treated tumor should not be histologically classified.

Nodular Ganglioneuroblastoma

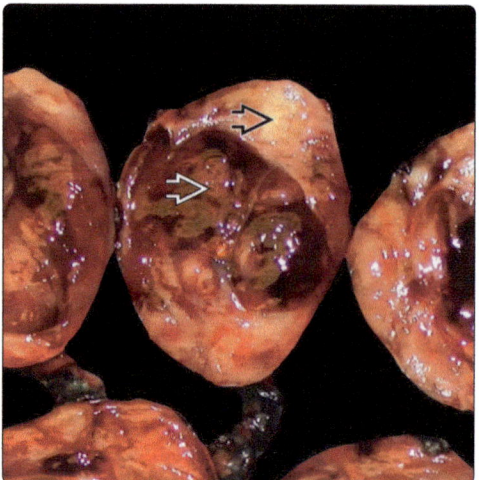

Nodular Ganglioneuroblastoma

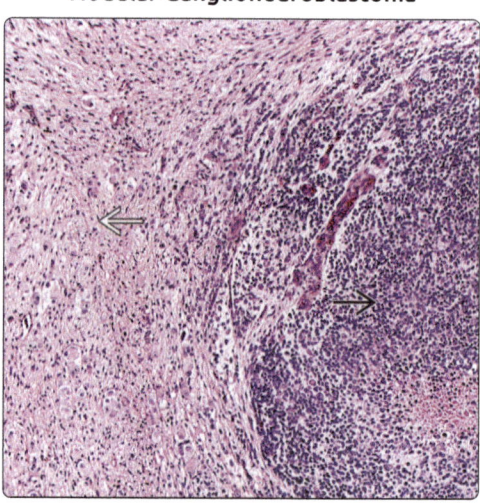

(Left) Typical gross appearance of nodular GNB is shown. The hemorrhagic nodule ➡ represents stroma-poor NB, whereas the tan, fleshy rim ➡ is either ganglioneuroma or intermixed GNB. (From DP: Endocrine.)
(Right) Nodular GNB shows a pushing border between the stroma-poor NB component ➡ and the ganglioneuroma component ➡. Even with this histologic picture, a grossly visible nodule is required to diagnose nodular GNB. (From DP: Endocrine.)

Neuroblastoma

Synaptophysin Expression

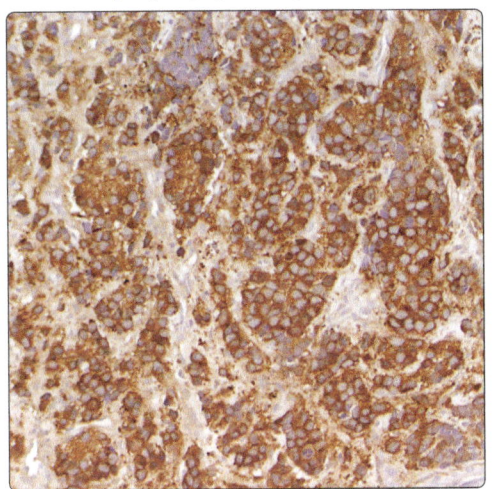

NSE Expression

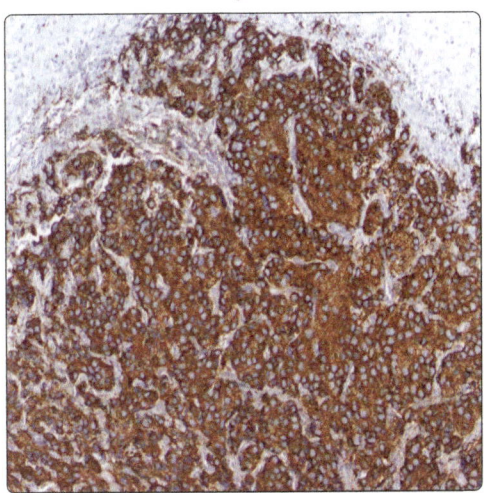

(Left) Synaptophysin shows membranous staining in this poorly differentiated NB. Such immunoreactivity, while nonspecific, is helpful in excluding other childhood small round cell tumors such as lymphoma, Ewing sarcoma, and rhabdomyosarcoma. (Right) NSE is a nonspecific but sensitive test for NB, shown here with strong diffuse cytoplasmic positivity. Other neuroendocrine markers, such as chromogranin and CD56, will also be positive.

ALK1 Expression

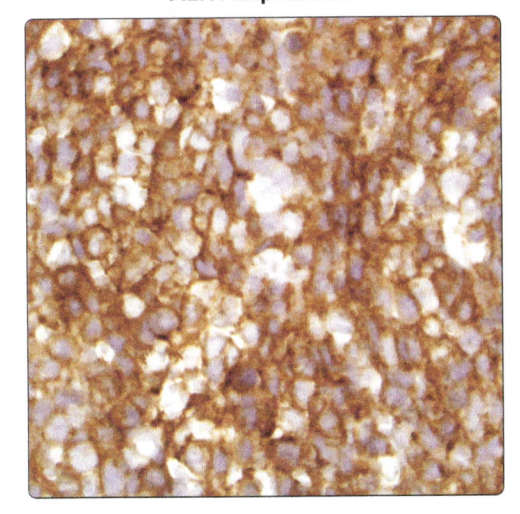

Chromosome 1p Deletion

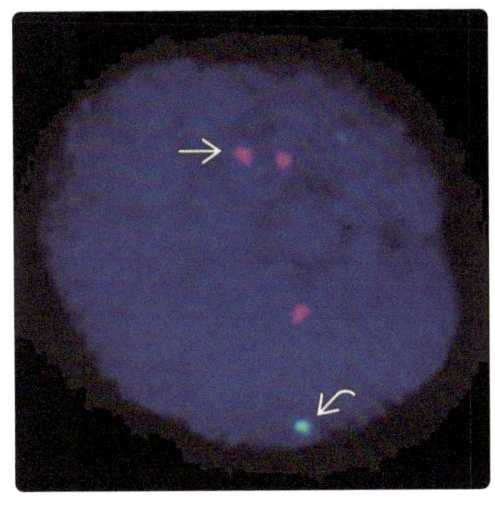

(Left) ALK1 shows strong membranous staining. Activating mutations in the ALK gene have been reported in NB and provide a potential therapeutic target. (From DP: Endocrine.) (Right) Deletion of 1p might be seen in 70-80% of NB. Here, red signals represent chromosome 1 centromere ➡, and green signal represents 1p36 ➡. Only 1 chromosomal copy is present. (From DP: Endocrine.)

Low-Level *MYCN* Amplification

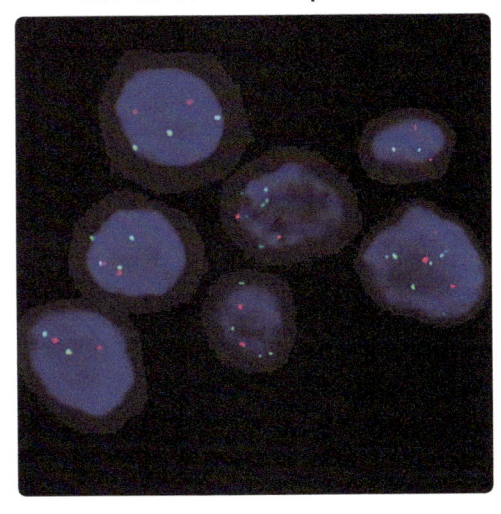

High-Level *MYCN* Amplification

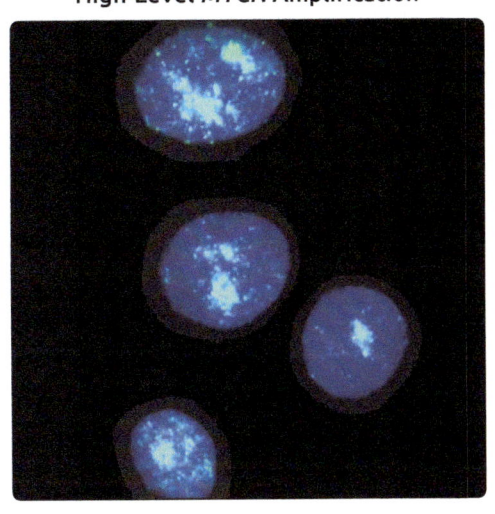

(Left) FISH shows tumor cells with low-level MYCN amplification in this case of NB. The presence of MYCN amplification is associated with poor prognosis and is often present in advanced disease. (From DP: Endocrine.) (Right) FISH shows marked amplification of MYCN (multiple confluent green signals) in this case of NB. (From DP: Endocrine.)

Adrenal Cortical Adenoma

KEY FACTS

TERMINOLOGY
- Benign neoplasm arising from adrenal cortical cells

ETIOLOGY/PATHOGENESIS
- Aldosterone- and cortisol-producing ACA arises from mutations involving ion channel genes or PKA signaling pathway
- Majority are considered sporadic
- Increased incidence in several tumor syndromes

MOLECULAR
- Molecular pathogenesis is poorly understood
- Adrenocortical adenoma and carcinoma share subset of known molecular alterations
- Frequently seen molecular alterations include
  - Somatic mutations in *PRKAR1A*
  - Mutations in *MEN1* and LOH
- Constitutive activation of Wnt/β-catenin pathway
  - Usually caused by mutations in *CTNNB1*

MICROSCOPIC
- Circumscribed lesions comprised of cells with well-defined borders
- Abundant cytoplasm ranges from compact and eosinophilic to foamy and lipid-rich

ANCILLARY TESTS
- Positive for SF1, inhibin, Melan A, and synaptophysin
- Aldosterone-producing ACA positive for CYP11B2
- Negative for chromogranin and weak to negative for cytokeratins
- Germline testing for patients with suspected germline mutation

TOP DIFFERENTIAL DIAGNOSES
- Adrenal cortical carcinoma
- Pheochromocytoma
- Renal cell carcinoma
- Metastatic carcinoma

Gross Appearance

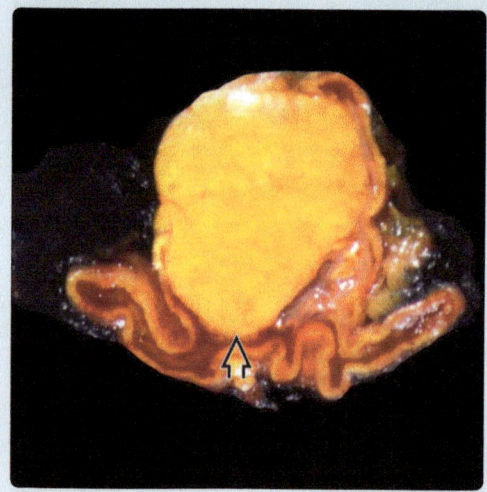

Radiologic Features

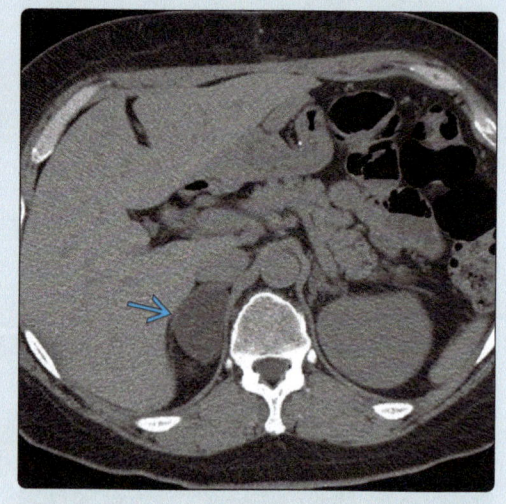

(Left) Adrenal mass shows the classic "canary yellow" color of an aldosterone-secreting adenoma. Another characteristic of these tumors is the pushing borders ➡. (From DP: Endocrine.) (Right) Axial CT in a 60-year-old woman shows a nonfunctioning, 3-cm adrenal cortical adenoma ➡ with low density (< 10 HU). (From DP: Endocrine.)

Interface of Adenoma and Normal Adrenal

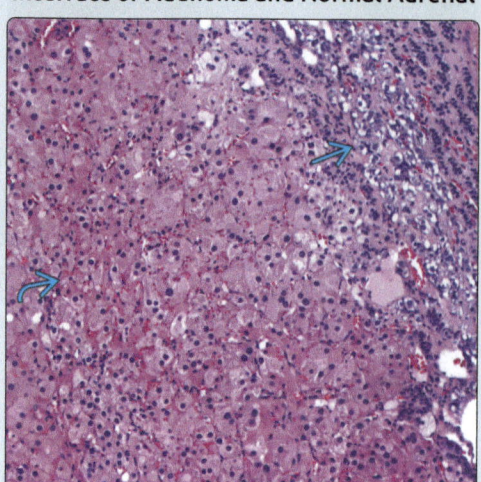

TP53 Mutation

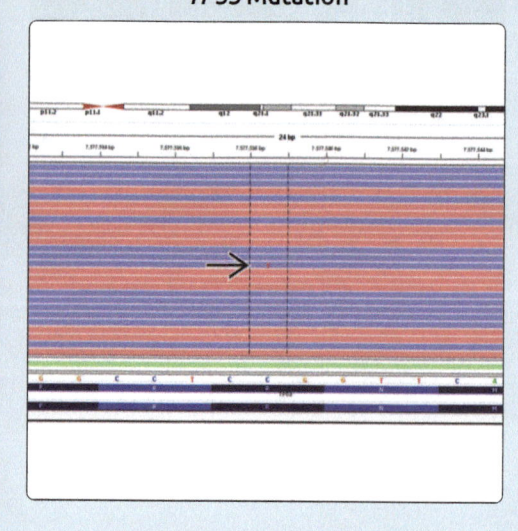

(Left) Low-power view shows the well-defined interface between a sex steroid-producing adenoma ➡ and the surrounding, slightly compressed adrenal gland ➡. The cytologic features of ACA overlap with those of the nonneoplastic adrenal cortex. (Right) NGS analysis of TP53 exon 7 shows c.743 G>A substitution resulting in a TP53 R248Q mutation ➡. (Courtesy H. Qureshi, MD.)

Adrenal Cortical Adenoma

TERMINOLOGY

Abbreviations
- Adrenal cortical adenoma (ACA)

Synonyms
- Adrenocortical adenoma

Definitions
- Benign neoplasm arising from cells of adrenal cortex

ETIOLOGY/PATHOGENESIS

Underlying Cause of ACA
- Aldosterone and cortisol producing ACA arises from mutations involving ion channel genes or PKA signaling pathway
  o Resulting in cell proliferation and excess hormone production
- Majority of adrenal cortical adenomas are sporadic

Subtypes
- Nonfunctional ACA
- Functional ACA
  o Cortisol-producing ACA
  o Aldosterone-producing ACA
  o Sex steroid-producing ACA

Syndrome Associations
- Multiple endocrine neoplasia type 1 (MEN1)
- Carney complex
- Others: Beckwith-Wiedemann syndrome, McCune-Albright syndrome, Congenital adrenal hyperplasia, and Carney triad

CLINICAL ISSUES

Epidemiology
- ACA is most common adrenal cortical tumor
- Present in ~ 1-5 % of general population

Presentation
- ACA can be separated on basis of hormone production
  o Nonfunctional tumors account for ~ 85% of cases
    – No measurable hormone production
    – Sometimes detected incidentally
  o Functional tumors account for ~ 15% of cases
    – Produce hormones, leading to clinical symptoms
- Presentation of functional tumors depends on specific hormone excess
  o Cortisol
    – Cushing syndrome; ~ 10% of cases due to ACA
      □ Protein wasting, striae, skin thinning, diabetes, hypertension, gonadal dysfunction, muscle atrophy, osteoporosis, central obesity, moon facies, and psychiatric disorders
  o Aldosterone
    – Conn syndrome with hypertension and hypokalemia
  o Androgens
    – Virilization in women
    – Excess testosterone in men
    – Precocious puberty in children
  o Estrogens
    – Gynecomastia and testicular atrophy in men
    – Menstrual irregularities, endometrial hyperplasia
    – Precocious puberty in children

Treatment
- Surgical excision via unilateral adrenalectomy

IMAGING

General Features
- Well-defined, homogeneous lesions with smooth borders

CT Findings
- Attenuation values less than normal adrenal tissue
- May enhance after contrast administration

MACROSCOPIC

General Features
- Typically unilateral and solitary
- Average diameter: ~ 3.6 cm (range: 1.5-6.0 cm)
- Cut surfaces are usually yellow or brown
- Darkly pigmented foci are occasionally seen
  o Due to lipofuscin deposition &/or lipid depletion of lesional cells
- Necrosis and cystic change are unusual
- Nonneoplastic adrenal parenchyma often atrophic in cortisol-secreting adenomas

MOLECULAR

In Situ Hybridization
- *CYP11B2* mRNA expression
  o Postoperative ISH analysis may help differentiate unilateral adenoma from bilateral adrenal hyperplasia
    – High *CYP11B2* mRNA expression is typically localized to dominant adrenal nodule in adenoma
    – Patients not cured by adrenalectomy may express *CYP11B1* or *CYP17A1* but typically lack *CYP11B2* mRNA expression
- *CYP11B1::CYP11B2* fusion fusion
  o Can be detected by FISH in familial hyperaldosteronism type 1 (FH1)
  o ~ 1% of primary aldosteronism due to aldosterone-producing adenoma or bilateral adrenal hyperplasia

Molecular Genetics
- Mutations in *KCNJ5, CACNA1D, ATP1A1, ATP2B3*, and *CLCN2* encoding ion channels
  o In > 90% of aldosterone-producing adenomas
  o Mutation disrupts regulation of aldosterone production
- *MEN1*
  o Heterozygous inactivating germline mutation
    – Found in 90% of families with MEN1
    – Adrenocortical tumors &/or hyperplasia found in 25-40% of MEN1 patients
  o Somatic mutation of *MEN1* is very rare in ACA
    – LOH at 11q13.1 can be seen in 20% of ACA
- *TP53*
  o Somatic *TP53* mutations are rare in ACA (0-6%)
  o Certain groups have much higher rates of *TP53* mutation
    – Up to 73% in specific Taiwanese populations with ACA
- *PRKAR1A*

Adrenal Cortical Adenoma

- Somatic mutations seen in ~ 10% of ACA, typical those that secrete cortisol
- Clinical and pathologic characteristics similar to primary pigmented nodular adrenal dysplasia
- Seen in cortisol-secreting adenomas in Carney complex
- PDE11A
  - Inactivating nonsense mutations in PDE11A initially described in micronodular adrenal cortical hyperplasia
  - Less deleterious germline mutations may play role in genetic predisposition to development of ACA
- Constitutive activation of Wnt/β-catenin pathway
  - Seen in both ACA and adrenal cortical carcinoma
    - Usually caused by mutations in CTNNB1 that encodes β-catenin
  - Seen in ~ 27% of adenomas

MICROSCOPIC

Histologic Features
- Usually unencapsulated with circumscribed pushing border
- Several architectural patterns including nests, cords, pseudoglandular, and solid areas
- Distinct cell borders mimicking cells of nonneoplastic adrenal cortical cells
- May have areas of lipomatous or myelolipomatous metaplasia
- Mitotic figures are uncommon; no atypical mitoses
- Degenerative changes may be seen (calcification, fibrosis, focal cystic change)
- Mixture of cells with pale, lipid-rich cytoplasm and cells with lipid-poor, compact cytoplasm
- Specific features of functional adenomas
  - Aldosterone-producing adenomas: Abundant, lipid-rich, microvesicular cytoplasm, mimicking cells of zona fasciculata
  - Cortisol-producing adenomas: Cytoplasmic lipofuscin pigment and varying amounts of lipid
  - Sex steroid-producing adenomas: Compact, eosinophilic cytoplasm mimicking cells of zona reticularis

Cytologic Features
- Cells usually larger than those of nonneoplastic adrenal, sometimes with increased levels of pleomorphism ("endocrine atypia")
- Abundant clear to eosinophilic cytoplasm, often finely vacuolated due to intracytoplasmic lipid accumulation
- Nuclei are generally single, round to oval, with relatively prominent nucleoli
  - Intranuclear cytoplasmic inclusions are frequently seen

ANCILLARY TESTS

Immunohistochemistry
- Positive for SF1, inhibin, Melan A, and synaptophysin
- Aldosterone-producing ACA positive for CYP11B2
- Negative for chromogranin
- Weak or negative for cytokeratins

Genetic Testing
- Germline testing for patients with suspected germline mutation

DIFFERENTIAL DIAGNOSIS

Adrenal Cortical Carcinoma
- Multiple classification systems are used to distinguish benign from malignant adrenocortical tumors (Hough, Weiss, van Slooten)
- Histologic features suggestive of malignancy
  - High-grade cytology
  - Increased mitotic activity (> 5/50 HPF), atypical mitoses
  - Confluent tumor necrosis
  - Lymphovascular and capsular invasion
  - Diffuse architecture in > 1/3 of tumor

Pheochromocytoma
- Positive for chromogranin and INSM1, negative for inhibin and Melan A
- S100(+) sustentacular cells highlight zellballen pattern

DIAGNOSTIC CHECKLIST

2022 WHO Classification ACA Pathological Correlates
- Characterized by different histologic, pathogenetic, and clinical presentation
  - Cortisol and APA are most frequent functional correlates of ACA
- APA cytomorphological features are reflected in their genotype-phenotype correlations
  - KCNJ5-mutant APA enriched in zona fasciculata like clear cells and have yellow gross appearance
  - KCNJ5-wildtype tumors are enriched in lipid-poor cells, zona reticularis-like
- WHO recommends CYP11B2 immunohistochemistry for all adrenalectomy specimens from patients with primary aldosteronism to distinguish between unilateral and bilateral disease
- Nonfunctioning ACA does not show characteristic histologic features
- ACA lacks morphologic features of malignancy
  - Endocrine atypia should not be mistaken for nuclear atypia
  - Predominant myxoid change or large size may indicate malignancy
- Nontumorous cortical atrophy is characteristic gross and microscopic feature of cortisol-secreting ACA
- Pigmented "black" ACA composed of tumor cells with lipofuscin pigment deposition
  - May show mild autonomous cortisol secretion
- Oncocytic ACA
  - Have characteristic mahogany brown appearance
  - Adrenal cortical origin should always be confirmed in
    - All nonfunctional adrenal lesions
    - ACA with oncocytic features to prevent clinically relevant misinterpretation

SELECTED REFERENCES

1. Erickson LA et al: Adrenal cortical adenoma. In: WHO Classification of Tumours Editorial Board. Endocrine and neuroendocrine tumours. IARC, 2022
2. Mete O et al: Overview of the 2022 WHO Classification of Adrenal Cortical Tumors. Endocr Pathol. 33(1):155-96, 2022
3. Altieri B et al: Adrenocortical incidentalomas and bone: from molecular insights to clinical perspectives. Endocrine. 62(3):506-16, 2018

Adrenal Cortical Adenoma

Adrenal Cortical Adenoma/Normal Adrenal Interface

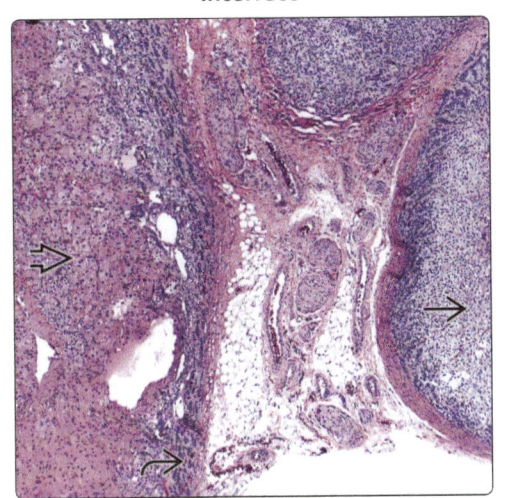

Cortisol-Producing Adrenal Cortical Adenoma

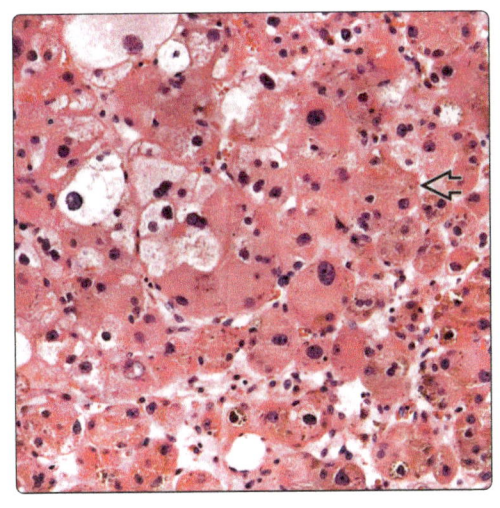

(Left) Low-power view shows the well-defined interface between a sex steroid-producing adenoma ⇒ and the surrounding adrenal gland ⇒. Additional compressed nonneoplastic adrenal parenchyma is seen at the tumor periphery ⇒. (Right) Tumor cells in cortisol-producing adrenal adenomas are arranged in a solid pattern with cytoplasmic lipofuscin pigment ⇒, a gradation in cell size, and a varying amount of lipid. (From DP: Endocrine.)

Mineralocorticoid-Producing Adrenal Cortical Adenoma

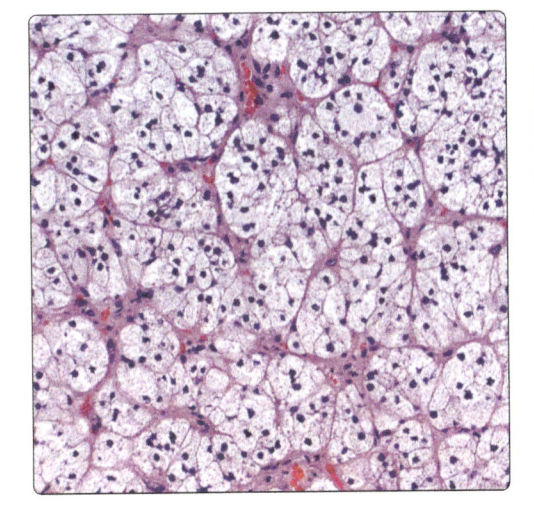

Sex Steroid-Producing Adrenal Cortical Adenoma

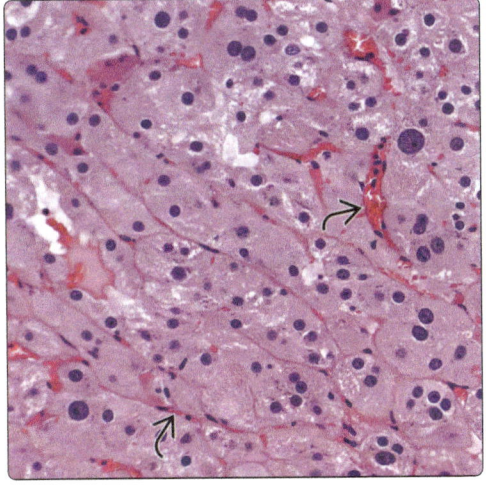

(Left) Mineralocorticoid-producing adrenal cortical adenomas have cells arranged in nests and cords, often with characteristic microvesicular, lipid-rich cytoplasm, which mimics the adrenal zona fasciculata. This gives the tumor its characteristic bright yellow color. (Right) Sex steroid-producing adenomas often show compact eosinophilic cytoplasm resembling that seen in the zona reticularis. The cells are arranged in a trabecular pattern, separated by delicate fibrovascular septa ⇒.

Adrenal Cortical Adenoma With Atypia

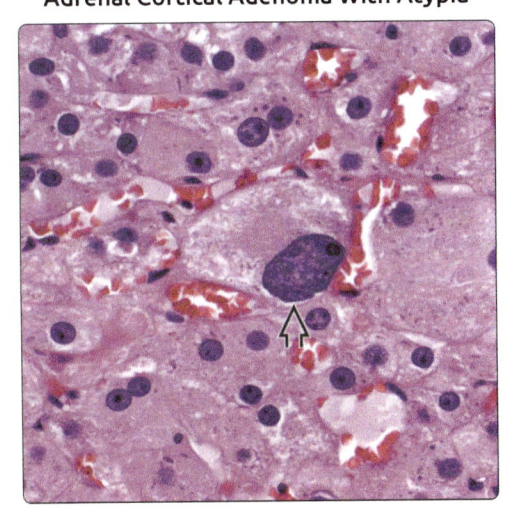

Adrenal Cortical Adenoma With Lipomatous Metaplasia

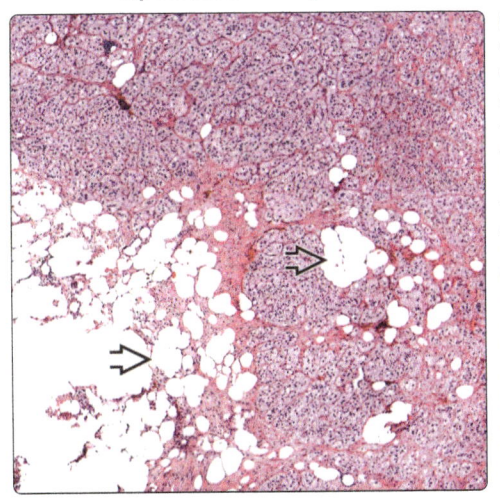

(Left) ACAs can show foci of cytologic atypia, demonstrated here by marked nuclear enlargement, a large nucleolus, and mild nuclear membrane irregularities ⇒. This "endocrine atypia" does not signify malignant potential in a lesion with otherwise benign features. (Right) ACA shows intimately admixed adipose tissue. This is lipomatous metaplasia ⇒, a benign feature of some adenomas, which should not be misinterpreted as extraadrenal extension. (From DP: Endocrine.)

Prostatic Adenocarcinoma, Acinar Type and High-Grade Prostatic Intraepithelial Neoplasia

KEY FACTS

TERMINOLOGY
- Prostatic adenocarcinoma, acinar type (PCa)

ETIOLOGY/PATHOGENESIS
- Combination of genetic and environmental factors

CLINICAL ISSUES
- Most frequent noncutaneous malignancy in men, 2nd most common cause of cancer deaths among men in USA
- Heterogeneous disease with highly variable clinical course

MOLECULAR
- *TMPRSS2* fusion with member of ETS transcription factor family in ~ 50% of cases
- ETS fusion-positive tumors appear biologically distinct from ETS-negative PCas
- Mutations in *SPOP*, *FLI1*, *FOXA1*, and *IDH1* mutually exclusive with ETS rearrangement and with each other
- *SPOP* mutations and *CHD1* deletions may be driver mutations in ETS-negative tumors
- Alterations in androgen receptor gene and pathway in hormone-refractory PCa
- Chromothripsis and chromoplexy common
- Other genetic alterations common in *MYC*, *PTEN*, *TP53*, and *NKX3-1*
- Alterations in PI3K-AKT-mTOR pathway more common in advanced tumors
- *PCA3* overexpressed in > 90% of prostate cancers
- Epigenetic changes common with hypermethylation of many genes, including *GSTP1*
- Mutations in DNA repair genes involved in homologous recombination repair or in mismatch repair in up to 20% of metastatic carcinomas

ANCILLARY TESTS
- NKX3.1, prostein, PSA, PSAP, and AMACR positive
- Invasive carcinoma lacks staining for basal cell markers p63, CK5, and 34βE12

High-Grade Prostatic Intraepithelial Neoplasia

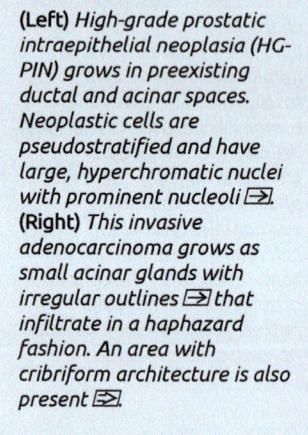

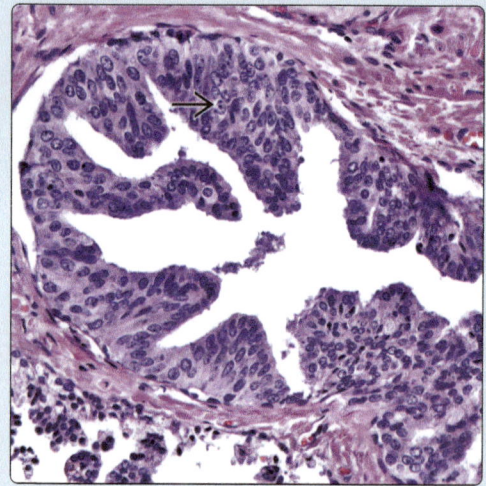

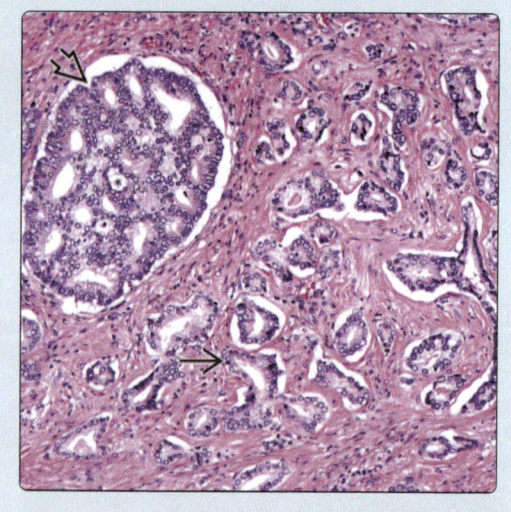

(Left) *High-grade prostatic intraepithelial neoplasia (HG-PIN) grows in preexisting ductal and acinar spaces. Neoplastic cells are pseudostratified and have large, hyperchromatic nuclei with prominent nucleoli ➡.* (Right) *This invasive adenocarcinoma grows as small acinar glands with irregular outlines ➡ that infiltrate in a haphazard fashion. An area with cribriform architecture is also present ➡.*

Invasive Acinar Adenocarcinoma

Invasive Acinar Adenocarcinoma

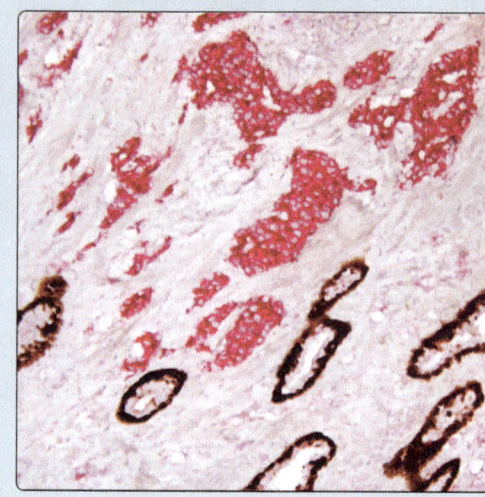

(Left) *Malignant glands of Gleason pattern 3 prostatic acinar adenocarcinoma ➡ are seen infiltrating between normal, benign glands ➡.* (Right) *Triple IHC stain for AMACR/p63/CK5 in the same case shows strong expression of AMACR by the invasive carcinoma (red staining). Normal, benign glands are highlighted by the p63/CK5-positive basal cell layer (brown staining) that is absent in the malignant glands.*

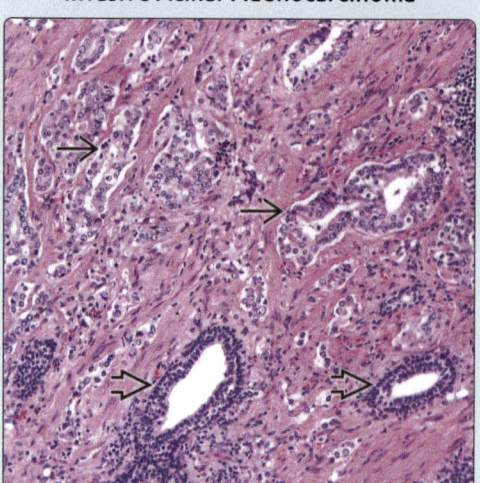

Triple IHC for AMACR/p63/CK5

Prostatic Adenocarcinoma, Acinar Type and High-Grade Prostatic Intraepithelial Neoplasia

TERMINOLOGY

Abbreviations
- Prostatic adenocarcinoma, acinar type (PCa)
- High-grade prostatic intraepithelial neoplasia (HG-PIN)

Definitions
- Acinar adenocarcinoma
  o Malignant neoplasm of prostatic epithelial origin
- HG-PIN
  o Noninvasive epithelial proliferation in preexisting acini and ducts with neoplastic cytologic features

ETIOLOGY/PATHOGENESIS

Etiologic and Pathogenetic Factors
- Acinar adenocarcinoma
  o Combination of genetic and environmental factors
  o Well-documented familial association
  o Role of infection &/or inflammation remains unclear
- HG-PIN
  o Commonly associated with invasive PCa
  o Shares multiple molecular genetic abnormalities with invasive carcinoma

CLINICAL ISSUES

Epidemiology
- Acinar adenocarcinoma
  o Most frequent noncutaneous malignancy in men
  o 2nd most common cause of cancer deaths among men in USA

Laboratory Tests
- Acinar adenocarcinoma
  o Serum PSA screening remains 1st-line biomarker
    – Lacks high sensitivity and specificity
    – Leads to overdetection of indolent disease and may lead to overtreatment in many cases
  o PSA indices include free PSA, PSA density, and PSA velocity

Treatment
- Acinar adenocarcinoma
  o Active surveillance (watchful waiting) with repeat biopsy in patients with low-grade, low-volume disease
  o Radical prostatectomy
  o Brachytherapy or external beam radiation
  o Androgen-deprivation therapy for systemic disease
    – Bilateral orchiectomy, luteinizing hormone-releasing hormone (LHRH) agonists, antiandrogens, or LHRH antagonists
  o Docetaxel or cabazitaxel chemotherapy
  o Palliative transurethral resection to relieve obstructive symptoms

Prognosis
- Acinar adenocarcinoma
  o Heterogeneous disease with highly variable clinical course
    – Many patients have indolent disease that will not threaten their health during lifetime
    – Other patients have aggressive disease with progression and metastases
  o Established prognostic factors
    – Preoperative serum PSA levels, histologic grade (Gleason score, grade group), tumor volume, pathologic stage, surgical margin status
  o Prognosis of hormone-refractory prostate cancer is poor with survival ~ 1 year
  o Development of new prognostic and predictive markers is major goal of ongoing research

Risk Factors
- Acinar adenocarcinoma
  o Positive family history
  o Risk low < age 50, rises steeply with older age
  o Ethnicity: Risk higher in Black populations with greater mortality, lower in Asian populations

MOLECULAR

Molecular Genetics
- Acinar adenocarcinoma
  o Fusion of androgen-regulated *TMPRSS2* with member of ETS family of transcription factors, including *ERG* or, less commonly, *ETV1*, *ETV4*, *ETV5*, and *FLI1*
    – Detected in ~ 50% of cases
    – *TMPRSS2::ERG* fusion by far most common, leads to ERG protein overexpression
    – Gene fusions detectable by break-apart FISH assay
    – ETS family fusion-positive tumors appear biologically distinct from ETS-negative PCa
    – ETS-positive tumors are enriched in mutations or deletions of *PTEN* and *TP53*
  o Mutations in *SPOP*, *FLI1*, *FOXA1*, *IDH1* mutually exclusive with ETS rearrangement and with each other
  o *SPOP* mutations detected in 5-15% of primary PCa
    – Mutually exclusive with *TP53* and *PTEN* alterations
    – *SPOP*-mutant tumors show distinct pattern of genomic alteration, specifically deletions of *CHD1*
    – *SPOP*-mutant tumors lack alterations in PI3K pathway
  o *CHD1* deletions in 10-25% of PCa
  o *SPOP* mutations and *CHD1* deletions may be driver mutations in ETS-negative tumors
  o *SPINK1* overexpression in ~ 10% of ETS-negative tumors, associated with aggressive disease
  o Other molecular genetic abnormalities
    – Alterations in androgen receptor gene (*AR*) and pathway in hormone-refractory PCas include *AR* amplification (~ 40%), point mutations (~ 10%), and splice variants
      □ Typically absent in clinically localized cancers but emerge during androgen-deprivation therapy
      □ If *AR* is not altered, genes that modulate AR function may be dysregulated
    – Chromothripsis (shattering and subsequent complex rearrangement of chromosomes) found in 20-23% of clinically significant PCa
    – Chromoplexy (balanced interweaving of interchromosomal translocations) in 50% of PCa
    – Loss of *PTEN* by deletion or mutation in ~ 40% of primary PCa, associated with higher Gleason score and poor prognosis

Prostatic Adenocarcinoma, Acinar Type and High-Grade Prostatic Intraepithelial Neoplasia

- *PTEN* genomic deletions and inactivating mutations
- *TP53* point mutations in up to 40%, deletions in 25-40% of PCa
- *TP53* alterations in 25-30% of clinically localized PCa, suggesting they are not exclusively late events
- *MYC* is commonly amplified &/or overexpressed
- *NKX3-1* deleted in 10-40% of cases
- Recurrent mutations in *FOXA1*, *CUL3*, *IDH1* found in < 10% of cases
- Amplification of *PIK3CA* in ~ 25% of PCa
  □ Alterations in PI3K-AKT-mTOR pathway more common in metastatic &/or hormone-refractory cases
- Genomic alterations in WNT/β-catenin pathway in ~ 10%
- RAS-RAF-MAPK signaling pathway alterations in ~ 5%
- Allelic loss of *NKX3-1* tumor suppressor gene
- Loss of *CDKN1B* associated with poor prognosis
- *PCA3* overexpressed in > 90% of PCa but not expressed in benign prostate
- *EZH2* has critical role in chromatin regulation, is overexpressed in PCa, associated with aggressive disease
- Epigenetic changes common with hypermethylation of many genes, including *GSTP1*
  □ Recurrent mutations in epigenetic regulators and chromatin remodelers
- Genome-wide association studies identified > 100 PCa susceptibility loci
- Germline or somatic mutations in DNA repair genes involved in homologous recombination repair (HRR) or in mismatch repair found in up to 20% of metastatic carcinomas
  □ HRR defects may be associated with sensitivity to poly (ADP-ribose) polymerase (PARP) inhibitors
  □ DNA mismatch repair defects may be associated with sensitivity to immune checkpoint inhibitors
  □ Germline &/or somatic testing for DNA repair defects recommended for aggressive primary and for metastatic tumors
  □ Most common actionable mutations in DNA repair genes in *BRCA2*, *ATM*, *CHEK2*, and *BRCA1*
- **HG-PIN**
  o *TMPRSS2* fusion with member of ETS transcription factor family detected in ~ 20%
  o *SPOP* mutations found in ETS-negative cases
  o *MYC* overexpression common

MICROSCOPIC

Histologic Features

- **Acinar adenocarcinoma**
  o Typically located in peripheral zone
  o Multifocal growth common
  o Architectural features
    - Haphazard growth of crowded acinar glands
    - Infiltrative pattern often with irregular gland outlines and sharp luminal borders
    - Basal cell layer absent
  - Characteristic but not diagnostic features include luminal blue mucin, pink amorphous luminal secretions, bright eosinophilic crystalloids
  - Features diagnostic of carcinoma are perineural invasion, mucinous fibroplasia, and glomerulations
  o Cytologic features
    - Amphophilic cytoplasm, nuclear enlargement with nuclear overlap, prominent nucleoli
  o Gleason grading system based on architectural features
    - Grade of primary and secondary patterns added to obtain Gleason score
  o Gleason patterns 1 and 2 rare
  o Gleason pattern 3
    - Small acinar glands infiltrate haphazardly between normal glands
    - Invasive glands vary in size and shape, often have angular shapes
  o Gleason pattern 4
    - Poorly defined fused glands, cribriform fused glands, or glomeruloid architecture
  o Gleason pattern 5
    - Absence of glandular lumina; grows as solid sheets, strands, or single cells
  o Grade groups 1-5 are reported in conjunction with Gleason scores
  o Histologic variants include foamy gland variant, mucinous (colloid), signet-ring cell, atrophic, and pseudohyperplastic
- **HG-PIN**
  o Acini and ducts lined by cells with neoplastic cytologic features
    - Enlarged, hyperchromatic nuclei with coarse chromatin and prominent nucleoli
  o 4 architectural patterns
    - Flat, tufting, micropapillary, and cribriform

ANCILLARY TESTS

Immunohistochemistry

- **Acinar adenocarcinoma**
  o NKX3.1, prostein (P501S), PSA, PSAP, AMACR (P504S), and MYC positive; subset positive for ERG or SPINK1
  o Absent staining for basal cell markers p63, CK5, and 34βE12 (CK903)
- **HG-PIN**
  o Luminal cells positive for AMACR (P504S) and MYC
  o Basal cells positive for p63, CK5, and 34βE12 (CK903)

SELECTED REFERENCES

1. Kulac I et al: Molecular pathology of prostate cancer. Surg Pathol Clin. 14(3):387-401, 2021
2. Sokolova AO et al: Genetic contribution to metastatic prostate cancer. Urol Clin North Am. 48(3):349-63, 2021
3. Vlajnic T et al: Molecular pathology of prostate cancer: a practical approach. Pathology. 53(1):36-43, 2021
4. Lotan TL et al: Report from the International Society of Urological Pathology (ISUP) Consultation Conference on Molecular Pathology of Urogenital Cancers. I. Molecular Biomarkers in Prostate Cancer. Am J Surg Pathol. 44(7):e15-29, 2020
5. Armenia J et al: The long tail of oncogenic drivers in prostate cancer. Nat Genet. 50(5):645-51, 2018
6. Espiritu SMG et al: The evolutionary landscape of localized prostate cancers drives clinical aggression. Cell. 173(4):1003-13.e15, 2018

Prostatic Adenocarcinoma, Acinar Type and High-Grade Prostatic Intraepithelial Neoplasia

High-Grade Prostatic Intraepithelial Neoplasia

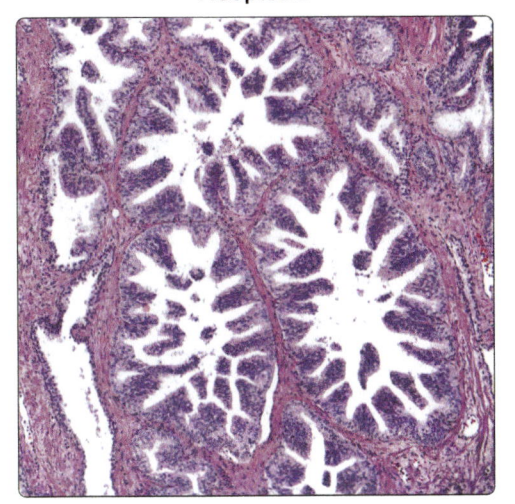

Triple IHC for AMACR/p63/CK5

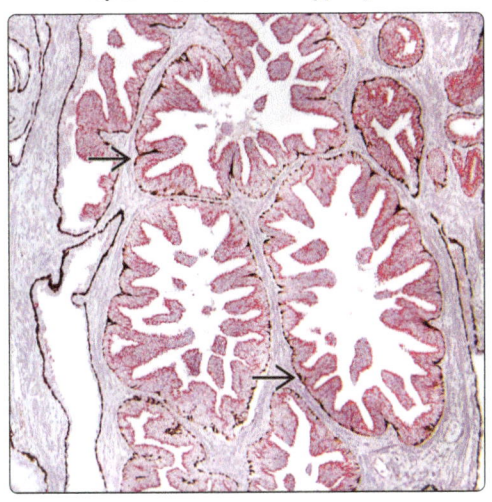

(Left) HG-PIN often stands out from the surrounding normal parenchyma with its micropapillary architecture. Neoplastic cells have a high nuclear:cytoplasmic ratio and hyperchromatic nuclei. (Right) In HG-PIN, triple IHC stain for AMACR/p63/CK5 typically labels the neoplastic cells red due to AMACR expression. The brown staining highlights the preserved basal cells that express CK5 and p63 ⇥.

Invasive Adenocarcinoma, Gleason Grade 5

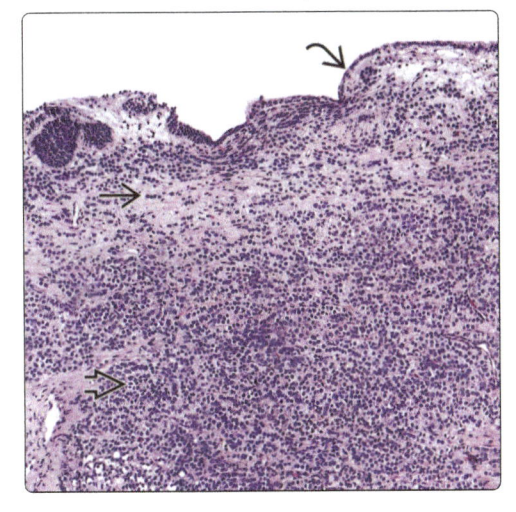

P501S Immunohistochemistry

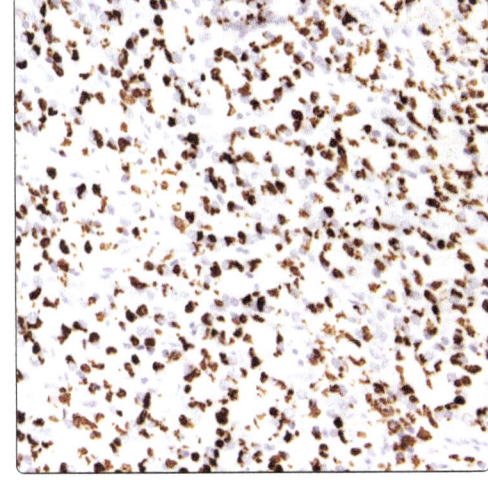

(Left) Poorly differentiated prostatic acinar adenocarcinoma grows as solid sheets ⇥ and in single files ⇥ without visible gland formation (Gleason pattern 5). This tumor is from a transurethral resection specimen that has a urothelial lining ⇥. (Right) Prostein (P501S) confirms the prostatic origin of this poorly differentiated carcinoma and can be helpful in identifying the origin of locally advanced or metastatic tumors.

PSA Immunohistochemistry

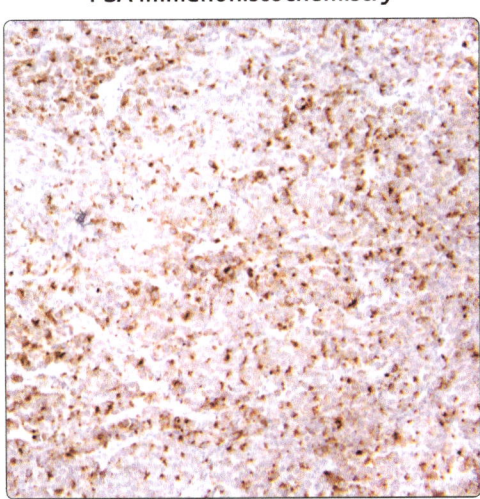

NKX3.1 Immunohistochemistry

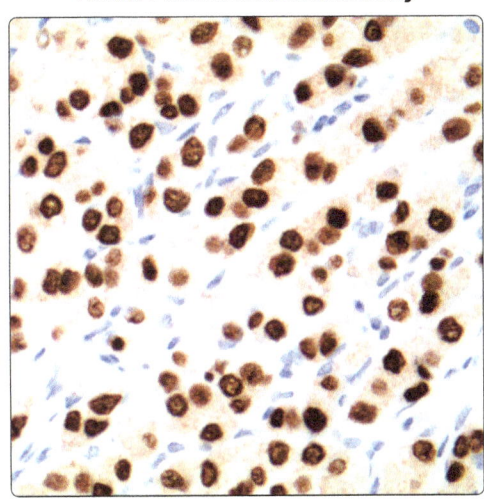

(Left) PSA is a widely used, sensitive and specific marker for prostatic adenocarcinoma but may be negative in a subset of high-grade carcinomas. (Right) NKX3.1 marks the nuclei of prostatic adenocarcinoma. This marker is often expressed in high-grade carcinomas that may be negative for PSA.

ADH and DCIS (Dysplastic, Premalignant)

KEY FACTS

ETIOLOGY/PATHOGENESIS

- Atypical ductal hyperplasia (ADH) likely represents early stage in low-grade breast neoplasia pathway
  - Increased risk of invasive and in situ carcinoma in both breasts
  - Flat epithelial atypia (FEA) and ADH have some of same genetic changes found in low-grade ductal carcinoma in situ (LGDCIS)
  - Genetic changes shared by other members of "low-grade breast epithelial neoplasia" family
- FEA and ADH may be precursors of low- to intermediate-grade DCIS

MOLECULAR

- Accumulating data suggest that FEA, ADH, and LGDCIS represent evolutionary continuum
  - Shared alterations include gains of 1q, loss of 16q
  - Losses at 16q particularly frequent in ADH and most frequent change shared with LGDCIS
- Distinctive patterns of genomic alterations in DCIS associated with tumor grade
  - LGDCIS: Frequent loss of 16q
  - High-grade DCIS: Complex genomic alterations; 13q loss and high-level amplification of 17q12 and 11q13
  - Genetic events and molecular changes necessary for transition to invasive carcinoma not yet understood
- ADH and LGDCIS have similar patterns of gene expression
  - Dominated by ER and ER-regulated genes
- Majority of DCIS strongly expresses ER (~ 80%)
  - Increased ER expression likely plays role in disease progression
- Overexpression of ERBB2 in DCIS associated with high grade, presence of central necrosis
- ERBB2 overexpression, absence of ER and PR, accumulation of TP53, and high Ki-67 expression strong predictors of local recurrence for DCIS
- Genetic events and molecular changes necessary for transition to invasive carcinoma not yet understood

---

Atypical Ductal Hyperplasia

Low-Grade Ductal Carcinoma In Situ

(Left) *Atypical ductal hyperplasia (ADH) is a clonal proliferation of luminal-type cells involving ducts and lobules. ADH has some (but not all) features of low-grade ductal carcinoma in situ (LGDCIS). Lesions are often detected due to calcifications ⇉.* (Right) *LGDCIS is also a clonal process. The involved duct spaces are widely distended by a monotonous proliferation showing low-grade atypia and architectural complexity with punched-out cribriform spaces ⇉.*

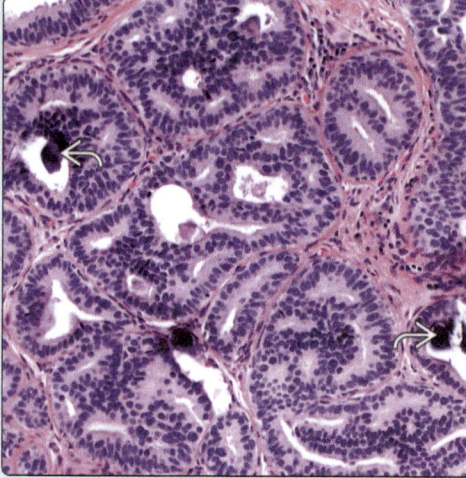

Mammary Carcinoma In Situ, Mixed Histology (Ductal and Lobular)

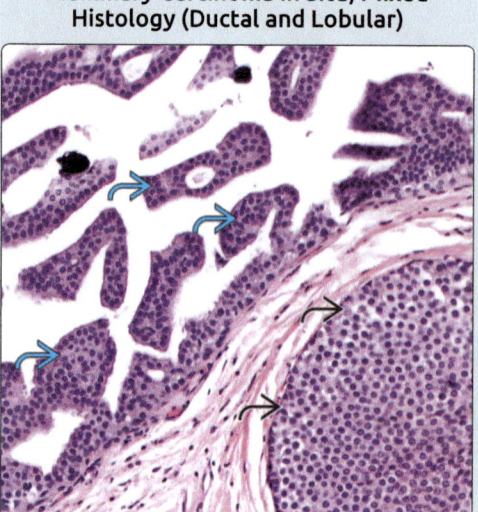

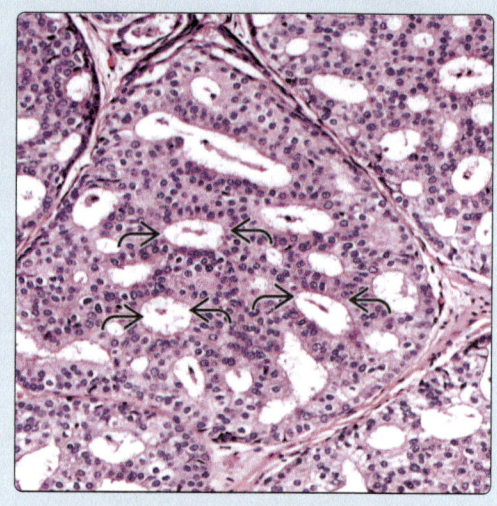

Variant-Type Lobular Carcinoma In Situ With Central Necrosis

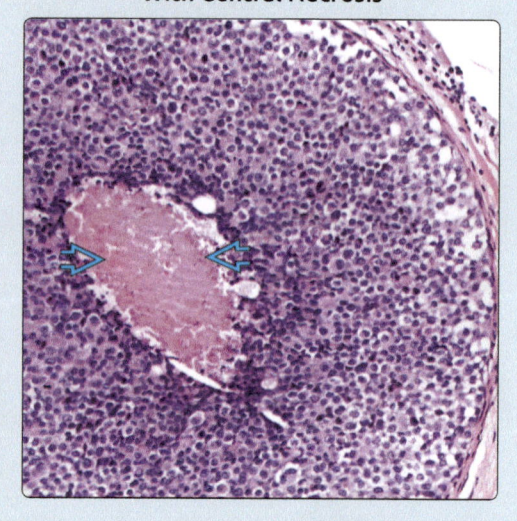

(Left) *Rarely, in situ breast cancers can show a mixed histology. The lesion shown here contains LGDCIS with a micropapillary pattern ⇉ as well as classic lobular carcinoma in situ (LCIS) ⇉.* (Right) *Variant types of LCIS are rare (< 5% of in situ lesions), and these lesions were likely classified as DCIS in the past. This case of LCIS shows central necrosis ⇉, which may show calcifications and mimic LGDCIS. Demonstrating the loss of E-cadherin expression is useful diagnostically.*

ADH and DCIS (Dysplastic, Premalignant)

TERMINOLOGY

Abbreviations
- Atypical ductal hyperplasia (ADH)
- Ductal carcinoma in situ (DCIS)
  - Low-grade DCIS (LGDCIS)
  - High-grade DCIS (HGDCIS)

Definitions
- ADH
  - Clonal intraductal proliferation with architectural and cytologic features approaching those seen in LGDCIS
    - Monotonous, uniform, evenly placed epithelial cells involving terminal-ductal lobular units
  - Associated with increased risk of developing invasive carcinoma in either breast
- DCIS
  - Clonal proliferation of cells confined to ducts and lobules with cohesive pattern that is E-cadherin positive
  - "Ductal" used as descriptor because involved spaces are generally large and resemble ducts
    - DCIS has expansile growth pattern causing lobules to unfold and form larger spaces
    - DCIS can be classified based on architectural patterns and nuclear grade of proliferating neoplastic cells

ETIOLOGY/PATHOGENESIS

ADH as Nonobligate Precursor
- ADH likely represents early stage in low-grade breast neoplasia pathway
  - Normal ductal epithelium composed of mixture of luminal and basal cells
  - ADH is clonal expansion of luminal compartment with nuclear &/or architectural atypia
  - Increased bilateral risk of invasive and in situ carcinoma
  - Often seen associated with LGDCIS and low-grade invasive ductal carcinoma (IDC)
- Majority of ADH does not progress to carcinoma
  - ADH associated with up to 30% lifetime risk of metachronous breast cancer
  - Factors responsible for progression from ADH to LGDCIS &/or possibly HGDCIS poorly understood
  - Active surveillance &/or endocrine therapy may be used to reduce risk of invasive breast cancer
  - Current guidelines support use of endocrine therapy for ER(+) DCIS

DCIS as Precursor Lesion
- LGDCIS considered precursor of low-grade invasive carcinoma; risk primarily in ipsilateral breast
- Precursor lesion for HGDCIS less clear
  - HGDCIS shows marked inter- and intratumoral heterogeneity; most likely part of distinct and separate pathway to neoplasia
- DCIS microenvironment
  - Cell types within DCIS microenvironment genetically and phenotypically altered compared to normal tissue
    - May play role in progression of DCIS to IDC
  - Immune microenvironment is important modulator of tumor progression
  - Assessment of tumor-infiltrating lymphocytes (TILs) provides prognostic and predictive information in IDC
  - Most DCIS show TILs prevalence of < 5%
  - DCIS with high TILs prevalence associated with larger size, higher nuclear grade, HER2(+), and high Ki-67
  - DCIS with high TILs prevalence have significant increased cumulative ipsilateral breast events compared with low TILs

Breast Neoplasia Pathways
- Model for breast cancer progression proposes independent low-grade and high-grade neoplastic pathways
  - LGDCIS progresses to low-grade and HGDCIS progresses to high-grade invasive cancer, respectively
- ADH has been considered general risk indicator and precursor of low-grade breast cancer pathway
  - Molecular studies looking at copy number alterations suggest that ADH may be multipotent with possible progression to either low- or high-grade carcinomas

CLINICAL ISSUES

Prognosis
- ADH
  - Marker of increased risk for developing invasive carcinoma (nonobligate precursor)
    - Associated with 4-5x increased relative risk or 13-17% lifetime risk of invasive carcinoma
    - Some (but not all) studies show increased risk for women with positive family history
    - Cancer risk is bilateral (~ 2:1 ratio of ipsilateral and contralateral)
  - Younger age at diagnosis of ADH significantly increases relative and absolute risk for breast cancer
- DCIS
  - Significant increase in diagnosis of DCIS due to uptake of mammography screening
  - Untreated DCIS has 8-10x increased relative risk of developing invasive carcinoma
    - Corresponds to ~ 1% of patients per year (or ~ 20-30% with invasive carcinoma at 20-30 years)
  - Risk of developing invasive carcinoma modified by treatment, including
    - Complete surgical excision with negative margins
    - Adjuvant radiation therapy &/or hormonal therapy
      - Reduces risk of recurrence to < 10%
- 5-10% of treated DCIS will develop subsequent IDC
  - Genomic analyses have shown that, in 75% of cases, invasive recurrence is clonally related to initial DCIS
    - 18% were clonally unrelated to DCIS (new independent lineage), and 7% were ambiguous

MOLECULAR

Molecular Overview
- Genomic technologies have made major contributions to defining subtypes of breast cancer
  - Molecular studies suggest that most dramatic transcriptome changes occur at transition from normal epithelium to DCIS
  - Genotypic analysis demonstrates that molecular heterogeneity already established in in situ lesions

ADH and DCIS (Dysplastic, Premalignant)

- Same chromosomal regions amplified with comparable frequencies in DCIS as in invasive disease
- High-tumor grade and presence of necrosis associated with greater gene expression variability and distinct transcriptional signatures
- Molecular profiling and histologic observations can help improve risk stratification for DCIS
  - Most preinvasive and invasive disease can be stratified into low- or high-grade molecular pathway

Chromosomal Microarray

- CGH-based studies support classic linear model of neoplastic progression in breast cancer
  - ADH can give rise to LGDCIS, which, in turn, is direct precursor to low-grade invasive carcinoma
  - Data support concept that early neoplastic stage of LGDCIS is direct precursor to invasive carcinoma
- Breast cancer progression may consist of several genetically distinct linear pathways, correlate with tumor grade

Molecular Genetics

- **ADH**
  - Accumulating data suggest that FEA, ADH, and LGDCIS represent evolutionary continuum
    - ADH has protein expression patterns supporting that it is clonal process
      - Diffuse expression of low molecular weight (luminal) cytokeratins and absences of high molecular weight (basal) cytokeratins
      - Diffuse expression of hormone receptors
    - Shared genomic alterations occur in ADH, LGDCIS, and invasive carcinoma from same breast
      - Shared alterations include gains of 1q, loss of 16q
    - Losses at 16q particularly frequent in ADH and most frequent change shared with LGDCIS
    - Loss of heterozygosity at 17p and 11q13 reported
- **DCIS**
  - Accumulating data suggest that DCIS, like invasive carcinoma, consists of 2 distinct genetic pathways
    - Nearly identical genetic changes found in DCIS found in synchronous and metachronous invasive carcinoma
    - Increased numbers of genomic changes correlate with increased nuclear grade
    - Genetic changes in LGDCIS and HGDCIS parallel changes seen in their invasive counterparts
      - Consistent with different molecular pathways (low and high grade) in breast neoplasia
    - Supporting direct precursor relationship between LGDCIS and HGDCIS and invasive carcinoma
  - Distinctive patterns of genomic alterations in DCIS seen and associated with tumor grade
    - LGDCIS: Frequent loss of 16q and 1q and overexpression of ER and PR
      - Lesions of this subgroup have been referred to as luminal
    - HGDCIS: Complex genomic alterations, including 13q loss and high-level amplification of 17q12 and 11q13
  - Genetic events and molecular changes necessary for transition to invasive carcinoma not yet understood
    - Identification of molecular mechanisms underlying progression to invasive carcinoma may help establish clinical biomarkers and potential therapeutic targets
- Alteration of DNA damage repair mechanisms are associated with invasive breast cancer
  - DNA polymerase β (POLβ) is enzyme involved in DNA base excision repair
  - Reduced expression of POLβ associated with DCIS and high nuclear grade, comedonecrosis, ER(-), HER2(+), and high Ki-67
  - Gradual reduction in POLβ expression from normal breast to DCIS to IDC
  - Low POLβ expression is independent predictor of recurrence in DCIS treated with breast conservation
  - POLβ expression in DCIS may provide additional feature for risk stratification
  - Flap endonuclease 1 (FEN1) plays key role in base excision repair and replication
  - High FEN1 expression in DCIS associated with higher nuclear grade, comedonecrosis, high proliferation, and triple-negative phenotype
  - High FEN1 may play role in DCIS progression to invasive disease

Gene Expression Profiling

- ADH and LGDCIS have similar patterns of gene expression
- Dominated by ER and ER-regulated genes
  - Differences seen in quantitative levels of expression
  - No significant qualitative differences in gene expression
- Distinct patterns and gene expression alterations associated with different breast cancer morphologic phenotypes and, in particular, tumor grade
  - Suggests that low- and high-grade tumors reflect distinct pathobiologic entities rather than direct continuum of cancer progression
  - HGDCIS and invasive tumors show gene expression patterns associated with increased mitotic activity and cell cycle processes
- Same gene expression molecular subtypes recognized with invasive carcinomas also seen in DCIS
  - Luminal A [ER(+), ERBB2(-)]: ~ 70%
    - Typically seen in LGDCIS
  - Luminal B [ER(+), ERBB2(+/-)]: ~ 10-20%
    - Typically seen in HGDCIS; may be LGDCIS
  - ERBB2 [ER(-), ERBB2(+)]: ~ 20-30%
    - Predominantly HGDCIS
  - Triple-negative or basal-like [ER/PR/ERBB2 (-)]: ~ 5-10%
    - Vast majority HGDCIS
- Gene expression analysis from microdissected samples show progressive loss in basal layer integrity during transition from DCIS to IDC
  - 2 epithelial to mesenchymal transitions identified; 1st early and 2nd coinciding with convergence of DCIS and IDC expression profiles
  - Reduced expression of *CAMK2N1*, *MNX1*, *ADCY5*, *HOXC11*, and *ANKRD22*; may be associated with progression of DCIS to IDC

Proprietary Recurrence Score (Oncotype DX Breast Cancer Assay for DCIS)

- Risk of developing ipsilateral breast event after surgical excision of DCIS without radiation therapy not well defined
- Multigene assays have been developed to help predict recurrence after surgery in patients not receiving radiation
  - Oncotype DX DCIS score assay

ADH and DCIS (Dysplastic, Premalignant)

- Assay includes assessment of 7 prognostic genes, including 5 proliferation genes, PR, and *GSTM1* by RT-PCR
- Assay was designed to quantify 10-year risk of local recurrence for both in situ and invasive carcinoma
- Assay results can be used to help determine local recurrence risk in patients with DCIS
- Clinical validation of Oncotype DX DCIS score
  - Retrospective study performed on 327 patient samples from ECOG E5197 clinical trial
  - Low- or intermediate-grade DCIS ≤ 2.5 cm (66% of patients) or HGDCIS ≤ 1 cm (34% of patients)
    – Surgical margins were at least 0.3 cm
    – Patients were not treated with radiation therapy
    – 30% received tamoxifen
    – Only 2.8% were ER(-), and 7.6% were ERBB2(+)
  - At 10 years, ipsilateral recurrence rates were 6% for invasive carcinoma and 8% for DCIS for entire group
  - Patients could be divided into 3 groups based on Oncotype DX DCIS recurrence score
    – Low risk (70% of patients): 3.7% invasive carcinoma and 7.2% DCIS recurrence risk
    – Intermediate risk (16% of patients): 12% invasive carcinoma and 16% DCIS recurrence risk
    – High risk (13% of patients): 19% invasive carcinoma and 8% DCIS recurrence risk
- Correlative studies have shown correlation between histopathologic feature and DCIS score
  - PR ≥ 90% ($P = 0.004$), mitotic count ≤ 1 ($P = 0.045$), ER ≥ 90% ($P = 0.046$) and low nuclear grade ($P < 0.0001$) associated with low score
  - Dense chronic inflammatory infiltrates surrounding DCIS associated with high score ($P = 0.034$)
  - Low score not observed in any case with at least 2 histopathologic features listed below
    – PR(-), > 1 mitosis, &/or presence of dense chronic inflammation surrounding DCIS (100% specificity)
- DCIS score quantifies ipsilateral breast event (IBE) risk and complements traditional clinical and pathologic factors in evaluating need for radiation therapy

Molecular Markers for Preinvasive Disease

- **Hormone receptors**
  - Majority of DCIS strongly expresses ER (~ 80%)
    – Almost all tumor cells show strong expression
    – Estrogen likely stimulates proliferation
      □ Likely plays role in pathogenesis and progression
    – Chemoprevention with tamoxifen reduces risk of ER(+) DCIS and other ER(+) cancers
      □ Treatment leads to significant reduction of subsequent breast cancer by 40-50%
  - Increased ER expression &/or increased sensitivity to estrogen likely plays role in pathogenesis and progression of ADH and LGDCIS
    – With ADH, chemoprevention with tamoxifen reduces risk of ER(+) cancers
  - Hormone receptor subtypes
    – ER(+)/PR(+) DCIS shows better prognosis than ER(+)/PR(-) DCIS in patients who receive tamoxifen therapy
    – Tamoxifen-treated patients show better survival than patient who did not receive tamoxifen only in ER(+)/PR(+) subtype
    – PR status is favorable prognostic factor in patient who receive tamoxifen independent of ER status
    – Testing for PR in addition to ER in DCIS is recommended to determine hormone receptor subtype
- **ERBB2 (HER2)**
  - Overexpression of ERBB2 primarily associated with high-grade, comedo-type DCIS
  - ERBB2 overexpression associated with gene amplification and protein overexpression, similar to ERBB2(+) invasive carcinoma
    – ERBB2 immunoreactivity has been reported to be significantly higher in DCIS compared with invasive carcinoma
  - DCIS with ERBB2 overexpression associated with significantly increased risk of in situ recurrence but not invasive recurrence
    – ERBB2 overexpression in DCIS predictive of radiotherapy benefit with greater reduction of in situ but not invasive recurrence
- *TP53*
  - Inactivating mutations of *TP53* have been reported in high percentage of cases of HGDCIS (40%)
  - LGDCIS does not exhibit any alterations in *TP53*
- **Molecular marker combinations**
  - Direct positive correlation has been observed for expression of ER, PR, and BCL2 for ADH and LGDCIS
  - ERBB2 overexpression, absence of ER and PR, accumulation of TP53, and high Ki-67 expression strong predictors of local recurrence for DCIS

Molecular Portrait: HGDCIS

- Full exome (tumor vs. matching normal) transcriptome, methylome analysis of HGDCIS has been performed
  - 62% of HGDCIS displayed mutations affecting cancer driver or potential driver genes
    – *PIK3CA* (21%), *TP53* (17%), *GATA3* (7%), *KMT2C* (7%)
  - 83% displayed numerous large chromosome copy number alteration
    – These changes might precede selection of cancer driver mutations
- Integrated pathway modeling identified 2 HGDCIS subgroups (DCIS-C1 and DCIS-C2)
  - More aggressive DCIS-C1 subtype (basal-like or *ERBB2*) displayed signature characteristic of activated Treg cells
- Studies suggest most HGDCIS displayed molecular profiles indistinguishable from high-grade invasive carcinomas

MICROSCOPIC

Histologic Features

- **ADH**
  - Clonal proliferation of luminal-type cells
  - May involve terminal ductal lobular units or interlobular ducts
  - Qualitative assessment of ADH
    – Most common architectural changes include cribriform spaces or arched bridges
    – Spaces formed not as uniform as seen in LGDCIS

ADH and DCIS (Dysplastic, Premalignant)

Differential Diagnosis: Intraductal Epithelial Proliferations

Features	Usual Hyperplasia	Atypical Ductal Hyperplasia	Low-Grade Ductal Carcinoma In Situ	High-Grade Ductal Carcinoma In Situ
Architectural pattern	Solid, cribriform, papillary, micropapillary	Cribriform, papillary, micropapillary	Solid, cribriform, papillary, micropapillary	Solid, cribriform, papillary, micropapillary, clinging
Nuclear grade	1 or 2	1 or 2	1 or 2	3
Epithelial cell population	Heterogeneous, mixed population	Partially monotonous population, monomorphic	Monotonous population, monomorphic low-grade atypia	Monotonous population, pleomorphic high-grade atypia
Necrosis	Very rare	Very rare	May be present, usually punctate	Often present; punctate or central necrosis
ER	Positive (> 99%), heterogeneous expression	Positive (> 99%), diffuse expression	Positive (> 99%), diffuse expression	Positive (~ 70%), usually diffuse expression
ERBB2 (HER2)	Negative	Negative	Rare (< 1%)	Frequently positive (~ 30-40%), usually associated with high-grade comedo-type ductal carcinoma in situ
High molecular weight cytokeratin	Positive, heterogeneous pattern	Negative	Negative	Usually negative (may be positive in basal-like high-grade ductal carcinoma in situ)

- Cells are uniform and luminal type; lack expression of high molecular weight cytokeratin (CK5/6)
- Some variability in architecture and cytology
- Involved spaces usually contain > 1 cell population; monomorphic atypical cells may merge with areas of usual hyperplasia
  o Quantitative assessment: Size &/or extent used to distinguish ADH from LGDCIS
- DCIS
  o Can be classified based on architectural patterns of proliferation and grade
    - Grade more important for prognosis; HGDCIS can have any architectural pattern
  o Architectural patterns include cribriform, papillary, micropapillary, comedo, solid, and clinging patterns
  o Nuclear grade for classifying DCIS
    - Same nuclear grading system used for invasive carcinoma can be used for DCIS
    - Low-grade monomorphic atypia: LGDCIS
    - Nuclear pleomorphism: HGDCIS

DIFFERENTIAL DIAGNOSIS

Lobular Carcinoma In Situ

- Also monomorphic population of neoplastic cells
- Cells lack cohesion and typically do not express E-cadherin
- LCIS cannot form architectural structures, such as papillae, micropapillae, or cribriform spaces
  o LCIS involving areas of ADH or collagenous spherulosis can closely mimic DCIS
- Rare cases of LCIS have high-grade nuclei &/or central necrosis (variant forms of LCIS)
  o Absence of E-cadherin has enhanced recognition of these cases as form of lobular neoplasia

Invasive Carcinoma

- Can infiltrate stroma as circumscribed nests of cells
  o Cribriform patterns of invasive carcinoma can closely mimic LGDCIS
- Arrangement generally haphazard rather than following normal pattern of ducts and lobules
- Desmoplastic stroma generally extends beyond cells rather than being circumferential as in some cases of DCIS
- IHC can be helpful in difficult cases for demonstrating presence or absence of myoepithelial cells

Lymphovascular Invasion

- Both DCIS and lymphovascular invasion (LVI) can present as circumscribed nests of tumor cells with no stromal response
- LVI follows vascular pattern and will be present between normal lobules and adjacent to veins and arterioles
- Location of DCIS will follow normal pattern of ducts and lobules

SELECTED REFERENCES

1. Lips EH et al: Genomic analysis defines clonal relationships of ductal carcinoma in situ and recurrent invasive breast cancer. Nat Genet. 54(6):850-60, 2022
2. Rebbeck CA et al: Gene expression signatures of individual ductal carcinoma in situ lesions identify processes and biomarkers associated with progression towards invasive ductal carcinoma. Nat Commun. 13(1):3399, 2022
3. Schiza A et al: Tumour-infiltrating lymphocytes add prognostic information for patients with low-risk DCIS: findings from the SweDCIS randomised radiotherapy trial. Eur J Cancer. 168:128-37, 2022
4. Wilson GM et al: Ductal carcinoma in situ: molecular changes accompanying disease progression. J Mammary Gland Biol Neoplasia. 27(1):101-31, 2022
5. Al-Kawaz A et al: The frequency and clinical significance of DNA polymerase beta (POLβ) expression in breast ductal carcinoma in situ (DCIS). Breast Cancer Res Treat. 190(1):39-51, 2021
6. Hwang KT et al: Hormone receptor subtype in ductal carcinoma in situ: prognostic and predictive roles of the progesterone receptor. Oncologist. 26(11):e1939-50, 2021
7. Thorat MA et al: Prognostic and predictive value of HER2 expression in ductal carcinoma in situ: results from the UK/ANZ DCIS randomized trial. Clin Cancer Res. 27(19):5317-24, 2021
8. Kader T et al: Atypical ductal hyperplasia is a multipotent precursor of breast carcinoma. J Pathol. 248(3):326-38, 2019

ADH and DCIS (Dysplastic, Premalignant)

Atypical Ductal Hyperplasia

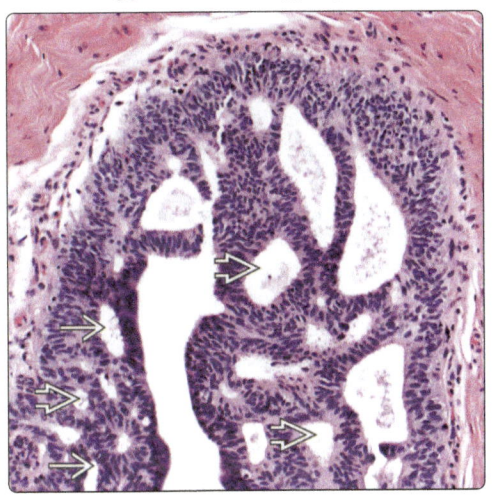

Luminal Cytokeratin Expression in Atypical Ductal Hyperplasia

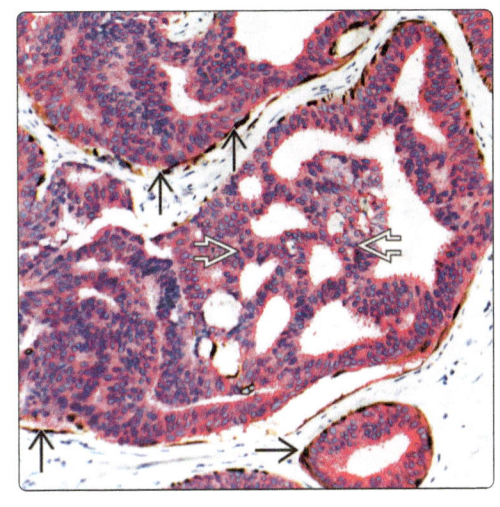

(Left) The cells in ADH appear more uniform than usual hyperplasia, but some variation in size and shape may be present. Although some spaces are round ⇨, there are also slit-like peripheral spaces ⇨. (Right) The clonal proliferation of luminal-type cells of ADH shows restricted expression of low molecular weight cytokeratins, including CK7/8/18 ⇨ (red chromogen). The cells do not express high molecular weight keratins or p63, which is seen in the myoepithelial cells ⇨.

Low-Grade Ductal Carcinoma In Situ: Round Luminal Spaces

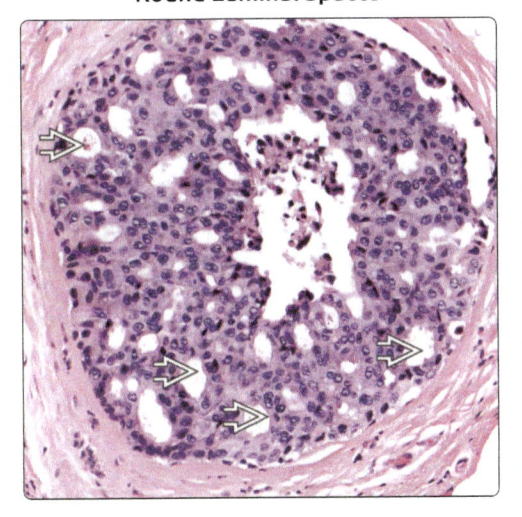

Low-Grade Ductal Carcinoma In Situ: Micropapillary

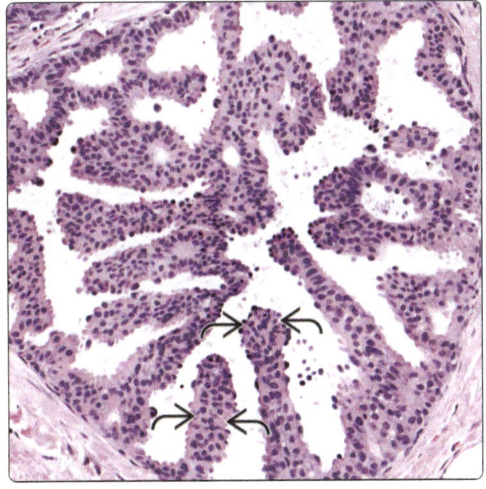

(Left) LGDCIS distends duct spaces and can show a number of architectural patterns, including cribriform growth, with luminal spaces that are round and appear punched out ⇨. The monotonous cells should be oriented around these lumina and evenly distributed in the involved duct. (Right) Micropapillary LGDCIS consists of narrow-based, elongated papillae extending into the duct space ⇨. The papillae are composed of monotonous cells and are solid without fibrovascular cores.

High-Grade Ductal Carcinoma In Situ With Central Necrosis

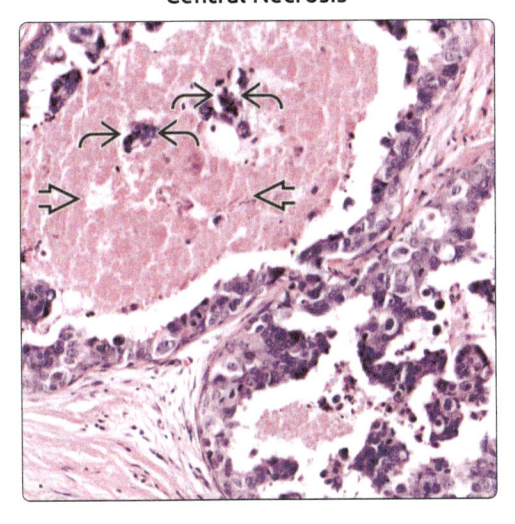

High-Grade Ductal Carcinoma In Situ

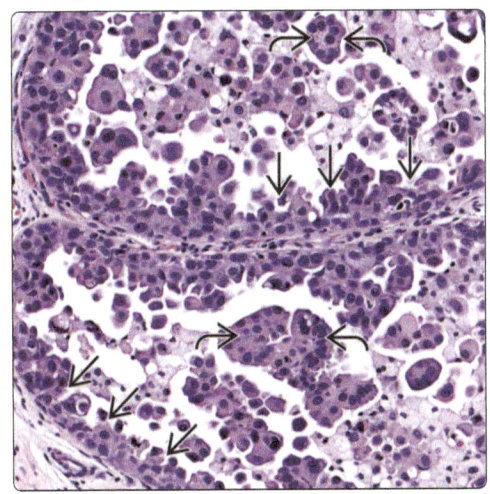

(Left) Prominent central necrosis ⇨, a.k.a. comedonecrosis, can be seen in high-grade DCIS (HGDCIS). Central necrotic areas tend to show calcification ⇨, which are detected mammographically. (Right) Nuclear grading is important for the classification of DCIS. HGDCIS will have complex genomic alterations, including 13q loss and high-level amplification of 17q12 and 11q13. The pleomorphic tumor cells show micropapillary ⇨ and clinging ⇨ architectural patterns in this case.

Ductal Carcinomas

KEY FACTS

TERMINOLOGY

- Invasive ductal carcinoma (IDC) is heterogeneous group of carcinomas with regards to clinical presentation, pathologic features, prognosis, clinical outcomes, and response to therapy
  - Multiple different treatment options available, including targeted therapies
  - Increasingly, clinical decisions on treatment options and targeted therapies require assessment of underlying tumor

ETIOLOGY/PATHOGENESIS

- Technical advances have made it possible to study tumor biology in clinical breast cancer samples
- Tumor tissue can be analyzed for DNA changes, gene expression profiling, and patterns of protein expression
- Clinically useful for breast cancer classification to help inform optimal patient management

MOLECULAR

- Molecular or intrinsic types of IDC
  - Global expression patterns can be used to group tumors into classes or groups with similar findings
- ER(+) luminal cancers (ER expression)
  - Luminal A (lower grade, low proliferation, indolent course) and luminal B (higher grade, more aggressive)
  - Most benefit from hormonal treatment; luminal B tumors may benefit from adding chemotherapy
- HER2-enriched cancer (HER2 overexpression)
  - Unfavorable prognosis; however, great benefit from chemotherapy and HER2-targeted therapy
- Basal-like carcinomas (triple-negative breast carcinoma)
  - Unfavorable prognosis but subset have good response to adjuvant or neoadjuvant chemotherapy
- Numerous multigene assays to predict prognosis and treatment benefit have been developed

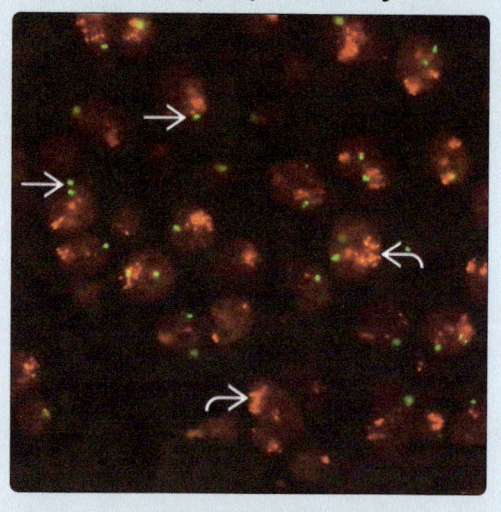

(Left) ERBB2 (HER2)-positive breast carcinomas are high nuclear grade and typically show increased mitotic activity ➡. Tumors with ERBB2 overexpression or gene amplification are eligible for targeted therapy. **(Right)** An increased number of ERBB2 (HER2) genes (red signals ➡) compared to 1 or 2 copies of chromosome 17 centromeric (green signals ➡) would be classified as marked ERBB2 gene amplification in this tumor.

High-Grade Invasive Ductal Carcinoma

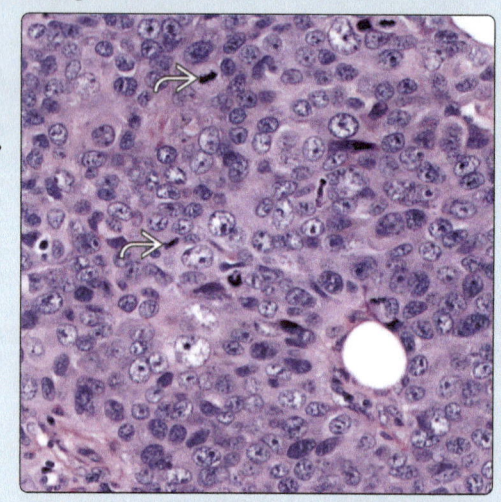

ERBB2 (HER2) Amplification by FISH

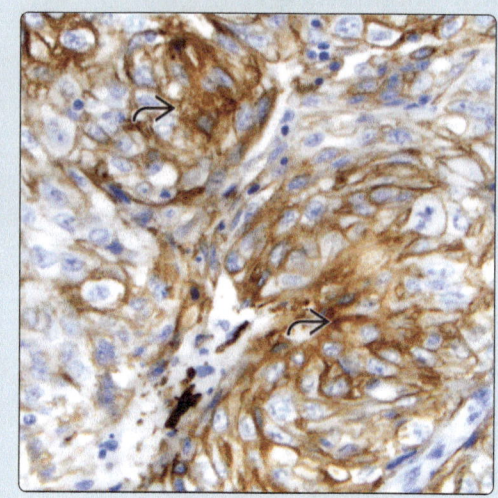

(Left) This high-grade invasive carcinoma shows sheets of tumor cells with a brisk mitotic rate ➡, suggestive of a basal-like carcinoma. While necrosis can be seen in other high-grade breast cancers, the necrosis in basal-like tumors tends to be sharply circumscribed and geographic ➡. **(Right)** Basal-like carcinoma typically shows expression of basal cytokeratins, CK5 in this case ➡. The expression of basal cytokeratins &/or EGFR can be used as an IHC surrogate for basal-like carcinomas.

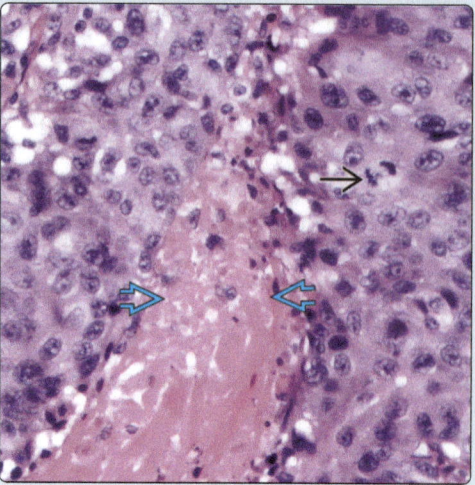

Basal-Like Carcinoma

Basal-Like Carcinoma: CK5

Ductal Carcinomas

TERMINOLOGY

Abbreviations
- Invasive ductal carcinoma (IDC)
  - IDC of no special type (IDCNST)
- Basal-like carcinoma (BLC)
- Triple-negative breast carcinoma (TNBC)

Definitions
- IDC includes all adenocarcinomas of breast that are not classified as special histologic type
  - Heterogeneous group of carcinomas with regards to clinical presentation, pathologic features, prognosis, clinical outcomes, and response to therapy
    - Multiple different treatment options available, including targeted therapies
    - Increasingly, clinical decisions on treatment options and targeted therapies require assessment of tumor biology/molecular drivers of disease progression
  - Need for clinically useful classification scheme to help assess prognosis, aid treatment decisions
    - Advances in molecular analysis that can be performed on clinical breast tumor tissue samples can help address these questions
    - Provides more comprehensive assessment of biologic characteristic of tumor tissue from clinical samples
    - Technologies are robust and reproducible
    - Can identify therapeutic targets in subsets of patients that could benefit from specific targeted therapies
    - Analysis serves as adjunct to standard clinical and pathologic assessment
  - Classification should help distinguish different prognostic groups among patients with similar features
    - Clinically useful breast cancer classification will help to inform optimal patient management

ETIOLOGY/PATHOGENESIS

Breast Cancer Biology and Classification
- Technical advances have made it possible to study tumor biology in clinical breast cancer samples
  - Tumor tissue can be analyzed for DNA changes, gene expression profiling (GEP), and patterns of protein expression
    - Each of these approaches can be used to classify tumors into different biologic subsets
    - Each approach has different specimen requirements
    - Most molecular studies have been adapted for use in formalin-fixed, paraffin-embedded tissue (FFPE)

MOLECULAR

Gene Expression Profiling
- **Molecular or intrinsic types of IDC**
- It has long been known that ER(+) and ER(-) cancers are fundamentally distinct tumors
  - Differ in risk factors, peak age incidence, histologic appearance, association with germline mutations, somatic mutations, patterns of metastasis, response to therapy, and clinical outcome
- GEP (mRNA) can be used to identify biologically distinct groups of carcinomas
  - Global expression patterns can be used to group tumors into classes or groups with similar findings
  - Identification of these subtypes is important, as they vary in morphology, expression of tumor markers, natural history, response to therapy, and prognosis
- ER(+) luminal cancers (ER expression)
  - Luminal A: Refers to most well-differentiated carcinomas of this group with low proliferation
  - Luminal B: Refers to higher grade carcinomas within this group with high proliferation
    - Gradation of proliferation and genomic changes with no discrete separation of A and B groups
    - Some luminal B cancers are HER2(+) (luminal HER2)
    - Chromosomal instability is strongly correlated with metastatic burden in ER(+)/HER2(+) tumors
- HER2-enriched cancer (HER2 overexpression)
  - Overall gene expression pattern is more similar to luminal cancers than to basal-like cancers
    - HER2-enriched carcinomas identified by GEP are typically ER(-)
  - *ERBB2* (HER2) amplification drives protein receptor overexpression, which in turn drives proliferation and more aggressive clinical course
  - HER2 overexpression can be effectively targeted by drugs like trastuzumab, pertuzumab, and TDM1
- BLCs (TNBC)
  - GEP dominated by proliferation, angiogenesis, expression of basal cytokeratins
    - Pattern of mutations is similar to that seen in high-grade serous ovarian carcinomas

Germline Mutations
- Inherited mutations can markedly elevate risk of developing breast cancer
  - *BRCA1* and *BRCA2* most common genes with highest risk
  - *TP53*, *CHEK2*, *PTEN*, *STK11*, and *ATM* mutations elevate risk to lesser degree
- These genes function in DNA repair and maintaining genomic integrity
- All of these mutations combined account for < 10% of all breast carcinomas
- Majority of resulting carcinomas are IDC

Multigene Assays
- Assessment for hormonal and HER2-targeted therapy is based on biomarker evaluation for ER/PR and HER2
  - Indication for adding chemotherapy to patients adjuvant treatment regimen is more challenging
    - Clinical tumor characteristics (size, grade, nodal involvement) are used to predict risk of recurrence and are considered in chemotherapy decision
    - Risk of recurrence is weighed against potential benefit (improved outcome) and drug toxicity
  - Molecular analysis of clinical samples provides new conceptual approach for evaluating risk and guiding chemotherapy decisions
    - Initial studies based on gene expression analysis but have been translated into RT-PCR multigene tests and other molecular methodologies
- **Oncotype DX assay**
  - Validated 21-gene quantitative RT-PCR assay

Ductal Carcinomas

- Developed for use in ER(+) breast cancer utilizing FFPE samples
- Quantitatively measures 16 cancer genes and 5 housekeeping genes to check RNA integrity
- Gene expression levels are used in algorithm to calculated numerical recurrence score (RS)
- RS is heavily weighted for proliferation genes as well as activated ER and HER2 pathways
  - RS is divided into low, intermediate, and high recurrence risk categories
    - Independently predictive of recurrence in multiple published studies
    - Has been show to be prognostic (predicts likelihood of recurrence at 10 years) and predictive of chemotherapy benefit for patient with high RS
    - Used clinically to help decide which ER(+) breast cancers need or can be spared adjuvant chemotherapy
    - Test was validated for ER(+)/node (-) tumor; may be informative for node (+) patients
  - Assay offered clinically as reference test by Genomic Health Incorporated
  - TAILORx clinical trial demonstrated that adjuvant endocrine and chemoendocrine had similar efficacy in women with midrange Oncotype DX assay scores
    - Found benefit of chemotherapy for some women ≤ 50 years of age with midrange score
  - RxPONDER trial shows no benefit for adjuvant chemotherapy + endocrine therapy for postmenopausal women with 1-3 positive lymph nodes and RS < 25
- **MammaPrint assay**
  - Involves gene expression analysis using microarray technology; has been adapted for FFPE tissue
    - 70-gene classifier is used to stratify patient into low-risk and high-risk categories for distant recurrence
      - Validation studies have shown that patient with good prognostic signature had < 15% risk of recurrence at 10 years
      - Patients with poor prognostic signature had 50% risk for distant metastases
      - Studies showed that risk predicted by MammaPrint is most likely associated with early recurrence
    - Originally required fresh or frozen tumor tissue, but test has been adapted for formalin-fixed samples
    - Function of 70 genes assayed is related to cellular pathways involving apoptosis, growth signaling, limitless potential to replicate, tissue invasion, and angiogenesis
  - Several clinical validation studies of MammaPrint have been conducted
    - Metaanalysis showed that MammaPrint is also predictive for chemotherapy benefit
  - Microarray in node (-) and 1-3 (+) lymph node disease may avoid chemotherapy (MINDACT randomized/prospective trial)
    - Randomized based on discordant risk assessment from MammaPrint vs. clinical risk based on Adjuvant! Online
    - Patients with high clinical risk but low genomic risk receiving no chemotherapy had 5-year survival that was 1.5% lower that those receiving chemotherapy
    - Concluded that ~ 46% of women at high clinical risk but low genomic risk based on MammaPrint might not require chemotherapy
- **Prosigna Breast Cancer Prognostic Gene Signature assay**
  - RT-PCR assay measuring expression levels of 50 genes
    - Results can classify breast tumors into intrinsic subtypes [luminal A and B, HER2(+), basal-like]
  - Risk of RS incorporates clinical treatment score data with gene expression data
    - Translates prognostic information from intrinsic subtypes into prognostic score
    - Useful for predicting late recurrence in ER(+) patients treated with endocrine therapy
    - Useful in identifying ER(+) patients with excellent outcome who may not benefit from chemotherapy
- **EndoPredict**
  - Multigene classifier to assess prognosis in ER(+)/HER2(-) cancer treated with endocrine therapy
    - Gene expression measured for 11 genes (8 cancer genes, 3 control genes)
    - Gene panel assesses proliferation and hormone receptor activity (does not include ER, PR, or HER2)
    - Results useful for low and high risk for recurrence
  - EndoPredict score significantly correlates with both early and late distant disease recurrence
    - Useful for assessing prognosis in ER(+)/HER2(-)/node (-) or node (+) postmenopausal cancer

Next-Generation Sequencing

- Permits simultaneous interrogation of genomic alterations present in panel of cancer genes, whole exomes, or entire genome
  - Most recurrently mutate genes in breast cancer: *PIK3CA* and *TP53* (30%)
  - *CCND1*, *FGFR1* mutations, and *HER2* amplification (15%)
  - Majority of other cancer genes and new potential driver mutations mutated at frequencies of < 5%
  - Mutations in *GATA3* and *RBFOX1* appear to be confined to ER(+) disease
  - Invasive ductal and lobular carcinomas characterized by different mutational landscapes
    - Enrichment of *CDH1*, *TBX3*, *FOXA1*, and *ERBB2* mutations in lobular carcinomas
  - Sequencing studies highlight important genomic diversity among breast tumors
- Genomic characterization of circulating tumor DNA (ctDNA) released from tumor cells shows promise for clinical applications
  - Noninvasive tumor genotyping
  - Surveillance and monitoring treatment response
  - Identification of residual disease in early-stage cancers
  - Identification of resistance-associated mutations, such as *ESR1* mutations, and endocrine resistance

MICROSCOPIC

Histologic Features

- **Histologic grade**
  - Elston and Ellis modification of Scarff-Bloom-Richardson histologic grade divides breast cancers into groups with different natural histories and biologic characteristics

Ductal Carcinomas

- Grading based on tumor differentiation and proliferation
  - Grade 1: Well differentiated; 20%; incidence higher in older women
  - Grade 2: Moderately differentiated; 30-35%
  - Grade 3: Poorly differentiated; 45-50%; incidence higher in younger women
- Histologic grade is strongly correlated with breast cancer-specific survival and disease-free survival
  - Significant association between grade and survival holds true for different tumor subgroups (tumor size and lymph node stages)
  - Grade correlates with overall length of survival regardless of clinical stage
- **Grade and genomic grade index (GGI)**
  - Developed using GEP comparing low- and high-grade carcinomas
    - 97-gene panel discriminates reproducibly between 2 ER(+) subgroups that correlate with grade and significantly different clinical outcome
    - GGI driven by proliferation and cell cycle-related genes
    - Only informative in ER(+), HER2(-) luminal tumors
    - Associated with prognosis and tumor grade
      - Grade 1 tumors: 85% low GGI; grade 3 tumors: 90% high GGI; grade 2 tumors: Split into low and high GGI categories
    - Predictive for recurrence in endocrine- and chemotherapy-treated patients and prognostic for neoadjuvant chemotherapy
- **Grade and DNA changes**
  - Number and pattern of genomic copy number alterations differ significantly when stratified by histologic grade
    - Average number of chromosomal changes increases with increasing grade
    - High-grade tumors: High genomic instability (gains at 5p, 8q, 10p, 17q12, and 19; losses at 3q, 4, 5q proximal, 9p, 11p, 18q, and 21)
    - Low-grade tumors: Low level of instability, deletion 16q and gain of 1q (80%)
  - Gains and losses occur at loci harboring oncogenes and tumor suppressor genes
  - Close correlation between DNA copy number changes and mRNA expression levels
  - Gene amplification may be common mechanism for driving GEP in breast carcinoma
- **IHC and breast cancer subtypes**
  - Groups similar to those defined by GEP can be defined based on expression of ER, PR, HER2, and proliferation index (IHC surrogate)
  - Subtypes defined by GEP and IHC overlap by 80-85%
    - Groups were originally defined by GEP; helpful to use same names to describe similar groups of cancers defined by IHC
    - Classification by IHC has advantage of organizing cancers according to therapeutic targets and likely response to chemotherapy
- **ER(+), HER2(-), low proliferation (luminal A)**
  - Invasive tumor: Well-formed tubules, cribriform nest
    - Majority are grade 1 or 2, small- to moderate-sized nuclei, minute or absent nucleoli
    - ER and PR generally present and highly expressed
  - $PIK3CA$ mutations (~ 35%); $TP53$ mutations rare
  - Favorable prognosis; most benefit from hormonal treatment; little benefit from chemotherapy
- **ER(+), HER2(+/-), high proliferation (luminal B)**
  - Poor acini formation; may invade as nests and sheets
    - Majority are grade 2 or 3; nuclei typically high grade with prominent nucleoli
    - ER is present but may be at low levels; PR may be absent; may be HER2(+)
  - Complex genomic changes, genetic instability, deletion 16q and gain 1q (50%); may have $TP53$ mutations
  - Less favorable prognosis, may benefit from endocrine and chemotherapy
- **ER(-), HER2(+) (HER2 enriched)**
  - Usually invade as nests or sheets of cells
    - Majority are grade 3; prominent nucleoli; may have abundant cytoplasm with apocrine features
    - May show necrosis (40%), lymphocytic infiltrates (60%), lymphatic invasion (45%)
  - Amplification of $ERBB2$ (HER2) and surrounding genes
  - $TP53$ mutations are common
  - Unfavorable prognosis; however, great benefit from chemotherapy and HER2-targeted therapy
- **ER(-), HER2(-) (basal-like, TNBC)**
  - Circumscribed border, syncytial-like growth
    - Most grade 3, pleomorphic nuclei, prominent nucleoli
    - Central fibrosis &/or geographic necrosis frequent
  - Genome highly unstable; numerous copy number changes; loss of function of DNA repair genes; majority have $TP53$ mutations
  - Unfavorable prognosis but subset has good response to adjuvant or neoadjuvant chemotherapy

ANCILLARY TESTS

Immunohistochemistry

- Breast cancer predictive assay used in clinical practice
- ER
  - Regulates growth and development of breast and other hormonally responsive tissues
    - After binding to its ligand (estrogen), ER is transported to nucleus where it functions as transcription factor
    - ER regulates expression of genes that are important in development and physiologic function, including proliferation
    - 70-80% of all invasive breast cancers express ER
    - ER drives tumor cell proliferation and disease progression in these tumors
  - ER expression in breast cancer can be detected by IHC
    - Tumor is considered ER(+) if as few as 1% of invasive tumor cells show moderate nuclear staining
    - Most low-grade breast cancers should be ER(+)
    - Endocrine therapies: Tamoxifen (ER antagonist) and aromatase inhibitors (block local estrogen production)
- HER2
  - Transmembrane growth factor receptor that regulates normal cell growth and development

Ductal Carcinomas

Molecular Subtypes of Invasive Ductal Carcinoma

Features	Luminal A	Luminal B	HER2 Enriched	Basal-Like
Percentage of breast cancers	55%	15%	15-20%	10-15%
Immunophenotype	ER(+), HER2(-), proliferation low	ER(+), [HER2(+) ~ 50%], proliferation high	ER(-), HER2(+), proliferation high	ER(-), HER2(-), proliferation high
Basal cytokeratins	Absent or low	Absent or low	May be present	40-85%
Common genomic changes	Low level of instability; 16q deletion and 1q gain (80%); PIK3CA mutations (~ 35%); TP53 mutations rare	Complex genomic changes; genetic instability; 16q deletion and 1q gain (50%); may have TP53 mutations	Amplification of ERBB2 and surrounding genes; may have TP53 mutations	Highly unstable; loss of function of DNA repair genes; majority have TP53 mutations
Prognosis	Favorable	Less favorable (improved with HER2-targeted therapy in positive cancers)	Less favorable (improved with HER2-targeted therapy)	Unfavorable (but subset will have good response to chemotherapy)
Systemic therapy	Majority benefit from hormonal treatment; benefit from chemotherapy less clear	May benefit from both hormonal therapy and chemotherapy	Benefit from chemotherapy and HER2-targeted therapy	Subset benefits from chemotherapy
Common patient characteristics	Older age, screen-detected cancers, associated with hormone replacement therapy	Younger age, BRCA2 carriers, TP53 carriers [if HER2(+)]	Younger age, BRCA2 carriers, TP53 carriers [if HER2(+)]	Relatively more common in young women; more common in African American and Hispanic women, BRCA1 carriers
Metastatic sites	Bone (70%), liver or lung (25%), brain (< 10%); survival with metastases possible	Bone (79%), liver or lung (30%), brain (10-15%)	Bone (60%), liver or lung (45%), brain (30%); long survival with metastases uncommon	Bone (40%), liver or lung (35%), brain (25%); long survival with metastases uncommon

Breast Cancer Histologic Grade and Molecular Characteristics

Histologic Grade	Hormone Receptors	HER2	Proliferation	TP53	DNA Copy Number Changes	Gene Expression Profiling
Low histologic grade	Typically ER and PR (+)	Typically HER2(-) (95%)	Low proliferation index, measured by IHC or gene expression	Normal function [p53 IHC (-)]	Fewer copy number changes; most common loss on 16q, gains on 1q	Most likely luminal A, some luminal B, low recurrence score, low genomic grade index
High histologic grade	Typically low or (-) for ER and PR	More likely HER2(+) (30%) or triple negative (15%)	High proliferation index, measured by IHC or gene expression	Frequent loss of function [p53 IHC (+)]	More frequent, extensive, and complex alterations; gains on 8q, 17q, 20q and loss on 17p, 1p, 19p, 19q	Luminal B, HER2 enriched, basal-like, high recurrence score, high genomic grade index

- ○ ERBB2 (HER2) located on chromosome 17, amplified (early oncogenic event) in 12-18% of invasive beast carcinomas
  - Gene amplification drives HER2 overexpression, increasing receptor activation and signaling
  - Activation of HER2 signaling drives proliferation, angiogenesis, and enhances cell survival pathways
- ○ HER2 can be assessed by IHC or in situ hybridization in clinical samples from breast cancer
  - Patients who test as HER2(+) are candidates for targeted therapies against HER2
  - HER2-targeted therapies include antibodies (trastuzumab, pertuzumab, and TDM1) and small molecule inhibitors (lapatinib)
  - HER2-targeted therapies are effective in metastatic, adjuvant, and neoadjuvant settings

SELECTED REFERENCES

1. Barrón-Gallardo CA et al: Transcriptomic analysis of breast cancer patients sensitive and resistant to chemotherapy: looking for overall survival and drug resistance biomarkers. Technol Cancer Res Treat. 21:15330338211068965, 2022
2. Nguyen B et al: Genomic characterization of metastatic patterns from prospective clinical sequencing of 25,000 patients. Cell. 185(3):563-575.e11, 2022
3. Kalinsky K et al: 21-gene assay to inform chemotherapy benefit in node-positive breast cancer. N Engl J Med. 385(25):2336-47, 2021
4. Sparano JA et al: Adjuvant chemotherapy guided by a 21-gene expression assay in breast cancer. N Engl J Med.12;379(2):111-21, 2018
5. Heng YJ et al: The molecular basis of breast cancer pathological phenotypes. J Pathol. 241(3):375-91, 2017
6. Krop I et al: Use of biomarkers to guide decisions on adjuvant systemic therapy for women with early-stage invasive breast cancer: American Society of Clinical Oncology Clinical Practice guideline focused update. J Clin Oncol. 35(24):2838-47, 2017
7. Rakha EA et al: Molecular classification of breast cancer: what the pathologist needs to know. Pathology. 49(2):111-9, 2017

Ductal Carcinomas

Invasive Ductal Carcinoma: Luminal A

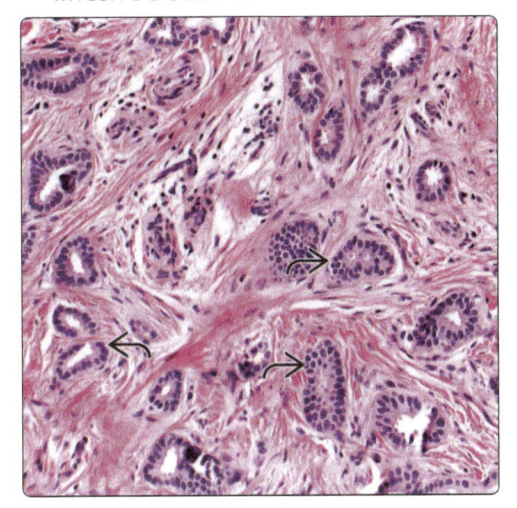

Luminal A Carcinoma: ER Expression

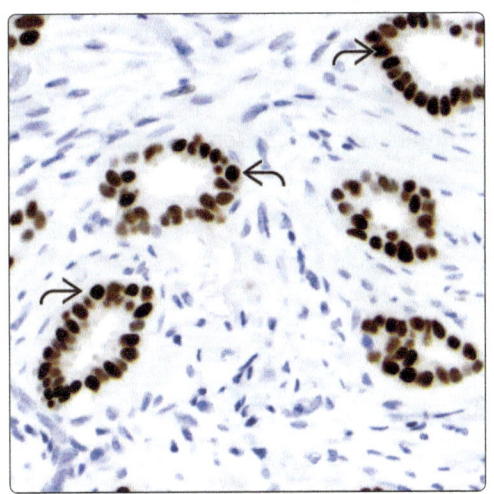

(Left) Luminal subtypes of breast cancer are defined by expression of ER and other genes regulated by an activated ER pathway. Luminal A cancers typically have a pattern of well-formed, infiltrating neoplastic tubules made up of cells that have a low nuclear grade ⇒ and infrequent mitotic figures. (Right) Luminal A cancers typically show strong ER expression ⇒ in the invasive tumor cells as well as PR expression. This level of ER expression is predictive for benefit from endocrine therapy.

Invasive Ductal Carcinoma: HER2

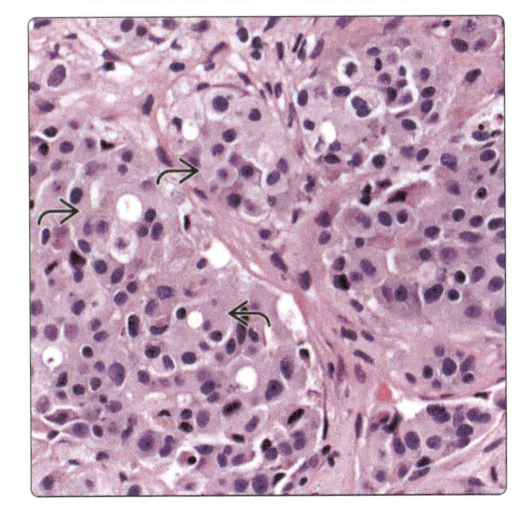

Invasive Ductal Carcinoma: HER2

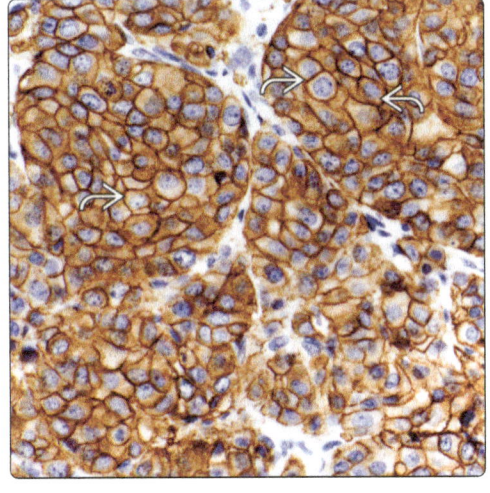

(Left) Breast cancers that fall into the HER2 subtype as defined by gene expression profiling are typically high grade and may show apocrine features ⇒. These tumors overexpress the HER2 protein by IHC and HER2 gene amplification by FISH. (Right) HER2 gene amplification (detected by in situ hybridization) results in increased expression of receptor protein in the membrane of tumor cells ⇒, which can be detected by IHC. Intense, circumferential membrane staining is considered a positive result.

Basal-Like Carcinoma: Geographic Necrosis

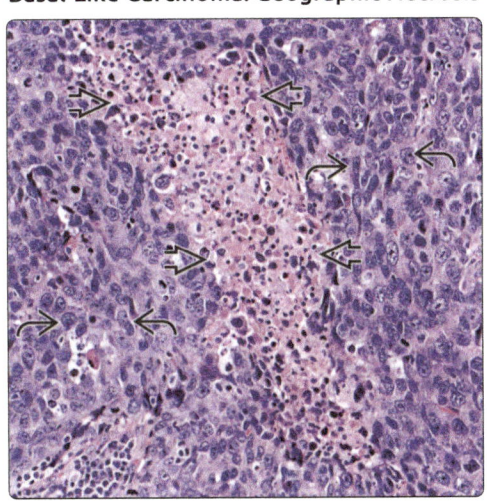

Basal-Like Carcinoma: EGFR

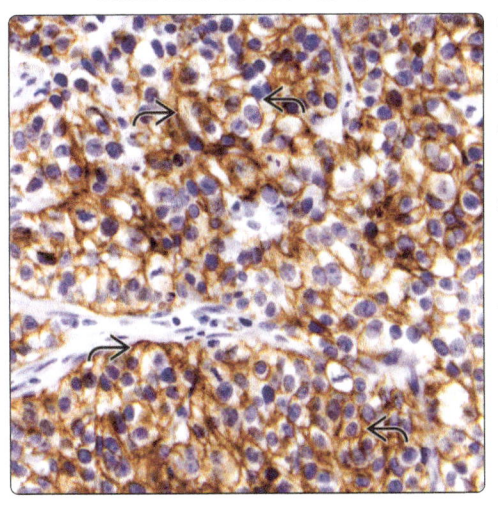

(Left) This poorly differentiated carcinoma shows pleomorphic tumor cells arranged in syncytial-like sheets ⇒ and no evidence of tubule formation. There are areas of geographic necrosis ⇒, a feature frequently associated with basal-like carcinomas. (Right) Basal-like carcinomas are typically negative for ER/PR and HER2 but frequently show expression for basal cytokeratin (CK5, CK14, CK17) and other growth factor receptors, such as EGFR ⇒.

Molecular Pathology of Solid Tumors

699

Lobular Carcinoma

KEY FACTS

TERMINOLOGY
- Group of invasive carcinomas with loss of normal cell adhesion and dysregulation of actin cytoskeleton

ETIOLOGY/PATHOGENESIS
- E-cadherin plays functional role in intercellular adhesion and cell polarity
  - Loss of E-cadherin expression (~ 85% of ILC)
  - 1 allele on 16q inactive by mutation (50-60% of ILC)
  - 2nd allele is inactivated by either loss of heterozygosity or by promoter hypermethylation
- Loss of E-cadherin affects cellular adhesion, cell motility, and possible cell division
- Responsible for characteristic morphology; plays role in detachment and invasion of neoplastic cells

CLINICAL ISSUES
- Prognosis for ILC similar to carcinomas of no special type if matched for grade and stage
- High-grade forms of ILC have more aggressive behavior

MOLECULAR
- ILC has fewer chromosomal abnormalities than carcinomas of no special type
  - Frequent and consistent changes in all ILC types have been described
  - Loss at 16q at location of *CDH1* (E-cadherin) at 6q22.1
- Majority of ILC are ER positive and of luminal molecular subtype
  - Show gene expression related to cell adhesion, cell-to-cell signaling, and actin cytoskeleton signaling
- Hereditary diffuse gastric cancer syndrome is due to germline mutation in *CDH1* (E-cadherin)
  - Risk of ILC for women is 40-50% by age 80
  - Risk of gastric carcinoma is 40-80% by age 80
- ILC of all grades are more similar to each other than to other breast cancer types

Single-File Growth

Loss of E-Cadherin Expression

(Left) The hallmark of invasive lobular carcinoma (ILC) is the presence of round, poorly cohesive cells in a single-file growth pattern ➔. The invasive tumor cells will often show circumferential growth around normal ducts ➔.
(Right) The majority of ILC lack expression of the cell adhesion protein E-cadherin ➔. Normal duct structures provide a good internal positive control, as they should show membrane staining ➔.

Pleomorphic Variant

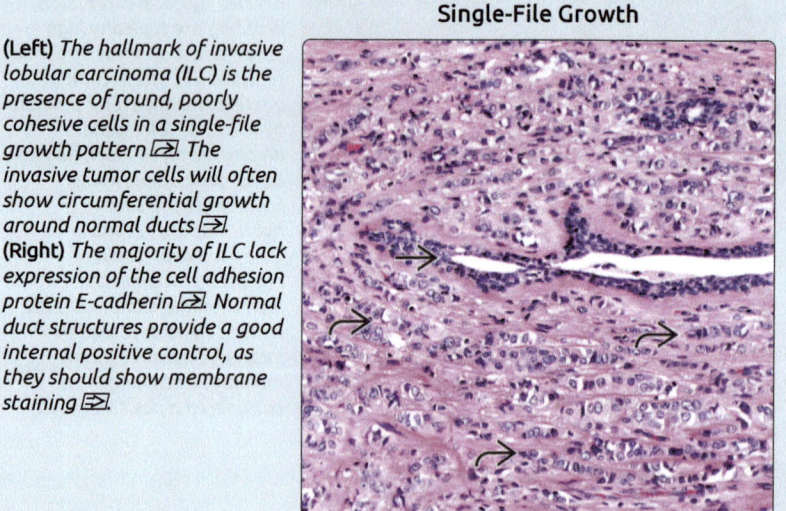

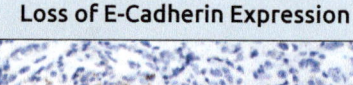

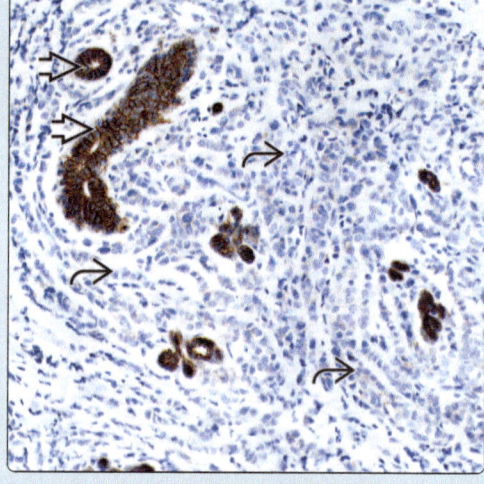

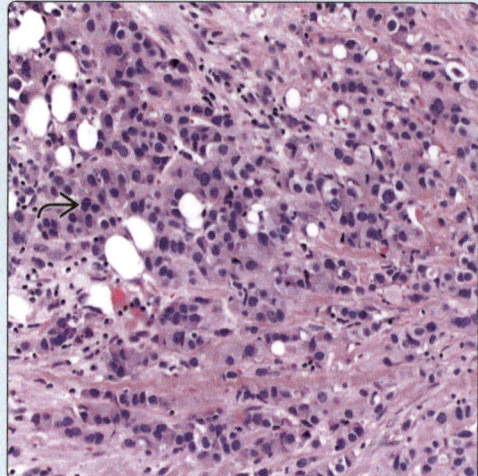

Pleomorphic Variant: HER2 Overexpression

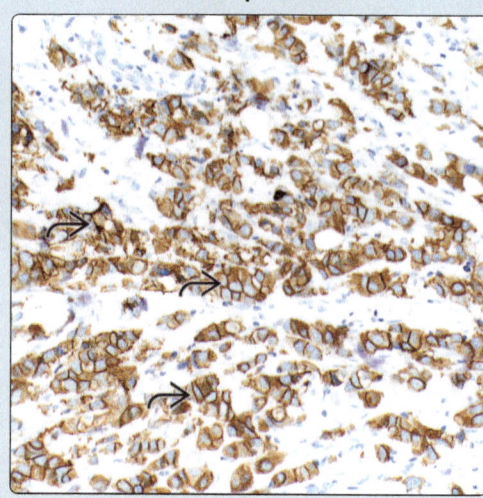

(Left) This poorly differentiated ILC contains pleomorphic nuclei ➔, abundant cytoplasm, and increased mitotic activity. Variant forms of ILC may be confused with ductal carcinoma. The loss of E-cadherin expression can be helpful diagnostically. (Right) Variant forms of lobular carcinoma show additional genomic changes compared with classic tumors, including TP53 mutations, amplification of ERBB2 and MYC, and overexpression of HER2 ➔, as shown here.

Lobular Carcinoma

TERMINOLOGY

Abbreviations
- Invasive lobular carcinoma (ILC)
- Lobular carcinoma in situ (LCIS)

Definitions
- ILC is group of invasive carcinomas characterized by loss of normal cell adhesion and dysregulation of actin cytoskeleton
  o Carcinomas show specific morphologic appearance, typically diffuse tissue infiltration and single-file growth
    – Pattern seen in breast and distant metastatic sites

Classification
- ILC originally defined as carcinoma having specific architectural and cytologic features (classic ILC)
  o Architecture: Single-file invasion of stroma (1 or 2 cells wide)
  o Cytologic grade 1 or 2 nuclei
- Later recognized that other invasive carcinomas not included in this definition also lacked cellular cohesion
  o Molecular studies support these carcinomas as part of family of lobular neoplasia
  o These carcinomas are classified as variants of ILC

ETIOLOGY/PATHOGENESIS

Cell Adhesion Protein Expression
- Characteristic dyscohesive growth pattern of ILC results from targeted disruption of E-cadherin
- Loss of E-cadherin gene (CDH1) expression in ~ 85% of ILC
  o Similar changes have been described in classic and variant forms of ILC
- E-cadherin is calcium-dependent transmembrane protein; has functional role in intercellular adhesion and cell polarity
  o Binds actin cytoskeleton through interactions with p120, α-, β-, and γ-catenin
- Loss of E-cadherin affects cellular adhesion, cell motility, and possible cell division
  o Plays role in detachment and invasion of neoplastic cells
  o Leads to loss of α-, β-, and γ-catenin
  o Leads to upregulation of p120 catenin and relocalization of protein from membrane to cytoplasm of tumor cells
    – Relocalization enables anoikis resistance of tumor cells, allowing survival independent from attachment
    – Promotes anchorage-independent growth and cell migration through Rho/Rock signaling
  o E-cadherin functions as negative regulator of insulin-like growth factor receptor 1 (IGF1R)
    – E-cadherin loss in ILC may sensitize cells to growth factor signaling and alter sensitivity to growth factor signaling inhibitors
    – Cell lines with CDH1 knock-out and ILC patient-derived organoids show increased sensitivity to IGFR1, PI3K, AKT, and MEK inhibitors
    – These targets require further exploration, as potential ILC treatment and CDH1 loss may be biomarker of response for patient stratification
  o Loss of E-cadherin promotes expression of DNA binding 2 (Id2), mediator of cell cycle progression in ILC
    – Id2 is essential for anchorage-independent survival
    – Loss of E-cadherin and subsequent expression of Id2 may contribute to indolence and dissemination of ILC
- Defect in cellular adhesion responsible for morphologic appearance of cells
  o Cells are rounded and dyscohesive
    – Cannot form cribriform spaces, tubules, or papillae
    – Cells infiltrate along path of least resistance between collagen bundles and along blood vessels
  o Phenotype in turn attributable to reduced stromal-epithelial crosstalk by transforming growth factor β

CLINICAL ISSUES

Epidemiology
- Incidence
  o ILC is most common special histologic type
    – Represents 5-15% of all invasive carcinomas
    – ILC variants are only 20-30% of all ILC

Prognosis
- Prognosis for ILC is similar to that for carcinomas of no special type if matched for grade and stage
  o Most studies suggest that classic ILC has better prognosis than variant forms of ILC
    – Patients with stage I classic ILC may show better recurrence-free survival
    – Trend toward late recurrence for ILC
  o Histologic grading (Nottingham grading) is recommended for all breast cancer, including ILC and variants
    – Histologic grade provides strong predictor of outcome for ILC and variants
  o High-grade forms of ILC have more aggressive behavior
  o Published studies show that histologic grading of ILC is associated with other prognostic markers
- ILC has distinctive patterns of metastatic spread
  o Serosal and mucosal involvement of GI and gynecologic tract and retroperitoneum
    – Metastatic ILC can occasionally be seen in GI mucosal biopsies and endometrial curetting
  o Leptomeninges and cerebrospinal fluid involvement
    – Carcinomatous meningitis is typically due to ILC
  o Bone metastases
    – Metastatic ILC can be very difficult to detect in bone marrow; may resemble hematopoietic cells
    – IHC for keratin can be very helpful to determine presence and extent of involvement
  o Pleural and pulmonary metastases are less common than for other histologic types of carcinoma

MOLECULAR

Mechanism of Loss of E-Cadherin
- E-cadherin plays functional role in intercellular adhesion and cell polarity
- 1 allele on 16q is inactivated by mutation (50-60% of ILC)
  o Most somatic CDH1 mutations in ILC are frameshift
    – Results in truncated, nonfunctional E-cadherin protein
  o CDH1 mutations are present in up to 80% of cases of ILC by whole-exome sequencing
- 2nd allele is inactivated by either loss of heterozygosity or by promoter hypermethylation

Lobular Carcinoma

- Leads to loss of E-cadherin protein expression, which can be detected by IHC
- Expression of E-cadherin but loss of other catenin complex proteins occurs in ~ 10-15% of ILC
  - If E-cadherin is expressed, then 1 or more catenins will show abnormal expression
  - p120 catenin will show abnormal cytoplasmic localization
- Some E-cadherin (+) ILC harbor CDH1 mutations, which preserve epitope recognized by commercial anti-E-cadherin antibodies

Molecular Genetics

- ILC more likely to be diploid than ductal tumors
- ILC has fewer chromosomal abnormalities than carcinomas of no special type
  - 3 frequent and consistent changes in all ILC types have been described
    - Loss at 16q at location of E-cadherin gene (CDH1) at 16q22.1, 16p, 17p, and 22q
    - Gains at 1q and 16q
- Poorly differentiated variant forms of ILC show additional genomic changes
  - TP53 mutations
  - Amplifications of ERBB2 (HER2), MYC, and MDM2
    - Mutations may help explain higher grade features and more aggressive clinical behavior
  - Pleomorphic ILC may demonstrate amplifications at loci 8q24, 17q12, and 20q13
    - These findings are also characteristic of high-grade invasive carcinomas of no special type

Gene Expression Profiling

- Majority of ILC are ER(+) and luminal subtype
  - ILC of all grades are more similar to each other than to other breast cancer types
    - Similar expression patterns related to cell adhesion, cell-to-cell signaling, and actin cytoskeleton signaling
  - Grade 1 and 2 ILC have distinct gene expression patterns compared to grade 1 and 2 carcinomas of no special type
- Variant ILC can be in luminal, molecular apocrine, or ERBB2-enriched subgroups by gene expression profiling
  - Basal-like subgroup is very rare
- Functional gene groups distinctive for lobular tumors
  - Adhesion; transforming growth factor β signaling; cell communication and trafficking; actin remodeling; lipid/prostaglandin synthesis
- 32-87% of ILC belong to luminal molecular subtype of breast cancer, and 50% are low risk by Oncotype DX
  - Lower percentage of patients with ILC vs. invasive ductal carcinoma (IDC) have high-risk Oncotype DX score (6.6% vs. 16%)
  - 11% of ILC patients are classified as high genomic risk by 70-gene signature test

Germline Mutations of CDH1 (E-Cadherin)

- Hereditary diffuse gastric cancer syndrome is due to germline mutation in CDH1
  - Risk of gastric carcinoma is 40-80% by age 80
  - Risk of ILC for women is 40-50% by age 80
- Gastric signet-ring cell carcinomas and ILC are morphologically similar
  - Both lack expression of E-cadherin protein
- Carcinomas have organ-specific gene expression patterns that differ between 2 sites
- Some affected families are detected by predominance of cases of ILC
- Vast majority of women with ILC do not carry germline mutation in CDH1
- Possibility of germline mutations in other cytoskeletal protein genes is under investigation

Precursor Lesion: LCIS

- LCIS is known risk factor of invasive carcinoma
  - Increasing data suggest nonobligate precursor relationship between LCIS and ILC
    - LCIS confers 8-10x increase in relative risk for subsequently developing invasive carcinoma
      - Annual rate of developing carcinoma is 2% with cumulative cancer incidence of 26% at 15 years
      - Cancers occurred in ipsilateral breast in 63%, contralateral breast in 25%, and in bilateral breasts in 12% of cases
    - LCIS and ILC are phenotypically and genetically similar
    - Most LCIS and ILC are luminal A molecular subtype, harboring recurrent gains of 1q and loss of 16q
    - Sequencing analyses focused on paired LCIS and ILC demonstrated comparable shared somatic mutations in CDH1, PIK3CA, and CBFB
  - 70-80% incidence of LCIS associated with cases of ILC
    - Similar to association between ductal carcinoma in situ and IDC
  - Invasive carcinoma arising in women with history of LCIS are 3x more likely to be ILC
  - Gene expression profiling studies separate classic LCIS into 2 groups
    - Differences between groups based on genes involved in proliferation, TGFB1, TP53, actin cytoskeleton, apoptosis, and Wnt signaling
    - Additional candidate precursor genes may play role in disease progression

Next-Generation Sequencing

- Technologic advances have led to ability to interrogate individual tumor genomes
  - Exome sequencing of ILC have demonstrated recurrent mutations in CDH1 and PIK3CA
    - PIK3CA mutation rate is similar to that observed overall in ER(+) breast cancers
    - Activation of PIK3CA by somatic mutations present in 30-50% of ILC
- Somatic mutations in ERBB2 are generally rare in breast cancer
  - ERBB2 mutations are significantly enriched in ILC
  - Activating ERBB2 somatic mutations associated with poorly differentiated, pleomorphic, and recurrent ILC
    - ERBB2 mutations preferentially affected tyrosine kinase activity domain
    - Frequent targetable ERBB2 mutation is p.L755S (57%)
  - ERBB2 is important clinically actionable target
    - Targeted sequencing analysis may aid in management of patient when planning therapy in future
    - ERBB2 mutation testing should be considered in all ILC with nuclear grade 3

Lobular Carcinoma

Invasive Lobular Carcinoma: Classic and Variant Forms

Features	Classic	Solid	Alveolar	Pleomorphic	Histiocytoid
Predominant growth pattern	Single file	Confluent sheets	Groups or round clusters	Single file	Single file
Nuclear grade	1 or 2	Usually 2 or 3	Usually 2 or 3	2 or 3	Usually 1 or 2
Cytoplasm	Scant	Scant	Scant	Abundant cytoplasm, eosinophilic (apocrine)	Foamy/pale or eosinophilic
Apocrine features (GCDFP-15)	(+/-)	(+/-)	(+/-)	(+++)	(+++)
E-cadherin	(-)	(-)	(-)	(-)	(-)
ER/PR	(+++)	(++)	(++)	(+) or (-)	(+)
HER2	(-)	(-)	(-)	(+) or (-)	(-)

- IDC and ILC are characterized by different mutational landscape
  o Enrichment for *CDH1*, *TBX3*, *FOXA1*, *AKT1*, *ERBB2*, and *ERBB3* mutations seen in lobular tumors
  o *PTEN* loss associated with increased AKT phosphorylation was highest in ILC among all breast cancer subtypes
  o Proliferation and immune-related signatures determine 3 ILC transcriptional subtypes associated with survival
  o Mixed IDC/ILC cases are molecularly classified as ILC-like and IDC-like with no true hybrid features

MICROSCOPIC

Histologic Features

- ILC has distinctive cytologic features
  o Cells are round in shape due to lack of cohesion
  o Nuclear grade can vary from grade 1 to grade 3
  o Cytoplasmic mucin vacuoles may be present
    – Prominent cells with signet-ring appearance have single vacuole with mucin droplet
- ILC has distinctive growth patterns
  o Classic growth pattern: Linear arrangement of dyscohesive cells in single file between collagen
    – Infiltration by bands of > 2 neoplastic cells across has been termed "trabecular" ILC
  o Single cells may be present
  o Skip lesions or patchy growth frequent
  o Desmoplastic stromal reaction may be absent
    – Correlates with absence of discrete mass by palpation or imaging in some cases
- ILC classic type (55% of cases)
  o Linear, single-file, invasive growth pattern
    – Single-file growth no more than 1-2 cells wide
    – Concentric pattern of growth around ducts
    – Focal alveolar or solid area may be present; should be < 20% of tumor
  o Nuclear grade 1 or 2 in vast majority of cases
- Architectural variants
  o Variants of ILC with distinctive tissue architecture and growth patterns
  o Solid variant (5-10% of cases)
    – Tumor forms large, usual circumscribed nests or sheets of poorly cohesive cells
    – Single-file growth may be present at periphery
    – 55% grade 3, 40% grade 2, 5% grade 1
  o Alveolar variant (5-20% of ILC)
    – Smaller, rounded aggregates of tumor cells arranged in clusters
    – 90% grade 2, 10% grade 3
    – Some cases may resemble LCIS but lack surrounding myoepithelial cell layer
  o ILC with extracellular mucin (ILCEM)
    – Rare histologic subtype demonstrating lobular morphology, extracellular mucin, and absent or reduced E-cadherin expression
    – ILCEM is typically moderate to poorly differentiated and frequently exhibits variant morphology
    – Distinct variant that often presents with higher grade and is associated with aggressive clinical course
- Cytologic variants
  o Signet-ring cell variant
    – Signet-ring cell morphology is prominent in ILC
  o Histiocytoid variant
    – Cells have abundant foamy cytoplasm and can closely resemble histiocytes
  o Pleomorphic variant
    – Cells have large, irregular nuclei (grade 2 or 3)
    – May have eosinophilic cytoplasm (apocrine)
    – Pleomorphic variant typically presents with greater tumor size, stage, fewer ER(+) and more HER2(+) cases

SELECTED REFERENCES

1. Elangovan A et al: Loss of E-cadherin induces IGF1R activation and reveals a targetable pathway in invasive lobular breast carcinoma. Mol Cancer Res. 20(9):1405-19, 2022
2. Jenkins JA et al: The 70-gene signature test as a prognostic and predictive biomarker in patients with invasive lobular breast cancer. Breast Cancer Res Treat. 191(2):401-7, 2022
3. Rätze MAK et al: Loss of E-cadherin leads to Id2-dependent inhibition of cell cycle progression in metastatic lobular breast cancer. Oncogene. 41(21):2932-44, 2022
4. Soong TR et al: Invasive lobular carcinoma with extracellular mucin (ILCEM): clinicopathologic and molecular characterization of a rare entity. Mod Pathol. 5(10):1370-82, 2022
5. Weiser R et al: Adjuvant chemotherapy in patients with invasive lobular carcinoma and use of the 21-gene recurrence score: a National Cancer Database analysis. Cancer. 128(9):1738-47, 2022

Lobular Carcinoma

Grade 1 ILC

Grade 3 ILC

(Left) In grade 1 ILC, the nuclei are small, round, and uniform in appearance ➔. Mitotic figures are typically absent, and the cytoplasm is scant. The cells can be mistaken for lymphocytes if sparse. (Right) Grade 3 ILC also shows poorly cohesive tumor cells with larger pleomorphic nuclei ➔. The cytoplasm is frequently abundant and eosinophilic, imparting an apocrine appearance. Lobular carcinomas with this appearance have been referred to as pleomorphic variant.

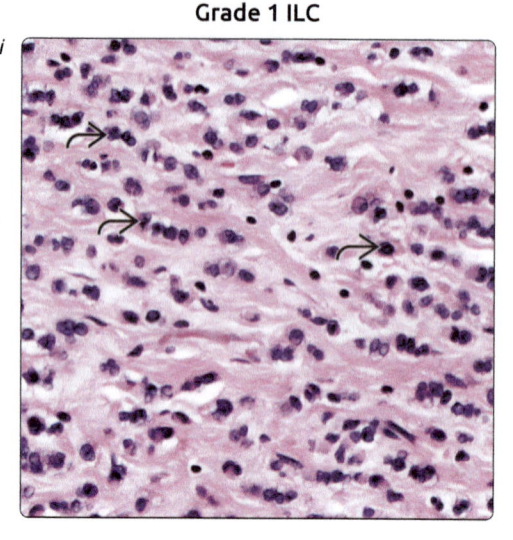

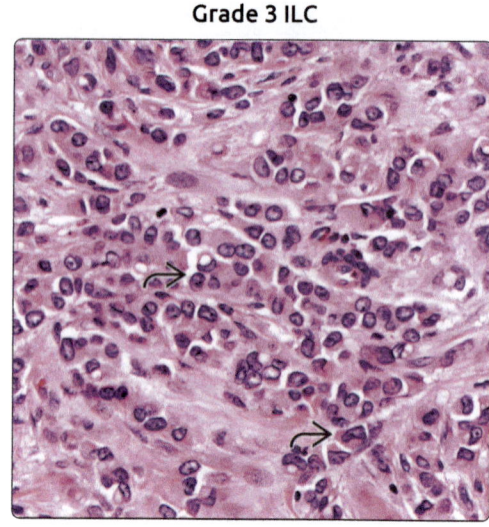

Bull's-Eye Appearance

Signet-Ring Cells

(Left) In ILC, tumor cell infiltration may be oriented in a circular fashion ➔ around normal ducts ➔, referred to as targetoid or bull's-eye appearance. (Right) This ILC also shows a circumferential growth pattern around normal ducts ➔. In addition, there are cytoplasmic mucin vacuoles ➔, which give the tumor cells a so-called signet-ring appearance, which is a common finding. Signet-ring cells in ILC typically have a single vacuole, which indents the nucleus.

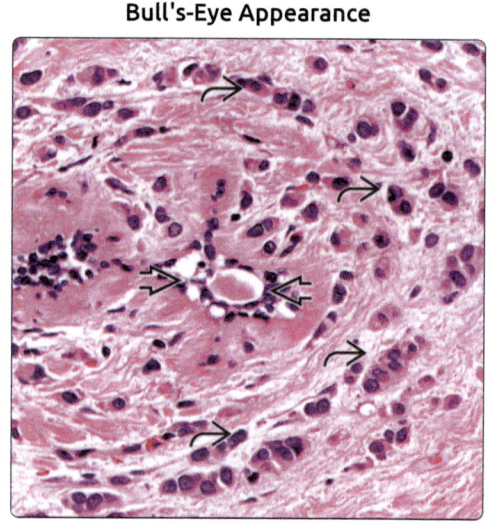

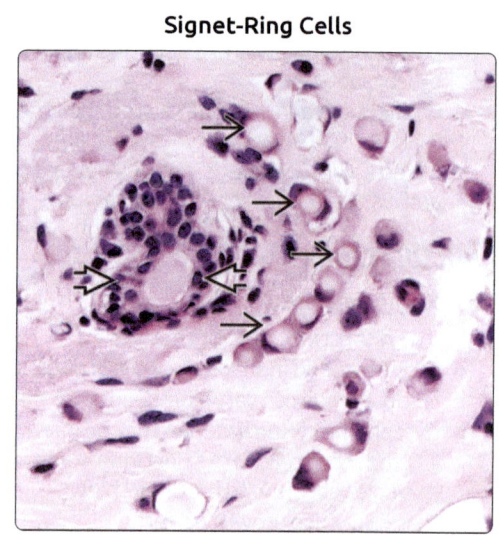

Alveolar Variant

Histiocytoid Variant

(Left) Alveolar ILC consists of clusters and nests of at least 20 tumor cells. These circumscribed nests can have an infiltrating pattern and can resemble lobular carcinoma in situ in some cases. The cells have a loose, poorly cohesive appearance and are cytologically identical to the cells of classic ILC. (Right) The histiocytoid variant of ILC consists of cells with eosinophilic foamy cytoplasm ➔ that can closely resemble histiocytes, particularly at metastatic sites or in areas of inflammation.

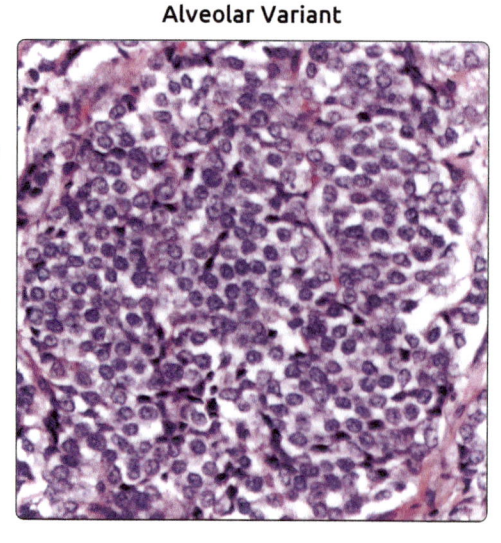

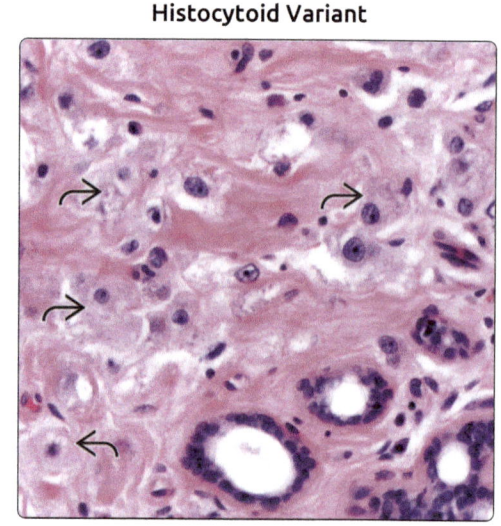

Lobular Carcinoma

Pleomorphic Variant

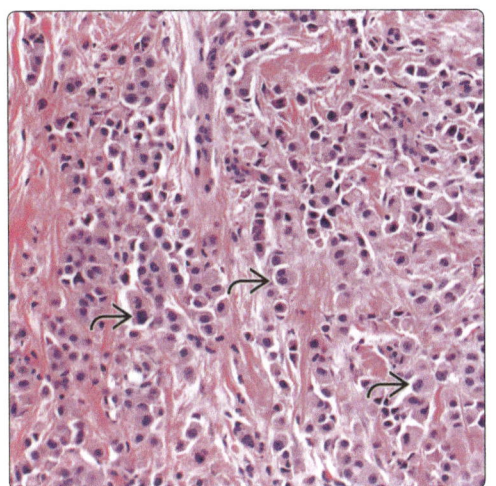

Pleomorphic Variant: ER

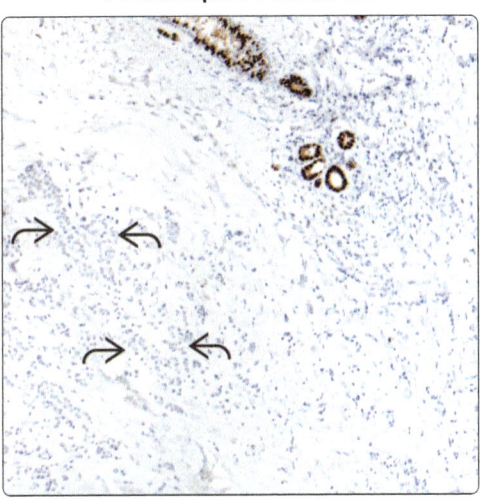

(Left) Variant forms of ILC differ from classic ILC with regard to architectural and cytologic features. The pleomorphic variant of ILC demonstrates marked nuclear atypia and frequently will have abundant eosinophilic cytoplasm ⊇ and an apocrine appearance. (Right) Variant forms of ILC may show an immunophenotype that differs markedly from classic ILC. Up to 10% of cases of pleomorphic ILC will show loss of ER expression ⊇, and 20-30% of cases may show HER2 overexpression.

H&E

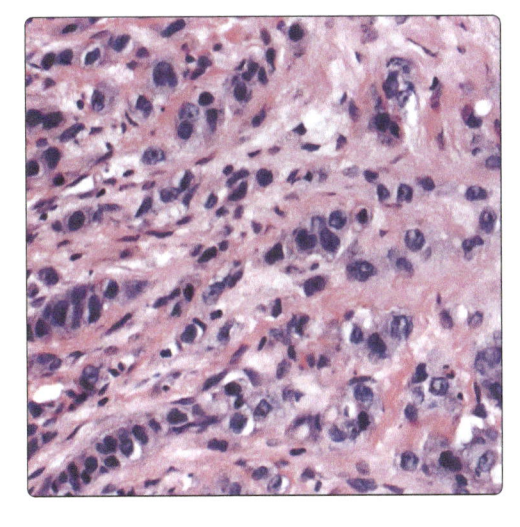

p120 Catenin

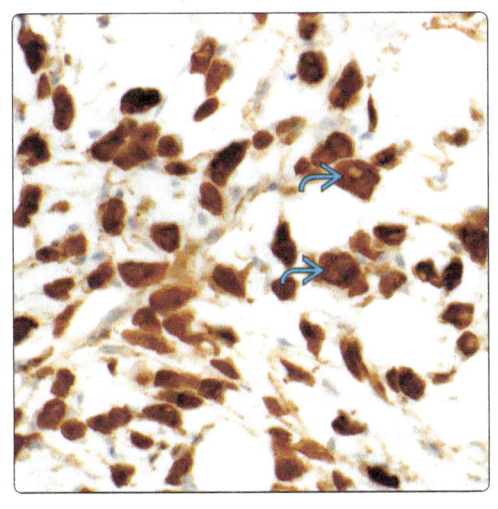

(Left) Loss of E-cadherin expression is seen in 85% of ILC cases. Some cases of ILC, such as the case shown here, retain E-cadherin expression but lack or have abnormal expression of 1 or more of the catenin complex proteins. (Right) Catenins attach E-cadherin to the actin cytoskeleton and are normally localized to the cell membrane. In ILC, p120 catenin is usually dispersed in the cytoplasm of tumor cells ⊇ instead of localized to the membrane and can be a useful diagnostic marker for difficult cases.

Histiocytoid Variant

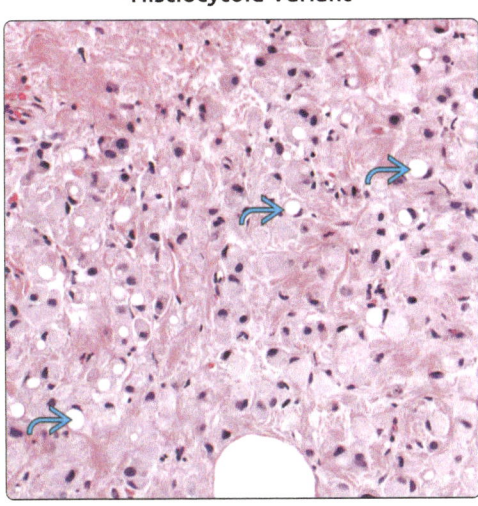

Histiocytoid Variant: *ERBB2* (HER2) Amplification

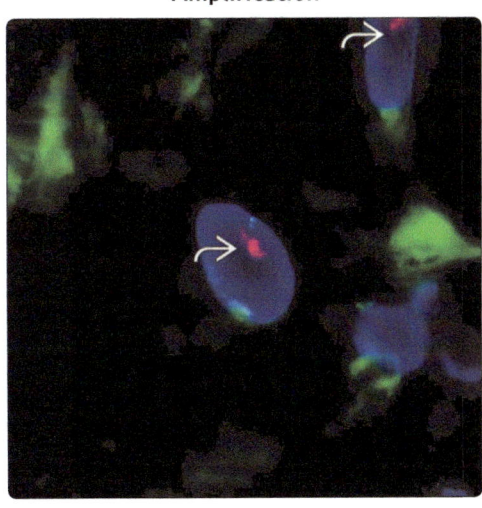

(Left) Histiocytoid ILC represents only 3% of variant tumors. The cells have copious foamy &/or eosinophilic cytoplasm and may resemble histocytes or the neoplastic cells of a granular cell tumor. The presence of signet-ring cells ⊇ is a clue to the correct diagnosis. (Right) Variant forms of ILC with histiocytoid or apocrine appearance that are high grade are more likely to be HER2(+). In this example, the *ERBB2* (HER2) gene is amplified by FISH ⊇.

705

Invasive Ductal Carcinoma of No Special Type With Medullary Features

KEY FACTS

TERMINOLOGY

- Historically described as medullary carcinoma, atypical medullary carcinoma, or carcinoma with medullary features
- In most recent WHO classification (5th edition), this entity is not considered separate histologic subtype and is now regarded as type of tumor-infiltrating lymphocyte (TIL)-rich invasive ductal carcinoma

CLINICAL ISSUES

- Targeted FDA-approved immunotherapy in breast cancer is attractive option for these patients given predictive role PD-L1 plays in triple-negative breast cancer (TNBC)
- Medullary pattern reported in 30-60% of breast tumor arising in patients with *BRCA1* germline mutations
  - Patients with germline BRCA mutations are candidates for treatment with PARP inhibitors
- Historically reported favorable prognosis is now considered to be secondary to TILs present in these tumors

MICROSCOPIC

- Invasive ductal carcinomas that display following features
  - Prominent lymphoplasmacytic infiltrates
  - Cohesive, expansile syncytial growth with circumscribed or pushing border
  - High-grade histology and proliferation

ANCILLARY TESTS

- Immunohistochemistry
  - Triple-negative profile in > 90% of cases
- Molecular genetics
  - Most tumors with *BRCA1* germline mutations have medullary pattern
- Gene expression profiling
  - 95% of cases exhibit basal-like phenotype
- *TP53* mutations are most common

Radiographic Appearance

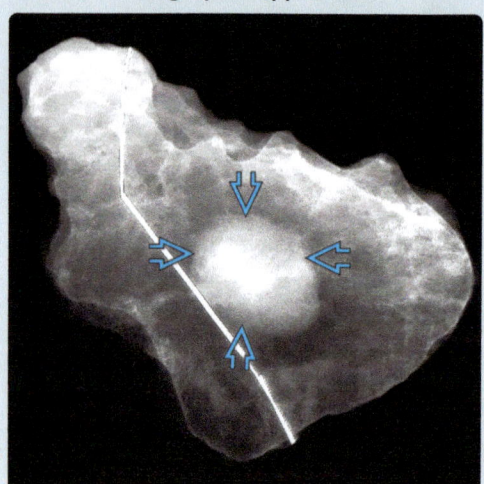

Gross Appearance

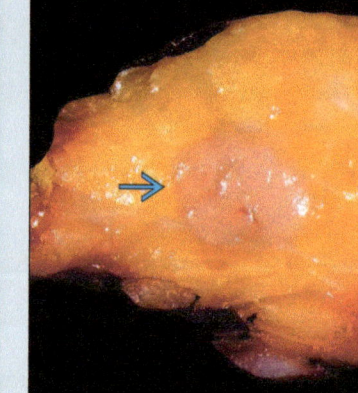

(Left) The typical mammographic appearance of invasive ductal carcinoma, medullary pattern (IDC-MP) is a mass with circumscribed borders ➡. (Right) IDC-MP usually presents as a well-circumscribed, soft to firm, lobulated mass ➡ by gross examination.

Pushing Borders

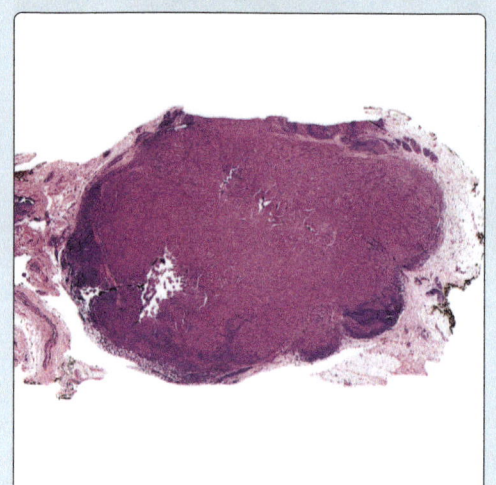

Medullary Pattern

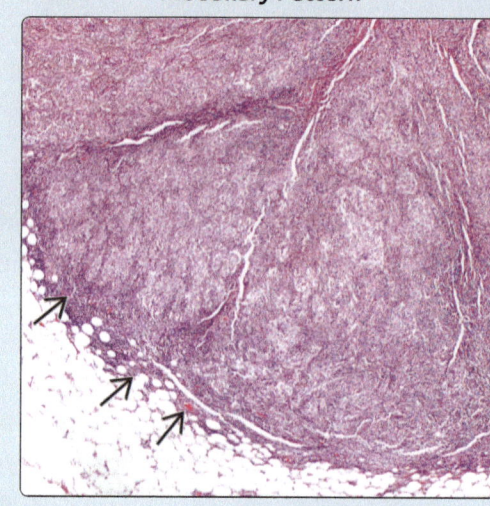

(Left) Well-circumscribed pushing borders can be appreciated in this whole-mount section. (Right) Inflammatory infiltrates are typically seen at the advancing edge ➡ of the tumor.

Invasive Ductal Carcinoma of No Special Type With Medullary Features

TERMINOLOGY

Abbreviations
- Invasive ductal carcinoma, medullary pattern (IDC-MP)
- Triple-negative breast cancer (TNBC)
- Tumor-infiltrating lymphocytes (TILs)

Definitions
- Historically described as medullary carcinoma, atypical medullary carcinoma, or carcinoma with medullary features
  - In most recent WHO classification (5th edition), this entity is not considered separate histologic subtype and is now regarded as type of TIL-rich invasive ductal carcinoma
- Typically has TNBC biomarker profile

ETIOLOGY/PATHOGENESIS

IDC-MP
- Basal-like molecular profile

CLINICAL ISSUES

Epidemiology
- Age
  - Most commonly observed in younger women
- Association with *BRCA1*
  - Medullary pattern reported in 30-60% of breast cancer arising in patients with *BRCA1* germline mutations
  - Medullary pattern reported in 25% of tumors with *BRCA1* somatic mutations

Treatment
- Treated similar to TNBC
  - Targeted FDA-approved immunotherapy in breast cancer is attractive option for these patients given predictive role PD-L1 plays in TNBC
  - Patients with germline BRCA mutations are candidates for treatment with PARP inhibitors

Prognosis
- Historically reported favorable prognosis is now considered to be secondary to TILs present in these tumors
- Dependent on stage of tumor like other TNBC
- TILs
  - Can be used both as prognostic and predictive immuno-oncologic biomarker
  - Predicts better response to chemotherapy (both in neoadjuvant and adjuvant setting)
  - Higher TILs in postneoadjuvant residual disease in TNBC are important independent predictor of improved survival
    - Improved metastasis-free survival and overall survival reported in postneoadjuvant TNBC patients with high TILs (> 60%)
- PD-L1 expression in TNBC
  - Compared to normal breast tissue, PD-L1 expression is upregulated in 38% of basal-like carcinomas (BLC)
  - Expression can serve significant prognostic biomarker of breast cancer
  - High PD-L1(+) TILs score (> 50%) is independently associated with better outcome in TNBC
  - Pathologic complete response after neoadjuvant chemotherapy is higher in case of PD-L1 upregulation
  - Can serve as important predictive biomarker
    - PD-L1 inhibitors + chemotherapy can prolong progression-free and overall survival among patients with metastatic TNBC

MICROSCOPIC

Histologic Features
- Invasive ductal carcinomas that display following features
  - Prominent intratumoral and peritumoral lymphoplasmacytic cell infiltrates
- Cohesive, expansile syncytial growth with circumscribed or pushing border
- High-grade histology and proliferation

ANCILLARY TESTS

Immunohistochemistry
- Prognostic and predictive biomarkers
  - ~ 90% of cases negative for ER, PR, and HER2 (triple-negative profile)
- Basal-like immunophenotype
  - CK5/6(+) in up to 94%
  - CK14(+) in ~ 12%
  - EGFR(+) in up to 71%
- p53
  - High rate of expression
- Lymphoid infiltrates

Genetic Testing
- Most tumors with *BRCA1* germline mutations have IDC-MP
- *TP53* mutations most common

Gene Expression Profiling
- Segregate for BLC in 95% of cases
  - Belongs to immunomodulatory (IM) subgroup in original 6-class system of TNBC and to BL1 subgroup in 4-class system
- Overexpressed genes are related to immune response

DIFFERENTIAL DIAGNOSIS

Intramammary Nodal Metastasis
- Metastases to intramammary lymph node may be difficult to distinguish from IDC-MP in come cases
  - Residual benign lymph node architecture usually present
  - No surrounding breast parenchyma

Lymphoma
- Lacks typical syncytial sheets of epithelial cell

SELECTED REFERENCES

1. Emens LA: Immunotherapy in triple-negative breast cancer. Cancer J. 27(1):59-66, 2021
2. Dieci MV et al: Update on tumor-infiltrating lymphocytes (TILs) in breast cancer, including recommendations to assess TILs in residual disease after neoadjuvant therapy and in carcinoma in situ: a report of the International Immuno-Oncology Biomarker Working Group on Breast Cancer. Semin Cancer Biol. 52(Pt 2):16-25, 2018
3. Romero P et al: Medullary breast carcinoma, a triple-negative breast cancer associated with BCLG overexpression. Am J Pathol. 188(10):2378-91, 2018

Invasive Ductal Carcinoma of No Special Type With Medullary Features

Syncytial Growth Pattern

Syncytial Growth Pattern

(Left) *Interconnecting ill-defined tongues and sheets of carcinoma cells ➡ are separated by thick, fibrous stoma septa infiltrated by inflammatory cells ➡.* (Right) *Higher power view of syncytial growth pattern ➡ shows ill-defined edges and indistinct cytoplasmic borders.*

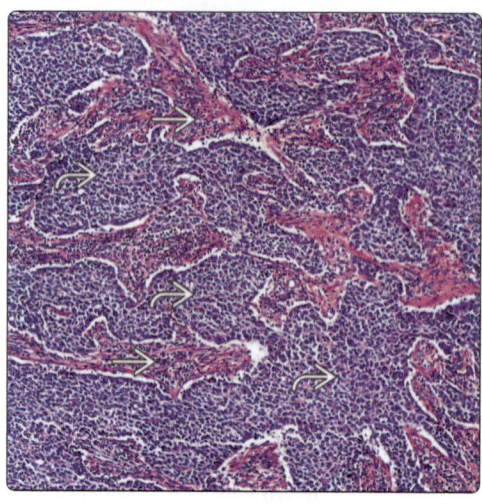

Prominent Tumor-Infiltrating Lymphocytes

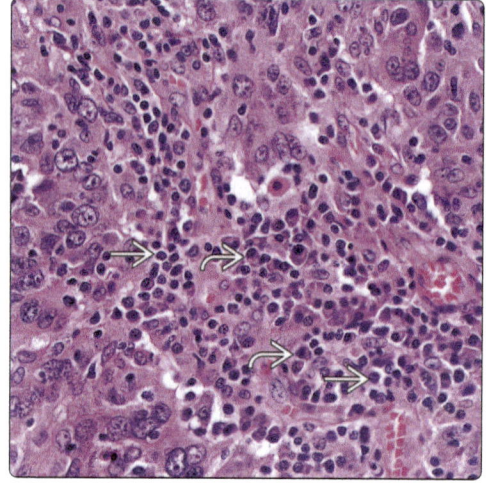

DCIS Associated With IDC-MP

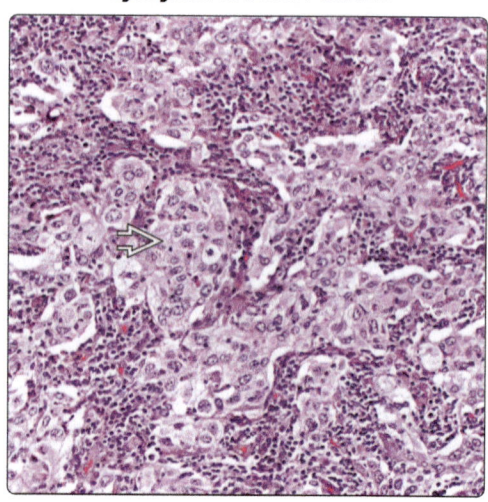

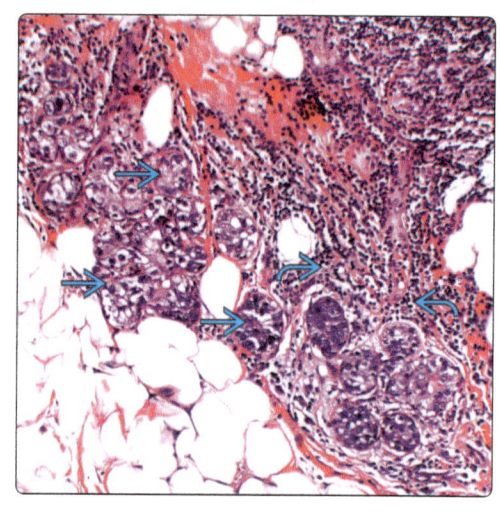

(Left) *Inflammatory cells can be observed mixed with carcinoma cells within the tumor. The inflammatory cells consist of mature lymphocytes ➡ and plasma cells ➡.* (Right) *Areas of ductal carcinoma in situ (DCIS) ➡, if present, are usually surrounded by an inflammatory infiltrate ➡. DCIS can form nodules that coalesce with the main tumor.*

Lymphocytic Lobulitis

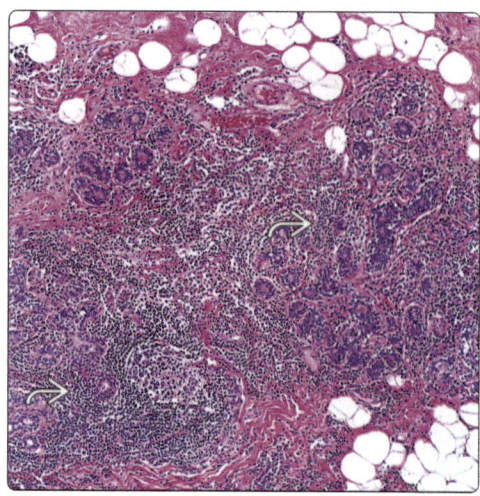

T-Cell Lymphocytic Lobulitis: CD43 Expression

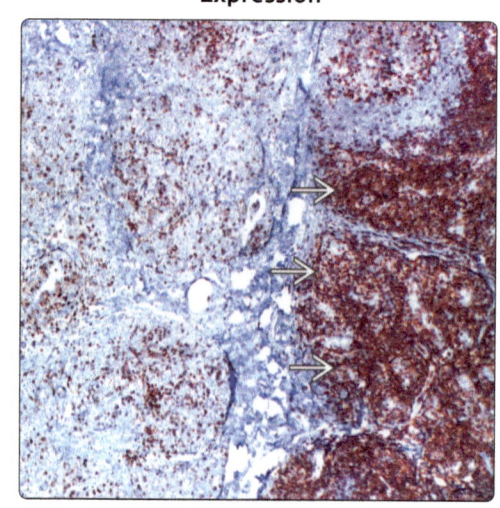

(Left) *Benign lobules can display chronic inflammation ➡. The lymphocytes surrounding these tumors and adjacent lobules are predominantly T cells. This lymphocytic lobulitis is typically present in women with germline BRCA1 mutations.* (Right) *The lymphocytic infiltrates are predominantly T cells. Benign lobules also display T-cell infiltrates ➡.*

Invasive Ductal Carcinoma of No Special Type With Medullary Features

IDC-MP Mimicking Lymph Node Metastasis

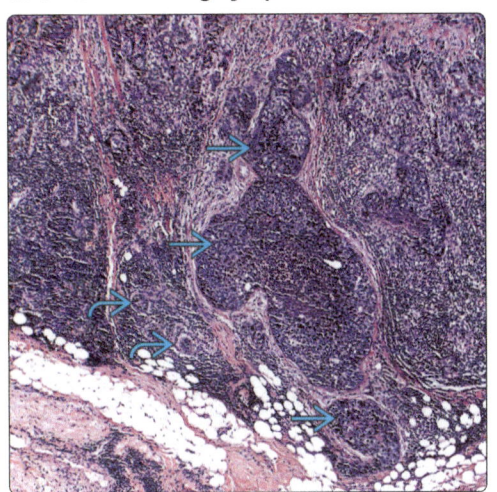

Metastatic Carcinoma to Lymph Node

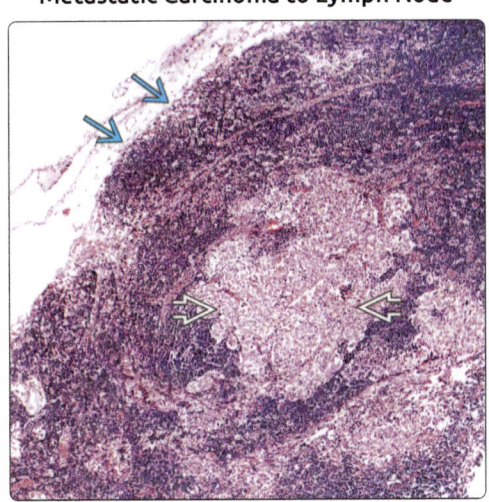

(Left) *Carcinomas occurring in the upper outer quadrant, associated with a dense lymphocytic infiltrate, can be confused with a lymph node metastasis. The presence of normal acini ➔ and DCIS ➔ help identify this lesion as a primary carcinoma.* **(Right)** *Metastatic carcinoma (MC) in a node ➔ can resemble IDC-MP. This may be challenging if the lesion is located in the upper outer quadrant. The lymphocytes in a node should be confined by a capsule ➔, while the lymphocytes associated with MC can infiltrate surrounding tissues.*

Lymphoid Aggregates

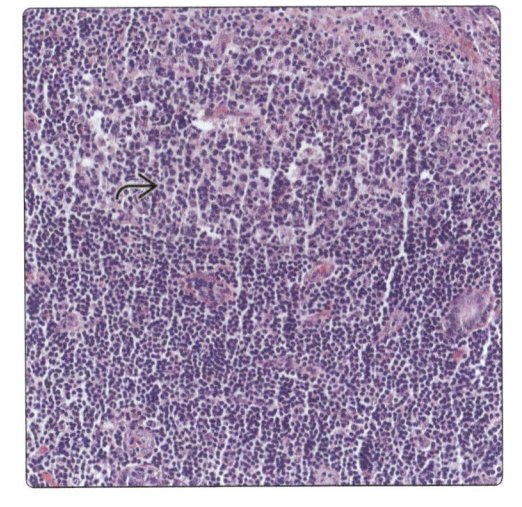

IDC-MP: Basal Cytokeratin Expression

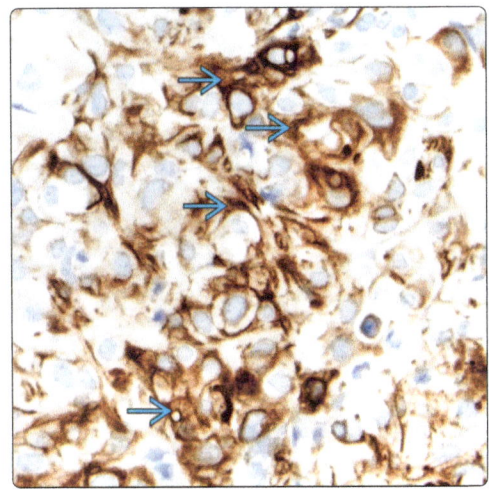

(Left) *High-power view shows one of the lymphoid aggregates at the periphery of IDC-MP. Frequently, these aggregates display prominent germinal centers ➔.* **(Right)** *Most IDC-MP belong to the basal-like group of tumors by gene expression profiling. Greater than 90% of these tumors show high levels of basal cytokeratins by IHC (CK5 ➔).*

EGFR Expression

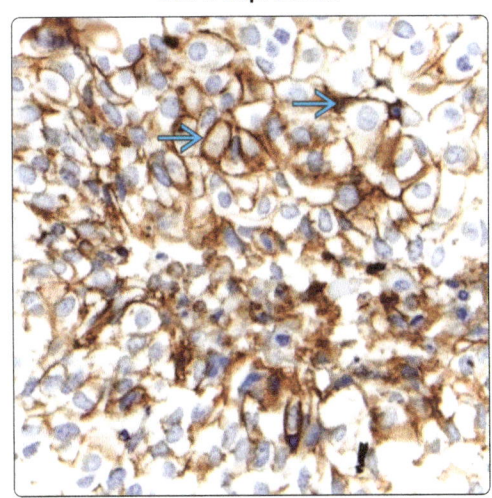

p53 Expression

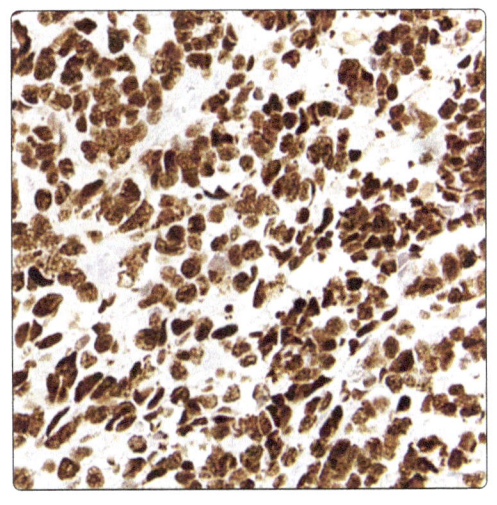

(Left) *In triple-negative breast cancer, the expression of basal cytokeratins &/or EGFR ➔ has been used as a surrogate for identifying tumors with a basal phenotype by gene expression profiling.* **(Right)** *Diffuse nuclear expression of p53 is shown.*

Metaplastic Breast Carcinoma

KEY FACTS

TERMINOLOGY
- Metaplastic breast carcinoma (MBC): Heterogeneous group of breast cancers characterized by differentiation of neoplastic epithelium to squamous &/or mesenchymal cells

CLINICAL ISSUES
- Higher rate of resistance to chemotherapy than other types of breast carcinoma, including triple-negative breast cancer (TNBC)
- Complete response reported in few patients with PD-L1 tumor expression
- MBC have been reported in gBRCA-positive patients with response to PARP inhibitors
- mTOR-based systemic therapy
  - Better long-term outcomes reported compared to other TNBC
- In general, poor prognosis, even when compared to other TNBC

MOLECULAR
- Basal gene profile
- Claudin-low profile
  - Share similar genetic features with claudin-low tumors
- MBC frequently harbors *TP53* mutations
  - TP53 protein overexpressed in up to 71% of cases
- *PIK3CA*
  - Mutations in up to 47% of cases
- TERT promoter mutations (25-33%)
- *MYC* amplification (more common in SqCC and SpCC)
- *EGFR* amplification (17.2%)

MICROSCOPIC
- Often mix of epithelial and mesenchymal components

ANCILLARY TESTS
- Frequent triple-negative biomarker profile (85%)
- Positive myoepithelial markers
- Cytokeratins usually positive, at least focally

Focal Keratinization

Malignant Epithelial and Stromal Components

(Left) *Metaplastic squamous carcinoma shows the characteristic appearance of squamous cells with a basal cell layer, abundant eosinophilic cytoplasm, and focal keratinization ➡.* (Right) *Malignant epithelial and stromal (spindle cell) components in metaplastic breast carcinoma are shown. Nuclear atypia is present in both the epithelial and stromal cells. Note the stromal mitotic figure ➡.*

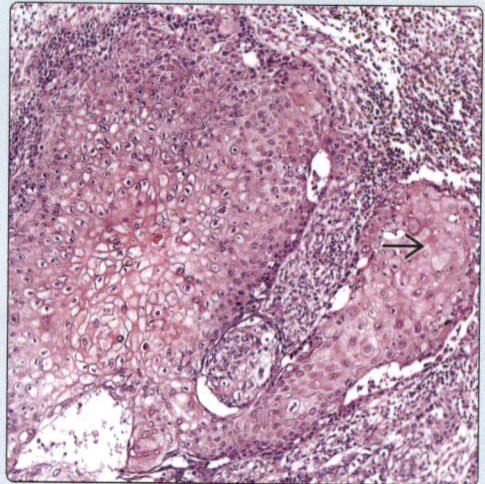

Heterologous Mesenchymal Differentiation

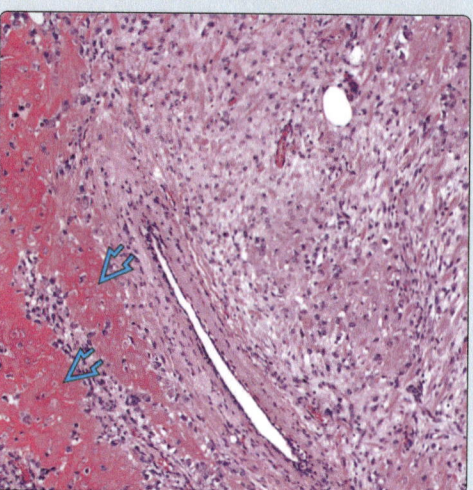

p63 Expression

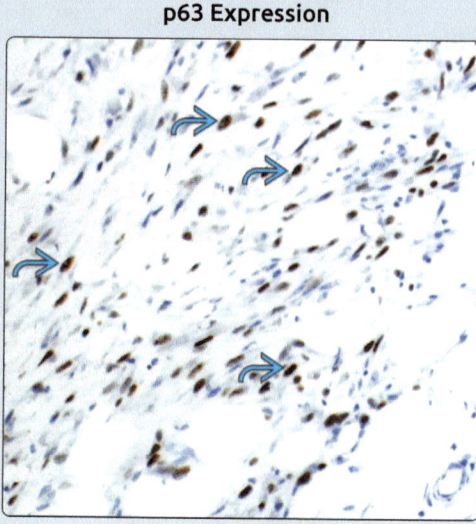

(Left) *Metaplastic carcinoma shows evidence of extracellular matrix production ➡, consistent with osteoid. It is important to rule out a metaplastic carcinoma or phyllodes tumor before diagnosing primary sarcoma.* (Right) *Expression of epithelial or myoepithelial markers can be helpful in distinguishing metaplastic carcinoma from other mesenchymal tumors. This spindle cell metaplastic carcinoma shows diffuse p63 expression ➡, supportive of the correct diagnosis.*

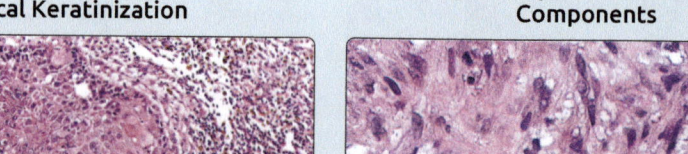

Metaplastic Breast Carcinoma

TERMINOLOGY

Abbreviations
- Metaplastic breast carcinoma (MBC)
- MBC with heterologous mesenchymal differentiation (MBCHMD)

Definitions
- Heterogeneous group of breast cancers characterized by
  o Differentiation of neoplastic epithelium toward squamous &/or mesenchymal elements with
    – Loss of intercellular adhesion
    – Downregulation of epithelial markers, including cytokeratins
    – Upregulation of mesenchymal markers vimentin, SMA, and myoepithelial markers, including p63
    – Increase in motility, invasiveness, and metastatic potential

CLASSIFICATION

World Health Organization (2019)
- Squamous cell carcinoma (SqCC)
- Spindle cell carcinoma (SpCC)
- Metaplastic carcinoma with heterologous mesenchymal differentiation
  o Chondroid differentiation
  o Osseous differentiation
  o Other types of mesenchymal differentiation
- Low-grade MBC
  o Low-grade adenosquamous carcinoma
  o Fibromatosis-like metaplastic carcinoma

ETIOLOGY/PATHOGENESIS

Cell of Origin
- All MBC show at least focal evidence of origin as epithelial malignancy
  o Cytokeratin expression should be present but may be focal and only high-molecular-weight basal keratins (5, 14, and 17)
- Many MBC have features of myoepithelial differentiation
  o 1/3 to 2/3 express markers typical of myoepithelial cells, including p63, SMA, P-cadherin, or CD10
  o Myoepithelial cells can produce basement membrane material that may resemble cartilage or bone matrix
  o Myoepithelial cells can be spindled in shape and closely resemble squamous cells
    – Myoepithelial cells can undergo squamous metaplasia
- Exome sequencing for paired metaplastic and adjacent conventional invasive carcinoma from same tumor has been reported
  o Tumor components have similar landscape of somatic mutation
  o Shared origin for tumors with differing histologies suggests that epigenetic or noncoding changes may mediate metaplastic phenotype in MBC
- EMT
  o Acquisition of mesenchymal phenotype by malignant epithelial cells
    – Cells acquire migratory and invasive properties that promote progression and induce chemoresistance
    – Characterized by switching of cadherins (E-cadherin to N-cadherin), downregulation of epithelial markers, including low-molecular-weight keratins and upregulation of mesenchymal markers
    – Pathways that can activate EMT include transforming growth factor β, Wnt, and tyrosine kinase receptors, resulting in activation of EMT transcription factors (SNAIL1/2, ZEB1/2, TWIST)
    – Enables cells to acquire different phenotypes due to secondary transdifferentiation
  o Evidence has shown that MBC is likely enriched in stem-cell-like cells

Immune Microenvironment
- PD-L1 is upregulated in EMT-activated human breast cancer cells; this may explain its upregulation in MBC
- Tumor-infiltrating lymphocytes (TILs) have been shown to be higher in MBC with high tumor mutation burden (TMB)
- Similarly, high PD-1 expression has been reported in inflammatory infiltrates

CLINICAL ISSUES

Epidemiology
- Incidence
  o 0.2-5.0% of all breast cancers

Presentation
- Large mass
- Median age: 59 years

Treatment
- Surgical resection
  o Usually total mastectomy, given commonly large tumor size
- Adjuvant radiation treatment
  o May improve overall and disease-related survival in some cases
- Traditional adjuvant chemotherapy
  o Higher rate of resistance to chemotherapy than other types of breast carcinoma, including TNBC
- Neoadjuvant chemotherapy
  o Chemoresistance to neoadjuvant regimens has been reported with complete pathologic response rate at 11.3% compared to 34% in TNBC
- mTOR-based systemic therapy
  o Better long-term outcomes reported compared to other TNBC
  o Secondary to high frequency of alterations in PI3K/AKT/mTOR pathway
- Immune checkpoint inhibitors (ICIs)
  o Complete response reported in few patients with PD-L1 tumor expression
  o FDA-approved ICIs available for treatment combined with chemotherapy for advanced/metastatic TNBC
- PARP1 inhibitors
  o MBC reported in *gBRCA*-positive patients with response

Prognosis
- In general, poor prognosis, even when compared to other TNBC
  o 5-year survival: 55% (vs. 85% and 75% for same-stage invasive ductal carcinomas and TNBC, respectively)

Metaplastic Breast Carcinoma

- Incidence of lymph node metastasis (35% of cases) is less than that seen in stage-matched invasive ductal carcinoma
- Distant visceral metastasis common at time of presentation (13%)
- Metastatic route may be primarily hematogenous to lung, brain, and liver
- Higher degree of chemoresistance in MBC compared to other TNBC
- Cases of low-grade adenosquamous carcinoma and fibromatosis-like metaplastic carcinoma with early-stage presentation have been associated with favorable clinical outcome and are considered low-grade variants of MBC, where patients have been adequately treated by complete surgical excision

IMAGING

General Features
- Commonly round or oval in shape
- Usually well circumscribed

MACROSCOPIC

General Features
- Mass lesion
  - Can be well circumscribed or may show ill-defined borders
- Firm or fleshy consistency
- Hemorrhage and necrosis common

Size
- Range: 1.2 to > 10 cm
- Mean: 3.9 cm

MOLECULAR

Gene Expression Profiling
- MBC has distinctive molecular signature, separating it from other molecular classes of breast carcinomas
  - Majority demonstrate transcriptional profile similar to but distinct from basal-like carcinomas
    - Transcriptional profiles suggest cells undergoing epithelial-to-mesenchymal transition
    - Profile is most similar to claudin-low group of carcinomas
- Basal gene profile
  - Overexpression of proliferation and basal-related genes encoding
    - EGFR protein
    - Basal/high-molecular-weight cytokeratins 5, 6, 14, and 17
- Claudin-low profile
  - Share similar genetic features with claudin-low tumors characterized by
    - Low to absent expression of GATA3 and E-cadherin proteins
    - Upregulation of mesenchymal antigens, e.g., vimentin
    - Downregulation of genes found in epithelial cells
    - Upregulation of genes found in fibroblasts
  - Claudin-low tumors show features similar to so-called cancer stem cells

Gene Mutations
- MBC frequently harbors *TP53* mutations
  - TP53 protein overexpressed in up to 71% of cases (median 58.7%) compared to 20-40% in conventional breast cancer
    - Hotspot mutations: R273H, R273C, and R273G (former two lead to more aggressive biology)
  - Frequency varies among MBC variants
    - More common in SqCC and MBCHMD
  - Less frequent when compared to other TNBC (87%)
- *PIK3CA*
  - Mutations seen in up to 47% of cases (median: 38.2%)
  - Hotspot mutation: H1047R most common
  - Frequency varies among MBC variants
    - More common in SpCC
  - More frequent when compared to other TNBC (13%)
- Other less common PI3K/AKT pathway gene mutations include
  - *PTEN* (12.7%, SqCC), *PIK3R1* (11.2%), *NF1* (9.8%), *HRAS* (8.5%), and *AKT1* (3%)
  - May respond to PI3K inhibitor drugs, such as mTOR inhibitors (temsirolimus)
- Mutations in genes that modulate Wnt pathway
  - *FAT1* (11%) and *APC* (5%)
- TERT promoter mutations (25-33%)
  - Through telomerase activation
  - Activation of WNT pathway through telomere-independent mechanisms
  - Detected in 80% of SpCC and 20% of SqCC but not in MBCHMD
- Compared with TNBC, MBC more frequently harbors mutations in PI3K/AKT/mTOR pathway (57% vs. 22%) and canonical Wnt pathway (51% vs. 28%)
  - MBC seems to be driven by repertoire of somatic mutations distinct from TNBC
  - Dysregulation of PI3K/AKT/mTOR pathway may provide rationale for metaplastic phenotype and response to PI3K/AKT/mTOR inhibitors
- Mutations in DNA repair pathway genes
  - *BRCA1* (3-15%), *BRCA2* (2-6%), and *ATM* (2-12%)
- Mutations in chromatin remodeling genes
  - *KMT2D* (17%) and *ARID1A* (6%)
- Concurrent mutations of *TP53*, *PIK3CA*, and *PTEN* have been recently described

Copy Number Variations
- Gene amplification (more common in SqCC and SpCC)
  - *MYC* (17.3%)
    - Other cell cycle control genes: *CCND1* (8.4%), *CCNE1* (5.9%), and *CDK4* (4%)
  - *EGFR* (17.2%)
    - Other tyrosine kinase receptors coding genes: *FGFR1* (5%) and *ERBB2* (4.8%)
- Gene loss
  - *CDKN2A*/*CDKN2B* locus (19%), *PTEN* (14.9%), and *RB1* (6.5%)

MICROSCOPIC

Histologic Features
- MBC comprises heterogeneous group of carcinomas

Metaplastic Breast Carcinoma

  - Commonly, mixture of epithelial and mesenchymal components

Squamous Cell Carcinoma

- Commonly cystic with cavity lined by neoplastic squamous cells
- Invasive edge of tumor composed of sheets or cords of squamous cells
  - Variable degrees of differentiation
  - Desmoplastic stroma
- Acantholytic variant may acquire pseudoglandular or pseudoangiomatous appearance
- Not uncommonly mixed with neoplastic spindle cells
- May be pure or mixed with conventional invasive ductal carcinoma

Spindle Cell Carcinoma

- Moderately or highly pleomorphic spindle cells
- Arranged in different patterns, including fascicular, storiform, or diffuse sheet-like
- Areas with epithelioid morphology or squamous differentiation can be found

Low-Grade Adenosquamous Carcinoma

- Infiltrative, well-formed, low-grade glandular and tubular structures mixed with nests of squamous cells
- Percolate between benign terminal duct-lobular units
- Radial scar-like background with low-grade spindle cell stroma with variable cellularity
- Prominent lymphoid aggregates may be present at periphery of tumor in cannonball pattern
- Osteocartilaginous elements may be detected rarely
- Coexisting ductal carcinoma in situ or conventional invasive ductal carcinoma usually absent
- May arise in association with complex sclerosing lesions and papillomas

Fibromatosis-Like Metaplastic Carcinoma

- Bland spindle cell proliferation arranged in wavy, interlacing fascicles in variably collagenized stroma
- Infiltrative, finger-like extensions into surrounding breast parenchyma
- Areas with epithelioid or squamous differentiation often found

Metaplastic Carcinoma With Heterologous Mesenchymal Differentiation

- Mesenchymal elements are usually chondroid, or osseous
  - Variable degrees of differentiation
  - Can mimic true soft tissue sarcomas
- Mixed with carcinomatous elements, which can be glandular or squamous
  - May be minor component
    - Extensive sampling is crucial to ensure adequate tissue component representation

ANCILLARY TESTS

Immunohistochemistry

- Frequent triple-negative biomarker profile (85%)
  - ER and PR negative
    - Reported positivity in 0-13%
  - HER2 (ERBB2) negative
    - Reported positivity in 0-10%
- Usually high Ki-67 proliferative index score
- Vimentin positive
- Positive myoepithelial markers
  - p63 positive, at least focal
- Calponin highlights lamellar cuffing around lesional glands in low-grade adenosquamous carcinoma
- Cytokeratins usually positive, at least focally
- May require use of > 1 cytokeratin marker in order to detect positive cells
- High-molecular-weight cytokeratins more often positive
  - CK5/6
  - CK14
  - CK17
- CD34 negative (usually positive in phyllodes tumor)

DIFFERENTIAL DIAGNOSIS

Metastatic Squamous Cell Carcinoma

- More common than primary SqCC of breast
- Primary SqCC of breast should be diagnosed only after exclusion of extension or metastasis from other sites, especially skin

Primary or Metastatic Soft Tissue Sarcomas

- Rare primary tumors in breast
  - Angiosarcoma is most common primary mammary sarcoma
    - Breast angiosarcoma can be secondary to prior radiation treatment or chronic lymphedema
- Soft tissue sarcoma should not be considered before MBC is ruled out
- Positivity for keratins and p63 favors metaplastic carcinoma
- Adequate sampling is crucial to identify mixture of epithelial and mesenchymal components in MBC

Phyllodes Tumors With Sarcomatous Overgrowth

- Immunohistochemical markers
  - p63 expressed in metaplastic carcinomas
    - Usually negative in sarcomatous component of phyllodes tumors
  - CD34 and BCL2 usually expressed in sarcomatous component of phyllodes tumors
    - Negative in metaplastic carcinomas
- Molecular testing may be helpful to detect some characteristic mutations associated with phyllodes tumors

SELECTED REFERENCES

1. González-Martínez S et al: Molecular features of metaplastic breast carcinoma: an infrequent subtype of triple negative breast carcinoma. Cancers (Basel). 12(7):1832, 2020
2. McCart Reed AE et al: Phenotypic and molecular dissection of metaplastic breast cancer and the prognostic implications. J Pathol. 247(2):214-27, 2019
3. Adams S: Dramatic response of metaplastic breast cancer to chemo-immunotherapy. NPJ Breast Cancer. 3:8, 2017
4. Avigdor B et al: Whole exome sequencing of metaplastic breast carcinoma indicates monoclonality with associated ductal carcinoma component. Clin Cancer Res. 23(16):4875-84, 2017
5. Edenfield J et al: Metaplastic breast cancer: molecular typing and identification of potential targeted therapies at a single institution. Clin Breast Cancer. 17(1):e1-10, 2017
6. Joneja U et al: Comprehensive profiling of metaplastic breast carcinomas reveals frequent overexpression of programmed death-ligand 1. J Clin Pathol. 70(3):255-9, 2017

Metaplastic Breast Carcinoma

Heterologous Mesenchymal Differentiation

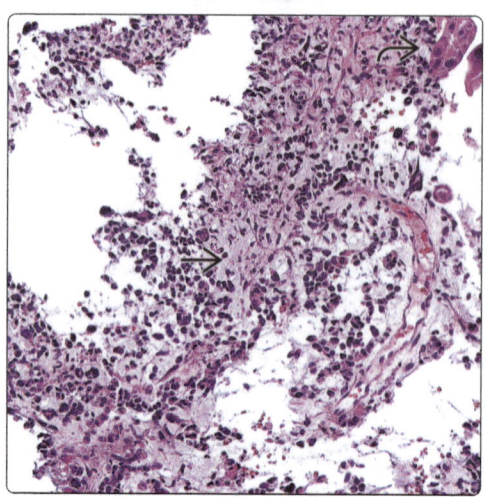

Spindle Cell Proliferation

(Left) Metaplastic carcinoma shows pleomorphic stromal cells with high N:C ratio producing myxoid matrix background ⇒ (historically "matrix-producing metaplastic carcinoma"). True chondroid differentiation was present in other fields. Note the pleomorphic epithelial cell component ⇒. (Right) Diffuse atypical spindle cell proliferation is shown. Storiform pattern ⇒ can mimic spindle cell sarcoma.

High Histologic Grade

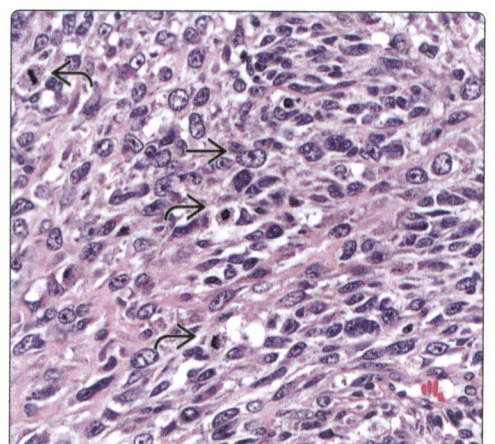

p53 Overexpression

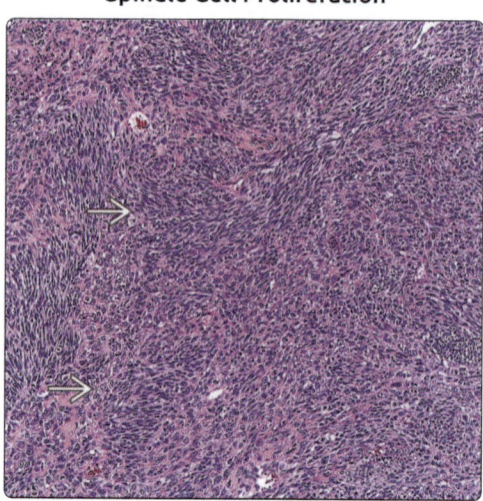

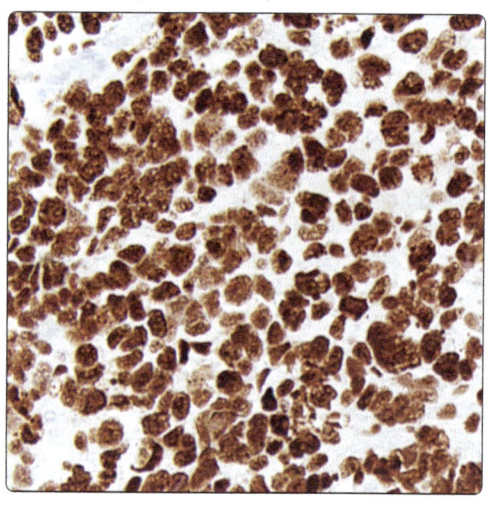

(Left) Spindle cell carcinoma of the breast shows prominent nuclear pleomorphism with variably enlarged, irregular nuclei with vesicular chromatin and prominent nucleoli ⇒. Mitotic figures are readily detectable ⇒. (Right) p53 overexpression is shown in up to 71% of metaplastic carcinomas, as evident in this representative section from a case of metaplastic spindle cell carcinoma of the breast.

p63 Expression

EGFR Amplification

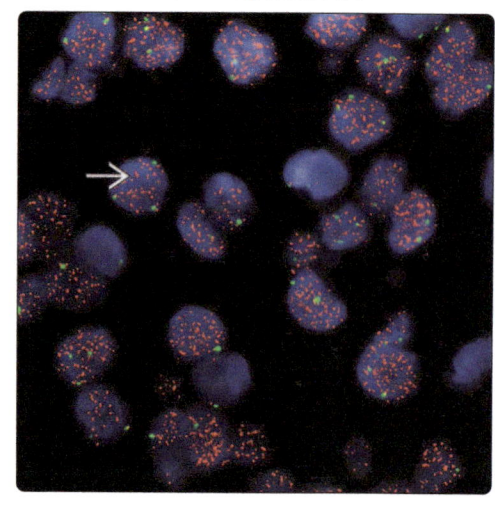

(Left) p63 shows diffuse and strong expression by epithelial tumor nest components ⇒ of this low-grade adenosquamous carcinoma. (Right) FISH using EGFR probes shows numerous EGFR signals (red) consistent with EGFR amplification ⇒ in this case of metaplastic breast carcinoma. EGFR is amplified in up to 70% of metaplastic breast carcinomas. Green signals represent centromeric chromosome 7 probes.

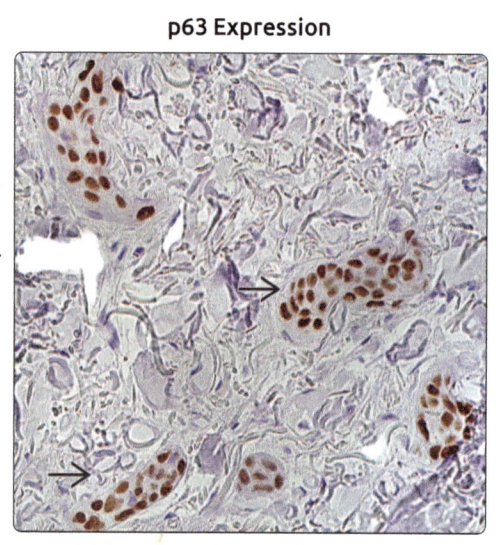

Metaplastic Breast Carcinoma

Fibromatosis-Like Disease

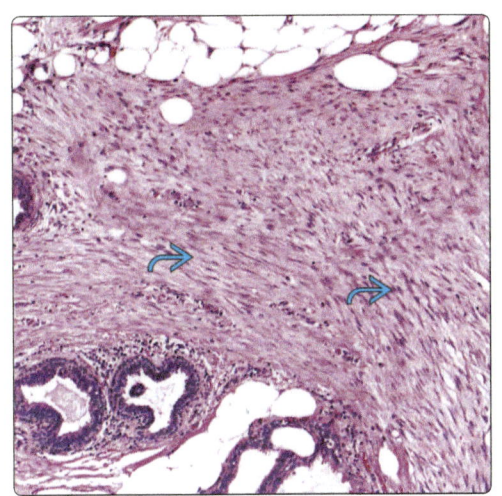

Epithelioid Nests

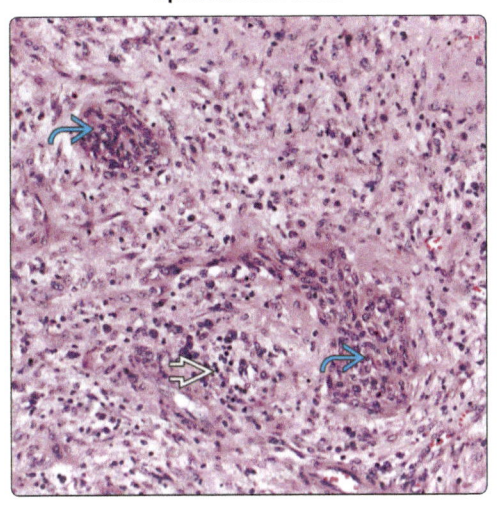

(Left) *Mildly cellular proliferation of low-grade atypical spindle cells ➡ resembling fibroblasts can closely resemble fibromatosis.* (Right) *In this metaplastic spindle cell carcinoma, epithelioid nests ➡ stand out against neoplastic spindle cells. The presence of inflammatory reaction ➡ is a characteristic feature of metaplastic carcinomas with spindle and squamous elements.*

High Histologic Grade

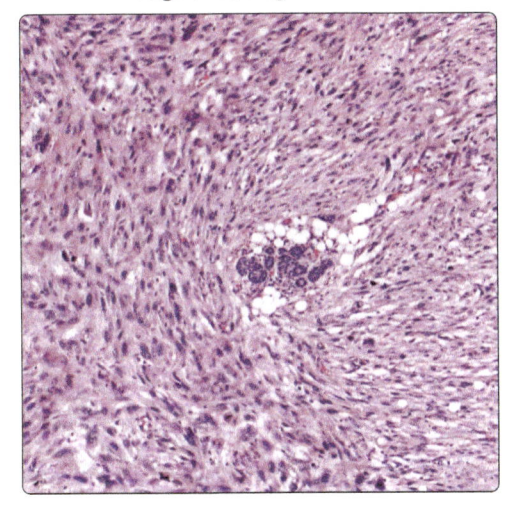

Heterologous Mesenchymal Differentiation

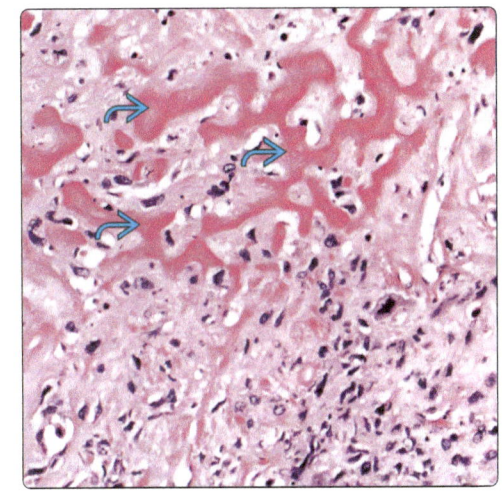

(Left) *Poorly differentiated spindle cell metaplastic carcinomas are highly cellular and have pleomorphic nuclei and frequent mitotic figures. Extensive sampling is sometimes needed to show areas with epithelial differentiation.* (Right) *Rarely, metaplastic carcinoma is associated with recognizable malignant mesenchymal elements. The most common sarcomatous component is osteosarcoma ➡.*

Angiosarcoma

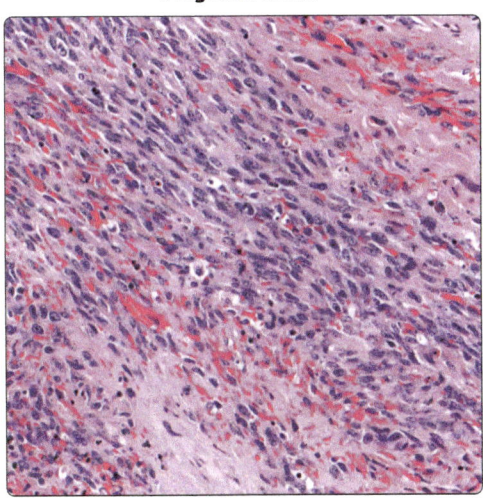

Rhabdomyosarcoma

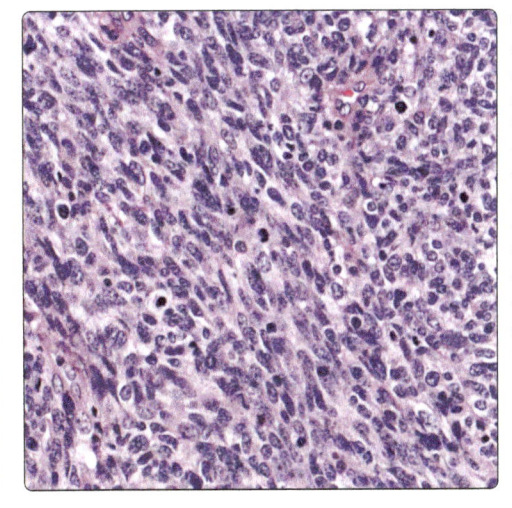

(Left) *Angiosarcomas are the most common type of primary breast sarcoma. This tumor has a predominant spindle cell appearance, and vascular spaces are poorly formed. This type of sarcoma may be difficult to distinguish from spindle cell carcinoma without IHC.* (Right) *Embryonal rhabdomyosarcoma can involve breast as either primary tumor or metastatic disease. High-grade spindle cell tumor showed strong desmin and myogenin expression, which was helpful in establishing the correct diagnosis.*

Phyllodes Tumors

KEY FACTS

TERMINOLOGY
- Phyllodes tumors (PT): Group of fibroepithelial tumors that consist of variable proportions of epithelial and stromal components
- Tumor consists of neoplastic clonal intralobular-type stromal cells and benign nonclonal epithelial cells

MOLECULAR
- Positive correlation between aneuploidy and malignant progression
- Average number of chromosome copy changes increases with histologic grade
- MED12 mutations
  - Missense mutations involving codon 44 within exon 2 detected in 80% of PT, regardless of tumor grade
  - Play critical role in pathogenesis of PT
- Malignant PT show increased mRNA levels of PAX3, homeobox protein SIX1, TGFB2, HMGA2, and HOXB13
- Strong evidence supporting monoclonality, especially of stromal component of PT
- High methylation of *RASSF1* and *TWIST1*
- Sequencing data has shown that *TERT* promoter mutations are frequent in PT (65%)
  - Mutations more common in borderline (87%) but also seen in benign (50%) and malignant (62%) PT
- Most common mutations: *TP53* (58%), *TERT* promoter (58%), *NF1* (46%), *MED12* (45%), *CDKN2A/CDKN2B* (33%)

MICROSCOPIC
- 3 histologic subtypes are classified according to degree of stromal overgrowth, nuclear atypia, mitotic activity, and invasiveness into surrounding benign breast tissue
  - Benign PT (60-75%)
  - Borderline PT (15-20%)
  - Malignant PT (10-20%)

ANCILLARY TESTS
- Stroma positive for CD34 and BCL2 and negative for p63

Leaf-Like Projections

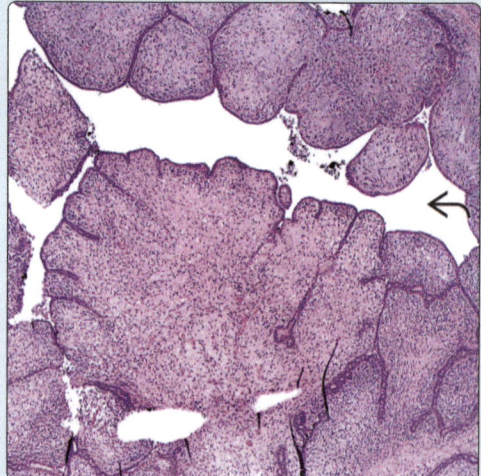

Malignant Phyllodes Tumor

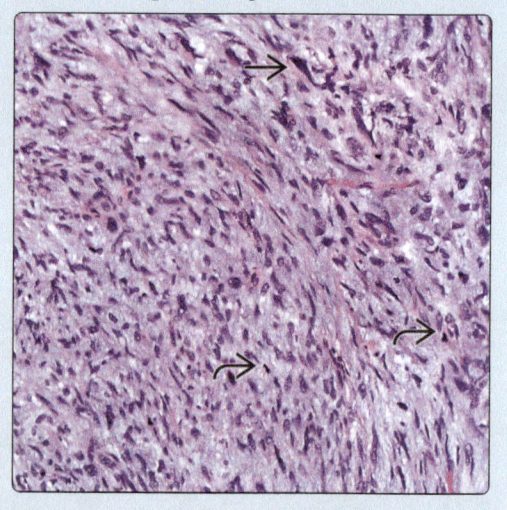

(Left) At low power, the pronounced intracanalicular growth of leaf-like projections into variably dilated ductal lumina ➡ is characteristic of phyllodes tumor (PT). (Right) Markedly cellular stroma and prominent stromal atypia ➡ are shown in malignant PT. Mitoses ➡ are readily detectable and can be ≥ 10 per 10 HPF.

Gross Appearance

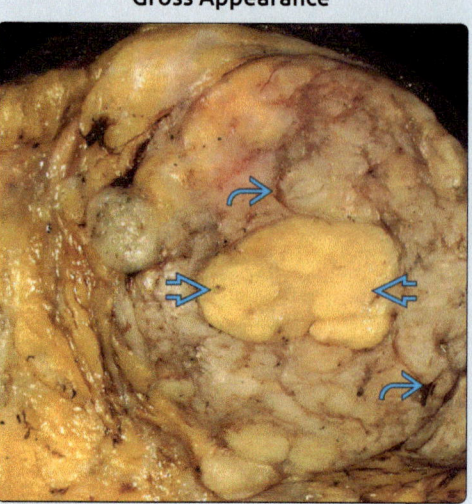

Heterologous Elements

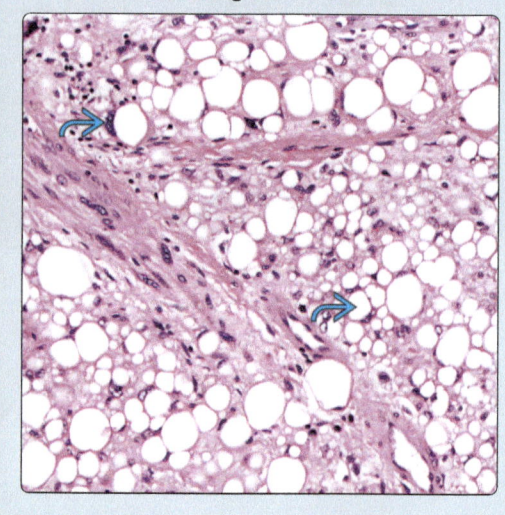

(Left) Gross photograph shows a 15-cm malignant PT with a tan-white, bosselated cut surface and cleft-like spaces ➡. In the center of the tumor is a homogeneous yellow nodule ➡ corresponding to liposarcoma. (Right) PT with malignant heterologous elements (except well-differentiated liposarcoma) is considered malignant. This area of liposarcoma was present in the center of a large PT. The presence of lipoblasts ➡ may be misinterpreted as invasion into benign adipose tissue.

Phyllodes Tumors

TERMINOLOGY

Abbreviations
- Phyllodes tumors (PT)

Definitions
- Fibroepithelial tumors with exaggerated intracanalicular pattern and leaf-like stromal fronds and hypercellular stroma

ETIOLOGY/PATHOGENESIS

Cell of Origin
- Thought to be derived from intralobular or periductal specialized stroma
- Associated epithelial cells are benign and are stimulated to proliferate by stroma

TP53 Germline Mutation
- Li-Fraumeni syndrome
- Significantly associated with increased risk of developing malignant PT

CLINICAL ISSUES

Epidemiology
- Incidence
  o 0.3-1.0% of all breast tumors
- Age
  o Middle-aged women (40-50 years)

Presentation
- Unilateral firm mass
- Bloody nipple discharge may occur
- Skin ulceration in large tumors

Prognosis
- Local recurrence (20-30% risk for malignant PT)
  o Recurrent tumors may display higher grade histology or dedifferentiation in 25-75% of cases
  o Positive margin of excision is most reliable predictive factors for local recurrence
- Distant metastasis (9% risk for malignant PT)
  o Lungs and bones most common sites for metastatic PT

MOLECULAR

Cytogenetics
- Positive correlation between aneuploidy and malignant progression

Chromosomal Microarray
- Rate of recurrent chromosomal imbalances
  o Increases with higher histologic grade
  o 55% in benign PT
  o 91% in borderline PT
  o 100% in malignant PT
- Most frequent gains
  o 1q, 2p, 3q, 7p, 8q, and 20
- Most frequent losses
  o 3p, 10, 13q, 15q, 16, 17p, 19, and X
- Malignant progression
  o Associated with gains of 1q and losses of 13q
- Deletion of 9p21
  o Involves *CDKN2A* locus
  o Malignant, some borderline and recurrent tumors
- High-level gains in 8q24
  o Results in amplification of *MYC*
  o Reported in stromal component
- Copy number analysis show intratumoral heterogeneity and evidence for divergent tumor evolution in malignant PT

Molecular Genetics
- *MED12*
  o Missense mutations involving codon 44
    - 80% of PT
      □ Lower rate in malignant PT compared to borderline and benign
      □ More cancer-related genes detected in malignant PT occurring without *MED12* mutations
  o Detected in fibroadenomas (62% of cases)
    - Suggests mutual genetic driver mutation in some cases
- *TERT* promoter mutations
  o Sequencing data has shown that *TERT* promoter mutations are frequent in PT (65%)
    - Mutations more common in borderline (87%) but also seen in benign (50%) and malignant (62%) PT
      □ *TERT* promoter mutations are uncommon in fibroadenomas (only 7%); therefore, detection may be useful diagnostically
  o All but one *TERT* promoter-mutated tumors also harbored *MED12* mutations, suggesting these mutations are strongly associated
- Comprehensive genomic profiling of malignant PT
  o All tumors studied were microsatellite stable
  o Most common mutated genes: *TP53* (58%), *TERT* promoter (58%), *NF1* (46%), *MED12* (45%), *CDKN2A/CDKN2B* (33%), *RARA* (32%), *KMT2D* (33%), *FLNA* (28%), *SETD2*, *BCOR*
    - Borderline and malignant PT show additional mutations in oncogenes with transforming ability (*NF1*, *RB1*, *PIK3CA*, *ERBB2*, *EGFR*, *KIT*) with potential targeted treatment implications
  o 16-gene mutation panel has been suggested by few studies in differentiating between malignant PT and other entities in differential diagnosis, such as metaplastic spindle cell carcinoma, and to differentiate between fibroadenomas and benign PT
    - *BCOR*, *EGFR*, *ERBB4*, *FLNA*, *IGF1R*, *KMT2D*, *MAP3K1*, *MED12*, *NF1*, *PIK3CA*, *PTEN*, *RARA*, *SETD2*, *TP53*, *RB1*, and *TERT* promoter mutations
  o Potential effective targeted treatments
    - Targetable kinase fusions, including *KIAA1549::BRAF* or *FGFR3::TACC3*, identified in 8.3% of tumors
    - Apatinib (TKI) has been recently reported to be effective in patient with metastatic malignant PT

Gene Expression Profiling
- Pattern of gene expression varies by PT grade
  o Supports separation of PT into 3 groups by grade
  o Majority of changes are in genes related to proliferation and stromal/epithelial interactions
- Malignant PT shows increased mRNA levels of
  o Paired box transcription factor 3 (PAX3)

Phyllodes Tumors

Classification of Phyllodes Tumors and Fibroadenoma

Features	Fibroadenoma	Benign Phyllodes Tumors	Borderline Phyllodes Tumors	Malignant Phyllodes Tumors
Incidence	Much more common than PT	60-75% of PT	10-26% of PT	8-20% of PT
Tumor borders	Well circumscribed	Well circumscribed, may be focally pushing	Well circumscribed or focally invasive	Usually widely invasive
Stromal cellularity	Low, can be mildly increased in cellular variant	Usually mildly increased, at least focally, subepithelial condensation** may be present	Moderately increased, subepithelial condensation may be prominent	High
Mitotic figures (per 10 HPF)	Absent or rare mitotic figures	< 5	5-9	≥ 10
Stromal atypia	Absent	Mild	Moderate	Marked
Stromal overgrowth*	Absent	Absent	Absent or focally present	Usually present
Malignant heterologous elements	Absent	Absent	Absent	May be present

PT = phyllodes tumor. *Defined as absence of epithelial component in at least 1 microscopic field at 40x total magnification (10x ocular objective and 4x microscopic lens objective). **Defined as increased stromal cellularity adjacent to epithelium.

- Involved in cell growth and development
  o Homeobox protein SIX1
    - Involved in cell growth and development
  o Transforming growth factor B2 (TGFB2)
    - Cytokine and downstream target of PAX3
  o High mobility group T-hook 2 (HMGA2)
    - Functional DNA transcription factor
  o Homeobox protein B13 (HOXB13)
    - Significantly correlates with stromal cellularity and atypia

Epigenetic Regulation by Gene Methylation
- PT displays high methylation of
  o Ras-association domain protein-1 gene (*RASSF1*)
  o Twist-related protein 1 gene (*TWIST1*)
    - Correlates with increasing malignancy

MICROSCOPIC

Histologic Features
- Pronounced intracanalicular growth
- Leaf-like projections into variably dilated ductal lumina
- Tumors classified into 3 histologic subtypes according to
  o Degrees of stromal overgrowth, nuclear atypia, mitotic activity, and invasiveness into surrounding benign breast tissue
  o **Benign PT**
    - 60-75% of cases
  o **Borderline PT**
    - 15-26% of cases
  o **Malignant PT**
    - 8-20% of cases
    - All features of malignancy should be present
- Malignant heterologous elements (chondrosarcoma, liposarcoma, osteosarcoma, rhabdomyosarcoma, angiosarcoma, and leiomyosarcoma) may be present (enough for diagnosis of malignant PT even in absence of other required features, except for well-differentiated liposarcoma)

ANCILLARY TESTS

Immunohistochemistry
- Stromal markers
  o Positive markers
    - CD34 (can be negative in some malignant PT)
    - BCL2 (variable)
    - Cytokeratins may be focally positive
  o Negative markers
    - p63 (can be focally positive)
- TP53
  o Positive stromal expression correlates with high-grade histology and reduced survival

DIFFERENTIAL DIAGNOSIS

Metaplastic Spindle Cell Carcinoma
- Positive for p63 and negative for CD34 and BCL2; however, PT can be focally positive for p63 and pancytokeratins; extensive sampling to find classic PT morphology may be helpful
- Molecular studies can be helpful

SELECTED REFERENCES

1. Ng CCY et al: Genetic differences between benign phyllodes tumors and fibroadenomas revealed through targeted next generation sequencing. Mod Pathol. 34(7):1320-32, 2021
2. Wang X et al: Apatinib treatment is effective for metastatic malignant phyllodes tumors of the breast: a case report. BMC Womens Health. 21(1):218, 2021
3. WHO Classification of Tumours Editorial Board: WHO Classification of Tumours: Breast Tumours. 5th ed. IARC Press, 2019

Phyllodes Tumors

Fibroadenoma

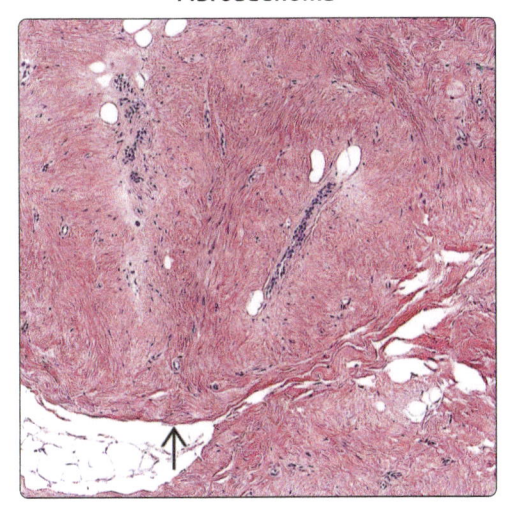

Low Grade (Benign)

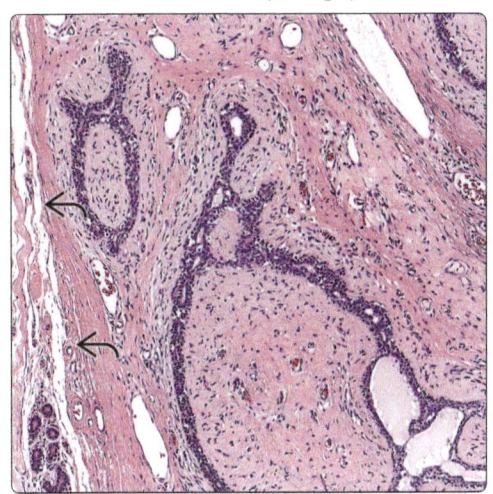

(*Left*) Fibroadenoma shows well-defined borders ➥, low stromal cellularity without atypia, and rare or absent mitotic figures. (*Right*) Benign PT is shown. The tumor borders are still predominantly well defined ➥. The stroma is only mildly cellular with subtle condensation around ductal epithelium. Atypical stromal cells may be seen. There is no significant increase in mitotic activity with < 5 mitotic figures/10 HPF.

Intermediate Grade (Borderline)

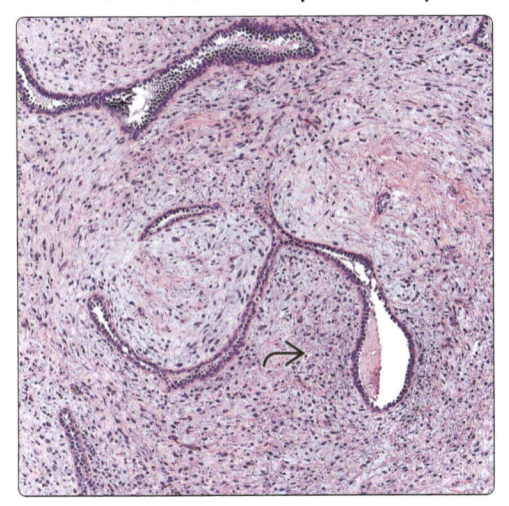

Intermediate Grade (Borderline)

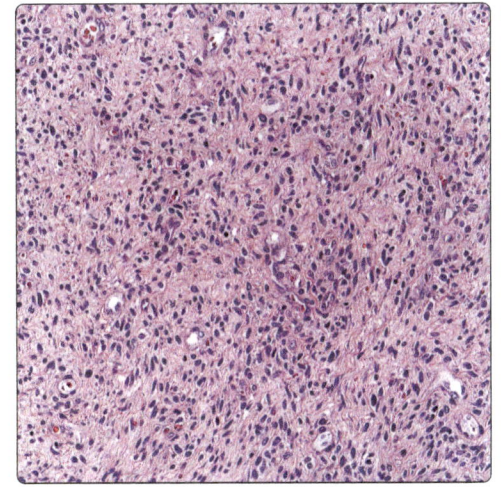

(*Left*) Borderline PT shows nonuniform, moderately cellular stroma with increased cellularity more prominent around ductal spaces ➥. Stromal atypia can be appreciated on this low-power view. (*Right*) High-power view of borderline PT is shown. Stromal atypia is more prominent compared to that of benign PT but not as pleomorphic as in malignant PT.

High Grade (Malignant)

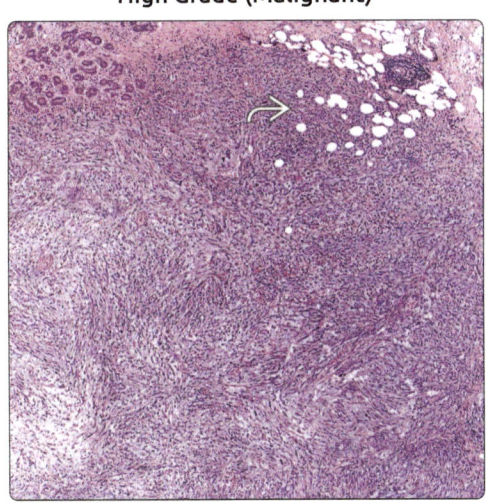

High Grade (Malignant)

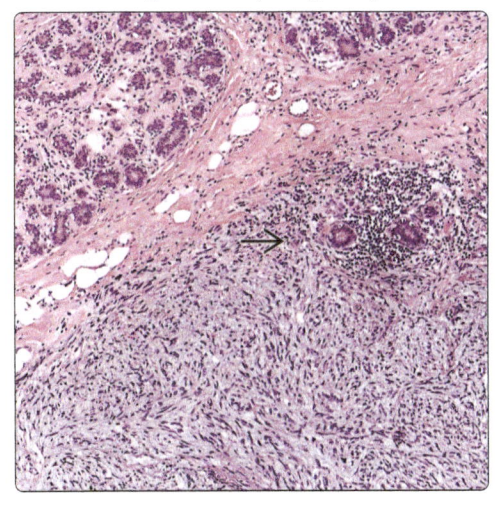

(*Left*) Low-power view of malignant PT is shown. Note the markedly cellular stroma with stromal overgrowth defined as absence of epithelial component in at least 1 microscopic field at 40x total magnification (10x ocular and 4x microscopic lens objectives). Note the infiltration into adipose tissue ➥. (*Right*) Infiltrative borders in malignant PT are shown. The sarcomatous stromal cells are invading into a nearby benign terminal duct lobular unit ➥.

Basal-Like and Triple-Negative Breast Carcinomas

KEY FACTS

TERMINOLOGY

- Basal-like carcinoma (BLC): Type of invasive breast cancer originally defined by gene expression profiling studies
- Triple-negative breast cancer (TNBC): Defined by lack of expression of hormone receptors and HER2 by IHC
  - 70-80% overlap between BLC and TNBC
- Important parameters of TNBC biology
  - High-grade and proliferative activity
  - Increased immune cell infiltrates
  - Deficiency in homologous recombination linked to loss of *BRCA1* function
- Knowledge of molecular alterations in TNBC has led to several promising clinical approaches
  - DNA damage response targeting, antiandrogens, immune checkpoint inhibitors

CLINICAL ISSUES

- Poor prognosis may be due to overexpression of genes promoting proliferation and migration

MICROSCOPIC

- Special histologic types of breast cancer classified as BLC
  - Medullary carcinoma, metaplastic carcinoma, adenoid cystic carcinoma, low-grade adenosquamous carcinoma

DIAGNOSTIC CHECKLIST

- 4 major classes of TNBC have been proposed with emerging therapeutic strategies for each
  - **Basal-like subtype**
    - Targeting DNA damage response with platinum salt and PARP inhibitors under investigation
  - **Mesenchymal subtype**
    - mTOR inhibitors under investigation
  - **Immune-enriched subtype**
    - Cytotoxic chemotherapy and immune checkpoint blockade under investigation
  - **Luminal androgen receptor subtype**
    - AR blockade and PIK3 inhibitors under investigation

TNBC/BLC: Gross Appearance

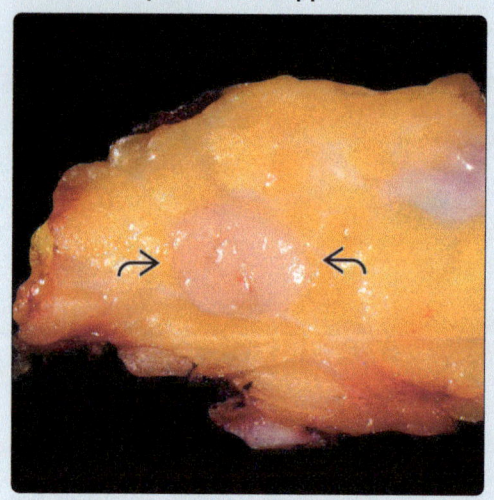

TNBC/BLC: Pushing Border

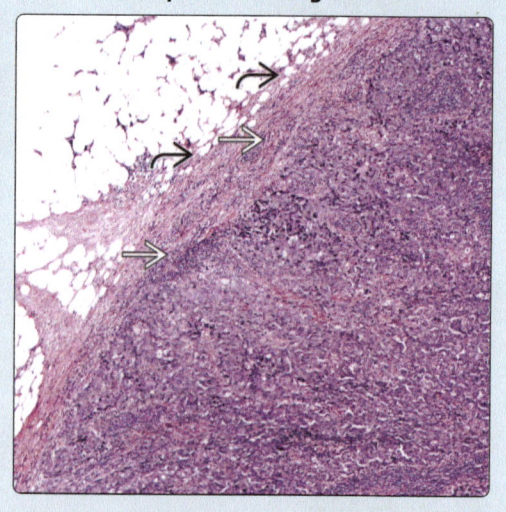

(Left) Triple-negative breast cancer (TNBC)/basal-like carcinoma (BLC) are frequently well circumscribed ⊋ and may mimic benign lesions grossly and radiographically. The subgroup of medullary carcinomas all have this gross appearance. (Right) TNBC/BLC typically grow as solid masses or sheets of cells with pushing borders ⊋ rather than infiltrating as small nests into the surrounding breast tissue. Immune cell infiltrates ⊋, central fibrosis, and necrosis are frequently present.

BLC: Invasive Pattern

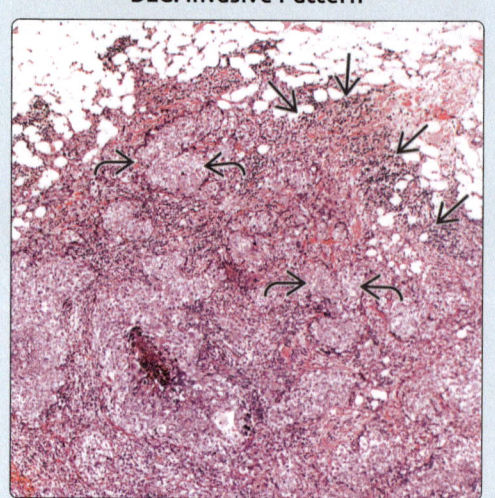

BLC: Cytokeratin 5/6

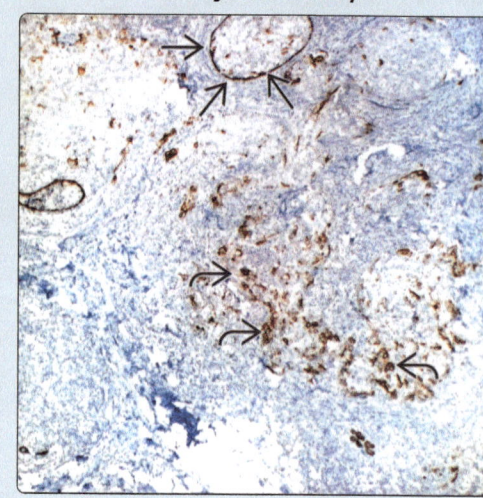

(Left) BLC and other triple-negative cancers will typically show a characteristic invasive pattern of nests of poorly differentiated cells ⊋ and a prominent lymphocytic infiltrate ⊋. (Right) This BLC is focally positive for cytokeratin 5/6 ⊋. Myoepithelial cells ⊋ in areas of ductal carcinoma in situ are also positive. Cytokeratin 5/6 expression in breast cancers that are triple negative (negative for ER, PR, and HER2) have been used as part of an IHC surrogate for identifying basal-like breast cancer.

Basal-Like and Triple-Negative Breast Carcinomas

TERMINOLOGY

Abbreviations
- Basal-like carcinoma (BLC)
- Triple-negative breast cancer (TNBC)

Definitions
- BLC: Type of invasive breast cancer originally defined by gene expression profiling studies
  o > 85% of breast cancers developing in *BRCA1* mutation carriers are TNBC
- TNBC: Defined by lack of expression of hormone receptors and HER2 by IHC
  o 70-80% overlap between BLC and TNBC
  o 11-19% of TNBC harbor *BRCA1* germline or somatic mutations
- Important parameters of TNBC biology
  o High proliferative activity
  o Increased immune cell infiltrates
  o Basal-like and mesenchymal phenotype
  o Deficiency in homologous recombination (HR) partly linked to loss of *BRCA1* function
  o Androgen receptor (AR) expression in subset of tumors
- Different molecular phenotypes observed in overlapping subsets of TNBC
- Knowledge of molecular alterations in TNBC has led to several promising clinical approaches
  o DNA damage response targeting, antiandrogens, immune checkpoint inhibitors

ETIOLOGY/PATHOGENESIS

BRCA1, BLC, and Hereditary Breast Cancer
- Majority of breast cancers occurring in *BRCA1* mutation carriers are in BLC group
  o Tumors arising in *BRCA1* carriers have many similarities to BLC sporadic breast tumors
    – Increased likelihood of being high grade, ER/PR(-), and HER2(-) with frequent *TP53* mutations
    – Basal keratins are expressed by both sporadic BLC and tumors with *BRCA1* mutations
  o *BRCA1* has many functions
    – DNA repair of double-strand breaks by HR
      □ Cells that lack *BRCA1* must rely on less reliable modes of repair and are genetically unstable
    – Cell cycle regulation, checkpoint control
    – Transcriptional control, ubiquitination, chromatin remodeling, and regulation of apoptosis
    – Required for transactivation of ER gene promoter; loss may result in ER negativity
    – Tumors with *BRCA1* mutation are deficient in HR
      □ Damage to DNA (double-strand breaks) cannot be repaired properly
  o *BRCA1* mutations lead to genetic instability and result in replication errors
    – Enables mutations in genes essential to cell cycle checkpoint activation
    – Accumulating mutations destabilizing genomic integrity predispose to tumor formation
- Many sporadic BLC also have altered *BRCA1* activity and loss of function
  o ~ 10-20% show hypermethylation of gene promoter
    – Hypermethylation associated with reduced BRCA protein by IHC and PD-L1 expression by tumor and immune cells
    – Promoter hypermethylation associated with benefit from adjuvant chemotherapy, basal-like features, and PD-L1 expression
  o Some BLC show decreased *BRCA1* mRNA
  o Mutations in *BRCA1* are rare in sporadic BLC/TNBC
  o Role of *BRCA1* in BLC as link between sporadic and hereditary tumors is still unclear

Progesterone Signaling, RANK and NFKB Pathways in Tumor Development
- Evidence points to amplification of progesterone signaling axis in precancerous breast tissue from *BRCA1* mutations carriers
  o Receptor activator of nuclear factor κ B ligand (RANKL) is important paracrine mediator of hormonal signaling in breast tissue
  o RANK and NFKB pathways are aberrantly activated in luminal progenitor cells resident in preneoplastic *BRCA1* mutation carriers
    – Augmented proliferation and predilection for DNA damage suggest that these cells are prime targets for basal-like cancer development
  o Hyperactive pathway, initiated by progesterone and amplified by DNA damage, induced NF-kB signaling
    – Likely accounts for susceptibility of *BRCA1*-mutant luminal progenitor cells to oncogenesis and breast tissue specificity for tumor formation

Homologous Recombination DNA Repair Deficiency
- With *BRCA1* mutations, defects in double-stranded DNA repair (DDR) and homologous recombination (HR) play role in pathogenesis of subset of TNBC
  o Several proteins involved in DDR and HR
  o Categories include sensors (*ATM*), mediators (*BRCA1* and *CHEK2*), effectors (*BRCA2* and *RAD51*), or facilitators of HR (*PALB2* and *BRIP1*)
  o In absence of *BRCA1*/*BRCA2* germline mutations, many TNBC still harbor BRCA-like HR-deficient phenotype
- Alteration of other HR genes have been shown to result in increased risk of breast cancer
  o Includes *PALB2*, *CHECK2*, *ATM*, and *NBN*
- Only biallelic (not monoallelic) inactivation of *BRCA1* and other HR genes is associated with genomic features of HR deficiency

CLINICAL ISSUES

Epidemiology
- Incidence
  o 10-15% of all invasive breast carcinomas
- Ethnicity
  o Frequency of TNBC varies by race and ethnicity
  o BLC is slightly more common in African American and Hispanic women compared to women of European descent

Treatment
- Adjuvant therapy

Basal-Like and Triple-Negative Breast Carcinomas

- No role for endocrine or HER2-targeted therapy due to lack of expression of hormone receptors and HER2
- Most patients treated with aggressive multiagent chemotherapy
  - Despite unfavorable prognosis, many TNBC are highly sensitive to chemotherapy compared with other breast cancer subtypes
  - Hypersensitivity to DNA-damaging agents due to abnormal DNA repair function
  - Anthracyclines and platinum agents
  - BLC may show resistance to mitotic spindle poisons (taxanes)
- BLC often shows good response after neoadjuvant chemotherapy
  - ~ 30-50% demonstrate pathologic complete response (CR) following neoadjuvant treatment
  - Pathologic CR is associated with good long-term survival
  - Tumors with high content of tumor-infiltrating lymphocytes (TILs) more likely to show good response to chemotherapy
  - Patients without pathologic CR to neoadjuvant chemotherapy have poor prognosis
- Targeted agents, such as inhibitors of poly (ADP-ribose) polymerase-1 (PARP inhibitors), mTOR, and immunomodulatory drugs, are in clinical testing
  - These agents target molecular signaling molecules that define TNBC and BLC
  - Improved outcomes have been observed for metastatic TNBC with germline *BRCA1/BRCA2* mutations treated with PARP inhibitors and platinum agents compared to standard chemotherapy
- Molecular analysis of TNBC has identified potential options for targeted therapeutic intervention
  - Approaches include targeting DNA damage response, angiogenesis inhibitors, immune checkpoint inhibitors, antiandrogens
  - Results of current trials based on evaluation of biologic alterations in TNBC are promising

- Immune checkpoint blockade (ICB)
  - Number of immune checkpoint inhibitors are approved for treatment of several cancer types (lung, melanoma, gastric, urothelial) by ICB
  - TNBC shows most robust immune cell infiltrates and higher PD-L1 expression among breast cancer subtypes
  - TILs are predictive of response to chemotherapy and improved survival
    - Presence of TILs in subset of TNBC raised hope for immunotherapies in these cancers
    - High TILs appears to correlate with response to ICB
    - Expression of PD-L1 occurs mainly on tumor-infiltrating immune cells and can inhibit anticancer immune responses
  - ICB that disrupts PD-1/PD-L1 interactions has shown promise in clinical trial for metastatic TNBC in combination with chemotherapy
    - Greater benefit for patients who receive treatment in 1st line as opposed to 2nd or 3rd
    - IMpassion 130 phase III trial showed prolonged progression-free survival with ICB + chemotherapy in 1st-line treatment of metastatic TNBC
      □ Patients whose tumors showed expression of PD-L1 (SP142) by IHC appeared to derive most benefit
    - KEYNOTE-355 trial showed increased progression-free survival with different ICB + chemotherapy in 1st-line treatment for metastatic TNBC
      □ Benefit was seen in tumors with expression of PD-L1 (22C3) by IHC (combined positive score > 10)
    - Trials investigating ICB + chemotherapy for neoadjuvant treatment of early-stage TNBC show promising benefit
      □ Long-term follow-up needed before ICB can be considered standard of care for early-stage TNBC
  - Novel biomarkers to help improve patient selection for ICB are under investigation
    - Multiplex IHC to profile immune cell subtypes, gene expression profiling to detect T-cell inflamed microenvironment
    - Next-generation sequencing to detect somatic mutations
    - New biomarker may provide more granular analysis of immune activity, may help personalize ICB therapies

- Antibody-drug conjugates (ADC)
  - Trophoblast cell-surface antigen-2 (Trop-2) is transmembrane calcium signal transducer overexpressed in many epithelial tumors, including breast cancer
    - Sacituzumab govitecan-hziy (SG) is anti-Trop-2 (ADC) that has shown significant survival benefit over chemotherapy for pretreated metastatic TNBC

Prognosis

- Most TNBC and BLC demonstrate aggressive clinical course and poor prognosis
  - Decreased disease-free interval, disease-specific survival, and overall survival compared with other breast cancers
    - Increased risk for early relapse/recurrence
    - Increased risk for visceral organs and CNS recurrence
    - Responsible for ~ 30% of breast cancer deaths
- However, some carcinomas within this group have exceptionally good prognosis
  - Adenoid cystic carcinoma, secretory carcinoma, and low-grade adenosquamous carcinoma
  - For these cancers, histologic classification is more important than expression profiling classification
  - Other special histologic types of BLC have poor prognosis
    - Metaplastic carcinoma, spindle cell carcinoma
    - These carcinomas are less likely to respond to chemotherapy
- BLC has specific pattern of metastases
  - Higher incidence of metastasis to brain (CNS) and lung
    - Metastases to these sites have poorer prognosis
  - Less likely to metastasize to bones or lymph nodes compared to ER(+) carcinoma
- TILs and TNBC
  - TILs are associated with favorable prognosis in TNBC
    - Median: ~ 20% TILs
    - 22% of TNBC have > 50% TILs (a.k.a. lymphocyte-predominant breast cancer)
  - TILs are significant predictor of better disease-free survival, distant disease-free survival, and overall survival

Basal-Like and Triple-Negative Breast Carcinomas

- TILs strongly predicted better survival, independent of age, nodal status, tumor size/grade, vascular invasion, and Ki-67 labeling index
  o TILs are associated with increased response to neoadjuvant chemotherapy
  o Focus on immune parameters in breast cancer is important for upcoming immunotherapy approaches
    - Data suggests that modulation of immune response with immune checkpoint inhibitors may increase therapy response in subgroups of TNBC
- Inhibitor of differentiation (ID) proteins
  o ID proteins are key regulators of development and tumorigenesis
  o One family member, ID4, controls lineage commitment during mammary gland development
    - Recent evidence supports emerging role for ID4 as lineage-dependent protooncogene
    - ID4 is overexpressed and amplified in subset of BLC, conferring poor prognosis
    - ID4 may suppress BRCA1 function in BLC patients and define set of BLC who may respond to therapies used in BRCA1-mutant cancers

MOLECULAR

Genomic Analysis, Mutations and Copy Number Changes

- Collectively, TNBC characterized by high levels of genomic instability, complex genomes, and recurrent TP53 mutations
- Comprehensive genomic analysis has not identified any mutations that are characteristic of TNBC
  o TNBC are mutationally heterogeneous from outset
  o Limited number of highly recurrent mutation genes; TP53 most frequently mutated
  o Total number of somatic mutations is higher in TNBC (median: 49) compared with luminal cancers (median: 27)
- Most frequent loss-of-function and gain-of-function alterations in TNBC involve genes associated with DNA damage repair and PI3K-signaling pathways
  o Alterations in DNA damage repair genes include loss of TP53, RB1, and BRCA1 function
  o Aberrant activation of PI3K pathway occurs due to loss of negative regulators, such as PTEN or INPP4B, or activating mutations in PIK3CA
- Mutations of TP53 are more common compared to all other breast cancer subtypes
  o BLC harbor TP53 mutations in up to 80% of cases, some contain oncogenic gain-of-function TP53
  o Mutation is thought to be early event in tumorigenesis and is related to both poor prognosis and resistance to chemotherapy
  o TP53 R273H gain-of-function mutation and PARP1 interact with DNA replication forks, may serve as biomarker for sensitivity to PARP inhibitors
- PIK3CA mutations in 10-20% of TNBC
  o PIK3CA mutations are increased in AR(+) TNBC
- Tumor mutation burden (TMB)
  o Gene mutations arising during carcinogenesis can result in altered proteins (neoantigens) that can be recognized by immune system
  o TNBC yield higher TMB compared with luminal subtypes
    - Resulting neoantigen expression promotes immune cell recruitment, expansion and is associated with local antitumor immunity
    - Part of rationale for immunotherapy trials in TNBC
- Copy number alterations are complex with many gains and losses across all chromosomes
  o Gains of 1q, 8q, and 10q; loss of 5q and 8p; amplifications of EGFR and FGFR2; loss of PTEN most frequent
  o Concurrent 1q gains and 16q losses, typical for ER(+) cancer, not found in TNBC

mRNA (Gene Expression Profiling)

- BLC and myoepithelial cells share expression of similar groups of genes
  o Term "basal" was chosen to include similarities with myoepithelial cells as well as possible precursor or progenitor cells
  o Mammary stem cells demonstrate basal-like gene expression profile
- Claudin-low breast cancer
  o Most of these tumors are TNBC and cluster close to BLC by gene expression profiling
    - Express markers of epithelial to mesenchymal transition and have cancer stem cell-like features
    - Response to chemotherapy is intermediate between that of BLC and luminal-type breast cancer
- Subtyping TNBC by gene expression profiling
  o Gene expression studies focusing on TNBC have identified additional disease subtypes
    - 2 basal-like subtypes (BL1 and BL2)
      □ BL1: Increased cell cycle and DNA damage response signature
      □ BL2: High expression of growth factor pathways and myoepithelial markers
    - Immunomodulatory subtype (IM): Enriched immune cell processes
    - Mesenchymal subtype (M): Upregulated genes associated with differentiation and growth factor signaling
    - Mesenchymal stem-like subtype (MSL): Upregulated genes associated with differentiation and growth factor signaling
    - Luminal AR subtype (LAR): Upregulated AR signaling
  o TNBC subtypes have different response rates to neoadjuvant chemotherapy
    - Highest response rates for BL1
    - Lower response rates for BL2, LAR, M subtypes
  o LAR subtype (15% of TNBC) may be candidate for antiandrogen therapy

Other Genomic Changes

- Angiogenesis-related genes
  o Vascular endothelial growth factor A (VEGFA) is located on chromosome arm 6p, region that is prone to gains in BLC
    - VEGFA overexpression drives angiogenesis and is associated with decreased survival
  o Angiogenesis is potential therapeutic target

Protein

- Protein expression patterns characteristic of BLC include

Basal-Like and Triple-Negative Breast Carcinomas

- Lack of hormone receptor and HER2 expression (or only very rare expression)
- High expression of basal cytokeratins 5, 14, and 17 (specific for BLC)
  - Most also express luminal cytokeratins 7, 8/18, and 19
  - Recent data suggest that expression of cytokeratins 5 and 17 may contribute to adverse behavior of BLC
  - Cytokeratins 5 and 17 knockdowns compared with control cells generated fewer lymph node and lung metastases in vivo
  - May be untapped source of therapeutic vulnerability in BLC
- High expression of proliferation-related genes
- High expression of EGFR in 45-75% of BLC
- p53 overexpression present in 50-60%
- CD117(+) in ~ 45% of BLC
  - Does not correlate with mutations indicative of sensitivity to tyrosine kinase inhibitors
- Poor prognosis may be due to overexpression of genes promoting proliferation and migration
  - EGFR activates signaling pathways involved in cell proliferation
  - Alpha-B-crystallin, heat shock protein, inhibits apoptosis
  - Fascin, cell motility protein, promotes tumor cell invasion
  - VEGFA promotes angiogenesis
  - Alterations in cell cycle regulation, including functional loss of RB and increased expression of cyclin-E and p16INK4a, have been described
    - Resulting high proliferation rates are involved in pathogenesis of BLC
      - May help to explain especially poor prognosis
  - AR expressed in normal breast epithelium and 60-90% of breast cancers
  - TNBC expressing AR referred to as LAR subtype
    - AR antagonism might be therapeutic target in this subtype

MICROSCOPIC

Histologic Features

- Most BLC have distinctive morphologic features
  - Circumscription with pushing borders
  - Sheets of pleomorphic tumor cells, syncytial-like growth pattern
  - High nuclear grade, high mitotic index
  - Areas of geographic necrosis or fibrosis
  - Brisk lymphocytic stromal reaction; may be related to cytokine production by tumor cells
- BLC with medullary features
  - Prominent lymphoplasmacytic infiltrate
  - Syncytial growth pattern
  - Associated with better prognosis compared with all other morphologic subtypes of BLC
- BLC with central fibrotic focus of > 30% associated with poorer prognosis compared with all other BLC
- Special histologic types with same gene expression profile as BLC have specific morphologic features
  - Medullary carcinoma, metaplastic carcinoma, adenoid cystic carcinoma
- Small subset of TNBC are low grade, often with indolent clinical behavior
- Secretory carcinomas harbor *ETV6::NTRK3* fusion
- Adenoid cystic carcinoma: Activation of MYB pathway through *MYB::NFIB* fusion, *MYBL1* rearrangement or amplification

ANCILLARY TESTS

Surrogate IHC Tests to Identify BLC

- Gene expression profiling requires fresh or frozen tissue and is not available for majority of breast cancers
- Panels of IHC markers have been developed to identify BLC as defined by gene expression profiling
  - Triple negative (negative for ER, PR, and HER2)
    - ~ 70% specific, as some TNBC are not BLC
    - ~ 90% sensitive, as majority of BLC are TNBC
    - Does not identify 15-45% of BLC that are not TNBC
  - Triple negative and positive for either cytokeratin 5/6 or EGFR ("5-marker method" or "core basal classification")
    - Any immunoreactivity for cytokeratin 5/6 or EGFR is considered positive result (100% specific, 76% sensitive)
  - Triple negative and positive for cytokeratin 14, cytokeratin 34BE12 (includes cytokeratins 1, 4, 10, and 14), and EGFR
    - 100% specific, 78% sensitive
    - Cytokeratin 5/6 was not used in this particular study, as < 10% of cases were positive, and EGFR positivity was not specific for BLC
    - Suggests that it may be difficult to reproduce BLC classification across institutions due to differences in IHC results
  - Triple negative and positive for 1 basal cytokeratin, EGFR, &/or CD117
    - 100% specific, 76% sensitive
  - Compared with TNBC that are negative for CK5/6 and EGFR, BLC (defined by expression of cytokeratin 5/6 or EGFR)
    - Is more likely to be high grade (87% vs. 64%)
    - Is more frequent in patients < 40 years of age (19% vs. 10%), and
    - Has decreased 10-year breast cancer survival (57% vs. 67%)

DIFFERENTIAL DIAGNOSIS

Basal-Like vs. Triple-Negative Carcinoma

- TNBC defined by absence of ER, PR, and HER2 by IHC
  - Accounts for 10-15% of all breast cancers
- 50-80% of TNBC are BLC by expression profiling
  - Therefore, these 2 categories of cancer have substantial overlap but are not identical
- Subtypes in 20-50% of TNBC that are not BLC have been identified
  - Claudin (-) breast cancer; low expression of basal markers and genes involved in tight junctions and cell adhesion
- Cancers that are TNBC and BLC have pathologic features described for BLC
  - High histologic grade and high proliferative rate
  - Metastases more frequent to brain and lung than to bone and lymph nodes compared to ER(+) cancer
  - Risk of early recurrence within 5 years and death

Basal-Like and Triple-Negative Breast Carcinomas

TNBC Subtypes Identified by Gene Expression Profiling and Hierarchical Clustering

TNBC Subtype	Molecular Features	Sensitivity to Therapeutic Agents in Representative Cell Lines and Neoadjuvant Trials
Basal like-1 (BL1)	Elevated cell cycle and DNA damage response gene expression [highest rate of *TP53* mutations (92%)], high gain/amplifications of *MYC*, *CDK6*, or *CCNE1*, and deletions in *BRCA2*, *PTEN*, *MDM2*, and *RB1*	Highest rates of pathologic CR (pCR) after neoadjuvant anthracycline and cyclophosphamide followed by taxane (ACT), mutations in AR/FOXA1 pathways are associated with sensitivity to ACT chemotherapy, and patients with mutations in these pathways had ~ 90% pCR rate
Basal like-2 (BL2)	Enriched in growth factor signaling, metabolic pathways, and myoepithelial marker expression	Highly proliferative phenotype that correlates with improved pathologic CR with mitotic inhibitors
Mesenchymal stem-like (MSL)	Increased growth factor signaling compared with (M), lower proliferation, enrichment of genes associated with angiogenesis and stem cells, low claudin expression	Very low levels of PD-1/PD-L1 expression, unlikely to respond to immunotherapy
Immunomodulatory (IM)	Genes involved in cytokine and core immune signal transduction pathways (e.g., JAK/STAT, TNF, and NFKB)	May be more likely to respond to immunotherapy than other triple-negative subtypes
Mesenchymal (M)	Augmented gene expression for EMT events, cell motility and differentiation (Wnt, ALK, TGF-beta), activation of PI3K pathway	Mesenchymal cell lines are more sensitive to multifamily tyrosine kinase inhibitor dasatinib and show some sensitivity to PI3K/mTOR inhibitors; FGFR and NOTCH gamma-secretase inhibitors might be promising
Luminal androgen receptor (LAR)	Increase in hormonally regulated pathways (e.g., high levels of FOXA1, GATA3, SPDEF, and XBP1), AR signaling, high rate of *PIK3CA*-activating mutations and *AKT1*, *NF1*, *CDH1*, and *GATA3* mutations	Sensitive to AR antagonist bicalutamide, PI3K inhibitors, and CDK4/6 inhibitors

TNBC subtypes have implications for pathologic complete response (CR) rates following neoadjuvant therapy and for disease-free survival following adjuvant chemotherapy pathologic CR.

- Cancers that are TNBC but not BLC have different pathologic features
  - Lower incidence of *TP53* mutations compared with BLC
  - No increased incidence of brain and lung metastases and decreased incidence of lymph node metastases
  - Better overall survival compared with BLC
- TNBC is more common in some ethnic groups
  - 20-25% of carcinomas in African American women are TNBC, compared with 10% in all women
  - 17% of carcinomas in Hispanic women are TNBC
- TNBC includes special histologic types of breast cancer
  - Medullary, adenosquamous, secretory, metaplastic (including spindle cell), squamous cell, adenoid cystic
  - Here, histologic classification may be more important than immunoprofile for predicting clinical behavior

DIAGNOSTIC CHECKLIST

Clinically Relevant Pathologic Features

- 4 major classes of TNBC have been proposed with emerging therapeutic strategies for each
  - **Basal-like subtype**
    - Activated cell cycle and DNA damage response pathways
    - Targeting DNA damage response with agents, including platinum salt and PARP inhibitors, under investigation
  - **Mesenchymal subtype**
    - Characterized by gene clusters involving cell motility, matrix interactions, growth factors, and epithelial to mesenchymal transition
    - mTOR inhibitors under investigation
  - **Immune-enriched subtype**
    - Enriched for gene involving immune cell processes
    - Cytotoxic chemotherapy and immune checkpoint blockade under investigation
  - **Luminal AR subtype**
    - Hormone regulations and ER/AR metabolism pathways are differently expressed compared with other subtypes
    - AR blockade and PIK3 inhibitors under investigation

SELECTED REFERENCES

1. Derakhshan F et al: Pathogenesis of triple-negative breast cancer. Annu Rev Pathol. 17:181-204, 2022
2. Kwapisz D: Sacituzumab govitecan-hziy in breast cancer. Am J Clin Oncol. 45(7):279-85, 2022
3. McGinn O et al: Cytokeratins 5 and 17 maintain an aggressive epithelial state in basal-like breast cancer. Mol Cancer Res. 20(9):1443-55, 2022
4. Isaacs J et al: Biomarkers of immune checkpoint blockade response in triple-negative breast cancer. Curr Treat Options Oncol. 22(5):38, 2021
5. Jacot W et al: BRCA1 promoter hypermethylation is associated with good prognosis and chemosensitivity in triple-negative breast cancer. Cancers (Basel). 12(4):828, 2020
6. Xiao G et al: Gain-of-function mutant p53 R273H interacts with replicating DNA and PARP1 in breast cancer. Cancer Res. 80(3):394-405, 2020
7. Rida P et al: First international TNBC conference meeting report. Breast Cancer Res Treat. 169(3):407-12, 2018
8. Schmid P et al: Atezolizumab and nab-paclitaxel in advanced triple-negative breast cancer. N Engl J Med. 379(22):2108-21, 2018
9. Nolan E et al: Out-RANKing BRCA1 in mutation carriers. Cancer Res. 77(3):595-600, 2017
10. Ahn SG et al: Molecular classification of triple-negative breast cancer. J Breast Cancer. 19(3):223-30, 2016

Basal-Like and Triple-Negative Breast Carcinomas

Invasive Carcinoma: Central Fibrotic Focus

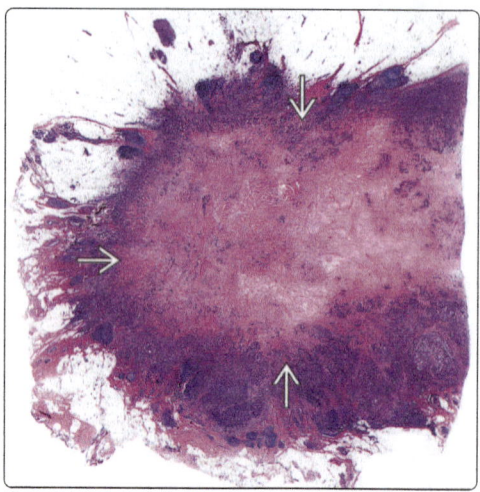

TNBC: Central Fibrotic Focus

(Left) Carcinomas with a central fibrotic focus ⇨ are typically high grade and negative for ER, PR, and HER2. Extensive central necrosis is also sometimes seen. Most will be TNBC/BLC. (Right) TNBC with a central fibrotic focus ⇨ and narrow peripheral rim of viable carcinoma ⇨ is shown. This pattern is likely due to rapid growth resulting in ischemia in the center of the tumor. Low perfusion and ischemia may allow some tumor cells to escape the toxic effects of chemotherapy.

TNBC/BLC: Necrosis

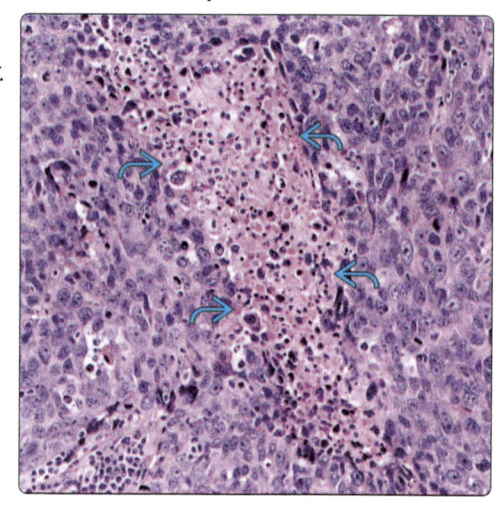

TNBC/BLC: Lymphoplasmacytic Infiltrate

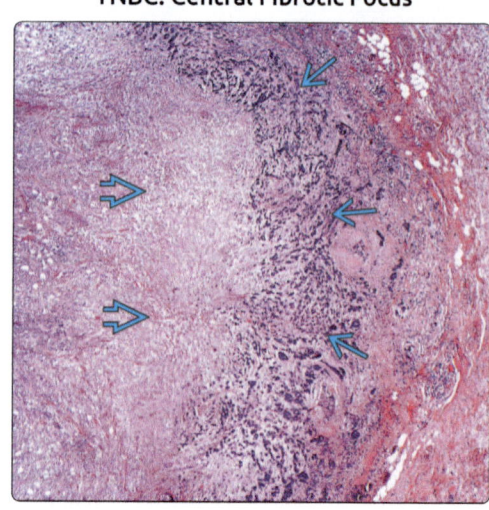

(Left) The presence of extensive necrosis ⇨ is a common feature of TNBC/BLC. These areas can be prominent and may give rise to a cystic appearance on ultrasound. Carcinomas with extensive necrosis have a high proliferation index and higher rate of response to chemotherapy. (Right) TNBC/BLC is often associated with a marked lymphoplasmacytic infiltrate ⇨ that may include germinal centers. Cancers with these infiltrates have a better response to chemotherapy.

TNBC/BLC: Proliferation

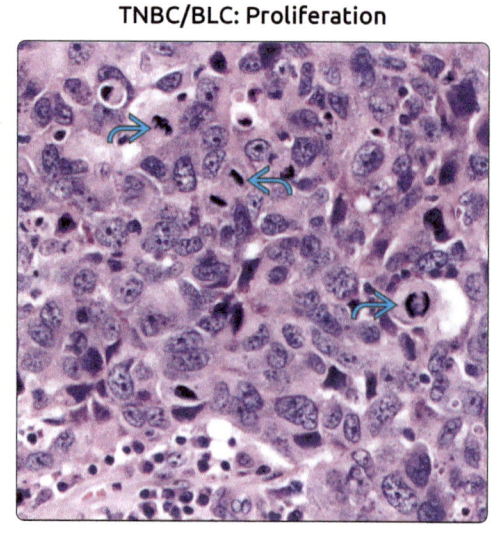

TNBC/BLC: EGFR

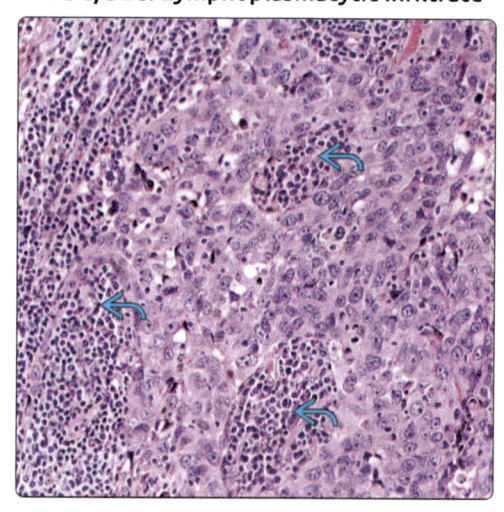

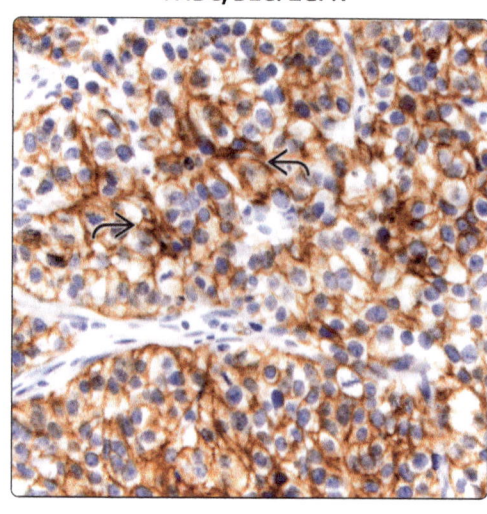

(Left) High-grade pleomorphic tumor cells arranged in syncytial-like sheets are typical of TNBC/BLC. Frequent mitotic figures are usually readily apparent ⇨, while indicators of proliferation by IHC, such as Ki-67, will also be highly expressed. (Right) IHC can be used to identify TNBC most likely to be BLC. This carcinoma is positive for EGFR ⇨ and was also positive for basal cytokeratins 5/6. It is highly likely that it would be classified as BLC by gene expression profiling.

Basal-Like and Triple-Negative Breast Carcinomas

TNBC/BLC: Proliferation

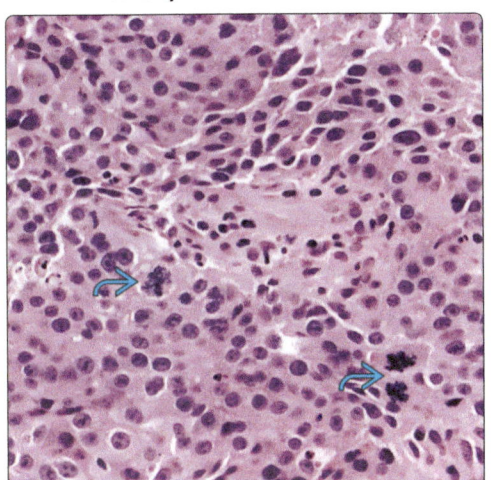

TNBC/BLC: Necrosis

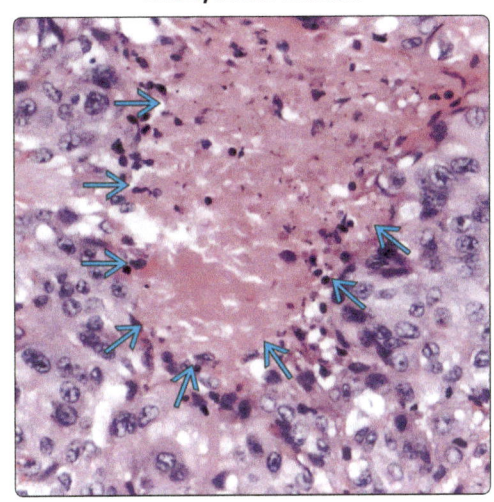

(Left) TNBC is typically of high grade and has a high mitotic rate ➡. In addition, abnormal mitotic figures are also present. The majority of TNBC are also BLC. It is not yet clear if it is clinically important to identify TNBC that is not BLC. (Right) While necrosis can be seen in other types of high-grade breast cancer, the necrosis in TNBC/BLC tends to be characteristically "geographic" or sharply circumscribed ➡.

TNBC/BLC: Core Needle Biopsy

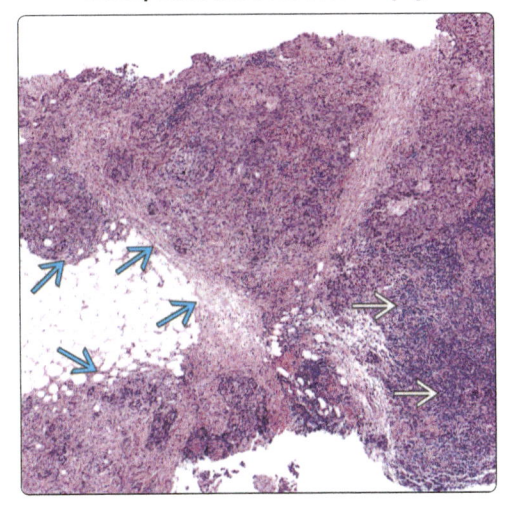

TNBC/BLC: Cytokeratin 5

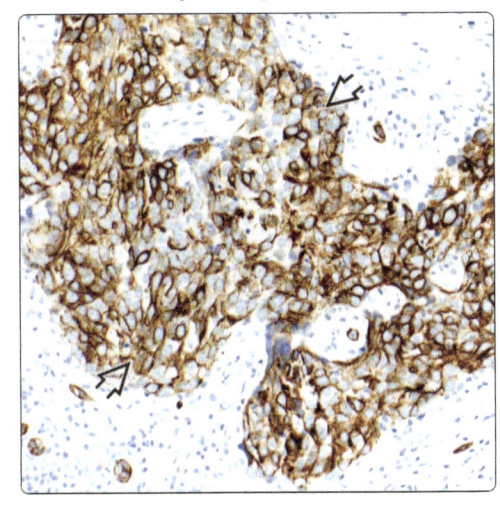

(Left) Patients may be diagnosed with TNBC/BLC on core needle biopsy. This patient was young and presented with a circumscribed mass on imaging. The circumscription is suggested by "pushing borders" in this biopsy ➡. A brisk lymphoplasmacytic infiltrate is also present ➡. (Right) Basal cytokeratin expression ➡ is seen in this TNBC/BLC. TNBC that express cytokeratin 5 are more likely to be high grade and are more aggressive compared with TNBC that are negative for cytokeratin 5 and EGFR.

TNBC/BLC: Proliferation (Ki-67)

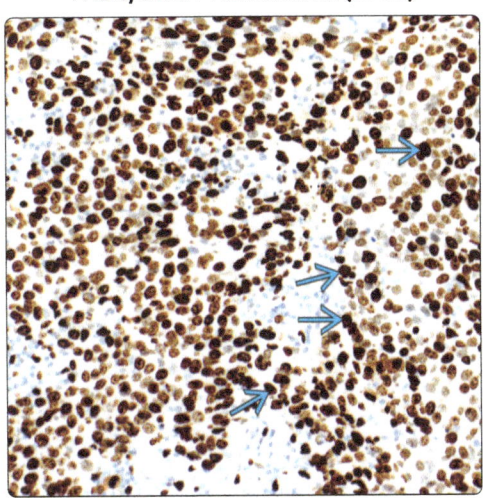

TNBC/BLC: EGFR

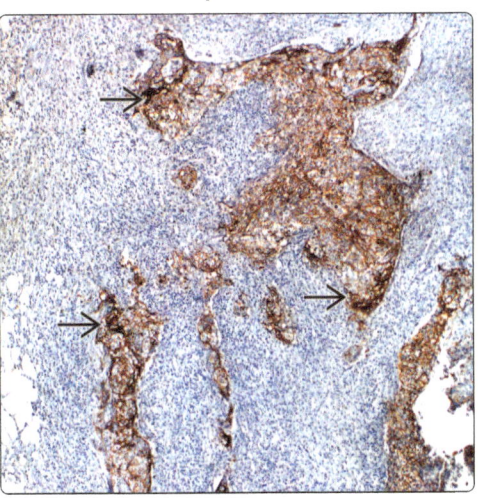

(Left) One of the hallmarks of TNBC/BLC is a high proliferation index, which can be demonstrated by high mitotic activity or a high Ki-67 proliferative index, as seen here ➡. Expression profiling also shows a high expression of proliferation-related genes in these tumors. (Right) This TNBC is focally positive for EGFR ➡. This increases the likelihood that the carcinoma would be classified as BLC by expression profiling. The poor prognosis seen in these tumors may be due to overexpression of genes promoting proliferation, such as EGFR.

Basal-Like and Triple-Negative Breast Carcinomas

TNBC, Tumor Cells: PD-L1

TNBC, Immune Cells: PD-L1

(Left) PD-L1 expression is used as a biomarker for ICB that targets PD-1/PD-L1 interactions in TNBC and other malignancies. This TNBC shows membrane staining for PD-L1 ➔ that is weak to moderate in intensity. (Right) In the clinical trial looking at the efficacy of ICB in TNBC, PD-L1 expression on tumor-infiltrating immune cells (IC) was found to predict benefit. Scoring was assessed as the proportion of tumor area occupied by PD-L1(+) IC ➔ of any intensity. A proportion of > 1% correlated with benefit.

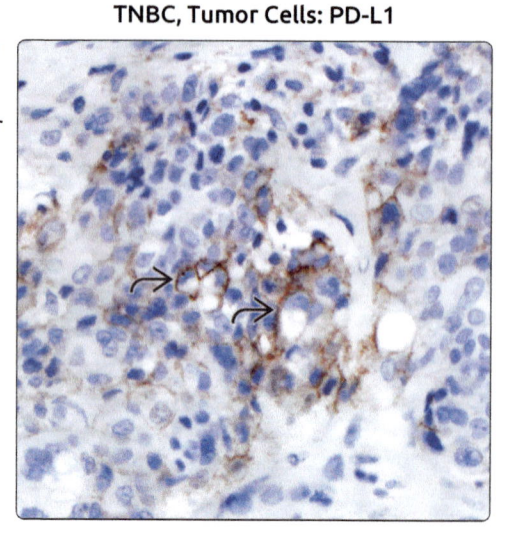

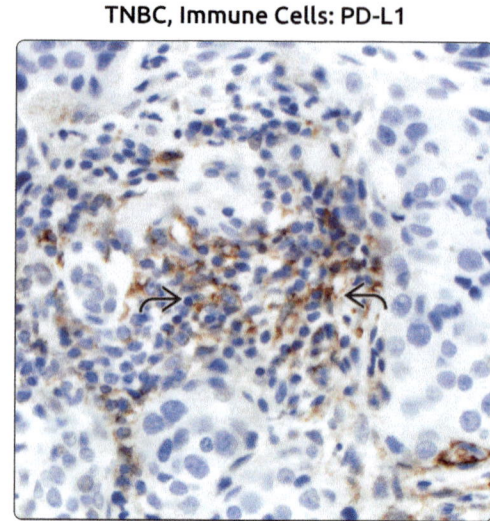

Secretory Carcinoma

Low-Grade Adenosquamous Carcinoma

(Left) Secretory carcinoma is a very rare type of TNBC associated with a t(12;15); ETV6::NTRK3 translocation. When it occurs in young women, the prognosis is favorable. (Right) Low-grade adenosquamous carcinoma is characterized by squamous cell nests with keratin formation ➔ in addition to well-formed tubules ➔. ER, PR, and HER2 are not expressed, and proliferation is low. Unlike the majority of TNBC, this special histologic type has a good prognosis.

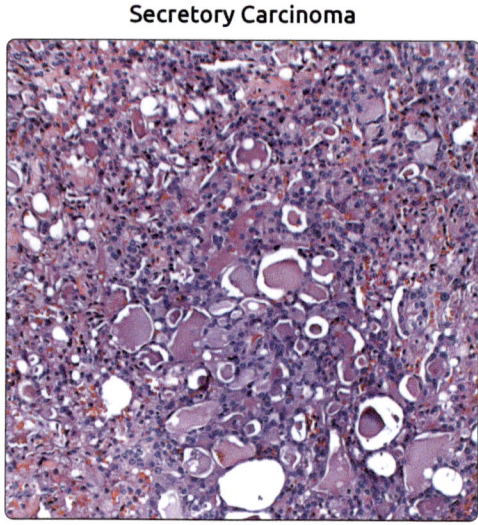

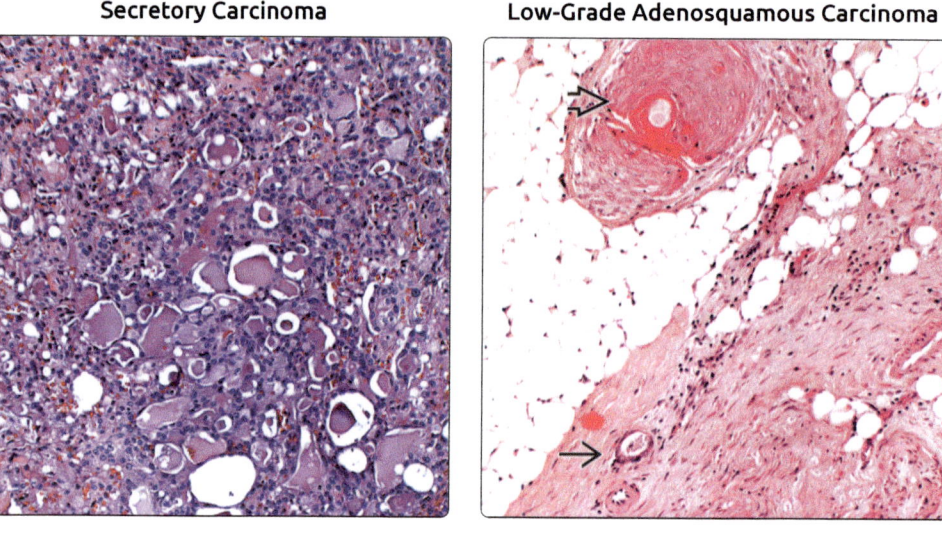

Carcinoma With Medullary Features

Adenoid Cystic Carcinoma

(Left) Carcinomas with medullary features are a subtype of TNBC/BLC. BRCA1-associated carcinomas often have this appearance. The better prognosis may be related to the dense lymphocytic infiltrate, which is predictive of a better response to chemotherapy. (Right) Adenoid cystic carcinomas are composed of 2 populations of luminal-like and myoepithelial-like cells. Although they cluster with BLC by gene expression profiling (GEP) and are a type of TNBC, prognosis is very favorable.

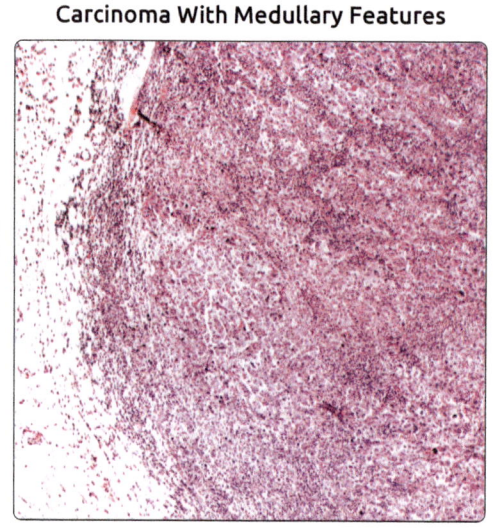

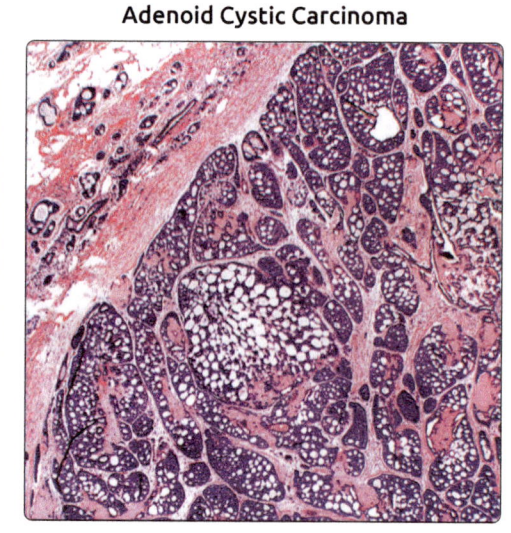

Basal-Like and Triple-Negative Breast Carcinomas

BRCA1-Associated Carcinoma

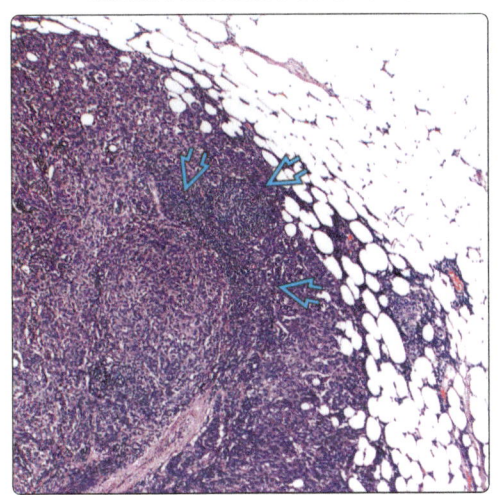

Metaplastic Spindle Cell Carcinoma

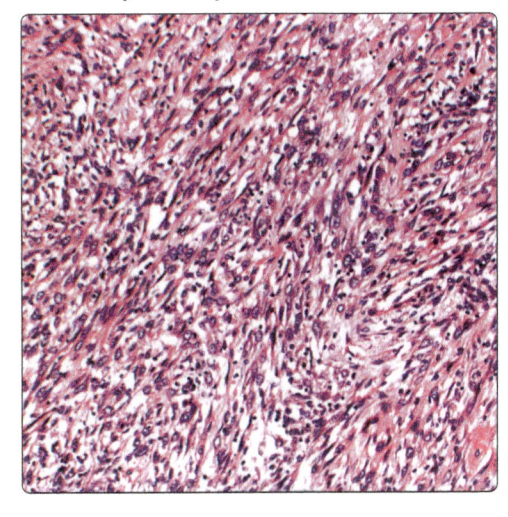

(Left) *BRCA1-associated cancers are usually high-grade and often associated with a dense lymphocytic infiltrate* ⇨. *They cluster with BLC by GEP. Some BLC may have reduced BRCA1 function, although specific mutations are rare.* (Right) *Metaplastic carcinomas, including spindle cell carcinomas, also cluster with BLC by GEP. They often have morphologic or tumor markers suggestive of squamous or myoepithelial differentiation, including frequent expression of p63 and basal keratins.*

Metaplastic Spindle Cell Carcinoma: Low Grade

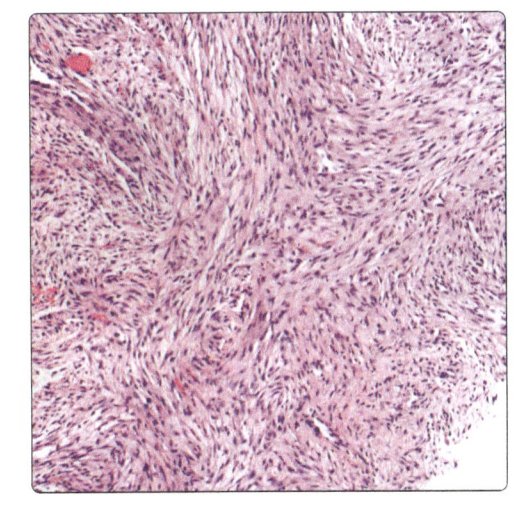

Metaplastic Spindle Cell Carcinoma: Cytokeratin Expression

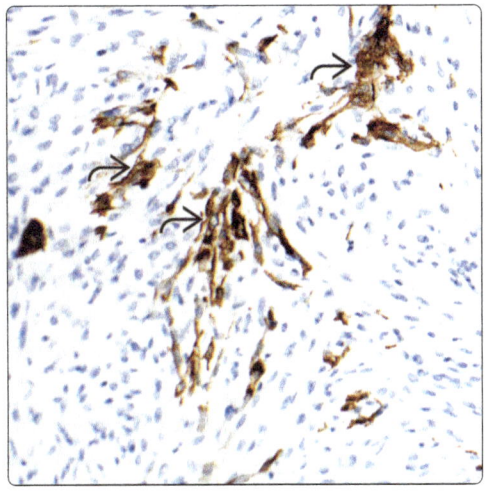

(Left) *Spindle cell carcinomas, a type of TNBC, can demonstrate a broad morphologic spectrum from cytologically bland spindle cell lesion (as seen here) to high-grade neoplasms resembling sarcomas. Confirmation of the diagnosis of carcinoma requires use of IHC markers.* (Right) *Confirmation of spindle cell carcinoma requires the use antibodies to high-molecular-weight basal cytokeratins 14, 17, and 5/6. In this case, the neoplastic spindle cells are positive for cytokeratin 5/6* ⇨, *which can show focal expression.*

Metaplastic Carcinoma: Extracellular Matrix

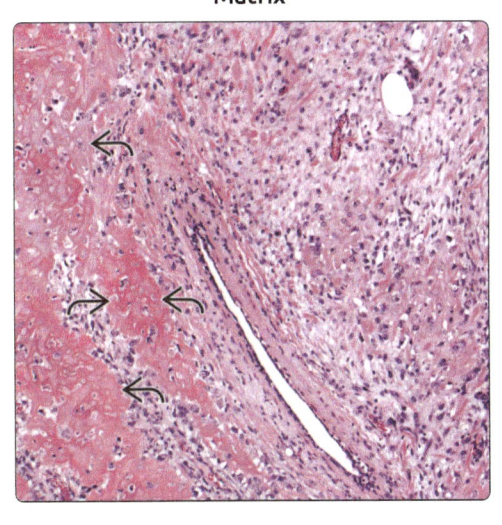

Metaplastic Carcinoma: p63 Expression

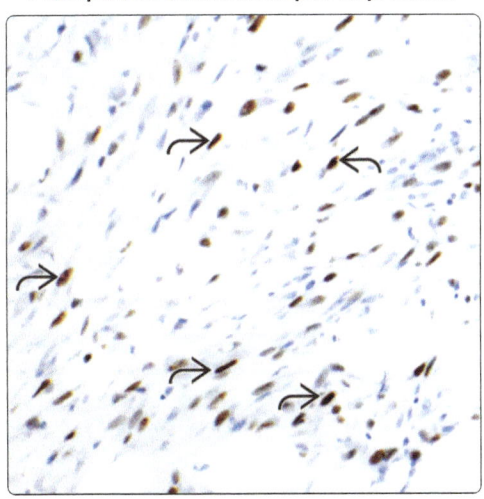

(Left) *In rare cases, metaplastic carcinoma is associated with recognizable malignant mesenchymal elements. The most common is osteosarcoma. Osteoid* ⇨ *can sometimes be seen as calcification on imaging. Primary sarcomas of the breast are exceedingly rare, and a diagnosis of metaplastic carcinoma should always be considered.* (Right) *Expression of p63* ⇨ *is seen in > 90% of metaplastic carcinomas and can be helpful in confirming the diagnosis of carcinoma in spindle cell breast lesions.*

Preneoplastic Conditions, Cervix/Vulva/Vagina

KEY FACTS

ETIOLOGY/PATHOGENESIS

- Cervix, vagina, and vulva (HPV-associated, HPV-A)
  - Persistent high-risk (HR)-HPV infection is single most important factor in development of precancerous lesions
  - HR-HPV in high-grade squamous intraepithelial lesion (HSIL) and most low-grade squamous intraepithelial lesions (LSIL)
- Viral integration into host genome often present in HSIL
  - Degrades p53 and RB1; p16 overexpressed
- Endocervical adenocarcinoma in situ (AIS)
  - HR-HPV infection in ~ 80-90% with increased HPV-18
- Differentiated vulvar intraepithelial neoplasm (HPV-independent HPV-I)
  - TP53 mutations detectable in most cases
- Extramammary Paget disease
  - 10-20% associated with adenocarcinoma from Bartholin gland or skin adnexa
  - 20% associated with invasive adenocarcinoma elsewhere

CLINICAL ISSUES

- Prevention of HPV-A disease
  - Primary prevention with nonavalent HPV vaccine for protection against HSIL and genital warts
  - Pap or primary HPV for initial screening options

MOLECULAR

- Common technique used for HR-HPV detection
- Signal amplification hybridization, real-time PCR, methylation status, amplification E6/E7 mRNA transcripts
- Extended genotyping of HR-HPV genotyping for assessment of squamous cell carcinoma risk

ANCILLARY TESTS

- Immunostain for p16 of value for histologic diagnosis of HSIL and adenocarcinoma in situ
- Cytology dual stain with CINtech Plus (p16 and Ki-67) for HSIL

Low-Grade Squamous Intraepithelial Lesion

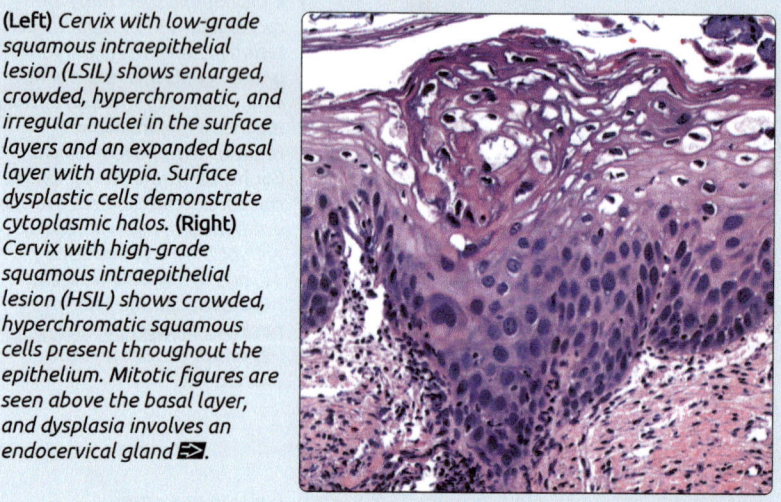

High-Grade Squamous Intraepithelial Lesion

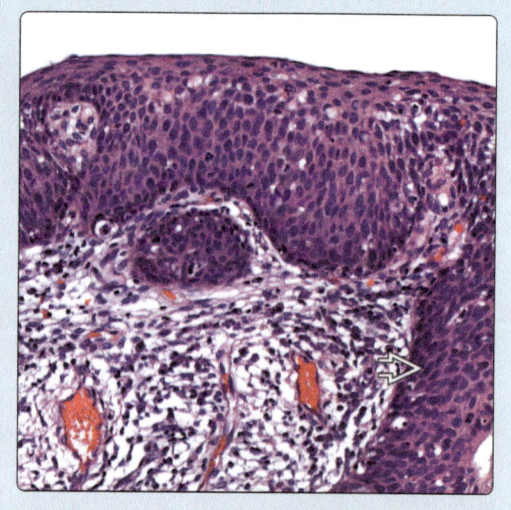

(Left) Cervix with low-grade squamous intraepithelial lesion (LSIL) shows enlarged, crowded, hyperchromatic, and irregular nuclei in the surface layers and an expanded basal layer with atypia. Surface dysplastic cells demonstrate cytoplasmic halos. (Right) Cervix with high-grade squamous intraepithelial lesion (HSIL) shows crowded, hyperchromatic squamous cells present throughout the epithelium. Mitotic figures are seen above the basal layer, and dysplasia involves an endocervical gland ➡.

Stratified Mucin-Producing Intraepithelial Lesion

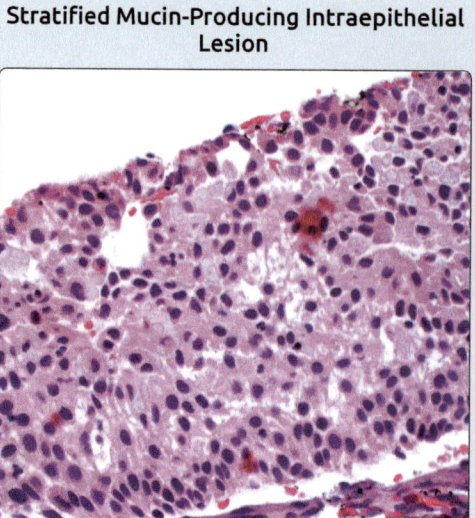

Extramammary Paget Disease

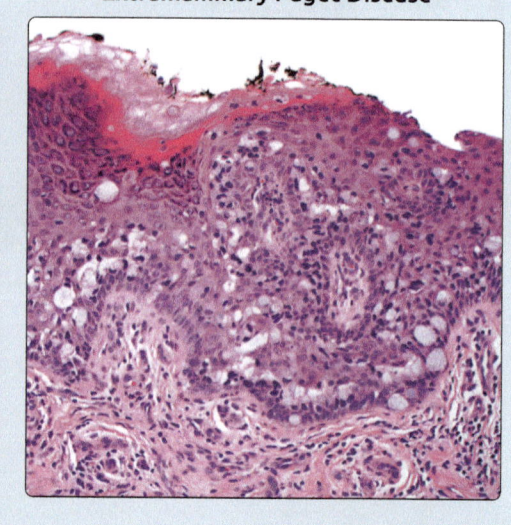

(Left) Cervix with stratified mucin-producing intraepithelial lesion (SMILE) shows dysplastic cells with intracellular mucin. This lesion was associated with HSIL elsewhere in the specimen. (Right) Vulva with extramammary Paget disease shows keratinized squamous mucosa with numerous intraepithelial cells with pale, mucinous cytoplasm. The cells are present singly and in small nests at all levels of the epithelium.

Preneoplastic Conditions, Cervix/Vulva/Vagina

TERMINOLOGY

Definitions
- Intraepithelial lesions of lower female genital tract in squamous and glandular mucosa of cervix, vagina, and vulva
- Classifications
  o Lower anogenital squamous terminology (LAST): Low- and high-grade squamous intraepithelial lesions (LSIL/HSIL) with intraepithelial neoplasia (WHO-IN)
  o Site-specific intraepithelial neoplasia (WHO)
    – Cervical intraepithelial neoplasia (CIN) 1-3
    – Vaginal intraepithelial neoplasia (VaIN) 1-3
    – Vulvar intraepithelial neoplasia (VIN) 1-3

ETIOLOGY/PATHOGENESIS

Cervix, Vagina, Vulva (HPV-Associated, HPV-A)
- Persistent oncogenic high-risk HPV (HR-HPV) infection is single most important factor in development of precancerous lesions
- HR-HPV in HSIL and most LSIL
  o HPV-16, -18, -45, and -31 highest risk
  o Viral integration into host genome often present in HSIL
    – HPV proteins E6 and E7 overexpressed and degrade tumor suppressor proteins p53 and pRB1
    – E6 upregulates telomerase with loss of replicative senescence
  o E7 upregulates genes necessary for S-phase progression and cellular proliferation; p16 overexpressed
  o Altered regulation of apoptosis-related factors
    – BCL2, FasL, survivin, MDM, TP53, BAX, and caspase-3
- Cervical adenocarcinoma in situ (AIS)
  o HPV infection in ~ 80-90% with increased HPV-18
- Other risk factors and cofactors
  o Cigarette smoking, nutritional deficiencies, other sexually transmitted infections, early sexual debut, high parity, lack of Pap screening
  o Immunosuppression (HIV, posttransplant)
- VaIN and VIN risk factors
  o Previous WHO-IN, previous pelvic irradiation (VAIN)

Vulva (HPV-Independent, HPV-I)
- Differentiated VIN (D-VIN)
  o High-grade squamous dysplasia associated with lichen sclerosus in postmenopausal women
  o *TP53* mutations detectable in most cases
  o Some cases associated with autoimmune disease
- Extramammary Paget disease (EPD)
  o Primary type originates from pluripotent epidermal stem cells of skin or skin adnexa
  o High frequency of mutations occurs in key genes of RAS/RAF and PI3K/AKT pathways
  o Secondary type (20%) associated with metastatic adenocarcinoma (e.g., bowel, urogenital tract, breast)

CLINICAL ISSUES

Epidemiology
- Incidence
  o Cervix
    – ~ 200,000 cases of HSIL diagnosed by Pap yearly per CDC (2022)
    – ~ 0.6 cases/100,000 endocervical AIS
  o Vagina
    – ~ 0.2 cases/100,000 VaIN among White women; ~ 0.3 cases/100,000 among Black women
  o Vulva
    – EPD primarily presents in postmenopausal women of European descent
- Age
  o Average: 25 years for CIN; peak at 25-34 years
  o Mean age of endocervical AIS: ~ 38 years
  o Mean age for VaIN: 53 years; peak at 60-70 years
  o 4th-5th decade for VIN; 7th-8th decade for D-VIN
  o After 4th decade for EPD, peak at 65 years

Presentation
- HSIL
  o Asymptomatic with abnormal squamous cells on Pap
  o Colposcopy: Acetowhite lesions, abnormal vessels, and mosaicism
- Endocervical AIS
  o Asymptomatic with abnormal glandular cells on Pap
  o Colposcopy: Acetowhite to red lesions and abnormal vessels; concurrent SIL 50-70%
- VaIN
  o Asymptomatic with normal or abnormal Pap test, sometimes vaginal bleeding
  o Colposcopy: Acetowhite to pink, raised lesions with abnormal vessels; upper 1/3 posterior wall
  o 50% multifocal, coexistent CIN or VIN in 10-30%
- HPV-A VIN
  o Vulvar irritation, pruritus, maculopapular or plaque, acetowhite to pigmented lesions
  o Found primarily on labia minora; 70% multifocal
- D-VIN
  o Symptomatic with pruritus in distribution of lichen sclerosus, dermatitis, eczema, and leukoplakia
- EPD
  o Symptomatic with pruritus, pain, erythematous or eczematous lesion, and moist, weepy surface
  o Localized to widespread; may involve perianus

Treatment
- HSIL
  o Laser electrocautery excision procedure (LEEP), cryotherapy, laser ablation, cold knife cone, observation if young
- Endocervical AIS
  o Cold knife cone, trachelectomy, or hysterectomy
- VaIN
  o Excision, partial vaginectomy, laser ablation, or topical 5-fluorouracil for VaIN 2-3
- VIN
  o Topical imiquimod for VIN 1, local excision, partial superficial vulvectomy, LEEP, or laser ablation for VIN 2-3
- EPD
  o Wide local excision or vulvectomy, topical 5-fluorouracil, laser ablation, or systemic retinoids
- Prevention

Preneoplastic Conditions, Cervix/Vulva/Vagina

- Primary: nonavalent HPV vaccine offers protection against HSIL and genital warts (HPV-16, -18, -31, -33, -45, -52, -58, -6, and -11)
- Secondary: Screening by Pap test at 21-25 years or primary HPV test at 25 years; cotesting 30-65 years

Prognosis
- CIN
  - LSIL: ~ 62% of LSIL regress in 24 months, 22% persist as LSIL, and 16% progress to HSIL
  - HSIL: ~ 50% of CIN 2 regress in 24 months
  - HSIL: ~ 20% of CIN 3 progress to squamous cell carcinoma (SCC) if untreated
- VaIN
  - ~ 5-10% of VaIN 3 progress to SCC after treatment
- VIN
  - ~ 10% of HPV-related VIN 3 progress to SCC untreated
  - ~ 80-90% of differentiated VIN progresses to SCC
- EPD
  - May persist for years as noninvasive lesion
  - 10-20% progress to invasive adenocarcinoma
  - Poor prognosis if metastatic from other sites

MOLECULAR

In Situ Hybridization
- Tissue detection of HPV E6 and E7 mRNA (IS-HPV)

PCR
- RT-PCR detects specific viral RNA and multiple HPV types
- Extended genotyping for risk stratification
  - HPV-16, -18, -31, -45, -51, and -52; 35/39/68; 56/59/66; 33/58
- Methylation status by pyrosequencing or methylation-specific PCR
  - *EPB41L3/L1, L2, CADM1/MAL, MAL/miR-124-2, FAM19A4/miR-124-2, SOX14*

Next-Generation Sequencing
- For HPV variants, novel HPV types, and integration sites
- *LINC00290, LINC02500*, and *LENG9* as possible driver genes

mRNA E6/E7 Oncoprotein Overexpression
- Upregulation of E6/E7 proteins with increased risk of SCC

Signal Amplification Hybridization
- DNA hybridization by hybrid capture or invader chemistry

Lateral Flow Immunochromatographic Test
- E6 protein from HPV-16, -18, and -45 detected in HSIL, AIS

Gene Expression Profiling
- Upregulation of *MCM, E2F1*, and DNA repair genes *BRCA2-BRIP1, FANCA*, and *CMYC*
- MAPK, JAK-STAT, transcriptional misregulation pathways

MICROSCOPIC

Histologic Features
- HPV-A cervical, vaginal, and vulva show similar histologic findings
  - LSIL
    - Expanded basal layer and surface with enlarged, irregular, hyperchromatic, and crowded nuclei
    - Mitotic figures in lower 1/3 of epithelium
  - HSIL
    - Near- to full-thickness epithelium with enlarged, irregular, hyperchromatic cells, increased N:C ratio
    - Mitotic figures in all levels of epithelium
  - Endocervical AIS
    - Hyperchromatic, pseudostratified nuclei, mitoses, apoptotic bodies, HSIL also seen in 50%
    - Subtypes: Intestinal, endometrioid, gastric, tubal
- D-VIN
  - Marked nuclear atypia in basal layer with some superficial maturation and differentiation
  - Basal nuclei with pleomorphism, dispersed chromatin, eosinophilic cytoplasm, prominent nucleoli, and mitoses
- EPD
  - Intraepithelial proliferation of atypical cells with enlarged nuclei, prominent nucleoli, and abundant cytoplasm

ANCILLARY TESTS

Immunohistochemistry
- Cervix, vagina, and vulva HR-HPV-A lesions
  - p16 strongly and diffusely (+), CINtec PLUS (+) (p16 and Ki-67), ProExC (+) (Top2a and MCM2), IS-HPV
- Endocervical AIS
  - p16 strongly and diffusely (+); CEA (+), ProExC (+), Ki-67 (+) > 75%; ER (-), vimentin (-)
  - Intestinal type CDX2 (+), may be p16 (-)
- EPD
  - Primary: CK7, CEA, GCDFP-15, GATA3, and BerEp4 (+)
    - ER, PR, HMB-45, and MART1/Melan-A (-)
  - Secondary: Shows site of origin-specific staining
- Differentiated VIN
  - p53 (+) in basal layer in > 50%, Ki-67 (+) over background, p16 (-), HR-HPV (-)

DIFFERENTIAL DIAGNOSIS

Atrophy, Reactive and Radiation Atypia
- Nuclear enlargement and atypia similar to CIN, VaIN, VIN
- All are negative for p16, IS-HPV

Mesonephric Remnants
- Glandular proliferation in deep lateral cervical wall
- PAS (+) luminal material, GATA3 (+), p16 (-), HR-HPV (-)

Tubal Metaplasia
- Endocervical glands with cilia, bland nuclei lacking mitoses
- ER/PR (+), p16 patchy (+), BCL2 (+), vimentin (+), and HPV (-)

Endometriosis
- Presence of endometrial glands and stroma in cervix
- ER, PR, BCL2, and vimentin (+), stroma CD10 (+), and p16 (-)

Melanoma, In Situ and Superficial Spreading
- Atypical basal cells with prominent nucleoli ± pigmented
- S100, A103, HMB45, MART1, and SOX10 (+)
- Cytokeratin (-) and GCDFP15 (-) help differentiate EPD

SELECTED REFERENCES
1. Olivas AD et al: Overview of ancillary techniques in cervical cytology. Acta Cytol. 67(2):119-28, 2023

Preneoplastic Conditions, Cervix/Vulva/Vagina

Cervix With High-Grade Squamous Intraepithelial Lesion

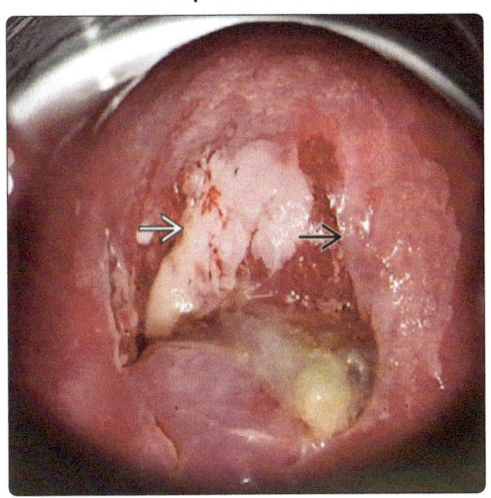

p16: Cervical High-Grade Squamous Intraepithelial Lesion

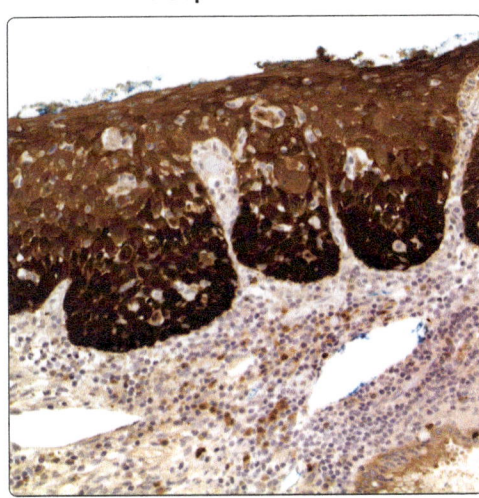

(Left) Colposcopy shows acetowhite lesions of HSIL ⇒ with dense, white plaque with sharp borders. Also note the paler lesion of LSIL with defined borders ⇒. (Courtesy A. Waxman, MD.) (Right) p16 shows strong and diffuse block positivity of HSIL throughout the epithelial layers.

Cervical Adenocarcinoma In Situ

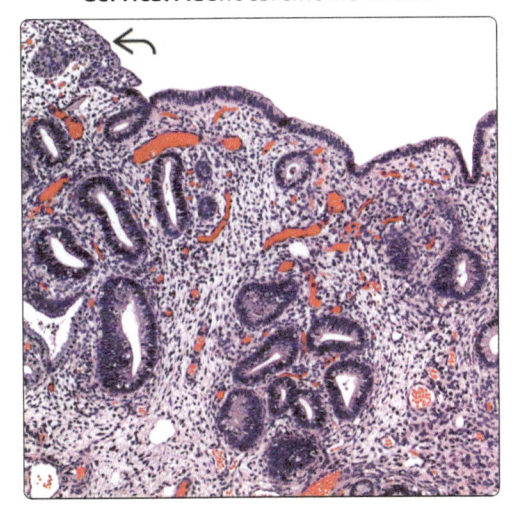

p16: Cervical Adenocarcinoma In Situ

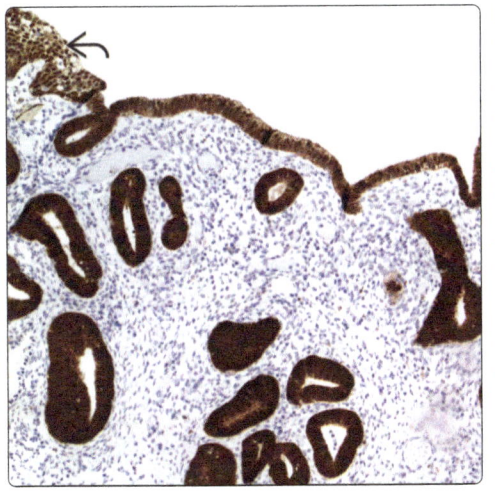

(Left) Cervical adenocarcinoma in situ shows replacement of normal mucinous glandular epithelium with dysplastic cells with nuclear pseudostratification, enlargement, and hyperchromasia. Concomitant HSIL is also present ⇒. (Right) Cervical adenocarcinoma in situ shows strong expression of p16 in dysplastic glandular cells. Concomitant HSIL also shows strong block p16 positivity ⇒.

Differentiated Vulvar Intraepithelial Neoplasm

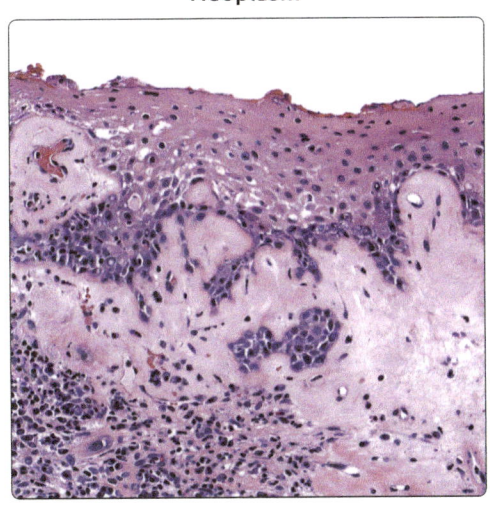

p53: Differentiated Vulvar Intraepithelial Neoplasm

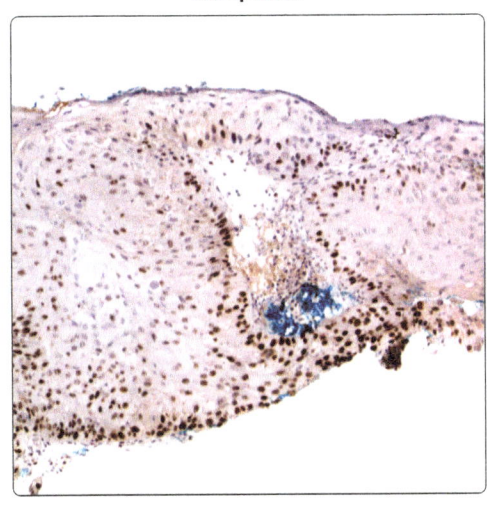

(Left) Differentiated vulvar intraepithelial neoplasm (VIN) shows atypical basal cells with nuclear enlargement and prominent nucleoli with surface maturation in a background of lichen sclerosus. (Right) p53 shows strong nuclear expression in basal and suprabasal layers in this differentiated VIN. p16 (not shown) was negative.

Squamous Cell Carcinoma, Cervix/Vulva/Vagina

KEY FACTS

ETIOLOGY/PATHOGENESIS

- Persistent infection by high-risk oncogenic HPV-16, -18, -31, -45, and others with viral integration into host genome
  - Single most important factor in multistep oncogenesis with 99.7% of squamous cell carcinoma (SCC) with high-risk human papillomavirus (HR-HPV)
  - Viral DNA integration into host genome is common
  - Leads to overexpression of viral E6 and E7 proteins, which interact with central regulators of cell cycle and apoptosis
- HPV infection not sufficient for carcinogenesis but requires other cofactors
  - Cigarette smoking, other microbial infections, nutritional deficiencies, hormonal factors, immunosuppression
- HPV-independent (HPV-I) vulvar SCC
  - ~ 60% of vulvar SCC associated with lichen sclerosus, other vulvar dermatoses, and differentiated vulvar intraepithelial neoplasia

ANCILLARY TESTS

- Immunohistochemistry in HPV-related SCC
  - Positive p16, Ki-76, ProExC, and CINtec PLUS
  - Non-HPV-related vulvar and vaginal SCC: Positive p53 (in 50%) and negative p16
- HPV genotyping methods
  - Hybrid capture or invader chemistry
  - RT-PCR or next-generation sequencing
  - Transcription-mediated amplification of E6/E7 mRNA transcripts
- Methylation status of host and viral genes of *EPB41L3/L1, L2, CADM1/MAL, MAL/miR-124-2,* and *FAM19A4/miR-124-2*

TOP DIFFERENTIAL DIAGNOSES

- Poorly differentiated endocervical adenocarcinoma, neuroendocrine carcinoma, melanoma, urothelial carcinoma with local extension, pseudoepitheliomatous hyperplasia

Cervical Squamous Cell Carcinoma

Invasive Squamous Cell Carcinoma

(Left) Gross photograph of cervical squamous cell carcinoma (SCC) is shown. The bulky exophytic tumor in the endocervical canal protrudes through the cervical os ➡ and involves the exocervix. (Right) Nonkeratinizing invasive SCC shows solid nests of malignant cells infiltrating through fibrous stroma.

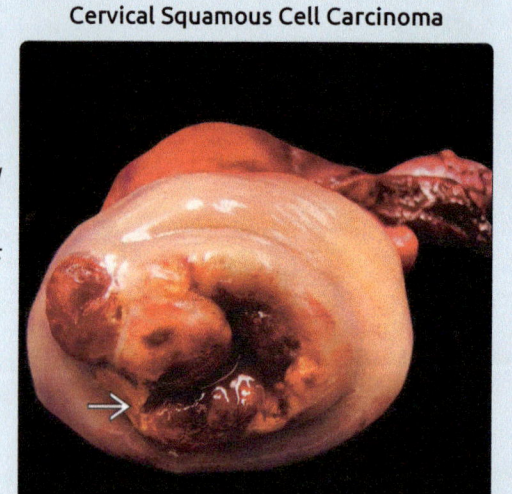

Invasive Squamous Cell Carcinoma, Spindle Cell Type

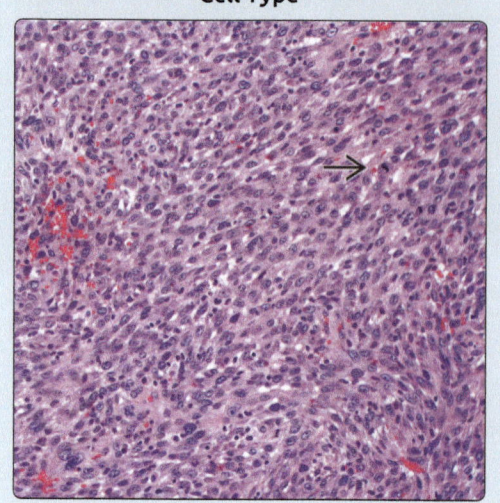

Superficially Invasive Squamous Cell Carcinoma

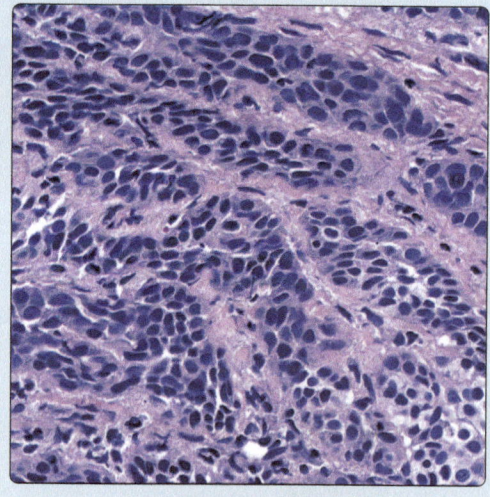

(Left) Invasive vaginal SCC with spindle cell morphology shows intersecting fascicles of spindle cells with mitotic activity ➡. Areas of conventional SCC were present elsewhere in the specimen. (Right) Cervix with superficially invasive SCC shows irregular nests of neoplastic squamous epithelium invading into the underlying stroma ➡. The tumor arises from an overlying high-grade squamous intraepithelial lesion.

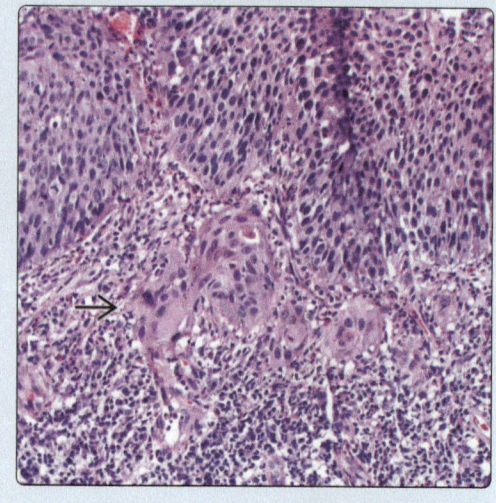

Squamous Cell Carcinoma, Cervix/Vulva/Vagina

TERMINOLOGY

Abbreviations
- Squamous cell carcinoma (SCC)

Definitions
- Primary malignant squamous neoplasms of female lower genital tract
  - ~ 75-80% of cervical carcinomas
  - ~ 85% of vaginal carcinomas
  - ~ 90% of vulvar carcinomas

ETIOLOGY/PATHOGENESIS

Persistent Infection by High-Risk Human Papillomavirus
- High-risk oncogenic human papillomavirus (HPV), including HPV-16, -18, -31, -45, and others
  - Preceded by HPV-associated (HPV-A) high-grade squamous intraepithelial lesions (HSIL) at all sites
- Persistent infection (99.7% cervix, > 60% vagina, ~ 40% vulva)
- Viral DNA integration into host genome with multistep oncogenesis
  - Interaction of viral E6 and E7 proteins with central regulators of cell cycle and apoptosis
  - Promotes cellular proliferation with clonal expansion of relatively undifferentiated squamous cells, immortalization, and malignant transformation
    - E6 and E7 overexpression inactivate tumor suppressor genes *TP53*, *RB1*, *STK11*, and *PTEN*
    - Activates telomerase with loss of normal replicative senescence
    - Removes suppression of p16 expression bypassing cell cycle arrest
  - Upregulation of genes critical for S-phase progression and cellular proliferation, including
    - *CDKN2A*, *MCM2*, *PCNA*, *CCNE1*, *CCND1*, *MIB1*, *TOP2A*, *HRAS*, *EGFR*, and *MYC*
  - Altered regulation of apoptosis-related factors
    - BCL2, FASLG, survivin, MDM2, p53, BAX, and caspase-3
  - Methylation of host promoter regions of *CADM1*, *MAL*, *DAPK1*, *RARB*, *UTF1*, *FAM19A4*, and *EPB41L3*
  - Significant mutated genes: *ERBB3* (HER3), *CASP8*, *HLA-A*, *SHKBP1*, *TGFBR2*, *PIK3CA*; APOBEC mutagenesis patterns
- HPV infection not sufficient for carcinogenesis; role of other risk factors and cofactors
  - Cigarette smoking, other sexually transmitted infections, early sexual debut, oral contraceptives, high parity, nutritional deficiencies, hormones
  - Immunosuppression (HIV, post transplantation)
- HPV-independent (HPV-I) vulvar SCC
  - ~ 60% associated with lichen sclerosus, other dermatoses, and differentiated vulvar intraepithelial neoplasia (D-VIN) with possible role of *TP53* mutations
    - 2-9% of lichen sclerosus patients progress to D-VIN; ~ 80-90% of D-VIN progress to SCC

CLINICAL ISSUES

Epidemiology
- Incidence
  - Cervix (2020, 2022)
    - USA: 14,100 cases per year; mortality: 4,280 per year; 7.8 cases per 100,000
    - Worldwide: 604,237 cases per year; mortality: 341,831 per year; 13.3 cases per 100,000
  - Vagina (2018)
    - USA: 5,170 cases per year; mortality: 1,330 per year; 0.5 cases per 100,000
    - Worldwide: 17,600 cases per year; mortality: 8,062
  - Vulva (2018)
    - USA: 6,020 cases per year; mortality: 1,150 per year; 2.5 cases per 100,000
    - Worldwide: 44,235 cases per year; mortality: 15,222
- Age
  - Cervical, HPV-A vaginal, and vulvar SCC
    - Mean: Cervix: 50.6 years; vagina: 66.1 years; vulva: 66.9 years
  - Vaginal HPV-I SCC: Mean: 73 years
  - Vulvar HPV-I SCC: Mean: 66.1 years

Presentation
- Cervix
  - Asymptomatic or may present with vaginal bleeding, dyspareunia, or cervical mass
  - Abnormal Pap test, abnormal colposcopic examination with discrete, acetowhite lesions with abnormal vessels
- Vagina
  - Asymptomatic or present with vaginal bleeding, mass, malodorous discharge, and urinary tract symptoms
  - HPV-A: Posterior upper 1/2 vagina; HPV-I: Lower vagina
  - Abnormal Pap test and colposcopy, indurated mucosa
- Vulva
  - Mass; red, brown, black to white macule/papule/plaque, most commonly on labia majora; 10% multifocal; Bartholin gland mass
  - HPV-I SCC may present with inflammatory dermatoses, pain, pruritus, dysuria, and dyspareunia

Treatment
- Cervix
  - Stage-dependent, ranging from conization, trachelectomy, simple to radical hysterectomy, sentinel lymph nodes ± pelvic and periaortic lymphadenectomy, brachytherapy to chemoradiation
- Vagina
  - Stage-dependent, ranging from partial vaginectomy to radical hysterectomy with upper vaginectomy ± inguinal &/or iliac lymph node dissection, brachytherapy to chemoradiation
- Vulva
  - Stage-dependent, ranging from wide local resection to radical local resection and radical vulvectomy, sentinel nodes ± inguinal and femoral lymph node dissection, radiation, chemotherapy

Prognosis
- Cervix

Squamous Cell Carcinoma, Cervix/Vulva/Vagina

- 5- to 10-year survival: Stage IA: 95%; stage IB: 90%; stage II: 50-70%; stage III: 30-50%; stage IV: 5-15%
- Vagina
  - 5-year survival: Stage I: 75-95%; stage II: 50-80%; stage III: 30-60%; stage IV: 15-50%
- Vulva
  - 5-year survival: Stage I: 85%; stage II: 60%; stage III: 40%; stage IV: 15%
  - 5-year survival: 60-80% with < 2-cm lesion; < 10% with > 2-cm lesion with lymph node metastases

MOLECULAR

In Situ Hybridization
- Tissue detection of HPV E6 and E7 mRNA
- FISH shows chromosomal gains at 3q25, 5p15, 20q13, cen7

PCR
- HPV-genotyping methods
  - RT-PCR can detect specific viral and multiple HPV types
  - Transcription-mediated amplification of E6/E7 mRNA
  - Extended genotyping for HPV-16, -18, -45, -31, -51, -52; 33/58; 35/39/68 and 56/59/66 for risk stratification
- Methylation-specific PCR and pyrosequencing technology
  - EPB41L3/L1, L2, CADM1/MAL, MAL/miR-124-2, FAM19A4/miR-124-2
- Microsatellite instability high in cervical SCC

HPV Signal Amplification DNA Hybridization
- DNA hybridization by hybrid capture and invader chemistry

mRNA E6/E7 Oncoprotein Overexpression
- Upregulation of E6/E7 oncoproteins in cervical SCC

Lateral Flow Immunochromatographic Test
- Detects E6, E7 oncoprotein from HPV-16, -18, and -45
- Amplification integrated assay detects HPV-16, -18 DNA

Chromosomal Microarray
- Cervical SCC
  - Chromosomal gains include 3q, 1q, and 5p regions; losses include 14p, 13q, 2q, 4q, and 6q regions
  - Loss of heterozygosity at 3p14.2, 3p21.3, 3p24.2, 1p32.3, 1p36.21, 4q11, 4q34, 6p21.2, and 8p23.3 by SNP array

Gene Expression Profiling
- 12 significantly mutated genes, suggesting APOBEC mutagenesis
  - EP300, HLA-B, PTEN, NFE2L2, ARID1A, KRAS, MAPK1, SHKBP1, ERBB3, CASP8, HLA-A, and TGFBR2
  - Amplification of CD274 (PD-L1) and PDCD1LG2 immune targets, also BCAR4
- Cell cycle, signaling pathways and c-MYC upregulation

Cytogenetics
- Numerical alterations in chromosomes 1q, 3p, 4q, 5p, 6p, 11q, and 17q in cervical SCC

Next-Generation Sequencing
- Detects HPV variants, novel HPV types, and integration events
- HPV-I cervical SCC with KRAS, ARID1A, and PTEN mutations
- HPV-I vulvar SCC with TP53 mutations
- TLINC00290, LINC02500, and LENG9 are potential driver genes

Multiomics
- Productive HPV integration with increased E6/E7 proteins, tumor aggressiveness, and immunoevasion

MICROSCOPIC

Histologic Features
- Cervix, vagina, vulva
  - Cohesive irregular nests and cords of malignant squamous cells invading into underlying stroma
  - Variable keratinization and necrosis and associated HSIL
- Histologic types, HPV-A, all sites
  - Verrucous, condylomatous (warty)
  - Papillary/squamotransitional
  - Spindle cell, basaloid
  - Lymphoepithelioma like: Cervix
- HPV-I vaginal SCC
  - Mostly keratinizing SCC
- HPV-I vulvar SCC
  - Keratinizing SCC; may be accompanied by D-VIN, lichen sclerosus, or lichen planus
  - Verrucous, sarcomatoid, acantholytic, warty, and basaloid

ANCILLARY TESTS

Immunohistochemistry
- Cervical, vaginal, and vulvar HPV-A SCC
  - Positive p16, Ki-67, CINtec PLUS (p16 and Ki-67), ProExC (Top2a and MCM2), CK5, CK7, p63, p40, and IS-HPV0
  - Negative for p53
  - EGFR overexpression in 70-90% of SCC
  - PD-L1 status important for treatment decisions
- Cervical, vaginal, and vulvar HPV-I SCC
  - Some p53 positivity; negative p16 and IS-HPV

DIFFERENTIAL DIAGNOSIS

Poorly Differentiated Endocervical Adenocarcinoma
- Cytoplasmic mucin; positive CEA and negative p63 and p40

Neuroendocrine Carcinoma
- Dark chromatin; positive chromogranin, synaptophysin, CD56

Urothelial Carcinoma With Local Extension
- Positive GATA3 and CK20; negative IS-HPV

Melanoma
- Positive S100, HMB-45, Melan-A/MART-1, SOX-10, and PRAME; negative cytokeratin, p16, and IS-HPV

Pseudoepitheliomatous Hyperplasia
- Reactive squamous epithelium; negative p16 and IS-HPV

SELECTED REFERENCES

1. Fan J et al: Multi-omics characterization of silent and productive HPV integration in cervical cancer. Cell Genom. 3(1):100211, 2023
2. Balasubramaniam SD et al: Gene expression profiling of HPV-associated cervical carcinogenesis in formalin-fixed paraffin-embedded (FFPE) tissues using the NanoString nCounter(TM) platform. Gene. 825:146385, 2022

Squamous Cell Carcinoma, Cervix/Vulva/Vagina

Invasive Squamous Cell Carcinoma

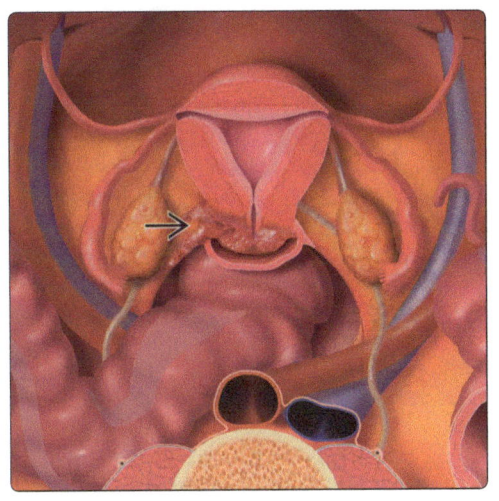

Molecular Pathogenesis of Squamous Cell Carcinoma

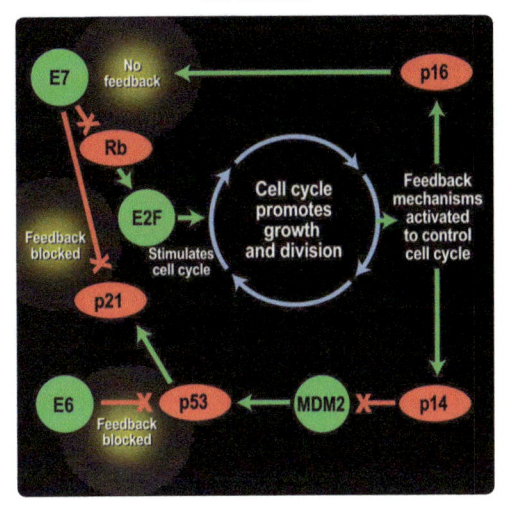

(Left) Graphic shows female pelvic organs with cross section of the uterus and cervix demonstrating SCC of the cervix with local extension of the tumor into pericervical soft tissue ⇨. (Right) High-risk human papillomavirus (HPV) infection and pathogenesis of SCC are driven by E6 and E7 viral gene products and disruption of central regulators of apoptosis (p53) and cell cycle (p21 and Rb). Upregulation of these genes is critical for S-phase progression and cellular proliferation.

Keratinizing Invasive Squamous Cell Carcinoma

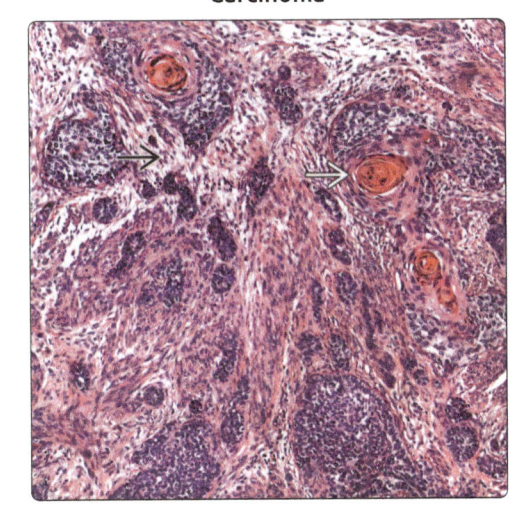

p16: Invasive Squamous Cell Carcinoma

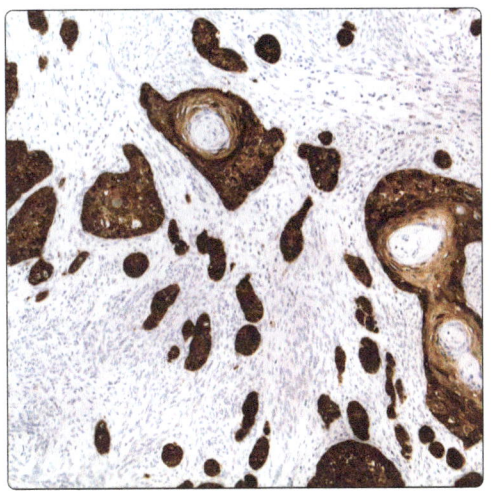

(Left) Cervix with keratinizing invasive SCC shows irregular nests of neoplastic squamous cells infiltrating the underlying stroma with reactive desmoplastic stromal response ⇨. Focal SCC nests show densely eosinophilic keratin pearls ⇨. (Right) p16 of invasive SCC shows strong, diffuse positivity in the islands of malignant squamous cells.

D-VIN and Invasive Squamous Cell Carcinoma

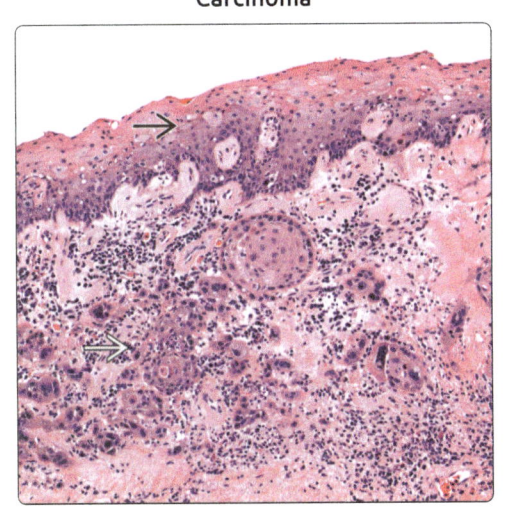

Lymphoepithelial-Like Variant Invasive Squamous Cell Carcinoma

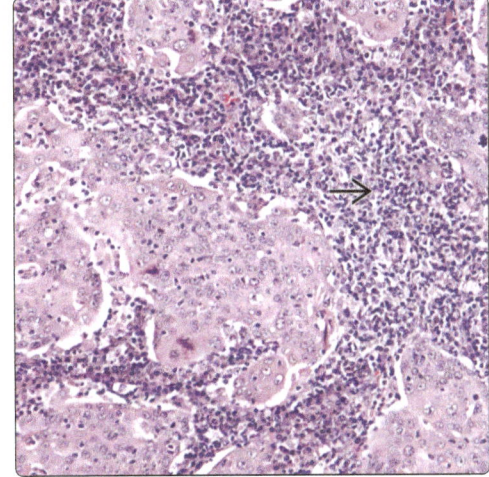

(Left) Vulvar skin shows surface epidermis with differentiated vulvar intraepithelial neoplasia (D-VIN) ⇨ and well-differentiated invasive SCC in the underlying dermis. Irregular nests of malignant squamous cells fill the superficial to mid dermis ⇨. (Right) Lymphoepithelial-like variant of cervical SCC with solid nests of tumor is shown. This is accompanied by a prominent circumferential lymphocytic infiltrate ⇨.

Adenocarcinoma, Cervix/Vulva/Vagina

KEY FACTS

ETIOLOGY/PATHOGENESIS

- Cervical adenocarcinoma (ADC)
  - Majority (90-95%) are HPV-associated (HPV-A); HPV-16 most prevalent with HPV-18 more highly represented than in SCC; also HPV-45
- Vagina ADC
  - Clear cell ADC is related to in utero exposure to DES pre-1970s, < 0.14% of DES-exposed females
- Vulvar ADC
  - Arises from Bartholin gland or vulvar skin appendages
  - EPD-related ADC either primary or secondary to metastasis from distant site

ANCILLARY TESTS

- Cervical ADC
  - HPV-A: p16, CINtec Plus, ProEX C, CEA, cyclin-A, and cyclin-B positive; ER, PR, and vimentin negative
  - HPV independent (HPV-I): CEA, PAX8, GATA3, some p53; IS-HPV negative; p16 usually negative
  - Testing for HPV includes hybrid capture, invader chemistry, PCR, NGS, and amplification of E6/E7 mRNA transcripts
- Minimal deviation and gastric-type cervical ADC
  - May have mutations of *STK11*, either sporadic or related to Peutz-Jeghers syndrome
- Vagina ADC
  - Clear cell type positive for CEA, EMA, cCK7; p53 (in some cases) and p16 negative
- Vulvar ADC of Bartholin gland
  - CEA, CAM 5.2, EMA, ER, and PR positive

TOP DIFFERENTIAL DIAGNOSES

- Cervix ADC: Endometrial adenocarcinoma, benign glandular proliferations, endometriosis, atypical lobular endocervical gland dysplasia
- Vaginal ADC: Vaginal adenosis, endometriosis, cervical ADC
- Vulvar ADC: Metastatic ADC, melanoma, endometriosis, dermatoses

(Left) Gross photograph shows a polypoid tumor that appears to arise in the endocervical canal. Histologic examination showed an invasive cervical adenocarcinoma. (Right) Invasive endocervical adenocarcinoma is shown. Tumor cells exhibit large, pleomorphic nuclei, prominent nucleoli, and pleomorphism.

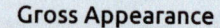

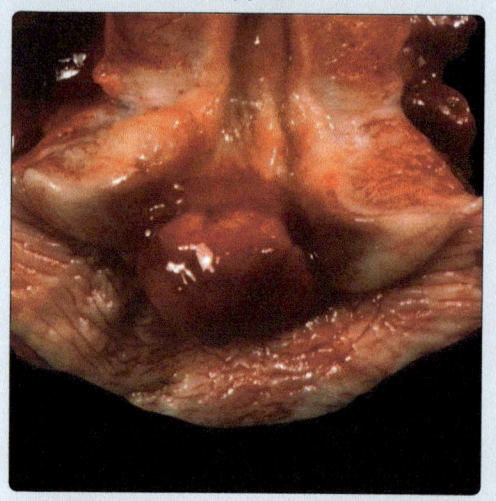

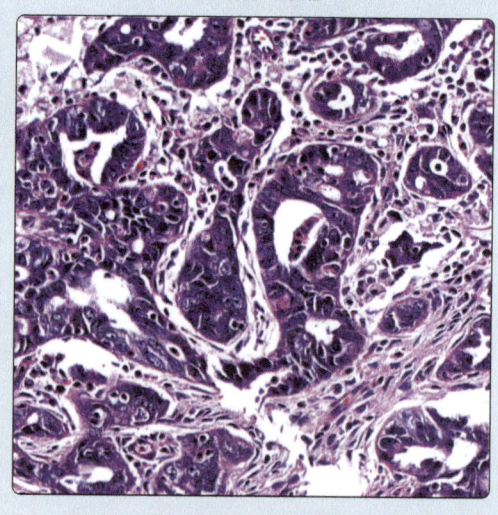

(Left) Cervix with exophytic villoglandular adenocarcinoma shows finger-like villous structures arising from the surface. The villous structures have fibrovascular cores, and the lining cells have mild nuclear atypia and few mitoses. (Right) Endocervix shows a focus of superficially invasive adenocarcinoma arising in a background of adenocarcinoma in situ. Neoplastic glandular cells infiltrate the stroma in small nests and single cells ➡.

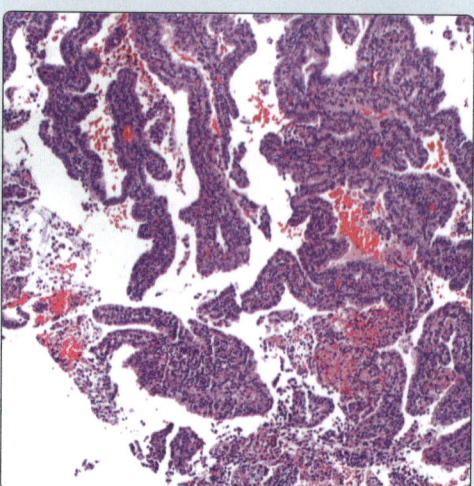

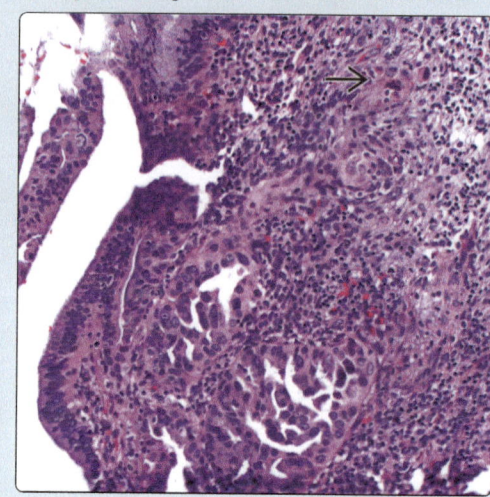

Adenocarcinoma, Cervix/Vulva/Vagina

TERMINOLOGY

Abbreviations
- Adenocarcinoma (ADC)
- Squamous cell carcinoma (SCC)

Definitions
- ADC: Malignant glandular neoplasms of female lower genital tract, including cervix, vagina, and vulva
  - 2nd most common primary cervical carcinoma after SCC

ETIOLOGY/PATHOGENESIS

Cervical Adenocarcinoma
- Heterogeneous group of tumors; 70-90% HPV-associated (HPV-A)
  - Persistent infection by high-risk oncogenic HPV (HR-HPV), including HPV-16, -18, -45, -45, -51, and -52
  - Single most important factor in multistep oncogenesis; similar pathogenesis to cervical SCC
- Viral integration into host genome is common
- Viral E6 and E7 proteins interact with central regulators of cell cycle and apoptosis
  - Promotes cellular proliferation with clonal expansion and malignant transformation
  - Suppression of tumor suppressor genes *TP53*, *RB1*, *STK11*, and *PTEN*
  - Activates telomerase with loss of normal replicative senescence
  - Inactivates cell cycle inhibitors p21 and p27
  - Altered regulation of apoptosis-related factors: BCL2, FasL, and survivin
- *KRAS* mutations common; CpG island methylator low and high phenotype; low and high APOBEC signatures
- Other risk factors and cofactors
  - Cigarette smoking, nutritional deficiencies, oral contraceptives, sexually transmitted infections, early sexual debut, no Pap test ever or in past 5 years
  - Immunosuppression (HIV, post transplant)
- Rare (~ 5%) ADC subtypes HPV-independent (HPV-I) with *KRAS*, *ARID1A*, and *PTEN* mutations
- Minimal deviation and gastric ADC associated with Peutz-Jeghers Syndrome and germ-line mutations in *TP53*

Vaginal Adenocarcinoma
- Clear cell adenocarcinoma
  - Rare cases (< 0.14%) related to in utero exposure to diethylstilbestrol (DES) pre-1970s (also seen in cervix)
  - Females with in utero DES exposure 40x more likely to develop clear cell ADC than nonexposed females
- Nonclear cell adenocarcinoma
  - Possible link to unopposed estrogen, adenosis and endometriosis; gastric type possibly with *TP53* mutation
- Adenocarcinoma, HPV-A types 16, 18, and 31

Vulvar Adenocarcinoma
- 5% of vulvar cancers; HPV-I; most are SCC at this site
- Extramammary Paget disease (EPD)-related ADC in 4-8%
  - Primary type originates in vulvar pluripotent stem cells of epidermis or skin adnexa
  - May see mutations in *PIK3CA* and *AKT1*
  - Secondary type metastatic from other sites (cervix, bowel, urogenital tract, breast, and others)

CLINICAL ISSUES

Epidemiology
- Incidence
  - Cervical ADC: 2.1 cases per 100,000
    - ~ 25% of all cervical carcinomas
    - Increased incidence in last few decades, particularly in younger women
  - Vaginal ADC: 0.1 cases per 100,000
    - ~ 5-10% of all vaginal carcinomas; most are SCC
  - Vulvar ADC: 0.04 cases/100,000
    - ~ 10% of all vulvar carcinomas; most are SCC
- Age
  - Cervical adenocarcinoma
    - 4th-5th decades (mean: 49 years of age); recent increase in women < 35 years of age
    - Villoglandular ADC: 23-55 years of age (average: 35 years of age)
  - Vaginal adenocarcinoma
    - DES-related clear cell type: Bimodal with 2 peaks, 2nd and 5th decades (mean: 19 years)
    - Non-DES-related, nonclear cell type: Uncommon; 4th-8th decades (mean: 55 years)
  - Vulvar adenocarcinoma
    - Invasive EPD-related ADC: Mean: 71.5 years
    - Bartholin gland ADC: Mean: 57 years

Presentation
- Cervical adenocarcinoma
  - Asymptomatic or vaginal bleeding, visible cervical mass
  - Abnormal Pap test with atypical glandular cells
  - Abnormal colposcopy with acetowhite or red lesions, enlarged gland openings, abnormal vessels
  - Minimal deviation ADC with mucoid or watery discharge
- Vaginal adenocarcinoma
  - Asymptomatic or with vaginal bleeding, dyspareunia
  - Abnormal Pap test with atypical glandular cells
  - Vaginal surface irregularity to discrete mass
- Vulvar adenocarcinoma
  - Asymptomatic or with vaginal bleeding, pruritus, pain, dyspareunia, vulvar mass
  - Bartholin gland mass
  - EPD-related ADC presents with erythematous and eczematous rash to discrete mass

Treatment
- Cervical adenocarcinoma
  - Stage dependent, conization, trachelectomy, simple to radical hysterectomy, ± pelvic lymphadenectomy, brachytherapy, chemoradiation
- Vaginal adenocarcinoma
  - Stage dependent; vaginectomy to radical hysterectomy ± pelvic lymph node dissection; advanced stage: Primarily radiation
- Vulvar adenocarcinoma
  - Wide local excision to radical vulvectomy if large ± inguinal lymph node dissection, radiation, and chemotherapy

Adenocarcinoma, Cervix/Vulva/Vagina

Prognosis
- Cervical adenocarcinoma, usual type
  - 5- to 10-year survival for stage 1A: ~ 95%; stage 1B: ~ 83%; stage 2: 50-59%; stage 3: 15-20%; stage 4: < 10%
- Cervical adenocarcinoma, other types
  - Villoglandular with excellent prognosis; minimal deviation with ~ 50% stage 1; gastric poor prognosis
- Vaginal adenocarcinoma
  - 5-year survival for all clear cell adenocarcinoma: ~ 93%; 10-year survival: 87%, 30% if metastases
  - Prognosis more favorable if DES-related with > 90% stage 1; non-DES-related 5-year survival: ~ 69%
- Vulvar adenocarcinoma
  - 5-year survival with negative lymph nodes: ~ 56-80%; < 2-cm lesion: ~ 70%; > 2 cm with positive nodes: < 10%

MOLECULAR

PCR
- Loss of heterozygosity at 19p13.2-13.3 region in minimal deviation ADC
- HR-HPV genotyping methods
  - RT-PCR
  - Transcription-mediated amplification of E6/E7 mRNA transcripts, hybrid capture, and invader chemistry
  - Extended HPV genotyping for risk stratification: HPV-16, -18, -31, -45, -51, -52; 33/58; 35/39/68; 56/59/66
- Methylation status by pyrosequencing or methylation-specific PCR
  - *EPB41L3/L1, L2, CADM1/MAL, MAL/miR-124-2, FAM19A4/miR-124-2, SOX14*
- Microsatellite instability in DES-related vaginal ADC

Array Comparative Genomic Hybridization
- Detects LOH at 4p15.3 in minimal deviation cervical ADC

Next-Generation Sequencing
- HPV-A ADC: Mutations in *HRAS*, *PIK4CA*, and *BRACA2*
- HPV-I ADC: Mutations in *TP53*, *KRAS*, *CDKN2A*, *STK11*, and *ARID1A*

In Situ Hybridization
- Tissue detection of HPV by viral E6 and E7 mRNA

MICROSCOPIC

Histologic Features
- Cervical adenocarcinoma
  - Simple to complex infiltrative glands with nuclear pseudostratification, hyperchromasia, and mitoses
  - Eosinophilic to mucinous cytoplasm, apoptotic bodies
  - Often with associated AIS and cervical high-grade squamous intraepithelial lesion (HSIL)
  - HPV-A subtypes: Usual type (conventional, endocervical) is 50%, villoglandular, endometrioid ADC
  - HPV-I subtypes: Minimal deviation, gastric, intestinal, mesonephric, clear cell, serous
- Vaginal adenocarcinoma
  - Clear cell ADC with hobnail cells and bulbous bland nuclei, low mitotic activity, pale to eosinophilic cytoplasm
  - Nonclear cell ADC subtypes: Endometrioid, mucinous gastric, intestinal, mesonephric, HPV-A
- Vulvar adenocarcinoma
  - Bartholin gland and ADC at other vulvar sites
    - Subtypes: Usual ADC, adenoid cystic, adenosquamous, mucoepidermoid
  - EPD-related ADC
    - Dermal invasion of malignant glands and nests
    - Secondary type resembles site of primary tumor

ANCILLARY TESTS

Immunohistochemistry
- Cervical adenocarcinoma
  - HPV-A: p16, CEA, CINtec PLUS (p16 and Ki-67), ProEx C (TOP2A and MCM2), Ki-67, and CK 7 positive; PAX8 variable; ER and PR negative/patchy; vimentin negative
  - HPV-I: CEA, PAX8, GATA3, some p53 and HNF-1B positive; p16 usually negative
  - PD-L1 with heterogeneous expression in HPV-A and HPV-I
- Vaginal adenocarcinoma
  - Clear cell ADC: CEA, EMA, PAX8, CK 7, HNF-1B, and Napsin A positive; p53 variable; p16 negative
- Vulvar adenocarcinoma
  - Bartholin gland ADC: CEA, CAM 5.2, EMA, ER, and PR positive
  - Primary EPD-related ADC: CK7, CEA, GCDFP-15, GATA3 and CAM5.2 positive; Her-2 variable; melanoma markers, ER, and PR negative
  - Secondary EPD-related ADC metastatic from extragenital tumors
    - CK20, CDX-2, and SATB2 positive in colorectal origin; CK7, CK20, GATA3 and uroplakin positive in genitourinary tract origin; cervix with p16, IS-HPV

In Situ Hybridization
- Positive IS-HPV mRNA for all HPV-A ADC all sites

DIFFERENTIAL DIAGNOSIS

Endometrial Adenocarcinoma
- Known endometrial ADC: Positive ER, PR, and vimentin; negative for p16, IS-HPV, and CEA

Other Glandular Proliferations: p16 and HPV-ISH Negative
- Microglandular and mesonephric hyperplasia
- Endometriosis: ER and PR positive; CD10 positive in stroma
- Florid vaginal adenosis
- Tubal metaplasia
- Atypical lobular endocervical gland hyperplasia

Vulvar Dermatoses
- EPD ADC presents with eczematous rash

SELECTED REFERENCES
1. Ren H et al: International endocervical adenocarcinoma criteria and classification (IECC): an independent cohort with clinical and molecular findings. Int J Gynecol Pathol. 40(6):533-40, 2021
2. Jenkins D et al: Molecular and pathological basis of HPV-negative cervical adenocarcinoma seen in a global study. Int J Cancer. 147(9):2526-36, 2020
3. Hodgson A et al: Cervical adenocarcinomas: a heterogeneous group of tumors with variable etiologies and clinical outcomes. Arch Pathol Lab Med. 143(1):34-46, 2019

Adenocarcinoma, Cervix/Vulva/Vagina

Cervical Adenocarcinoma

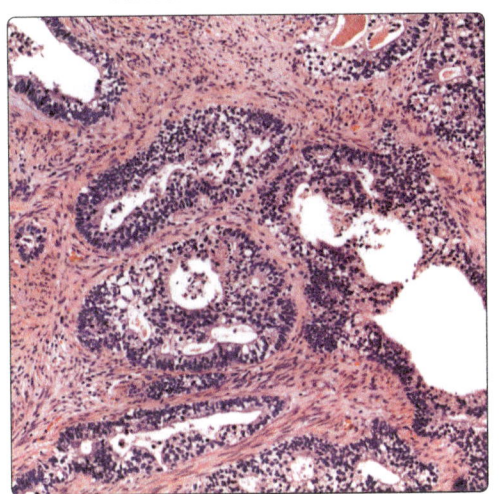

p16 Immunohistochemistry

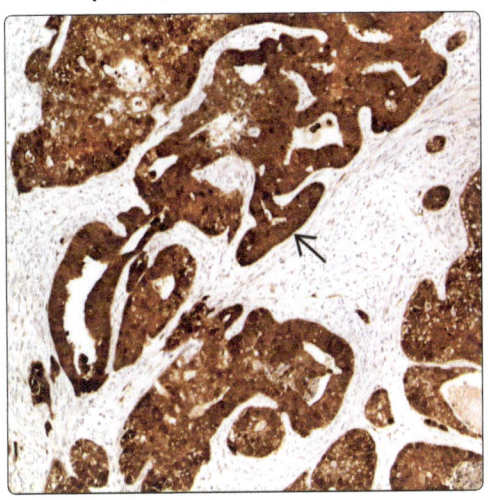

(Left) Invasive endocervical adenocarcinoma shows small to large, irregular, malignant glands infiltrating a reactive and inflamed desmoplastic stroma. Some glands show cribriform architecture with glands within glands. *(Right)* p16 shows strong and diffuse expression by neoplastic cells ➡ of invasive endocervical adenocarcinoma.

CEA Immunohistochemistry

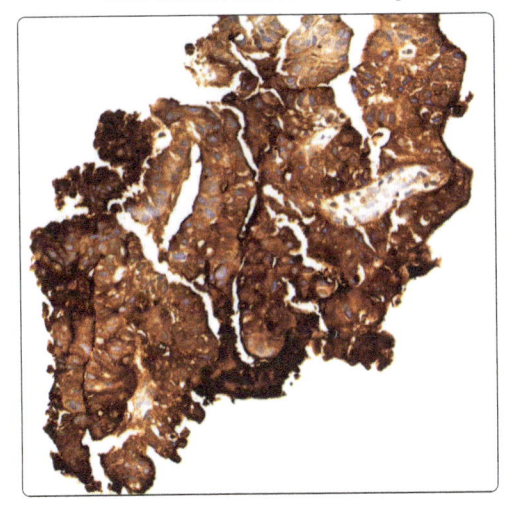

Gastric-Type Adenocarcinoma

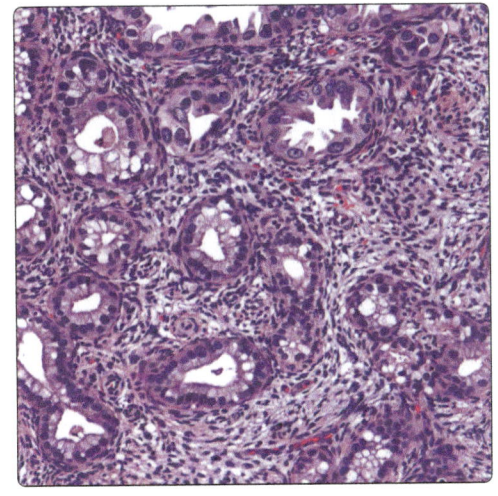

(Left) CEA shows diffuse expression by neoplastic cells in fragmented endocervical adenocarcinoma identified in this endocervical curettage specimen. *(Right)* Gastric-type invasive endocervical adenocarcinoma shows glands with pale or clear, mucinous cytoplasm in mostly simple glands with desmoplasia. Mild to moderate nuclear pleomorphism and prominent nucleoli are present. This is an HPV-independent tumor and is negative for p16.

Vaginal Clear Cell Adenocarcinoma

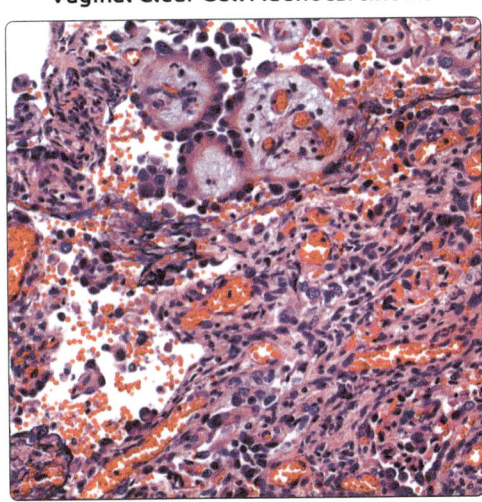

Vulvar Paget Disease

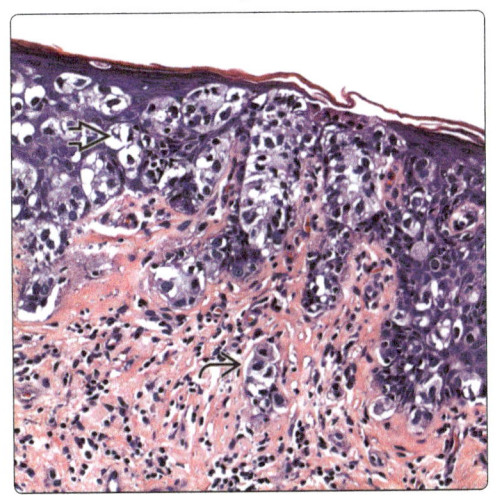

(Left) Vaginal clear cell adenocarcinoma shows papillary tufts of surface tumor with small cells with protruding nuclei. The tumor invades into stroma with slit-like spaces. *(Right)* Vulvar extramammary Paget disease shows intraepidermal nests of tumor cells ➡ and an invasive component of adenocarcinoma infiltrating into the underlying dermis ➡.

Endometrial Intraepithelial Neoplasia

KEY FACTS

TERMINOLOGY
- Endometrioid intraepithelial neoplasia (EIN)
  - Premalignant lesion often preceding endometrial endometrioid carcinoma (EEC)

ETIOLOGY/PATHOGENESIS
- Hormonal effects
  - Exogenous hormonal therapy (unopposed estrogen)
  - Elevated endogenous estrogen levels

MOLECULAR
- Most frequent mutations include those seen in EEC (*PTEN*, *CTNNB1*, *KRAS*, *ARID1A*, *PIK3CA*)
- *PAX2*-inactivating mutations
- Hypermethylation of *MLH1*
- Studies analyzing paired EIN and carcinoma cases support presence of clonal evolution of EIN and histologically indistinct pre-EIN lesions
  - Large copy number alterations (CNA) with at least 1 shared CNA in each pair and identical TCGA subtypes by NGS
  - Progressive accumulation of microsatellite instability of EIN compared with EEC in MMR-deficient cohort by NGS
  - Concordance of MMR protein status and similar driver mutations in EIN as found in EEC (*PTEN*, *ARID1A*, *PIK3CA*, *CTNNB1*, *KRAS*) by whole-exome sequencing
  - Identification of ≥ 1 recurring mutation in biopsies preceding diagnosis of EIN in up to 52% of paired cases subjected to serial genomic analysis via high-throughput screening
    - High correlation with abnormal expression patterns by immunohistochemistry for PTEN, ARID1A, and CTNNB1 (β-catenin)

Evolution of Normal Endometrium to EIN

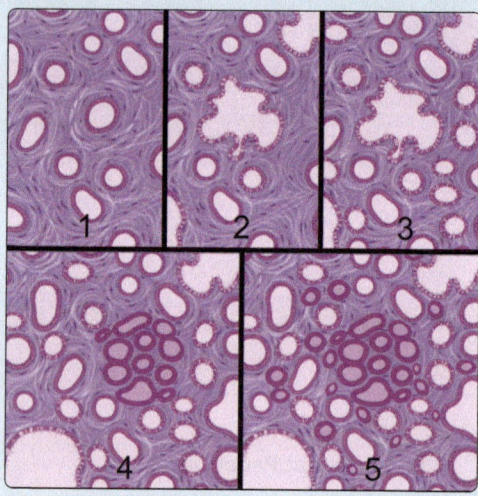

EIN Involving Polyp

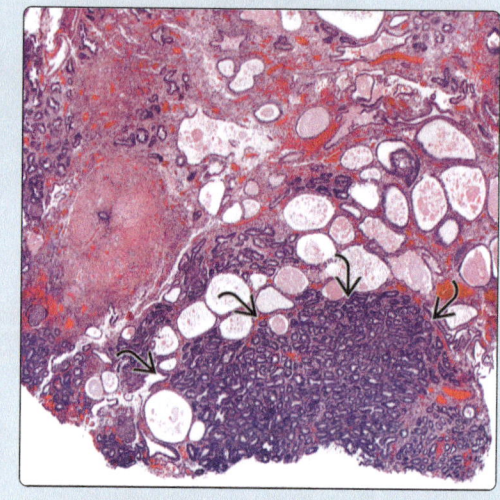

(Left) Benign endometrium (1), cystic change following estrogen exposure (2), increased glands compatible with hyperplasia without atypia (3), localized lesion of endometrioid intraepithelial neoplasia (EIN) (4), and expanded EIN (5) are shown. (Right) Localized EIN involving an endometrial polyp is shown. In this case, the EIN ➡ is easily appreciated at low power.

Background Endometrial Glands

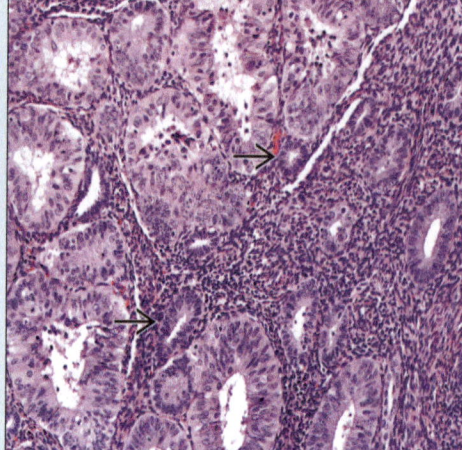

Extensive Morular Metaplasia

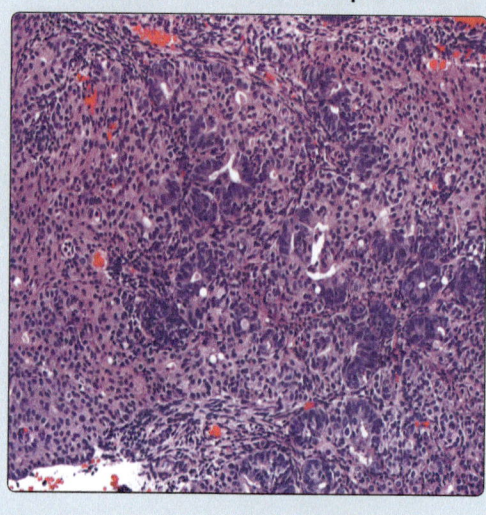

(Left) EIN represents a clonal localizing lesion with increased gland:stroma ratio, which differs from background endometrial glands ➡. (Right) EIN with extensive morular metaplasia is shown. The diagnosis should be made based on the morphology of the glandular component.

Endometrial Intraepithelial Neoplasia

TERMINOLOGY

Abbreviations
- Endometrioid intraepithelial neoplasia (EIN)

Definitions
- Premalignant endometrial lesion often preceding development of endometrial endometrioid carcinoma (EEC)

ETIOLOGY/PATHOGENESIS

Hormonal Effects
- Exogenous hormonal therapy (unopposed estrogen)
- Endogenous abnormal estrogen sources
  - Obesity
    - Peripheral aromatase in adipose tissue converts circulating androstenedione to estradiol
  - Persistent or prolonged anovulatory cycles
  - Polycystic ovarian syndrome
  - Estrogen-producing tumors

CLINICAL ISSUES

Epidemiology
- Age
  - Average: 50-55 years

Presentation
- Abnormal vaginal bleeding

Treatment
- Progestin therapy to preserve fertility or spare surgery for inoperable patients
- Total hysterectomy in majority of cases

Prognosis
- Excellent in absence of concurrent adenocarcinoma

MOLECULAR

Molecular Genetics
- *PTEN*-inactivating mutations in up to 55%
- *PAX2*-inactivating mutations in 71%
  - Concurrent *PTEN* and *PAX2* mutations in ~ 31%
- *KRAS* mutations in ~ 15%
- *CTNNB1* mutations in ~ 25-30%
- *ARID1A* mutations in ~ 16%
- Microsatellite instability
  - Epigenetic inactivation of *MLH1* in 15-20%
- Studies analyzing paired EIN and carcinoma cases
  - 83% with large copy number alterations (CNA) (CNA > 10 genes in length) with at least 1 shared CNA in each pair and identical TCGA subtypes by NGS
  - Progressive accumulation of microsatellite instability of EIN compared with EEC in MMR-deficient cohort by NGS
  - Close concordance of MMR protein status and similar driver mutations in EIN as found in EEC (*PTEN*, *ARID1A*, *PIK3CA*, *CTNNB1*, *KRAS*) by whole-exome sequencing
  - Identification of ≥ 1 recurring mutation in biopsies preceding diagnosis of EIN in up to 52% of paired cases subjected to serial genomic analysis via high-throughput screening
  - High correlation with abnormal expression patterns by immunohistochemistry for PTEN, ARID1A, and CTNNB1 (β-catenin)

MICROSCOPIC

Histologic Features
- Discrete, localizing lesion large enough to exclude artifact
- No architectural complexity, solid growth, or myoinvasion

Cytologic Features
- Low- to intermediate-grade cytologic atypia in endometrial glands morphologically distinct from nonlesional background endometrium
  - Benign mimics should be excluded

ANCILLARY TESTS

Immunohistochemistry
- Loss of staining for PTEN, PAX2, or mismatch repair proteins

DIFFERENTIAL DIAGNOSIS

Mechanical Artifacts
- Telescoping artifact: Gland within gland
- Push artifact: Apparent gland crowding due to mechanical shearing of tissue

Endometrial Polyp
- Disorganized abnormal glands and stroma lacking cytological atypia and architectural complexity

Atypical Polypoid Adenomyoma
- Lobulated growth of endometrial glands associated with squamous metaplasia within fibromuscular stroma

Endometrial Hyperplasia Without Atypia
- Disordered proliferative endometrium contains exaggerated proliferative endometrium with low gland:stroma ratio
- Benign endometrial hyperplasia contains variably shaped glands with preserved to increased gland:stroma ratio

Endometrial Endometrioid Adenocarcinoma
- Cytologically atypical glandular proliferation with architectural complexity ± myoinvasion

Endocervical Adenocarcinoma In Situ
- Mildly to moderately atypical glandular proliferation with apical mitoses and apoptotic bodies
- p16 strongly and diffusely positive by immunohistochemistry and positive for high-risk HPV subtypes by PCR or in situ hybridization

SELECTED REFERENCES

1. Aguilar M et al: Reliable identification of endometrial precancers through combined pax2, β-catenin, and Pten immunohistochemistry. Am J Surg Pathol. 46(3):404-14, 2022
2. Aguilar M et al: Serial genomic analysis of endometrium supports the existence of histologically indistinct endometrial cancer precursors. J Pathol. 254(1):20-30, 2021
3. Li L et al: Genome-wide mutation analysis in precancerous lesions of endometrial carcinoma. J Pathol. 253(1):119-28, 2021

Uterine Endometrioid Carcinoma

KEY FACTS

TERMINOLOGY
- Endometrial endometrioid carcinoma (EEC)
- Historically classified as prototypical type I tumor, TCGA analysis now illuminates groups with distinct and prognostically significant molecular profiles

MOLECULAR
- Sporadic EEC
  - Frequent mutations in *PTEN*, *KRAS*, *CTNNB1*, and *PIK3CA*
  - MSI due to epigenetic *MLH1* promoter hypermethylation in up to 40%
- Lynch syndrome-associated EEC
  - MSI due to germline mutations in DNA MMR genes
  - *MSH6* > *MSH2* > *MLH1* > *PMS2*
  - *MSH6* germline mutations associated with later age of cancer onset (> 50 years); cumulative lifetime risk of endometrial carcinoma substantially higher than for CRC
- EECs (particularly grade 3) segregate into all 4 TCGA prognostically significant molecular groups
- Simplified molecular classifier facilitates classification into analogous molecular groups
  - *POLE* ultramutated: Very favorable prognostic group identified via targeted sequencing of hotspot mutations
  - MMR deficient: Identified via MMR IHC, corresponding to TCGA MSI hypermutated group; intermediate prognosis
  - p53 mutated: Identified via p53 mutant pattern of IHC staining, corresponding to TCGA copy number high group; poorer prognosis
  - No specific molecular profile (NSMP): Absence of *POLE* mutation, p53 wildtype IHC pattern and MMR-proficient corresponding to TCGA copy number low group; intermediate prognosis
- Prominent immune microenvironment in both ultramutated *POLE*-mutant and MSI hypermutated groups
  - Increased CD8(+) tumor-infiltrating lymphocytes (TILs) compared to MSS tumors
  - PD-1 and PD-L1 significantly overexpressed in TILs and peritumoral lymphocytes compared to MSS tumors

Confluent Growth Pattern and Architectural Complexity

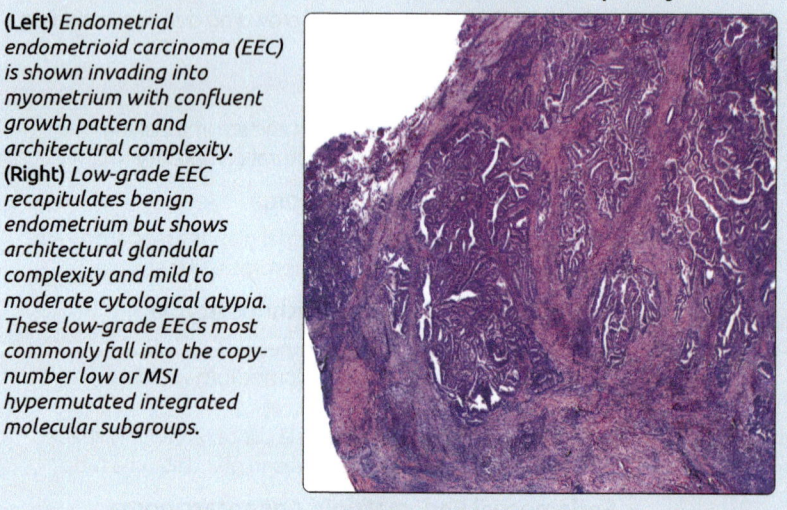

Endometrioid Architecture and Low to Intermediate Cytologic Atypia

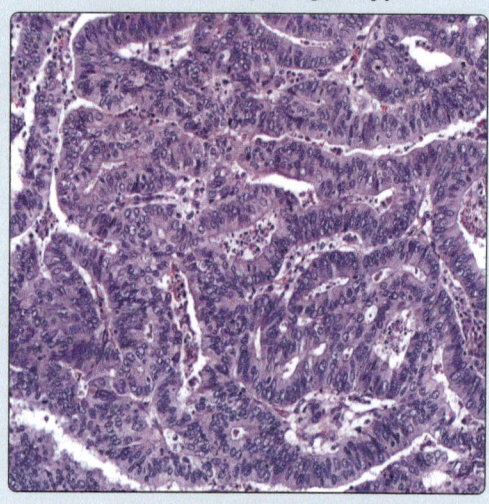

(Left) *Endometrial endometrioid carcinoma (EEC) is shown invading into myometrium with confluent growth pattern and architectural complexity.* (Right) *Low-grade EEC recapitulates benign endometrium but shows architectural glandular complexity and mild to moderate cytological atypia. These low-grade EECs most commonly fall into the copy-number low or MSI hypermutated integrated molecular subgroups.*

High-Grade EEC

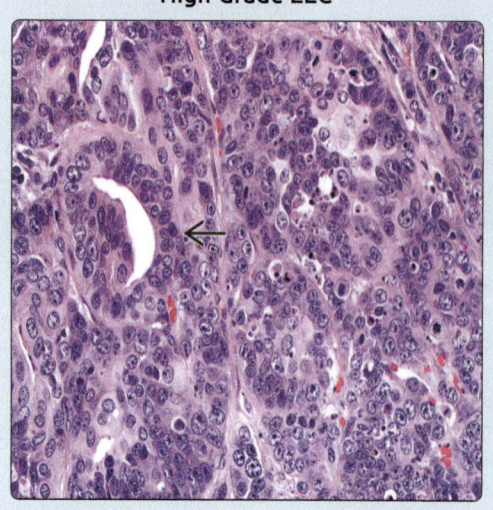

Wildtype p53 Staining Pattern

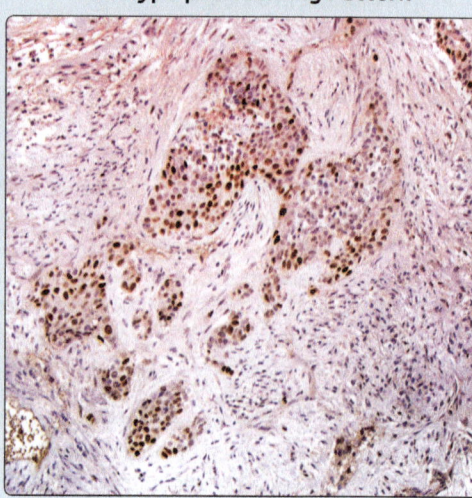

(Left) *High-grade EEC shows a mainly solid growth pattern and marked cytological atypia. However, at least focally, there is endometrioid differentiation ➡, and the tumor lacks the marked nuclear pleomorphism characteristic of serous carcinoma.* (Right) *Weak, patchy p53 staining is consistent with wildtype TP53 expression, supportive of grade 3 EEC. Such tumors have been found to segregate into all 4 of the integrative molecular subgroups of endometrial carcinoma.*

Uterine Endometrioid Carcinoma

TERMINOLOGY

Abbreviations
- Endometrial endometrioid carcinoma (EEC)

Definitions
- Glandular malignancy usually due to estrogen stimulation and acquisition of genetic &/or epigenetic alterations

ETIOLOGY/PATHOGENESIS

Diverse Group of Tumors
- Historical prototypical type I (estrogen-driven) carcinoma
  o Exogenous administration of estrogen-predominant hormonal replacement therapy
  o Elevated endogenous sources
  o Endometrioid intraepithelial neoplasia (EIN/atypical endometrial hyperplasia) as precursor lesion
- TGCA analysis since revealed groups with distinct and prognostically significant molecular profiles

Genetic Predisposition Syndromes
- Lynch syndrome (LS)
  o Germline mutations in DNA mismatch repair (MMR) genes resulting in microsatellite instability
- Cowden syndrome
  o Multiple hamartoma syndrome due to germline mutations in *PTEN*
  o Lifetime risk of endometrial cancer approaches 28%

CLINICAL ISSUES

Epidemiology
- Incidence
  o 13-20 per 100,000 worldwide
  o Endometrioid type comprises most endometrial carcinomas (~ 75%)
- Age
  o Perimenopausal and postmenopausal women
    - Mean age: ~ 60 years in sporadic EEC
    - Mean age: ~ 50 years in LS-associated EEC

Presentation
- Abnormal uterine bleeding or atypical glandular cells on Pap smear

Treatment
- Total hysterectomy and bilateral salpingo-oophorectomy
- Pelvic/paraaortic lymphadenectomy if high-risk features present (FIGO grade 3, ≥ 50% myometrial invasion, > 2 cm in size)
- Adjuvant radiation therapy if at least 2 adverse risk factors present [age > 60, FIGO grade 3, ≥ 50% myoinvasion, lymphovascular invasion (LVI)]
- Adjuvant chemotherapy in advanced stages

Prognosis
- Dependent upon stage
  o 5-year survival for stage I (tumor limited to endometrium): ~ 95%
  o 5-year survival for stage III (serosal/adnexal invasion or metastasis to vagina/pelvis or paraaortic lymph nodes): ~ 54%
  o 5-year survival for stage IV (distant metastasis): < 20%

MOLECULAR

Sporadic EEC
- Characteristic genetic mutations
  o *PTEN* in 52-78%
  o *PIK3CA* in 36-52%
  o *PIK3R1* in 21-43%
  o *KRAS* in 15-43%
  o *CTNNB1* in 20-24%
  o *ARID1A* in 25-48%
  o *TP53* in up to 24%
- Microsatellite instability
  o Seen in ~ 28-40% of sporadic EEC due to
    - Epigenetic hypermethylation of promoter *MLH1*
    - Acquired biallelic somatic mutations
  o MSI leads to progressive accumulation of secondary alterations in downstream regulatory genes

LS-Associated EEC
- Clinical features
  o 2-3% of all endometrial carcinomas and up to 9% of endometrial carcinoma in patients < 50 years of age
  o Most common non-colorectal cancer (CRC) in LS
    - Confers 40-60% lifetime risk of EC, which equals or exceeds risk of CRC
  o In patients with metachronous cancers, 51% present with endometrial carcinoma as their sentinel cancer
  o Median interval between endometrial carcinoma and CRC: ~ 11 years
- Molecular features
  o MSI due to germline mutations in 1 DNA MMR gene followed by acquired mutation in 2nd allele
  o Frequency of gene mutations
    - *MSH6* > *MSH2* > *MLH1* > *PMS2*
    - *MSH6* mutations associated with later age of cancer onset (> 50 years), and lifetime risk of endometrial carcinoma substantially higher than for CRC
  o Lifetime risks associated with MMR gene mutations
    - *MSH2*: 21-49%
    - *MLH1*: 20-54%
    - *MSH6*: 16-71%
    - *PMS2*: 15%
  o Germline *EPCAM* deletion mutation
    - Deletion of 3' end results in epigenetic silencing of *MSH2*

Cancer Genome Atlas Molecular Subtypes
- EECs (particularly grade 3) segregate into all 4 molecular categories identified in TCGA project
  o Ultramutated subgroup with mutated *POLE* accounts for ~ 7% of EECs (grade 3 > grade 1-2)
    - Hotspot mutations in exons 9-14 of DNA polymerase epsilon (*POLE*) exonuclease domain facilitate identification via targeted sequencing
    - Very high somatic mutation rates (232 x 10^{-6} mutations/Mb) and increased frequency of C>A transversions
    - Younger age at presentation (< 60 years)
    - Frequent mutations in *PTEN*, *PIK3CA*, *PIK3R1*, *FBXW7*, *KRAS*, and *ARID1A*

Uterine Endometrioid Carcinoma

- Highly favorable clinical outcomes despite frequent high-grade histology and occasional *TP53* mutations
  - MSI hypermutated subgroup (grades 1-3 EEC, clinically intermediate risk)
    - Identification facilitated via MMR immunohistochemistry (MMR-deficient EEC)
    - High mutation rates (18×10^{-6} mutations/Mb)
    - MSI often due to *MLH1* promoter hypermethylation
    - Missense and indels with frameshift mutations in *RPL22* identified in ~ 12.5% of EEC in TCGA project
  - Copy-number high subgroup (serous and serous-like, clinically high risk)
    - Mainly serous carcinomas, but 25% of grade 3 EECs fall into this subgroup
    - High rate of *TP53* mutations and corresponding aberrant p53 IHC staining (p53-mutant EEC)
    - Extensive somatic copy number alterations
    - Low mutation rate (2.3×10^{-6} mutations/Mb)
    - Recurrent *FBXW7*, *PPP2R1A* mutations
    - Infrequent *PTEN* and *KRAS* mutations
    - Microsatellite stable
  - Copy-number low subgroup (grades 1-2 EEC, clinically low to intermediate risk)
    - Lacking *TP53* or *POLE* mutations and microsatellite stable (no specific molecular profile = NSMP)
    - Low mutation rates (2.9×10^{-6} mutations/Mb)
- Immune modulatory pathways
  - Prominent immune microenvironment in both ultramutated *POLE*-mutant and MSI hypermutated subgroups
    - Increased CD8(+) tumor-infiltrating lymphocytes (TILs) compared to MSS tumors
    - PD-1 and PD-L1 significantly overexpressed in TILs and peritumoral lymphocytes compared to MSS tumors

MICROSCOPIC

Histologic Features

- Conventional EEC with typical type I tumor histology recapitulates proliferative phase endometrium
  - Distinct endometrioid architecture with architectural complexity; grade dependent on extent of nonsquamous solid growth pattern
- LS-associated EEC
  - Histologic features described not as consistently associated with MSI as with CRC counterparts
    - Dense peritumoral lymphocytes apparent at low-power magnification
    - Prominent TILs (> 40 per 10 HPF)
    - Tumor heterogeneity with 2 distinct tumors comprising at least 10% of overall tumor volume adjacent to but not admixed with each other
- Integrated histomolecular groups
  - *POLE* ultramutated: High grade, prominent TILs
  - MMR deficient: High grade, prominent TILs, microcystic elongated fragmented (MELF)-type invasion, frequent LVI
  - p53 mutant: High grade with marked cytologic atypia
  - NSMP: Predominantly low grade with frequent squamous differentiation or squamous morules; TILs absent

ANCILLARY TESTS

Immunohistochemistry

- Positive for ER, PR, and vimentin; p53 typically wildtype pattern but can show mutant pattern
- Loss of PTEN and nuclear PAX2 staining
- MSI tumors show loss of MMR expression

Surrogate Testing for Integrated Histomolecular EEC Classification

- *POLE*-ultramutated EEC
  - Hotspot analysis: p.Pro286Arg, p.Val411Leu, p.Ser297Phe, p.Ala456Pro, p.Ser459Phe
- MMR-deficient EEC
  - Immunohistochemistry for MLH1, PMS2, MSH2, and MSH6
  - Absence of nuclear staining indicates MMR deficiency only when staining is intact in internal control cells (stromal cells, adjacent nonneoplastic epithelium, inflammatory cells)
  - Loss of MLH1 ± PMS2 should be followed by *MLH1* promoter hypermethylation testing
    - Likely sporadic EEC
  - Isolated loss of MSH2, MSH6, or PMS2, or loss of MSH2 and MSH6 should trigger recommendation for genetic testing
- p53-mutated EEC
  - Aberrant p53 staining includes strong diffuse positivity (overexpression) or complete loss of staining (null pattern)
- No specific molecular profile (NSMP)
  - Absence of *POLE* mutations, p53 wildtype and MMR protein expression intact

MSI Testing

- 3 dinucleotide and 2 mononucleotide repeats, or 5 mononucleotide repeats loci are typically analyzed
- May not detect subset of *MSH6*-mutated tumors
- Should be reflexed to *MLH1* promoter hypermethylation assay in MSI cases
  - Presence of hypermethylation essentially excludes germline mutation in MMR genes
  - *MLH1* promoter gene nonmethylated cases should be reflexed to MMR protein testing by IHC
    - Will narrow down potential candidate genes for further sequencing

SELECTED REFERENCES

1. National Comprehensive Cancer Network. NCCN Clinical Practice Guidelines in Oncology (NCCN Guidelines): Uterine Neoplasms. Version 2.2023. Accessed July 2023. https://www.nccn.org/professionals/physician_gls/pdf/uterine.pdf
2. IARC: WHO Classification of Tumours: Female Genital Tumours, 5th ed. IARC, 2020
3. Bosse T et al: Molecular classification of grade 3 endometrioid endometrial cancers identifies distinct prognostic subgroups. Am J Surg Pathol. 42(5):561-8, 2018
4. Hussein YR et al: Molecular insights into the classification of high-grade endometrial carcinoma. Pathology. 50(2):151-61, 2018
5. Jones NL et al: Distinct molecular landscapes between endometrioid and nonendometrioid uterine carcinomas. Int J Cancer. 140(6):1396-404, 2017
6. Billingsley CC et al: Polymerase ε (POLE) mutations in endometrial cancer: clinical outcomes and implications for Lynch syndrome testing. Cancer. 121(3):386-94, 2015

Uterine Endometrioid Carcinoma

Low-Grade EEC

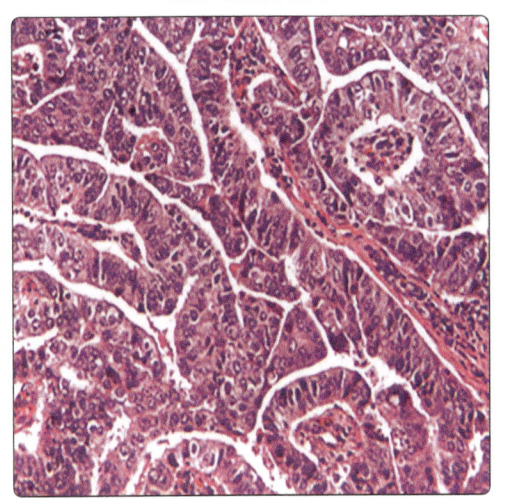

Low-Grade EEC With Aberrant p53 Staining Pattern

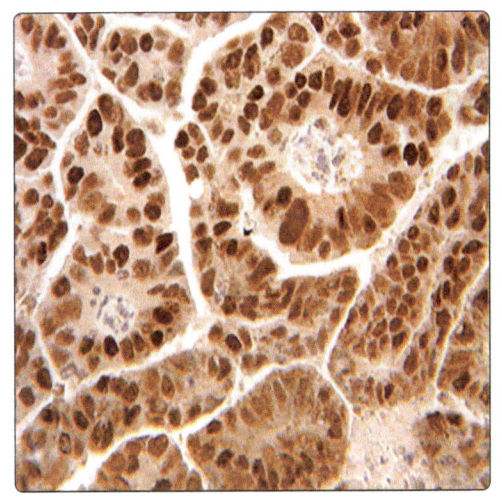

(Left) EEC shows distinct endometrioid architecture and predominantly low nuclear grade. (Right) Low-grade EEC shows strong, diffuse p53 expression, indicative of TP53 mutation. Aberrant p53 can also present as complete loss of staining due to missense or frameshift mutations. A small proportion of such EECs may fall into either the POLE-EDM (excellent prognosis) or copy-number high molecular subgroup (clinically aggressive).

Peritumoral Lymphocytes

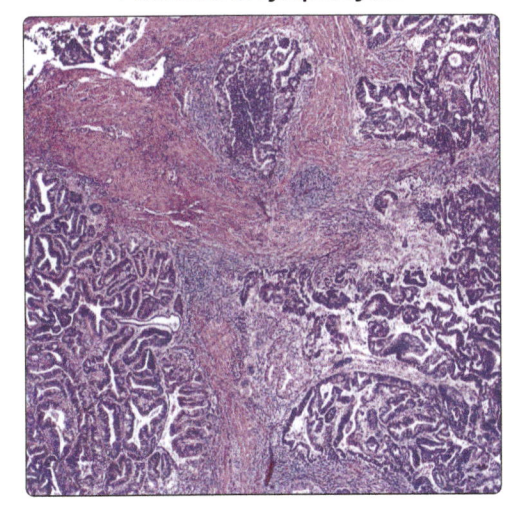

Tumor-Infiltrating Lymphocytes

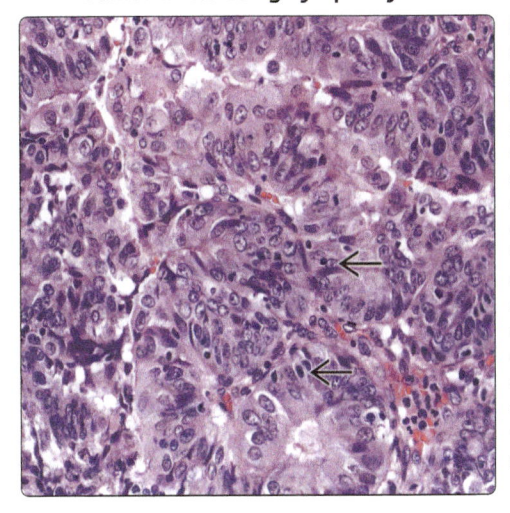

(Left) At low power, this invasive EEC shows associated peritumoral lymphocytes. (Right) EEC with MSI may also bear increased intratumoral lymphocytes ⇨. Such histological features are not as frequently seen in MSI-associated EECs compared with their colorectal carcinoma counterparts. TILs and peritumoral lymphocytes are also seen in ultramutated tumors with POLE mutation, suggesting that these 2 subgroups may be amenable to immune modulatory pathway targeting.

Negative MLH1

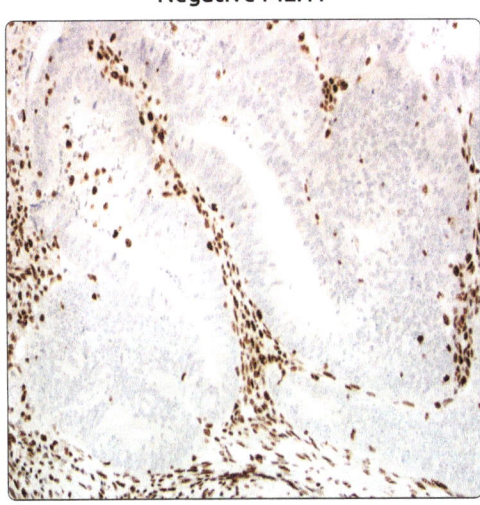

Negative MSH6

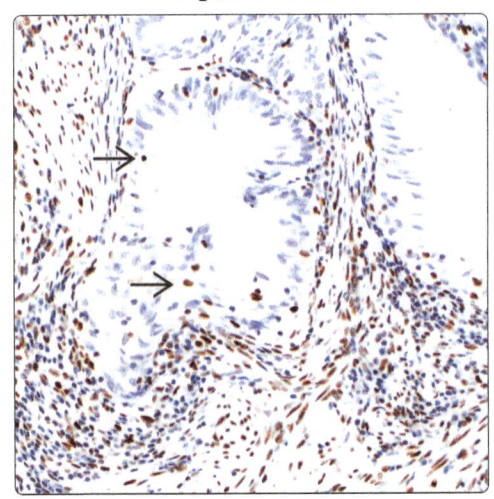

(Left) Low-grade EEC is negative for MLH1 and was also negative for PMS2 (not shown). However, MLH1 methylation assay was positive, excluding a germline MMR gene mutation. (Right) Low-grade EEC shows isolated loss of MSH6 expression. Staining is present in the stroma, TILs ⇨, peritumoral lymphocytes and stroma, but neoplastic epithelium is negative. Such findings should prompt additional testing to identify germline vs. acquired somatic MSH6 mutations.

Uterine Serous Carcinoma

KEY FACTS

TERMINOLOGY
- High-grade nonendometrioid endometrial carcinoma typically presenting at advanced stage and clinically aggressive

CLINICAL ISSUES
- < 10% of all endometrial carcinomas but accounts for up to 40% of deaths from endometrial cancer

MOLECULAR
- Uterine serous carcinoma (USC) segregates into TCGA copy number high genomic classification
  - Extensive somatic copy number alterations
  - Low mutation rate (2.3 x 10^{-6} mutations/Mb)
  - Recurrent *TP53*, *FBXW7*, *PPP2R1A*, and *PIK3CA* mutations
  - Infrequent *PTEN* and *KRAS* mutations
  - Microsatellite stable
- *TP53* mutations in 60-90%
- HER2 amplification/overexpression in 25-30%

MICROSCOPIC
- Papillary, solid, or glandular growth patterns
- Distinction between USC and grade 3 endometrial endometrioid carcinoma often diagnostically challenging

ANCILLARY TESTS
- p53 aberrant patterns include strong diffuse positivity (overexpression) or complete lack of staining (null pattern)
- Positive for p16 (strong, diffuse), PAX8, IMP2, IMP3
- Hormone receptor expression variable
- HER2 overexpression typically in lateral or basolateral distribution rather than completely membranous
- No consensus guidelines for reporting of HER2 testing, but application of modified ASCO-CAP breast carcinoma guidelines proposed

Papillary Pattern

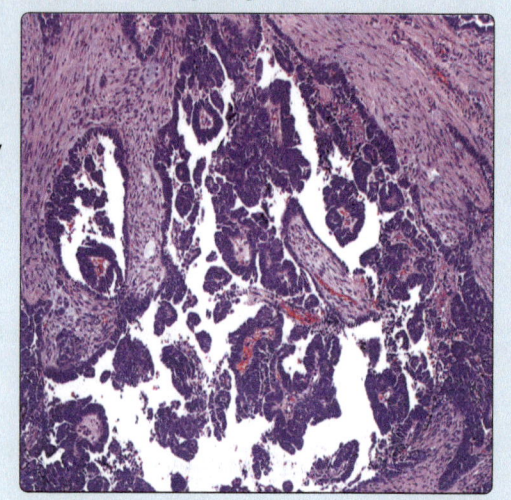

High-Grade Cytology

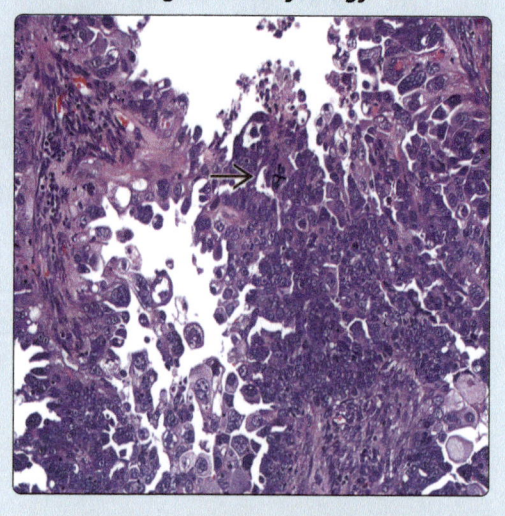

(Left) *Endometrial serous carcinoma shows a papillary architecture in this example, but solid or glandular growth patterns can also be seen.* (Right) *Serous carcinoma is, by definition, a high-grade malignancy with marked cytologic atypia characterized by nuclear pleomorphism and frequent mitoses, including abnormal forms* ➔.

p53 Immunohistochemistry

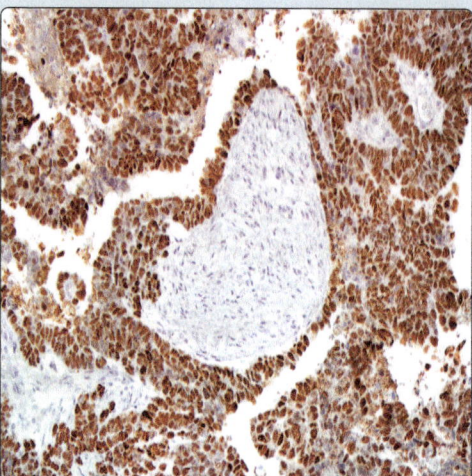

p16 Immunohistochemistry

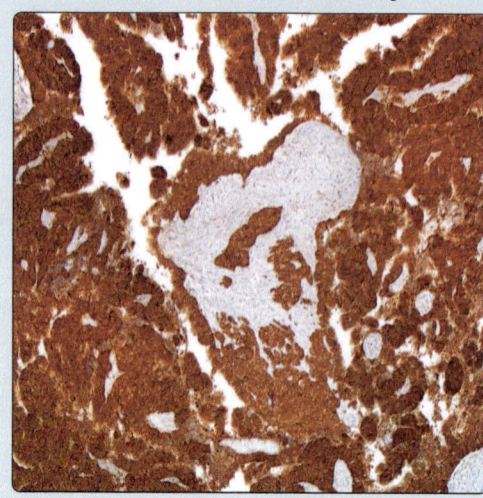

(Left) *Serous carcinoma typically shows diffuse and strong expression of p53.* (Right) *Serous carcinoma is strongly and diffusely positive for p16. The mechanism for p16 overexpression is non-HPV related. Grade 3 endometrial endometrioid carcinoma may also be p53 and p16 positive in a subset of cases, but serous carcinoma usually lacks squamous or mucinous metaplasia, shows variable hormone receptor positivity, and is typically MMR-proficient.*

Uterine Serous Carcinoma

TERMINOLOGY

Abbreviations
- Uterine serous carcinoma (USC)

Definitions
- High-grade epithelial malignancy of endometrium with multiple growth patterns and severe cytologic atypia

ETIOLOGY/PATHOGENESIS

Prototypical Type II Endometrial Carcinoma
- High-grade nonendometrioid endometrial carcinoma typically presenting at advanced stage and clinically aggressive
- Typically estrogen independent

Genetic Predisposition
- Can arise in patients with *BRCA1* and *BRCA2* mutations
- Can also arise in Lynch syndrome

CLINICAL ISSUES

Epidemiology
- Incidence
  - < 10% of all endometrial carcinomas yet accounts for up to 40% of deaths from endometrial cancer
- Age
  - Postmenopausal women (mean age: Late 60s)

Presentation
- Abnormal uterine bleeding or atypical glandular cells on Pap smear
- Extrauterine involvement in ~ 60-70% of cases

Treatment
- Total hysterectomy and bilateral salpingo-oophorectomy with surgical staging
- Adjuvant chemotherapy ± radiation therapy; anti-HER2 therapy in advanced stage or recurrent HER2(+) USC

Prognosis
- Poor prognosis with 5-year overall survival of ~ 18-27%
- Poor progression-free survival

MOLECULAR

Recurrent Genetic Alterations
- *TP53* mutations in 60-90%
  - Missense mutations in hotspot residues most frequent
  - Subset with frameshift or nonsense mutations (complete loss of p53 expression = null pattern)
- *PIK3CA* mutations in 24-42%
- *PPP2R1A* mutations in 15-43%
- *FBXW7* mutations in 12-33%
- *ERBB2* (HER2) amplification in 17-44%
  - Randomized phase 2 clinical trial of advanced-stage and recurrent HER2(+) USC patients treated with standard chemotherapy + trastuzumab showed prolonged progression-free survival vs. those treated with chemotherapy alone
  - HER2 testing endorsed by National Comprehensive Cancer Network Guidelines for advanced-stage and recurrent HER2(+) USC patients

Cancer Genome Atlas Molecular Classification
- USC segregates into copy number high genomic classification
  - Extensive somatic copy number alterations
  - Low mutation rate (2.3 x 10^{-6} mutations/Mb)
  - Commonly mutated genes per TCGA data: *TP53*, *PPP2R1A*, *PIK3CA*, and *FBXW7*
  - Infrequent *PTEN* and *KRAS* mutations
  - Microsatellite stable
- Overlaps with high-grade serous ovarian carcinomas and basal-like breast carcinomas

MICROSCOPIC

Histologic Features
- Papillary, solid, or glandular growth patterns

Cytologic Features
- Severe cytologic atypia, including marked nuclear pleomorphism, hyperchromasia, and high mitotic activity

ANCILLARY TESTS

Immunohistochemistry
- p53 aberrant patterns include strong diffuse positivity (overexpression) or complete lack of staining (null pattern)
- Up to 60% ER, 32% PR, and 27% AR positivity reported
- HER2 overexpression in 20-30%
  - Staining pattern typically in lateral or basolateral distribution rather than completely membranous
  - No consensus guidelines for reporting of HER2 testing, but assessment of complete or basolateral/lateral staining pattern using a modification of ASCO-CAP guidelines for breast carcinoma proposed
    - Negative (0): No staining observed
    - Negative (1+): Incomplete membrane staining that is faint/barely perceptible in any proportion of cells or weak complete staining in < 10% tumor cells
    - Equivocal (2+): Intense complete or basolateral/lateral membrane staining in ≤ 30% tumor cells or weak to moderate staining in ≥ 10% tumor cells
    - Positive (3+): Intense complete or basolateral/lateral membrane staining in > 30% tumor cells

In Situ Hybridization
- No recommendations to perform FISH instead of IHC testing; reflex FISH testing of equivocal HER2 IHC result proposed
- Based on data from a large clinical trial, reporting of HER2 FISH testing is proposed as follows
  - Negative: FISH HER2/CEP17 ratio < 2.0 and average HER2 copy number < 6 per nucleus
  - Positive: FISH HER2/CEP17 ratio ≥ 2.0 **or** FISH HER2/CEP17 ratio < 2.0 with average HER2 copy number ≥ 6 per nucleus
- Detection of *ERBB2* amplification by next-generation sequencing reported to be concordant with IHC and FISH

SELECTED REFERENCES
1. Buza N: HER2 Testing in endometrial serous carcinoma: time for standardized pathology practice to meet the clinical demand. Arch Pathol Lab Med. 145(6):687-91, 2021

Clear Cell Carcinoma, Uterus

KEY FACTS

TERMINOLOGY
- High-grade carcinoma with clear to eosinophilic cytoplasm and distinctive growth patterns

CLINICAL ISSUES
- Rare tumor presenting with abnormal bleeding in postmenopausal women
- Behavior intermediate between grade 3 endometrioid carcinoma and serous carcinoma
- Overall 5-year survival: 40-60%

MOLECULAR
- Clear cell carcinoma (CCC) distributes among TCGA 4 molecular subtypes of endometrial carcinoma
  - Most frequently falls into *TP53*-mutated or *TP53*-wildtype (no specific molecular profile) groups
  - Microsatellite instability-high uncommon and ultramutated cases with *POLE* mutations rare
- Mutational profile overlaps with that of endometrial serous carcinomas (*TP53* and *PPP2R1A* mutations frequent)
- *PTEN*, *KRAS* mutations uncommon
- PI3K pathway alterations: *PIK3CA* up to 36%, *PIK3R1* up to 22%
- *ARID1A* mutations in up to 75%
- *TERT* promoter mutations in 21% but not associated with other clinicopathologic factors

MICROSCOPIC
- Tubulocystic, papillary, or solid growth patterns of hobnail or polygonal tumor cells with clear/eosinophilic cytoplasm and high-grade nuclear atypia
- Frequently admixed with serous or endometrioid subtypes; pure CCC uncommon

ANCILLARY TESTS
- ER/PR typically negative
- HNF-1β, napsin A, and AMACR (P504S) positive

Solid Growth Pattern

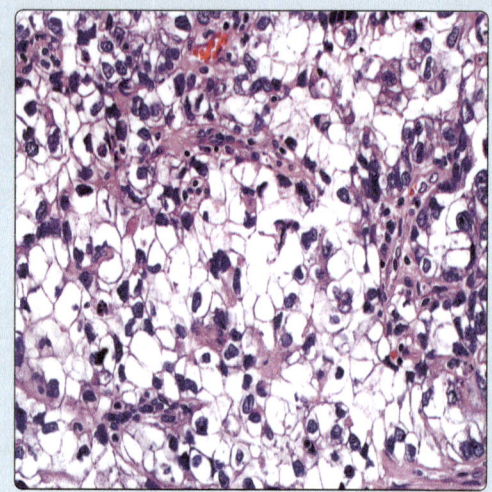

Papillary Growth Pattern

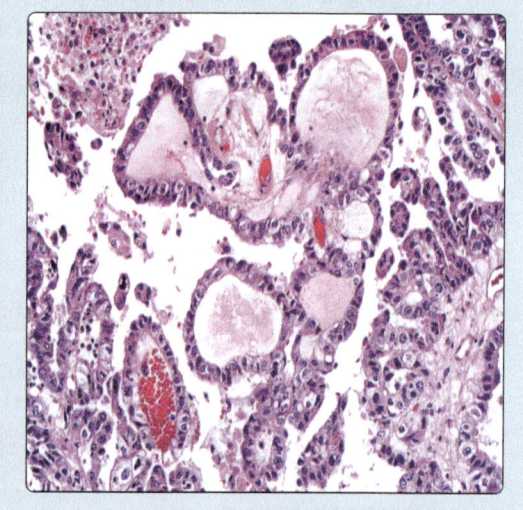

(Left) Endometrial clear cell carcinoma (CCC) shows distinctive architectural growth patterns and cytologic features. Cells with clear cytoplasm bear enlarged, irregular, hyperchromatic nuclei with prominent nucleoli. (Right) Papillary structures with stromal hyalinization are lined by a single layer of markedly atypical tumor cells with more eosinophilic cytoplasm in this case of CCC.

Napsin A Positivity

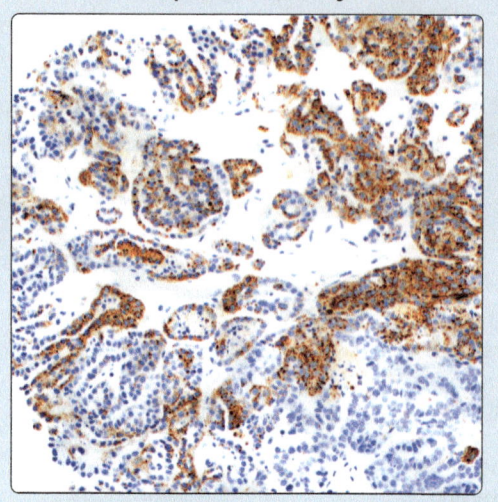

ER Negativity

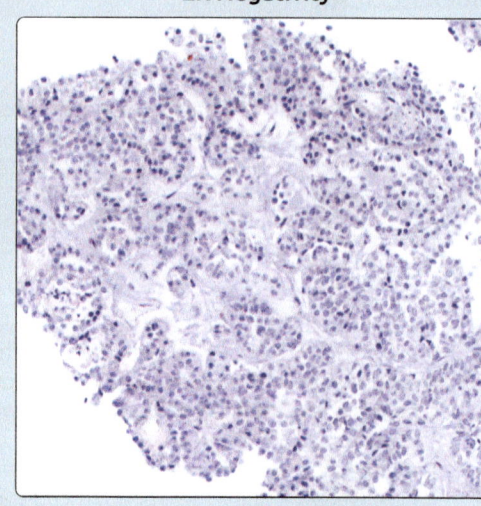

(Left) Napsin A shows immunohistochemical pattern of endometrial CCC, which is positive in a cytoplasmic distribution. (Right) ER shows immunohistochemical pattern of endometrial CCC, which is typically negative.

Clear Cell Carcinoma, Uterus

TERMINOLOGY

Synonyms
- Clear cell adenocarcinoma

Definitions
- Clear cell carcinoma (CCC): High-grade endometrial carcinoma with pure population of markedly atypical cells with clear to eosinophilic cytoplasm
- Distinctive architectural growth patterns
  o Tubulocystic
  o Papillary
  o Solid

ETIOLOGY/PATHOGENESIS

Environmental Exposure
- Historically classified as type II endometrial carcinoma
  o Estrogen independent
  o Not associated with diethylstilbestrol exposure

Genetic Predisposition
- May develop in patients with Lynch syndrome

CLINICAL ISSUES

Epidemiology
- Incidence
  o 1-5% of all endometrial carcinomas
  o Increased incidence in African American women
- Age
  o Postmenopausal women

Presentation
- Abnormal uterine bleeding or atypical glandular cells on cervical Pap smear
- Can be associated with thromboembolic events
- Paraneoplastic hypercalcemia may be seen

Natural History
- Behavior intermediate between stage-matched grade 3 endometrioid carcinoma and serous carcinoma
- Recurrence commonly in pelvis, paraaortic lymph nodes, and distant sites
  o Decreased propensity for peritoneal dissemination

Treatment
- Total hysterectomy, bilateral salpingo-oophorectomy with surgical staging ± adjuvant radiation therapy ± chemotherapy

Prognosis
- 5-year overall survival: 40-60%
- 5-year disease-free survival: ~ 43%
- Stage is most important prognostic factor

MACROSCOPIC

General Features
- May exhibit polypoid or diffuse growth pattern
- No distinctive gross features

MICROSCOPIC

Histologic Features
- Distinctive architectural growth patterns
  o Tubulocystic pattern
    – May include intraluminal mucin or eosinophilic material
  o Papillary pattern
    – Usually short, small, round papillae with hyalinized stroma
  o Solid pattern
    – Tumor in sheets or nests
- Frequently arises in atrophic endometrial background
- Can arise within endometrial polyps
- May coexist with endometrial endometrioid or serous carcinoma
- Interobserver variability in morphologic diagnosis
  o Greater for endometrial vs. ovarian CCC
- Recent studies have examined cohorts rigorously selected by consensus diagnosis by gynecologic pathologists

Cytologic Features
- Hobnail, polygonal, or cuboidal cells
- Enlarged, irregular, hyperchromatic nuclei and prominent nucleoli
- Clear cytoplasm due to glycogen, but cytoplasm may also be eosinophilic
- Intracellular eosinophilic hyaline globules or inclusions can be seen
- Psammoma bodies may be present

ANCILLARY TESTS

Immunohistochemistry
- Usually ER and PR negative
  o Can be focally weakly positive
- Aberrant p53 staining (overexpression or null patterns) in up to 72%
- HNF-1β positive
  o Not as sensitive or specific marker as for ovarian CCC
- Napsin A, AMACR (P504S) positive
- Ki-67 proliferative index intermediate between endometrioid and serous carcinomas

Genetic Testing
- Studies limited due to small numbers of pure endometrial CCC
- Tumors distribute among The Cancer Genome Atlas (TCGA) 4 molecular subtypes of endometrial carcinoma
  o *TP53* mutated: 29-59%
  o *TP53* wildtype [no specific molecular profile (NSMP)]: 46-54%
  o Microsatellite instability-high (MSI-H): 9-12%
    – Mismatch repair protein deficient (MMRd): Up to 33%
      □ MMRd tumors associated with more favorable prognosis than either p53-aberrant or p53-wildtype tumors
  o Ultramutated tumors with mutations in exonuclease domain of *POLE*: Rare (2-7%)
- Mutational profile overlaps with that of endometrial serous carcinoma

Clear Cell Carcinoma, Uterus

- ○ *PPP2R1A* missense mutations: 9-36%
- ○ *PIK3CA* mutations: 11-36%
- ○ *FBXW7* missense mutations: 4-8%
- ○ Gene amplifications
  - *CCNE1*: 18%
  - *ERBB2*: 11%
- Genetic alterations usually associated with endometrial endometrioid carcinomas infrequent
  - ○ *PTEN* mutations: 6-21%
  - ○ *KRAS* mutations: 8-11%
- Mutations in PI3K pathway genes other than *PTEN*
  - ○ *PIK3R1* mutations: 16-22%
  - ○ No mutations in *PIK3R2* reported
- *ARID1A*
  - ○ Encodes member of SWI/SNF family (BAF250A)
  - ○ Missense mutations: Up to 75%
  - ○ BAF250A protein expression lost in 22%
    - Appears not prognostically significant
- Other mutations
  - ○ *SPOP* (involved in ubiquitin-mediated proteolysis): 14-29%
  - ○ *ZFHX3*: 14%
  - ○ *CSMD3*: 14%
  - ○ *TSPYL2*: 7%
  - ○ *ARHGAP35*: 7%
  - ○ *ABCC9*: 7%
- *TERT*
  - ○ Encodes telomerase protein subunit
  - ○ Mutated in 21%
    - Mutations in promoter gene results in enhanced telomerase activity
    - Not associated with any clinicopathologic factors
    - No impact on prognosis

Gene Expression Profiling

- Given small numbers, CCC often included with serous carcinomas in most studies
- Similar expression profile to other CCC
- Upregulated genes
  - ○ Genes involved in increasing apoptotic signals
    - *MAP3K5*
    - *GLRX*
  - ○ Inhibition of cellular proliferation
    - *TFPI2*
  - ○ Increased resistance to chemotherapeutic agents
    - *ANXA4*
    - *UGT1A1*

DIFFERENTIAL DIAGNOSIS

Endometrioid Carcinoma With Squamous Differentiation

- Cytoplasmic clearing due to intracellular glycogen accumulation in cells with squamous differentiation
- Areas of more readily identifiable squamous metaplasia usually present
- Minimal cytologic atypia present

Endometrioid Carcinoma, Secretory Variant

- Resembles day 17 secretory endometrium
- Mild cytologic atypia present

- Characteristic architectural patterns of CCC absent

Papillary Serous Carcinoma

- Solid areas may show cytoplasmic clearing, but nuclear atypia is usually marked to severe
- Papillae are more variably sized
- Typically strongly and diffusely positive for p53 but may be completely negative in p53-null variant

Endometrioid Carcinoma With Clear Cell Changes, Not Otherwise Specified

- Clear cell changes comprise foamy granular or empty cytoplasm or contain prominent cytoplasmic vacuoles
- Changes attributed to intracellular accumulation of lipid, mucin, or glycogen or secondary to hydropic changes
- Generally negative for napsin A and positive for ER

Arias-Stella Reaction

- Focal clear cell change with degenerative atypia
- Background endometrium with preserved architecture and progestin effect
- Minimal proliferative activity

Reactive Superficial Epithelial Changes

- Papillary or eosinophilic metaplasia in reactive states or with endometrial breakdown
- p53 negative or only focally weakly positive

SELECTED REFERENCES

1. Ackroyd SA et al: Molecular portraits of clear cell ovarian and endometrial carcinoma with comparison to clear cell renal cell carcinoma. Gynecol Oncol. 169:164-71, 2023
2. Irshaid L et al: Molecular landscape of mullerian clear cell carcinomas identifies The Cancer Genome Atlas-like prognostic subgroups. Mod Pathol. 36(5):100123, 2023
3. Travaglino A et al: Diagnostic accuracy of HNF1β, Napsin A and P504S/alpha-methylacyl-CoA racemase (AMACR) as markers of endometrial clear cell carcinoma. Pathol Res Pract. 237:154019, 2022
4. Travaglino A et al: Clear cell endometrial carcinomas with mismatch repair deficiency have a favorable prognosis: a systematic review and meta-analysis. Gynecol Oncol. 162(3):804-8, 2021
5. Kim SR et al: Molecular subtypes of clear cell carcinoma of the endometrium: opportunities for prognostic and predictive stratification. Gynecol Oncol. 158(1):3-11, 2020
6. Travaglino A et al: Clear cell endometrial carcinoma and the TCGA classification. Histopathology. 76(2):336-8, 2020
7. Baniak N et al: Targeted molecular and immunohistochemical analyses of endometrial clear cell carcinoma show that POLE mutations and DNA mismatch repair protein deficiencies are uncommon. Am J Surg Pathol. 43(4):531-7, 2019
8. Zannoni GF et al: Clear cell carcinoma of the endometrium: an immunohistochemical and molecular analysis of 45 cases. Hum Pathol. 92:10-7, 2019
9. DeLair DF et al: The genetic landscape of endometrial clear cell carcinomas. J Pathol. 243(2):230-41, 2017
10. Le Gallo M et al: Somatic mutation profiles of clear cell endometrial tumors revealed by whole exome and targeted gene sequencing. Cancer. 123(17):3261-8, 2017
11. Bae HS et al: Should endometrial clear cell carcinoma be classified as type II endometrial carcinoma? Int J Gynecol Pathol. 34(1):74-84, 2015
12. Hoang LN et al: Targeted mutation analysis of endometrial clear cell carcinoma. Histopathology. 66(5):664-74, 2015
13. Huang HN et al: Molecular alterations in endometrial and ovarian clear cell carcinomas: clinical impacts of telomerase reverse transcriptase promoter mutation. Mod Pathol. 28(2):303-11, 2015

Clear Cell Carcinoma, Uterus

Solid Growth Pattern

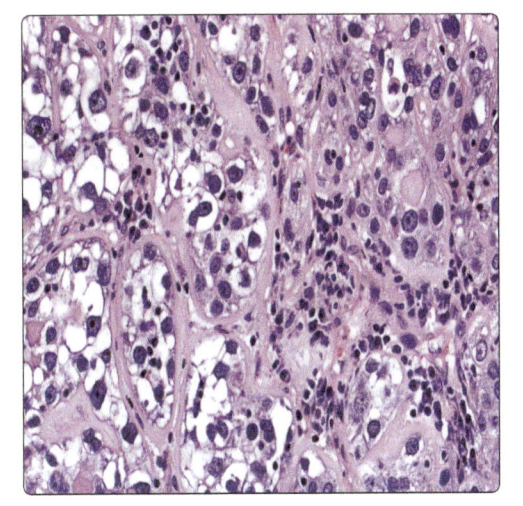

Intracytoplasmic Hyaline Bodies

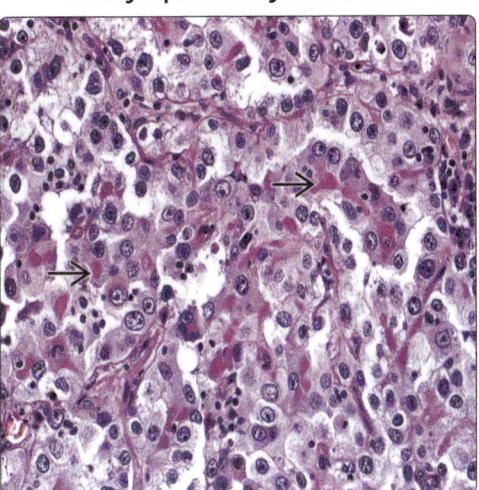

(Left) Solid CCC contains characteristic polygonal cells bearing enlarged, irregular, hyperchromatic nuclei with prominent nucleoli. At left, cells contain distinctively clear cytoplasm but are adjacent to a population with more eosinophilic cytoplasm at right. *(Right)* Tumor cells in this case of CCC contain more eosinophilic cytoplasm and intracytoplasmic hyaline bodies ➡.

Papillary Growth Pattern

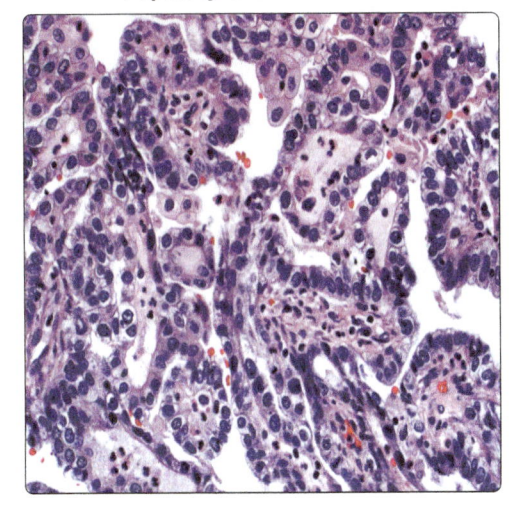

Papillae and Tubules

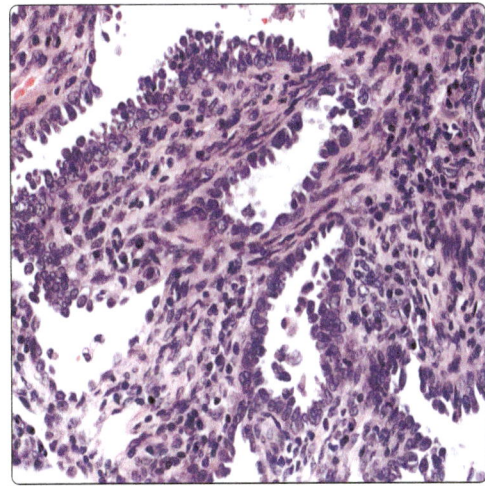

(Left) CCC shows a papillary growth pattern lined by a single layer of cuboidal cells with clear to eosinophilic cytoplasm and central, round to irregular, hyperchromatic nuclei. *(Right)* Endometrial CCC shows papillae and tubules lined by neoplastic cells with somewhat smaller cells, hobnail morphology, and less conspicuous cytologic atypia.

Tubulocystic Growth Pattern

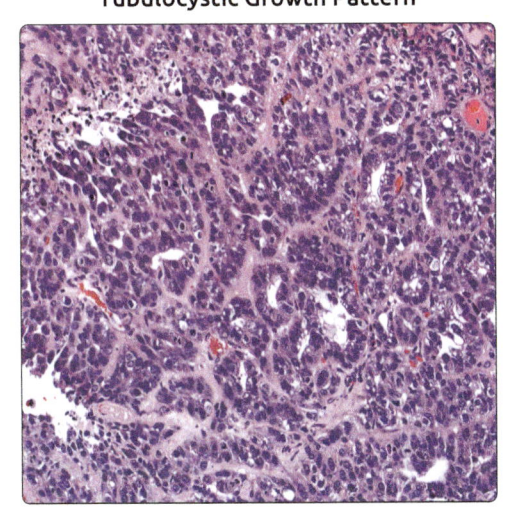

Tubulocystic Pattern

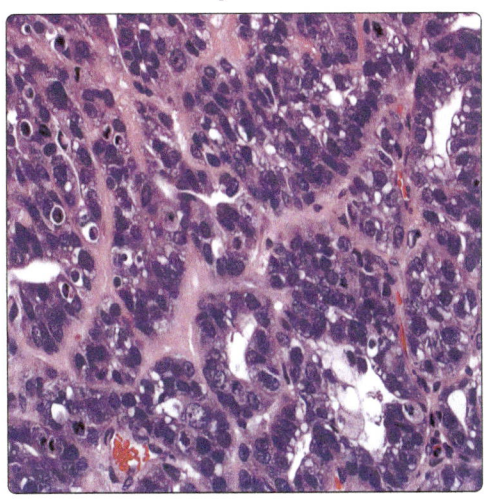

(Left) The tubulocystic pattern is less common in CCC of the endometrium compared with ovarian CCC. This tumor shows focal tubule formation and stromal hyalinization. *(Right)* High-power view of the same case shows the tumor cells to be cuboidal to polygonal with eosinophilic cytoplasm. While the nuclear atypia is high grade, CCC typically does not exhibit the marked nuclear pleomorphism characteristic of serous carcinomas.

Uterine Sarcomas

TERMINOLOGY

Definitions
- This chapter covers malignant mesenchymal tumors primary to uterus
- WHO 2020 classification
  - Endometrial stromal sarcomas (ESS)
    - Low-grade ESS (LG-ESS)
    - High-grade ESS (HG-ESS)
  - Undifferentiated uterine sarcoma (UUS)
  - Uterine leiomyosarcoma (uLMS)
- Other primary uterine sarcomas
  - Rare: Perivascular epithelioid cell tumor (PEComa), inflammatory myofibroblastic tumor (IMFT), Ewing sarcoma, rhabdomyosarcoma, and other sarcomas
  - Recently characterized uterine sarcomas: *SMARCA4*-deficient uterine sarcoma and NTRK-rearranged fibrosarcoma-like uterine sarcoma

EPIDEMIOLOGY

General
- Risk factors
  - Hormone exposure may play role
    - Prolonged estrogenic stimulation
    - Tamoxifen
  - Certain hereditary syndromes: Hereditary retinoblastoma, Li-Fraumeni syndrome
  - Prior pelvic radiation
  - Preceding tumor: Only rarely does uLMS develop from leiomyoma or UUS from LG-ESS/HG-ESS
  - Obesity and diabetes are associated with increased risk for ESS
  - HPV infection: Exceptional cases of uLMS associated with HPV-51
- Incidence
  - Primary uterine sarcomas make up ~ 3% of primary malignant uterine tumors overall
  - uLMS makes up 80% of uterine sarcomas
  - ESS makes up ~ 15% of uterine sarcomas
  - USS only represents ~ 5% of uterine sarcomas

Low-Grade Endometrial Stromal Sarcoma
- Age: Premenopausal; 40s most commonly
- Behavior
  - Tumor stage is best predictor of survival
    - FIGO I and II: > 90% 5-year survival
    - FIGO III and IV: 38-50% 5-year survival
  - 30% have lymph node metastases

High-Grade Endometrial Stromal Sarcoma
- Age: Premenopausal; 40s most commonly
- Behavior
  - Prognosis is intermediate between LG-ESS and UUS
  - Higher proportion of patients present with advanced-stage disease than for LG-ESS

Undifferentiated Uterine Sarcoma
- Age: Postmenopausal women most commonly
- Behavior: Aggressive with < 20% 5-year survival

Leiomyosarcoma
- Age: 45-55 years most commonly
- Behavior: Tumor stage best predictor of survival; 25-75% 5-year survival

MICROSCOPIC

Low-Grade Endometrial Stromal Sarcoma
- Architecture
  - Classic: Sheets of monotonous cells mixed with spiral arterioles and capillaries
  - Variant features: Sclerosis, myxoid change, scattered benign glands, sex cord-like differentiation, foamy histiocytes
- Cells
  - Classic cells are uniform, small, oval to fusiform with high nuclear:cytoplasmic ratio
    - Mitotic rate may be low (< 5/10 HPF most commonly) or high (high mitotic rate does **not** exclude diagnosis of LG-ESS)
    - High mitotic rate does not impart worse prognosis

Leiomyosarcoma: Morphologic Appearance

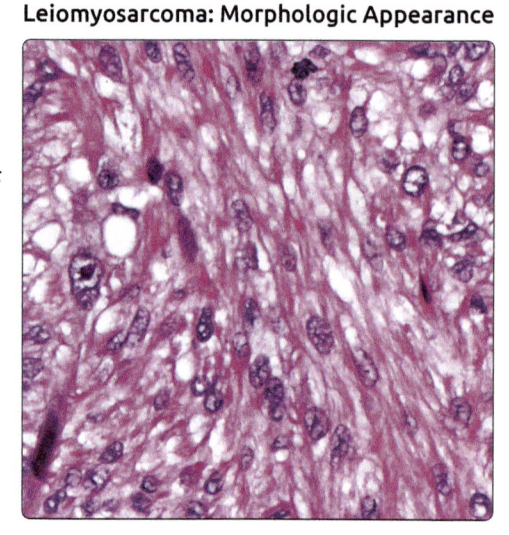

Epithelioid Leiomyosarcoma

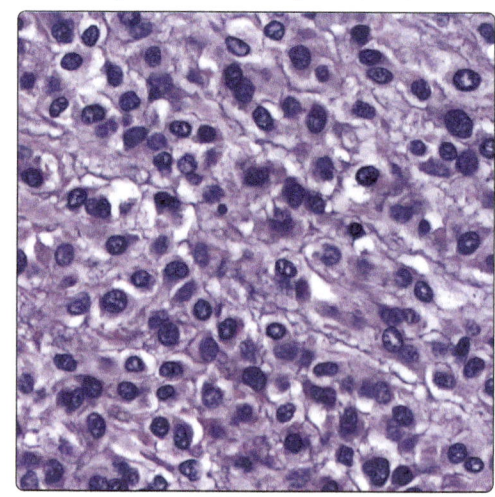

(Left) *The most common histologic variant of uterine leiomyosarcoma (LMS) consists of spindled eosinophilic cells with moderate to marked cytologic atypia. Note the ragged cytoplasmic vacuolation.* (Right) *Uterine LMS may have various histologic appearances. This tumor exhibits an epithelioid morphology.*

Uterine Sarcomas

- Other cell types
  - Smooth muscle cells (45% of cases); may be spindled or epithelioid
  - Sex cord-like epithelioid cells with eosinophilic or foamy cytoplasm (25% of cases)
  - Skeletal muscle cells
  - Rhabdoid cells
- Immunohistochemistry
  - Positive
    - CD10: Usually strongly diffusely positive
    - Muscle markers (SMA, desmin, caldesmon): Usually only positive in areas of smooth muscle differentiation
    - β-catenin: Often shows nuclear reactivity
    - Sex cord-like areas likely to express inhibin, calretinin
    - Hormone receptors: ER and PR usually strongly, diffusely positive
  - Negative: Cyclin-D1
- Genetic tests
  - FISH for translocations, such as *JAZF1::SUZ12*, present in ~ 60%
    - Not specific for LG-ESS: Also found in ~ 65% of endometrial stromal nodules

High-Grade Endometrial Stromal Sarcoma

- Architecture
  - 50% are similar to LG-ESS
  - 50% are composed of mixture of round cell and fibroblastic (low-grade spindle cell) components
  - Necrosis and vascular space invasion more common than in LG-ESS
  - May have variant features as noted for LG-ESS
- Cells
  - Round cells: Tumor nuclei larger, more angulated and irregular than in LG-ESS
    - Mitotic rate often > 10/HPF
  - Fibroblasts: Bland spindled cells
- Immunohistochemistry
  - Round cells: Cyclin-D1 is often strongly positive; CD10, ER, PR negative or patchy
  - Spindled cells: Usually strongly and diffusely positive for CD10, ER, PR
  - May have patchy positivity for desmin, SMA, EMA or diffuse BCOR positivity in *BCOR*-altered cases
- Genetic tests
  - *YWHAE::NUTM2B* fusion found on FISH or PCR (> 90% of cases)
  - *BCOR* or *BCORL1* alterations in few cases

Undifferentiated Uterine Sarcoma

- Architecture
  - Sheets of cells with destructive rather than permeative myometrial invasion
  - Lacks uniform vascular pattern of ESS
  - Necrosis usually prominent
  - Few cases may have LG-ESS component
  - Heterologous components may be present
    - Rhabdomyosarcoma and osteosarcoma most commonly
- Cells: Often markedly pleomorphic
  - Usually high mitotic rate ± atypical mitotic figures
- Immunohistochemistry
  - Often positive: p53
  - Sometimes positive: CD10 (patchy), cyclin-D1, ER/PR (patchy)
  - Negative: Keratins, desmin, caldesmon, CD34

Uterine Leiomyosarcoma

- Architecture
  - Classic: Long, sweeping fascicles of spindled tumor cells intersecting at right angles
    - Diagnostic criteria: Must have at least 2 of following: 2-3+ cytologic atypia, tumor cell necrosis, ≥ 4 mitoses/mm² (~ ≥ 10 mitoses/10 HPF)
  - Other variants
    - Myxoid: Prominent myxoid matrix; must have 2 or more of 2-3+ cytologic atypia, tumor necrosis, ≥ 0.4 mitoses/mm² (~ > 1 mitoses/10 HPF)
    - Epithelioid: Epithelioid cells; must have 1 or more of 2-3+ cytologic atypia, tumor cell necrosis, ≥ 1.6 mitoses/mm² (~ ≥ 4 mitoses/10 HPF)
    - Dedifferentiated: Conventional low-grade fascicular spindled leiomyosarcoma with pleomorphic undifferentiated areas
    - uLMS with other sarcoma components: Can include osteosarcoma, chondrosarcoma, rhabdomyosarcoma
- Cells
  - Spindled tumor cells
    - Lower grade cells have train car- or cigar-shaped nuclei
    - Higher grade cells have more irregularly shaped nuclei; may be multinucleated
    - Ragged cytoplasmic clearing reminiscent of normal contraction bands of smooth muscle often present
  - Epithelioid tumor cells: Rounded with discrete cell borders and round nuclei ± nucleoli
  - Dedifferentiated tumor cells
    - Pleomorphic spindled and tumor giant cells lacking myogenic differentiation
- Immunohistochemistry
  - Positive
    - Muscle markers (desmin, caldesmon, SMA) usually diffusely positive (at least desmin or caldesmon), except in epithelioid or myxoid variants
  - Sometimes positive
    - CD10 sometimes positive, usually patchy if present
    - ER/PR positive in ~ 60%
    - Keratins, EMA
- Genetic tests
  - Negative for ESS translocations
  - Usually negative for *MED12* (Xq13.1) somatic mutations that are present in ~ 70% of leiomyomas
    - Only ~ 20% show *MED12* mutations

Other Rare Uterine Sarcomas

- PEComa
  - Epithelioid cells often arranged radially around blood vessels
  - May be benign (uniform cells) or malignant (pleomorphic cells ± necrosis, high mitotic rate)
- Liposarcoma
  - Adipocytic cells, including lipoblasts and atypical stromal cells
- Rhabdomyosarcoma

Uterine Sarcomas

- Pure population of rhabdomyoblasts at varying stages of differentiation
- IMFT with atypia
  - Usually composed of low-grade fascicular smooth muscle component with areas of cytologically atypical IMFT (atypical spindled to epithelioid tumor cells with inflammation)
  - ALK fusion positive in > 95% with various partners
- Uterine tumor resembling ovarian sex cord tumor (UTROSCT)
  - Epithelioid cells arranged in multiple patterns, including glands, tubules, cords, or may show spindle cell fascicular or round cell sheet-like growth
  - ESR1 or GREB1 fusions: Tumors with GREB1 fusions more likely to show spindled cell fascicular growth
  - May be related to LG-ESS according to gene expression profiling

DIFFERENTIAL DIAGNOSIS

DDx for Low-Grade Endometrial Stromal Sarcoma

- Endometrial stromal nodule
  - Histologically, can look identical to LG-ESS
  - Limited to < 3-mm myoinvasion and < 3 interdigitations at tumor interface with myometrium
  - Lacks vascular invasion
  - Genetics not discriminatory: Majority have JAZF1::SUZ12 fusion
- Cellular leiomyoma
  - Cells bigger with more abundant cytoplasm
  - Strong, diffuse reactivity for at least 1, and usually 2, muscle markers
  - Negative for ESS-associated gene fusions
- Adenosarcoma
  - Leaf-like (phyllodes) processes
  - Glands often atypical, cystically dilated with periglandular stromal condensation

DDx for High-Grade Endometrial Stromal Sarcoma

- Undifferentiated carcinoma
  - Sheets of dyscohesive high-grade cells that lack fine capillary network of ESS
  - Lacks round cell bland fibroblastic mixture, as in 50% of HG-ESS
  - Epithelial markers usually positive but may be focal (EMA, keratin 18)
  - Lacks reactivity for CD10
- SMARCA4-deficient uterine sarcoma: High-grade epithelioid to rhabdoid cells; loss of SMARCA4 expression

DDx for Undifferentiated Uterine Sarcoma

- Undifferentiated carcinoma
  - May have lower grade carcinoma elements
  - Lacks spindle cell component
  - Negative for muscle markers and CD10
  - Epithelial markers usually positive but may be focal
- Malignant mixed müllerian tumor (MMMT) (sarcomatoid carcinoma)
  - Contains malignant epithelial component
  - At least patchy positivity for epithelial markers

DDx for Leiomyosarcoma

- Malignant PEComa
  - Granular or clear epithelioid cells ± spindled cells
  - Melanocytic markers positive (HMB-45, melan-A) in more than rare cells
  - Genetics: TSC1/TSC2 alterations or RAD51B fusions or TFE3 rearranged
- Smooth muscle tumor of uncertain malignant potential (STUMP)
  - May be cellular with atypia but lacks > 10 mitoses/10 HPF and tumor necrosis
  - uLMS usually positive for at least 2 of following: p53, Rb, and PTEN by immunohistochemistry, while STUMP is negative or positive for 1 only
- Mitotically active leiomyoma: No cytologic atypia, no tumor-type necrosis
- Cellular leiomyoma: No cytologic atypia and no tumor-type necrosis; mitotic rate < 10 mitoses/10 HPF
- IMFT: Usually has at least mild inflammation; some cells with features of myofibroblasts; positive for ALK fusions; often positive for ALK by immunohistochemistry
- NTRK-rearranged uterine sarcoma: Positive for pan-TRK, and usually positive for S100 and CD34 with only focal SMA; NTRK fusions

SELECTED REFERENCES

1. Momeni-Boroujeni A et al: Molecular-based immunohistochemical algorithm for uterine leiomyosarcoma diagnosis. Mod Pathol. 36(4):100084, 2023
2. Costigan DC et al: NTRK-rearranged uterine sarcomas: clinicopathologic features of 15 cases, literature review, and risk stratification. Am J Surg Pathol. 46(10):1415-29, 2022
3. Kertowidjojo EC et al: Update on uterine mesenchymal neoplasms. Surg Pathol Clin. 15(2):315-40, 2022
4. Williams EA et al: HPV51-associated leiomyosarcoma: a novel class of TP53/RB1-wildtype tumor with predilection for the female lower reproductive tract. Am J Surg Pathol. 46(6):729-41, 2022
5. Choi J et al: Integrated mutational landscape analysis of uterine leiomyosarcomas. Proc Natl Acad Sci U S A. 118(15):e2025182118, 2021
6. Selenica P et al: Genomic profiling aids classification of diagnostically challenging uterine mesenchymal tumors with myomelanocytic differentiation. Am J Surg Pathol. 45(1):77-92, 2021
7. Croce S et al: Uterine and vaginal sarcomas resembling fibrosarcoma: a clinicopathological and molecular analysis of 13 cases showing common NTRK-rearrangements and the description of a COL1A1-PDGFB fusion novel to uterine neoplasms. Mod Pathol. 32(7):1008-22, 2019
8. Arias-Stella JA 3rd et al: Novel PLAG1 gene rearrangement distinguishes a subset of uterine myxoid leiomyosarcoma from other uterine myxoid mesenchymal tumors. Am J Surg Pathol. 43(3):382-8, 2018
9. Chiang S et al: NTRK fusions define a novel uterine sarcoma subtype with features of fibrosarcoma. Am J Surg Pathol. 42(6):791-8, 2018
10. Dickson BC et al: Uterine tumor resembling ovarian sex cord tumor: a distinct entity characterized by recurrent NCOA2/3 gene fusions. Am J Surg Pathol. 43(2):178-86, 2018
11. Kolin DL et al: SMARCA4-deficient undifferentiated uterine sarcoma (malignant rhabdoid tumor of the uterus): a clinicopathologic entity distinct from undifferentiated carcinoma. Mod Pathol. 31(9):1442-56, 2018
12. Mohammad N et al: ALK is a specific diagnostic marker for inflammatory myofibroblastic tumor of the uterus. Am J Surg Pathol. 42(10):1353-9, 2018
13. Bennett JA et al: Inflammatory myofibroblastic tumor of the uterus: a clinicopathological, immunohistochemical, and molecular analysis of 13 cases highlighting their broad morphologic spectrum. Mod Pathol. 30(10):1489-503, 2017
14. Chiang S et al: BCOR is a robust diagnostic immunohistochemical marker of genetically diverse high-grade endometrial stromal sarcoma, including tumors exhibiting variant morphology. Mod Pathol. 30(9):1251-61, 2017
15. Sciallis AP et al: High-grade endometrial stromal sarcomas: a clinicopathologic study of a group of tumors with heterogenous morphologic and genetic features. Am J Surg Pathol. 38(9):1161-72, 2014

Uterine Sarcomas

Genetic Features of Selected Uterine Mesenchymal Tumors

Entity	Main Genetic Finding	Histology Highlights	Immunohistochemistry
Low-grade endometrial stromal sarcoma	JAZF1::SUZ12 (60%); JAZF1::PHF1 (11%); EPC1::PHF1 (6%); others, including MEAF6::PHF1; MBTD1::EZHIP	Permeative hypercellular growth of uniform small cells with scant cytoplasm; often with smooth muscle areas; may have minor sex-cord like foci	Positive: CD10; IFITM1, often smooth muscle markers; ER diffuse, nuclear β-catenin, focal inhibin and calretinin in sex cord foci
High-grade endometrial stromal sarcoma	YWHAE::NUTM2A/NUTM2B; ZC3H7A::BCOR; EPC1::BCOR; EPC1::SUZ12; BCORL1 fusions; other alterations of BCOR and BCORL1: Tandem duplications, deletions, truncating mutations	Hypercellular infiltrative or pushing growth of cytologically atypical cells, necrosis and ↑ mitoses are typical; may have LG-ESS component BCOR-altered cases commonly show myxoid background	Positive: Cyclin-D1, CD10, BCOR in some, SMA (sometimes positive) Negative: Desmin and caldesmon are usually negative or very focal
Uterine tumor resembling ovarian sex cord tumor	NCOA1/NCOA2 with GREB1, NR4A3, SS18, ESR1, and GTF2A1	ESR1 fusion cases show sex cord-like features; GREB1 fusion cases more fascicular with sparse to absent sex cord features	Positive: SMA, desmin, inhibin, calretinin, keratins Negative: Inhibin, calretinin focal to absent in GREB1 fusion cases
Uterine leiomyosarcoma, classic morphology	Complex aneuploidy; mutations of TP53, PTEN, RB1, ATRX, CDKN2A, DAXX, FH, MED12, and others	Fascicular growth of spindled cells often with scattered pleomorphic cells; varying cell grades, including pleomorphic and deceptively bland	Positive: Smooth muscle markers, p16, and p53 commonly Negative: HMB-45 (absent or only scattered cells)
Uterine leiomyosarcoma, myxoid morphology	PLAG1 fusions (25%)	Hypocellular proliferation of spindled cells embedded in prominent myxoid matrix	Positive: SMA most commonly; desmin, caldesmon, and CD10 often; PLAG1 (50%) Negative: ALK, strong BCOR
Uterine leiomyosarcoma, epithelioid morphology	Complex aneuploidy; mutations as for classic uterine leiomyosarcoma; PGR fusions in subset	Epithelioid cells arranged in nodules, nests, cords, sheets; PGR fusion cases may also have spindled cells and ↓ atypia	Positive: SMA, desmin, caldesmon, EMA, and keratins commonly Negative: PGR fusion cases may be negative for caldesmon
Undifferentiated uterine sarcoma	Complex aneuploidy; no consistent findings; very few cases reported	Hypercellular uniform or hypercellular pleomorphic; both patterns with ↑ mitoses	Positive: p53, p16, and CD10 (sometimes positive) Negative: Diffuse expression of smooth muscle markers
SMARCA4-deficient uterine sarcoma	SMARCA4 mutations SMARCB1 mutations (rare)	Infiltrative hypercellular sheets of large epithelioid (rhabdoid) cells	Positive: SMARCA4 loss Negative: Keratins, EMA, and claudin-4 negative or only focally positive
NTRK-rearranged fibrosarcoma-like uterine sarcoma	NTRK1 (1q23) or NTRK3 (15q25) fusions; NTRK1/NTRK3 fusion partners include TPM3 (1q21), LMNA (1q22), RBPMS (8p12), and TPR (1q31)	Herringbone, fascicular hypercellular arrangement of spindled cells with ↑ mitoses	Positive: Pan-TRK, CD34, and S100 commonly; SMA (focal) in 33% Negative: Desmin
Inflammatory myofibroblastic tumor	Predominantly ALK fusions (~80%) with numerous partners; rarely ROS1, ETV6, and RET fusions	Spindled and polygonal cells in varying proportions of myxoid, fascicular, and sclerotic areas with inflammation	Positive: ALK, smooth muscle markers, CD10, hormone receptors variable Negative: S100, CD34
Perivascular epithelioid cell tumor	Inactivating mutations of TSC1 or TSC2 (most common); TFE3 fusions; inactivating TSC2 mutation + RAD51B	Epithelioid cells with granular cytoplasm in sheets and nests with prominent vascular network (most commonly)	Positive: HMB-45, TFE3, desmin, caldesmon, SMA, cathepsin K Negative: Muscle markers in some TFE3 fusion cases

The classification of uterine mesenchymal tumors continues to evolve with ongoing molecular genetic discoveries.

Uterine Sarcomas

Leiomyosarcoma: Fascicles

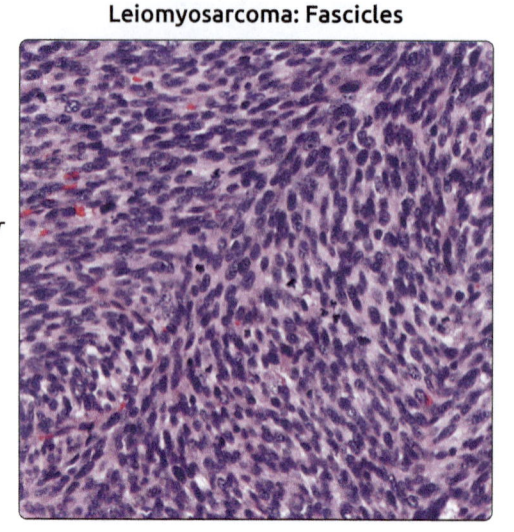

Leiomyosarcoma: Nuclear Features

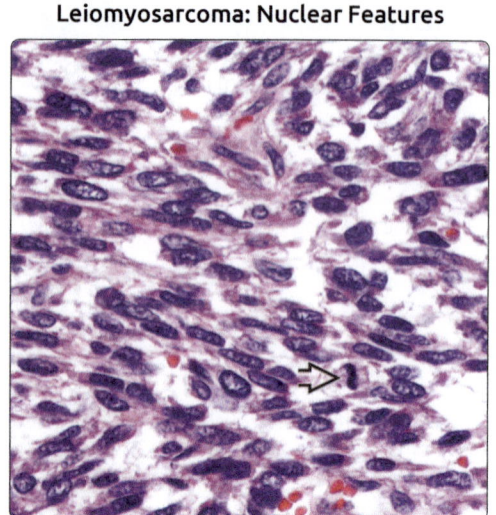

(Left) The most common arrangement of tumor cells in uterine LMS shows long, sweeping fascicles that intersect at right angles. (Right) The nuclei of at least some of the tumor cells in a uterine LMS have a tram car or cigar shape with squared off or rounded ends, respectively. Although the tumor cells are uniform, the nuclei feature coarse chromatin, and a mitotic figure ➡ is present. Other areas showed tumor-type necrosis.

Leiomyosarcoma: Pleomorphism

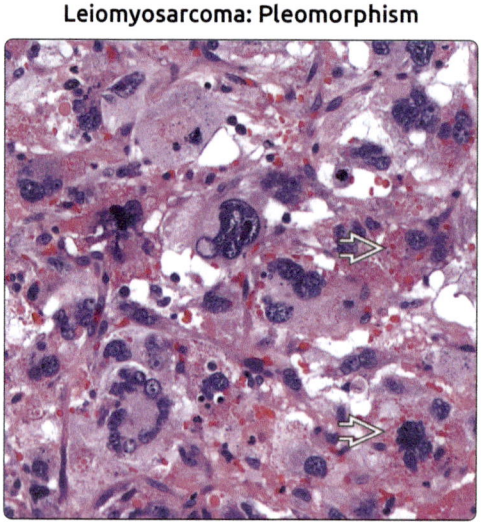

Epithelioid Leiomyosarcoma

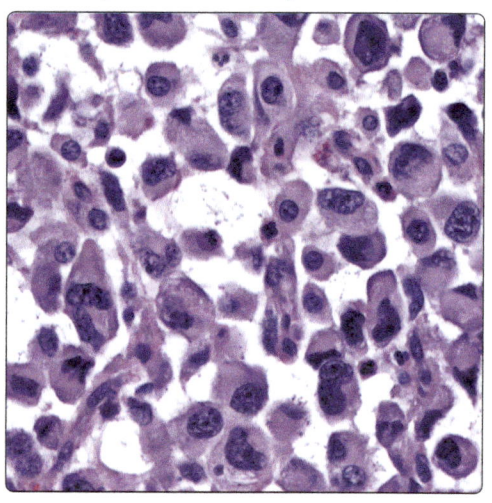

(Left) LMS shows markedly pleomorphic tumor giant cells. Many cells contain degenerative red cytoplasmic inclusions ➡. This tumor also had lower grade areas, suggestive of dedifferentiated LMS. The low-grade areas diffusely expressed SMA and desmin. (Right) LMS shows an epithelioid morphology characterized by round rather than spindled tumor cells. The histologic differential diagnosis includes undifferentiated uterine sarcoma (UUS) and undifferentiated carcinoma.

Myxoid Leiomyosarcoma Arising From Leiomyoma

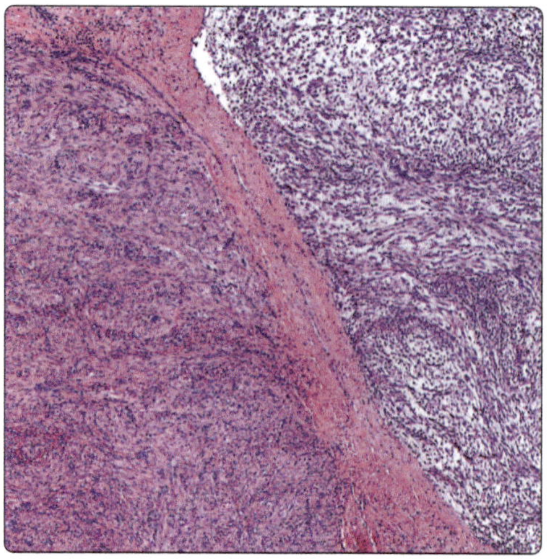

Myxoid Leiomyosarcoma

(Left) This myxoid LMS arose from leiomyoma, a rare event in uterine LMS. The leiomyoma is on the left and abruptly transforms to myxoid LMS on the right. The great majority of uterine LMS are de novo malignant. (Right) High-power view of myxoid LMS shows abundant gray-blue matrix, spindled to polygonal mildly atypical tumor cells, and a mitotic figure ➡.

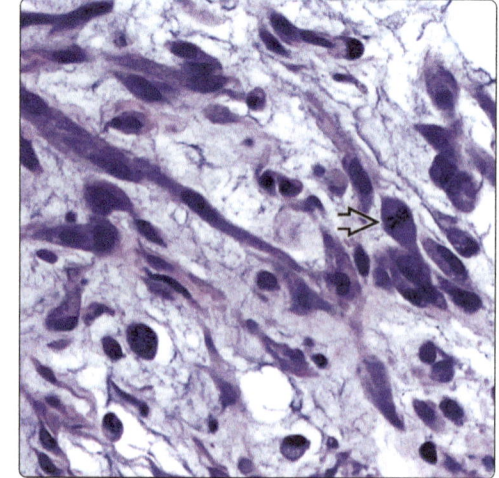

Uterine Sarcomas

Low-Grade Endometrial Stromal Sarcoma

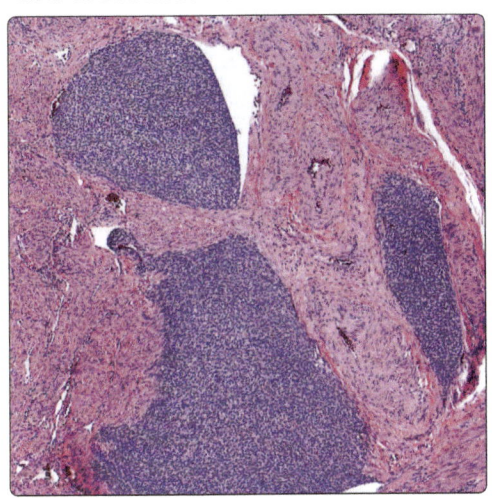

Low-Grade Endometrial Stromal Sarcoma: Cellular Morphology

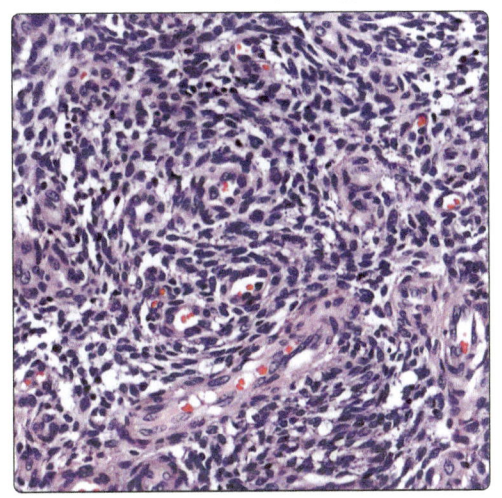

(Left) The tumor cells of low-grade endometrial stromal sarcoma (LG-ESS) can look identical to an endometrial stromal nodule. However, endometrial stromal nodule shows only limited permeative invasion (if any) of the myometrium and lacks vascular invasion. (Right) The tumor cells of LG-ESS are relatively small, uniform, and typically swirl around spiral arterioles, as seen here.

Smooth Muscle in Low-Grade Endometrial Stromal Sarcoma

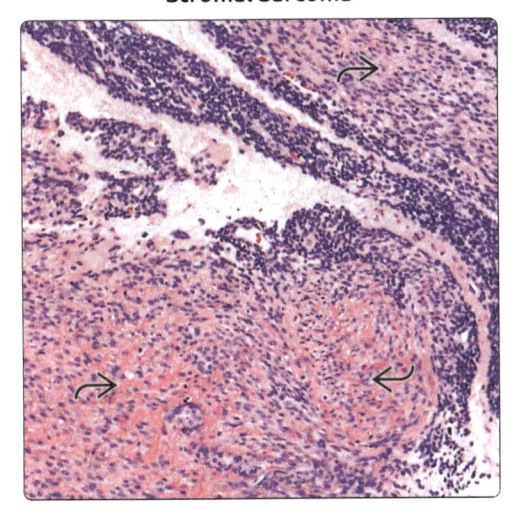

Collagen Balls in Low-Grade Endometrial Stromal Sarcoma

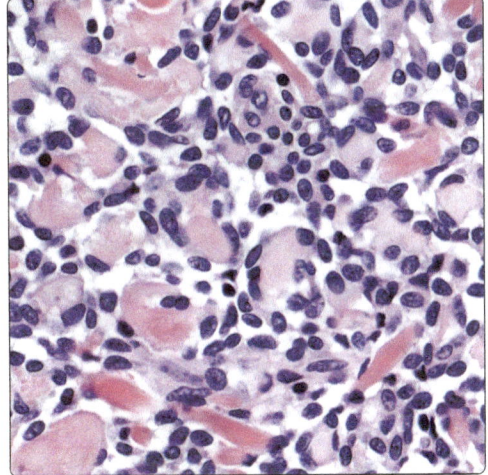

(Left) Approximately 45% of LG-ESS contain areas of smooth muscle differentiation ⮕. The behavior of these mixed tumors is driven by the stromal cell component, and, thus, these tumors are still diagnosed as LG-ESS. (Right) Many morphologic variants of LG-ESS can occur. This tumor features balls of collagen surrounded by uniform, ovoid, bland spindle cells. The tumor was diffusely and strongly CD10(+) with nuclear β-catenin, consistent with LG-ESS.

ER Expression in Low-Grade Endometrial Stromal Sarcoma

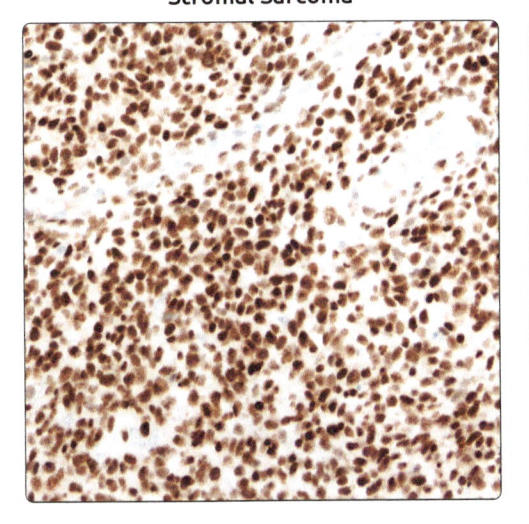

β-Catenin Expression in Low-Grade Endometrial Stromal Sarcoma

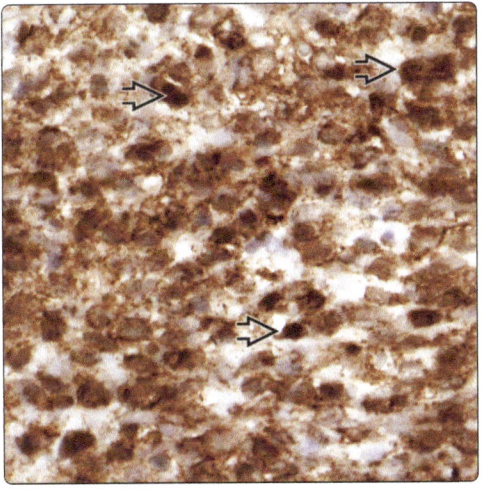

(Left) LG-ESS is characteristically diffusely and strongly ER(+), as seen here. (Right) β-catenin is usually expressed in at least some of the nuclei of LG-ESS ⮕.

Uterine Sarcomas

High-Grade Endometrial Stromal Sarcoma

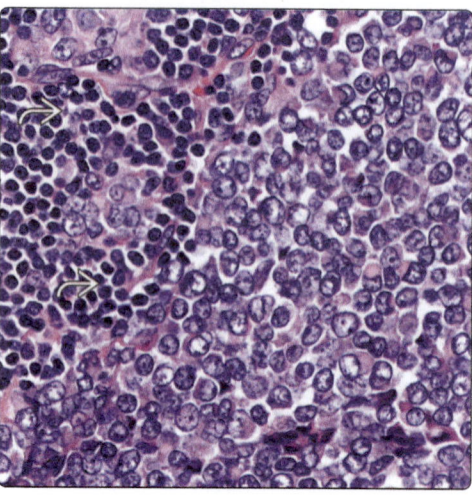

Nuclear Features of High-Grade Endometrial Stromal Sarcoma

(Left) High-grade ESS (HG-ESS) shows different nuclear features compared to LG-ESS. For example, the nuclei of the round cell component are larger (2-3x the size of a lymphocyte). Note the relatively large size of the tumor cells compared to the plasma cells/lymphocytes ⇨. (Right) The cells of HG-ESS are more variable than those seen in LG-ESS with slightly irregular nuclear contours as well as an overall larger nuclear size. Mitoses are often numerous ⇨.

Biphasic Appearance of High-Grade Endometrial Stromal Sarcoma

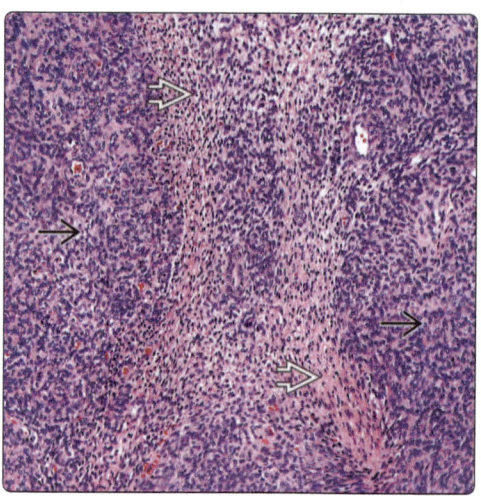

Vasculature

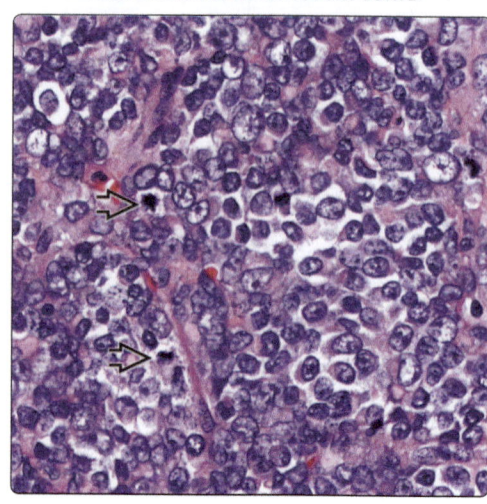

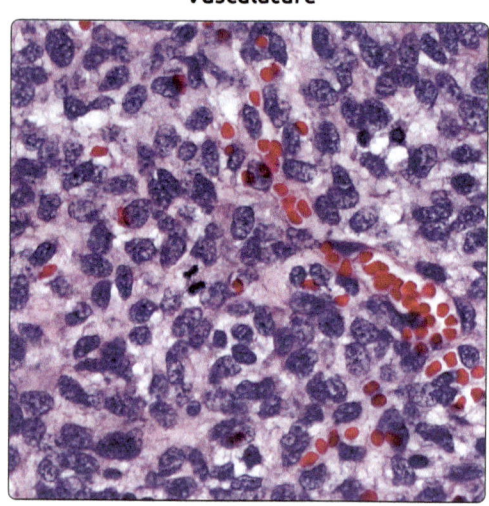

(Left) ~ 50% of HG-ESS are characterized by a biphasic population of round blue cells ⇨ mixed with areas of bland, spindled fibroblastic cells set in a collagenous or fibromyxoid matrix ⇨. This duality can be a clue to the diagnosis at low power. (Right) HG-ESS shows subtle nuclear atypia, mitotic activity, and a small capillary. The vascular network in HG-ESS is typically composed of a mesh of small, delicate capillaries.

Blood Vessel Invasion

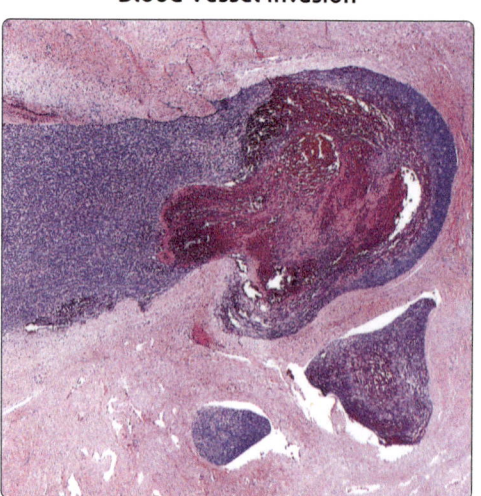

Cyclin-D1 Expression

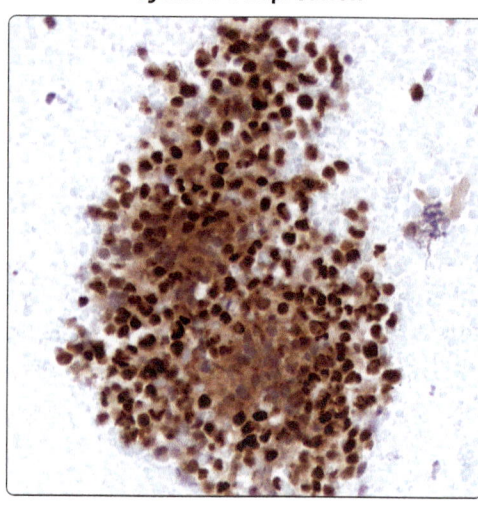

(Left) HG-ESS invades blood vessels more often than LG-ESS. Both LG- and HG-ESS invade the myometrium in a permeative manner. However, HG-ESS contains necrotic areas more often than LG-ESS. (Right) Cyclin-D1 is positive in most cases of HG-ESS, and diffuse nuclear expression supports the diagnosis. It is typically not expressed in LG-ESS but can be focally expressed in UUS.

Uterine Sarcomas

Undifferentiated Uterine Sarcoma

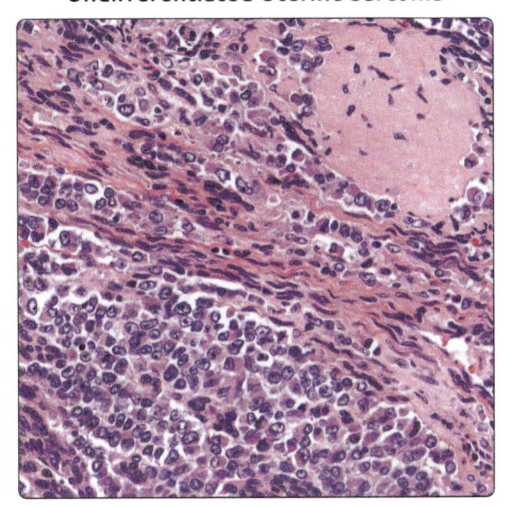

Undifferentiated Uterine Sarcoma With Rhabdoid Cells

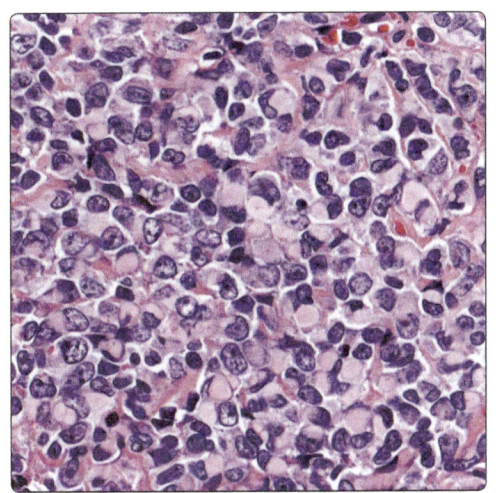

(Left) Like LMS and ESS, UUS has a variety of histologic appearances. In all cases, it lacks endometrial stromal differentiation and usually invades the myometrium destructively. Tumor cells are usually markedly pleomorphic with a high mitotic rate. This example shows mixed epithelioid and spindled cell components with focal dense collagen production. (Right) Rhabdoid cells are present in this UUS but had intact SMARCB1 by IHC.

CD10 Expression

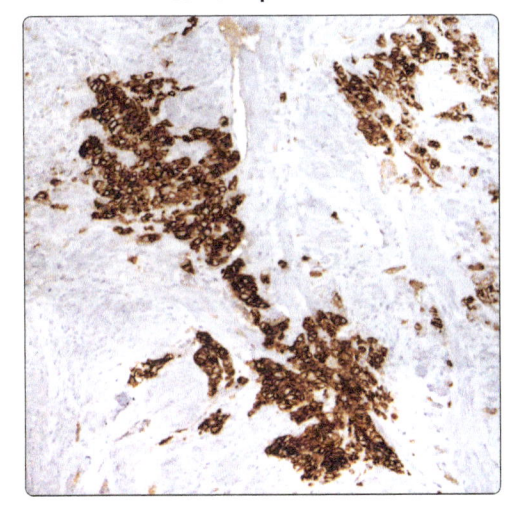

Epithelioid and Polygonal Cells

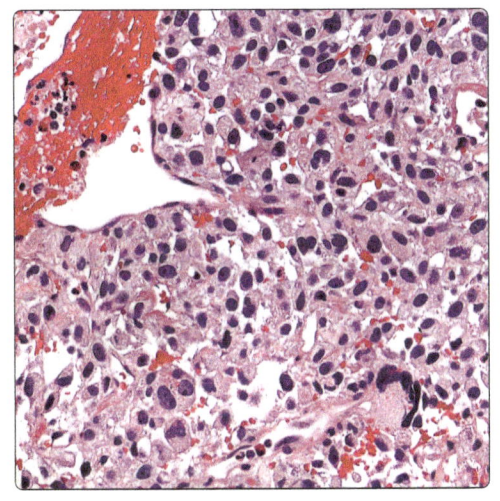

(Left) UUS commonly shows patchy reactivity for CD10, as seen here. Other proteins that may be expressed include cyclin-D1, ER, and PR. Cases with heterologous differentiation, such as osteosarcoma or rhabdomyosarcoma, will express proteins specific to those components. (Right) UUS shows epithelioid to polygonal cells with a moderate nuclear:cytoplasmic ratio and scattered tumor giant cells.

Alveolar Pattern

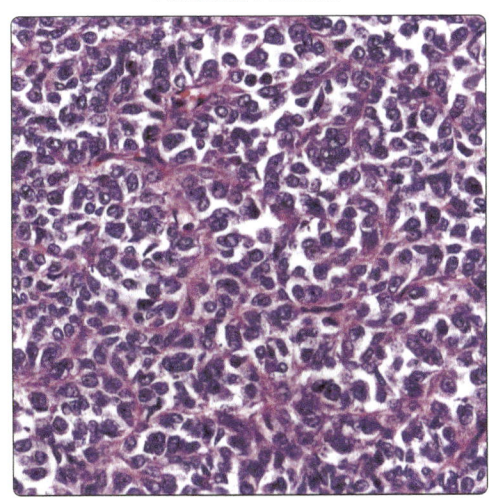

WT1 Expression

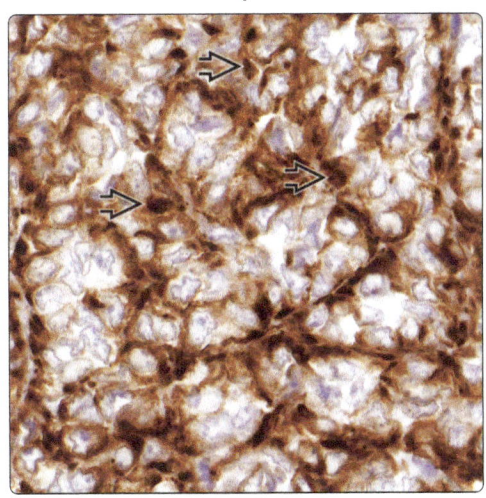

(Left) UUS shows an unusual nested or alveolar pattern with central cellular dyscohesion. Other entities that must be excluded include undifferentiated carcinoma, HG-ESS, LMS, and rare sarcomas, such as perivascular epithelioid cell tumor (PEComa). (Right) UUS with pseudoalveoli shows an unusual pattern of cytoplasmic and nuclear WT1 staining ⇒ at the periphery of tumor nests. WT1 is also expressed in ESS and LMS in a nuclear, cytoplasmic, or combined pattern.

Serous Tumors of Ovary and Fallopian Tube

KEY FACTS

TERMINOLOGY
- Benign serous tumors (BST)
- Serous borderline tumors (SBT)
- Low-grade serous carcinoma (LGSC)
- High-grade serous carcinoma (HGSC)
  - 2nd most common gynecologic malignancy in USA, as well as most lethal in this group

CLINICAL ISSUES
- LGSC and SBT with invasive implants are treated by primary cytoreductive surgery and secondary cytoreduction (for recurrence)
  - Do not respond to platinum-based combination chemotherapy
  - Prognosis is generally dependent on clinical stage with excellent prognosis for stage I
- HGSC is treated by aggressive surgical debulking followed by platinum-based combination chemotherapy
  - PARP inhibitors for homologous recombination-deficient (HRD) tumors regardless of germline BRCA1/BRCA2 mutation status
  - Immune checkpoint inhibitors
  - Stage and debulking status are still major prognostic factors

MOLECULAR
- Low-grade tumors (SBT and LGSC)
  - Most common mutations: KRAS or BRAF
- HGSC
  - TP53 mutations or inactivation are most common and detected in nearly all tumors (> 96%)
  - Gene alterations in homologous recombination pathway, resulting in HRD with secondary lethal accumulation of DNA repair defects (50% of tumors)
    - BRCA1 and BRCA2 (better survival than patients with wildtype BRCA1 and BRCA2)
      □ Germline or somatic mutations and epigenetic alterations in 22%
    - Mutations in non-BRCA homologous recombination genes: ATM, BARD1, BRIP1, CHEK1, CHEK2, ABRAXAS1, MRE11, NBN, PALB2, RAD51C, and RAD51D
  - Widespread somatic copy number alterations resulting in genomic instability and gene mutations in multiple signaling pathways involved in cell cycle regulation
  - mRNA and miRNA expression analysis
    - At least 4 robust expression profile subtypes exist in HGSC (immunoreactive, differentiated, proliferative, and mesenchymal)
      □ Better prognosis observed in immunoreactive subtype, which is associated with BRCA1 disruptions and high tumor-infiltrating lymphocytes (TILs)
- Currently actionable molecular genomic alterations
  - KRAS mutations
    - Predicts sensitivity to MEK inhibitors
  - BRCA1 or BRCA2 mutations and other homologous recombination genes
    - Predicts sensitivity to PARP inhibitors

ANCILLARY TESTS
- BRCA1/BRCA2 test
- Multigene panel tests
- HRD tests

TOP DIFFERENTIAL DIAGNOSES
- Metastatic colorectal adenocarcinoma
- High-grade endometrioid adenocarcinoma
- Clear cell carcinoma
- Germ cell tumors, e.g., embryonal carcinoma and yolk sac tumor
- Diffuse malignant mesothelioma

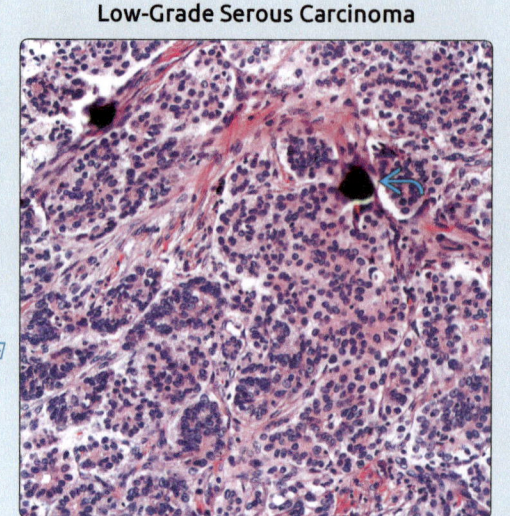

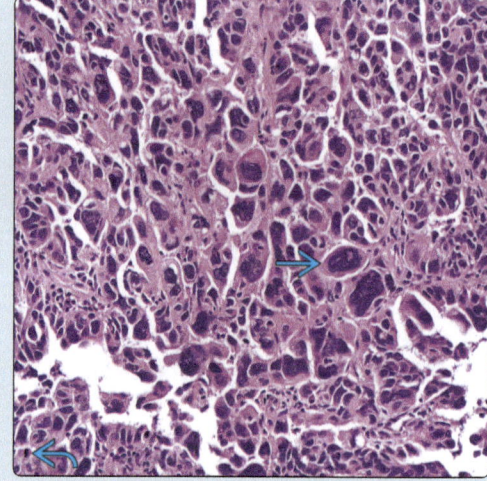

(Left) Low-grade serous carcinoma is characterized by complex papillary clusters of low-grade cells with small nuclei, inconspicuous nucleoli, and few mitoses. Psammoma bodies can be observed ➡. (Right) High-grade serous carcinoma is characterized by high-grade bizarre nuclei with marked variation in nuclear size and prominent vesicular nucleoli ➡. Mitotic figures ➡ can be readily observed.

Serous Tumors of Ovary and Fallopian Tube

TERMINOLOGY

Abbreviations
- Benign serous tumors (BST)
- Serous borderline tumor (SBT)
- Low-grade serous carcinoma (LGSC)
- High-grade serous carcinoma (HGSC)

Synonyms
- SBT
  - Micropapillary/cribriform subtypes

Definitions
- BST (~ 78% of serous tumors)
  - Composed of benign epithelium resembling fallopian tube epithelium
  - Serous cystadenoma and cystadenofibroma most common histologic subtypes
- SBT (~ 2% of serous tumors)
  - Noninvasive, low-grade, proliferative serous epithelial neoplasms exhibiting complex architecture without stromal invasion
  - SBT with microinvasion
    - Early stromal invasion by single cells or small clusters of neoplastic cells cytologically similar to those in noninvasive component in ≥ 1 areas, each < 5 mm
- Serous carcinoma
  - Invasive epithelial carcinoma composed of
    - Neoplastic cells resembling those of fallopian tube epithelium in LGSC (~ 5% of ovarian carcinomas)
    - Highly anaplastic-appearing cells with brisk mitotic activity in HGSC (~ 70% of ovarian carcinomas)
  - Ovarian serous carcinomas represent 95% of ovarian cancer
    - 2nd most common gynecologic malignancy in USA, as well as most lethal in this group (2021)
    - 8th most common cancer diagnosis and cause of death in women with estimated 313,959 cases and 207,252 deaths worldwide (2020)

ETIOLOGY/PATHOGENESIS

General Risk Factors for High-Grade Serous Carcinoma
- Family history of breast/ovarian carcinoma
  - Hereditary ovarian cancer accounts for ~ 15% of cases
    - *BRCA1* &/or *BRCA2* germline mutations
    - 30-70% risk of developing HGSC by age of 70
- Advancing age
- Nulliparity

Site of Origin
- Tubal-type epithelium
  - Fallopian tube fimbria
    - Less commonly, tubal-type epithelium on ovarian surface or lining cortical inclusion cysts

CLINICAL ISSUES

Presentation
- BST
  - Wide age range with pelvic mass-related symptoms or incidental
- SBT
  - Median age: 50 years ± pelvic mass-related symptoms
- LGSC
  - Median age: 43 years with history of SBT in small subset ± pelvic mass-related symptoms/ascites
- HGSC
  - Median age: 65 years with nonspecific symptoms, including abdominal pain or distention secondary to abdominopelvic organ involvement and ascites
    - Advanced stage in ~ 80% of cases

Treatment
- BST
  - Unilateral salpingo-oophorectomy or ovarian cystectomy
- SBT without invasive implants
  - Conservative surgical resection with intraoperative surgical staging (i.e., cystectomy or salpingo-oophorectomy)
- LGSC and SBT with invasive implants
  - Primary cytoreductive surgery and secondary cytoreduction for recurrences
  - Do not respond to platinum-based combination chemotherapy
- HGSC
  - Aggressive surgical debulking followed by platinum-based combination chemotherapy
  - PARP inhibitors for homologous recombination-deficient (HRD) tumors regardless of germline *BRCA1/BRCA2* mutation status
  - Immune checkpoint inhibitors

Prognosis
- BST
  - Excellent prognosis but may recur if incompletely excised
- SBT, excluding micropapillary variants
  - Excellent prognosis for stage I disease
- LGSC
  - Generally dependent on clinical stage with excellent prognosis for stage I
  - Not responsive to chemotherapy in most cases
- HGSC
  - Stage and debulking status are still major prognostic factors
  - Most patients have poor 5-year survival and suffer from recurrence &/or development of chemoresistance
  - Better prognosis observed in tumors with germline *BRCA1/BRCA2* mutations

MACROSCOPIC

BST
- Unilocular or multilocular cysts lined by flat smooth lining and filled with clear watery or serous fluid
- Adenofibromas usually solid with interspersed glandular spaces

SBT
- Intracystic proliferation in form of papillary excrescences or exophytic with surface involvement

Serous Tumors of Ovary and Fallopian Tube

- Bilateral in 2/3 of cases especially in micropapillary and cribriform subtypes

Serous Carcinomas

- Often bilateral, multilocular, cystic, and solid with soft, friable papillae filling cyst cavity containing serous, turbid bloody fluid
- Hemorrhage, solid areas, and necrosis common in HGSC
- Fallopian tube is often partially or entirely embedded within ovarian mass and difficult to grossly visualize

MOLECULAR

Molecular Carcinogenesis

- 2 broad categories of different histologic subtypes of ovarian serous neoplasms based on characteristic molecular pathologic features
  - Low-grade tumors (SBT and LGSC)
    - *KRAS* or *BRAF* mutation
      - Account for most common mutations
  - HGSC
    - Most common mutations involve *TP53*

SBT

- Activating mutations in ERBB2/RAS/RAF/MAPK pathway in 82% of tumors
  - *KRAS* codon 12 mutations in 37%
  - *BRAF* V600E variant in ~ 39%
  - *BRAF* non-V600E variants in 3.5%
    - Less frequent in advanced stage
  - *ERBB2* (HER2) exon 20 in 5%
- Genomic copy number aberrations (CNAs) and copy number loss of heterozygosity (CNLOH) in 61% of tumors

LGSC

- Activating mutations in RAS/RAF/MAPK pathway in 63% of tumors
  - *KRAS* codon 12 mutations (21%)
    - Associated with tumor recurrence
  - *BRAF* V600E mutation (16%)
    - Less common in advanced-stage LGSC
  - *NRAS* (26%)
  - Loss of p16/ARF/p15 activity that may be potentially integral to progression from SBT to LGSC
    - *CDKN2A* homozygous deletions detected in 53% of tumors
    - Increased rate of loss of 9p/9p21.3 (not reflected by p16 overexpression by immunohistochemistry)
  - Other driver gene mutations
    - *EIF1AX, USP9X*

HGSC

- *TP53* mutations or inactivation are most common and detected in nearly all tumors (> 96%)
  - Gene alterations in FOXM1 signaling pathway, resulting in cell cycle progression and DNA repair defects (84% of tumors)
    - *TP53* inhibits FOXM1 pathway
      - High rate of *TP53* mutation in HGSC plays significant role in FOXM1 overexpression
      - *AURKB, CCNB1, BIRC5*, and *PLK1* are consistently overexpressed

- Gene alterations in homologous recombination pathway, resulting in HRD with secondary lethal accumulation of DNA repair defects (50% of tumors)
  - *BRCA1* and *BRCA2* mutations better survival than patients with wildtype *BRCA1* and *BRCA2*
    - Germline or somatic mutations/epigenetic alterations in 22%
    - Loss of expression due to epigenetic silencing of *BRCA1* in 11%
  - Mutations in non-*BRCA1*/*BRCA2* homologous recombination genes
    - *ATM, BARD1, BRIP1, CHEK1, CHEK2, ABRAXAS1, MRE11, NBN, PALB2, RAD51C*, and *RAD51D*
- Widespread somatic CNAs resulting in genomic instability and gene mutations in multiple signaling pathways involved in cell cycle regulation
  - Gene alterations in RB1 signaling pathway, resulting in cell cycle progression (67% of tumors)
    - *CDKN2A, CCNE1, CCND2, RB1*
      - *CCNE1* amplification reported to be associated with poor prognosis and chemotherapy resistance
  - Gene alterations in PI3K/RAS signaling pathway, resulting in cell proliferation and survival (45% of tumors)
    - *PTEN, PIK3CA, AKT1, NF1, KRAS*
  - Gene alterations in Notch signaling pathway, resulting in cell proliferation (22% of tumors)
- mRNA and miRNA expression analysis
  - At least 4 robust expression profile subtypes, including immunoreactive, differentiated, proliferative, and mesenchymal, exist in HGSC
    - Better prognosis observed in immunoreactive subtype, which is associated with *BRCA1* disruptions and high tumor-infiltrating lymphocytes (TILs)
- Promoter methylation involving ~ 168 genes is detected

Actionable Genomic Alterations

- Currently actionable
  - *KRAS* mutations
    - Predicts sensitivity to MEK inhibitors
  - *BRCA1* or *BRCA2* mutations and other homologous recombination genes
    - Predicts sensitivity to PARP inhibitors
- Potentially actionable
  - PI3K pathway mutations
    - May predict sensitivity to mTOR inhibitors
  - *CCNE1* mutations
    - CDK inhibitors may be useful to sensitize *CCNE1*-amplified tumors to chemotherapy

MICROSCOPIC

Histologic Features

- BST
  - Cyst lined by single layer of flattened to cuboidal cells or pseudostratified tubal epithelium without atypia or mitosis
- SBT
  - Hierarchical branching with successively smaller papillae emanating from larger more centrally located papillae
  - Epithelial stratification and tufting with detachment of individual cells and cell clusters
  - Mitoses uncommon (rarely exceed 4/10 HPF)

Serous Tumors of Ovary and Fallopian Tube

- No stromal invasion but foci of stromal microinvasion (< 5 mm each) can be seen
- Can be associated with peritoneal implants
- Cribriform &/or micropapillary subtypes
- LGSC
  - Invasive clusters, small/inverted papillae, mircopapillae, or slit-like glands surrounded by clear space
  - Mild to moderate cytologic atypia with variation in nuclear size < 3x and occasional prominent nucleoli
  - Mitosis present and can be up to 12/10 HPF
  - Frequently associated with coexisting SBT
  - Psammoma bodies often present
- HGSC
  - Solid, papillary, labyrinthine, slit-like, glandular, or cribriform architecture
    - HRD tumors
      - Frequently exhibit solid, endometrial-like, and transitional (SET) variant histology
      - Often associated with geographic necrosis and increased TILs
    - Areas with cytoplasmic clearing may be observed
  - Marked cytologic atypia, smudgy chromatin, prominent nucleoli, and marked variation in nuclear size
  - High mitotic index (> 12/10 HPF) with abnormal mitotic figures

ANCILLARY TESTS

Immunohistochemistry

- LGSC
  - Positive markers
    - CK7, PAX8, WT1, and ER (typically strong and diffuse)
    - PR variable
    - p16 focal/patchy positive (or negative)
  - Negative markers
    - CK20, calretinin, napsin A
    - p53
- HGSC
  - Positive markers
    - CK7, PAX8, WT1 (typically strong and diffuse)
    - p16 strongly and diffusely positive in most cases
    - ER is positive in 88-95% of cases, PR variable
  - PTEN and ARID1A retained
  - Negative markers
    - CK20, napsin, HNF-1β, CDX2, SATB2
  - Variable p53 expression pattern (absent, overexpressed as strong and diffuse in ≥ 80% of cells or rarely cytoplasmic)

Genetic Testing

- *BRCA1/BRCA2* test performed on blood or saliva sample
  - Germline mutations
- Multigene panel tests
  - Next-generation sequencing (NGS) based
  - Detects mutations (somatic, including those with germline implications) involving multiple genes implicated in homologous recombination repair pathway, including *BRCA1/BRCA2*
  - Formalin-fixed, paraffin-embedded (FFPE) tissue sample typically used for detection of somatic mutations
- HRD/genomic scar assays
  - Detects HRD-positive tumors regardless of type or location of genetic mutation and genomic alteration
    - HRD score
      - NGS dosage analysis
      - Measure of LOH, telomeric allelic imbalance, and large-scale transitions
      - FFPE tumor tissue is typical sample used for detection
    - Functional HRD assays
      - RAD51 redistribution assay for compounds inducing replication-associated DNA double-stranded breaks
      - Immunofluorescence assay
  - Predict sensitivity to PARP inhibitors
  - Functional assays may help predict drug resistance

DIFFERENTIAL DIAGNOSIS

DDx for HGSC

- Metastatic colorectal adenocarcinoma
  - Positive for CK20, CDX2, SATB2
- High-grade endometrioid adenocarcinoma
  - Diffuse and strong ER and PR positivity
  - WT1 negative or focal, patchy positivity
  - p53 usually negative
- Clear cell carcinoma
  - Characteristic histomorphologic features usually helpful
  - Positive for napsin A, HNF-1β
  - Negative for WT1, PR, p53
- Germ cell tumors (e.g., embryonal carcinoma and yolk sac tumor)
  - Markers useful to separate germ cell tumors include PLAP, CD30, glypican 3, SALL4, and AFP
- Diffuse malignant mesothelioma
  - Positive for calretinin
  - Negative for claudin-4, MOC31, and Ber-EP4

SELECTED REFERENCES

1. Hada T et al: Comparison of clinical behavior between mucinous ovarian carcinoma with infiltrative and expansile invasion and high-grade serous ovarian carcinoma: a retrospective analysis. Diagn Pathol. 17(1):12, 2022
2. De Leo A et al: What is new on ovarian carcinoma: integrated morphological and molecular analysis following the new 2020 World Health Organization classification of female genital tumors. Diagnostics (Basel). 11(4):697, 2021
3. Konstantinopoulos PA et al: Germline and somatic tumor testing in epithelial ovarian cancer: ASCO guideline. J Clin Oncol. 38(11):1222-45, 2020
4. Miller RE et al: ESMO recommendations on predictive biomarker testing for homologous recombination deficiency and PARP inhibitor benefit in ovarian cancer. Ann Oncol. 31(12):1606-22, 2020
5. WHO Classification of Tumours Editorial Board: WHO Classification of Tumours: Female Genital Tumours. 5th ed. IARC Press. 2020
6. Cancer Genome Atlas Research Network: Integrated genomic analyses of ovarian carcinoma. Nature. 474(7353):609-15, 2011

Serous Tumors of Ovary and Fallopian Tube

Serous Cystadenofibroma

Serous Borderline Tumor

(Left) Serous cystadenofibroma is characterized by proliferation of hypocellular fibrous stromal projections lined by a single layer of bland cells resembling fallopian tubal epithelium. Note the absence of complex papillary architecture and mitotic activity. **(Right)** Serous borderline tumor is characterized by the complex papillary hierarchical architecture with detached floating papillary clusters ➡. Note the absence of stromal invasion.

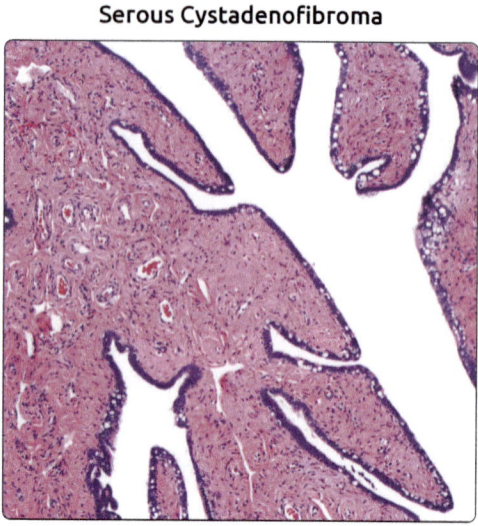

Micropapillary Serous Carcinoma

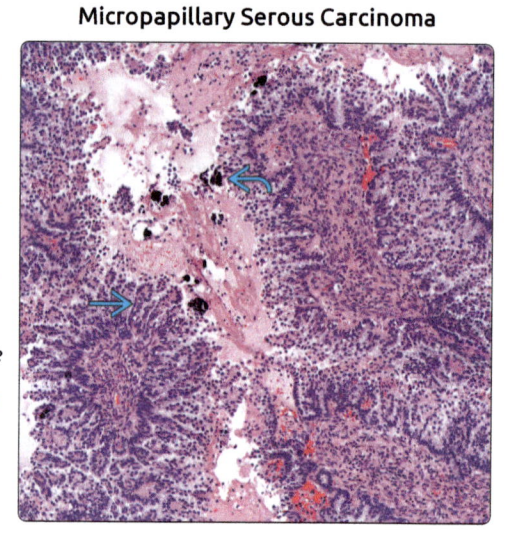

Stromal Invasion in Low-Grade Serous Carcinoma

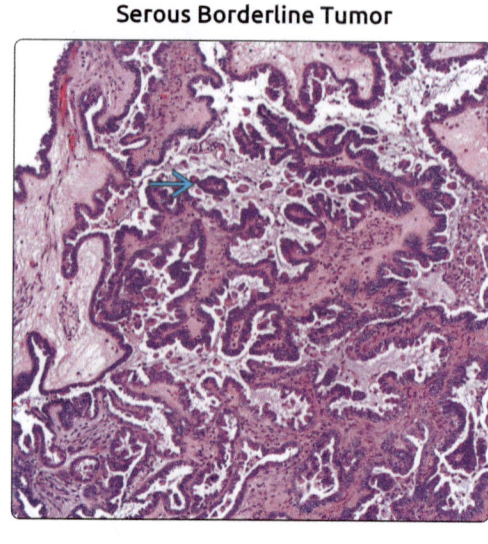

(Left) Micropapillary serous carcinoma is characterized by elongated, thin micropapillae. The length of each micropapillary projection is ~ 5x its width ➡. Psammomatous calcifications can also be observed ➡. **(Right)** Low-grade serous carcinoma is characterized by invasive micropapillary nests of low-grade serous cells in a desmoplastic stroma. Note the nonepithelialized clear space surrounding invasive nests ➡. The nuclei are small and uniform.

High-Grade Serous Carcinoma

Pleomorphic Cells

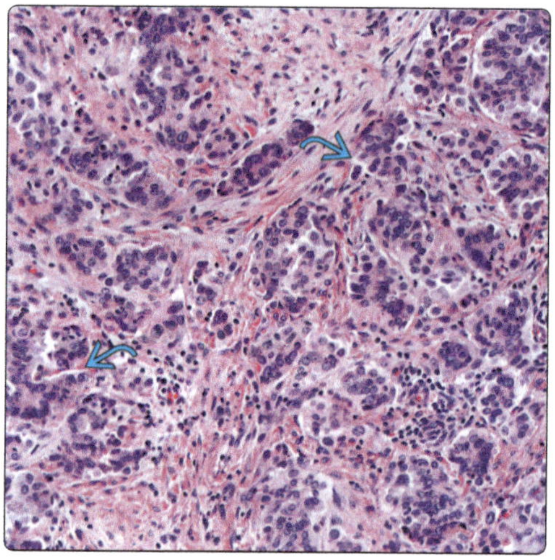

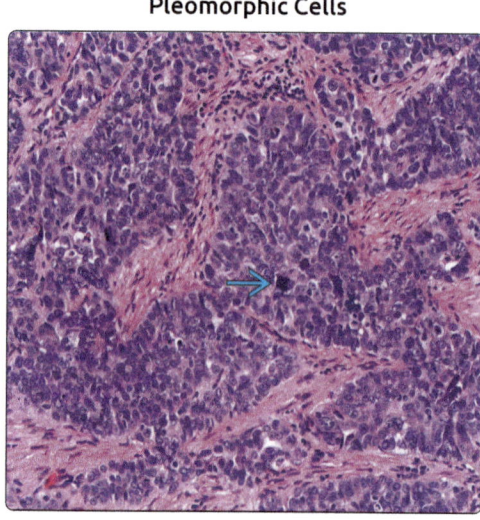

(Left) High-grade serous carcinoma shows a vague papillary architecture ➡ with very little intervening stroma. **(Right)** This high-grade serous carcinoma is characterized by diffuse and solid sheets of highly pleomorphic cells with nuclei displaying smudgy chromatin ➡. Note the absence of the classic papillary architecture.

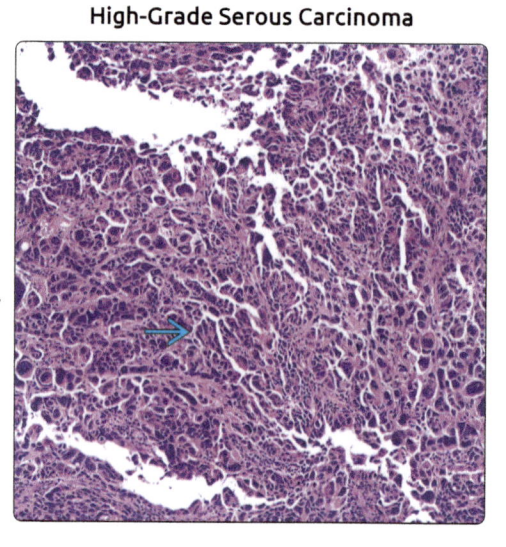

Serous Tumors of Ovary and Fallopian Tube

p53 Immunohistochemical Staining

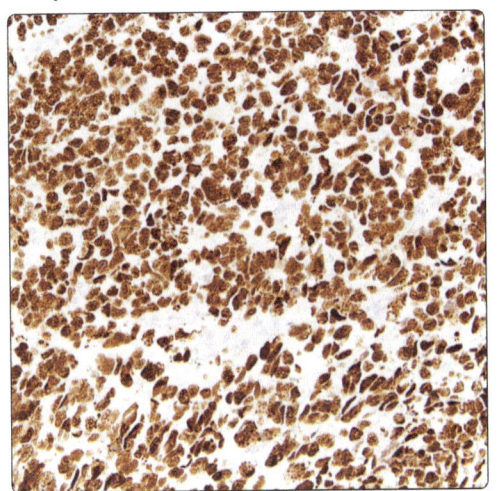

KRAS Mutation

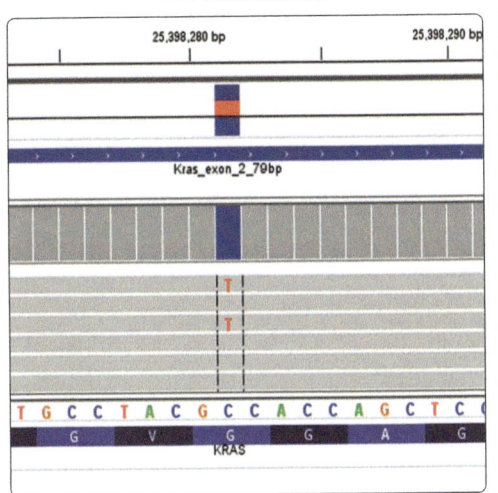

(Left) p53 demonstrates strong and diffuse nuclear expression in this high-grade serous carcinoma of the ovary. (Right) Massive parallel sequencing [next-generation sequencing (NGS)] of DNA extracted from a low-grade serous carcinoma shows a G>A base substitution in codon 13 of the KRAS gene, resulting in G13D mutation. Most KRAS mutations in low-grade serous carcinomas involve codon 12 and, less commonly, codon 13.

BRAF Mutation

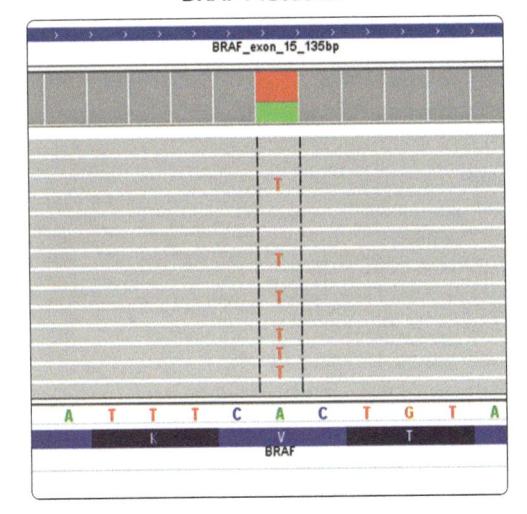

Serous Cystadenoma

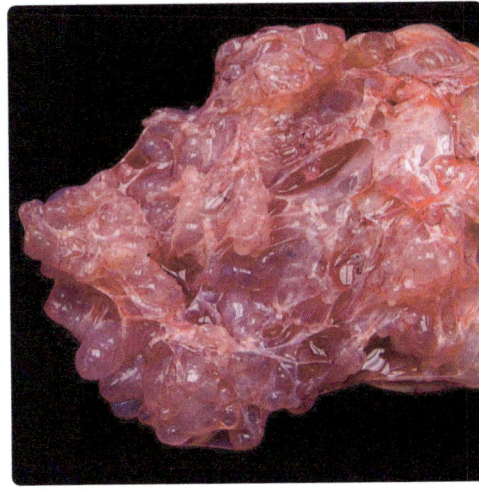

(Left) Massive parallel sequencing (NGS) detects a codon 600 BRAF mutation (V600E) in this serous borderline tumor. This mutation is more common in borderline tumors than in low-grade serous carcinomas. (Right) Gross photograph shows a serous cystadenoma. Note the multiloculated nature of this cystic neoplasm. Each cystic space is lined by a smooth cyst wall without nodular, papillary, or solid areas. These cysts are frequently filled with clear serous fluid.

Serous Borderline Tumor

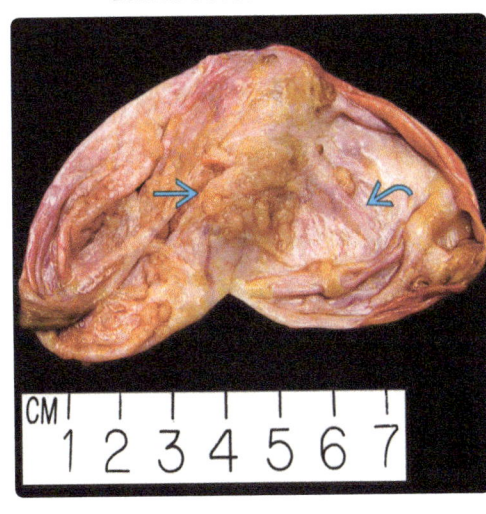

High-Grade Serous Carcinoma

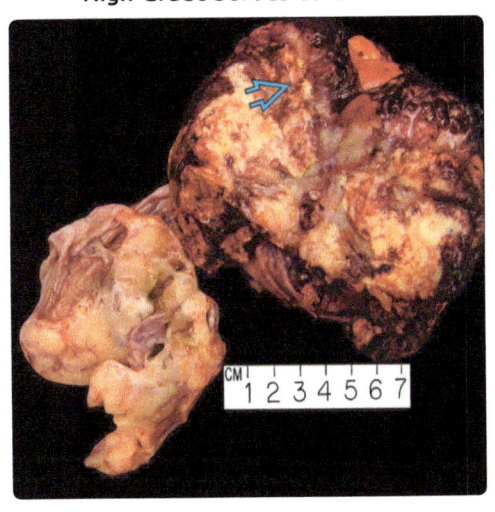

(Left) Gross photograph shows a serous borderline tumor. Note the cystic nature of the tumor where the cyst lining is predominantly smooth ➡ with foci of papillary growth ➡. Thorough sampling of these papillary areas is important to demonstrate the complex papillary architecture characteristic of serous borderline tumors and to rule out areas of stromal invasion. (Right) Gross photograph shows a high-grade serous carcinoma. Note the solid, necrotic, and hemorrhagic appearance ➡.

767

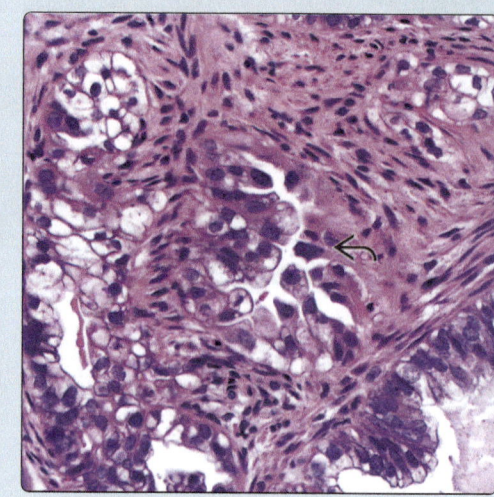

Other Surface Epithelial Tumors of Ovary

KEY FACTS

TERMINOLOGY
- Benign tumors
- Borderline tumors
- Malignant tumors
- WHO 5th edition classification (2020)
  - Mucinous tumors
  - Endometrioid tumors
  - Clear cell tumors
  - Seromucinous tumors
  - Brenner tumors
  - Other carcinomas
    - Mesonephric-like carcinoma
    - Undifferentiated and dedifferentiated carcinoma
    - Carcinosarcoma
    - Mixed carcinoma

ETIOLOGY/PATHOGENESIS
- Mucinous tumors
  - Possible germ cell origin in tumors associated with teratomas or epithelial origin in tumors associated with Brenner tumors
- Endometriosis-associated tumors
  - Endometrioid tumors and clear cell tumors most common
- Brenner tumors
  - Possibly Walthard rests or germ cell origin
- Lynch syndrome
  - Accounts for 6-12% of epithelial ovarian cancers
  - Most common histologic subtypes include
    - Endometrioid and clear cell carcinoma
  - Autosomal dominant tumor syndrome
  - Results in microsatellite instability and increased cancer risk

CLINICAL ISSUES
- Borderline tumors
  - Salpingo-oophorectomy with peritoneal washing, peritoneal biopsies, and possibly omentectomy
  - Chemotherapy has not been proven to significantly improve survival in advanced stage or microinvasive borderline tumors
- Malignant tumors
  - Surgical tumor debulking, staging, and chemotherapy
- Borderline tumors
  - Stage I tumors: > 95% survival
- Malignant tumors
  - Most patients with advanced-stage disease die of disease
  - Clear cell carcinomas characterized by poor responsiveness to platinum-based chemotherapy

MOLECULAR
- Mucinous carcinoma
  - *KRAS* mutations in up to 75%
  - *ERBB2* (HER2) amplification reported in ~ 15-26%
  - Copy number loss of *CDKN2A* in ~ 76%
  - *TP53* mutations in ~ 64%
- Endometrioid carcinoma
  - Mutations in *ARID1A* detected in ~ 30%
  - *CTNNB1* mutations result in β-catenin-mediated signaling deregulation in 53%
  - *PTEN* mutations in ~ 17%
  - *PIK3CA*-activating mutations in ~ 40%
  - *KRAS* mutations in ~ 33%
  - *TP53* mutations in up to 9-13%
  - MMR deficiency in 13%
- Clear cell carcinoma
  - *ARID1A* mutations in 46-57%
  - *PIK3CA*-activating mutations in ~ 40%
  - Associated with Lynch syndrome
    - Germline mutations in *MSH2*
- Malignant Brenner tumor
  - Alterations in *CDKN2A* reported
- Undifferentiated carcinoma
  - Deficient mismatch repair proteins in 50%
  - *ARID1A/ARID1B*, *SMARCA2/SMARCA4*, and *SMARCB1* inactivation

Borderline Endometrioid Tumor

Clear Cell Carcinoma

(Left) Borderline endometrioid tumor shows a complex architecture with papillary projections ⊞ and < 5-mm foci of complex glandular crowding without intervening stroma ⊞. (Right) Clear cell carcinoma shows invasive pleomorphic cells with hyperchromatic apical nuclei with nuclear hobnailing ⊞ without significant mitotic figures despite the high nuclear grade.

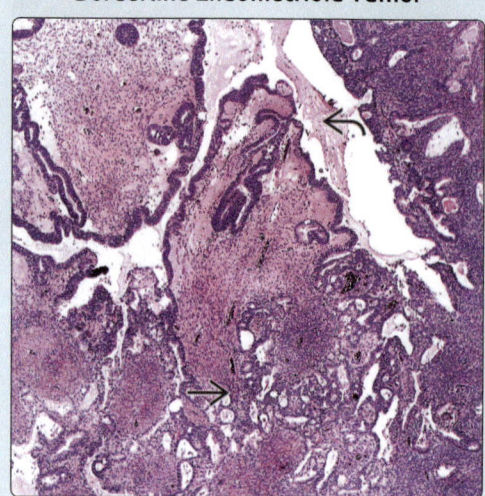

Other Surface Epithelial Tumors of Ovary

TERMINOLOGY

Definitions
- **Benign tumors**
  - Cystadenomas, adenofibromas
- **Borderline tumors**
  - Proliferative atypical lining epithelium with complex architecture
  - Absent stromal invasion
- **Malignant tumors**
  - Invasion into surrounding stroma
- **WHO classification of tumors (5th edition)**
  - Mucinous tumors
  - Endometrioid tumors
  - Clear cell tumors
  - Brenner tumors
  - Seromucinous tumors
  - Other carcinomas
    - Mesonephric-like carcinoma
    - Undifferentiated/dedifferentiated carcinoma
    - Carcinosarcoma

ETIOLOGY/PATHOGENESIS

Mucinous Tumors
- Possible germ cell origin in tumors associated with dermoid cysts/teratomas
- Possible epithelial origin in tumors associated with Brenner tumors

Endometriosis-Associated Tumors
- Endometrioid tumor
- Clear cell tumors
- Seromucinous tumors
- Mesonephric-like carcinoma

Brenner Tumors
- May be associated with Walthard nests
- Possible germ cell origin in rare cases associated with dermoid cysts/teratomas

Lynch Syndrome
- Accounts for 6-12% of epithelial ovarian cancers
- Women with Lynch syndrome (LS) have 6-12% cumulative lifetime risk of developing ovarian cancer
- Most common histologic subtypes
  - ~ 65% are nonserous epithelial carcinomas
    - Endometrioid and clear cell carcinomas contribute to ~ 67% of *MSH6*-mutated tumors than in *MLH1/MSH2*-mutated tumors (44%)
- Autosomal dominant tumor syndrome
  - Germline mutation in one of DNA mismatch repair (MMR) genes (*MLH1, PMS2, MSH2, MSH6*)
  - Results in microsatellite instability (MSI) and ↑ cancer risk
- Ovarian cancer preceded diagnosis of other LS-related synchronous &/or metachronous (extraovarian) cancers in majority of cases

Undifferentiated/Dedifferentiated Carcinoma
- Association with low-grade endometrioid carcinoma in dedifferentiated tumors suggest origin from endometrioid carcinoma

Carcinosarcoma
- Common monoclonal epithelial cell (likely serous) origin for both epithelial and sarcomatous components

CLINICAL ISSUES

Epidemiology
- **Mucinous tumors**
  - Benign mucinous tumors
    - 80% of all ovarian mucinous tumors
  - Mucinous borderline tumor
    - 2nd most common borderline tumor in Western world (30-50%) and most common in Asia (70%)
  - Mucinous carcinoma
    - 3-4% of all primary epithelial carcinomas of ovary
- **Endometrioid tumors**
  - Benign endometrioid tumors
    - Most likely represent endometriotic cysts in which stromal component is not distinct
  - Endometrioid borderline tumor
    - Concomitant endometrial hyperplasia or endometrial endometrioid carcinoma in 39% of reported cases
  - Endometrioid carcinoma
    - ~ 10% of ovarian epithelial carcinomas
    - Most arise in endometriosis (~ 85-90%)
- **Clear cell tumors**
  - Clear cell borderline tumor
    - < 1% of all borderline tumors
  - Clear cell carcinoma
    - Arises from ovarian endometriosis in up to 70% of cases
- **Brenner tumors**
  - Benign Brenner tumor
    - ~ 5% of benign epithelial tumors of ovary
    - ~ 95% of Brenner tumors
  - Malignant Brenner tumor
    - < 5% of Brenner tumors
- **Seromucinous tumors**
  - Benign seromucinous tumors
    - Rare
  - Seromucinous borderline tumor
    - Uncommon
    - 31-35% associated with endometriosis
- **Other carcinomas**
  - Carcinosarcoma
    - ~ 2% of ovarian cancer

Presentation
- **Benign tumors**
  - Usually incidental unilateral pelvic mass
  - Pain secondary to torsion or bleeding into underlying endometriotic cyst
- **Borderline tumors**
  - Most commonly unilateral mass confined to ovary
- **Malignant tumors**
  - Abdominal distension and pain
  - Clear cell carcinomas
    - Pelvic endometriosis
    - Paraneoplastic hypercalcemia
    - Venous thromboembolism

Other Surface Epithelial Tumors of Ovary

Treatment
- **Benign tumors**
  - Simple cystectomy or unilateral salpingo-oophorectomy
- **Borderline tumors**
  - Salpingo-oophorectomy with peritoneal washing, peritoneal biopsies, and possibly omentectomy
  - Chemotherapy has not been proven to significantly improve survival in advanced stage or microinvasive borderline tumors
- **Malignant tumors**
  - Surgical tumor debulking (cytoreductive surgery) and staging
  - Chemotherapy
    - Platinum-based chemotherapeutic regimen for advanced-stage disease

Prognosis
- **Benign tumors**
  - Excellent prognosis with adequate surgical excision
- **Borderline tumors**
  - Stage I tumors > 95% survival
- **Malignant tumors**
  - Favorable prognosis in early FIGO stage I disease
  - Most patients with advanced-stage disease die of disease
  - Carcinosarcoma and undifferentiated carcinoma are characteristically clinically aggressive and present with advanced stage
  - Mesonephric-like carcinoma behaves aggressively and presents with advanced stage
  - Depending on type of carcinoma, confluent pattern of invasion is associated with better prognosis than destructive stromal pattern of invasion
  - Recurrence usually occurs early with development of chemoresistance
  - Clear cell carcinomas are characterized by poor responsiveness to platinum-based chemotherapy

MACROSCOPIC

Benign Tumors
- Unilateral (> 95% of cases) with smooth outer surface
- Cystic unless solid adenofibromatous component present

Borderline Tumors
- Usually unilateral, can be up to 50 cm
- Usually smooth outer surface with solid or friable papillary excrescences or solid mural nodules
- Thorough sampling (especially in mucinous tumors) essential to exclude stromal invasion

Malignant Tumors
- Usually unilateral, large with complex solid and cystic masses, friable papillary excrescences
- Rupture common ± surface involvement

MOLECULAR

Mucinous Tumors
- *KRAS* mutations detected in all types of mucinous tumors
- Benign mucinous tumors
  - *KRAS* mutations reported in subset of cases
- Mucinous borderline tumor
  - *KRAS* mutations reported in 30-75% of cases
  - Less commonly *TP53* mutations
- Mucinous carcinoma
  - Copy number loss of *CDKN2A* in ~ 76% of cases
  - *KRAS* mutations in ~ 64% of cases
  - *TP53* mutations in ~ 64%
  - *ERBB2* (HER2) gene amplification reported in ~ 15-26% of cases
    - Occurs almost exclusively in association with *TP53* mutations
    - *KRAS* mutations usually absent in *ERBB2*-amplified cases

Endometrioid Tumors
- Endometrioid carcinoma
  - WNT/β-catenin signaling pathway
    - Most common molecular alterations
    - *CTNNB1* mutations
      - Result in β-catenin-mediated signaling deregulation in 53% of endometrioid carcinomas
      - Present in ~ 90% of endometrioid borderline tumors
  - PI3K pathway
    - *PIK3CA*-activating mutations in ~ 40%
    - *PTEN* mutations in ~ 17%
      - *PTEN* and *PIK3CA* mutations often coexist
  - MAPK pathway
    - *KRAS* mutations in ~ 33%
  - SWI/SNF pathway
    - Mutations in *ARID1A* in ~ 30%
  - Molecular subtypes analogous to endometrial endometrioid carcinoma by The Cancer Genome Atlas (TCGA)
    - Hypermutated due to mismatch repair deficiency (~ 13%)
      - Lower incidence of *MLH1* hypermethylated tumors compared to endometrial endometrioid carcinoma
    - Hypermutated due to *POLE* exonuclease domain mutations (5%)
    - *TP53* mutation (~ 9-13%)
      - Uncommon in tumors with mutations in WNT/β-catenin &/or PI3K signaling pathways
      - Associated with higher histologic grade
    - No specific molecular profile (69-73%)

Clear Cell Tumors
- Clear cell carcinoma
  - *ARID1A* loss-of-function mutations in ~ 46-57%
    - Also detected in borderline tumors
  - *PIK3CA*-activating mutations in ~ 40%
    - Can occur with *ARID1A* loss
  - Associated with LS
    - Germline mutations in *MSH2* most common
  - *TERT* promoter mutations in 16%
  - *KRAS* mutations in 10%
  - *TP53* mutations in < 10%

Brenner Tumors
- Borderline malignant Brenner tumor
  - Alterations in *CDKN2A* reported with loss of p16 expression by immunohistochemistry

Other Surface Epithelial Tumors of Ovary

- ○ *KRAS* mutations
- ○ *PIK3CA* mutations
- ○ *MDM2* mutations

Seromucinous Borderline Tumor
- *ARID1A* mutations in 30%
- *KRAS* mutations in 69%

Undifferentiated Carcinoma
- SWI/SNF pathway
  - ○ *ARID1A/ARID1B*, *SMARCA2/SMARCA4*, and *SMARCB1* inactivation
- Deficient MMR proteins in ~ 50% of cases

Mesonephric-Like Carcinoma
- Tumors associated with serous borderline tumors or low-grade serous carcinomas show common genetic alterations in *KRAS* or *NRAS*
- *PIK3CA* mutations have been described

Carcinosarcoma
- *TP53* mutations
- Amplification of chromosomal segments containing *PIK3CA*, *CCNE1*, *TERT*, and *MYC*
- Other reported gene mutations/amplifications include *CDKN1B*, *CTNNB1*, *FBXW7*, *PPP2R1A*, *BCOR*, and *CDH4*

MICROSCOPIC

Histologic Features
- **Mucinous tumors**
  - ○ Benign mucinous tumors
    - Lined by bland, nonstratified gastrointestinal-type or müllerian-type mucinous epithelium
    - Associated dermoid cysts or Brenner tumors in 10%
  - ○ Mucinous borderline tumor
    - Glands lined by mild to moderately atypical gastrointestinal-type mucinous cells
    - Variable nuclear stratification, tufting, or filiform papillae
    - Mitotic figures easily detected
    - If associated with teratoma, prominent mucin extravasation in ovarian stroma and peritoneum can occur
    - Mucin granulomas
    - Intraepithelial carcinoma
      □ Highly atypical nuclei with vesicular chromatin, prominent nucleoli, and loss of polarity
      □ High N:C ratio with mucin depletion
      □ Increased mitotic activity with apical mitotic figures
    - Microinvasion
      □ Single cells or small clusters < 5 mm in greatest extent with same degree of atypia as rest of tumor
    - Mural nodules
      □ Sarcoma-like: Relatively noninfiltrative, mitotically spindled and epithelioid, mononuclear stromal proliferation with exuberant histiocytic, inflammatory cells and multinucleated, Epulis-type giant cells
      □ Sarcomatous: Rare, infiltrative, most commonly rhabdomyosarcomatous or leiomyosarcomatous
      □ Anaplastic carcinoma: Infiltrative proliferation of variably shaped, mitotically active, highly atypical cells with rhabdoid/spindle or pleomorphic morphology
  - ○ Mucinous carcinoma
    - Invasive, highly atypical gastrointestinal-type mucinous cells
    - Confluent glandular expansile pattern of invasion with markedly crowded glands with little intervening stroma
    - Less commonly, destructive stromal invasive pattern with prominent desmoplastic reaction
- **Endometrioid tumors**
  - ○ Benign endometrioid tumors
    - Lined by bland endometrioid epithelial cells without underlying stroma
    - Usually develop in association with endometriotic cyst
    - Squamous morules and calcifications may be present
  - ○ Endometrioid borderline tumor
    - Crowded, irregular glands with mild to moderate atypia (reminiscent of atypical endometrial hyperplasia) with lobular architecture in background adenofibromatous stroma
  - ○ Endometrioid carcinoma
    - Invasive, highly atypical endometrial cells
    - Resembles endometrioid carcinoma of uterus with cribriforming/papillary formation
    - Expansile pattern of invasion characterized by back-to-back glands without intervening stroma > 5 mm
    - Less commonly, destructive stromal invasion
    - Squamous and mucinous differentiation and clear cell/secretory change can occur
    - Sex cord-stromal-type pattern may occur
    - Seromucinous carcinoma
      □ Mixed müllerian type epithelial lining, predominantly serous and endocervical-type mucinous epithelium, foci containing clear cells with areas of endometrioid with squamous differentiation
- **Clear cell tumors**
  - ○ Benign clear cell tumors
    - Consist of glands or cystic spaces lined by bland, cuboidal to flattened cells with clear cytoplasm widely spaced in fibrous stroma
  - ○ Clear cell borderline tumor
    - Crowded glands or cysts lined by atypical clear cells
  - ○ **Clear cell carcinoma**
    - Invasive, uniformly atypical cells with areas of nuclear pleomorphism
    - Clear or eosinophilic cytoplasm
    - Hyperchromatic apical nuclei (nuclear hobnailing)
    - Tubulocystic, papillary with hyalinized cores, or solid architecture
    - Mitotic figures are uncommon
- **Brenner tumors**
  - ○ Benign Brenner tumor
    - Solid or hollow nests of bland, urothelial-type epithelium filled with mucinous or eosinophilic secretions
    - Dense, fibrous stroma
    - Ovoid nuclei that may show longitudinal grooves

Other Surface Epithelial Tumors of Ovary

- Borderline Brenner tumor
  - Displays more urothelial-type epithelial noninvasive papillary proliferation with larger epithelial nests than those seen in benign Brenner tumor
  - Less intervening stroma
- Malignant Brenner tumor
  - Invasive, highly atypical, mitotically active, urothelial-like cells
  - Resembles urothelial carcinoma of urinary bladder
  - Often benign or borderline Brenner component present nearby
  - Mucinous glandular component or, less commonly, invasive mucinous carcinoma may coexist
- **Seromucinous tumors**
  - Benign seromucinous tumors
    - Ciliated serous, low cuboidal, hobnail, nondescript eosinophilic cells and endocervical-type mucinous epithelial cell lining cells
  - Borderline seromucinous tumor
    - Proliferative atypical epithelial cells
    - Complex architecture with broad edematous papillae
- **Undifferentiated carcinoma**
  - Highly pleomorphic, often noncohesive cells
  - No specific differentiation characteristic of any müllerian cell type
  - Areas of geographic necrosis common
- **Mesonephric-like carcinoma**
  - Tubular, glandular (pseudoendometrioid), ductal with slit-like angulated glands, papillary and solid patterns
  - Nuclei with dense or vesicular chromatin with inconspicuous nucleoli and nuclear overlap
- **Carcinosarcoma**
  - High-grade carcinomatous epithelial (most commonly serous) and sarcomatous stromal components
  - Heterologous elements (rhabdomyosarcoma, chondrosarcoma, or osteosarcoma) may be present

ANCILLARY TESTS

Immunohistochemistry

- **Mucinous tumors**
  - Positive markers include CK 7, PAX8, CK20, and CDX2 in ~ 40%; SATB2 positive in teratoma-associated tumors
  - Mural nodules
    - Cytokeratins show variable positivity in sarcoma-like and anaplastic carcinoma nodules and are negative in sarcomatous nodules
    - CD68 highlights histiocytes and giant cells present in abundance in sarcoma-like nodules
    - Anaplastic carcinoma
      - Loss of expression of SWI/SNF signaling pathway proteins has recently been described
      - Claudin-4 positivity detected in ~ 40%
    - p53 is typically negative
    - Other negative markers include WT1, napsin A, ER, PR, and vimentin
- **Endometrioid tumors**
  - Positive markers include ER and PR in ~ 85%, vimentin, PAX8 in ~ 85%
  - p53 usually shows wildtype expression; can be mutant in up to 15% of cases, associated with high histologic grade
  - Negative markers include WT1, napsin A, CDX2, and SATB2
- **Clear cell tumors**
  - Positive markers include PAX8, napsin A, and HNF-1β (not specific)
  - Negative markers include WT1, ER, and PR (can be positive in 5-7%)
  - p53 negative in majority of the cases
- **Brenner tumors**
  - Positive markers include TP63, GATA3, uroplakin, thrombomodulin (more commonly positive in benign and borderline tumors than in malignant tumors), and CK7; CK20 variable
  - Negative markers include PAX8, WT1, and ER/PR (may be focal positive)
  - p53 negative
- **Mesonephric-like carcinoma**
  - Positive markers include GATA3, TTF-1, CD10 (luminal), and PAX8
  - Negative markers include ER/PR and WT1
  - p53 negative
- **Undifferentiated/dedifferentiated carcinoma**
  - Loss of SMARCA4 (BRG-1) and SMARCB1 (INI-1)
  - Only focal EMA and pancytokeratin positivity
  - Negative markers include PAX8 (can be only focal positive), ER/PR, and WT1
  - p53 negative
- **Mismatch repair (MMR) protein expression**
  - MLH1, PMS2, MLH-2, and MLH-6
  - Used as screening tool for LS as well as for eligibility for immunotherapy

Molecular Testing

- MLH-1 hypermethylation testing
  - Should be performed in all cases with with MMR protein loss to separate sporadic tumors from potential LS
  - MMR gene mutational analysis testing for *MLH1* promoter region unmethylated tumors

DIFFERENTIAL DIAGNOSIS

Metastatic Mucinous Carcinomas to Ovary

- Usually bilateral with destructive invasion, ovarian surface and extraovarian involvement

Metastasis From Uterine Endometrial Endometrioid Carcinoma

- Findings favoring metastasis of endometrial endometrioid carcinoma to ovary include
  - Large, deeply invasive tumor in uterus in background of complex atypical hyperplasia
  - Positive lymphovascular invasion

SELECTED REFERENCES

1. Ran X et al: The clinical features and management of Lynch syndrome-associated ovarian cancer. J Obstet Gynaecol Res. 48(7):1538-45, 2022
2. Talia KL et al: Ovarian mucinous and seromucinous neoplasms: problematic aspects and modern diagnostic approach. Histopathology. 80(2):255-78, 2022
3. WHO Classification of Tumors Editorial Board: WHO Classification of Tumours: Female Genital Tumours. 5th ed. IARC Press. 2020

Other Surface Epithelial Tumors of Ovary

Benign Brenner Tumor

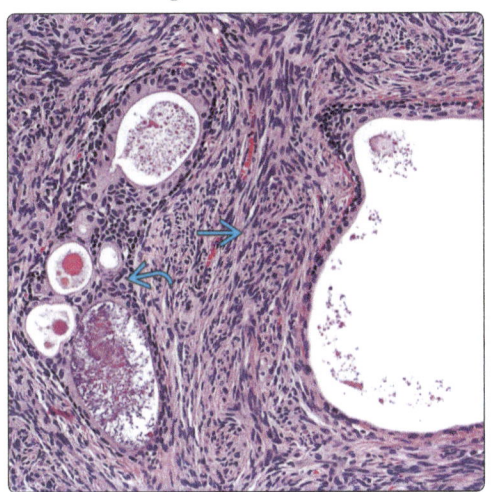

Malignant Brenner Tumor

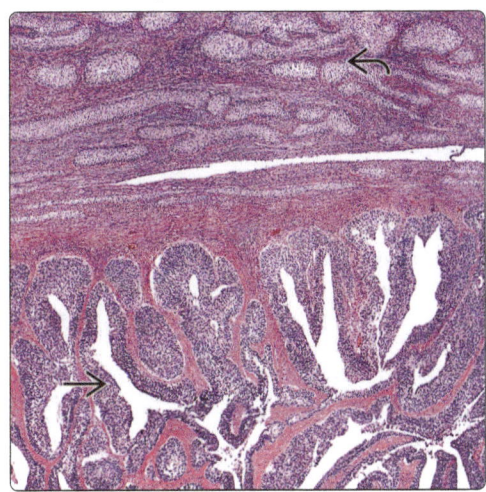

(Left) Benign Brenner tumor shows nests of bland, urothelial-type cells filled with mucinous and eosinophilic secretions ⇨. These nests are typically embedded in abundant dense, fibrous stroma ⇨. (Right) Malignant Brenner tumor shows papillary, urothelial-like projections ⇨ adjacent to the borderline Brenner area with crowded urothelial nests embedded in dense, fibrous stroma ⇨. GATA3 was positive and WT1 was negative.

Carcinosarcoma

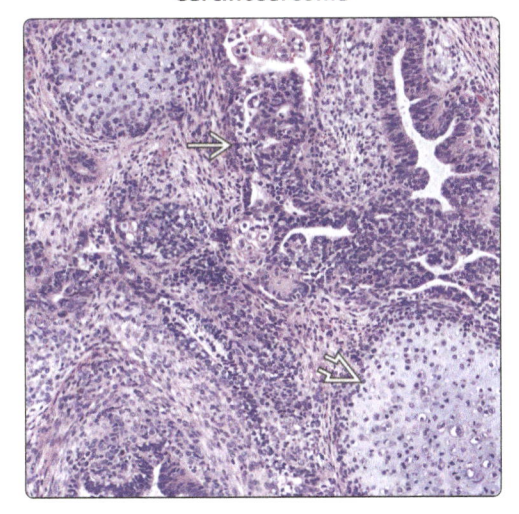

Mesonephric-Like Carcinoma

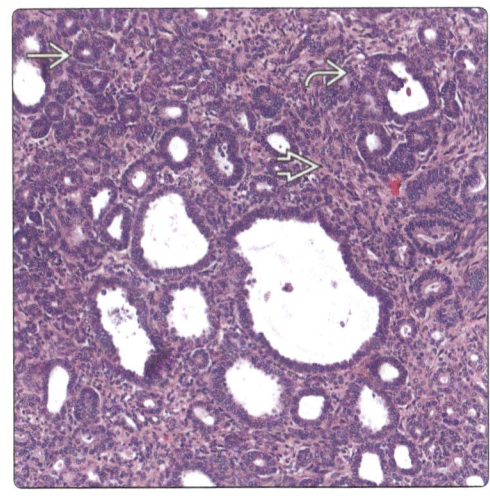

(Left) Note the biphasic nature of this tumor. The carcinoma component is usually high grade with serous carcinoma being most common ⇨. The sarcomatous component shows heterologous elements in the form of chondrosarcoma ⇨. (Right) Note the heterogeneous morphology of this tumor with areas of tubule formation ⇨ and gland formation ⇨ admixed with spindled tumor cells ⇨. ER was negative and p53 showed no significant expression.

Mucinous Carcinoma

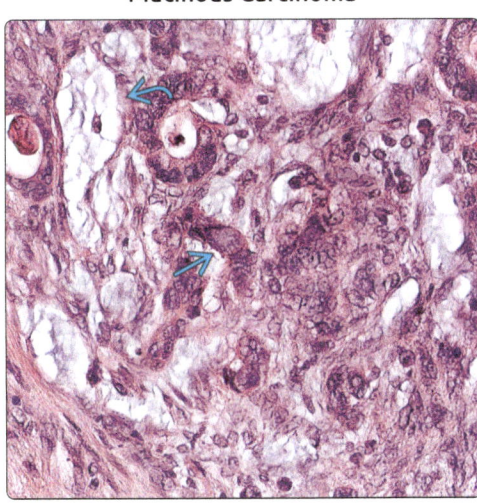

Mucinous Borderline Tumor

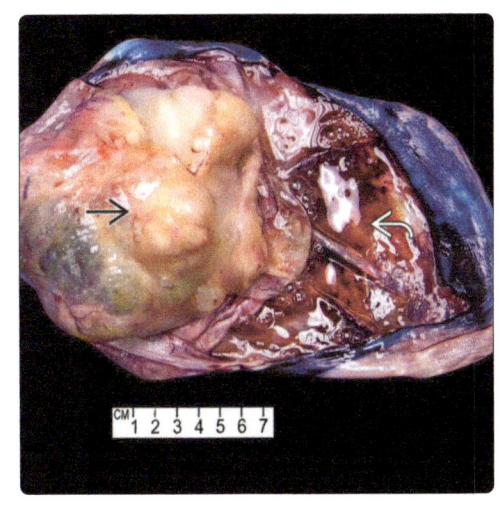

(Left) Pleomorphic gastrointestinal-type mucinous cells with goblet cells ⇨ and mucin pools ⇨ are present in this mucinous carcinoma. Mucinous carcinoma may show a confluent glandular, expansile pattern with markedly crowded glands and little intervening stroma or a destructive stromal invasive pattern with prominent desmoplastic reaction. (Right) Gross photograph shows a mucinous borderline tumor with complex solid ⇨ and cystic ⇨ areas.

773

Sex Cord-Stromal Tumors of Ovary

KEY FACTS

TERMINOLOGY

- Sex cord-stromal tumor (SCST): Ovarian tumors composed of different cell types, singly or in variable combinations, at variable degrees of differentiation
  - Granulosa cells, fibroblasts, theca cells and their luteinized variants, Sertoli cells, Leydig cells

CLINICAL ISSUES

- **Adult granulosa cell tumor**
  - Concurrent endometrial hyperplasia in 1/3 of cases and, rarely, endometrial endometrioid adenocarcinoma
- **Juvenile granulosa cell tumor**
  - Associated with Ollier disease (enchondromatosis) and Maffucci syndrome (enchondromatosis and hemangiomatosis)
- **Sex cord tumor with annular tubules**
  - Associated with Peutz-Jeghers syndrome, commonly bilateral
- **Sertoli-Leydig cell tumor**
  - These hereditary cases are associated with *DICER1* syndrome

MOLECULAR

- **Microcystic stromal tumor**
  - *CTNNB1* mutation
  - *APC* mutation
- **Adult granulosa cell tumor**
  - *FOXL2* mutation c.402C>G mutation (p.Cys134Trp) detected in almost all tumors (~ 97%)
- **Juvenile granulosa cell tumor**
  - *GNAS* mutations (30%)
  - *AKT1* mutation (60%)
  - *IDH1/IDH2* mutations in tumors associated with Ollier disease and Maffucci syndrome
- **SCST with annular tubules**
  - Germline mutations in *STK11*
- **Sertoli-Leydig cell tumors**
  - 3 molecular subtypes
    - *DICER1* mutant (majority of cases)
    - *FOXL2* mutant (0-22%)
    - *DICER1/FOXL2* wildtype

ANCILLARY TESTS

- Most SCST positive for at least 1 sex cord marker, including inhibin, calretinin, SF1
- Reticulin surrounds individual tumor cells in thecoma
- Most SCST negative for EMA
- **Microcystic stromal tumor**
  - Positive for diffuse nuclear β-catenin, WT-1, cyclin-D1, and SF1
- **Adult granulosa cell tumor**
  - Positive for inhibin, calretinin, FOXL2, SF1, WT1 pancytokeratin, and ER
  - Less commonly positive for SMA, desmin, CD99, and CD10
  - Negative for EMA, PAX8, CK7, and CK5/6
- **Juvenile granulosa cell tumor**
  - Positive for inhibin, calretinin, SF1, CD56, CD99, and low-molecular-weight keratins
  - Variably positive for FOXL2 (without associated mutation)
  - Majority negative for EMA and CK5/6
- **SCST with annular tubules**
  - Positive for FOXL2, SF1, WT1, CD56, and broad-spectrum keratins
- **Sertoli-Leydig cell tumors**
  - Positive for inhibin, calretinin, DICER1, vimentin, pancytokeratin, SF1, WT1, and CD56, and 50% express CD99 (Sertoli cells only) and FOXL2
    - Retiform and poorly differentiated tumors likely to be negative
  - Heterologous elements show immunohistochemical expression that reflects their cell of origin

---

Adult Granulosa Cell Tumor Morphology

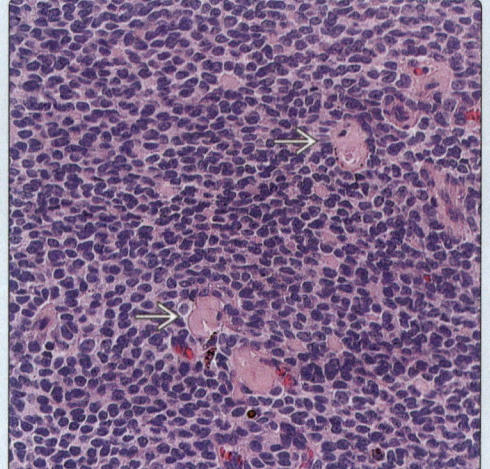

Grooved Nuclei

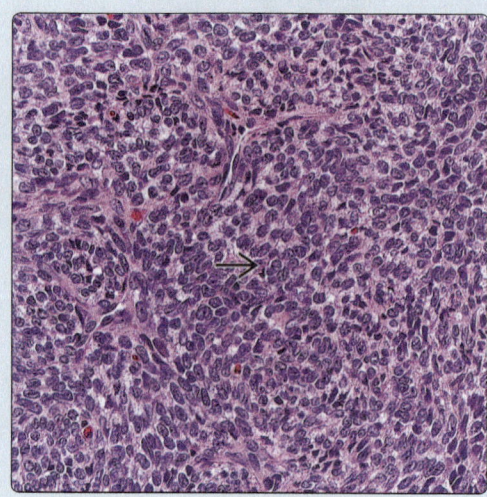

(Left) Adult granulosa cell tumor (AGCT) grows in a variety of patterns. The microfollicular pattern (most common) is depicted with Call-Exner bodies filled with eosinophilic material ➡. (Right) Neoplastic cells in this case of AGCT show scant cytoplasm and low-grade, round to ovoid nuclei with longitudinal nuclear grooves ➡. Mitotic activity rarely exceeds 1-2 per 10 HPF.

Sex Cord-Stromal Tumors of Ovary

TERMINOLOGY

Abbreviations

- Sex cord-stromal tumor (SCST)
  - Adult granulosa cell tumor (AGCT)
  - Juvenile granulosa cell tumor (JGCT)
  - Sertoli-Leydig cell tumor (SLCT)

World Health Organization Classification (5th Edition)

- Pure stromal tumors
  - Fibroma, not otherwise specified (NOS)
  - Thecoma, NOS
  - Luteinized thecoma associated with sclerosing peritonitis
  - Sclerosing stromal tumor
  - Signet ring stromal tumor
  - Microcystic stromal tumor
  - Leydig cell tumor, NOS
  - Steroid cell tumors
  - Fibrosarcoma, NOS
- Pure sex cord tumors
  - AGCT
  - JGCT
  - Sertoli cell tumor, NOS
  - Sex cord tumor with annular tubules (SCTAT)
- Mixed SCSTs
  - SLCT, NOS
  - SCSTs, NOS
  - Gynandroblastoma

CLINICAL ISSUES

Epidemiology

- Incidence
  - SCST accounts for 8% of all ovarian tumors
- Fibroma
  - Most common pure ovarian stromal tumor
  - Occurs in 75% of patients with nevoid basal cell carcinoma syndrome (Gorlin syndrome)
- AGCT
  - Most common SCST
  - Wide age range but most common in perimenopausal women
- JGCT
  - Accounts for 5% of all granulosa cell tumors
  - Most common during first 3 decades of life
- SLCT
  - < 0.5% of ovarian neoplasms
  - Mean age: 25 years
  - Retiform pattern or germline DICER1 mutation present at younger age
- Microcystic stromal tumor
  - May rarely present as extracolonic manifestation of familial adenomatous polyposis syndrome

Presentation

- Fibroma
  - Bilateral if associated with Gorlin syndrome
  - Ascites and pleural effusion (Meigs syndrome) in 1% of cases
- Thecoma
  - Unilateral mass in majority of cases
  - Commonly estrogenic
    - Patients may have hormone-related changes, most commonly endometrial proliferative lesions
  - Luteinized thecoma
    - Associated with sclerosing peritonitis
    - Bilateral
    - Premenopausal women
- Leydig cell tumor and steroid cell tumor
  - Most commonly, unilateral mass with androgenic manifestations
    - Steroid cell tumor may be associated with estrogenic symptoms in 10% of cases, Cushing syndrome, or, occasionally, von Hippel-Lindau syndrome
- AGCT
  - Unilateral abdominal mass with ascites in 10% of cases (hemoperitoneum and rupture)
  - Can occur at any age but most common in perimenopausal women who present with menstrual irregularities, or postmenopausal women who present with bleeding
    - Concurrent endometrial hyperplasia in 1/3 of cases and, rarely, endometrial endometrioid adenocarcinoma
  - JGCT
    - Associated with Ollier disease (enchondromatosis) and Maffucci syndrome (enchondromatosis and hemangiomatosis)
    - Most common in young women
    - Estrogenic manifestation in form of menstrual irregularities and precocious puberty in prepubertal girls
- Sex cord tumor with annular tubules
  - Associated with Peutz-Jeghers syndrome, commonly bilateral
- SLCT
  - Androgenic manifestations in majority of patients; may present with ascites or ruptured tumor masses
  - These hereditary cases may also have familial multinodular goiter and other rare tumors, e.g., cervical rhabdomyosarcoma, and other tumors of kidney, thyroid, ovary, cervix, testicle, brain, eye, and lining of lung (DICER1 syndrome)

Treatment

- Granulosa cell tumor
  - Unilateral salpingo-oophorectomy (in younger women desiring fertility, cystectomy should be avoided)
  - Total hysterectomy with bilateral salpingo-oophorectomy (in menopausal or postmenopausal women)
  - Adjuvant chemotherapy
    - Advanced-stage disease
    - Ruptured or recurrent tumors (following aggressive cytoreductive surgery)
- SLCT
  - Unilateral salpingo-oophorectomy in younger women desiring fertility
  - Total hysterectomy with bilateral salpingo-oophorectomy in menopausal or postmenopausal women

Sex Cord-Stromal Tumors of Ovary

- Adjuvant chemotherapy indicated in
  - Poorly differentiated tumors
  - Tumors with mesenchymal heterologous elements
  - Ruptured tumors of intermediate differentiation
  - Tumors with any degree of differentiation presenting at advanced clinical stage or with recurrence (following aggressive cytoreductive surgery)

Prognosis

- **Fibroma**
  - Mostly benign
  - Cellular variants may rupture or present with extraovarian involvement with increased risk of recurrence
- **Thecoma**
  - Almost always benign
- **Fibrosarcoma**
  - Poor prognosis secondary to aggressive behavior
- **Steroid cell tumor**
  - Malignant behavior seen in 1/3 of cases
- **Granulosa cell tumors**
  - Tumor stage is most important prognostic factor
    - 90% of patients present at stage I with > 90% survival rate
    - Survival drops to 60% for similar stage with ruptured tumors
  - 10-30% develop recurrences
    - As late as 20-30 years
    - Associated with poor prognosis (> 80% of patients typically die of disease)
    - Present with disseminated peritoneal metastasis
- **Sex cord tumor with annular tubules**
  - Benign course if associated with Peutz-Jeghers syndrome
  - Non-Peutz-Jeghers syndrome-related tumors show low-grade malignant course with incidence of extraovarian involvement in 20% of patients
- **SLCT**
  - Impact of histologic grade on prognosis
    - Poorly differentiated tumors are malignant and recur in peritoneal cavity within 2 years
    - ~ 10% of moderately differentiated tumors exhibit malignant behavior
  - Tumors with retiform pattern
    - Associated with adverse effect in early stage or well- to moderately differentiated SLCT
    - ~ 25% of stage I moderately differentiated SLCT with retiform pattern behave in malignant fashion as opposed to only 10% without retiform pattern
  - Other poor prognostic factors
    - Presence of heterologous elements
    - Clinical stage II and higher

MACROSCOPIC

General Features

- Usually solid
- Steroid cell content or degree of luteinization usually reflected by yellow cut surface

MOLECULAR

Cytogenetics

- **Fibroma**
  - Trisomy &/or tetrasomy 12
- **Fibrosarcoma**
  - Trisomy 12 and 8
- **Sclerosing stromal tumor**
  - Trisomy 12
- **AGCT**
  - Trisomy 12 and 14
  - Monosomy 22 and 16
  - Deletion of 16q
- **JGCT**
  - Trisomy 12
- **SLCTs**
  - Trisomy 8, 6, and 12
  - Aberrations affecting sex chromosomes, chromosomal rearrangements of chromosomes 5 and 18

Chromosomal Microarray

- Loss of heterozygosity at 9q22.3 (*PTCH1*) and 19p13.3 (*STK11*) in cellular fibromas

Molecular Genetics

- **AGCT**
  - *FOXL2* mutations
    - c.402C>G mutation (p.Cys134Trp) detected in almost all tumors (~ 97%)
    - Sensitive and specific biomarker
    - Induces estrogenic manifestations
  - *TERT* promoter mutations
    - More frequent in recurrent tumors (64% vs. 26% in primary)
  - *TP53*, *MED12*, and *TET2* additionally reported in recurrent tumors only
- **JGCT**
  - *GNAS* mutations
    - Common mutations include R201C or R201H
    - Detected in 30% of cases
    - Associated with aggressive behavior in up to 77% of cases
  - *AKT1* mutation (60%)
  - *IDH1*/*IDH2* mutations
    - In tumors associated with Ollier disease and Maffucci syndrome
  - Rarely, germline *TP53*, *PTEN* and tuberous sclerosis, *DICER1* syndrome
- **SLCT**
  - 3 molecular subtypes
    - *DICER1* mutant
      - Detected in majority of cases
      - Present at younger age (1st-2nd decades)
      - Moderately/poorly differentiated histology
      - Can serve as relatively specific biomarker
      - Hotspot mutations in RNase IIIb domain of *DICER1*, resulting in global gene expression alteration and induction of androgenic symptoms
      - Also detected in other Sertoli cell tumors
      - 69% occur as germline mutation

Sex Cord-Stromal Tumors of Ovary

- Retiform differentiation and heterologous elements are highly predictive
  - *FOXL2* mutant
    - c.402C>G mutation (p.Cys134Trp)
    - Postmenopausal
    - Moderately/poorly differentiated histology
    - Less frequent (0-22%)
    - Estrogenic manifestations
    - Mutually exclusive of *DICER1* mutation
  - *DICER1/FOXL2* wildtype
    - Reproductive patient age
    - Includes all well-differentiated tumors
- **Microcystic stromal cell tumor**
  - WNT/β-catenin signaling pathway
    - *CTNNB1* mutations
      - Point mutation in codon 33 (S33C)
      - Aberrant nuclear immunoreactivity for β-catenin
    - *APC* mutation
      - Less frequent
      - Aberrant nuclear Cyclin-D1 expression
- **Sex cord tumor with annular tubules**
  - *STK11* mutations in 19p13.3
    - Germline mutations in tumors associated with Peutz-Jeghers syndrome
    - Detected in ~ 30% of cases
- **Sclerosing stromal tumor**
  - *FHL2::GLI2* fusion (65%)
- **Fibrosarcoma**
  - Case report with syndromic *DICER1* mutation
- **Gynandroblastoma**
  - Tumors with SLCT and JGCT
    - *DICER1* mutations
    - Likely represent pure SLCT with variant morphology
  - Tumors with mixed SCLT and AGCT
    - *FOXL2* wildtype
    - Different from pure AGCT

MICROSCOPIC

Histologic Features

- **Fibroma**
  - Spindled to ovoid nuclei with scant cytoplasm that may rarely contain hyaline globules
  - Arranged in intersecting bundles, occasionally with storiform appearance
  - Collagen bands or hyaline plaques
  - Mitotic figures are uncommon
  - Cellular (mitotically active) fibroma
    - ~ 10% of fibromas show increased stromal cellularity, sometimes associated with high mitotic activity with no or only mild nuclear atypia
    - Hemorrhage, infarction-type necrosis, and rupture of ovarian capsule may occur
  - Calcifications common in tumors associated with Gorlin syndrome
- **Thecoma**
  - Oval to round nuclei with pale pink (pale grayish) cytoplasm and ill-defined borders arranged in sheets
  - Little to no atypia with infrequent mitotic figures
  - Common hyaline plaques and calcifications
  - Prominent luteinization, spindled cells, and brisk mitotic activity characterize luteinized thecoma associated with sclerosing peritonitis
- **Fibrosarcoma**
  - Hypercellularity with prominent nuclear atypia (moderate to severe)
  - Increased mitotic figures (> 4/10 HPF)
  - Hemorrhage and necrosis
- **Sclerosing stromal tumor**
  - Pseudolobular architecture
  - Round and spindled cells arranged in cellular nodules with low mitotic activity
  - Background of hypocellular edematous or collagenous stroma
  - Thin, dilated (hemangiopericytoma-like) vessels
- **Signet-ring stromal tumor**
  - Signet-ring cells with eccentric nuclei and large cytoplasmic vacuoles in background reminiscent of cellular fibroma
- **Microcystic stromal tumor**
  - Variable amounts of microcysts mixed with solid cellular areas and collagenous stroma with occasional hyaline plaques
- **Leydig cell tumor**
  - Round nuclei with single prominent nucleoli and abundant lipid-rich cytoplasm with lipochrome pigments
  - Reinke crystals may be seen in cytoplasm (rod-shaped elongated eosinophilic inclusions) specific to Leydig cells
- **Steroid cell tumors**
  - Typically sheets of lipid-rich cells with intracytoplasmic lipochrome pigments
  - Nuclear atypia and increased mitotic activity in malignant types
  - Factors predicting malignant behavior
    - > 7 cm, increased mitotic activity, marked nuclear atypia, hemorrhage, and necrosis
- **AGCT**
  - Scant cytoplasm, longitudinal nuclear grooves (absent in luteinized tumors)
  - Low mitotic activity (rarely exceeds 1-2/10 HPF)
  - Luteinized variants acquire abundant pink cytoplasm and nuclei loose their characteristic grooves
  - Variety of architectural patterns (diffuse, insular, gyriform/watered silk, macrofollicular, sarcomatoid, and pseudopapillary)
    - Most characteristically microfollicular with Call-Exner bodies (dense eosinophilic secretions)
    - Diffuse pattern is most commonly encountered in clinical practice
    - Can be cystic
  - Less common histologic features include increased mitotic figures, bizarre nuclei, mucinous epithelium, hepatic differentiation, and minor component resembling JGCT
- **JGCT**
  - Macrofollicles filled with eosinophilic or basophilic fluid
  - Cytomegaly with bizarre nuclei and macronuclei
  - Absent nuclear grooves
  - Abundant mitotic figures
  - Occasional pseudopapillary architecture or extensive sclerosis

Sex Cord-Stromal Tumors of Ovary

- **Sertoli cell tumor**
  - Tubular growth pattern of cells
  - Small round nuclei with pink/pale cytoplasm
- **Sex cord tumor with annular tubules**
  - Nodules with annular tubules filled with eosinophilic hyaline material and lined by cells with antipodal nuclear arrangement in fibrous stroma
- **SLCT**
  - Well-differentiated tumors
    - Sertoli cell arranged in well-formed tubules
    - Delicate stroma displaying clusters or cords of Leydig cells
  - Moderately differentiated tumors
    - Sertoli cells in nested or solid tubular pattern punctuated by varying degrees of scattered, less well-formed hollow tubules
    - Leydig cells can be found in clusters at periphery or intermixed with other elements
    - Nuclear atypia may be prominent but of no prognostic value
    - Mitotic activity averages 5/10 HPF
  - Poorly differentiated tumors
    - Sarcomatoid stroma with primitive features
    - Brisk mitotic activity, up to 20/10 HPF
    - Minor, moderately differentiated component is usually present
  - Retiform tubules pattern
    - Anastomosing slit-like spaces resembling rete testis/ovarii
    - Not present in well-differentiated tumors
    - May be associated with slightly worse prognosis if detected in moderately differentiated or early-stage tumors
  - Heterologous elements (20% of cases)
    - Can be epithelial or mesenchymal (more common)
      - Benign enteric mucinous epithelium is most common (borderline or malignant features may be seen)
      - Carcinoid tumors rarely
      - Cartilage or skeletal muscle
    - In moderately or poorly differentiated tumors
- **Sex cord tumors, NOS**
  - No distinctive histologic features
  - Usually detected during pregnancy
- **Gynandroblastoma**
  - Mixture of female elements (AGCT or JGCT) and male elements (SLCT or Sertoli cell tumor)
- **Microcystic stromal tumor**
  - Cellular islands with coalescing microcysts intersected by bands of hyalinized stroma

ANCILLARY TESTS

Histochemistry

- Reticulin surrounds individual tumor cells in thecoma
  - Helpful in separating thecomas from granulosa cell tumors that may show overlapping histologic features

Immunohistochemistry

- Most SCST positive for at least 1 sex cord marker, including
  - Inhibin, calretinin, and SF-1
- Most SCST negative for EMA
- **Microcystic stromal tumor**
  - Positive for diffuse nuclear β-catenin, WT-1, cyclin-D1, and SF1
  - Typically negative for inhibin and calretinin
- **AGCT**
  - Positive for inhibin, calretinin, FOXL2, steroidogenic factor 1, WT1 pancytokeratin, and ER
    - May be used as prognostic biomarker for risk of recurrence, especially in early-stage disease
  - Less commonly positive for SMA, desmin, CD99, and CD10
  - Negative for EMA, PAX8, CK7, and CK5/6
- **JGCT**
  - Positive for inhibin, calretinin, steroidogenic factor 1, CD56, CD99, and low-molecular-weight keratins
  - Variably positive for FOXL2 protein (without associated mutation)
  - Majority negative for EMA and CK5/6
- **SLCT**
  - Positive for inhibin, calretinin, DICER1, vimentin, pancytokeratin, steroidogenic factor 1, WT1, and CD56, and 50% express CD99 (Sertoli cells only) and FOXL2
    - Retiform and poorly differentiated tumors likely to be negative
  - Heterologous elements show immunohistochemical expression that reflects their cell of origin

DIFFERENTIAL DIAGNOSIS

Small Cell Carcinoma

- JGCT may mimic hypercalcemic-type small cell carcinoma
- Both tumors may show follicle-like spaces containing luminal eosinophilic or basophilic material, nuclear atypia, and brisk mitotic activity
  - Sex cord immunohistochemical markers negative in small cell carcinoma
  - Small cell carcinoma positive for EMA and neuroendocrine markers

Endometrioid Adenocarcinoma

- Adequate sampling may help by revealing areas with typical SLCT elements or gonadal-type stroma
- IHC markers for EMA and those specific for SCSTs helpful

Yolk Sac Tumors

- May resemble retiform subtype of SLCT
- IHC markers specific for SCSTs, EMA, and yolk sac tumor markers helpful

SELECTED REFERENCES

1. Yasukawa M et al: Management of recurrent granulosa cell tumor of the ovary: contemporary literature review and a proposal of hyperthermic intraperitoneal chemotherapy as novel therapeutic option. J Obstet Gynaecol Res. 47(1):44-51, 2021
2. Rabban JT: Practical roles for molecular diagnostic testing in ovarian adult granulosa cell tumour, Sertoli-Leydig cell tumour, microcystic stromal tumour and their mimics. Histopathology. 76(1):11-24, 2020
3. WHO Classification of Tumors Editorial Board: WHO Classification of Tumours: Female Genital Tumours. 5th ed. IARC Press. 2020
4. Lim D et al: Ovarian sex cord-stromal tumours: an update in recent molecular advances. Pathology. 50(2):178-89, 2018

Sex Cord-Stromal Tumors of Ovary

Cystic Adult Granulosa Cell Tumor

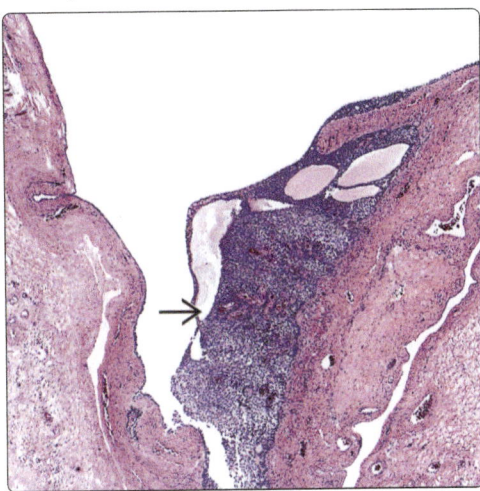

Calretinin Immunohistochemistry

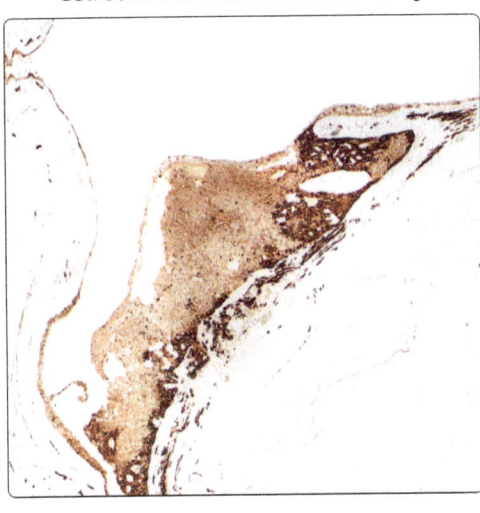

(Left) Cystic pattern of AGCT is shown. Not uncommonly, these tumors present as cystic ovarian masses. Note the characteristic granulosa cells with Call-Exner bodies lining the cyst cavity ➡. (Right) Calretinin shows positive expression in tumor cells lining the cyst. Positive calretinin and inhibin characterize sex cord-stromal tumors, including this cystic granulosa cell tumor.

Trisomy 12 Karyotype in Adult Granulosa Cell Tumor

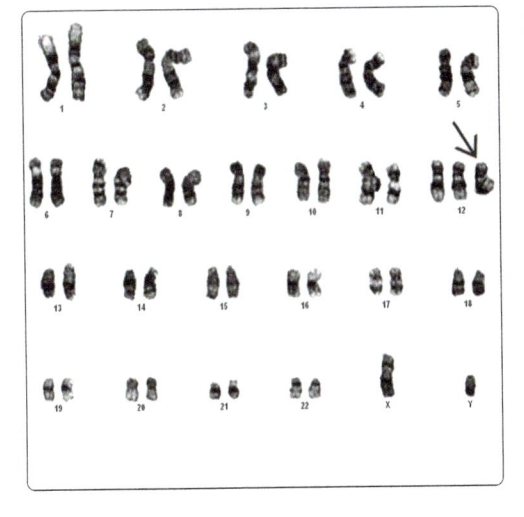

***FOXL2* Mutation in Adult Granulosa Cell Tumor**

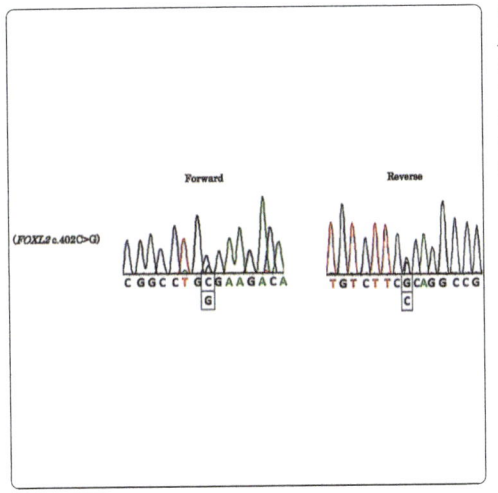

(Left) Cytogenetic analysis of AGCT shows an extra copy of chromosome 12 ➡. Trisomy 12 is detected in up to 33% of cases. (Right) FOXL2 mutation c.402C>G is a driver gene alteration in AGCT.

Sclerosing Stromal Tumor

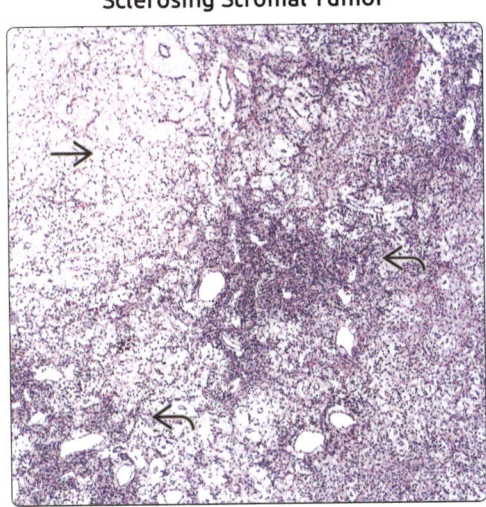

Sertoli-Leydig Cell Tumor

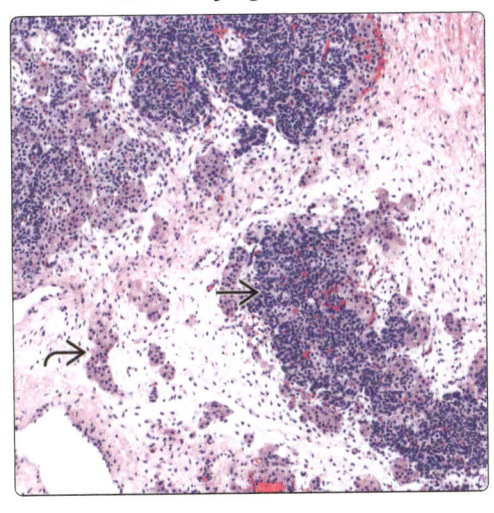

(Left) Sclerosing stromal tumor shows characteristic pseudolobular architecture with neoplastic round and spindled cells arranged in vaguely cellular nodules ➡ in a background of hypocellular and edematous stroma ➡. (Right) Moderately differentiated Sertoli cells form compressed tubules, cords, and focal sheets and have hyperchromatic, oval or spindled nuclei ➡. Small clusters of Leydig cells with round nuclei and abundant eosinophilic cytoplasm ➡ are noted.

Germ Cell Tumor, Ovary

KEY FACTS

TERMINOLOGY
- Germ cell tumors (GCTs) of ovary
  - Group of tumors arising from germ cells at different stages of development that are capable of differentiating into embryonic and extraembryonic elements

ETIOLOGY/PATHOGENESIS
- Derived from primordial germ cells, which migrate into gonadal ridge at 6 weeks of embryonic life

CLINICAL ISSUES
- Median age of presentation is 18 years
- GCTs account for ~ 30% of primary ovarian tumors
- In USA, overall survival is good (95%), attributed to advancement in therapy

MOLECULAR
- GCTs typically have 1 or more additional copies of chromosome 12p or other chromosome 12 abnormalities
  - Most common is isochromosome 12 [i(12p)]
  - Found in most dysgerminomas and embryonal carcinomas
  - Not usually in immature teratomas
- Activating *KIT* mutations in 8% of GCTs, mostly in dysgerminomas
- Complex karyotypes have been reported in yolk sac tumor
- Wnt signaling pathway genes can differentiate dysgerminoma from yolk sac tumor
- *CCND2*, *RB1*, and *PRDM14* are also altered in GCTs

ANCILLARY TESTS
- Important immunostains include OCT3/4, CD117, CD30, AFP, and glypican-3

TOP DIFFERENTIAL DIAGNOSES
- Clear cell carcinoma
- Undifferentiated carcinoma

Dysgerminoma

Dysgerminoma

(Left) At low power, dysgerminoma shows irregular nests of tumor cells separated by thin, fibrous septa ➡ containing lymphocytes ➡. (Right) At high power, dysgerminoma shows clear cells ➡ with prominent cytoplasmic borders and no overlapping. The nuclei are large with variably prominent nucleoli ➡.

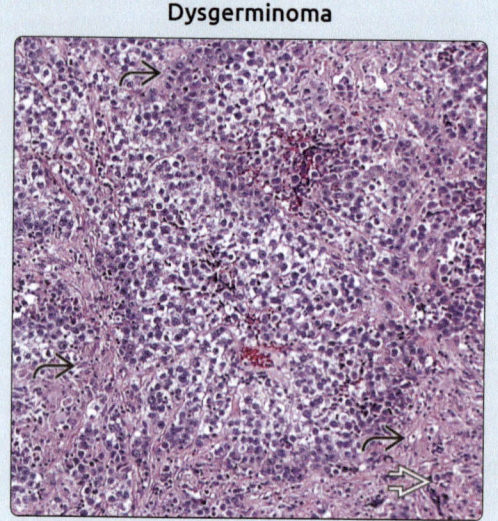

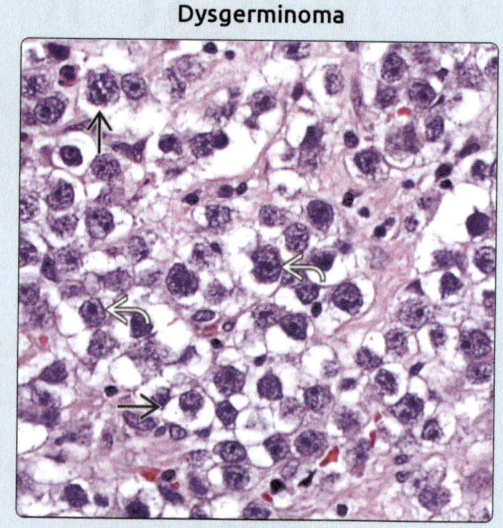

Teratoma

Yolk Sac Tumor

(Left) Teratomas can contain ectodermal, endodermal, and mesodermal tissue. This case showed prominent neural tissue and palisading of atypical cells. (Right) Yolk sac tumor shows cystic ➡ as well as solid ➡ areas. The cells can be flat or cuboidal.

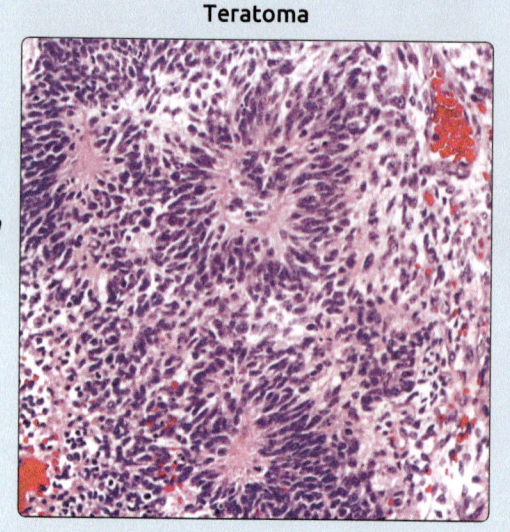

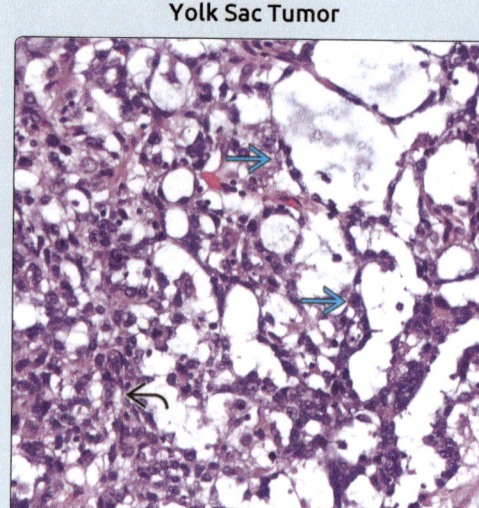

Germ Cell Tumor, Ovary

TERMINOLOGY

Abbreviations
- Germ cell tumors (GCTs)

Definitions
- Group of tumors arising from primitive germ cells at different stages of development

ETIOLOGY/PATHOGENESIS

Cell of Origin
- Derived from primordial germ cells, which migrate into gonadal ridge at 6 weeks of embryonic life

Associations
- Dysgerminoma is rarely associated with gonadal dysgenesis, Cowden syndrome, and Down syndrome

CLINICAL ISSUES

Epidemiology
- Incidence
  - ~ 20% of primary ovarian tumors
    - 95% of GCTs are mature cystic teratomas
    - Malignant GCTs constitute 5% of all ovarian malignancies
    - Embryonal carcinoma is much less common in ovaries than in testes
- Age
  - Young women
    - ~ 60% of ovarian tumors in women < 21 years of age are GCTs
    - Median: 18 years

Presentation
- Typically painless ovarian mass

MACROSCOPIC

Mature Cystic Teratoma
- Often circumscribed, solid &/or cystic mass
- Cysts may contain keratinous debris or mucinous fluid
- May have hairs, teeth, bone, or cartilage

MOLECULAR

Cytogenetics
- Chromosome 12 abnormalities
  - GCTs typically have 1 or more copies of 12p or other chromosome 12 abnormalities
  - Isochromosome 12 [i(12p)] is most common abnormality
    - Found in most dysgerminomas (82%) and embryonal carcinomas
    - Detected in ~ 50% of yolk sac tumors, ~ 40% of mixed GCTs
    - Not found in immature teratomas, but extra copies of chromosome 12 have been reported
    - If i(12p) is detected in tumor suspected to be immature teratoma, tumor is most likely mixed GCT, so carefully look for other tumor types
  - 12p amplification also seen
- Trisomy 14
  - Detected in ~ 33% of GCTs
- Complex karyotypes have been reported in yolk sac tumor
- Chromosome 3q27 aberration
  - Single case report in mixed GCT showed 46, XX, t(3;20)(q27;q13.3)
    - Mixed GCT contained teratoma and yolk sac tumor

Chromosomal Microarray
- Gains of 12p (typically [i(12p)] or 12p amplification) are detected
  - More associated with dysgerminoma (80%) as compared to yolk sac tumor and immature teratoma
- Other abnormalities reported
  - Loss of distal 1p and gain of 2q
  - Deletion of 4q and 6q
  - Gain of 20q

Molecular Genetics
- *KIT* mutations
  - Activating *KIT* mutations in 8% of GCTs
  - Mostly in dysgerminomas
    - 33% of dysgerminomas
    - Not reported in yolk sac tumors or immature teratomas
  - Often involve codon 816 of exon 17 (30-50% of dysgerminomas)
  - Few mutations reported in exon 11
  - Also described in extragonadal sites, including mediastinum
  - Prognosis
    - *KIT* mutations associated with advanced pathologic stage
    - *KIT* mutations do not appear to be increased risk factors for bilateral gonadal involvement
- *KIT* amplification
  - Also detected in 30% of dysgerminomas
  - Not related to stage of disease
- Immature teratomas usually diploid (92%)
- *CCND2*, *RB1*, and *PRDM14* also altered in GCTs

Gene Expression Profiling
- Wnt signaling pathway genes can differentiate dysgerminoma from yolk sac tumor
  - Utilizing 8 genes from Wnt pathway
  - Highlights importance of Wnt pathway for GCT pathogenesis

MicroRNA
- MiR-302-367 and miR-371-373 are overexpressed in GCT

MICROSCOPIC

Dysgerminoma
- Nests of polygonal cells compartmentalized by thin fibrosis in alveolar pattern
  - Cells have vesicular chromatin, large central nuclei; cells typically do not overlap
  - Abundant granular eosinophilic or clear cytoplasm and distinct membranes
- Fibrous septa typically contain lymphocytes
  - Mostly T cells
  - Can form germinal centers and extend beyond septa

Germ Cell Tumor, Ovary

- Insular, corded, pseudoglandular, and diffuse patterns also seen
- May have granulomas, necrosis, or calcification

Yolk Sac Tumor
- Variable patterns, including reticular (80%, micro-/macrocystic), endodermal sinus pattern (Schiller-Duval bodies), solid, festoon, papillary, polyvesicular vitelline, cribriform-tubular, glandular, parietal, hepatoid, and mixed
  - Reticular pattern has multiple channels, which expand to form microcysts lined by primitive cells
  - Schiller-Duval bodies have papillary fibrovascular structures with central blood vessel mantled by tumor cells
- Primitive cells with varied shape; can be cuboidal, columnar, flattened, or spindled
- Clear to eosinophilic cytoplasm, may have hyaline globules, overlapping border, and relatively regular nuclei with no to mild atypia
- Stroma is hypocellular, loose, or myxoid

Teratoma
- **Mature cystic teratoma**
  - Composed of structures from all 3 germ cell layers
    - Mixture of ectodermal (e.g., epidermis, neural tissue), endodermal (e.g., gastrointestinal or respiratory mucosa, thyroid), and mesodermal (e.g., cartilage, smooth muscle, fat, bone) tissues
  - Ectodermal are most abundant component
- **Immature teratoma**
  - Presence of immature neuroectoderm
- Secondary tumors occur in teratomas
  - Squamous cell carcinomas most common (80%)

Nongestational Choriocarcinoma
- Malignant GCT composed of cytotrophoblast and syncytiotrophoblast cells
  - Syncytiotrophoblasts are giant multinucleated cells
  - Cytotrophoblasts are smaller mononuclear polygonal cells with prominent membrane and uniform nuclei
- Dilated vascular sinusoids and blood lakes
  - Hemorrhage invariably present, forming pseudocystic hemorrhagic nodules
- Stromal luteinization
- Lymphovascular invasion common

Mixed Germ Cell Tumor
- Combination of any of germ cell neoplasms, including dysgerminoma, yolk sac tumor, embryonal carcinoma, teratoma, or nongestational choriocarcinoma in varying proportions
- 10-20% of all malignant germ cell tumors
- Most common combinations are dysgerminoma and yolk sac tumor, but any combination may occur
- Usually exhibits hemorrhages and necrosis

Embryonal Carcinoma
- Mainly exhibits sheets, nests, glandular, or papillary growths
- Large, high-grade, monomorphic to markedly pleomorphic cells with indistinct cytoplasmic border, modest amphophilic cytoplasm, large nuclei, and prominent irregular nucleoli; cells usually overlap
- Ovarian embryonal carcinoma is often mixed with other GCTs

ANCILLARY TESTS

Immunohistochemistry
- Majority of GCTs express SALL4, at least focally
- Dysgerminoma
  - Positive markers include SALL4, OCT3/4, and CD117
  - Cytokeratin may be focal, cytoplasmic, and have dot- or rim-like staining, but EMA is negative
- Yolk sac tumor
  - Positive markers include SALL4, AFP (often focal), glypican-3, Hep-Par1 (hepatoid pattern), CDX2 (intestinal pattern), and TTF-1 (foregut/respiratory pattern)
    - AE1/3(+/-), PAX8(+/-)
- Immature teratoma
  - Immature neuroectoderm can be positive for SALL4, OCT 3/4, and glypican-3
  - GFAP, NSE, NF, and S100 are positive in mature and immature neuroepithelium
  - AFP may be positive in immature gastrointestinal-type glands
- Nongestational choriocarcinoma
  - hCG is positive in syncytiotrophoblasts
- Embryonal carcinoma
  - Positive markers include CD30, OCT 3/4, SALL4, and AE1/3
  - Negative for EMA

DIFFERENTIAL DIAGNOSIS

Clear Cell Carcinoma
- Morphology similar to dysgerminoma sometimes
  - Tubulocystic and papillary patterns
  - Rarely associated with endometriosis; negative for SALL4(-)
  - Positive for PAX8, HNF-1β, EMA, napsin A, and AMACR

Undifferentiated Carcinoma
- Similar to embryonal carcinoma
- Negative for OCT4 and SALL4; focally positive for EMA

SELECTED REFERENCES

1. Pinto MT et al: Molecular biology of pediatric and adult ovarian germ cell tumors: a review. Cancers (Basel). 15(11):2990, 2023
2. Vang R et al: WHO Classification of Tumours: Female Genital Tumours. 5th ed. IARC, 119-20, 2020
3. Huang X et al: Recent advances in molecular biology and treatment strategies for intracranial germ cell tumors. World J Pediatr. 12(3):275-82, 2016

Germ Cell Tumor, Ovary

Reticular Pattern of Yolk Sac Tumor

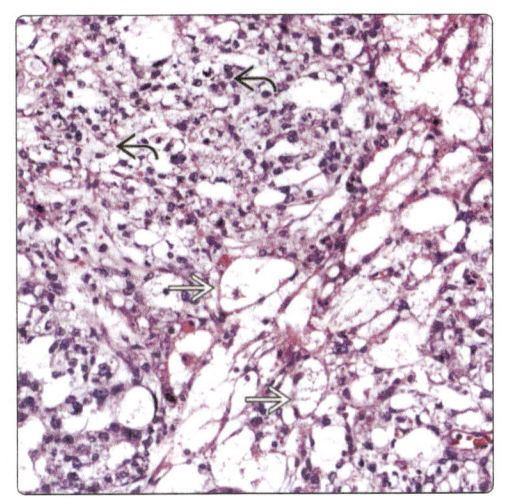

Schiller-Duval Body

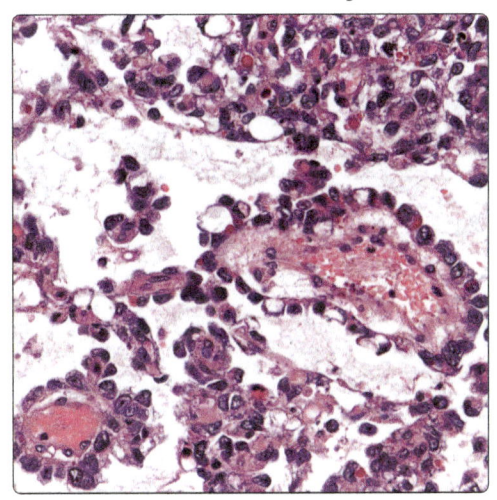

(Left) Yolk sac tumor shows a reticular pattern ⇨ with interanastomosing channels as well as a microcystic pattern ⇨. The microcystic pattern often merges with the reticular pattern. (Right) Schiller-Duval body from a yolk sac tumor is characterized by a central fibrovascular core surrounded by primitive neoplastic cells imparting a papillary appearance. (From DP: GYN.)

Choriocarcinoma

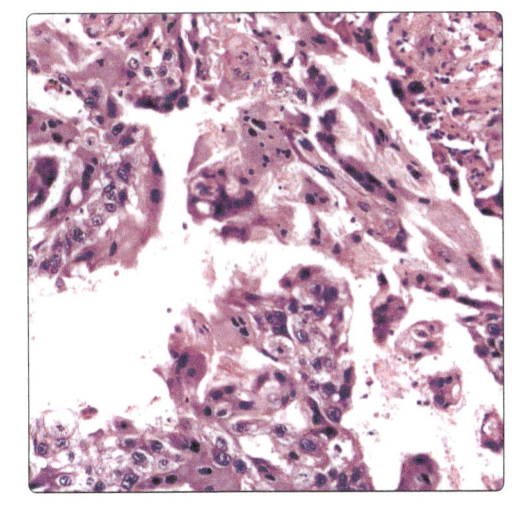

Immature Teratoma

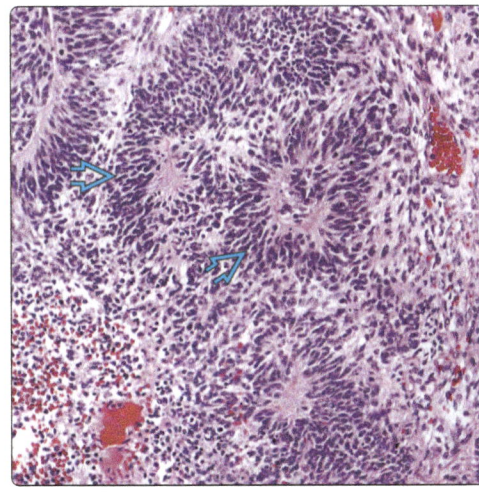

(Left) Nongestational choriocarcinoma shows proliferation of cytotrophoblasts, intermediate trophoblasts, and syncytiotrophoblasts. The latter are larger with dense, eosinophilic cytoplasm and are often multinucleate with smudgy nuclear chromatin. (Right) Immature teratoma shows immature neuroectodermal tubules ⇨ with admixed glial tissue. The tumor cells are hyperchromatic with scant tissue.

Mature Cystic Teratoma

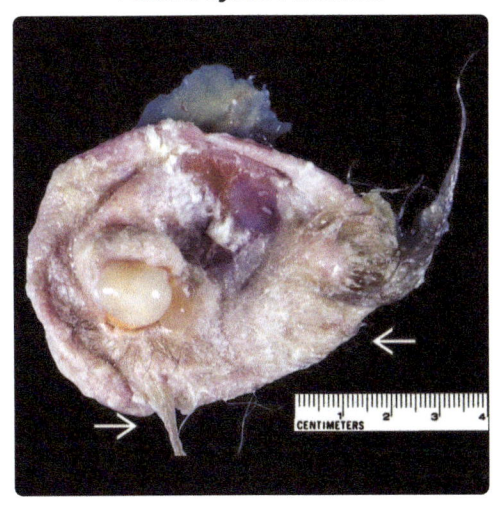

Mature Cystic Teratoma

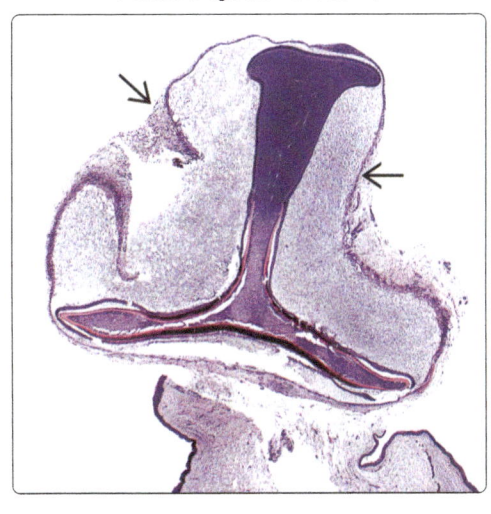

(Left) Gross photograph of a mature cystic teratoma shows a unilocular cyst with abundant hair ⇨ and yellow sebaceous material. (Right) Mature cystic teratomas will show tissue structures from each of the 3 germ layers: Endoderm, mesoderm, and ectoderm. Here, teeth ⇨ are present. (From DP: GYN.)

Premalignant Conditions, Skin

KEY FACTS

TERMINOLOGY
- Premalignant lesions: Atypical proliferations/tumors that may progress to malignancy in some cases

CLINICAL ISSUES
- Surgical excision is most common treatment for most lesions/tumors, except for atypical lymphoid infiltrates
- Excellent prognosis in most cases; only low risk of malignant transformation, except for atypical vascular lesions

MOLECULAR
- Actinic keratosis (AK): Most show mutations in *TP53*, associated with UVB irradiation and increased activation or levels of EGFR, MYC, and ATF3
- Atypical (dysplastic) nevi (AN): Most nevi show mutations in *BRAF* but lack other genetic abnormalities
- Atypical lymphoid infiltrate (ALI): Most do not show clonal T-cell receptors (*TRB*, *TRG*) or *IGH* rearrangements
- Atypical vascular lesions (AVL): Lack *MYC* amplification (in contrast to angiosarcoma)

MICROSCOPIC
- AK: Proliferation of atypical basilar keratinocytes in epidermis
- AN: Atypical melanocytes forming irregular nests with bridging across rete ridges, increased single lentiginous cells, and shouldering
- ALI: Atypical lymphoid proliferation that does not meet criteria for lymphoma
- AVL: Proliferation of dilated, irregularly shaped blood vessels in dermis

ANCILLARY TESTS
- AK: Atypical cells are positive for p53 and Ki-67
- AN: PRAME is typically (-) in nevi (in contrast to melanoma)
- AVL: Low levels of Ki-67 and p53 expression compared to angiosarcoma

Acantholytic Actinic Keratosis

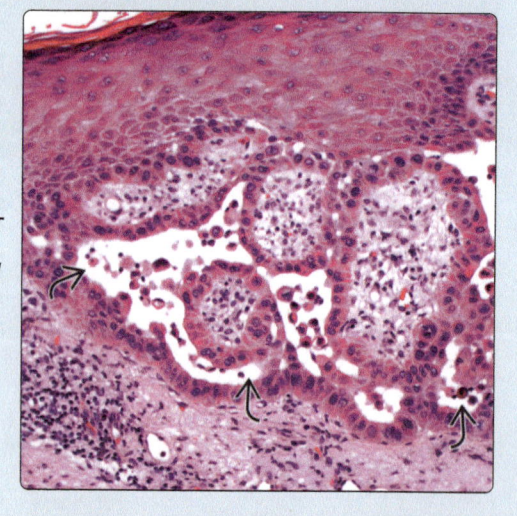

Actinic Keratosis: Ki-67

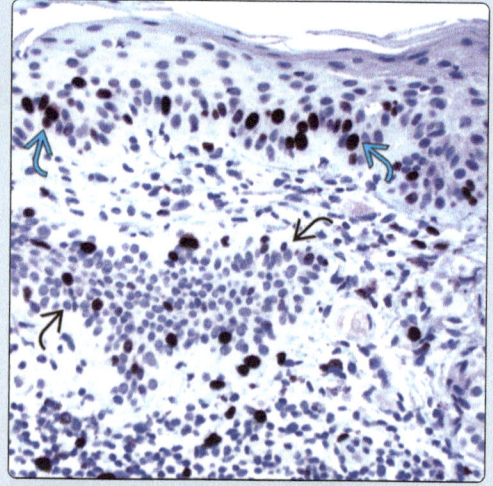

(Left) *Acantholytic actinic keratosis shows intraepidermal acantholysis ⊞ above the atypical basilar keratinocytes.* (Right) *Ki-67 in actinic keratosis shows strong nuclear staining within many of the atypical intraepidermal keratinocytes ⊞ in the basilar 1/3 of the epidermis. There is also a superficial dermal basal cell carcinoma ⊞ present in this case.*

Atypical Vascular Lesion in Superficial Dermis

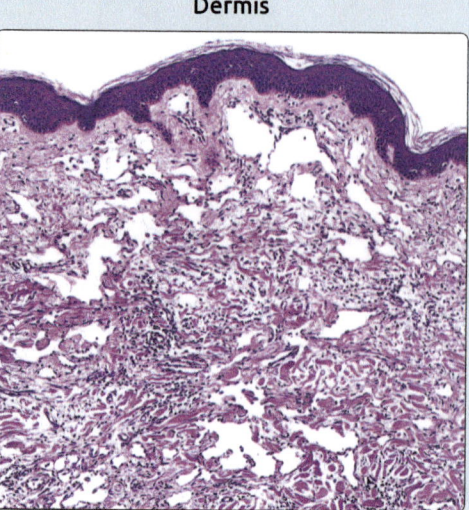

Atypical Vascular Lesion: Ki-67

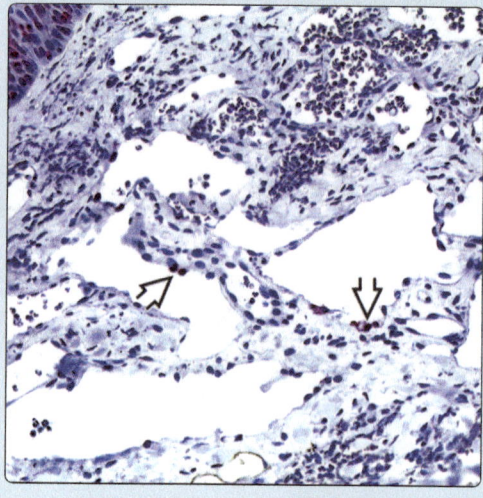

(Left) *Atypical vascular lesion (AVL) shows a superficially located, lymphangioma-like lesion composed of dilated vascular structures lined by relatively small endothelial cells.* (Right) *The presence of scattered Ki-67(+) endothelial cells ⊞ represents an atypical finding in cases of AVL after radiotherapy; however, the levels of staining are typically much higher in angiosarcoma, and MYC is not amplified in AVL.*

Premalignant Conditions, Skin

TERMINOLOGY

Synonyms
- Atypical/borderline tumors

Definitions
- Premalignant proliferations/tumors that may progress to malignancy in some cases
  - Actinic keratosis (AK)
  - Atypical nevi (AN)/dysplastic nevi (DN)
  - Atypical vascular lesions (AVL)
  - Atypical lymphoid infiltrate (ALI)

ETIOLOGY/PATHOGENESIS

Etiology
- Unknown in most cases
- Solar damage
  - Clearly associated with AK
  - May be involved in pathogenesis of AN/DN
- Radiation therapy associated with AVL

CLINICAL ISSUES

Presentation
- Signs and symptoms depend on specific condition

Treatment
- Surgical approaches
  - Surgical excision is typical treatment for most lesions/tumors other than ALI

Prognosis
- Depends on specific type of lesion
  - Excellent in most cases; only low risk of malignant transformation
  - AK has very low risk for transformation to invasive squamous cell carcinoma (SCC)
  - AN have very low risk for transformation to melanoma (controversial if any greater risk than conventional nevi)
  - AVL shows significant risk for development of angiosarcoma (AS), particularly in breast (post radiation)

MOLECULAR

Cytogenetics
- AK
  - Genetic alterations have been identified involving 3p, 9p, 9q, 13q, 17p, and 17q chromosomal regions
- AN
  - Typically do not show identifiable alterations
  - May show isolated chromosomal abnormalities
- ALI
  - Usually does not show karyotypic abnormalities
- AVL
  - Lacks chromosomal translocations or amplifications seen in angiosarcoma

Polymerase Chain Reaction
- AK
  - Most cases show mutations in *TP53*
- AN
  - Most nevi (up to 80%) show mutations in *BRAF*
  - Typically only abnormality present, unlike melanoma, which shows multiple mutations and rearrangements
- ALI
  - Mostly do not show clonal *TRB* or *TRG* or *IGH* rearrangements
    - B-cell clonality only rarely seen in reactive conditions
    - T-cell clonality can be seen in many reactive conditions
- AVL
  - Lacks *MYC* amplification that could be seen in angiosarcoma

Molecular Genetics
- AK
  - *TP53* is often mutated in AK, associated with UVB irradiation
    - Many similar pathways activated as in SCC, supporting association between AK and SCC
    - Increased activation or levels of EGFR, MYC, and ATF3 also identified
- AN
  - Most nevi show mutations in *BRAF* but lack other genetic abnormalities
  - Some congenital nevi show mutations in *NRAS* but lack *BRAF* mutations
- ALI
  - In reactive conditions
  - Typically lack mutations and clonality
- AVL
  - Lacks identifiable genetic abnormalities

MICROSCOPIC

Histologic Features
- AK
  - Proliferation of atypical basilar keratinocytes in epidermis
  - Atypical cells often show budding, nuclear crowding, hyperchromasia, and overlying parakeratosis
  - Typically spare adnexal structures
  - Subtypes include
    - Lichenoid (with associated dense dermal inflammatory infiltrate)
    - Acantholytic (with suprabasilar/intraepidermal acantholysis)
    - Hypertrophic (with associated epidermal hyperplasia, dense hyperkeratosis, and parakeratosis)
    - Bowenoid (atypical keratinocytes involving lower 1/2 to 2/3 of epidermis)
- AN
  - Melanocytes forming irregular nests and often showing bridging across rete ridges, increased single lentiginous cells, and shouldering (extension of junctional component beyond intradermal component)
  - Typically graded based on degree of cytologic atypia (mild, moderate, or severe)
  - Junctional mitoses can be seen, but dermal mitoses should be rare or absent
  - Pagetoid scatter into upper levels of epidermis is only rarely seen and should be very focal
    - Usually in severely atypical lesions but may also be secondary to irritation/trauma or previous biopsy

Premalignant Conditions, Skin

- ALI
  - Atypical lymphoid proliferations that do not meet criteria for lymphoma
  - Can be intradermal &/or intraepidermal (epidermotropic)
  - Reactive infiltrates that may be considered in differential diagnosis with lymphoma include
    - Lymphomatoid drug reactions, pityriasis lichenoides chronica, pityriasis lichenoides et varioliformis acuta, pigmented purpuric dermatoses, persistent arthropod bite or scabies reactions, and lupus
- AVL
  - Proliferation of dilated, irregularly shaped blood vessels in dermis
  - Often show low-grade cytologic features
  - Lack anastomosing features, increased atypia and mitoses, or endothelial multilayering of angiosarcoma

ANCILLARY TESTS

Immunohistochemistry

- AK
  - Atypical cells are positive for p53 and Ki-67
- AN
  - PRAME is typically negative in nevi
    - In contrast, PRAME is typically strongly and diffusely positive in melanoma
  - p16 is typically (+) in nevi
    - In contrast, p16 is typically (-) in melanomas
  - HMB-45 usually (+) in junctional cells but weak to (-) in dermal cells
  - Ki-67 shows low proliferative rate in nevi (< 5%), elevated in most melanomas (> 15-20%)
    - In contrast, Ki-67 index is high in most melanomas (> 15-20%)
- ALI
  - Mixed T- and B-cell infiltrates in most cases often with scattered other cell types, including histiocytes, eosinophils, neutrophils, mast cells, and plasma cells
  - T-cell population should be composed of mixture of CD4(+) and CD8(+) T-cell subsets
    - Most T-cell lymphomas are either CD4(+) or CD8(+) or occasionally CD4/CD8 double positive or double negative
- AVL
  - Low levels of MYC, Ki-67, and p53 staining compared to angiosarcoma

DIFFERENTIAL DIAGNOSIS

DDx of Actinic Keratosis

- SCC in situ: Full-thickness epidermal atypia
  - Can be difficult to distinguish from bowenoid AK, especially if there is epidermal erosion/ulceration and inflammation
- Invasive SCC: At least focal dermal involvement by atypical squamoid cells
  - Can be difficult to diagnose in small, superficial biopsies with scant amounts of dermis

DDx of Atypical (Dysplastic) Nevi

- Melanoma: Greater architectural and cytologic atypia
  - Junctional component shows more lentiginous hyperplasia and often pagetoid spread
  - Dermal component in melanoma lacks maturation with dermal descent, shows dermal mitotic figures, often deep &/or atypical

DDx of Atypical Lymphoid Infiltrates

- Mycosis fungoides (MF) and other epidermotropic T-cell lymphomas
  - Atypical epidermotropic T-cells usually show predominance of CD4(+) cells by IHC but CD8(+) variants also described, including hypo-/hyperpigmented MF
  - Other rare, more aggressive epidermotropic T-cell lymphomas, including primary cutaneous aggressive epidermotropic cytotoxic CD8(+) T-cell lymphoma and γδ T-cell lymphoma [CD4/CD8 double negative, CD56(+), βF1(-)]
- B-cell lymphomas and other dermal-based lymphomas
  - Usually composed of larger, nodular to sheet-like aggregates of monomorphous-appearing B cells
    - Less of mixed background infiltrate, except for marginal zone lymphoma (MZL), which often has prominent mixed infiltrate and reactive germinal centers
    - IHC shows BCL6 and CD10 staining in primary cutaneous follicle center lymphoma, BCL2(-/+)
    - IHC in primary cutaneous MZL shows BCL2 coexpression and light chain restriction

DDx of Atypical Vascular Lesions

- Kaposi sarcoma
  - Proliferation of spindle cells associated with slit-like blood vessels, hemosiderin deposition, and plasma cells
  - HHV8(+) [(-) in AVL]
    - HHV8 is negative in AVL
- Angiosarcoma
  - Larger, more deeply infiltrative proliferation of irregular, anastomosing blood vessels with endothelial atypia
  - Elevated levels of MYC, Ki-67, and p53 staining compared to AVL

SELECTED REFERENCES

1. Kim HN et al: Factors for risk stratification of patients with actinic keratosis using integrated analysis of clinicopathological features and gene expression patterns. Australas J Dermatol. 64(1):80-91, 2023
2. Maher NG et al: Biology and genetics of acquired and congenital melanocytic naevi. Pathology. 55(2):169-77, 2023
3. Spaccarelli N et al: Dysplastic nevus part II: dysplastic nevi: molecular/genetic profiles and management. J Am Acad Dermatol. 88(1):13-20, 2023
4. Etesami I et al: Drug-induced cutaneous pseudolymphoma: a systematic review of the literature. Australas J Dermatol. 64(1):41-9, 2023
5. Kim YS et al: Targeted deep sequencing reveals genomic alterations of actinic keratosis/cutaneous squamous cell carcinoma in situ and cutaneous squamous cell carcinoma. Exp Dermatol. 32(4):447-56, 2023
6. Craddock AP et al: Use of ultrasensitive RNA in situ hybridization for determining clonality in cutaneous B-cell lymphomas and lymphoid hyperplasia decreases subsequent use of molecular testing and is cost-effective. Am J Surg Pathol. 46(7):956-62, 2022
7. Khalil S et al: Cutaneous reactive B-cell lymphoid proliferations. J Cutan Pathol. 49(10):898-916, 2022
8. Zhao J et al: Benign and intermediate-grade melanocytic tumors with BRAF mutations and spitzoid morphology: a subset of melanocytic neoplasms distinct from melanoma. Am J Surg Pathol. 46(4):476-85, 2022
9. Motaparthi K et al: MYC gene amplification by fluorescence in situ hybridization and MYC protein expression by immunohistochemistry in the diagnosis of cutaneous angiosarcoma: systematic review and appropriate use criteria. J Cutan Pathol. 48(4):578-86, 2021

Premalignant Conditions, Skin

Atypical Halo Compound Nevus

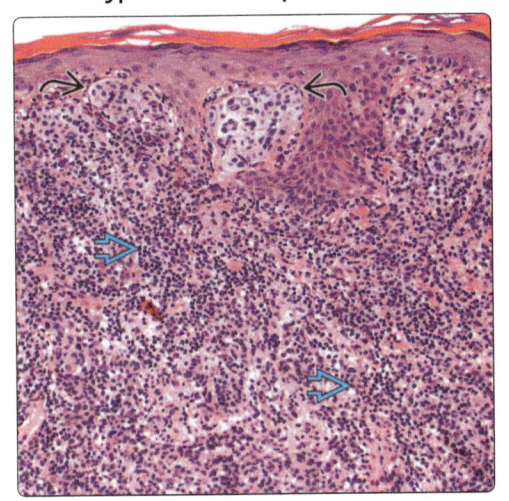

Atypical Halo Compound Nevus: p16

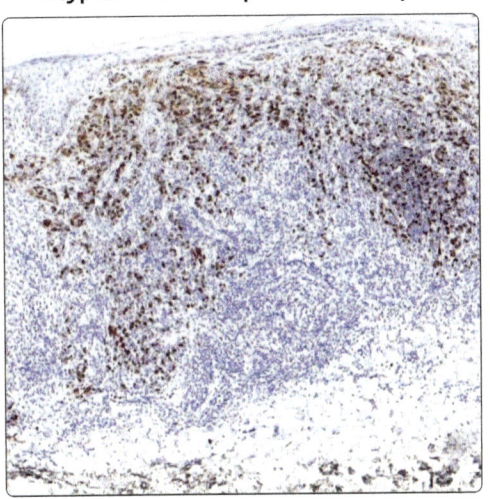

(Left) This atypical/dysplastic halo nevus is composed of irregular junctional nests ➡ and scattered single atypical junctional lentiginous cells. There is a dense dermal lymphocytic infiltrate ➡ associated with scattered smaller, more bland-appearing nevoid cells. (Right) p16 shows strong positivity in most of the atypical compound nevus cells. This marker is often positive in nevi and lost (weak or negative) in invasive melanomas.

Atypical Compound Nevus: HMB-45

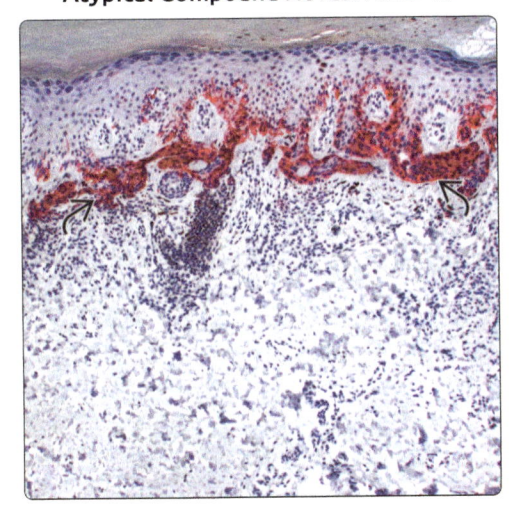

Atypical Lymphoid Infiltrate

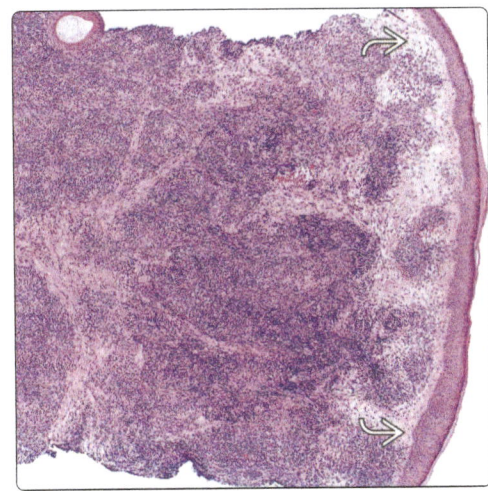

(Left) HMB-45 in an atypical compound nevus shows strong staining of the junctional cells, highlighting the bridging across multiple rete ridges ➡. However, the superficial dermal nests are negative for this marker, consistent with the pattern of maturation typically seen in nevi but not in melanoma. (Right) Atypical lymphoid infiltrate is shown. The epidermis is uninvolved, and there is a grenz zone ➡ in the superficial dermis. IHC showed a mixed infiltrate, consistent with reactive process.

Atypical Lymphoid Infiltrate

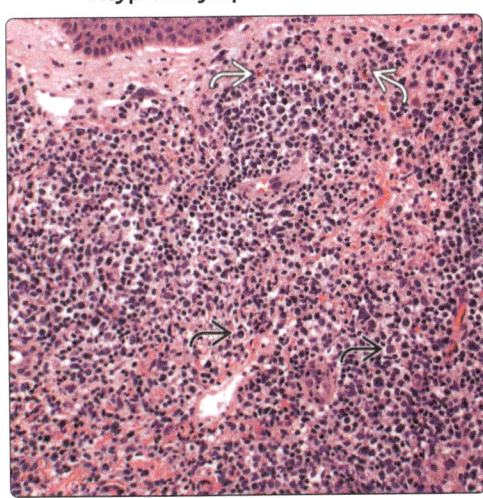

Atypical Lymphoid Infiltrate: CD4

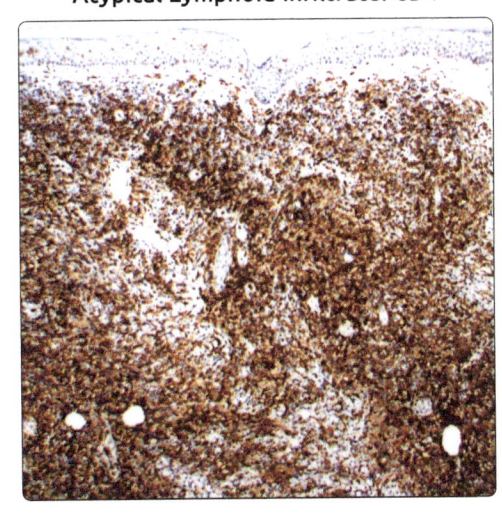

(Left) Higher power shows an infiltrate composed of many lymphocytes, histiocytes, and scattered plasma cells ➡, neutrophils, and eosinophils ➡. The mixed nature of the infiltrate favors a reactive process. (Right) CD4 in the same case highlights many B cells, and there were also many CD8(+) T cells present (not shown), consistent with reactive mixed B-cell and T-cell lymphoid infiltrate.

Melanoma

KEY FACTS

TERMINOLOGY
- Proliferation of atypical melanocytes often present both as irregular nests and single cells

CLINICAL ISSUES
- 6th most common malignancy in United States; continuously increasing in incidence

MOLECULAR
- *BRAF* mutations are most common aberration in sporadic melanoma
  - PCR for *BRAF* V600E mutation is often performed to assess for treatment responsiveness to BRAF inhibitors
- FISH is typically done with 4 probes for known genes often altered in melanoma
- Complex rearrangements with multiple amplifications and deletions are typically seen by chromosomal microarray
- Familial cases often show mutations of *CDKN2A* on chromosome 9p21
- *PTEN* mutations are relatively common (up to 30-40% of cases)
- *NRAS* mutations are next most common (up to 15% of cases)
- *HRAS* mutations seen in some Spitz nevi
- *KIT* mutations are seen in cases of acral lentiginous and lentigo maligna melanoma
- *GNAQ* mutations are rare in cutaneous melanomas; commonly seen in uveal melanomas and blue nevi
- *ALK* fusions recently described in some Spitz nevi and atypical Spitz tumors
- *BAP1* mutations described in some familial melanoma kindreds and sporadic tumors
- *TERT* mutations recently described in many melanomas; associated with worse prognosis

TOP DIFFERENTIAL DIAGNOSES
- Atypical (dysplastic) nevi
- Spitz nevi and atypical Spitz nevi/tumors

Recurrent Invasive Lentigo Maligna Melanoma

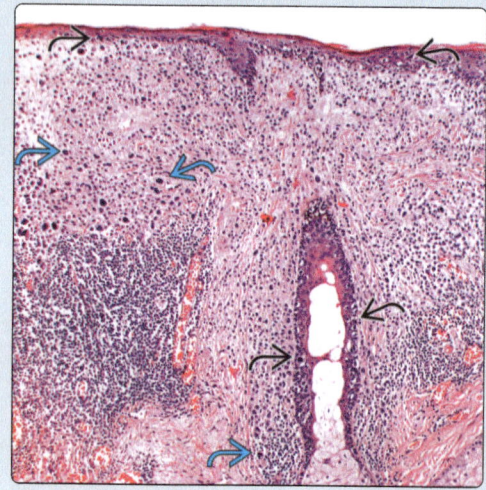

PRAME Expression

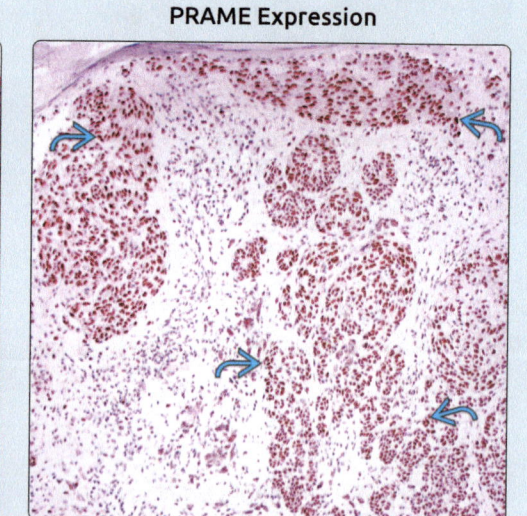

(Left) Recurrent invasive lentigo maligna melanoma is shown. A previous biopsy several years prior showed melanoma in situ (residual is this biopsy ➡). However, now there is a diffusely invasive tumor in the dermis with scattered markedly enlarged, atypical cells ➡. (Right) PRAME typically shows strong and diffuse nuclear staining in melanoma ➡ (> 50-75% of cells). Most cases of nevi are negative or only show focal/weak staining of a few cells.

FISH Study

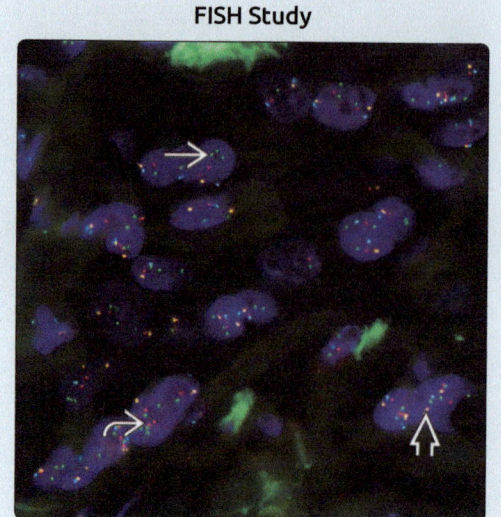

***KIT* Exon 17 Mutation**

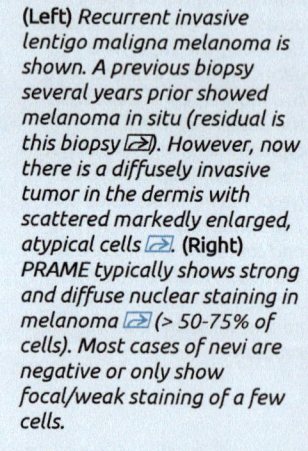

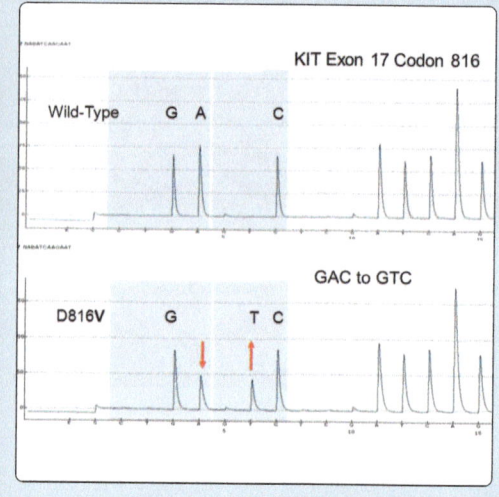

(Left) FISH study of melanoma shows multiple chromosomal gains, including amplification of red (RREB1, 6p25) ➡, yellow (MYB, 6q23) ➡, and green (CCND1, 11q13) ➡ probes. (Courtesy S. Billings, MD.) (Right) KIT exon 17 codon 816 gene sequencing study in a case of acral melanoma shows a c.2447A>T mutation corresponding to KIT D816V pathogenic mutation (wildtype on top, mutation on bottom).

Melanoma

TERMINOLOGY

Abbreviations
- Melanoma in situ (MIS)
- Lentigo maligna melanoma (LMM)
- Superficial spreading melanoma (SSM)
- Desmoplastic melanoma (DM)
- Acral lentiginous melanoma (ALM)

Definitions
- Proliferation of atypical melanocytes, often present both as irregular nests and single cells
  o MIS: Lesions confined to epidermis (or mucosal epithelium)
  o Invasive melanoma: Tumor cells infiltrating into dermis or stroma; can be as single cells, nests, nodules, or sheet-like collections

CLINICAL ISSUES

Epidemiology
- Incidence
  o 6th most common malignancy in United States; continuously increasing in incidence
- Age
  o Usually occurs in older patients in chronically sun-damaged skin
  o Familial melanoma typically occurs at younger age; autosomal dominant inheritance in most cases
- Ethnicity
  o Most cases occur in White populations; lighter skin types and red hair confer higher risk
  o ALM tends to occur more in Asian, Hispanic, and African populations

Presentation
- Macular, papular, or nodular lesion often with irregular color, shape, and borders

Treatment
- Surgical approaches
  o Surgical excision with clear margins remains standard treatment and can be curative for early-stage lesions
- Adjuvant therapy
  o Immunotherapies targeting specific molecules and mutations being used more commonly in metastatic melanoma
    – Anti-BRAF therapy may be utilized in tumors showing *BRAF* V600E mutation
    – MEK inhibitors block growth and induce cell death in *BRAF*- and *NRAS*-mutated melanomas
      □ Combined BRAF and MEK inhibitors often used together
    – Anti-PD-1/PD-L1 (CD152) inhibitors are being used against tumors showing PD-1/PD-L1 expression
    – Anti-CTLA4 monoclonal antibodies are immune checkpoint inhibitors
      □ Typically given in combination with other adjuvant therapies, such as anti-PD-1/PD-L1 inhibitors

Prognosis
- Depends on size (Breslow depth), presence or absence of ulceration, lymphovascular invasion, and dermal mitotic index
- Molecular findings are increasingly being utilized to attempt to predict prognosis and treatment responsiveness

MOLECULAR

Cytogenetics
- Not typically done for melanoma but show complex alterations in most cases

In Situ Hybridization
- FISH is typically done with 4-6 probes for known genes often altered in melanoma
  o Probes most commonly used include 6p24 (*RREB1*), 6p23 (*MYB*), 11q13 (*CCND1*), and centromeric chromosome 6 probe
    – Newer probes of potential utility include 8q24 and 9p21 (*CDKN2A*)
  o Relatively high sensitivity (up to 85-90%) and specificity (up to 95%) reported, but histologically ambiguous cases have not been as well characterized
    – Severely atypical Spitz nevi, atypical/dysplastic nevi, and atypical cellular blue nevi do not always show unambiguous results
    – Studies have not shown good sensitivity for DM

PCR
- PCR studies for *BRAF* V600 mutation are often performed to assess for treatment responsiveness to BRAF inhibitors
  o *BRAF* V600E mutation most common (up to 80% of cases); *BRAF* V600K next most common variant (up to 20% of cases)
- Some newer tests utilize NGS panels for multiple genes, which may be mutated, up- or downregulated in melanoma

Chromosomal Microarray
- Complex rearrangements with multiple amplifications and deletions are typically seen
- 96% of melanomas reportedly show at least 1 aberration; most nevi, including Spitz nevi, show no abnormalities

Molecular Genetics
- Familial cases often show mutations of *CDKN2A* on chromosome 9p21
  o Encodes for p16 and p14 proteins; p16 is tumor suppressor protein, which inhibits CDK4 (which regulates G1-S transition via RB phosphorylation)
- *BRAF* mutations are most common aberration in sporadic melanoma
  o Seen in up to 50% of cases, tend to correlate with superficial spreading type histologically
  o Often in younger patients and in skin with less chronic sun damage
  o Part of RAS/RAF/MAPK pathway; mutations lead to activation of this cascade
- *PTEN* mutations are relatively common (up to 30-40% of cases)
  o Acts as inhibitor of PI3K/AKT pathway

Melanoma

- *NRAS* mutations are next most common (up to 15% of cases)
  - Less commonly seen in SSM, more common in nodular melanoma
  - Increase MAPK and PI3K pathways signaling
- *HRAS* mutations seen in some Spitz nevi
  - Up to 17% of Spitz nevi (usually desmoplastic type); not identified in spitzoid melanomas
  - Often associated with 11p amplifications
- *KIT* mutations are seen in some cases of melanoma
  - More commonly seen in LMM, ALM, and mucosal melanomas, not in SSM
  - *KIT* encodes stem cell factor receptor tyrosine kinase
  - Leads to activation of MAPK, PI3K, and JAK/STAT pathways
- *ALK* fusions recently described in some Spitz nevi and atypical Spitz tumors
  - Reportedly correlate with predominantly dermal tumors showing plexiform morphology
  - Fusion partners include *TPM3* and *DCTN1*
- *GNAQ* and *GNA11* mutations are rare in cutaneous melanomas but commonly seen in uveal melanomas and blue nevi
  - ~ 50% of uveal melanomas show *GNAQ* or *GNA11* mutations
  - Also seen in cellular blue nevi and atypical and malignant blue nevi (melanoma arising in or mimicking blue nevus)
- *BAP1* mutations described in some familial melanoma kindreds and sporadic tumors
  - Associated with epithelioid spitz nevi/tumors, uveal melanomas, and mesotheliomas
  - Spitz tumors are often cytologically atypical but clinically benign
  - Often associated with *BRAF* V600E mutations
- *TERT* mutations described in many melanomas; may confer worse prognosis
  - Encodes for telomerase; mutations may lead to increased transcriptional activity and immortalization of tumor cells
  - Also identified in some atypical/malignant spitzoid tumors; reportedly associated with worse prognosis

MICROSCOPIC

Histologic Features

- MIS: Proliferation of atypical junctional lentiginous or nested melanocytes with foci of confluence and pagetoid upward scatter
  - LMM in situ: Single cells predominate over nests; often show spindle cell features, peripheral trailing off of single cells, and adnexal involvement
  - SSM in situ: Nests predominate over single cells; often show epithelioid cell features with prominent pagetoid spread
- Invasive melanoma: Extension of atypical single cells &/or nests into dermis
  - LMM: Invasion of dermis by atypical oval to spindle-shaped cells; often with associated DM
  - SSM: Invasion of dermis by nests of atypical epithelioid-shaped cells; no evidence of maturation with dermal descent; dermal mitoses often present
  - Spindle cell/DM: Proliferation of mostly single atypical, infiltrative spindle cells associated with prominent stromal sclerosis (desmoplasia)
  - ALM: Acral site, lentiginous junctional proliferation of atypical cells overlying infiltrative dermal spindle cell proliferation
  - Nodular-type melanoma: Large, predominantly dermal-based, nodular to sheet-like proliferation of markedly atypical cells; often only small junctional component

Cytologic Features

- Enlarged atypical and pleomorphic-appearing cells, often with prominent red nucleoli
- Mitoses usually easily identified in invasive and metastatic melanomas

DIFFERENTIAL DIAGNOSIS

Atypical (Dysplastic) Nevi

- Show symmetry, circumscription, dermal maturation in most cases
- Lack significant pagetoid spread and mitoses (rare junctional or superficial dermal ones may be seen)
- Severely atypical nevi can be very difficult to distinguish from melanoma in some cases, especially in partial biopsies
  - Additional studies, including immunohistochemistry &/or molecular studies, may be useful in such cases

Spitz Nevi and Atypical Spitz Nevi/Tumors

- Cells are usually large, mixed spindled and epithelioid cell types, and show some degree of atypia, pleomorphism, and pagetoid spread
- May have dermal mitoses but should be superficial and nonatypical
- Severely atypical Spitz nevi/tumors very difficult, if not impossible, to distinguish from spitzoid melanoma by histologic features alone in some cases
  - FISH, chromosomal microarray, and NGS studies may be helpful in differential diagnosis with melanoma

SELECTED REFERENCES

1. Boutko A et al: TERT promoter mutational analysis as an ancillary diagnostic tool for diagnostically challenging melanocytic neoplasms. Am J Dermatopathol. 5(5):289-99, 2023
2. Roy SF et al: Spectrum of melanocytic tumors harboring BRAF gene fusions: 58 cases with histomorphologic and genetic correlations. Mod Pathol. 36(6):100149, 2023
3. Saad M et al: Neoadjuvant therapy in melanoma: where are we now? Curr Oncol Rep. 25(4):325-39, 2023
4. Wang W et al: Identification of a novel immune-related gene signature for prognosis and the tumor microenvironment in patients with uveal melanoma combining single-cell and bulk sequencing data. Front Immunol. 14:1099071, 2023
5. Birkeälv S et al: Mutually exclusive genetic interactions and gene essentiality shape the genomic landscape of primary melanoma. J Pathol. 259(1):56-68, 2022
6. Hanna J et al: Cutaneous melanocytic tumor with CRTC1::TRIM11 translocation: an emerging entity analyzed in a series of 41 cases. Am J Surg Pathol. 46(11):1457-66, 2022
7. Sabag N et al: Novel biomarkers and therapeutic targets for melanoma. Int J Mol Sci. 23(19):11656, 2022
8. Wagstaff W et al: Melanoma: molecular genetics, metastasis, targeted therapies, immunotherapies, and therapeutic resistance. Genes Dis. 9(6):1608-23, 2022
9. Nassar KW et al: The mutational landscape of mucosal melanoma. Semin Cancer Biol. 61:139-48, 2020
10. Darmawan CC et al: Early detection of acral melanoma: a review of clinical, dermoscopic, histopathologic, and molecular characteristics. J Am Acad Dermatol. 81(3):805-12, 2019

Melanoma

Invasive Melanoma With Blue Nevus-Like Features

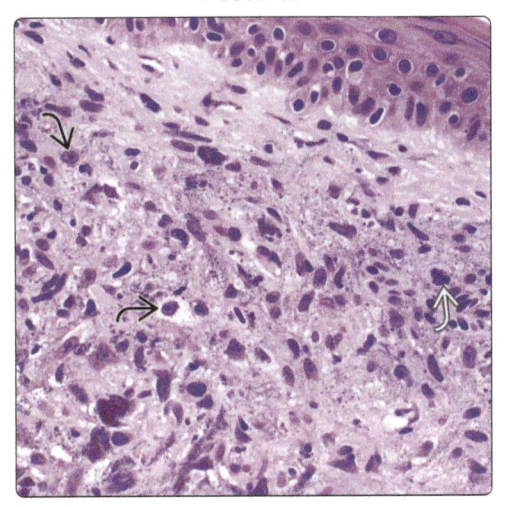

Loss of p16 Expression in Malignant Blue Nevus

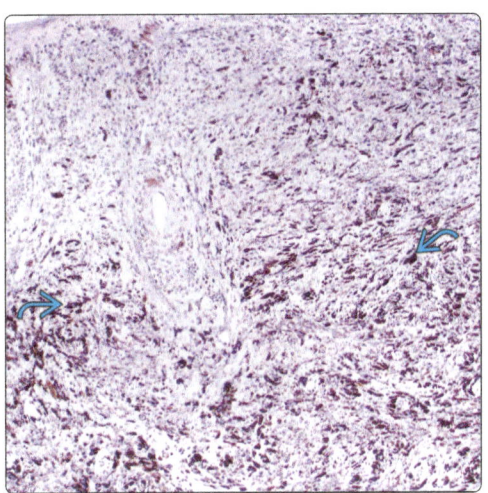

(Left) *Invasive melanoma arising in or mimicking a blue nevus is shown. The cells are enlarged, markedly atypical and pleomorphic-appearing, with nuclear hyperchromasia and prominent nucleoli ➡. A mitotic figure is also identified ➡.* **(Right)** *Loss of p16 expression is often seen in invasive melanoma, including this malignant blue nevus with abundant melanin pigment ➡.*

BRAF V600 Mutation

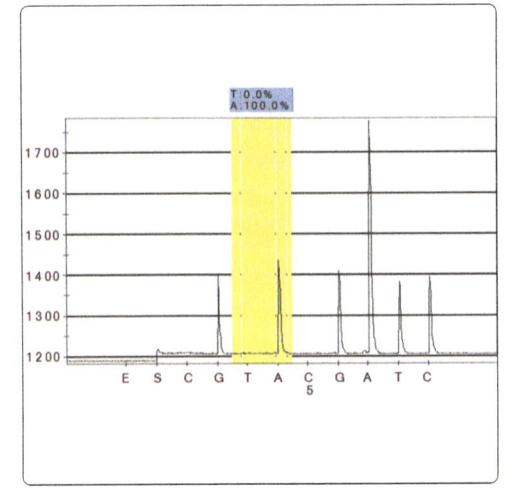

BRAF Codon V600 Wildtype Sequence in Nevus

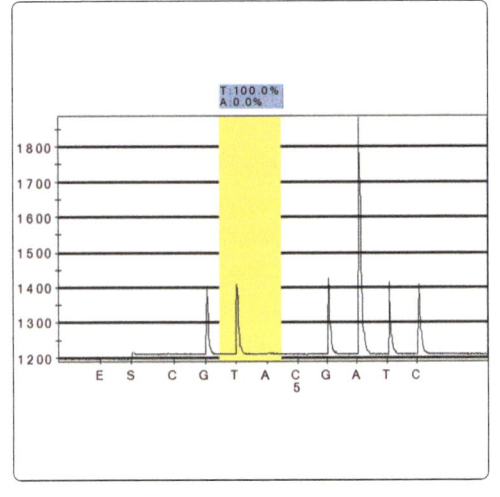

(Left) *Pyrosequencing shows a c.1799T>A substitution in codon 600 of BRAF corresponding to BRAF V600E variant in this case of malignant melanoma.* **(Right)** *Pyrosequencing shows BRAF wildtype gene sequence at codon 600 with 100% T, 0% A in a melanocytic nevus.*

FISH Study

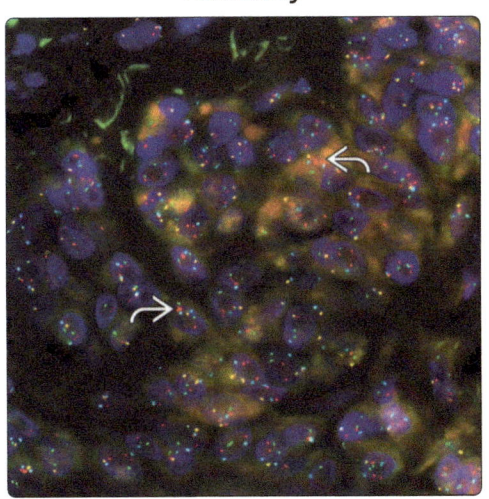

Cluster Analysis of miRNAs

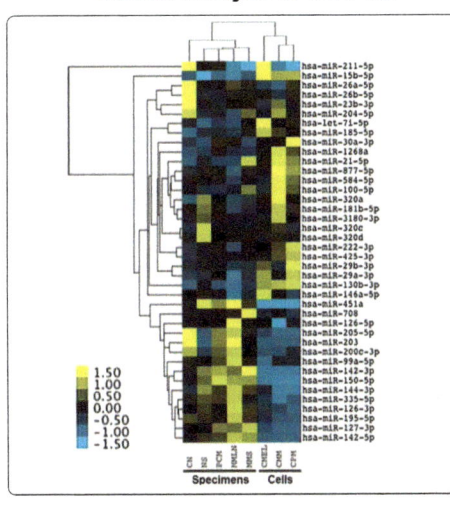

(Left) *FISH study of melanoma shows an amplification of the red (RREB1, 6p25) signal probe ➡ with multiple loci staining in each nucleus. (Courtesy S. Billings, MD.)* **(Right)** *Cluster analysis of miRNAs by NGS separates primary cutaneous melanoma (PCM), normal skin (NS), common nevus (CN), metastatic melanoma to lymph node (MMLN), metastatic melanoma to skin (MMS), cultured primary melanoma (CPM), cultured metastatic melanoma (CMM), and cultured melanocytes (CMEL).*

Squamous Cell Carcinoma, Skin

KEY FACTS

ETIOLOGY/PATHOGENESIS
- Most cases are related to ultraviolet (UV) radiation-induced *TP53* mutations

CLINICAL ISSUES
- Good prognosis in superficial and well-differentiated cases
- Worse prognosis with poorly differentiated, deeply invasive, or aggressive subtypes

MOLECULAR
- Comparative genome hybridization (CGH): Highly aberrant karyotypes are usually seen
- Next-generation sequencing
  - Mutations in *TP53*, especially UV-induced mutations, identified as early events
  - *NOTCH1* mutations are found in up to 75% of cases
- EGFR, RAS, and p16INK4A signaling have been implicated in pathogenesis of squamous cell carcinoma (SCC)
- MAPK pathway is more highly active in SCC than in actinic keratoses

MICROSCOPIC
- SCC in situ shows full-thickness atypia of epidermis, often with prominent mitoses and apoptotic cells
- Invasive lesions are composed of infiltrating nests, sheets, and cords of cells, often with areas of keratinization and squamous eddies
- Cytologically, cells show abundant eosinophilic cytoplasm and large nucleus with vesicular chromatin and prominent nucleoli
- Multiple variants of differing malignant potential described

TOP DIFFERENTIAL DIAGNOSES
- Basal cell carcinoma
- Atypical fibroxanthoma
- Poorly differentiated carcinoma (including metastatic)
- Pseudoepitheliomatous hyperplasia
- Keratoacanthoma

Overlying Serum Crust and Hemorrhage

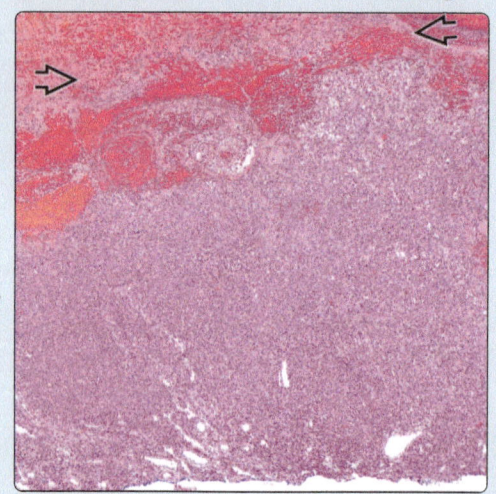

Numerous Mitotic Figures

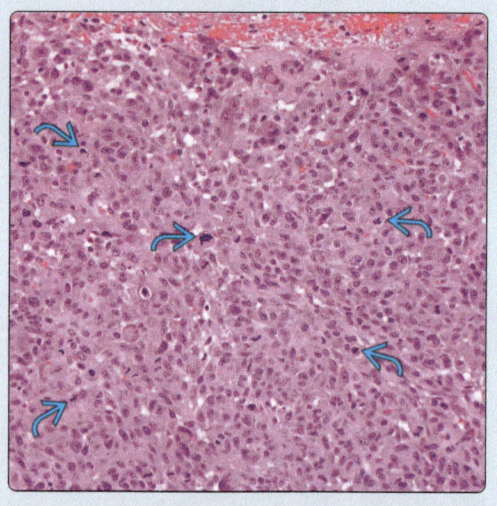

(Left) Invasive, poorly differentiated squamous cell carcinoma (SCC) is ulcerated with dense overlying serum crust and hemorrhage ⇨ and infiltrates throughout the superficial and deep dermis in diffuse, sheet-like collections of cells. *(Right)* Invasive, poorly differentiated SCC shows many large, atypical, epithelioid to oval-shaped cells with abundant eosinophilic-staining cytoplasm. Note the numerous mitotic figures ⇨.

Comparative Genome Hybridization

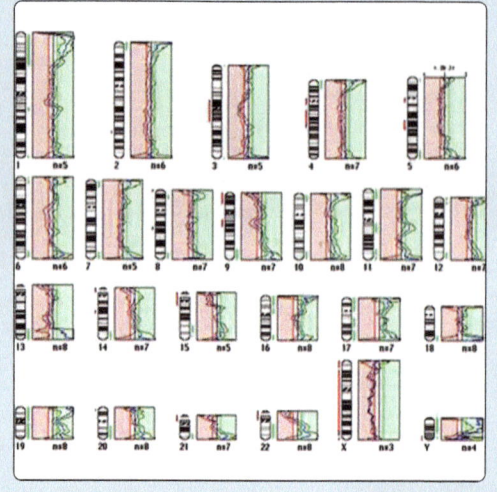

p63 Immunohistochemistry

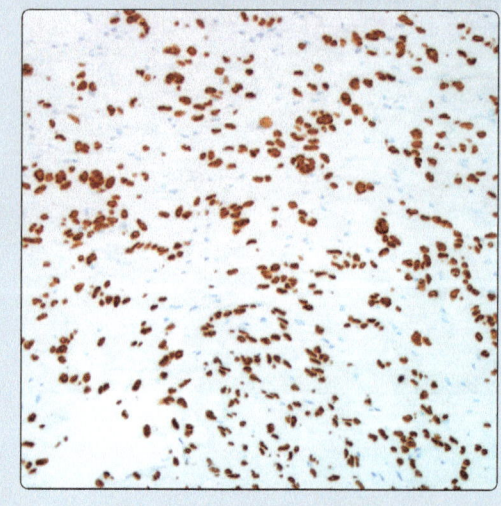

(Left) Comparative genome hybridization (CGH) of SCC shows chromosomal alterations compared to normal skin. The red and green bars on the right show where the gains/losses fall. (Courtesy M. Carless, PhD.) *(Right)* p63 shows strong and diffuse nuclear staining in a poorly differentiated, infiltrating SCC.

Squamous Cell Carcinoma, Skin

TERMINOLOGY

Abbreviations
- Squamous cell carcinoma (SCC)

Definitions
- Malignant tumor of squamous keratinocytes

ETIOLOGY/PATHOGENESIS

Environmental Exposure
- Most cases are related to ultraviolet (UV) radiation, which induces mutations in genes, including *TP53*
- Previous radiation therapy is implicated in some cases, usually associated with more aggressive SCC
- Human papillomavirus (HPV) is associated with some cases
  - Especially anogenital carcinomas, and SCC in immunosuppressed patients

Classification
- Acantholytic/adenoid/pseudoglandular SCC
- Verrucous carcinoma (well-differentiated variant)
- Keratoacanthoma (KA) (very well-differentiated variant, regresses spontaneously)

CLINICAL ISSUES

Epidemiology
- Age
  - Usually in older patients, especially solar-related lesions
  - Wide range (34-95 years)
  - Rare cases in children
    - Should prompt genetic studies

Presentation
- Slow-growing, papular, nodular, or plaque-like lesion
- Often arises in sun-damaged skin, including head and neck tumors
- Vast majority of cases associated with preexisting actinic keratosis (AK)
- May be ulcerated or bleeding

Treatment
- Surgical approaches
  - Complete surgical excision is optimal and definitive therapy
    - Mohs surgery has been shown to be highly effective for most tumors
- Drugs
  - If patients are not surgical candidates, topical chemotherapeutics or immunomodulators may be used
- Radiation
  - May be used for very advanced cases where surgical therapy is not curative

Prognosis
- Excellent in most cases
- Worse prognosis with poorly differentiated, deeply invasive, or rare aggressive subtypes
- Site of tumor is important for prognosis
  - Lip and ear tumors are more aggressive, regardless of degree of differentiation

MACROSCOPIC

General Features
- Papular to nodular or plaque-like lesion; can be exophytic
  - May be ulcerated or hemorrhagic

MOLECULAR

Cytogenetics
- Highly aberrant karyotypes are usually seen

In Situ Hybridization
- Various types of HPV can be detected in some cases

Array Comparative Genome Hybridization
- Numerous abnormalities are reported in comparison to normal skin and pseudoepitheliomatous hyperplasia; gains more common than losses
- Fewer abnormalities in comparison to AK

Molecular Genetics/Next-Generation Sequencing
- Mutations in *TP53*, especially UV-induced mutations
  - *TP53* mutations have been identified as early events
- *CDKN2A* mutations are related to shorter disease-specific survival in metastatic SCC
- *NOTCH1* mutations are found in up to 75% of cases
- Many other pathways also implicated in pathogenesis of SCC, including
  - Epidermal growth factor receptor (EGFR), RAS, FYN, and p16INK4A pathways
- MAPK pathway is more highly active in SCC than in AK
- Loss-of-function mutations in tumor suppressor gene *DLC1*

MICROSCOPIC

Histologic Features
- Proliferation of atypical keratinocytes
  - Associated atypical basilar keratinocytes (AK) is very common
  - SCC in situ (SCCis) is defined as full-thickness atypia of epidermis, often with prominent mitoses and apoptotic cells
  - Invasive cases are composed of cells present in nests, sheets, and infiltrative cords in dermis
  - Often show areas of keratinization (keratin pearls) and squamous eddies
  - Cytologically, cells show abundant eosinophilic cytoplasm and large nucleus with vesicular chromatin and prominent nucleoli
  - Intercellular bridges (desmosomes) should be present on high-power examination
  - Presence of dyskeratotic cells (apoptotic keratinocytes) is reliable sign of squamous differentiation
  - If no definite squamous differentiation is present, immunohistochemistry should be used to confirm diagnosis
- Degree of differentiation is variable, ranging from well- to moderately to poorly differentiated
  - Amount of keratinization typically decreases and cytologic atypia increases with higher grades
- Multiple variants of differing malignant potential described

Squamous Cell Carcinoma, Skin

- o Low-risk variants include well-differentiated SCC arising in AK, KA, verrucous carcinoma, and trichilemmal (variant of clear cell) carcinoma
- o Intermediate-risk variants include acantholytic (adenoid/pseudoglandular) and lymphoepithelioma-like carcinoma of skin
- o High-risk variants include spindle cell/sarcomatoid, basaloid, adenosquamous, and desmoplastic
  – Also radiation, burn scar, and immunosuppression-related SCCs

ANCILLARY TESTS

Immunohistochemistry

- Not necessary in well-/moderately differentiated cases, but may be needed in poorly differentiated and spindle cell cases
- Cytokeratins are most important markers, especially high-molecular-weight cytokeratins (HMWCKs)
  - o HMWCKs are most sensitive markers for poorly differentiated and spindle cell/sarcomatoid SCC
    – Pankeratin can be lost in poorly differentiated and spindle cell cases
  - o p63/p40 are also very sensitive markers and can be used in addition to HMWCKs to confirm diagnosis
- Expression of p16 is often seen, especially in SCCis in genital cases
  - o Correlates with HPV infection in most cases
- Negative staining for other markers, including
  - o S100, SOX10, MART-1/Melan-A, and HMB-45 (positive in melanoma)
  - o CD10, CD68, and CD99 [positive in atypical fibroxanthoma (AFX), pleomorphic sarcoma]
  - o Ber-EP4 [positive in basal cell carcinoma (BCC)], AR, and adipophilin (positive in sebaceous carcinoma)

DIFFERENTIAL DIAGNOSIS

Basal Cell Carcinoma

- Cells are typically smaller, more hyperchromatic-staining, and show peripheral palisading, mucinous stroma, and retraction artifact
- Cytokeratins do not distinguish BCC from SCC, but Ber-EP4 and AR are almost always positive in BCC and negative in SCC

Atypical Fibroxanthoma

- Usually large, ulcerated nodular lesions in heavily sun-damaged (typically head and neck) skin
- Immunohistochemistry is essential in excluding poorly differentiated SCC
  - o SCC is typically positive for HMWCKs and p40/p63; AFX is negative for these markers and often CD10 and CD99 positive

Poorly Differentiated Carcinoma (Including Metastatic)

- Clinical history and imaging studies are paramount, as immunohistochemistry may not be able to distinguish some cases from primary SCC
- Adenocarcinomas may show varying degree of ductal/glandular differentiation
  - o If present, ductal spaces can be highlighted with markers, such as EMA and CEA

Pseudoepitheliomatous Hyperplasia

- Can mimic SCC, especially SCCis, but does not show infiltrative features or high-grade cytologic atypia
- Molecular abnormalities should not be present

Keratoacanthoma

- Essentially very well-differentiated variant of SCC that spontaneously regresses in most cases
- Typically composed of large, crateriform (cup-like) lesion filled with abundant keratin debris
- Cells are enlarged with abundant glassy-appearing/hyalinized cytoplasm
- Most cases regress, but giant KA and subungual KA can be aggressive; some may metastasize in immunosuppressed patients

DIAGNOSTIC CHECKLIST

Clinically Relevant Pathologic Features

- Degree of differentiation
- Depth of invasion
  - o Deeply invasive tumors have much higher rates of recurrence and metastasis
- Perineural invasion
  - o Tumors with perineural invasion have high rates of local recurrence and increased risk of metastasis
- Location of tumor important (i.e., lip, mucosal lesions more aggressive)

Pathologic Interpretation Pearls

- Invasive proliferation of epithelioid cells with areas of keratinization (keratin pearls) and squamous eddies
  - o Intercellular bridges (desmosomes) and dyskeratotic cells confirm squamous differentiation in poorly differentiated cases

SELECTED REFERENCES

1. Cozma EC et al: Update on the molecular pathology of cutaneous squamous cell carcinoma. Int J Mol Sci. 24(7):6646, 2023
2. Tsang DA et al: Molecular alterations in cutaneous squamous cell carcinoma in immunocompetent and immunosuppressed hosts-a systematic review. Cancers (Basel). 15(6):1832, 2023
3. Win TS et al: Keratinocytic skin cancers-update on the molecular biology. Cancer. 129(6):836-44, 2023
4. Beebe E et al: Defining the molecular landscape of cancer-associated stroma in cutaneous squamous cell carcinoma. J Invest Dermatol. 142(12):3304-12.e5, 2022
5. Biao T et al: From Bowen disease to cutaneous squamous cell carcinoma: eight markers were verified from transcriptomic and proteomic analyses. J Transl Med. 20(1):416, 2022
6. Geidel G et al: Emerging precision diagnostics in advanced cutaneous squamous cell carcinoma. NPJ Precis Oncol. 6(1):17, 2022
7. Hedberg ML et al: Molecular mechanisms of cutaneous squamous cell carcinoma. Int J Mol Sci. 23(7):3478, 2022
8. Su W et al: Exploring potential biomarkers, ferroptosis mechanisms, and therapeutic targets associated with cutaneous squamous cell carcinoma via integrated transcriptomic analysis. J Healthc Eng. 2022:3524022, 2022
9. Droll S et al: Oh, the mutations you'll acquire! A systematic overview of cutaneous squamous cell carcinoma. Cell Physiol Biochem. 55(S2):89-119, 2021
10. Azimi A et al: Investigating proteome changes between primary and metastatic cutaneous squamous cell carcinoma using SWATH mass spectrometry. J Dermatol Sci. 99(2):119-27, 2020
11. Mulvaney PM et al: Molecular prediction of metastasis in cutaneous squamous cell carcinoma. Curr Opin Oncol. 32(2):129-36, 2020

Squamous Cell Carcinoma, Skin

Clinical Appearance

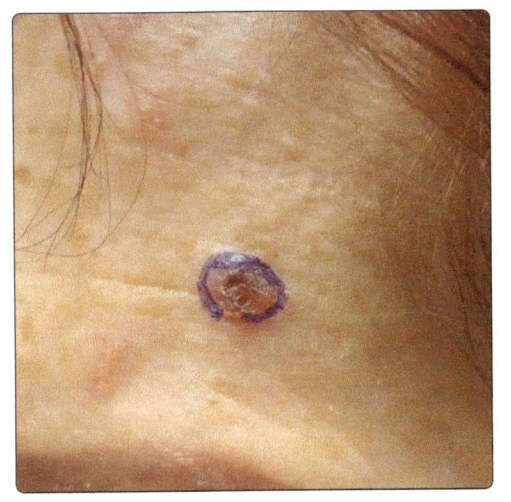

Chromosomal Changes

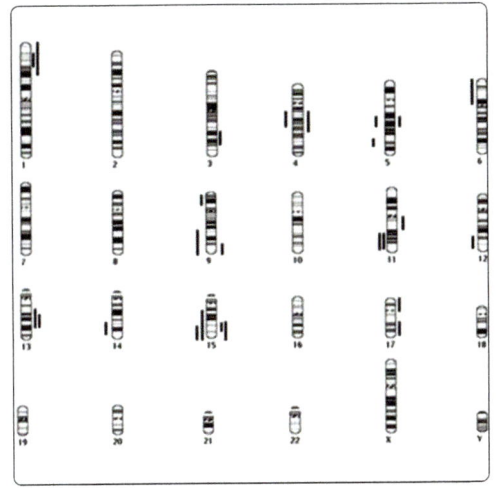

(Left) An ulcerated, invasive cutaneous SCC arising on the forehead of an older adult patient is shown. (Right) Schematic karyogram shows a summary of chromosomal alterations seen in SCC (keratoacanthoma type) compared to normal skin. (Courtesy M. Carless, PhD.)

Poorly Differentiated Spindle Cells

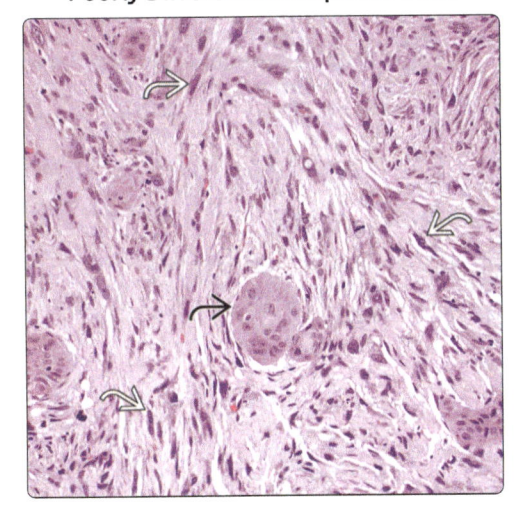

Multiple Lymphatics

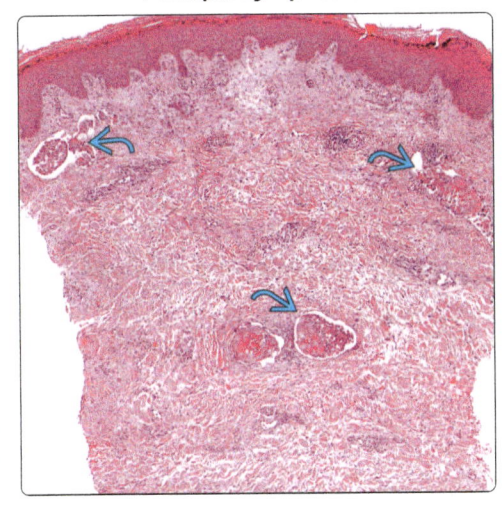

(Left) This tumor consists mostly of invasive, poorly differentiated spindled cells ⊒, although focal areas of more squamoid-appearing cells ⊒ are also seen. The spindle cells should raise a differential diagnosis with spindle cell melanoma, AFX, pleomorphic sarcoma, and other spindle cell tumors. (Right) This is a metastatic SCC to the skin from a primary cutaneous SCC. Note the involvement of multiple lymphatics ⊒. The patient was an organ transplantation recipient who had multiple cutaneous SCCs and BCCs.

CK903 Immunohistochemistry

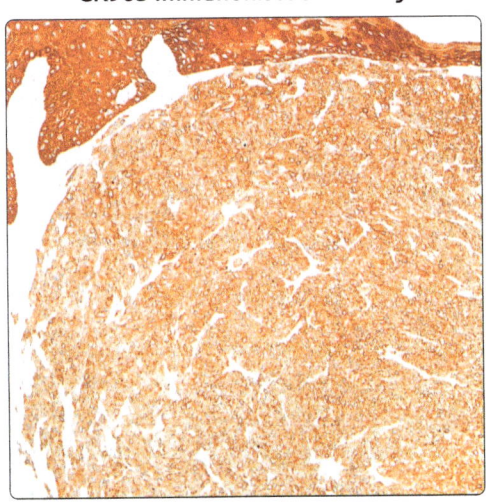

CK5/6 Immunohistochemistry

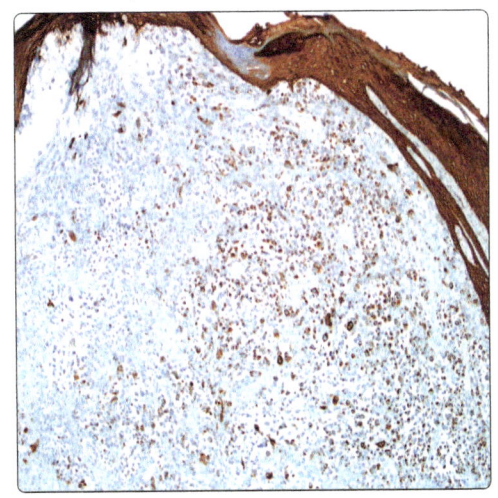

(Left) CK903 (HMWCK) shows diffuse staining of an invasive, poorly differentiated SCC with strong internal control staining of the overlying epidermis. (Right) CK5/6 (HMWCK) shows strong staining of the epidermis and many single cells in this poorly differentiated SCC.

Basal Cell Carcinoma, Skin

KEY FACTS

ETIOLOGY/PATHOGENESIS
- Related to sun exposure, radiation, immunosuppression
- May be derived from follicular stem cells

CLINICAL ISSUES
- Very common: Most common cancer in humans
- Prognosis usually excellent, most cases cured by excision
- More aggressive subtypes include infiltrative, micronodular, desmoplastic, and basosquamous
- Treated by complete excision or electrodesiccation and curettage

MOLECULAR
- Recurrent aberrations of chromosomes 6, 7, 9, and X reported
- Mutations in *TP53* typically detected
- Constitutive activation of Sonic Hedgehog signaling pathway by acquired mutations in *PTCH1* and *SMO*

MICROSCOPIC
- Proliferation of nodules, nests, and cords of small basaloid cells with peripheral palisading, stromal retraction artifact, and mucinous material
- Numerous mitotic and apoptotic figures typically present
- Cells show enlarged hyperchromatic nuclei with inconspicuous nucleoli and scant amounts of eosinophilic cytoplasm

ANCILLARY TESTS
- Greater staining for BCL2, TP53, and Ki-67 compared to benign follicular tumors

TOP DIFFERENTIAL DIAGNOSES
- Squamous cell carcinoma
- Actinic keratosis (on superficial shave biopsy)
- Follicular neoplasms (trichoepithelioma and trichoblastoma)
- Merkel cell carcinoma

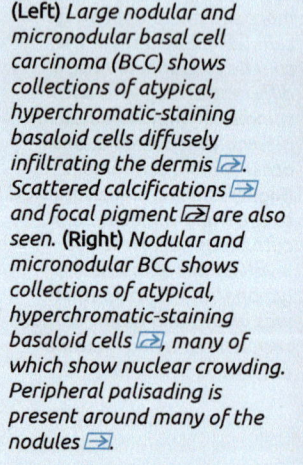

Nodular and Micronodular Basal Cell Carcinoma

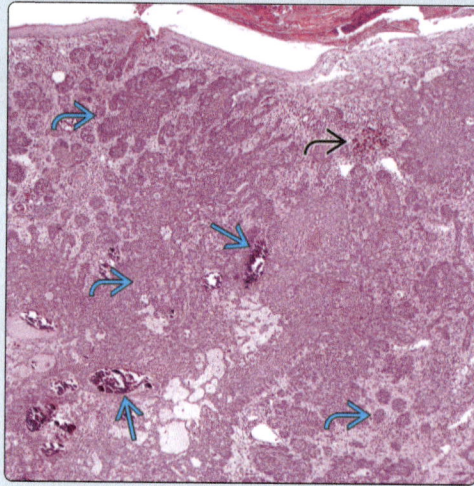

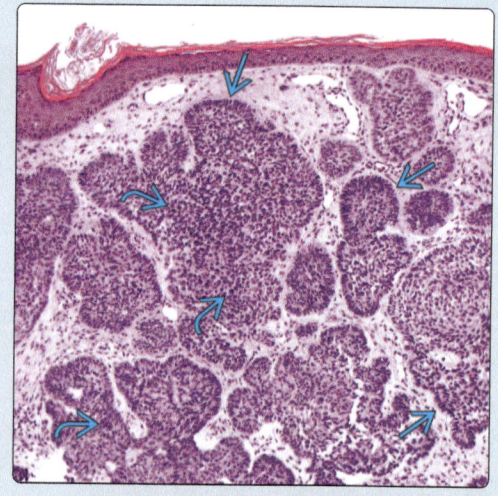

(Left) Large nodular and micronodular basal cell carcinoma (BCC) shows collections of atypical, hyperchromatic-staining basaloid cells diffusely infiltrating the dermis ⇒. Scattered calcifications ⇒ and focal pigment ⇒ are also seen. **(Right)** Nodular and micronodular BCC shows collections of atypical, hyperchromatic-staining basaloid cells ⇒, many of which show nuclear crowding. Peripheral palisading is present around many of the nodules ⇒.

Ber-EP4/CD326 Immunohistochemistry

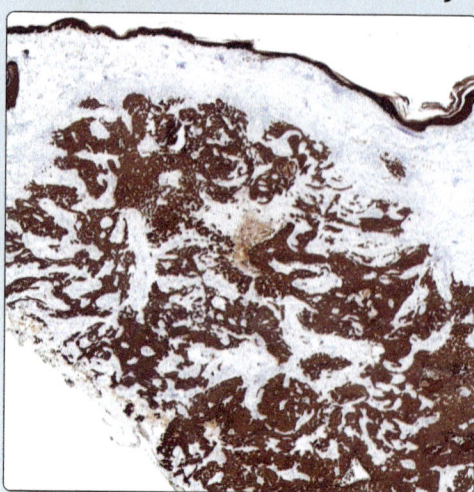

p53 Immunohistochemistry

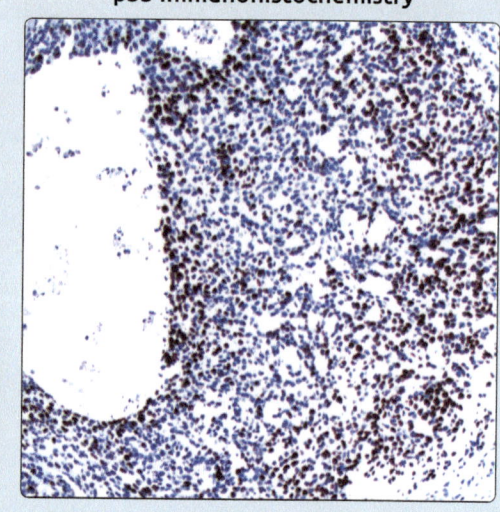

(Left) Ber-EP4 shows strong and diffuse staining of many of the tumor cells. This marker is typically negative in squamous cell carcinoma and most other tumors in the differential diagnosis. **(Right)** Nodular and cystic BCC shows relatively strong nuclear p53 staining in many of the tumor cells. This marker is typically negative in benign tumors, such as trichoepithelioma and trichoblastoma, which may be considered in the differential diagnosis.

Basal Cell Carcinoma, Skin

TERMINOLOGY

Abbreviations
- Basal cell carcinoma (BCC)

Synonyms
- Basal cell epithelioma (older term, not preferred)

Definitions
- Low-grade malignancy of basaloid keratinocytes

ETIOLOGY/PATHOGENESIS

Multifactorial
- Related to sun exposure (vast majority of cases), often with UV-induced *TP53* mutations
  o Some cases may also be associated with radiation, immunosuppression (organ transplantation), and burn scars
    – These tumors tend to be more aggressive
- May actually be derived from follicular stem cells

Genetics
- Rare cases are associated with genetic syndromes, including nevoid BCC syndrome (Gorlin syndrome), xeroderma pigmentosum, Bazex syndrome, Rombo syndrome, and metaphyseal chondrodysplasia, McKusick type
  o Genes implicated include *PTCH1* (Gorlin syndrome), *TP53*, *SOX9*, *BMI1*, *BAX*, and *RMRP*

CLINICAL ISSUES

Epidemiology
- Incidence
  o Extremely common: Most common cancer in humans when skin cancers are included
    – Accounts for 70% of primary cutaneous malignancies
- Age
  o Typically older adults; few cases in young adults
    – If in child, should consider genetic syndrome
- Sex
  o Slightly greater incidence in males
- Ethnicity
  o White/light-skinned individuals
  o Rare in darker skin types

Site
- Most common in head and neck region (up to 80% of cases)
  o ~ 15% occur on trunk and shoulders
  o Very rare cases involve lips, breast, axillae, groin, inguinal region, and genitalia

Presentation
- Typically papular, plaque-like, or nodular lesion
  o Often present as pearly, translucent papule with telangiectasia
  o Larger lesions often ulcerated with bleeding &/or overlying crusting

Treatment
- Surgical approaches
  o Complete excision or electrodesiccation and curettage (ED & C)
  o Mohs micrographic surgery often used in facial cases

Prognosis
- Usually excellent, cured by local excision
- More aggressive subtypes, including micronodular, infiltrative, desmoplastic, and basosquamous, have higher rate of recurrence and increased risk of metastasis
  o Overall risk of metastasis estimated at 0.05%

MACROSCOPIC

Size
- Variable, small (few mm) to large (several cm)

MOLECULAR

Cytogenetics
- Typically show multiple alterations
  o Recurrent aberrations of chromosomes 6, 7, 9, and X reported

Molecular Genetics
- Mutations in *TP53* typically detected
- Constitutive activation of Sonic Hedgehog signaling pathway by acquired mutations in *PTCH1* and *SMO* genes
  o Hedgehog signaling is highly conserved pathway in vertebrates, composed of hedgehog, PTCH1, SMO, and GLI proteins
  o Mutations of *PTCH1* include frameshift, missense, and nonsense mutations
- *BAP1* mutations (associated with some familial melanomas and Spitz nevi) have also been described
- *TERT* promoter mutations (often seen in melanomas) also reported in > 50% of cases of BCC
- Mutations in *STAT5B*, *CRNKL1*, and *NEBL* also reported in some cases

MICROSCOPIC

Histologic Features
- Tumor is composed of nodules, nests, &/or infiltrative cords
  o Overlying ulceration and serum crust often present in large tumors
- Proliferation of small basaloid cells with peripheral palisading
- Stromal retraction artifact
  o Between tumor cells and stroma
- Mucinous material may be present
- Numerous mitotic and apoptotic figures present
- Cells show enlarged hyperchromatic nuclei with inconspicuous or small nucleoli and scant eosinophilic cytoplasm

Variants
- **Superficial multicentric**: Superficial nests attached to epidermis separated by areas of uninvolved epidermis
- **Nodular**: Large, rounded predominantly dermal-based nests with prominent peripheral palisading
- **Micronodular**: Predominantly dermal infiltrative proliferation of small nests

Basal Cell Carcinoma, Skin

- **Infiltrative**: Small cords and nests, often deeply invasive and can have perineural invasion; more aggressive subtype
- **Desmoplastic/sclerosing/morpheaform**: Infiltrative strands and nests associated with dense sclerotic stroma; more aggressive variant
- **Infundibulocystic**: Mature folliculocystic spaces containing keratinous material and often calcifications
- **Basosquamous/metatypical**: Prominent areas of squamous differentiation [may mimic squamous cell carcinoma (SCC)]; less peripheral palisading present
  - Squamous differentiation often seen in large, ulcerated tumors, but if only associated with area of ulceration, should not be diagnosed as basosquamous type
- **Fibroepithelioma of Pinkus**: Numerous small, anastomosing cords of basaloid cells attached to epidermis; low-grade variant
- Rare variants include adenoid, clear cell, signet-ring cell, plasmacytoid/myoepithelial, and BCC with neuroendocrine differentiation

ANCILLARY TESTS

Immunohistochemistry

- Not necessary in most cases except when unusual features present
- BCC vs. trichoepithelioma and trichoblastoma
  - BCC shows greater staining for BCL2, TP53, and Ki-67
  - BCC shows loss of intratumoral Merkel cells by CK20
- BCC vs. SCC
  - BCC is positive for Ber-EP4 (MOC31); SCC is almost always negative

DIFFERENTIAL DIAGNOSIS

Squamous Cell Carcinoma

- Most cases are easily separated; however, basosquamous type of BCC shows prominent squamous differentiation
  - Usually, areas of more typical BCC are present, especially at periphery of tumor
  - Overlying actinic keratosis (AK) or Bowen disease often seen in association with SCC
  - Ber-EP4 strongly positive in BCC, almost always negative in SCC
- Superficial shave biopsies of ulcerated and inflamed cases may be very difficult or impossible to accurately separate

Actinic Keratosis

- Can be difficult to distinguish on very small, superficial shave biopsies
  - Typically shows basilar budding of atypical squamous cells and overlying parakeratosis
  - No mucinous stroma, peripheral palisading, or tumor-stromal retraction artifact should be seen
  - Numerous apoptotic and mitotic figures favor BCC

Follicular Neoplasms (Trichoepithelioma and Trichoblastoma)

- Dermal-based basaloid adnexal neoplasms; may be large and nodular (trichoblastoma)
  - Usually symmetric and well circumscribed at scanning magnification
- Typically lack degree of cytologic atypia, mitoses, and apoptotic figures of BCC
- May show peripheral palisading but mucinous stroma and tumor-stromal retraction artifact typically lacking

Merkel Cell Carcinoma

- Nodular to sheet-like proliferation of highly atypical basaloid cells
- Nuclei typically show speckled (salt and pepper) chromatin pattern or nuclear clearing
- Perinuclear, dot-like staining with CK20, pancytokeratin, and CAM5.2
- Positive immunoreactivity with neuroendocrine markers, such as INSM1, chromogranin, and synaptophysin

Sebaceous Carcinoma

- Can show prominent areas of basaloid differentiation
- Focal atypical clear/multivacuolated cells with nuclear indentations usually present
- Lacks peripheral palisading, mucinous stroma, and stromal retraction artifact
- Immunohistochemistry may be useful
  - Androgen receptor and adipophilin positive; may also be positive in some BCC (usually focal)
  - CAM5.2 and CK7 (+/-); typically negative in BCC
  - EMA often positive in clear cells, although it is often lost in poorly differentiated cases
  - Strong Ber-EP4 and BCL2 favor BCC but are positive in some sebaceous carcinomas

DIAGNOSTIC CHECKLIST

Clinically Relevant Pathologic Features

- Aggressive subtypes (micronodular, infiltrative, sclerosing/morpheaform, and basosquamous)
- Deep subcutaneous invasion
- Perineural invasion

Pathologic Interpretation Pearls

- Proliferation of nodules, nests, and cords of small basaloid cells with peripheral palisading, stromal retraction artifact, and mucinous material

SELECTED REFERENCES

1. Gibson F et al: Epigenetics and cutaneous neoplasms: from mechanism to therapy. Epigenomics. 15(3):167-87, 2023
2. Vergara IA et al: Genomic profiling of metastatic basal cell carcinoma reveals candidate drivers of disease and therapeutic targets. Mod Pathol. 36(4):100099, 2023
3. Win TS et al: Keratinocytic skin cancers-update on the molecular biology. Cancer. 129(6):836-44, 2023
4. Ciążyńska M et al: Risk factors and clinicopathological features for developing a subsequent primary cutaneous squamous and basal cell carcinomas. Cancers (Basel). 14(13):3069, 2022
5. Gambini D et al: Basal cell carcinoma and hedgehog pathway inhibitors: focus on immune response. Front Med (Lausanne). 9:893063, 2022
6. Guerrero-Juarez CF et al: Single-cell analysis of human basal cell carcinoma reveals novel regulators of tumor growth and the tumor microenvironment. Sci Adv. 8(23):eabm7981, 2022
7. Hoashi T et al: Molecular mechanisms and targeted therapies of advanced basal cell carcinoma. Int J Mol Sci. 23(19):11968, 2022
8. Xie D et al: Prediction of diagnostic gene biomarkers associated with immune infiltration for basal cell carcinoma. Clin Cosmet Investig Dermatol. 15:2657-73, 2022
9. Nawrocka PM et al: Profile of basal cell carcinoma mutations and copy number alterations - focus on gene-associated noncoding variants. Front Oncol. 11:752579, 2021
10. Boeckmann L et al: Molecular biology of basal and squamous cell carcinomas. Adv Exp Med Biol. 1268:171-91, 2020

Basal Cell Carcinoma, Skin

Clinical Appearance

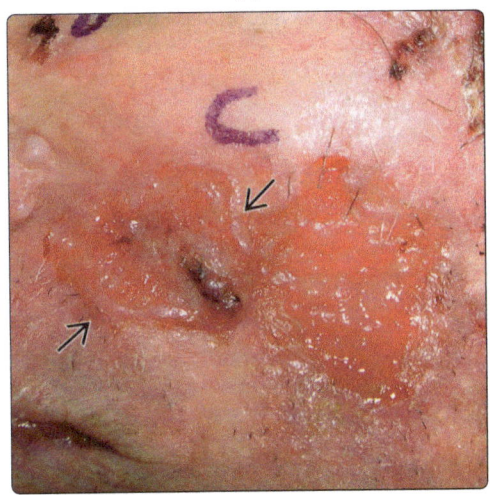

Fibroepithelioma of Pinkus-Type Basal Cell Carcinoma

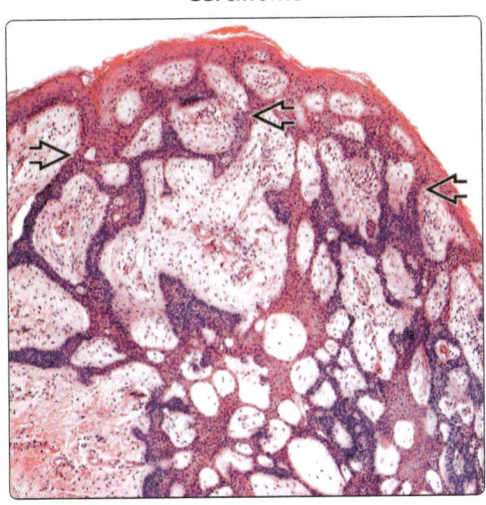

(Left) Clinical photograph of a large facial BCC shows areas of ulceration and granulation-like tissue surrounded by a raised border ⇨. (Courtesy S. Yashar, MD.) (Right) Fibroepithelioma of Pinkus-type BCC is characterized by numerous small, anastomosing cords of basaloid cells with multiple epidermal connections ⇨.

Basosquamous-Type Basal Cell Carcinoma

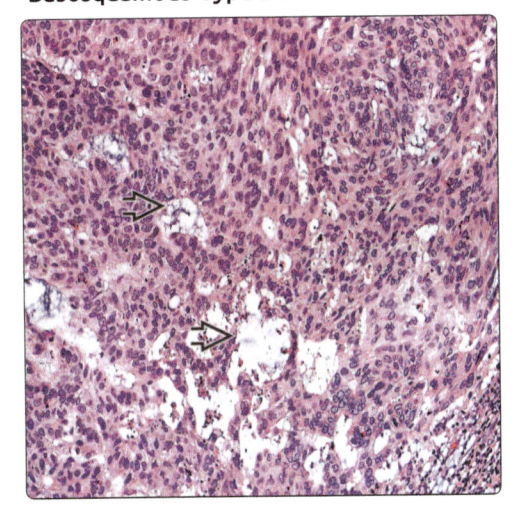

Metastatic Basal Cell Carcinoma

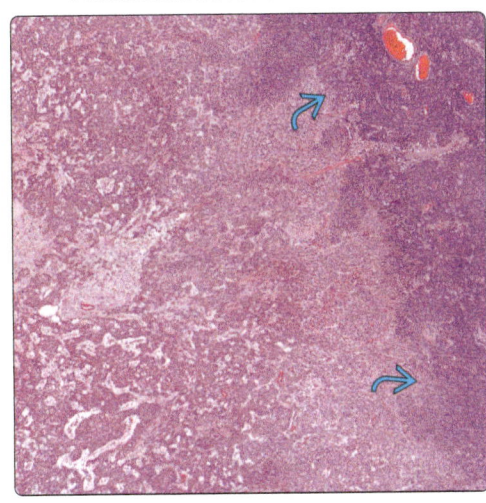

(Left) Basosquamous-type BCC shows a proliferation of large, atypical, squamoid-appearing cells with abundant eosinophilic cytoplasm and focal mucin collections ⇨. (Right) Rare example of metastatic BCC involving lymph node is shown. Note the peripheral nodal tissue ⇨ surrounding the basaloid tumor, which was a deeply invasive, nodular and micronodular BCC.

Ki-67 Immunohistochemistry

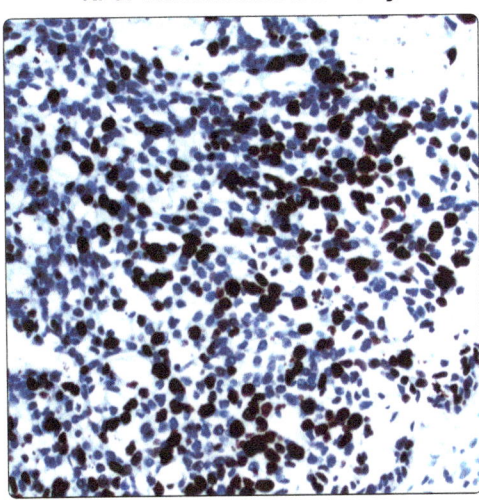

BCL2 Immunohistochemistry

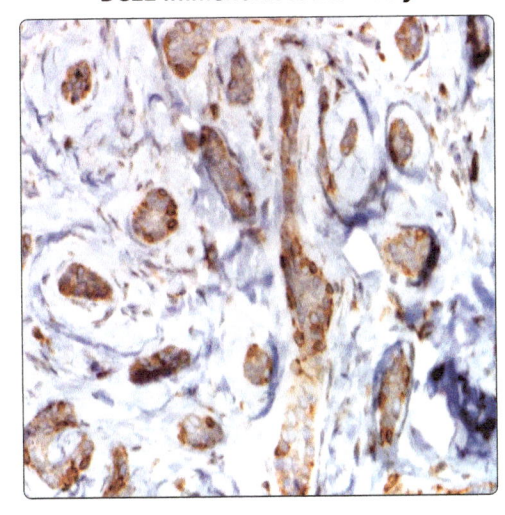

(Left) Strong and diffuse nuclear Ki-67 staining is seen in BCC, consistent with the elevated proliferative rate of this tumor. This marker is usually low or negative in benign tumors. (Right) BCL2 in micronodular BCC shows moderate to strong cytoplasmic staining of the tumor cells. This marker is typically weak or negative in benign follicular tumors.

Sebaceous Tumors

KEY FACTS

TERMINOLOGY
- Sebaceous carcinoma (SC)
  - Proliferation of atypical sebaceous clear cells with multivacuolated cytoplasm
- Sebaceous adenoma (SA)
  - Benign sebaceous tumor composed of bland clear cells with abundant multivacuolated cytoplasm
- Sebaceoma
  - Benign sebaceous tumor composed mostly of small basaloid cells with focal collections of clear cells

ETIOLOGY/PATHOGENESIS
- SC, SA, and sebaceoma all may be associated with Muir-Torre syndrome (MTS)
- MTS is autosomal dominant disease due to mutations in mismatch repair (MMR) genes: *MLH1*, *MSH2* (most common), *MSH6*, or *PMS2* (rare)
  - Can be screened for by IHC for MMR proteins or PCR for microsatellite instability assays followed by sequencing for mutation detection
    - Sequencing of involved MMR gene(s) for detection of mutations

MOLECULAR
- SC, SA, and sebaceoma: NGS for detection of mutations in *MLH1*, *MSH2*, *MSH6*, or *PMS2* in MTS cases
  - Mutations in *TP53* also reported in many SC cases
  - *ERBB2* (HER2) amplification reported in some SC cases

MICROSCOPIC
- SC: Nodular, dermal-based proliferation of atypical clear cells with multivacuolated cytoplasm

ANCILLARY TESTS
- AR, adipophilin, FXIIIA (AC-1A1 clone only), CK7, EMA, and CD10 are often positive in both benign and malignant tumors

Sebaceoma With Cystic/Mucinous Features Associated With MTS

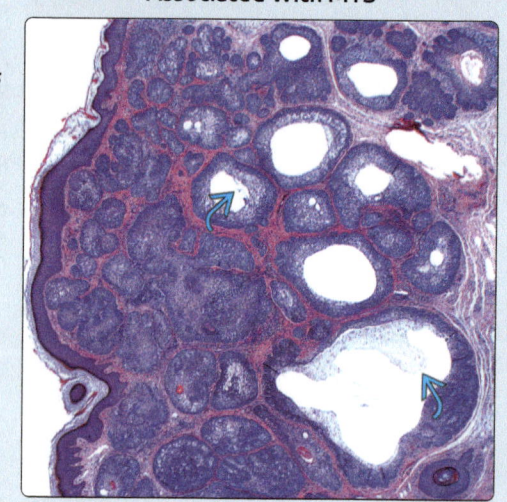

Pedigree of Muir-Torre Syndrome Family

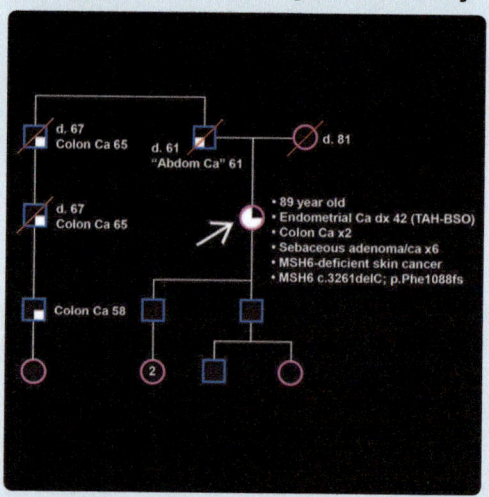

(Left) Sebaceoma shows multiple cystic areas containing mucin ⇨, features which are strongly associated with Muir-Torre syndrome (MTS). (Right) Genetic pedigree of MTS family with MSH6 mutation is shown. The index patient ⇨ had multiple sebaceous adenomas, a sebaceous carcinoma, and history of colon cancer and endometrial carcinoma.

p53 in Sebaceous Carcinoma

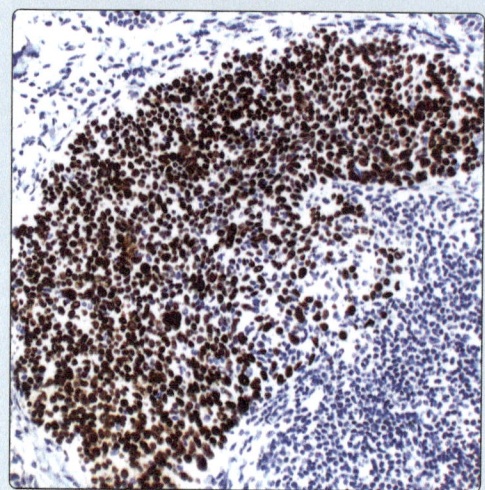

Loss of MMR Protein MSH6

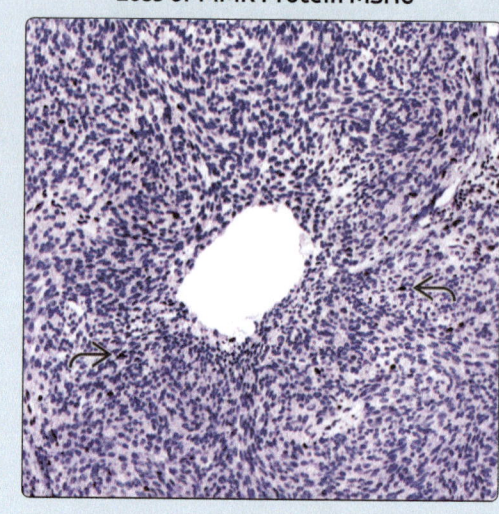

(Left) p53 is positive in most sebaceous carcinomas and shows strong and diffuse nuclear staining in the majority of the tumor cells. Sebaceoma and adenomas are typically weak/negative for p53. (Right) Loss of MMR protein expression is often seen in sebaceous tumors in MTS patients. MSH6 in the same patient from the MTS family showing loss of MSH6 shows only scattered lymphocytes staining ⇨, serving as positive internal control.

Sebaceous Tumors

TERMINOLOGY

Definitions
- Sebaceous carcinoma (SC)
  - Proliferation of atypical sebaceous cells with abundant pale/clear to multivacuolated cytoplasm
- Sebaceous adenoma (SA)
  - Benign sebaceous tumor composed mostly of bland clear cells with abundant multivacuolated cytoplasm
- Sebaceoma
  - Benign sebaceous tumor composed mostly of small basaloid cells with more focal collections of clear cells

ETIOLOGY/PATHOGENESIS

Genetics
- SC, SA, and sebaceoma all may be associated with Muir-Torre syndrome (MTS)
  - Autosomal dominant disease due to mutations in mismatch repair (MMR) genes *MLH1*, *MSH2* (most common), *MSH6*, or *PMS2* (rare)
  - Mutations in MMR genes lead to genomic instability
  - Can be screened for by IHC for MMR proteins or PCR for microsatellite instability detection
    - Sequencing for mutation detection after narrowing down involved gene on MMR proteins testing by IHC

CLINICAL ISSUES

Presentation
- Dermal mass lesion
  - SC usually presents as ocular/periocular nodular lesion; may be ulcerated, hemorrhagic

Treatment
- Surgical approaches
  - SC
    - Complete excision with wide margins
    - May be followed by chemotherapy or radiation therapy for aggressive or metastatic cases
    - Mohs surgery may be best option for complete removal with narrowest margins, especially for eyelid and other facial lesions
  - SA and sebaceoma
    - Conservative excision (narrow margins) is adequate for removal

Prognosis
- SC: Aggressive carcinoma with significant rate of metastasis
- SA and sebaceoma: Benign tumors with very low rate of malignant transformation

MOLECULAR

Polymerase Chain Reaction
- SC: NGS for detection of mutations in *MLH1*, *MSH2*, *MSH6*, or *PMS2* in MTS cases
  - Mutations in *TP53* also reported in many cases
  - *ERBB2* (HER2) amplification reported in some cases

Molecular Genetics
- SC: Mutations in MMR genes in MTS cases lead to genomic instability with acquisition of multiple additional mutations
  - Acquired *CDKN2A* promoter hypermethylation has been reported in many cases
  - Activation of Shh and Wnt signaling pathways reported to correlate with more aggressive behavior

MICROSCOPIC

Histologic Features
- SC
  - Nodular to sheet-like, dermal-based proliferation of large, atypical clear cells
  - Pale to clear-staining cells with abundant vacuolated cytoplasm, nuclear indentations, and prominent nucleoli
  - May show basaloid or squamoid features in some cases, making differential diagnosis with basal cell carcinoma (BCC) and squamous cell carcinoma difficult
- SA
  - Lobular or nodular dermal proliferation of mostly large, bland-appearing clear cells with multivacuolated cytoplasms
  - Smaller component of basaloid cells (by definition, < 50% of tumor) at periphery of tumor lobules or nodules
  - Few mitoses may be seen, but not numerous or atypical; no necrosis or infiltrative features should be seen
- Sebaceoma
  - Lobular or nodular dermal proliferation of mostly basaloid cells with few collections of clear/multivacuolated cells
  - Smaller component of clear cells (by definition, < 50% of tumor)
  - Increased mitoses may be seen but not atypical forms; no necrosis or infiltrative features

ANCILLARY TESTS

Immunohistochemistry
- SC, SA, and sebaceoma
  - IHC for MMR proteins (MLH1, MSH2, MSH6, or PMS2) can be done to screen for MTS
    - Most commonly lost is MSH2/MSH6, followed by MLH1; PMS2 loss is rare
  - AR, adipophilin, FXIIIA (AC-1A1 clone only), CK7, and EMA are often positive in both benign and malignant tumors

SELECTED REFERENCES

1. Morawala A et al: Sebaceous gland carcinoma: analysis based on the 8th edition of American Joint Cancer Committee classification. Eye (Lond). 37(4):714-9, 2023
2. Seger EW et al: Adnexal and sebaceous carcinomas. Dermatol Clin. 41(1):117-32, 2023
3. Plotzke JM et al: Molecular pathology of skin adnexal tumours. Histopathology. 80(1):166-83, 2022
4. Zhao H et al: Overexpression of miR-651-5p inhibits ultraviolet radiation-induced malignant biological behaviors of sebaceous gland carcinoma cells by targeting ZEB2. Ann Transl Med. 10(9):517, 2022
5. Kaliki S et al: Malignant eyelid tumors: are intra-operative rapid frozen section and permanent section diagnoses of surgical margins concordant? Int Ophthalmol. 39(10):2205-11, 2019
6. Bladen JC et al: MicroRNA and transcriptome analysis in periocular sebaceous gland carcinoma. Sci Rep. 8(1):7531, 2018
7. North JP et al: Cell of origin and mutation pattern define three clinically distinct classes of sebaceous carcinoma. Nat Commun. 9(1):1894, 2018

Dermatofibroma and Dermatofibrosarcoma Protuberans

KEY FACTS

TERMINOLOGY
- Dermatofibroma (DF)
  - Benign dermal spindle cell proliferation composed of fibrohistiocytic cells
- Dermatofibrosarcoma protuberans (DFSP)
  - Monomorphic, low-grade, malignant spindle tumor involving dermis and subcutaneous adipose tissue

ETIOLOGY/PATHOGENESIS
- DFSP: Harbors *PDGFB::COL1A1* rearrangements
- DF: Most do not show recurrent genetic abnormalities

CLINICAL ISSUES
- DF: Excellent prognosis; local recurrences relatively common (more in cellular lesions); metastases rare
- DFSP: Local recurrences common; metastasis very rare (only in cases with fibrosarcomatous transformation)
- Complete excision for DFSP
- Complete excision usually not necessary for DF, unless for more cellular or atypical variants

MOLECULAR
- DFSP: t(17;22) leading to fusion of *PDGFB* and *COL1A1*

MICROSCOPIC
- DF: Benign dermal spindle cell proliferation composed of fibrohistiocytic cells
  - Many variants described, including cellular, hemosiderotic, aneurysmal, histiocytoid, clear cell, granular cell, and atypical DF
- DFSP: Monomorphic low-grade malignant spindle tumor
  - Often based in deep dermis and invades into subcutaneous fat with honeycombing fat entrapment

ANCILLARY TESTS
- DFSP is usually strongly and diffusely positive for CD34; weak/negative for CD10 and FXIIIa

Cellular Dermatofibroma

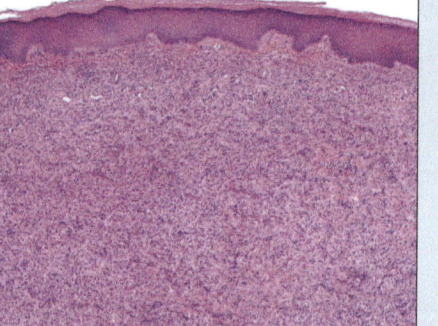

Dermatofibroma: CD163 Expression

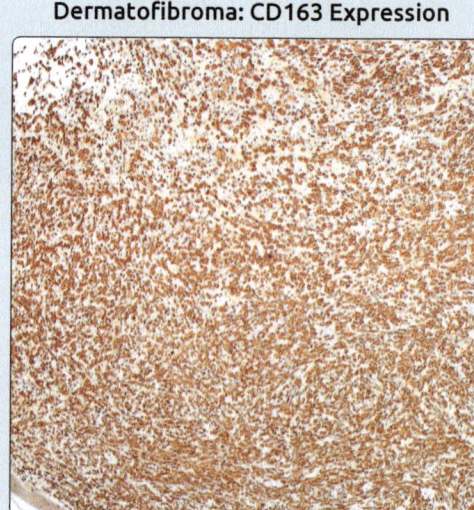

(Left) Large, cellular dermatofibroma (DF) shows a diffuse proliferation of spindled and histiocytoid cells filling the dermis. The overlying epidermis shows irregular acanthosis. (Right) CD163 is strongly and diffusely positive in DF. This marker, along with CD10 and FXIIIA, is usually positive in DF and negative in dermatofibrosarcoma protuberans (DFSP).

DFSP With Fat Entrapment

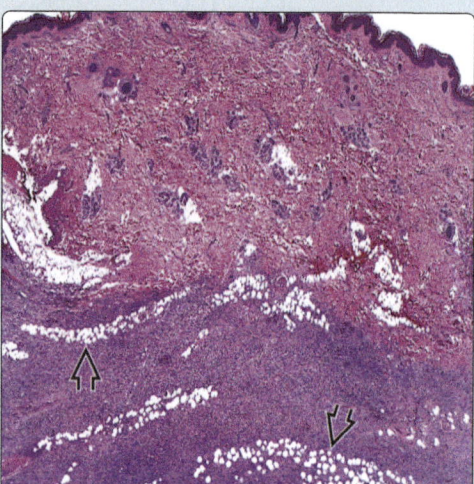

FISH Analysis of DFSP

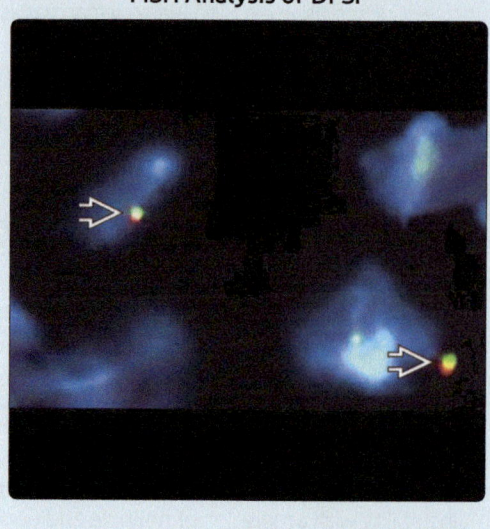

(Left) DFSP shows deep dermal and subcutaneous involvement by a cellular spindle cell tumor with fat entrapment ⇨. The epidermis and superficial dermis are uninvolved. (Right) FISH analysis of DFSP shows the characteristic 17;22 translocation. Green BACs labeling the region on chromosome 22 are fused with red BACs labeling the region on chromosome 17 ⇨. (From DP: Soft Tissue.)

Dermatofibroma and Dermatofibrosarcoma Protuberans

TERMINOLOGY

Definitions
- Dermatofibroma (DF)
  - a.k.a. fibrous histiocytoma (FH)
  - Benign dermal spindle cell proliferation composed of fibrohistiocytic cells
- Dermatofibrosarcoma protuberans (DFSP)
  - Monomorphic, low-grade, malignant spindle tumor involving dermis and subcutaneous adipose tissue

ETIOLOGY/PATHOGENESIS

Genetics
- DF: Most do not show recurrent genetic abnormalities
  - Some cellular, atypical, and metastatic tumors have shown chromosomal aberrations
  - ALK rearrangements in epithelioid FH (EFH)
- DFSP: Rearrangements of PDGFB and COL1A1
  - t(17;22)(q21; q13); COL1A1::PDGFB

CLINICAL ISSUES

Presentation
- Dermal mass lesion
  - DF: Often small, papular to nodular tumor with overlying hyperpigmentation
  - DFSP: Large, nodular to multinodular tumor

Treatment
- Surgical approaches
  - Complete excision for DFSP; usually not necessary for DF, unless more cellular or atypical variant

MOLECULAR

Cytogenetics
- DFSP: t(17;22) leading to fusion of PDGFB and COL1A1
  - FISH targeted probes directed to PDGFB::COL1A1 may be used
- DF: Some cases have been reported to show chromosomal abnormalities
  - Epithelioid FH harbors ALK rearrangement
  - Isolated loss of 5q and gain in chromosome 20 in cellular FH

MICROSCOPIC

Histologic Features
- DF
  - Benign dermal spindle cell proliferation composed of fibrohistiocytic cells
  - Many variants described, including cellular, hemosiderotic, aneurysmal, histiocytoid, clear cell, granular cell, and atypical FH (AFH)
    - Most do not show more aggressive behavior, although cellular and aneurysmal have relatively high local recurrence rate, and AFH can rarely metastasize
- DFSP
  - Monomorphic, low-grade, malignant spindle tumor involving dermis and subcutaneous adipose tissue
  - Often based in deep dermis and invades into subcutaneous fat with honeycombing fat entrapment

ANCILLARY TESTS

Immunohistochemistry
- DF
  - Typically positive for nonspecific markers, such as CD10, CD68, CD163, and FXIIIa; negative for CD34
- DFSP
  - Usually strongly and diffusely positive for CD34; weak/negative for CD10, CD68, CD163, and FXIIIa

DIFFERENTIAL DIAGNOSIS

DF
- Main differential diagnosis is with DFSP (which is usually deeper, more cellular, and monotonous-appearing)
- Negative for CD34 (positive in DFSP)
- Strong and diffuse CD10 staining usually seen; CD68 and FXIIIa may be more focal and weak

DFSP
- Main differential diagnosis is with cellular DF (can be deep, but typically does not show more than focal fat involvement)
- Positive for CD34 (negative in DF)
- Negative for CD10, FXIIIa, and CD68 (some staining may be seen in background dermis)
- Other potential differential diagnosis include AFH

Angiomatoid FH
- Soft tissue tumor with intermediate behavior per 2020 WHO soft tissue tumors
- Harbors fusion genes, including EWSR1::ATF1, EWSR1::CREM, and EWSR1::CREB1
- DF is superficial within dermis and lacks recurrent genetic abnormalities

SELECTED REFERENCES

1. Dai Z et al: Head and neck dermatofibrosarcoma protuberans: survival analysis and immunohistochemical indicators. Oral Dis. ePub, 2023
2. Georgantzoglou N et al: Molecular investigation of ALK-rearranged epithelioid fibrous histiocytomas identifies CLTC as a novel fusion partner and evidence of fusion-independent transcription activation. Genes Chromosomes Cancer. 61(8):471-80, 2022
3. Han Q et al: Dermatofibrosarcoma protuberans of the face: a clinicopathologic and molecular study of 34 cases. J Dtsch Dermatol Ges. 20(11):1463-73, 2022
4. Lee PH et al: Molecular characterization of dermatofibrosarcoma protuberans: the clinicopathologic significance of uncommon fusion gene rearrangements and their diagnostic importance in the exclusively subcutaneous and circumscribed lesions. Am J Surg Pathol. 46(7):942-55, 2022
5. Lu Y et al: Coamplification of 12q15 and 12p13 and homozygous CDKN2A/2B deletion: synergistic role of fibrosarcomatous transformation in dermatofibrosarcoma protuberans with a cryptic COL1A1-PDGFB fusion. Virchows Arch. 481(2):313-9, 2022
6. Peng C et al: Genomic alterations of dermatofibrosarcoma protuberans revealed by whole-genome sequencing. Br J Dermatol. 186(6):997-1009, 2022
7. Kazlouskaya V et al: Spindle cell variant of epithelioid cell histiocytoma (spindle cell histiocytoma) with ALK gene fusions: cases series and review of the literature. J Cutan Pathol. 48(7):837-41, 2021

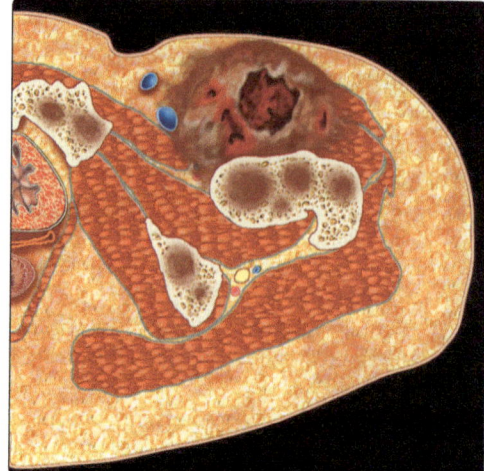

Overview of Molecular Pathology of Bone and Soft Tissue Tumors

TERMINOLOGY

WHO Classification of Tumors of Bone and Soft Tissue, 2020 Edition

- Soft tissue tumor types
  - Total number of entities: 135
  - Largest tumor categories: Fibroblastic/myofibroblastic (38 entities), tumors of uncertain differentiation (31 entities)
  - Classified according to resemblance to specific normal mesenchymal cell
  - Bone tumor types
    - Total number of entities: 51
    - Largest tumor categories: Chondrogenic (17 entities), osteogenic (9 entities)
    - Classified according to resemblance to specific normal skeletal mesenchymal cell
    - Caveat: Soft tissue tumors of almost any type can also originate in skeleton
- Some tumors have multiple histologic variants
  - Variants may or may not have different prognosis
    - e.g., liposarcoma in order of good to poor prognosis: Well-differentiated, myxoid, dedifferentiated, round cell, pleomorphic
- New tumors still being described and added to WHO classification
  - For example: *EWSR1::SMAD3*-positive fibroblastic tumor and superficial CD34-positive fibroblastic tumor
  - Proposed new tumors must be histologically and clinically distinctive
  - Massively parallel sequencing helps to identify potential new mesenchymal tumor types
- Some tumors previously considered distinct entities now recognized to be 1 tumor with different histologic appearances
  - e.g., hemangiopericytoma, giant cell angiofibroma, solitary fibrous tumor = all types of solitary fibrous tumor
  - Clues: Same genetic findings ± some cases show overlapping histopathology encompassing both entities
- Some tumors have multiple genetic variants
  - e.g., epithelioid hemangioendothelioma can have *WWTR1::CAMTA1* fusion or *YAP1::TFE3* fusion

Behavior

- Benign
  - Majority of bone and soft tissue tumors
- Intermediate (locally aggressive) can locally recur
  - Recurrences can be destructive/difficult to excise
- Intermediate (rarely metastasizing) can locally recur and can rarely metastasize (1-5%)
- Malignant can locally recur and can metastasize (> 5%)

General Diagnostic Approach

- Clinical characteristics
  - Age, sex helpful in probability assessment for particular sarcoma type
  - Location in soft tissues: Superficial (suprafascial) vs. deep, body site including viscera
- Imaging characteristics
  - Especially important in bone tumor diagnosis
  - Location in long bone: Epiphysis, apophysis, metaphysis, diaphysis
  - Acral, axial, appendicular, flat bones, cranial bones
- Histopathology
  - Soft tissue tumors
    - Cytologic features assist in narrowing differential diagnosis
  - Bone tumors
    - Matrix features assist in narrowing differential diagnosis
  - IHC often essential to make correct diagnosis
- Genetic findings
  - Tumors divided into 4 broad categories
    - Normal karyotype
    - Specific chromosomal translocation
    - Complex aneuploid karyotype
    - Unknown genetics
  - Genetic findings becoming increasingly important in diagnosis ± prognosis ± prediction to treatment response

---

Primary Bone Sarcoma

Soft Tissue Sarcoma

(Left) Graphic of primary bone sarcoma shows aggressive features, including irregular marrow permeation and penetration through the bone cortex into adjacent soft tissue ➡. (Right) Graphic of soft tissue sarcoma highlights the heterogeneity that may occur with areas of hemorrhage and necrosis. Note that the tumor is deep but extends into the subcutis.

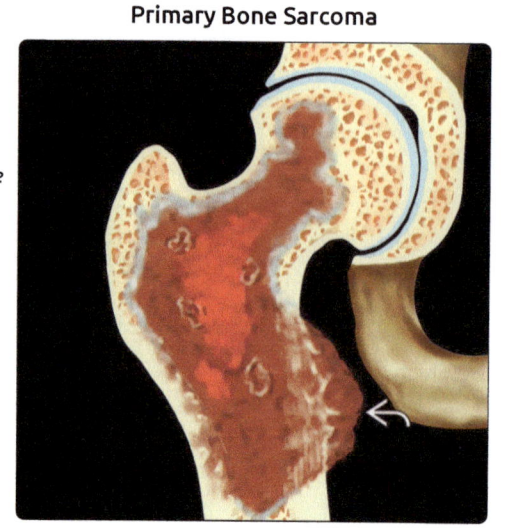

Overview of Molecular Pathology of Bone and Soft Tissue Tumors

- New fusion genes and molecular pathway alterations reported every year

EPIDEMIOLOGY

Age Range
- Tumors with narrow age range
  - General rule: Primitive blastic-type tumors occur typically in children to young adults
    - e.g., Ewing sarcoma, desmoplastic small round cell tumor, alveolar rhabdomyosarcoma
  - General rule: Pleomorphic tumors with complex aneuploid karyotypes typically occur in middle-aged to older adults
    - e.g., dedifferentiated liposarcoma, pleomorphic undifferentiated sarcoma, leiomyosarcoma
- Tumors with broad or biphasic age range
  - e.g., osteosarcomas
    - Most occur in late childhood/adolescence
    - 2nd peak in middle-aged to older adults

Sex
- Males usually more affected than females in general for sarcomas
  - Sex disparity usually small

Incidence
- Clinically significant tumors rare compared to malignancies like melanoma, lung, colon, prostate, and breast cancer
  - Sarcomas annual incidence: 1.8-5 per 100,000 individuals per year
- Benign tumors, however, are very common (e.g., lipomas, hemangiomas, dermatofibromas, schwannomas)

Ethnicity Relationship
- Few tumors show increased prevalence in certain ethnicities
  - e.g., Ewing sarcoma, synovial sarcoma more common in White populations

ETIOLOGY/PATHOGENESIS

Specific Genetic Abnormalities
- Translocation-specific tumors: ~ 40% of bone and soft tissue tumor types, but more discovered annually
- Complex aneuploid tumors: ~ 40% of bone and soft tissue tumor types

Genetic Syndromes
- Many syndromes predispose to sarcomas ± benign mesenchymal tumors
- Li-Fraumeni syndrome
  - Germline TP53 mutation
  - May be more common than previously estimated
    - Consider genetic testing for germline TP53 mutation in patient with sarcoma at young age (< 50 years), multiple sarcomas, or multiple malignant tumors
    - TP53 germline mutation found in ~ 3.5% of 1 adult sarcoma cohort (n = 559 patients tested)
  - Most common sarcomas: Rhabdomyosarcoma (most patients < 5 years of age), osteosarcoma (most patients < 20 years of age), leiomyosarcoma (most patients > 20 years of age)
    - Type of sarcoma may be related to specific type of TP53 mutation
- Hereditary retinoblastoma
  - Germline mutation in tumor suppressor gene RB1 (13q14)
  - Most common associated sarcomas: Osteosarcoma, rhabdomyosarcoma
- Neurofibromatosis type 1
  - Germline mutation in tumor suppressor gene NF1 (17q11)
  - Most common associated sarcomas: Gastrointestinal stromal sarcoma (GIST), malignant peripheral nerve sheath tumor, rhabdomyosarcoma, soft tissue sarcoma not otherwise specified
- Neurofibromatosis type 2
  - Germline mutation in tumor suppressor gene NF2 (22q12)
  - Most common associated soft tissue tumors: Vestibular schwannoma (usually bilateral), cranial nerve schwannoma
- Familial adenomatous polyposis
  - Germline mutation of tumor suppressor gene APC (5q22)
  - Site of APC mutation determines risk for deep fibromatosis (desmoid)
    - Severe desmoid phenotype occurs with mutations at 3' end of APC
  - Most sporadic desmoid tumors harbor CTNNB1 mutations
- Many other syndromes reported to increase risk but affect small number of patients

Environmental Exposures
- Of unknown significance in most sarcomas
- Infectious agents
  - Implicated in few tumors
    - HHV-8 in Kaposi sarcoma
    - EBV in muscle and myopericytic tumors in immunocompromised patients
- Ionizing radiation therapy: Poses risk for sarcoma development
  - e.g., postradiation sarcoma developing 10-20 years after treatment of Ewing sarcoma
- Preceding localized conditions
  - Bone infarct, fibrous dysplasia, chronic osteomyelitis: Increased risk of osteosarcoma
- Metal medical implants: Increased risk of high-grade pleomorphic sarcoma

CLINICAL IMPLICATIONS

Clinical Presentation
- Soft tissue tumors
  - Asymptomatic
  - Slowly growing mass
- Bone tumors
  - Pain
  - Pathologic fracture
  - Incidental finding on imaging performed for other indication, such as trauma

Overview of Molecular Pathology of Bone and Soft Tissue Tumors

Imaging Findings
- Most common modalities
  - CT, MR imaging performed for most deep lesions
- Soft tissue tumors
  - Usually nonspecific findings
  - Can identify fatty component
  - Can identify areas of possible necrosis, hemorrhage, calcifications
- Bone tumors
  - Imaging findings can be diagnostically essential
  - Some tumors with more characteristic features
    - Giant cell tumor of bone
    - Nonossifying fibroma
    - Ewing sarcoma in long bone location
  - Musculoskeletal radiology subspecialty training/experience especially helpful for bone tumors
    - Helps narrow differential diagnosis
    - Helps prevent misdiagnosis in lesions with similar histologic features

MACROSCOPIC

General Features
- Soft tissue tumors
  - Sarcomas may show deceptively sharp margin
- Bone tumors
  - Matrix components may be grossly visible (bone, cartilage)

Specimen Handling
- Rapid fixation
  - Important for ancillary studies, such as IHC, and RNA analysis
  - Minimize exposure to decalcifying solutions in bone tumors
    - If possible, process at least 1 section without decalcification
    - Use EDTA as decalcifying agent to best preserve antigenicity and nucleic acids
- Critical features to describe
  - Percent necrosis, hemorrhage, gross margin status
- Tumor necrosis mapping
  - Required in patients with neoadjuvant therapy for osteosarcoma and Ewing sarcoma
  - Determines response to neoadjuvant therapy
- Collect fresh specimen for research tumor banking when possible
- Additional specimens beyond primary tumor
  - Metastases: May require molecular testing, such as NGS, to identify potential new targetable mutations/alterations
  - Peripheral blood: Circulating tumor DNA (ctDNA), RNA, and exosomes may be prognostic or predictive
    - e.g., presence of ctDNA in osteosarcoma and Ewing sarcoma patients is poor prognostic finding
      - Results reported in multiinstitutional Children's Oncology Group (COG) study

DIAGNOSTIC STEPS

Step 1: Identify Cell Shapes
- Cell shape: Spindled, polygonal, epithelioid, small round blue cells, pleomorphic, vacuolated, mix of cells types
- Automatically creates defined lists of possibilities

Step 2: Note Architectural Features
- Cell organization: Fascicles, solid sheets, storiforming packets, balls, alveolar, microcystic, vasoformative, etc.
- Matrix: No matrix, thick sclerotic matrix, calcifications, bone formation, cartilage formation, myxoid matrix, etc.
- Necrosis: Absent, present, geographic, apoptotic or both; percentage of necrotic tumor

Step 3: Assess Nuclei
- Nuclear size, shape, variation, presence/absence of multinucleation, macronucleoli
- Nuclear grade
- Mitotic rate
- Atypical mitotic figures: Absent/present

Step 4: Consider Histopathologic Features in Context of Nonpathology Findings
- Clinical history and imaging findings: Generate pretest probabilities for histologic differential
- Imaging findings particularly important with bone tumors

Step 5: Perform Ancillary Tests
- Perform selected diagnostic ancillary studies if necessary
- IHC often useful
  - Most common panels
    - Muscle markers: SMA, desmin, caldesmon, myogenin, MYOD1
    - Neural markers: S100, SOX10
    - Epithelial markers (positive in some bone and soft tissue tumors), broad spectrum keratins, keratins 8 and 18, EMA
    - Vascular markers: CD34, CD31, ERG, podoplanin (D2-40)
  - Many tumors show range of reported reactivity for IHC proteins
    - Caution advised in interpreting results
  - Nearly every commercial antibody can react with multiple tumor types
    - Caution advised in interpreting results
- FISH helpful for particular differentials, such as fusion sarcomas (such as Ewing sarcoma) and gene amplified tumors (such as well-differentiated/dedifferentiated LPS)
- Massively parallel sequencing increasingly used; can confirm diagnosis, provide tumor mutation burden, tumor neoantigen burden; discover novel recurrent abnormalities

Step 6: Consult With Expert
- Consult with expert if findings are ambiguous or ancillary studies confusing
  - Advised especially in cases where specific diagnosis impacts treatment
  - Expert consultants often have access to esoteric ancillary testing
- Expert consultation enables accrual of enough cases for meaningful aggregated study by experts

Overview of Molecular Pathology of Bone and Soft Tissue Tumors

Examples of Genetic Alterations in Bone and Soft Tissue Tumors

Tumor	Main Karyotype Finding	Chromosomal Findings in More Detail	Additional Molecular Genetic Findings	Additional Epigenetic Findings	Additional Microenvironment Findings
Lipoma	Mildly abnormal karyotype in 60%	Translocations 6p21-23 rearrangement 13q loss	Various gene fusions mostly involving *HMGA2*	None reported	None reported
Low-grade osteosarcoma	Ring chromosome	Rings composed of amplified 12q	*MDM2*, *CDK4* amplification corresponding to ring chromosomes	None reported	None reported
High-grade osteosarcoma	Complex aneuploid karyotype	Some recurrent changes, including lengthened telomeres	*TP53*, *RB1*, *RECQL4*, *RUNX2* changes; many other genes (> 900) and pathways altered	Numerous hypo- and hypermethylated sites; altered miRNAs	Complex immune cell interactions with tumor cells prompt role for immunotherapy
Ewing sarcoma	Karyotype with variety of translocations; most common: t(11;22); *EWSR1::FLI1* ± additional changes	Secondary changes present, some recurrent	Hundreds of genes abnormally upregulated or downregulated by fusion transcript; somatic mutation rate fairly low	Altered miRNAs; histones abnormally modulated; epigenetic population variation increases risk	Complex immune cell interactions with tumor cells prompt role for immunotherapy

MOLECULAR GENETICS

Complex Molecular Pathobiology
- Commonly found
- Includes epigenetic as well as genetic abnormalities
- Even translocation-specific sarcomas often show additional changes
    - At chromosomal level with additional insertions, deletions, fusions
    - At molecular pathway level with some pathways hyperactive, others repressed or rerouted
    - At gene level with additional genes showing LOH, mutations of various types

Molecular Pathways Altered
- Overlap many of those altered in carcinomas
- *TP53* gene pathway interactions to include *MYCN*, *MDM2*, and *CDK4*
- Cell cycle: *RB1*, *CDKN2A*
- PI3K/mTOR signaling pathway
- Wnt pathway
- MAPK pathway
- Many others

Research in Sarcomas
- Hampered by relative rarity and high diversity of bone and soft tissue tumors
- Multiinstitutional collaborations often required to collect enough cases for study
- Some tumors have < 30 reported examples
    - Difficult to characterize completely

New Therapies for Sarcomas
- Developed with knowledge of molecular genetic and epigenetic findings
    - Targeted therapies may be most effective if combined to address multiple dysregulated pathways
    - May require systems biology approach
    - Metastases, recurrences, and residual disease may require repeated genetic/epigenetic testing
        - Resistant subclones: Identification of these subclones may guide alternative therapeutic options

Role of Stromal Microenvironment in Sarcomas
- Incompletely known

Role of Inflammation and Immune Response in Sarcomas
- Incompletely known: Many sarcomas are immunologically "cold" (evoke minimal immune response)
- Immunotherapy: Trials are ongoing combining immune checkpoint inhibitors with chemotherapy and other approaches

SELECTED REFERENCES

1. Moreno Tellez C et al: Immunotherapy in sarcoma: where do things stand? Surg Oncol Clin N Am. 31(3):381-97, 2022
2. Roulleaux Dugage M et al: Improving immunotherapy efficacy in soft-tissue sarcomas: a biomarker driven and histotype tailored review. Front Immunol. 12:775761, 2021
3. WHO Classification of Tumours Editorial Board: Soft tissue and bone tumors. IARC, 2020
4. Kandel RA et al: Molecular analyses in the diagnosis and prediction of prognosis in non-GIST soft tissue sarcomas: a systematic review and meta-analysis. Cancer Treat Rev. 66:74-81, 2018
5. Shulman DS et al: Detection of circulating tumour DNA is associated with inferior outcomes in Ewing sarcoma and osteosarcoma: a report from the Children's Oncology Group. Br J Cancer. 119(5):615-21, 2018
6. Szurian K et al: Role of next-generation sequencing as a diagnostic tool for the evaluation of bone and soft-tissue tumors. Pathobiology. 84(6):323-38, 2017

Overview of Molecular Pathology of Bone and Soft Tissue Tumors

Leiomyosarcoma: Gross Appearance

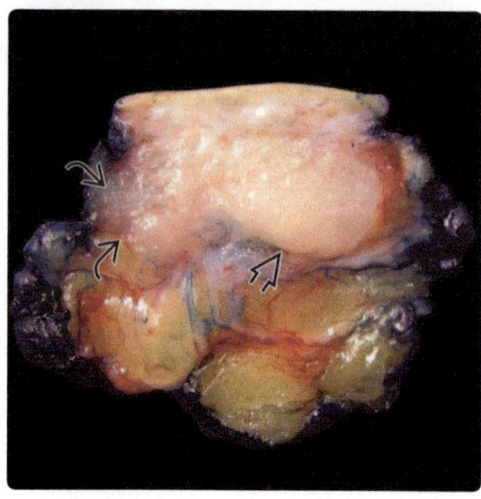

Primary Bone Sarcoma: Gross Appearance

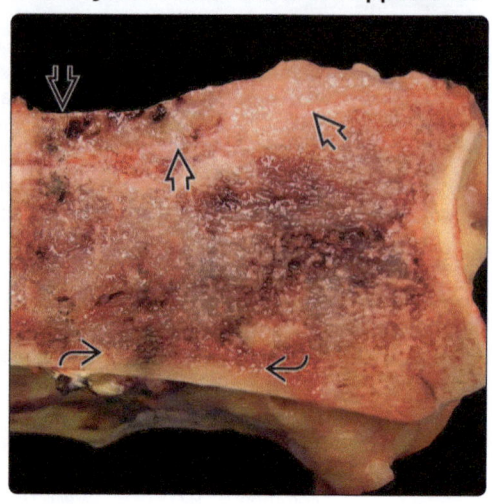

(Left) Superficial leiomyosarcoma expands the dermis and shows both sharp ⇒ and irregular margination ⇒ with the subcutaneous fat. Because it extends into subcutaneous fat, the tumor is capable of metastasis. Muscle tumors entirely confined to the dermis do not metastasize. (Right) Primary bone sarcoma shows irregular, mottled infiltration of bone marrow, extraosseous extension at top ⇒, and preserved cortical bone at bottom ⇒.

Sarcoma With Spindled Tumor Cells

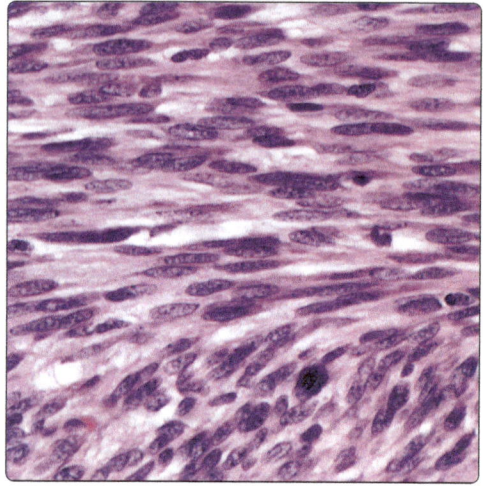

Small Round Blue Cell Sarcoma

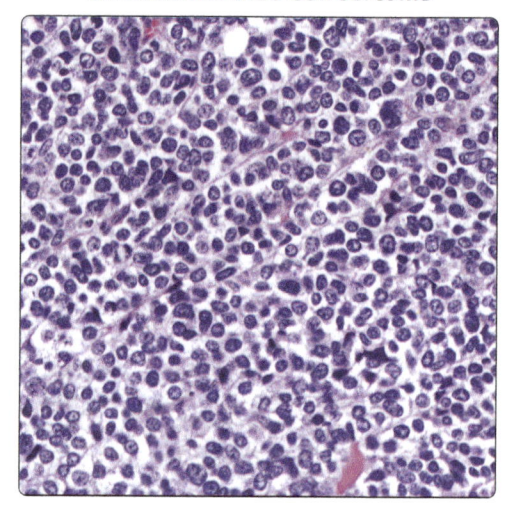

(Left) Spindled tumor cells are commonly found in soft tissue tumors. Typically, the nuclei are also spindle shaped. Some tumors are entirely composed of spindled cells. Others, such as high-grade leiomyosarcoma, may have pleomorphic regions with lower grade regions formed by spindled cells. (Right) Small round blue cell sarcomas (SRBCS) may occur in soft tissue and bones. Some SRBCS can contain spindled cells as well (e.g., alveolar rhabdomyosarcoma).

Sarcoma With Epithelioid Cells

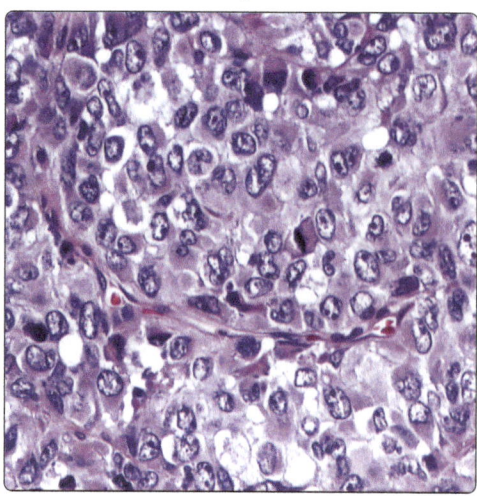

Sarcoma With Pleomorphic Polygonal Cells

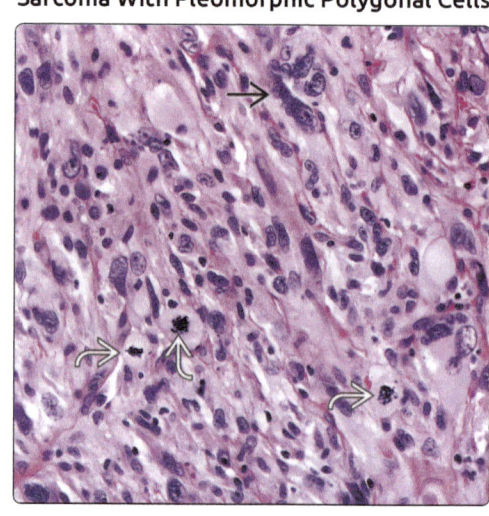

(Left) This epithelioid-appearing sarcoma consists of vague nests of round cells with fairly well-defined cell borders and round to oval nuclei. The differential diagnosis in epithelioid tumors includes various sarcomas, carcinomas, and melanoma. Immunohistochemistry, clinical history, and sometimes genetic testing may be required to make the correct diagnosis. (Right) Sarcoma shows polygonal cells with marked nuclear pleomorphism ⇒ and high mitotic rate ⇒.

Overview of Molecular Pathology of Bone and Soft Tissue Tumors

Rhabdomyosarcoma With Strap Cells

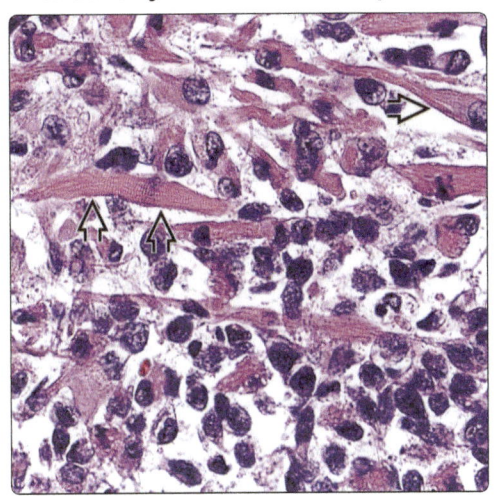

Lipoblasts With Malignant Nuclei

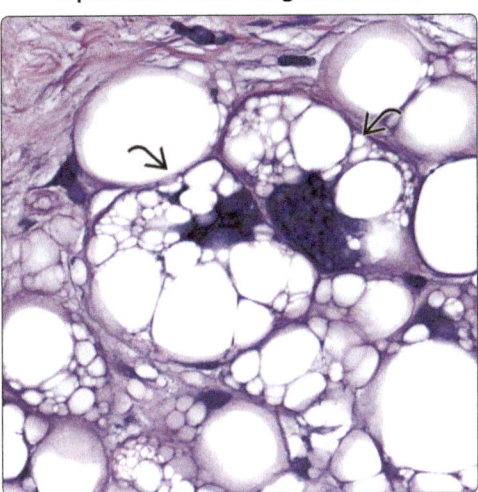

(Left) Some tumors contain cells with very specific and diagnostically helpful features. For example, the cross striations ⇒ in the strap-shaped rhabdomyoblasts of this rhabdomyosarcoma are indicative of skeletal muscle differentiation. (Right) Another specific cell type, the lipoblast, is unfortunately not limited to one tumor type. Nuclear atypia varies in lipoblasts, but those with marked atypia, such as these 2 cells ⇒, are only found in sarcomas.

Osteoid

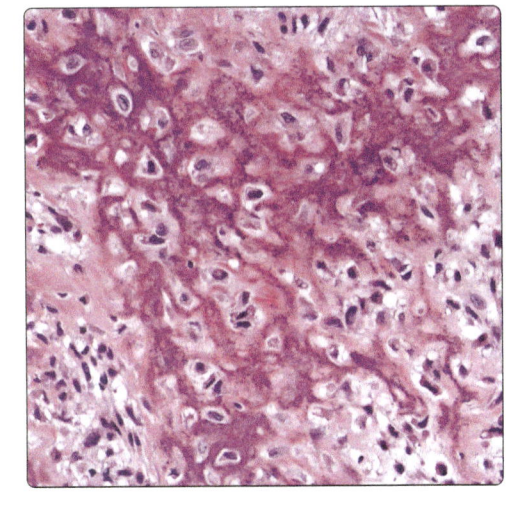

Myxoid Matrix

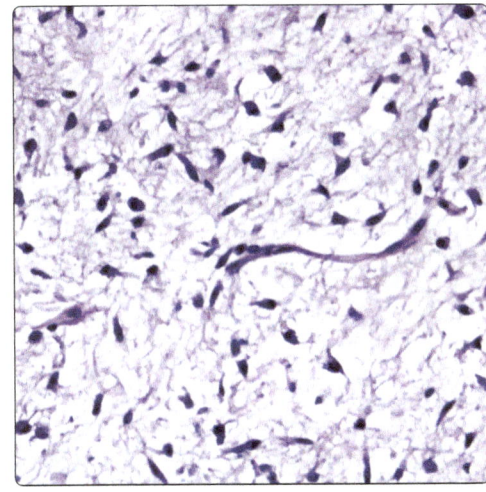

(Left) The presence or absence of matrix can help narrow the differential diagnosis in bone and soft tissue tumors. This matrix is osteoid. Osteoid can be found in soft tissue tumors as well as bone tumors. It may be reactive (metaplastic) or an integral part of the tumor. It may exhibit a variety of appearances and can be confused with sclerotic collagen. SATB2 expression can be confirmatory. (Right) Myxoid matrix is another common type of matrix in bone and soft tissue tumors.

Permeative Growth of Chondrosarcoma

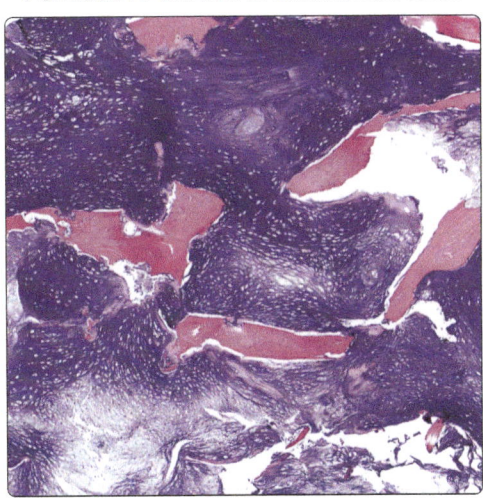

CD31 Immunohistochemistry

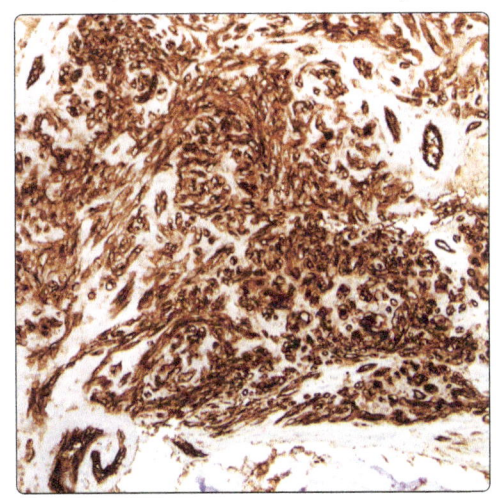

(Left) This low-grade chondrosarcoma destroys and engulfs preexisting bone. Cartilaginous proliferations may also occur as a metaplasia similar to osseous metaplasia. (Right) CD31 is expressed in this angiosarcoma. IHC is currently more commonly performed than genetic testing; however, some sarcomas require molecular testing for diagnosis, prognosis, and therapy response prediction.

Osteosarcomas

TERMINOLOGY

Abbreviations
- Osteosarcoma (OS)

Definitions
- Sarcomas that show phenotypic differentiation toward osteoblasts/osteocytes
  - By definition, these sarcomas must produce neoplastic osteoid

EPIDEMIOLOGY

Conventional Central Osteosarcoma
- Age
  - 10-20 years most common (~ 70% of cases)
  - 2nd smaller peak in middle age (~ 20% of cases)
- Location
  - Metaphysis of long bones
    - Distal femur, proximal tibia, and proximal humerus most common
    - Few cases centered in diaphysis (~ 8-10%) or epiphysis (1-2%)
  - Axial and craniofacial bones more commonly affected in older adults

Telangiectatic Osteosarcoma
- Age
  - 10-20 years
- Location
  - Metaphysis of long tubular bones
    - Tumors may extend into epiphysis
    - Distal femur, proximal tibia, proximal humerus, and proximal femur most common

Periosteal Osteosarcoma
- Age
  - 10-20 years (90%)
  - > 50 years (10%)
- Location
  - Diaphysis most common
  - Distal femur, proximal tibia (80%), humerus, fibula, ulna, others
  - Tumor forms sessile cortical mass and may wrap around bone

Parosteal Osteosarcoma
- Age
  - 20s most common
- Location
  - Metaphysis of long bones
  - Distal femur (70%), proximal tibia, and proximal humerus most common

Low-Grade Central Osteosarcoma
- Age
  - 20s most common
- Location
  - Metaphysis or diaphysis of long bones
  - Distal femur and proximal tibia most common
    - Flat bones and acral bones in few cases

Small Cell Osteosarcoma
- Age
  - 10-20s most common but broad range
- Location
  - Metaphysis of long bones most common

ETIOLOGY/PATHOGENESIS

Conventional Central Osteosarcoma
- Sporadic cases
  - Genome-wide association studies (GWAS) reveal increased risk for OS with single-nucleotide polymorphism (SNP) variants of few genes
  - Variants thus far described increase risk no more than 1.5-3.0x
    - Chromosome 9p21 genetic variants
    - MicroRNA processing machinery gene polymorphisms
    - Others, including *RECQL5*, *VEGFA*, and *GRM4* variants and variant in gene desert at 2p25.2

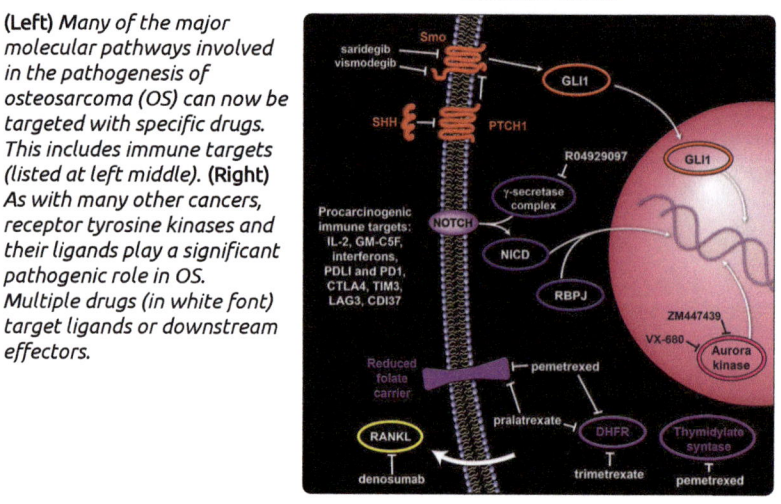

Targets for Therapy in Conventional Osteosarcoma

Targets for Therapy in Conventional Osteosarcoma

(Left) *Many of the major molecular pathways involved in the pathogenesis of osteosarcoma (OS) can now be targeted with specific drugs. This includes immune targets (listed at left middle).* (Right) *As with many other cancers, receptor tyrosine kinases and their ligands play a significant pathogenic role in OS. Multiple drugs (in white font) target ligands or downstream effectors.*

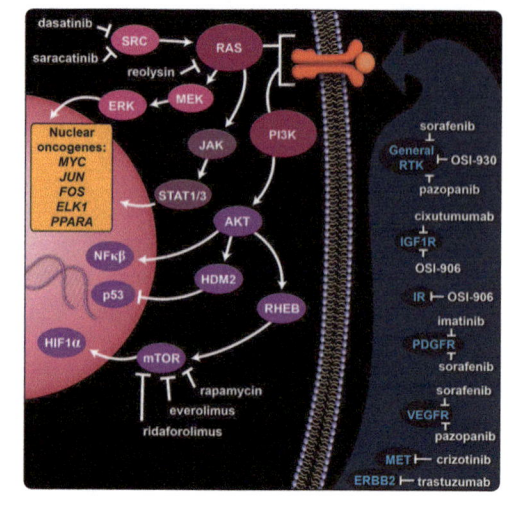

Osteosarcomas

- Susceptibility highest during periods of marked bone growth
  - Late childhood → adolescence = puberty
  - Older patients in setting of Paget disease
  - High level of stimulatory growth factors
  - Increased numbers of proliferating osteoblast progenitor cells
  - Increased level of bone remodeling
- Genetic and epigenetic changes account for pathogenesis
  - High-grade OS shows complex and numerous changes
  - Low-grade (parosteal, central) OS shows simple changes
- Germline syndromes
  - Many syndromes show increased risk for OS
    - Neurofibromatosis type 1
    - Diamond-Blackfan anemia
    - McCune-Albright syndrome
    - Mazabraud syndrome
    - Multiple osteochondroma (hereditary exostoses)
  - Hereditary retinoblastoma
    - *RB1* germline mutation
    - Autosomal dominant
    - Increases risk for OS (several 100x)
  - Li-Fraumeni syndrome
    - *TP53* germline mutation
    - Autosomal dominant
    - Found in up to 3% of children with OS
    - ~ 12% of Li-Fraumeni patients develop OS
  - Rothmund-Thomson syndrome
    - *RECQL4* mutations in ~ 2/3 of cases
    - Autosomal recessive
  - Some abnormal genes found in syndromes often altered in sporadic OS
    - *RB1* inactivated in ~ 35% of sporadic high-grade OS
    - *TP53* loss of heterozygosity (LOH), deletion, or mutation in ~ 40% of sporadic high-grade OS
    - *RECQL4* increased copy number and overexpression common in sporadic high-grade OS
- Secondary OS
  - Ionizing radiation
    - 2nd most common postradiation sarcoma
  - Chronic osteomyelitis
  - Benign bone tumors
    - Fibrous dysplasia
    - Osteochondroma
    - Enchondroma
    - Liposclerosing myxofibrous tumor
  - Paget disease
    - ~ 1% of patients with Paget disease develop OS
    - Most cases are sporadic
    - Familial and some sporadic cases associated with mutations in *SQSTM1*
  - Metal implant/prosthesis related
  - Bone infarct

Telangiectatic Osteosarcoma

- Most cases sporadic

Parosteal and Low-Grade Central Osteosarcomas

- Episomal ring neochromosomes
  - *MDM2*, *CDK4*, and *FRS2* amplifications
- No association with syndromes

Periosteal and Small Cell Osteosarcomas

- Pathogenesis presumed same as for conventional central OS

General Comments

- Low-grade central and parosteal OS: Driven by 12q13-15 amplification
- High-grade OS
  - Chromothripsis: Thousands of clustered chromosomal rearrangements occurring in single event
    - Found in ~ 25% of OS
    - Chromosomal structural variations and copy number alterations > > single nucleotide variations
  - p53 pathway altered in ~ 95% of non-low-grade OS
    - Alterations often occur by inactivating rearrangements of *TP53* in addition to some cases with point mutations

CLINICAL IMPLICATIONS

Treatment

- Conventional central, telangiectatic, and small cell OS
  - Surgery and neoadjuvant multiagent chemotherapy
    - Additional chemotherapy if neoadjuvant chemotherapy necrosis is < 90%
    - Standard chemotherapy regimen includes doxorubicin and cisplatin ± high-dose methotrexate
    - Additional regimens in clinical trials use kinase inhibitors, PARP inhibitors, and others
- Periosteal, parosteal, and low-grade central OS
  - Surgery alone
- Immunotherapy
  - Some OS express PD-L1 in tumor cells (up to 25%)
    - Higher levels of PD-L1 usually associated with more aggressive behavior and worse prognosis
    - However, single-agent immune checkpoint inhibitor generally ineffective
  - Combination of immunotherapy with chemotherapy &/or radiotherapy in clinical trials
  - Other approaches selectively boost antitumoral cell populations: Adoptive T-cell therapy, dendritic cell therapy, and others

Outcome After Treatment

- Conventional central OS
  - Overall cure rate: ~ 70%
  - 5-year survival for relapsed or metastatic: ~ 20%
  - Poor prognostic factors
    - Axial location, > 40 years of age, overt metastatic disease at diagnosis
  - Specific SNPs may predict lower progression-free survival
    - 5-year progression-free survival significantly decreases with increasing number of risk alleles in *FASLG*, *MSH2*, *CASP3*, *ABCC5*, and *CYP3A4* from 100% (0-1 allele) to 42% (all 5 risk alleles)
- Telangiectatic OS

Osteosarcomas

- Slightly higher survival compared to conventional OS when treated with multiagent neoadjuvant therapy
- Periosteal OS: Overall 10-year survival ~ 85%
- Parosteal OS: Overall 10-year survival ~ 100%
  - Rarely, cases that dedifferentiate on recurrence have worse prognosis
- Low-grade central OS: Overall 5-year survival ~ 90%
  - Uncommonly, cases may dedifferentiate on recurrence and have worse prognosis
- Small cell OS: May have slightly worse survival than conventional OS

MOLECULAR PATHOLOGY

Conventional Central Osteosarcoma

- Cytogenetics
  - Complex aneuploid karyotype
    - Many numerical and structural chromosome aberrations
  - Massive clustered chromosomal rearrangements in localized genomic region in 1 or few chromosomes
    - Found in ~ 33% of high-grade OS
  - Alternative lengthening of telomeres due to homologous recombination that prevents normal telomere attrition during DNA replication
    - Found in ~ 85% of high-grade OS
    - Enables infinite replicative potential of tumor cells
- Chromosomal microarray
  - Recurrent amplification and copy number gains
    - 1p36, 1q21-22, 6p12-21, 8q21-24, 12q11-14, 17p11-13, 19q12-13
  - Recurrent losses
    - 3q13, 8p21, 9p13, 13q14
- Gene alterations
  - Localized hypermutation (kataegis) colocalized with somatic genome rearrangements
    - Found in 50% of high-grade OS
  - *TNFSF11*
    - Overexpression in some high-grade OS
  - Overexpression of bone development genes
    - *IHH*
    - *PTCH1*
    - *GLI1*
    - *NOTCH1, NOTCH2, NOTCH3*
    - *RUNX2*
  - Genes with underexpression, deletion, or LOH
    - *DKK3*
    - *LSAMP* deletion or LOH in ~ 60% of high-grade OS
    - *CDKN2A* deleted in ~ 15% of high-grade OS
    - *TP53* deletion or LOH in ~ 40% of high-grade OS
    - *APC* LOH in ~ 60%
    - *MET* deleted in ~ 40% of high-grade OS; other studies report *MET* overexpression
    - *PTEN* deleted in ~ 40% of high-grade OS
    - Allelic loss of *BUB3* and *FGFR2* in ~ 60%
  - Overexpression of receptor tyrosine kinases (TKs) or TK ligands
    - *PDGFA/PDGFB* and *PDGFRA/PDGFRB* receptors overexpression variably reported in ~ 75% of OS
    - *VEGFA* amplified in ~ 60% of high-grade OS
    - *IGF1* and *IGF2R*
    - *ERBB2* (HER2)
  - Overexpression of intracellular signaling molecules
    - *SRC* kinase
    - *AURKA, AURKB*
    - *MYC* amplified in ~ 10-50% of high-grade OS
    - *CDK4* amplified in ~ 10%
    - *RUNX2* amplified or mutated or hypermethylated in ~ 20-55% of high-grade OS
    - *MDM2* amplified in ~ 10% of high-grade OS
  - Mutated genes
    - *TP53* mutated in ~ 85% of high-grade OS
    - *RB1* mutated in 10-40% of high-grade OS
    - *ATRX* mutated in ~ 30%
    - *DLG2* mutated in ~ 50% of high-grade OS
- Epigenetic alterations
  - Abnormal patterns of hypo- and hypermethylation
    - *WIF1* hypermethylated
    - *HIC1* hypermethylated in ~ 20%
  - Histone modifications
    - Abnormally enhance or repress gene expression, depending on location of hypermethylation
  - miRNAs dysregulated
    - miR-21, miR-34, miR-125b, miR-340, miR-240, mir-208a, and others differentially regulated
    - Dysregulated miRNAs act as tumor suppressors or oncogenes
  - lncRNAs dysregulated
    - DANCR, HIF1A-AS2, TTN-AS1 and others differentially regulated
    - When located in the cytoplasm: Inhibit interaction between miRNAs and mRNAs
      - Cytoplasmic lncRNAs that "sponge" miRNAs are also termed competing endogenous RNAs (ceRNAs)
- Major pathways dysregulated
  - Pathways normally involved in bone development
    - Hedgehog
    - Wnt
    - Notch
  - mTOR pathway
  - Cell cycle
  - Crosstalk among altered pathways may require multiagent targeted therapy

Telangiectatic Osteosarcoma

- Karyotype
  - May have less complex karyotypes than conventional high-grade OS
- Additional genetic findings lacking due to paucity of cases

Periosteal Osteosarcoma

- Karyotype
  - Aneuploid karyotype that may be as complex as conventional central OS
- *TP53* point mutations in ~ 40%
- Additional genetic findings lacking due to paucity of cases

Parosteal Osteosarcoma

- Karyotype
  - Simple karyotype with giant ring chromosomes

Osteosarcomas

- Gene alterations as in low-grade central OS

Low-Grade Central Osteosarcoma
- Karyotype
  - Simple karyotype with giant ring chromosomes of amplified chromosome 12q13-15
- Gene amplifications at 12q13-15 resulting in supernumerary ring and giant rod chromosomes
  - *MDM2* amplification
  - *CDK4* amplification
  - *FRS2* amplification
    - Normally interacts with various receptor TKs
    - Involved in cell differentiation, proliferation, and tumorigenesis
  - These genes are also amplified in atypical lipomatous tumor/well-differentiated and dedifferentiated liposarcoma

Small Cell Osteosarcoma
- Karyotype
  - No consistent findings in very few cases studied
- Detailed genetic findings lacking due to rarity of subtype
  - Lacks *EWSR1* translocations in few cases assessed

MICROSCOPIC

Conventional Central Osteosarcoma
- Tumor cells
  - Heterogeneous: Epithelioid to polygonal to spindled or mixed
  - Moderate to marked nuclear atypia = grade 2 or 3
    - Pleomorphic
    - Macronucleoli
    - Moderate to high mitotic rate
- Matrix/background
  - Osteoid present with embedded tumor cells (not metaplastic)
  - Osteoid appearances
    - Lace-like, most commonly
    - Large, solid, expansile, fusing nodules
    - All tumor bone is woven (immature), except rare cases of low-grade OS
- Histologic variants with no difference in treatment and outcome
  - Osteoblastic comprises ~ 75% of all variants
    - Osteoid is main matrix component
    - Tumor composed almost entirely of osteoid = "sclerosing variant"
  - Chondroblastic accounts for ~ 15% of all variants
    - Hyaline cartilage also present identical to grade 2 or 3 chondrosarcoma
    - Uncommonly, cartilaginous component is more myxoid
    - Tumor must contain large amounts of cartilaginous matrix to be considered chondroblastic OS
  - Fibroblastic comprises ~ 10% of all variants
    - Tumor cells are entirely or predominantly spindled
    - Architecture is storiforming or fascicular
  - Giant cell rich
    - Numerous reactive osteoclastic giant cells present
    - Giant cells may be dispersed evenly throughout tumor, mimicking giant cell tumor of bone at low power
  - Epithelioid
    - Tumor cells are large, round to polygonal with distinct cell borders
  - Clear cell
    - Very rare epithelioid variant composed of cells with clear cytoplasm
  - Osteoblastoma-like
    - Tumor cells cuff neoplastic osteoid as in osteoblastoma
    - Permeative growth, unlike osteoblastoma
    - More cytologic atypia than osteoblastoma
  - Chondroblastoma-like
    - Resembles chondroblastoma with epithelioid cells with clefting, filigree calcifications, and pink chondroid
    - Permeative growth, unlike chondroblastoma
    - More cytologic atypia than chondroblastoma

Telangiectatic Osteosarcoma
- Tumor cells
  - Heterogeneous: Epithelioid to polygonal to spindled or mixed
  - Grade 2 &/or grade 3 nuclei
  - May have prominent reactive osteoclasts
- Matrix/background
  - Osteoid usually sparse
  - Large, blood-filled, unlined cystic spaces
  - Tumor cells directly abut bloody cysts

Periosteal Osteosarcoma
- Tumor cells
  - Heterogeneous: Epithelioid to polygonal to spindled or mixed
  - Usually grade 2 nuclei
- Matrix
  - Hyaline cartilage-like matrix in addition to neoplastic osteoid
    - Abundant
    - Nuclei are identical to those of grade 2 or 3 chondrosarcoma
  - Chondroid matrix occasionally more myxoid

Parosteal Osteosarcoma
- Tumor cells
  - Spindled tumor cells
  - Grade 1 nuclei in most cases
    - 20% have focal grade 2 nuclei
- Matrix
  - Osteoid
    - Abundant parallel trabeculae
    - ± osteoblastic rimming
    - ± bone maturation
  - Chondroid areas
    - Hyaline cartilage that is mildly cellular with mild atypia
    - Some cases show cap of hyaline cartilage
- Dedifferentiation
  - 10-15% of cases
  - Appearance of dedifferentiated areas

Osteosarcomas

- High-grade spindle cell sarcoma, not otherwise specified (NOS)
- High-grade conventional OS

Low-Grade Central Osteosarcoma
- Tumor cells
  - Cellularity low to moderate
  - Usually spindled
  - Nuclear grade 1
- Matrix
  - Sparse to abundant osteoid
  - Various appearances
    - Fibrous dysplasia-like
    - Long, parallel trabecular, as in parosteal OS
    - Nonspecific lacy to expansive areas
  - Hyaline cartilage may be present
    - Minor component if present

Small Cell Osteosarcoma
- Tumor cells
  - High cellularity
  - Round to oval tumor cells with moderate to high N:C ratio
    - Rare tumors have short, plump spindle cells
  - Nuclei
    - Round to oval to spindled (in spindle cell variant)
    - Fine to coarse chromatin
    - Nucleoli usually small and single or absent
- Matrix
  - Osteoid
    - Must be present
    - Usually lace-like in configuration

ANCILLARY STUDIES

Immunohistochemistry
- Conventional central OS
  - Tumor cells express nuclear SATB2, p53(+/-)
- Telangiectatic OS
  - Tumor cells express SATB2, p53(+/-)
- Periosteal OS
  - Neoplastic cells express SATB2, p53(+/-)
- Parosteal OS
  - Tumor cells express MDM2 and CDK4
- Low-grade central OS
  - Tumor cells express MDM2 and CDK4
- Small cell OS
  - Neoplastic cells express SATB2, CD99(+/-), CD334(+/-), and SMA(+/-)

Karyotype
- Conventional central and telangiectatic OS
  - Complex aneuploid
- Periosteal OS
  - Abnormal but not usually as aneuploid as with conventional OS
- Small cell OS
  - No consistent findings (only rare cases with karyotype reported)

DIFFERENTIAL DIAGNOSIS

DDx for Conventional Central Osteosarcoma
- Dedifferentiated chondrosarcoma with malignant OS component
  - *IDH1/IDH2* mutations present in chondrosarcoma and absent in most cases of OS
- High-grade pleomorphic sarcoma, NOS
  - Lacks tumor osteoid
- Fracture callus
  - Clinical history and imaging helpful
  - Lacks genetic abnormalities
  - ± more organized pattern of bone formation

DDx for Telangiectatic Osteosarcoma
- Aneurysmal bone cyst
  - Imaging may be helpful
  - Lacks marked atypia of lesional cells

DDx for Periosteal Osteosarcoma
- Periosteal chondrosarcoma
  - Lacks tumor osteoid
  - *IDH1/IDH2* mutations present

DDx for Parosteal Osteosarcoma
- Fibrous dysplasia
  - Only rarely grows as parosteal tumor
  - "Chinese character" irregular neoplastic trabeculae
  - CDK4 and MDM2 (-)
- Reactive periostitis
  - Imaging and clinical history helpful
  - CDK4 and MDM2 (-)
  - Usually small lesion

DDx for Low-Grade Central Osteosarcoma
- Fibrous dysplasia
  - "Chinese character" irregular neoplastic trabeculae
  - Lacks permeative growth
  - *CDK4*, *MDM2*, and *FRS2* amplification (-) by FISH
    - CDK4, MDM2, and FRS2 IHC results not as sensitive or specific
  - *GNAS* mutations (+)

DDx for Small Cell Osteosarcoma
- Ewing sarcoma family of tumors
  - Nearly all lack tumor osteoid
  - SATB2(-)
  - (+) for fusion transcripts, such as *EWSR1::FLI1*, by RNAseq or *EWSR1* break-apart probe (+) by FISH
- Other small round cell sarcomas
  - Rarely occur as primary tumor in bone
  - Lack tumor osteoid
  - Many show characteristic fusion transcripts lacking in small cell OS

SELECTED REFERENCES

1. Nacev BA et al: Clinical sequencing of soft tissue and bone sarcomas delineates diverse genomic landscapes and potential therapeutic targets. Nat Commun. 13(1):3405, 2022
2. Wen Y et al: Immune checkpoints in osteosarcoma: recent advances and therapeutic potential. Cancer Lett. 547:215887, 2022
3. Yang G et al: The role of noncoding RNAs in the regulation, diagnosis, prognosis and treatment of osteosarcoma (Review). Int J Oncol. 59(3), 2021

Osteosarcomas

Conventional Osteosarcoma

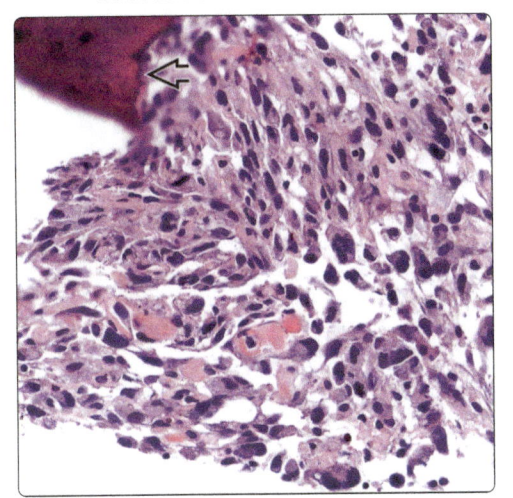

Conventional High-Grade Osteosarcoma

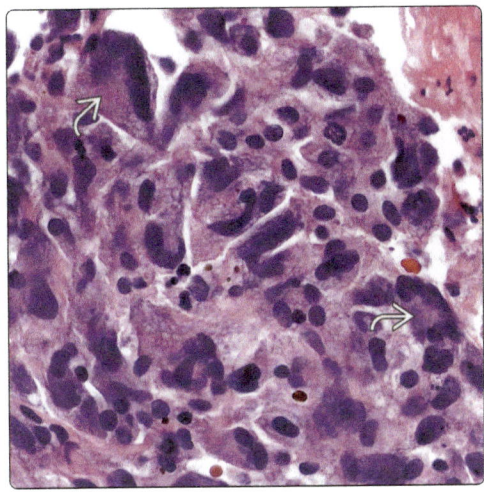

(Left) Aggressive metaphyseal tumor from an 11-year-old girl shows scant pink, globular material suspicious for osteoid. The tumor is eroding adjacent host bone ⇒, typical of an aggressive bone tumor. *(Right)* The majority of OS occurring in children are conventional central high-grade OS, as shown here. The tumor cells are large, pleomorphic, and include multinucleated tumor giant cells ⇒.

SATB2 Expression in High-Grade Osteosarcoma

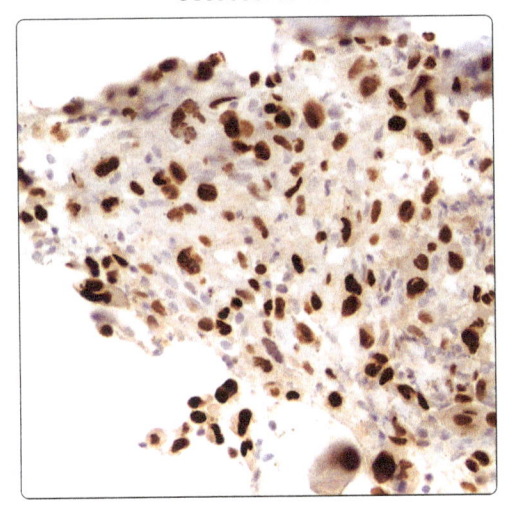

Small Cell Osteosarcoma

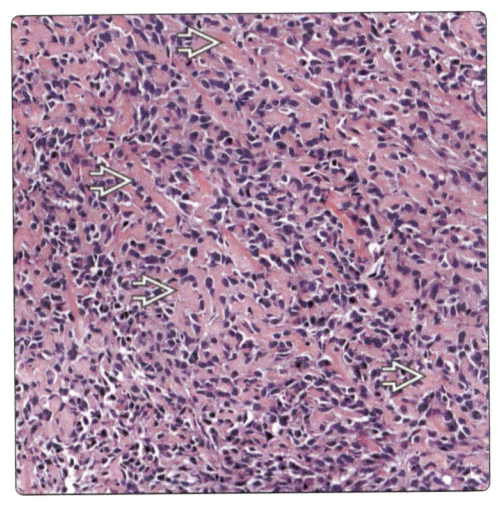

(Left) High-grade OS shows strong, diffuse nuclear expression of SATB2, which is found in cells of osteoblastic differentiation and can confirm the diagnosis of OS in the correct clinical, imaging, and histopathologic settings. It is especially helpful in small biopsies when osteoid is absent or ambiguous. *(Right)* Small cell OS is one of the rarest subtypes of OS. Tumor osteoid is a key diagnostic feature ⇒.

Giant Cell-Rich Osteosarcoma

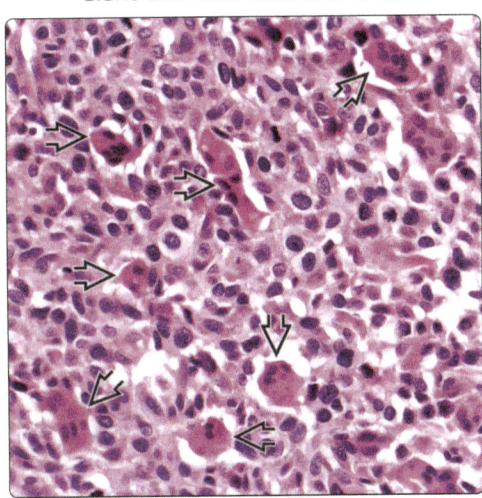

Osteoclastic Giant Cell

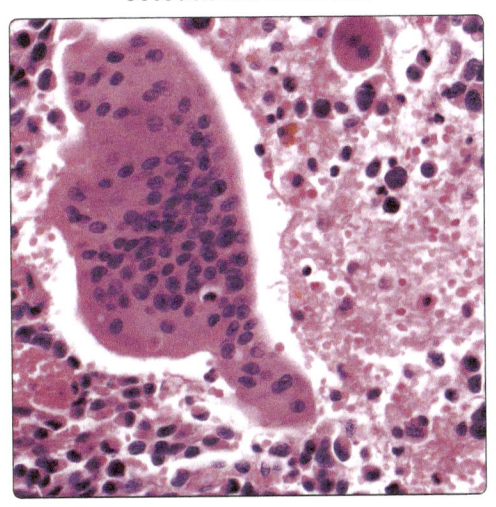

(Left) Giant cell-rich OS is shown. Multiple osteoclastic giant cells are dispersed throughout the tumor ⇒. Cursory examination could lead to misdiagnosis of giant cell tumor of bone (GCTB). However, the neoplastic cells are more atypical than those of GCTB, and they display a prominent epithelioid morphology. *(Right)* Osteoclastic giant cell in this case of OS shows the extremely large size often found in GCTB but which also may occur in OS.

Osteosarcomas

Chondroblastic Osteosarcoma

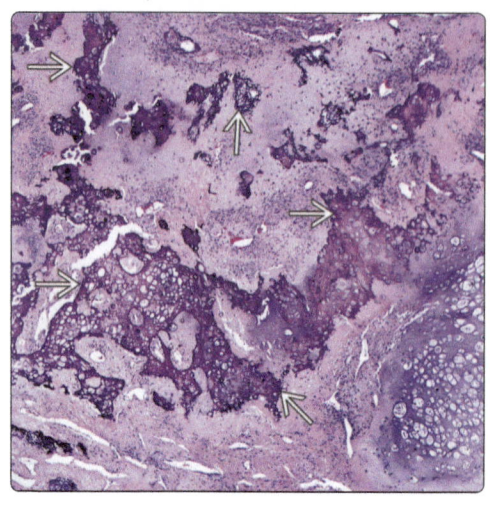

Tumor Osteoid in Chondroblastic Osteosarcoma

(Left) Chondroblastic OS is recognizable even at low power due to extensive irregular tumor bone ⇒ intermixed with fibrous and hyaline cartilage-like areas. The neoplastic cartilage exhibits the appearance of grade 1 or 2 chondrosarcoma. (Right) High-grade chondroblastic OS shows cytologically atypical osteocytes embedded in tumor osteoid. Filigree-like pericellular osteoid is also present ⇒.

Gross Appearance of Periosteal Osteosarcoma

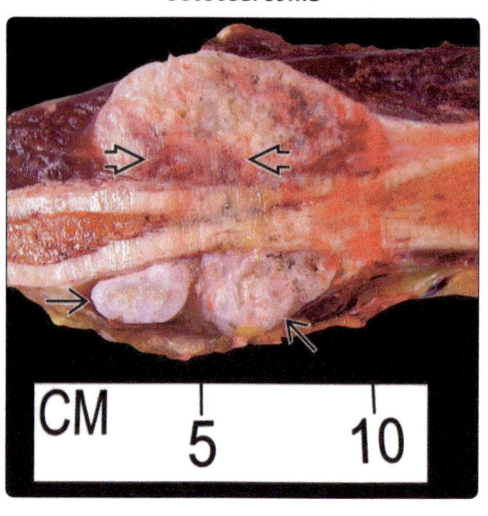

Periosteal Osteosarcoma

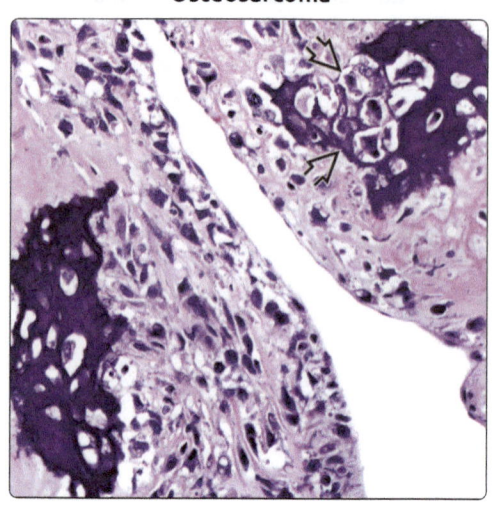

(Left) Periosteal OS of the femur wraps around the diaphysis and sits on the femoral cortex without invading into the medullary canal. The base of the tumor is ossified ⇒, but most of the tumor is composed of semitranslucent, gray, glistening malignant cartilage ⇒. Typically, rays of calcified tumor fan out into the tumor from the cortical base. (Right) The ossified base and overlying cap of tumor cartilage is clearly seen in this case of periosteal OS.

Fibrous and Cartilaginous Matrix Types

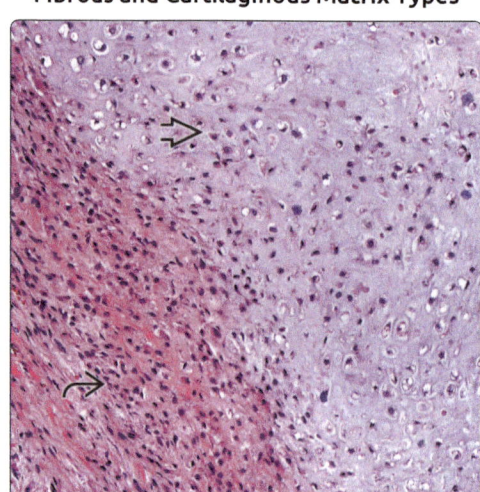

Tumor Osteoid

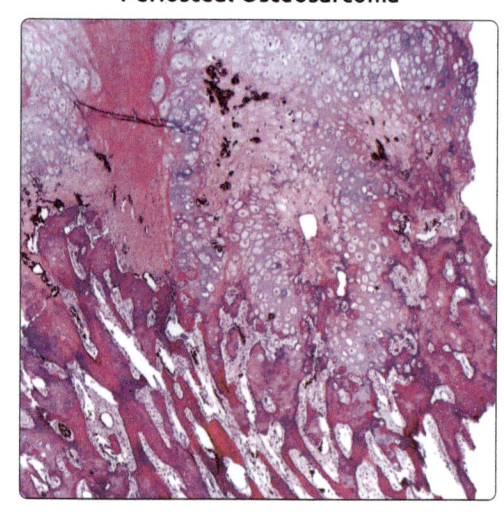

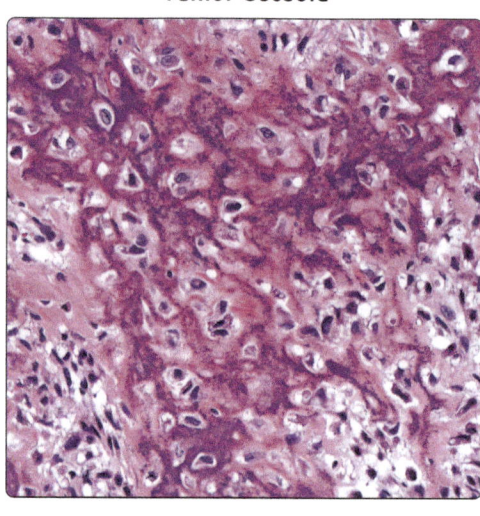

(Left) High-grade OS shows 2 matrix types: Fibrous ⇒ and cartilaginous ⇒. Most OS contain varying amounts of fibrous, cartilaginous, or osseous matrix, but if one strongly predominates in a given tumor, it is often described by that matrix, as for example, fibroblastic OS, chondroblastic OS, or osteoblastic OS. (Right) Tumor osteoid may or may not show "normalization" (i.e., contain fewer atypical cells than in the intervening stroma).

Osteosarcomas

Telangiectatic Osteosarcoma

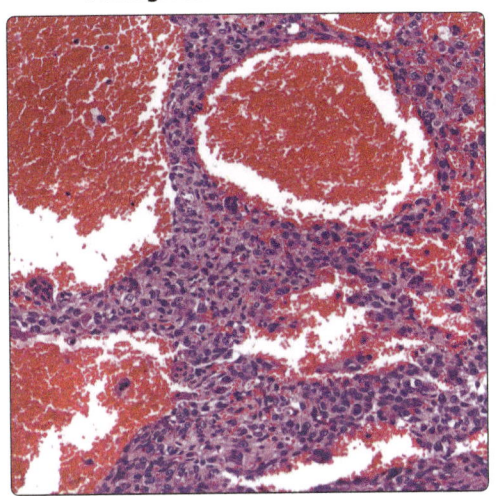

Telangiectatic Osteosarcoma

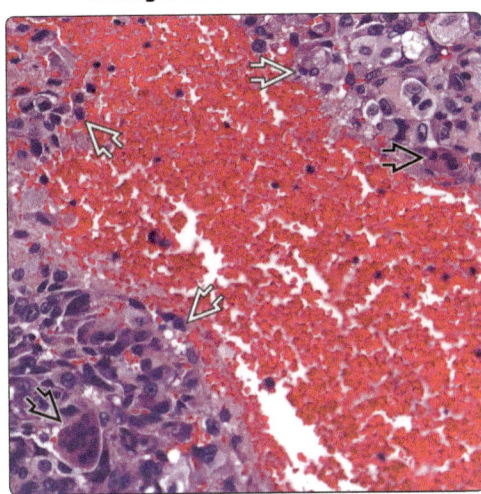

(Left) Telangiectatic OS contains large, blood-filled sinuses surrounded by tumor cells. The blood lakes can be appreciated on imaging and may somewhat mimic an aneurysmal bone cyst. (Right) Telangiectatic OS shows marked pleomorphism of tumor cells. Osteoclastic giant cells ➤ may be numerous and may aggregate around the blood lakes. Note the lack of endothelial lining with direct apposition of tumor cells to the hemorrhagic focus ➤.

Parosteal Osteosarcoma

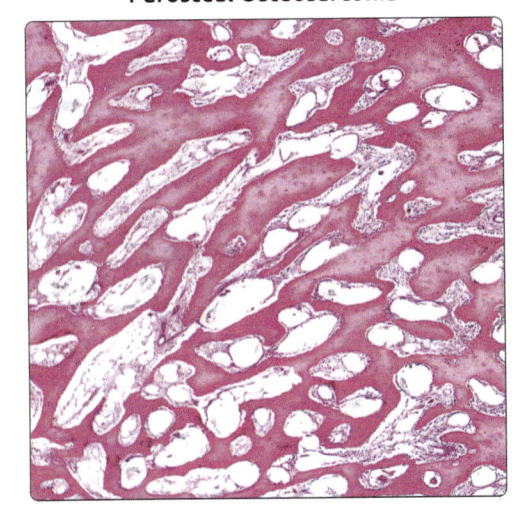

Parosteal Osteosarcoma

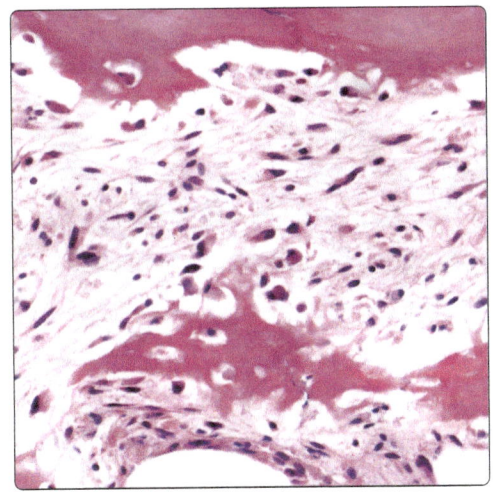

(Left) Parosteal OS shows the parallel arrays of tumor osteoid typical of this type of low-grade OS. (Right) Parosteal OS shows low-grade features of only mild atypia of tumor cells in hypocellular interosseous areas and "normalization" of osteocytes embedded in bone matrix, consistent with low-grade, pure parosteal OS, which carries an excellent prognosis.

Low-Grade Central Osteosarcoma

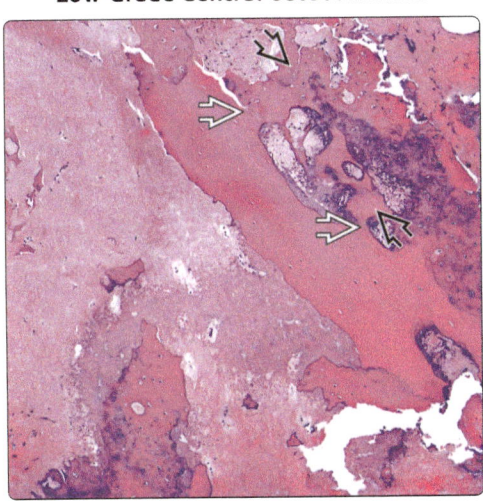

Low-Grade Central Osteosarcoma

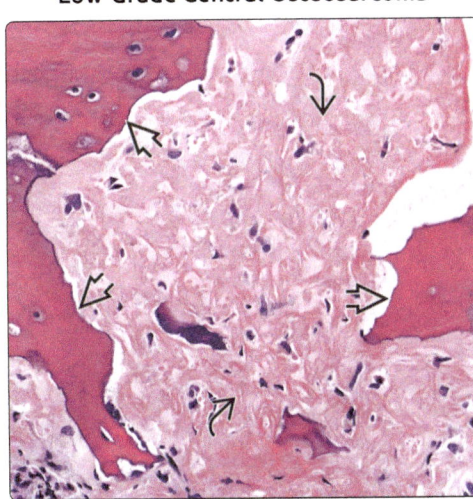

(Left) This low-grade central OS was located in the metatarsal of a 34-year-old woman who had symptoms related to the tumor for > 10 years. Note that the tumor bone ➤ uses the patient's native trabecular bone partially as a scaffold ➤, a common finding in OS. (Right) Low-grade OS produces pale osteoid ➤, is hypocellular, and erodes native bone ➤.

Ewing Sarcoma

KEY FACTS

TERMINOLOGY
- Ewing sarcoma (ES): Peripheral neuroectodermal tumor

ETIOLOGY/PATHOGENESIS
- FET family gene fuses to ETS family gene, creating aberrant transcription factor
  - FET gene family: *EWSR1*, *FUS*, and *TAF15*
  - ETS gene family: *FLI1*, *ERG*, *ETV1*, *ETV4*, and *FEV*
- *EWSR1::FLI1* fusion
  - Encodes protein that directly affects chromatin remodeling
  - Causes widespread profound changes in gene expression
  - This translocation is found in ~ 85% of ES
- White populations most commonly affected
  - 10x higher incidence of ES than in Black populations
  - White populations may have higher percentage of permissive GGAA microsatellite repeats in transcriptionally important sites
- Cell of origin: Mesenchymal stem cell or neural crest stem cell

CLINICAL ISSUES
- ES generally considered "immune desert" or "cold" tumor that provokes minimal immune response

MOLECULAR
- Major pathways disrupted
  - EGFR pathway
  - IGF-1 (insulin-like growth factor type 1) pathway
  - Pi3K/AKT/mTOR pathway
  - Cell cycle
  - Degree and variety of disruptions varies by patient
  - Targeted therapy may require testing of each patient's tumor for specific alterations
- Abnormal expression of various genes appear prognostic but not clinically validated

Hypercellular Sacral Tumor

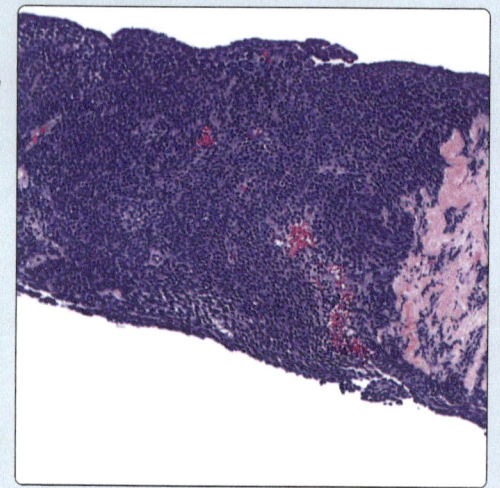

Classic Appearance

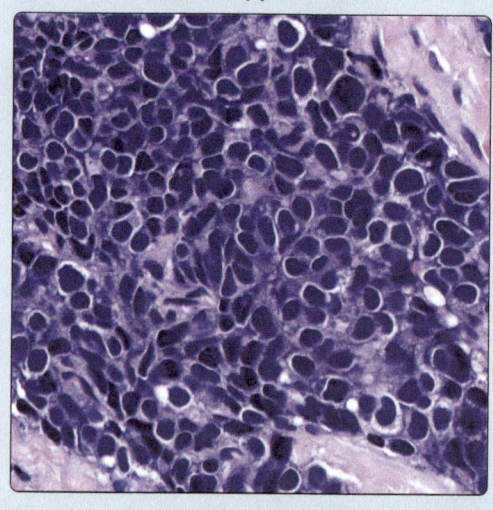

(Left) Core needle biopsy of sacral tumor from a 12-year-old girl is hypercellular and monotonous with interspersed areas of fibrosis. (Right) High-power view of core needle biopsy shows classic Ewing sarcoma (ES) histology: Uniform small round cells with high N:C ratio, inconspicuous nucleoli, and low mitotic rate.

Adamantinoma-Like Ewing Sarcoma

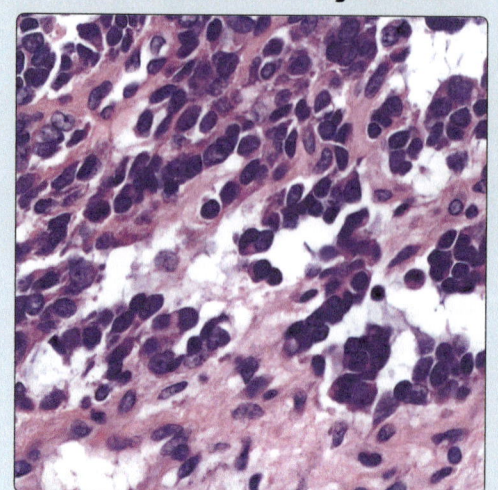

Adamantinoma-Like Ewing Sarcoma: Keratin

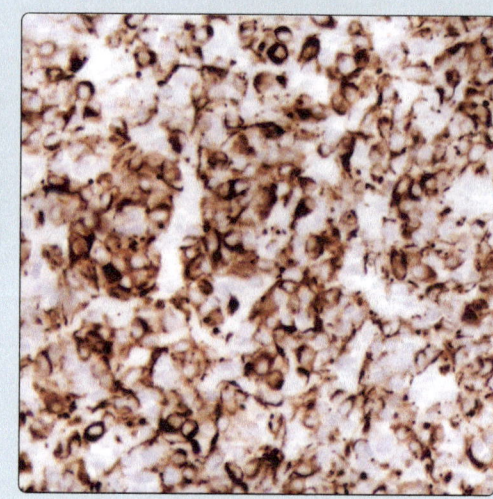

(Left) Adamantinoma-like ES does not always show overt squamous differentiation. In this case, the tumor cells contain more cytoplasm than usual and show a pseudoalveolar growth pattern. (Right) Characteristically, adamantinoma-like ES shows diffuse positivity for AE1/AE3 keratins. The diagnosis was confirmed by identification of *EWSR1::FLI1* fusion.

Ewing Sarcoma

TERMINOLOGY

Abbreviations
- Ewing sarcoma (ES)

Synonyms
- Peripheral neuroectodermal tumor (PNET)

Definitions
- Primitive mesenchymal sarcomas of bone and soft tissue characterized by
  o Small round blue cell morphology
  o Rearrangements of FET (TET) family gene with ETS family gene: FET::ETS
    – Most common rearrangement: EWSR1::FLI1 (70-80% of cases)
    – Others: EWSR1/FUS::ERG (15%), EWSR1/FUS::FEV (5%), and EWSR1::ETV1/ETV4 (1%)

ETIOLOGY/PATHOGENESIS

Putative Cell of Origin
- Mesenchymal stem cell or neural crest stem cell

FET Family Gene Rearrangements
- Rearrangements of FET family gene (most commonly EWSR1) with ETS family gene (most commonly FLI1)
  o FET gene family: EWSR1, FUS, and TAF15
  o ETS gene family: FLI1, ERG, ETV1, ETV4, FEV, E1AF, and 21 others
- Fusion protein acts as aberrant transcription factor to dysregulate numerous pathways
  o Cell differentiation is repressed
  o Cell cycle is disrupted
  o Cell migration and proliferation are disrupted
- EWSR1::FLI1 fusion protein
  o Encoded protein aberrantly affects chromatin remodeling
  o Creates novel enhancers at GGAA repeats
    – Abnormally activates numerous genes
  o Represses normal enhancers by competing with ETS proteins
    – Abnormally represses numerous genes
  o Represses miRNAs including miRNA-145 low levels of which impair differentiation

Genetic Predisposition
- Germline mutation of PTPRD
  o PTPRD encodes tyrosine phosphatase protein
  o Normally inhibits STAT3 activation
    – STAT3 highly overexpressed in ES
- NR0B1 overexpression
  o Specific susceptibility alleles at 1p36, 10q21, 15q15
    – White populations show highest frequency
    – Associated with mild increase in ES risk
- Inactivating variants or mutations in DNA damage repair genes found in ~ 13% of patients
- CD99 germline polymorphisms reported to increase risk of developing ES
  o Encodes CD99 protein
- 6 candidate susceptibility loci identified by genome wide association studies (GWAS)
  o Genes include some downstream targets of EWSR1::FLI1 fusion protein, genes involved in centrosome stabilization and in apoptosis
  o Most risk alleles are more common in White populations

CLINICAL ISSUES

Epidemiology
- Incidence
  o Annual USA incidence: 250-400 patients (~ 3 patients/million/year)
- Age
  o Patients with bone tumors: 90% < 30 years
    – Peak: 15 years
  o Patients with soft tissue tumors: Broader age range than for primary bone ES
- Ethnicity
  o White populations most commonly affected
    – 10x higher incidence than Black populations
    – Higher percentage of permissive GGAA microsatellite repeats present in White populations increases risk for ES

Site
- Bone (80%)
- Soft tissue and skin (~ 20%)

Presentation
- Mass, usually painful, sometimes with systemic symptoms
  o Pathologic fracture (~ 15% of patients)

Natural History
- 80% have localized disease
  o ~ 70% 5-year survival
- 20% have metastases
  o ~ 20% 5-year survival
  o Patients with isolated pulmonary metastases do better than patients with bone/bone marrow involvement

Treatment
- Complete surgical excision ± radiation ± intense induction chemotherapy for resectable tumors
- Radiation ± chemotherapy for unresectable tumors
- New treatment approaches
  o Immunotherapy
  o Targeted therapy to downstream effector proteins

Prognosis
- Unfavorable prognostic indicators (representative)
  o Metastatic disease is worst predictor of outcome
  o 1q gain (30% of patients)
  o TP53 mutations (7-13% of patients): Controversial in terms of worsening prognosis
  o CDKN2A deletions (~ 12% of patients)
  o HDGF overexpression
  o STAG2 loss-of-function mutations (15-21% of patients)
  o Detectable or high levels of circulating tumor DNA (ctDNA) may predict higher risk for relapse
- Favorable prognostic indicators (representative)
  o Few (< 3) to no copy number alterations (CNA)

Ewing Sarcoma

MOLECULAR

Cytogenetics
- Karyotype can detect translocations
- Additional chromosomal abnormalities often present

In Situ Hybridization
- Commercial *EWSR1* break-apart probe
  - ~ 90% of ES tumors
  - Split signal found in all tumors with *EWSR1* translocations
  - Not specific for ES
    - Many other tumors besides ES family have *EWSR1* rearrangements

Chromosomal Microarray
- ~ 80% of ES have copy number alterations
- Gains: 1q (30%), 8 (35%), 12 (25%), 20q most common
  - Patients with 1q gains have inferior overall survival
- Deletions/LOH: 10q, 11p, 16q, 17p most common
  - Patients with 16q loss have inferior survival

Molecular Genetics
- Fusion of FET family member gene with ETS family member gene to create novel *FET::ETS* fusion protein
  - *EWSR1* is FET partner for ~ 99% of Ewing sarcoma gene fusions
- t(11;22)(q24;q12) *EWSR1::FLI1*
  - Most common translocation found in ES (~ 85% of cases)
  - Number of splice variants: Multiple (at least 18)
    - Site of gene fusion not prognostic or predictive
  - Common feature
    - 5' end of *EWSR1* joined to 3' end of *FLI1* or other ETS family gene members
  - Expression levels of *EWSR1::FLI1* protein in individual tumor cells correlates with invasive capacity
    - Tumor cells with lower expression (minority of tumor) show enhanced migration, invasion, and metastasis
    - By contrast, tumor cells with higher expression (most of tumor) are more proliferative and show high cell-cell adhesion propensity
- Major genes upregulated
  - *DKK2*
  - *ERBB4*
  - Others: *CCND1, EZH2, SOX2, NKX2-2, VRK1, PTK2*
- Major genes downregulated
  - *ERRFI1, CABLES1, TGFβ1, SNAI2, TRPS1, NT5E, FOXO1, STAG2*

Gene Expression Profiling
- Major pathways disrupted
  - EGFR pathway
  - IGF-1
  - Pi3K/AKT/mTOR pathway
  - Cell cycle
  - p53 protein pathways
- Degree of disruption varies among patients
  - Targeted therapy may require testing of each patient's tumor for specific alterations

Molecular Immunopathology
- *CTLA4* polymorphisms associated with ES
  - CTLA4 expressed on cytotoxic T lymphocytes
    - Reduces T-cell antitumor response by regulating effector T cells
  - *CTLA4* 49G/A genotype: ↑ risk and ↑ metastatic rate
    - Correlated with high expression of CTLA4 protein
    - Also associated with other cancers and some autoimmune diseases
  - *CD86* 1057G/A genotype: ↑ risk
    - CD86 is binding partner of CTLA4
    - Also increases risk for osteosarcoma
- Immune suppressive myeloid cells
  - Arise from myeloid-derived suppressor cells and ↑ in pediatric sarcomas
    - Present in peripheral blood and tumor microenvironment
  - Express SMA and CD34, but not CD163, consistent with nascent fibrocyte phenotype

Epigenetics
- Differential expression of microRNAs (miRNAs)
  - Tumor suppressor effect of miRNA-31
    - Diminished due to ↓ expression in ES (1 study)
  - Tumor suppressor effect of miRNA-34
    - ↓ expression in primary tumor of patients with metastasis at presentation or within 1 year of diagnosis
- Hypermethylation of specific genes
  - 8 genes silenced in > 20% of cases tested
    - *CTHRC1, DNAJA4, ECHDC2, NEFH, NPTX2, PHF11, RARRES2, CEP41*
    - *NPTX2* or *PHF11* hypermethylation → ↓ prognosis
    - Most of these genes also show > 20% hypermethylation frequency in osteosarcomas
  - Hypermethylation of *RASSF2*
- Abnormalities of long noncoding RNAs (lncRNAs)
  - At least 12 lncRNAs reported to be abnormally upregulated in ES
    - Could serve as druggable targets in ES
  - One lncRNA example: *EWSAT1* (Ewing sarcoma-associated transcript 1)
    - Originally described in ES
    - Promotes tumor proliferation

MICROSCOPIC

Histologic Features
- Classic (conventional) ES
  - Architecture: Sheets to vague lobules ± prominent perivascular cuffing in areas of necrosis
  - Small round blue cells with round nuclei, inconspicuous nucleoli, low mitotic rate
  - Cytoplasm may be clear due to glycogen
- Tumors with neural differentiation
  - Same features as classic ES but also with Homer Wright rosettes
  - Neural markers positive
  - Previously called primitive neuroectodermal tumor (PNET)
- Atypical (large cell) ES
  - Architecture: Similar to classic ES

Ewing Sarcoma

- Cells: Larger than classic ES with more nuclear pleomorphism, vesicular nuclei ± macronucleoli, and ↑ mitoses
- Unusual features
  - Architecture: Adamantinoma-like, sclerotic, hemangioendothelioma-like
  - Extensive component of spindled tumor cells

ANCILLARY TESTS

Immunohistochemistry

- CD99
  - Strong membranous reactivity in ~ 95% of ES
    - Cytoplasmic reactivity much less specific finding
  - Other tumors can be CD99 positive
    - e.g., rhabdomyosarcoma, synovial sarcoma, others
- FLI-1
  - Positive in most cases of ES, regardless of fusion type
  - Not specific antibody for ES
- ERG
  - Positive in tumors with EWSR1::ERG fusions but expressed in multiple other non-Ewing sarcomas
- NKX2.2
  - Highly sensitive but only moderately specific for ES
- Keratin
  - Usually focal, positive in ~ 33% of cases
- Neural differentiation markers: S100, NSE, CD57 (+/-)
- Desmin: Rarely positive

DIFFERENTIAL DIAGNOSIS

Lymphoma

- Different phenotype, including CD45 reactivity
  - CD45 negative in ES
- Lymphoblastic lymphoma
  - Often negative for CD45, CD20, and CD3, like ES
  - Positive for CD99 and FLI-1, like ES
  - Positive for CD43, CD19, CD10, CD79A, and TdT; supports B lymphoblastic lymphoma
  - Negative for EWSR1::FLI1 rearrangements

Mesenchymal Chondrosarcoma

- Biphasic with small round blue cells and cartilage matrix
- CD99 can be positive
- SOX9 positive
- FLI-1, ERG negative
- FISH negative for EWSR1 translocation

Small Cell Osteosarcoma

- Biphasic with small round blue cells and osteoid matrix
- CD99 can be positive
- FLI-1 negative
- FISH negative for EWSR1 translocation

Desmoplastic Small Round Cell Tumor

- Soft tissue tumor composed of small round blue cells, epithelioid like areas, and sclerotic matrix
- IHC
  - CD99 can be positive
  - Polymorphous expression of keratins, desmin (paranuclear dot-like in many cases), WT1, and NSE
- FISH positive for EWSR1 translocation

Poorly Differentiated Synovial Sarcoma

- Sheets of small round blue cells, but classic components often present
- IHC
  - TLE-1 sensitive and relatively specific for synovial sarcoma
  - FLI-1 and CD99 may be present in synovial sarcoma, and CD99 rarely can show membranous expression pattern, like ES
  - SSX highly sensitive and specific for synovial sarcoma
- FISH
  - Positive for t(X;18) in ~ 95% of cases
  - Negative for EWSR1 translocation

Rhabdomyosarcoma

- Alveolar RMS
  - Alveolar architecture may be absent or focal
  - Small round blue cells but also multinucleated tumor cells and positive rhabdomyoblasts
  - IHC
    - Similar to ES: CD99 positive, keratins focally positive
    - Dissimilar to ES: Positive for myogenin, MYOD1
    - Desmin positive (rare in ES)
  - FISH
    - Positive for PAX3 or PAX7 translocations
    - Negative for EWSR1 translocation
- Embryonal RMS
  - Usually spindled cells and rhabdomyoblasts
  - IHC
    - Similar to ES: May be CD99 positive
    - Dissimilar to ES: Myogenin, MYOD1 positive
  - FISH
    - Negative for EWSR1 translocation

Ewing-Like Sarcomas

- May be histologically and clinically very similar
- IHC: CD99 often positive
- FISH: Negative for EWSR1 translocation, except for EWSR1::NFATC2 sarcoma and EWSR1::PATZ1 sarcoma

SELECTED REFERENCES

1. Aryee DNT et al: Zooming in on long non-coding RNAs in Ewing sarcoma pathogenesis. Cells. 11(8), 2022
2. Shulman DS et al: An international working group consensus report for the prioritization of molecular biomarkers for Ewing sarcoma. NPJ Precis Oncol. 6(1):65, 2022
3. Riggi N et al: Ewing's sarcoma. N Engl J Med. 384(2):154-64, 2021
4. Anderson ND et al: Rearrangement bursts generate canonical gene fusions in bone and soft tissue tumors. Science. 361(6405), 2018
5. Baldauf MC et al: Are EWSR1-NFATc2-positive sarcomas really Ewing sarcomas? Mod Pathol. 31(6):997-9, 2018
6. Machiela MJ et al: Genome-wide association study identifies multiple new loci associated with Ewing sarcoma susceptibility. Nat Commun. 9(1):3184, 2018
7. Antonescu CR et al: Promiscuous genes involved in recurrent chromosomal translocations in soft tissue tumours. Pathology. 46(2):105-12, 2014
8. Monument MJ et al: Clinical and biochemical function of polymorphic NR0B1 GGAA-microsatellites in Ewing sarcoma: a report from the Children's Oncology Group. PLoS One. 9(8):e104378, 2014
9. Riggi N et al: EWS-FLI1 utilizes divergent chromatin remodeling mechanisms to directly activate or repress enhancer elements in Ewing sarcoma. Cancer Cell. 26(5):668-81, 2014

Ewing Sarcoma

Perivascular Tumor Preservation

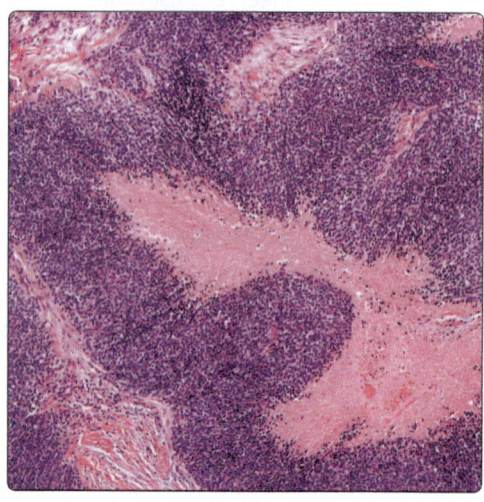

PAS-D Highlighting Glycogen

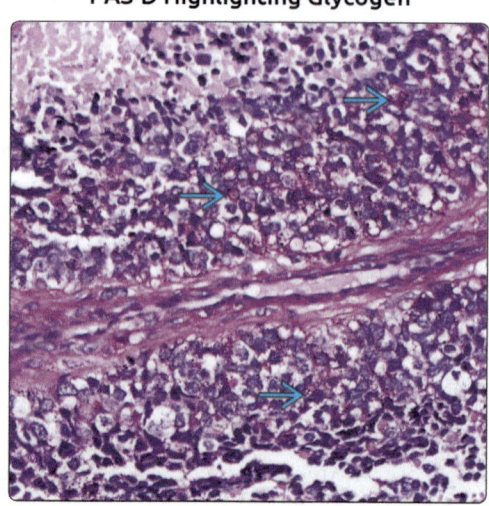

(Left) A common finding in ES is perivascular cuffing, which imparts a serpiginous appearance to the tumor at low power. Tumor cells retain viability only within close proximity to blood vessels. This would be an unusual histologic feature for lymphoma, an entity in the histologic differential. (Right) PAS without diastase highlights purple granules of intracytoplasmic glycogen ➡ in viable perivascular tumor cells.

Representative Karyotype

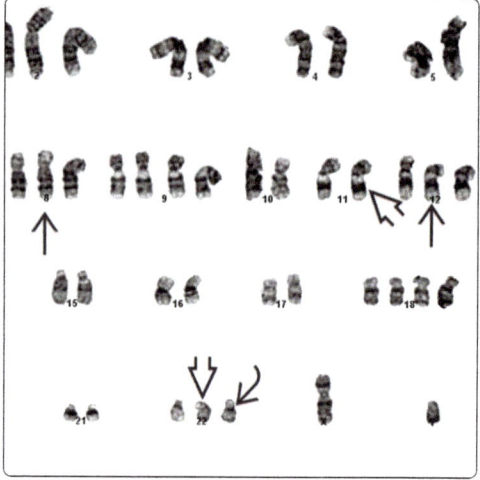

FISH

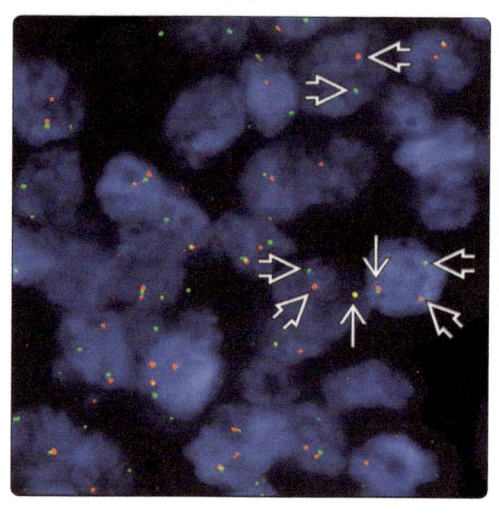

(Left) ES partial karyotype shows t(11;22) ➡, derivative 22 ➡, trisomies of 8 and 12 ➡, and other changes. (Right) Soft tissue ES shows rearrangement of EWSR1 in 92% of cells analyzed using a dual-color, break-apart probe. Fused signal ➡ is yellow or has touching signals, while 5' and 3' split signals are red and green ➡, indicating rearrangement. There is generally 1 normal EWSR1 allele and 1 split allele per nucleus.

CD99 Membranous Expression

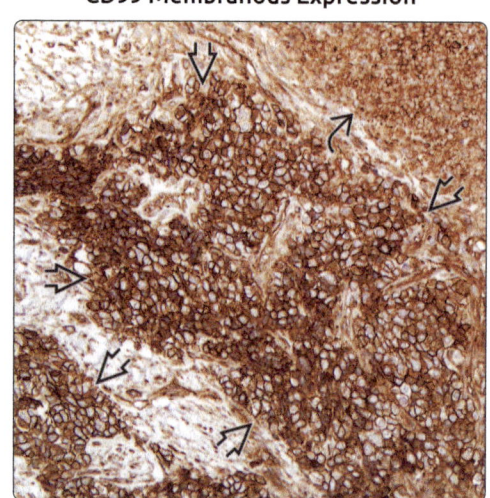

Synaptophysin Variably Present

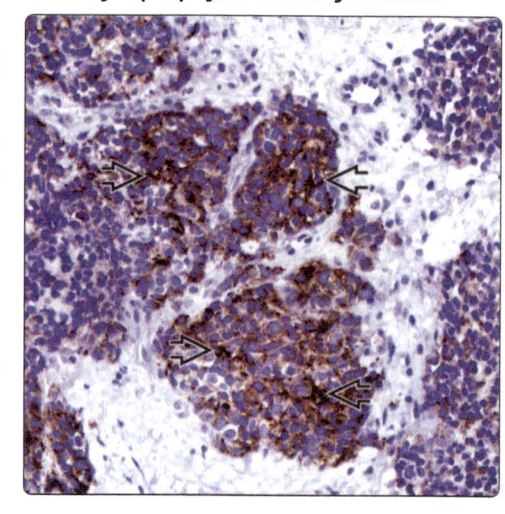

(Left) Membranous expression of CD99 is characteristic of ES and seen in ~ 95% of cases. The viable cells ➡ show typical expression, while the nonviable cells show nonspecific granular expression ➡. It is important to assess the viable areas only. (Right) Neuroendocrine marker expression, such as synaptophysin ➡, can be present even in tumors without overt neuroectodermal features.

Ewing Sarcoma

EWSR1 or FUS Fusions Tumors

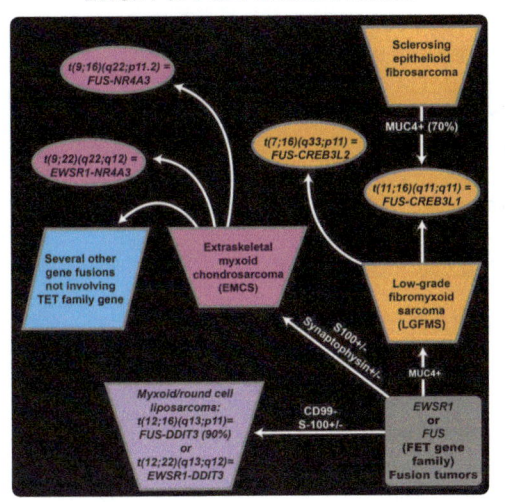

FET Gene Family Fusion Tumors

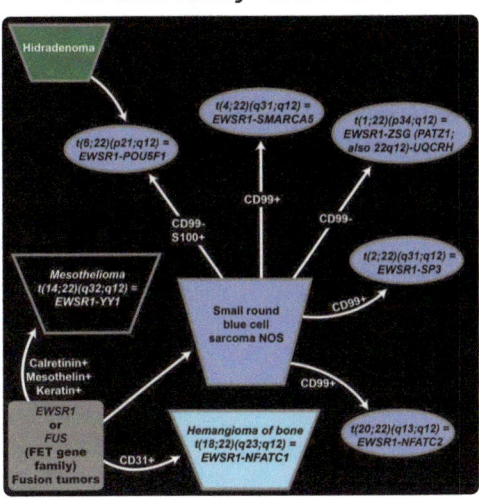

(Left) EWSR1 or FUS fusion partner tumors include extraskeletal myxoid chondrosarcoma, a tumor with multiple gene fusions, including some non-TET gene family fusions, and 2 related tumors: Low-grade fibromyxoid sarcoma and its higher grade counterpart, sclerosing epithelioid fibrosarcoma. Although all tumors in this graphic can have myxoid regions, they are not otherwise histologically similar. (Right) Several TET (FET) gene family fusion tumors are shown.

Ewing Sarcoma Family of Tumors

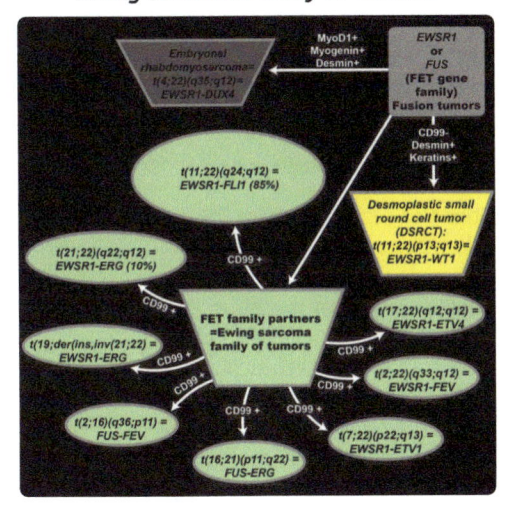

Same Fusions Found in Different Tumors

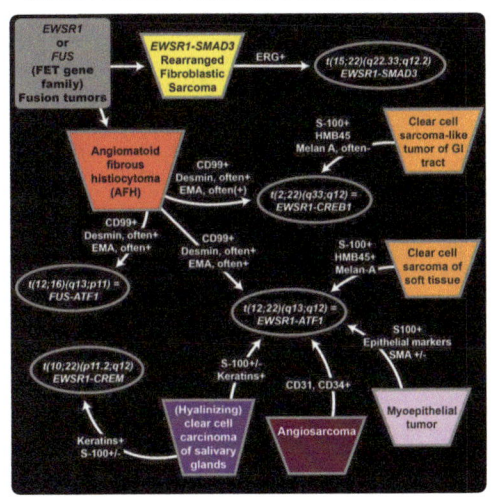

(Left) Ewing sarcoma family of tumors is defined by fusion of an FET family member (EWSR1, FUS, or TAF15) with an ETS family member (such as FLI1, ERG, or FEV). (Right) In some cases, the same fusion occurs in distinctly different tumors that have different clinicopathologic characteristics. Note, for example, that AFH and clear cell sarcomas share fusions.

Ewing Sarcoma Mimicking Lymphoma

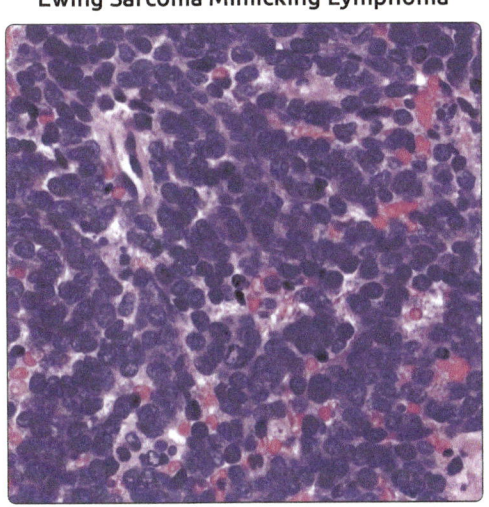

Atypical Ewing Sarcoma

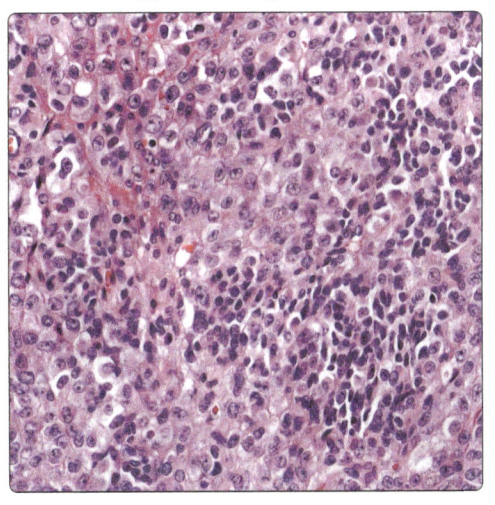

(Left) This case of ES lacks defined cell borders. At low power, due to extremely high N:C ratio and streaming of tumor cells, this could be mistaken for a lymphoma. In many cases, IHC, molecular analysis, and clinical and imaging findings are required to render the correct diagnosis. (Right) Atypical (large cell) variant of ES is composed of larger cells containing more cytoplasm, vesicular nuclei, and macronucleoli.

Other Small Round Blue Cell Sarcomas

TERMINOLOGY

Definition
- Small round cell sarcomas with specific gene fusions that are not Ewing sarcoma
- Tumors
  - Desmoplastic small round cell tumor (DSRCT): Classified as "tumor of uncertain differentiation" by WHO
  - *CIC*-rearranged sarcomas: Classified as "undifferentiated round cell sarcomas" by WHO
  - Sarcoma with *BCOR* genetic alterations: Classified as "undifferentiated round cell sarcoma" by WHO
  - Round cell sarcoma with *EWSR1*::non-ETS gene family fusions: Classified as "undifferentiated round cell sarcomas" by WHO

EPIDEMIOLOGY

Incidence
- Overall rare: May represent ~ 5-10% of small round blue cell sarcomas occurring in pediatric age group
- DSRCT
  - Age: Adolescents most common
  - Sex: M:F = 5:1
- CIC-rearranged sarcomas
  - Accounts for ~ 70% of *EWSR1* fusion-negative undifferentiated small round cell sarcomas
  - Age: Young adults most common
  - Sex: M slightly > F
- Sarcoma with BCOR genetic alterations
  - Age: Adolescents most common; 90% of patients < 20 years of age
  - Sex: M > > F
- Round cell sarcoma with EWSR1-non-ETS fusions
  - *EWSR1/FUS*::*NFATC2* tumors: Broad age range; M:F = 5:1
  - *EWSR1*::*PATZ1* tumors: Broad age range; M = F

Body Site
- DSRCT
  - Deep peritoneal-lined spaces
  - Abdominal cavity most common
  - Organs, such as kidneys, testis, and ovaries
- CIC-rearranged sarcomas
  - Deep soft tissue (86%), viscera (12%), and bone (3%)
- Sarcoma with BCOR genetic alterations
  - Skeleton: Long bones and pelvis most common
  - Soft tissue sites: Deep intramuscular
- Round cell sarcoma with EWSR1::non-ETS fusions
  - *EWSR1/FUS*::*NFATC2* tumors: Bone most commonly but also soft tissue (4:1 ratio)
  - *EWSR1*::*PATZ1* tumors: Soft tissue

ETIOLOGY/PATHOGENESIS

Desmoplastic Small Round Cell Tumor
- *EWSR1*::*WT1*; t(11;22)(p13;q12)
- Abnormal fusion transcript upregulates numerous genes
  - *BAIAP3*, *SLC29A4*, and *EGR1*
  - Upregulates specific tyrosine kinases and ligands, including *IGF1R*, *KDR*, and *PDGFA*

CIC-Rearranged Sarcomas
- t(4;19)(q35;q13); *CIC*::*DUX4* or t(10;19)(q26;q13)
  - Fusion protein causes ↑ expression of PEA3 transcription factors (ETV1, ETV4, ETV5)
- *CIC* (19q13)
  - Transcriptional repressor involved in normal development of CNS
  - Abnormalities also reported in rare CNS primitive neuroectodermal tumors and others
- *DUX4* (4q35)
  - Encodes double homeobox protein that increases global H3 acetylation at lysine 18 (H3K18) and lysine 27 (H3K27)
- Abnormal fusion transcript acts to increase activity of *CIC*
  - Fusion protein deregulates many of same genes as *EWSR1*::*FLI1* (Ewing sarcoma) transcript
- Other rare fusion partners for CIC-rearranged sarcomas: ~ 5% of cases
  - *DUX4L*, *FOX04*, *LEUTX*, *NUTM1*, *NUTM2A*, *AXL*, *CITED1*, and *SYK*

Peritoneal DSRCT

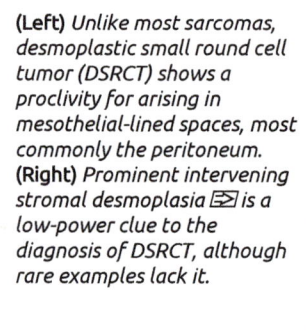

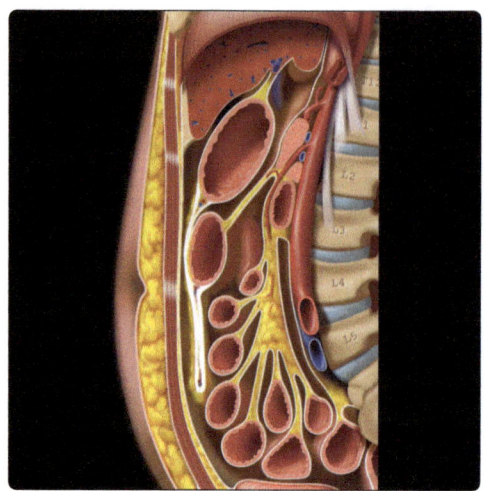

Stromal Desmoplasia in DSRCT

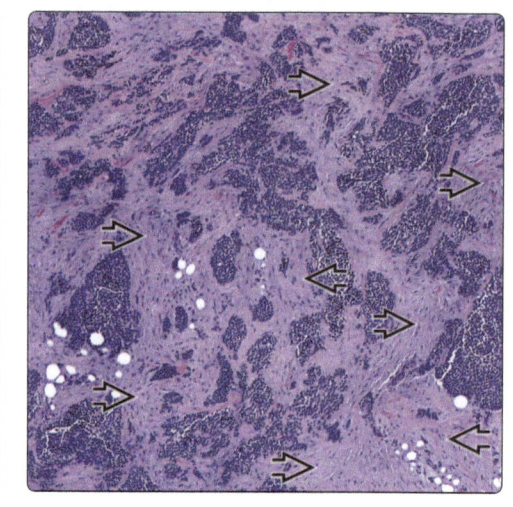

(Left) Unlike most sarcomas, desmoplastic small round cell tumor (DSRCT) shows a proclivity for arising in mesothelial-lined spaces, most commonly the peritoneum. (Right) Prominent intervening stromal desmoplasia ➡ is a low-power clue to the diagnosis of DSRCT, although rare examples lack it.

Other Small Round Blue Cell Sarcomas

- t(X;19)(q13;q13); *CIC::FOXO4*: Rare alternate translocation reported in head and neck

Sarcoma With *BCOR* Genetic Alterations
- *BCOR::CCNB3* involves paracentric inversion of X chromosome
  - Fusion protein has decreased BCOR activity
- *BCOR* (BCL6 interacting corepressor)
  - Normally functions as transcriptional repressor
- *CCNB3* (cyclin B3)
  - Normally functions in meiosis
- Other tumors with *BCOR* alterations
  - Some leukemias, myelodysplastic syndrome (as N-terminal partner: *BCOR::RARA*)
  - Endometrial stromal sarcoma (with t(X;22), as C-terminal partner)
  - Ossifying fibromyxoid tumor (as C-terminal partner)
  - Clear cell sarcoma of kidney
  - Primitive myxoid mesenchymal tumor of infancy
  - High-grade neuroepithelial tumor with *BCOR* alterations

Round Cell Sarcoma With *EWSR1*::Non-ETS Fusions
- *EWSR1/FUS::NFATC2* tumors: Fusion protein acts as abnormal transcription factor
- *EWSR1::PATZ1* tumors: Fusion protein acts as abnormal transcriptional activator
  - Other tumors with *EWSR1::PATZ1* fusion: CNS glioneuronal tumors, thyroid-like follicular renal cell carcinoma

CLINICAL IMPLICATIONS

Clinical Behavior
- DSRCT
  - Aggressive with death occurring within 1.5 years in majority
  - Rare cases may have longer survival
    - May show unusual morphology, such as spindled tumor cells
    - Most cases with prolonged survival are low stage at presentation
- CIC-rearranged sarcomas
  - Aggressive with death occurring within 1.5 years in majority
- Sarcoma with BCOR genetic alterations
  - Appears to behave similarly to stage-matched Ewing sarcoma
- Round cell sarcoma with *EWSR1*::non-ETS fusions
  - *EWSR1/FUS::NFATC2* tumors can recur, metastasize, and cause death
    - Solid hypercellular tumors (sarcomas) can behave aggressively and cause death
    - Simple bone cysts and vascular lesions of bone that contain these fusions can recur locally in nondestructive manner
  - *EWSR1::PATZ1* tumors can behave aggressively and cause death

MICROSCOPIC

Desmoplastic Small Round Cell Sarcoma
- Low magnification
  - Solid, irregular nests embedded in prominent paucicellular desmoplastic stroma
  - Squamous-like nests, glands, or rosettes may be present
  - Rare cases lack desmoplastic stroma
- High magnification
  - Small round blue cells predominant component
    - Nuclei usually hyperchromatic
  - Some cases contain foci of larger cells with more cytoplasm
  - Necrosis usually ↑
  - Mitoses usually ↑

CIC-Rearranged Sarcomas
- Low magnification
  - Solid sheets or nodules
  - Myxoid background relatively common
  - Geographic necrosis usually present
- High magnification
  - Round cells
    - Some cases contain intermixed spindled cells and rhabdoid/plasmacytoid cells
  - Cytoplasm clear to eosinophilic
  - Nuclei vesicular with nucleoli in most cases
    - Few cases may have hyperchromatic nuclei
  - Mitoses usually ↑ (> 10/10 HPF)

Sarcoma With BCOR Genetic Alterations
- Low magnification
  - Hypercellular and dyscohesive without specific architecture in nearly all cases
    - Minority may be mixed hyper- and hypocellular
  - Edematous to myxoid stroma
  - Highly vascular with meshwork of thin-walled ectatic vessels ± intravascular thrombi (~ 80% of cases)
  - ± geographic necrosis
- High magnification
  - Small round cells with ↑ N:C ratio and scant pale to eosinophilic cytoplasm
    - Nuclei: Hyperchromatic ± angulated without prominent nucleoli in most cases
    - Nuclei in few cases: Vesicular with small nucleoli with fine, evenly dispersed chromatin
  - Short spindle cells in some cases
    - Some tumors contain predominantly or exclusively spindle cells
  - ↑ mitotic rate and ↑ apoptotic rate in most cases
- Recurrences or metastases
  - Often becomes more pleomorphic ± more spindled
  - May show osteoblastic differentiation and tumor osteoid
  - Retains CCNB3 nuclear IHC expression in almost all specimens
- Postchemotherapy changes
  - Often shows at least partial to complete response
  - Partial response: Hypocellular, bland spindle cells
  - CCNB3 nuclear IHC expression often retained but may be patchy
  - RT-PCR assay for *BCOR::CCNB3* transcript remains positive

Round Cell Sarcoma With *EWSR1*::Non-ETS Fusions
- Low magnification

Other Small Round Blue Cell Sarcomas

- o *EWSR1/FUS::NFATC2* sarcoma: Cords, trabeculae, nests with scant to abundant hyaline ± chondroid ± myxoid stroma
- o *EWSR1/FUS::NFATC2* intraosseous cyst: Simple or complex cysts with thin to thick lining and central cyst debris
- o *EWSR1::PATZ1* tumors: Sheets &/or nests often with fibrous or myxohyaline stroma
- High magnification
  - o *EWSR1/FUS::NFATC2* tumors: Round to plump spindled cells; may be more atypical in sarcomatous examples
  - o *EWSR1::PATZ1* tumors: Round to spindled cells

MOLECULAR GENETICS

Desmoplastic Small Round Cell Sarcoma

- *EWSR1::WT1* fusion
  - o Only gene fusion described thus far for DSRCT
  - o Chimeric fusion protein acts as strong transcription factor
    - – Binds to promoter regions of BAIAP3, EGR1, and others
    - – Induces upregulation of genes encoding some tyrosine kinase receptors and ligands
- Copy number gains/amplifications of *MDM2* &/or *MDM4*
  - o Abnormally represses *TP53*
- Pathways dysregulated
  - o Wnt pathway upregulated

CIC-Rearranged Sarcomas

- t(4;19)(q35;q13); *CIC::DUX4*
  - o *CIC::DUX4*: Accounts for ~ 95% of *CIC*-rearranged sarcomas
  - o Fusion may not be detectable in karyotype or by FISH due to cryptic rearrangements
  - o Other rare fusion partners include *DUX4L, FOXO4, LEUTX, NUTM1, NUTM2A, AXL, CITED1,* and *SYK*
    - – *CIC::NUTM1* sarcomas most commonly occur in axial skeleton
  - o Deregulates panel of genes distinct from those dysregulated by *EWSR1::FLI1* fusion in Ewing sarcoma
- Copy number alterations (CNA)
  - o Present but too few cases to confirm recurrent findings
  - o May have extra copies of 19q13 region

Sarcoma With *BCOR* Genetic Alterations

- BCOR protein function: Involved in epigenetic regulation of transcription
  - o Subunit of noncanonical polycomb repressive complex 1
  - o Interacts with BCL6: BCOR = "BCL6 corepressor"
- *BCOR::CCNB3*: Paracentric inversion on chromosome X of *BCOR* (Xp11.4; full length) and *CCNB3* (Xp11.22; C-terminus)
- Other *BCOR* alterations in soft tissue sarcomas
  - o *BCOR::MAML3*
    - – *MAML3* (4q31) encodes transcriptional coactivator in mastermind-like (MAML) group
  - o *BCOR::ITD*: BCOR with internal tandem duplications (ITDs)
    - – Also found in intracranial tumors and primitive myxoid mesenchymal tumor of infancy
  - o *ZC3H7B::BCOR*
    - – *ZC3H7B* (22q13) encodes nuclear protein
  - o Histologically similar to *BCOR::CCNB3* sarcoma
  - o Transcription signature similar to *BCOR::CCNB3* sarcoma
  - o Other rare *BCOR*-rearranged sarcoma fusions: *BCOR::CIITA, BCOR::CHD9,* and *KTM2D::BCOR*
- Recurrent CNA of *BCOR::CCNB3* cases
  - o Deletions at 17p, 10q
  - o Lacks recurrent CNA of Ewing sarcoma: 8q gain (50% of ES), 1q, 12 gain (~ 25% of ES), loss of 16q (~ 25% of ES)
- Genes overexpressed in *BCOR::CCNB3* and *BCOR::MAML3* cases
  - o HOX homeobox genes: Involved in development, especially of skeleton
- Hyperactivated pathways in *BCOR::CCNB3* cases
  - o Wnt signaling pathway
  - o Hedgehog signaling pathway

Round Cell Sarcoma With *EWSR1*::Non-ETS Fusions

- *EWSR1/FUS::NFATC2* lesions
  - o *EWSR1/FUS::NFATC2* fusion is amplified with more complex karyotype (more CNVs) in sarcomas than benign lesions with this fusion
    - – ↑ fusion gene dosage effect may result in sarcoma rather than benign lesion
    - – FET fusion partner effect
      - □ *EWSR1::NFATC2* and *FUS::NFATC2* tumors significantly differ in gene transcription profiles
- *EWSR1::PATZ1* tumors
  - o PATZ1
    - – Transcription factor that helps regulate cell differentiation
    - – Gene Location: 22q12 close to *EWSR1*
      - □ Fusion most likely results from intrachromosomal paracentric inversion
  - o Effect of fusion: Overexpression of PATZ1 → aberrant gene transcription
  - o Recurrent secondary genetic findings: *CDKN2A/CDKN2B* loss or partial deletion, *MDM2* amplification

ANCILLARY STUDIES

Desmoplastic Small Round Cell Tumor

- IHC: Characteristic mix of reactivity for NSE, desmin (often paranuclear), keratins, WT1 (nuclear)
  - o Majority of cases may also express AR (androgen receptor): Possibly indicates therapeutic target
- FISH: Commercial *EWSR1* break-apart probe diagnostically helpful
  - o Requires correlation with morphology, IHC, and clinical findings

CIC-Rearranged Sarcomas

- IHC
  - o Diffuse ETV4 + at least focal nuclear WT1: Relatively sensitive and specific
  - o CD99: May show membranous reactivity; usually focal
  - o Others: May express CD31, ERG
- FISH
  - o *CIC* break-apart probes available but less sensitive than diffuse nuclear ETV4 IHC expression

Other Small Round Blue Cell Sarcomas

 - Lack of *EWSR1* rearrangement by FISH in setting of small round cell tumor with expression of WT1 and ETV: Highly supportive of *CIC::DUX4* fusion sarcoma diagnosis

Sarcoma With *BCOR* Genetic Alterations
- IHC
  - Diffuse strong nuclear expression of CCNB3 protein: Helps confirm diagnosis of *BCOR::CCNB3* sarcoma in appropriate setting
  - Diffuse strong nuclear expression of BCOR is supportive of *BCOR*-rearranged sarcoma in appropriate clinicopathologic context
    - Diffuse, strong nuclear expression also seen in some high-grade endometrial sarcomas, synovial sarcomas, and others
  - Other commonly positive antigens (> 80%) include SATB2, TLE1, BCL2, cyclin D1, and pan-TRK
- Sequencing: Can confirm diagnosis

Round Cell Sarcoma With *EWSR1*::Non-ETS Fusions
- *EWSR1/FUS::NFATC2* tumors
  - IHC: CD99 (50%); variably positive for NKX2-2, AE1/AE3 keratins, and CD138
    - NKX3-1 may be relatively specific but also is positive in mesenchymal chondrosarcoma, primitive component only
      - Requires use of low-level positive control to validate antibody, such as Sertoli cells rather than prostate epithelial cells
  - FISH or sequencing identifies diagnostic fusion
- *EWSR1::PATZ1* tumors
  - IHC: Described as often "polyphenotypic"; varying dual expression of muscle markers (desmin, MYOD1, myogenin) and neural markers (S100, SOX10, GFAP, MITF)
  - Sequencing identifies diagnostic fusion
  - FISH using break-apart *EWSR1* probe may be falsely negative due to adjacent locations of *EWSR1* and *PATZ1* at 22q12

DIFFERENTIAL DIAGNOSIS

DDx for Desmoplastic Small Round Cell Tumor
- Biphasic synovial sarcoma
  - Usually lacks desmoplastic stroma; positive for t(X;18) by FISH or RT-PCR
- Mesothelioma
  - Different age group; negative for NSE, S100; negative for t(11;22) by FISH or RT-PCR
- Rare Ewing sarcoma with epithelial differentiation
  - May require sequencing for diagnosis
- Metastatic germ cell tumor
  - Often more polymorphic on histology; positive for germ cell markers; negative for t(11;22) by FISH or PCR

DDx for *CIC*-Rearranged Sarcomas
- Ewing sarcoma
  - May appear similar on histology; WT1 negative by IHC; positive for FET::ETS gene fusion by FISH or sequencing
- Other small round cell sarcomas of pediatric age group
  - Different by histology (such as RMS, lymphoma), IHC; negative for *CIC::DUX4* fusion

DDx for Sarcoma With *BCOR* Genetic Alterations
- Ewing sarcoma
  - Most cases lack spindle cells common in *BCOR::CCNB3* sarcomas; lack CCNB3 or BCOR nuclear IHC expression, express NKX2.2 and diffuse membranous CD99
- Other small round cell sarcomas of pediatric age group
  - Different by histology (such as rhabdomyosarcoma, lymphoma); differing IHC reactivity, including lack of nuclear CCNB3
- Other spindle cell sarcomas of pediatric age group
  - Lack of nuclear CCNB3 IHC expression; lack of *BCOR::CCNB3* by sequencing

DDx for Round Cell Sarcoma With *EWSR1*::Non-ETS Fusions
- Ewing sarcoma
  - Most cases lack spindle cells common in *EWSR1*::non-ETS fusion tumors; usually more sheet-like growth; negative for specific non-ETS fusions
- High-grade myxoid liposarcoma
  - May grow in cords or trabeculae but may also have lower grade areas or lipoblasts; does not express muscle markers; will be positive for *DDIT3* fusion and often DDIT3 protein by IHC
- Synovial sarcoma (SS)
  - May mimic *EWSR1*::non-ETS fusion sarcomas histologically; IHC reactivity may overlap but SS also expresses TLE1, EMA, and SSX
  - Nearly all cases positive for *SS18::SSX1/SSX2/SSX4* fusion
- Other small round cell tumors (lymphoma, alveolar RMS, metastatic small cell carcinoma, neuroblastoma etc): differ by IHC in some cases; negative for *EWSR1*::non-ETS fusion

SELECTED REFERENCES

1. Linos K et al: Expanding the molecular diversity of CIC-rearranged sarcomas with novel and very rare partners. Mod Pathol. 36(5):100103, 2023
2. Yoshida A: Ewing and Ewing-like sarcomas: a morphological guide through genetically-defined entities. Pathol Int. 73(1):12-26, 2023
3. Brcic I et al: Implementation of copy number variations-based diagnostics in morphologically challenging EWSR1/FUS::NFATC2 neoplasms of the bone and soft tissue. Int J Mol Sci. 23(24), 2022
4. Cidre-Aranaz F et al: Small round cell sarcomas. Nat Rev Dis Primers. 8(1):66, 2022
5. Kojima N et al: Co-expression of ERG and CD31 in a subset of CIC-rearranged sarcoma: a potential diagnostic pitfall. Mod Pathol. 35(10):1439-48, 2022
6. Lamhamedi-Cherradi SE et al: The androgen receptor is a therapeutic target in desmoplastic small round cell sarcoma. Nat Commun. 13(1):3057, 2022
7. Le Loarer F et al: Advances in the classification of round cell sarcomas. Histopathology. 80(1):33-53, 2022
8. Kallen ME et al: From the ashes of "Ewing-like" sarcoma: a contemporary update of the classification, immunohistochemistry, and molecular genetics of round cell sarcomas. Semin Diagn Pathol. 39(1):29-37, 2022
9. Ong SLM et al: Expanding the spectrum of EWSR1-NFATC2-rearranged benign tumors: a common genomic abnormality in vascular malformation/hemangioma and simple bone cyst. Am J Surg Pathol. 45(12):1669-81, 2021
10. Yoshida A et al: Confirmation of NKX3-1 expression in EWSR1-NFATC2 sarcoma and mesenchymal chondrosarcoma using monoclonal antibody immunohistochemistry, RT-PCR, and RNA in situ hybridization. Am J Surg Pathol. 45(4):578-82, 2021

Other Small Round Blue Cell Sarcomas

Irregular Nest of Tumor Cells in DSRCT

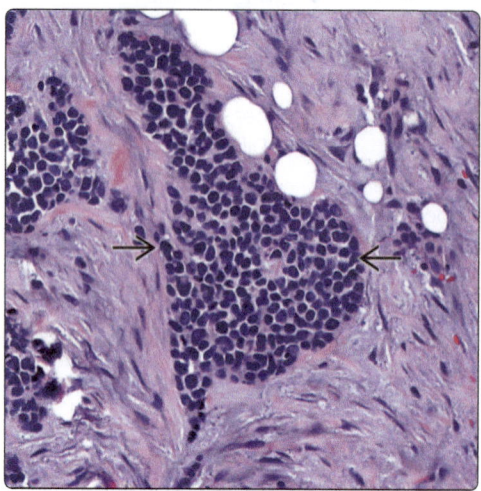

Primitive Blastic Cell in DSRCT

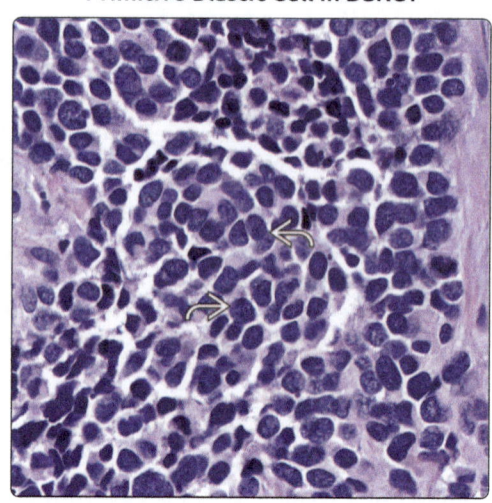

(Left) DSRCT shows an irregularly shaped nest of tumor cells ➡ embedded in myxoid to collagenized stroma. The tumor effaces most of the normal tissue, which in this case consists of a few residual adipocytes. (Right) The most common cell type in DSRCT is a primitive blastic cell ➡ with a high N:C ratio and round to oval, normochromatic to hyperchromatic nuclei without macronucleoli.

Epithelial-Appearing Cells in DSRCT

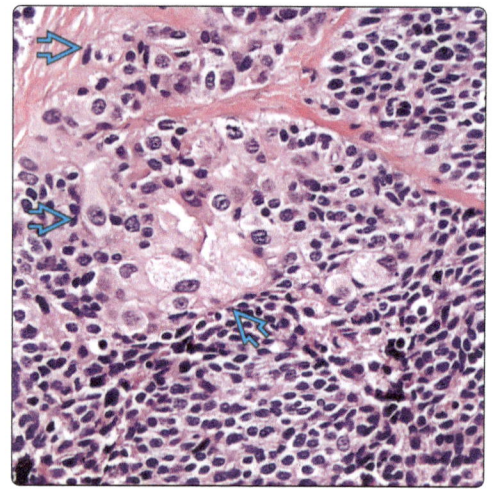

Glomeruloid Hypervascularity in DSRCT

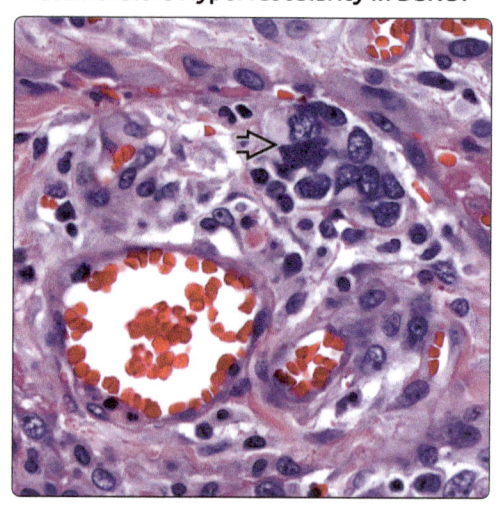

(Left) While the majority of tumor cells in DSRCT are blastic small round blue cells, nests of epithelial-appearing cells ➡ are common. Actual squamous cell and glandular differentiation may also occur. (Right) DSRCT may elicit a prominent neovascular response in the surrounding tissue. In this field, a small nest of tumor cells ➡ abuts reactive, thin-walled ectatic vessels.

DSRCT With NSE Expression

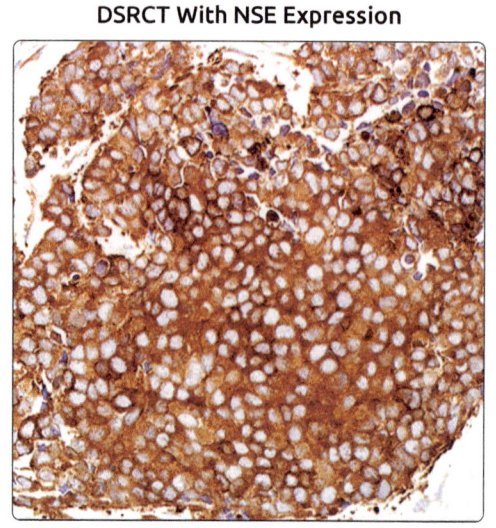

DSRCT With Paranuclear Desmin Expression

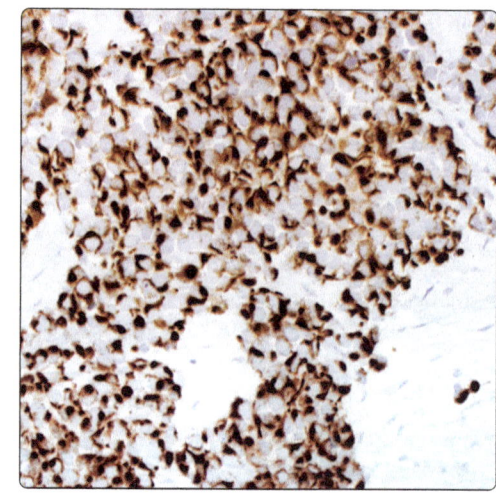

(Left) DSRCT is characterized by polyphenotypic IHC expression. Here, tumor cells strongly and diffusely express NSE. (Right) Many cases of DSRCT show a peculiar paranuclear, dot-like expression pattern of desmin, as seen here.

Other Small Round Blue Cell Sarcomas

CIC::DUX4 Fusion Sarcoma

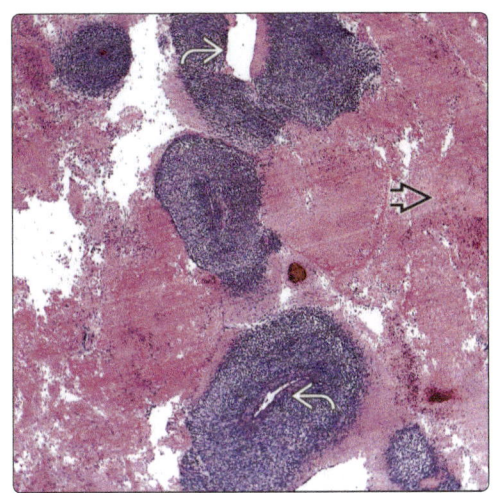

CIC::DUX4 Fusion Sarcoma

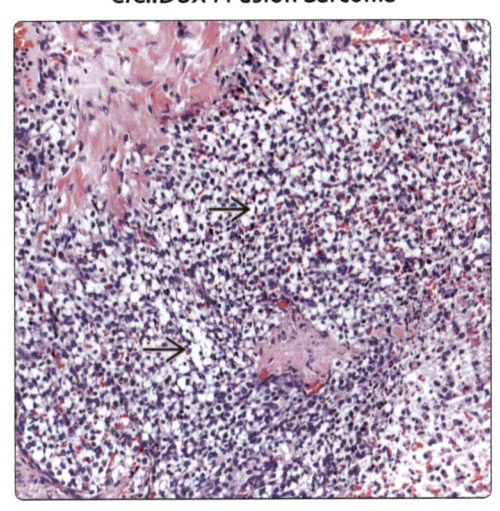

(Left) This 14-year-old boy had deep soft tissue CIC::DUX4 fusion sarcoma in his knee. There is abundant geographic necrosis ⇨ and preservation around blood vessels ⇨, as seen in rapidly growing sarcomas. (Right) The tumor cells of CIC::DUX4 fusion sarcoma may have clear cytoplasm ⇨.

CIC::DUX4 Fusion Sarcoma

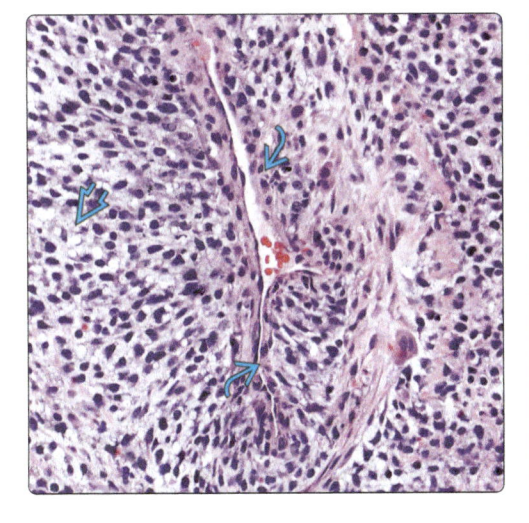

CIC::DUX4 Fusion Sarcoma

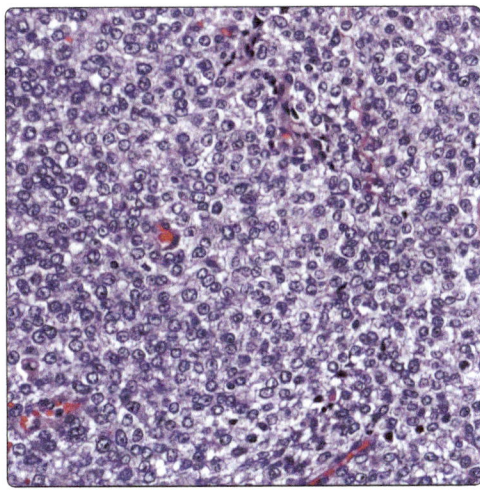

(Left) Tumor cells invade the wall of an intratumoral blood vessel ⇨. Note the myxoid background ⇨. (Right) The nuclei of the tumor cells are typically vesicular and may exhibit small nucleoli. The cytoplasm may also be amphophilic, as seen here.

CIC::DUX4 Fusion Sarcoma Expressing Nuclear WT1

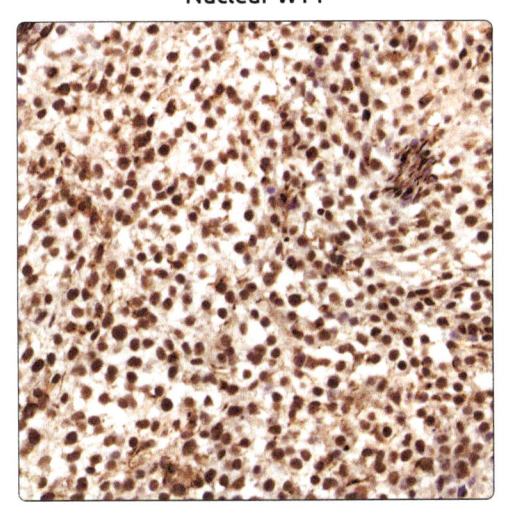

CIC::DUX4 Fusion Sarcoma Expressing CD99

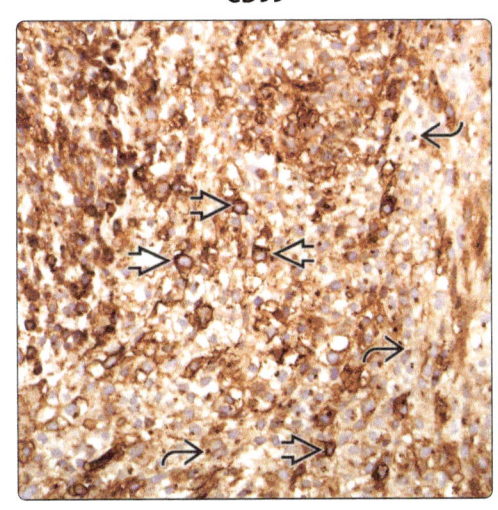

(Left) WT1 is diffusely and strongly expressed in CIC::DUX4 fusion sarcomas, as in this case with virtually all cells showing nuclear WT1. (Right) CD99 can be expressed in CIC::DUX4 fusion sarcoma, but it is usually patchy. Some cells show membranous reactivity ⇨, identical to the pattern seen in Ewing sarcoma. Most Ewing sarcomas exhibit strong, diffuse, and monotonous membranous CD99, not the mottled pattern seen here. Note also the nonspecific paranuclear reactivity ⇨.

Other Small Round Blue Cell Sarcomas

(Left) The vascular pattern in BCOR::CCNB3 fusion sarcoma contains thin-walled branching vessels ➡ that delicately invest the tumor. **(Right)** BCOR::CCNB3 fusion sarcoma shows sheets of dyscohesive small round blue cells with vesicular chromatin and small nucleoli. More commonly, the tumor nuclei are hyperchromatic and ovoid or angulated.

BCOR::CCNB3 Fusion Sarcoma

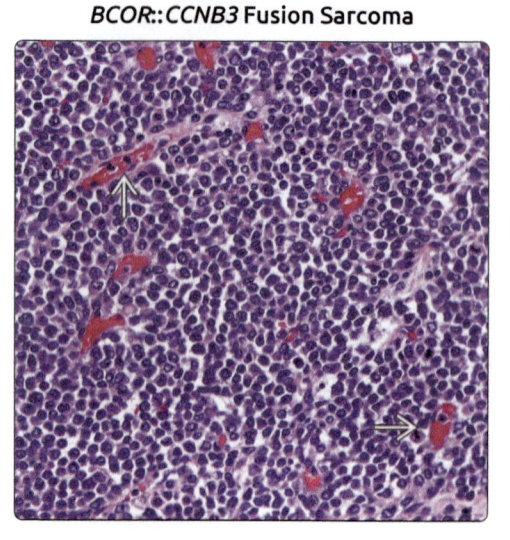

BCOR::CCNB3 Fusion Sarcoma

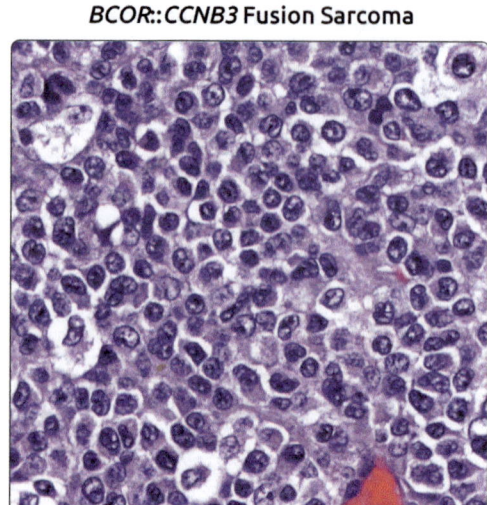

(Left) A substantial percentage of BCOR::CCNB3 fusion sarcomas feature a spindle cell component. In rare cases, the entire tumor may consist of plump spindled cells. **(Right)** A histologic clue to the diagnosis of BCOR::CCNB3 fusion sarcoma is a mixed round cell-spindle cell sarcoma lacking muscle marker expression. Synovial sarcoma and malignant peripheral nerve sheath tumor may also have spindled and small round cells.

BCOR::CCNB3 Fusion Sarcoma

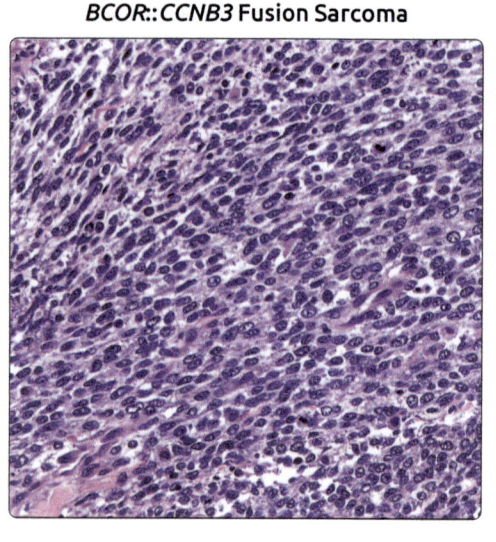

BCOR::CCNB3 Fusion Sarcoma

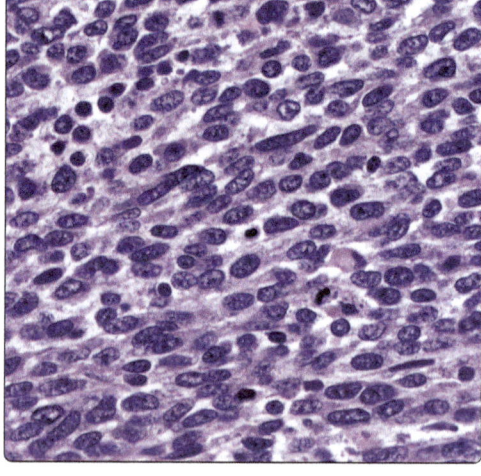

(Left) Some BCOR::CCNB3 fusion sarcomas express CD99 in a membranous pattern, mimicking Ewing sarcoma family of tumors. This example shows convincing membranous expression ➡. **(Right)** Nuclear reactivity ➡ for CCNB3 is specific and sensitive for the diagnosis of BCOR::CCNB3 fusion sarcoma but only in the appropriate clinical and morphologic setting. Staining is usually strong and diffuse but may become patchy in treated tumors.

BCOR::CCNB3 Fusion Sarcoma With Membranous CD99 Expression

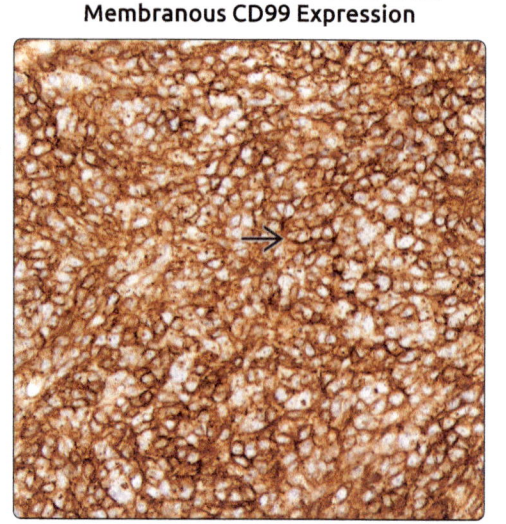

BCOR::CCNB3 Fusion Sarcoma With Nuclear CCNB3 Expression

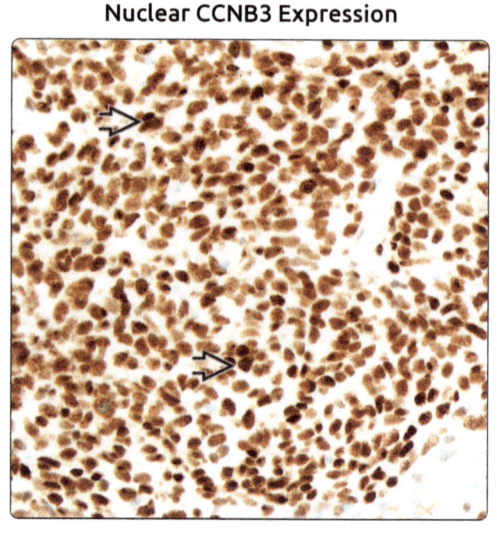

Other Small Round Blue Cell Sarcomas

EWSR1/FUS::NFATC2 Sarcoma

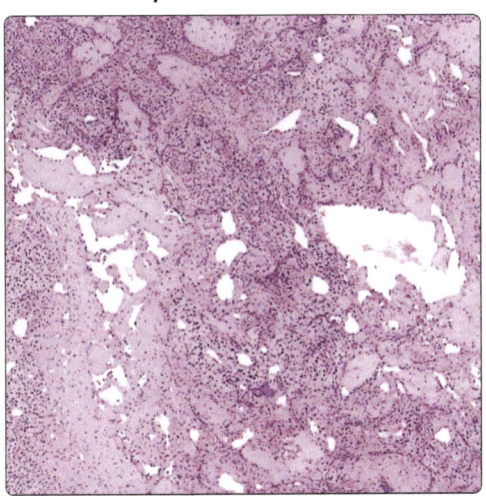

EWSR1/FUS::NFATC2 Sarcoma

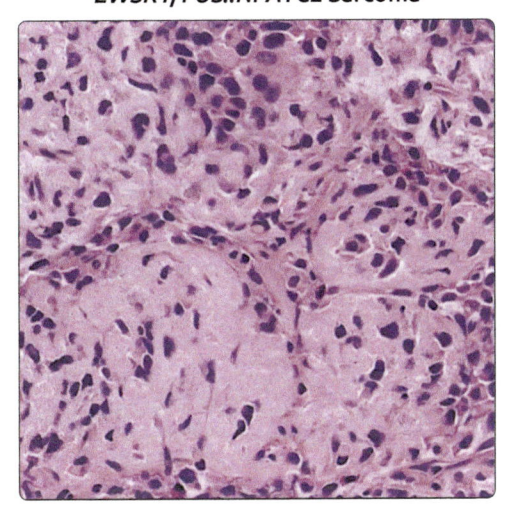

(Left) *EWSR1/FUS::NFATC2* sarcoma arose in the femur of a man in his 30's. The tumor is variably cellular with HPC-like blood vessels and sclerotic stroma. A prominent, fibrous, hyaline or myxoid stroma often occurs in this tumor. (Courtesy MG Evans, MD.) (Right) At high magnification, tumor cells are uniform, round to oval and embedded in hyaline matrix. Cellular atypia is usually minimal in this tumor. (Courtesy MG Evans, MD.)

EWSR1/FUS::NFATC2 Fusion-Positive Intraosseous Hemangioma

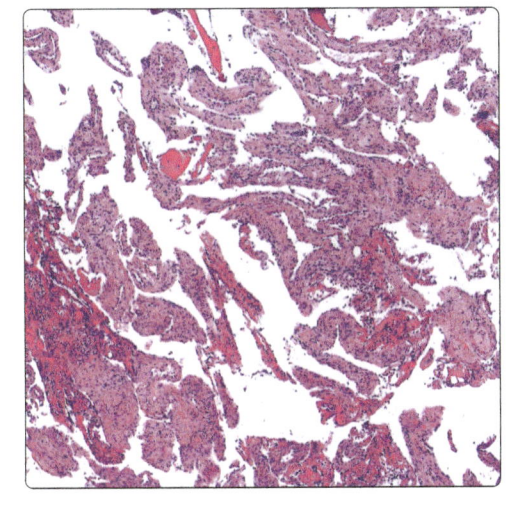

EWSR1/FUS::NFATC2 Fusion-Positive Intraosseous Cyst

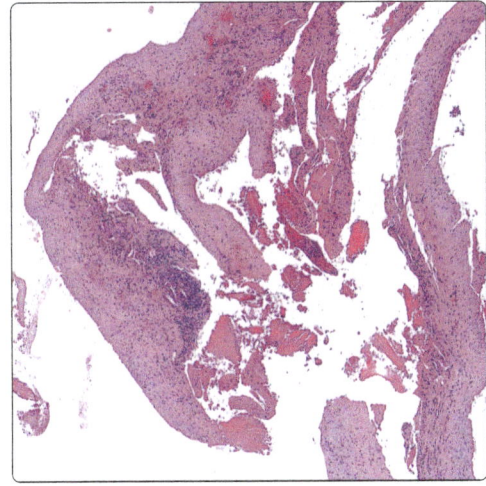

(Left) Intraosseous hemangiomas may feature *EWSR1/FUS::NFATC2* fusion. These fusion-positive hemangiomas are histologically indistinguishable from nonfusion cases. NKX2.2 is not expressed in these cases, unlike most *EWSR1/FUS::NFATC2* sarcomas. (Right) Many simple bone cysts (SBCs) harbor *EWSR1/FUS::NFATC2* fusion. Benign behavior of fusion-positive SBCs may be related to lower expression level of the fusion transcript &/or absence of secondary genetic events.

EWSR1::PATZ1 Sarcoma

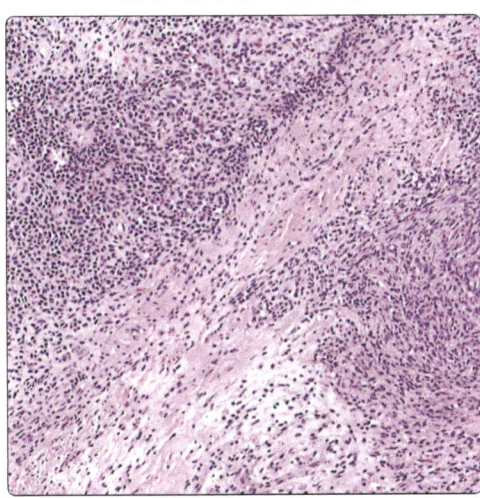

EWSR1::PATZ1 Sarcoma

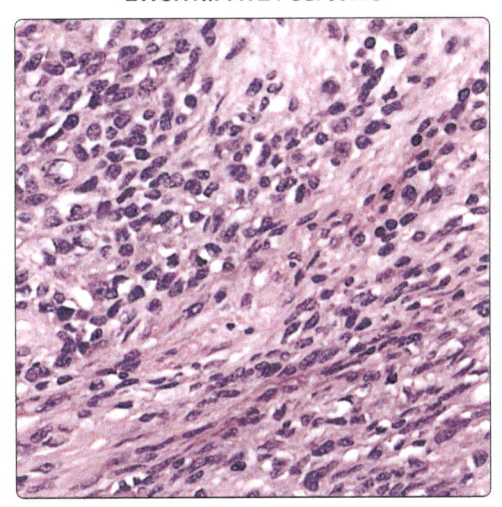

(Left) This tumor arose in the retroperitoneum of a 31-year-old man. It is variably cellular with sheets of cells and a fibrous background. (Courtesy MG Evans, MD.) (Right) Tumor cells appear undifferentiated and are round to oval in shape. (Courtesy MG Evans, MD.)

Giant Cell Tumor of Bone

KEY FACTS

TERMINOLOGY

- Primary, locally aggressive, rarely metastasizing mesenchymal tumor of bone characterized by mononuclear stromal cells, macrophages and osteoclast-like giant cells
- Multiple cell types form tumor
  - Monocytes and fused monocytes = osteoclasts
  - Stromal spindle cells are clonal tumor cell

ETIOLOGY/PATHOGENESIS

- *H3F3A* mutation found in 96% of GCTB
  - Codes for H3 family histone protein
  - Exact oncogenic function in GCTB not yet elucidated

CLINICAL ISSUES

- High risk of recurrence (18-35%)
- Malignant transformation rare (~ 4% of GCTB)

MOLECULAR

- Polyclonal tumor by cytogenetic karyotyping
  - Includes numerous types of monoclonal aberrations
  - Telomeric associations in 70% of karyotypes
- Epigenetic changes: Hypermethylation of promoter regions of *DLK1-DIO3* cluster at 14q32
  - Hypermethylation at 14q32 common → downregulation of 3 tumor suppressors
  - Some miRNAs downregulated
- Pathways dysregulated in GCTB
  - Notch and Wnt signaling pathways
  - Various abnormal pathway effects on p53 production, including ↑ MDM2

ANCILLARY TESTS

- H3F3A G34W monoclonal antibody
  - Nuclear expression helps confirm diagnosis of giant cell tumor
  - Most rare variant mutations are negative for antibody

Distal Radius Tumor

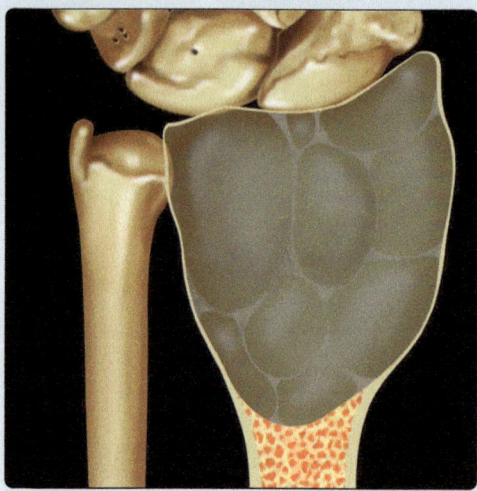

Gross Appearance

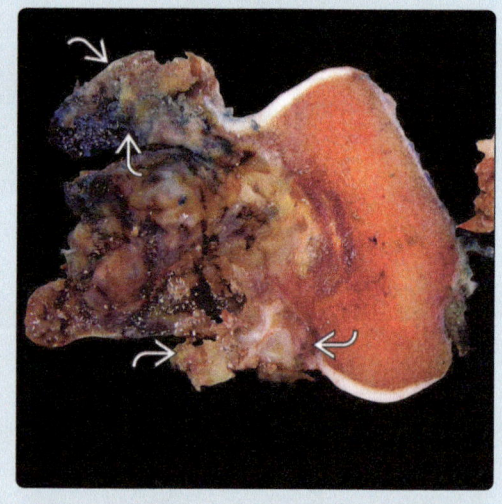

(Left) Graphic shows a common location for giant cell tumor of the bone (GCTB), the distal radius. The tumor expands the epiphysis and metaphysis of this skeletally mature bone. (Right) Gross photograph of recurrent GCTB shows the typical shaggy, hemorrhagic appearance. This tumor perforates the cortex and extends into soft tissue ➡.

Osteoid Formation Post Denosumab Therapy

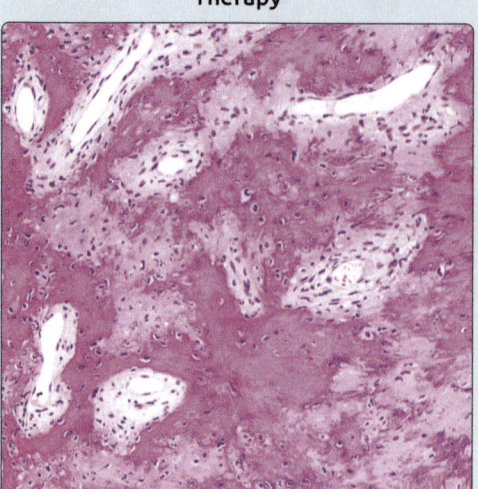

Hypercellularity Post Denosumab Therapy

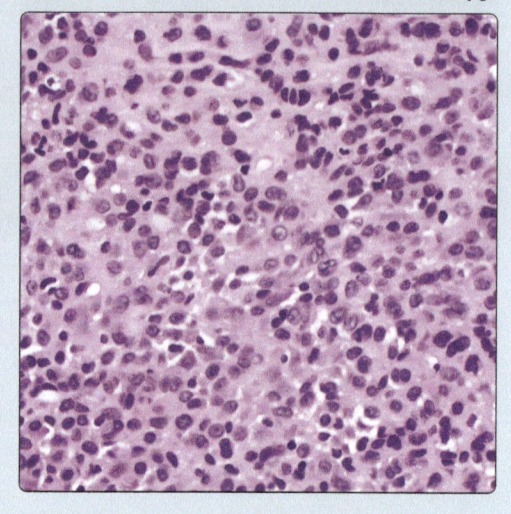

(Left) Changes induced by denosumab therapy include abundant osteoid-woven bone production. (Right) Tumors that respond to denosumab lack osteoclasts. The underlying, unaffected tumor cells may proliferate, leading to a hypercellular, mitotically active appearance that should not be mistaken as malignant transformation.

Giant Cell Tumor of Bone

TERMINOLOGY

Abbreviations
- Giant cell tumor of bone (GCTB)

Synonyms
- Osteoclastoma

Definitions
- Primary, locally aggressive, rarely metastasizing mesenchymal tumor of bone with recurrent *H3F3A* mutations characterized by diffuse infiltrates of reactive multinucleated osteoclasts

ETIOLOGY/PATHOGENESIS

Cell of Origin
- 3 main cell types form tumor
  - Stromal spindle cells are thought to be tumor cells
    - Only cell type with *H3F3A* mutation
  - Osteoclasts: May be abnormal but are not neoplastic
  - Monocytes: Recruited to tumor; some fuse to form osteoclasts

H3F3A Mutation
- Chromosome 1q42.12
- Found in > 95% of cases
- Codes for H3.3, replication-independent histone protein
- Alteration of glycine 35 amino acid
  - Switch glycine to tryptophan (95% of cases)
  - Switch glycine to leucine amino acid (5% of cases)

H3 Histone Family Mutations in Other Tumors
- Chondroblastoma
  - ~ 95% of cases
  - Mutations in *H3F3B* (17q25.1) or *H3F3A*
    - Different amino acid changes in H3.3 protein
    - H3.3 protein encoded by both *H3F3B* and *H3F3A*
- Chondrosarcomas and osteosarcomas show rare mutations
  - *H3F3B* or *H3F3A* mutations in 1-7% of cases
  - Specific mutation correlates with osteoblastic vs. chondroblastic differentiation
- Some pediatric brain gliomas

CLINICAL ISSUES

Epidemiology
- Incidence
  - Rare: Comprises ~ 6% of primary bone tumors
    - ~ 20% of benign bone tumors
  - Annual incidence: ~ 1-2 per million
- Age
  - Young to middle-aged adults most commonly (20-45 years)
  - Up to 10% may occur in patients < 18 years
    - Up to 20% arise in metaphysis without epiphyseal involvement
    - Typical histologic features may comprise minority of tumor
      - Poses diagnostic challenges on needle core biopsy
    - May contain reactive new bone simulating osteosarcoma
- Sex
  - Slightly F > M in Western countries

Site
- Intraosseous
  - Epiphysis/apophysis of long bones
  - Pelvic bones, especially sacrum, spine, cranial bones next most common
  - Occurs in skeletally mature bone (bone with closed growth plate)
    - Rarely occurs in bone with open physis (2-10% of cases)

Natural History
- Local effects
  - Pathologic fracture
  - Soft tissue extension
  - Recurrence risk is relatively high at 18-35%
- "Benign metastases"
  - Otherwise conventional GCTB can spread as nodular lung implants
  - Lung "metastases" usually indolent; may regress; may convert to mature bone
- Malignant transformation
  - Incidence: ~ 4%
  - Radiation associated
    - Secondary malignancy in GCTB
  - Spontaneous malignant transformation
    - Histologic features of preceding GCT do not predict risk for sarcoma development

Treatment
- Surgical approaches
  - Extensive curettage preferred where possible
  - Wide resection reduces local recurrence risk but may impair functionality
- Drugs
  - Bisphosphonates
  - Denosumab
    - Monoclonal antibody that inhibits RANKL pathway
    - Denosumab responsive tumors lack osteoclasts but may become hypercellular with osteoid &/or chondroid matrix
      - Do not misdiagnose hypercellular changes as osteosarcoma or sarcoma, not otherwise specified
    - Rare denosumab-treated tumors undergo malignant transformation (< 5%): Most commonly resembles osteosarcoma
- Radiation
  - Radiation used for treating cases not amenable to surgery
  - Poses risk for malignant transformation

MOLECULAR

Cytogenetics
- Polyclonal tumor at level of karyotype
  - Insertions, deletions, translocations common
  - But not clonal
- Telomeric associations
  - Common but not specific for GCTB
    - Found in 70%

Giant Cell Tumor of Bone

- Most common chromosome arms involved
  - 11p, 15p, 19q, 20q
- Often associated with 11p deletion

In Situ Hybridization

- Can divide GCTB into 5 groups corresponding to clinical behavior (one study of 52 cases)
  - Diploid nonrecurrent and recurrent
  - Tetraploid nonrecurrent and recurrent
    - Increased aneusomy compared to nonrecurrent groups
- Ploidy may change during clinical course

Molecular Genetics

- *H3F3A*
  - Driver mutation for GCTB
  - Changes occur at glycine 35 amino acid
    - Majority comprise G35W mutation
    - Minority includes G35L, G35M, G35V, and others
- *TNFSF11*
  - Overexpressed in multiple cell types, including monocytes, osteoclasts, and tumor stromal cells
  - Activation leads directly to osteoclastogenesis from mononuclear precursors
- *CSF1*
  - Overexpressed and synthesized by tumor stromal cells
  - Promotes osteoclastogenesis
- Other growth factors that can substitute for CSF1 protein in inducing osteoclastogenesis
  - VEGFA
  - FLT3 ligand
  - Placental growth factor (PlGF)
  - Hepatocyte growth factor (HGF)
- Other genes overexpressed in GCTB involved in osteoclastogenesis
  - *NFATC1*
  - *DCSTAMP*
    - Reduced cell surface expression in some monocytes → large osteoclasts characteristic of many GCTB
  - *CEBPB*
    - May result in larger osteoclasts
    - Promotes ↑ RANKL expression in both tumor stromal cells and osteoclasts
  - *PTH1R*
    - Overexpressed in osteoclasts in GCTB and in osteoclasts in hyperparathyroidism
    - Promotes ↑ RANKL expression
  - Monocyte recruitment by tumor stromal cells
    - *CXCL12*
    - *VEGFA*
- *TP53*
  - Role controversial in nonsarcomatous giant cell tumor
  - Mutations in tumor stromal cells may be associated with more aggressive behavior
  - Protein may be decreased due to ↑ MDM2

Gene Expression Profiling

- Pathways dysregulated in GCTB
  - Notch signaling pathway
- Recurrent GCTB
  - Differentially expresses some genes compared to primary GCTB
  - Pathways involved
    - p53 signaling
    - Osteoclast differentiation
    - Wnt signaling
  - Genes overexpressed in recurrent GCTB
    - *MDM2*: MDM2 protein also overexpressed by IHC
    - *IGF1* (12q23)
    - *STAT1* (2q32.2)
    - *RAC1* (7p22.1)
    - *GPX1*: GPX1 protein also overexpressed by IHC
  - Gene underexpressed in recurrent GCTB
    - *DPT*: Protein also ↓ in recurrent GCTB compared to nonrecurrent
- Metastatic GCTB
  - Differentially expresses some genes compared to primary GCTB
  - Underexpressed
    - *LUM* (12q21.3-q22): Protein also ↓
    - *DCN* (12q21.33): Protein also ↓
  - Overexpressed
    - *TP53* may also be mutated; p53 protein overexpression reportedly higher in malignant GCTB

Epigenetics

- Hypermethylation at promoter region of *DLK1-DIO3* cluster at 14q32
  - Downregulates tumor suppressor genes: *DLK1*, *MEG3*, *MEG8*
  - Abnormally silences specific microRNAs at this site
- miR30A abnormally downregulated
  - *RUNX2* consequently overexpressed
    - Involved in osteoblastogenesis
- miR126 abnormally downregulated in GCTB
  - Parathyroid hormone-related protein (PTHrP) consequently overexpressed
    - Stimulates osteoclastic bone resorption
    - Causes proliferation of tumor stromal cells
- miR136 abnormally downregulated in metastatic GCTB compared to nonmetastatic GCTB
  - *NFIB* consequently overexpressed

Tumor Immunology

- Complex interactions between monocyte populations and tumor stromal cells cause osteoclast formation

MICROSCOPIC

Histologic Features

- Low magnification
  - Hypercellular sheets of cells with diffuse distribution of large osteoclasts
  - Other features often present in varying proportions
    - Secondary aneurysmal bone cyst (ABC) changes
    - Geographic necrosis
    - Fibrosis/fibroplasia
    - Focal reactive osteoid
- High magnification
  - 3 main cell populations
    - Osteoclasts: Often large with ≥ 20 nuclei

Giant Cell Tumor of Bone

- – Mononuclear stromal cells: Precursors to osteoclasts
- – Tumor stromal cells: Round to plump spindle cells
- o Nuclear features
  - – Atypia usually absent
    - □ Rare cases may show marked nuclear atypia = "symplastic/pseudoanaplastic change"
    - □ Symplastic/pseudoanaplastic GCT may have specific H3F3A mutation [p.Gly35Trp (G35W)]
  - – Mitotic rate may be high
  - – Negative for atypical mitoses
- Post denosumab therapy
  - o Osteoclasts and mononuclear cells absent to sparse
  - o Stromal neoplastic cells continue to proliferate
- GCTB with malignant transformation
  - o May arise de novo with intermixed histologically conventional GCTB
  - o Most common morphologies in malignant component
    - – Osteosarcoma
    - – Undifferentiated pleomorphic sarcoma
    - – Fibrosarcoma

ANCILLARY TESTS

Immunohistochemistry

- H3F3A G34W monoclonal antibody
  - o Nuclear expression helps confirm diagnosis of GCT
  - o Found in > 95% of giant cell tumors
    - – Most of rare variant mutations (~ 5%) occur in small bones of hands, feet, patella, and axial skeleton
- Nonspecific but sensitive markers
  - o p63: Nuclear expression
  - o SATB2: Nuclear expression
    - – Indicates tumor stromal cells are osteoblastic

DIFFERENTIAL DIAGNOSIS

Giant Cell-Rich Osteosarcoma

- Imaging features
  - o Metaphyseal or metadiaphyseal
    - – Not epiphyseal as in most GCTB
- Histologic features
  - o Unequivocal cytologic atypia present
  - o Atypical mitoses ± absent in GCT B
- Genetic features
  - o Complex aneuploid karyotype
  - o Rare subarticular giant-cell rich osteosarcoma may represent actual malignant giant cell tumor
    - – These cases harbor H3F3A mutations

Nonossifying Fibroma

- Histologic features
  - o Storiform arrangement of fibroblasts
  - o Irregular distribution of small osteoclasts
  - o Mononuclear cells inconspicuous compared to GCTB
- Genetic features
  - o Lacks H3F3A mutation
  - o Lacks telomeric associations, which are detected in 70% of GCTB

Aneurysmal Bone Cyst

- Histologic features
  - o Solid and cystic components
  - o Irregular distribution of small osteoclasts (usually < 20 nuclei)
- Genetic features
  - o 70% of primary ABC show USP6 rearrangements by FISH or PCR
  - o Primary ABC: Rearrangements of chromosome 16 or 17 on karyotype
  - o Lack H3F3A mutations

Giant Cell Tumor of Bone With Malignant Transformation

- Histologic features
  - o Marked nuclear atypia with coarse chromatin, pleomorphism
  - o ± atypical mitotic figures
  - o May have diffuse strong ↑ expression of p53
- Genetic features
  - o H3.3 mutation usually but not always identified on molecular test or IHC
  - o May have additional driver mutations and higher tumor mutation burden compared to nonmalignant GCTB

Chondroblastoma

- Histologic features
  - o Epithelioid tumor cells with clefted nuclei
  - o Irregular distribution of small osteoclasts
  - o ± chicken-wire calcifications
  - o S100, keratins, DOG1 positive
- Genetic features
  - o H3F3A or H3F3B mutations at sites distinct from GCTB H3F3A mutation

Giant Cell-Rich Bone Tumor With HMGAT2::NCOR2 Fusion

- Rare tumor that histologically mimics GCTB or nonossifying fibroma
- Lacks H3.3 mutation

SELECTED REFERENCES

1. Panagopoulos I et al: Recurrent fusion of the genes for high-mobility group AT-hook 2 (HMGA2) and nuclear receptor co-repressor 2 (NCOR2) in osteoclastic giant cell-rich tumors of bone. Cancer Genomics Proteomics. 19(2):163-77, 2022
2. Vari S et al: Malignant transformation of giant cell tumour of bone: a review of literature and the experience of a referral centre. Int J Mol Sci. 23(18), 2022
3. Fittall MW et al: Drivers underpinning the malignant transformation of giant cell tumour of bone. J Pathol. 252(4):433-40, 2020
4. Yoshida KI et al: Absence of H3F3A mutation in a subset of malignant giant cell tumor of bone. Mod Pathol. 32(12):1751-61, 2019
5. Amary F et al: H3F3A (Histone 3.3) G34W immunohistochemistry: a reliable marker defining benign and malignant giant cell tumor of bone. Am J Surg Pathol. 41(8):1059-68, 2017
6. Righi A et al: Histone 3.3 mutations in giant cell tumor and giant cell-rich sarcomas of bone. Hum Pathol. 68:128-35, 2017
7. Broehm CJ et al: Two cases of sarcoma arising in giant cell tumor of bone treated with denosumab. Case Rep Med. 2015:767198, 2015
8. Behjati S et al: Distinct H3F3A and H3F3B driver mutations define chondroblastoma and giant cell tumor of bone. Nat Genet. 2013 Dec;45(12):1479-82. Epub 2013 Oct 27. Erratum in: Nat Genet. 46(3):316, 2014

Giant Cell Tumor of Bone

Representative Karyotype

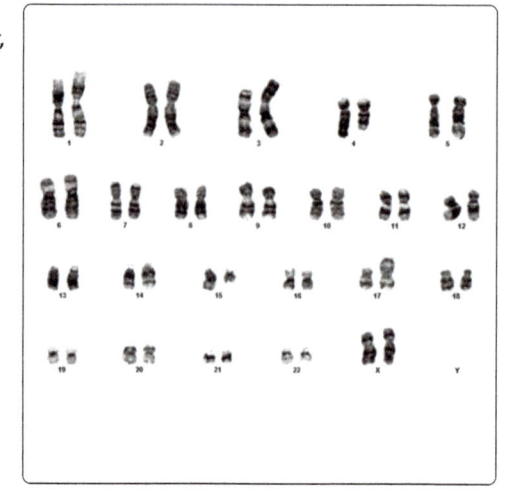

(Left) Karyotype shows the characteristic, but not specific, telomeric associations common in GCTB. (Right) Karyotype of the same GCTB shows another distinct, but nonclonal, telomeric association.

Additional Subclones Common

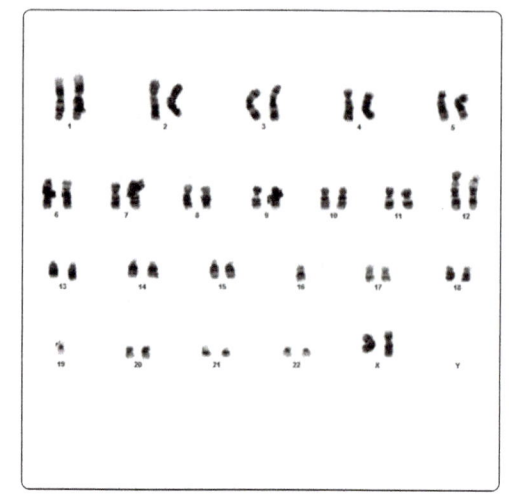

Common Complexity of Karyotypes

Nonclonal Aberration(s):
46,XX,add(16)(p13.3)(1)/
46,XX,t(1;4)(p32;q31)(1)/
44,X,dic(X;21)(q28;q22),dic(12;17)
 (p13;p13),dic(12;19)(p13;q13.4)[1]/
44,XX,dic(12;16)p13;p13.3),dic(12;19)
 (p13;q13.4)(1)/
45,X,del(X)(q24), del(19)(q13.1),-22[1]/
45,X,dic(X;6)(q28;q27)(1)/
46,XX,-2,-4,+2mar[1]/
46,XX,-17,add(19)(p13.3),+mar[1]/
45,XX,dic(16;19)(p13.3;q13.4)(1)
9 cells with nonclonal karyotypic changes (above) were included in the 20 metaphases analyzed.

(Left) Cytogenetics report lists the numerous nonclonal changes found in GCTB. The karyotypes can be complex, as in this case with multiple different nonclonal changes, or can be diploid ± telomeric associations. (Right) At low power, classic areas of GCTB show an even distribution of osteoclastic giant cells.

Classic Appearance

Gigantic Giant Cells

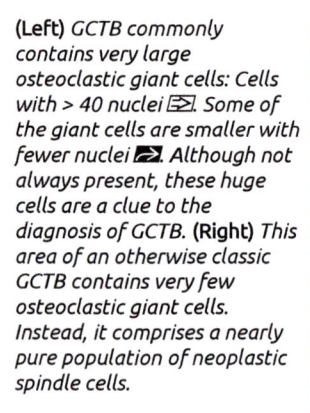

Spindle Cells

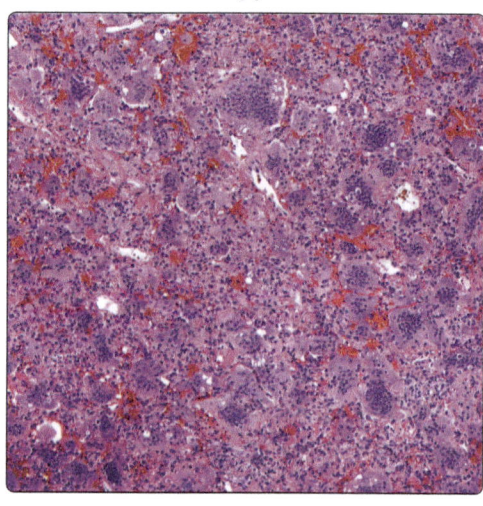

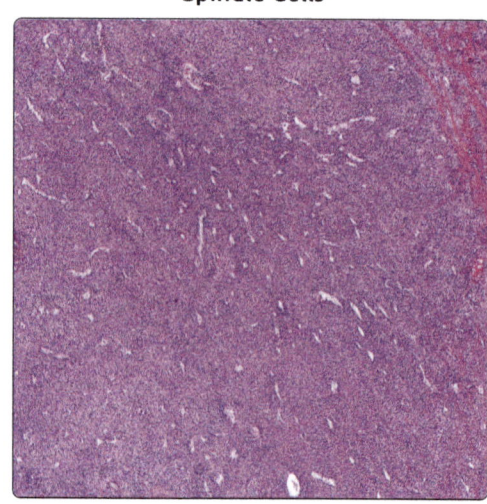

(Left) GCTB commonly contains very large osteoclastic giant cells: Cells with > 40 nuclei. Some of the giant cells are smaller with fewer nuclei. Although not always present, these huge cells are a clue to the diagnosis of GCTB. (Right) This area of an otherwise classic GCTB contains very few osteoclastic giant cells. Instead, it comprises a nearly pure population of neoplastic spindle cells.

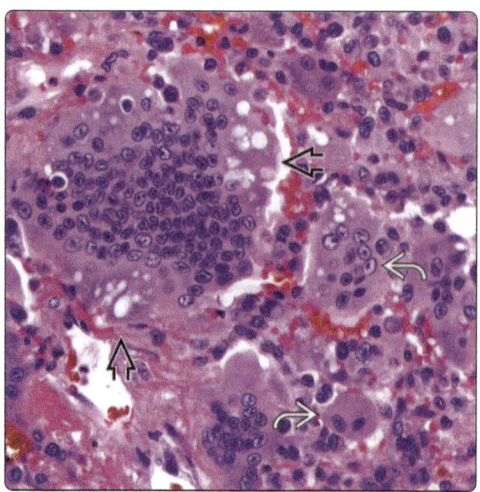

Giant Cell Tumor of Bone

CD68: Reactive Monocytes and Giant Cells

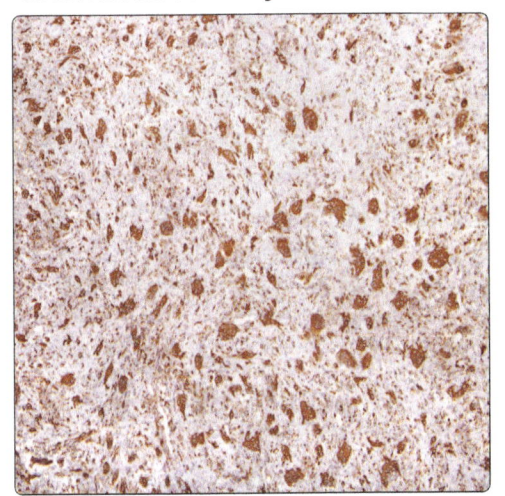

H3G34W Antibody Expression

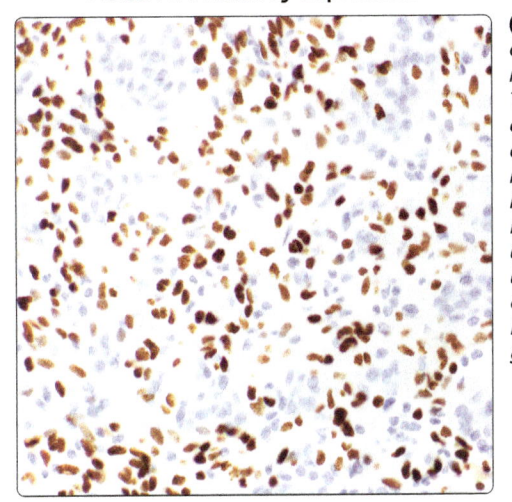

(Left) CD68 is expressed in the cells of histiocytic lineage, but many cells lack expression. This latter group of CD68(-) cells are the true neoplastic cells. (Right) Diffuse strong nuclear expression of anti-histone H3.3 antibody identifies the mononuclear tumor cells of this giant cell tumor of bone. Note the lack of expression of the antibody in the multinucleated, reactive giant cells.

Malignant Tumor With Spindle Cells

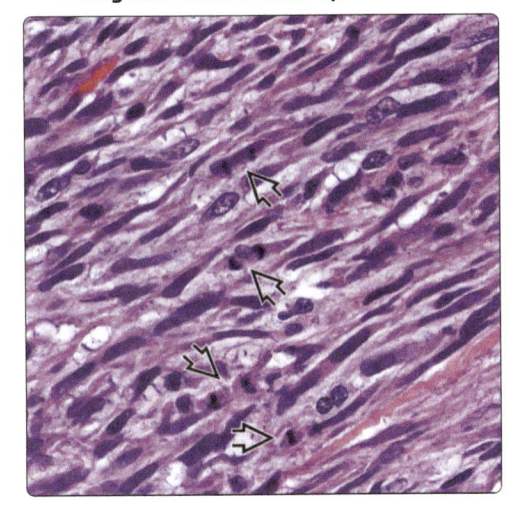

Malignant Tumor With Chondroid

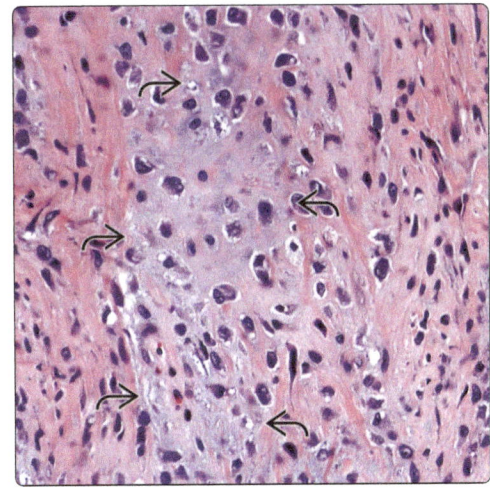

(Left) GCTB with malignant transformation shows a common morphology to the sarcomatous element and often shows high-grade, nonspecific spindle cell sarcoma. Note the numerous mitotic figures ⇨. (Right) GCTB with malignant transformation frequently shows a chondroid-appearing matrix ⇨ in the sarcomatous areas.

Malignant Tumor With Osteosarcomatous Component

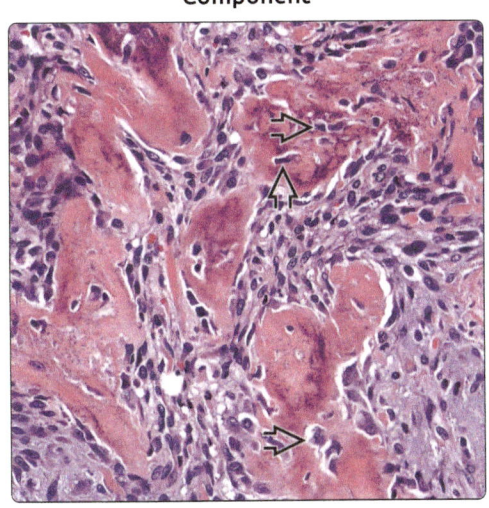

Malignant Tumor With Epithelioid Cells

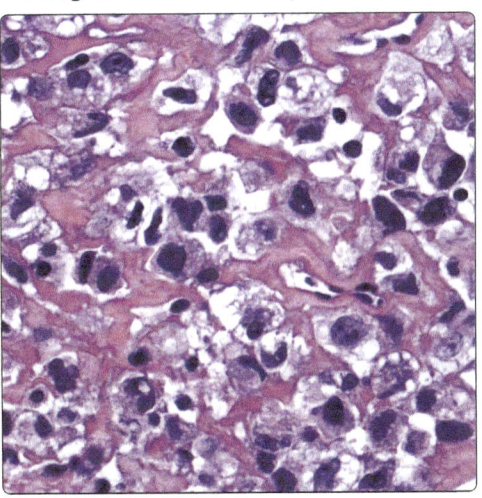

(Left) Malignant transformation of GCTB can also commonly include osteosarcoma, as in this example. Note the neoplastic osteoid contains atypical osteocytes ⇨. (Right) Osteosarcoma arising in nonirradiated GCTB contains large, epithelioid-appearing, malignant osteoblasts that form interconnecting strands of nonmineralized osteoid.

Intermediate and Malignant Cartilaginous Tumors of Bone

TERMINOLOGY

Definitions

- Cartilage-forming tumors of bone with intermediate or malignant behavior
  - Central chondrosarcoma (CS), including central atypical cartilaginous tumor (ACT/CS) grade 1
    - Intramedullary sarcoma of chondrocytes with 3 grades
  - Secondary peripheral CS, including peripheral ACT/CS grade 1
    - Cortically located sarcoma of chondrocytes arising in osteochondroma
    - Usually grade 1 or 2
  - Periosteal CS
    - Cortically located sarcoma of chondrocytes
    - Usually grade 1 or 2
  - Dedifferentiated CS
    - Biphasic sarcoma composed of low-grade conventional CS or enchondroma plus high-grade sarcoma
  - Clear cell CS
    - Low-grade sarcoma of clear to eosinophilic round cells with intermixed osteoid nodules and osteoclastic giant cells
  - Mesenchymal CS
    - Biphasic sarcoma composed of small round blue cells plus conventional CS, usually grade 1 or 2
  - Chondroblastoma
    - Intermediate chondroid tumor composed of round epithelioid tumor cells with clefted nuclei and intermixed osteoclastic giant cells
  - Chondromyxoid fibroma (CMF)
    - Benign but potentially locally aggressive, multilobulated tumor

EPIDEMIOLOGY

Central CS

- Incidence
  - Accounts for ~ 85% of all malignant cartilaginous tumors
  - Grades 1 and 2 account for ~ 70% of CS
  - 2nd most common bone sarcoma
- Age: 5th to 7th decade most commonly
- Sex: M slightly > F
- Location
  - Most common: Pelvis > femur > humerus > ribs > others
  - In long bones, metaphysis or diaphysis

Secondary Peripheral CS

- Incidence: Develops in 1% of patients with sporadic osteochondroma (OC) and 5% of patients with multiple OCs
- Age: Middle-aged adults in sporadic OC; slightly younger in patients with multiple OCs
- Sex: M slightly > F
- Location: Flat bones and long bones

Periosteal CS

- Incidence: Rare; 2.5% of all CS
- Age: 3rd to 4th decade most common but broad range, including children
- Sex: M > F
- Location: Long bones; femur > humerus > others

Dedifferentiated CS

- Incidence
  - Rare; ~ 5-10% of patients with conventional CS
- Age: 6th to 8th decade most common
- Sex: M > F
- Location: Pelvis > femur > humerus > others

Clear Cell CS

- Incidence: Rare; 2% of all CS
- Age: 3rd to 5th decade most common
- Sex: M > F
- Location: Epiphysis/apophysis of long bones, most commonly femur, humerus

Mesenchymal CS

- Incidence: Rare; 2% of all CS

Metaphyseal Location

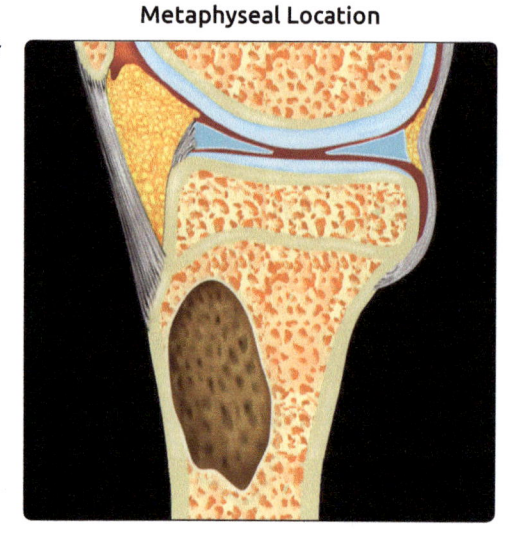

Epiphyseal Location

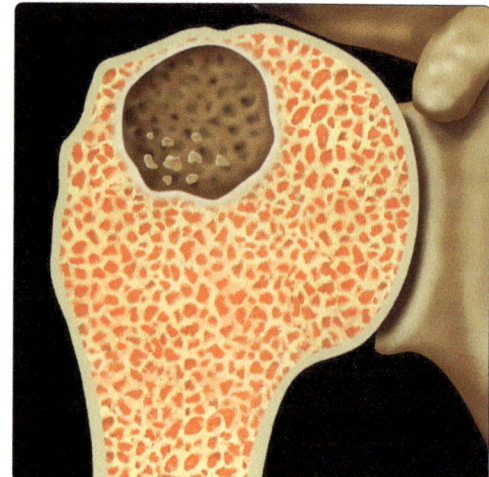

(Left) *Graphic shows the most common location of many cartilaginous tumors: The metaphysis of a long bone, such as at the knee.* (Right) *Relatively few primary bone tumors involve the epiphysis, as depicted here. Two cartilaginous tumors that do so almost exclusively are chondroblastoma and clear cell chondrosarcoma (CS).*

Intermediate and Malignant Cartilaginous Tumors of Bone

- Age: 3rd to 4th decade most common
- Sex: M = F
- Location
  o Skeletal
    – Craniofacial > spine > ribs > pelvis > long bones
    – In long bones, diaphysis
  o Extraskeletal
    – 20-33% of all mesenchymal CS
    – In soft tissue, meninges, deep soft tissues of trunk and extremities, and rarely viscera

Chondroblastoma

- Incidence: Uncommon to rare
- Age: Prepubertal children → young adults most common
- Sex: M > F
- Location
  o Open epiphysis (75%) or open apophysis (25%) of long bones most common
    – Commonly extends into metaphysis as well
  o Hands/feet: ~ 10%
  o In older adults, craniofacial bones most common

CMF

- Incidence: Rare; 1/4 as common as chondroblastoma
- Age: Younger adults, most commonly teens → 4th decade
- Sex: M > F
- Location
  o Metaphysis of long bones (50%), tibia, femur, fibula, humerus, flat bones (30%), feet (15%), craniofacial (5%), hands (3%)

ETIOLOGY/PATHOGENESIS

Central CS

- *IDH1/IDH2* gain-of-function mutations (50-90%)
- *COL2A1* mutations (~ 50%)
- Additional genetic alterations as grade increases

Secondary Peripheral CS

- *EXT1/EXT2* mutations in syndromic and nonsyndromic cases
- Additional genetic alterations as grade increases, usually involving p53 and RB1 pathways

Periosteal CS

- *IDH1/IDH2* and *COL2A1* mutations in some patients similar to central CS

Dedifferentiated CS

- Similar to high-grade central CS for central cases and high-grade peripheral CS for peripheral cases

Clear Cell CS

- Aberrations of *RB1* signaling: 95% of cases
- Loss of p16 expression (majority)

Mesenchymal CS

- *HEY1::NCOA2*: ~ 90% of cases
- *IRF2BP2::CDX1*: Single case report

Chondroblastoma

- *H3F3B* (majority) or *H3F3A* mutations: 95% of cases

CMF

- *GRM1* mutations: ~ 80% of cases

CLINICAL IMPLICATIONS

Treatment

- Surgery mainstay of treatment
  o Ranges from aggressive curettage to en bloc resection to amputation
- Chemotherapy/adjuvant therapy
  o Used in patients with high-grade metastatic CS
  o Conventional chemotherapy generally ineffective
  o Targeted therapies in trials (2022) include inhibitors to IDH1, histone deacetylase, LSD1, SUMO, and BET proteins

Outcome

- Central CS
  o ACT/grade 1 CS
    – Does not metastasize but can locally recur as higher grade tumor with metastatic capability
  o Grade 2, 3 CS
    – 5-year survival: ~ 55%
    – Only grades that metastasize
- Secondary peripheral CS
  o Most cases grade 1 or 2 with relatively good outcomes
    – 5-year survival: ~ 83% overall for grades 1 and 2
- Dedifferentiated CS
  o 5-year survival: < 10%
- Clear cell CS
  o 5-year survival: > 90%
  o Local recurrence: ~ 25%
- Mesenchymal CS
  o 5-year survival: ~ 55%
  o 10-year survival: ~ 27%
- Chondroblastoma
  o 5-year survival: ~ 98%
  o Local recurrence: 14-18%
- CMF
  o 5-year survival: 100%

MICROSCOPIC

Central CS

- ACT/grade 1 CS
  o Hypocellular often lobulated ± peripheral cuffs of osteoid
  o Matrix composed of hyaline cartilage ± myxoid degenerated areas
  o Nuclei relatively uniform, often dark, but may be open with small nucleoli
- Grade 2
  o Moderately cellular
  o Matrix may include myxoid regions containing suspended tumor cells
  o Nuclei larger than in grade 1 CS, open with coarse chromatin and rare to absent mitotic figures
  o Vascularity increased
- Grade 3
  o Hypercellular
  o Matrix often focally myxoid, containing suspended tumor cells
    – Some tumor cells may be spindled
    – Hyaline cartilage may be sparse

Intermediate and Malignant Cartilaginous Tumors of Bone

- Nuclei pleomorphic with coarse chromatin and mitoses often present
- Vascularity increased
- IHC
  - Not typically used for diagnosis
  - Positivity for Ki-67 may help distinguish lower grade CS from enchondroma
    - Indicates active proliferation, which should be absent in enchondroma
- Genetic testing
  - Karyotype progressively more complex proceeding from ACT (may be normal) to grade 3 CS (complex aneuploidy)
  - *IDH1/IDH2* mutations often present (~ 80%)

Secondary Peripheral CS

- Grading
  - Same as for central CS
- IHC
  - Same as for central CS
- Molecular genetic testing not usually performed

Periosteal CS

- Grading
  - Same as for central CS
- Often shows peripheral metaplastic bone at edges of cartilaginous nodules as in central ACT/grade 1 CS

Dedifferentiated CS

- Histology
  - Low-grade component
    - Includes grade 1 (rarely grade 2) CS, enchondroma, or rarely osteochondroma
  - High-grade component
    - Most common: High-grade spindle cell sarcoma, NOS
    - Others: Osteosarcoma (OS), rhabdomyosarcoma, leiomyosarcoma
    - Abrupt transition from low-grade and high-grade components
- IHC
  - Low-grade areas show S100 expression
  - High-grade areas express markers consistent with morphology, such as SATB2 for osteosarcomatous component
- Molecular genetic testing not usually performed

Mesenchymal CS

- Histology
  - Small round blue cell component
    - May include some short spindled cells
    - Often shows hemangiopericytomatous vessels
  - Cartilaginous areas
    - Usually grade 1 or 2 CS
    - Abrupt &/or blended interface with small round blue cell areas
  - Matrix may include calcified or ossified cartilage ± osteoid like regions
- IHC
  - Small round blue cell component
    - Negative for FLI-1
    - ± strong membranous reactivity for CD99
  - Low-grade areas show S100 expression

- Molecular genetic testing
  - *HEY1::NCOA2* assessed by PCR, FISH
  - Rare other fusions detected by RNASeq

Chondroblastoma

- Histology
  - Hypercellular
    - Few cases may be prominently cystic with residual diagnostic tumor in cyst walls
  - Cells
    - Medium-sized, eosinophilic epithelioid cells with clefted or reniform, pale nuclei
    - Osteoclastic giant cells usually present and irregularly distributed
    - ± mitoses
  - Matrix
    - Chicken-wire calcifications (33%)
    - Pink chondroid that resembles woven bone usually present
    - Basophilic chondroid often present
    - ± geographic necrosis
- IHC
  - H3F3 K36M
    - Most specific marker for chondroblastoma: Diffuse nuclear positivity in ~ 96% of cases
    - Does not stain giant cell tumor of bone, which most commonly harbors *H3F3A* p.G34W mutation
  - CK8 (90%), CK18(90%), CK19(90%), DOG1(90%), SMA(90%), S100 (100%)
- Molecular genetic testing
  - *H3F3A* (7%) or *H3F3B* (93%) mutations assessed by PCR, NGS

CMF

- Histology
  - Classic cases usually easily diagnosed on histology
    - Biopsy specimen may contain cellular areas only mimicking chondroblastoma
  - Rare cases may lack lobulation and hypercellular areas = "fibromyxoma"
- IHC
  - GRM1 antibody is specific and sensitive for diagnosis
  - Mix of collagens relatively specific: Collagen types I, II, III, VI
- Genetic testing: Not usually performed

MOLECULAR PATHOLOGY

Central CS

- Primary central CS
  - *IDH1* (2q) or *IDH2* (15q) gain-of-function mutations
    - Found in 50% of tumors
    - Causes ↑ 2HG (2-hydroxyglutarate) = metabolite with oncogenic properties = "oncometabolite"
    - Leads to abnormal CpG island hypermethylation at key genes involved in cellular differentiation
    - Causes abnormal ongoing persistence of proliferative progenitor cell that fails to differentiate
  - Pathways dysregulated by *IDH1/IDH2* mutations
    - ↓ retinoic acid receptor activation pathway

Intermediate and Malignant Cartilaginous Tumors of Bone

- – ↓ pathways involving osteoblast, osteoclast, and chondrocyte functions
  - ○ COL2A1 (12q)
    - – Mutations found in ~ 50%
    - – May have oncogenic role
  - ○ Additional dysregulated pathways
    - – ↑ insulin-like growth factor signaling
    - – ↓ RB1 and ↑ cell cycle
    - – ↑ PI3K-AKT pathway
    - – ↑ SRC pathway
    - – ↑ IHH pathway
    - – ↑ PTHLH signaling
    - – ↑ COX2 signaling
    - – ↑ BMP signaling, especially in high-grade CS
    - – ↑ TGFβ signaling, especially in high-grade CS
    - – ↑ CCN signaling
- Secondary central CS
  - ○ Most common scenario: Ollier disease or Maffucci syndrome
    - – Somatic mosaicism of IDH1/IDH2 mutations in most cases
- Additional genetic alterations in high-grade central CS
  - ○ Complex aneuploid karyotype
    - – Uniparental disomy (loss of 1 chromosome) with repeated duplication = polyploidization of hyperhaploid-hypodiploid initial chromosome set
    - – Additional gains, losses, and rearrangements occur subsequently
    - – Chromosomes 5, 7, 19, 20, 21 frequently retained heterozygosity
  - ○ TP53 mutations
  - ○ MDM2 amplification
  - ○ Loss of 9p21 (CDKN2A)
    - – Loss of functional p16 may contribute to polyploidization of hyperhaploid-hypodiploid clones
  - ○ NRAS mutations (~ 20-33%)

Secondary Peripheral CS

- EXT1 or EXT2 mutations (germline in syndromic cases)
  - ○ Proportion of EXT-wild type neoplastic cartilaginous cells increases with grade
- High-grade (grades 2 and 3) additional mutations
  - ○ Additional alterations in p53-related pathways
  - ○ Additional alterations in RB1-related pathways

Periosteal CS

- Relatively few cases studies
- IDH1/IDH2 mutations reported with varying frequencies from low to high
- CDKN2A: Homozygous deletion
- Downregulated signaling pathways: ↓ Wnt (90%), ↓ RB1 (50%)

Dedifferentiated CS

- Arising centrally
  - ○ Karyotype
    - – Aneuploid
  - ○ Array-CGH findings
    - – Recurrent deletions: 5q14-q21, 6q16-q25, 9p24-q12, 9p21
  - ○ IDH1/IDH2 mutations
  - ○ COL2A1 mutations
  - ○ Alterations of TP53 and MDM2, as in high-grade CS
- Arising peripherally
  - ○ Aneuploid karyotype
  - ○ ↓ PTHLH signaling pathway
  - ○ CDKN2A: Mutations/deletions
  - ○ PDGF-Rβ: ↑ expression

Clear Cell CS

- Pathways altered
  - ○ RB1 (~ 95%) of cases
- Other genes/proteins altered
  - ○ p53 overexpressed without mutations at exons 5-9 in TP53
  - ○ H3F3B mutation in ~ 7%: Same mutation as in chondroblastoma
  - ○ p16 expression lost in most cases without CDKN2A point mutations
    - – However, loss or rearrangements of chromosome 9p are common (CDKN2A is located at 9p)

Mesenchymal CS

- HEY1::NCOA2 in most cases (~ 80-90%)
  - ○ HEY1 (8q21.13)
  - ○ NCOA2 (8q13.3)
  - ○ Fusion arises via interstitial deletion or t(8;8)(q13;q21)
  - ○ Other tumors with NCOA2 fusions
    - – Some childhood leukemias
    - – Other mesenchymal tumors including soft tissue angiofibroma and rare rhabdomyosarcomas
- Other rare fusion reported
  - ○ IRF2BP2::CDX1 t(1;5)
- Karyotype
  - ○ Chromosome 8 structural or numerical changes
  - ○ Robertsonian translocation: der(13;21)(q10;q10) reported in 2 cases
  - ○ t(1;5)(q41;q32) reported in 1 case
- Other genes/proteins altered
  - ○ p53 overexpressed (60%) without mutations at exons 5-9 in TP53

Chondroblastoma

- H3F3B (chromosome 17) or H3F3A (chromosome 1) mutations
  - ○ Both genes code for identical H3.3 histone protein
  - ○ Mutations found in 96% of chondroblastomas studied
    - – Change comprises p.Lys36Met alteration with majority occurring in H3F3B
  - ○ Giant cell tumor of bone also shows H3F3A mutation (~ 92% of cases)
    - – Change most commonly comprises p.GLY34Trp alteration

CMF

- Karyotype and CGH findings
  - ○ Recurrent rearrangements of chromosome 6 at 6p23-25, 6q12-15, 6q23-27
    - – Includes variety of translocations, inversions, hemizygous loss
  - ○ Secondary changes include inconsistent additional translocations, telomeric associations, chromosome losses and deletions

Intermediate and Malignant Cartilaginous Tumors of Bone

- Driver gene mutation
  - *GRM1* (6q)
    - *GRM1* upregulated by fusion of coding region to promoters of other genes
    - Fusion partners include *COL12A1* (6q), *TBL1XR1* (3q), *BCLAF1* (6q), and *MEF2A* (15q)
    - Additional fusion partners likely to be described in future
    - *GRM1* upregulation by promoter swapping and other means found in 90% of cases
  - GRM1 protein function
    - G protein-coupled receptor
    - Activates phospholipase C
    - Pathways activated include PIK3CA-AKT1-MTOR, MAPK
  - Other tumors with abnormal ↑ GRM1 levels
    - Melanoma
    - Breast carcinoma
  - Other gene drivers account for remaining 10% of cases

DIFFERENTIAL DIAGNOSIS

DDx for Central CS
- Enchondroma
  - Lacks permeative growth
  - Can be impossible to distinguish from ACT/grade 1 CS on curettage
- Chondroblastic OS
  - Contains tumor osteoid
  - SATB2-reactive cells present, consistent with malignant osteoblasts

DDx for Secondary Peripheral CS
- Osteochondroma
  - Cartilaginous cap is thin
  - No soft tissue nodules
  - No significant atypia and no increased cellularity
  - Bony base
- Periosteal (juxtacortical) chondroma
  - May erode or scallop underlying bone but does not permeate bone like CS
  - Most cases hypocellular without atypia

DDx for Periosteal CS
- Secondary peripheral CS
  - Associated with preexisting OC
- Periosteal OS
  - Contains cytologically atypical (neoplastic) osteoid as well as lobules of atypical cartilage
- Periosteal (juxtacortical chondroma)

DDx for Dedifferentiated CS
- OS
  - Lacks grade 1 CS-like areas
  - Biopsy specimen accurate diagnosis; may require testing for *IDH1*/*IDH2* mutations
- Undifferentiated pleomorphic sarcoma
  - Lacks biphasic appearance of grade 1 or 2 CS component

DDx for Clear Cell CS
- Chondroblastoma
  - Osteoid absent in most cases
  - Chondroblasts show clefted nuclei
    - Positive for H3F3 K36M, DOG1, and keratins in many cases
  - Chicken-wire calcifications present in 33%
- OS
  - Seldom occurs in epiphysis (< 5%)
  - Negative for S100
  - Often shows marked cytologic atypia

DDx for Mesenchymal CS
- Other small round blue cell sarcomas
  - Lack grade 1 or 2 CS component
  - Biopsy specimen accurate diagnosis; may require molecular testing, such as *EWSR1* break-apart FISH for Ewing sarcoma

DDx for Chondroblastoma
- Clear cell CS
  - Cells larger without clefted nuclei
  - Osteoid often dolloped evenly throughout tumor
  - ± low-grade conventional CS elements
  - Negative for DOG1 and usually negative for H3F3 K36M

DDx for CMF
- Chondroblastoma
  - Epiphyseal location
  - Lacks lobules of myxoid tumor
  - Pink chondroid material often abundant
  - ± chicken-wire calcifications
  - IHC: Positive for H3F3 K36M, keratins, and DOG1; negative for GRM1

SELECTED REFERENCES

1. Tlemsani C et al: Biology and management of high-grade chondrosarcoma: an update on targets and treatment Options. Int J Mol Sci. 24(2), 2023
2. Miwa S et al: Therapeutic targets and emerging treatments in advanced chondrosarcoma. Int J Mol Sci. 23(3), 2022
3. Toland AMS et al: GRM1 immunohistochemistry distinguishes chondromyxoid fibroma from its histologic mimics. Am J Surg Pathol. 46(10):1407-14, 2022
4. Hameed M: Malignant cartilage-forming tumors. Surg Pathol Clin. 14(4):605-17, 2021
5. de Andrea CE et al: Integrating morphology and genetics in the diagnosis of cartilage tumors. Surg Pathol Clin. 10(3):537-52, 2017
6. Amary MF et al: The H3F3 K36M mutant antibody is a sensitive and specific marker for the diagnosis of chondroblastoma. Histopathology. 69(1):121-7, 2016
7. Cleven AH et al: Periosteal chondrosarcoma: a histopathological and molecular analysis of a rare chondrosarcoma subtype. Histopathology. 67(4):483-90, 2015
8. Behjati S et al: Distinct H3F3A and H3F3B driver mutations define chondroblastoma and giant cell tumor of bone. Nat Genet. 2013 Dec;45(12):1479-82. Epub 2013 Oct 27. Erratum in: Nat Genet. 46(3):316, 2014
9. Chen PC et al: The CCN family proteins: modulators of bone development and novel targets in bone-associated tumors. Biomed Res Int. 2014:437096, 2014
10. Nord KH et al: GRM1 is upregulated through gene fusion and promoter swapping in chondromyxoid fibroma. Nat Genet. 46(5):474-7, 2014
11. Lu C et al: Induction of sarcomas by mutant IDH2. Genes Dev. 27(18):1986-98, 2013
12. Tarpey PS et al: Frequent mutation of the major cartilage collagen gene COL2A1 in chondrosarcoma. Nat Genet. 45(8):923-6, 2013
13. Nakayama R et al: Detection of HEY1-NCOA2 fusion by fluorescence in-situ hybridization in formalin-fixed paraffin-embedded tissues as a possible diagnostic tool for mesenchymal chondrosarcoma. Pathol Int. 62(12):823-6, 2012
14. Amary MF et al: IDH1 and IDH2 mutations are frequent events in central chondrosarcoma and central and periosteal chondromas but not in other mesenchymal tumours. J Pathol. 224(3):334-43, 2011

Intermediate and Malignant Cartilaginous Tumors of Bone

Bone Entrapment in ACT/Grade 1 CS

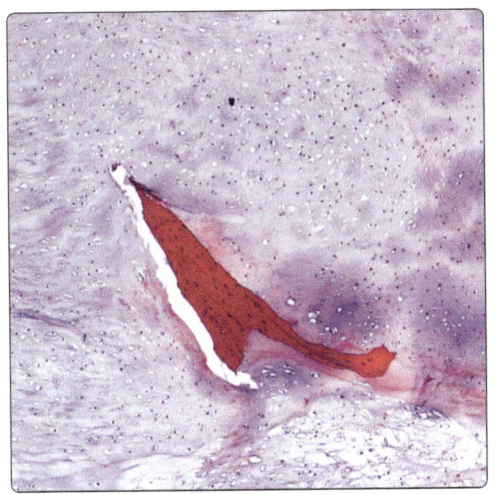

Uniform Differentiated Cells of ACT/Grade 1 CS

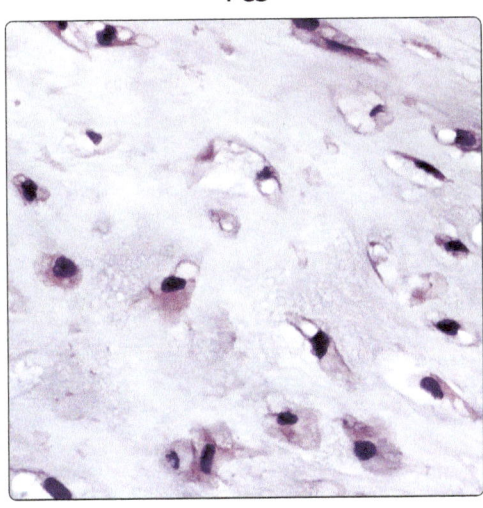

(Left) Atypical cartilaginous tumor (ACT)/low-grade CS is hypocellular and composed of vague lobules of hyaline cartilage. Unlike enchondroma, it surrounds and destroys native trabecular bone, a key diagnostic feature. (Right) High-power view of ACT/low-grade CS shows uniform chondrocytes with dark nuclei. A few low-grade CS are composed of chondrocytes with more open nuclei.

Grade 2 Chondrosarcoma

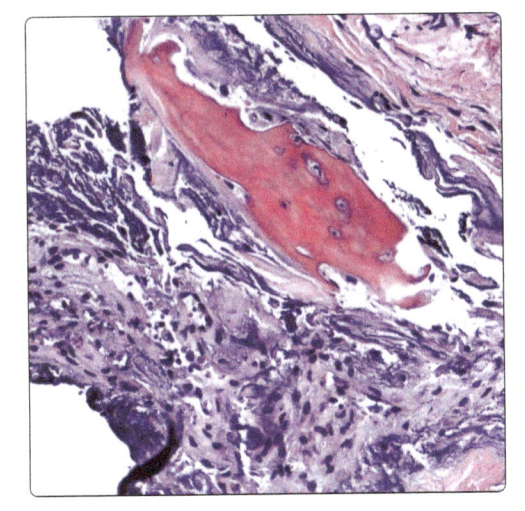

Grade 2 Chondrosarcoma

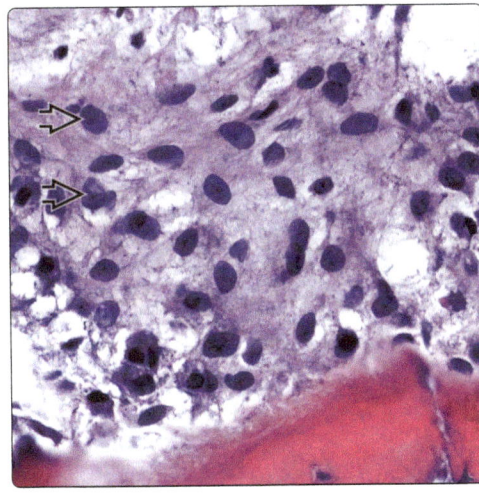

(Left) Grade 2 CS also permeates trabecular bone. It is more cellular than grade 1 CS and may show myxoid change. (Right) High-power view of grade 2 CS reveals cells with larger nuclei than in grade 1 CS. Usually, the nuclei in grade 2 CS are vesicular with visible nucleoli ➡.

Multiple Coexisting Grades in Chondrosarcoma

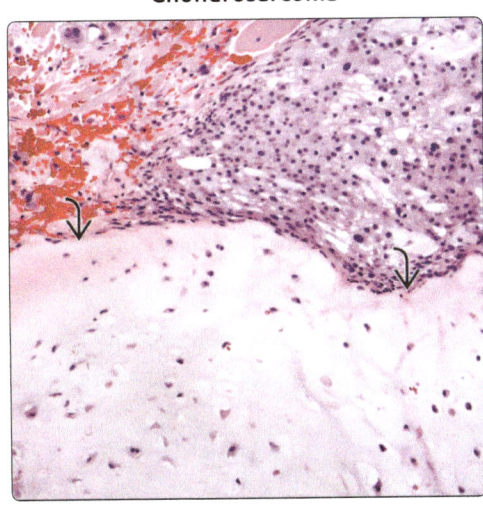

Grade 3 Chondrosarcoma

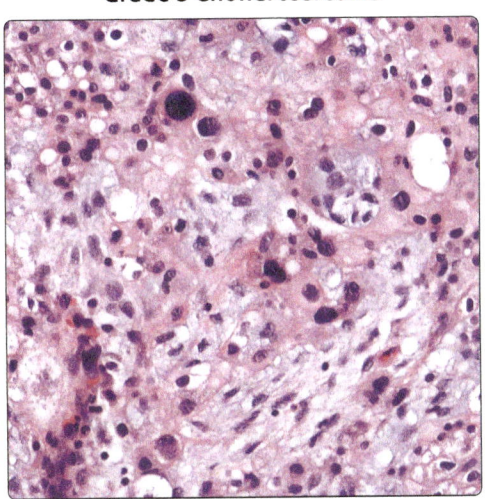

(Left) Grade 2 and 3 CS may contain grade 1 foci ➡, as seen in this case of grade 3 CS. The low-grade focus consists of hypocellular neoplastic hyaline cartilage. (Right) High-power view of grade 3 CS shows typical features of hypercellularity, marked nuclear pleomorphism, and lack of hyaline cartilage differentiation.

Intermediate and Malignant Cartilaginous Tumors of Bone

Ki-67 Reactivity in Low-Grade Chondrosarcoma

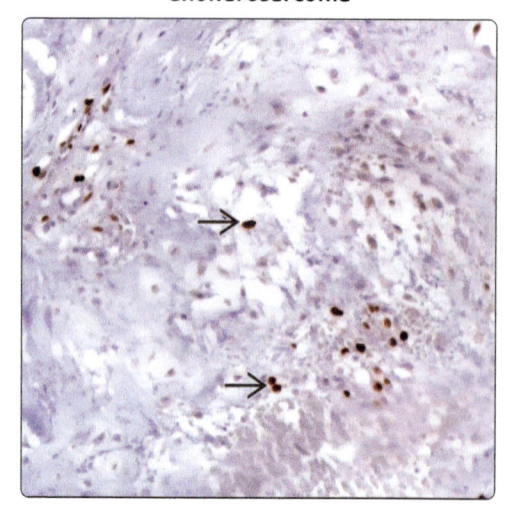

Karyotype of High-Grade Chondrosarcoma

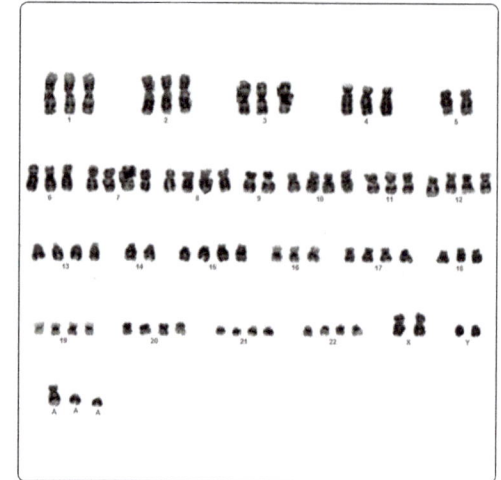

(Left) Ki-67 shows scattered proliferating neoplastic chondrocytes ⇨ in a low-grade CS. Expression of Ki-67 can support diagnosis of CS rather than enchondroma, since the latter should not be continuing to grow when found in an adult patient. (Right) This near-tetraploid karyotype derives from a case of high-grade CS. Additional testing would reveal polyploidization of haploidy.

Dedifferentiated Chondrosarcoma

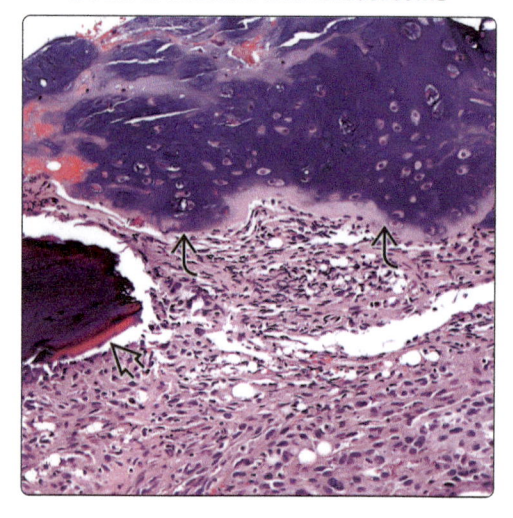

Dedifferentiated Chondrosarcoma

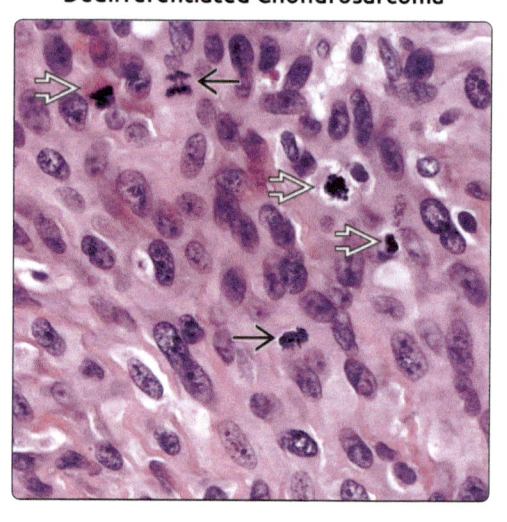

(Left) Dedifferentiated CS shows the required biphasic appearance of low-grade CS ⇨ juxtaposed against high-grade sarcoma. Normal trabecular bone ⇨ is eroded and surrounded by sarcoma. (Right) At higher power, the dedifferentiated area reveals plump spindle cell sarcoma, NOS with a high mitotic rate ⇨ and apoptosis ⇨.

Dedifferentiated Chondrosarcoma With Spindled Cells

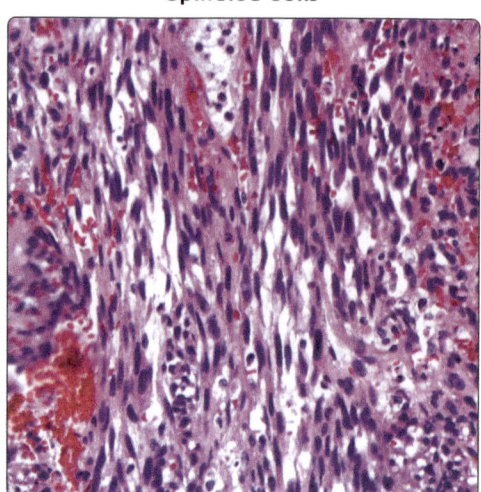

Dedifferentiated Chondrosarcoma With Variable Morphology

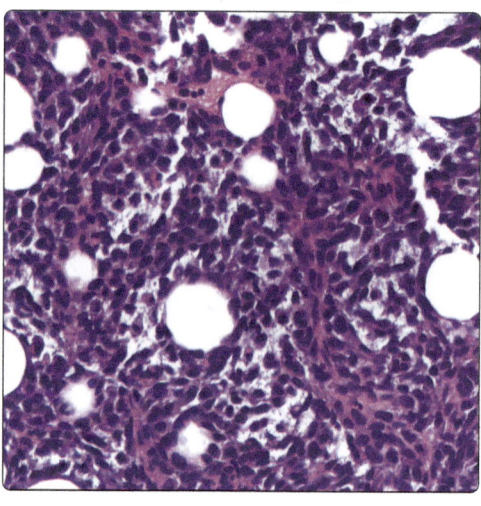

(Left) High-grade component of dedifferentiated CS contains cellular fascicular sarcoma. The spindled cells are eosinophilic and resemble malignant smooth muscle cells. (Right) The same dedifferentiated CS that produced a fascicular spindle cell sarcoma also shows an unusual small round cell high-grade area with a variably myxoid matrix. The tumor cells in this component infiltrate the marrow fat (fat cells appear as clear spaces).

Intermediate and Malignant Cartilaginous Tumors of Bone

Clear Cell Chondrosarcoma

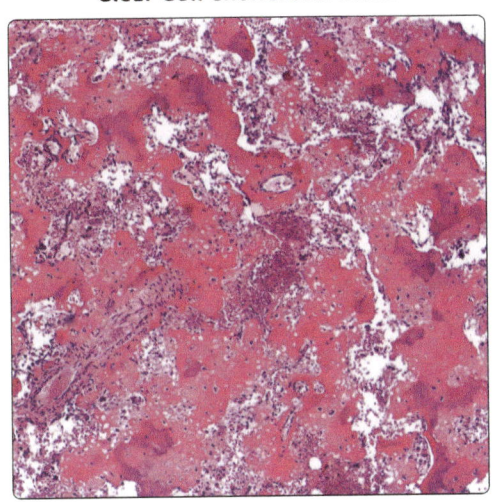

Clear Cell Chondrosarcoma

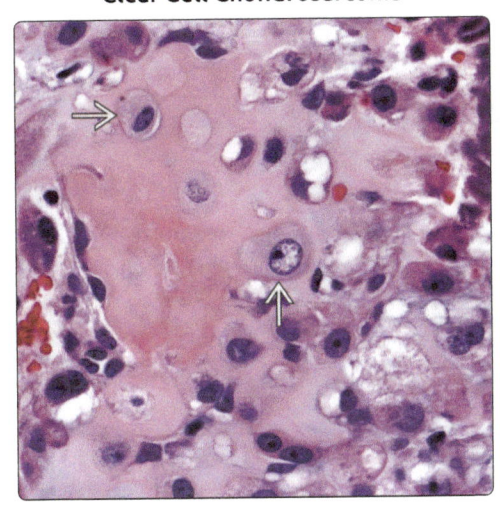

(Left) At low power, clear cell CS can easily mimic osteosarcoma due to the abundant tumor osteoid typically present in this low-grade sarcoma. (Right) At high power, the intimate association of the tumor cells and osteoid is readily apparent, with malignant cells embedded in the osteoid ➡.

Clear Cell Chondrosarcoma: Cell Types

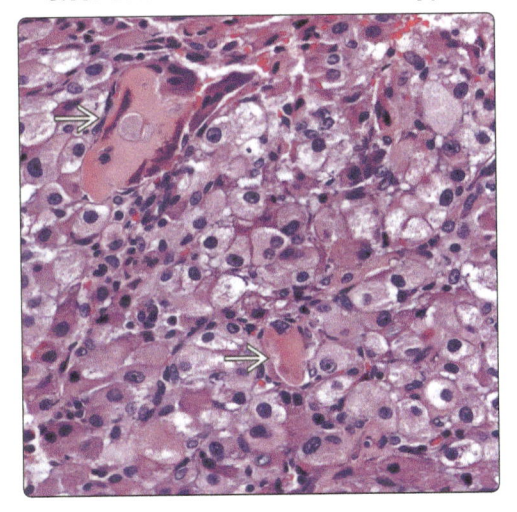

Clear Cell Chondrosarcoma With Glycogen

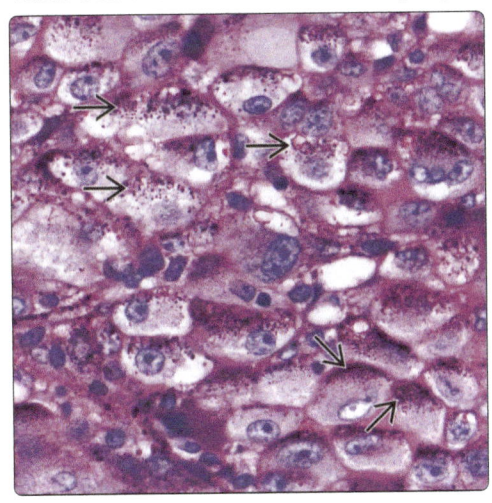

(Left) Despite the name, the tumor cells of clear cell CS are often eosinophilic and slightly granular, although clear cells may also be seen. Notice the small, globular deposits of osteoid ➡. This relatively even distribution of nodular osteoid closely encircled by tumor cells is the most common architectural pattern of clear cell CS. (Right) Cytoplasmic glycogen ➡ accounts for some of the eosinophilic granular appearance of the tumor cells.

Clear Cell Chondrosarcoma With S100 Expression

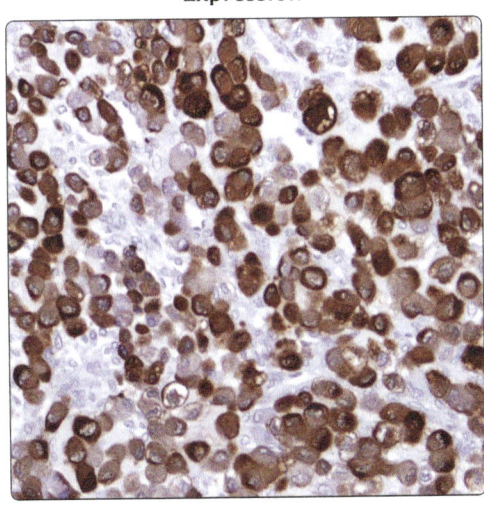

Recurrent Clear Cell Chondrosarcoma

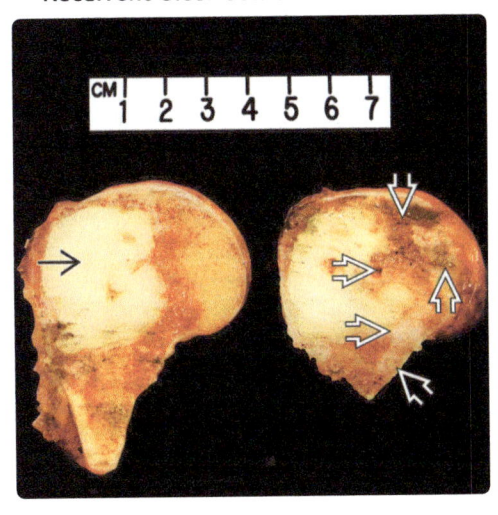

(Left) S100 is positive in clear cell CS, as S100 is often immunoreactive in cartilaginous lesions. (Right) Recurrent clear cell CS required en bloc resection of the distal femur. Bone cement from a curettage 3 years prior ➡ is partly eroded by soft tan to hemorrhagic recurrent tumor ➡. Clear cell CS is prone to local recurrence, especially after curettage.

Intermediate and Malignant Cartilaginous Tumors of Bone

(Left) At low power, most CS are cellular and may feature prominent hemorrhage. **(Right)** Tumor cells are described as histiocytoid or epithelioid with pale eosinophilic cytoplasm, a round shape, and pale nuclei that are often clefted, grooved ⇨, or reniform ⇨.

Chondroblastoma

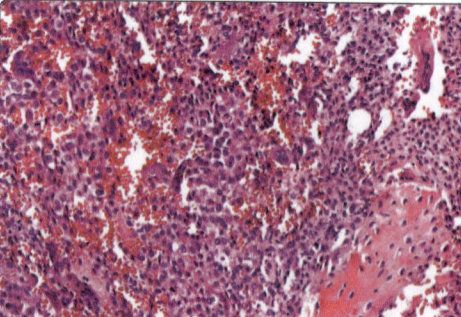

Chondroblastoma

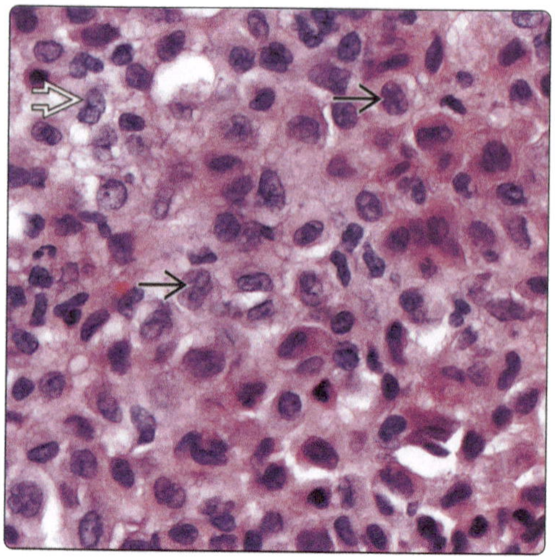

(Left) Chicken-wire calcifications are a distinctive feature found in 33% of CS. These are a helpful and relatively specific diagnostic clue. **(Right)** Chondroblastoma shows strong expression of DOG1. Few tumors other than gastrointestinal stromal tumor and CS express this antigen. Most CS have at least focal reactivity. DOG1 expression is a helpful diagnostic adjunct.

Chondroblastoma With Chicken-Wire Calcifications

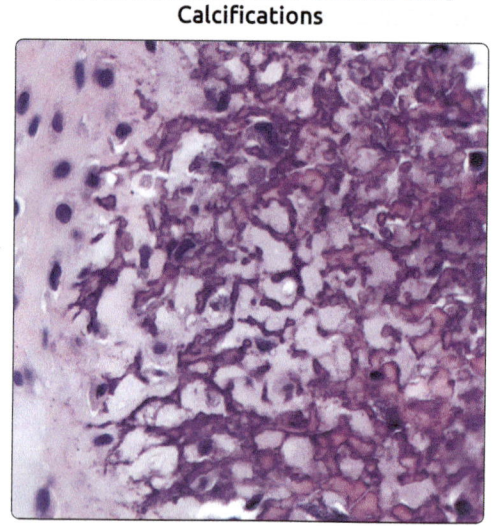

Chondroblastoma With DOG1 Expression

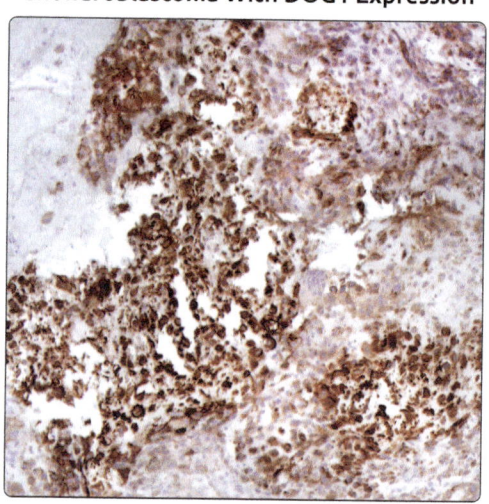

(Left) Tumor located in the patella ⇨ is shown. CS almost always arises in the epiphysis or apophysis of the bone. Although the large long bones are most commonly affected, in this case it is the apophysis of the patella that is involved. In young patients, the most common tumor of the patella is CS. The most common patellar tumor in adults is giant cell tumor of bone. **(Right)** CS contains large areas of pink matrix ⇨.

Plain Film of Chondroblastoma

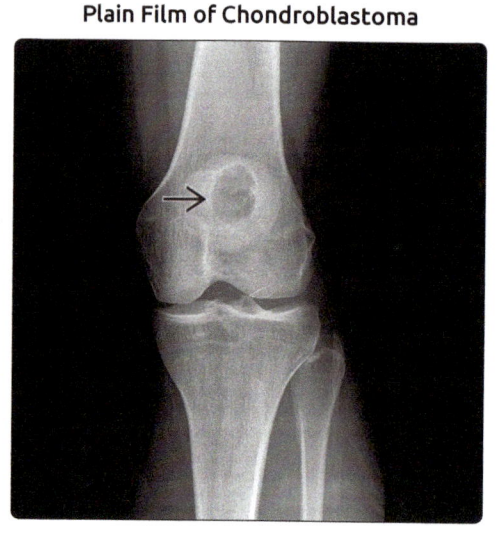

Chondroblastoma With Pink Matrix

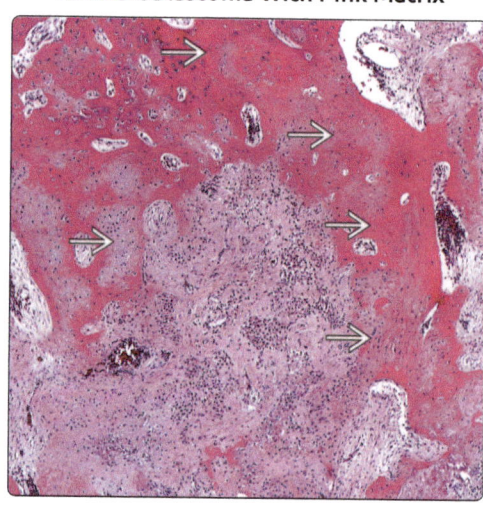

Intermediate and Malignant Cartilaginous Tumors of Bone

MR of Chondromyxoid Fibroma

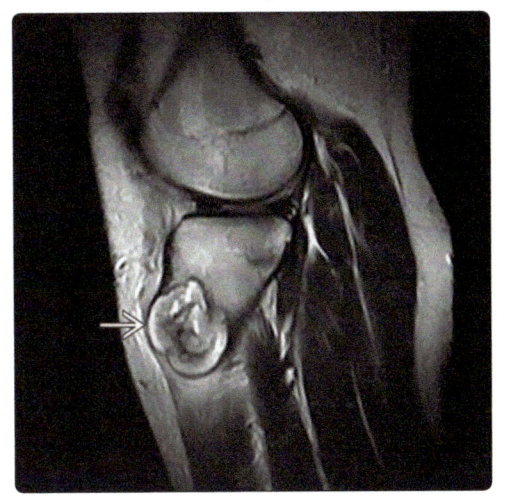

Chondromyxoid Fibroma

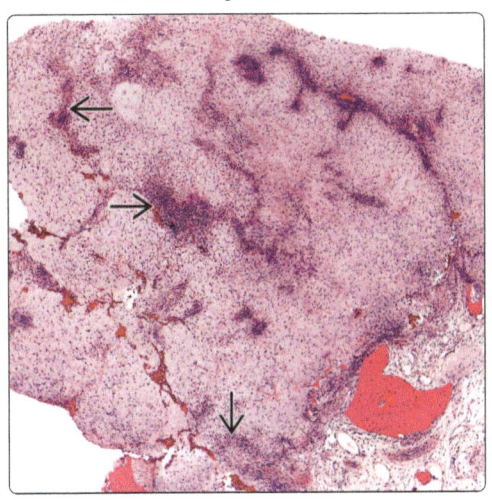

(Left) Sagittal MR through the knee shows a large metaphyseal tumor of the proximal tibia ➡, a common location for chondromyxoid fibroma (CMF). (Right) Histologically classic CMF shows vague lobulation at low power with hypercellularity at the periphery of some of the lobules ➡.

Chondromyxoid Fibroma

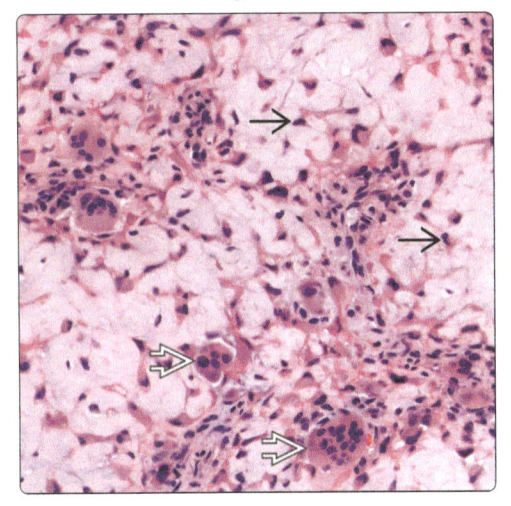

Chondromyxoid Fibroma With Cartilage

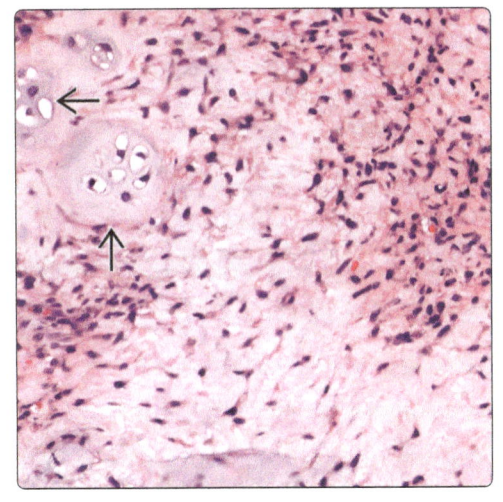

(Left) Peripheral hypercellular areas may contain osteoclasts ➡. Cells with the appearance of chondroblasts (as in CS) may also be prominent but are absent in this example. The tumor cells floating in the myxoid matrix are spindled to stellate ➡. (Right) Hyaline cartilage nodules ➡ can be found in CMF but are usually absent to rare.

Chondromyxoid Fibroma

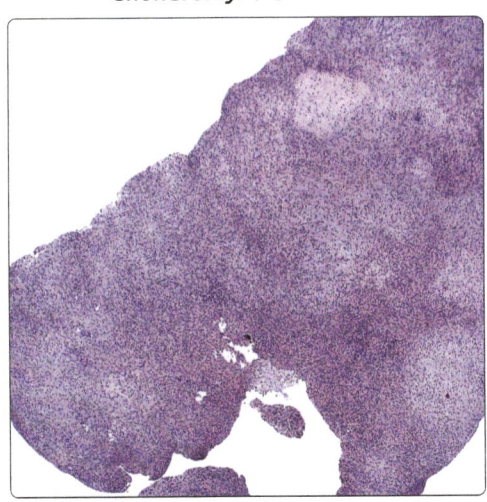

Chondromyxoid Fibroma: Hypercellularity

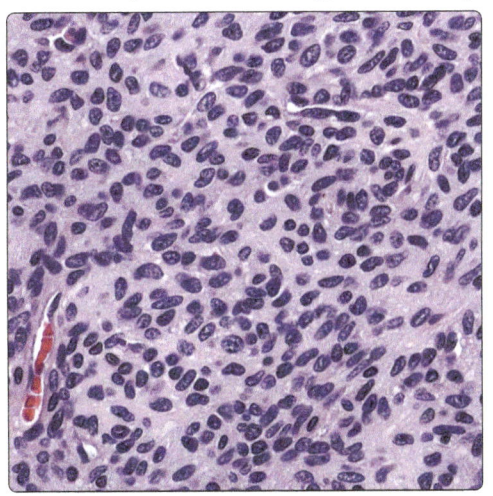

(Left) Core needle core biopsy of a femur CMF retains the vague lobularity of most CMF, but distinct hypercellular peripheral rims are absent. (Right) High-power view of CMF shows an area of hypercellularity composed of cells with indistinct borders and plump spindled nuclei. By molecular genetic testing, this tumor showed a GRM1 mutation, supporting the diagnosis of CMF.

Molecular Pathology of Solid Tumors

847

Intermediate and Malignant Myofibroblastic/Fibroblastic Tumors

TERMINOLOGY

Definitions

- Intermediate and malignant myofibroblastic/fibroblastic tumors (IMFT)
  - Mesenchymal tumors that show differentiation toward fibroblasts &/or myofibroblasts and have intermediate or malignant behavior

CLINICAL IMPLICATIONS

Desmoid Fibromatosis

- Age: Children to middle-aged adults
- Sex: M = F (except in abdominal wall, where F > > M)
- Location
  - Sporadic
    - Deep soft tissue of shoulder, chest and back, thigh, head and neck, mesentery
  - Familial/hereditary
    - Intraabdominal
- Behavior
  - Varies but can be locally aggressive; may be multifocal in hereditary/familial cases
    - 20-30% regress, mostly abdominal wall cases
    - Cases with *CTNNB1* S45F mutations show increased risk of local recurrence after resection
- Treatment
  - Favored treatment varies by tumor location, whether tumor is growing &/or symptomatic
    - Medical therapy (kinase inhibitors or cytotoxic agents) or cryotherapy most commonly employed
    - Surgery for superficial lesions or progressive nonmedically responsive cases
    - Radiotherapy only in select cases

Inflammatory Myofibroblastic Tumor

- Age: Children to young adults
- Sex: F > M
- Location
  - Lung, mesentery, omentum > soft tissues, mostly head and neck > bone
  - Rare epithelioid variant of IMFT is almost exclusively intraabdominal
- Behavior
  - Most cases benign; 25% local recurrence rate; rare metastases
  - Intraabdominal epithelioid IMFT aggressive with high mortality rate
- Treatment
  - Marginal resection; wide resection in aggressive cases; radiotherapy, ALK inhibitors, and ICIs also used

Low-Grade Myofibroblastic Sarcoma

- Age: Adults > children
- Location
  - Extremities, head and neck, oral cavity, tongue
- Behavior
  - Can locally recur or, rarely, metastasize
- Treatment
  - Complete conservative resection

Dermatofibrosarcoma Protuberans

- Age: Adults (3rd-5th decades); giant cell fibroblastoma variant mostly in children
- Sex: M > F
- Location
  - Superficial tissues of trunk, proximal upper extremity, proximal lower extremity > others
- Behavior
  - High rate of local recurrence (~ 50%); cases with high-grade sarcoma have ~ 15% metastasis rate
- Treatment
  - Wide resection ± adjuvant therapy

Solitary Fibrous Tumor

- Age: Young to older adults
- Sex: M = F (except for fat-forming type, where M > F)
- Location
  - 60% in deep soft tissue of trunk, extremities, and head and neck; many visceral and mesothelial-lined spaces
  - 40% in superficial tissue
- Behavior

Gross Appearance of Myxofibrosarcoma

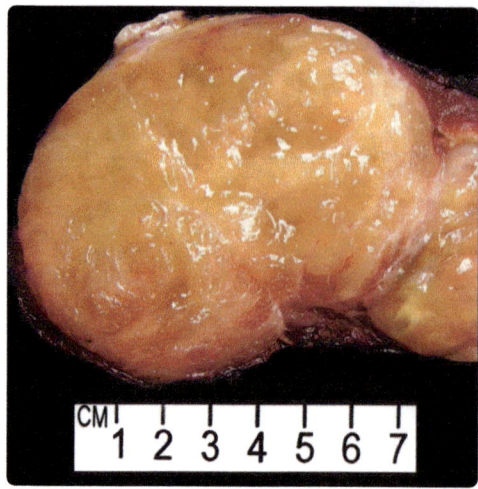

Intermediate-Grade Myxofibrosarcoma

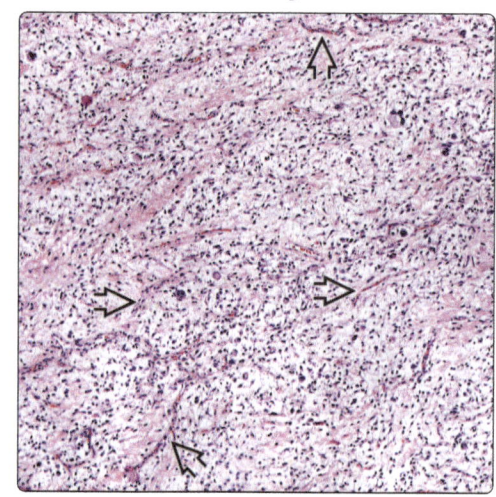

(Left) This relatively large, deep myxofibrosarcoma shows a glistening, semitranslucent appearance, consistent with myxoid tumor. (Right) Corresponding tissue section shows intermediate-grade myxofibrosarcoma with characteristic curvilinear vessels ⇨ coursing throughout the tumor.

Intermediate and Malignant Myofibroblastic/Fibroblastic Tumors

- Classic: 85% benign, but 10% may metastasize, sometimes after many years
- Malignant: Commonly metastasizes
- Dedifferentiated: Aggressive
- *TERT* promoter mutations associated with larger tumor, older age, and more aggressive behavior
- Treatment
  - Surgical resection ± adjuvant therapy

Myxoinflammatory Fibroblastic Sarcoma
- Age: Adults >> children
- Sex: M = F
- Location
  - Acral >> elbow, knee
- Behavior
  - High local recurrence rate; rarely metastasizes
- Treatment
  - Complete resection

Myxofibrosarcoma
- Age: Older adults (≥ 6th decade) >> young adults > children
- Sex: M slightly > F
- Location
  - 60% in deep soft tissues of extremities > trunk > head and neck > acral
  - 40% in superficial soft tissue
- Behavior
  - Grade 2 and 3 tumors can metastasize; grade 1 recurrences can transform to higher grade; better prognosis for smaller and superficial tumors; 5-year survival rate: 70%
- Treatment
  - Complete resection ± adjuvant therapy

Low-Grade Fibromyxoid Sarcoma
- Age: Young to middle-aged adults
- Sex: M slightly > F
- Location
  - Deep soft tissue of proximal extremities, trunk >> other sites
  - Rarely may occur in superficial soft tissue (more commonly in children)
- Behavior
  - High rate of local recurrences and ~ 40% disease-related mortality; often after many years
- Treatment
  - Complete resection

Sclerosing Epithelioid Fibrosarcoma
- Age: Middle-aged to older adults
- Sex: M = F
- Location
  - Deep soft tissue of lower extremity, limb girdle > upper extremity > trunk > head and neck; rare reports in viscera, bone
- Behavior
  - High local recurrence rate (~ 50%); up to 80% metastatic rate
- Treatment
  - Complete resection ± adjuvant therapy

MICROSCOPIC

Desmoid Fibromatosis
- Architecture
  - Long, sweeping fascicles of cells
  - Infiltrative tumor front
  - Variably collagenized background to point of appearing keloidal; rarely myxoid
  - Thin-walled vessels that are squeezed shut or ectatic
    - ± perivascular congeries of chronic inflammatory cells
- Cells
  - Bland, plump to elongate, spindled myofibroblasts
    - Cytoplasm often amphophilic
  - Vesicular nuclei ± small nucleoli
  - Mast cells (average: ~ 1 per HPF)
- Ancillary studies
  - IHC
    - β-catenin nuclear (+) in ~ 70%
      - Nuclear expression may be focal
    - SMA often (+), S100 may be patchy (+)

Inflammatory Myofibroblastic Tumor
- Architecture
  - 4 patterns
    - Pattern 1: Granulation tissue-like or nodular fasciitis-like
    - Pattern 2: Hypercellular spindled fascicular
    - Pattern 3: Hypocellular scar-like or desmoid-like
    - Pattern 4: Hypercellular sheets of predominantly epithelioid cells in usually myxoid stromal background
  - Inflammation always present
    - Patterns 1-3: Usually lymphocytes, eosinophils, plasma cells
    - Pattern 4: Many neutrophils or eosinophils, few lymphocytes, uncommonly plasma cells
- Cells
  - Myofibroblasts with plump, spindled to polygonal shape
    - Reed-Sternberg-like or ganglion-like cells may be present
    - Pattern 4 epithelioid cells are large with vesicular nuclei and often single macronucleoli
    - Cytoplasm is usually amphophilic but may be eosinophilic
- Ancillary studies
  - IHC
    - Patterns 1-3 IMFT: 50% ALK(+), variable positivity for SMA and CAM5.2; few desmin (+); caldesmon (-); may be MDM2(+)
    - Pattern 4 IMFT: ALK(+) (usually cell membrane or paranuclear), desmin, CD30, SMA(+/-); keratins/EMA, S100, caldesmon (-)
  - FISH: *ALK* rearrangement (+)
    - Aggressive epithelioid IMFT usually shows *RANBP2::ALK* fusion

Low-Grade Myofibroblastic Sarcoma
- Architecture
  - Long, sweeping fascicles of spindled tumor cells
    - Storiform pattern less common
  - Usually no fibrosis
  - ± thin-walled capillaries

Intermediate and Malignant Myofibroblastic/Fibroblastic Tumors

- Cells
  - Elongate spindled cells but may be plump
  - Nuclei vary mildly in size and are hyperchromatic
- Ancillary studies
  - IHC: Variable positivity for SMA, desmin; few cases may be CD34(+), h-caldesmon (-)

Dermatofibrosarcoma Protuberans

- Architecture
  - Storiform or cartwheel whorls with characteristic "honeycomb" infiltration of subcutaneous fat
  - Higher grade foci consist of fibrosarcomatous herringbone or fascicular arrangements
  - Focal myoid differentiation uncommon [nest of eosinophilic, actin (+) myofibroblastic cells]
  - Giant cell fibroblastoma is hypocellular myxoid or fibrotic ± pseudovascular clefts
- Cells
  - Ovoid to spindled with pale nuclei without atypia
  - Higher grade areas usually contain elongated spindled cells with hyperchromasia and increased mitoses
    - Rare high-grade areas may resemble high-grade pleomorphic undifferentiated sarcoma
  - Contain melanin pigment in Bednar variant
  - Giant cell fibroblastoma has scattered giant cells, which are mostly multinucleated
- Ancillary studies
  - IHC: Usually CD34(+) except in high-grade areas
  - FISH: *PDGFB* rearrangement

Solitary Fibrous Tumor

- Architecture
  - Classic: Patternless pattern of hypocellular and hypercellular zones haphazardly arranged
  - Cellular: Hypercellular with hemangiopericytomatous growth pattern
  - Fat forming: Classic features with many interspersed adipocytes
  - Giant cell rich: Contains multinucleated giant cells ± pseudovascular spaces
  - Malignant: Increased cellularity, mitoses (> 4/10 HPF), and hyperchromasia of tumor nuclei, ± necrosis ± infiltrative margins
  - Dedifferentiated: Abrupt transition from classic to high-grade sarcoma
- Cells
  - Low grade: Ovoid to plump spindled cells with relatively uniform ovoid and slightly vesicular nuclei
  - Dedifferentiated: Marked nuclear pleomorphism in large and variably shaped tumor cells in dedifferentiated areas
  - Giant cell rich: Scattered multinucleated giant cells without marked atypia
- Ancillary studies
  - IHC: Diffusely CD34(+) in most cases; high-grade areas may lack CD34; STAT6(+)
  - PCR: *NAB2::STAT6* (+)

Myxoinflammatory Fibroblastic Sarcoma

- Architecture
  - Intermixed myxoid and fibrotic lobules, which are intensely inflamed (acute and chronic)
  - ± hemosiderin deposition
  - Multilobulated, predominantly subcutaneous with infiltrative borders
  - Some cases have areas resembling hemosiderotic fibrolipomatous tumor (HSFLT) or pleomorphic hyalinizing angiectatic tumor (PHAT)
  - Few cases may progress to myxofibrosarcoma morphologically
- Cells
  - Mononuclear epithelioid fibroblasts, plump spindled fibroblasts most common
  - Large Reed-Sternberg-like or virocyte-like fibroblasts scattered throughout
  - Cytoplasmic vacuolation common, mimicking lipoblasts in some cases
  - Marked inflammation
- Ancillary studies
  - IHC: Vimentin (+); variable CD34/CD68; usually actins (-)
  - FISH: (+) for t(1:10) in almost all cases

Myxofibrosarcoma

- Architecture
  - 3 grades, all featuring myxoid lobules with incomplete fibrous septa and thin-walled, curvilinear vessels, often with perivascular hypercellularity ± inflammation
    - Grade 1: Hypocellular
    - Grade 2: Moderately cellular
    - Grade 3: Sheets of cells
  - Many cases contain mixtures of lower and higher grade tumor
- Cells
  - Spindled to polygonal, large, pleomorphic, multinucleated tumor giant cells
    - Nuclei are mildly to markedly atypical (hyperchromatic, coarse irregular chromatin, macronucleoli) depending on grade
    - Necrosis and mitoses increase with grade
  - Rare epithelioid cell variant
  - Pseudolipoblasts (vacuolated tumor cells containing mucin) common
- Ancillary studies
  - IHC: ~ 50% CD34(+), ± scattered actin positivity
  - Karyotype: Complex aneuploid in almost all cases

Low-Grade Fibromyxoid Sarcoma

- Architecture
  - Myxoid and fibrous areas, usually with abrupt interface
    - Whorls and fascicles of spindled cells form entire tumor
  - Fibrous areas usually similar to desmoid tumor in cellularity
  - Myxoid areas usually contain waterfall- or arcade-like arrangements of blood vessels
  - 20% of cases may contain hypercellular areas
  - Giant rosettes with central collagenous cores uncommonly occur
- Cells
  - Spindled cells with ovoid or blunt-ended nuclei
  - Nuclei usually show minimal variation in shape and size with few mitoses
- Ancillary studies

Intermediate and Malignant Myofibroblastic/Fibroblastic Tumors

- o IHC: MUC4(+) in almost all cases, EMA(+) in 80%, ± focal actins
- o FISH: (+) for *FUS* rearrangement in almost all cases

Sclerosing Epithelioid Fibrosarcoma

- Architecture
  - o Prominently sclerotic to myxohyaline tumor
  - o ± osteochondroid metaplasia
  - o ± areas resembling low-grade fibromyxoid sarcoma or fibrosarcoma with fascicles of spindled cells
- Cells
  - o Small epithelioid often with clear cytoplasm
  - o Round nuclei with little variation; usually low mitotic rate
- Ancillary studies
  - o Shares same IHC and FISH findings as in low-grade fibromyxoid sarcoma

DIFFERENTIAL DIAGNOSIS

DDx for Desmoid Fibromatosis

- Superficial fibromatosis: Location helpful; often more cellular than desmoid-type fibromatosis; can show nuclear β-catenin
- Exuberant scar: Noninfiltrative margin; more variable histologically with scattered inflammation, macrophages; nuclear β-catenin (-)

DDx for Inflammatory Myofibroblastic Tumor

- Nodular fasciitis: Small, rapidly growing; acute hemorrhage; often more mitoses than IMFT; (-) for *ALK* fusion
- Inflamed smooth muscle tumor: Eosinophilic, spindled cells with cigar-shaped nuclei present at least focally; strong, diffuse reactivity for 2 muscle markers, often including caldesmon

DDx for Low-Grade Myofibroblastic Sarcoma

- Leiomyosarcoma: Eosinophilic cells have features of smooth muscle, including contraction band-like clearing; strongly caldesmon (+) in many cases

DDx for Dermatofibrosarcoma Protuberans

- Adult fibrosarcoma: Diagnosis of exclusion; CD34(-)
- Fibrous histiocytoma: More variable cell population than DFSP; lacks honeycomb invasive pattern
- Plaque-like CD34(+) dermal fibroma: Usually less cellular than DFSP; (-) for *PDGFB* fusion

DDx for Solitary Fibrous Tumor

- Malignant peripheral nerve sheath tumor: Usually more cytologically atypical with infiltrative borders; S100(+) in ~ 60%; usually CD34 and STAT6 (-)
- Synovial sarcoma: Often more monotonous in appearance ± epithelial differentiation; usually CD34 and STAT6 (-), TLE1 diffusely (+); (+) for t(X;18) in almost all cases

DDx for Myxoinflammatory Fibroblastic Sarcoma

- Hodgkin lymphoma: Classically CD30 and CD115 (+); (-) for t(1;10)
- HSFLT: May be closely related to MIFS; spindled fibroblasts mixed with adipocytes, macrophages, osteoclastic giant cells, and hemosiderin
- PHAT: May be closely related to MIFS; prominent hyalinized ectatic vessels and pleomorphic cells

DDx for Myxofibrosarcoma

- High-grade pleomorphic undifferentiated sarcoma: Lacks prominent myxoid matrix, often CD34(-)
- Intramuscular myxoma: No atypia, usually less cellular than myxofibrosarcoma

DDx for Low-Grade Fibromyxoid Sarcoma

- Low-grade myxofibrosarcoma: More cytologic atypia, pseudolipoblasts; MUC4(-); (-) for *FUS* fusion
- Perineurioma: Fibrosis usually absent; MUC4(-), EMA(+); (-) for *FUS* fusion
- Intramuscular myxoma: Usually lacks fibrosis; MUC4(-)

DDx for Sclerosing Epithelioid Fibrosarcoma

- Epithelioid sarcoma: Not usually so sclerotic; may show loss of SMARCB1; CK8 and CK19 (+); MUC4(-); (-) for *FUS* fusion
- Spindle cell/sclerosing rhabdomyosarcoma: Often includes spindled tumor cells; muscle markers (+); (-) for *FUS* fusion
- High-grade pleomorphic undifferentiated sarcoma with epithelioid cells: Usually more cytologically atypical, higher mitotic rate; (-) for *FUS* fusion
- Metastatic carcinoma: Usually more cytologically atypical; (-) for *FUS* fusion

SELECTED REFERENCES

1. Gros L et al: Inflammatory myofibroblastic tumour: state of the art. Cancers (Basel). 14(15):3662, 2022
2. Prendergast K et al: The evolving management of desmoid fibromatosis. Surg Clin North Am. 102(4):667-77, 2022
3. Puls F et al: Overlapping morphological, immunohistochemical and genetic features of superficial CD34-positive fibroblastic tumor and PRDM10-rearranged soft tissue tumor. Mod Pathol. 35(6):767-76, 2022
4. Takeuchi Y et al: The landscape of genetic aberrations in myxofibrosarcoma. Int J Cancer. 151(4):565-77, 2022
5. Bieg M et al: Gene expression in solitary fibrous tumors (SFTs) correlates with anatomic localization and NAB2-STAT6 gene fusion variants. Am J Pathol. 191(4):602-17, 2021
6. Suster D et al: Myxoinflammatory fibroblastic sarcoma: an immunohistochemical and molecular genetic study of 73 cases. Mod Pathol. 33(12):2520-33, 2020
7. Liu H et al: The t(1;10)(p22;q24) TGFBR3/MGEA5 translocation in pleomorphic hyalinizing angiectatic tumor (PHAT), myxoinflammatory fibroblastic sarcoma (MIFS), and hemosiderotic fibrolipomatous tumor (HFLT). Arch Pathol Lab Med. 143(2):212-21, 2019
8. Ogura K et al: Integrated genetic and epigenetic analysis of myxofibrosarcoma. Nat Commun. 9(1):2765, 2018
9. Kao YC et al: Recurrent BRAF gene rearrangements in myxoinflammatory fibroblastic sarcomas, but not hemosiderotic fibrolipomatous tumors. Am J Surg Pathol. 41(11):1456-65, 2017
10. Bahrami A et al: TERT promoter mutations and prognosis in solitary fibrous tumor. Mod Pathol. 29(12):1511-22, 2016
11. Antonescu CR et al: Molecular characterization of inflammatory myofibroblastic tumors with frequent ALK and ROS1 gene fusions and rare novel RET rearrangement. Am J Surg Pathol. 39(7):957-67, 2015
12. Akaike K et al: Distinct clinicopathological features of NAB2-STAT6 fusion gene variants in solitary fibrous tumor with emphasis on the acquisition of highly malignant potential. Hum Pathol. 46(3):347-56, 2015
13. Arbajian E et al: Recurrent EWSR1-CREB3L1 gene fusions in sclerosing epithelioid fibrosarcoma. Am J Surg Pathol. 38(6):801-8, 2014
14. Carter JM et al: TGFBR3 and MGEA5 rearrangements in pleomorphic hyalinizing angiectatic tumors and the spectrum of related neoplasms. Am J Surg Pathol. 38(9):1182-992, 2014
15. Ieremia E et al: Myxoinflammatory fibroblastic sarcoma: morphologic and genetic updates. Arch Pathol Lab Med. 138(10):1406-11, 2014

Intermediate and Malignant Myofibroblastic/Fibroblastic Tumors

Chromosome and Gene Alterations in Various Fibroblastic/Myofibroblastic Tumors

Tumor	Chromosomal Abnormality	Genes Involved	Proportion of Tumors With Abnormality
Dermatofibrosarcoma protuberans	Giant rod or marker chromosomes t(17;22)	COL1A1::PDGFB; rarely COL6A3 or EMILIN2::PDGFD	Almost all cases have t(17;22)
Gardner fibroma	LOH or mutations at 5q	APC LOH or mutation	Most patients have Gardner syndrome, familial adenomatous polyposis, or familial desmoid fibromatosis
Desmoid-type fibromatosis	Trisomies of 8 and 20, loss of Y	Sporadic cases: Activating mutations of CTNNB1; mostly cases associated with FAP: Inactivating germline mutations of APC	Majority of cases show mutations or LOH of CTNNB1 (90%) or APC (~ 10%); CTNNB1 mutations in codons 32-45 most common
Solitary fibrous tumor	Recurrent breakpoints at 12q13; trisomy 21; 4q13 and 12q rearrangements in some cases	Intrachromosomal inversion rearrangement at 12q13; NAB2::STAT6; overexpression of some genes: IGF2, DDR1, ERBB2, and FGFR1; TERT promoter mutations	Majority (> 90%) have NAB2::STAT6; specific exon breakpoints associated with morphology and gene up-/downregulation profile; most cases with TERT promoter mutations behave aggressively
Inflammatory myofibroblastic tumor	ALK (2p23) rearrangements with various partners ROS1 (6q22), PDGFRB (5q32), or RET (10q11) rearrangements or t(12;15); ETV6::NTRK3 fusions in some ALK fusion-negative cases	ALK::TPM3, TPM4, CLTC, ATIC, SEC31A1, CARS, RANBP2, RRBP1, TFG, DCTN1, EML4 ROS1 or ETV6::NTRK3 fusions	~ 80%: Type of translocation affects pattern of ALK protein expression in tissue sections (e.g., nuclear, cytoplasmic, or membranous reactivity); ALK::RANBP2 and ALK::RRBP1 restricted to aggressive epithelioid variant
Low-grade myofibroblastic sarcoma	Alterations of 12p11 and 12q13-q22 in some cases	Unknown	Unknown
MIFS	t(1;10) or der10 (1;10) 7q34 rearrangements, including t(7;17)	TGFBR3::OGA; TEAD1::MRTFB in one case; BRAF::OM1L2 and other BRAF partners; BRAF amplification VGLL3 amplification	TGFBR3::OGA: (5-30%); BRAF rearrangements or amplification (~ 22%); VGLL3 amplification (40%); cooccurs with above rearrangements
Pleomorphic hyalinizing angiectatic tumor	t(1;10)	TGFBR3 &/or OGA (MGEA5) rearrangements	Some cases have same translocation as in MIFS and HSFLT; relationship to MIFS and HSFLT unresolved
Infantile fibrosarcoma	t(12;15); trisomies of 8, 11, 17, and 20	ETV6::NTRK3; rarely other fusions	~ 100% (same translocation also present in several other nonsarcoma tumors)
Myxofibrosarcoma	Complex heterogeneous aneuploid karyotype; may have 7q and 12q gains more frequently than gains and losses at other sites; ring chromosomes may be present	TP53 biallelic alterations; some cases have MET overexpression; p53 pathway gene alterations; cell cycle checkpoint alterations, 3 methylation clusters	Majority of low-grade cases and all high-grade cases have complex aneuploid karyotype; ~ 90% of cases have p53 or cell cycle checkpoint alterations
LGFMS	t(7;16); may have ring forms also containing these genes; t(11;16)	FUS::CREB3L2 translocation; FUS::CREB3L1 or rarely EWSR1::CREB3L1	95% have FUS::CREB3L2 translocation or ring forms; few cases have FUS::CREB3L1 translocation
SEFS	Same translocations as in LGFMS; also rearrangements of 10p11, 17q11, and 1p31 described in single case reports	EWSR1::CREB3L1, EWSR1::CREB3L2; rarely FUS::CREB3L2; DMD intragenic microdeletions; CD24 upregulated in both SEFS and LGFMS	EWSR1::CREB3L1: 80-90%; rare other fusions; more genetic alterations compared to LGFMS DMD: ~ 30%; CD24 upregulated in majority of SEFS and LGFMS
Superficial CD34(+) fibroblastic tumor	Various translocations of PRDM10 at 11q24.3	PRDM10 rearrangements; most with MED12 or CITEDD2	~ 90%

LOH = loss of heterozygosity; MIFS = myxoinflammatory fibroblastic sarcoma; LGSFMS = low-grade fibromyxoid sarcoma; SEFS = sclerosing epithelioid fibrosarcoma.

Intermediate and Malignant Myofibroblastic/Fibroblastic Tumors

Desmoid Fibromatosis

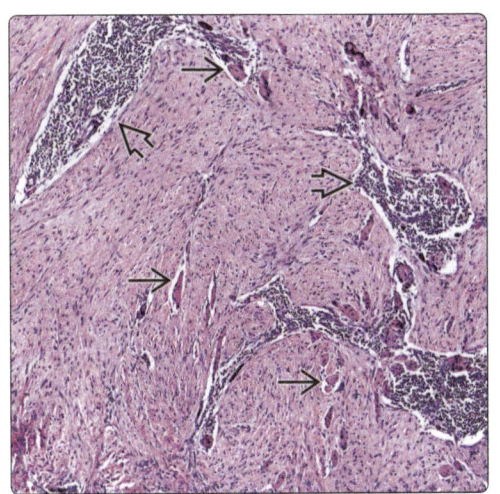

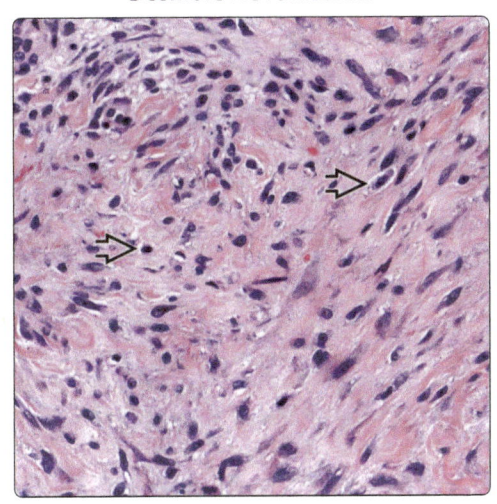

Desmoid Fibromatosis

(Left) Desmoid-type fibromatosis shows prominent perivascular inflammation ⇨ and infiltrates skeletal muscle, causing atrophy of residual muscle fibers ⇨. Permeative, destructive growth helps distinguish desmoid-type fibromatosis from exuberant scar tissue. (Right) Most desmoid-type fibromatoses are only mildly cellular with little to no nuclear overlap. The cells show minimal atypia and contain pale nuclei with fine chromatin. Mast cells ⇨ are present.

Nuclear β-Catenin Immunohistochemistry

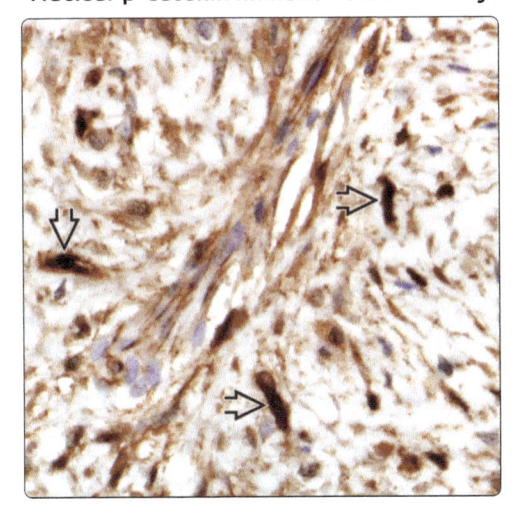

Inflammatory Myofibroblastic Tumor

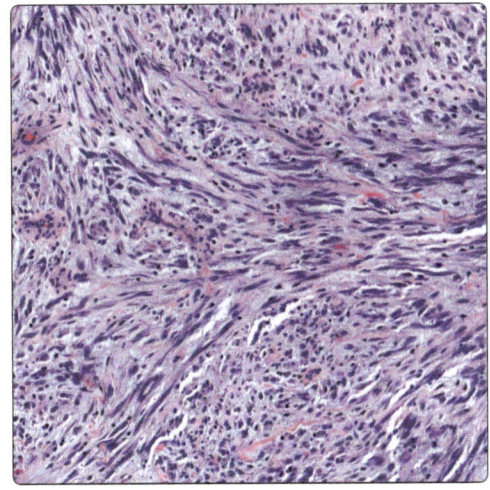

(Left) Abnormal nuclear accumulation of β-catenin ⇨ is a common and characteristic finding in desmoid-type fibromatosis but is also found in plantar and palmar fibromatoses. (Right) Inflammatory myofibroblastic tumor shows an almost nodular fasciitis-like appearance at low power with a pale gray myxoid background and sprinkles of lymphocytes. Tumor cells are spindled and arranged in loose fascicles.

Early Microcyst Formation

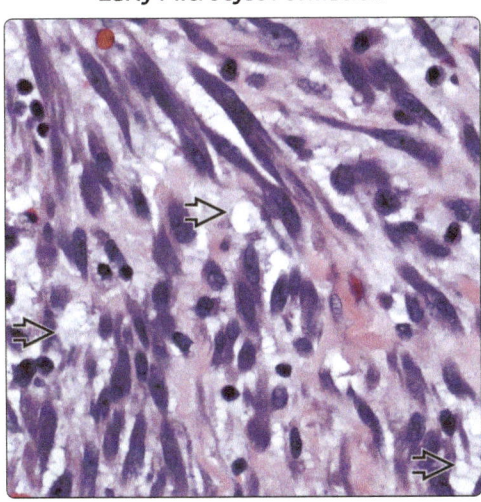

Myocardial Inflammatory Myofibroblastic Tumor With Necrosis

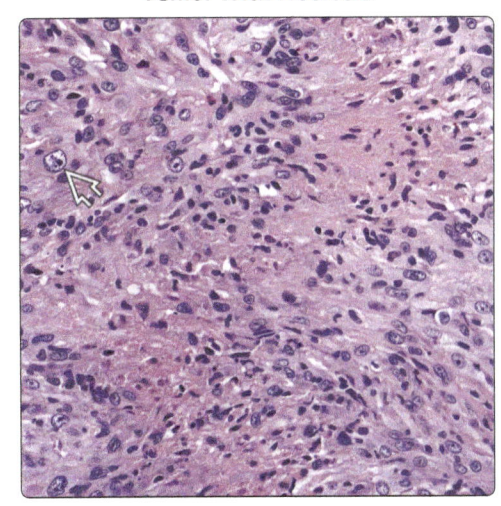

(Left) At high power, the plump to elongate tumor myofibroblasts show classic features of amphophilic cytoplasm and pale, somewhat vesicular, ovoid nuclei with small nucleoli. The background is myxoid with a hint of early microcyst formation ⇨. This could easily be mistaken for nodular fasciitis. (Right) Necrosis, here forming a serpiginous band, is an unusual feature in IMFT, which occurred in the heart of a 24-year-old woman. Nuclear atypia ⇨ is noted.

Intermediate and Malignant Myofibroblastic/Fibroblastic Tumors

(Left) *Myxoinflammatory fibroblastic sarcoma (MIFS) is a predominantly acral tumor composed of fibrous and myxoid areas with marked secondary inflammation ⇒.* **(Right)** *The periphery of this MIFS contains tendrils of fibroblasts mixed with macrophages and strongly resembles hemosiderotic fibrolipomatous tumor (HSFLT). MIFS, HSFLT, and pleomorphic hyalinizing angiectatic tumor (PHAT) share an acral body site preference and some histologic and genetic findings.*

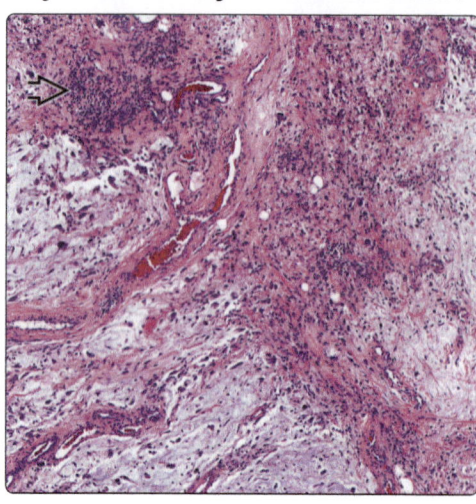

Myxoinflammatory Fibroblastic Sarcoma

MIFS Resembling Hemosiderotic Fibrolipomatous Tumor

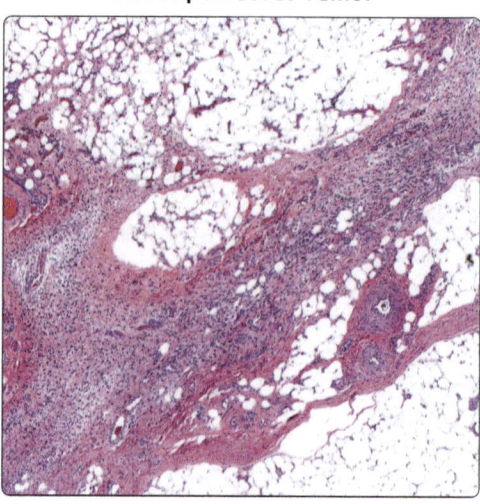

(Left) *Although nuclear atypia is often striking and commonly resembles the atypia of virocytes or Reed-Sternberg cells, the scattered pleomorphism of MIFS does not confer an aggressive behavior. Note the hemosiderin ⇒ in tumor cells, a feature that can be found in MIFS, HSFLT, and PHAT.* **(Right)** *Low-grade myxofibrosarcoma shows ongoing proliferation ⇒ and subtle, diagnostically helpful nuclear atypia consisting of nuclear hyperchromasia and coarse chromatin ⇒.*

Hemosiderin-Laden Tumor Cells

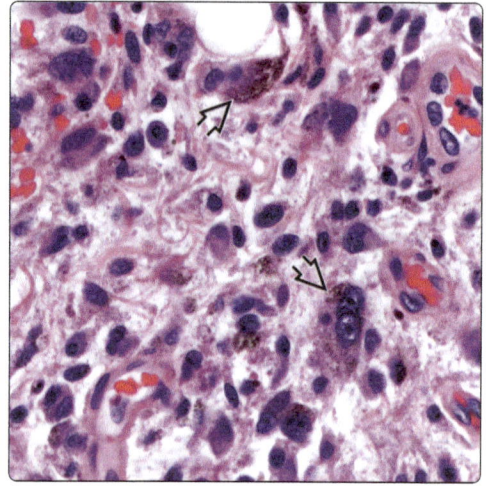

Low-Grade Myxofibrosarcoma

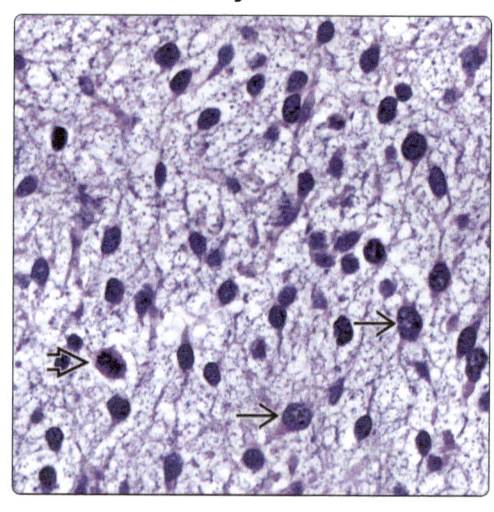

(Left) *Approximately 50% of myxofibrosarcoma expresses CD34, as in this case. This is a high-grade area of tumor with diffuse, strong expression.* **(Right)** *Some myxofibrosarcomas contain cells that can mimic lipoblasts with clear cytoplasmic vacuoles ⇒ and even signet-ring cells ⇒. Other areas of tumor showed classic low-grade myxofibrosarcoma.*

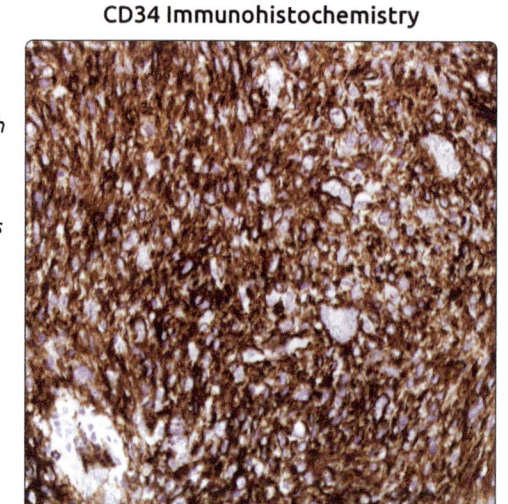

CD34 Immunohistochemistry

Pseudolipoblasts

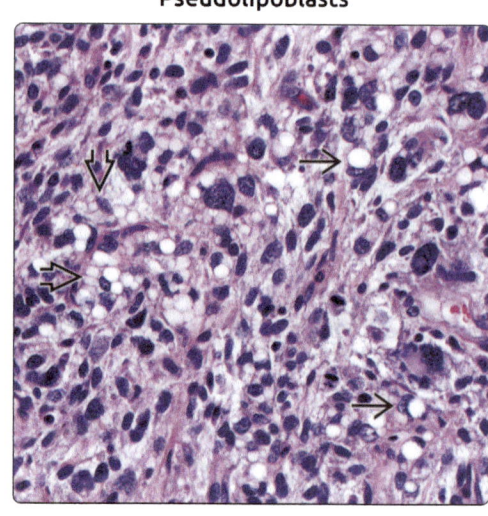

Intermediate and Malignant Myofibroblastic/Fibroblastic Tumors

Dermatofibrosarcoma Protuberans

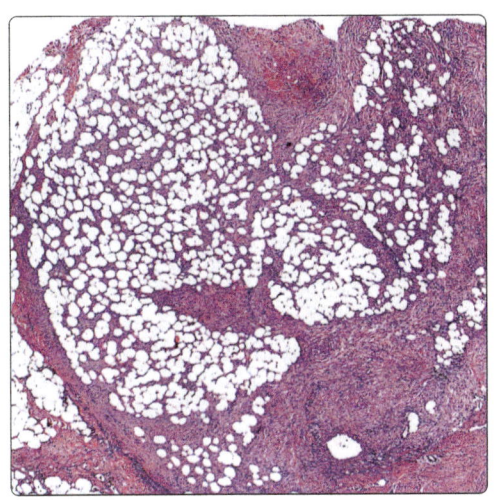

Dermatofibrosarcoma Protuberans

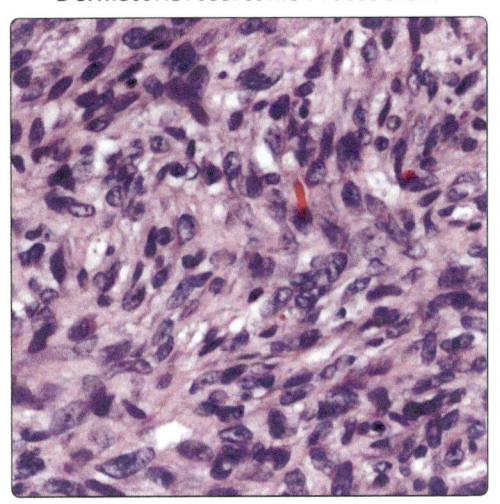

(Left) Dermatofibrosarcoma protuberans (DFSP) shows a typical pattern of infiltration into the subcutaneous fat that is described as a sandwich or layering pattern. The tumor permeates between the adipocytes rather than completely destroying and replacing them, a low-power clue to the diagnosis. (Right) Most DFSP consist of storiforming swirls of plump spindle cells with minimal nuclear atypia.

Bednar Tumor

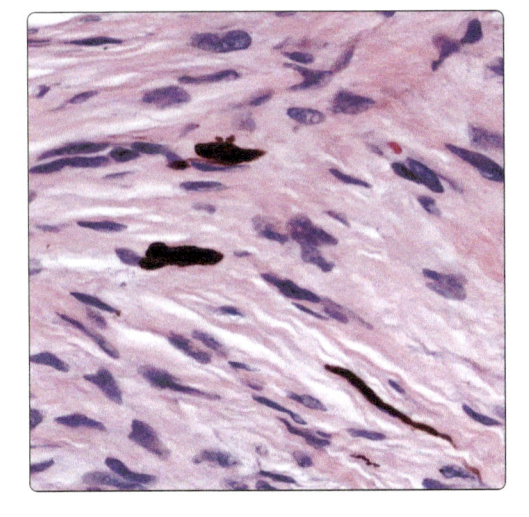

Sarcomatous Transformation

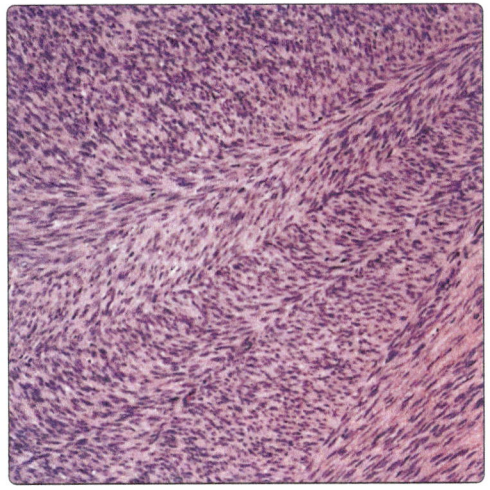

(Left) Rarely, DFSP contains cytoplasmic melanin. These behave as classic DFSP and have been called Bednar tumors. (Right) This high-grade area of DFSP shows the most common morphology of sarcomatous progression, which consists of long, sweeping fascicles of spindled cells flowing in a herringbone pattern, mimicking adult-type fibrosarcoma. Increased mitotic figures and loss of CD34 expression were also noted.

Low-Grade Myofibroblastic Sarcoma

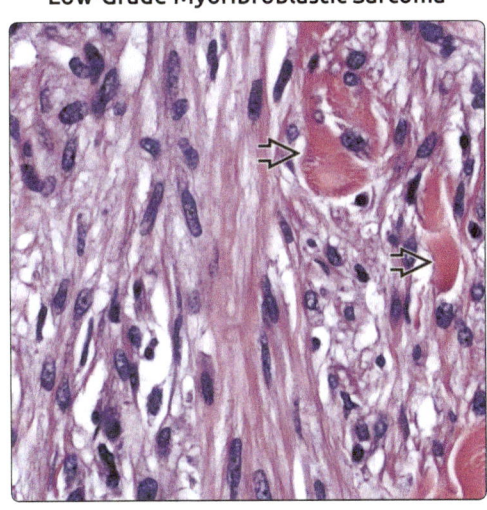

SMA Immunohistochemistry

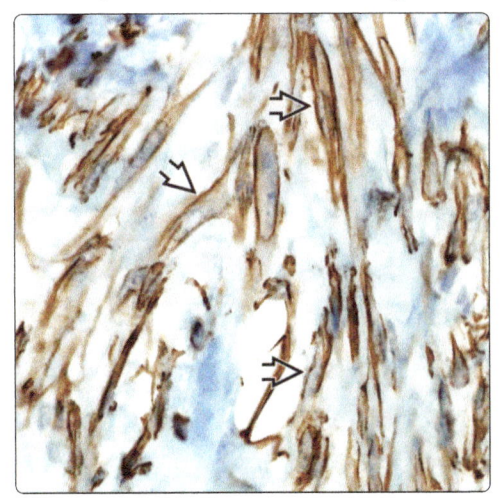

(Left) Low-grade myofibroblastic sarcoma contains long fascicles of spindled cells with pale to eosinophilic cytoplasm, which may mimic that seen in smooth muscle tumors. This tumor, centered in subcutaneous fat, extends into the dermis, where it dissects between dermal collagen bundles ⇒. (Right) Tram-track staining for SMA ⇒ in low-grade myofibroblastic sarcoma is more consistent with myofibroblasts than smooth muscle cells.

Intermediate and Malignant Myofibroblastic/Fibroblastic Tumors

Classic Solitary Fibrous Tumor

Cellular Solitary Fibrous Tumor

(Left) Classic solitary fibrous tumor (SFT) shows tumor cells haphazardly growing in a slightly fibrotic matrix. Note the sprinkles of inflammatory cells and lack of nuclear atypia. Clear spaces or clefts in the fibrous stroma ⇨ can become very prominent in heavily sclerosed areas. (Right) Cellular SFT, previously known as soft tissue hemangiopericytoma, shows the typical crowded, smaller round cells and staghorn vessels of this type.

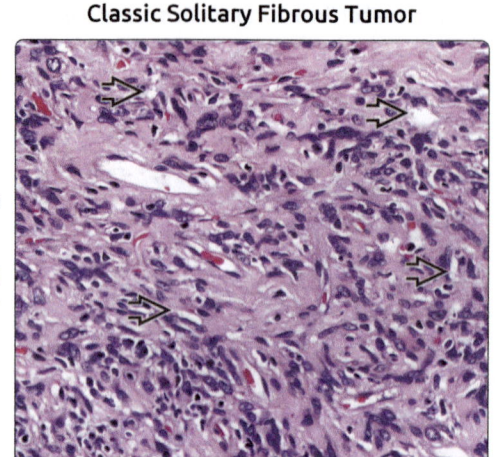

Mixed Classic and Cellular Solitary Fibrous Tumor

Solitary Fibrous Tumor With Unusual Metaplasia

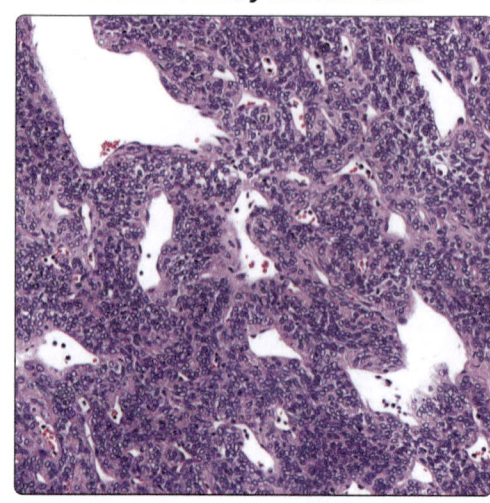

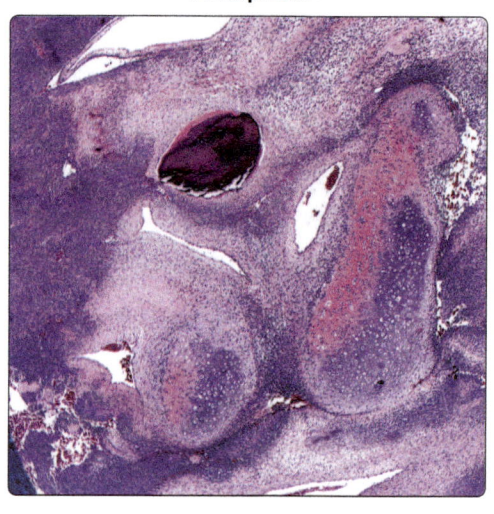

(Left) Some tumors contain a mixture of cellular SFT ⇨ and classic SFT ⇨. Such mixed tumors were an early clue suggesting that soft tissue hemangiopericytoma was a subtype of SFT. Note that the staghorn vascular pattern is present in both regions of this tumor. (Right) Striking osteochondroid metaplasia, which is an uncommon finding in these tumors, is present in this case of SFT.

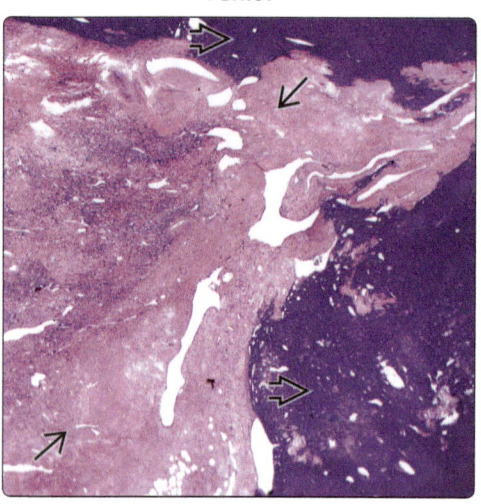

Solitary Fibrous Tumor With Giant Cell Angiofibroma Histology

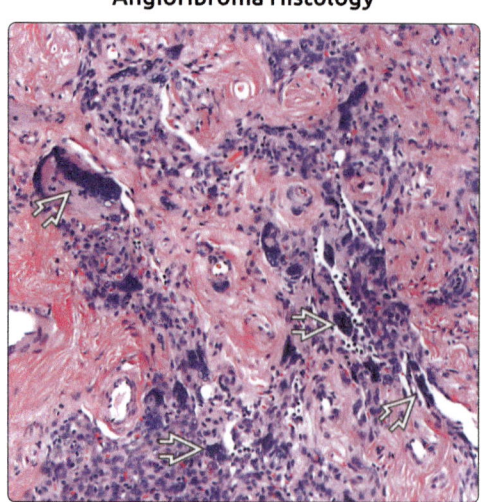

STAT6 Immunohistochemistry

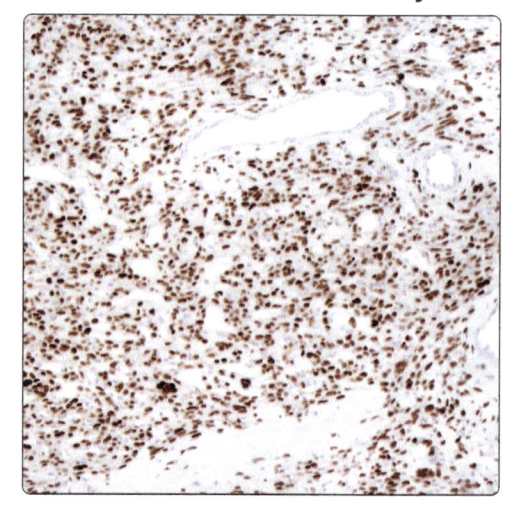

(Left) Subcutaneous SFT of the scalp shows the giant cell angiofibroma pattern with multinucleated tumor cells dispersed throughout the tumor and also arranged next to pseudovascular spaces or clefts ⇨. (Right) SFT shows strong, diffuse nuclear reactivity for STAT6, correlating with the NAB2::STAT6 fusion that is pathognomonic of this tumor.

Intermediate and Malignant Myofibroblastic/Fibroblastic Tumors

Low-Grade Fibromyxoid Sarcoma

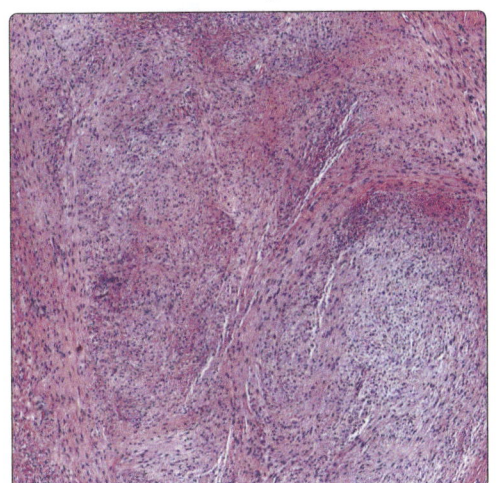

Low-Grade Fibromyxoid Sarcoma

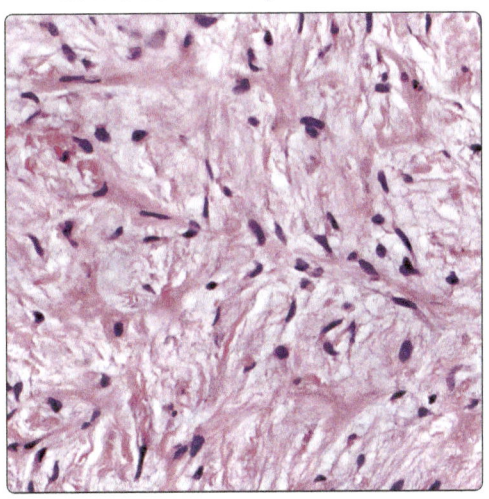

(Left) Low-grade fibromyxoid sarcoma usually has distinct alternating fibrous and myxoid areas, as seen here. Tumor cells are cytologically similar in both areas. (Right) High-power view of a myxoid area shows the minimally atypical fibroblasts arranged haphazardly in a gray myxoid matrix. Collagen fibers splay off from the tumor cells.

Sclerosing Epithelioid Fibrosarcoma

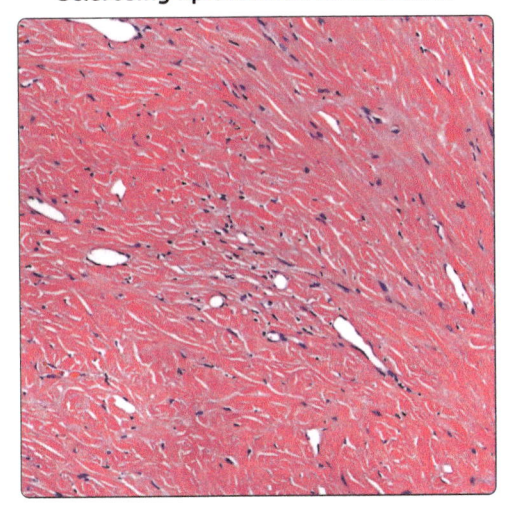

Sclerosing Epithelioid Fibrosarcoma

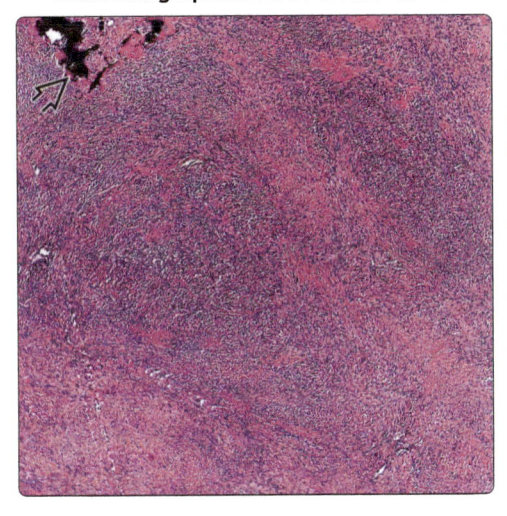

(Left) This case of sclerosing epithelioid fibrosarcoma (SEFS) could be mistaken for scar tissue or some type of benign fibroma. Other areas of this particular tumor were more cellular. (Right) SEFS shows alternating hypo- and hypercellular regions. Metaplastic bone ⇨ is present and is associated with hypocellularity. SEFS can be irregularly heterogeneous in terms of cellularity.

Sclerosing Epithelioid Fibrosarcoma With MUC4 Expression

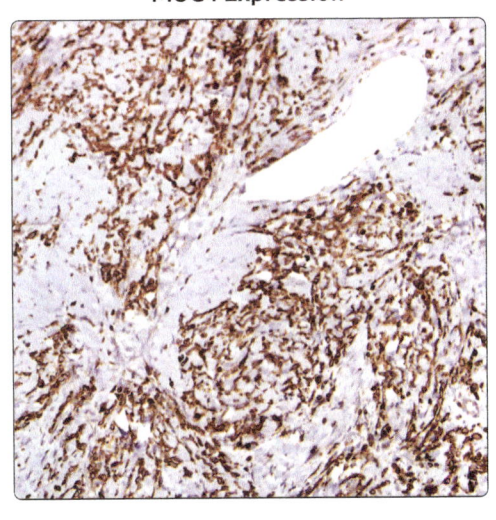

Sclerosing Epithelioid Fibrosarcoma

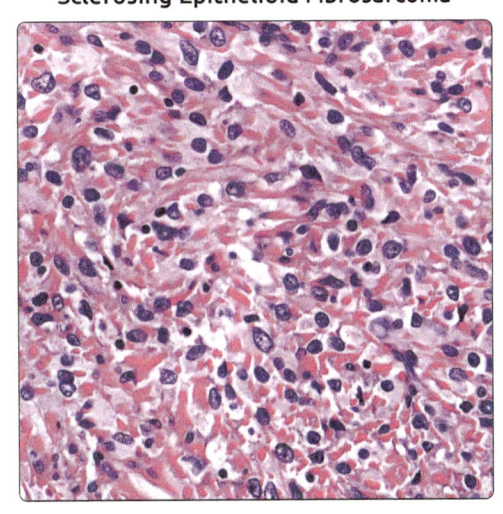

(Left) SEFS shows strong cytoplasmic expression of MUC4, which is found in ~ 70% of cases. Low-grade fibromyxoid sarcoma is also usually positive for MUC4. Expression of MUC4 is helpful diagnostically if the morphologic features are also supportive. (Right) Pale to clear, round epithelioid cells of SEFS can be arranged in cords, nests, clusters, or in an alveolar pattern. Here, the cells show a less organized, sheet-like growth with intervening condensed collagen.

Liposarcomas

TERMINOLOGY

Abbreviations
- Liposarcoma (LPS)
- Well-differentiated LPS (WDLPS)
- Atypical lipomatous tumor (ALT)
- Atypical spindle cell/pleomorphic lipomatous tumor (ASC/P-LT)

Definitions
- LPS are locally aggressive and metastasizing sarcomas of adipose tissue
- Intermediate tumors have risk for local recurrence and no risk for metastasis: ALT and ASC/P-LT

Classification of Intermediate and Malignant Fatty Tumors
- ASC/P-LT: Benign but has low risk for local recurrence
- ALT/WDLPS
  o ALT is morphologically and genetically identical to WDLPS
  o Term ALT is used when this tumor occurs in easily surgically resectable sites
    – Sites include superficial and deep soft tissue of extremities, trunk, head and neck
  o WDLPS is designation when this tumor occurs in not easily resectable sites
    – These sites include retroperitoneum, abdominal cavity, mediastinum, and spermatic cord region
    – At these sites, this tumor usually eventually causes death due to multiple permeative local recurrences
  o ALT has much better prognosis than WDLPS, which is due to site of tumor
    – Both tumors exhibit locally aggressive (infiltrative) growth
    – Both tumors can dedifferentiate (transform to higher grade), acquiring metastatic potential
- Dedifferentiated LPS
- Myxoid LPS
  o High-grade myxoid LPS contains > 5% round cell component
- Pleomorphic LPS
  o Epithelioid LPS
- Myxoid pleomorphic LPS

EPIDEMIOLOGY

ASC/P-LT
- Incidence: Uncommon type of benign, well-differentiated lipomatous tumor
- Age: Middle-aged to older adults
- Sex: M = F
- Location
  o Limbs or limb girdles > trunk, back > head and neck > > deep body cavities
    – Acral locations most common
  o Subcutis slightly > subfascial

ALT/WDLPS
- Incidence
  o 2nd most common sarcoma in adults
  o ~ 50% of all LPSs
- Age: Middle-aged to older adults
- Sex: M = F
- Location
  o ALT
    – Deep (subfascial) tissue of extremities (thigh most common), uncommon in subcutis, trunk, head and neck
  o WDLPS
    – Retroperitoneum most commonly, abdominal cavity, mediastinum, paratesticular soft tissue

Dedifferentiated LPS
- Occurs in ~ 10% of WDLPS and less commonly in ALT
- Incidence
  o ~ 10-15% of undifferentiated pleomorphic sarcomas (UPS) of extremities are actually dedifferentiated LPS
    – UPS also show identical overexpression and amplification of *MDM2* ± *CDK4*
    – UPS show similar, relatively better behavior, identical to dedifferentiated LPS

Myxoid LPS: Gross Appearance

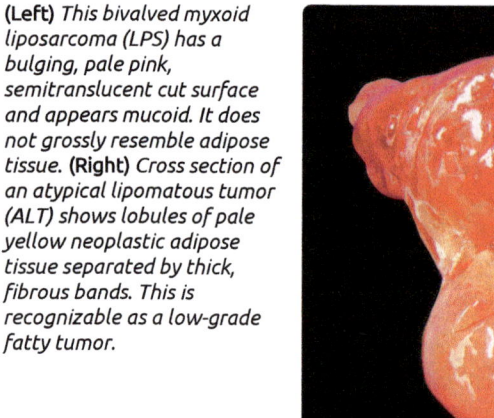

ALT: Gross Appearance

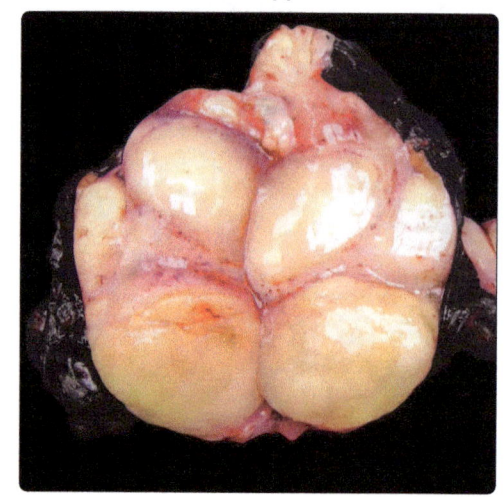

(Left) This bivalved myxoid liposarcoma (LPS) has a bulging, pale pink, semitranslucent cut surface and appears mucoid. It does not grossly resemble adipose tissue. (Right) Cross section of an atypical lipomatous tumor (ALT) shows lobules of pale yellow neoplastic adipose tissue separated by thick, fibrous bands. This is recognizable as a low-grade fatty tumor.

Liposarcomas

- Age: Middle-aged to older adults
- Sex: M = F
- Location: Retroperitoneum, abdominal cavity > extremities > trunk > head and neck

Myxoid LPS

- Incidence
  - 3rd most common LPS after ALT (#1) and dedifferentiated LPS (#2)
  - ~ 10% of adult sarcomas
- Age: Younger adults (3rd to 6th decade most common)
- Sex: M = F
- Location: Deep (subfascial) tissue of extremities (thigh most common)

Pleomorphic LPS

- Incidence: Rare; 5% of all LPS
- Age: Older adults (≥ 6th decade)
- Sex: M = F
- Location: Deep (subfascial) tissues of extremities > > trunk, retroperitoneum > paratesticular, mediastinum, head and neck

Myxoid Pleomorphic LPS

- Incidence: Very rare
- Age: Young adults > adolescents > children
- Sex: F > M
- Location: Mediastinum > > other deep locations of extremities, trunk, head and neck

ETIOLOGY/PATHOGENESIS

ASC/P-LT

- Loss of *RB1*; monosomy of chromosome 7 (~ 40-60% each)

ALT/WDPLS

- Amplification of genes at 12q13-15

Dedifferentiated LPS

- Amplification of genes at 12q13-15, + additional changes

Myxoid LPS

- Driver event: 1 of 2 specific gene fusions

Pleomorphic LPS

- Multiple chromosomal abnormalities with some recurrent findings

Myxoid Pleomorphic LPS

- Some show 13q14 losses (loss of *RB1* and flanking *RCBTB2*, *DLEU1*, *ITM2B*) (12 cases studied)
- Marked loss of heterozygosity of 80% of genome combined with *TP53* mutations (8 cases studied)

Tumor-Immune Microenvironment in LPS

- May play role in pathogenesis or transformation to higher grade tumor

CLINICAL IMPLICATIONS

Treatment

- ASC/P-LT
  - Complete surgical excision (~ 10-13% risk of local recurrence)
  - Does not appear to dedifferentiate or metastasize
- ALT
  - Complete surgical excision
    - Difficult or impossible to achieve negative margins at some sites
  - Recurrent tumor can dedifferentiate
    - Treatment of dedifferentiated LPS is surgery ± multiagent therapy
- Myxoid LPS
  - Complete excision for smaller, lower grade tumors with localized disease
  - Radiation therapy can be effective for local control
  - Chemotherapy for high-grade, disseminated disease
- Pleomorphic LPS
  - Complete excision for small, localized tumors with negative margins
  - Radiation ± chemotherapy for large tumors with disseminated disease or positive margins
- Myxoid pleomorphic LPS: Complete excision with radiation ± chemotherapy

Prognosis

- ASC/P-LT
  - ~ 100% 10-year disease-specific survival
- ALT/WDLPS
  - Extremity tumors: ~ 98% 10-year disease-specific survival
  - Body cavity tumors: ~ 20% 10-year disease-specific survival
- Dedifferentiated LPS
  - Extremity tumors: ~ 40% local recurrence rate > 10 years, 15% metastasis rate, 60-70% overall 5-year survival
  - Body cavity tumor: < 10% 10-year survival
  - Low-grade dedifferentiated component does not improve outcome
- Myxoid LPS
  - Low-grade myxoid LPS: < 10% metastatic rate
  - Higher grade (including > 5% round cell component): Worse outcome
  - Overall 10-year disease-specific survival for localized disease: 87%
  - Poor outcome associated with male sex, age > 45 years, higher grade, recurrent tumor
  - Genetic prognostic indicators under study
- Pleomorphic LPS
  - 30-50% metastatic rate
  - 60% overall 5-year survival
- Myxoid pleomorphic LPS: High rates of local recurrence and distant metastasis

GENETIC FINDINGS

ASC/P-LT

- Karyotype
  - Lacks giant ring and marker chromosomes (which is characteristic of ALT)
  - Monosomy 7 occurs in some cases
- Major gene abnormalities
  - *RB1* shows heterozygous deletion (currently ~ 70%)
    - 13q14 deletions also involve deletions in genes adjacent to *RB1*
      - *RCBTB2*, *DLEU1*, and *ITM2B*
  - Lacks *MDM2* amplification (which is characteristic of ALT)

Liposarcomas

ALT/WDLPS
- Identical genetic findings between ALT and WDLPS
- Karyotype
  - Supernumerary giant ring or marker (rod) chromosomes
    - These are true neochromosomes: Contain centromeres ± telomeres
    - Consist predominantly of amplified regions of 12q13-15
    - 1q21-25: Additional region commonly amplified in ring/marker chromosome
  - Otherwise karyotype is diploid, near diploid, or, uncommonly, tetraploid
  - Telomeric associations are common
- Chromosomal microarray
  - Gain of 12q13-15
- Major genes altered = genes predominantly at 12q13-15
  - *MDM2*, *CDK4*
    - FISH for *MDM2* amplification can be used as confirmatory diagnostic test
  - Other amplified genes that may be contributory to oncogenesis: *HMGA2*, *TSPAN31*, *YEATS4*, *CPM*, *FRS2*, *HOXC13*, *AKT1*
- Major pathways dysregulated
  - Cell cycle
    - *MDM2* inactivates *TP53*

Dedifferentiated LPS
- Karyotype
  - Similar findings to ALT
    - May have more structural and numeric changes
    - Giant ring/marker neochromosomes
    - Neochromosomes identical to those in ALT
    - Double-minute chromosomes common
- Chromosomal microarray
  - Recurrent gains
    - 12q13-15 (97%), 12q24 (46%), 20q13 (41%), 6q22-q24 (24%), 9q33-q34 (24%)
  - Recurrent losses
    - 13q14-q21 (35%), 11q22-q23 (22%)
- Major genes altered
  - Amplified genes found in 12q13-q15 (as in ALT/WDLPS)
    - *MDM2* and *CDK4* amplification detected in ~ 90%
      - High copy numbers (> 38 *MDM2*; > 30 *CDK4*) may portend more aggressive course
    - *FRS2* abnormally activated and expressed in most cases
  - Genes commonly mutated: *MAPKAP1*, *PTPN9*, *DAZAP2*
  - Genes commonly overexpressed: *JUN*, *CALR*, *CDK11B*, *SDC1*
  - Genes commonly amplified &/or hyperactivated: *JUN*, *MAP3K5*, *AKT1*
  - *RB1* loss or loss of heterozygosity
- Major pathways dysregulated
  - Cell cycle
  - Apoptosis signaling
  - Adipogenesis/differentiation
  - PI3K/AKT pathway
  - Cellular RNA transcription and processing
  - β-catenin signaling
- Epigenetic abnormalities
  - *CEBPA* methylated → loss of expression (24%)
  - *HDAC1* mutated (~ 9%)
  - Many genes abnormally methylated (~ 700)
  - miR-193b hypermethylated; miR-155 overexpressed

Myxoid LPS
- Fusion genes
  - t(12;16); *FUS::DDIT3* (95% of cases)
  - t(12;22); *EWSR1::DDIT3* (~ 5% of cases)
  - *FUS* and *EWSR1* are members of TET gene family = encode RNA-binding proteins
    - Multifunctional proteins
    - Help regulate gene expression, genomic integrity, and mRNA and miRNA processing, among others
    - *FUS* and *EWSR1* are involved in other gene fusions in multiple tumors, predominantly mesenchymal
  - *DDIT3*: Transcription factor that normally prevents differentiation of adipocytes
    - Fusion protein also blocks differentiation
- Karyotype
  - Diploid to near diploid most commonly
  - Rare cases hyperdiploid to near triploid
- Chromosomal microarray
  - Recurrent gains: 8p21-p23, 8q24 (29%), 13q, 20q13 (29%), 1q21-24 (21%)
- Major genes altered in addition to fused genes
  - *PIK3CA* activating mutations (~ 18%)
  - *PTEN* homozygous loss
    - Mutually exclusive with *PIK3CA* activating mutations
  - Genes overexpressed: *RET*, *IGF1R*, *IGF2*, *CTAG1B*, *PRAME*
  - *TERT* mutated (~ 74%)
- Major pathways dysregulated
  - PI3K/AKT pathway
  - RAS/RAF/ERK/MAPK pathway
  - Cell cycle

Pleomorphic LPS
- Karyotype
  - Complex aneuploid
- Chromosomal microarray
  - Recurrent gains
    - 5p13-p15 (54%), 20q13 (60%), 6p21 (45%), 17p11.2-p12 (45%), 9q33-q34 (40%), 1p12-p21 (35%), 1q21-q24 (35%), 22q13 (35%), 12q24 (30%), 1p31 (30%), 13q33-q34 (30%), 21q21-q22 (30%)
  - Recurrent losses
    - 11q22-q23 (30%), 1q42-q43 (30%), 2q33-q36 (25%), 13q14-q21 (25%)
- Major genes altered
  - *TP53* mutated (~ 17%) or commonly deleted (~ 60%)
  - *NF1* mutated (~ 9%)
  - 5p13-5p15 amplified genes: *TRIO*, *IRX2*, *NKD2*
  - *CTAG1B* upregulated: Produces NY-ESO-1 protein, cancer-testis antigen
- Segmental acquired uniparental disomy (aUPD)
  - 13q13.2-q13.3 (~ 74%): Codes for *RB1*, *TNFSF11*, *SMAD9*, and others
- Major pathways dysregulated
  - Cell cycle
  - Adipogenesis/cell differentiation

Liposarcomas

Myxoid Pleomorphic LPS
- RB1 inactivation in majority (20 cases studied) generally through loss of 13q14
- Recurrent chromosomal gains: 1, 6-8,18-21
- Recurrent chromosomal losses: 13,16,17

MICROSCOPIC

ASC/P-LT
- Architecture
  - Subcutaneous with infiltrative margins
  - Intermixed spindle cells and adipocytic cells with myxoid &/or fibrotic background
  - Broad range of cellularity from hypo- to hypercellular
- Cells
  - Spindle cells short and plump, as in spindle cell lipoma, or more elongate and neural-like
  - Lipoblasts and mature fat cells often present
  - Atypia is usually mild
- Ancillary studies
  - IHC: CD34 positive in spindle cells; RB1 protein expression completely or partially lost in ~ 60%, desmin positive in 20% (positive in spindle cells); may show focal MDM2 but negative for *MDM2* amplification

ALT/WDLPS
- Identical morphology for ALT and WDLPS
- Architecture
  - Lipoma-like variant: Mimics lipoma but with great variation in adipocyte size (10x or more) and fibrous trabeculations
  - Sclerosing variant: Large areas of relatively hypocellular fibrosis, usually with increase in stromal cells
  - Inflammatory variant: Abundant chronic inflammatory cells ± fibrosis
- Cells
  - Rare to scattered atypical stromal cells, which often occur in fibrous septa; lipoblasts often sparse
- Ancillary studies
  - IHC: ~ 90% MDM2 overexpression ± CDK4 overexpression
  - Genetic tests: > 90% show *MDM2* ± *CDK4* amplified by FISH

Dedifferentiated LPS
- Architecture
  - Often contains areas of ALT
  - Dedifferentiated areas are usually high grade but may include low-grade sarcoma
  - Dedifferentiated components can include
    - Nonspecific high-grade sarcoma
    - Specific sarcoma subtypes, such as leiomyosarcoma, osteosarcoma
    - Dedifferentiated component can uncommonly consist of pleomorphic LPS
- Cells
  - Lipoblasts are usually present
  - Other cell types correlate with type of dedifferentiated sarcoma present, such as malignant smooth muscle cells, myofibroblastic cells, osteoblasts, etc.
- Ancillary studies
  - IHC: > 90% MDM2 overexpression ± CDK4 overexpression
  - Genetic tests: > 90% show *MDM2* ± *CDK4* amplified by FISH
    - More specific for diagnosis than MDM2 overexpression

Myxoid LPS
- Architecture
  - Usually lobular with peripheral hypercellularity
  - Chicken-wire branching vasculature
  - Myxoid stroma
  - ± pulmonary edema pattern
- Cells
  - Lipoblasts include signet-ring-like, monovacuolated, and multivacuolated (less common)
    - Lipoblasts often found in clusters or sheets
  - Round to oval to plump spindled cells
    - Uniform, small cells with normochromatic to hyperchromatic nuclei
    - These cells may form higher grade "round cell" component but only when they are tightly crowded together
- Ancillary studies
  - IHC: Negative for MDM2/CDK4
  - Genetic studies: FISH positive for *DDIT3* translocations

High-Grade Myxoid LPS
- Architecture
  - Hypercellular solid sheets or lobules
  - Transitional areas of low to moderate cellularity common
    - Transitional areas can include low-grade myxoid LPS with gradually increasing cellularity culminating in back-to-back, highly cellular round cell areas
- Cells
  - Back-to-back primitive small cells with increased nuclear:cytoplasmic ratio and vesicular to hyperchromatic nuclei
    - Some cases contain larger cells with eosinophilic cytoplasm
  - Lipoblasts usually present but may be sparse
- Ancillary studies
  - Same as for myxoid LPS

Pleomorphic LPS
- Architecture
  - Diffuse sheets of markedly atypical cells, often with necrosis
- Cells
  - Markedly atypical "pleomorphic" lipoblasts
    - Always present but may be sparse
    - Nuclei are enlarged, hyperchromatic with coarse chromatin ± nucleoli
    - Nuclear atypia > > than lipoblasts in other LPSs, except dedifferentiated LPS when it contains pleomorphic LPS
  - Spindled, polygonal, or large, epithelioid-appearing, nonlipoblastic cells often predominate
- Ancillary studies: Negative for MDM2 and CDK4 overexpression and gene amplification

Liposarcomas

Myxoid Pleomorphic LPS
- Mixture of myxoid LPS architecture/cells **and** pleomorphic LPS architecture/cells

DIFFERENTIAL DIAGNOSIS

General Comments
- Classification of adipocytic tumors continues to evolve: Expect changes
- Molecular genetic testing: Maintain low threshold for ordering because entities overlap histologically
  - Treatment varies substantially depending on diagnosis: Rendering correct diagnosis is critical

DDx for ASC/P-LT
- Pleomorphic/spindle cell lipoma
  - Discrete pushing margin rather than infiltrative
  - Prominent ropy collagen fibers
  - By IHC, both are CD34 positive, and both may show loss of RB1 protein expression by IHC
- ALT with prominent spindled stromal cells
  - Usually deep soft tissue location or in body cavity
  - Positive for MDM2 ± CDK4 on examination and gene amplification

DDx for ALT/WDLPS
- Lipoma
  - Lacks marked variation in adipocyte size (except in areas of fat necrosis)
    - "Dysplastic lipoma" shows marked variation in adipocyte size but is negative for *MDM2* amplification
  - Negative for atypical stromal cells
  - Negative for MDM2 and CDK4 overexpression and gene amplification
- Pleomorphic/spindle cell lipoma
  - Subcutaneous with pushing, noninvasive margin
  - Negative for MDM2 and CDK4 overexpression and gene amplification
  - Shows loss of RB1 protein on IHC
- Hibernoma, lipoma-like variant
  - Microvacuolated fat cells are relatively common and dispersed in tumor (can have few in some ALT)
  - Negative for MDM2 and CDK4 overexpression and gene amplification
  - Karyotype shows 11q13 deletions or translocations

DDx for Dedifferentiated LPS
- Pleomorphic LPS
  - Markedly atypical "pleomorphic" lipoblasts
  - Negative for low-grade ALT areas
  - Negative for MDM2/CDK4 overexpression and gene amplification
- Sclerosing variant of ALT: Not as hypercellular, although atypical cells are identical to scattered atypical stromal cells of ALT
  - Hypocellular rather than hypercellular
  - Atypical stromal cells are often less atypical than malignant cells in dedifferentiated LPS
- UPS
  - UPS lacks *MDM2* amplification and usually lacks MDM2 overexpression
  - UPS lacks low-grade ALT areas that are found in some dedifferentiated LPS

DDx for Myxoid LPS
- Lipoblastoma
  - Occurs in infants → young children
  - Negative for *DDIT3* fusions by FISH
  - Positive for *PLAG1* rearrangements by FISH
- ALT with prominent myxoid stroma
  - Usually (but not always) lacks prominent chicken-wire vasculature
  - Negative for *DDIT3* fusions by FISH
  - Positive for MDM2 ± CDK4 overexpression and gene amplification

DDx for High-Grade Myxoid LPS
- Other small round cell sarcomas
  - Lack lipoblasts
  - Lack transitional myxoid LPS-like areas
  - Lack *DDIT3* fusions by FISH
  - Often positive for other specific fusions by FISH

DDx for Pleomorphic LPS
- Dedifferentiated LPS with pleomorphic LPS component ("homologous dedifferentiation")
  - Lower grade ALT component often present
  - *MDM2* ± *CDK4* amplified

DDx for Myxoid Pleomorphic LPS
- Pleomorphic LPS: Lacks areas resembling myxoid LPS
- ASC/P-LT: Lacks true cytologic pleomorphism of myxoid pleomorphic LPS
- Myxoid LPS: Lacks architecture and markedly atypical lipoblasts of pleomorphic LPS

SELECTED REFERENCES

1. Dermawan JK et al: Myxoid pleomorphic liposarcoma is distinguished from other liposarcomas by widespread loss of heterozygosity and significantly worse overall survival: a genomic and clinicopathologic study. Mod Pathol. 35(11):1644-55, 2022
2. Thway K: What's new in adipocytic neoplasia? Histopathology. 80(1):76-97, 2022
3. Anderson WJ et al: Atypical pleomorphic lipomatous tumor: expanding our current understanding in a clinicopathologic analysis of 64 cases. Am J Surg Pathol. 45(9):1282-92, 2021
4. Creytens D et al: Myxoid pleomorphic liposarcoma-a clinicopathologic, immunohistochemical, molecular genetic and epigenetic study of 12 cases, suggesting a possible relationship with conventional pleomorphic liposarcoma. Mod Pathol. 34(11):2043-9, 2021
5. Michal M et al: Dysplastic Lipoma: a distinctive atypical lipomatous neoplasm with anisocytosis, focal nuclear atypia, p53 overexpression, and a lack of MDM2 gene amplification by FISH; a report of 66 cases demonstrating occasional multifocality and a rare association with retinoblastoma. Am J Surg Pathol. 42(11):1530-40, 2018
6. Mariño-Enriquez A et al: Atypical spindle cell lipomatous tumor: clinicopathologic characterization of 232 cases demonstrating a morphologic spectrum. Am J Surg Pathol. 41(2):234-44, 2017
7. Ricciotti RW et al: High amplification levels of MDM2 and CDK4 correlate with poor outcome in patients with dedifferentiated liposarcoma: a cytogenomic microarray analysis of 47 cases. Cancer Genet. 218-219:69-80, 2017

Liposarcomas

ALT With Marked Variation in Adipocytes

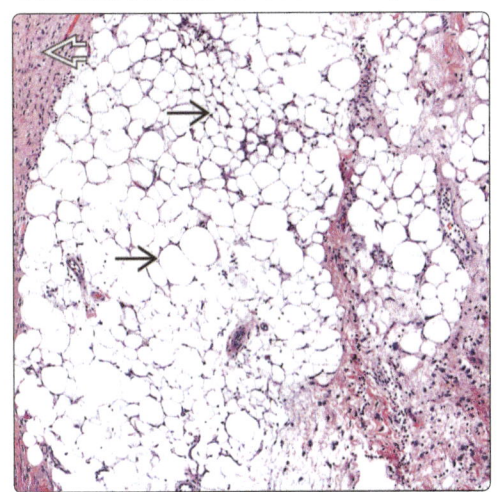

Sclerosing Variant of ALT

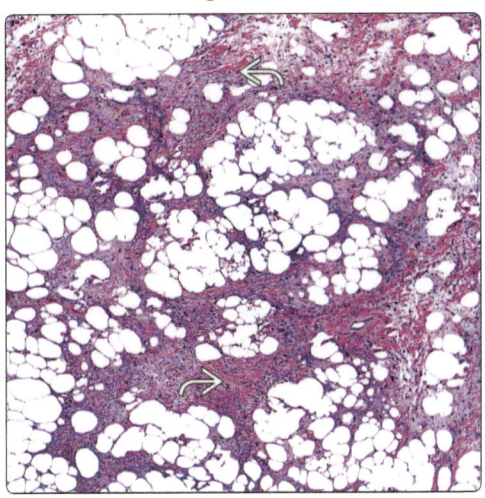

(Left) ALT shows the marked variation ⇒ of adipocyte size characteristic of this tumor. Fibrous bands ⇒ irregularly course through the lesion. (Right) The sclerosing variant of ALT/well-differentiated LPS (WDLPS) features expansion of the fibrous bands ⇒ to form large areas of the tumor. Atypical stromal cells are often concentrated in the sclerotic regions.

Atypical Stromal Cells of ALT/WDLPS

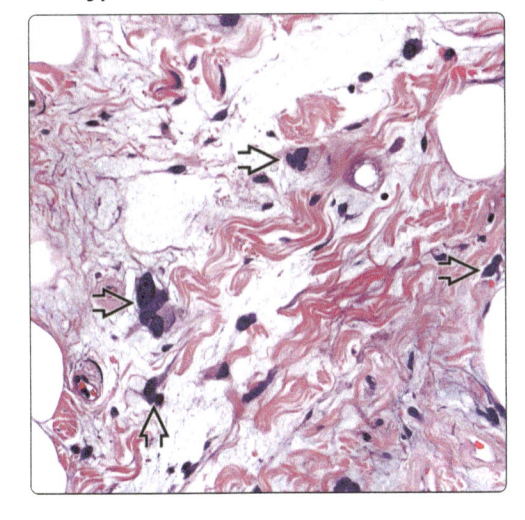

Dedifferentiated LPS

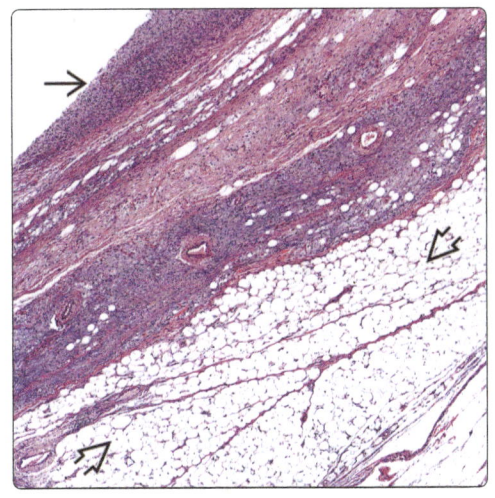

(Left) Higher power view of a sclerotic band reveals the atypical stromal cells ⇒, which are hyperchromatic and may be mono- or multinucleated. The nuclei are more hyperchromatic than the nuclei of cells of Lockhern. (Right) Dedifferentiated LPS shows a layered look with the low-grade component ⇒ at the bottom and progressively more cellular layers on top. The high-grade dedifferentiated component ⇒ is hypercellular and lacks adipocytes.

MDM2 Amplification by FISH in ALT

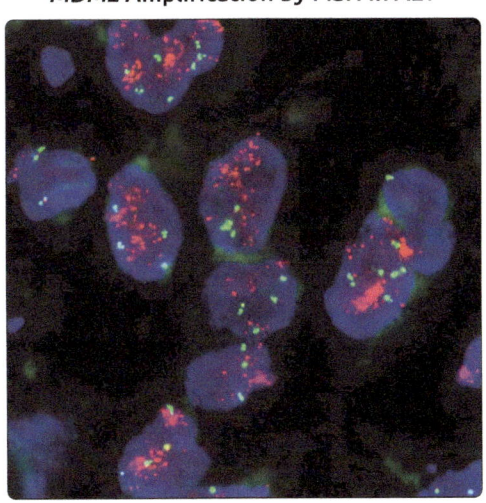

Dedifferentiated LPS With Low-Grade Region

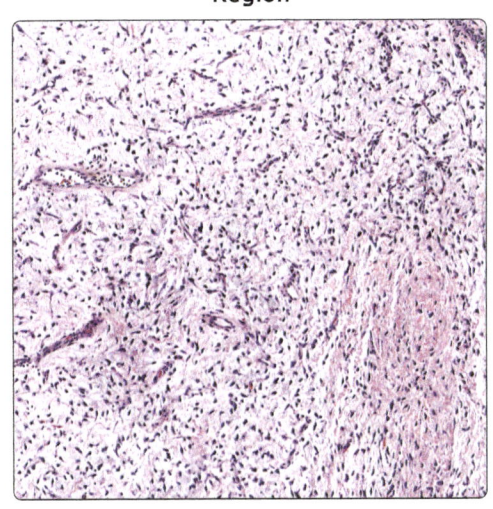

(Left) MDM2 FISH in a case of ALT shows MDM2 probed in red. Numerous red signals per cell indicates amplification of MDM2. (Right) Dedifferentiated LPS containing low-grade differentiated areas is shown. The cells are hyperchromatic, but cellularity is modest, and marked atypia is absent. Dedifferentiated LPS with only low-grade areas may be indistinguishable from hypercellular WDLPS.

Liposarcomas

Dedifferentiated LPS: Gross Appearance

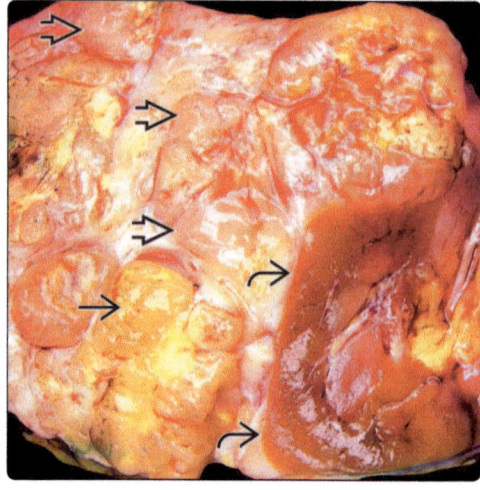

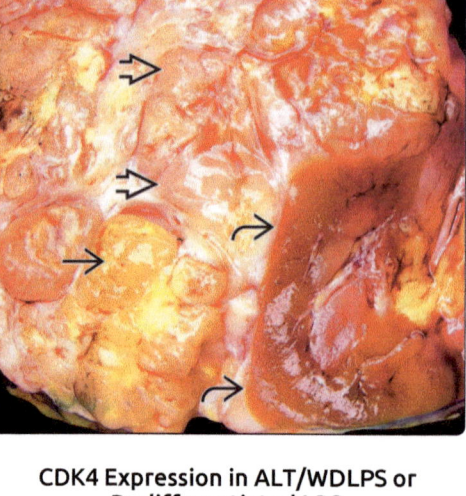

Dedifferentiated LPS: Karyotype

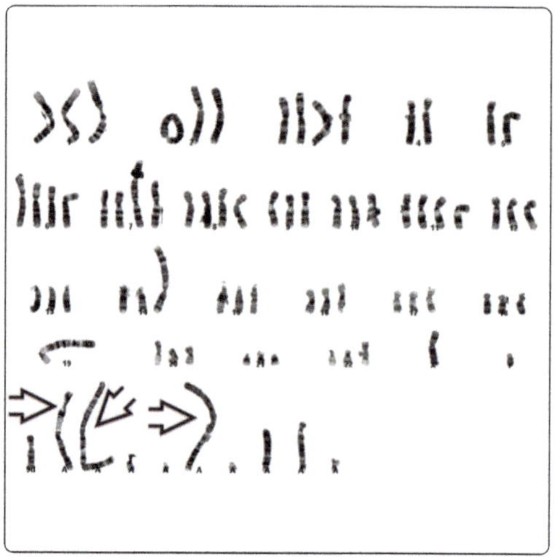

(Left) This dedifferentiated LPS is heterogeneous on cut section. Most areas show a lobulated fish-flesh appearance ⇨ and only focal hints of fat differentiation ➡. Necrosis is present, and the tumor is firmly annealed to the kidney ➡. The retroperitoneum is the most common location of the tumor. (Right) Karyotype of dedifferentiated LPS shows giant marker chromosomes ⇨, such as ALT/WDLPS, but also near tetraploidy.

CDK4 Expression in ALT/WDLPS or Dedifferentiated LPS

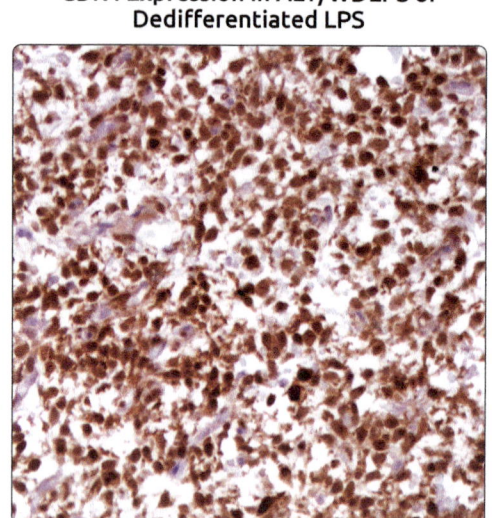

MDM2 Expression in ALT/WDLPS and Dedifferentiated LPS

(Left) CDK4 may be overexpressed in ALT/WDLPS and in dedifferentiated LPS. Often, there are only scattered positive cells, but most tumor cells are reactive in this case. (Right) MDM2 is also overexpressed in most ALT/WDLPS and dedifferentiated LPS. MDM2 overexpression helps distinguish ALT from deep lipomas and myxoid LPS. Overexpression is also demonstrated by amplification of MDM2 by FISH.

Dedifferentiated LPS: Inflammation

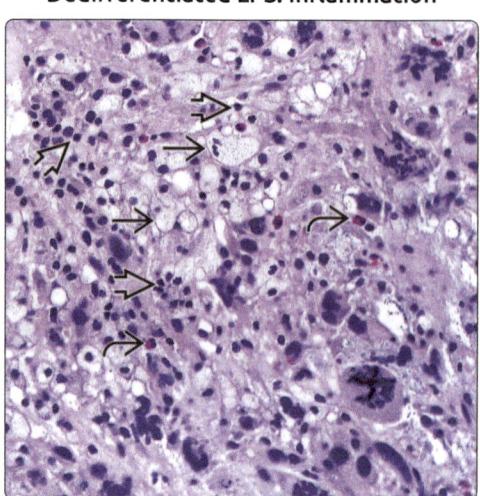

ALT/WDLPS With Abnormal Vessel

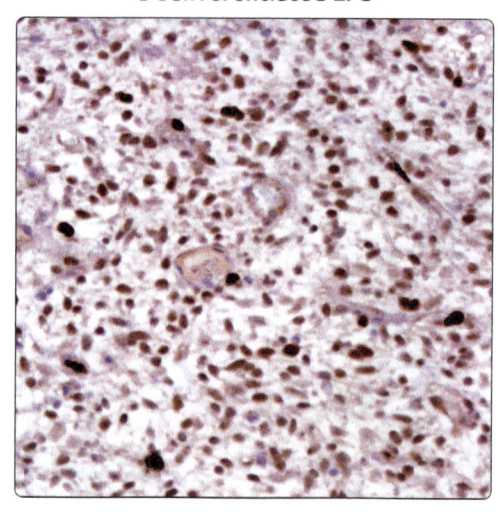

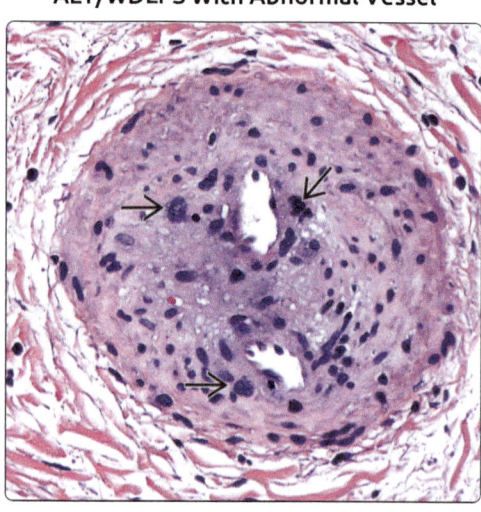

(Left) Many LPS contain inflammatory infiltrates. This example of a dedifferentiated LPS contains intermixed lymphocytes ➡, eosinophils ➡, and lipophages ➡. Inflammation may play a role in LPS development. Usually, the inflammation is lymphoplasmacytic and may obscure the tumor cells. (Right) Many ALT/WDLPS and differentiated LPS contain thick-walled vessels with intramural atypical cells ➡.

Liposarcomas

Myxoid LPS With Low-Grade Features

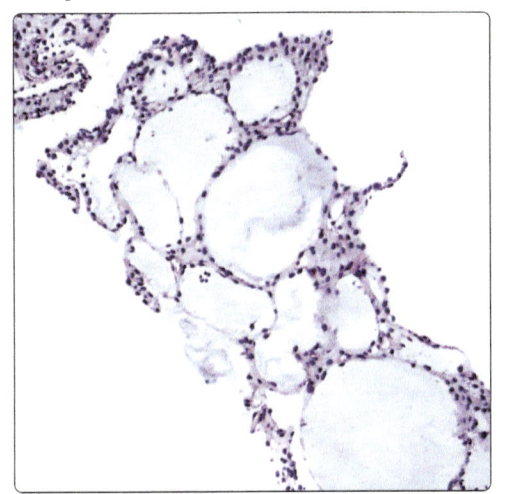

Myxoid LPS

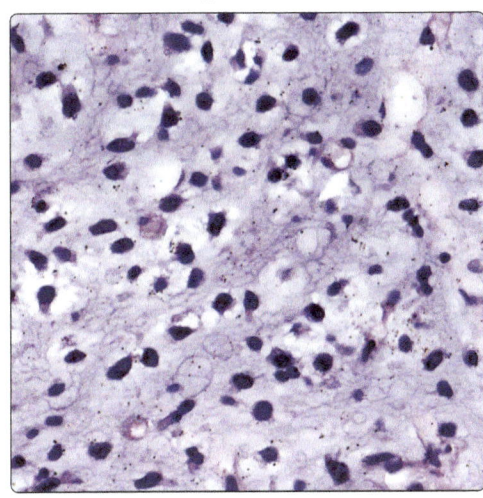

(**Left**) Core needle biopsy of low-grade myxoid LPS from a 15-year-old boy shows a common pulmonary edema-like pattern of small, cystic pools of myxoid matrix. (**Right**) Low-grade myxoid LPS contains short, plump stromal cells with a moderate N:C ratio. The nuclei are normo- to mildly hyperchromatic, and pleomorphism is absent. Cellularity is relatively low.

Myxoid LPS With Hypercellular Region

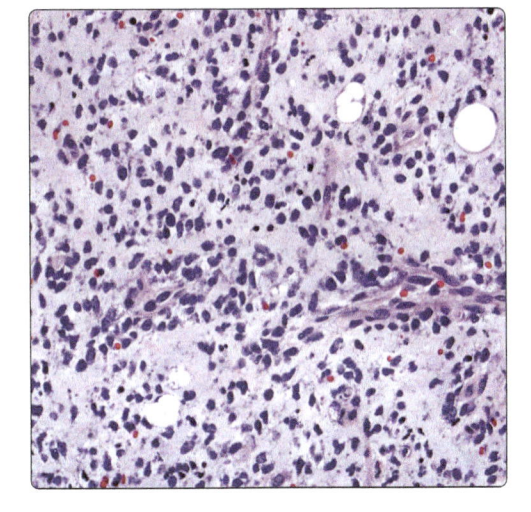

Myxoid LPS: High Grade

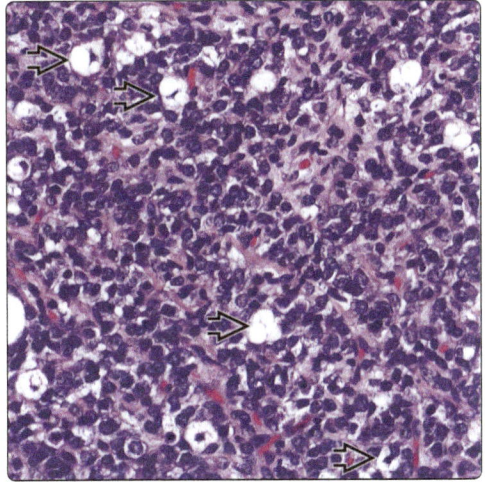

(**Left**) Transitional region in myxoid LPS features increased cellularity, but the myxoid matrix is still discernible. This would not yet be considered a round cell component. (**Right**) High-grade myxoid LPS shows a hypercellular, back-to-back arrangement of small round cells with a few intermixed lipoblasts ⇒. A round cell component of > 5% equates with more aggressive behavior and is considered minimum criterion for high-grade designation.

Myxoid LPS: Typical Vascular Network

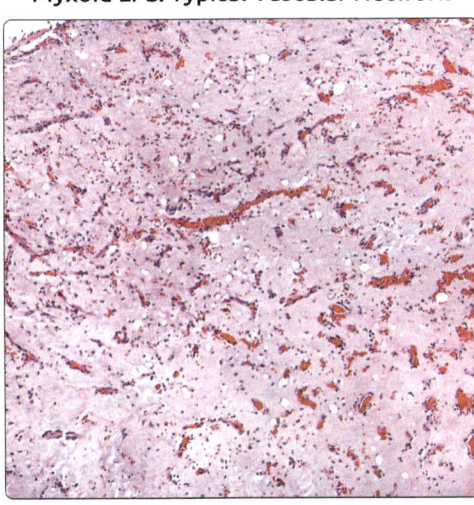

Myxoid LPS With Signet-Ring Lipoblasts

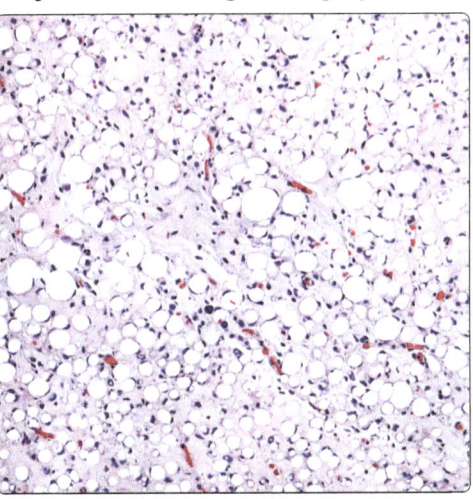

(**Left**) Low-power view of myxoid LPS shows ectatic blood vessels forming a chicken-wire-like network in the tumor. Although typical of myxoid/round cell LPS, this vascular pattern is not entirely specific and can be seen in a few ALT/WDLPS with myxoid stroma. (**Right**) Many myxoid LPS show an abundance of univacuolated to signet-ring cell lipoblasts, as seen here.

Liposarcomas

Myxoid LPS With CD34 Highlighting Chicken-Wire Vessels

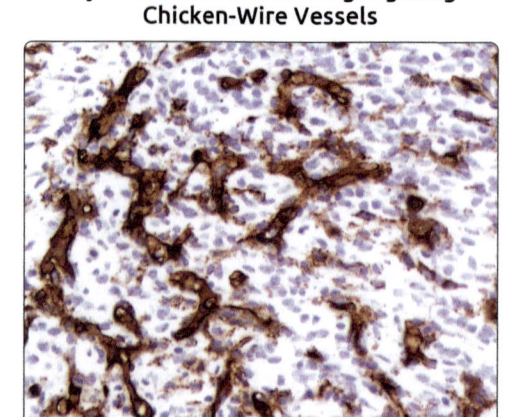

Pleomorphic LPS

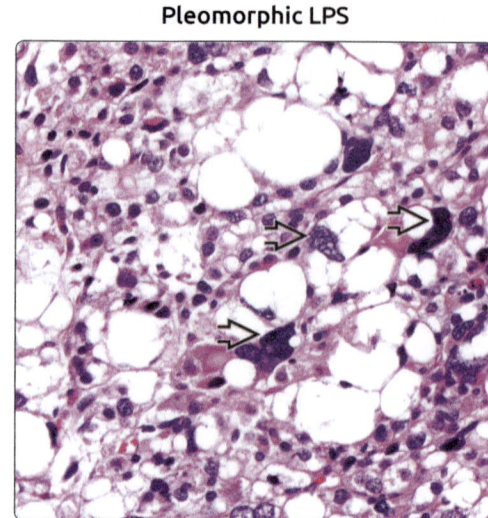

(Left) CD34 can be helpful in highlighting the chicken-wire vascular pattern of myxoid/round cell LPS. This is especially useful in round cell LPS and is a diagnostic clue. (Right) Pleomorphic LPS is composed of a mixture of high-grade sarcoma, not otherwise specified, and intermixed pleomorphic lipoblasts ⇨ that show more nuclear atypia than the lipoblasts of ALT/WDLPS, dedifferentiated LPS, and myxoid/round cell LPS.

Metastatic Pleomorphic LPS

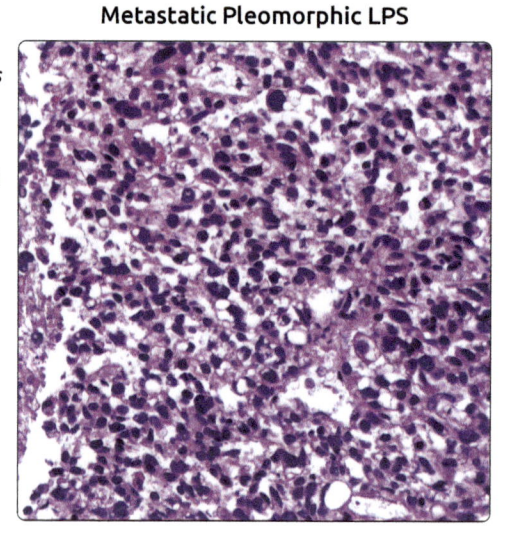

ASC/P-LT

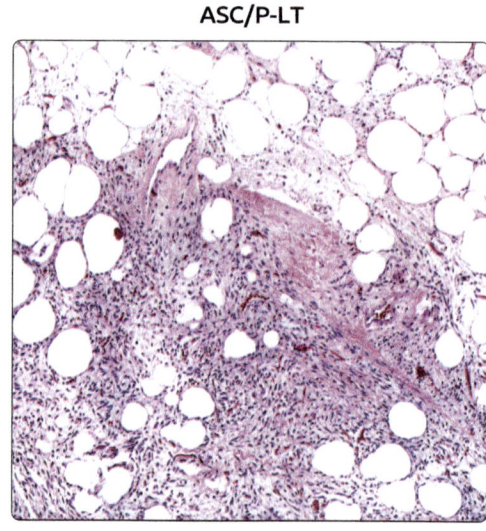

(Left) Pleomorphic LPS that has metastasized to the liver is shown. Many examples of pleomorphic LPS contain only sparse pleomorphic lipoblasts, as seen here. Multiple sections may be required to find the diagnostic cells. The nonadipogenic cells may be spindled, polygonal, or round to epithelioid. (Right) ASC/P-LT comprises adipocytes of varying size and interspersed short spindle cells. Lipoblasts are usually also found, but they are not seen here.

Spindle Cells of ASC/P-LT

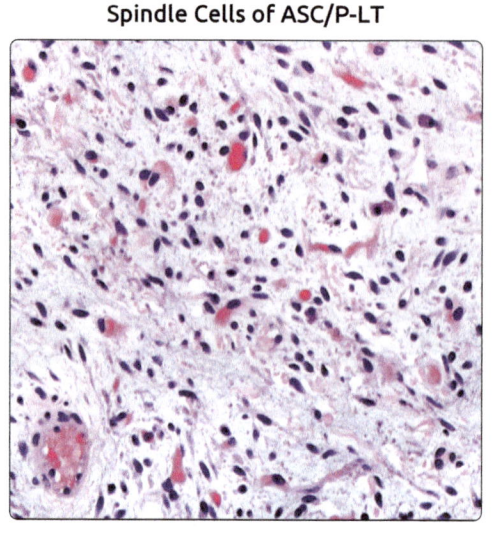

ASC/P-LT With Diffuse CD34 Expression

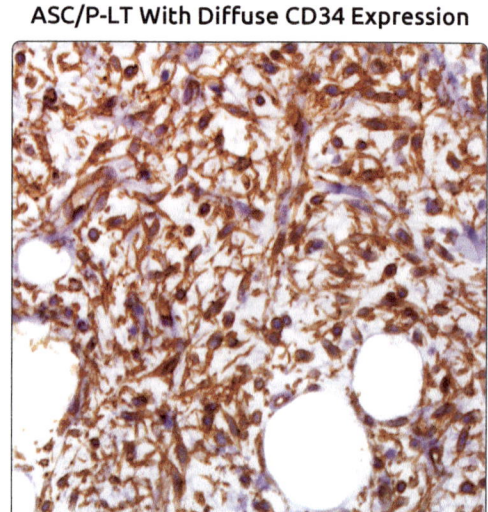

(Left) Spindle cells can be short or elongate and resemble elongate Schwann cells. The nuclei are often slightly hyperchromatic, but pleomorphism is absent. Although vessels are conspicuous, a chicken-wire pattern typical of myxoid LPS is lacking. (Right) Spindle cells are often diffusely strongly reactive for CD34. Both atypical spindle cell/pleomorphic lipomatous tumor (ASC/P-LT) and spindle cell/pleomorphic lipoma contain CD34-reactive stromal cells. Other features distinguish the 2 tumors.

Liposarcomas

IML

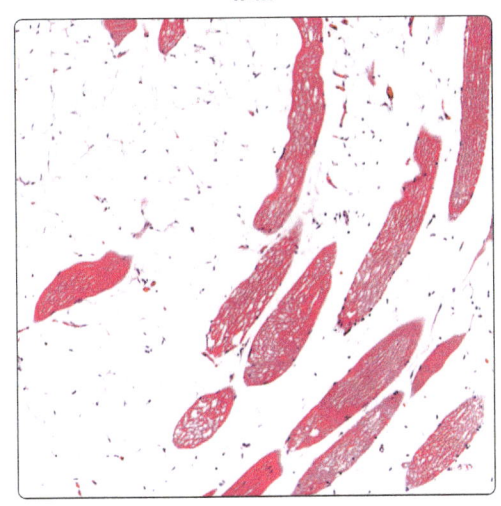

Spindle Cell/Pleomorphic Lipoma

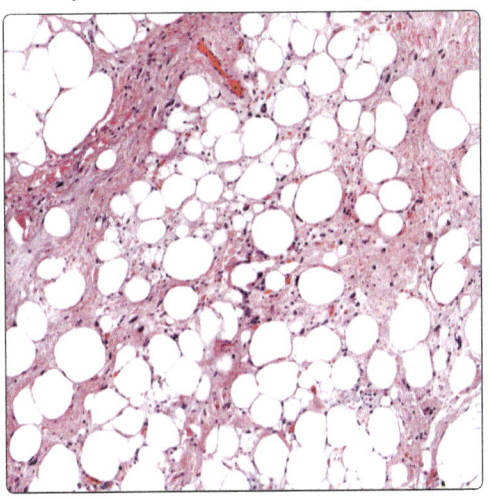

(Left) Intramuscular lipoma (IML) may mimic ALT because it is deeply located and can often attain a size > 10 cm. Histologic examination reveals a permeative tumor that dissects between skeletal muscle fibers, as seen here. This intercalating growth between skeletal muscle cells is a clue to the diagnosis. Additionally, IML lacks marked variation in adipocyte size, atypical stromal cells, and lipoblasts. (Right) Spindle cell/pleomorphic lipoma mimics ALT at low power.

Spindle Cell/Pleomorphic Lipoma

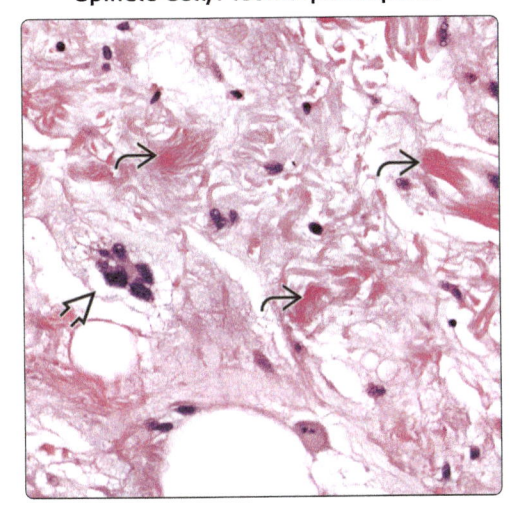

Lipoblastoma

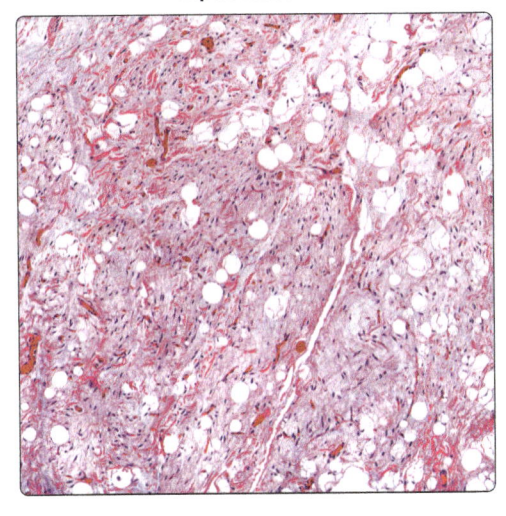

(Left) High-power view of spindle cell/pleomorphic lipoma reveals atypical cells that can resemble florets ⇒, which can simulate atypical stromal cells of ALT. Ropy collagen fibers ⇒, lack of MDM2 or CDK4 expression, loss of RB1 expression, and superficial location with pushing margins are clues to the diagnosis. (Right) Lipoblastoma can be histologically indistinguishable from myxoid LPS.

Lipoblastoma With Signet-Ring Lipoblasts

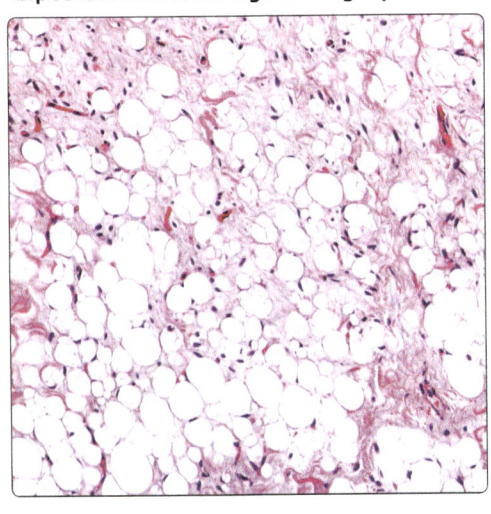

Lipoblastoma With Chicken-Wire Vascular Network

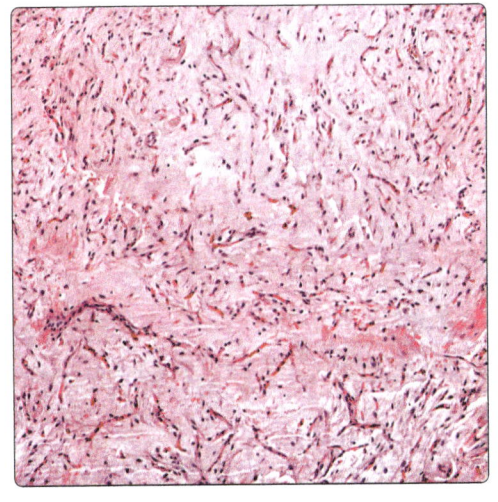

(Left) Lipoblastomas may contain numerous monovacuolated and signet-ring lipoblasts, as in myxoid LPS. (Right) A chicken-wire vascular network is well developed in this area of lipoblastoma, mimicking myxoid LPS. Fortunately, the 2 tumors seldom overlap in age (lipoblastoma occurs in young children, while myxoid LPS occurs in young to middle-aged adults). Lipoblastoma shows chromosome 8 changes, distinctly different from the gene fusions of myxoid LPS.

Muscle Sarcomas

TERMINOLOGY

Definitions
- Sarcomas phenotypically showing differentiation to smooth muscle or skeletal muscle

ETIOLOGY/PATHOGENESIS

Leiomyosarcoma
- Sporadic
  - Most common type
  - Complex genetic alterations with fairly consistent findings
- Syndrome associated
  - Li-Fraumeni syndrome: Mutation in *TP53*
  - Hereditary leiomyomatosis and renal cell cancer (HLRCC)
    - Germline loss of function of fumarate hydratase (*FH*) (1q)
- Epstein-Barr virus (EBV) association
  - Almost always occurs in setting of immunosuppression
  - Rare cause of leiomyosarcoma (LMS) and leiomyoma
  - Usually excellent prognosis

Alveolar Rhabdomyosarcoma
- Specific *FOXO1* translocations are driver event in at least 90%
- Additional rare fusions also reported: PAX3::FOXO4/NCOA1/INO80D or FOXO1::FGFR1

Embryonal Rhabdomyosarcoma
- Sporadic
  - Complex genetic alterations with some relatively consistent findings
- Syndrome associated
  - Neurofibromatosis type 1 (NF1)
    - Rhabdomyosarcoma (RMS) develops in 1.5-6% of NF1 patients
  - Li-Fraumeni syndrome
    - RMS in setting of *TP53* germline mutation often show diffuse anaplasia
  - Hereditary retinoblastoma syndrome
    - Germline *RB1* mutation
  - Beckwith-Wiedemann syndrome
    - Methylation abnormalities of *GF2* and *H19* at 11P locus
    - Genes at this site also important in sporadic embryonal RMS (ERMS)
- May rarely arise from germ cell tumor of testis, ovary, or mediastinum

Spindle Cell/Sclerosing Rhabdomyosarcoma
- 3 groups of specific genetic alterations

Pleomorphic Rhabdomyosarcoma
- Complex genetic alterations

CLINICAL IMPLICATIONS

Clinical Presentation
- LMS
  - Age: Middle-aged to older adults most commonly
  - Sex
    - F > M for retroperitoneal and large vessel tumors
    - M > F for deep soft tissue tumors
    - M = F for superficial tumors
  - Location
    - Retroperitoneum most common site
    - Uterine and other müllerian sites
    - Large vessel-associated tumors include inferior vena cava and its branches > large leg veins > others
    - Deep soft tissues of extremities account for 10-15% of extremity sarcomas
    - Dermal and subcutaneous tumors occur most commonly on extremities
    - May also occur as primary bone sarcoma
- Alveolar RMS (ARMS)
  - Age: Adolescents to young adults most commonly
  - Sex: M = F
  - Location
    - Extremities (most common location) > trunk/pelvis > retroperitoneum

Alveolar Rhabdomyosarcoma With Solid Growth

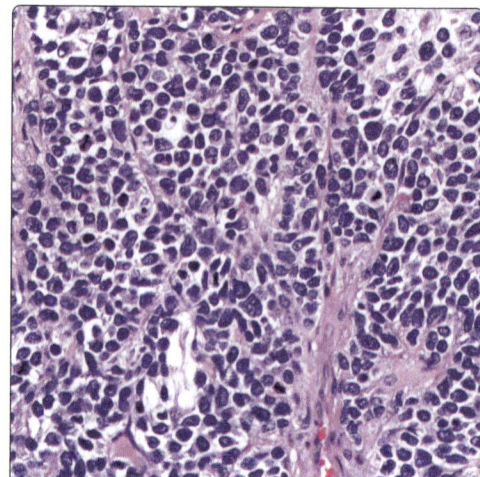

FOXO1 Break-Apart ISH in Alveolar Rhabdomyosarcoma

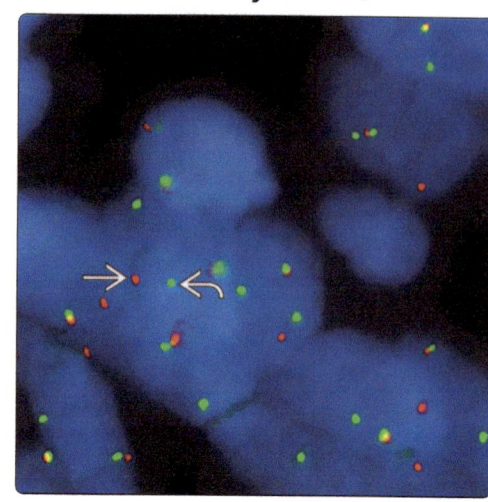

(Left) Some alveolar rhabdomyosarcomas (ARMS) show little to no evidence of an alveolar growth pattern, as in this case. Many of these solid-type ARMS (but not all) are FOXO1 fusion negative. *(Right)* Dual-color break-apart probes for FOXO1 on chromosome 13q14 show split red ➔ and green ➔ signals, indicating translocation involving FOXO1. (From DP: Soft Tissue.)

Muscle Sarcomas

- Head and neck; most commonly nasopharynx, sinuses, or parameningeal
- Rare patients present with diffuse bone marrow involvement and no known primary site
- ERMS
  o Age: Children < 10 years most commonly
  o Sex: M (slightly) > F
  o Location
    - Head and neck = genitourinary region (~ 85% of cases) > trunk/extremities (~ 9% of cases) > other visceral locations
- Spindle cell/sclerosing RMS
  o Age
    - Bimodal distribution in children and adults
    - Cases in infants (< 1 year) show specific genetic alterations and usually nonaggressive behavior
  o Sex
    - M > F ~ 6:1 for adult group
  o Location
    - Head and neck: Most common location for spindle cell examples in adults with *MYOD1*-mutant tumors
    - Paratesticular soft tissues: Most common site for non-*EWSR1*/*FUS*::*TFCP2* spindle cell examples in children
    - Extremities: Most common site for sclerosing examples
    - Rarely may occur elsewhere: Retroperitoneum and viscera or craniofacial bones for *EWSR1*/*FUS*::*TFCP2* cases
- Pleomorphic RMS
  o Age: Middle-aged to older adults
  o Sex: M > F
  o Location
    - Extremities (especially lower) > trunk > abdomen/retroperitoneum > paratesticular > head and neck
    - Rarely reported at other sites, such as uterus

Treatment

- Surgery ± radiation for local control
  o Complete surgical excision may be curative in small stage I tumors
- Chemotherapy used for higher stage tumors with surgery ± radiation
- New therapies under study: PARP inhibitors + cytotoxic agents, MEK inhibitors + IGFR1 inhibitors, HDAC inhibitors, and novel cytotoxic agents
- Specific treatment regimen may be driven by genetic findings rather than morphology in future

Outcome

- Muscle sarcomas in adults tend to behave more aggressively than most other sarcomas
- Stage is best predictor of outcome
- Many genetic markers are reportedly prognostic
  o But none have been prospectively validated in large series except for ARMS translocations
- LMS
  o Dermal tumors do not metastasize unless invading subcutaneous fat
  o Extremity tumors
    - Larger tumor size (> 5 cm), deep location, and grade > 1 are adverse prognostic factors
  o Retroperitoneal tumors
    - Nearly all patients succumb to disease due to recurrences &/or metastases
  o Tumors associated with large vessels
    - Generally poor prognosis
  o EBV-related LMS
    - Favorable prognosis (only 5% death rate)
- ARMS
  o ARMS generally behave worse than similarly staged ERMS
    - *PAX7*::*FOXO1* tumors behave better than *PAX3*::*FOXO1* tumors
- ERMS
  o Age is factor: Prognosis better for young children (to 9 years) > older children > adults
  o Prognosis also varies by histologic variant
    - Botryoid ERMS has relatively good prognosis
    - Anaplastic ERMS has worse prognosis
  o Prognosis also varies by site
    - Orbital and paratesticular better than extremity and parameningeal tumors
- Spindle cell/sclerosing RMS
  o Age: Prognosis better in children than in adults
    - However, pediatric cases with *MYOD1* mutations behave as aggressively as adult cases with *MYOD1* mutations
    - Congenital/infantile type with *NCOA2* or *VGLL2* rearrangements has high overall 5-year survival
    - *EWSR1*/*FUS*::*TFCP2* fusion-positive RMS: Behaves aggressively
- Pleomorphic RMS
  o Poor prognosis with metastatic rate of ~ 50%

MICROSCOPIC

Leiomyosarcoma

- Architecture
  o Conventional subtype
    - Long, sweeping fascicles intersecting at 90° angles
    - Ragged cytoplasmic clearing reminiscent of contraction bands in normal smooth muscle
  o Myxoid subtype
    - Gray-blue myxoid matrix reduces cellularity and can obscure fascicular architecture
  o Other variants: Inflammatory, osteoclastic giant-cell rich, pleomorphic, epithelioid
    - Epithelioid subtype grows as solid sheets
- Cell morphology
  o Conventional subtype
    - Eosinophilic plump spindle cells with cigar-shaped or train car-shaped nuclei
    - Nuclear pleomorphism increases with grade
  o Myxoid subtype
    - Plump spindle cells, similar to those in conventional subtype, but also may include polygonal or stellate cells
  o Epithelioid subtype
    - Large, round epithelioid tumor cells with vesicular nuclei and macronucleoli

Muscle Sarcomas

- Usually mixed with conventional areas
- Pleomorphic (poorly differentiated) subtype
  - Nonspecific, high-grade, poorly differentiated areas with marked cellular and nuclear pleomorphism
  - Usually mixed with conventional areas
- Ancillary studies
  - IHC
    - Muscle markers positive: SMA, desmin, MSA, caldesmon
    - Negative markers: MYOD1 and myogenin, except in rare cases of mixed LMS/RMS
    - Positivity for at least 2 muscle markers is more supportive of diagnosis than just 1, because other tumor types may express SMA, MSA, or desmin

Alveolar Rhabdomyosarcoma

- Architecture
  - Conventional subtype
    - Alveolar-like spaces created by tumor cells falling off into central space, leaving single layer of attached lining cells
  - Solid subtype
    - Solid sheets or nests separated by dense, fibrous stroma
- Cell morphology
  - Medium-sized round cells with high N:C ratio
  - Spindle cells or clear cells may rarely be present
  - "Wreath cells" = tumor giant cells with peripheral ring of nuclei
    - Relatively common and clue to diagnosis
  - Rhabdomyoblasts
    - Eosinophilic cells ± cross striations = more differentiated tumor cells
- Ancillary studies
  - IHC
    - Muscle markers: Myogenin (usually diffusely strongly positive), MYOD1 in more differentiated rhabdomyoblasts; CD56, desmin also positive
    - Other markers uncommonly positive: Keratins, chromogranin, synaptophysin
  - FISH for specific translocations
    - Break-apart probe for FOXO1 positive in ~ 90% of cases with FOXO1 translocations

Embryonal Rhabdomyosarcoma

- Architecture
  - Conventional subtype
    - Alternating hypercellular and hypocellular areas often with myxoid background
    - Cellular fascicles and sheets
  - Botryoid subtype
    - Cambium layer: Band of hypercellular tumor running under epithelial surface
    - Lobules usually myxoid and sparsely cellular
  - Dense pattern subtype
    - Mimics solid-type ARMS
    - Solid sheets of round blue cells
  - Anaplastic subtype
    - Diffuse or focal distribution of markedly pleomorphic tumor cells
- Cell morphology
  - Conventional and botryoid ERMS
    - Round to ovoid to stellate, less differentiated cells
    - Cells showing more myogenic features, including brightly eosinophilic cytoplasm ± cross striations
  - Dense pattern subtype
    - Predominantly primitive round blue cells packed tightly together
  - Anaplastic ERMS
    - Markedly pleomorphic with irregular enlarged and multilobated, hyperchromatic nuclei and coarse chromatin
    - Mitoses (including atypical forms) common
    - Conventional cells also often present
- Ancillary studies
  - IHC
    - Muscle markers usually show patchy positivity for myogenin in contrast to ARMS, which almost always shows diffuse strong reactivity; CD56, desmin also positive; MYOD1 in more differentiated tumor cells; SMA sometimes positive
    - Other markers: Membranous expression of CD99 in some cases; cytoplasmic expression of WT1 in some cases; rarely keratins, S100, and NFP
  - FISH: FOXO1 is intact by break-apart probe testing

Spindle Cell/Sclerosing Rhabdomyosarcoma

- Architecture
  - Congenital/infantile group: Crowded fascicles of spindled cells ± fibrotic background ± areas of conventional ERMS
  - Adult group: Fascicles of spindled cells often with dense, collagenized background, sometimes imparting clefted pseudovascular appearance
  - EWSR1/FUS::TFCP2 RMS group: Sheets and fascicles of spindled and epithelioid tumor cells
- Cell morphology
  - Spindled cells are plump to elongate with vesicular to hyperchromatic spindled nuclei
    - Epithelioid cells also present in EWSR1/FUS::TFCP2 RMS
  - Primitive (blastic) cells &/or more differentiated rhabdomyoblasts may be present
  - Pleomorphic cells may be present
    - Especially in adult cases
- Ancillary studies
  - IHC
    - Muscle markers: Myogenin often only focally positive in scattered cells; desmin and (often) SMA positive
    - Other markers: EMA and keratins may be positive (keratins and ALK usually positive in EWSR1/FUS::TFCP2 RMS)
  - ISH
    - Congenital/infantile type may show specific NCOA2 or VGLL2 rearrangements
    - TFCP2 rearrangements in EWSR1/FUS::TFCP2 RMS
  - PCR/Sanger sequencing or next-generation sequencing
    - Adult group: MYOD1 mutations

Pleomorphic Rhabdomyosarcoma

- Architecture
  - Sheets and fascicles of pleomorphic cells

Muscle Sarcomas

- Cell morphology
  - Pleomorphic spindled tumor cells with irregular, hyperchromatic nuclei
  - Tumor giant cells
  - Few cells may have marked cytoplasmic eosinophilia, suggesting diagnosis
  - High mitotic rate with atypical mitotic figures
  - Differentiated rhabdomyoblasts with cross striations are usually absent
- Ancillary studies
  - Desmin positive; reactivity for myogenin may be focal; MYOD1 usually negative

GENETIC FINDINGS

Leiomyosarcoma

- Karyotype
  - Complex aneuploid karyotype found in majority of cases
- Chromosomal microarray
  - Copy number losses > gains
  - Specific gain or loss is usually seen in ≤ 20% of cases, except for 13q loss (~ 60% of cases)
- Major genes altered
  - *TP53*: Mutated or lost (~ 90%)
  - *RB1*: Lost (~ 95%)
  - *CDKN2A*: Lost or hypermethylated
    - Inactivation may independently impart worse prognosis
  - *PTEN*: Lost or inactivating mutation (~ 60%); rarely gain-of-function mutation
  - *MYOCD*: Amplified in 70%
  - *ATRX*: Loss of expression in ~ 33%
  - *DMD*: Mutated in ~ 50%
- Major pathways dysregulated
  - Cell cycle
  - PI3K/AKT pathway
  - Telomere maintenance
    - Alternative lengthening of telomeres (ALT) found in ~ 60% of cases
  - Muscle development pathways
  - Cell assembly and organization pathways
  - DNA replication, recombination, and repair pathways
  - CD44/AKT pathway
- Gene expression profiling results identify distinct subsets of LMS
  - Transcriptionally distinctive subsets vary by investigator
    - 4 studies each divided LMS into 3 subsets based on differential gene expression
      - Proposed subsets were not independently prognostic
    - Most recent attempt at transcriptional subtyping divided LMS into sets based on gene expression in distinct smooth muscle tumor cell lineages
      - Dedifferentiated, abdominal, abdominal or extremity, gynecologic
  - *SRC* overexpressed in most LMS
  - LMS of retroperitoneum may have distinct gene expression profile compared to LMS of other sites (based on results of 2 studies)
- Epigenetics
  - miRNAs upregulated that are involved in smooth muscle differentiation and in mesenchymal stem cell proliferation

Alveolar Rhabdomyosarcoma

- ~ 90% of ARMS contain specific gene fusion as driver event
- Fusion genes
  - t(2;13); *PAX3::FOXO1*
    - Accounts for ~ 65-75% of fusion-positive ARMS
  - t(1;13); *PAX7::FOXO1*
    - Accounts for ~ 20-25% of fusion-positive ARMS
  - Other rare fusions reported include either *PAX3* or *FOXO1* with novel partners
  - Fusion proteins act as potent and highly expressed transcriptional activators that affect
    - Proliferation pathways
    - Apoptosis pathways
    - Myogenic differentiation
    - Motility pathways
- Chromosomal microarray
  - Shares some of copy number losses with ERMS but generally at lower frequency
  - Commonly amplified sites include 1p36, 2p24, 12q13-q14, 13q14, 13q31
    - ARMS has higher rate of amplifications than ERMS
- Additional genes altered beyond fusion genes
  - Few genes are mutated in ARMS compared to ~ 30% of ERMS cases
  - Fibroblast growth factors overexpressed or upregulated
  - *MYC* and *MYCN* overexpressed
  - Genes close to *PAX* commonly altered: *NRAS*, *KRAS*, *FGFR4*, *PIK3CA*, *CTNNB1*, *FBXW7*, and *BCOR*
  - *ALK* overexpressed in most cases
  - *SMARCA4* overexpressed in most cases
- Epigenetic alterations include overexpression of *PRC2*, which hypermethylates histone H3

Embryonal Rhabdomyosarcoma

- Karyotype
  - Complex aneuploid karyotype found in most cases
  - Mild hyperdiploidy in subset (tetraploidy is rare)
- Major genes altered or differentially expressed
  - Inactivation of tumor suppressor gene at 11p15.5
  - Genes
    - RAS pathway genes: Mutated in ~ 50% of cases (*NRAS*, *KRAS*, *HRAS*, *FGFR4*, *NF1*, *PIK3CA*)
    - Other mutated genes: *TP53* (~ 10%), *BCOR* (~ 15%), *DICER1* (especially in RMS of female genital tract)
    - Genes amplified: *MYCN*, *CDK4*
  - Fibroblast growth factors often overexpressed
  - *SNAI2* highly overexpressed
    - SNAIL family transcription factor: Acts as oncogene to inhibit MYOD-driven differentiation and instead promote tumor growth
    - Represses expression of myogenic differentiation regulators: *MYOD1*, *MYOG*, *MEF* family TEFs, and *CDKN1A*
  - *SIX1* highly overexpressed
    - SIX family transcription factor: Acts as oncogene to inhibit muscle cell differentiation at early point in cell differentiation

Muscle Sarcomas

- Major pathways dysregulated: PI3K/AKT and other downstream pathways of FGF and IGF signaling and WNT/β-catenin signaling
- Epigenetic alterations are distinct from those in ARMS
  - Epigenetic changes in both ARMS and ERMS include hypermethylation of various tumor suppressor and cell differentiation genes

Spindle Cell/Sclerosing Rhabdomyosarcoma

- 3 genetic groups now recognized
- Spindle cell/sclerosing RMS adult group
  - Most common in adolescents → adults
  - Complex aneuploid karyotype, including gains and losses of whole and partial chromosomes
  - Genes altered
    - *MYOD1* mutations in ~ 60%
    - *PIK3CA* mutations in ~ 30%
      - Dual *MYOD1* and *PIK3CA* mutations appear to correlate with sclerosing morphology
- Congenital/infantile group
  - Most cases show specific rearrangement
  - *NCOA2* fusions
    - t(8;11); *TEAD1::NCOA2*
    - t(6;8)(p21;q13); *SRF::NCOA2*
    - t(6;8)(q22'q13); *VGLL2::NCOA2*
  - Additional *VGLL2* (6q22) rearrangement
    - t(6;6); *VGLL2::CITED2*
      - Chromosome 6q22-23 breaks and inverts, resulting in fusion of 3' *CITED2* to 5' *VGLL2*
  - Normal role of *NCOA2*: Transcriptional coactivator for nuclear hormone receptors, including vitamin D, thyroid, steroid, and retinoid receptors
    - Forms pathogenic fusions in some cases of acute myeloid leukemia, acute lymphoblastic leukemia, and most cases of mesenchymal chondrosarcoma (fusing with *HEY1*)
  - Normal roles of *TEAD1*, *SRF*, *VGLL2*: Help control skeletal muscle-specific gene transcription
- *EWSR1/FUS::TFCP2* group
  - Occurs in all age groups
  - Most commonly craniofacial bones (intraosseous)
  - *MEIS1::NCOA2* cases: Included with *EWSR1/FUS::TFCP2* cases as aggressive, intraosseous RMS

Pleomorphic Rhabdomyosarcoma

- Karyotype
  - Complex aneuploid karyotype: Most commonly loss of chromosomes 2, 13, 14, 15, 16, and 19

DIFFERENTIAL DIAGNOSIS

DDx for Leiomyosarcoma

- Other fascicular spindle cell sarcomas
  - Malignant peripheral nerve sheath tumor
    - Negative muscle markers except malignant triton tumor, which also expresses neural markers, such as patchy S100 and SOX10
  - Low-grade myofibroblastic sarcoma
    - Usually desmin negative
  - Synovial sarcoma
    - Negative muscle markers; positive for TLE1; positive for t(X;18)
  - Fibrosarcoma arising in dermatofibrosarcoma protuberans
    - May have lower grade areas present; usually negative for 2 muscle markers; positive for t(17;22)
- Desmoplastic or spindle cell melanoma
  - May show reactivity for melanoma markers, almost always negative for muscle markers

DDx for Alveolar Rhabdomyosarcoma and Dense Pattern Embryonal Rhabdomyosarcoma

- Other small round blue cell tumors
  - Ewing sarcoma family of tumors
    - Lacks rhabdomyoblasts; positive for *EWSR1* or *FUS* fusions
  - Metastatic Wilms tumor
    - Biphasic or triphasic in many cases; lacks rhabdomyoblasts, WT1 nuclear positivity by IHC
  - Metastatic neuroblastoma
    - Neurofibrillary matrix and rosettes often present; lacks muscle marker expression

DDx for Embryonal Rhabdomyosarcoma

- Pediatric spindle cell tumors
  - Congenital fibrosarcoma
    - May have multiple histologic patterns, lacks muscle markers; positive for t(12;15)(p13;q25)
  - Inflammatory myofibroblastic tumor
    - More prominent inflammation, usually ALK positive (in children)

DDx for Spindle Cell/Sclerosing Rhabdomyosarcoma

- Includes those for LMS
- Osteosarcoma: True osteoid and malignant osteoblasts present; positive for SATB2

DDx for Pleomorphic Rhabdomyosarcoma

- Pleomorphic undifferentiated sarcoma: Lacks rhabdomyoblasts and lacks skeletal muscle marker expression

SELECTED REFERENCES

1. Kerrison WGJ et al: The biology and treatment of leiomyosarcomas. Crit Rev Oncol Hematol. 184:103955, 2023
2. Agaram NP: Evolving classification of rhabdomyosarcoma. Histopathology. 80(1):98-108, 2022
3. Bharathy N et al: SMARCA4 biology in alveolar rhabdomyosarcoma. Oncogene. 41(11):1647-56, 2022
4. Hsu JY et al: SIX1 reprograms myogenic transcription factors to maintain the rhabdomyosarcoma undifferentiated state. Cell Rep. 38(5):110323, 2022
5. Apellaniz-Ruiz M et al: DICER1-associated embryonal rhabdomyosarcoma and adenosarcoma of the gynecologic tract: pathology, molecular genetics, and indications for molecular testing. Genes Chromosomes Cancer. 60(3):217-33, 2021
6. Pomella S et al: Interaction between SNAI2 and MYOD enhances oncogenesis and suppresses differentiation in fusion negative rhabdomyosarcoma. Nat Commun. 12(1):192, 2021
7. Shern JF et al: Genomic classification and clinical outcome in rhabdomyosarcoma: a report from an international consortium. J Clin Oncol. 39(26):2859-71, 2021
8. Agaram NP et al: MYOD1-mutant spindle cell and sclerosing rhabdomyosarcoma: an aggressive subtype irrespective of age. A reappraisal for molecular classification and risk stratification. Mod Pathol. 32(1):27-36, 2019
9. Groisberg R et al: Clinical genomic profiling to identify actionable alterations for investigational therapies in patients with diverse sarcomas. Oncotarget. 8(24):39254-67, 2017

Muscle Sarcomas

Leiomyosarcoma

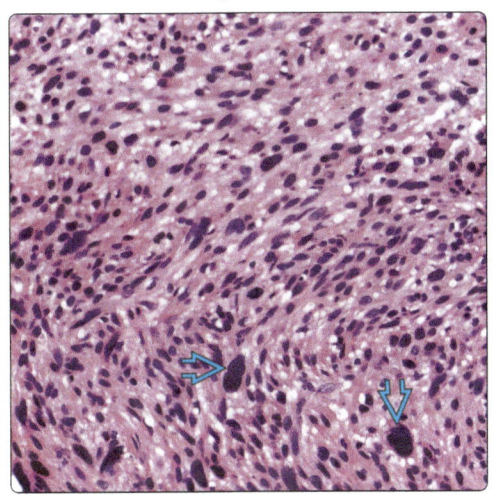

Leiomyosarcoma: Most Common Nuclear Shape

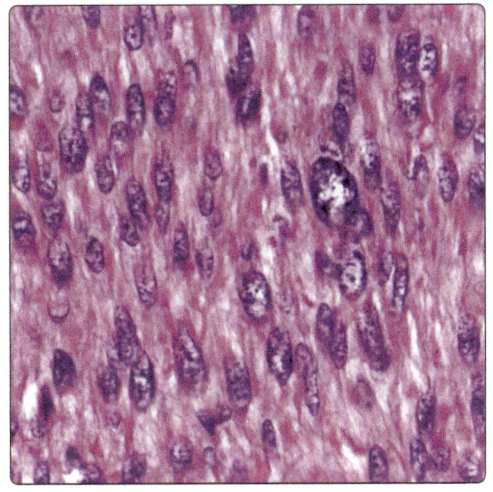

(Left) Deep leiomyosarcoma (LMS) of the lower leg shows scattered, more pleomorphic nuclei that are much larger and more hyperchromatic than the surrounding tumor nuclei ⇨. Such scattershot distribution of markedly pleomorphic nuclei popping out among fascicles of eosinophilic spindle cells is a clue to the diagnosis of LMS, although not entirely specific. (Right) Many LMS feature cigar-shaped or train car-shaped nuclei, as in this case.

Leiomyosarcoma: Cytoplasmic Clearing Mimicking Contraction Bands

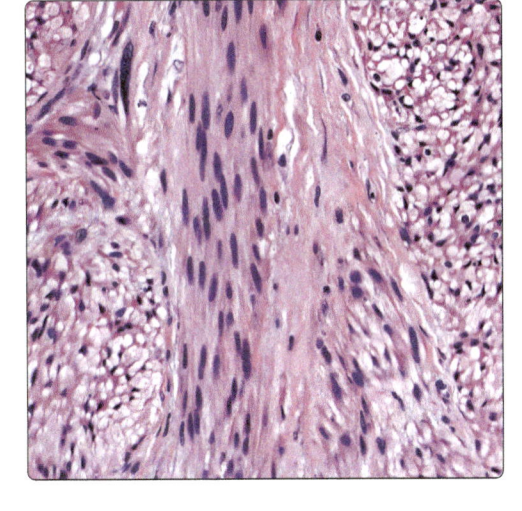

Leiomyosarcoma: Desmin Expression

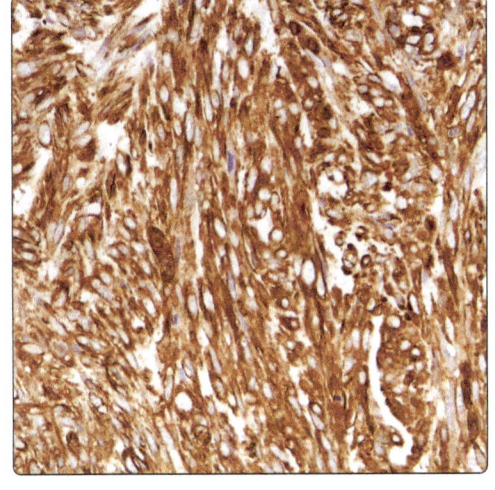

(Left) Dermal LMS shows the classic growth pattern of long fascicles of spindle cells intersecting at right angles. Notice the cytoplasmic clearing in many cells, reminiscent of contraction bands in normal smooth muscle. Although not entirely specific, contraction band-like clearing should prompt including a smooth muscle tumor in the differential diagnosis. (Right) Desmin is usually strongly expressed in LMS, as is notable here.

Myxoid Leiomyosarcoma

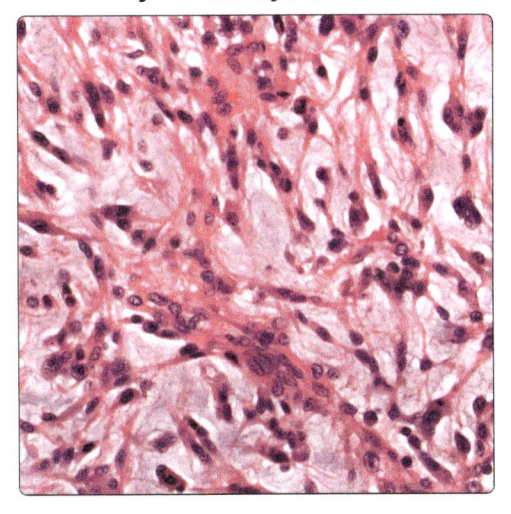

Epithelioid Leiomyosarcoma

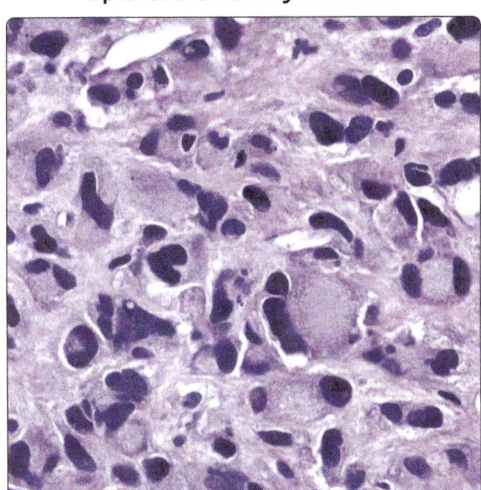

(Left) LMS of deep soft tissue may contain myxoid areas, but myxoid LMS is more common in gynecologic sites. The matrix may be variable in amount and ranges in color. (Right) LMS shows a focal multinucleate and epithelioid cytomorphology. LMS comes in several histologic variants; in the soft tissues, the classic variant is by far the most common.

Muscle Sarcomas

Embryonal Rhabdomyosarcoma

Embryonal Rhabdomyosarcoma With Spindle Cells

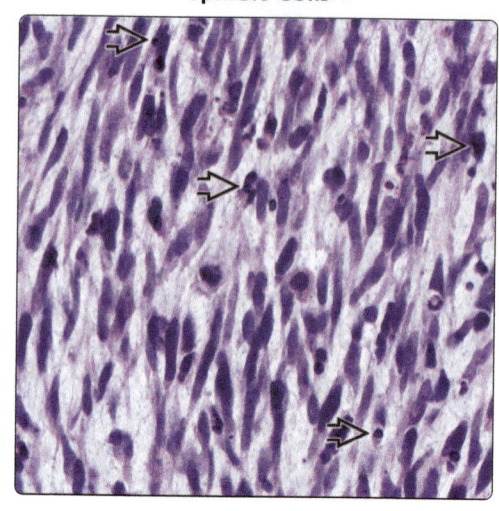

(Left) Many examples of embryonal rhabdomyosarcoma (ERMS) show zones of alternating hyper- and hypocellularity, as in this example from the orbital area of a 6-year-old boy. (Right) This case of ERMS is primarily composed of elongate, relatively uniform spindle cells set in a gray myxoid matrix. Note the relatively high apoptotic rate ⇨. Eosinophilic cytoplasm is absent, and the tumor is nondescript in histologic appearance.

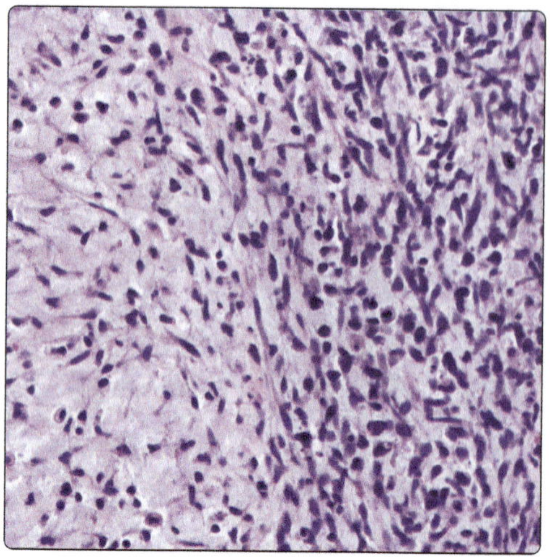

Embryonal Rhabdomyosarcoma: Desmin Expression

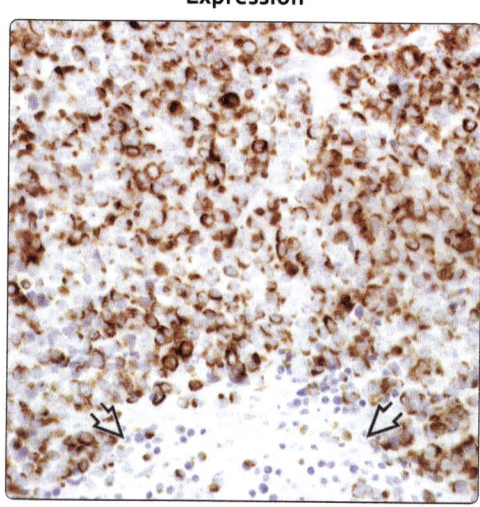

Dense Pattern Embryonal Rhabdomyosarcoma: Focal Myogenin

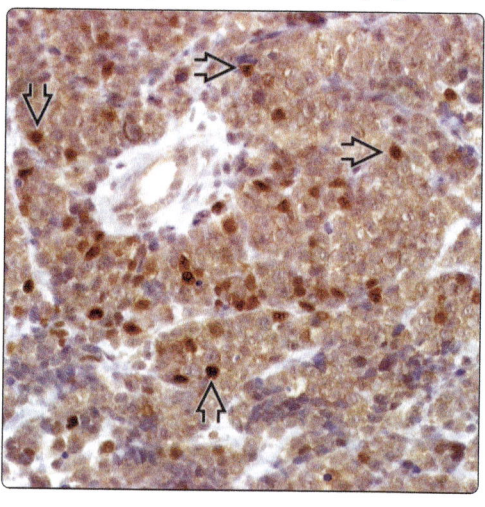

(Left) Desmin expression is usually diffuse and strong in ERMS; however, only viable cells that show some muscle differentiation will express the antigen. Note the negative area ⇨ composed of necrotic tumor cells. (Right) Dense pattern ERMS expresses myogenin in only a few scattered cells ⇨. Sparse myogenin reactivity is characteristic of ERMS and many fusion-negative ARMS.

Dense Pattern Embryonal Rhabdomyosarcoma

Dense Pattern Embryonal Rhabdomyosarcoma

(Left) Dense pattern ERMS can mimic many other small round blue cell tumors, especially if more differentiated rhabdomyoblasts are absent. (Right) Touch imprint of dense pattern ERMS reveals a relatively uniform population of small round blue cells. Tumor cell cytoplasm is scant but eosinophilic, suggesting possible muscle differentiation.

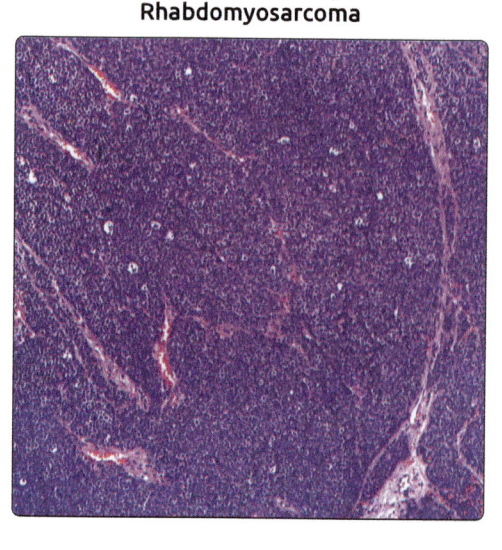

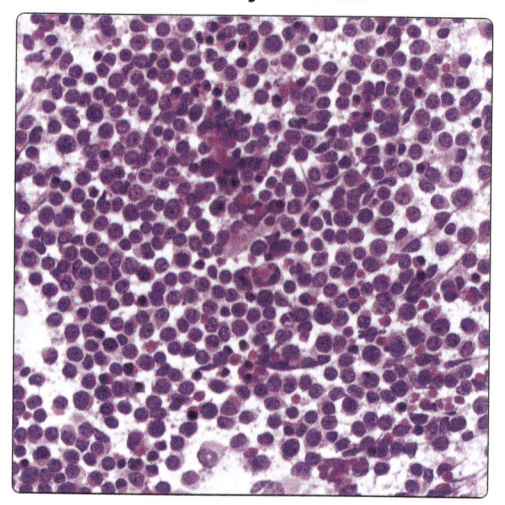

Muscle Sarcomas

Embryonal Rhabdomyosarcoma With Ovoid Nuclei

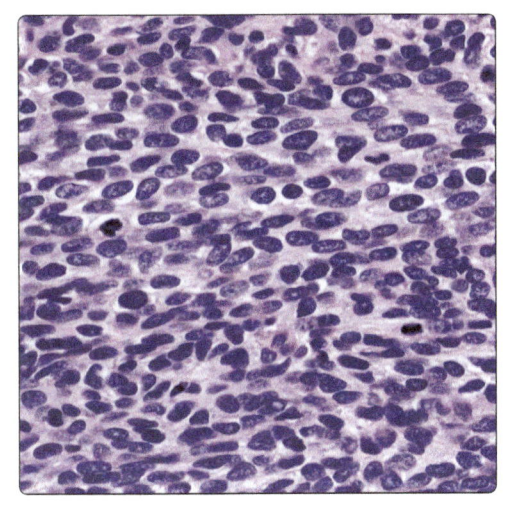

Embryonal Rhabdomyosarcoma: Maturation Post Chemotherapy

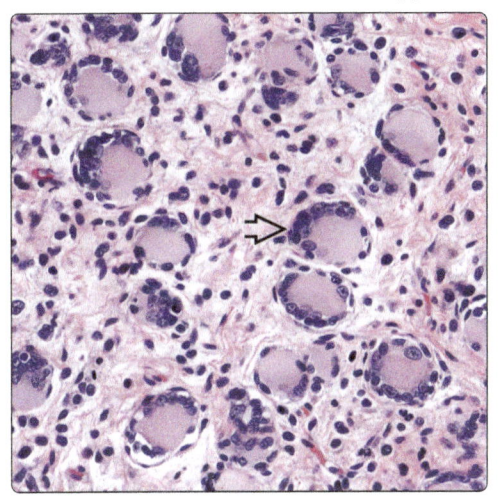

(Left) ERMS shows cellular areas containing cells with ovoid nuclei. Ovoid nuclei are usually absent in ARMS. (Right) Maturation of rhabdomyoblasts is often seen in postchemotherapy resections. Here, ERMS shows striking differentiation toward myotubes ⇨. The preneoadjuvant treatment biopsy contained only primitive small round cell and spindled cells without overt muscle differentiation.

Embryonal Rhabdomyosarcoma: Strong Membranous CD99 Reactivity

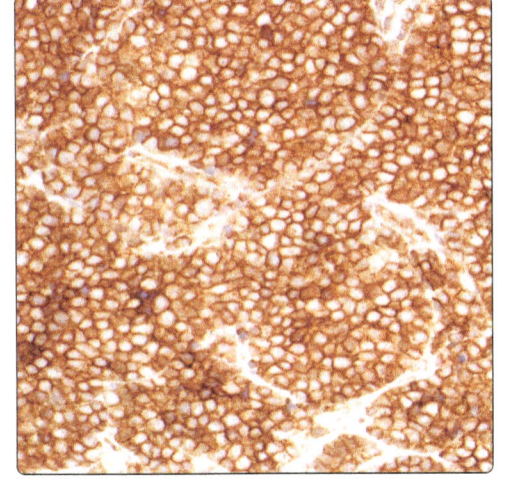

Alveolar Rhabdomyosarcoma Karyotype

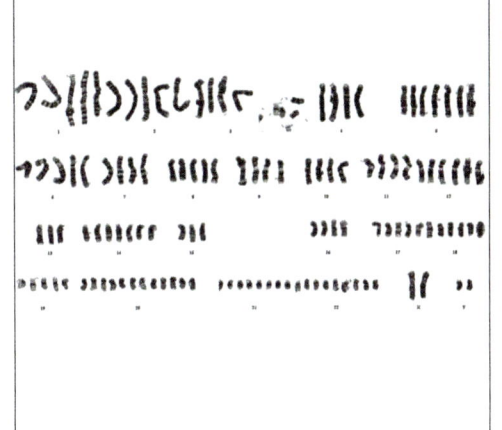

(Left) ERMS shows diffuse membranous expression of CD99. Typically, membranous CD99 reactivity is considered fairly specific for Ewing sarcoma family of tumors; however, membranous expression is found occasionally in other sarcomas, including rhabdomyosarcoma (RMS). (Right) ARMS is known for fusions involving PAX3 or PAX7 and FOXO1; however, other genetic abnormalities occur, as in this rare example of near pentaploidy.

Alveolar Rhabdomyosarcoma With Classic Alveolar Growth Pattern

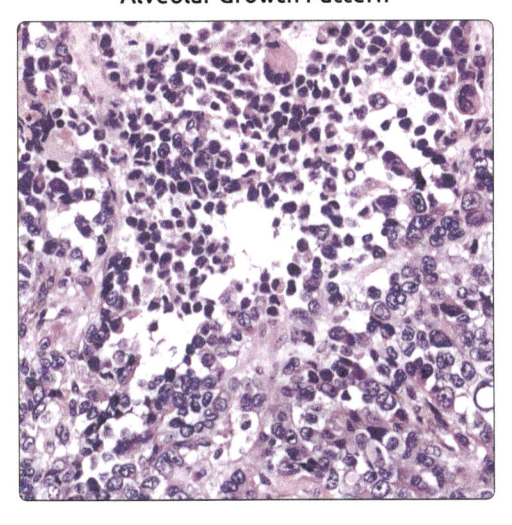

Alveolar Rhabdomyosarcoma With Strap Cells

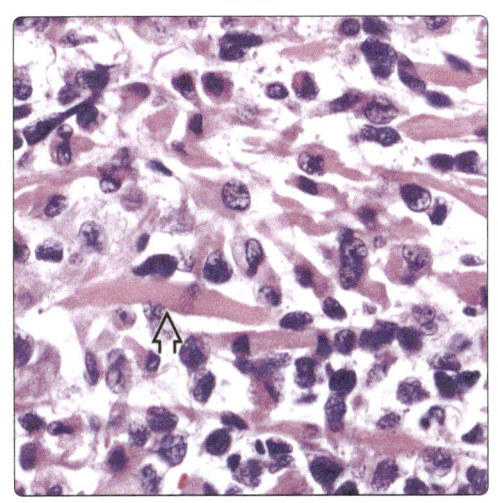

(Left) The classic appearance of ARMS consists of spaces lined by a single residual layer of tumor cells created by drop-off and subsequent necrosis of central cells. This pattern can be appreciated at relatively low power and (although not entirely specific) is a clue to the diagnosis. (Right) ARMS shows many strap cells, some with obvious cross striations ⇨. All types of RMS can contain such diagnostically helpful differentiated cells.

875

Muscle Sarcomas

(Left) ARMS shows classic areas of alveolar spaces. Note the prominent eosinophilia of the cytoplasm of the tumor cells and the round nuclear shape. **(Right)** This area of ARMS in an otherwise histologically classic tumor shows pleomorphic multinucleate tumor cells. Such marked anaplasia may occur in ARMS but is more common in ERMS.

Alveolar Rhabdomyosarcoma

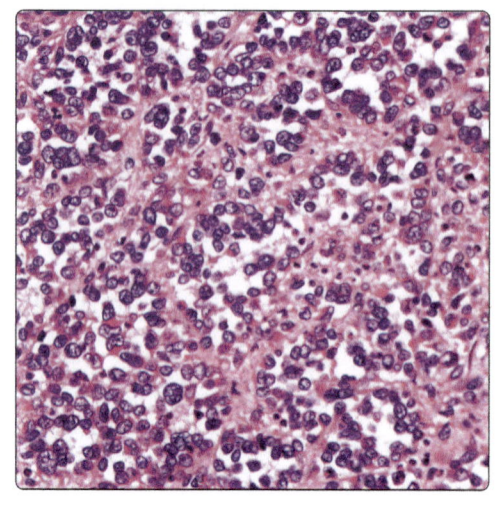

Alveolar Rhabdomyosarcoma With Unusual Marked Anaplasia

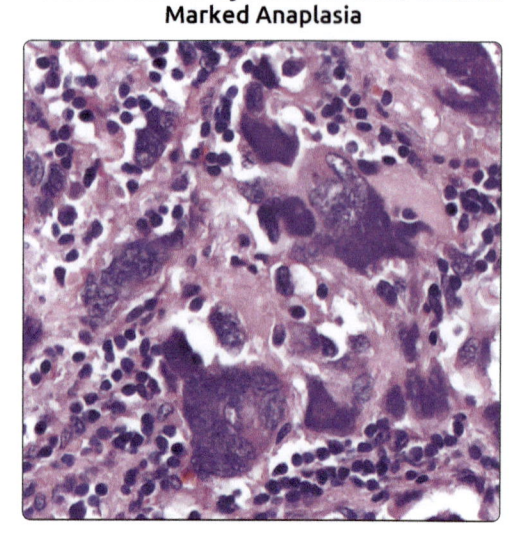

(Left) This patient's leg tumor metastasized to the testis (note seminiferous tubule ➔). Myogenin is diffusely expressed in tumor cells, typical of fusion-positive ARMS. **(Right)** Wreath-like multinucleate giant cells ➔ can be scattered among mononuclear tumor cells in ARMS and are rare to absent in nonanaplastic ERMS.

Alveolar Rhabdomyosarcoma: Typical Diffuse Myogenin Expression

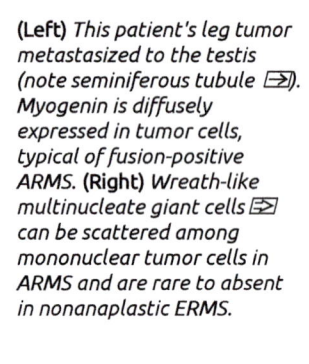

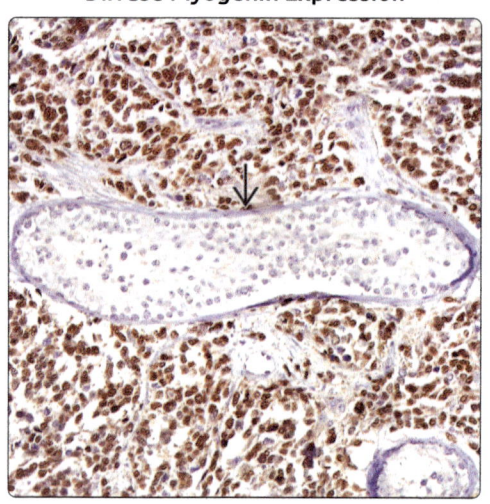

Wreath Cells in Alveolar Rhabdomyosarcoma

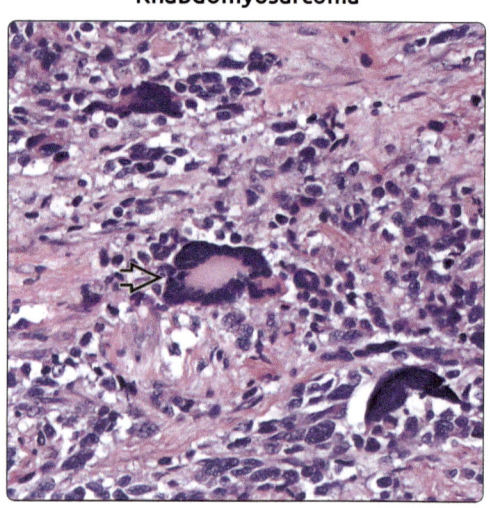

(Left) Bone marrow is a relatively common site of metastasis for ARMS. Here, the tumor cells completely efface normal marrow constituents. Rare ARMS can simulate the presentation of leukemia. **(Right)** Clot section from involved marrow reveals a loose cluster of less-differentiated rhabdomyoblasts that mimic other small round cell tumors. IHC &/or FISH would be needed to establish the diagnosis of metastatic ARMS.

Alveolar Rhabdomyosarcoma With Bone Marrow Involvement

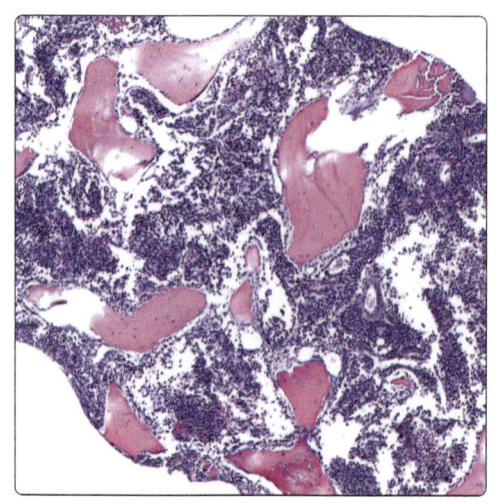

Alveolar Rhabdomyosarcoma

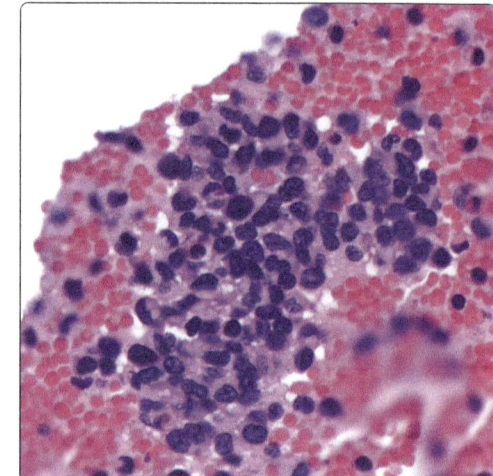

Muscle Sarcomas

Spindle Cell/Sclerosing Rhabdomyosarcoma

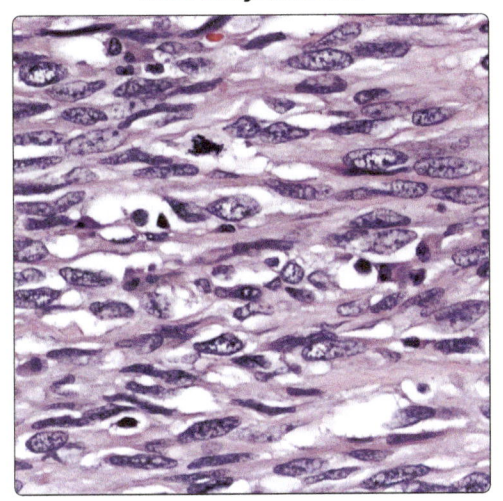

Spindle Cell/Sclerosing Rhabdomyosarcoma: Desmin Expression

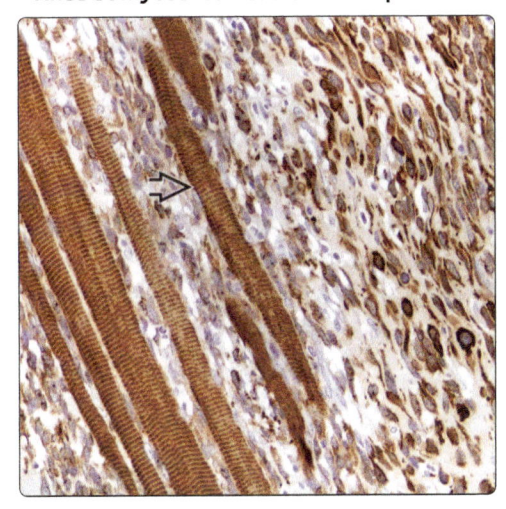

(Left) This spindle cell area of a spindle cell/sclerosing RMS mimics the features of LMS or other spindle cell sarcoma. (Right) Desmin stain is strongly reactive in the tumor cells of this spindle cell/sclerosing RMS. Note the deep location of the tumor infiltrating around normal skeletal muscle fibers, which also serve as an internal positive control ➡.

Sclerosed Region of Spindle Cell/Sclerosing Rhabdomyosarcoma

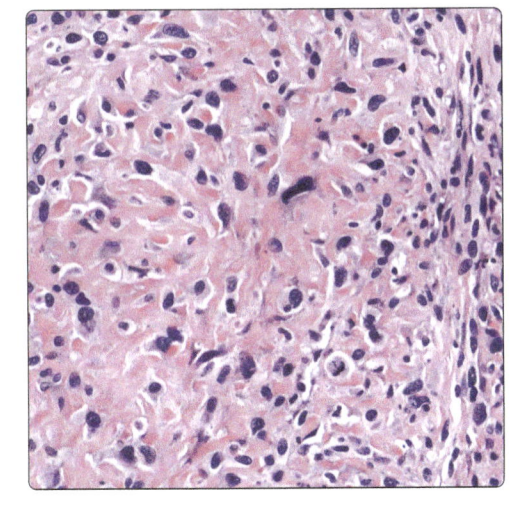

Spindle Cell/Sclerosing Rhabdomyosarcoma: Diffuse Actin

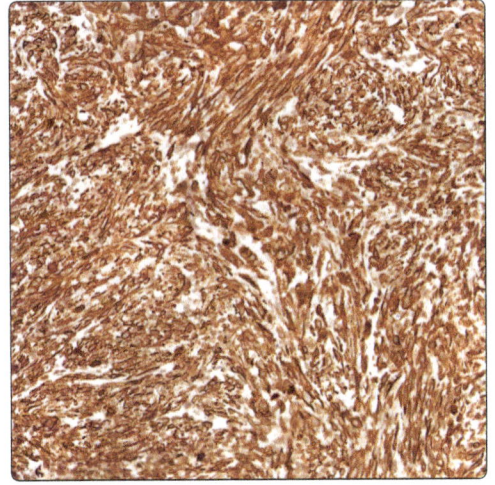

(Left) This collagenized area of a spindle cell/sclerosing RMS contains epithelioid to polygonal cells embedded in dense hyaline fibrosis. Most spindle cell/sclerosing RMS contain both fascicles of spindled cells and dense, fibrotic regions. The latter can impose a pseudovascular pattern on the encased rhabdomyoblasts. (Right) Spindle cell/sclerosing RMS shows strong diffuse SMA expression, a relatively common finding in this type of RMS.

Pleomorphic Rhabdomyosarcoma

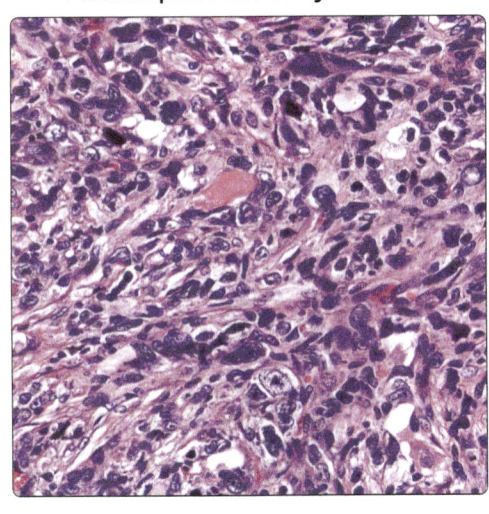

Pleomorphic Rhabdomyosarcoma

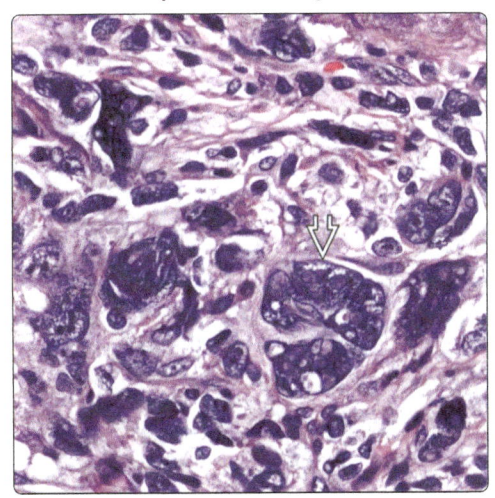

(Left) Pleomorphic RMS mimics other high-grade pleomorphic sarcomas, such as pleomorphic undifferentiated sarcoma, dedifferentiated liposarcoma, and dedifferentiated LMS. In most cases of pleomorphic RMS, myogenin expression is sparse but present and helps confirm the diagnosis. (Right) Note the prominent multinucleation ➡ in this case of pleomorphic RMS. Some cases contain cells with eosinophilic cytoplasm, but cross striations are almost always absent.

Intermediate and Malignant Vascular Tumors

TERMINOLOGY

Definitions
- Mesenchymal tumors that show differentiation toward endothelial cells with intermediate or malignant behavior
  - Angiosarcoma (AS), epithelioid hemangioendothelioma (EHE), Kaposi sarcoma (KS), and other hemangioendotheliomas (HE), including retiform, composite, and kaposiform, and papillary intralymphatic angioendothelioma (PILA)

ETIOLOGY/PATHOGENESIS

Angiosarcoma
- Possible causes
  - Complex genomic changes
  - *CIC* rearrangements &/or missense mutations in ~ 9%
  - Neurofibromatosis type 1 or Maffucci syndrome increases risk
  - Excessive sun exposure
  - Specific chemical exposures
- Further associations
  - Chronic lymphedema
  - Ionizing radiation
  - Longstanding vascular graft

Epithelioid Hemangioendothelioma
- Gene fusion: t(1;3); *WWTR1::CAMTA1* or t(11;X) *YAP1::TFE3*
- Rare other *WWTR1* fusions reported, including *WWTR1::MAML2* and *WWTR1::ACTL6A*

Other Hemangioendotheliomas and PILA
- Retiform, composite, and kaposiform HE and papillary intralymphatic AE
  - Specific molecular alterations found in some to all cases
- Pseudomyogenic hemangioendothelioma
  - Specific gene fusions are driver events
    - *FOSB* fusions: *SERPINE1::FOSB*, *ACTB::FOSB*, *CLTC::FOSB*

Kaposi Sarcoma
- KS-associated herpesvirus (KSHV), a.k.a. human herpesvirus 8 (HHV-8)
  - HHV-8 infection is causative in conjunction with altered host immune response
  - Host risk factors
    - Immune suppression
    - Higher levels of inflammatory cytokines
  - Human papillomavirus subtypes (HPV-14, HPV-12, HPV-24) detected in some tumors
    - Unknown if this superinfection contributes to tumorigenesis
- 5 clinical/epidemiologic scenarios

CLINICAL IMPLICATIONS

Clinical Presentation
- AS
  - Age
    - Cutaneous AS: Most commonly older adults
    - Soft tissue and bone AS: Any age, but older adults more frequent
    - Breast AS: Primary breast AS in younger women than secondary AS
  - Sex: M > F, except for breast location
  - Location
    - Cutaneous AS: Head and neck (scalp) most common site
    - Soft tissue AS: Deep tissue of extremities > trunk > head and neck > body cavities
- EHE
  - Age: Usually young adults to 6th decade
  - Sex: F > M
  - Location
    - Subcutis and deep soft tissues of extremities, trunk, head and neck
    - Visceral locations include liver, spleen, and lungs
- Other hemangioendotheliomas and PILA
  - Retiform HE: Most commonly middle-aged adults; also in children and young adults; M = F

Soft Tissue Angiosarcoma

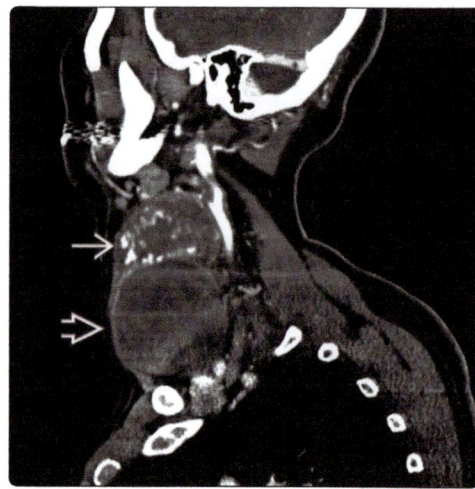

Soft Tissue Angiosarcoma

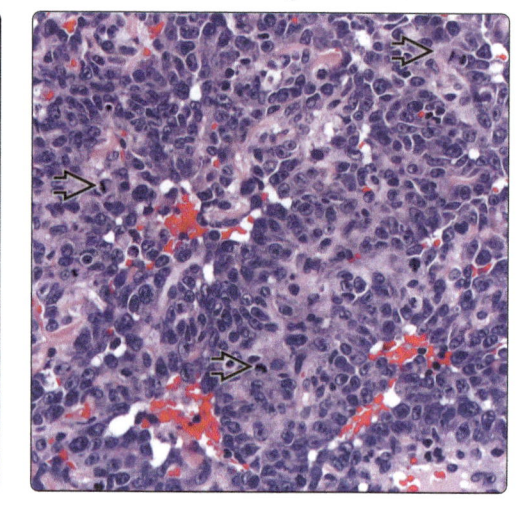

(Left) Sagittal and slightly oblique MR in a 46-year-old man shows a deep 7-cm angiosarcoma (AS) of the neck with cystic ➡ and calcified solid components ➡, which grew rapidly over several months. (Right) Resection of the same case shows high-grade AS containing poorly formed vascular channels and comprising epithelioid-appearing pleomorphic tumor cells. Mitoses are numerous ➡.

Intermediate and Malignant Vascular Tumors

- o Composite HE: Young adults; also in children; F > M
- o Kaposiform HE: Young children (Usually < 1 year); M > F
- o Papillary intralymphatic AE: Adults; F slightly > M; ~ 60 cases reported
- o Pseudomyogenic HE: Young adults; M > F
  - Presents as crops of dermal and deep soft tissue ± bone nodules
- KS
  - o Age and sex vary with epidemiologic form
  - o Location: Skin and oral mucosa, lymph nodes, lungs, GIT, other viscera

Treatment

- AS
  - o Surgery ± radiation ± chemotherapy
  - o Targeted therapies in clinical trials or under development
- EHE
  - o Surgery ± radiation ± chemotherapy
  - o Complete surgical excision
- Other HE and PILA
  - o Surgery for all types
  - o Kaposiform HE also treated with chemotherapy
- KS
  - o Treat immunosuppressive host state
  - o ± surgery ± radiation ± chemotherapy

Prognosis

- AS
  - o Cutaneous AS
    - ↑ rate of local recurrences
    - 20% 5-year survival
  - o Secondary AS: Poor 5-year survival
  - o Primary breast AS
    - Improved 5-year survival compared to other AS
    - Controversial whether low grade predicts improved outcome
  - o Soft tissue AS
    - 30% local recurrence rate
    - 50% distant metastasis rate
    - 30% 5-year survival
- EHE
  - o Classic EHE
    - ~ 15% local recurrence rate
    - 15-30% metastasis rate
    - ~ 20% disease-specific death rate
  - o Malignant EHE
    - Follows more aggressive course than classic EHE
- Other HE and PILA
  - o Retiform HE: High local recurrence rate; only rare regional lymph node metastases; overall excellent survival
  - o Composite HE: 50% local recurrence rate; ~ 10% metastasis rate (usually to regional lymph nodes)
  - o Kaposiform HE: High local recurrence rate; rare regional lymph node metastases; 10% mortality, mostly due to Kasabach-Merritt syndrome
  - o Papillary intralymphatic AE: Excellent outcome with complete excision; exceptionally may metastasize
  - o Pseudomyogenic HE: ~ 60% local recurrence rate; uncommon regional lymph node metastases; presumed excellent overall survival
- KS
  - o Prognosis depends on clinical subtype and stage
  - o Multivisceral involvement portends poor outcome

MICROSCOPIC

Angiosarcoma

- Architecture
  - o Neoplastic vessels present but may be sparse
    - Common tumor vessel features: Interanastomosis, multilayering, hobnailing, intraluminal papillary tufts
  - o Background may be hemorrhagic
  - o Solid growth common
  - o Necrosis frequent
- Cells
  - o Polygonal to epithelioid most commonly
  - o Nuclear atypia varies from minimal to marked
  - o Higher grades often show macronucleoli and ↑ mitotic rate
- Ancillary studies
  - o IHC: Positive for at least 1 vascular marker (CD34, CD31, ERG, FLI-1)
    - Tumors with epithelioid features often express keratins
  - o FISH: *MYC* amplification common in secondary AS
    - *MYC* amplification rare in primary AS

Epithelioid Hemangioendothelioma

- Architecture
  - o Strands, cords, clusters, and isolated tumor cells
  - o Solid growth sometimes present especially in higher grade tumors
  - o Absent to very sparse neoplastic vessels, except in *YAP1::TFE3* fusion variant
  - o 25-33% associated with large vessel growing through and around it
  - o Myxohyaline to chondroid stroma almost always present but may be focal
- Cells
  - o Epithelioid to slightly spindled with mild variation in size and shape
  - o Blister cells have single cytoplasmic vacuoles, which are considered incipient vessel lumina
    - Vacuoles may also contain red blood cells
  - o High-grade "malignant" variant
    - "Malignant EHE" accounts for ~ 33% of all EHE
    - Increased nuclear atypia, including macronucleoli, pleomorphism, increased mitoses
- Ancillary studies
  - o IHC: CD31, CD34, and FLI-1 (+); pankeratin (+) in ~ 33%; actin (+) in ~ 25%
    - TFE3 nuclear expression may be present in EHE of either fusion type but more common in *YAP1::TFE3* fusion
    - CAMTA1: Diffuse nuclear expression in *WWTR1::CAMTA1* fusion
      - Relatively specific marker for EHE of CAMTA1 fusion
  - o FISH: Positive for *WWTR1::CAMTA1* (~ 90-95%) or *YAP1::TFE3* (5-10%) fusions

Intermediate and Malignant Vascular Tumors

Other Hemangioendothelioma and PILA
- Retiform HE: Dermal growth of thin-walled, angulated, anastomosing vessels resembling rete testis often with lymphocytic inflammation
- Composite HE: Mixed pattern most often composed of retiform HE and EHE, but also may include overt AS-like areas
- Kaposiform HE: Multinodular with spindled areas resembling KS and areas with capillary hemangioma features
- Papillary intralymphatic angioendothelioma (PILA): Noncircumscribed proliferation of lymphatic channels ± hobnailing ± intraluminal tufts without atypia
- Pseudomyogenic HE: Epithelioid to spindled cells forming nodules, sheets, short fascicles without vessel formation
  - Some cells may mimic rhabdomyoblasts (large strap shaped with brightly eosinophilic cytoplasm)
  - Blister cells absent or rare
  - IHC
    - FOSB: Diffusely positive in tumor nuclei in ~ 90%
    - Vascular markers variable: ERG and FLI-1 positive in ~ 100%; CD31 positive in 50%; CD34 negative
    - Keratin: Typically diffusely strongly positive
  - FISH
    - Positive for SERPINE1::FOSB fusion: ~ 60%
    - Positive for ACTB::FOSB fusion: Perhaps up to 40-50%
    - FOSB fusions are not specific for pseudomyogenic HE; also occur in epithelioid hemangiomas
      - Epithelioid hemangioma fusions: FOS, FOSB, or FOX01 with various partners

Kaposi Sarcoma
- Architecture
  - Initial patch stage
    - Subtle pattern of increased vessels infiltrating dermis
  - Developed lesions
    - Fascicles of spindled cells with embedded slit-like vascular channels
    - Vascular channels often contain red blood cells
  - Multiple variants described
- Cells
  - Spindled with minimal atypia but high mitotic rate
  - Inflammation prominent
  - Eosinophilic hyaline bodies commonly present
- Ancillary studies
  - Positive for HHV8, CD31, CD34, and FLI-1

GENETIC FINDINGS

Angiosarcoma
- Karyotype: Complex aneuploid
- Major genes altered
  - CIC rearrangements ± missense mutations in ~ 9%
    - Patients with CIC alterations: Typically younger than most AS patients (average age: 41 years)
  - Upregulation of vascular-specific tyrosine kinase genes
    - TIE1, KDR, TEK, FLT1
  - KDR mutations (10%)
    - KDR strongly expressed in breast AS (primary and secondary)
  - MYC amplified in secondary AS and only rarely in primary AS
  - FLT4 amplified in ~ 25% of secondary AS
  - PTPRB mutated in 26%
    - Encodes tyrosine phosphatase that inhibits angiogenesis
    - Expressed normally exclusively in endothelial cells
    - All mutations disrupt PTPRB function
  - PLCG1 mutated in ~ 10%
  - TP53 mutated (20%) and p53 overexpressed (~ 50%)
  - KDM6A mutated (13%)
  - RAS genes (HRAS, KRAS, NRAS) mutated (~ 14%)
  - PTEN expression decreased (~ 40% of primary bone AS)
  - KIT overexpressed (~ 90% of soft tissue AS and in secondary AS)
  - RET overexpressed in many secondary AS
- Major pathways dysregulated
  - Angiogenesis pathways
  - Cell cycle
    - RB1 pathway disturbed in 55% of primary bone AS but not in extraosseous AS
    - CDKN2A expression lost in 50% of primary osseous AS
  - Apoptosis
  - AKT/PI3K pathway hyperactivated
  - TGF-β1 pathway hyperactivated in primary intraosseous AS
  - MAPK pathway hyperactivated (~ 50%)

Epithelioid Hemangioendothelioma
- Fusion genes
  - t(1;3); WWTR1::CAMTA1 in ~ 90% of cases
    - Creates novel transcription factor with overexpression of C-terminus of CAMTA1
  - t(11;X); YAP1::TFE3 in ~ 10% of cases
    - Causes over expression of TFE3
    - YAP1 similar to WWTR1: Both encode for WW-domain containing transcriptional coactivators
    - EHE with this gene fusion may have better prognosis than tumors with WWTR1::CAMTA1 fusions
  - Other rare WWTR1 fusions: with MAML2 or ACTL6A as partner
    - Heart: preferred site of occurrence

Other Hemangioendotheliomas and PILA
- Pseudomyogenic hemangioendothelioma (epithelioid sarcoma-like hemangioendothelioma)
  - t(7;19)(q22;q13); SERPINE1::FOSB
    - Results in overexpression of FOSB → abnormal transcription of multiple genes
  - t(7;19)(p22;q13); ACTB::FOSB fusion
    - Also results in overexpression of FOSB
- Retiform HE: YAP1::MAML2 fusion
- Composite HE: PTBP1::MAML2 and EPC1::PHC2 fusions
- Kaposiform HE: GNA14 or PIK3CA mosaics
- Papillary intralymphatic angioendothelioma (PILA): PIK3CA mutations

Kaposi Sarcoma
- Karyotype: Oligoclonal or polyclonal in most cases
- Viral genes important in pathogenesis

Intermediate and Malignant Vascular Tumors

- Latent and lytic (active) gene expression contribute to pathogenesis
  - Actively infected cells (which eventually lyse) induce release of viral and cellular cytokines with proliferative, angiogenic, immune-regulatory activities
- LANA-1
  - Nuclear latency protein of KS virus
  - Inhibits p53 and RB1
  - Increases transcription of *MYC*
- Viral cytokines trigger Th2 inflammatory response and inhibit Th1 response
  - Depresses host immune surveillance
- vGPCR (viral G-protein coupled receptor)
  - Expressed early in actively infected lytic cells (~ 5% of tumor cells in tumor)
  - Works in paracrine manner to enhance angiogenesis
- Major host genes altered
  - *PTGS2* upregulated
    - Recruits activated immune cells that release proangiogenic factors, growth factors
    - Matrix metalloproteinase secreted by tumor cells
  - *HEY1* upregulated and overexpressed
    - Downstream effector of Notch pathway
  - *KRAS* mutated
  - *NFKB1* constitutively activated
  - *STAT3* constitutively activated
  - *PDLIM2* (negative controller of NFKB1 and STAT3) repressed in KS via epigenetic promoter methylation
  - *MAP4K4* overexpressed
    - Promotes reactivation of HHV-8 virus
    - Enhances invasiveness of tumor spindle cells
- Major pathways dysregulated
  - Cell cycle hijacked
  - Apoptosis suppressed
  - Angiogenesis augmented
  - NOTCH pathway hyperactivated
  - AKT-PI3K pathway hyperactivated
  - mTOR pathway hyperactivated

DIFFERENTIAL DIAGNOSIS

Angiosarcoma

- Hemangioma
  - Spindle cell hemangioma
    - Often arises in association with medium-sized vessel
    - No significant atypia of spindled tumor cells
    - Bland blister cells often present
  - Epithelioid hemangioma
    - Lobulated and circumscribed
    - Well-formed vessels with plump lining endothelial cells with usually only minimal nuclear atypia
    - Absent to sparse spindled tumor cells
    - *FOS* or *FOSB* rearrangements detectable by FISH
- Atypical vascular proliferation
  - Occurs in dermis of irradiated tissue
  - Retiform slit-like anastomosing vessels dissect collagen
  - Cytologic atypia minimal
  - FISH: Negative for *MYC* amplification
- Pseudoangiomatoid carcinoma
  - May have conventional areas forming glands/tubules
  - IHC: Negative for vascular markers; often positive for CEA, MOC-31
- Other spindle cell sarcomas: Lack neoplastic vessels; usually lack specific vascular marker expression, such as CD31 and ERG
- Other sarcomas with epithelioid cells
  - Lack neoplastic vessel formation
  - Usually lack vascular markers
    - Exception is epithelioid sarcoma: Often expresses CD34 and ERG
      - Most epithelioid sarcomas also show loss of INI1 expression (diagnostically helpful)

Epithelioid Hemangioendothelioma

- Epithelioid hemangioma
  - Well-formed vessels
  - Lack translocations of EHE
- AS
  - May be difficult to distinguish "malignant" (high-grade) EHE from AS
    - AS lacks translocations of EHE
    - AS lacks CAMTA1 or TFE3 IHC reactivity
- Extraskeletal myxoid chondrosarcoma
  - Lacks blister cells
  - Lobulated growth with peripheral hypercellularity
  - FISH shows break-apart of *NR4A3*
- Myoepithelioma
  - Lacks relationship to large vessel
  - Negative for blister cells
  - Negative for vascular markers

Kaposi Sarcoma

- AS
  - Usually more cytologically atypical
  - Commonly has epithelioid cell morphology
  - IHC: Negative for HHV8
- Other spindle cell sarcomas: Often lack slit like vascular channels; negative for HHV8

SELECTED REFERENCES

1. Diaz-Perez JA et al: Benign and low-grade superficial endothelial cell neoplasms in the molecular era. Semin Diagn Pathol. 40(4):267-83, 2023
2. Torrence D et al: The genetics of vascular tumours: an update. Histopathology. 80(1):19-32, 2022
3. Antonescu CR et al: Recurrent YAP1 and MAML2 gene rearrangements in retiform and composite hemangioendothelioma. Am J Surg Pathol. 44(12):1677-84, 2020
4. Suurmeijer AJH et al: Variant WWTR1 gene fusions in epithelioid hemangioendothelioma-a genetic subset associated with cardiac involvement. Genes Chromosomes Cancer. 59(7):389-95, 2020
5. Agaram NP et al: Expanding the spectrum of genetic alterations in pseudomyogenic hemangioendothelioma with recurrent novel ACTB-FOSB gene fusions. Am J Surg Pathol. 42(12):1653-61, 2018
6. Hung YP et al: FOSB is a useful diagnostic Marker for pseudomyogenic hemangioendothelioma. Am J Surg Pathol. 41(5):596-606, 2017
7. Huang SC et al: Recurrent CIC gene abnormalities in angiosarcomas: a molecular study of 120 cases with concurrent investigation of PLCG1, KDR, MYC, and FLT4 gene alterations. Am J Surg Pathol. 40(5):645-55, 2016
8. Doyle LA et al: Nuclear expression of CAMTA1 distinguishes epithelioid hemangioendothelioma from histologic mimics. Am J Surg Pathol. 40(1):94-102, 2016
9. Gramolelli S et al: The role of Kaposi sarcoma-associated herpesvirus in the pathogenesis of Kaposi sarcoma. J Pathol. 235(2):368-80, 2015

Intermediate and Malignant Vascular Tumors

Breast Angiosarcoma

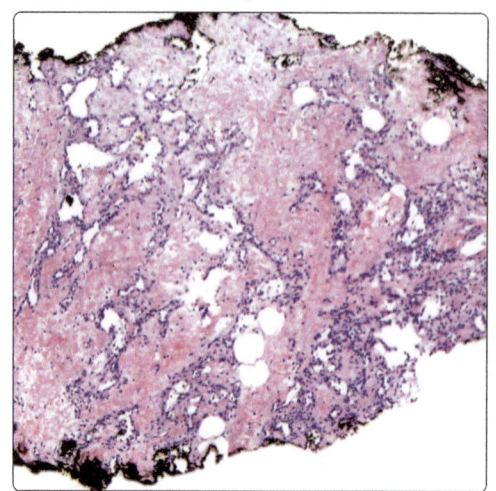

Low-Grade Angiosarcoma

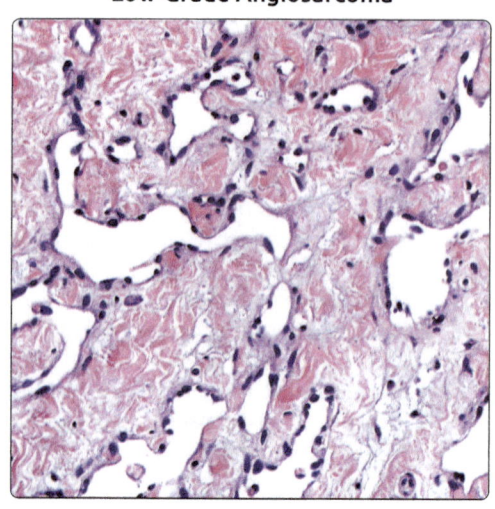

(Left) Low-grade AS arose in the breast of a 17-year-old girl with no known risk factors. **(Right)** Breast AS in the same case shows gaping, thin-walled vessels with minimal nuclear atypia other than hyperchromasia and subtle hobnailing. The diagnosis of AS was supported by a diffusely infiltrative growth pattern.

Metastatic Angiosarcoma to Soft Tissue

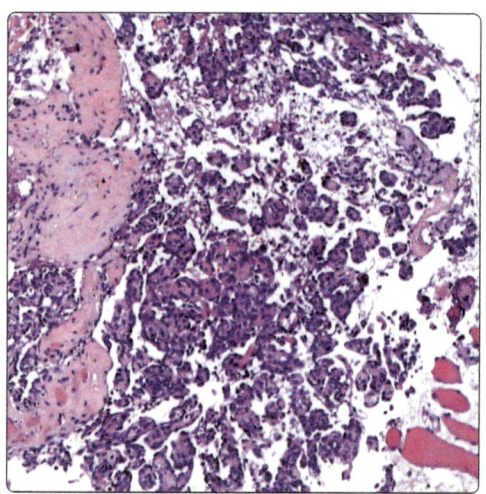

Intermediate-Grade Angiosarcoma

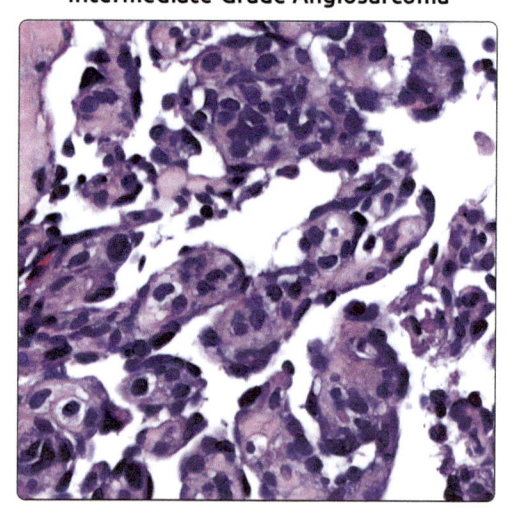

(Left) In the same case, metastasis to the deep soft tissue of the forearm from low-grade breast AS is shown. Metastasis occurred 7 years after initial presentation. The tumor forms vascular channels, is partly fibrotic, and infiltrates skeletal muscle. **(Right)** Metastatic AS in the same case shows increased cellularity and nuclear pleomorphism, consistent with intermediate-grade AS. The prognostic impact of grade in breast AS is controversial.

Scalp Angiosarcoma

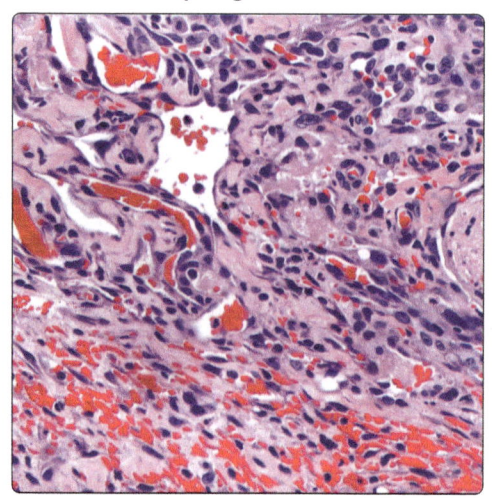

Poorly Differentiated Angiosarcoma

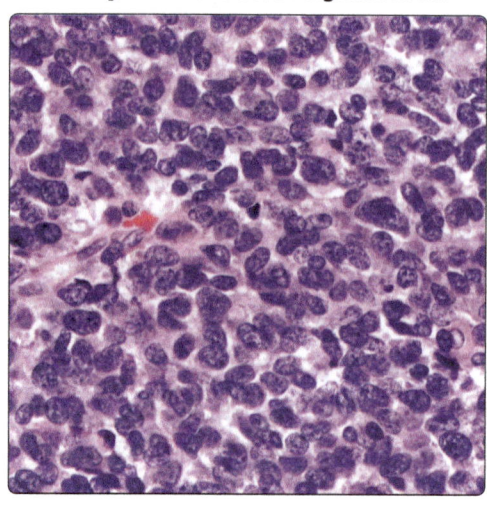

(Left) The vascular nature of this high-grade scalp AS is evident by anastomosing channels of irregular shape lined by atypical endothelial cells. Hemorrhage is present and is commonly a feature of higher grade AS. **(Right)** Poorly differentiated scalp AS contains areas that do not form vessels and lack intracytoplasmic lumina. However, other regions showed classic vasculogenesis. The cells in this area also strongly expressed CD31.

Intermediate and Malignant Vascular Tumors

Epithelioid Angiosarcoma

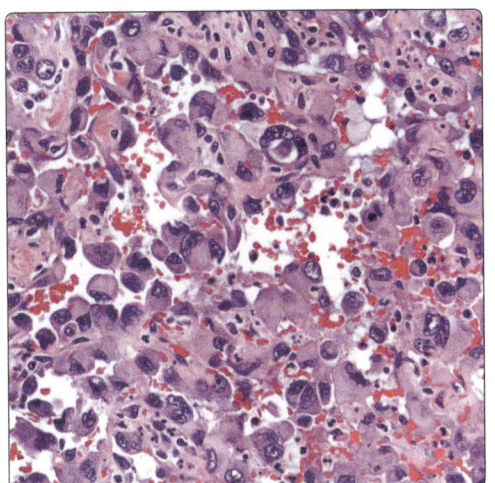

Epithelioid Angiosarcoma

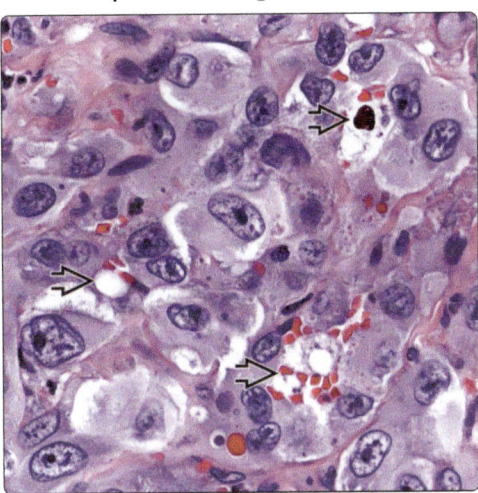

(Left) High-grade AS of deep soft tissue shows an epithelioid cell morphology with dyscohesion. Well-formed vascular channels are absent. (Right) High-grade AS with epithelioid-appearing tumor cells shows marked nuclear pleomorphism, prominent nucleoli, and rare cytoplasmic or paracellular nascent blood vessel lumina that variably contain whole or fragmented red blood cells or hemosiderin ⇨.

CK-PAN Expression in Angiosarcoma

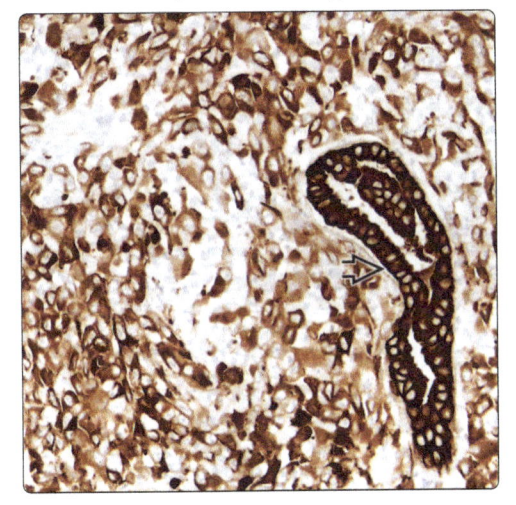

CD31 Expression in Angiosarcoma

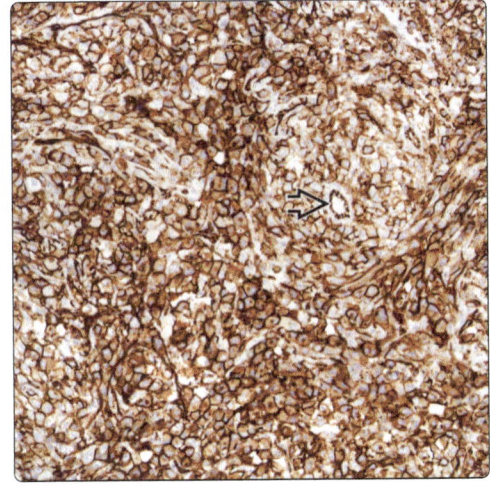

(Left) AS of the scalp shows strong diffuse expression of CK-PAN. An eccrine duct ⇨ serves as a strong internal control. ~ 50% of epithelioid AS express keratins, a possibly confusing finding. (Right) Most AS express CD31, as in this case of epithelioid AS. The reactivity pattern can be membranous, cytoplasmic, or mixed. Here, it is predominantly membranous. A normal vessel ⇨ provides a good internal control.

Kaposi Sarcoma

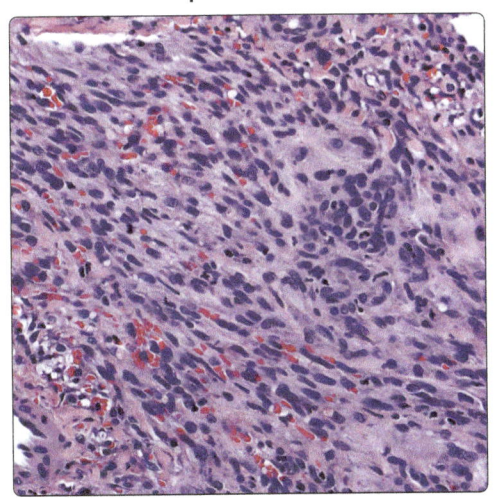

HHV8 Expression in Kaposi Sarcoma

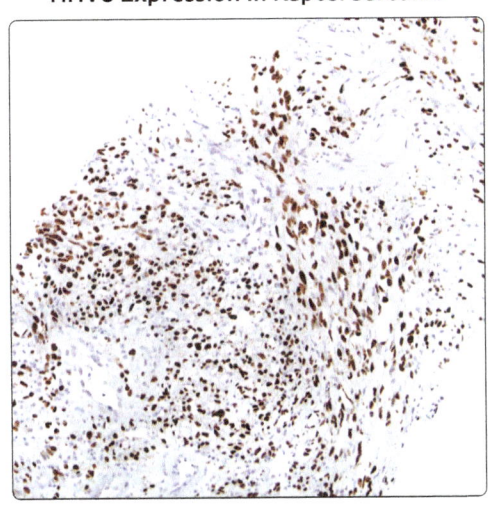

(Left) Kaposi sarcoma (KS) shows the characteristic proliferation of bland spindle cells with embedded slit-like vessels. Note the hemorrhage and scattered lymphocytes, common features in KS. (Right) Core needle biopsy of a soft tissue lesion shows diffuse nuclear expression of HHV8, a helpful diagnostic finding in KS. Spindled tumor cells of KS also usually express CD31, CD34, and D2-40.

Intermediate and Malignant Vascular Tumors

Epithelioid Hemangioendothelioma

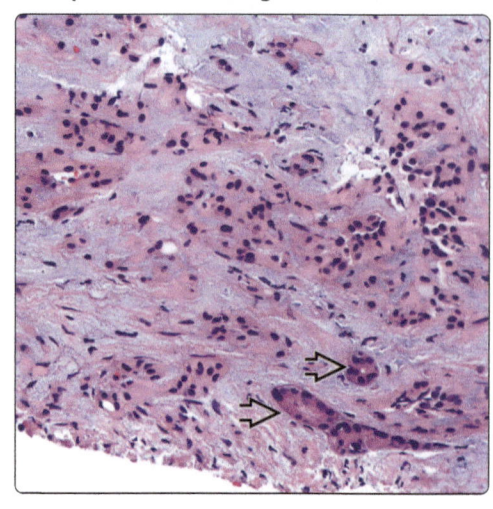

Epithelioid Hemangioendothelioma Matrix

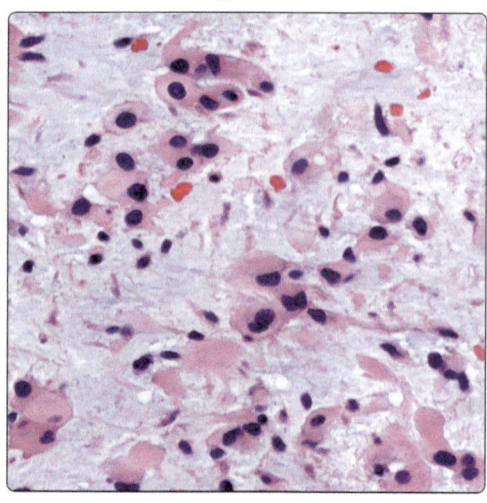

(Left) Core needle biopsy of a liver mass in a 31-year-old man reveals epithelioid hemangioendothelioma (EHE). A few residual hepatocyte groups ⇒ are surrounded by tumor. The liver is a relatively common primary site for EHE. (Right) The characteristic myxohyaline matrix of EHE ranges from gray to pink. In this tumor, it assumes a blue-gray color.

Blister Cells in Epithelioid Hemangioendothelioma

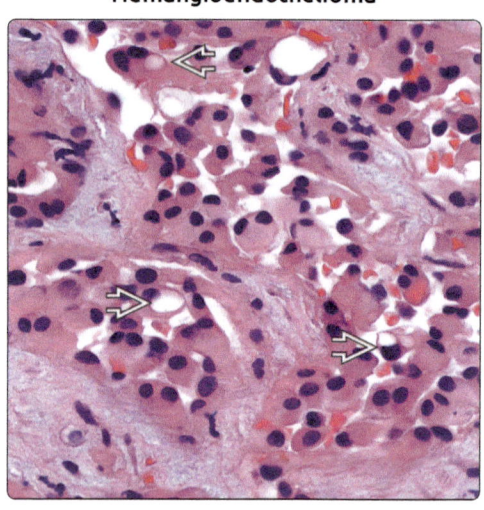

CD31 Expression in Epithelioid Hemangioendothelioma

(Left) Most cases of EHE lack well-formed tumor blood vessels. However, clues to the possible diagnosis of a vascular tumor seen here include tumor cell dyscohesion with intermixed red blood cells filling the ragged open spaces, and blister cells ⇒ (cells with cytoplasmic vacuoles that indent the nucleus and which may represent early vessel formation). (Right) CD31 is expressed in the epithelioid tumor cells of EHE in a crisp membranous pattern ➡.

Pseudomyogenic Hemangioendothelioma

Pseudomyogenic Hemangioendothelioma

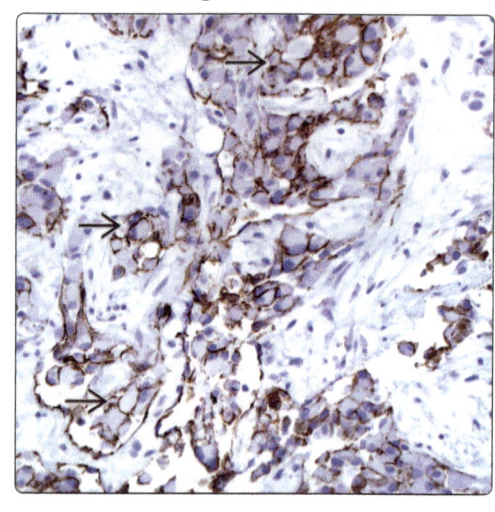

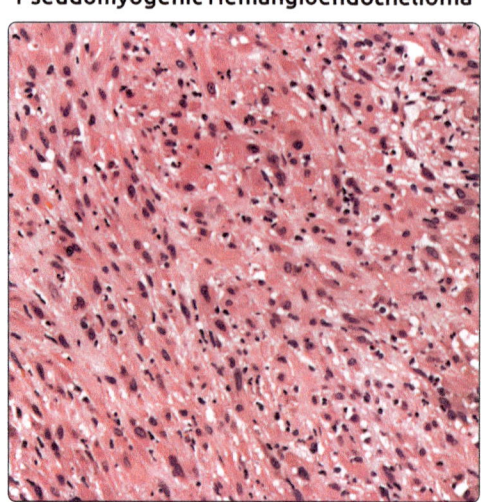

(Left) Pseudomyogenic HE shows epithelioid tumor cells with relatively abundant eosinophilic cytoplasm. The tumor transitions from epithelioid areas to more spindled areas in the left side of the image. (From DP: Soft Tissue.) (Right) At high magnification, the pseudomyogenic HE cells have large but not pleomorphic nuclei. On H&E, this low-grade vascular tumor can mimic a smooth muscle tumor or epithelioid sarcoma. (From DP: Soft Tissue.)

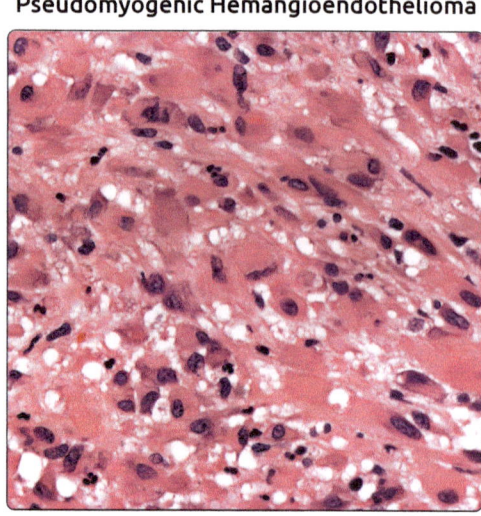

Intermediate and Malignant Vascular Tumors

Kaposiform Hemangioendothelioma

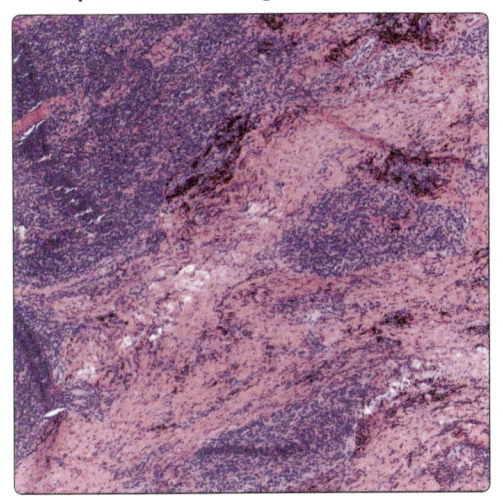

Kaposiform Hemangioendothelioma With Kaposi-Like Features

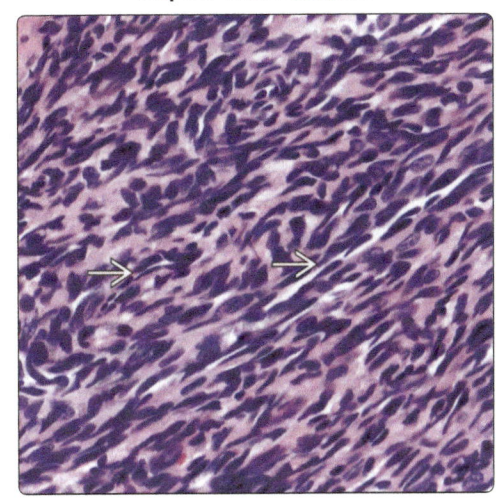

(Left) Kaposiform HE shows characteristic multilobularity at low magnification. In this example, hemosiderin is deposited next to islands of tumor. (Right) KS-like areas of kaposiform HE are composed of fascicles of spindled cells with intermingled slit-like blood vessels ➡. Unlike KS, the tumor cells lack HHV8 expression.

CD31 Expression in Kaposiform Hemangioendothelioma

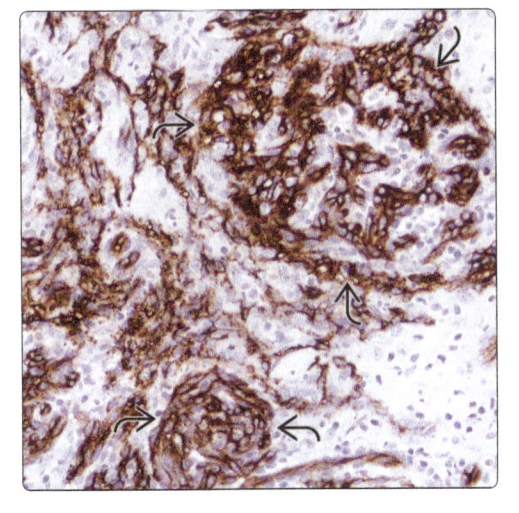

Composite Hemangioendothelioma

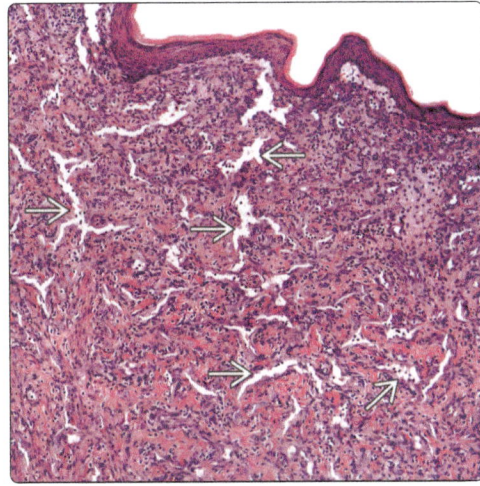

(Left) A common feature in the capillary hemangioma-like areas of kaposiform HE are balls of vessels reminiscent of renal glomeruli ➡. CD31 highlights these glomeruloid arrangements. (Right) Composite HE shows a dissecting dermal proliferation of ragged, thin-walled branching vessels resembling retiform HE ➡. Most composite HE are centered in the dermis, as is the case with this example.

Composite Hemangioendothelioma With AS-Like Vascular Channels

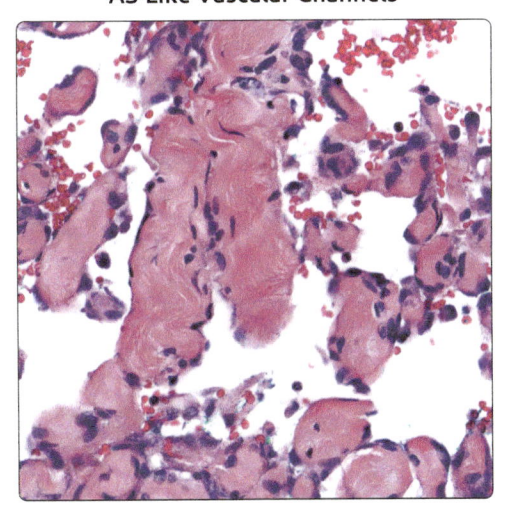

Composite Hemangioendothelioma With Epithelioid Hemangioma-Like Area

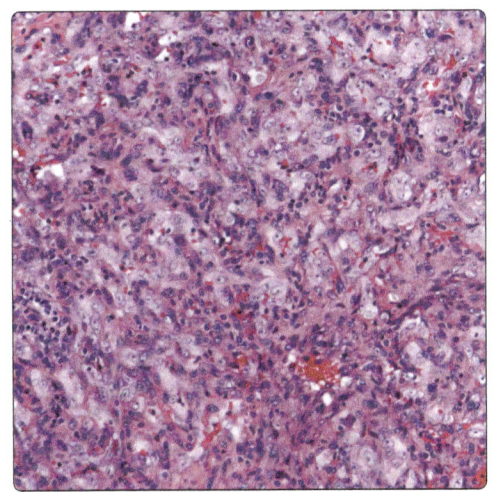

(Left) Composite HE mimics low-grade AS with irregular, poorly formed vascular channels with superimposed Masson change lined by a single layer of endothelial cells with nuclear hyperchromasia. An AS-like component does not worsen the outcome. (Right) Composite HE mimics epithelioid hemangioma. The most common patterns in composite HE are retiform and epithelioid HE, but it can also resemble epithelioid or spindle cell hemangioma.

Malignant Peripheral Nerve Sheath Tumor

KEY FACTS

TERMINOLOGY
- Sarcoma often arising from nerve, from benign nerve sheath tumor, or in association with neurofibromatosis type 1 (NF1)

ETIOLOGY/PATHOGENESIS
- 50% associated with NF1
  - Lifetime incidence: 2-16%
- 40% sporadic
- 10% associated with radiation
- NF1-related and most sporadic MPNST require biallelic inactivation of *NF1* + additional alterations to develop
- Epithelioid variant **not** usually associated with NF1 and driven by *SMARCB1* (22q) mutations

CLINICAL ISSUES
- Mostly adults (20-50 years)
- Most (70%) arise in major nerve trunks
- Local recurrence: > 40%
- Metastasis: 30-60%
- 5-year survival: 15-34%

MOLECULAR
- Deficiency of neurofibromin (NF1 protein) leads to abnormal activation of numerous cell pathways, primarily RAS related
- Common but inconsistent additional genetic aberrations include *CDKN2A* (early event), *TP53*, *RB1* (25%), *PTEN*, *EGFR*, and PRC2 genes modulating histone methylation
- Many genes are up- or downregulated with subsequent oncogenic effects

MICROSCOPIC
- Mostly high-grade sarcoma
- Conventional (spindle cell) MPNST (80%)
  - Long fascicles of closely spaced hyperchromatic spindle cells ± pleomorphic cells ± small round cells
- Epithelioid MPNST (5%)
- Heterologous differentiation (15%)

Deep MPNST

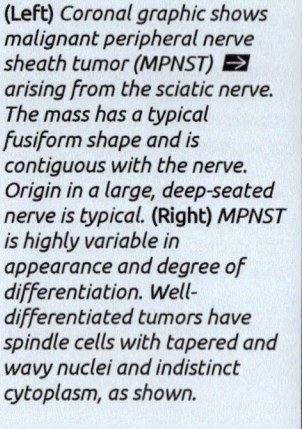

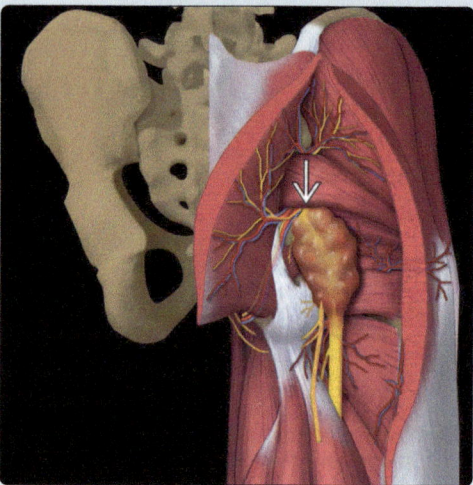

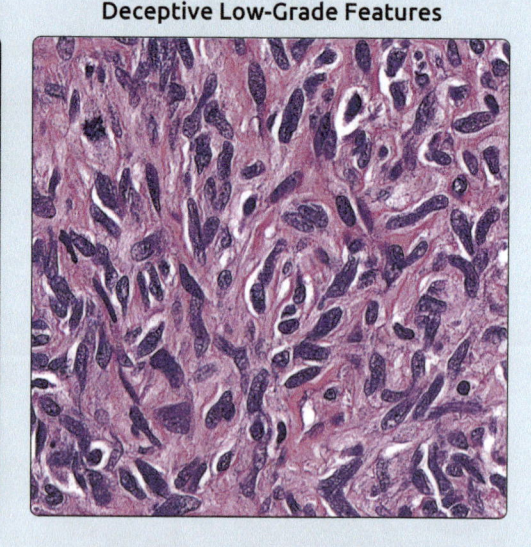

Deceptive Low-Grade Features

(Left) Coronal graphic shows malignant peripheral nerve sheath tumor (MPNST) ➡ arising from the sciatic nerve. The mass has a typical fusiform shape and is contiguous with the nerve. Origin in a large, deep-seated nerve is typical. (Right) MPNST is highly variable in appearance and degree of differentiation. Well-differentiated tumors have spindle cells with tapered and wavy nuclei and indistinct cytoplasm, as shown.

MPNST Arising in Plexiform Neurofibroma

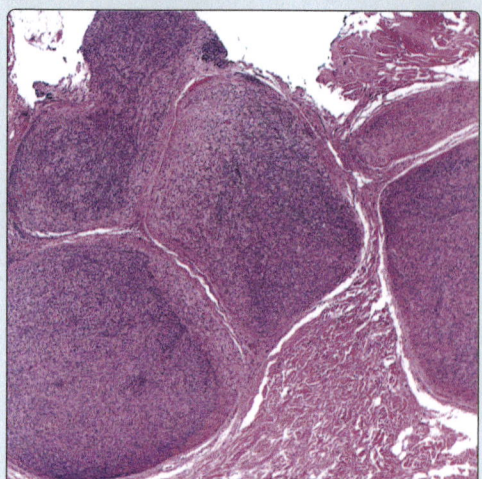

MPNST in Plexiform Neurofibroma

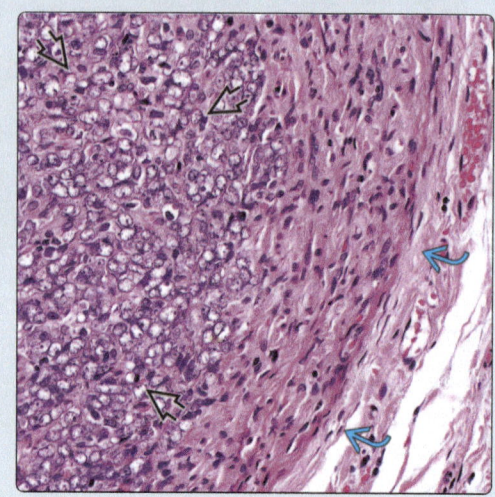

(Left) Plexiform neurofibroma undergoing transformation to MPNST is shown. This patient presented in early childhood with diagnostic features of neurofibromatosis type 1 (NF1). (Right) This case of MPNST is epithelioid, hypercellular, and markedly atypical ➡. It is entirely confined within the margins of involved plexiform neurofibroma ➡. Not all transformed cases are so obvious.

Malignant Peripheral Nerve Sheath Tumor

TERMINOLOGY

Abbreviations
- Malignant peripheral nerve sheath tumor (MPNST)

Definitions
- Spindle cell sarcoma often arising from nerve, from benign nerve sheath tumor, or in association with neurofibromatosis type 1 (NF1)

ETIOLOGY/PATHOGENESIS

Genetic Predisposition
- 50% associated with NF1
  - Lifetime incidence: 2-16%
- 40% sporadic

Environmental Exposure
- 10% associated with radiation

Molecular Pathogenesis
- NF1: Caused by germline mutation of *NF1* tumor suppressor gene (17q)
  - Additional somatic loss of 2nd *NF1* allele required for tumorigenesis + additional genetic/epigenetic changes
- Epithelioid MPNST is usually **not** associated with NF1
  - May arise from schwannoma or nonsyndromic neurofibroma
  - Associated with functional loss of *SMARCB1* locus (22q) in many cases
    - *SMARCB1* is located adjacent to *NF2* (22q12)
- NF1-related and most sporadic MPNST require biallelic inactivation of *NF1* + additional alterations to develop
  - Neurofibromin functions as tumor suppressor
    - *RAS* GTPase activity inactivates RAS pathways
      - Loss of neurofibromin dysregulates cell proliferation, survival, migration, and differentiation
  - Neurofibromin involves cytoskeleton, calcium- and cAMP-modulated pathways, and others
- MPNST has more primitive stem cell-like tumor cells than neurofibroma
  - These cells are enriched for *ZEB1* expression and are most similar to neural crest mesenchymal-like cells
    - May represent drug target

CLINICAL ISSUES

Epidemiology
- Incidence: Rare (~ 5-10% of soft tissue sarcomas); mostly adults 20-50 years; M = F

Site
- Common sites: Thigh, buttock, trunk, upper arm, retroperitoneum, head and neck
  - Mostly deep: 70% arise in major nerve trunks

Prognosis
- Poor (5-year survival: 15-34%)
  - NF1 patients have worse overall prognosis

MOLECULAR

Cytogenetics: Complex Aneuploid Karyotype
- Complex aneuploid karyotypes most commonly
  - Any chromosome can be affected
  - Near triploidy present in some cases

Molecular Genetics
- Genes commonly overexpressed or amplified (> 15% of cases) in conventional (spindled cell) MPNST
  - Growth factor receptors or interacters: *EGFR, PDGFRA, IGF1R, MET*
  - Cell cycle genes: *CDK4, FOXM1, TOP2A*
  - Angiogenesis gene: *PTGS2*
  - Mitotic regulators: *BUB1B, PBK, NEK2*
- Genes commonly lost or mutated (> 15% of cases) in conventional MPNST include *TP53, PTEN, CDKN2A, RB1,* PRC2 (polycomb repressor complex 2) genes, and *BRAF*

Gene Expression Profiling in Conventional MPNST
- NF1 deficiency → RAS hyperactivation → AKT/mTOR and RAF/MEK/ERK pathways hyperactivation
- ↑ angiogenesis occurs in MPNST due to overexpression of angiogenesis factors, such as VEGFA

Epigenetic Findings in Conventional MPNST
- PRC2 is impaired (~ 80% of conventional MPNST)
  - Normally modulates histone methylation by trimethylating H3K27 histone 3 protein
  - *SUZ12, EED, EPC1,* and *CHD4* encode proteins in complex and commonly show LOF mutations in MPNST
    - Leads to lack of normal methylation of histone H3 protein expression (loss of H3K27me3)
    - Abnormally nonmethylated (instead acetylated) H3 proteins enable *BRD4* to bind and thereby activate transcription of oncogenic factors
- Hypermethylation of *RASSF1* in MPNST arising in NF1 patients independently confers worse prognosis
- Downregulation of miR-210 promotes proliferation and invasion

Tumor Immune Microenvironment
- Cases with H3K27 loss show protumorigenic immune microenvironment

MICROSCOPIC

Histologic Features
- Wide spectrum of cytoarchitectural patterns
  - High-grade sarcoma appearance: Hypercellular, pleomorphic or coarse chromatin, high mitotic rate and geographic necrosis
  - Only ~ 15% are histologically low grade
  - Diffuse sarcomatous proliferation with no evidence of nerve or nerve sheath origin common
  - Nerve sheath differentiation: Nuclear palisades or tactoid or Wagner-Meissner-like foci uncommon
  - Intraneural tumor shows intraneural microscopic extension usually within preexisting plexiform neurofibroma
  - Tumors arising from preexisting benign nerve sheath tumor

Malignant Peripheral Nerve Sheath Tumor

- Neurofibroma most common; transitional areas; usually in NF1 patients
- New consensus criteria: Distinguish atypical neurofibroma and neurofibroma with uncertain malignant potential from intraneural MPNST
- Conventional or spindle cell MPNST (80%)
  - Long fascicles of uniform, closely spaced, hyperchromatic spindle cells
  - Alternating cellular fascicles and hypocellular areas ("tapestry" or "marbled" pattern)
  - Other findings may include storiforming, small round blue cells, and pleomorphic tumor giant cells
  - Extensive necrosis with perivascular preservation common
- Epithelioid MPNST (5%)
  - Large epithelioid cells arranged in nodules, cords, clusters
  - Spindle cells also often present
- Heterologous differentiation in spindle cell MPNST (15%)
  - Most common is benign or malignant bone but also benign or malignant cartilage, others
  - Rhabdomyosarcomatous (triton tumor) imparts worse prognosis; most occur in NF1 patients

ANCILLARY TESTS

Immunohistochemistry
- S100(+) &/or SOX10(+) in ~ 70%; typically focal except in epithelioid cases where more commonly diffuse
- SMARCB1/INI1 expression lost in ~ 75% of epithelioid MPNST
- H3K27me3 lost in ~ 80% of conventional MPNST; normal expression in epithelioid MPNST
  - Relatively specific for spindle cell MPNST but also commonly lost in synovial sarcoma, rhabdomyosarcoma, and few other histologic mimics

Genetic Testing
- Karyotype: Complex structural and numeric chromosomal abnormalities (complex aneuploidy)

Serologic Testing
- MPNST circulating cell-free DNA (cfDNA): Could be prognostic and track patient status

DIFFERENTIAL DIAGNOSIS

Monophasic or Poorly Differentiated Synovial Sarcoma
- Nuclei have finer chromatin and usually lower mitotic rate
- TLE1(+), usually diffusely and strongly
  - MPNST uncommonly diffusely and strongly positive
- Usually EMA and keratin (+)
  - MPNST usually (-) except for biphasic cases
- S100 can be (+) in 15% and patchy as in MPNST
- t(X;18); SS18 break-apart probe positive by FISH
  - SSX(+); specific and sensitive marker of fusion

Cellular Schwannoma
- Exclusively Antoni A areas; often lacks Verocay bodies
- Mitotic figures can be present but importantly lacks malignant cytologic atypia

- IHC results supporting cellular schwannoma compared to MPNST
  - Strong, diffuse S100 expression
    - MPNST usually has only focal expression except in epithelioid variant
  - Ki-67 (MIB-1) expression < 20%

Atypical Neurofibroma
- Large, hyperchromatic spindle cells some with smudgy (degenerated) chromatin with absent to very rare mitoses
- Usually retains cytoarchitectural features of neurofibroma

Malignant Melanoma
- Spindle cell/sarcomatoid melanoma
  - Diffusely S100(+)
    - MPNST S100(-) (40%) or shows only focal staining
  - Usually HMB-45 and melan-A (-)
- Epithelioid melanoma
  - Usually HMB-45 and melan-A (+)

Clear Cell Sarcoma
- Multinodular, vague, nested architecture
- Uniform epithelioid and spindle cells often with prominent nucleoli
- Diffuse S100(+/-), HMB-45(+/-), melan-A staining in most
- EWSR1 break-apart FISH (+) due to EWSR1::ATF1 or EWSR1::CREB1 fusions

Ewing Sarcoma
- Usually primary bone tumor but may present as soft tissue primary
- Small round blue cell tumor
  - Diffusely CD99(+), usually S100d(-)
    - MPNST sometimes CD99(+) but usually weak/focal and nonmembranous
  - EWSR1 break-apart FISH (+) due to t(11;22), t(7;22), t(21;22), or t(2;22)

Embryonal Rhabdomyosarcoma
- Small round blue cells and spindle cells ± rhabdomyoblasts
- S100(-); desmin and myogenin (+)

Other Round Cell Sarcomas
- Include EWSR1::non-ETS fusion tumors, CIC-rearranged sarcomas, and sarcomas with BCOR genetic alterations
- Distinguishable by IHC and molecular genetic testing

SELECTED REFERENCES

1. Cortes-Ciriano I et al: Genomic patterns of malignant peripheral nerve sheath tumor (MPNST) evolution correlate with clinical outcome and are detectable in cell-free DNA. Cancer Discov. 13(3):654-71, 2023
2. Somatilaka BN et al: Malignant peripheral nerve sheath tumor: models, biology, and translation. Oncogene. 41(17):2405-21, 2022
3. Wu LMN et al: Single-cell multiomics identifies clinically relevant mesenchymal stem-like cells and key regulators for MPNST malignancy. Sci Adv. 8(44):eabo5442, 2022
4. Le Guellec S et al: Malignant peripheral nerve sheath tumor Is a challenging diagnosis: a systematic pathology review, immunohistochemistry, and molecular analysis in 160 patients from the French Sarcoma Group Database. Am J Surg Pathol. 40(7):896-908, 2016

Malignant Peripheral Nerve Sheath Tumor

Focal "Tigroid" Appearance

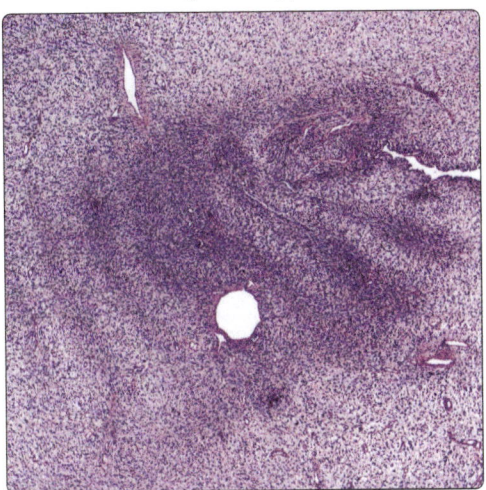

MPNST Invading Intratumoral Blood Vessel Walls

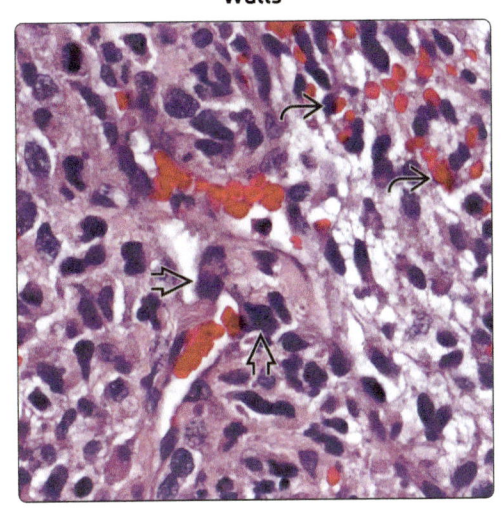

(Left) Note the alternating hypo- and hypercellular bands in this case of MPNST. This creates a striped or "tigroid" pattern and is a common but not exclusive pattern in MPNST that is appreciated at low power. (Right) Another typical finding in MPNST is invasion or undermining of the walls of tumor blood vessels. Note the close apposition of tumor cells to vessel lumen ⇥. One vessel has been breached with subsequent acute hemorrhage ⇥.

Spindle Cell MPNST and Plexiform Neurofibroma

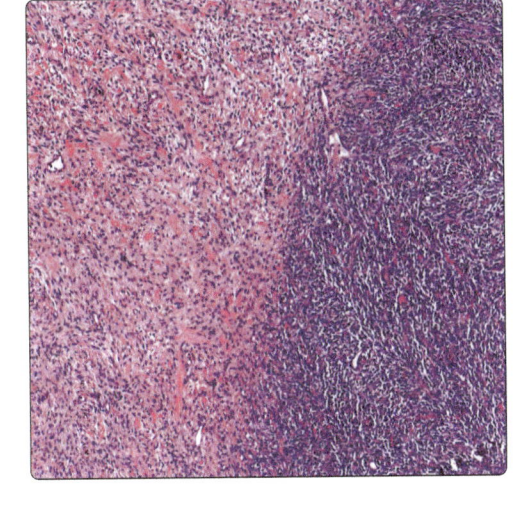

MPNST Karyotype

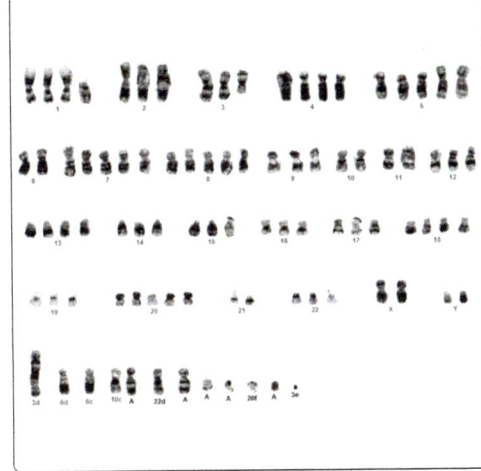

(Left) Benign nerve sheath tumor (left) and hypercellular MPNST (right) are shown. MPNST may arise from a benign nerve tumor, such as neurofibroma, but most commonly involves a deep plexiform neurofibroma in patients with NF1. (Right) Complex aneuploid karyotype of MPNST shows polyploidy and numerous marker chromosomes (bottom row). Most MPNST karyotypes contain multiple chromosomal abnormalities like this one but lack highly consistent, recurrent findings.

Typical Histopathology

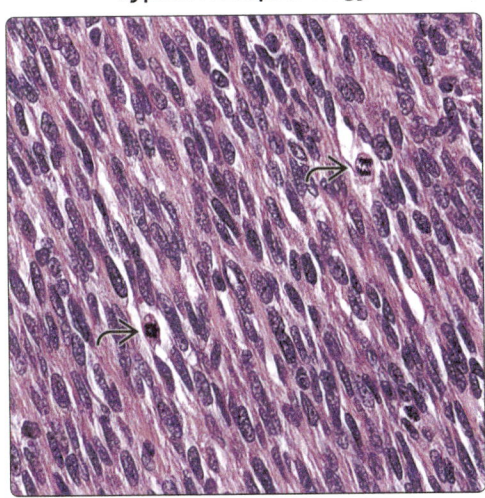

Marked Pleomorphism

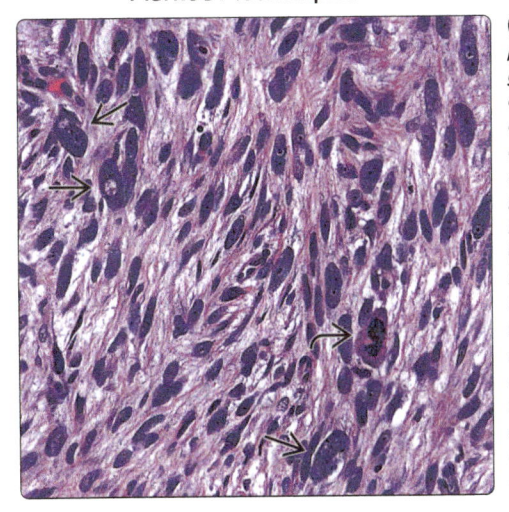

(Left) The most common pattern of MPNST is high-grade spindle cell sarcoma composed of long fascicles of closely spaced, uniform spindle cells with ill-defined cytoplasmic borders, coarse nuclear hyperchromasia, and brisk mitotic activity ⇥. (Right) MPNST can sometimes have a pleomorphic spindle cell pattern with marked nuclear enlargement ⇥ and atypical mitotic figures ⇥, mimicking pleomorphic undifferentiated sarcoma. More typical areas or nerve connection are helpful diagnostic clues.

Malignant Peripheral Nerve Sheath Tumor

Malignant Triton Tumor

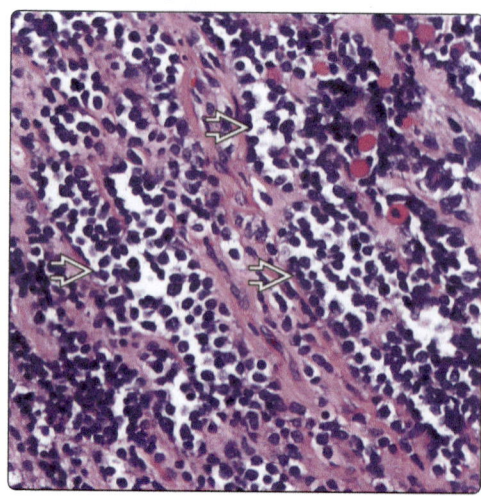

Rhabdomyoblasts in Malignant Triton Tumor

(Left) Malignant triton tumor with rhabdomyosarcoma component contains areas identical to alveolar rhabdomyosarcoma with pseudoalveolar spaces lined by a single layer of small round blue cells with luminal dyscohesion and drop-off ➡. (Right) Malignant triton tumor most often occurs in MPNST arising in NF1 and contains rhabdomyoblasts with marked eosinophilic cytoplasm ➡ mixed with primitive blastic tumor cells.

Neoplastic Glands

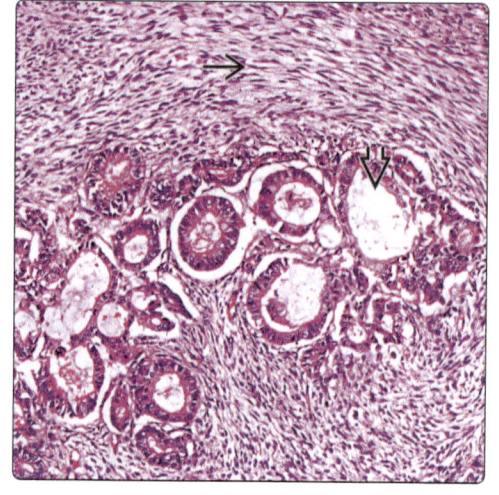

Myxoid Stroma

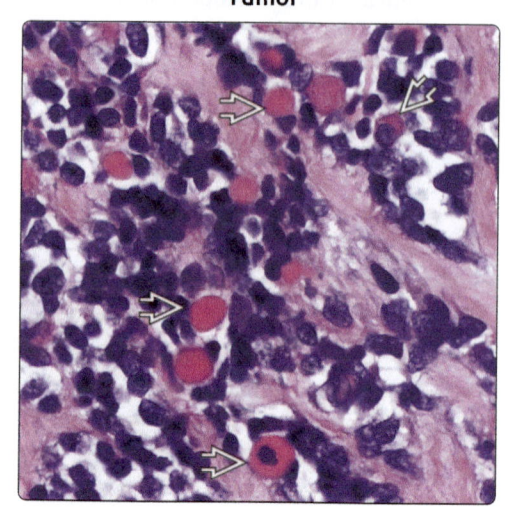

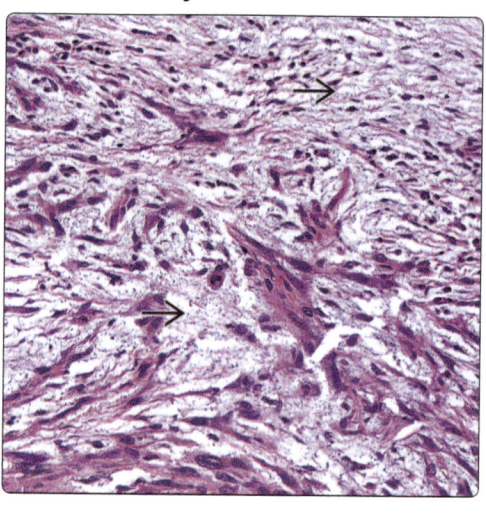

(Left) Rarely, MPNST ➡ can have heterologous glandular elements. In this tumor, the glands secrete mucin ➡ and can have focal neuroendocrine differentiation. This tumor must not be mistaken for biphasic synovial sarcoma. (Right) Myxoid stroma ➡ is common in MPNST. It usually accounts for only a portion of a given tumor with solid areas predominating, but this can occasionally lead to diagnostic difficulty on core biopsy.

Small Round Blue Cells

Multinucleated Giant Cells

(Left) MPNST can have prominent small round blue cell areas, mimicking Ewing sarcoma or poorly differentiated synovial sarcoma. Appropriate IHC and molecular genetic investigation can resolve these differential diagnoses in most instances. (Right) Markedly enlarged pleomorphic cells, including multinucleated giant cells ➡, are occasionally seen in MPNST, exemplified in this resected thigh tumor in a case of NF1.

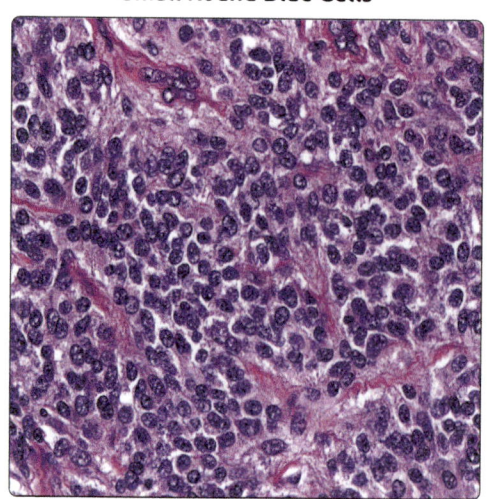

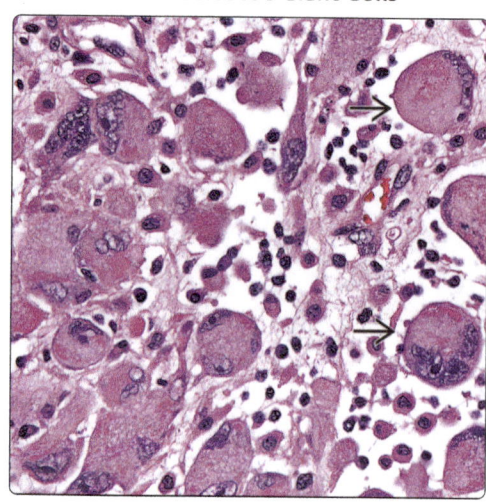

Malignant Peripheral Nerve Sheath Tumor

Verocay Body

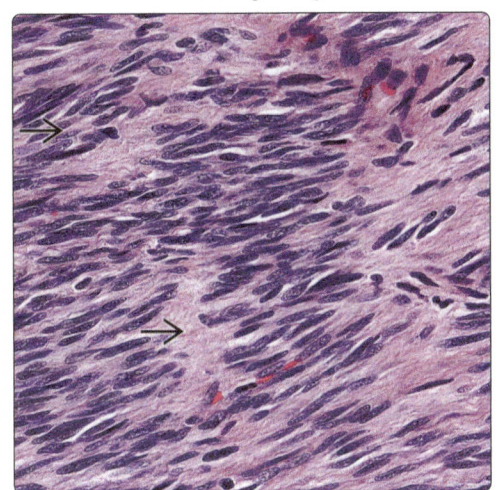

Tactoid-Like Bodies

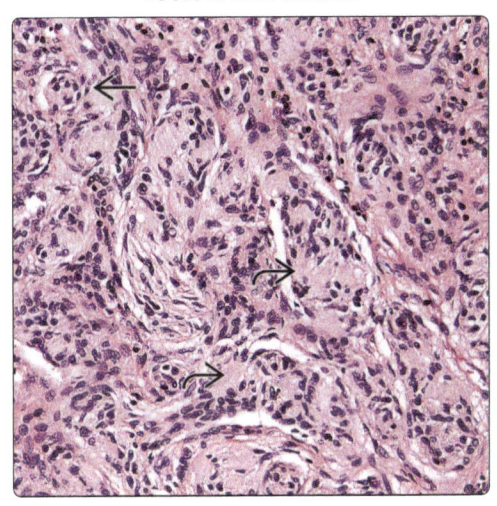

(Left) Microscopic evidence of nerve sheath differentiation is uncommon in MPNST. For example, nuclear palisading with Verocay body ➡ is seen in only 15% of MPNST, and it is usually a focal finding. (Right) Tactoid differentiation is also uncommon in MPNST. Here, cell clusters with vague whorling growth pattern ➡ and hyaline matrix ➡ mimic tactoid or Wagner-Meissner-like bodies.

Epithelioid Tumor Cells

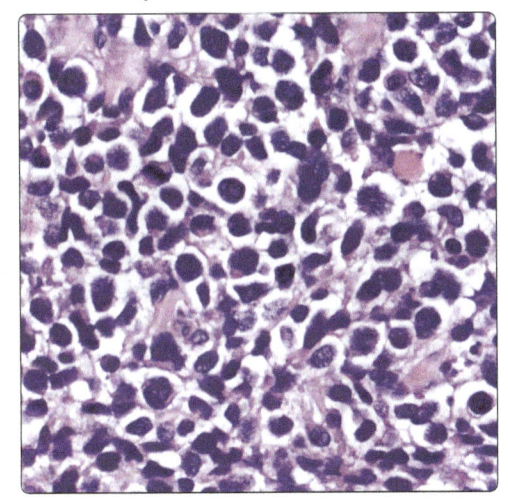

Epithelioid MPNST Diffusely Reactive for S100

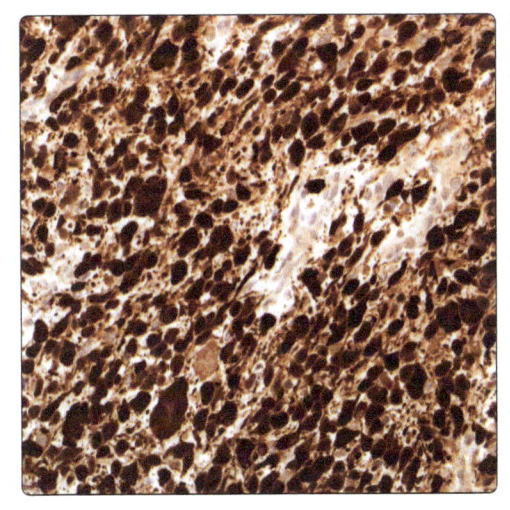

(Left) Some MPNST consist of malignant epithelioid tumor cells, as in this example. Such tumors may arise from schwannoma, which is otherwise a very rare occurrence with typical, spindled, fascicular MPNST. Epithelioid MPNST may also show loss of RB1 expression, and, correlatively, some schwannomas have patchy loss of RB1. (Right) S100 is often diffusely strongly expressed in epithelioid MPNST (DAB is the chromogen here). It is negative or patchy in most nonepithelioid MPNST.

Perivascular Viability Pattern

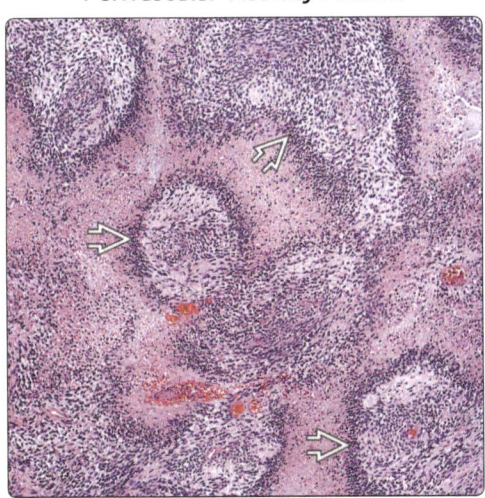

Intraneural Involvement

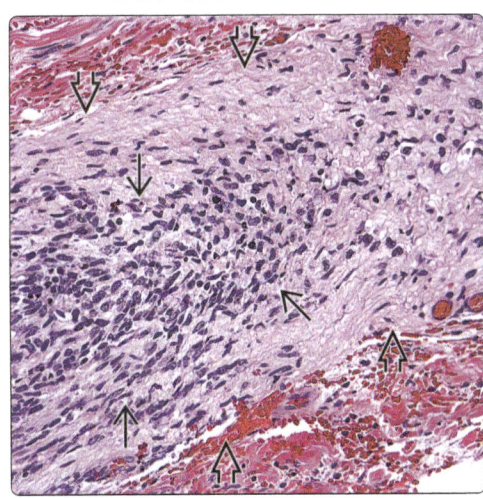

(Left) A common low-power growth pattern in MPNST is perivascular preservation ➡, which leads to a serpiginous pattern of viable tumor areas surrounded by pink necrotic bands, located further away radially from blood vessels. (Right) Intraneural extension beyond the grossly visible mass is depicted here by hyperchromatic spindle cells ➡ infiltrating within a peripheral nerve ➡. This can result in a positive surgical margin and local recurrence.

Representative Genetic Findings in Bone and Soft Tissue Tumors

Soft Tissue Tumors or Lesions

Tumor or Lesion	Genetic Finding	Ancillary Testing &/or Prevalence of Genetic Abnormality
Alveolar soft part sarcoma	1) *ASPSCR1::TFE3*, t(X;17) 2) Other *TFE3* fusions with *DVL2*, *HNRNPH3*, *PRCC*	1-2) Diffuse nuclear TFE3 Ab(+) 1) Majority 2) Rare
Angiomatoid fibrous histiocytoma	1) *EWSR1::CREB1*, t(2;22) 2) *FUS::ATF1* 3) *CDKN2A/CDKN2B* homozygous deletions	1-2) FISH for *EWSR1* or *FUS* rearrangements 1-2) Sequencing to identify specific partners 3) Only found in metastasizing cases
Angiosarcoma	1) Complex aneuploidy 2) *NUP160::LC43A3*, t(11;11) 3) *CIC* rearrangements, including *CIC::LEUTX*, t(19;19) or mutations 4) *TP53* mutations 5) *CDKN2A* deletions 6) RAS gene family mutations, *BRAF*, *MAPK1*, *NF1*	1) Majority of cases 2) Few cases 3) ~ 10%; young adults; epithelioid morphology and solid growth 4) ~ 50% 5) ~ 25% 6) Subset
Atypical lipomatous tumor/well-differentiated liposarcoma	Supernumerary ring and giant marker chromosomes containing amplified 12q14-15 region = overexpression and amplification of *MDM2* and other genes (*CDK4* in ~ 85%)	~ 100% show *MDM2* amplification by FISH
Biphenotypic sinonasal sarcoma	*PAX3* (2q) fusions with *MAML3* (4q), *NCOA2* (8q), or *FOXO1* (13q)	~ 100%
Cellular angiofibroma	*RB1* (13q) ± 16q partial monosomy	~ 100%
Chondroid lipoma	*ZFTA::MRTFB*, t(11;16)	~ 100%
CIC-rearranged sarcoma	1) *CIC::DUX4*, t(4;19) 2) *CIC::FOXO4*, t(X;19) 3) *CIC* fusions with other partners, including *AXL*, *CITED1*, *SYK*, and *LEUTX*	1) WT1 cTER Ab(+) in most cases; nuclear DUX4 Ab(+) in *DUX4* fusion cases, ETV4 Ab(+) in all *CIC*-rearranged cases 2) Rare; WT1 Ab(+) in most cases; new CIC Ab(+) 3) Rare 1-3) May express ERG ± CD31
Clear cell sarcoma	1) *EWSR1::ATF1*, t(12;22) 2) *EWSR1::CREB1*, t(2;22) 3) *EWSR1::CREM*, t(10;22) 4) *CDKN2A* or *TERT* promoter mutations	1) ~ 70% 2) ~ 15% 3) Rare 4) 50%; mutually exclusive; associated with worse outcome
Composite hemangioendothelioma	1) *YAP1::MAML2* 2) *PTBP1::MAML2* 3) *EPC1::PHC2*	1) More common in acral sites 2-3) Positive for synaptophysin as well as vascular markers
Dedifferentiated liposarcoma	*MDM2*, *CDK4*, *HMGA2*, and others amplified in giant ring &/or marker chromosomes (12q14-15) Coamplification of *JUN*, *MAP3K5*	~ 100% Can use FISH to identify amplified *MDM2*
Deep (aggressive) angiomyxoma	*HMGA2* rearrangements (12q14)	Majority
Dermatofibrosarcoma protuberans	1) *COL1A1::PDGFB*, t(17;22) 2) *COL6A3::PDGFD* 3) *EMILIN2::PDGFD*	1) ~ 90% identified by FISH 2) Predilection for breast location 3) ~ 4%
Desmoid-type fibromatosis	1) *CTNNB1* (3p), β-catenin mutations 2) Trisomy 8, trisomy 20 3) *APC* loss, 5q21-22	1) Nuclear β-catenin Ab(+) (~ 70%) 2) Common 3) Uncommon
Desmoplastic fibroblastoma	1) *FOSL1* rearrangements (11q13) 2) *FOS* rearrangements (14q24)	1) Majority 2) Minority
Desmoplastic small round cell tumor	1) *EWSR1::WT1*, t(11;22) 2) *EWSR1::ERG*, t(21;22) 3) Androgen receptor O/E and pathway upregulation	1) Diffuse nuclear WT1 cTER Ab(+) 2) Rare 3) 40-60%
Epithelioid hemangioendothelioma	1) *WWTR1::CAMTA1*, t(1;3) 2) *YAP1::TFE3*, t(11;X) 3) *WWTR1::MAML2*, *WWTR1::ACTL6A*, *WWTR1* rearranged with unknown partners	1) 90%; nuclear CAMTA1 Ab(+) 2) 5%; nuclear TFE3 Ab(+) 3) Rare; predilection for heart
Epithelioid hemangioma	1) *FOS* rearrangements with various partners 2) *FOSB* rearrangements, including *ZFP36::FOSB*, t(19;19); *WWTR1::FOSB*, t(3;19)	~ 33% show *FOS* or *FOSB* rearrangements 1) Predilection for bone 2) Some cases show nuclear FOSB Ab(+)

Representative Genetic Findings in Bone and Soft Tissue Tumors

Soft Tissue Tumors or Lesions (Continued)

Tumor or Lesion	Genetic Finding	Ancillary Testing &/or Prevalence of Genetic Abnormality
	4) GATA6::FOXO1	3) Nuclear FOSB Ab(+) 4) Predilection for head and neck
Epithelioid sarcoma	1) SMARCB1 homozygous deletions: 22q11 abnormalities 2) SMARCB1 intact cases may show abnormalities of other SWI/SNF genes, such as SMARCA4, SMARCC1, or SMARCC2	1) ~ 95%; SMARCB1 Ab(-) 2) Extremely rare
EWSR1::SMAD3-positive fibroblastic tumor	EWSR1::SMAD3, t(15;22)	~ 100%; acral location
Extraskeletal myxoid chondrosarcoma	EWSR1::NR4A3, t(9;22)(q31;q12) TAF15::NR4A3, t(9;15) TCF12::NR4A3, t(9;17) TFG::NR4A3, t(3;9) FUS::NR4A3, t(9;16)	NR4A3 rearrangement by FISH; EWSR1::NR4A3 in majority
Fibroma of tendon sheath	USP6 (17p13) fusions	Found in "cellular" examples
Gastrointestinal stromal tumor	1) KIT (4q) mutation (majority) 2) PDGFRA (4q) mutation (minority) 3) SDHB, SDHC, SDHD mutations or SDHC epimutation (minority)	1) C-kit Ab(+) and DOG1 Ab(+) 2) DOG1 Ab(+) 3) Loss of SDH Ab(-); nodular epithelioid histology; young patients
Giant cell tumor of soft tissue	1) Lack H3F3 mutations in giant cell tumor of bone 2) HMGA2::NCOR2 in keratin-expressing tumors	1) 100% 2) Minority; may represent distinct tumor
Glomus tumor	1) NOTCH1/NOTCH2/NOTCH3 fusions, most commonly NOTCH2::MIR143 2) GLMN-inactivating mutations 3) PDGFRB mutations	1) ~ 50% overall; benign glomus tumor in extremities but not subungual cases; malignant glomus tumor in viscera 2) Found in familial glomus tumor 1, 3) Also found in other pericytic (perivascular) tumor types
Hibernoma	11q13-21 rearrangements leading to deletions of MEN1 and AIP	~ 100%
Infantile fibrosarcoma	1) ETV6::NTRK3, t(12;15) 2) Other NTRK fusions: NTRK1 (1q), NTRK2 (9q), NTRK3 (15q)	1) Pan-TRK Ab(+) 2) NTRK3 fusions: Pan-TRK Ab(+) nuclear ± cytoplasmic reactivity NTRK1/NTRK2 fusions: Pan-TRK Ab(+) cytoplasmic reactivity
Inflammatory myofibroblastic tumor	ALK (2p) fusions or ROS1 fusions: 1) TPM3::ALK, t(1;2) 2) TPM4::ALK, t(2;19) 3) CLTC::ALK, t(2;17) 4) RANBP2::ALK, t(2;2) 5) YWHAE::ROS1, t(6;17) 6) FG::ROS1, t(3;6)	1-6) ALK or ROS1 Ab(+) or FISH for ALK, ROS1 rearrangements 1-5) ALK Ab(+): Reactivity pattern varies by fusion 6) Rare; ROS1(+)
Intramuscular myxoma	GNAS (20q) point mutations	Majority
Classic leiomyosarcoma	1) Complex aneuploidy, including inactivation of TP53 (17p13) and RB1 (13q) 2) MYOCD (17p) copy number gain/amplification	1) Majority 2) Relatively common
Myxoid leiomyosarcoma	PLAG1 (8q12) rearrangements with TRPS1 (8q23.3) or RAD51B (14q24.1)	~ 25% of myxoid leiomyosarcoma show rearrangement and diffuse nuclear PLAG1 Ab(+)
Inflammatory leiomyosarcoma	Near-haploid genotype with NF1 (17q) mutations	Rare variant
Lipoblastoma	PLAG1 (8q) rearrangements	~ 100%
Lipoma, conventional	HMGA2 (12q) rearrangements HMGA1 (6p) rearrangements	~ 100%
Low-grade fibromyxoid sarcoma	1) FUS::CREB3L2, t(7;16) 2) FUS::CREB3L1, t(11;16) 3) EWSR1::CREB3L1, t(11;22)	1) ~ 95%; MUC4 Ab(+) 2-3) Rare; MUC4 Ab(+)
Malignant peripheral nerve	1) Complex aneuploidy	1) Majority

Representative Genetic Findings in Bone and Soft Tissue Tumors

Soft Tissue Tumors or Lesions (Continued)

Tumor or Lesion	Genetic Finding	Ancillary Testing &/or Prevalence of Genetic Abnormality
sheath tumor	2) *NF1* (17q) biallelic alterations 3) *CDKN2A* (9p) mutations 4) *SUZ12* (17q) microdeletions/mutations 5) *EED* (11q) mutations	2) *NF1* loss in all 3) Majority (and in precursor lesion) 4-5) Relatively common; at least 50% of cases have PRC2 (polycomb repressive complex 2) gene alterations All cases H3K27me3 Ab(-)
Malignant peripheral nerve sheath tumor, epithelioid variant	*SMARCB1* (22q11) abnormalities	SMARCB1 Ab(-) in some cases; can be patchy loss
Mammary-type myofibroblastoma	*RB1* (13q) ± 16q partial monosomy	Partial to complete loss of RB1 Ab expression in some cases
Myoepithelial carcinoma of soft tissue	1) *EWSR1::PBX1*, t(1;22) 2) *EWSR1::ZNF444*, t(19;22)(q13;q12) 3) *EWSR1::POU5F1*, t(6;22) 4) *FUS::*unknown gene, 16p11 rearrangement 5) *SMARCB1* (22q11) homozygous deletions	1-3) FISH for *EWSR1* rearrangement 4) FISH for *FUS* rearrangement 5) SMARCB1 Ab(-) (~ 50%)
Myxofibrosarcoma	Complex aneuploidy	Majority
Myxoid/round cell liposarcoma	1) *FUS::DDIT3*, t(12;16) 2) *EWSR1::DDIT3*, t(12;22)	FISH for fusion: 1) ~ 90% of cases 2) ~ 5% of cases
Myopericytoma	1) *PDGFRB* mutations 2) *NOTCH1/NOTCH2/NOTCH3* rearrangements 3) *ACTB::GLI1*, t(7;12)	1) Minority 2) Minority 3) Minority
Myxoinflammatory fibroblastic sarcoma	1) *TGFBR3::OGA* (MGEA5), t(1;10) 2) *BRAF* (7q) rearrangement with *TOM1L2* (17p) or *BRAF* amplification	1) FISH or sequencing; same fusion found in phosphaturic mesenchymal tumor and HSFLT 2) FISH or sequencing (~ 40%)
Neurofibroma	*NF1* (neurofibromin 1; 17q11) monoallelic or biallelic loss	100%
Nodular fasciitis	*USP6* rearrangements with *MYH9::USP6*, t(17;22) most common	~ 40%
NTRK-rearranged spindle cell neoplasm	*NTRK1/NTRK2/NTRK3* fusions with various partners, including *TPR*, *TPM3*, *LMNA*, and others	100% Majority are *NTRK1* fusions Frequent dual expression of S100 and CD34
Ossifying fibromyxoid tumor	1) *EP400::PHF1*, t(6;12) 2) *EPC1::PHF1*, t(6;10) 3) *MEAF6::PHF1*, t(1;6) 4) *ZC3H7B::BCOR*, t(X;22) 5) *KDM2A::WWTR1*, t(3;11) 6) *CREBBP::BCORL1*, t(16;X)	1) ~ 45% 2) Uncommon 3-6) Rare 4) BCOR Ab(-)
Perineurioma	1) 10q22-24 deletions, rearrangements (in sclerosing perineurioma) 2) 22q11.2 alterations in some cases of both types	1, 2) Majority
Perivascular epithelioid cell tumor	1) *TSC2* (16p) or *TSC1* (9q) inactivations 2) *TFE3* (Xp) rearrangements with *SFPQ* (1p) or *DVL2* (17p)	1) Majority 2) Minority; diffuse nuclear TFE Ab(+)
Phosphaturic mesenchymal tumor	*FN1::FGFR1*, t(2;8;)	~ 60%
Pleomorphic hyalinizing angiectatic tumor of soft tissue	*TGFBR3* (1p) &/or *OGA* (10q) rearrangements	~ 60%
Pleomorphic liposarcoma	1) Complex aneuploidy 2) Mutations/deletions in *TP53*, *RB1*, *NF1*	1) ~ 100% 2) Common
Pleomorphic myxoid liposarcoma	1) Focal copy number changes 2) Methylation profiling shows epigenetic overlap with pleomorphic liposarcoma 3) 13q deletion affecting *RB1*, *RCBTB2*, *ITM2B*, *DLEU1*	1) ~ 100% 2) ~ 100% 3) 50-60%
Pseudomyogenic	1) *SERPINE1::FOSB*, t(7;19)	1) FISH or sequencing (~ 60%)

Representative Genetic Findings in Bone and Soft Tissue Tumors

Soft Tissue Tumors or Lesions (Continued)

Tumor or Lesion	Genetic Finding	Ancillary Testing &/or Prevalence of Genetic Abnormality
hemangioendothelioma	2) *ACTB::FOSB*, t(7;19) 3) *FOSB* fusions with *WWTR1*, *EGFL7*, *CLTC*	2) FISH or sequencing (~ 30%) 3) Rare
Retiform hemangioendothelioma	*YAP1* rearrangements to *MAML2* and others	~ 40%
Rhabdoid tumor of soft tissue (extrarenal rhabdoid tumor)	*SMARCB1* del22q11	SMARCB1 Ab(-)
Alveolar rhabdomyosarcoma	1) *PAX3::FOXO1*, t(2;13) 2) *PAX7::FOXO1*, t(1;13) *PAX3::FOX04*, t(2;X) *PAX3::NCOA1*, t(2;2)	1) FISH or sequencing (majority of alveolar rhabdomyosarcoma) 2) FISH or sequencing (~ 20% of alveolar rhabdomyosarcoma)
Embryonal rhabdomyosarcoma	Complex aneuploidy with some fairly recurrent point mutations	100%
Infantile rhabdomyosarcoma	*NCOA2* (8q) or *VGLL2* (6q) fusions	Common under 1 year of age
Spindle cell/sclerosing rhabdomyosarcoma	*MYOD1* (11p) mutations	Majority of pediatric and adult cases
Pleomorphic rhabdomyosarcoma	Complex aneuploidy	100%
Schwannoma	*NF2* (merlin, schwannomin, 22q12) loss	Majority
Sclerosing epithelioid fibrosarcoma	*FUS::CREB3L2*, t(7;16) *FUS::CREB3L1*, t(11;16) *FUS::CREM*, t(10;16) *PAX5::CREB3L1*, t(9;11)	Majority are *FUS::CREB3L2*
SMARCA4-deficient thoracic sarcoma	*SMARCA4* (19p) inactivating mutations	~ 100%
Soft tissue angiofibroma	*AHRR::NCOA2*, t(5;8)	
Solitary fibrous tumor	*NAB2::STAT6*, 12q13 intrachromosomal rearrangement; partial deletions at 13q, 14q	~ 100%; diffuse nuclear STAT6 Ab(+)
Spindle cell lipoma/pleomorphic lipoma	16q13-qter rearrangements; monosomy 13 or partial del(13q)	~ 100% Partial to complete loss of RB1 Ab expression
Superficial CD34-positive fibroblastic tumor	*PRDM10* rearrangements	100% express CD34 50-70% express keratins
Synovial sarcoma	*SS18::SSX1*, t(X;18) *SS18::SSX2*, t(X;18) *SS18::SSX4*, t(X;18) *SS18L1::SSX1*, t(X; 20) Other SS18 rearrangements	*SS18::SSX1*, t(X;18) most common Diffuse nuclear TLE1 Ab(+), SSX Ab(+) for all fusions
Tenosynovial giant cell tumor, diffuse or localized	*CSF1::COL6A3*, t(1;2); trisomy 5, trisomy 7	Majority
Undifferentiated pleomorphic sarcoma	Complex aneuploidy	~ 100%

References for all tables in this chapter are listed in the online version.

Bone Tumors or Lesions

Tumor or Lesion	Genetic Finding	Utility
Aneurysmal bone cyst	*USP6* (17p) translocations: *CDH11::USP6*, t(16;17) *THRAP3::USP6*, t(1;17) *CNBP::USP6*, t(3;17) *OMD::USP6*, t(9;17) *COL1A1::USP6*, t(17;17)	~ 100%
BCOR-rearranged tumors	1) *BCOR::CCNB3* X chromosome paracentric inversion; *BCOR* (Xp); *CCNB3* (Xp) 2) *BCOR::MAML3*, t(X;4)	1) Majority; diffuse BCOR Ab(+) 2) Minority; diffuse BCOR(+) 3) Minority; diffuse BCOR Ab(+)

895

Representative Genetic Findings in Bone and Soft Tissue Tumors

Bone Tumors or Lesions (Continued)

Tumor or Lesion	Genetic Finding	Utility
	3) *BCOR* internal tandem duplications (Xp)	
Chondroblastoma	1) *H3F3B* (17q) mutations 2) Heterogeneous rearrangements	1) 95% 2) 5% 1-2) H3F3 K36M Ab(+)
Chondromyxoid fibroma	*GRM1* (6q) rearrangements; rare other translocations	
Chordoma	*TBXT* (6q) and *EGFR* (7p) copy number gains	~ 90% of cases Diffuse brachyury Ab(+)
Poorly differentiated chordoma	*SMARCB1* (22q11) homozygous deletions	Rare; pediatric age group Brachyury Ab(+); Loss (-) of SMARCB1 Ab expression
Clear cell chondrosarcoma	May have extra copies of 20, or 9p loss or rearrangement; RB1 pathway commonly altered	
Chondrosarcoma, low-grade central	More complex karyotype than most enchondromas *IDH1* (2q) or *IDH2* (15q) mutations	*IDH* mutations in majority
Chondrosarcoma, high-grade central	1) Complex aneuploidy 2) *TP53*, *COL2A1* mutations 3) *CDKN2A/CDKN2B* deletions	1) ~ 100% 2) Common 3) Common
Chondrosarcoma, dedifferentiated	1) Complex aneuploidy 2) *IDH1* (2q) or *IDH2* (15q) mutations	1) 100% 2) *IDH1/IDH2* mutations (50%)
Chondrosarcoma, peripheral	1) *EXT1/EXT2* mutations Additional alterations	1) 80%
Enchondroma	Usually normal karyotype *IDH1* or *IDH2* mutations	*IDH1/IDH2* mutations; 40% sporadic; 90% syndromic
Ewing sarcoma	FET::ETS fusions: 1) *EWSR1::FLI1*, t(11;22) 2) *EWSR1::ERG*, t(21;22) 3) *EWSR1::ETV1*, t(7;22) 4) *EWSR1::ETV4*, t(17;22) 5) *EWSR1::FEV*, t(2;22) 6) *FUS::ERG*, t(16;21) 7) *FUS::FEV*, t(2;16)	1) 90% 2) ~ 5% 3-7) Rare CD99 Ab(+) diffuse membranous expression in most cases
Round cell sarcoma with *EWSR1*::non-ETS fusions	1) *EWSR1::PATZ1*, inv(22) 2) *EWSR1::SP3*, t(2;22) 3) *EWSR1::NFATC2*, t(20;22) 4) *EWSR1::SMARCA5*, t(4;22)	1-4) Rare
Fibrous dysplasia	*GNAS* (20q) mutations	~100%
Giant cell tumor of bone	1) *H3F3A* (1q) mutations (92%) 2) Telomeric associations	1) ~ 95% H3F3A Ab(+)
Mesenchymal chondrosarcoma	1) *HEY1::NCOA2*, del(8)(q13.;q21) 2) *IRF2BP2::CDX1*, t(1;5)	1) 80% 2) Rare
Osteoblastoma and osteoid osteoma	1) *FOS* (14q) rearrangements or 2) *FOSB* (19q) rearrangements	~ 95%
Osteochondroma	*EXT1* (8q) or *EXT2* (11p) mutations	~ 90%
Osteosarcoma, low grade	*MDM2* (12q) and *CDK4* (12q) amplification	~ 100%
Osteosarcoma, high grade	Complex aneuploidy	~ 100%
Spindle cell rhabdomyosarcoma of bone	1) *FUS::TFCP2*, t(12;16) 2) *EWSR1::TFCP2*, t(12;22) 3) *FET::TFCP2* 4) *MEIS1::NCOA2* 5) *EWSR1::UBP1*	1-3) Very rare 3) May also be prominently epithelioid 4) May be separate variant; purely spindle cell growth; lacks ALK and keratin expression seen in 1-3

References for all tables in this chapter are listed in the online version.

Representative Genetic Findings in Bone and Soft Tissue Tumors

Recently Described Provisional Bone and Soft Tissue Tumors With Specific Genetic Findings*

Tumor Description	Location	Histologic Description	Genetic Finding
CIC::NUTM1 sarcoma	Head and neck	Round epithelioid to rhabdoid cells with mixed chondroid, myxoid, hyaline matrix	CIC::NUTM1, t(15;19)
NUTM1-fusion positive undifferentiated nonmidline tumors	Soft tissue and viscera	Nonpleomorphic round cells to epithelioid/rhabdoid cells arranged in nests, sheets, cords ± myxoid, fibrotic background or perivascular rosettes: Pankeratin (+) in 4/6; ± NUT IHC	NUTM1 (15q) fusion with BRD4 (19p), BRD3 (9q), MXD1 (2p), and BCORL1 (Xq) 2 fusions same as NUT midline carcinoma (BRD4 and BRD3)
Pseudoendocrine sarcoma	Soft tissue, often paravertebral	Sheets, cords, trabeculae with pseudoglandular structures common and uniform, epithelioid to oval cells	CTNNB1 mutations; 95% show nuclear β-catenin expression
Undifferentiated round cell sarcoma of infancy (subset)	Deep soft tissue	Heterogeneous with epithelioid cells or small round blue cells or clear cells ± myxoid matrix	BCOR (Xp11.4) internal tandem duplications (~ 40%) YWHAE::NUTM2B, t(10;17); same changes as renal clear cell sarcoma
CRTC1::SS18 undifferentiated round cell sarcoma	Deep soft tissue	Round cells to epithelioid cells with fibrous background; NTRK1(+)	CRTC1::SS18, t(18;19); expression profiling results similar to clear cell sarcoma of soft tissue
GAB1::ABL1 spindle cell neoplasm	Superficial or deep soft tissue	Perineurioma-like or low-grade fibromyxoid sarcoma-like; claudin-1 frequently positive; MUC4(-)	GAB1::ABL1
GLI1 epithelioid sarcoma	Soft tissue (5/6 cases); bone (1 case)	Epithelioid cells in sheets, cribriform nests, cords, or solid nests; S100(+); SOX10/SMA/EMA (-)	GLI1 (12q) fusions with ACTB (7p), MALAT1 (11q), or PTCH1 (9q)
Distinctive nested glomoid neoplasm	Diverse	Nested glomoid cells ± microcysts, clear cells	GLI1 alterations, including fusions or amplification; partners include ACTB, PTCH1, and others
Spindle cell tumors defined by S100 and CD34 coexpression	Soft tissue	Uniform hypercellular spindle cell proliferation with stromal and perivascular collagen; S100 and CD34 (+); SOX10(-); retained H3K27me3	RAF1 (3p), BRAF (7q) alterations
Infantile spindle cell sarcoma with neural features	Soft tissue	Fascicular and patternless growth of spindled cells; S100(+); retained H3K27me3; SOX10(-)	TFG::MET, t(3;7)
Adult fibrosarcoma with CD34 expression and NTRK fusions	Soft tissue	Long spindle cells arranged in long fascicles; diffuse CD34(+); diffuse pan-TRK(+); focal SMA(+)	NTRK3::STRN, t(2;15) NTRK3::STRN3, t(14;15)
Adult superficial spindle cell sarcoma resembling fibrosarcomatous dermatofibrosarcoma protuberans	Superficial soft tissue	Monomorphic spindle cells storiforming and invading fat like dermatofibrosarcoma protuberans (honeycomb fashion) with focal increased mitoses; CD34 patchy (+)	EML4::NTRK3, t(2;15) Same fusion as in congenital fibrosarcoma, mesoblastic nephroma, glioblastoma
Novel myxoid mesenchymal tumor	Intracranial (predominantly)	Oval to round cells in cords; reticular pattern with myxoid background; "sunburst" amianthoid fibers common; EMA(+); desmin (+) in 3/5	EWSR1::CREB family member (ATF1, CREB1, CREM) fusion CREM (10p) ATF1 (12q) CREB1 (2q)
TRAF7-mutated fibromyxoid spindle cell tumor	Deep soft tissue	Mixed myxoid and fibrous architecture with mild to moderate numbers of bland spindle cells	TRAF7 missense mutations
Cellular myofibroma/myopericytoma	Soft tissue	Heterogeneous but commonly spindle cells in fascicles and round to oval cells arranged in nests or syncytium; SMA, desmin, caldesmon (+); myogenin (-)	SRF::RELA, t(6;11)

*Not WHO designated. These are potential new distinct tumors. Most have only been described by 1 or 2 groups of investigators with 1-20 cases each.

References for all tables in this chapter are listed in the online version.

Rare Sarcomas of Uncertain Differentiation With Specific Molecular Alterations

TERMINOLOGY

Definitions
- Sarcomas or intermediate-grade tumors that **do not** differentiate toward known cell type but have specific genetic and histologic findings

EPIDEMIOLOGY

Synovial Sarcoma
- Age: 3rd to 6th decade > older > children
- Sex: M > F
- 2nd most common pediatric sarcoma
- Behavior
  - ~ 50% local recurrence rate; 40-80% 5-year survival

Epithelioid Sarcoma
- Age: 3rd to 4th decade but broad range
- Sex: M > F
- Behavior
  - Classic type: ~ 70% local recurrence rate; 45% metastasis rate; 50-80% 5-year survival
  - Proximal type: ~ 70% local recurrence rate; 35% 5-year survival

Alveolar Soft Part Sarcoma
- Age: 2nd to 3rd decade > other ages
- Sex: F slightly > M in patients under 30 years of age
- Behavior
  - < 10% local recurrence rate; ~ 80% metastasis rate; 60% 5-year survival dropping to ~ 35% at 10 years

Clear Cell Sarcoma of Soft Tissue
- Age: Young adults > other ages
- Behavior
  - ~ 20% local recurrence rate; ~ 60% metastasis rate; 50-60% 5-year survival

Extraskeletal Myxoid Chondrosarcoma
- Age: Middle-aged to older adults > other adults
- Behavior
  - ~ 45% local recurrence rate; ~ 45% metastasis rate; ~ 90% 5-year survival; ~ 70% 10-year survival

Extrarenal Rhabdoid Tumor
- Age: Infants to young children > > young adults > middle-aged adults
- Behavior
  - ~ 30% local recurrence rate; ~ 10% 5-year survival; ~ 0% 10-year survival

Intimal Sarcoma
- Age: Middle-aged to older adults > others
- Sex: F = M
- Behavior
  - < 2-year overall survival

Perivascular Epithelioid Cell Tumor
- Age: 3rd to 6th decade > others
- Sex: F > > M (6:1)
- Behavior
  - Tumors without atypia, necrosis, high mitotic rate, infiltrative growth rarely metastasize or cause death (majority of cases)
  - Malignant-appearing PEComas can metastasize and cause death

ETIOLOGY/PATHOGENESIS

Synovial Sarcoma
- Fusion driven: *SS18* fusion with *SSX1/SSX2/SSX3/SSX4* → abnormal transcription or repression of specific genes
  - Fusion protein abnormally links to SWI/SNF protein complex (chromatin remodeling complex that promotes transcription epigenetically by opening up nucleosomes)
    - Abnormal complex then hones in on and preferentially dislodges polycomb repressive complex PRC1.1
      - Genes normally repressed are now accessible for transcription: ↑ phosphorylated CREB, for example, drives proliferation
      - Dislodged PRC1.1 complex now free to abnormally repress other specific genes

(Left) PAS-D stain of alveolar soft part sarcoma (ASPS) highlights red granules and rod-like crystals ➡ typical of this tumor but not seen in all cases. **(Right)** ASPS is characterized by der(17) t(X;17)(p11;q25) = ASPSCR1-TFE3 fusion. Here, TFE3 FISH break-apart probe shows split signal ➡, which represents the translocation.

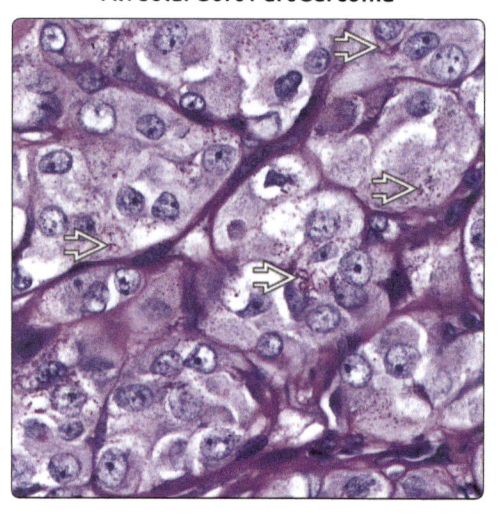

Alveolar Soft Part Sarcoma

ASPS With *TFE3* Split Signal

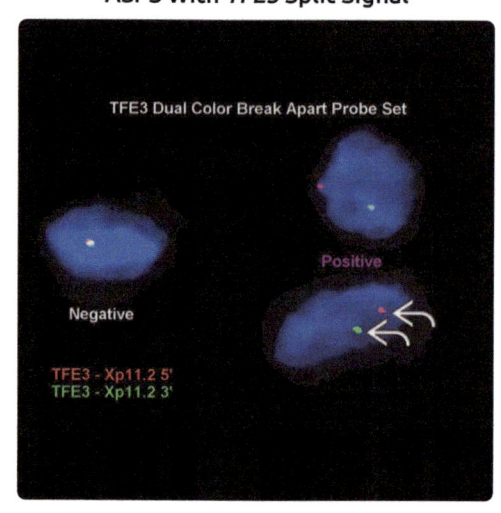

Rare Sarcomas of Uncertain Differentiation With Specific Molecular Alterations

- □ KDM2B protein (part of PRC1.1) directly mediates interaction between *SS18::SSX1/SSX2/SSX3/SSX4* fusion, SWI/SNF complex and PRC1.1
- Consequently, unique transcriptional profile of synovial sarcoma is due to combined abnormal transcription or repression of specific genes
  - □ Genes with altered expression include many neurogenic genes and transcription factors
  - □ High expression of TLE1 may support stem cell-like nature of tumor cells by assisting in repressing *ATF2* target genes
- Pathways dysregulated: Insulin-like GF, PI3K/Akt, WNT and HIPPO among others
- Rare noncanonical fusions: Rare fusions with *SSX1* (< 5%) that show histologic features and IHC of synovial sarcoma include *EWSR1::SSX1* and *SS18L1::SSX1*

Epithelioid Sarcoma
- INI1 (SMARCB1) biallelic deletions/mutations in ~ 92%
  - Lack of INI1 protein → SWI/SNF complex cannot normally evict polycomb repressive complex from specific gene sites → tumor suppressor genes cannot be normally transcribed
- Loss of other SWI/SNF chromatin remodeling complex proteins in ~ 5%
- Genes affected by defective SWI/SNF complex: ↑ *MYC* expression, ↑ *GLI1* expression, ↑ *EZH2* expression, ↑ *EGFR* expression, ↓ *PTEN* expression

Alveolar Soft Part Sarcoma
- Fusion driven: *TFE3* fusions; most commonly t(X;17); *ASPSCR1::TFE3* unbalanced translocation
  - Fusion protein induces MET expression → abnormally activates MET downstream pathways, including PI3/AKT and MAPK
  - Other genes targeted by fusion protein: Genes in cell cycle, cell adhesion, lysozymes, autophagy and angiogenesis-related pathways
  - *TFE3*: Member of microphthalmia transcription factor (MiT) gene family (*TFE3, TFEB, TFEC, MITF*)
  - *ASPSCR1::TFE3* also occurs in variant of Xp11 renal cell carcinoma

Clear Cell Sarcoma
- Fusion driven: *EWSR1::ATF1* in most cases
  - Rare alternative fusions: t(2;22); *EWSR1::CREB1* or t(10;22); *EWSR1::CREM*
  - Other tumors with *EWSR1::ATF1* &/or *EWSR1::CREB1*: Angiomatoid fibrous histiocytoma (AFH), malignant gastrointestinal neuroectodermal tumor (MGNET)
  - Effect of EWSR1-ATF1 protein
    - Compels SOX10, TFAP2, MITF transcription factors to bind to EWSR1-ATF binding sites
      - □ Leads to persistent, immature neural crest precursor cell phenotype

Extraskeletal Myxoid Chondrosarcoma
- Fusion driven: *NR4A3* fusions; t(9;22)(q31;q12) *EWSR1::NR4A3* accounts for ~ 65% of cases
  - Alternative fusions involve *TAF15* and *FUS* (like *EWSR1*, members of FET or TET family of genes that bind RNA and DNA), or, exceptionally, *TCF12, TFG, HSPA8*
    - *TAF15::NR4A3* cases often show high-grade, rhabdoid morphology or, rarely, biphasic appearance with p63 expression
  - All fusion proteins function as abnormal, strong transcriptional activators
- *NR4A3* = nuclear receptor subfamily 4 group A member: Transcription activator involved in proliferation, survival, differentiation, metabolism, and inflammation
  - Other tumors with *NR4A3* fusions: Mesenchymal chondrosarcoma and epithelial-myoepithelial carcinoma

Extrarenal Rhabdoid Tumor
- INI1 (SMARCB1) lost through biallelic inactivation
  - Losses occur through diverse mechanisms, including whole-gene or partial-gene deletions, indels, splice site and nonsense mutations
  - Specific pathways affected by INI1 loss (and in all tumors characterized by INI1 loss) include cell cycle, sonic hedgehog pathway, Wnt/β-catenin pathway, and *MYC* target genes
  - SMARCB1 loss → polycomb repressive complex able to freely bind to genes responsible for cell differentiation → genes cannot be expressed → rhabdoid tumor cell

Intimal Sarcoma
- **Complex aneuploidy**
  - Activating mutations/amplification of *PDGFRA*, *PDGFRB*, *EGFR*, and *MDM2* common

Perivascular Epithelioid Cell Tumor
- *TSC2* or *TSC1* inactivating mutations: ~ 65% of cases
  - mTOR pathway abnormally upregulated
- *TFE3* fusions: ~ 20% of cases
  - Fusion proteins increase *TFE3* expression → increased abnormal gene transcription
  - Most common partners: *SFPQ* (majority) and *DVL2*
  - Exceptional cases occurring in viscera show *ASPSCR1::TFE3* fusions (n = 3 cases reported)
    - These rare cases highlight close kinship of ASPS, PEComa, and Xp11 translocation renal cell carcinoma

MICROSCOPIC
Synovial Sarcoma
- Architecture
  - Classic
    - Monophasic: Plump spindle cells in streaming fascicles or sheets ± tigroid (striped alternating hypo- and hypercellular bands)
    - Biphasic: Plump spindle cells and epithelial cells in nests, cords, glands dispersed among fascicles of plump spindle cells
    - Stroma: Usually scant but can be fibrotic or myxoid
    - Calcifications sometimes, including osseous metaplasia present in ~ 33%
  - Poorly differentiated: Hypercellular ± geographic necrosis
- Cells
  - Classic
    - Spindled cells: Plump with relatively uniform, often overlapping nuclei, moderate N:C ratio, normo- to hyperchromatic; inconspicuous nucleoli

Rare Sarcomas of Uncertain Differentiation With Specific Molecular Alterations

- Epithelial cells: Pale, eosinophilic with round nuclei; may form intraluminal mucin, rarely show granular or squamous features
- Poorly differentiated
  - Can have 3 cell shapes but all are characterized by crowding, increased mitoses ± apoptosis
  - 3 cell shapes include small round blue cell, mimicking Ewing sarcoma, spindled cells with increased nuclear atypia compared to conventional areas, or epithelioid with macronucleoli, irregular chromatin distribution
- Ancillary studies
  - Immunohistochemistry
    - SSX antibody: Nuclear expression is 95% sensitive and highly specific for synovial sarcoma
    - Spindled and epithelial areas positive for EMA and often keratins (7, 8, 14, 18, and 19 most commonly)
    - Many cases show diffuse strong expression of TLE1 (many MPNST also express TLE1, usually not diffusely)
    - CD99 often positive and can show membranous reactivity, mimicking Ewing sarcoma family of tumors
    - Others: Only rarely positive (< 5%) for CD34; up to 40% focally S100 reactive
  - Genetic tests
    - Break-apart FISH for t(X;18) helps confirm diagnosis (Fusion occurs in > 95% of cases)
    - RT-PCR or NGS for fusion transcript also used

Epithelioid Sarcoma
- Architecture
  - Classic/conventional
    - Oval to sinuous nests of tumor cells seen at low power with central necrosis mimics caseating granulomas
    - Some tumors may have solid growth without classic pseudogranulomas
    - Epithelioid cells often present in central portion of tumor with spindled cells at periphery
  - Proximal type
    - Sheets or nodules of tumor cells
    - Mixed classic and proximal type comprise rare cases
  - Uncommon patterns
    - Angiomatoid: Tumor has prominent intermingled blood-filled cysts
    - Fibrous: Tumor has prominent fibrotic stroma, usually with spindled tumor cells
    - Myxoid: Tumor has prominent mucin-rich stroma
    - Dystrophic calcifications ± metaplastic bone (20%)
- Cells
  - Classic/conventional
    - Epithelioid cells: Large ovoid to polygonal with mild atypia of vesicular nuclei and small nucleoli; eosinophilic cytoplasm
    - Spindled cells: Plump spindled cells with ovoid vesicular nuclei and small nucleoli
    - Chronic inflammation common, especially at periphery of tumor nodules
    - Rhabdoid cells may occur
    - Mitotic rate usually ↓
  - Proximal type
    - Large, round to polygonal cells with round, vesicular nuclei and macronucleoli
    - Mitotic rate may be ↑
- Ancillary studies
  - Immunohistochemistry
    - Positive: SMARCB1 (INI1) lost in ~ 95%, keratins 8/18, often keratin 19 (95%); EMA, CD34 (50%), ERG (~ 30%)
    - Rarely positive: Desmin (focal), CD99 (25%), SMA (in spindled cells primarily, ~ 20%)
  - Genetic tests
    - FISH shows *SMARCB1* (INI1) homozygous deletions in ~ 90% of cases

Alveolar Soft Part Sarcoma
- Architecture
  - Classic/conventional
    - Nests with central sloughing of tumor cells resembling lung alveoli, &/or organoid growth of solid nests separated by thin vascular septa, &/or solid sheet-like growth (less common)
- Cells
  - Round to polygonal cells with eosinophilic to amphophilic granular cytoplasm
    - Nuclei usually fairly uniform, round with prominent nucleoli
    - Mitotic rate usually ↓
  - Cytoplasmic crystals commonly present but may be sparse
    - PAS positive/diastase resistant
    - Range from granular to rod shaped
- Ancillary studies
  - Immunohistochemistry
    - Positive: Strong diffuse TFE3 nuclear reactivity; focal desmin (50%), S100 in few cases
  - Genetic tests
    - FISH for *TFE3* rearrangement is diagnostically helpful
    - RT-PCR or NGS methods can also be used to detect *ASPSCR1::TFE3* fusion

Clear Cell Sarcoma of Soft Tissue
- Architecture
  - Most common pattern: Nests of cells separated by fibrous septa
  - Other patterns: Sheets of tumor cells; cutaneous examples often have dense sclerotic stroma
- Cells
  - Most common: Round to polygonal with eosinophilic to amphophilic cytoplasm
    - Multinucleated tumor cells with wreath-like array of nuclei relatively common and diagnostic clue
    - Nuclei usually uniform, vesicular with macronucleoli
    - Mitotic rate: Usually ↓
    - Melanin usually not detectable on H&E but present in ~ 66% on Fontana stain
  - Other tumor cell variants
    - Spindled tumor cells: Relatively common as small component but may be predominant or sole component
    - Plasmacytoid cells: Uncommon
    - Rhabdoid cells: Uncommon
    - Small round blue cells: Rare
- Ancillary studies
  - Immunohistochemistry

Rare Sarcomas of Uncertain Differentiation With Specific Molecular Alterations

- – Positive: Strongly positive for at least 1 melanocytic marker (S100, HMB-45, MITF, Melan-A, etc.)
  - o Genetic tests
    - – FISH shows *EWSR1* rearrangement in ~ 100% of cases
    - – RT-PCR or NGS methods also show t(12;22); *EWSR1::ATF1* or t(2;22); *EWSR1::CREB1*

Extraskeletal Myxoid Chondrosarcoma
- Architecture
  - o Myxoid lobules with cords, clusters, and cribriform arrays of small tumor cells
- Cells
  - o Classic/conventional
    - – Round to plump spindled cells with finely granular eosinophilic to amphophilic to vacuolated cytoplasm
    - – Nuclei usually relatively uniform, round to ovoid, vesicular with small nucleolus
    - – Mitotic figures usually ↓
  - o Poorly differentiated or high grade
    - – Hypercellular epithelioid or rhabdoid morphology with ↑ nuclear pleomorphism, ↑ mitoses ± necrosis
- Ancillary studies
  - o Immunohistochemistry
    - – Positive: Vimentin (100%), C-kit (30%), S100 (20%); few cases positive for synaptophysin
    - – SMARCB1 (INI1) may be completely absent in few cases (especially with rhabdoid cells) or show patchy pattern of nuclear reactivity
  - o Genetic tests
    - – FISH positive for *NR4A2* rearrangement (~ 90%); diagnostically helpful and specific for this sarcoma

Extrarenal Rhabdoid Tumor
- Architecture
  - o Sheets often with cellular dyscohesion
- Cells
  - o Small to medium-sized round cells with round to reniform nuclei, macronucleoli, and glassy, globoid cytoplasmic inclusion
  - o Small round blue cell component may be present
  - o Mitotic rate usually ↑
- Ancillary studies
  - o Immunohistochemistry
    - – Loss of SMARCB1 nuclear expression (> 95% of cases); EMA, keratins often positive in inclusions, which are intermediate filaments; vimentin, synaptophysin, and CD99 positive
  - o Genetic tests
    - – RT-PCR detects *SMARCB1* alterations that include mutations or homozygous deletions
    - – ~ 35% of patients have germline *SMARCB1* alterations
    - – Rarely, *SMARCA4* somatic ± germline mutations account for pathogenesis

Intimal Sarcoma
- Architecture
  - o Intravascular tumor most commonly composed of sheets of cells but also can be fascicular
  - o Stroma may be myxoid or include neoplastic bone if osteosarcomatous component present
- Cells
  - o Diverse array of cell types reported from large polygonal to epithelioid to spindled
  - o Usually at least moderate nuclear pleomorphism
  - o Specific differentiation can be present, such as osteosarcoma or rhabdomyosarcoma
- Ancillary studies
  - o Immunohistochemistry
    - – 70% positive for MDM2; other positive markers can include SATB2 (if osteosarcoma present), myogenin (if rhabdomyosarcoma present), desmin, and SMA
  - o Genetic tests: Nonspecific high-level amplification of *PDGFRA* (~ 80%), *MDM2* (~ 65%), *EGFR* (~ 70%) by FISH

Perivascular Epithelioid Cell Tumor
- Architecture
  - o Classic/conventional: Nests of cells usually with at least some centered on thin-walled blood vessels ± subendothelial growth
    - – Cell nests girded by thin-walled vessel or slips of collagen
  - o Malignant PEComa: Nests and sheets of pleomorphic cells ± perivascular arrangement
  - o Sclerosing variant (~ 15% of cases): Marked stromal sclerosis with corded or trabecular arrangement of tumor cells
  - o *TFE3* translocation-associated PEComa: Nests or sheets of cells ± central dyscohesion; no spindled areas; no subendothelial growth
- Cells
  - o Classic/conventional and sclerosing variant: Uniform bland epithelioid cells with relatively ↓ N:C ratio
    - – Cytoplasm: Abundant, pale eosinophilic and slightly granular to clear
  - o Malignant PEComa: Increased nuclear pleomorphism often with ↑ mitotic rate, necrosis ± atypical mitotic figures
  - o *TFE3* translocation-associated PEComa: Clear epithelioid cells with low or high nuclear atypia ± spindled tumor cells (uncommon)
- Ancillary studies
  - o Immunohistochemistry
    - – Myoid markers positive in *TSC2*/*TSC1*-altered cases: SMA, caldesmon
    - – Melanocytic markers positive in *TSC2*/*TSC1*-altered cases: HMB-45, Melan-A, MiTF, SOX10, S100 (10%)
    - – *TFE3* translocation-associated PEComa: Strong diffuse nuclear TFE3, HMB-45, and cathepsin-K; myoid markers and MiTF usually negative
  - o Genetic tests
    - – Conventional and sclerotic PEComas: *TSC2* loss of heterozygosity (LOH) with rare cases showing *TSC1* LOH
    - – *TFE3*-rearranged PEComas (~ 20% of cases): *TFE3* rearrangement detectable by FISH

SELECTED REFERENCES
1. Tanaka M et al: ASPSCR1::TFE3 orchestrates the angiogenic program of alveolar soft part sarcoma. Nat Commun. 14(1):1957, 2023
2. Warmke LM et al: TAF15::NR4A3 gene fusion identifies a morphologically distinct subset of extraskeletal myxoid chondrosarcoma mimicking myoepithelial tumors. Genes Chromosomes Cancer. 62(10):581-8, 2023

Rare Sarcomas of Uncertain Differentiation With Specific Molecular Alterations

Genetics of Soft Tissue Sarcomas of Uncertain Differentiation

Tumor	Genes Involved	Additional Molecular Genetic Findings	Abnormality Prevalence (%)
Synovial sarcoma	*SS18* (18q11)::*SSX1*, *SSX2*, *SSX3*, or *SSX4* (all Xp11) *SS18L1* (20q13)::*SSX1* ~ 66% have *SS18*::*SSX1* fusion ~ 33% have *SS18*::*SSX2* fusion All fusions expel SMARCB1 from SWI/SNF complex	Patients with multiple changes on karyotype or aCGH are at increased risk for ProgDse; O/E *KIF18A*, *CDCA2*, and *AURKA* in primary tumor are associated with ProgDse	~ 96% have *SS18*::*SSX1* or *SS18*::*SSX2* translocations
Epithelioid sarcoma	*SMARCB1* (INI1) (22q11) loss or translocation	PTEN expression lost leading to overactivation of mTOR pathway Rare cases show LOE of SMARCA4, SMARCC1, SMARCC2	~ 90% of epithelioid sarcoma, conventional and proximal types, have *SMARCB1* (INI1) abnormalities
Alveolar soft part sarcoma	*ASPSCR1*::*TFE3*	O/E MET leads to overactivation of MAPK and PI3K/AKT pathways; upregulation of JAG1 and MDK promotes angiogenesis Cathepsin-K O/E	~ 100% have gene fusion
Clear cell sarcoma of soft tissue	*EWSR1*::*ATF1* *EWSR1*::*CREB1*	Rare cases reported to have *BRAF* or *KIT* mutations in addition to *EWSR1* rearrangement; overactivation of PI3K/AKT and mTOR pathways IGF1R (15q26) O/E	~ 100% (same translocations as in angiomatoid fibrous histiocytoma)
Extraskeletal myxoid chondrosarcoma	*EWSR1*::*NR4A3* *TAF15*::*NR4A3* *TCF12*::*NR4A3* *TFG*::*NR4A3* *FUS*::*NR4A3* *HSPA8*::*NR4A3*	Cases with non-*EWSR1* fusions more likely to be high grade and aggressive; SMARCB1 (INI1) expression lost or patchy in some cases	~ 100% [t(9;22) most common]
Extrarenal rhabdoid tumor	*SMARCB1* (INI1) deleted on 22q11; *SMARCA4* (19p13) mutation or loss in rare cases	*TP53* mutations common; ~ 33% of patients have germline deletion or truncating mutation in *SMARCB1* as sporadic event or in setting of familial rhabdoid predisposition syndrome 1	~ 99% (*SMARCB1* abnormalities)
Perivascular epithelioid cell tumor (PEComa)	*TSC2*, *TSC1*: Altered tuberous sclerosis complex genes *TFE3* fusions to *SFPQ* or DVL2	Cathepsin-K O/E, TFE3 O/E; mTOR pathway hyperactivated in cases with *TSC2*/*TSC1* alterations	Majority may have *TSC2* LOH; rare cases have both *TSC2* and *TSC1* LOH
Intimal sarcoma	*PDGFRA*, *PDGFRB*, *MDM2*, *EGFR* amplified/gained and O/E	Loss of *CDKN2A*/*CDKN2B* *KIT* amplification	~ 40-80% have *PDGFRA* amplification; ~ 65-75% have *MDM2*, *EGFR* amplification

*In karyotype &/or aCGH. O/E = overexpressed; LOH = loss of heterozygosity; ProgDse = progressive disease; aCGH = array comparative genomic hybridization.

3. Argani P et al: PEComa-like neoplasms characterized by ASPSCR1-TFE3 fusion: another face of TFE3-related mesenchymal neoplasia. Am J Surg Pathol. 46(8):1153-9, 2022
4. Cyra M et al: SS18-SSX drives CREB activation in synovial sarcoma. Cell Oncol (Dordr). 45(3):399-413, 2022
5. Del Savio E et al: Beyond SMARCB1 loss: recent insights into the pathobiology of epithelioid sarcoma. Cells. 11(17):2626, 2022
6. Drosos Y et al: NSD1 mediates antagonism between SWI/SNF and polycomb complexes and is required for transcriptional activation upon EZH2 inhibition. Mol Cell. 82(13):2472-89.e8, 2022
7. Möller E et al: EWSR1-ATF1 dependent 3D connectivity regulates oncogenic and differentiation programs in Clear Cell Sarcoma. Nat Commun. 13(1):2267, 2022
8. Yoshida A et al: Identification of novel SSX1 fusions in synovial sarcoma. Mod Pathol. 35(2):228-39, 2022
9. Baranov E et al: A novel SS18-SSX fusion-specific antibody for the diagnosis of synovial sarcoma. Am J Surg Pathol. 44(7):922-33, 2020
10. Banito A et al: The SS18-SSX oncoprotein hijacks KDM2B-PRC1.1 to drive synovial sarcoma. Cancer Cell. 33(3):527-41.e8, 2018
11. Morgan MA et al: Epigenetic conFUSION: SS18-SSX fusion rewires BAF complex to activate bivalent genes in synovial sarcoma. Cancer Cell. 33(6):951-3, 2018
12. Waterfall JJ et al: A non-canonical polycomb dependency in synovial sarcoma. Cancer Cell. 33(3):344-6, 2018
13. Davis EJ et al: Next generation sequencing of extraskeletal myxoid chondrosarcoma. Oncotarget. 8(13):21770-7, 2017
14. Fu X et al: Activating mutation of PDGFRB gene in a rare cardiac undifferentiated intimal sarcoma of the left atrium: a case report. Oncotarget. 8(46):81709-16, 2017

Rare Sarcomas of Uncertain Differentiation With Specific Molecular Alterations

Synovial Sarcoma

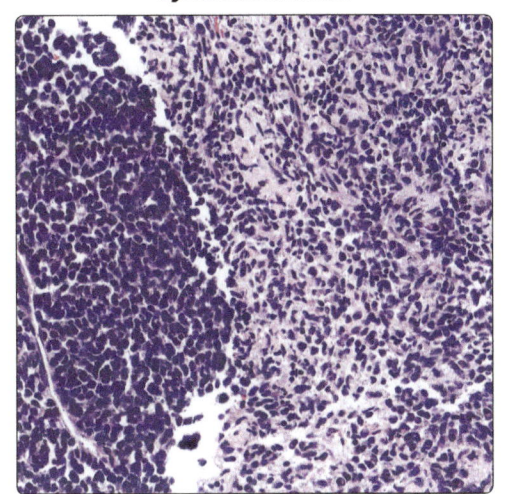

Synovial Sarcoma

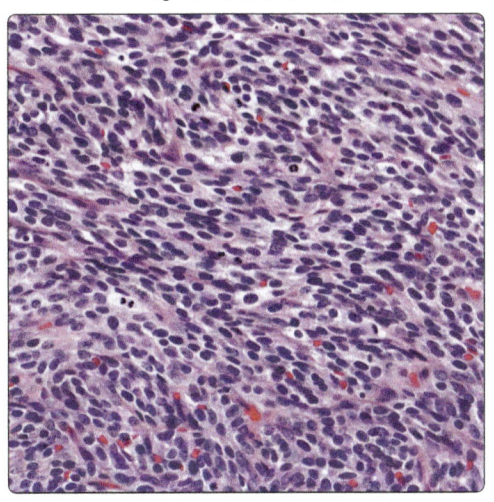

(Left) Even the monophasic variant of synovial sarcoma (SS) can appear heterogeneous microscopically with areas of hyper- and hypocellularity, as seen here. (Right) Although by definition SS is a high-grade tumor, many cases contain relatively bland, plump spindled cells with uniform ovoid nuclei, fine chromatin, inconspicuous nucleoli, and a relatively low mitotic rate.

Poorly Differentiated Synovial Sarcoma

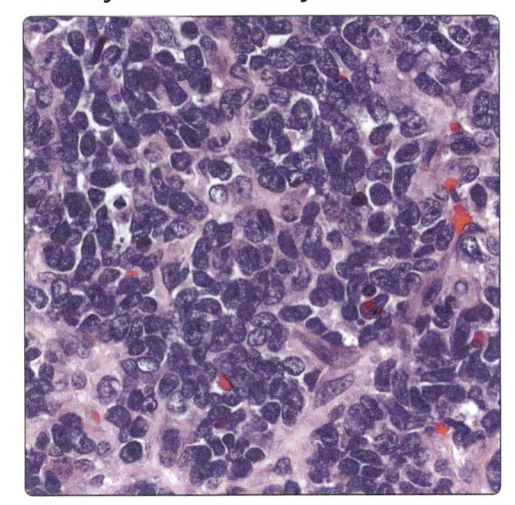

Synovial Sarcoma With Diffuse TLE1 Expression

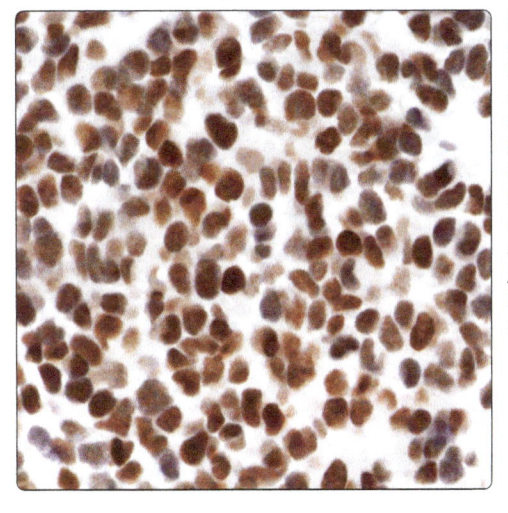

(Left) Poorly differentiated SS consists of tightly packed tumor cells with scant cytoplasm, high N:C ratio, and ovoid hyperchromatic nuclei. Most poorly differentiated SS have classic areas as well, helping to confirm the diagnosis. However, IHC and sometimes FISH are required for diagnosis in many cases. (Right) TLE1 is usually strongly and diffusely expressed in SS.

Biphasic Synovial Sarcoma

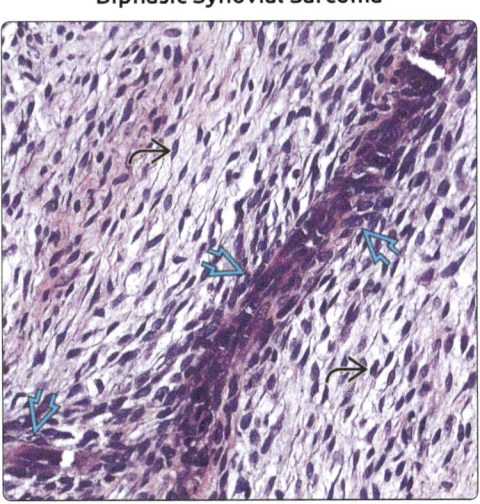

Biphasic Synovial Sarcoma With Keratin Expression

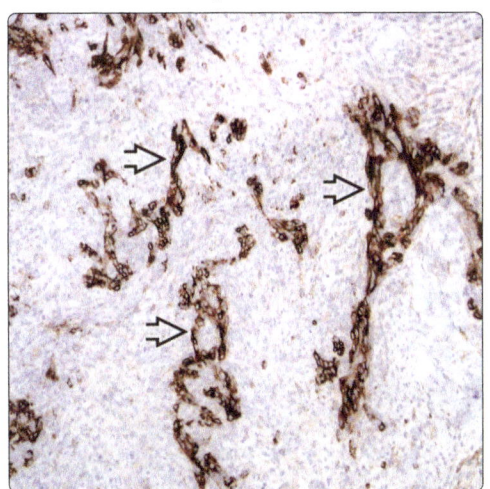

(Left) Biphasic SS is primarily composed of plump spindled cells ⇨. The epithelioid component in this tumor consists of cohesive, eosinophilic round cells that form cords or arcades ⇨. Some biphasic tumors have overt glandular or rarely squamous differentiation. (Right) The epithelial cords and arcades of this biphasic SS strongly express keratins 8/18 ⇨. At least some spindled cells usually also express EMA or keratin.

Rare Sarcomas of Uncertain Differentiation With Specific Molecular Alterations

Epithelioid Sarcoma

Epithelioid Sarcoma

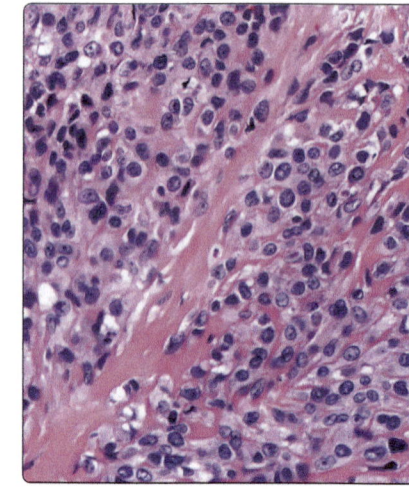

(Left) Classic epithelioid sarcoma mimics granulomatous inflammation at low power. Epithelioid tumor cells ➡ surround central foci of necrosis and imitate caseating granulomas. (Right) At high power, the tumor cells also vaguely resemble histiocytes, further mimicking granulomatous inflammation. However, the tumor cells have a higher N:C ratio and more nuclear atypia than histiocytes.

Epithelioid Sarcoma With Keratin Expression

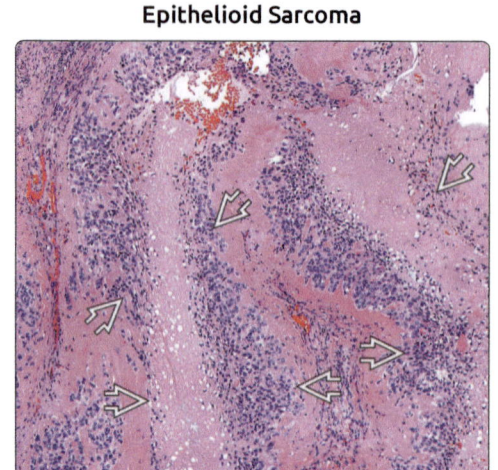

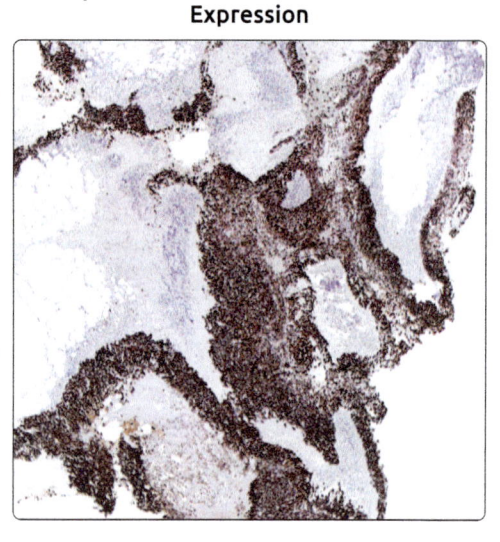

Proximal-Type Epithelioid Sarcoma

(Left) The tumor cells of epithelioid sarcoma are diffusely reactive for AE1/AE3. (Right) Proximal-type epithelioid sarcoma shows much greater cellular atypia than classic type. Here, the tumor cells show marked variation in size, coarse, irregularly distributed chromatin, and prominent enlarged nucleoli. A plasma cell reveals the relatively large size of the tumor cells ➡. Most proximal epithelioid sarcomas behave aggressively.

Alveolar Soft Part Sarcoma

Alveolar Soft Part Sarcoma

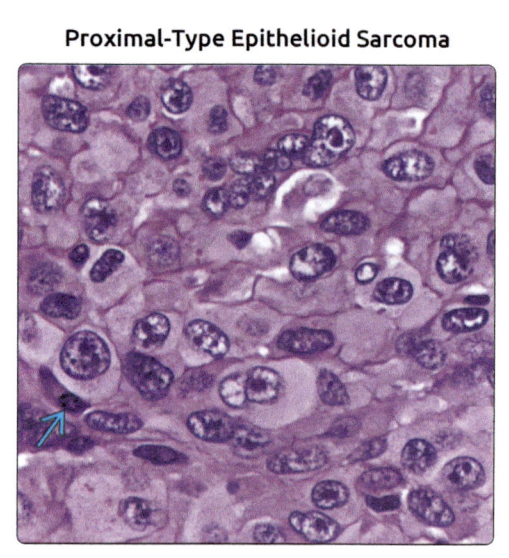

(Left) Alveolar soft part sarcoma shows the classic nested or organoid growth pattern. Central dyscohesion and cell lysis can impart a pulmonary alveolar appearance to the nests. Some cases also simply grow as solid sheets of cells. For these latter tumors, a high index of suspicion is needed in order to make the correct diagnosis. (Right) Alveolar soft part sarcoma at high power shows cells with usually only mild nuclear atypia and a low mitotic rate.

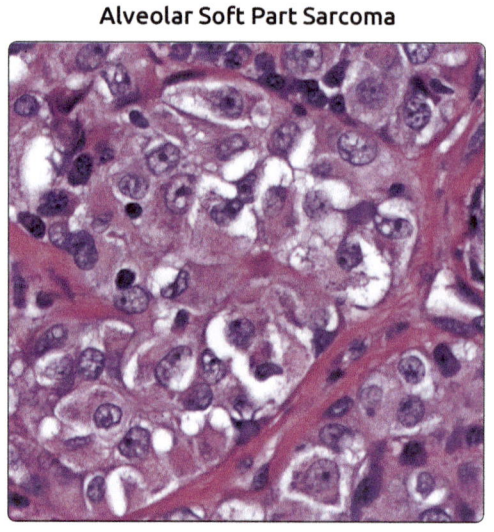

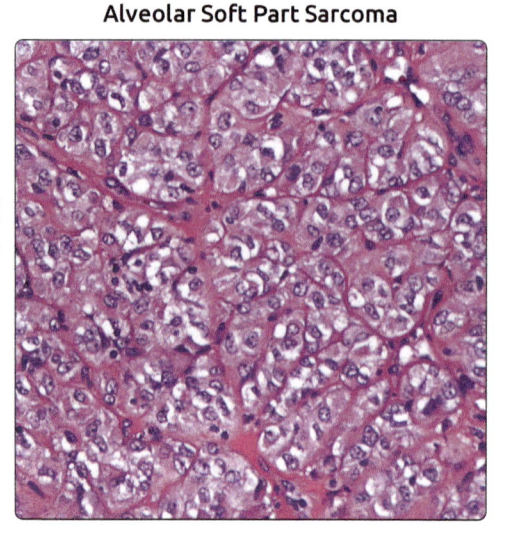

Rare Sarcomas of Uncertain Differentiation With Specific Molecular Alterations

Clear Cell Sarcoma

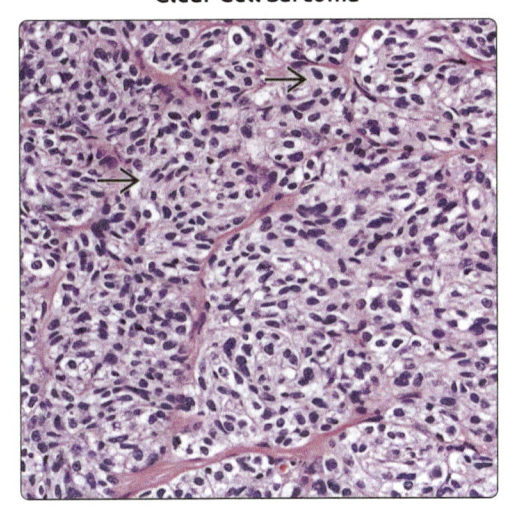

Dermal Sclerosing Clear Cell Sarcoma

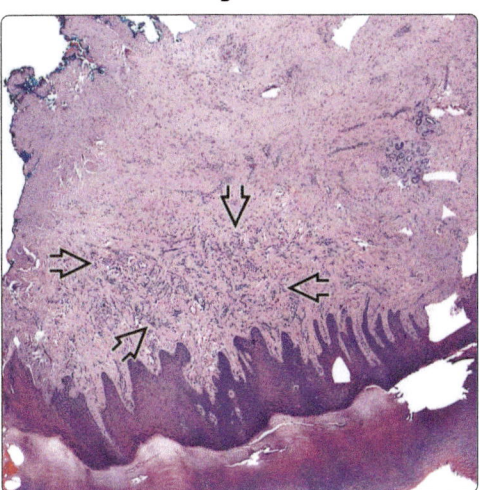

(Left) *Clear cell sarcoma most commonly grows in a back-to-back nested pattern with thin, intervening fibrous trabeculae. Note that very few of the cells have clear cytoplasm. Instead, most have pale eosinophilic cytoplasm ➡. Clear cells are typically uncommon or absent in clear cell sarcoma.* (Right) *A diagnostically challenging variant is dermal sclerosing clear cell sarcoma ➡, which can be relatively hypocellular and induces a marked fibrotic reaction.*

Sclerosing Clear Cell Sarcoma

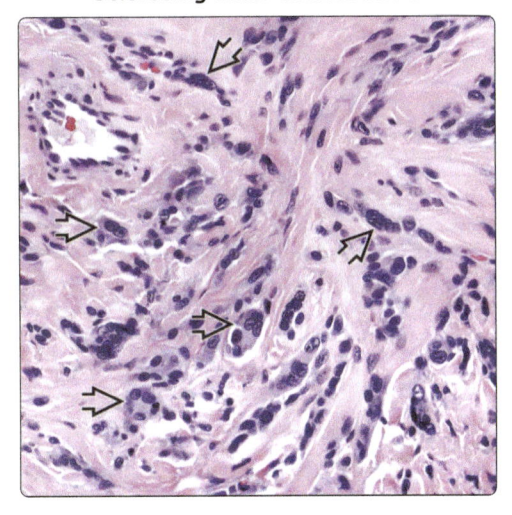

Clear Cell Sarcoma With S100 Expression

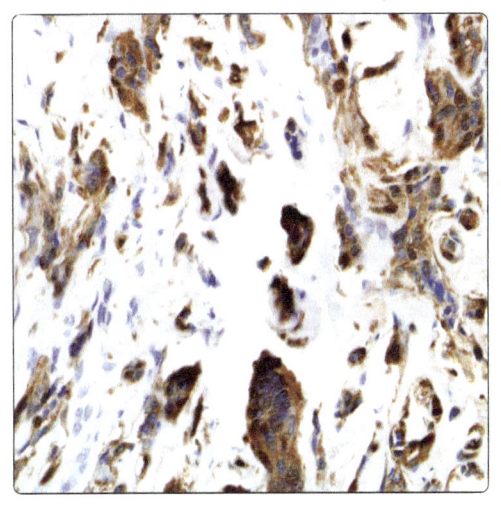

(Left) *Sclerosing clear cell sarcoma shows strands of mononucleated cells and interspersed multinucleated tumor cells ➡. Multinucleated tumor cells are a common finding and can suggest the diagnosis if other histologic and clinical features are concordant.* (Right) *Clear cell sarcoma expresses one or more melanocytic markers. This tumor shows diffuse expression of S100.*

Extraskeletal Myxoid Chondrosarcoma

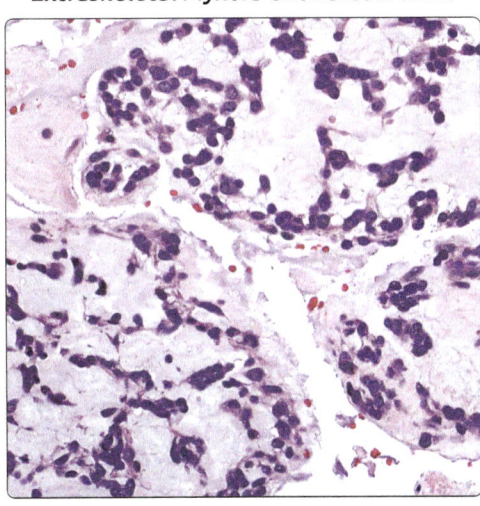

Extraskeletal Myxoid Chondrosarcoma With Cytologic Atypia

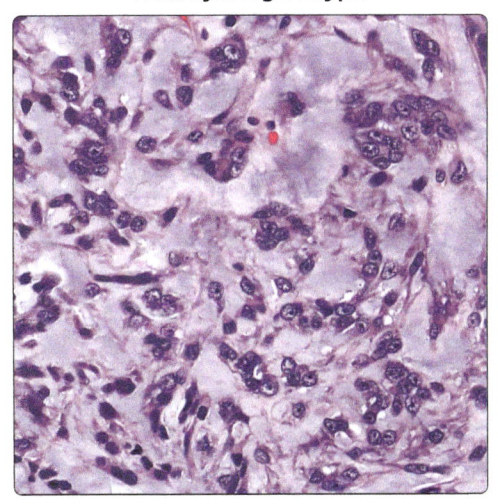

(Left) *Extraskeletal myxoid chondrosarcoma (ESMCS) consists of lobules of intermixed cords, clusters, and lattices of small round tumor cells set in a myxoid matrix. The tumor does not make hyaline cartilage and is not a chondrosarcoma, despite the name.* (Right) *This case of ESMCS has increased nuclear atypia with prominent nucleoli and more anisonucleosis compared to most cases. Tumors with marked nuclear atypia may behave more aggressively and can include rhabdoid cell morphology.*

Rare Sarcomas of Uncertain Differentiation With Specific Molecular Alterations

(Left) Extrarenal rhabdoid tumor (ERRT) most often grows as solid sheets of cells. Dyscohesion is sometimes notable ⇒, even at low power. **(Right)** In this ERRT, a subtle rhabdoid appearance is conferred by prominent paranuclear hyaline globules. Nuclei are vesicular with macronucleoli. Some cases may have spindled cells &/or small round cells, and the rhabdoid part may be focal. Note the high mitotic rate ⇒, which is typical of this tumor.

Extrarenal Rhabdoid Tumor

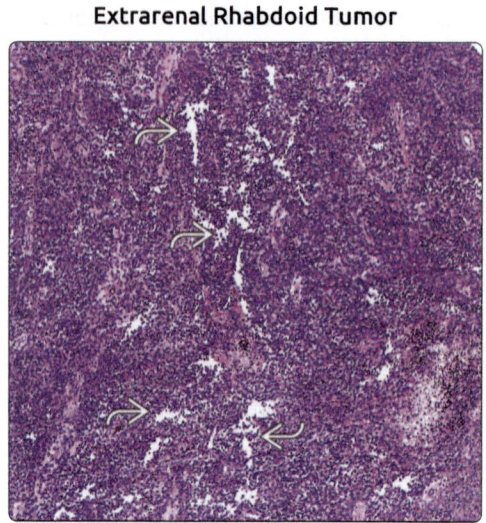

Extrarenal Rhabdoid Tumor

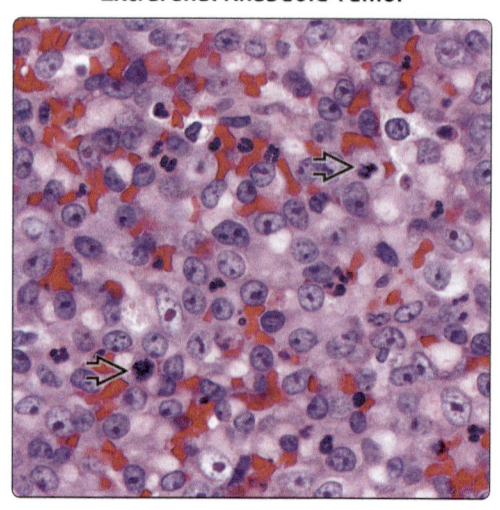

(Left) The cytoplasmic inclusions of this ERRT strongly express keratins, a common finding. **(Right)** The rhabdoid appearance of ERRT tumor cells is often most conspicuous in areas of dyscohesion. The cells resemble rhabdomyoblasts and can express SMA, but they are neither smooth muscle nor skeletal muscle in differentiation. Due to the eccentric nuclei and hyaline globules, the cells also resemble osteoblasts or plasma cells.

Extrarenal Rhabdoid Tumor With Cytoplasmic Globular Keratin Expression

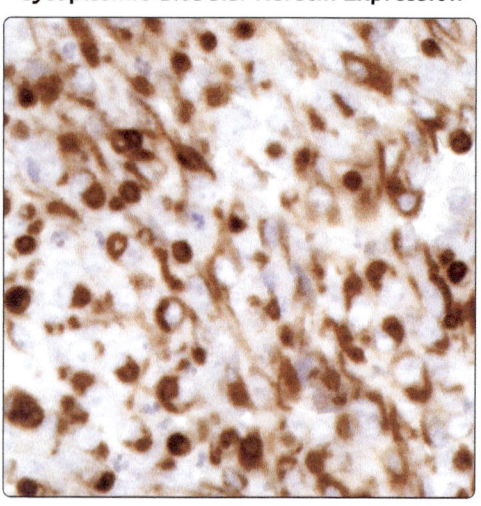

Extrarenal Rhabdoid Tumor With Classic Rhabdoid Cells

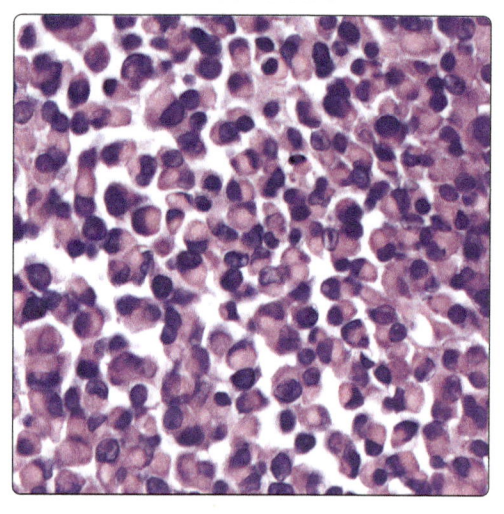

(Left) Tumor cells in this PEComa are arranged in nests or trabeculae separated by thin, interconnecting fibrous bands. Other growth patterns include a diffuse sheet-like growth, radial arrangement of tumor cells around blood vessels, and subendothelial undermining by tumor cells. **(Right)** ~ 15% of PEComas exhibit a markedly sclerotic matrix. This sclerosing PEComa also includes psammoma bodies ⇒. The tumor cells are clear to slightly amphophilic.

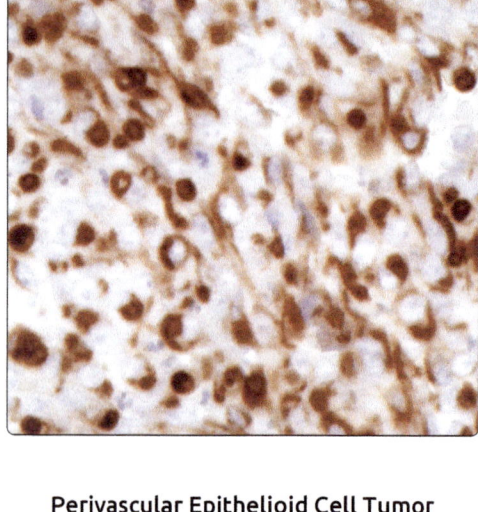

Perivascular Epithelioid Cell Tumor

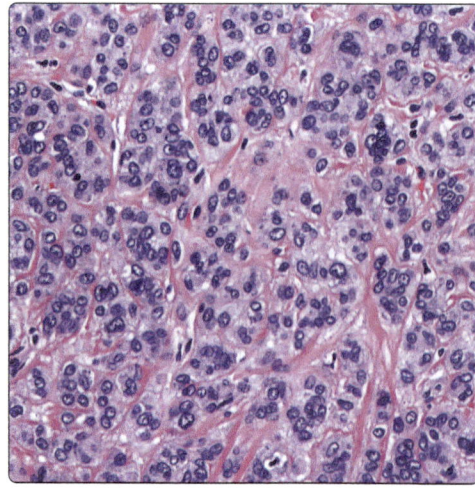

Perivascular Epithelioid Cell Tumor With Sclerotic Matrix

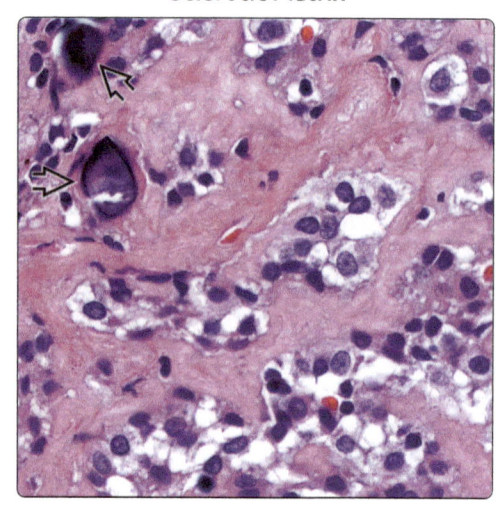

Rare Sarcomas of Uncertain Differentiation With Specific Molecular Alterations

Malignant Perivascular Epithelioid Cell Tumor

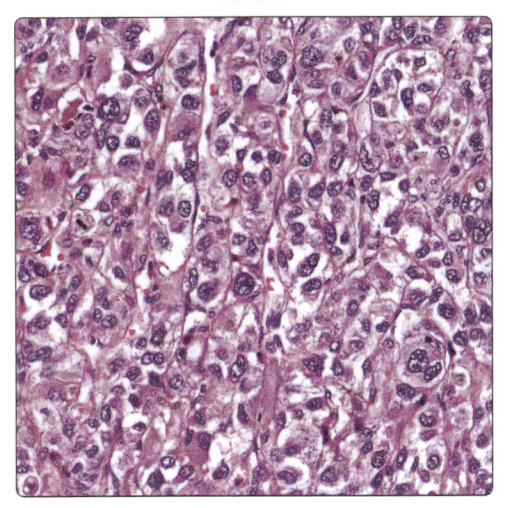

Malignant Perivascular Epithelioid Cell Tumor

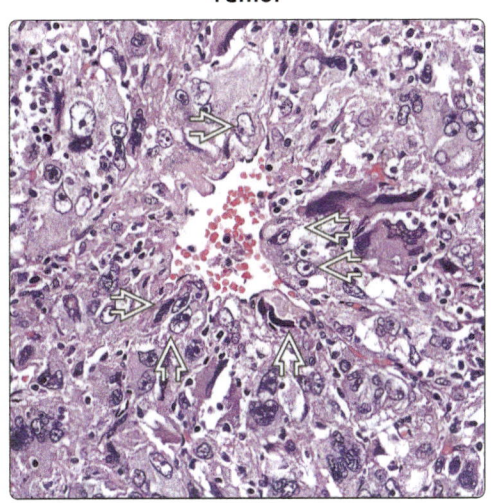

(Left) Malignant PEComa shows only minimal pleomorphism in this field. Other fields showed loss of trabecular architecture and marked nuclear pleomorphism with necrosis and a high mitotic rate. Both benign and malignant PEComas are composed of cells that usually have clear or eosinophilic granular cytoplasm. (Right) Tumor cells of this highly pleomorphic malignant PEComa deeply invade into the vessel wall ⇨. This is called subendothelial growth and is common in PEComas.

Intimal Sarcoma

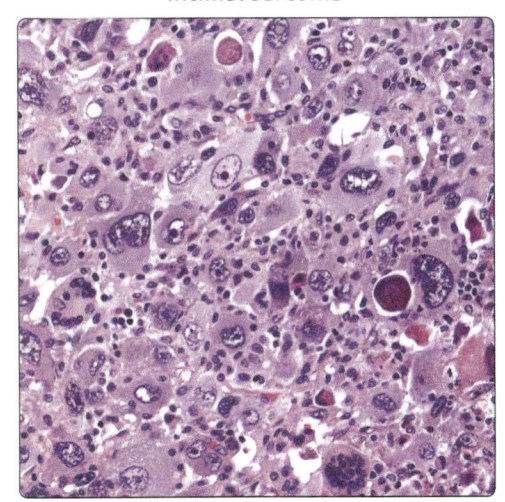

Intimal Sarcoma With Reactive Giant Cells

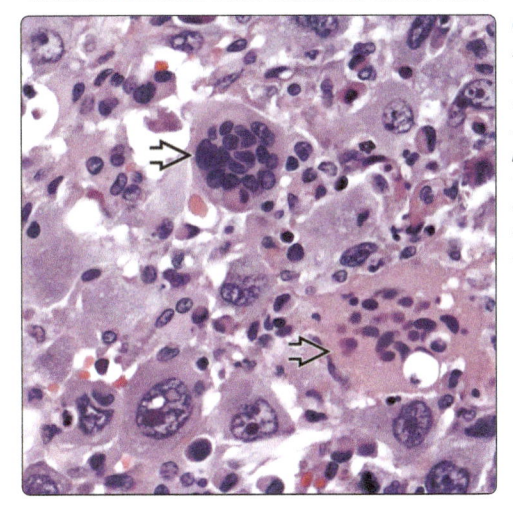

(Left) Intimal sarcoma can have a variety of cell types, including spindled, polygonal, and rarely epithelioid. This intimal sarcoma is highly pleomorphic and somewhat chronically inflamed. (Right) Reactive, osteoclast-like multinucleated giant cells ⇨ infiltrate this intimal sarcoma.

Intimal Sarcoma

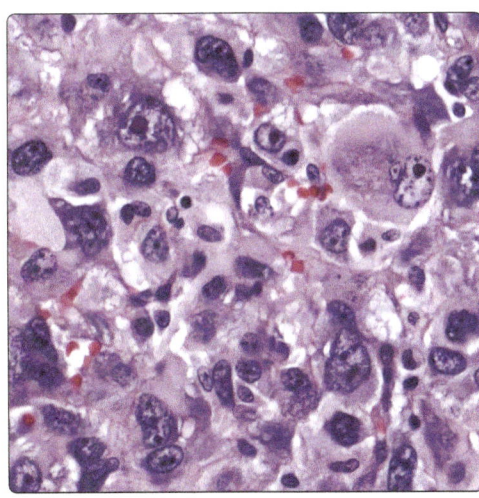

Intimal Sarcoma With MDM2 Expression

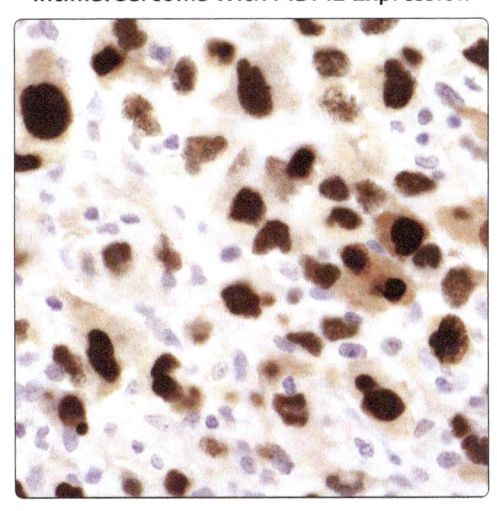

(Left) The degree of atypia in intimal sarcoma is at least moderate. This tumor is markedly pleomorphic with marked anisonucleosis, coarse chromatin, and macronucleoli. Fresh hemorrhage, the somewhat epithelioid appearance of tumor cells, and location at a blood vessel raised the differential of epithelioid angiosarcoma. (Right) Many intimal sarcomas show strong nuclear expression of MDM2, as seen here.

Rare Sarcomas of Uncertain Differentiation With Specific Molecular Alterations (Continued)

TERMINOLOGY

Definitions

- Sarcomas or intermediate-grade tumors that **do not** differentiate toward known cell type but have specific genetic and histologic findings

EPIDEMIOLOGY

Myoepithelial Carcinoma

- Age: Children > 4th to 5th decade > older
- Sex: M = F
- Location: Subcutis > deep; extremities > trunk > head and neck > bone and viscera > skin
- Behavior: 50% recurrence and metastasis

Pleomorphic Hyalinizing Angiectatic Tumor of Soft Parts

- Age: Middle-age adults > others
- Sex: F slightly > M
- Location: Subcutis of ankle > > deep ST of buttock, perineum, arm
- Behavior: 50% recurrence rate; exceptionally dedifferentiates to frank sarcoma, such as spindle cell sarcoma NOS, myxofibrosarcoma, or SMARCA4-deficient sarcoma

Phosphaturic Mesenchymal Tumor

- Age: Middle-aged adults > others
- Sex: M = F
- Location: Soft tissue > bone; Soft tissue and bone > > > viscera, mediastinum, retroperitoneum
- Behavior: Benign except for exceptional cases, which metastasize and may cause death
  - Tumor-induced osteomalacia (TIO) caused by even small, superficial tumors

Ossifying Fibromyxoid Tumor

- Age: Adults > others (broad range)
- Sex: M slightly > F
- Location: Subcutis > deep; leg > head and neck, trunk
- Behavior: Ranges based on degree of atypia (benign, atypical, and malignant variants) from 0-60% metastasis
  - However, rare cytologically "benign" OFMT may metastasize after many years

Angiomatoid Fibrous Histiocytoma

- Age: 1st to 2nd decade > other ages
- Sex: M = F
- Location: Subcutis of extremities > trunk and head and neck > nonsomatic deep sites
  - Many (2/3) occur at sites of lymph node aggregates, such as groin, axilla, or neck
- Behavior: Superficial tumors show 15% recurrence, 2-5% metastasis; deep tumors seem to be more aggressive

NTRK-Rearranged Spindle Cell Neoplasm

- Age: ~ 60% in children > other ages
- Location: Subcutis = deep; extremities or trunk
- Behavior: Low-grade tumors may locally recur; high-grade tumors may metastasize and cause death

ETIOLOGY/PATHOGENESIS

Myoepithelial Carcinoma

- Fusion driven or SMARCB1 loss
  - Fusions comprise 50% of cases: *EWSR1* or rarely *FUS* with multiple partners including *POU5F1*, *PBX1*, *PBX3*, *KLF15*, *KLF17*, *ZNF44*, *ATF1*, others
  - Specific fusion may correlate with histology
    - *EWSR1::POU5F1*: Nests of clear, epithelioid cells (deep soft tissue of children most commonly)
    - *EWSR1::PBX1*: Bland spindle cells embedded in fibrotic stroma (commonly intraosseous)
    - *EWSR1::PBX3*: Syncytial growth of bland spindled, ovoid, and histiocytoid cells (cutaneous syncytial myoepithelioma)
    - *EWSR1::KLF15*: Biphasic with small round cell component ± focal clear cell features
    - *FUS::KLF17*: Chordoma-like pattern comprising strands of epithelioid cells embedded in myxoid to myxohyaline matrix

Phosphaturic Mesenchymal Tumor

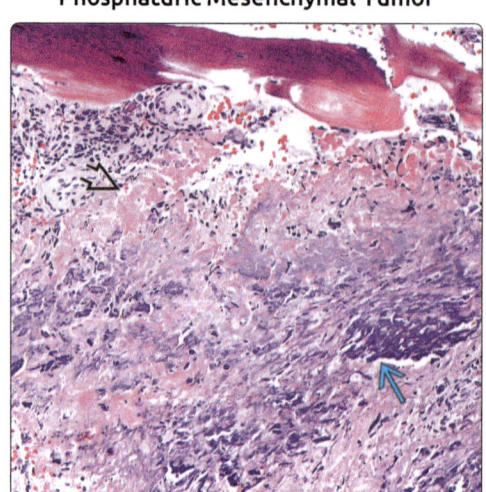

Phosphaturic Mesenchymal Tumor With SATB2 Expression

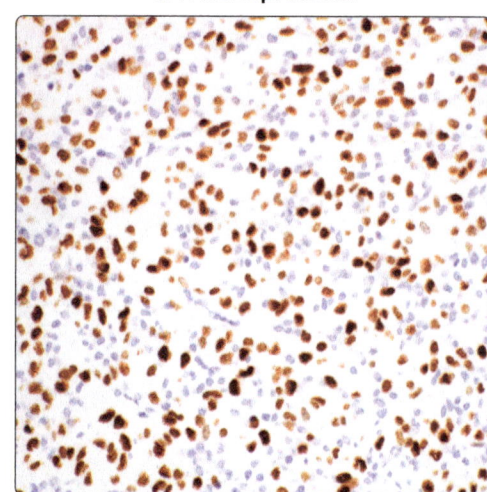

(Left) Phosphaturic mesenchymal tumor (PMT) usually contains "grungy" calcifications ➡ and osteoid ➡ when arising within bone, as in this case from the distal fibula. (Right) Nuclear expression of SATB2 is common in PMT. Other proteins commonly expressed include CD56, ERG, D2-40, and FGFR1.

Rare Sarcomas of Uncertain Differentiation With Specific Molecular Alterations (Continued)

- ○ SMARCB1 loss comprises 10-40% of cases: Homozygous deletions occur in 60% of MECa that lack fusions
- PLAG1 rearrangements in acral dermal tumors, which feature nests of eosinophilic, epithelioid cells ± ducts (50%) ± myxoid change ± angiectatic vessels
  - ○ Likely represents distinctive subset of cutaneous mixed tumor
  - ○ Metastasizing cases may exhibit bland cytologic features or marked atypia and infiltrative growth
  - ○ Most cases with nonatypical cytology appear to be benign

Pleomorphic Hyalinizing Angiectatic Tumor of Soft Parts

- Rearrangement driven: Rearrangements of TGFBR3 (1p22) &/or OGA (MGEA5); 10q24
  - ○ Results in transcriptional upregulation of FGF8 and NPM3
  - ○ Does not result in transcribed fusion protein
- Coinciding amplification of VGLL3 (3p11-12)
- Other tumors with these rearrangements and amplification of VGLL3: Hemosiderotic fibrolipomatous tumor (HFLT), hybrid HFLT-myxoinflammatory fibroblastic sarcoma, myxoinflammatory fibroblastic sarcoma (MIFS)
  - ○ Relationship or overlap of PHAT, HFLT, and MIFS still being resolved
    - – MIFS: Categorized by WHO 2020 as myofibroblastic tumor, not tumor of uncertain differentiation
      - □ MIFS also may show rearrangements of BRAF thus far not identified in HFLT

Phosphaturic Mesenchymal Tumor

- Fusion driven: FN1::FGFR or FN1::FGF1 (50% of cases); other abnormalities may be detected in non-FN1 fusion cases
  - ○ Fusion protein (aberrant tyrosine kinase functionality) → ↑ FGF23 (phosphaturic hormone) → tumor-induced osteomalacia (TIO)
  - ○ Rare cases causing TIO do not show elevated FGF23
  - ○ Rare cases do not cause TIO

Ossifying Fibromyxoid Tumor

- Fusion driven: PHF1 fusions involving EP400 (most common), MEAF6, EPC1, TFE3, and rare others
  - ○ Additional rare fusions involve BCOR, BCOR1, CREBBP, and KDM2A
    - – Occur preferentially in malignant OFMT
  - ○ Mechanism of action of PHF1 fusion: Dysregulates transcription of specific genes through altering histones
- SMARCB1 diminished expression: Patchy loss (75% of cases)
  - ○ Contributes to dysregulated transcription by altering activity of SWI/SNF complex

Angiomatoid Fibrous Histiocytoma

- Fusion driven: FET family gene and CREB family gene, including EWSR1::CREB1 > EWSR1::ATF1 > FUS::ATF1 > > EWSR1/FUS::CREM
- Other tumors with ≥ 1 of above-listed fusions
  - ○ Clear cell sarcoma of soft tissue
    - – EWSR1::ATF1: Exon 8 of EWSR1 fuses to exon 4 of ATF1
      - □ Fusion protein → acts as unregulated transcriptional activator → ↑ transcription of MITF → tumor shows melanocytic differentiation
    - – EWSR1::CREB1: Fusion protein functions similarly as EWSR1::ATF1 fusion
  - ○ Hyalinizing clear cell carcinoma of salivary gland
  - ○ Primary pulmonary myxoid sarcoma
  - ○ Intracranial mesenchymal FET::CREB fused tumors
    - – May represent spectrum of tumors, including intracranial AFH and 2nd group with different, distinctive gene expression profile
  - ○ Malignant gastrointestinal neuroectodermal tumor
  - ○ AFH-like tumor of peritoneal-lined spaces
    - – Predominantly epithelioid morphology, often expressing keratins ± EMA
    - – Most cases behave aggressively (few cases reported to date)
  - ○ Others: Rare cases of angiosarcoma, myoepithelial tumors, mesothelioma

NTRK-Rearranged Spindle Cell Neoplasm

- Rearrangement/fusion driven: NTRK1/NTRK2/NTRK3 with multiple partners
  - ○ Representative fusion partners: TPM3, LMNA, TPM4, SQSTM1, STRN3, IRF2BP2, TPR, TFG, EML4, ETV6
- Other tumors with ETV6::NTRK3 fusion: Infantile fibrosarcoma, congenital mesoblastic nephroma, subset of inflammatory myofibroblastic tumors, secretory carcinomas of breast and salivary gland

MICROSCOPIC

Myoepithelial Carcinoma

- Architecture
  - ○ Low power: Multinodular or lobular
  - ○ Medium power: Diversity of patterns ranging from solid, nested, and streaming to reticular and trabecular; often mixed patterns
  - ○ Stroma: Diverse, from myxoid to myxochondroid to fibrotic/hyalinized
  - ○ Heterologous differentiation: Uncommon (15%) and usually chondrosarcomatous but also squamous carcinoma
- Cells
  - ○ Range from epithelioid (most common) to undifferentiated small round blue cells (more common in pediatric cases) ± rhabdoid cells, clear cells, and plasmacytoid cells
  - ○ Nuclear atypia: Must be present and differentiates MECa from myoepithelioma
- Ancillary studies
  - ○ IHC: Range of expression as in morphology
    - – Most commonly positive antibodies: S100, broad spectrum keratins, calponin
    - – May be positive: p63, SOX10, GFAP, SMA, desmin
    - – INI1 (SMARCB1): Lost in some MECa

Pleomorphic Hyalinizing Angiectatic Tumor of Soft Parts

- Architecture

Rare Sarcomas of Uncertain Differentiation With Specific Molecular Alterations (Continued)

- Sheets of tumor cells and inflammation mixed with thin-walled, ectatic blood vessels of irregular shapes featuring fibrinoid mural deposits in walls ± thrombi
- Cells
  - Mixed spindled to epithelioid cells with some cells showing marked nuclear pleomorphism; rare to absent mitoses; intracellular hemosiderin; inflammation often present
- Ancillary studies
  - IHC: CD34 expressed in tumor cells
  - Genetic studies: May show rearrangements of *TGFBR3* &/or *MGEA5* and *VLL3* amplification
    - Malignant PHAT (with high-grade transformation) may show additional genetic abnormalities

Phosphaturic Mesenchymal Tumor

- Architecture: Broad variety of appearances in some cases related to location
  - Most cases: Hypocellular to moderately cellular with prominent vascular network comprising small, branching capillaries or HPC-like pattern
  - Matrix: Ranges from basophilic deposits to flower-like crystals to "grungy" calcifications to chondroid or osteochondroid regions
    - Malignant PMT do not produce matrix but may be associated with benign PMT
  - Intraosseous cases may show ABC-like changes &/or abundant osteoid
  - Intranasal cases may contain fat and thick-walled vessels
  - Intramandibular cases may contain epithelial elements (may be reactive and not neoplastic)
- Cells
  - Benign cases: Mix of bland spindled and stellate cells + epithelial elements in craniofacial bones
  - Malignant cases: Marked cytologic atypia ± mitoses ± necrosis
  - Other nonneoplastic intermixed cells: Chronic inflammatory cells, multinucleated giant cells, spindled fibroblasts, adipocytes
- Ancillary studies
  - IHC: CD56, ERG, FGF1, SATB2, D2-40, and CD99 usually expressed
  - Genetic studies: *FN1::FGFR1* or *FN1::FGF1* detected in 50%

Ossifying Fibromyxoid Tumor

- Architecture
  - Multinodular with pushing borders ± pseudocapsule, often with peripheral reactive bone
  - Variable tumor cell patterns: Solid, cords, nests, trabeculae with intermixed fibrous to myxoid stroma
- Cells
  - Uniform spindled to round cells with inconspicuous cell borders, uniform oval nuclei, and absent to very rare mitoses
  - OFMT more likely to behave aggressively: "Malignant" OFMT" (more hypercellular with > 2 mitoses/10 mm² ± high nuclear grade)
- Ancillary studies
  - IHC: SMARCB1 mosaic pattern of lost expression (75%), S100 (~ 66%), desmin (~50%); uncommonly keratins, SMA, EMA, and MUC4
  - Genetic studies: *PHF1* fusions

Angiomatoid Fibrous Histiocytoma

- Architecture
  - Nodular proliferation containing pseudoangiomatoid spaces surrounded by lymphoplasmacytic cuff
  - Common cell arrangements: Syncytia > storiforming bundles, whorls
  - Variant architectures: Solid growth only, extensive myxoid change, prominent sclerosis, hemosiderin deposition
- Cells
  - Usually plump spindled to eosinophilic epithelioid with nonatypical, ovoid nuclei
  - Less common features: Scattered atypical cells, clear cells, small round cells with high N:C ratio, scattered osteoclast-like cells
- Ancillary studies
  - IHC: Desmin focal or diffuse (50%), TLE (majority); may also express CD99, EMA, CD68, and ALK
  - Genetic studies: *EWSR1* rearrangements identified in majority

NTRK-Rearranged Spindle Cell Neoplasm

- Architecture
  - Diverse, but some cases exhibit perivascular collagen rings
  - Lipofibromatosis neural tumor-like pattern
  - Cellular spindle cell MPNST or fibrosarcoma-like pattern
  - Small round cell sarcoma-like pattern
  - Rare cases have heterologous elements, such as liposarcoma, rhabdomyosarcoma
- Cells
  - Most commonly ovoid to spindled
  - Cell lineage: Most likely fibroblastic/myofibroblastic (4 recent studies)
- Ancillary studies
  - IHC: Most tumors express pan-TRK antibody (10% of NTRK3 fusions tumors are negative) relatively nonspecific antibody; many express S100, CD34, and CD30; some cases express SMA ± desmin
  - Genetic studies: Positive for *NTRK1/NTRK2/NTRK3* rearrangements or fusions

SELECTED REFERENCES

1. Fischer GM et al: Gene fusions in superficial mesenchymal neoplasms: emerging entities and useful diagnostic adjuncts. Semin Diagn Pathol. 40(4):246-57, 2023
2. Kojima N et al: Frequent CD30 expression in an emerging group of mesenchymal tumors with NTRK, BRAF, RAF1, or RET Fusions. Mod Pathol. 36(4):100083, 2023
3. Tauziède-Espariat A et al: NTRK-rearranged spindle cell neoplasms are ubiquitous tumours of myofibroblastic lineage with a distinct methylation class. Histopathology. 82(4):596-607, 2023
4. Trecourt A et al: CREB fusion-associated epithelioid mesenchymal neoplasms of the female adnexa: three cases documenting a novel location of an emerging entity and further highlighting an ambiguous misleading immunophenotype. Virchows Arch. 482(6):967-74, 2023
5. Ulici V et al: Extraenteric malignant gastrointestinal neuroectodermal tumor- A clinicopathologic and molecular genetic study of 11 cases. Mod Pathol. 36(7):100160, 2023
6. Agaimy A et al: Rapidly fatal SMARCA4-deficient undifferentiated sarcoma originating from hybrid hemosiderotic fibrolipomatous tumor/pleomorphic hyalinizing angiectatic tumor of the foot. Virchows Arch. 480(5):1115-20, 2022

Rare Sarcomas of Uncertain Differentiation With Specific Molecular Alterations (Continued)

Genetics of Soft Tissue Sarcomas of Uncertain Differentiation

Tumor	Genes Involved	Additional Molecular Genetic Findings	Abnormality Prevalence (%)
Myoepithelial carcinoma (MECa)	*EWSR1* (rarely *FUS*) fusions; fusion partners include *POU5F1*, *PBX1/PBX3*, *ZNF44*, *KLF15/KLF17*, and *ATF1*; *INI1* (SMARCB1) homozygous deletions; *PLAG1* rearrangements in rare acral dermal MECa	Sparse data to date: Chromoplexy (specific mechanism of breakage of chromosomes) reported in one case; *GGNBP2::ASCC2* fusion reported in single case with *SMARCB1* loss	Fusions: ~ 50% of MECa; *SMARCB1* deletions: 10-30% of MECa; *PLAG1* rearrangements rare; confined to acral dermal sites
Pleomorphic hyalinizing angiectatic tumor of soft parts (PHAT)	Rearrangements of *TGFB3* &/or *OGA* (MGEA5), usually in cases with peripheral HFLT-like appearance	Rearrangement of *FBXW14* (10q24.2); *FGF8* overexpressed consistent with *TGFBR3::MGEA5* rearrangement; amplification of *VGLL3*; *SMARCA4* loss	Subsets of PHAT show listed genetic findings; *SMARCA4* loss in malignant PHAT reported in one recent case
Phosphaturic mesenchymal tumor (PMT)	*FN1::FGFR1* or *FN1::FGF* fusions	*NIPBL2::BEND2* fusion reported in one intraosseous case with TIO	50% of cases show *FN1* fusions
Ossifying fibromyxoid tumor (OFMT)	*PHF1* fusions to *EP400*, *MEAF6*, *EPC1*, and *TFE3*	*SMARCB1* loss; rare other fusions involve *BCOR*, *BCOR1*, *CREBBP*, and *KDM2A*	85% show *PHF1* fusions; 75% show patchy SMARCB1 loss; rare additional fusions preferentially occur in malignant OFMT
Angiomatoid fibrous histiocytoma (AFH)	FET family-CREB family fusions: *EWSR1::CREB1*, *EWSR1::ATF1*, *EWSR1/FUS::CREM*	*CDKN2A* or *CDKN2B* deletions; *TERT* promoter amplification; *XAF1* and *S100A4* upregulation	90% show *EWSR1::CREB1* fusion; *EWSR1/FUS::CREM* fusions rare; *CDKN2A/CDKN2B* deletions in cases with metastases
NTRK-rearranged spindle cell neoplasm	*NTRK1/NTRK2/NTRK3* rearrangements or fusions with many partners, including *LMNA*, *TPM3*, *STRN3*, and *ETV6*	*TGF::MET* fusion spindle cell tumors may be related (based on DNA methylation profiling); *CDKN2A* deletion	By definition, 100% have *NTRK1*, *NTRK2*, or *NTRK3* fusions; 33-55% show *CDKN2A* deletions

7. Agaimy A et al: Intra-abdominal EWSR1/FUS-CREM-rearranged malignant epithelioid neoplasms: two cases of an emerging aggressive entity with emphasis on misleading immunophenotype. Virchows Arch. 480(2):481-6, 2022
8. Cyrta J et al: Whole-genome characterization of myoepithelial carcinomas of the soft tissue. Cold Spring Harb Mol Case Stud. 8(7), 2022
9. Dermawan JK et al: Comprehensive genomic profiling of EWSR1/FUS::CREB translocation-associated tumors uncovers prognostically significant recurrent genetic alterations and methylation-transcriptional correlates. Mod Pathol. 35(8):1055-65, 2022
10. Klubíčková N et al: RNA-sequencing of myxoinflammatory fibroblastic sarcomas reveals a novel SND1::BRAF fusion and 3 different molecular aberrations with the potential to upregulate the TEAD1 gene including SEC23IP::VGLL3 and TEAD1::MRTFB gene fusions. Virchows Arch. 481(4):613-20, 2022
11. Mehta A et al: Cutaneous myoepithelial neoplasms on acral sites show distinctive and reproducible histopathologic and immunohistochemical features. Am J Surg Pathol. 46(9):1241-9, 2022
12. Shibayama T et al: Cytokeratin-positive malignant tumor in the abdomen with EWSR1/FUS-CREB fusion: a clinicopathologic study of 8 cases. Am J Surg Pathol. 46(1):134-46, 2022
13. Sloan EA et al: Intracranial mesenchymal tumors with FET-CREB fusion are composed of at least two epigenetic subgroups distinct from meningioma and extracranial sarcomas. Brain Pathol. 32(4):e13037, 2022
14. Surrey LF et al: NTRK-Rearranged soft tissue neoplasms: a review of evolving diagnostic entities and algorithmic detection methods. Cancer Genet. 260-1:6-13, 2022
15. Tsai JW et al: Adult NTRK-rearranged spindle cell neoplasms of the viscera: with an emphasis on rare locations and heterologous elements. Mod Pathol. 35(7):911-21, 2022
16. Tauziède-Espariat A et al: An integrative histopathological and epigenetic characterization of primary intracranial mesenchymal tumors, FET:CREB-fused broadening the spectrum of tumor entities in comparison with their soft tissue counterparts. Brain Pathol. 32(1):e13010, 2022
17. Sloan EA et al: Intracranial mesenchymal tumor with FET-CREB fusion-A unifying diagnosis for the spectrum of intracranial myxoid mesenchymal tumors and angiomatoid fibrous histiocytoma-like neoplasms. Brain Pathol. 31(4):e12918, 2021
18. Arbajian E et al: Deep sequencing of myxoinflammatory fibroblastic sarcoma. Genes Chromosomes Cancer. 59(5):309-17, 2020
19. Argani P et al: EWSR1/FUS-CREB fusions define a distinctive malignant epithelioid neoplasm with predilection for mesothelial-lined cavities. Mod Pathol. 33(11):2233-43, 2020
20. Chang B et al: Malignant gastrointestinal neuroectodermal tumor: clinicopathologic, immunohistochemical, and molecular analysis of 19 cases. Am J Surg Pathol. 44(4):456-66, 2020
21. Jo VY: Soft Tissue special issue: myoepithelial neoplasms of soft tissue: an updated review with emphasis on diagnostic considerations in the head and neck. Head Neck Pathol. 14(1):121-31, 2020
22. Suster D et al: Myxoinflammatory fibroblastic sarcoma: an immunohistochemical and molecular genetic study of 73 cases. Mod Pathol. 33(12):2520-33, 2020
23. Suurmeijer AJH et al: A morphologic and molecular reappraisal of myoepithelial tumors of soft tissue, bone, and viscera with EWSR1 and FUS gene rearrangements. Genes Chromosomes Cancer. 59(6):348-56, 2020
24. Folpe AL: Phosphaturic mesenchymal tumors: a review and update. Semin Diagn Pathol. 36(4):260-8, 2019
25. Thway K et al: Mesenchymal tumors with EWSR1 gene rearrangements. Surg Pathol Clin. 12(1):165-90, 2019
26. Wu H et al: Phosphaturic mesenchymal tumor with an admixture of epithelial and mesenchymal elements in the jaws: clinicopathological and immunohistochemical analysis of 22 cases with literature review. Mod Pathol. 32(2):189-204, 2019
27. Cheah AL et al: ALK expression in angiomatoid fibrous histiocytoma: a potential diagnostic pitfall. Am J Surg Pathol. 43(1):93-101, 2019
28. Liu H et al: The t(1;10)(p22;q24) TGFBR3/MGEA5 translocation in pleomorphic hyalinizing angiectatic tumor (PHAT), myxoinflammatory fibroblastic sarcoma (MIFS), and hemosiderotic fibrolipomatous tumor (HFLT). Arch Pathol Lab Med. 143(2):212-21, 2019
29. Boland JM et al: Hemosiderotic fibrolipomatous tumor, pleomorphic hyalinizing angiectatic tumor, and myxoinflammatory fibroblastic sarcoma: related or not? Adv Anat Pathol. 24(5):268-77, 2017
30. Kao YC et al: EWSR1 fusions with CREB family transcription factors define a novel myxoid mesenchymal tumor with predilection for intracranial location. Am J Surg Pathol. 41(4):482-90, 2017

Rare Sarcomas of Uncertain Differentiation With Specific Molecular Alterations (Continued)

Myoepithelial Carcinoma

Myoepithelial Carcinoma

(Left) Although myoepithelial carcinomas can show a variety of growth patterns and variable matrix production, numerous mitoses ⇨ are typical. (Right) Tumor cell nuclei of myoepithelial carcinoma characteristically exhibit prominent nucleoli, as in this example.

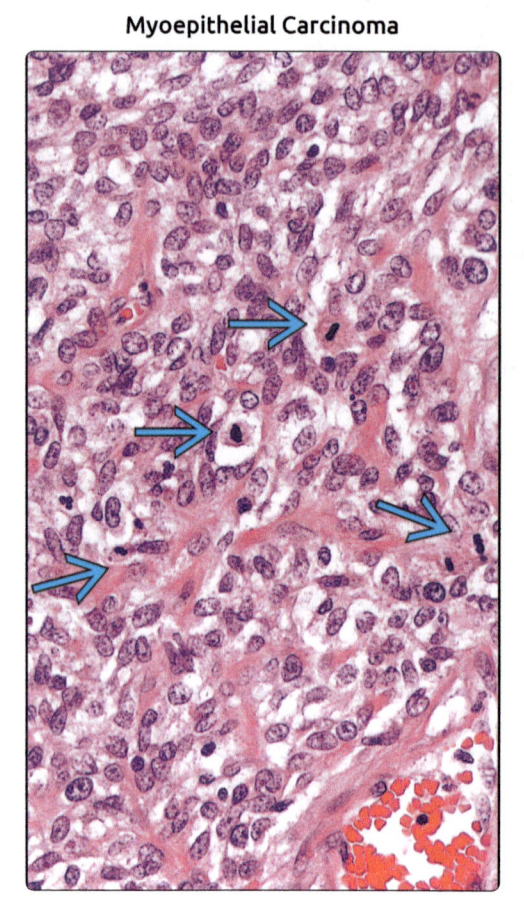

Mixed Tumor of Soft Tissue

Mixed Tumor of Soft Tissue

(Left) Mixed tumor of soft tissue is related to myoepithelial carcinoma but benign. By definition, mixed tumors include a ductal/epithelial component ⇨. (Right) Mild nuclear size variation is notable. However, in contrast to myoepithelial carcinoma, nuclear atypia in the form of prominent nucleoli is absent.

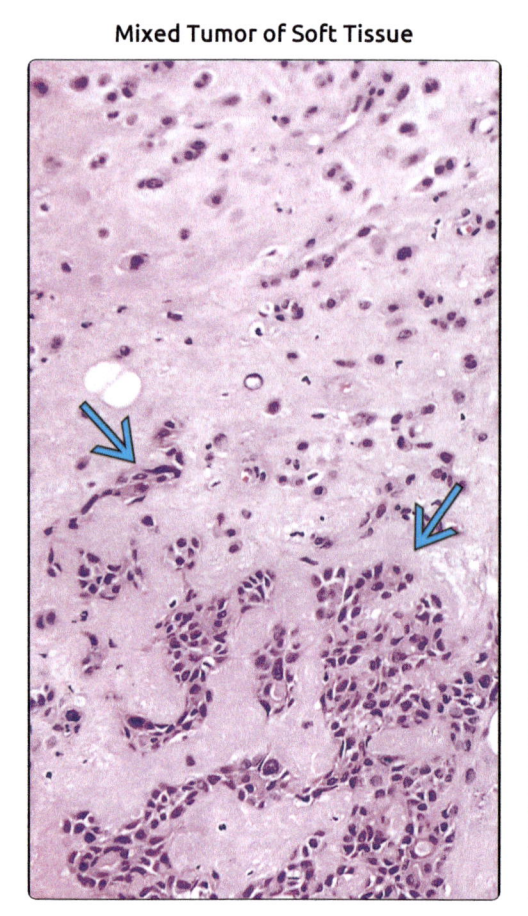

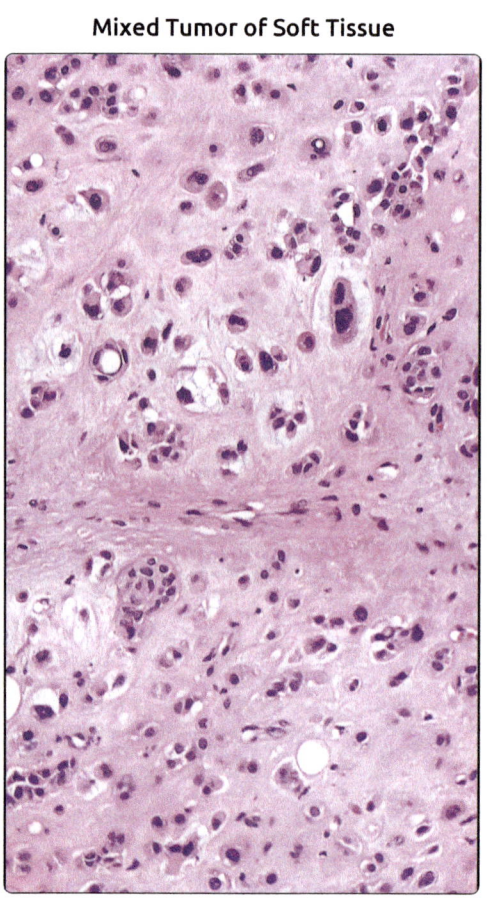

Rare Sarcomas of Uncertain Differentiation With Specific Molecular Alterations (Continued)

PHAT Classic Features

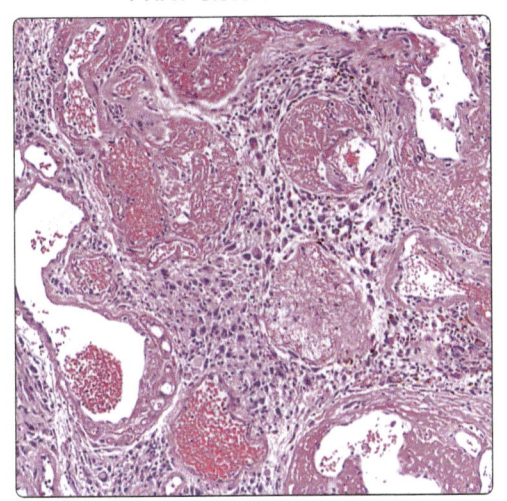

PHAT With Hemosiderin Deposits

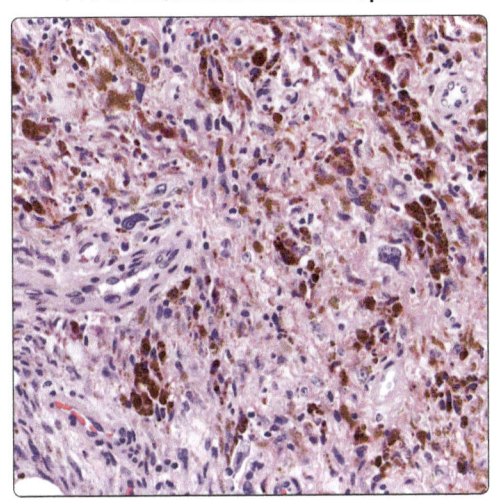

(Left) Classic features of PHAT include thin-walled ectatic blood vessels with thick collars of amorphous eosinophilic material. Thromboses may be present. The intervening tissue contains sheets of tumor cells, inflammation, and hemosiderin. (Right) The periphery of PHAT resembles that of a closely related tumor: Hemosiderotic fibrolipomatous tumor (HFLT). These peripheral regions consist of spindle cells infiltrating adipose tissue associated with prominent intermixed hemosiderin.

PHAT With Inflammation

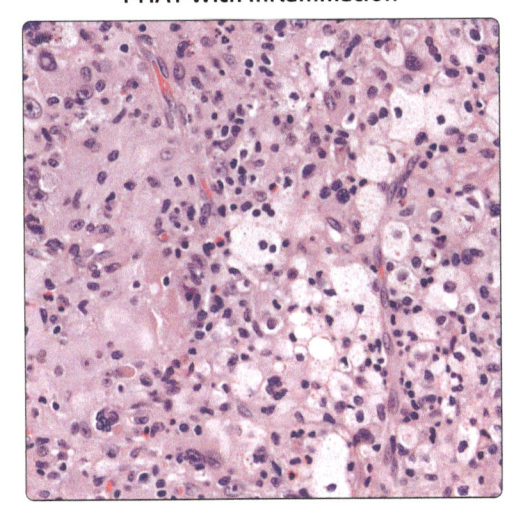

PHAT With Classic Nuclear Pleomorphism

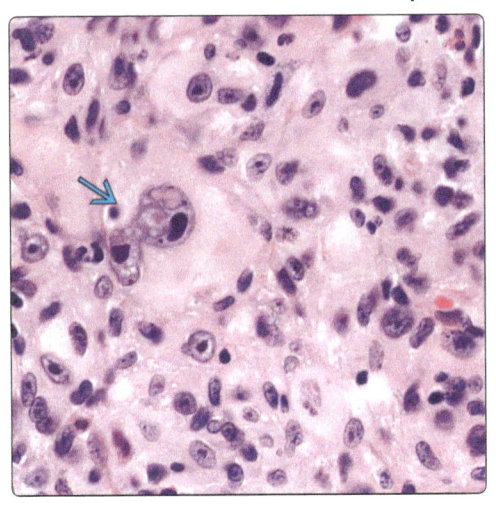

(Left) Reactive inflammation is common in PHAT and is usually mixed. Here, lymphocytes and histiocytes mingle with the larger polygonal tumor cells. (Right) PHAT usually contains scattered tumor cells showing striking nuclear atypia that have been previously described as comparable to the nuclear atypia of Reed-Sternberg cells or virally infected cells ➡. Despite the pleomorphism, classic PHAT shows little mitotic activity.

PHAT With High-Grade Transformation Mimicking MIFS

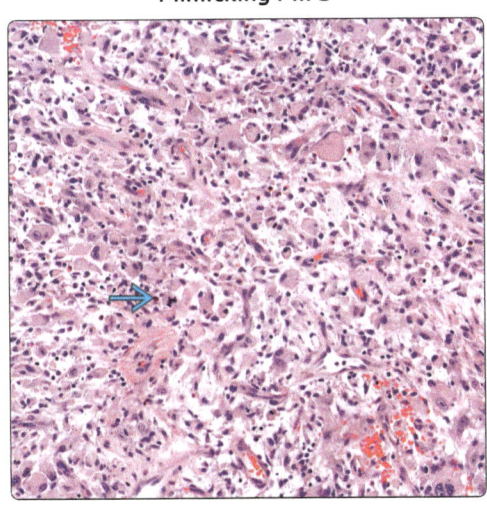

PHAT With High-Grade Transformation

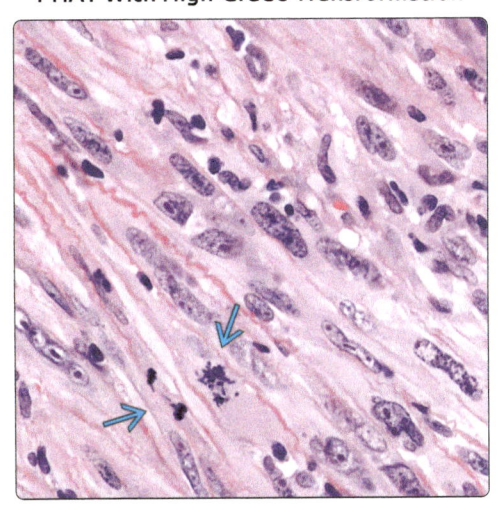

(Left) Atypical epithelioid and polygonal tumor cells floating in a myxoid matrix with intermingled inflammation are shown. Mitotic figures ➡ are present. This high-grade transformation occurred in a recurrent PHAT in an older man. (Right) Another area of the tumor consists of atypical spindled cells with increased mitoses ➡. The tumor also demonstrated invasion of large veins indicative of aggressive behavior incompatible with classic PHAT. Malignant transformation is rare.

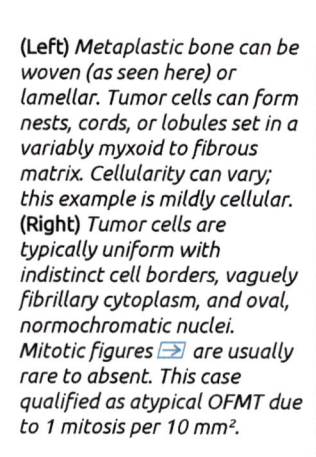

Rare Sarcomas of Uncertain Differentiation With Specific Molecular Alterations (Continued)

Phosphaturic Mesenchymal Tumor With Prominent Osteoid

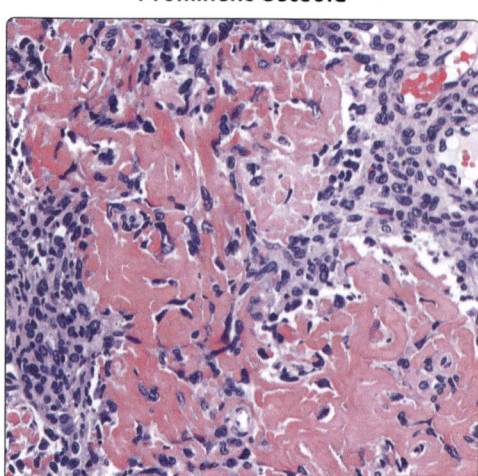

Phosphaturic Mesenchymal Tumor

(Left) Some PMT produce abundant osteoid. Since the cells also express SATB2, the differential diagnosis can include bone-forming tumors, such as osteosarcoma and osteoblastoma. (Right) Hypercellular regions of PMT may mimic sarcoma. Clinical findings, including hypophosphatemia, hyperphosphaturia and tumor-induced osteomalacia, are diagnostically helpful. However, phosphate levels quickly return to normal soon after resection.

Ossifying Fibromyxoid Tumor of Peripheral Bone

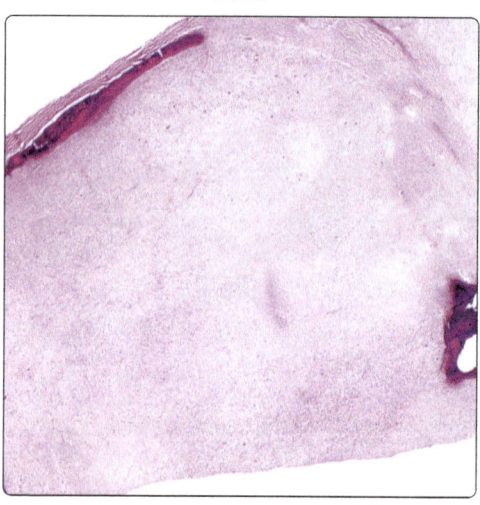

Ossifying Fibromyxoid Tumor With Pushing Border

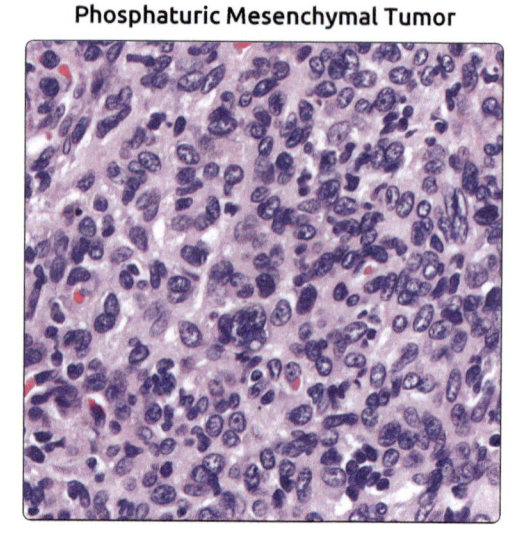

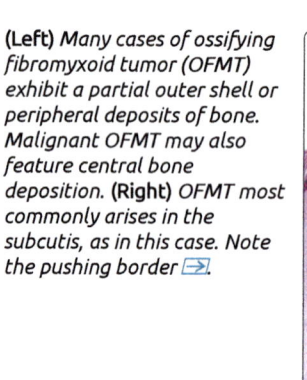

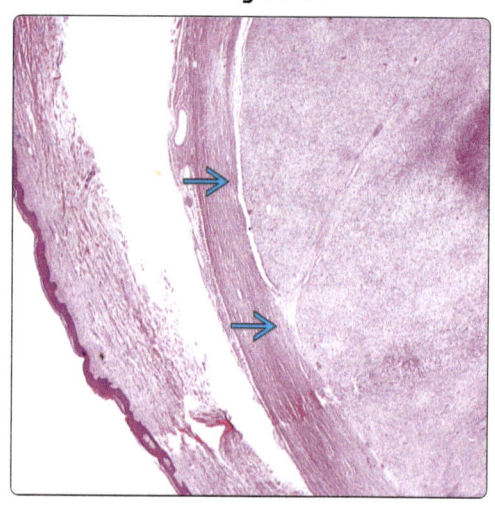

(Left) Many cases of ossifying fibromyxoid tumor (OFMT) exhibit a partial outer shell or peripheral deposits of bone. Malignant OFMT may also feature central bone deposition. (Right) OFMT most commonly arises in the subcutis, as in this case. Note the pushing border ➡.

Ossifying Fibromyxoid Tumor With Metaplastic Bone

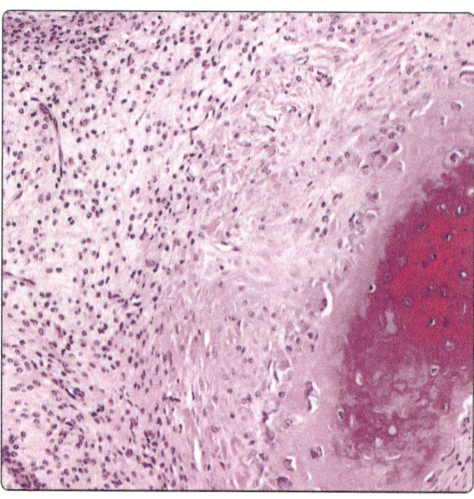

Atypical Ossifying Fibromyxoid Tumor

(Left) Metaplastic bone can be woven (as seen here) or lamellar. Tumor cells can form nests, cords, or lobules set in a variably myxoid to fibrous matrix. Cellularity can vary; this example is mildly cellular. (Right) Tumor cells are typically uniform with indistinct cell borders, vaguely fibrillary cytoplasm, and oval, normochromatic nuclei. Mitotic figures ➡ are usually rare to absent. This case qualified as atypical OFMT due to 1 mitosis per 10 mm².

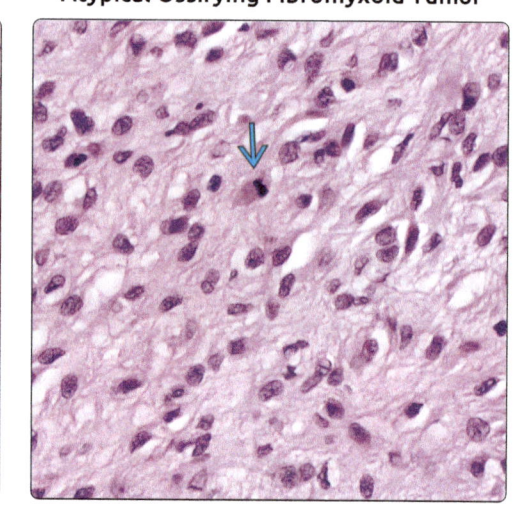

Rare Sarcomas of Uncertain Differentiation With Specific Molecular Alterations (Continued)

Angiomatoid Fibrous Histiocytoma Classic Features

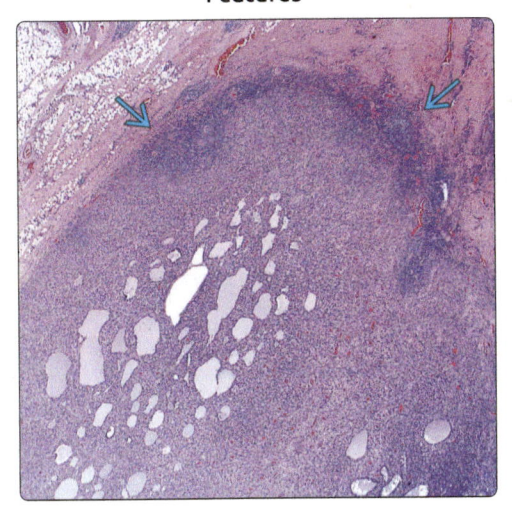

Angiomatoid Fibrous Histiocytoma

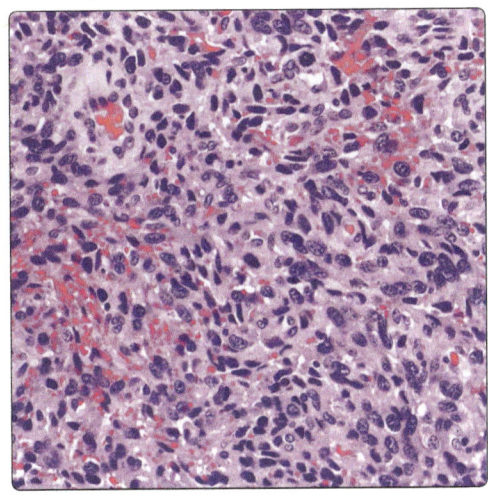

(Left) The most common low-power appearance of angiomatoid fibrous histiocytoma (AFH) comprises a nodular, variably cystic tumor with pushing margins cuffed by prominent lymphoplasmacytic aggregates ➡ that can even form germinal centers and erroneously suggest lymph node metastasis. *(Right)* The tumor cells of AFH typically are plump and spindled and arranged in irregular, tangled mats. Nuclear atypia is usually mild. Mitoses are usually sparse. Note the hemorrhage.

Angiomatoid Fibrous Histiocytoma With Desmin Expression

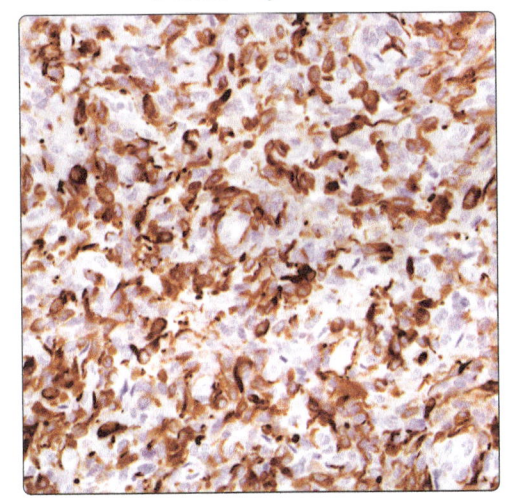

NTRK-Rearranged Spindle Cell Neoplasm

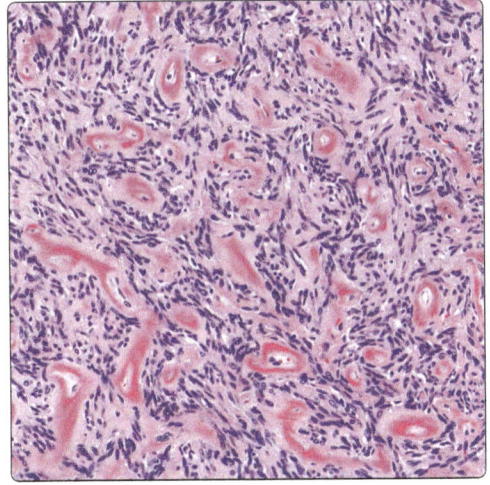

(Left) Desmin is expressed in ~50% of cases. Expression may be very focal, patchy, or diffuse. *(Right)* Perivascular collagen rings are a striking feature found in some NTRK-rearranged spindle cell tumors. In this example, the tumor cells swirl around the vessels and exhibit minimally atypical nuclei.

NTRK-Rearranged Spindle Cell Neoplasm: S100 Positive

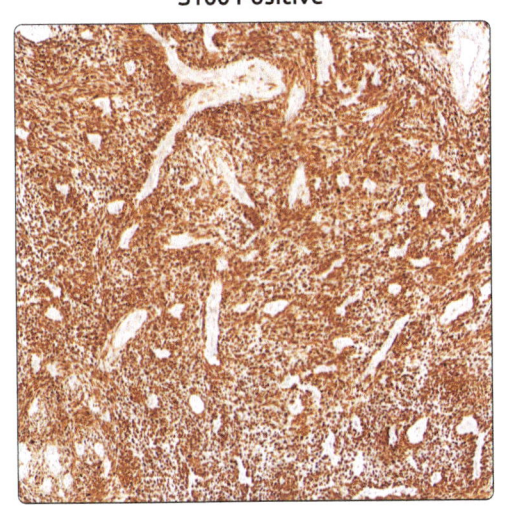

NTRK-Rearranged Spindle Cell Neoplasm: CD34 Positive

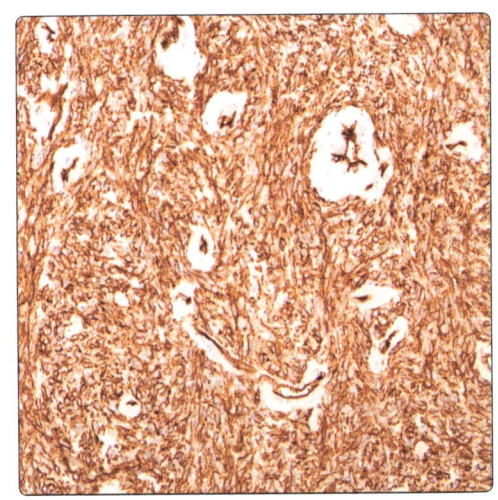

(Left) The tumor shows diffuse strong expression of S100. *(Right)* Reactivity for CD34 is also strong and diffuse. Dual expression of S100 and CD34 is common in this tumor type.

Glioblastoma, IDH Wildtype

KEY FACTS

TERMINOLOGY
- Glioblastoma, IDH wildtype
  - Diffuse astrocytic glioma that is IDH and H3 (*H3C14*) wildtype and has one or more of following histologic or genetic features
    - Microvascular proliferation, necrosis, *TERT* promoter mutation, *EGFR* amplification, +7/-10 chromosome copy number changes
- Subtypes
  - Giant cell glioblastoma, gliosarcoma, epithelioid glioblastoma

CLINICAL ISSUES
- Most common malignant brain tumor in adults
- Accounts for 45-50% of all primary malignant brain tumors
- Small numbers are inherited as part of genetic tumor syndromes, including
  - Lynch syndrome, constitutional mismatch repair deficiency syndrome, Li-Fraumeni syndrome, and neurofibromatosis type 1

IMAGING
- Ring enhancing on T1 C+ MR

MOLECULAR
- Epigenetic alterations
  - *MGMT* promoter hypermethylation
    - Improved response to alkylating agents
  - *EZH2* overexpression
- Frequently mutated genes
  - *EGFR* alterations in ~ 60% of cases
  - *PTEN* mutations in 40% of cases
  - *PIK3CA*, *PIK3R1*, or other PI3K pathway gene mutations in 25-30% of cases
  - *PDGFRA* alterations in 10-15% of cases
  - *TP53* mutations or deletions in 25% of cases

Pseudopalisading Necrosis

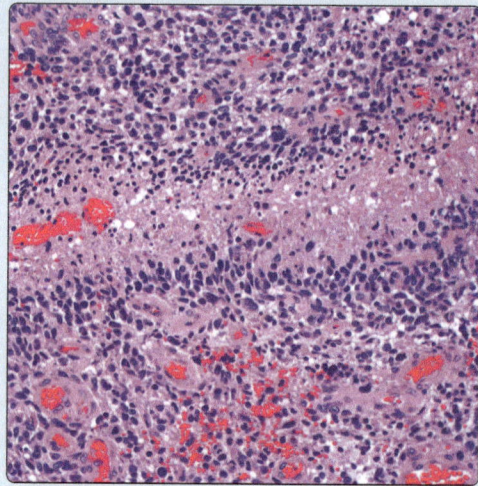

Infiltrating Edge of Glioblastoma

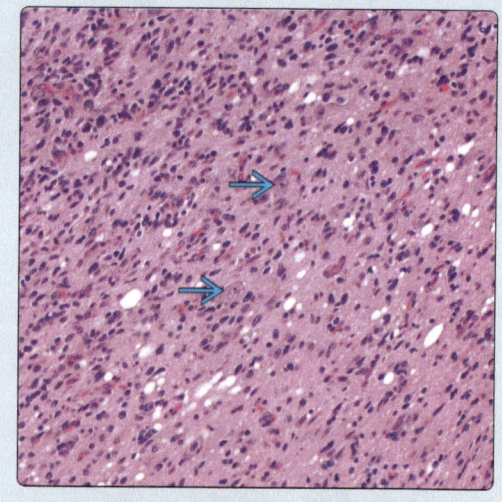

(Left) *Molecularly documented IDH wildtype glioblastoma shows classic pseudopalisading necrosis.* (Right) *Infiltrating edge of glioblastoma is shown. Grading can be difficult when only the edge of a high-grade tumor is sampled surgically. Molecular criteria can facilitate grading. Trapped neurons ➡ are present.*

Anaplasia and Mitotic Activity

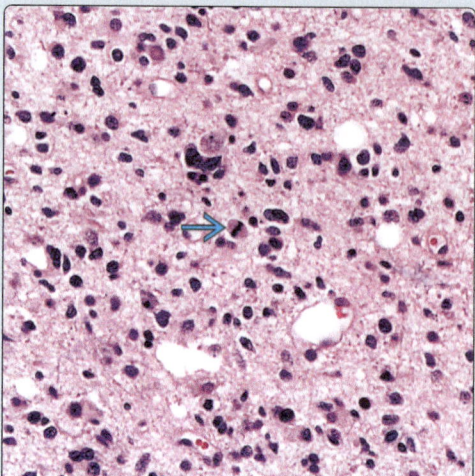

Cellular Anaplasia

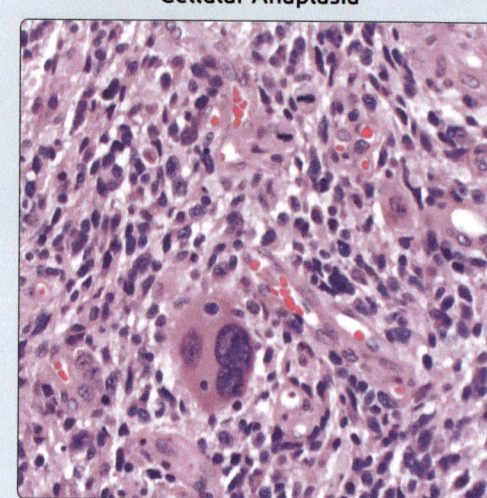

(Left) *Highly pleomorphic cells and mitotic figures ➡ are shown. Definitive grading depends on IDH1/IDH2 mutation status and molecular criteria. (From DP: Neuro.)* (Right) *Highly pleomorphic cells, mitotic figures, and vascular proliferation are shown. Giant cells are often associated with mismatch repair deficiency and TP53 mutations.*

Glioblastoma, IDH Wildtype

TERMINOLOGY

Synonyms
- Glioblastoma multiforme (not recommended)

Definitions
- Glioblastoma, IDH wildtype
  ○ Diffuse astrocytic glioma that is IDH and H3 (*H3C14*) wildtype and has one or more of following histologic or genetic features
    – Microvascular proliferation, necrosis, *TERT* promoter mutation, *EGFR* amplification, +7/-10 chromosome copy number changes
  ○ Subtypes
    – Giant cell glioblastoma, epithelioid glioblastoma, gliosarcoma

CLINICAL ISSUES

Epidemiology
- Most common malignant brain tumor in adults
- Accounts for 45-50% of all primary malignant brain tumors
- Peak incidence in patients 55-85 years of age
- Small numbers are inherited as part of genetic tumor syndromes, including
  ○ Lynch syndrome, constitutional mismatch repair deficiency syndrome, Li-Fraumeni syndrome, and neurofibromatosis type 1
  ○ Reported association with genomic variants in *TERT*, *EGFR*, *CCDC26*, *CDKN2B*, *PHLDB1*, *TP53*, and *RTEL1*

Presentation
- Symptoms depend on tumor location
- Seizure, mass effect, headache, focal neurologic deficits
- Behavioral and neurocognitive changes are common

Treatment
- Surgical resection
  ○ Provides tissue for diagnosis and relieves mass effect
  ○ Resection may not be possible if eloquent brain involved
- Some patients benefit from radiation, alkylating chemotherapy, and bevacizumab

Prognosis
- 5-year survival of 6-7%
- Improved survival in patients with younger age, high performance status, complete tumor resection, and MGMT promoter hypermethylation

IMAGING

MR Findings
- Ring enhancing on T1 C+ MR

MACROSCOPIC

General Features
- Usually supratentorial: Cerebral cortex > other brain location > spinal cord
- Intraaxial
- May appear circumscribed in gliosarcoma subtype
- Variegated with areas of hemorrhage and necrosis
- Enlarged, thrombosed vessels common
- Usually unilateral; may cross corpus callosum (butterfly); 10% multifocal

MOLECULAR

Cytogenetics
- Trisomy 7 and monosomy 10 are most frequent numerical alterations
- Less common alterations include 7q gain &/or 10q loss
- Loss of 9p, including homozygous deletion of *CDKN2A* &/or *CDKN2B* locus
- 13q, 22q, and sex chromosome loss and gains of chromosome 19 and 20
- Most common gene amplification involves *EGFR*

Molecular Genetics
- Genetic alterations associated with glioblastoma, IDH wildtype
  ○ *IDH1*/*IDH2*
    – Wildtype by definition
  ○ Epigenetic alterations
    – *MGMT* promoter hypermethylation
      □ Present in 30-40% of cases
      □ Improved response to alkylating agents
  ○ Other epigenetic modifier alterations
    – IDH wildtype glioblastomas harbor one or more mutations affecting chromatin organization
    – *EZH2* overexpression
      □ Presumably contributes to silencing of tumor suppressor genes
    – *ATRX* mutations
      □ Detected in ~ 4.5% of cases
    – *SETD2* mutations
      □ Occurs in only 2% of IDH wildtype glioblastoma
    – *KMT2B*, *KMT2C*, and *KMT2D* mutations
      □ Detected in rare cases
  ○ PI3K-AKT-mTOR pathway alteration
    – *EGFR* alterations present in ~ 60% of cases
      □ Alterations include amplification, mutation, rearrangement, or splice site mutations
      □ *EGFR* amplification is most frequent alteration seen in ~ 40% of all cases
      □ *EGFR* amplification are often associated with 2nd *EGFR* alteration, such as *EGFR* variant III mutation or deletion
    – Alterations in PI3K, RTK pathway genes and *PTEN* in ~ 90% of cases
    – *PTEN* mutations in ~ 40%
      □ PI3K and *PTEN* mutations appear mutually exclusive
    – *PIK3CA*, *PIK3R1*, or other PI3K pathway gene mutations in 25-30% of cases
    – *PDGFRA* alterations in 10-15% of cases
    – *MET* or *FGFR3* alterations in ~ 3% of cases
    – *NF1* mutations in 10% of cases
  ○ p14ARF-p53-MDM2-MDM4 pathway
    – Genetic alteration of this pathway occurs in ~ 90% of cases
    – *TP53* mutations or deletions in 25% of cases
    – Genetic alterations involving *CDKN2A*, *MDM2* or *MDM4*, and *TP53* are typically exclusive of one another

Glioblastoma, IDH Wildtype

- CDK4/6, CDKN2A/B-RB1 cell cycle pathway
  - One or more genetic alterations in CD4/6-RB1 pathway detected in ~ 80% of cases
  - *CDKN2A* deletions are most common and often involve *CDKN2B* as well
  - *CDK4* and *CDK6* amplification detected in ~ 15% of cases
  - *RB1* mutations/deletions present in ~ 8% of cases
  - *RB1* alterations and *CDKN2A* deletions are mutually exclusive
- Gene fusions in IDH wildtype glioblastoma
  - Mostly involve receptor tyrosine kinase family, including *EGFR, MET, NTRK1, NTRK2,* or *NTRK3*
    - *EGFR* fusions occurs as part of complex rearrangements
  - Fusion partners are often genes at proximity of *EGFR*
    - *SEPTIN14, PSPH, SEC61G, SDK1*
    - Fusions results in truncation of *EGFR* c-terminal domain
    - *EGFR* fusions typically co-occur with *EGFR* amplification
  - *FGFR3::TACC3* fusions
    - ~ 3% frequency in IDH wildtype glioblastoma
    - Associated with *CDK4* and *MDM2* amplifications
    - Mutually exclusive of *EGFR* amplifications
  - *MET* fusions
    - Fusion partners include *PTPRZ1* and various others
    - More common in high-grade, IDH-mutant astrocytoma and diffuse pediatric-type high-grade glioma, H3 and IDH wildtype
    - May also occur in adult-type, IDH wildtype glioblastomas
  - *NTRK1, NTRK2,* and *NTRK3* fusions
    - Various fusion partners
    - ~ 1-2% frequency in IDH wildtype glioblastoma
  - *PDGFRA* fusions
    - Reported but are exceedingly rare
  - Other reported, potentially relevant fusions
    - *PTPRZ1::ETV1, KLHL7::BRAF, CEP85L::ROS1, CCDC127::TERT*

MICROSCOPIC

Histologic Features

- Diffusely infiltrating, densely cellular tumor composed of pleomorphic astrocytes
  - Mitotic figures present
  - Vascular proliferation &/or necrosis
- Gliosarcomas appear circumscribed
  - Mixed glial and sarcomatous (reticulin-rich, spindle cell) components
  - Molecular profile identical in both components
- Giant cell glioblastoma subtype
  - Reserved to those in which bizarre, multinucleated giant cells are dominant histologic finding
  - Glioblastomas in setting of mismatch repair deficiency often show severe atypia and multinucleation
- Epithelioid glioblastoma subtype
  - Loosely cohesive aggregates of large epithelioid cells, often circumscribed, sometimes rhabdoid cells
  - May mimic metastatic carcinoma or melanoma
  - Overlaps with pleomorphic xanthoastrocytoma
- Occasional oligodendrocyte-like clear cells mimicking oligodendroglioma may be seen
- Primitive neuronal component
  - Discrete foci with Homer Wright rosettes, cells with high N:C ratio, increased mitotic rate

ANCILLARY TESTS

Immunohistochemistry

- Variable expression of GFAP and preserved nuclear ATRX expression in majority of cases
- p53 positivity in 25-30% of cases, more frequent in giant cell subtype
- OLIG2 and S100 (+)
  - OLIG2 is highly specific glioma marker
- GFAP and OLIG2 (-) in sarcomatous component of gliosarcoma
- AE1/AE3(+), CK7/CK20(-)
  - Positivity reflects cross-reactivity
- Ki-67 proliferation index ≥ 20%
- *BRAF* V600E mutation specific antibody (+) in subset of epithelioid subtype

DIFFERENTIAL DIAGNOSIS

Oligodendroglioma, WHO Grade 3

- Associated with 1p19q co-deletions

Lymphoma

- CD45(+); usually B lineage CD20(+)

Diffuse Hemispheric Glioma, H3G34 Mutant

- OLIG2(-), ATRX loss of nuclear expression, MAP2(+), p53 strongly (+)

Astrocytoma, IDH Mutant

- *IDH1* or *IDH2* mutated by definition
- ATRX nuclear expression lost in tumor cells

Pediatric-Type, Diffuse High-Grade Glioma

- H3 wildtype and IDH wildtype
- *PDGFRA* amplification or mutation, *TP53* mutation, *NF1* alterations, *EGFR* mutation or amplification
- Diagnosis requires DNA methylation profiling

SELECTED REFERENCES

1. Gritsch S et al: Diagnostic, therapeutic, and prognostic implications of the 2021 World Health Organization classification of tumors of the central nervous system. Cancer. 128(1):47-58, 2022
2. Louis DN et al: The 2021 WHO Classification of Tumors of the Central Nervous System: a summary. Neuro Oncol. 23(8):1231-51, 2021
3. Suwala AK et al: Glioblastomas with primitive neuronal component harbor a distinct methylation and copy-number profile with inactivation of TP53, PTEN, and RB1. Acta Neuropathol. 142(1):179-89, 2021
4. Capper D et al: Practical implementation of DNA methylation and copy-number-based CNS tumor diagnostics: the Heidelberg experience. Acta Neuropathol. 136(2):181-210, 2018
5. Korshunov A et al: Epithelioid glioblastomas stratify into established diagnostic subsets upon integrated molecular analysis. Brain Pathol. 28(5):656-62, 2018

Glioblastoma, IDH Wildtype

Chromosomal Microarray

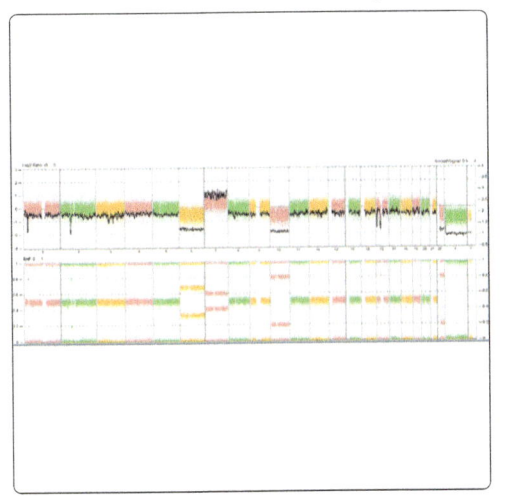

Vascular Proliferation

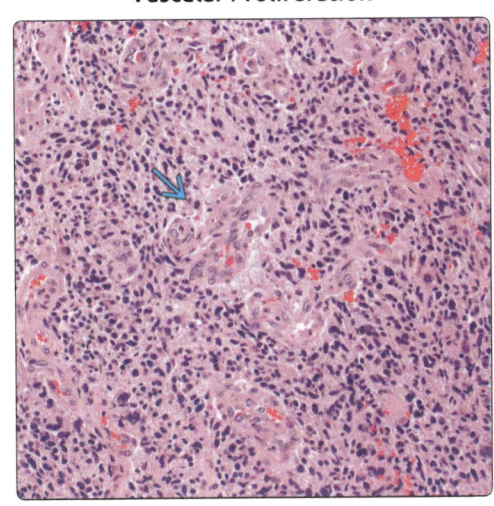

(Left) Chromosome copy number alterations, +7/-10, often in combination, are commonly detected in glioblastoma, even in the absence of necrosis &/or vascular proliferation. (Right) Abundant microvascular proliferation is shown. The blood vessels toward the center have a somewhat glomeruloid pattern ➡.

Hypercellularity and Atypia

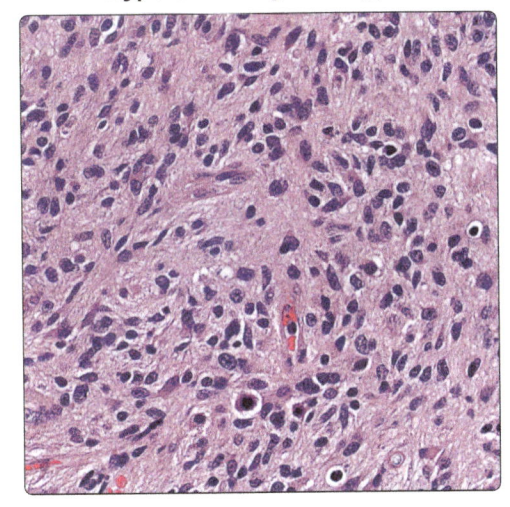

Increased Mitotic Figures

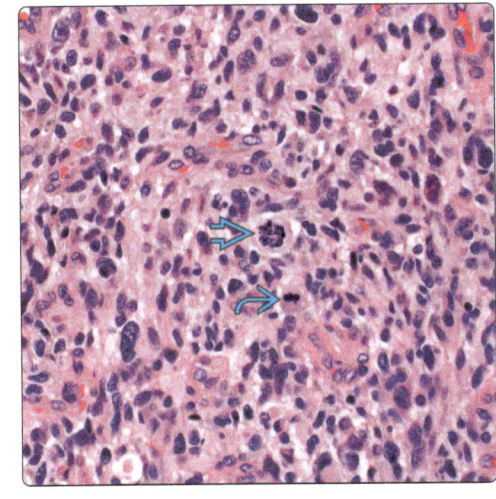

(Left) Small cell anaplastic astrocytomas demonstrate hypercellularity similar to the cellularity of glioblastoma, and they typically evolve into glioblastoma. (From DP: Neuro.) (Right) Large, atypical mitotic figure ➡ and occasional additional mitotic figures ➡ are shown. Microvascular proliferation can also be appreciated.

Vascular Proliferation and Necrosis

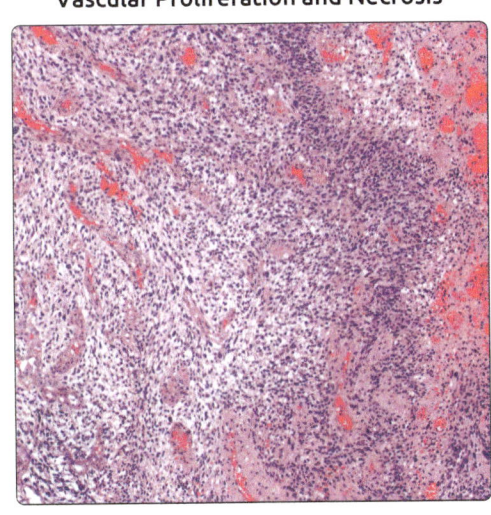

FISH Testing of *EGFR* Amplification

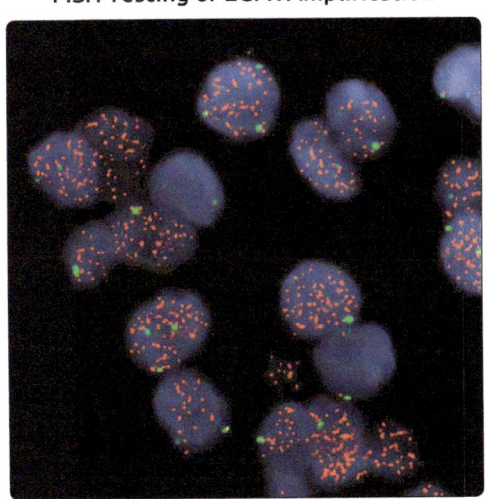

(Left) Classic features of glioblastoma are shown, including vascular proliferation (left) and pseudopalisading necrosis (right). Clear cell, oligodendroglial-like cells are also present. (Right) FISH demonstrates EGFR gene amplification (red signals) in a documented case of IDH wildtype glioblastoma.

Astrocytoma, IDH-Mutant

KEY FACTS

TERMINOLOGY

- Astrocytoma, IDH-mutant (WHO classification of CNS tumors, 5th edition)
  - Diffusely infiltrating *IDH1* or *IDH2*-mutant glioma
  - Frequent *ATRX* &/or *TP53* mutations
  - Absence of 1p/19q codeletion
  - Subtyped as CNS WHO grades 2, 3, and 4
    - Glioblastoma is no longer applied to grade 4 IDH-mutant astrocytoma

CLINICAL ISSUES

- Localization
  - Any region of CNS, including brainstem and spinal cord
  - Most common location is supratentorial compartment
  - Usually centered near or within frontal lobes
  - Similar localization to IDH-mutant and 1p/19q-codelted oligodendroglioma

MOLECULAR

- *IDH1* and *IDH2* mutations
  - By definition, present in IDH-mutant astrocytomas
  - Absent in oligodendrogliomas
  - Absent in reactive astrocytosis/gliosis
- *ATRX* mutations
  - Present in ~ 87-97% of IDH-mutant astrocytomas
  - *ATRX* alterations lead to loss of encoded protein expression
  - *ATRX* mutations are mutually exclusive of activating *TERT* promoter mutations
  - ATRX mutations are absent in oligodendrogliomas

MICROSCOPIC

- Diffusely infiltrating, fibrillary or gemistocytic astrocytoma
- Microvascular proliferation &/or necrosis correspond to WHO grade 4 tumors

Imaging Appearance

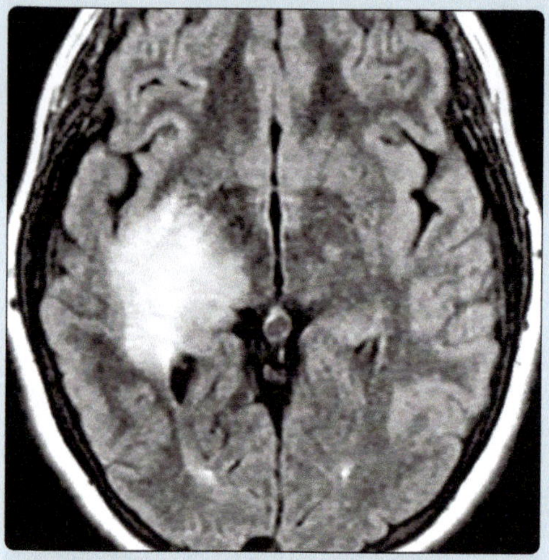

Astrocytoma, WHO Grade 2

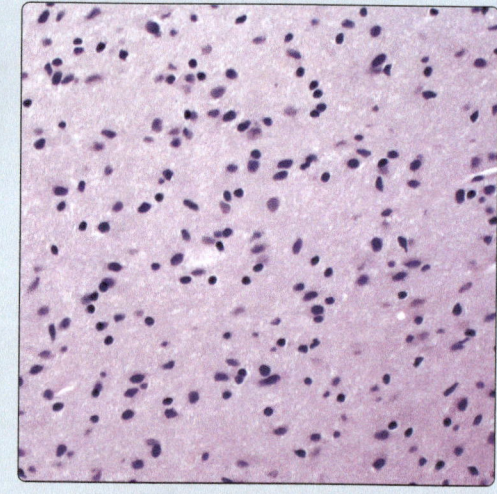

(Left) *Axial FLAIR MR shows a hyperintense, infiltrative right temporal mass extending medially into the basal ganglia and thalamus in this patient with WHO grade 2 fibrillary astrocytoma. (From DI2: Brain.)* (Right) *High-power view of an infiltrating glioma shows a mild increase in cellularity characterized by excess astrocytes with minimal cytologic atypia.*

IDH1 Expression

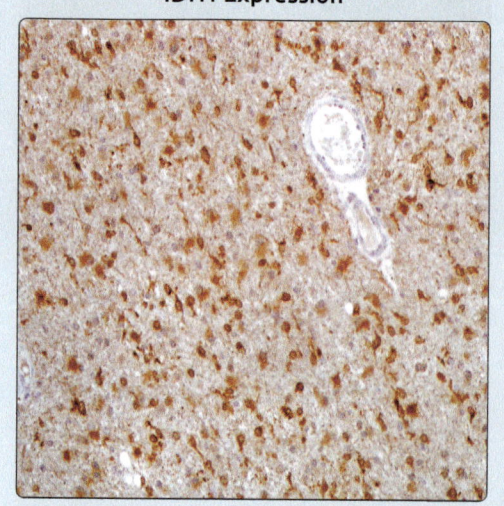

Retained ATRX Expression in Glioblastoma, IDH Wildtype

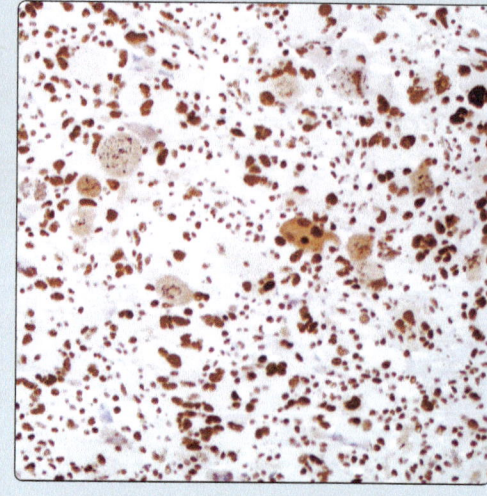

(Left) *IHC using IDH1 R132H mutation-specific antibody shows positive staining of neoplastic cells in this case of astrocytoma, IDH-mutant. R132H is the most common IDH1 mutation variant among cases of IDH-mutant astrocytoma.* (Right) *ATRX shows retained expression in neoplastic cells in this case of IDH-wildtype glioblastoma. In contrast, IDH-mutant astrocytoma shows loose expression of this antigen due to commonly detected ATRX gene mutations.*

Astrocytoma, IDH-Mutant

TERMINOLOGY

Synonyms
- Related terminology (not recommended per WHO 5th edition)
  - Diffuse astrocytoma, IDH-mutant
  - Anaplastic astrocytoma, IDH-mutant
  - Low-grade astrocytoma
  - High-grade astrocytoma
  - Infiltrating astrocytoma
  - Diffuse glioma

Definitions
- Astrocytoma, IDH-mutant
  - Diffusely infiltrating *IDH1* or *IDH2*-mutant glioma
  - Frequent *ATRX* &/or *TP53* mutations (WHO grades 2-4)
  - Absence of 1p/19q codeletion
  - Glioblastoma is no longer applied to grade 4 IDH-mutant astrocytoma
- Astrocytoma, IDH-mutant subtypes
  - Astrocytoma, IDH-mutant, CNS WHO grade 2
  - Astrocytoma, IDH-mutant, CNS WHO grade 3
  - Astrocytoma, IDH-mutant, CNS WHO grade 4

CLINICAL ISSUES

Presentation
- Localization
  - Any region of CNS, including brainstem and spinal cord
  - Most common location is supratentorial compartment
    - Usually centered near or within frontal lobes
    - Similar localization to IDH-mutant and 1p/19q-codelted oligodendroglioma
- Signs and symptoms
  - Seizures (most common)
  - Headache, mass effect, focal deficits
  - Incidental finding in small subset of cases following neuroimaging performed post trauma or for headache
  - Neurocognitive function is relatively preserved
  - Behavioral or personality changes with frontal tumors
    - May be initial clinical presentation feature

Treatment
- Surgical approaches
  - Biopsy generally for diagnosis or to reduce mass effect
  - Chemotherapy and radiation often deferred until recurrence/histologic progression

Prognosis
- Younger age at presentation correlates with better survival
- Other prognostic indicators
  - Size and extent of resection
  - Karnofsky performance score (KPS)
  - Homozygous deletion of *CDKN2A* &/or *CDKN2B* associated with shorter survival
    - Correspond with CNS WHO grade 4 disease
- Impact of WHO grades 2-3 on prognosis less clear

IMAGING

Radiographic Findings
- Infiltrative and expansile
- T2 FLAIR mismatch sign (T2 hyperdensity, FLAIR hypodensity) favors astrocytoma over oligodendroglioma

MOLECULAR

In Situ Hybridization
- 1p/19q status can be assessed with FISH probes targeting these chromosomal regions
  - Not recommended due to false-positive results with partial chromosome arm deletion

Molecular Genetics
- Clinically relevant tests
  - *IDH1* and *IDH2* mutational analysis
    - IDH (isocitrate dehydrogenases) catalyze oxidative decarboxylation of isocitrate to α-ketoglutarate
    - Accumulation of D2-hydroxyglutarate (oncometabolite)
      - Leads to epigenetic reprogramming with global DNA hypermethylation
      - Glioma CpG island methylator phenotype (G-CIMP)
    - Immunohistochemistry and sequencing techniques can be used for detection of *IDH1/IDH2* mutations
      - *IDH1* c.395G>A, p.R132H variant detected in up to 91% of IDH-mutant gliomas by IHC or sequencing
      - *IDH1* R132C, R132G, R132S, or R132L variants in ~ 3-4% of cases, detected by sequencing
      - *IDH2* mutations localized to codon R172 with p.R172K variant being most frequent
      - *IDH1/IDH2* mutations absent in reactive gliosis
  - *TP53* mutations
    - Present in > 90% of IDH-mutant grade 2 astrocytoma
    - Uncommon in glioblastoma
  - *ATRX* mutations
    - Induces abnormal telomere maintenance, a.k.a. alternative lengthening telomeres
    - Present in ~ 87-97% of IDH-mutant astrocytoma, but absent in oligodendrogliomas
    - Mutually exclusive of activating *TERT* promoter mutations
  - *PTEN* mutations and *EGFR* amplification
    - Rarely detected in IDH-mutant astrocytoma
  - Noncanonical *IDH1* mutations (non-R132H variants) in posterior fossa tumors
    - *IDH1* mutations other than R132H, including
      - *IDH1* R132C, *IDH1* R132G, *IDH1* R132S, and *IDH1* R132L variants
    - Longer survival time reported in patients with noncanonical *IDH1* mutation

DNA Methylation Profiling
- Unsupervised hierarchical clustering analyses separate IDH-mutant astrocytomas from other gliomas
- Low-grade and high-grade IDH-mutant astrocytomas form separate clusters
- Supratentorial and infratentorial IDH-mutant astrocytomas form distinct clusters
- Overall copy number variability increases with WHO grade
  - Measure of chromosomal instability that correlates with poor clinical outcome

Astrocytoma, IDH-Mutant

MGMT Promoter Methylation
- *MGMT* encodes DNA repair protein
- *MGMT* promoter methylation is commonly observed in IDH-mutant gliomas
  - Patients with methylated *MGMT* promoter region demonstrate better response to temozolomide therapy

Genetic Alterations Associated With Disease Progression
- Homozygous deletion of *CDKN2A* &/or *CDKN2B*
  - Corresponds to WHO grade 4 regardless of histological features
  - Associated with shorter survival
- *CDK4* amplification and *RB1* mutation or homozygous deletion
  - May be associated with accelerated growth
- *PDGFRA* amplification and *MET* alterations
  - Associated with shorter survival
- *PIK3R1* and *PIK3CA* mutations and *MYCN* amplification
  - Also associated with shorter survival

MICROSCOPIC

Histologic Features
- Astrocytoma, IDH-mutant
  - Infiltration of gray and white matter by variably atypical fibrillary astrocytes
  - Cellularity increases across tumor grades, from low in CNS WHO grade 2 to markedly hypercellular in grade 4 tumors
  - Nuclear features of neoplasia include irregular nuclear contours
  - Mitotic activity increases from low to absent in WHO grade 2 to brisk in WHO grade 4 tumors
    - Mitotic thresholds between WHO grades not clearly established
  - Microvascular proliferation &/or necrosis correspond to WHO grade 4 tumors
- Gemistocytic astrocytes with abundant eosinophilic cytoplasm may be present
  - Focal gain of chromosome 12p encompassing *CCND2*
- Primary mismatch repair-deficient IDH-mutant astrocytomas often histologically high-grade

ANCILLARY TESTS

Immunohistochemistry
- GFAP, S100, and vimentin (+)
  - Naked nuclei may be essentially negative
- Ki-67
  - Varies according to tumor grade
- IDH1 R132H (+)
- OLIG2
  - Nuclear positivity confirms glial lineage in GFAP(-) cases
- ATRX
  - Loss of nuclear staining on IHC
    - > 90% in supratentorial IDH-mutant astrocytomas
    - ~ 50% in infratentorial IDH-mutant astrocytoma
- p53 nuclear positivity

DIFFERENTIAL DIAGNOSIS

Reactive Astrocytosis/Gliosis
- Astrocytes typically more evenly distributed
- Fibrillary, reactive-appearing, GFAP-positive
- *IDH1* immunostaining and *IDH1/IDH2* mutation analysis negative
- Ki-67 proliferation index low or negative
- *TP53* mutations generally absent

Oligodendroglioma
- 1p19q codeleted
- ATRX nuclear staining retained

Glioblastoma, IDH Wildtype
- *IDH1/IDH2* negative
- ATRX protein retained

Diffuse Midline Glioma, H3 K27-Altered
- Immunohistochemistry for H3 (*H3C14*), p.K27M is negative
- Rarely coexpressed

Diffuse Hemispheric Glioma, H3 G34 Mutant
- Immunohistochemistry &/or molecular analyses
- Tumor cells typically lack nuclear OLIG2 expression

Diffuse Astrocytoma, *MYB*- or *MYBL1*-Altered
- A rare, low-grade, often pediatric-onset astrocytoma
- *IDH1/IDH2* wildtype
- Common fusion partners include *MAML2*, *MMP16*, *PCDHGA1*

Diffuse Low-Grade Glioma, MAPK Pathway-Altered
- Requires DNA methylation profiling or next generation sequencing

High-Grade Astrocytoma With Piloid Features
- Requires DNA methylation profiling

DIAGNOSTIC CHECKLIST

Clinically Relevant Pathologic Features
- Diffuse infiltration
- Necrosis &/or vascular proliferation in WHO grade 4 tumors
- IDH1 R132H positive in most cases
- Loss of ATRX nuclear staining
- Positive p53 nuclear staining

SELECTED REFERENCES

1. WHO Classification of Tumours Editorial Board: WHO Classification of Central Nervous System Tumours. 5th ed. International Agency for Research on Cancer, 2022
2. Wenger A et al: Methylation profiling in diffuse gliomas: diagnostic value and considerations. Cancers (Basel). 14(22), 2022
3. Ahrendsen JT et al: IDH-mutant gliomas with additional class-defining molecular events. Mod Pathol. 34(7):1236-44, 2021
4. Morshed RA et al: Molecular features and clinical outcomes in surgically treated low-grade diffuse gliomas in patients over the age of 60. J Neurooncol. 141(2):383-91, 2019
5. Capper D et al: DNA methylation-based classification of central nervous system tumours. Nature. 555(7697):469-74, 2018
6. Nandakumar P et al: The role of ATRX in glioma biology. Front Oncol. 7:236, 2017

Astrocytoma, IDH-Mutant

Diffuse Astrocytoma With Microcystic Features

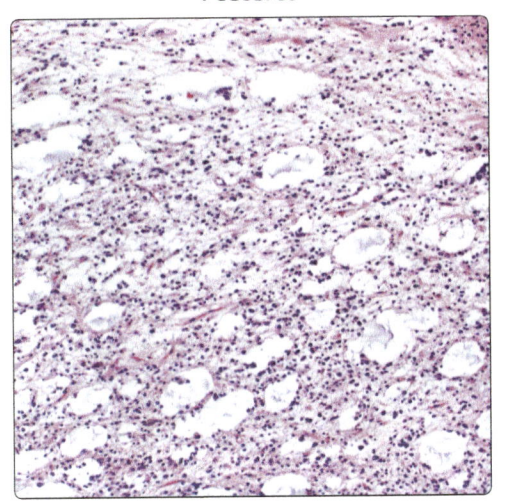

Atypical Glial Cells in Infiltrating Astrocytoma

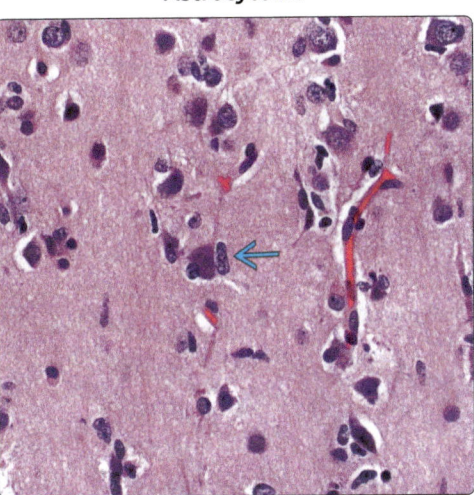

(Left) Diffuse astrocytoma with extensive microcystic features and cobweb-like architecture has been described as protoplasmic. Microcyst formation in the tumor stroma is a frequent feature of astrocytoma (CNS WHO grade 3). (Right) Although mitotic figures were present elsewhere in this specimen, this infiltrating edge shows the typical features of a low-grade astrocytoma with mildly atypical astrocytes surrounding neurons ⇒.

Diffuse Astrocytoma

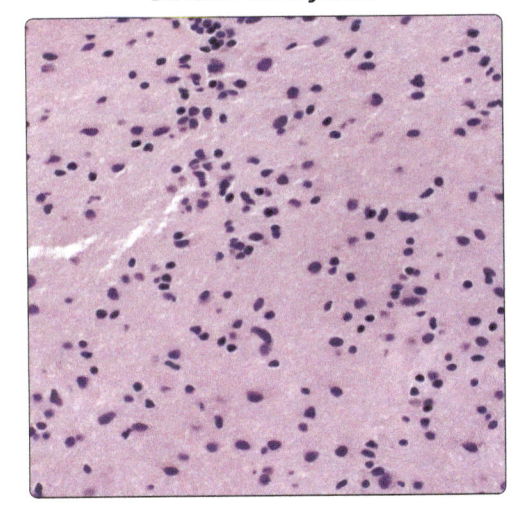

Isolated Mitotic Figure

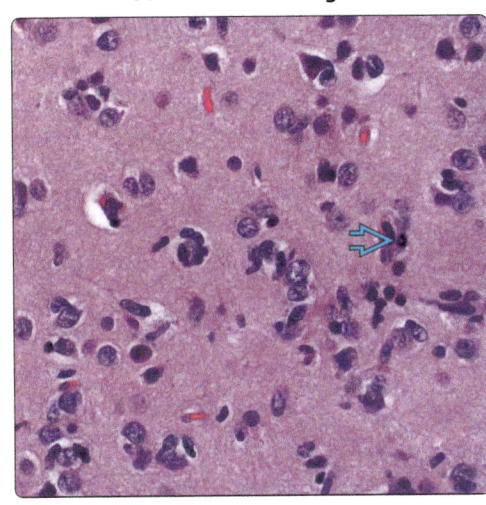

(Left) The degree of hypercellularity in this case is typical for infiltrating glioma; however, the distinction from a reactive gliosis can be difficult in some cases. Ki-67 and IDH1 R132H immunostains can be helpful in separating these entities. (Right) The single isolated mitotic figure ⇒ seen in this biopsy is not necessarily predictive of a higher grade lesion; however, if frequent mitotic figures are present, a diagnosis of astrocytoma (CNS WHO grade 3) should be considered.

Reactive Perineuronal Satellitosis

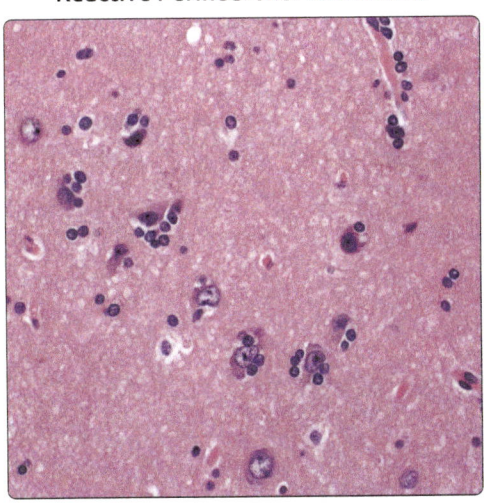

IDH1 R132C Mutation

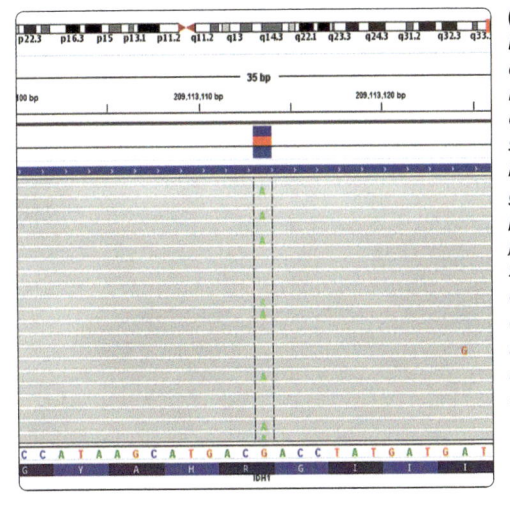

(Left) Perineuronal satellitosis by bland cells with oligodendroglial morphology is a nonspecific finding that can sometimes be seen in seizure resections. (Right) Massive parallel next-generation sequencing performed on DNA extracted from low-grade astrocytoma shows a G>A base change in codon 132 of the IDH1 gene corresponding to R132C mutation variant. IDH1/IDH2 mutations are absent in reactive gliosis.

Pilocytic Astrocytoma

KEY FACTS

TERMINOLOGY
- WHO grade I astrocytic tumor with biphasic morphology
  - Variable amounts of compact bipolar cells with Rosenthal fibers and loose multipolar cells with cysts and eosinophilic granular bodies

CLINICAL ISSUES
- Excellent prognosis with complete surgical resection
- Optic pathway gliomas often associated with NF1

IMAGING
- Classic appearance is cyst with enhancing mural nodule; lateral cerebellar hemisphere
- Well circumscribed; may be solid or macrocystic
- Circumscribed, amenable to complete surgical resection

MOLECULAR
- Activation of MAPK pathway with different gene mutations
  - Includes *KIAA1549-BRAF*, *NF1*, *BRAF* V600E, *FGFR1*, and *NTRK*
- *KIAA1549*::*BRAF* fusion is most common genetic abnormality
  - May be diagnostically useful, detected by FISH, PCR, NGS, DNA methylome analysis
  - Often in cerebellar tumors
- *FAM131B*::*BRAF* and *SRGAP3*::*RAF1* fusions rare
- *BRAF* V600E mutation rarely occurs

MICROSCOPIC
- Biphasic morphologic pattern with both compact fibrillar tissue and sometimes with spongy, myxoid, oligodendroglial-like areas
- Rosenthal fibers and eosinophilic granular bodies

ANCILLARY TESTS
- GFAP, Olig2, synaptophysin (variable), SOX2, and MAP2 (+) but IDH1(-) and H3 p.K28M (K27M) (-)

Microcystic Appearance

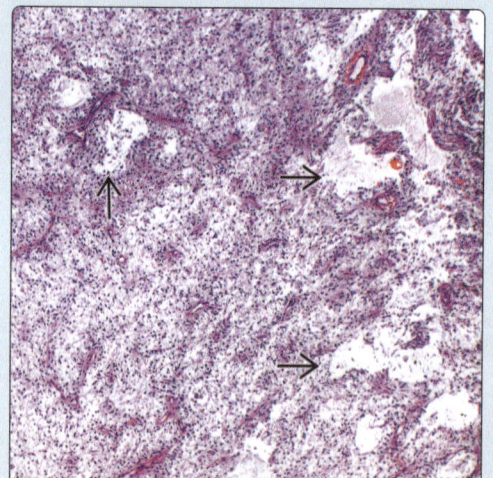

Rosenthal Fibers

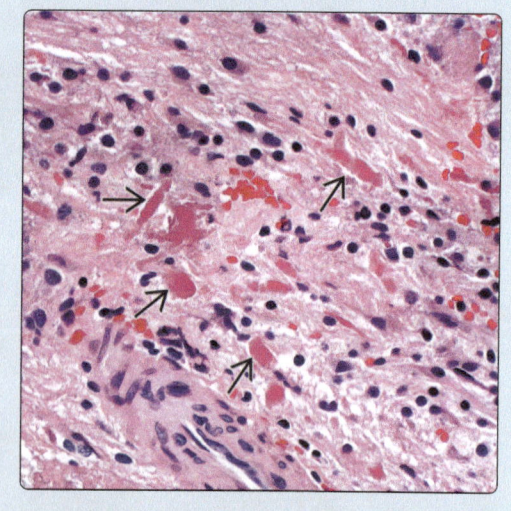

(Left) Pilocytic astrocytoma (PA) removed from the posterior fossa of a 7-year-old shows the microcystic nature ➡ of this neoplasm at low power. (Right) Rosenthal fibers ➡ are eosinophilic, irregular, elongated, "corkscrew" aggregates, which are characteristic for PA.

Astrocytic Processes

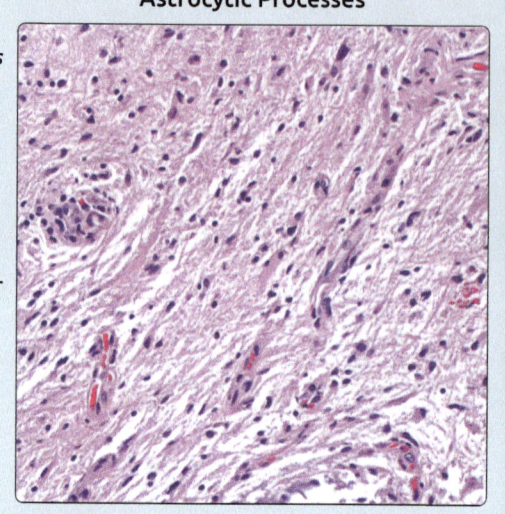

***KIAA1549*::*BRAF* Fusion**

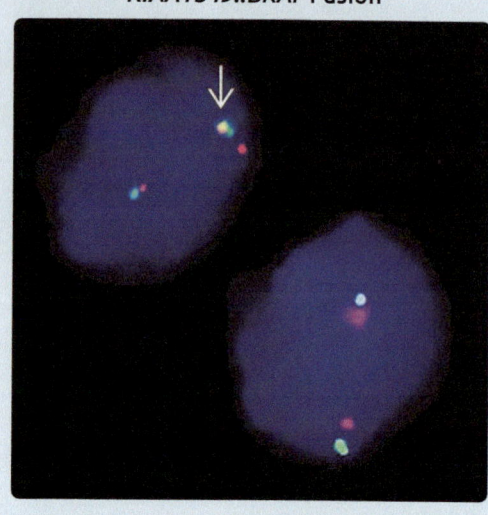

(Left) Elongated astrocytic processes are shown. Most PAs show fibrillary or hair-like (piloid) areas. (Right) A tumor cell (upper left) has 1 normal chromosome and 1 with a KIAA1549::BRAF fusion (red and green signals overlap so as to appear yellow ➡). This genetic abnormality is especially common in posterior fossa and optic pathway tumors. (Courtesy V. P. Collins, MD.)

Pilocytic Astrocytoma

TERMINOLOGY

Abbreviations
- Pilocytic astrocytoma (PA)

Synonyms
- Juvenile PA (JPA) no longer recommended

Definitions
- WHO grade I astrocytic tumor with biphasic morphology with variable amounts of compact bipolar cells with Rosenthal fibers (RF) and loose, multipolar cells with cysts and eosinophilic granular bodies; MAPK pathway alterations (especially *KIAA*1549::*BRAF*) are present

ETIOLOGY/PATHOGENESIS

Sporadic Pilocytic Astrocytoma
- Constitutive activation of MAPK signaling pathway appears to play critical role in pathogenesis of PA
  - Pathway activation is due to *BRAF* fusion gene in most PA cases
- No known environmental risk factors

Neurofibromatosis 1-Associated Pilocytic Astrocytoma
- Neurofibromatosis 1 (NF1)
  - Common autosomal dominant disorder with frequency of 1 in 3,000 live births
- NF1-associated tumors demonstrate mutation or loss of wildtype *NF1* allele
  - *NF1* is tumor suppressor gene located at 17q11.2
- 15-20% of all PA cases occur in setting of NF1
  - Up to 70% of optic pathway/hypothalamic PAs are in NF1 patients
- Optic pathway is most frequent location (75%); most of remaining are in brainstem
- Optic pathway tumors in NF1 may stabilize
  - Regression uncommon
- Up to 15% of children with hereditary tumor syndrome NF1 develop PA
- Biallelic inactivation of *NF1* in NF1 patients but not sporadic cases
- *NF1* encodes neurofibromin 1 (a.k.a. NF-related protein NF1)
  - Neurofibromin 1 protein is negative regulator of RAS in MAPK/ERK pathway
  - Expression is reduced in NF1-related PA
  - Loss of neurofibromin 1 results in constitutive activation of RAS and downstream hyperactivation of mTOR pathways

CLINICAL ISSUES

Epidemiology
- Incidence
  - 1/100,000
- Age
  - 5-19 years; peak incidence at 5-9 years
  - Most common glioma of childhood

Presentation
- Most common site (sporadic tumors) is cerebellum, typically lateral (not midline) location
  - Presentation correlates with site; headache, nausea, vomiting, ataxia common with cerebellar tumors
- Optic pathways, hypothalamus, dorsal brainstem, and spinal cord also common
  - Optic pathway and brainstem tumors are commonly NF1 associated
  - Typically exophytic rather than infiltrative in brainstem
- Supratentorial locations less common
- ~ 80% of cases are sporadic

Treatment
- Surgical resection often curative for cerebellar tumors
- Optic pathway/hypothalamic, deep midline, and brainstem gliomas generally nonresectable
- MAPK inhibitors for progressive or recurrent tumors
- 2nd-line radiotherapy sometimes considered
  - Controversial due to side effects in children

Prognosis
- Excellent with 20-year survival in > 80% of cases
  - Indolent growth; rarely show histologic progression
    - Cyst recurrence frequent after incomplete resection
  - Progression-free survival 70% in adults
- Supratentorial tumors, optic pathway tumors, nonresectable and spinal cord tumors have less favorable prognosis
- Midline, hypothalamus, and dorsal brainstem tumors are least favorable and often inoperable

IMAGING

General Features
- Best diagnostic clue
  - Classic appearance is cyst with enhancing mural nodule
  - Almost always well circumscribed; may be solid or macrocystic
  - Infiltrative in optic nerve
  - Exophytic in brainstem

MACROSCOPIC

General Features
- Well-circumscribed, soft, gray, discrete tumors
- ~ 50% are cystic

MOLECULAR

Molecular Genetics
- *KIAA1549::BRAF* fusion
  - Most common mutation (> 70% of tumors)
  - Tandem duplication resulting in fusion between 5' end of *KIAA1549* and 3' end of *BRAF*
  - Fusion gene transcripts contain amino terminus of KIAA1549 and BRAF kinase domain but lack autoregulatory domain of BRAF
    - This results in activation of MAPK signaling pathway
  - Detected by FISH, PCR, NGS
  - Common in PAs, usually cerebellar, rare in other gliomas

Pilocytic Astrocytoma

- Not entirely specific, also seen in leptomeningeal glioneuronal tumor
- *BRAF* and various other gene fusions
  - Deletions or translocations resulting in BRAF fusion proteins, which lack BRAF regulatory domain and activates MAPK pathway
  - *FAM131B::BRAF* fusion
    - Less frequent
    - Occurs after interstitial deletion that removes *BRAF* N-terminal inhibitory domain
  - *SRGAP3::RAF1* fusion
    - Rare fusion
    - Tandem duplication at 3p25 results in fusion between *SRGAP3* and *RAF1* genes
  - Other rare fusion partners include *RNF130*, *CLCN6*, *NKRN1*, *GNA11*, *QKI*, *FXR1*, and *MACF1*
- *NF1* mutations, *BRAF* V600E mutation, *FGFR1* and *NTRK* genes are all part of MAPK pathway
  - *FGFR1* mutations are mostly in midline structures
  - *BRAF* V600E and *NTRK* gene mutations are usually supratentorial tumors
- *KRAS* mutations rare
- Gene mutations common in infiltrating astrocytoma are uncommon in PA
  - *TP53* mutations, *PTEN* mutations, *EGFR* amplification, and 9p21 deletion are all extremely uncommon in PA
- NF1-associated PA is distinct from sporadic cases
  - Allelic loss of *NF1* and reduced neurofibromin 1 expression

DNA Methylation Array
- Copy number profile if narrow gain of 7q34 region is seen

MICROSCOPIC

Histologic Features
- Astrocytes have piloid (hair-like) appearance
- Biphasic architecture
  - Compact piloid areas (often with RF)
  - Areas with loose, microcystic appearance, sometimes with round, oligodendrocyte-like astrocytes [often with eosinophilic granular bodies (EGB)]
- May have multinucleated astrocytes, which look like horseshoes, a.k.a. "pennies on plate"
- RF and EGB
  - EGB highlighted by PAS with diastase and trichrome
  - RF may be coated by GFAP and ubiquitin and α-B-crystallin (+)
  - Protein droplets (similar to EGB)
- Glomeruloid vascular endothelial proliferation is common and not useful for grading
- Mitotic figures uncommon and not useful for grading
- Necrosis uncommon but not clinically relevant

Cytologic Features
- Hair-like cells (piloid) create finely fibrillar background; nuclei are bland, uniform
- May see RF, EGB in smear preparations

ANCILLARY TESTS

Immunohistochemistry
- GFAP(+), Olig2(+), especially in oligodendroglioma-like and spongy areas
- Synaptophysin variable (+), more in pilomyxoid variant
- pERK(+), especially for tumors with BRAF duplication
- Other (+) markers include SOX2, S100, vimentin, and MAP2
- Ki-67 generally shows low proliferation index (1-3%)
- p53(-)
- IDH1 R132H (-)
- H3 p.K28M (K27M) (-)
- CD34(-) compared to ganglioglioma (+) or other glioneuronal tumor

DIFFERENTIAL DIAGNOSIS

Pilomyxoid Astrocytoma
- Subtype of PA
- Tends to occur in very young children (mean age: 18 months), hypothalamic region common
- No RF; EGB extremely rare
- Myxoid background with fibrillary processes arranged perpendicularly to blood vessels (angiocentric)
- Similar MAPK pathway gene alterations

Reactive Processes
- Piloid gliosis lacks biphasic features
- Correlation with imaging can be helpful

Infiltrating Astrocytoma
- Growth is infiltrating rather than circumscribed
  - Some infiltration may be seen at edges of PA
  - Correlation with imaging can prove helpful
- No RF or EGB
- *IDH1* and *IDH2* mutations common
- *TP53* mutation common
- Diffuse midline gliomas, H3K27 altered
  - H3 p.K28M (K27M) IHC (-)

Oligodendroglioma
- IDH mutant, 1p19q codeleted

High-Grade Astrocytoma With Piloid Features
- High-grade piloid &/or glioblastoma-like histology
- Distinct DNA methylation profile combined with alterations of MAPK pathway genes
  - *CDKN2A/CDKN2B* deletions &/or *ATRX* mutation or loss of nuclear ATRX expression

SELECTED REFERENCES

1. WHO Classification of Tumours Editorial Board. World Health Organization Classification of Tumours of the Central Nervous System. 5th ed. IARC, 2021
2. Stichel D et al: Accurate calling of KIAA1549-BRAF fusions from DNA of human brain tumours using methylation array-based copy number and gene panel sequencing data. Neuropathol Appl Neurobiol. 47(3):406-14, 2021
3. Khater F et al: Recurrent somatic BRAF insertion (p.V504_R506dup): a tumor marker and a potential therapeutic target in pilocytic astrocytoma. Oncogene. 38(16):2994-3002, 2019
4. Maraka S et al: BRAF alterations in primary brain tumors. Discov Med. 26(141):51-60, 2018

Pilocytic Astrocytoma

Uniform Round Cells

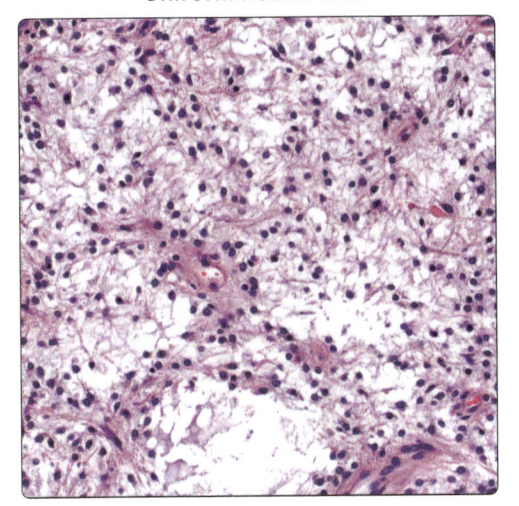

Hair-Like Astrocytes and Rosenthal Fibers

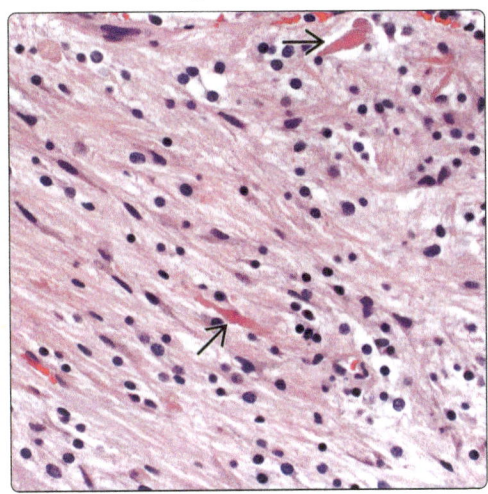

(Left) Myxoid area shows microcysts and tumor cells with a round, evenly spaced, oligodendroglial-like appearance. (Right) Classic hair-like, elongated fibrillary processes that are typically seen in more compact regions are shown. Note the scattered Rosenthal fibers ⇒.

Eosinophilic Granular Body

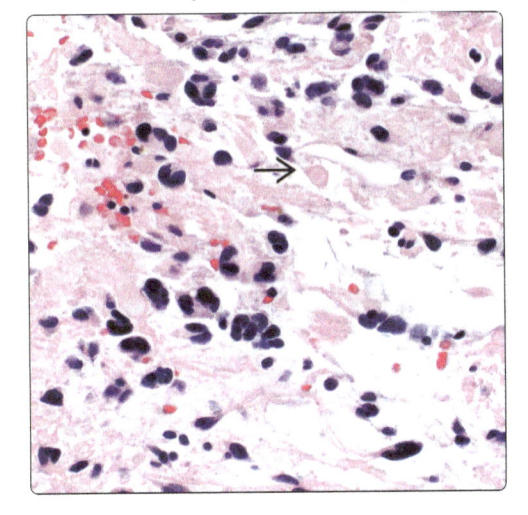

Eosinophilic Granular Body

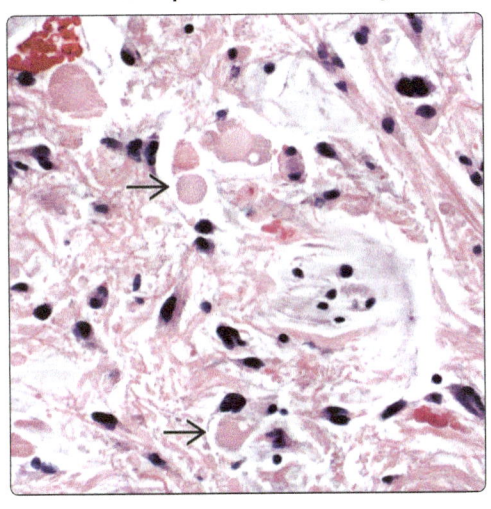

(Left) A region of tumor where the cells appear multinucleated ("pennies on a platter") is shown. Several scattered eosinophilic granular bodies ⇒ are also present. (Right) PA shows abundant eosinophilic granular bodies ⇒. Similar structures can be seen in ganglioglioma, which is in the differential diagnosis of PA.

GFAP Immunohistochemistry

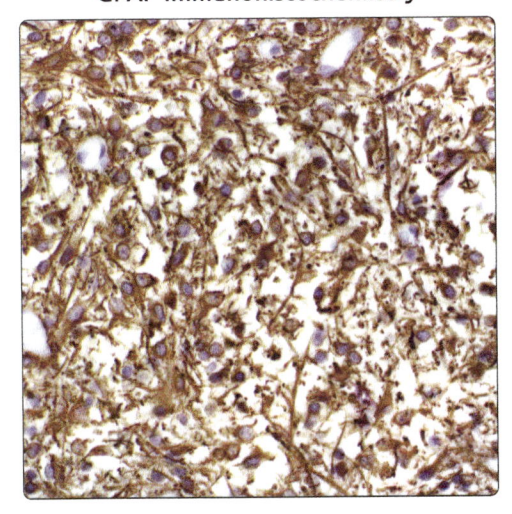

Ki-67 Immunohistochemistry

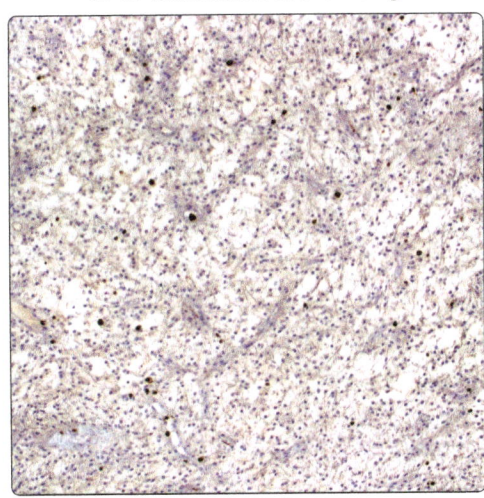

(Left) Fibrillary processes are highlighted with GFAP in a region that had myxoid, microcystic, oligodendroglial-like features on H&E. This pattern of GFAP(+) fibrillarity would be uncommon for oligodendroglioma. (Right) Ki-67 generally shows a very low proliferation index in PA. Here, there is positive nuclear staining in < 5% of tumor cell nuclei.

Oligodendroglioma, IDH Mutant, and 1p/19q Codeleted

KEY FACTS

TERMINOLOGY
- Diffusely infiltrating glioma with *IDH1* or *IDH2* alterations and codeletion of chromosome arms 1p and 19q

CLINICAL ISSUES
- Adults (30-50 years of age)
- Frequently involve cerebral hemispheres
- Surgery involves gross total resection when possible
- Most patients receive chemotherapy
- Clinical trials of IDH1 inhibitors and IDH1 vaccination in *IDH1*-mutant cases
- Average survival for WHO grade 2 is 10-15 years, with PCV chemotherapy, and 14 years in grade 3

IMAGING
- Low-grade tumor typically nonenhancing
- T2 and FLAIR hyperintense
- Occasionally more circumscribed than infiltrating astrocytoma

MOLECULAR
- Balanced 1p19q (whole chromosome) codeletions
- *IDH1* and *IDH2* mutations
  - Identified in all cases
- *CIC* and *FUBP1* mutations may indicate poor prognosis
- *TERT* promoter region mutations
- Hypermethylation of multiple CpG islands, glioma CpG island methylator phenotype (G-CIMP)

MICROSCOPIC
- Round, uniform glial cells with perinuclear halos
- Microcalcifications common (albeit nondiagnostic)
- Minigemistocytes

ANCILLARY TESTS
- IDH-R132H immunohistochemistry (+)

Next-Generation Sequencing for *IDH1* Mutation

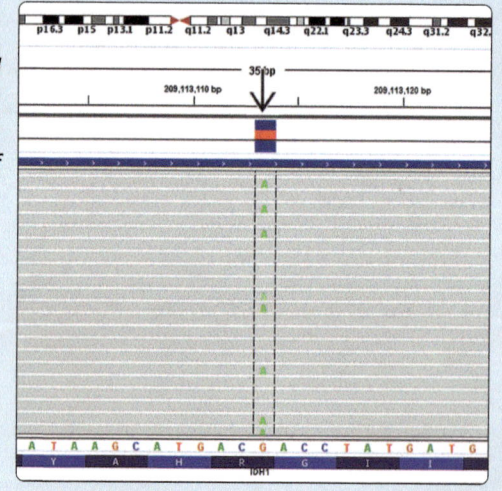

Classic Appearance

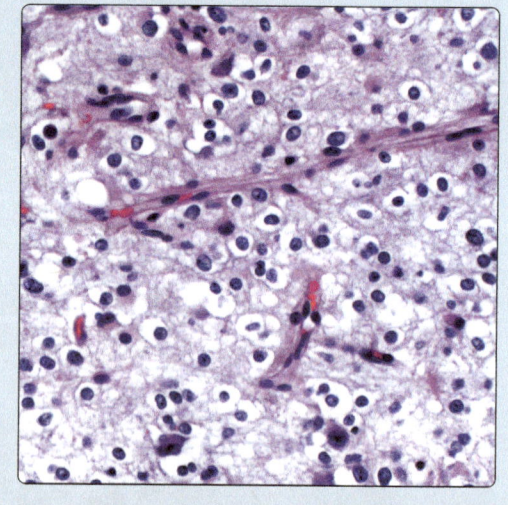

(Left) Next-generation sequencing pileup of PCR-amplified IDH1 exon 2 shows a G>A base substitution in codon 113 (c.113G>A) ➡ corresponding to an IDH1 R132C mutation in this case of oligodendroglioma. (Right) Classic appearance of uniform cells with round nuclei, scant cytoplasm, distinct nucleoli, and artificial perinuclear halos is shown. There is also a delicate chicken-wire arcuate vascular network.

Uniform Cells

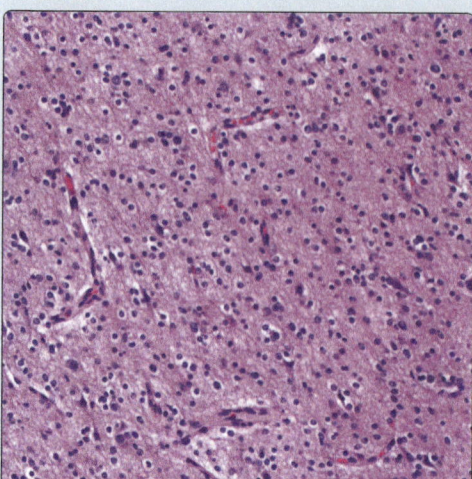

IDH-1 Immunohistochemistry

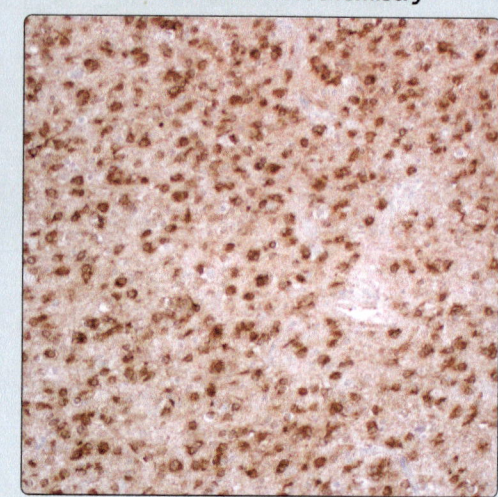

(Left) At low power, there are uniform cells with a classic fried egg appearance of tumor cells and a chicken-wire vascular pattern. (Right) IDH-1 is positive with nuclear and cytoplasmic staining pattern in oligodendroglioma. Neurons and reactive astrocytes are IDH-1(-).

Oligodendroglioma, IDH Mutant, and 1p/19q Codeleted

TERMINOLOGY

Synonyms
- Oligodendroglioma, IDH mutant, 1p19q codeleted (WHO grade 2)
- Oligodendroglioma, IDH mutant (WHO grade 3)

Definitions
- Diffusely infiltrating glioma with *IDH1* or *IDH2* alterations and codeletion of chromosome arms 1p and 19q

CLINICAL ISSUES

Epidemiology
- Incidence
  - Accounts for 15-20% of infiltrating gliomas
- Age: Typically present at 30-50 years

Presentation
- Seizures most common; focal neurological deficits, focal deficits

Treatment
- Surgical approaches
  - Aim is for complete resection when possible
- Drugs
  - Most patients receive chemotherapy
    - Temozolomide is most commonly used
    - PCV (procarbazine, lomustine, vincristine)
  - IDH1 inhibitors
    - In phase 1, clinical trials to evaluate suppression of 2-HG in *IDH1*-mutated gliomas
  - IDH1 vaccination
    - In phase 1, clinical trials to evaluate IDH1R132H 20-mer peptide vaccine in newly diagnosed patients
- Radiation
  - Radiotherapy common with subtotal resection

Prognosis
- Average survival for WHO grade 2 is 10-15 years and even 14 years in grade with PCV chemotherapy

IMAGING

MR Findings
- Low-grade tumors typically nonenhancing
- T2 and FLAIR hyperintense

MACROSCOPIC

General Features
- Sometimes described as gelatinous or mucinous

MOLECULAR

Fluorescence In Situ Hybridization
- 1p and 19q codeletions
  - Characteristic of oligodendrogliomas
- False-positives, less reliable than PCR

Molecular Genetics
- *IDH1* and *IDH2* mutations
  - Detected in all cases
  - 90% canonical *IDH1* p.R132H mutation with more *IDH2* mutations than in astrocytomas
- *CIC* and *FUBP1* mutations are common
  - Poor prognostic indicator
- *TERT* promoter region mutations stable throughout disease
  - *IDH* mutant, Ip19q codeleted oligodendrogliomas in teenagers may lack p*TERT* mutations
- *PIK3CA*, *PIK3R1*, *NOTCH1* mutations
- Homozygous *CDKN2A* deletion with tumor progression

Epigenetic changes
- Hypermethylation of multiple CpG islands, glioma CpG island methylator phenotype (G-CIMP)
  - DNA methylation classifier differs from IDH mutant astrocytoma
- *MGMT* promoter methylated in most oligodendrogliomas

MICROSCOPIC

Histologic Features
- Cells infiltrate diffusely with perineuronal satellitosis, perivascular and subpial accumulations
- Round, uniform glial cells with artificial perinuclear halos giving fried egg appearance
- Microcalcifications not specific; sometimes (mini)gemistocytes

ANCILLARY TESTS

Immunohistochemistry
- IDH-1(+)
  - In ~ 90% of adults, but usually (-) in children
  - Nuclear and cytoplasmic staining
- GFAP variable, Olig2 uniformly (+), synaptophysin (+) with neurocytic differentiation
- Lack strong nuclear p53(+) &/or loss of nuclear ATRX

DIFFERENTIAL DIAGNOSIS

Central Neurocytoma
- Typically intraventricular, often septum pellucidum
- Distinct DNA methylation cluster

Clear Cell Ependymoma
- Frequent *ZFTA* (C11orf95) fusions
- Olig2(-) and IDH(-), EMA(+) dots

Dysembryoplastic Neuroepithelial Tumor
- Mucin-rich nodules containing floating neurons
- FGFR1 alterations

Astrocytoma, IDH Mutant
- ATRX nuclear loss, p53 accumulation
- Lack 1p19 codeletion

SELECTED REFERENCES

1. WHO Classification of Tumours Editorial Board. World Health Organization Classification of Tumours of the Central Nervous System. 5th ed. IARC, 2021
2. Hassanudin SA et al: Determination of genetic aberrations and novel transcripts involved in the pathogenesis of oligodendroglioma using array comparative genomic hybridization and next generation sequencing. Oncol Lett. 17(2):1675-87, 2019

Oligodendroglioma, IDH Mutant, and 1p/19q Codeleted

(Left) FISH using chromosomal enumeration probe (CEP1) as a control probe (green) and marker on chromosome 1p (red) shows 2 green signals in most cells and only 1 red signal in most cells, consistent with 1p deletion. **(Right)** FISH using chromosomal enumeration probe (CEP1) as a control probe (green) and marker on chromosome 19q (red) shows 2 green signals in most cells and only 1 red signal in most cells, consistent with 19q deletion.

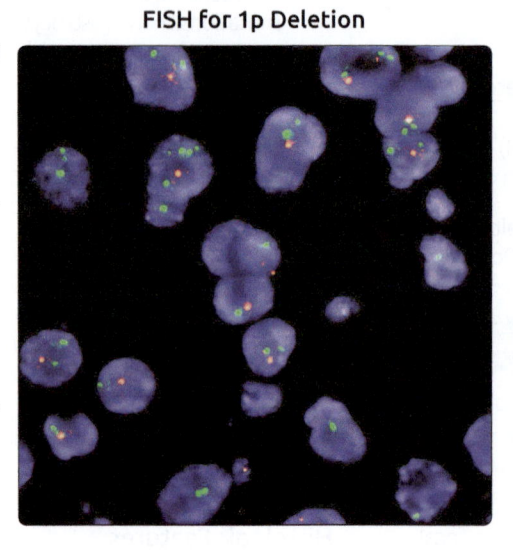

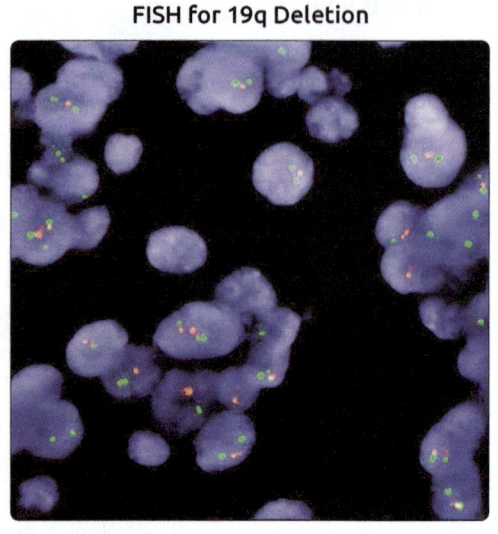

FISH for 1p Deletion

FISH for 19q Deletion

(Left) Oligodendroglioma shows some cells with vaguely astrocytic features and a single punctate microcalcification ➡. New definitions strongly discourage a mixed oligodendroglial diagnosis. **(Right)** The delicate capillary pattern (sometimes described as chicken-wire or arcuate vasculature) can be seen nicely here, although the capillaries are more straight than arched in this example.

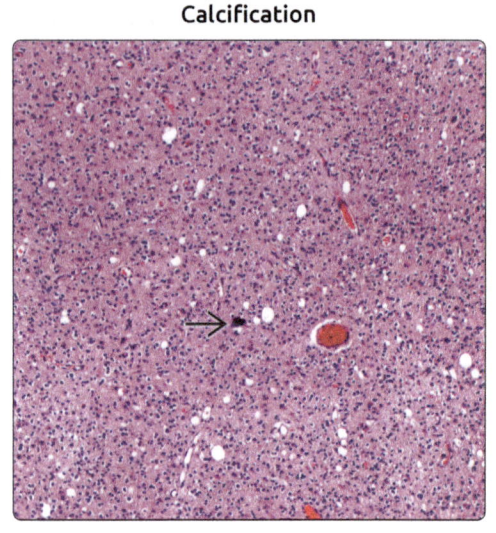

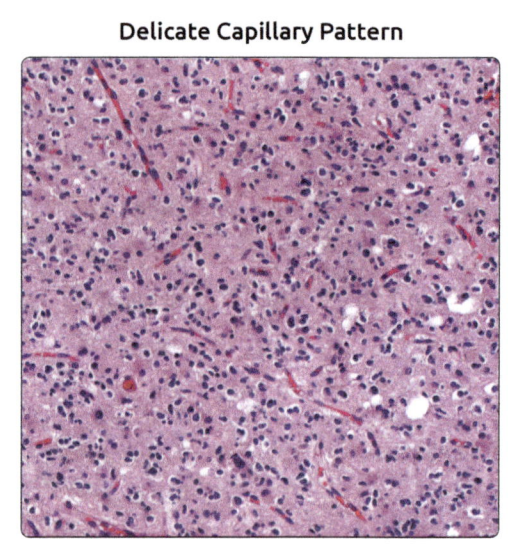

Calcification

Delicate Capillary Pattern

(Left) Primarily grade 2 oligodendroglioma shows the classic fried egg appearance of oligodendroglial cells and the round, evenly spaced nature of tumor cell nuclei. In contrast, astrocytomas are usually less uniform and have less distinct nucleoli. **(Right)** Typical low-grade oligodendroglioma is shown. Microcalcifications or calcospherites are more common in oligodendroglial tumors than in other glial tumors and, when extensive, can be seen radiographically.

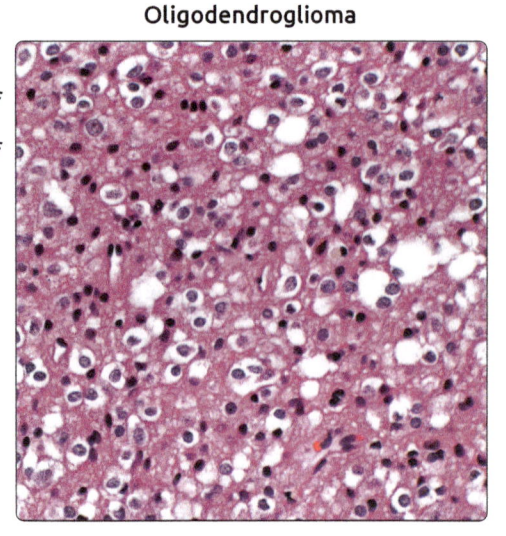

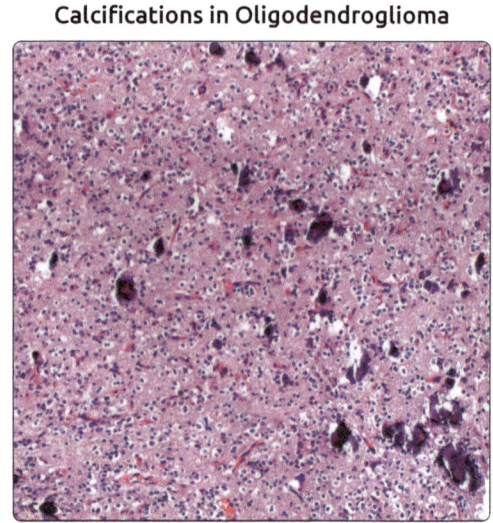

Oligodendroglioma

Calcifications in Oligodendroglioma

Oligodendroglioma, IDH Mutant, and 1p/19q Codeleted

Higher Grade Tumor

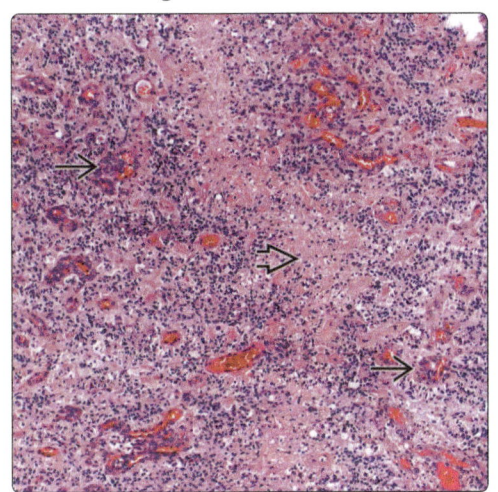

Glioblastoma

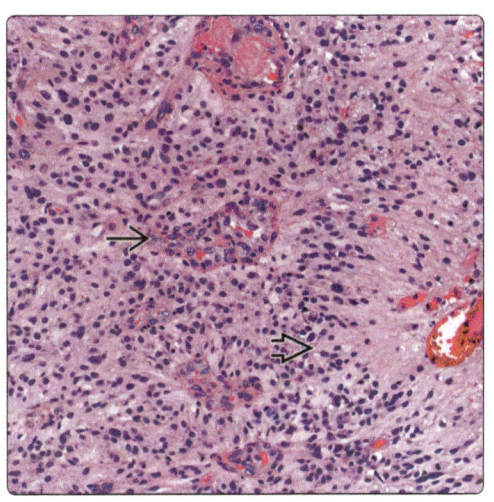

(Left) *Higher grade tumor in an otherwise low-grade-appearing glioma is shown. There is abundant microvascular proliferation ➡ on both sides of a region of necrosis ➡. IDH and 1p19q mutation status is needed for further classification/grading.* (Right) *Glioblastoma, IDH wildtype with some oligodendroglial features shows vascular proliferation ➡ with pseudopalisading of nuclei ➡ without obvious necrosis.*

Uniform Cells

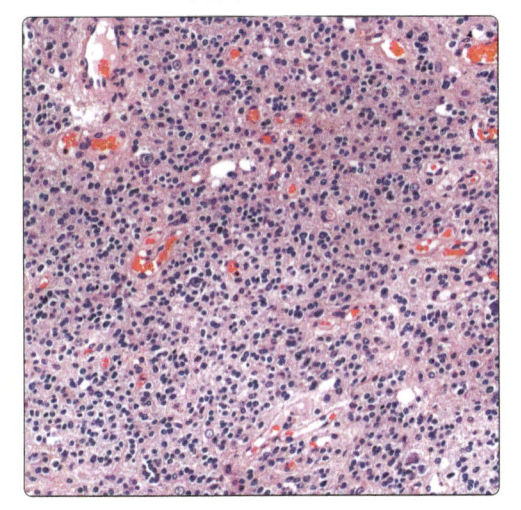

Hypercellular Oligodendroglioma

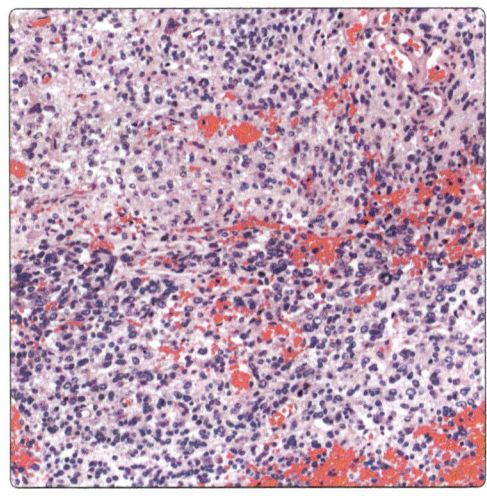

(Left) *Oligodendroglioma, IDH mutant, 1p19q codeleted shows uniform-appearing, low-grade cells with oligodendroglial features. Microvascular proliferation and brisk mitotic activity, defined as ≥ 2.5 mitoses/mm² (≥ 6 mitoses/10 HPF), correspond to grade 3 disease.* (Right) *Oligodendroglioma shows a focus of hypercellularity and some tumor cells with astrocytic features.*

Minigemistocytes

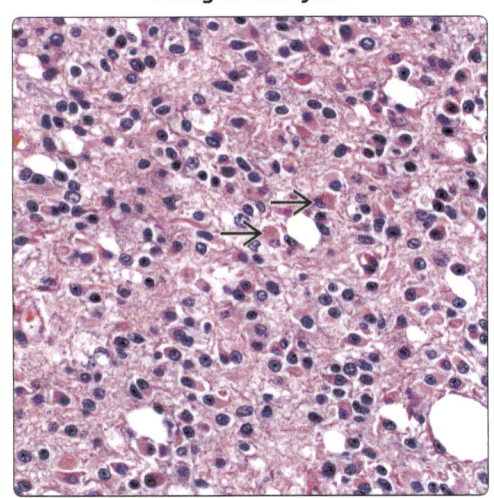

Minigemistocytes

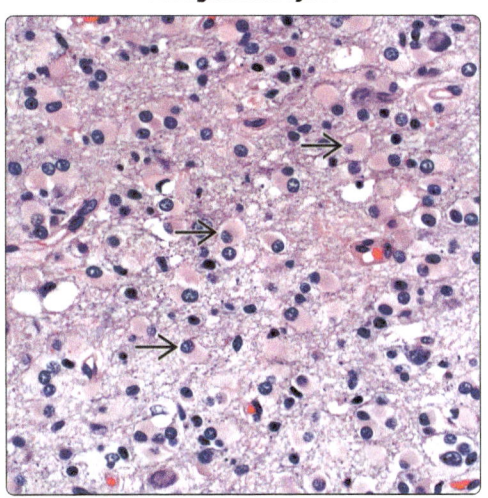

(Left) *Abundant mini- (or micro-) gemistocytes ➡ are a common feature in oligodendroglioma and are GFAP(+).* (Right) *Oligodendroglioma with abundant classic minigemistocytes ➡ is shown.*

Ependymal Tumors

KEY FACTS

TERMINOLOGY
- Circumscribed CNS neoplasm with dual glial and epithelial differentiation
- 2021 WHO classification of ependymal tumors is based on combination of histopathological features, molecular findings, and anatomical site

CLASSIFICATION
- **Updated 2021 WHO classification of ependymal tumors**
  - Supratentorial ependymoma
  - Supratentorial ependymoma, *ZFTA* fusion positive
  - Supratentorial ependymoma, *YAP1* fusion positive
  - Posterior fossa ependymoma
  - Posterior fossa group A (PFA) ependymoma
  - Posterior fossa group B (PFB) ependymoma
  - Spinal ependymoma, *MYCN*-amplified
  - Myxopapillary ependymoma
  - Subependymoma

CLINICAL ISSUES
- Ependymomas may arise anywhere in neuraxis
- Most frequent primary spinal cord neoplasm
- Prognosis depends on anatomic site (spinal cord excellent), extent of resection, and molecular subtype

MICROSCOPIC
- Perivascular pseudorosettes are present in most ependymomas
- True ependymal rosettes
- Usually sharp interface with CNS parenchyma

TOP DIFFERENTIAL DIAGNOSES
- Schwannoma
- Meningioma
- Astrocytoma
- Paraganglioma
- Metastatic carcinoma
- Oligodendroglioma

Spinal Cord Ependymoma

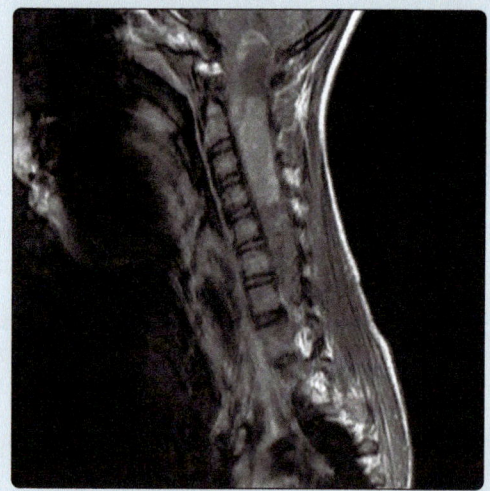

Posterior Fossa Ependymoma

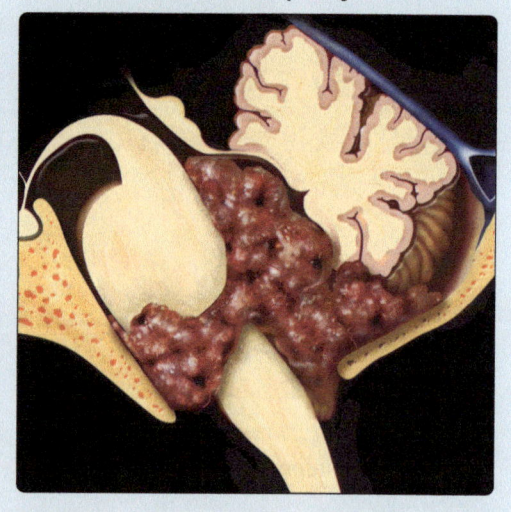

(Left) As this T1 MR shows, ependymomas form well-circumscribed masses, and most demonstrate contrast enhancement. The spinal cord represents a favored anatomic site for ependymoma. *(Right)* Posterior fossa ependymomas typically fill the 4th ventricle and represent a surgical challenge.

Perivascular Pseudorosettes

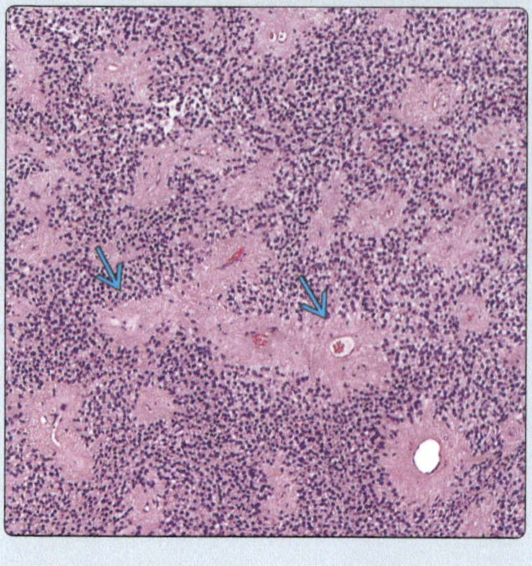

Microvascular Proliferation

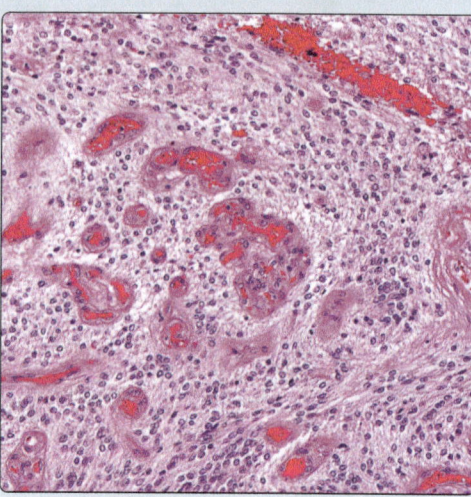

(Left) Among the main architectural features of ependymomas at low power are perivascular pseudorosettes, which impart an anuclear area around intratumoral vessels ➡. *(Right)* Microvascular proliferation is a worrisome feature in ependymomas and usually one of the histologic properties ascribed to anaplastic histology (WHO grade 3).

Ependymal Tumors

TERMINOLOGY

Definitions
- Circumscribed CNS neoplasm with dual glial and epithelial differentiation, properties resembling ependymal lining of ventricular system/central spinal cord canal
- 2021 WHO classification of ependymal tumors is based on combination of histopathological features, molecular findings, and anatomical site

Updated 2021 WHO Classification of Ependymal Tumors
- Supratentorial ependymoma, *ZFTA* fusion positive
- Supratentorial ependymoma, *YAP1* fusion positive
- Posterior fossa group A (PFA) ependymoma
- Posterior fossa group B (PFB) ependymoma
- Spinal ependymoma, *MYCN*-amplified
- Myxopapillary ependymoma
- Subependymoma

DNA Methylation Profiling of Ependymal Tumors
- Divides ependymal tumors into molecular groups across 3 main CNS anatomical sites
  - Supratentorial, posterior fossa, spine

CLINICAL ISSUES

Site
- May arise anywhere in neuraxis
  - Predilection for spinal cord in adults and posterior fossa/supratentorial compartment in children
- Most frequent primary spinal cord neoplasm in adults
- Predilection for cervical cord/cervicomedullary junction in patients with neurofibromatosis type 2 (NF2)

Presentation
- Mass effect (supratentorial), obstructive hydrocephalus (posterior fossa), pain/neurologic deficit (spinal)
- NF2-associated ependymomas are multiple in most patients
  - Predilection for spinal cord

Treatment
- Goal of surgery is complete surgical resection, if feasible
- Clinical follow-up is indicated for asymptomatic tumors in NF2

Prognosis
- Depends on anatomic site, extent of resection, and molecular subtype
  - Excellent prognosis in spinal cord tumors
- Most NF2-associated ependymomas are indolent

IMAGING

MR Findings
- Well-circumscribed neoplasms
- ↑ T2 signal, homogeneous contrast enhancement
- Heterogeneous enhancement in necrotic tumors
- Associated cyst/spinal cord syrinx may be present
- Leptomeningeal dissemination in subset of cases (intracranial tumors)

MICROSCOPIC

Histologic Features
- Perivascular pseudorosettes
  - Present in majority of ependymomas to variable extent
  - Glial processes surrounding vessels create anuclear zone
  - More accentuated in ependymomas but may be present to lesser extent in astrocytic and neuronal neoplasms
- True ependymal rosettes
  - Well-defined lumina resembling ependymal linings
  - When large, known as ependymal canals
  - May be minute and recognized by EMA with dot-like pattern or by electron microscopy
  - Less frequent than pseudorosettes but essentially diagnostic in right context
- Usually sharp interface with CNS parenchyma
  - Gliosis with Rosenthal fibers may be present
  - Infiltration is rare but may be found in supratentorial/recurrent tumors
- Neuropil islands and sarcomatous components rarely may develop

Cytologic Features
- Uniform, bland oval cells with relatively short processes
- Aggregation/clinging of cells around vessels (pseudorosettes) is characteristic

Updated Histologic Patterns of Ependymoma
- Papillary, clear cell, and tanycytic morphologic patterns
  - No longer listed as subtypes of ependymoma in updated 2021 WHO CNS classification
  - Included as patterns in histopathologic description of classic tumors
- Anaplastic ependymoma
  - No longer listed in updated 2021 WHO CNS classification
- Myxopapillary ependymoma and subependymoma remain listed as tumor types
  - Current molecular classification does not provide added clinicopathological utility for these 2 tumors
  - Updated WHO classification lists these 2 histologically defined diagnosis at any of 3 anatomic sites

Ependymal Tumors Subtypes
- Supratentorial ependymoma, *ZFTA* fusion positive
  - *ZFTA::RELA* most common fusion
  - Circumscribed supratentorial glioma that focally demonstrates pseudorosettes or ependymal rosettes
  - Uniform small cells with round nuclei embedded in fibrillary matrix
- Supratentorial ependymoma, *YAP1* fusion positive
  - *YAP1::MAMLD1* most common fusion
- Supratentorial ependymoma, NOS
  - Reserved for cases with undetectable *ZFTA* or *YAP1* fusion
- Posterior fossa group A (PFA) ependymoma
  - Circumscribed posterior fossa glioma
  - Identified by loss of nuclear H3 p.K28me3 (K27me3) expression in tumor cells or by DNA methylation profiling
- Posterior fossa group B (PFB) ependymoma

Ependymal Tumors

- PFB group is identified by DNA methylation profiling and retention of nuclear H3 p.K28me3 (K27me3) expression
- PFB ependymomas exhibit widespread cytogenetic abnormalities, most common of which include loss of 22q, monosomy 6, and trisomy 18 (50-60% of cases)
- Posterior fossa ependymoma, NOS
  - Circumscribed glioma in posterior fossa
  - This diagnosis should be used when molecular analysis either cannot assign molecular group or is not feasible
- Spinal ependymoma, *MYCN*-amplified
  - Well-demarcated spinal glioma demonstrating pseudorosettes or ependymal rosettes, necrosis, and high mitotic rate
  - By definition, *MYCN* amplification is demonstrated in tumor cells
  - Aggressive tumor associated with poor progression-free and overall survival
- Spinal ependymoma
  - Frequent loss of chromosome 22q and mutations of *NF2* are characteristic of spinal ependymomas
    - More frequently in patients with neurofibromatosis type 2 with germline nonsense and frameshift mutations in *NF2*
    - By definition, *MYCN* amplification is absent
- Myxopapillary ependymoma
  - Easily recognized with classic morphology
    - Radial arrangement of spindled or epithelioid tumor cells around blood vessels with microcyst formation
  - Unique DNA methylation profile
  - Gains of chromosome 16 and losses of chromosome 10 have been documented
  - Generally favorable behavior when totally resected
- Subependymoma
  - Distinctive architecture with clusters of neoplastic cells (low-power diagnosis)
  - Familial cases, including examples in monozygotic twins, are well documented but rare
    - These include examples associated with trichorhinophalangeal syndrome type 1 and germline *TRPS1* mutation
    - Subset of sporadic subependymomas also harbor *TRPS1* mutations
    - Isolated cases have also been described in patients with hereditary aniridia and *PAX6* mutation, as well as Noonan syndrome with germline *PTPN11* mutation
    - Patients with craniopharyngiomas have been reported to develop rare 3rd ventricular subependymomas
    - Losses of chromosomes 19 and 6, latter restricted to infratentorial tumors, appear to play role in many sporadic cases

ANCILLARY TESTS

Genetic Testing

- Molecular subgroups of ependymal tumors based on transcriptome and methylome analysis
- *ZFTA* and *YAP1* fusions in supratentorial ependymomas
- *MYCN* amplification testing to identify *MYCN*-amplified spinal ependymoma
- Alterations in *NF2* frequent in spinal cord ependymomas
- *NF2* mutations in spinal ependymoma

Gene Expression Profiling

- Relevant subtypes cluster according to anatomic site and clinical behavior

DIFFERENTIAL DIAGNOSIS

Schwannoma

- Almost always extramedullary, nerve root association
- S100(+) but EMA(-)

Meningioma

- Extramedullary location
- Membranous (rather than dot-like) EMA expression, GFAP(-)

Astrocytoma

- May be difficult to distinguish from ependymoma
- Rosenthal fibers and microcysts (pilocytic) or tissue infiltration (diffuse astrocytomas) not features of ependymoma
- Astrocytomas demonstrate strong GFAP expression
- Lack microlumina by EMA or electron microscopy

Paraganglioma

- Clinical and histologic overlap with myxopapillary ependymoma in filum terminale
- Strong synaptophysin and chromogranin positivity

Metastatic Carcinoma

- Rare in spinal cord proper
- Increased pleomorphism, strong cytokeratin expression

Oligodendroglioma

- Main differential diagnosis with clear cell histology pattern in ependymoma
- OLIG2(+), *IDH* mutations and 1p/19q codeletion, infiltrative growth

Choroid Plexus Tumors

- Main differential diagnosis for ependymomas with papillary histologic pattern
- Cytokeratin expression to greater extent in choroid plexus tumors
- Microlumina is feature of ependymoma

SELECTED REFERENCES

1. Horbinski C et al: Clinical implications of the 2021 edition of the WHO classification of central nervous system tumours. Nat Rev Neurol. 18(9):515-29, 2022
2. Kurokawa R et al: Major changes in 2021 World Health Organization classification of central nervous system tumors. Radiographics. 42(5):1474-93, 2022
3. Louis DN et al: The 2021 WHO classification of tumors of the central nervous system: a summary. Neuro Oncol. 23(8):1231-51, 2021
4. Pagès M et al: Diagnostics of pediatric supratentorial RELA ependymomas: integration of information from histopathology, genetics, DNA methylation and imaging. Brain Pathol. 29(3):325-35, 2019
5. Cavalli FMG et al: Heterogeneity within the PF-EPN-B ependymoma subgroup. Acta Neuropathol. 136(2):227-37, 2018
6. Fukuoka K et al: Significance of molecular classification of ependymomas: C11orf95-RELA fusion-negative supratentorial ependymomas are a heterogeneous group of tumors. Acta Neuropathol Commun. 6(1):134, 2018

Ependymal Tumors

Spinal Cord Ependymoma With Cystic Change

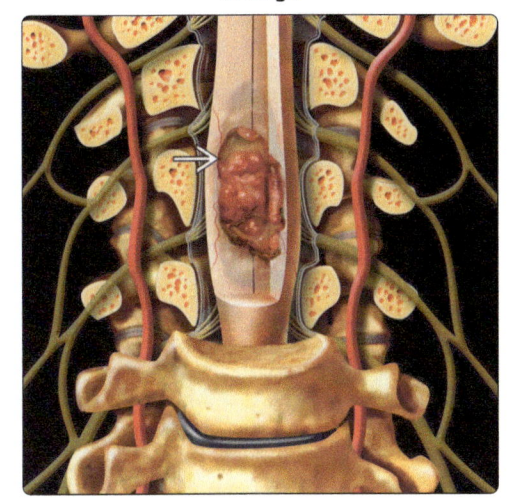

Perivascular Pseudorosettes

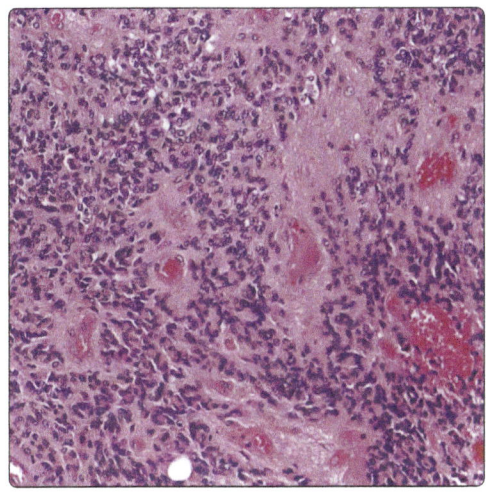

(Left) Ependymomas are well-circumscribed neoplasms that may develop anywhere along the neural axis but with a predilection for the spinal cord, particularly in adults and NF2 patients. Associated cystic changes ⇒ are not uncommon. (Right) Perivascular pseudorosettes are a hallmark of ependymoma, appearing as anucleate zones around blood vessels. They may be found in other tumors, but when conspicuous in a primary solid CNS tumor and composed of glial processes, they are highly supportive of the diagnosis.

Perivascular Pseudorosette

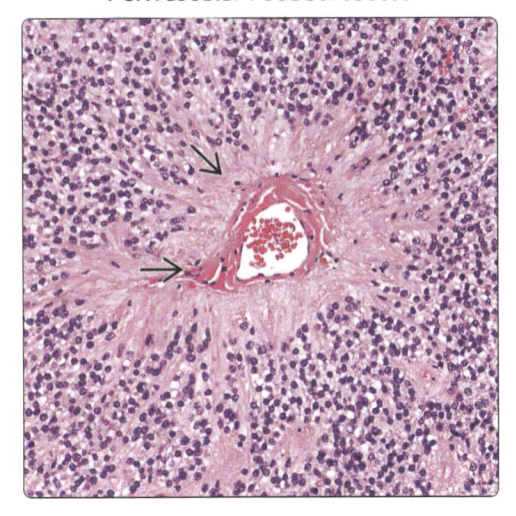

Ependymal Rosettes and Canals

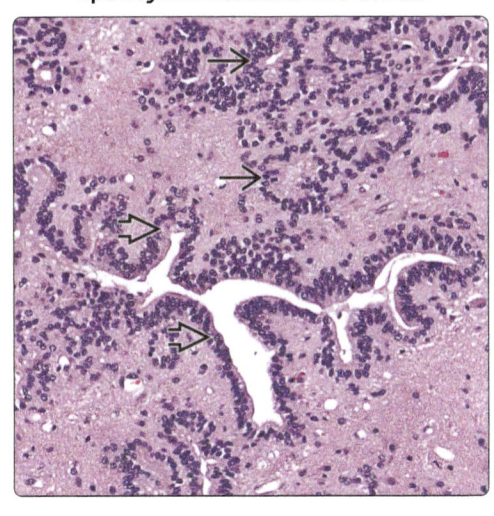

(Left) Perivascular pseudorosettes are frequent in ependymomas. They are composed of anuclear perivascular zones containing numerous neoplastic glial cell processes ⇒. (Right) A more specific histologic feature of ependymoma is the presence of well-developed epithelial surfaces resembling the lining of the ventricular system and central canal of the cord. These surfaces may be conspicuous in some tumors and include ependymal rosettes ⇒ as well as larger, elongated ependymal canals ⇒.

Circumscribed Architecture

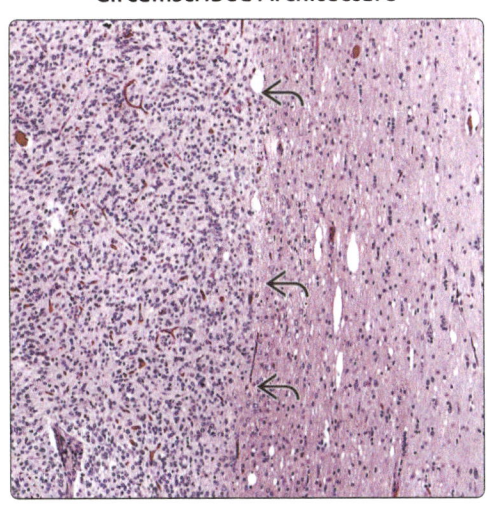

Clear Cells

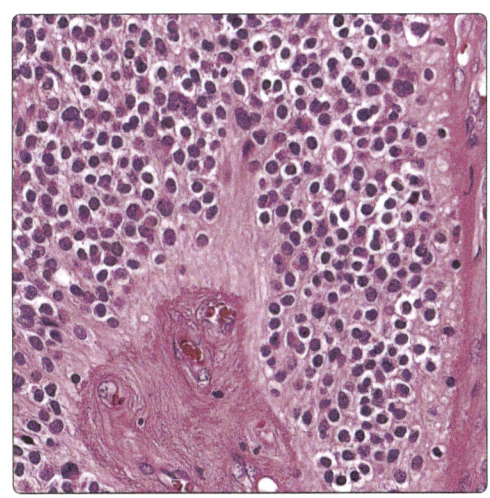

(Left) Among primary CNS neoplasms, ependymomas tend to be the most well-circumscribed tumors. A sharp interface with brain parenchyma ⇒ is seen in most cases. (Right) Ependymoma with clear cell histology shows round/oval nuclei and cytoplasmic clearing. The latter property raises the differential with oligodendroglial and neurocytic tumors.

Molecular Pathology of Solid Tumors

935

Ependymal Tumors

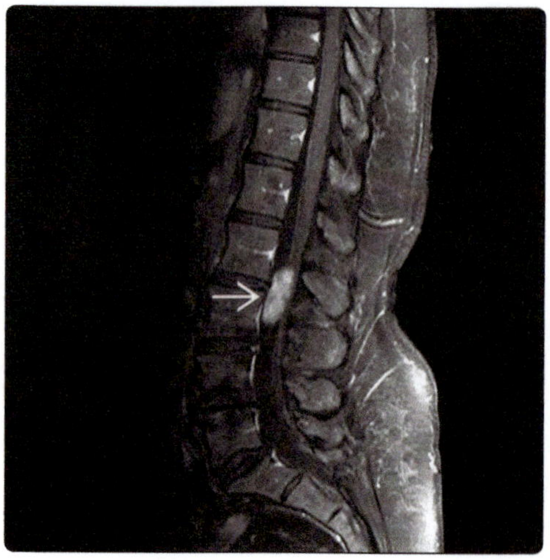

Myxopapillary Ependymoma

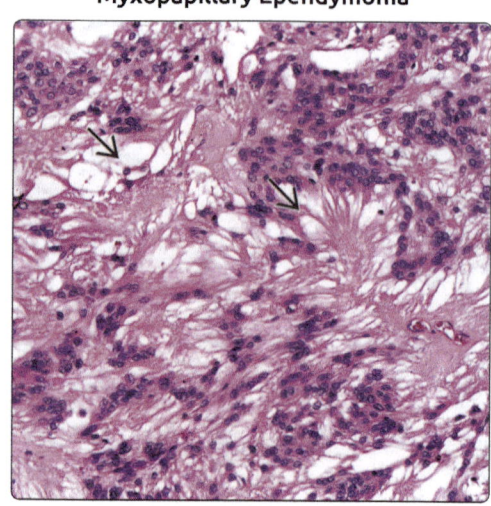

(Left) *Myxopapillary ependymomas form well-circumscribed masses and are almost always located in the distal cord, in the area of the conus medullaris/filum terminale ➡.* (Right) *Myxopapillary ependymoma is a distinctive subtype containing myxoid cuffs in pseudorosettes and stroma ➡. These tumors have a predilection for the distal cord/filum terminale region and are assigned grade 1 under the current WHO classification.*

Myxopapillary Ependymoma / High-Grade Histology

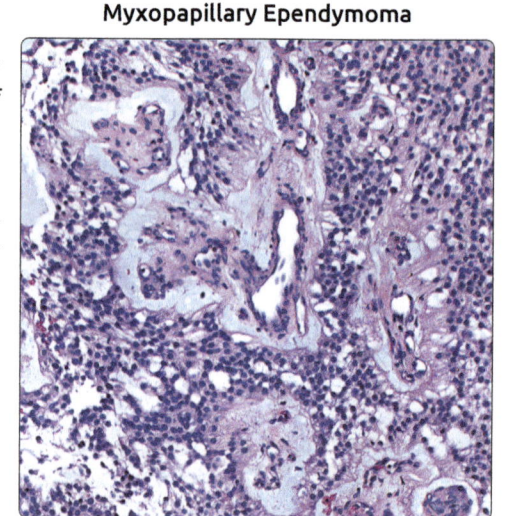

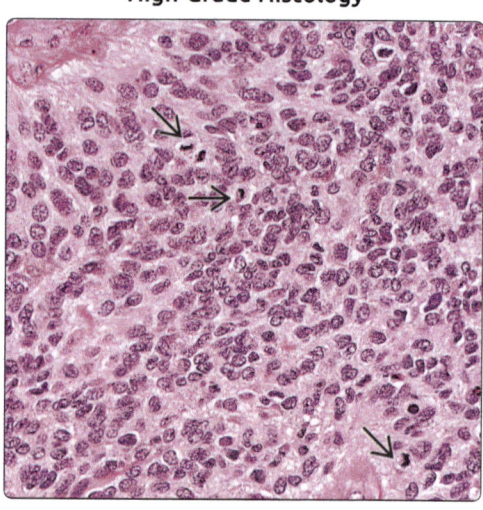

(Left) *Myxopapillary ependymomas may have focal solid areas, but when a cuff of myxoid material is present around vessels, at least focally, the diagnosis is strongly suggested.* (Right) *This ependymoma shows brisk mitotic activity and anaplastic histology. There are at least 3 mitoses ➡ in this single high-power field.*

Brisk Ki-67 Proliferation Index / GFAP Immunohistochemistry

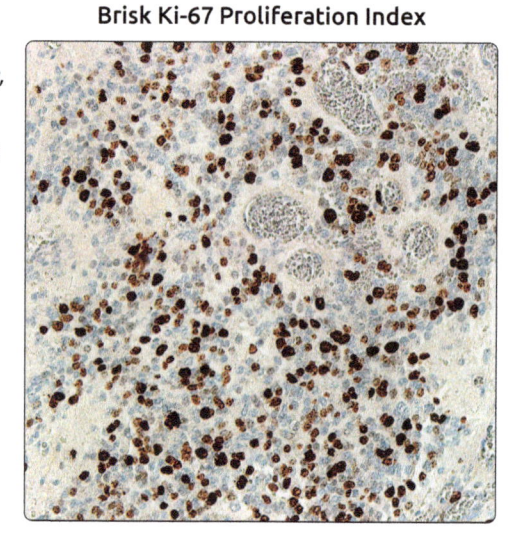

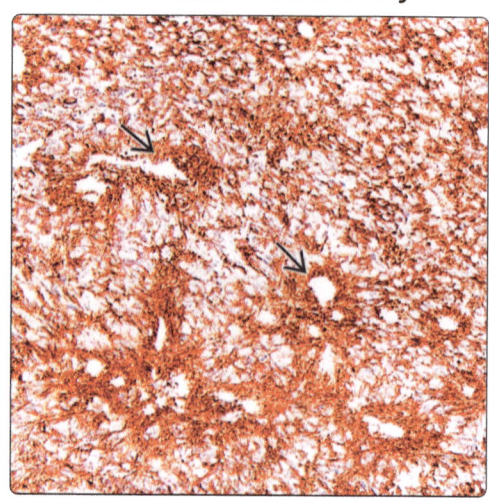

(Left) *Ki-67 labeling index is very high in this ependymoma, consistent with its anaplastic histologic features.* (Right) *GFAP expression is variable in ependymomas but usually accentuated around vessels, highlighting perivascular pseudorosettes ➡. This pattern of staining is not surprising, as pseudorosettes are rich in GFAP-containing glial processes.*

Ependymal Tumors

Dot-Like EMA Positivity in Microlumina

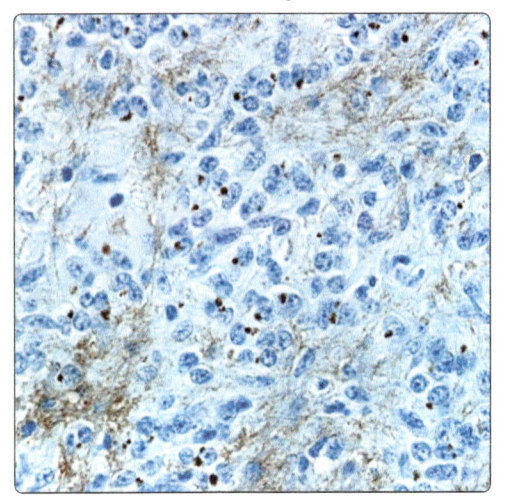

CD99 Immunohistochemistry

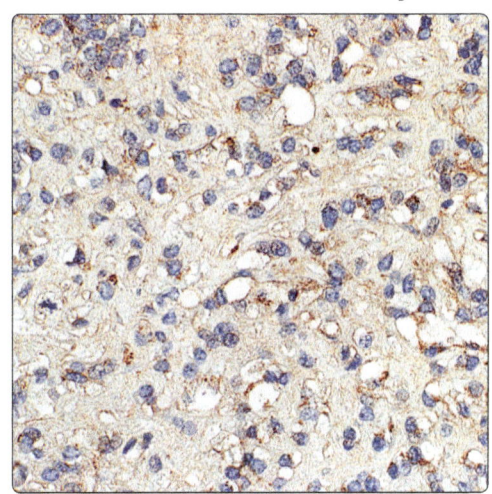

(Left) A useful IHC marker in the evaluation of ependymoma is EMA, which stains with a characteristic paranuclear/intercellular dot-like pattern. This pattern of staining is attributed to microlumina rich in microvilli, which may be demonstrated by electron microscopy. (Right) CD99 also frequently labels microlumina in ependymoma.

Microlumina

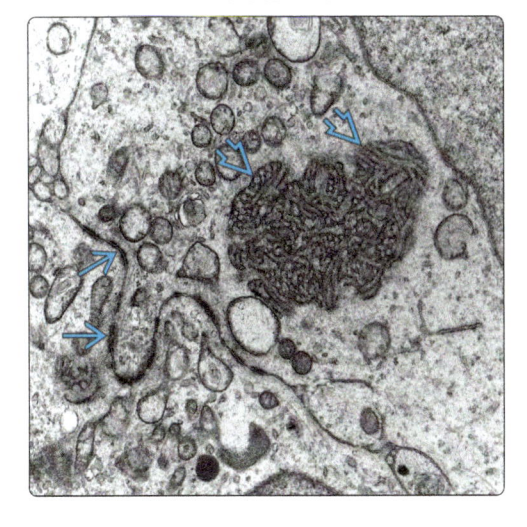

Clear Cells

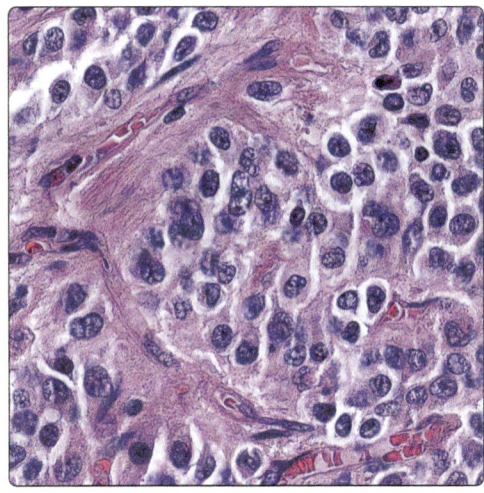

(Left) Electron microscopy is still a useful ancillary technique in the diagnosis of ependymoma. Features include well-formed intercellular junctions ➡ and microlumina ➡. (Right) Clear cell ependymomas are frequently supratentorial tumors. Recently they have also been associated with the RELA-fusion molecular subtype.

ZFTA::RELA Fused Ependymoma

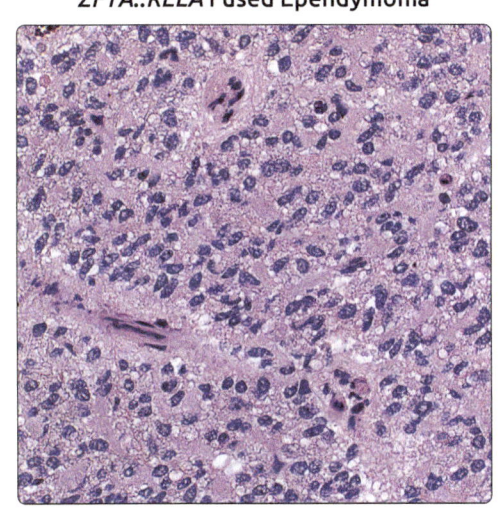

Cyclin-D1 Immunohistochemistry

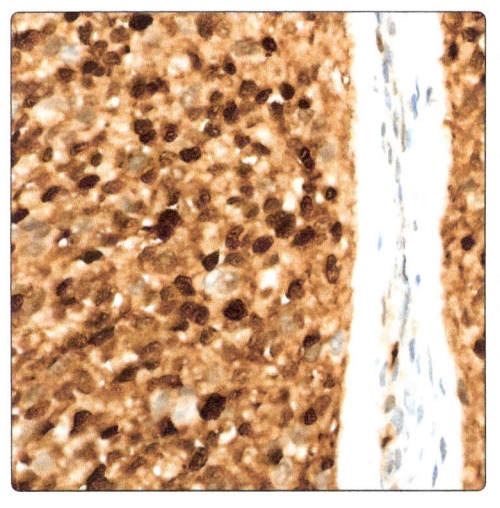

(Left) Not all ZFTA::RELA-fused ependymomas show clear cell histology, as seen here. There should be a high index of suspicion for this subtype in all supratentorial ependymomas, particularly in infants. (Right) Strong cyclin-D1 positivity is typical of ependymomas with ZFTA::RELA fusion. Strong positivity for this marker, although not diagnostic, may suggest the diagnosis in the right clinical and pathologic context and lead to further molecular testing.

Medulloblastoma

KEY FACTS

TERMINOLOGY

- **Medulloblastoma**
  - Malignant embryonal neoplasm with predominant neuronal differentiation arising in CNS parenchyma
    - CNS WHO grade 4
- **Molecularly defined medulloblastoma (WHO, 5th edition)**
  - Medulloblastoma, WNT-activated
    - Activation of WNT signaling pathway
  - Medulloblastoma, SHH-activated and *TP53*-wildtype
    - Activation of sonic hedgehog (SHH) signaling pathway
    - Germline or somatic mutations in *PTCH1*, *SMO*, and *SUFU*
  - Medulloblastoma, SHH-activated and *TP53*-mutant
    - Activation SHH signaling pathway combined with *TP53* mutation
  - Medulloblastoma, non-WNT/non-SHH
    - Classified as group 3 or group 4 tumors
    - Comprise 8 molecular subgroups
- **Histologically defined medulloblastoma (WHO, 5th edition)**
  - Classic medulloblastoma
  - Desmoplastic/nodular medulloblastoma
  - Medulloblastoma with extensive nodularity
  - Large cell/anaplastic medulloblastoma

ETIOLOGY/PATHOGENESIS

- Vast majority of medulloblastomas and CNS-embryonal tumors are sporadic
- Tumor predisposition syndromes associated with medulloblastoma
  - Nevoid basal cell carcinoma syndrome (Gorlin syndrome)
    - Germline mutations in *PTCH1* and *SUFU*
  - Li-Fraumeni syndrome
    - Germline *TP53* mutations
  - Familial adenomatous polyposis
    - Germline *APC* mutations

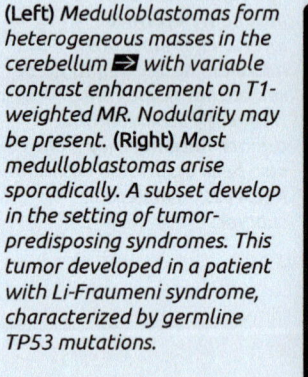

Contrast Enhancement

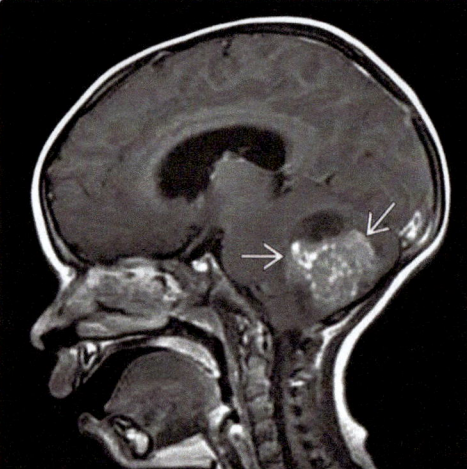

Li-Fraumeni Syndrome

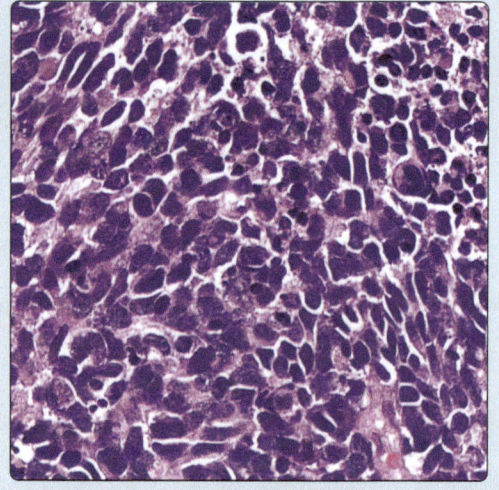

(Left) Medulloblastomas form heterogeneous masses in the cerebellum ➡ with variable contrast enhancement on T1-weighted MR. Nodularity may be present. (Right) Most medulloblastomas arise sporadically. A subset develop in the setting of tumor-predisposing syndromes. This tumor developed in a patient with Li-Fraumeni syndrome, characterized by germline TP53 mutations.

Desmoplastic/Nodular Medulloblastoma

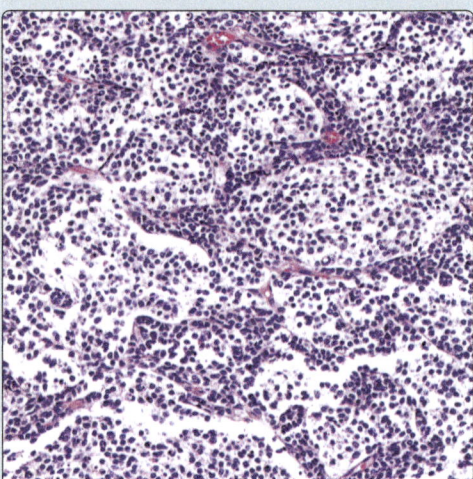

Medulloblastoma Metastatic to Bone

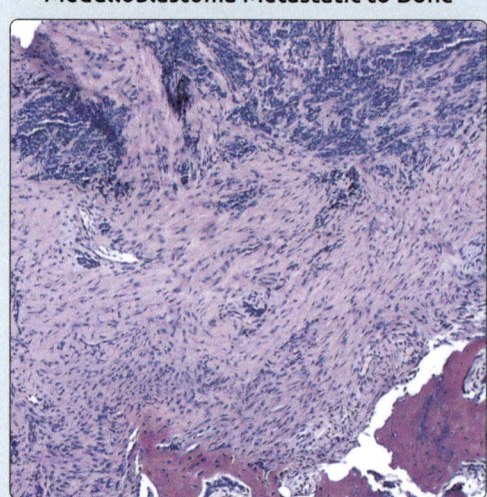

(Left) Desmoplastic/nodular medulloblastoma is characterized by pale nodules surrounded by mitotically active, more primitive cells in a desmoplastic stroma. (Right) Medulloblastomas are malignant neoplasms and, as other embryonal tumors, have a propensity for dissemination. Biologically aggressive examples may metastasize outside the CNS. This medulloblastoma spread to bone.

Medulloblastoma

TERMINOLOGY

Definitions
- Malignant embryonal neoplasms with predominant neuronal differentiation arising in CNS parenchyma
- WHO grade 4

Molecularly Defined Medulloblastoma (WHO, 5th Edition)
- Medulloblastoma, WNT-activated
  - Activation of WNT signaling pathway
  - Somatic mutations in *CTNNB1* in up to 89%
  - *APC* mutations among *CTNNB1* wildtype pediatric cases
  - Other somatically mutated genes include *SMARCA4, ARID1A, ARID2, DDX3X, CSNK2B, TP53, KMT2D,* and *PIK3CA*
  - Monosomy chromosome 6 in > 80% of cases
- Medulloblastoma, SHH-activated and *TP53*-wildtype
  - Activation of sonic hedgehog (SHH) signaling pathway
  - Germline or somatic mutations in *PTCH1* (40%), *SMO* (10%), and *SUFU* (10%)
  - Other genes commonly mutated include *DDX3X, KMT2D,* and *CREBBP*
  - *TERT* promoter mutations detected in most adult tumors (> 80%)
- Medulloblastoma, SHH-activated and *TP53*-mutant
  - Activation SHH signaling pathway combined with *TP53* mutation
    - > 1/2 of *TP53* mutations in this subtype are germline
  - *MYCN* amplification common
  - In noninfant children and adults, *TP53* mutation with *MYCN* amplification associated with very poor outcome
- Medulloblastoma, non-WNT/non-SHH
  - Lack of molecular signature associated with activation of WNT or SHH signaling pathway
  - Classified as group 3 or group 4 tumors and comprise 8 molecular subgroups
    - Subgroups 1-8 are characterized by DNA methylation profiling of group 3 and group 4
  - Overexpression of *MYC* in group 3
  - *MYC* amplification often accompanied by *PVT1::MYC* fusion in 17% of group 3
  - Other recurrently mutated genes include *SMARCA4, CTDNEP1,* and *KMT2D*
  - Recurrently amplified genes include *MYC* and *OTX2*
  - Chromosome 17 copy number alterations in up to 85% of group 4 and 58% of group 3
  - Other most frequently mutated or amplified genes in group 3 and 4 include
    - *KDM6A, ZMYM3, KMT2C, KBTBD4, MYCN, ZIC1, CDK6, KMT2D,* and *TBR1*
  - Deleterious heterozygous germline mutations in *BRCA2* and *PALB2* in 1-2% of cases

Histologically Defined Medulloblastoma (WHO, 5th Edition)
- Subtypes include
  - Classic medulloblastoma
  - Desmoplastic/nodular medulloblastoma
  - Medulloblastoma with extensive nodularity
  - Large cell anaplastic medulloblastoma

Integrated Diagnosis (Encouraged)
- Combination of molecular analysis and morphological interpretation
  - Provides optimal prognostic and predictive information
- Incorporation of other genetic alterations currently used in risk stratification but not included in classification
  - *MYC* amplification and other genetic alterations that could also be included in integrated report

ETIOLOGY/PATHOGENESIS

Sporadic Tumors
- Vast majority of medulloblastomas and CNS-embryonal tumors are sporadic

Inherited Cancer Syndromes Associated With Medulloblastoma
- Nevoid basal cell carcinoma syndrome (Gorlin syndrome)
  - Germline mutations in *PTCH1* and *SUFU*
- Li-Fraumeni syndrome
  - Germline *TP53* mutations
- Familial adenomatous polyposis
  - Germline *APC* mutations
- Rubinstein-Taybi syndrome
  - Germline *CREBBP* mutations
- Nijmegen-Breakage syndrome
  - Germline mutations in *NBN*
- Other syndromes associated with germline mutations (e.g., *BRCA2, PALB2,* etc.)
  - Germline mutations account for ~ 6% of medulloblastoma

CLINICAL ISSUES

Epidemiology
- Age
  - Predominantly childhood neoplasms
    - ~ 20-30% of medulloblastomas develop in adults (usually 2nd-3rd decades)

Site
- Involves posterior fossa
  - Cerebellar vermis, cerebellar hemispheres > 4th ventricle

Presentation
- Medulloblastoma
  - Ataxia, nausea, vomiting, headache
- CNS embryonal tumors
  - Symptoms secondary to mass effect, hydrocephalus

Treatment
- Craniospinal irradiation and chemotherapy

Prognosis
- Aggressive neoplasms with propensity for CSF dissemination
- Potentially curable tumors with aggressive therapy
- Prognosis better for medulloblastoma than CNS-embryonal tumors as group

Medulloblastoma

IMAGING

MR Findings
- Relatively well-circumscribed tumors
- Variable enhancement
- Spinal MR usually performed to assess for CSF dissemination

MICROSCOPIC

Histologically Defined Medulloblastoma (WHO, 5th Edition)
- Classic medulloblastoma
  - Prototypical embryonal round blue cell tumor; most frequent medulloblastoma subtype
- Desmoplastic/nodular medulloblastoma
  - Bicompartmental arrangement of nodular, reticulin-free zones (pale islands) surrounded by densely packed, poorly differentiated proliferative cells
- Medulloblastoma with extensive nodularity
  - Expanded lobular architecture due to larger reticulin-free zones and rich in neuropil-like matrix
- Large cell/anaplastic medulloblastoma
  - Characterized by nuclear enlargement (anaplasia) or large nuclei with macronucleoli (large); histologic marker of poor prognosis

ANCILLARY TESTS

Immunohistochemistry
- Synaptophysin expression present in almost all medulloblastomas
- Other markers of neuronal differentiation (e.g., neurofilament protein, chromogranin, NeuN) may also be positive but less consistent
- GFAP may also be expressed, usually around vessels or nodules in desmoplastic/nodular medulloblastoma variant

Genetic Testing
- Medulloblastoma, WNT-activated
  - *CTNNB1* mutations in up to 89% and monosomy chromosome 6
  - *APC* mutations among *CTNNB1* wildtype pediatric cases
- Medulloblastoma, SHH-activated and *TP53*-wildtype
  - Germline or somatic mutations in *PTCH1*, *SMO*, and *SUFU*
  - Other genes commonly mutated include *DDX3X*, *KMT2D*, and *CREBBP*
  - *TERT* promoter mutations detected in most adult tumors (> 80%)
- Medulloblastoma, SHH-activated and *TP53*-mutant
  - Activation SHH signaling pathway combined with *TP53* mutation
    - > 50% of *TP53* mutations in this subtype are germline
  - *TP53* mutation with *MYCN* amplification associated with very poor outcome in noninfant children and adults
- Medulloblastoma, non-WNT/non-SHH
  - Lack of molecular signature associated with activation of WNT or SHH signaling pathway
  - Classified as group 3 or group 4 tumors
    - Comprise 8 subgroups characterized by DNA methylation profiling of group 3 and group 4
  - *MYC* amplification often accompanied by *PVT1::MYC* fusion in 17% of group 3
  - Other most frequently mutated or amplified genes in group 3 and 4 include
    - *KDM6A*, *ZMYM3*, *KMT2C*, *KBTBD4*, *MYCN*, *ZIC1*, *CDK6*, *KMT2D*, and *TBR1*

DIFFERENTIAL DIAGNOSIS

Neurocytic Tumors
- Better differentiated, low proliferation

Lymphoma
- Primary CNS lymphoma almost always are large B cell
- CD45(+), CD20(+), synaptophysin (-)

Glial Neoplasms
- May arise at any age and any location in neuraxis
- Poorly differentiated astrocytomas may be difficult to separate from CNS-embryonal tumors
- High-grade oligodendrogliomas may resemble embryonal tumors and express neuronal markers
  - IDH1(+), OLIG2(+), 1p19q codeleted
- In adults, high-grade gliomas may develop primitive neuronal component
  - Infiltrating glial and neuronal components distinct
- Anaplastic ependymoma: EMA(+), perivascular pseudorosettes, true ependymal rosettes

Atypical Teratoid Rhabdoid Tumor
- May contain predominant undifferentiated round blue cell component
- Polyphenotypic pattern by immunohistochemistry [EMA, GFAP, SMA, and CK(+)], INI1 loss

Metastasis
- Metastatic embryonal tumors
- Small cell carcinoma should be considered in adults

Pineoblastoma
- By definition, arises in pineal gland region

Olfactory Neuroblastoma (Esthesioneuroblastoma)
- Tumor of adults; cribriform plate involvement

SELECTED REFERENCES

1. Choi JY: Medulloblastoma: Current perspectives and recent advances. Brain Tumor Res Treat. 11(1):28-38, 2023
2. Fang FY et al: New developments in the pathogenesis, therapeutic targeting, and treatment of pediatric medulloblastoma. Cancers (Basel). 14(9):2285, 2022
3. Louis DN et al: The 2021 WHO classification of tumors of the central nervous system: a summary. Neuro Oncol. 23(8):1231-51, 2021
4. Waszak SM et al: Spectrum and prevalence of genetic predisposition in medulloblastoma: a retrospective genetic study and prospective validation in a clinical trial cohort. Lancet Oncol. 19(6):785-98, 2018
5. Sturm D et al: New brain tumor entities emerge from molecular classification of CNS-PNETs. Cell. 164(5):1060-72, 2016
6. Zhukova N et al: Subgroup-specific prognostic implications of TP53 mutation in medulloblastoma. J Clin Oncol. 31(23):2927-35, 2013
7. Northcott PA et al: Rapid, reliable, and reproducible molecular sub-grouping of clinical medulloblastoma samples. Acta Neuropathol. 123(4):615-26, 2012
8. Ellison DW et al: Medulloblastoma: clinicopathological correlates of SHH, WNT, and non-SHH/WNT molecular subgroups. Acta Neuropathol. 121(3):381-96, 2011

Medulloblastoma

Well-Circumscribed Mass

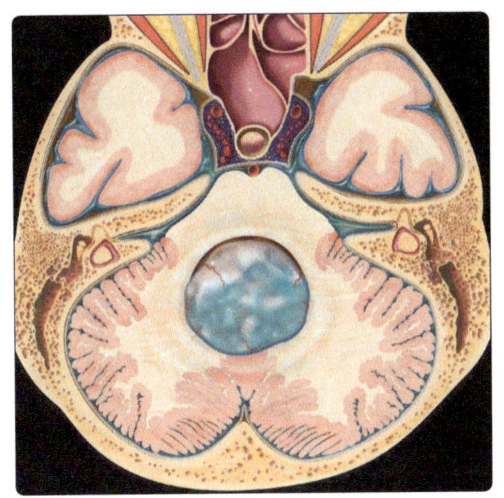

Gross Appearance

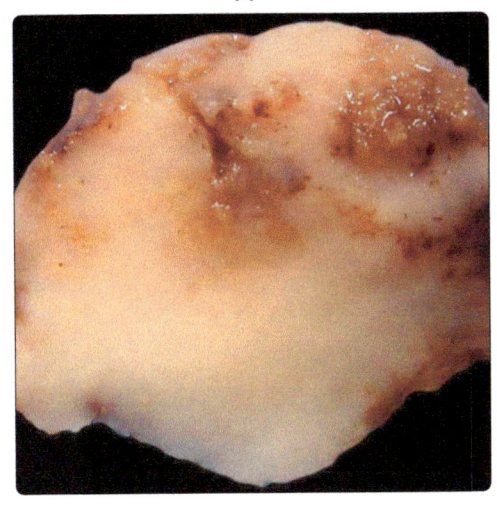

(Left) Medulloblastomas generally form well-circumscribed masses that, by definition, are centered in the cerebellum/4th ventricle region. Although they may appear well circumscribed, they have a propensity for CSF dissemination. Therefore, not only intracranial imaging but also spinal imaging is recommended for appropriate evaluation. (Right) Medulloblastomas are highly cellular neoplasms and may demonstrate a gray-white appearance on gross cut surface.

Classic Medulloblastoma

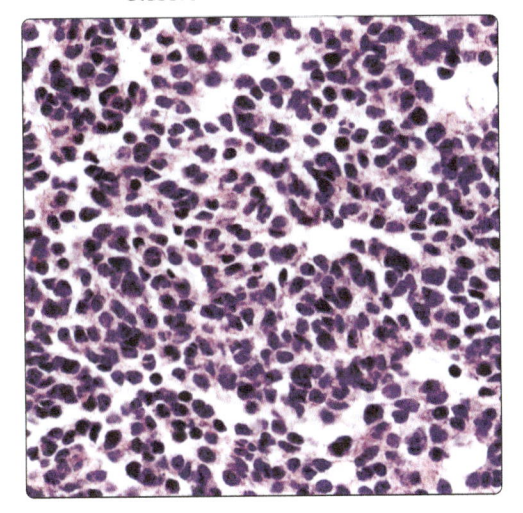

Desmoplastic/Nodular Medulloblastoma

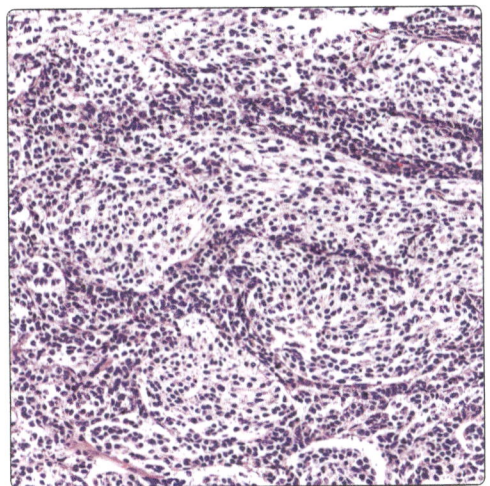

(Left) Classic medulloblastoma represents the main histologic subtype, characterized by sheets of packed round cells with apoptotic bodies and mitotic activity. Nuclear size varies from small to moderate. (Right) Desmoplastic/nodular medulloblastoma is characterized by pale nodules alternating with a proliferative desmoplastic cellular infiltrate. Molecularly, they demonstrate sonic hedgehog (SHH) activation and are overrepresented in Gorlin syndrome.

Desmoplastic/Nodular Medulloblastoma

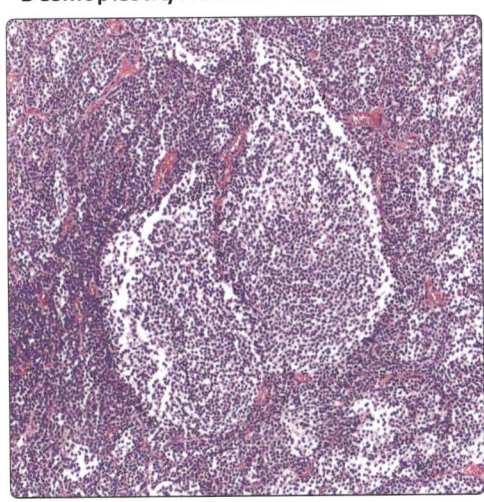

Internodular Reticulin

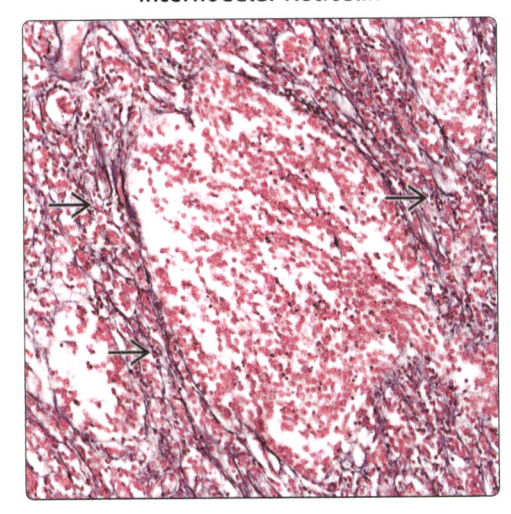

(Left) Nodules in the desmoplastic/nodular medulloblastoma variant are characterized by variable sizes and shapes. They may be ill defined or well circumscribed, appearing as an area of pallor, as shown here. They reflect neuronal differentiation in any embryonal tumor. (Right) Nodules of desmoplastic/nodular medulloblastoma are reticulin poor, which contrasts with the dense, pericellular, reticulin-rich internodular areas ➡.

Medulloblastoma

Anaplastic Medulloblastoma

Large Cell Medulloblastoma

(Left) *Anaplastic medulloblastoma is defined mainly on the basis of nuclear enlargement. Cell-to-cell wrapping ➡, apoptotic bodies, and increased mitotic activity are frequent.* (Right) *Large cell medulloblastoma is a unique variant recognized on the basis of cytologic features. The cells are large, round, and contain prominent nucleoli. Areas of anaplastic and large cell medulloblastoma may coexist.*

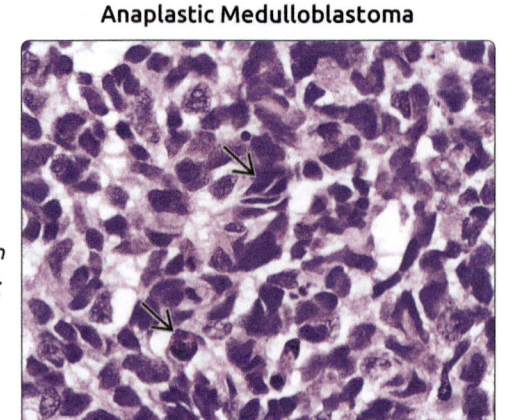

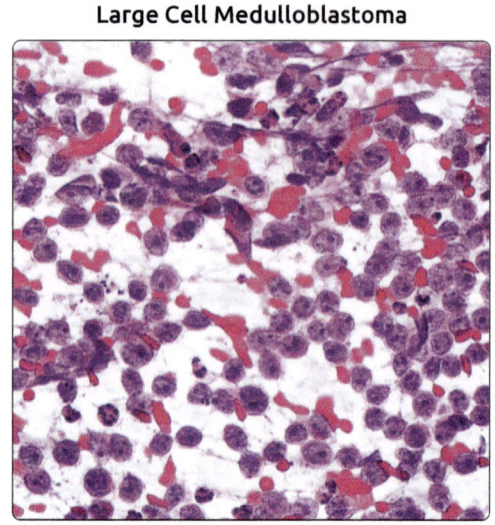

Synaptophysin Expression

GFAP Expression

(Left) *Synaptophysin expression is frequent in medulloblastomas and CNS embryonal tumors. Strong expression is evident in this example, but it varies from strong to weak.* (Right) *GFAP expression may also be present in medulloblastomas and CNS embryonal tumors, although to a limited extent. Labeling tends to be more frequent and stronger around intratumoral vessels ➡. GFAP expression is also frequent around nodules of nodular/desmoplastic medulloblastoma.*

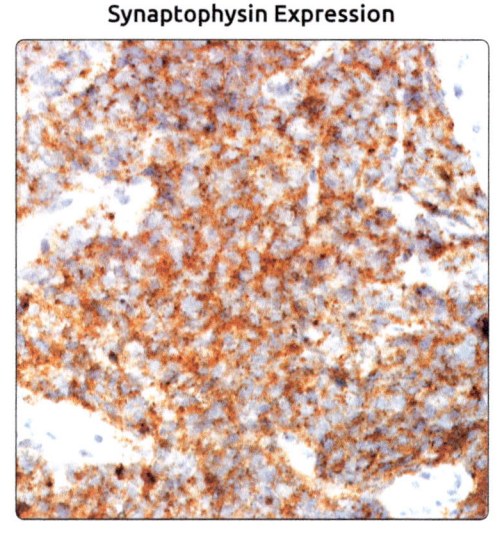

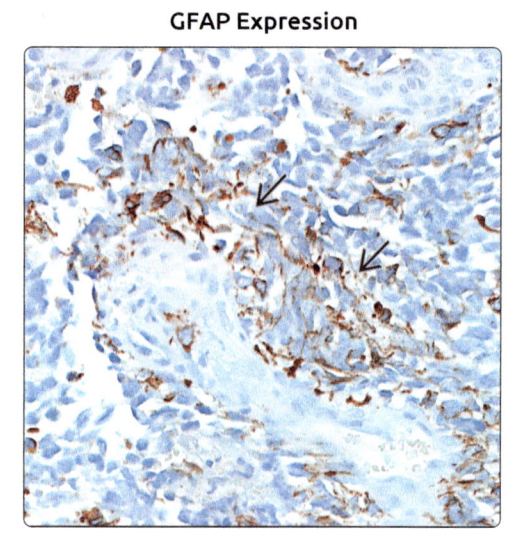

β-catenin Expression

Preserved INI1 Immunoreactivity

(Left) *β-catenin shows a membranous/cytoplasmic pattern in most medulloblastomas. When staining is nuclear, it identifies the diagnostically favorable WNT molecular subgroup.* (Right) *Nuclear INI1 labeling is a feature of all medulloblastomas. INI1 loss by neoplastic cells characterizes atypical teratoid rhabdoid tumor, which is an important entity in the differential diagnosis, particularly of the anaplastic/large cell variant.*

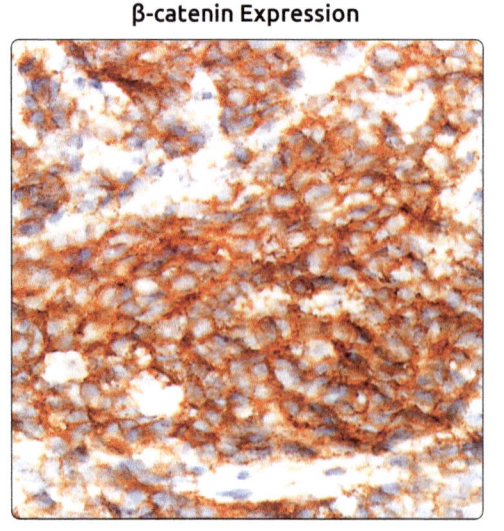

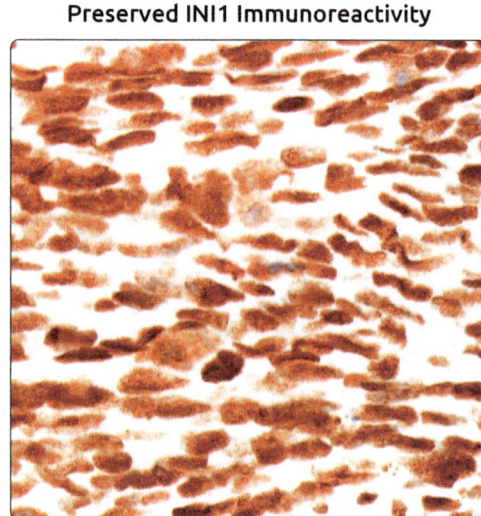

Medulloblastoma

CNS Embryonal Tumor

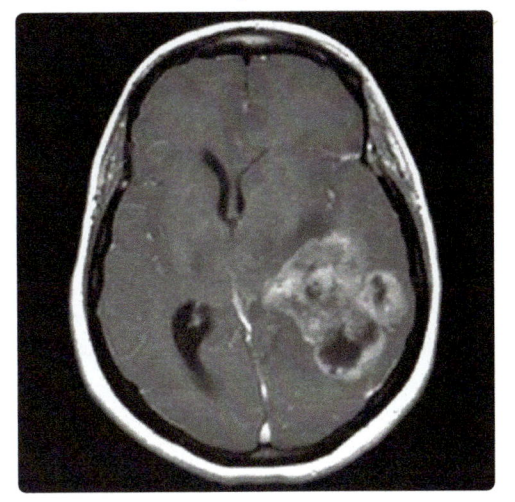

CNS Embryonal Tumor

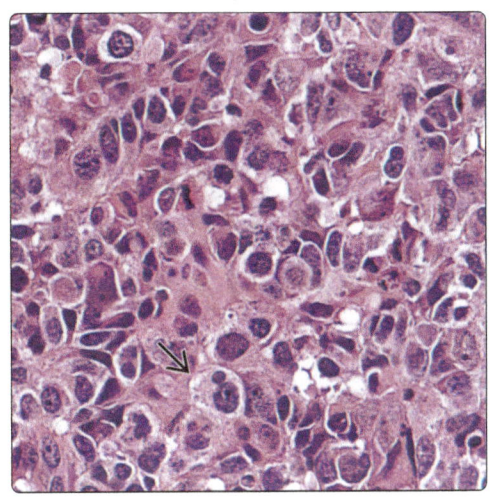

(Left) CNS embryonal tumors represent malignant embryonal neoplasms usually developing in the supratentorial compartment. This example developed in a patient with familial adenomatous polyposis (i.e., Turcot type 2 syndrome). (Right) Supratentorial CNS embryonal tumors can arise in familial adenomatous polyposis (FAP) syndrome. This example has considerable nuclear variability and large cells with a ganglioid appearance ⇒.

Nuclear β-catenin Staining

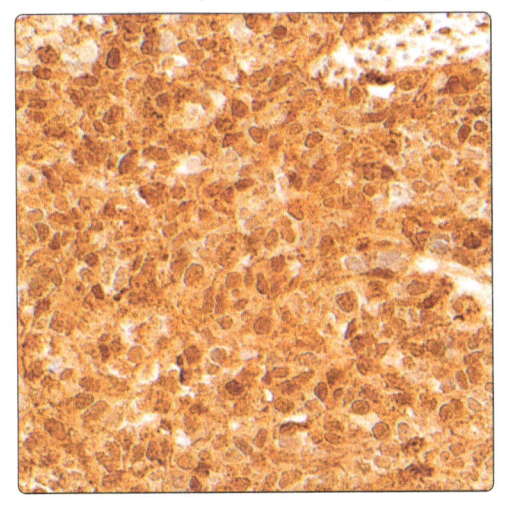

CNS Embryonal Tumor

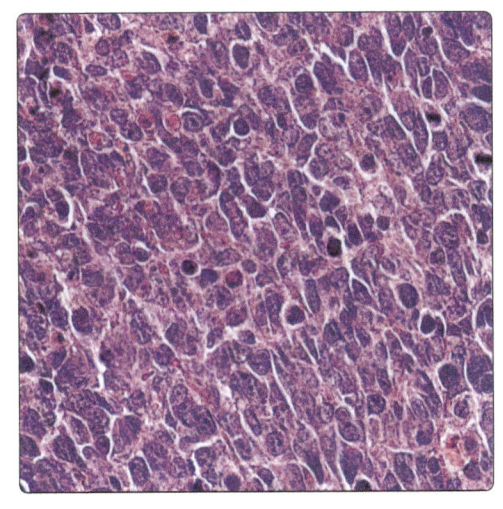

(Left) Nuclear β-catenin staining, seen in this CNS-embryonal tumor in a patient with familial adenomatous polyposis, reflects activation of the WNT signaling pathway. This pathway is also operational in a subset of medulloblastomas. (Right) CNS embryonal tumors are highly cellular neoplasms composed of sheets of cells with high N:C ratio, frequent apoptotic bodies, and increased mitotic activity. They are distinct from medulloblastoma at the molecular level.

Embryonal Tumor With Multilayered Rosettes

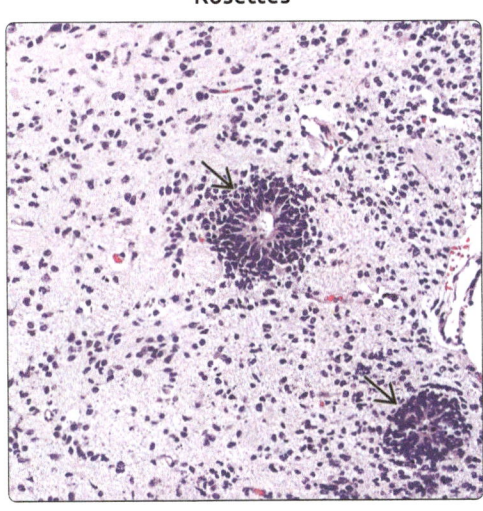

Primitive Neuronal Component

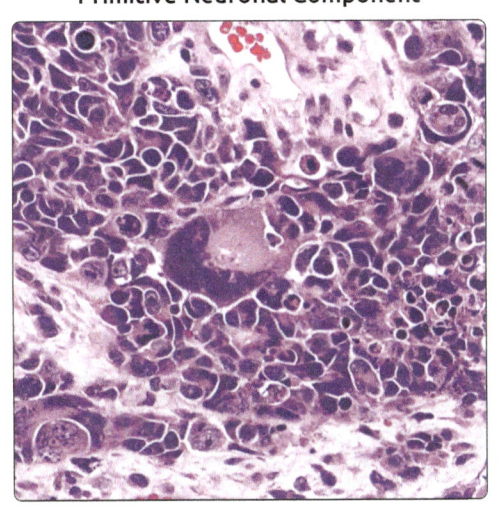

(Left) A distinctive subtype of CNS embryonal tumors are embryonal tumors with multilayered rosettes (ETMR), which may contain large areas of neuropil as well as distinctive rosettes with central lumina ⇒. The prognosis of this tumor is poor. (Right) Primitive neuronal component may be a dominant feature in a subset of high-grade gliomas. Careful histologic and immunohistochemical analysis must be done to identify the glial component of any presumed embryonal tumors in adults.

Choroid Plexus Tumors

KEY FACTS

TERMINOLOGY
- Spectrum of neoplasms arising in ventricular locations with anatomic, morphologic, and immunophenotypic similarities with choroid plexus

ETIOLOGY/PATHOGENESIS
- Most are sporadic
  - Choroid plexus carcinomas are strongly associated with germline *TP53* mutations
- Li-Fraumeni syndrome: Most CNS neoplasms are astrocytomas, but some are also choroid plexus tumors (carcinoma > papilloma)
- Rhabdoid predisposition syndrome: Reported cases of choroid plexus carcinoma may in fact be atypical teratoid/rhabdoid tumors (AT/RT)
- Aicardi syndrome: Associated with choroid plexus papillomas and cysts

MICROSCOPIC
- Papilloma: Papillary architecture with fibrovascular cores lined by cuboidal to columnar epithelium; mitotic activity rare to absent
- Atypical papilloma: Mitotic activity ≥ 2 per 10 HPF
- Carcinoma: Overtly malignant histology, brisk mitotic activity

ANCILLARY TESTS
- *TP53* alterations associated with poorer prognosis in choroid plexus tumors in some studies
- Notch pathway activation induces choroid plexus tumors in mice and is present in subset of human choroid plexus tumors

GRADING
- Papilloma (WHO grade 1), atypical papilloma (WHO grade 2), and carcinoma (WHO grade 3)

Imaging Appearance

Papillary Architecture

(Left) Choroid plexus carcinomas are malignant neoplasms that almost always develop in young children and demonstrate variable contrast enhancement ➡. (Courtesy T. Vanegas, MD.) (Right) Choroid plexus carcinomas usually have papillary architecture and variable pleomorphism. This young patient also developed a rhabdomyosarcoma, which strongly suggests Li-Fraumeni syndrome.

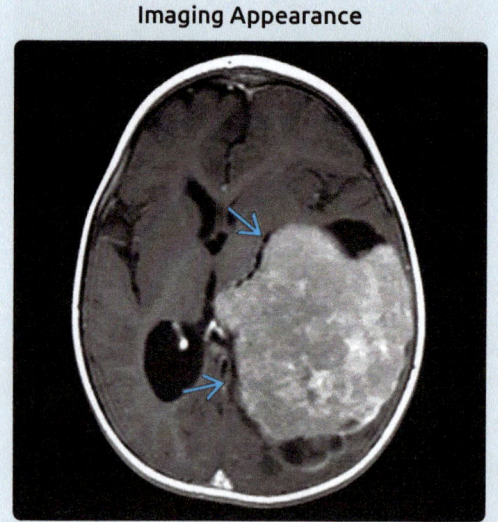

Pleomorphism

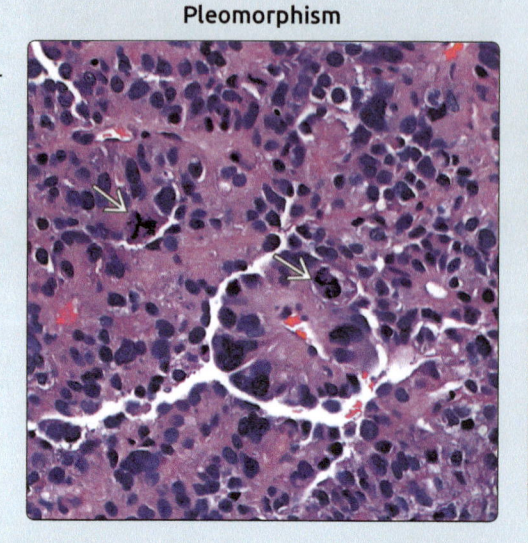

Cytokeratin Expression

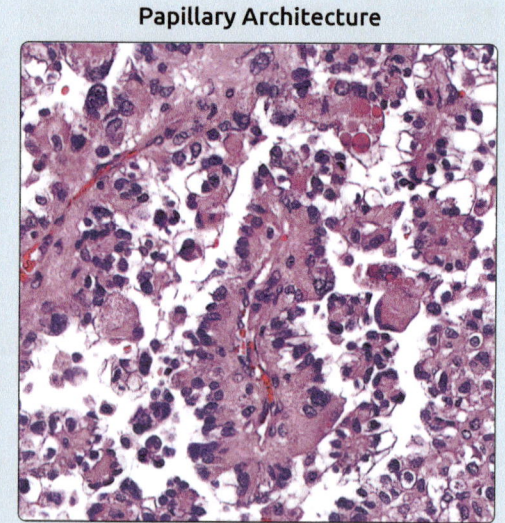

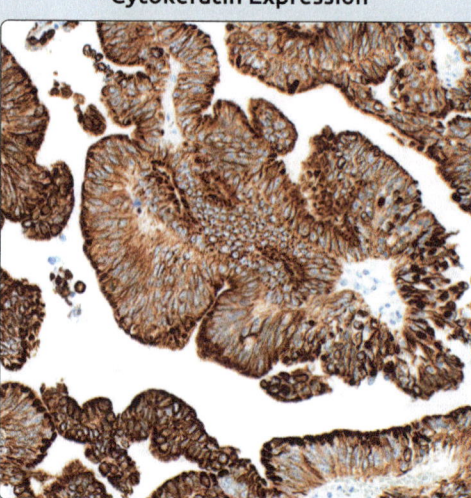

(Left) Choroid plexus carcinomas are typically high-grade malignant tumors and may display significant pleomorphism and brisk mitotic activity, including atypical mitoses ➡. (Right) CK8/18/CAM5.2 shows positive immunoreactivity in this choroid plexus tumor. All choroid plexus tumors consistently express cytokeratins.

Choroid Plexus Tumors

TERMINOLOGY

Definitions
- Spectrum of neoplasms arising in ventricular locations with anatomic, morphologic, and immunophenotypic similarities with choroid plexus that encompass
  - Choroid plexus papilloma (CNS WHO grade 1)
  - Atypical choroid plexus papilloma (CNS WHO grade 2)
  - Choroid plexus carcinoma (CNS WHO grade 3)

ETIOLOGY/PATHOGENESIS

Sporadic Tumors
- Most choroid plexus tumors are sporadic, but choroid plexus carcinomas are strongly associated with germline *TP53* mutations

Li-Fraumeni Syndrome
- Tumor predisposition syndrome most commonly secondary to germline *TP53* mutations
- Most CNS neoplasms in Li-Fraumeni patients are astrocytomas (~ 60%)
- Also develop medulloblastomas and choroid plexus tumors (carcinomas > papillomas)

Rhabdoid Predisposition Syndrome
- Choroid plexus carcinomas reported in some patients, but there is morphologic and immunophenotypic overlap with atypical teratoid/rhabdoid tumors (AT/RT)

Aicardi Syndrome
- Associated with choroid plexus papillomas
- Presumably X-linked dominant, exclusively in females, lethal in males

CLINICAL ISSUES

Epidemiology
- Incidence
  - Rare brain tumors overall (< 1%)
  - Relatively high proportion of brain tumors in infants

Presentation
- Symptoms attributable to hydrocephalus and increased intracranial pressure

Prognosis
- Varies from excellent in choroid plexus papilloma to poor in choroid plexus carcinoma

MICROSCOPIC

Histologic Features
- Choroid plexus papilloma
  - Papillary architecture with fibrovascular cores lined by single layer of cuboidal to columnar epithelium
  - Pleomorphism, sheet-like growth, and necrosis are rare
  - Mitotic activity rare to absent
- Atypical choroid plexus papilloma
  - Mitotic activity ≥ 2 per 10 HPF
  - ↑ cellularity, nuclear pleomorphism, solid growth, &/or necrosis may be present
- Choroid plexus carcinoma
  - Invasive growth pattern, may appear solid, hemorrhagic, or necrotic with brisk mitotic activity
  - Brain invasion may be present

ANCILLARY TESTS

Immunohistochemistry
- Positive for CK8/18/CAM5.2, vimentin, and S100; negative for CK7
- GFAP and EMA may be expressed (weak or focal)
- Frequent p53 immunopositivity in carcinomas
- KIR7.1 and stanniocalcin-1 expression retained in most choroid plexus papillomas and in ~ 50% of choroid plexus carcinomas

Genetic Testing
- *TP53* mutations in ~ 50% of choroid plexus carcinomas
  - Associated with poorer prognosis in choroid plexus tumors in some studies
- *TP53* mutational status was only significant prognostic variable in pediatric patients with choroid plexus carcinoma in SJYC07 trial
- Chromosomal instability frequent in choroid plexus tumors
- *TAF12*, *NFYC*, and *RAD54L* within chromosomal gains at 1p35.3 may play role in disease initiation and progression

DIFFERENTIAL DIAGNOSIS

Normal Choroid Plexus
- Cobblestone appearance, less cellularity than papilloma, microcalcifications

Cribriform Neuroepithelial Tumor
- Very rare low-grade intraventricular neoplasm with cribriform/trabecular architecture
- Surface EMA staining, INI1 loss

Ependymoma
- May have papillary pattern (papillary or myxopapillary ependymoma)
- Prominent pseudorosettes, true rosettes
- Dot-like or surface EMA immunopositivity

Papillary Tumor of Pineal Region
- Similar morphologic and immunophenotypic features
- Pineal gland location not feature of choroid plexus tumors
- Lacks KIR7.1 and stanniocalcin-1 positivity

Atypical Teratoid/Rhabdoid Tumor
- May have morphologic and immunophenotypic overlap with choroid plexus carcinoma
- INI1 loss

Metastatic Carcinoma
- Usually not seen in children but main consideration in adult patients

SELECTED REFERENCES

1. Liu APY et al: Outcome and molecular analysis of young children with choroid plexus carcinoma treated with non-myeloablative therapy: results from the SJYC07 trial. Neurooncol Adv. 3(1):vdaa168, 2021
2. Louis DN et al: The 2021 WHO classification of tumors of the central nervous system: a summary. Neuro Oncol. 23(8):1231-51, 2021

Choroid Plexus Tumors

(Left) Sagittal T1 MR shows choroid plexus papilloma involving the 4th ventricle ⇨, a common location in adults. Choroid plexus tumors almost always arise within the ventricular system. **(Right)** Choroid plexus tumors encompass a spectrum ranging from benign (CNS WHO grade 1) to malignant (CNS WHO grade 3). This grade 1 choroid plexus papilloma contains numerous papillae lined by cuboidal to columnar cells.

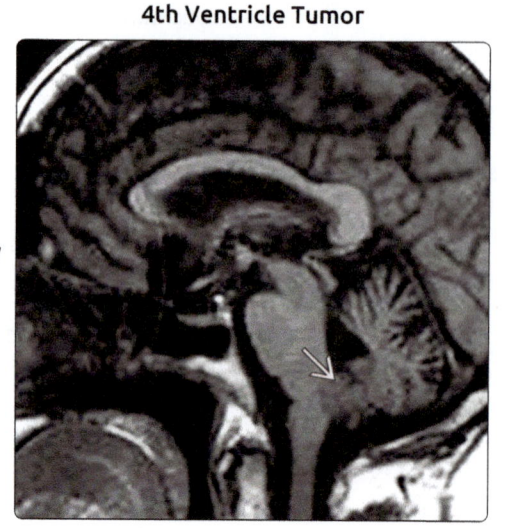

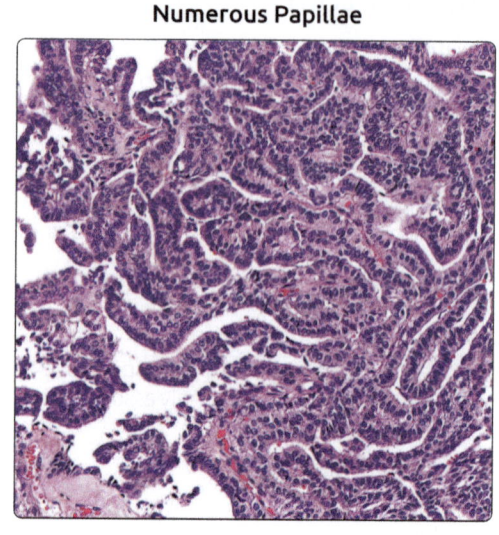

4th Ventricle Tumor

Numerous Papillae

(Left) Distinctive fibrovascular cores ⇨ are a hallmark of choroid plexus tumors. This choroid plexus papilloma has bland cytology and lacks mitotic activity and necrosis, consistent with CNS WHO grade 1 neoplasm. **(Right)** This choroid plexus tumor has a more solid pattern of growth, which may be a feature of a subset of tumors. Mitotic activity is not subtle ⇨, consistent with an atypical choroid plexus papilloma, indicating CNS WHO grade 2.

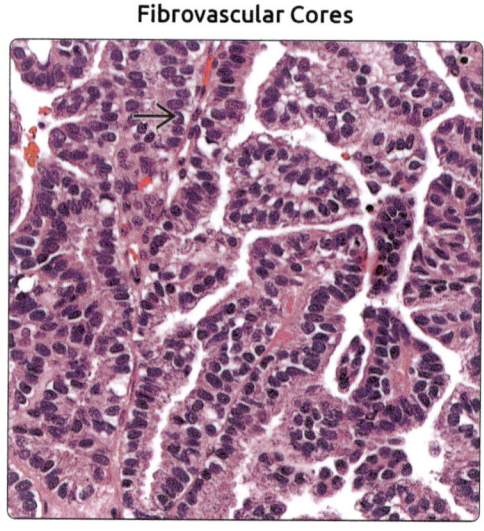

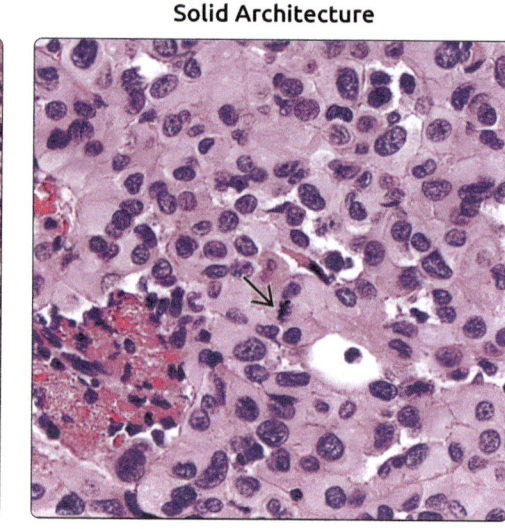

Fibrovascular Cores

Solid Architecture

(Left) Keratin expression is a universal feature of choroid plexus tumors. Strong labeling with cytokeratin CAM5.2 is strongly supportive of the diagnosis in the right context. **(Right)** Choroid plexus tumors may also express a variety of markers. This example expresses S100 with a nuclear and cytoplasmic pattern.

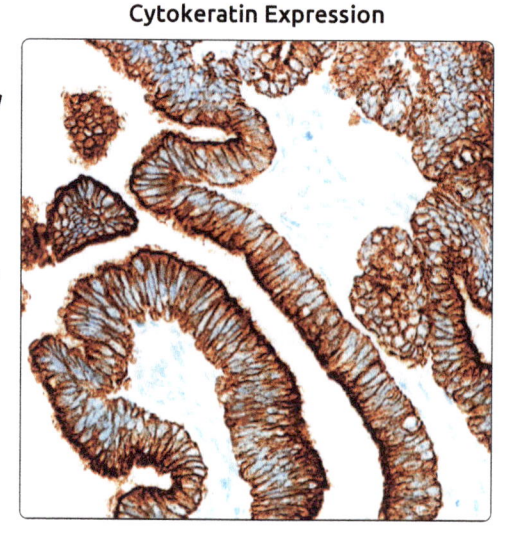

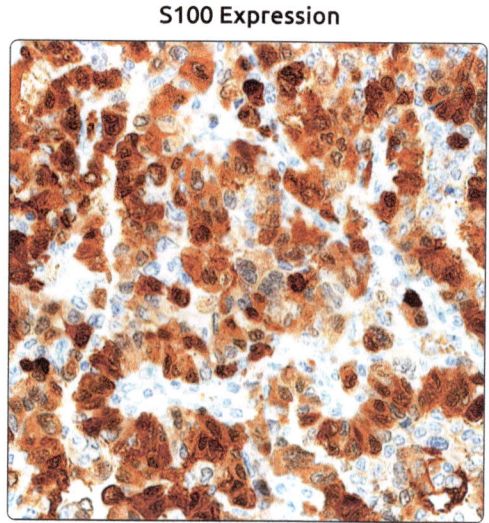

Cytokeratin Expression

S100 Expression

Choroid Plexus Tumors

Gross Appearance

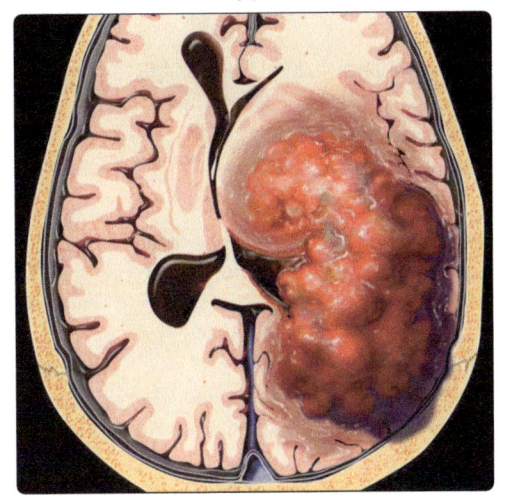

Pleomorphism

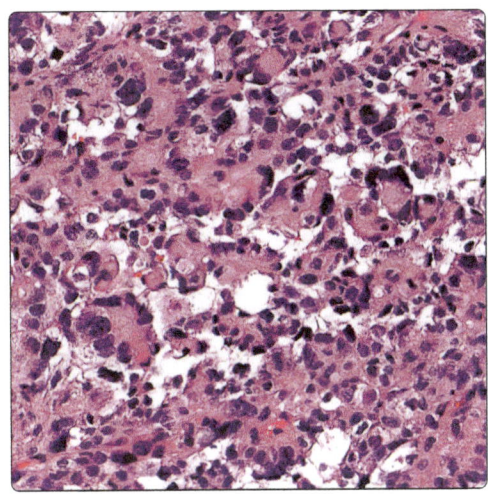

(Left) Choroid plexus carcinomas are highly malignant neoplasms and may form huge, fleshy masses with associated edema and mass effect in infants. (Right) Many choroid plexus carcinomas demonstrate cytologic features of malignancy, particularly nuclear enlargement, hyperchromasia, and pleomorphism. In this example, a papillary architecture is still evident.

Well-Differentiated Architecture

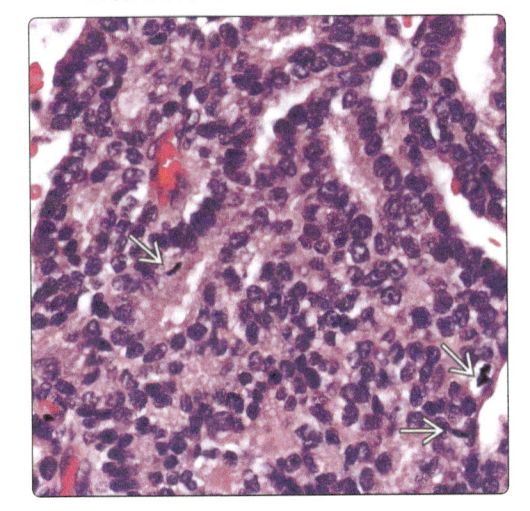

Necrosis

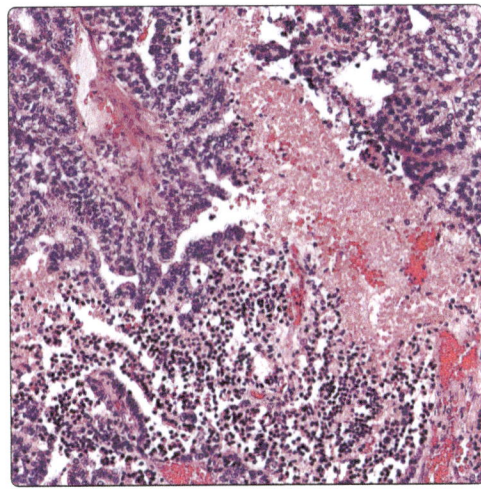

(Left) A subset of choroid plexus carcinomas may contain minimal atypia and are well differentiated at the architectural level. However, the presence of brisk mitotic activity ➡ in a choroid plexus tumor is very worrisome and consistent with carcinoma. (Right) Sheets of coagulative necrosis are not uncommon in choroid plexus carcinomas. In combination with brisk mitotic activity, this strongly supports the diagnosis.

Posttreatment Rhabdomyosarcoma

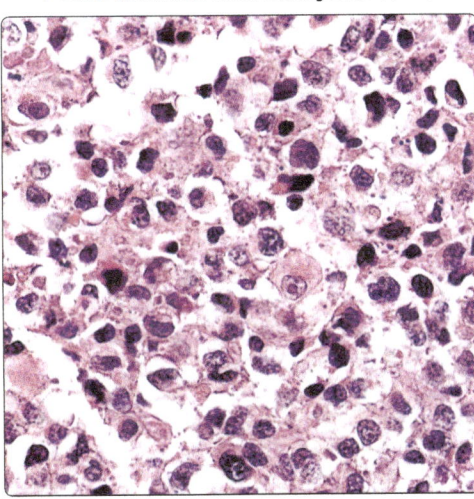

Myogenin Expression in Posttreatment Rhabdomyosarcoma

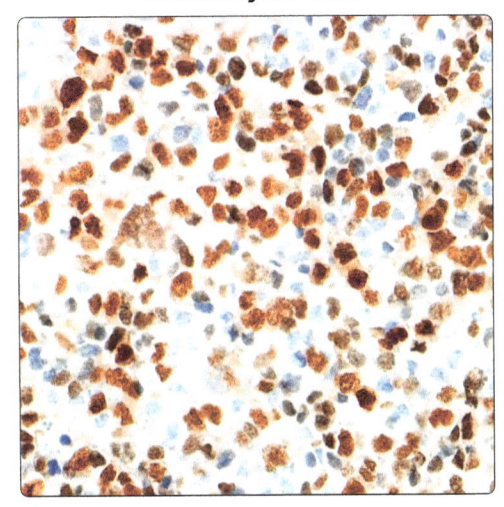

(Left) This tumor developed in a young patient after treatment for choroid plexus carcinoma and had morphologic and immunophenotypic features of rhabdomyosarcoma. The combination of choroid plexus carcinoma and sarcoma in a young patient is strongly suggestive of a tumor predisposition syndrome, particularly Li-Fraumeni. (Right) Strong nuclear myogenin labeling confirmed the diagnosis of rhabdomyosarcoma in this young patient treated for choroid plexus carcinoma.

Meningioma

KEY FACTS

TERMINOLOGY
- Dural-based tumor with features of meningothelial derivation
- Proposed histogenesis is from arachnoidal mater
- CNS WHO grade 1, 2, or 3

ETIOLOGY/PATHOGENESIS
- Ionizing radiation is risk factor with latency period of 20-35 years

CLINICAL ISSUES
- Accounts for ~ 37% of CNS tumors
- Higher incidence in women
- Headaches, weakness, and seizure are common but not specific
- Complete resection often curative
- 5-year survival: > 80%
- Associated with neurofibromatosis 2 (NF2)
  - Sporadic cases are not NF2 associated
- Mean age at diagnosis is 7th decade

IMAGING
- Isodense, contrast-enhancing dural mass on MR
- Contrast-enhancing dural tail sign is frequent imaging feature

MOLECULAR
- Chromosome 22q abnormalities
  - Most common mutation, more in higher grade tumors
  - More in meningothelial and transitional subtypes, less in radiation induced meningiomas
- *NF2*, *AKT1*, *SMO*, and *TRAF7* alterations
- *TIMP3* promoter hypermethylation
  - More often seen in high-grade meningiomas
- *SMARCE1* mutation exclusively in clear cell meningiomas

ANCILLARY TESTS
- EMA(+), SSTR2A(+), E-cadherin/D2-40(+), vimentin (+), CK18(+)

Psammoma Bodies

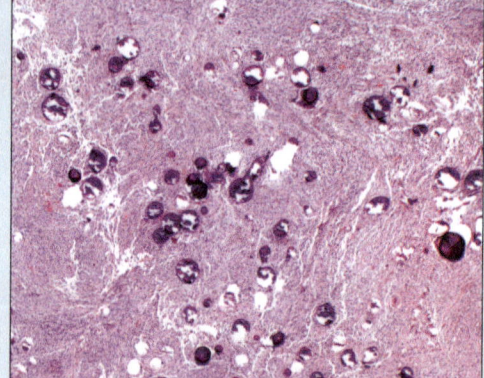

Meningothelial Features

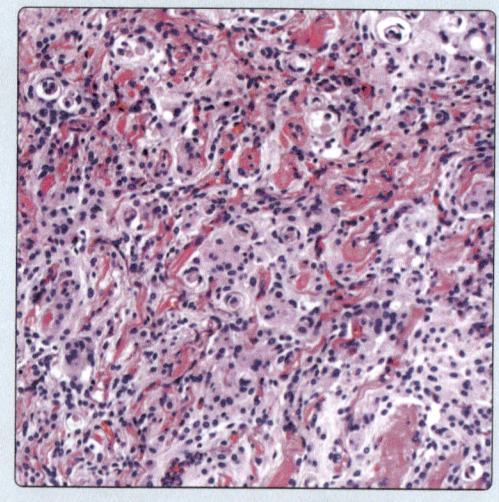

(Left) *Retromastoid low-grade meningioma in a 62-year-old woman shows abundant psammomatous mineralization. Psammoma bodies, which are concentric lamellated calcified structures, are seen in some (but certainly not all) meningiomas.* (Right) *WHO grade 1 meningioma shows both syncytial and meningothelial (whorling) patterns.*

Mitotic Figures

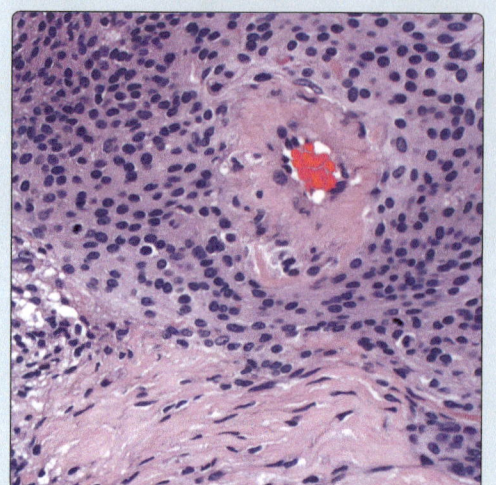

Atypical Meningioma

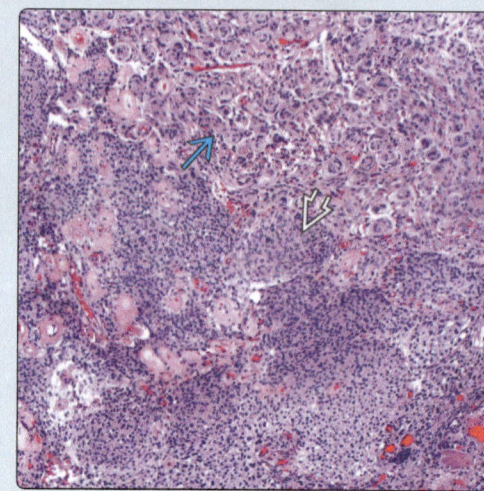

(Left) *This atypical meningioma had > 5 mitotic figures per 10 HPF.* (Right) *Although much of this tumor has a classic meningothelial appearance ➡, there are many more patternless-appearing foci ➡.*

Meningioma

TERMINOLOGY

Definitions
- Family of neoplasms that are likely derived from meningothelial cells of arachnoid matter
- WHO grades 1, 2 (atypical), or 3 (anaplastic)

ETIOLOGY/PATHOGENESIS

Environmental Exposure
- Ionizing radiation is primary established risk factor with latency period of 20-35 years
  - Risk is higher if exposure was in childhood
  - Strong evidence of genetic susceptibility to develop meningioma after radiation exposure
  - Association between endogenous or exogenous hormone use and current smoking and meningioma risk also reported

Syndromic Associations
- Neurofibromatosis 2 (NF2)
  - Microdeletion involving *NF2* at 22q12.2
  - Associated with predisposition to development of multiple meningiomas
- Families with germline defects/mutations in
  - *NF1*, *VHL*, *PTEN*, *PTCH1*, *BAP1*, *SUFU*, *SMARCE1*, and *CREBBP*

CLINICAL ISSUES

Epidemiology
- Incidence
  - Annual age-adjusted rate of ~ 8.6 per 100,000 population
  - Accounts for ~ 37% of CNS tumors
- Age
  - Median: 66 years at diagnosis
- Sex
  - Higher incidence in women
    - Symptoms may be exacerbated by progesterone/pregnancy
    - Female predominance not seen with pediatric and higher grade tumors

Site
- Arise in intracranial, intraspinal, or orbital locations
- Most common sites
  - Cerebral convexities, parasagittal, falx, olfactory grooves, sphenoid ridges, parasellar/suprasellar regions, optic nerve sheath, petros ridges, tentorium, and posterior fossa
  - Uncommon locations include intraventricular and epidural
  - Convexity meningiomas and majority of spinal meningiomas often carry 22q deletion &/or *NF2* mutations
  - Skull base meningiomas harbor mutations in *AKT1*, *TRAF7*, *SMO* &/or *PIK3CA*

Presentation
- Headaches, weakness, and seizure common but not specific
- Neurological deficit that varies depending on tumor location
- May be found incidentally with imaging (or at autopsy)
- Usually slow-growing, but high-grade and aggressive tumors progress more rapidly

Treatment
- Complete resection often curative
- May "watch and wait" if asymptomatic
- Conventional irradiation and radiosurgery, if resection incomplete or surgery not feasible

Prognosis
- 5-year survival: > 80%
- 10-year survival: ~ 75%
- 5-year survival for atypical meningioma: ~ 57%
- Incomplete resection associated with recurrence

IMAGING

MR Findings
- Isodense, contrast-enhancing dural mass

CT Findings
- Contrast-enhancing dural tail sign is frequent imaging feature
- Calcifications and hyperostosis in ~ 20% of cases

MOLECULAR

Cytogenetics
- Monosomy of chromosome 22
  - Most common known molecular alteration (~ 50% of cases)
  - Loss of heterozygosity (LOH) at 22q12.2 also seen in 40-70% of sporadic meningiomas
  - LOH at 22q12.2 in most NF2-associated meningiomas
  - More common in fibroblastic, transitional, and psammomatous types (80%) than in meningothelial (25%)
- Losses of 1p, 6q, 9p, 10, 14q, and 18q
- Less frequently losses on 2p/q, 3p, 4p/q, 7p, and 8p/q, and deletions of *CDKN2A* &/or *CDKN2B*
  - Associated with higher grade meningiomas
- Gains or amplifications involving 1q, 9q, 12q, 15q, 17q, and 20q are less common

Molecular Genetics
- *NF2*
  - Mutated in all CNS WHO grades supportive of early events in meningioma development
- *AKT1*
  - Mutation in ~ 13%
  - *AKT1* p.E17K hotspot mutation also found in breast and bladder cancer
  - Suggestive of oncogenic driver mutation
- *TRAF7*
  - Mutations detected in ~ 25% of meningiomas
  - May occur concurrently with *KLF4* mutation
- *SMO*
  - Mutations detected in ~ 5% of meningiomas
- *PIK3CA*
  - *PIK3CA* mutations activate several signaling pathways in meningiomas

Meningioma

- Mutations are more common in women with meningioma with history of prolonged progestin therapy
- APC
  - Tumor suppressor gene and component of Wnt signaling pathway
  - LOH of *APC* detected in ~ 47% of meningiomas
- *CDKN2A*
  - Interacts with *TP53* and regulates transition from G1 to S phase
  - Allelic losses or homozygous deletions at 9p21
  - Seen in higher grade meningiomas
- *TERT* promoter mutations
  - Associated with malignant progression
- *SMARCE1* mutation found nearly exclusively in clear cell meningiomas
- Epigenetic modifiers genes
  - *KDM5C*, *KDM6A*, and *SMARCB1* mutations
    - Detected in ~ 8% of meningiomas
- *TIMP3* promoter hypermethylation
  - More often seen in high-grade meningiomas
  - Associated with allelic loss on 22q12

MICROSCOPIC

Histologic Features
- 15 histologic subtypes
- Grading is based in subtype, mitotic rate, and invasion
- Circumscribed pushing border with brain (low grade)
- Skull infiltration with hyperostosis (low and high grades)
- Nuclear pseudoinclusions
- Syncytial: Lobules and whorls of cells with indistinct cell borders
- Fibroblastic: Spindle cells in fascicles, collagen, and reticulum
- Transitional (most common): Syncytial and fibroblastic features with meningothelial whorls

Histologic Subtypes
- 15 histologic subtypes (WHO 5th edition)
  - Meningothelial meningioma
  - Fibroblastic (fibrous) meningioma
  - Transitional (mixed) meningioma
  - Psammomatous meningioma
  - Angiomatous meningioma
  - Microcystic meningioma
  - Secretory meningioma
  - Lymphoplasmacyte-rich meningioma
  - Metaplastic meningioma
  - Chordoid meningioma
  - Clear cell meningioma
  - Rhabdoid meningioma
  - Papillary meningioma
  - Atypical meningioma
  - Anaplastic (malignant) meningioma
    - Fibroblastic, meningothelial, and transitional subtypes most common
- Features of more aggressive growth can arise in any of above morphologic patterns
  - Choroid and clear cell meningiomas have higher likelihood of recurrence and have therefore been assigned to CNS WHO grade 2
  - Brain invasive meningioma qualifies for CNS WHO grade 2
  - Historically, papillary and rhabdoid morphology have been qualified for CNS WHO grade 3

ANCILLARY TESTS

Immunohistochemistry
- EMA(+) (may be weak or focal), membranous pattern
- SSTR2A(+), dual E-cadherin/D2-40(+), vimentin (+), CK18(+), S100(+/-)
- CK20(-)

DIFFERENTIAL DIAGNOSIS

Solitary Fibrous Tumor-Hemangiopericytoma Spectrum
- Lack meningothelial whorls
- Characteristic collagen strips
- STAT6(+), CD34(+); EMA(-)

Schwannoma
- Verocay bodies and Antoni A and B patterns
- S100(+); EMA(-)
- Located in nerve sheath

Metastatic Carcinoma
- Carcinomas express keratin

GRADING

WHO Grade 2
- 4-19 mitotic figures in 10 consecutive HPF or
- Unequivocal brain invasion or
- Specific morphologic subtype (choroid or clear cell) or
- At least 3 of following
  - Sheeting architecture (uninterrupted patternless or sheet-like growth)
  - Small cell with high N:C ratio
  - Increased cellularity
  - Prominent nucleoli
  - Spontaneous necrosis (noniatrogenic necrosis)

WHO Grade 3
- ≥ 20 mitotic figures in 10 consecutive HPF or
- Frank anaplasia (sarcoma, carcinoma, or melanoma-like histology) or
- *TERT* promoter mutation or
- Homozygous deletion of *CDKN2A* &/or *CDKN2B*

SELECTED REFERENCES

1. Figarella-Branger D et al: The 2021 WHO classification of tumours of the central nervous system. Ann Pathol. 42(5):367-82, 2022
2. Lu VM et al: The prognostic significance of TERT promoter mutations in meningioma: a systematic review and meta-analysis. J Neurooncol. 142(1):1-10, 2019
3. Pereira BJA et al: Molecular alterations in meningiomas: literature review. Clin Neurol Neurosurg. 176:89-96, 2019
4. Gupta A et al: A simplified overview of World Health Organization classification update of central nervous system tumors 2016. J Neurosci Rural Pract. 8(4):629-41, 2017
5. Brastianos PK et al: Genomic sequencing of meningiomas identifies oncogenic SMO and AKT1 mutations. Nat Genet. 45(3):285-9, 2013
6. Clark VE et al: Genomic analysis of non-NF2 meningiomas reveals mutations in TRAF7, KLF4, AKT1, and SMO. Science. 339(6123):1077-80, 2013

Meningioma

Low-Grade Meningioma

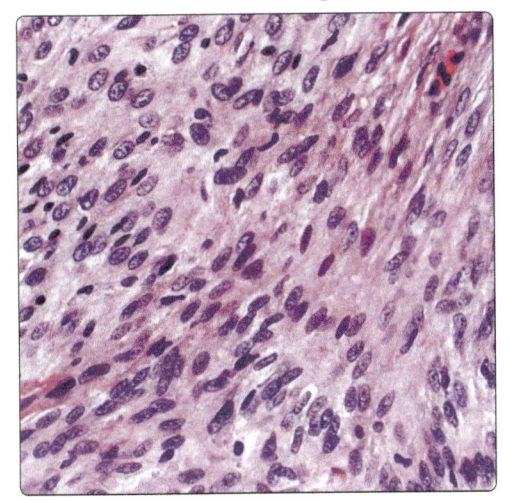

Syncytial Features

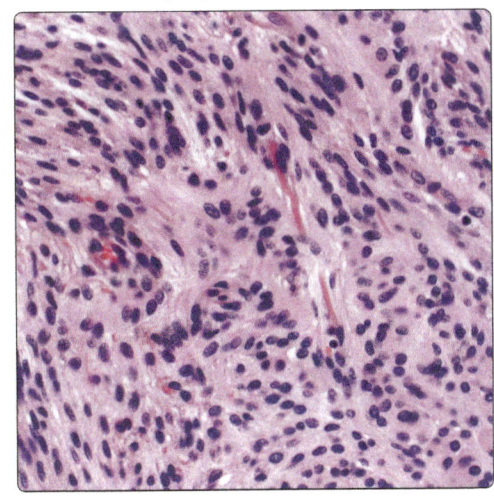

(Left) Low-grade meningioma shows the loss of distinction between cell borders characteristic of syncytial pattern. Although nucleoli are present, they are not a prominent feature. (Right) Low-grade meningioma shows a characteristically syncytial pattern but with hints of whorling.

Fibroblastic Features

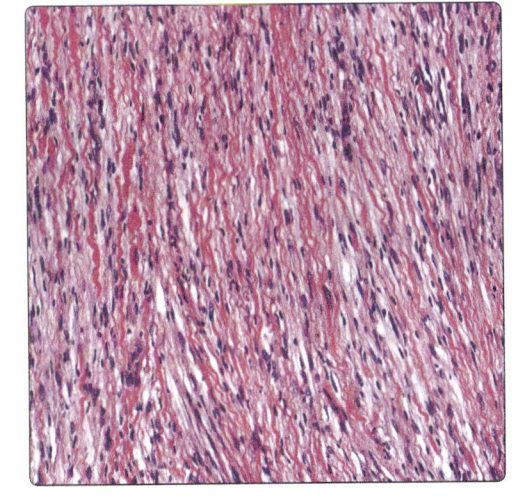

Prominent Nucleoli

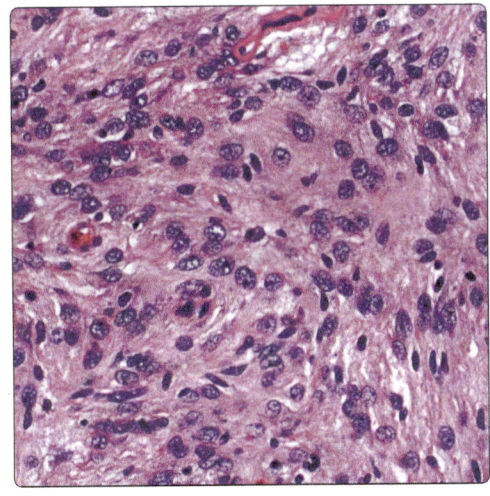

(Left) Low-grade meningioma in a 49-year-old woman shows the characteristic features of fibroblastic growth pattern with abundant wavy collagen between fibroblast-like cells. In certain locations, neurofibroma might have been a consideration. (Right) Nucleoli are prominent focally in this WHO grade 1 meningioma; however, there is no significant mitotic activity, and no additional atypical features are present.

Embolization Beads

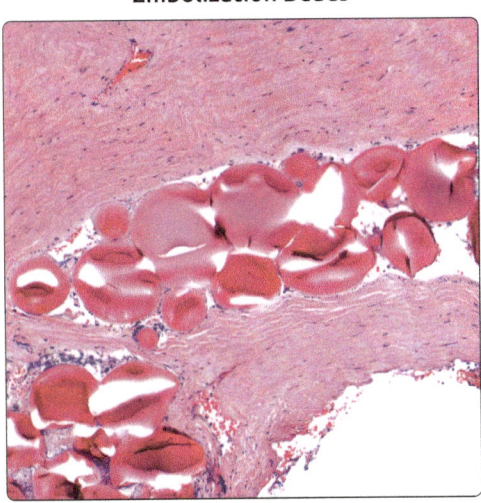

Iatrogenic Necrosis

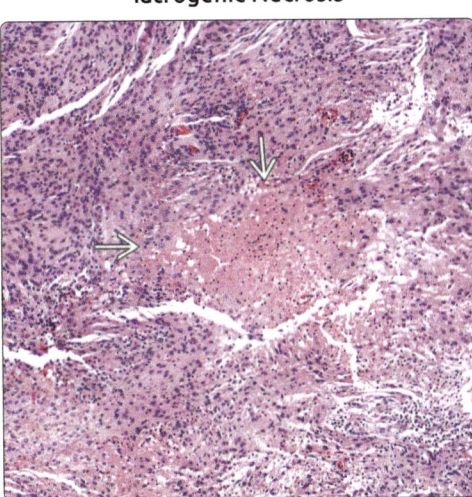

(Left) Materials used for therapeutic embolization include beads (microspheres), glues, and onyx. Embolic material, such as these beads, has a characteristic appearance within blood vessels. (Right) Foci of necrosis ➡ are common in meningiomas that have been embolized and should not be overinterpreted in grading. This case had no additional atypical features and was therefore WHO grade 1.

Retinoblastoma

KEY FACTS

TERMINOLOGY
- Familial retinoblastoma (RB) caused by germline *RB1* pathogenic mutations
- Rare cases of nonhereditary RB results from amplification of *MYCN* amplification without *RB1* mutations

ETIOLOGY/PATHOGENESIS
- Loss or inactivation of both alleles of *RB1*
- *MYCN* amplification accounts for 2% of all RB cases

CLINICAL ISSUES
- Most common intraocular malignancy in children
- Average age at diagnosis: 18-24 months
- ~ 40% have de novo or inherited germline pathogenic variants that are transmissible as autosomal dominant trait
- 2nd cancers common in patients with *RB1* mutations
  - Osteosarcoma, soft tissue sarcoma, melanoma, Hodgkin lymphoma, breast carcinoma
- Leukocoria is most common clinical presentation

IMAGING
- Calcified intraocular mass
- Diagnosis often made by imaging only

MICROSCOPIC
- RB is mitotically active small blue cell tumor composed of primitive neuroblastic cells
- Calcifications common
- Flexner-Wintersteiner rosettes
- Homer Wright rosettes

TOP DIFFERENTIAL DIAGNOSES
- Primitive neuroectodermal tumor
- Leukemia/lymphoma
- Astrocytoma
- Medulloepithelioma

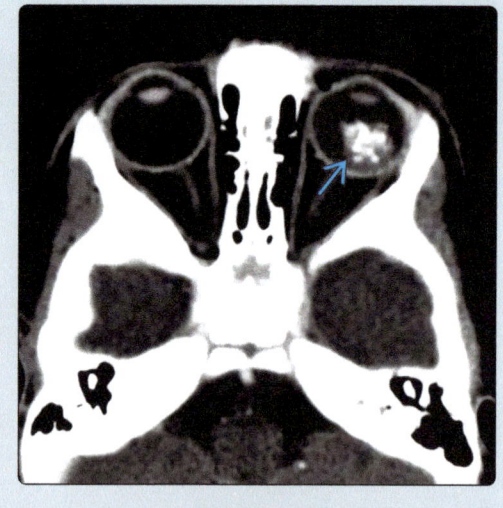

(Left) Retinoblastoma (RB) may have lobulated contours and extend through the limiting membrane into the vitreous. Punctate calcifications ⇨ are characteristic. (Right) Axial CT shows a large, lobulated, partially calcified left intraocular mass ⇨, typical of RB.

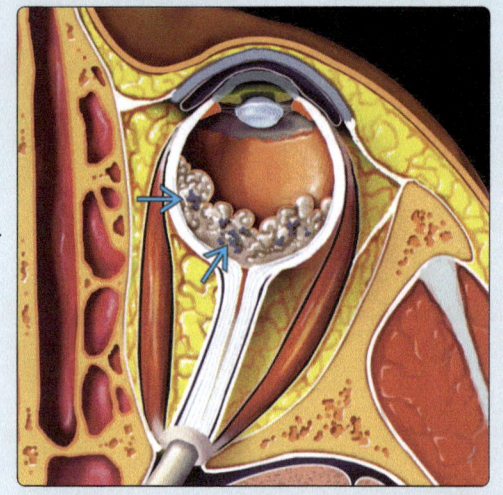

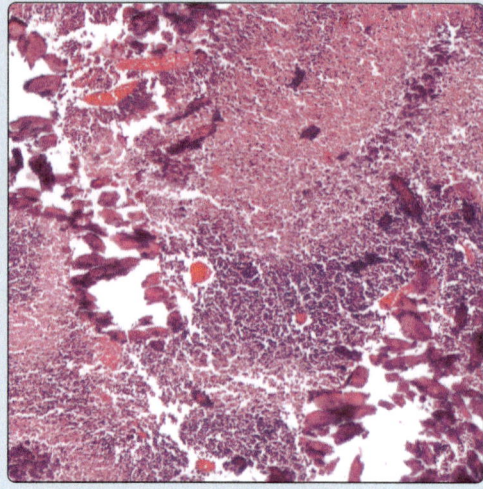

(Left) RB is a cellular malignant neoplasm composed of cells forming sheets with high N:C ratios. (Right) Calcifications may be prominent in some cases and are a useful diagnostic finding on radiograph-based imaging studies.

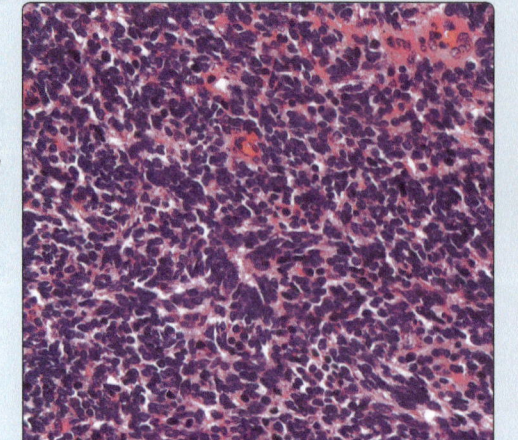

Retinoblastoma

TERMINOLOGY

Abbreviations
- Retinoblastoma (RB)

Definitions
- RB: Malignant pediatric retinal neoplasm
- Familial RB caused by germline *RB1* pathogenic mutations
  - ~ 40% have de novo or inherited germline pathogenic variants that are transmissible as autosomal dominant trait
- Rare cases of nonhereditary RB result from amplification of *MYCN* amplification without *RB1* mutations
  - *MYCN* amplification accounts for 2% of all RB cases

ETIOLOGY/PATHOGENESIS

Developmental Anomaly
- Loss or inactivation of both alleles of *RB1*
- RB results from 2 independent mutations
  - 1st mutation may be either somatic (sporadic) or inherited (germline)
  - 2nd mutation is sporadic
- *RB1*
  - Located at 13q14.2 locus
  - Tumor suppressor gene
  - Encodes RB1 protein
    - Negative regulator of cell cycle
    - Binds transcription factor E2F1, which controls cell cycle
    - Also stabilizes heterochromatin to maintain chromatin structure

CLINICAL ISSUES

Epidemiology
- Incidence
  - Most common intraocular malignancy in children
  - Average age at diagnosis is 18-24 months but younger in bilateral/familial cases

Site
- RB is intraocular tumor of retina
- Sporadic RB is usually unilateral
- Familial RB syndrome
  - Synchronous or metachronous malignant intracranial tumors (pineal or suprasellar) may develop
    - Combination of intraocular RB and similar brain tumor, most commonly in pineal gland, is called trilateral RB

Presentation
- Leukocoria (white pupillary reflex) and strabismus caused by visual loss
- Up to 40% have genetic predisposition
  - 5-10% have family history of RB
  - Remainder are new germline mutations

Treatment
- Depends on tumor size, intraocular location, and histopathologic risk factors

Prognosis
- If untreated, invariably fatal
- Poor prognosis if direct scleral invasion or invasion of optic nerve
- 90% cure rate if noninvasive
- 2nd cancers common in patients with *RB1* mutations
  - Osteosarcoma, soft tissue sarcoma, melanoma, Hodgkin lymphoma, breast carcinoma
  - Incidence is higher in inherited RB

IMAGING

General Features
- Calcified intraocular mass
- Diagnosis often made by imaging only

MOLECULAR

Chromosomal Microarray
- Gains of 6p and 1q in ~ 50% of RB cases

Molecular Genetics
- Inherited (germinal) RB
  - 1 copy or mutated *RB1* is inherited in autosomal dominant pattern
  - Mutation or deletion of other *RB1* copy must occur in retinal cells for RB to develop
- Acquired RB
  - Both copies of *RB1* in retinal cells acquire mutations or are deleted
    - Genetic testing is required to separate germinal from acquired form of RB

MICROSCOPIC

Histologic Features
- RB is mitotically active small blue cell tumor composed of primitive neuroblastic cells
- Perivascular cuffs of viable cells, tumor necrosis, and dystrophic calcification common
- Flexner-Wintersteiner rosettes
- Homer Wright rosettes
- Photoreceptor differentiation in 15-20% of RB cases
  - Aggregates of neoplastic photoreceptors called fleurettes
- May invade optic nerve and extend to brain or CSF
- *MYCN*-amplified cases have distinctive histologic features
  - Macronucleoli, undifferentiated cells, necrosis, frequent apoptosis, no calcifications

SELECTED REFERENCES

1. Schaiquevich P et al: Treatment of retinoblastoma: what is the latest and what is the future. Front Oncol. 12:822330, 2022
2. Torp SH et al: The WHO 2021 classification of central nervous system tumours: a practical update on what neurosurgeons need to know-a minireview. Acta Neurochir (Wien). 164(9):2453-64, 2022
3. Louis DN et al: The 2021 WHO classification of tumors of the central nervous system: a summary. Neuro Oncol. 23(8):1231-51, 2021
4. Fabian ID et al: Classification and staging of retinoblastoma. Community Eye Health. 31(101):11-13, 2018

Retinoblastoma

Leukocoria

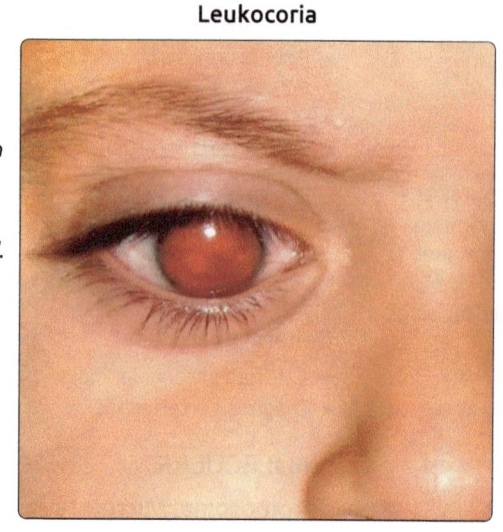

White Fluffy Tumor

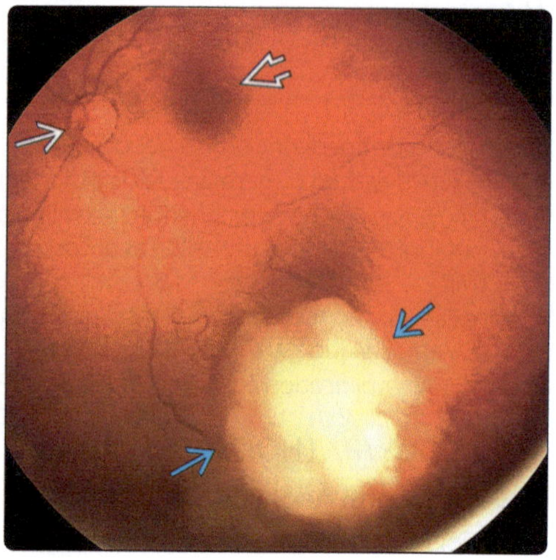

(Left) Leukocoria, or white pupil, is a common presentation of RB. (Courtesy D. Shatzkes, MD.) (Right) RB forms variably sized masses on funduscopic examination. Tumors are usually white and fluffy ➡. The optic nerve ➡ and macula ➡ are uninvolved. (Courtesy D. Dries, MD.)

Calcified Intraocular Mass

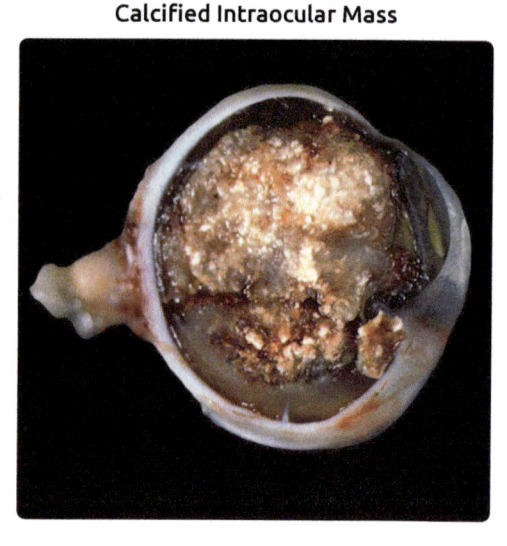

Necrosis

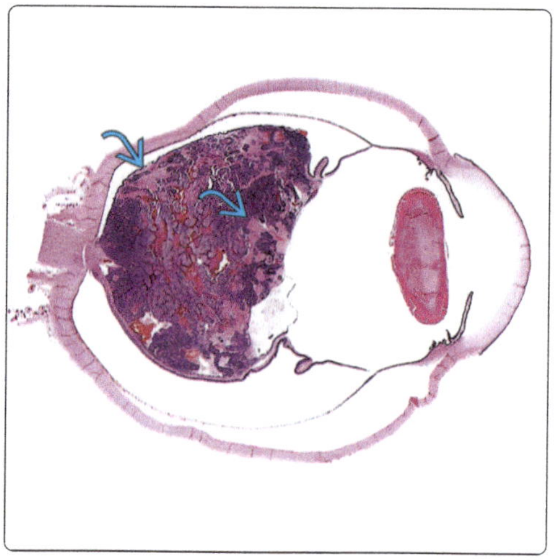

(Left) Gross pathology shows the macroscopic appearance of the eye after exenteration. This RB forms a calcified mass that fills the vitreous cavity. (Courtesy B. Ey, MD.) (Right) RB may form large intraocular masses, which block the normal retinal light reflex. Necrosis is a frequent finding ➡ and may be identified on low magnification.

Optic Nerve Invasion

Knudsen "2-Hit" Hypothesis

(Left) Optic nerve invasion ➡ is a negative prognostic factor and must be carefully searched for in surgical specimens. Invasion beyond the lamina cribrosa ➡ in particular is associated with an ominous prognosis. (Right) In the Knudsen "2-hit" hypothesis, the 1st hit may be either inherited (germline, bottom) or sporadic (somatic, top). The 2nd hit is always sporadic. Red chromosome 13 contains a mutant copy of a tumor suppressor gene, e.g., RB1.

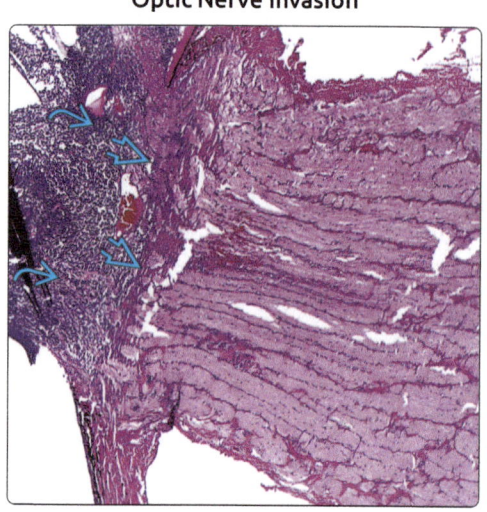

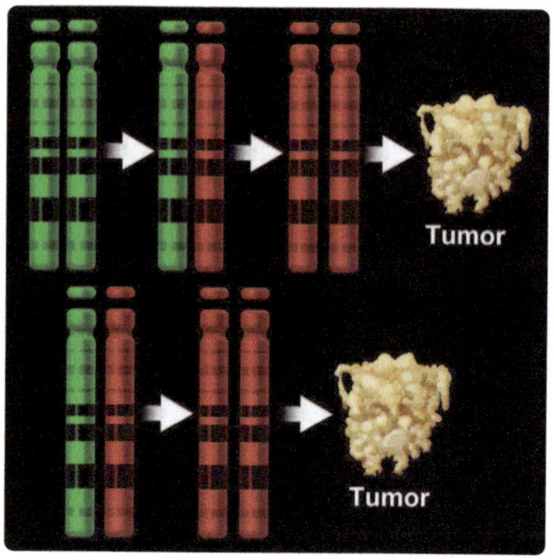

Retinoblastoma

Poorly Differentiated Retinoblastoma

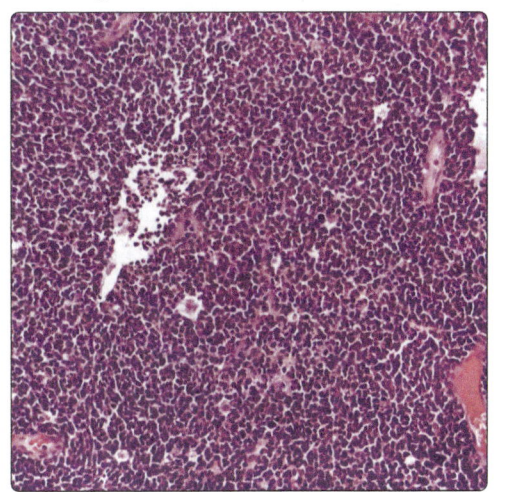

Necrosis and Calcifications

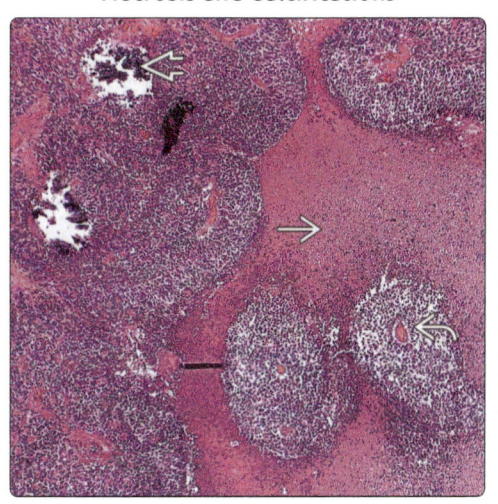

(Left) Sheets of small round blue cells make up this poorly differentiated RB. This field could be mistaken for primitive neuroendocrine tumor/embryonal neoplasm if the location was not known. (Right) Necrosis ➡ and calcifications ➡ are very common in RB. The necrosis is often seen sparing tumor cells around vascular spaces ➡ as the tumor outgrows its blood supply. Calcifications are an important marker in radiologic studies.

Flexner-Wintersteiner Rosettes

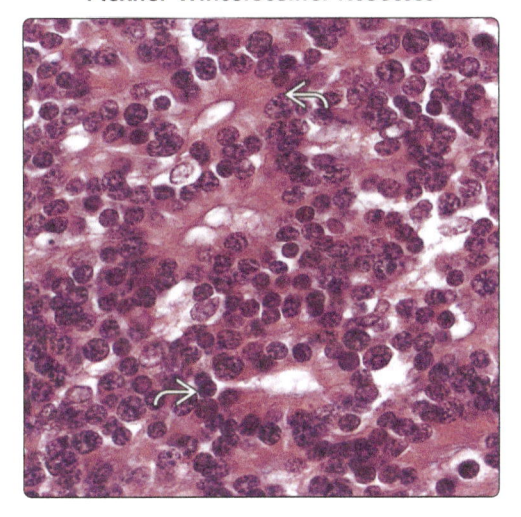

Homer Wright Rosettes

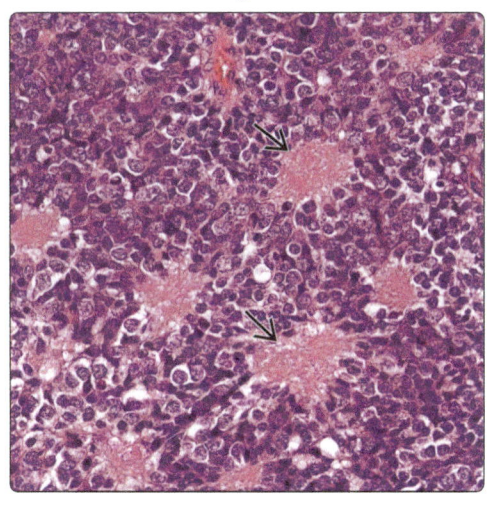

(Left) Flexner-Wintersteiner rosettes ➡ are seen in moderately differentiated RB. They have central lumina filled with mucopolysaccharide, and the surrounding tumor cells have their nuclei located away from the lumina. (Right) Homer Wright rosettes ➡ are less specific structures characterized by an anuclear center lacking lumina. They may be encountered in a variety of tumor types.

MYCN Amplification

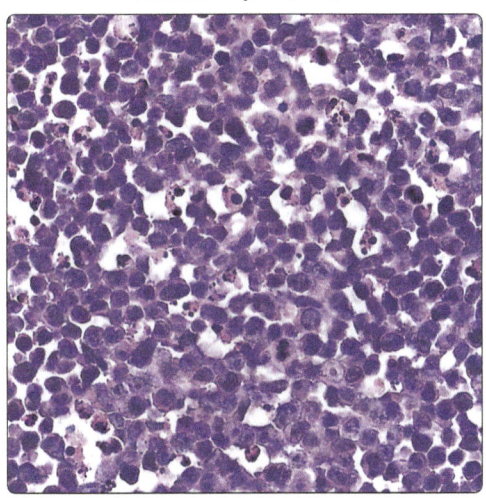

MYCN Amplification

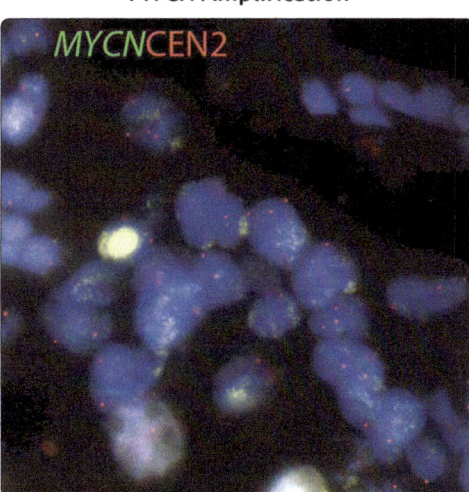

(Left) RB with MYCN amplification has distinctive histologic features, including nuclear enlargement with macronucleoli and numerous apoptotic bodies. (Right) Approximately 2% of RB cases have MYCN amplification, which may be recognized by FISH studies as numerous (green) copies of the gene locus. These tumors usually lack RB1 mutations.

955

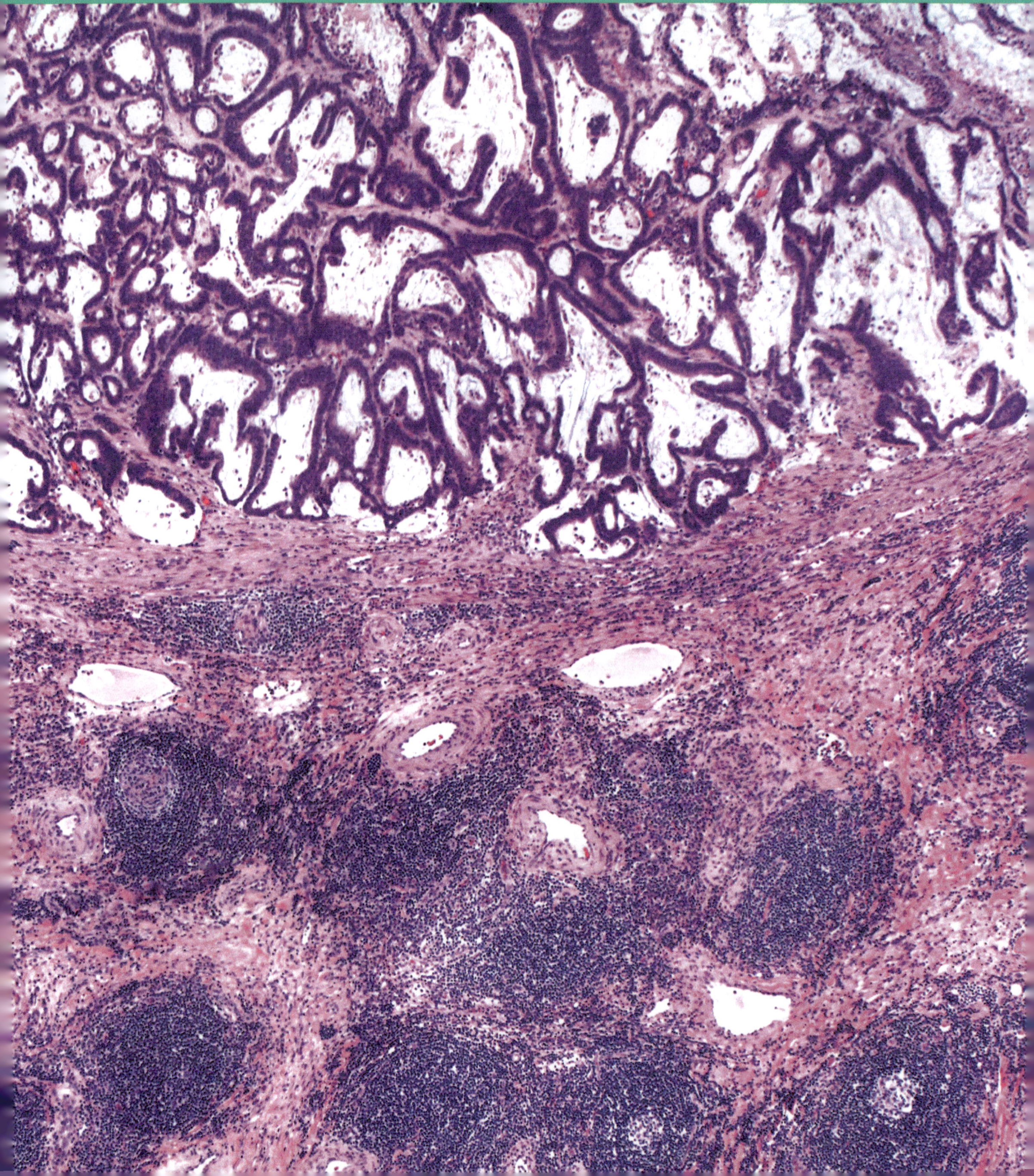

SECTION 9
Quality Assurance and Regulatory Issues

Federal Agencies and Regulation of Laboratories	958
FDA Regulations	960
Proficiency Testing and Accreditation	966

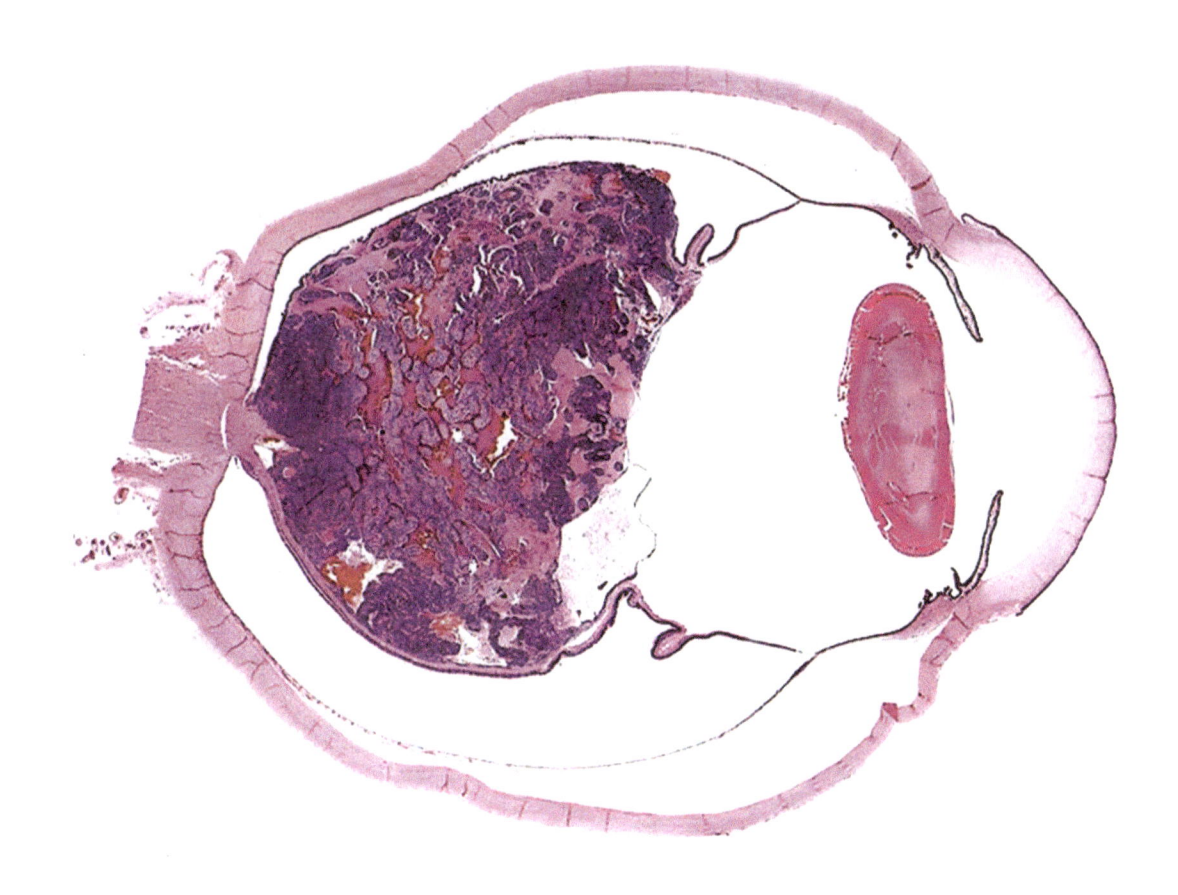

Federal Agencies and Regulation of Laboratories

TERMINOLOGY

Abbreviations
- Centers for Medicare and Medicaid Services (CMS)
- Clinical Laboratory Improvement Amendments (CLIA)
- Centers for Disease Control and Prevention (CDC)
- Food and Drug Administration (FDA)
- In vitro diagnostics (IVD)
- U.S. Department of Health and Human Services (HHS)

CMS

Overview
- CMS is federal agency under HHS that runs Medicare program and works with states to run Medicaid program
- CMS is also responsible for clinical laboratory quality standards through CLIA
  - CLIA requires secretary of HHS to certify laboratories that perform clinical testing
    - CMS administers CLIA certification program for secretary along with CDC and FDA
- Certification by CMS involves 2 main steps
  - On-site survey to ensure lab adheres to quality standards set by CMS
  - Lab participation in approved proficiency testing program to measure performance and ensure accuracy

Clinical Laboratory Improvement Amendments
- Law passed in 1988 by congress to establish quality standards for laboratory testing
  - Applies only to specimens derived from humans
  - Applies only to testing performed in clinical setting
    - Providing information for diagnosis, prevention, or treatment of any disease or impairment of health
    - Providing information for assessment of health of humans
- Requires all facilities that perform even 1 clinical test to meet certain federal requirements
  - Extent of federal requirements depends on complexity of test
- Laboratories exempt from CLIA
  - Labs that only perform testing for forensic purposes
  - Research laboratories that test human specimens but do not report patient-specific results
  - Laboratories certified by Substance Abuse and Mental Health Services Administration (SAMHSA)
- CLIA-defined roles
  - Defines certain roles that must be fulfilled by qualified individual in laboratory
  - Roles are based on test complexity
    - Waived: Laboratory director, testing personnel
    - Moderate: Laboratory director, clinical consultant, technical consultant, testing personnel
    - High: Laboratory director, clinical consultant, technical supervisor, general supervisor, testing personnel
  - Each role has certain requirements and assigned specific duties
    - Example of requirements: Technical consultants and supervisors should have minimum of bachelor degree
    - Example of duties: Competency assessment is performed by technical supervisor or general supervisor for high complexity tests and by technical consultant for moderate complexity tests

Certificates
- Under CLIA, CMS issues 5 types of certificates for laboratories
  - Certificate of waiver
    - Permits laboratory to perform only waived tests
    - Routine on-site surveys are not required unless there is complaint
    - Laboratory enrolls in CLIA program and pays fee
    - Laboratory follows manufacturer's instructions for specific tests
  - Certificate for provider-performed microscopy procedures
    - Permits laboratory to perform only microscopy
      - Classified as moderate complexity testing
      - Test must be performed by physician, dentist, or midlevel practitioner
      - Examples: Urine microscopy, potassium hydroxide smear
    - Routine on-site surveys are not required unless there is complaint
    - Laboratory enrolls in CLIA program and pays fee
    - Rules regarding moderate complexity tests apply
  - Certificate of registration
    - Temporary certification for laboratory to conduct moderate- and high-complexity tests
      - Issued when laboratory applies for CLIA certificate but before being inspected
    - Expires after 2 years or when laboratory meets certification requirements
  - Certificate of compliance
    - Issued to laboratory after inspection that finds laboratory to be in compliance with all applicable CLIA requirements
  - Certificate of accreditation
    - Issued to laboratory on basis of laboratory's accreditation by accreditation organization approved by CMS
- Separate CLIA certificate is required for each location in which testing is performed, with following exceptions
  - Mobile laboratory units
  - Not-for-profit or federal, state, or local government labs that engage in limited public health testing
  - Labs within hospital that are located at contiguous buildings on same campus and under common direction may file single application
- CLIA certificates include 10-digit unique number
  - Utilized to identify and track laboratory throughout its entire history

FOOD AND DRUG ADMINISTRATION

Overview
- Federal agency responsible for protecting and promoting public health through regulation and supervision of multiple categories
  - Medical devices is category relevant to laboratory
    - Includes IVD

Federal Agencies and Regulation of Laboratories

- □ Includes nucleic acid-based tests and companion diagnostic devices
- o Example of other categories include food, drugs, vaccines, blood, cosmetics, and tobacco
- FDA is empowered by United States Congress to enforce Federal Food, Drug, and Cosmetic Act

In Vitro Diagnostic Devices

- FDA regulates laboratory tests through its IVD devices program
  - o Reagents, instruments, and systems used in clinical laboratory
  - o Products intended for use in collection, preparation, and examination of specimens taken from human body
- FDA classifies IVDs into 3 categories according to level of regulatory control that is necessary to assure safety and effectiveness
  - o Class I: Subject to set of general controls
  - o Class II: Subject to general controls in addition to special controls
  - o Class III: Subject to general control in addition to premarket approval
- General purpose reagent
  - o Chemical reagent that has general laboratory use
  - o Used to collect, prepare, and examine specimens from human body for diagnostic purposes
  - o Not labeled or otherwise intended for specific diagnostic application
  - o e.g., tissue processing reagents, pH buffers
  - o Classified as class I IVD
- Analyte-specific reagent (ASR)
  - o Reagent that undergoes **specific** binding or chemical reaction with substances in specimen
    - e.g., antibodies (both polyclonal and monoclonal), specific receptor proteins, nucleic acid sequences
  - o Intended for use in diagnostic application for identification and quantification of individual chemical substance or ligand in biological specimens
  - o Majority of ASRs are class I
    - Exceptions include those used by blood banks to screen for infectious diseases or used to diagnose certain contagious diseases, such as HIV and TB
  - o If laboratory performs patient testing using class I ASRs that are not purchased as part of kit, federal regulations require that specific disclaimer accompany test result

Test Complexity

- FDA classifies laboratory tests into 3 main categories by evaluation of 7 criteria
  - o Knowledge required to perform test
  - o Training and experience required to perform test
  - o Difficulty of preparing reagents and materials
  - o Operational steps of test
  - o Calibration, quality control, and proficiency testing materials
  - o Test system troubleshooting and equipment maintenance
  - o Interpretation and judgment involved in test
- Levels of test complexity
  - o Waived tests
    - Simple laboratory examinations and procedures that have insignificant risk of erroneous result
    - e.g., fecal occult blood
  - o Moderate complexity
    - Laboratory tests with score of ≤ 12 based on FDA complexity scoring system
    - e.g., provider-performed microscopy
  - o High complexity
    - Laboratory tests with score of > 12 based on FDA complexity scoring system
  - o Moderate and high complexity tests are called nonwaived tests
  - o Complexity of certain test can be looked up using following URL
    - https://www.accessdata.fda.gov/scripts/cdrh/cfdocs/cfCLIA/search.cfm

Regulation of Laboratory Tests

- Laboratory-developed tests (LDTs)
  - o Type of IVD test that is designed, manufactured, and used within single laboratory
  - o Historically, FDA did not enforce premarket review and other applicable FDA requirements on LDTs, but this may change in future
    - H. R. 4128 (VALID act) is bill that was introduced by 117th congress in 2021 that could have significant consequences for LDTs by requiring some level of FDA review
      - □ Ultimately, bill did not pass, but FDA signaled it may use its administrative rule-making power to enact guidelines to revamp regulation of lab-based testing
- FDA-cleared tests
  - o Tests that FDA has determined to be substantially equivalent to another legally marketed test
  - o Premarket notification, referred to as 510(k), must be submitted to FDA for clearance
- FDA-approved tests
  - o Tests for which FDA has approved premarket approval (PMA) application prior to marketing
  - o Generally reserved for high-risk tests and involves more rigorous premarket review than 510(k) pathway
- Companion diagnostic devices
  - o IVD device or imaging tool that provides information that is essential for safe and effective use of corresponding therapeutic product
- FDA maintains searchable database of all cleared and approved medical devices, including laboratory tests

SELECTED REFERENCES

1. 117th Congress (2021-2022): VALID Act of 2021, H.R.4128, 117th Congress. Published June 2021. Accessed July 2023. https://www.congress.gov/bill/117th-congress/house-bill/4128/text
2. Centers for Medicare & Medicaid Services. CLIA Brochures. Updated Nov 28, 2018. Accessed Dec 23, 2018. http://www.cms.gov/Regulations-and-Guidance/Legislation/CLIA/CLIA_Brochures.html
3. U.S. Food and Drug Administration. CLIA Categorizations. Updated March 22, 2018. Accessed Dec 23, 2018. http://www.fda.gov/MedicalDevices/DeviceRegulationandGuidance/IVDRegulatoryAssistance/ucm393229.htm

FDA Regulations

TERMINOLOGY

Abbreviations and Acronyms
- Centers for Disease Control and Prevention (CDC)
- Centers for Medicaid and Medicare Services (CMS)
- Clinical Laboratory Improvement Amendments of 1988 (CLIA '88)
- Food and Drug Administration Modernization Act of 1997 (FDAMA)
- Food, Drug and Cosmetic Act of 1938 (FD&C Act)
- In vitro diagnostic products (IVDs)
- Laboratory developed tests (LDTs)
- Medical Device Amendment of 1976 (MDA '76)
- Public Health Service Act of 1944 (PHS Act)
- Tile 21 of Code of Federal Regulations (21 CFR)
- 21st Century Cures Act of 2016 (Cures Act)
- United States Code (U.S.C.)
- U.S. Department of Health and Human Services (HHS)
- U.S. Food and Drug Administration (FDA)

Definitions
- IVDs
    - Reagents, instruments, and systems intended for use in diagnosis of disease or other conditions, including determination of state of health, to cure, mitigate, treat, or prevent disease or its sequelae
    - Intended for use in collection, preparation, and examination of specimens taken from human body
    - Medical devices as defined in section 201(h) of FD&C Act or biological products subject to section 351 of PHS Act
    - Subject to premarket and postmarket controls by FDA
- LDTs
    - Type of IVD test that is designed, manufactured, and utilized within single laboratory
    - FDA has generally not enforced premarket review and other applicable requirements for LDTs
- FD&C Act
    - Federal law enacted by Congress in 1938
    - Primary statute that authorizes FDA's regulation and oversight of medical products
    - Authority for factory inspections
    - Can be found in U.S.C., beginning at 21 U.S.C. 301
- PHS Act
    - Federal law enacted by Congress in 1944
    - Covers broad spectrum of health concerns, including regulation of biologics and control of communicable diseases
    - Established certification of laboratories
- MDA '76
    - Amendment to FD&C Act in 1976 to ensure safety and effectiveness of medical devices, including IVDs
    - Created 3-class, risk-based classification system for all medical devices
    - Established regulatory pathways for new medical devices (after May 28, 1976) to get to market [premarket approval (PMA) and premarket notification 510(k)]
    - Created regulatory pathway to investigate new investigational medical devices in patients [investigational device exemptions (IDEs)]
    - Established several essential postmarket requirements [e.g., good manufacturing practices (GMPs)]
    - Authorized FDA to ban devices
- CLIA '88
    - Amendment to PHS Act in 1988, in which Congress revised federal program for certification and oversight of clinical laboratory testing
    - Has incorporated 2 subsequent amendments after 1988
        - FDAMA amended CLIA '88's criteria for waived testing
        - Takes Essential Steps for Testing Act of 2012 amended CLIA '88's certificate requirements and enforcement options related to proficiency testing (PT) referral
- FDAMA
    - Amendment to FD&C Act and PHS Act in 1997
    - Established De Novo program
    - Created "least burdensome" provisions for premarket review
- Cures Act
    - Amendment to FD&C Act in 2016
    - Helps accelerate medical product development and bring new innovations and advances to patients
- 21 CFR
    - Codification of general and permanent final rules or regulations published in Federal Register by federal executive departments and agencies
        - 21 CFR is for FDA regulations
- U.S.C.
    - Consolidation and codification by subject matter of general and permanent laws of USA
    - Divided by broad subjects into 53 titles and prepared by Office of Law Revision Counsel of U.S. House of Representatives

FDA REGULATION OF IN VITRO DIAGNOSTIC PRODUCTS

Key Federal Laws on In Vitro Diagnostic Products
- FD&C Act, PHS Act, MDA '76, and CLIA '88

FDA Regulations
- FDA develops regulations (21 CFR) according to laws set forth in FD&C Act and other federal laws under which FDA operates
    - 21 CFR interprets FD&C Act, PHS Act, and other related federal laws
- FDA regulations applicable to IVDs
    - 21 CFR 50: Protection of Human Subjects
    - 21 CFR 56: Institutional Review Boards (IRBs)
    - 21 CFR 312: Investigational New Drug Application (IND)
    - 21 CFR 600-680: Biologics Regulations
    - 21 CFR 807 Subpart E: 510(k)
    - 21 CFR 809: IVDs for Human Use
    - 21 CFR 812: Investigational Device Exemptions (IDEs)
    - 21 CFR 814 Subparts A-E: Premarket Approval (PMA) of Medical Device
    - 21 CFR 814 Subpart H: Humanitarian Use Devices (HUDs)
    - 21 CFR 820: Quality System Regulation (QSR)
    - 21 CFR 860: Medical Device Classification Procedures
    - 21 CFR 860 Subpart D: De Novo Classification

FDA Guidance
- FDA issues guidance based on procedures required by its Good Guidance Practice regulation (21 CFR 10.115)

FDA Regulations

- Describes agency's current thinking on regulatory issue and should be reviewed only as recommendations
- Does not establish legal binding on public or FDA

FDA Regulatory Responsibilities

- Center for Biologics Evaluation and Research (CBER)
  - Approves IVDs through Biologics License Application (BLA) under PHS Act
    - Blood grouping and phenotyping reagents
    - Donor screen assays for infectious pathogens and HIV diagnostic assays
  - Clears or approves IVDs associated with blood collection and processing procedures and cellular therapies under FD&C Act
    - 510(k): IVDs used by blood banking industry, including blood establishment computer software, etc.
    - PMA and humanitarian device exemption (HDE): IVDs associated with blood donor screen testing
- Center for Devices and Radiological Health (CDRH)
  - Clears or approves IVDs under FD&C Act
    - Clinical chemistry and clinical toxicology
    - Immunology and microbiology
    - Hematology, molecular genetics, and pathology
  - 21 CFR 862, 864, and 866 have listed classification of existing IVDs

In Vitro Diagnostic Product Classifications

- Section 513 (a) of FD&C Act established risk-based device classification system
  - Regulatory controls increase as device class increases from class I-III IVDs
- IVD classification determines appropriate premarket process
  - **Class I** (low to moderate risk to users): General controls
    - With and without exemptions
  - **Class II** (moderate to high risk to users): General and special controls
    - With and without exemptions
  - **Class III** (high risk to users): General controls and PMA

Regulatory Controls

- General controls
  - Basic provisions (sections 501, 502, 510, 516, 518, 519, and 520 of FD&C Act)
  - Apply to all IVDs and other medical devices, unless exempted by FD&C Act or regulations
  - Only level of controls applying to class I IVDs
- Special controls
  - Regulatory requirements for class II IVDs
  - Usually IVDs specific and include
    - Performance standards and postmarket surveillance
    - Patient registries and special labeling requirements
    - Premarket data requirements and guidelines
  - Special and general controls are necessary to ensure safety and effectiveness of class II IVDs
- PMA: General controls and PMA apply to class III IVDs

Premarketing Approval Process for In Vitro Diagnostic Products

- Presubmission (presub) process for IVD
  - Presub is formal written request from sponsor (applicant) as initial contact with FDA prior to premarket device submission, generally including
    - Cover letter, table of contents, and description of product
    - Overview of product development (e.g., outline of planned nonclinical and clinical studies)
    - Proposed intended use and indications for users
    - Previous discussions or submissions as appropriate
    - Any specific questions that sponsor wants FDA to answer and method for feedback
  - Methods for feedback from FDA
    - Formal written response, in-person meeting, or teleconference (documenting feedback in meeting minutes)
    - FDA and sponsor agree on whether IVD will require 510(k), PMA, De Novo request submission, or another investigational application
    - Any recommendations made in review of presub meeting package or meeting are not binding on sponsor or FDA
  - Recommendations from FDA
    - Presub is appropriate when FDA's feedback on specific questions is needed to guide product development &/or application preparation
    - Sponsors can use presub program before conducting nonclinical, analytical, and clinical studies or submitting marketing application
    - Before preparing for presub, sponsor should review all relevant FDA IVD-specific guidance documents
  - Potential benefits of submitting presub
    - Begin dialogue with FDA and promote greater understanding
    - Reduce cost of research studies by focusing on critical information needed for FDA approval, or clearance
    - Facilitate review process for future marketing application
  - Presub and feedback from FDA are strictly voluntary
- PMA submission
  - Can be submitted to FDA to request approval to market or continue to market class III IVDs
    - IVDs have unique link between safety and effectiveness, as safety of IVDs is not generally related to contact between IVDs and patients
    - Safety of IVD relates to impact of device's performance (i.e., impact of false-negative and false-positive results on patient's health)
  - Generally includes complete record of nonclinical and clinical studies performed and information on how IVD is designed and manufactured
    - Nonclinical studies demonstrate that IVD can accurately and reproducibly measure analytes under controlled conditions
    - Clinical studies are testing performed on specimens from users who meet predefined enrollment criteria
  - FDA reviews PMA application in 180-day timeline
    - FDA will approve it if application provides sufficient valid scientific evidence demonstrating that IVD is safe and effective for its intended use(s)

- Approval requires review of manufacturing processes, inspection of manufacturing facility, bioresearch-monitoring audit of clinical data sites, and comprehensive review of premarket data
- If FDA finds that IVD is safe and effective
  - Sponsor will receive official approval order for marketing IVD in USA
- Suppose PMA application has yet to address scientific issues
  - In that case, FDA can ask for additional information and put it temporarily on hold
- Suppose IVD is first of its kind or presents unusual safety and effectiveness issues
  - In that case, FDA will generally seek decision-making advice from outside experts appointed to FDA's Advisory Committee
- Class III device failing to meet PMA requirements is considered to be adulterated under section 501(f) of FD&C Act and cannot be marketed

- 510(k) submission
  - To market class I-III IVD intended for human use but not subject to PMA, sponsor can submit 510(k) to FDA, demonstrating that IVD is as safe and effective as legally marketed IVD [i.e., substantially equivalent (SE)], unless IVD is exempt from 510(k) requirements of FD&C Act, and does not exceed limitations of exemptions detailed in 21 CFR
    - Review of 510(k) is based on evaluation of analytic performance characteristics of new IVD compared to legally marketed IVD, including
      - Accuracy, precision, and analytical specificity and sensitivity of new IVD
    - Legally marketed IVDs [21 CFR 807.92 (a) (3)] are
      - IVDs legally marketed before May 28, 1976 (preamendments IVD)
      - Or IVD that has been reclassified from class III to class II or class I (predicate)
      - Or IVD recently cleared under 510(k)
    - IVD is SE, as compared to legally marketed IVD if it has
      - Same intended use **and**
      - Same technological characteristics, **or**
      - Differences in technological characteristics that do not raise different questions regarding safety and effectiveness; **and**
      - Information submitted to FDA, demonstrating that IVD is at least as safe and effective as legally marketed IVD
    - Studies required to demonstrate SE include
      - Analytical studies using clinical samples (most cases) or carefully selected artificial samples (some cases)
      - Clinical information required for IVDs that have no clearly defined link between analytical and clinical performances
      - FDA rarely requires prospective clinical studies for IVDs but regularly requests clinical samples with sufficient laboratory &/or clinical characterization to allow assessment of clinical validity of new IVD
    - Before marketing IVD, each sponsor must receive SE decision letter from FDA stating that IVD can be marketed in USA
    - FDA does not perform 510(k) preclearance facility inspections, but sponsor should be ready for FDA quality system inspection at any time after 510(k) clearance
    - If there are unaddressed scientific issues, FDA can ask for additional information and put submission temporarily on hold
    - If FDA determines that IVD is not SE, another submission [e.g., 510(k) with new data, De Novo petition, PMA, or HDE] is required
  - 3 types of 510(k) programs
    - Traditional
      - Can be used for any IVD that needs 510(k)
      - Relies on demonstration of SE
    - Special
      - Can only be used if certain criteria are met
      - Intended to facilitate submission, review, and clearance of change to manufacturer's own legally marketed IVD
    - Abbreviated
      - Can only be used if certain criteria are met
      - Relies on use of guidance documents, special controls, &/or voluntary consensus standards
  - FDA reviews traditional and abbreviated 510(k) submissions in 90-day timeline
  - FDA reviews special 510(k) submissions in 30-day timeline

- IDE submission
  - Allows investigational IVD to be used in clinical study to collect safety and effectiveness data
    - Clinical studies are conducted to support PMAs and small percentage of 510(k) applications
    - Approved IDE permits IVD to be shipped lawfully for purposes of conducting investigations without complying with other requirements of FD&C Act
    - Sponsors do not need to submit PMA or 510(k), register their establishment, or list IVD while IVD is under investigation
    - Sponsors are also exempt from QSR, except for requirements for design controls
  - 3 types of studies
    - Significant risk (SR) studies must follow 21 CFR 812, and have IDE application approved by FDA before it may proceed
    - Non-SR studies must follow abbreviated requirement [21 CFR 50, 56, 812.2(b), and 812.5] and do not have to have IDE application approved by FDA
    - Studies exempt from 21 CFR 812 may or may not be exempt from requirements for IRB approval and obtaining informed consent
  - FDA may approve, approve with modification, or disapprove IDE application
  - FDA reviews IDE in 30-day timeline

- De Novo request
  - Provides pathway for new types of IVDs with low to moderate risk to obtain marketing authorization as class I or class II IVDs based on reasonable assurance of safety and effectiveness but not SE
    - Requester first submits De Novo request for IVD to FDA according to statutory criteria (21 CFR 860.220)

FDA Regulations

- FDA then completes classification determination for De Novo IVD by issuance of written order within 150 FDA days
- FDA will grant De Novo request for IVD [21 CFR 860.260 (a)] if requester can demonstrate that IVD meets criteria outlined in section 513(a)(1)(A) or (B) of FD&C Act
  - Allows IVD to be marketed immediately
  - Creates classification regulation and special controls (if class II) for new IVD type
  - Permits De Novo IVD to serve as predicate for future 510(k) submissions
- If FDA declines De Novo request [21 CFR 860.260(c)], IVD remains in class III and may not be marketed, unless
  - IVD is found SE to existing legally marketed class I, class II, or preamendments IVD, IVD is reclassified under section 513(f)(3) of FD&C Act, PMA is approved, or new De Novo request is granted
- FDA will also consider De Novo request to be withdrawn in certain situations [21 CFR 860.250(a)(1)]
- HUD submission
  - IVDs intended to benefit patients in diagnosis of diseases or conditions that affect or are manifested in ≤ 8,000 individuals in USA per year (Section 3052 of Cures Act)
  - Marketing approval for HUD involves 2 steps
    - Submit HUD designation request and obtain approval from FDA's Office of Orphan Products Development (45-day timeline)
    - Submit HDE application to CDRH or CBER after HUD designation is granted
  - HUD approved for marketing under HDE has specific labeling requirements
    - HDE is premarketing application for HUD submitted to FDA (21 CFR 814 Subpart A)
      - Similar in both form and content to PMA application, but exempt from effectiveness requirements of PMA (sections 514 and 515 of FD&C Act)
      - Subject to certain profit and use restrictions
      - No comparable legally marketed IVD is available to diagnose same disease or condition
      - Should be approved by IRB or appropriate local committee with exception of emergency use
    - FDA actions: Approval letter, approvable letter pending resolution of minor deficiencies, major deficiency letter, not approvable letter, denial letter, and acknowledgement of voluntary withdrawal
    - FDA reviews HDE application in 75-day timeline
- Class I/II exemptions
  - 510(k) exemptions
    - Most class I and some class II IVDs are exempt from 510(k), subject to certain limitations on exemption
      - Do not require FDA review before marketed
      - Not required to provide reasonable assurance of safety and effectiveness
      - Most low-risk IVDs
    - Devices exempt from 510 (k):
      - Preamendments IVDs that have not been significantly changed or modified
      - Class I IVDs specifically exempted by FDA regulation or classified as class I under section 513 (with certain exceptions)
      - Class II IVDs specifically exempted by FDA regulation
    - Class I/II exempt IVDs from 510(k) are still needed to meet other requirements for marketing, such as
      - Suitability for intended use
      - Adequately packaged and properly labeled
      - Establishment registration and device listing forms on file with FDA
      - Manufactured under quality system
      - With exception of small number of class I devices that are subject only to complaint files and general record-keeping requirements
  - QSR/GMP exemptions
    - All IVDs are subject to QSR, including "GMP" unless there is exception or exemption noted in 21 CFR 820
  - Cures Act exemptions
    - Section 3054 of Cures Act amended section 510(l) and 510(m) of FD&C Act
      - Requires FDA to identify and determine any class I and class II IVDs that can be exempted from 510(k) requirements within certain timeframe and through publication in federal register notice
- Class I IVDs without exemption (reserved devices)
  - Meet reserved criteria in section 206 of FDAMA
  - Remain subject to premarket notification under new section 510(I) added to FD&C Act
  - May be intended for use of substantial importance in preventing impairment of human health or presenting potential unreasonable risk of illness or injury
- BLA submission
  - Request for permission to introduce, or deliver for introduction, biological product into interstate commerce (21 CFR 601.2)
    - Licensing IVD through BLA is very similar to approval process for other new human biologics
    - Sponsor who intends to conduct clinical investigation should submit IND to CBER for review and approval (21 CFR 312.23)
    - If data from Chemistry, Manufacturing and Controls, and nonclinical and clinical studies demonstrate that IVD is safe and effective for intended use, data can be submitted to CBER as part of BLA for approval for marketing
- Companion diagnostic (CDx)
  - Can be IVD or image tool that provides information essential for safe and effective use of corresponding drug or biologic product
  - Therapeutic product and its corresponding CDx are codeveloped contemporaneously or separately
  - FDA reviews CDx and therapeutic product collaboratively among relevant FDA centers
    - CDRH: Uses risk-based approach to determine regulatory pathway for CDx as defined in section 201(h) of FD&C Act
    - CBER: Reviews and approves for biological therapeutic products under section 351 of PHS Act

FDA Regulations

- Center for Drug Evaluation and Research: Reviews and approves for drug therapeutic products under section 505 of FD&C Act
- Breakthrough Devices Program
  - Voluntary program for certain IVDs and IVD-led combination products that provide for more effective diagnosis of life-threatening or irreversibly debilitating diseases or conditions
  - IVDs subject to PMA, 510(k) or request for De Novo designation are eligible for this program if IVDs meet designation criteria
  - Not only speeds up development, assessment, and review of IVDs, but also preserves statutory standards for PMA, 510(k) clearance and De Novo marketing authorization
- Emergency use authorizations (EUAs) for IVDs
  - HHS secretary must first make declaration that public health emergency exists under section 319 of PHS Act, justifying authorization of emergency use for IVD
  - HHS secretary also must issue EUA declarations under section 564 of FD&C Act to enable issuance of EUAs
    - EUA authority allows FDA to help strengthen nation's public health protections against chemical, biological, radiological, and nuclear threats
      - FDA can issue EUA to allow use of unapproved or uncleared IVDs to diagnose serious or life-threatening diseases when certain statutory criteria for issuance are met
      - Declaration generally lasts for 90 days but HHS secretary may extend it every 3 months until terminating it

REGULATIONS OF LABORATORY DEVELOPED TESTS

History of Laboratory Developed Test Regulations

- CLIA of 1967 provided first attempt to regulate laboratories by federal government
- Under MDA '76, FDA
  - First obtained comprehensive authority to regulate all IVDs as devices, including LDTs
  - Exercised enforcement discretion for LDTs
  - Did not provide assurance of analytic and clinical validity for test results
- Under CLIA '88, CMS regulates all LDTs (except research) performed on human specimens to ensure accurate and reliable test results in USA
  - Regulations established 3 categories of laboratory testing based on complexity of testing methodology
    - Waived tests and tests of moderate and high complexities
  - CLIA '88 mainly regulates operations of laboratories but not specifically LDTs
- FDA has had authority to implement CLIA test complexity categorization provisions since 2003
  - Interprets CLIA provisions related to complexity categorization
  - Holds public workshops and meetings on CLIA complexity
  - Develops and issues implementing rules and guidance for CLIA complexing categorization
- Current status in LDT oversight by FDA
  - LDTs have evolved and proliferated dramatically due to advances in technology and business models
  - Certain LDTs are now more complex, used in various USA facilities, and exhibit high risks (e.g., detection of risk for breast cancers and Alzheimer diseases)
  - FDA has identified some problems with several high-risk LDTs
    - Claims that are not adequately supported with evidence
    - Lack of appropriate controls yielding erroneous results
    - Falsification of data
  - FDA reconsidered its policy of enforcement discretion for LDTs to avoid patients being exposed to inappropriate therapies due to using faulty LDTs (2010)
    - FDA published draft guidance document entitled "Framework for Regulatory Oversight of Laboratory Developed Tests (LDTs)" (2014)
    - FDA also issued discussion paper on LDTs (2017) with hope that it can advance public discussion on future LDT oversight

Clinical Laboratory Improvement Amendment Regulations and Guidelines Pertaining to Laboratory Developed Tests

- CLIA regulations
  - Standards and Certification: Laboratory Requirements (42 CFR 493)
  - Established quality standards for laboratory testing performed on human specimens for purpose of diagnosis, prevention, or treatment of disease, or assessment of health
- CLIA interpretive guidelines to CLIA regulations
  - Published in CMS State Operations Manual (SOM)
  - State offices use SOM to administer various federal programs (e.g., clinical laboratory certification under CLIA regulations and enforced by CMS)
  - SOM is also source of guidance to laboratories for interpreting CLIA regulations

Clinical Laboratory Improvement Amendment Program

- CDC, CMS, and FDA within HHS support national CLIA program and clinical laboratory quality
  - CDC
    - Provides analysis, research, and technical assistance
    - Develops technical standards and laboratory practice guidelines
    - Conducts laboratory quality improvement studies
    - Monitors proficiency testing (PT) practices
    - Develops and distributes professional information and educational resources
    - Manages CLIA Advisory Committee
  - CMS
    - Issues laboratory certificates and collects user fees
    - Conducts inspections and enforces regulatory compliance
    - Approves private accreditation organizations for performing inspections and state exemptions
    - Monitors laboratory performance on PT, approves PT programs, and publishes CLIA rules and regulations
  - FDA

FDA Regulations

- Categorizes tests based on complexity
- Reviews requests for CLIA waiver by application
- Develops rules and guidance for CLIA complexity categorization

Regulatory Landscape for Laboratory Developed Tests

- CLIA currently covers ~ 320,000 laboratory entities
  - Laboratory should obtain specific type of CLIA certificate depending upon complexity of tests it will perform
    - Waive tests
      - e.g., fecal occult blood-non-automated [42 CFR 493.15(c)]
    - Tests of moderate complexity (42 CFR 493.17)
      - e.g., provider-performed microscopy procedure for fecal leukocyte examination
    - Tests of high complexity (42 CFR 493.17)
      - e.g., molecular test for detecting DNA variations to diagnose genetic disease
  - Laboratories only performing waived tests
    - Must have CLIA certificate and follow manufacturer's instructions
  - Laboratories performing moderate- or high-complexity testing or both
    - Must have CLIA certificate and be inspected
    - Must meet CLIA quality standards outlined in 42 CFR 493 subparts H, J, K, and M
    - Regulatory requirements between moderate- and high-complexity testing differ mainly in standards for quality control and personnel
  - Laboratory may perform 1 or any combination of 3 categorized tests
    - More complex test to be performed, more stringent requirements are
  - CLIA and its implementing regulations do not affect FDA's authority under FD&C Act to regulate LDTs or other IVDs used by laboratories

Centers for Medicaid and Medicare Services and FDA Regulatory Schemes for Laboratory Developed Tests

- Different in focus, scope, and purpose but complementary
  - CMS regulates laboratories that perform LDTs to ensure accurate and reliable test results in USA through CLIA '88
    - CLIA prohibits release of any LDT results before laboratory establishes specific performance characteristics relating to analytical validity for use of this LDT on its site
      - Analytical validation is limited to specific conditions, staff, equipment, and patient population of laboratory, so findings of this laboratory-specific analytic validation are not meaningful outside laboratory that performed analysis
      - Laboratory's analytical validation of LDTs is reviewed during its routine biennial survey after laboratory has already started testing
    - CLIA requirements for LDTs address laboratory's testing process (i.e., ability to perform LDTs in accurate and reliable manner)
    - CLIA program does not address clinical validity of any LDT
    - CLIA program alone may not ensure that LDTs are appropriately designed, consistently manufactured, and safe and effective for patients or users
  - FDA regulates manufacturers and IVDs to ensure that IVDs are reasonably safe and effective under FD&C Act or PHS Act
    - FDA reviews analytical validity before marketing testing system and, thus, before use of IVD on patient specimens in clinical diagnosis and treatment context
    - FDA assesses analytical validity of IVD in greater depth and scope through its premarket clearance or approval processes
    - FDA evaluates clinical validity of IVD as part of review that is focused on safety and effectiveness of IVD

SELECTED REFERENCES

1. CLIA, CMS, HHS. https://www.cms.gov/regulations-and-guidance/legislation/clia. Updated January 23, 2023. Accessed July 12, 2023
2. IVDs regulated by CBER, FDA, HHS. https://www.fda.gov/vaccines-blood-biologics/blood-blood-products. Updated March 7, 2023. July 12, 2023
3. CLIA, CDC, HHS. https://www.cdc.gov/clia/law-regulations.html. Updated November 14, 2022. Accessed July 12, 2023
4. De Novo Classification Request, FDA, HHS. https://www.fda.gov/medical-devices/premarket-submissions-selecting-and-preparing-correct-submission/de-novo-classification-request. Updated October 4, 2022. Assessed July 12, 2023
5. Premarket Notification 510 (k), FDA. HHS. https://www.fda.gov/medical-devices/premarket-submissions-selecting-and-preparing-correct-submission/premarket-notification-510k. Updated October 3, 2022. Accessed July 12, 2023
6. CLIA, FDA, HHS. https://www.fda.gov/medical-devices/ivd-regulatory-asssitance/clinical-laboratory-improvement-amendments-clia. Updated September 13, 2021. Accessed July 12, 2023
7. Guidance for Industry and Food and Drug Administration Staff: Requests for Feedback and Meetings for Medical Device Submissions: The Q-Submission Program, 2021
8. Overview of IVD Regulation, FDA, HHS. https://www.fda.gov/medical-devices/ivd-regulatory-assistance/overview-ivd-regulation. Updated October 18, 2021. Accessed July 12, 2023
9. Premarket Approval (PMA), FDA, HHS. https://www.fda.gov/medical-devices/premarket-submissions-selecting-and-preparing-correct-submission/premarket-approval-pma. Updated May 16, 2019. Accessed July 12, 2023
10. FD&C Act, FDA Regulations, and FDA Guidance. https://www.fda.gov/about-fda/fda-basics/what-difference-between-federal-food-drug-and-cosmetic-act-fdc-act-fda-regulation-fda-guidance. Updated March 29, 2018. Accessed July 12, 2023
11. LDTs, FDA, HHS. https://www.fda.gov/medical-devices/in-vitro-diagnostics/laboratory-developed-tests. Updated September 27, 2018. Accessed July 12, 2023
12. Guidance for Industry and FDA Staff: In Vitro Diagnostic (IVD) Device Studies -Frequently Asked Questions (June 25, 2010)

Proficiency Testing and Accreditation

TERMINOLOGY
Abbreviations
- Proficiency testing (PT)
- Clinical Laboratory Improvements Amendments (CLIA)
- Centers for Medicare and Medicaid Services (CMS)
- U.S. Department of Health and Human Services (HHS)
- College of American Pathologists (CAP)

FEDERAL REGULATIONS
Clinical Laboratory Improvements Amendments
- Law passed by Congress in 1988 for certification and oversight of clinical laboratory testing

ACCREDITATION
Overview
- Accreditation: Determination that lab has successfully met standards set by accreditation organization
- Laboratories performing testing for clinical purposes in USA must have CLIA certificate issued by CMS
- Laboratories can be accredited by another organization that is approved by CMS
    - In order to be approved by CMS, accreditation organization must meet or exceed standards of CLIA
    - List of approved accreditation organizations under CLIA
        - CAP
        - Joint Commission (JC)
        - American Association for Laboratory Accreditation (A2LA)
        - Association for Advancement of Blood and Biotherapies (AABB)
        - Accreditation Commission for Health Care (ACHC)
        - American Society for Histocompatibility and Immunogenetics (ASHI)
        - Commission on Office Laboratory Accreditation (COLA)
- Laboratories are required to meet quality laboratory standards set by CLIA

COLLEGE OF AMERICAN PATHOLOGY ACCREDITATION
Programs
- CAP has multiple accreditation programs
- Laboratory accreditation program (LAP) is most common
    - Covers broad spectrum of disciplines, including molecular
- CAP 15189 is special voluntary nonregulated accreditation program
    - Based on ISO 15189:2012 standard published by International Organization for Standardization
    - Aims to reduce risk, optimize performance, and lower costs
    - Provides proof of integrated quality management system throughout organization

Laboratory Director and Core standards
- Core principles of CAP accreditation program ensure that accredited laboratories meet needs of patients, physicians, and other health care practitioners
- 4 main standards relating to laboratory director, physical resources, quality management, and administrative requirements
- Qualifications of laboratory director
    - Qualifications include academic degree, license to practice medicine, training and certification
    - Qualifications required depend on complexity of testing performed
    - For high-complexity testing, director must have any of following qualifications
        - MD, DO, or DPM licensed to practice (if required) in jurisdiction where laboratory is located, and have one of following
            - Certification in anatomic or clinical pathology, or both, by American Board of Pathology or American Osteopathic Board of Pathology, or possess qualifications equivalent to those required for certification
            - MD, DO, or DPM with active license and 1 year of laboratory training during residency or 2 years of experience supervising high-complexity testing
            - Have at least 2 years of experience supervising high-complexity testing
        - Doctoral degree in chemical, physical, biological, or clinical laboratory science from accredited institution, and have current certification by board approved by HHS
    - For moderate-complexity testing, director must have any of following qualifications
        - Qualify for high-complexity testing
        - MD, DO, or DPM, licensed to practice in jurisdiction where laboratory is located (if required) and have one of following
            - At least 20 hours of continuing medical education credit hours in laboratory medicine
            - Equivalent training during medical residency/fellowship
            - At least 1 year of experience supervising nonwaived laboratory testing
        - Doctoral degree in chemical, physical, biological, or clinical laboratory science from accredited institution with one of following
            - At least 1 year of experience supervising nonwaived laboratory testing
            - Current certification by board approved by HHS
    - For waived testing with annual volume not exceeding 500,000 tests, director must have any of following qualifications
        - MD, DO, or DPM, licensed to practice in jurisdiction in which laboratory is located
        - Doctoral degree in chemical, physical, biological, or clinical laboratory science from accredited institution
- Responsibilities of laboratory director
    - Given enough authority to match his/her responsibility
    - Provide consultations as needed for clinicians regarding test ordering and interpretation
    - Laboratory personnel
        - Ensures number of personnel is sufficient
        - Ensures adequate education and training of personnel
        - Ensures personnel work in safe environment
    - Delegation of functions

Proficiency Testing and Accreditation

- Lab director can delegate some of his/her functions to other personnel
  - Must ensure that persons performing these functions are qualified to do so
  - Must follow-up that these functions have been carried out properly
  - Must be in writing
- Following functions cannot be delegated
  - Initial approval of new procedures, policies, individualized quality control plans (IQCPs), and subsequent significant changes
  - Periodic on-site visits to ensure physical and environmental safety and adequacy of staffing
  - Ensuring supervisory and technical staff are appropriately trained and their responsibilities are identified
- Approval of laboratory policies and procedures
  - Should be completed within 3 months of change of directorship
  - Must be documented with signature and date
- Cannot direct > 5 laboratories

Other Standards

- **Physical resources of laboratory**
  - Adequate space that does not compromise quality of work or safety of personnel
  - Adequate working environment
    - Adequate lighting, ventilation, electricity, and water
    - Controlled room temperature and humidity
    - Minimized exposure to direct sunlight
  - Safe working environment
    - Policies regarding safety, accidents, and occupational injuries
    - Disaster preparedness
    - Protection against blood-borne pathogens
    - Fire prevention and protection
    - Electrical and chemical safety
    - Proper storage of hazardous material
  - Well-maintained instrumentation
- **Quality management**
  - Must ensure continuous monitoring and evaluation of quality within laboratory
  - Monitoring of quality indicators that cover preanalytic, analytic, and postanalytic steps of testing
  - Laboratory director is responsible for making sure program is implemented across all sections of lab
  - Lab must have procedure to encourage employees to communicate any concerns or complaints about quality to proper authorities
- **Administrative requirements**
  - Complying with requirements specified in standards, terms of accreditation, and checklists

College of American Pathology Commissioners

- Pathologists who volunteer to work with CAP to implement its accreditation program
- Regional commissioners are responsible for accreditation activities of specified group of laboratories, timely assignment of inspectors, review of inspection findings and presentation of them to accreditation committee
- State commissioners assist regional commissioners
  - Validate proposed inspectors match for laboratories in their geographic regions
  - Available to provide guidance for team leaders

College of American Pathology Inspections

- On-site surveys to determine whether laboratory has fulfilled and maintained standards of LAP
- Inspections are performed by team of active laboratorians
  - Leader of team is usually pathologist
  - Majority of inspectors are volunteers who have expertise in section of laboratory they are inspecting
    - Laboratories accredited by CAP are required to provide team of volunteer inspectors to inspect similar-sized lab 1x every 2 years
  - Inspectors of certain areas of laboratory (e.g., flow cytometry, molecular) must be approved by CAP prior to participation in inspection
  - Professional inspectors employed by CAP also participate in inspections
  - Inspectors must complete online training course
- Multiple types of inspections
  - Initial inspection
    - 1st time laboratory gets inspected by CAP to determine whether or not accreditation will be granted
    - Inspection is announced
  - Routine inspection
    - Performed every 2 years after initial inspection to ensure continuous adherence of laboratory to CAP standards
    - Inspection is unannounced (hospital-based labs) or with short notice of 14 days (nonhospital-based labs)
  - Nonroutine inspection
    - Inspection performed in addition to routine inspection
    - Performed for variety of reasons
      - Change in location, director, or ownership of laboratory
      - Added discipline, usually anatomic pathology, cytology, or histocompatibility
      - Secondary on-site inspection usually requested by regional commissioner if profound deficiencies found on routine inspection
      - Repeated noncompliance with proficiency testing performance standards
      - Complaint against laboratory
    - May be announced or unannounced
    - May include professional CAP inspectors
  - Self-inspection
    - Laboratories accredited by CAP are required to perform self-inspection in year between on-site inspections
    - Laboratory must document findings from self-inspection and corrective actions taken

College of American Pathologists Checklists

- Detailed lists of requirements that inspector uses to determine whether laboratory meets required standards
- Each discipline of laboratory has its own checklist along with common checklist
- Laboratories enrolled in CAP accreditation program receive customized checklists

Proficiency Testing and Accreditation

- o Lab provides information about its scope of testing and lists all reportable assays
  - Sum of this information for each particular section of lab is called activity menu
  - Lab must ensure that its activity menu is up to date and reflects tests being done by that lab
  - If, at time of inspection, inspector notices discrepancy between activity menu and tests offered, deficiency will be cited
    - □ If this discrepancy causes significant mismatch between checklist and tests offered by lab, nonroutine inspection might follow
  - o Checklist is customized to meet each lab's accreditation needs based on its activity menu
- CAP periodically reviews checklist and issues new checklist versions
  - o CAP sends new checklist to lab before each on-site inspection and during self-inspection year
  - o Inspectors use same checklist version that was sent to lab by CAP, even if newer version of checklist is available

Deficiencies

- Noncompliance with requirement of accreditation checklist
- Deficiencies are cited at time of inspection, when inspector makes assessment that lab is noncompliant
  - o If laboratory is compliant but there is room for improvement, inspector might issue recommendation instead of citing deficiency
    - Laboratory is not obligated to respond to or implement recommendation
    - Recommendation that should have been cited as deficiency will be changed to deficiency by CAP staff or regional commissioner
- 2 types of deficiencies
  - o Phase 1
    - Compromises quality but does not endanger health and safety of patients and personnel
    - Correction and written response to CAP is required
  - o Phase 2
    - May have serious impact on quality or may endanger health or safety of patients or personnel
    - Lab must provide plan of action to correct deficiency and supporting documentation that plan has been implemented
- Lab must respond to deficiencies within 30 days
- Lab can challenge deficiency if it disagrees with it
  - o Lab should clearly indicate on response form its intent to challenge deficiency
  - o Lab should provide documentation showing it was in compliance prior to inspection
  - o If challenge is accepted by regional commissioner, deficiency will be removed and will not appear in permanent record
- Deficiencies can be corrected on-site during inspection
  - o Only applies to minor corrections
    - e.g., editing procedure to match current practice that is already compliant, or signing 1 or 2 procedures
  - o Inspector will cite deficiency and indicate it was corrected on-site
  - o Deficiency will remain on lab's permanent record
- o CAP might request additional documentation to indicate how deficiency was corrected on site

Probation

- Accreditation status assigned by accreditation committee for any of following reasons
  - o Documentation is insufficient to determine compliance
  - o Accreditation committee wants to monitor progress of deficiency correction by laboratory
  - o Laboratory engaged in conduct contrary to CAP policies but not significant enough to warrant revocation of accreditation
- Laboratory is allowed to continue testing as accredited laboratory during probation
- Agencies accepting CAP accreditation, such as CMS and JC, are notified of probation
- Lab may undergo nonroutine inspection to determine if conditions leading to probation have been corrected
- Laboratory that is on probation will remain on probation until accreditation committee revokes or denies accreditation or removes probation and accredits laboratory

Probation With Immediate Jeopardy

- Accreditation status assigned to laboratory when circumstances are identified that necessitate immediate corrective action
  - o These circumstances caused, are causing, or are likely to cause serious injury, harm, or death to individuals served by laboratory, laboratory workers, or visitors
- This status is reported to CMS and regulatory partners within 10 days

Probation With Suspension

- In addition to accreditation status of probation, laboratory or sections of it that are suspended might not perform testing as accredited laboratory
- Might lose accreditation if it fails to address issues that lead to suspension within 45 days

Denial or Revocation of Accreditation

- Laboratory is denied accreditation if it fails to meet any standards of accreditation program and is unable to correct this within time allowed
  - o e.g., laboratory is cited for numerous significant deficiencies after inspection, which cannot be corrected within reasonable period of time

PROFICIENCY TESTING

Definition

- Testing of unknown samples sent to laboratory by CMS-approved PT program to determine laboratory testing performance by means of interlaboratory comparisons

Clinical Laboratory Improvements Amendment Regulations

- CMS requires labs conducting moderate- and high-complexity testing (nonwaived testing) to participate in PT for certain analytes
  - o These analytes are listed in Subpart I (Proficiency Testing Programs for Nonwaived Testing) of CLIA regulations
  - o These analytes are called **regulated analytes**

Proficiency Testing and Accreditation

- While PT is not required for unregulated analytes, CLIA requires that labs verify accuracy of testing at least 2x annually
- CMS-approved PT programs
  - List of CMS-approved PT providers is available on CMS website (www.cms.hhs.gov/clia)
  - CMS annually evaluates PT providers and updates list
- CMS-approved PT program sends laboratory set of unknown samples ~ 3x per year
  - Laboratory tests these specimens in manner similar to way it tests patient specimens
    - PT sample must never be sent out of laboratory for any reason even if lab routinely sends out patient samples for confirmation
  - Results of testing are reported back to PT provider before certain deadline
  - PT provider grades results according to CLIA grading criteria and sends laboratory back its scores
  - Laboratory performance in PT impacts its accreditation status and type of tests it is allowed to do
- While CLIA does not require PT for waived tests, accreditation organization might have more strict requirements
- PT enrollment per analyte is required for each CLIA certificate (i.e., if lab performs testing for same analyte at multiple sites under 1 CLIA certificate, it should only enroll 1x and not for each site)
- Sending PT sample to another laboratory for testing is considered PT referral and will result in serious consequences, such as
  - Loss of laboratory's CLIA certificate for at least 1 year
  - Director cannot direct laboratory for 2 years
  - Laboratory owner may not own or operate laboratory for 2 years
- If analyte is tested using 2 different test systems under same CLIA certificate, PT testing is required for only 1 test system that is considered primary method for patient testing during PT event

College of American Pathology Proficiency Testing

- CAP requires participation in PT for most tests for which laboratory reports patient results
  - CAP maintains list of all analytes for which it requires PT on its website, which is more than what is required by CMS
- CAP-accepted PT providers
  - CAP does not accept all CMS-approved PT providers
  - CAP accepts PT providers on analyte-by-analyte basis
    - Each PT provider maintains list of accepted analytes
- PT challenges
  - Specimens are sent out in cycles throughout year, mostly 3x each year by PT provider
    - In most cases, 5 challenges per analyte per cycle
    - In general, labs must get at least 4 out of 5 correct (80%) or challenge will be considered unsatisfactory
  - Laboratory must treat PT specimen exactly as it treats patient samples
  - Testing should be run by same personnel that run patient specimens
    - Lab director or designee and person who performed testing must **physically sign** attestation form
    - Listing of typed names of personnel who performed test **is not** enough
  - Laboratory must send results back before deadline
- Alternative assessment
  - Determination of laboratory testing performance by means other than participation in CAP-approved PT program
  - Required when PT is not available for particular laboratory test (e.g., PT program is oversubscribed) or PT was available but could not be scored for various reasons
  - Lab director determines appropriate alternative assessment
  - Examples of alternative assessment
    - Participation in ungraded/education PT program
    - Split sample analysis with another lab or within same lab using different method
    - Clinical validation by reviewing patient chart and ensuring that lab results are consistent with clinical presentation
- PT failure
  - PT score < 80% in particular challenge, failure to submit results by deadline, or failure to enroll in PT
  - Failing 1 PT is called unsatisfactory performance
    - Lab must investigate cause, take corrective action, and determine whether patient results were affected
  - Failing PT for specific analyte or for specific specialty in 2 consecutive cycles or in 2 out of 3 cycles is called unsuccessful performance
    - If this happens for 1st time, CMS might permit technical assistance or retraining
    - If this is repeated occurrence for certain analyte or specialty, CMS will require lab to cease testing for that analyte or specialty
  - Cease testing
    - Laboratory is required to immediately discontinue testing
    - Medicare and Medicaid reimbursement will be suspended for 6-month period
    - Laboratory must identify and correct reasons of unsuccessful performance
    - Laboratory must perform 2 consecutive PT events successfully prior to resume testing

Proficiency Testing Material Referral

- CAP requires labs to have PT policy that specifically states that referral of PT material is prohibited

SELECTED REFERENCES

1. CLIA Approved PT Programs. http://www.cms.gov/Regulations-and-Guidance/Legislation/CLIA/Downloads/ptlist.pdf. Updated April 2019. Accessed April 2019
2. CLIA Proficiency Testing and PT Referral. http://www.cms.gov/Regulations-and-Guidance/Legislation/CLIA/downloads/cliabrochure8.pdf. Published September 2017. Accessed April 2019
3. CLIA Regulations. http://www.cms.hhs.gov/clia. Updated April 2019. Accessed April 2019
4. Ford A: New push to strengthen interim self inspections. CAP Today. 27(1): 5-8, 2013
5. Clinical laboratory improvement amendments of 1988; final rule. Fed Register. 42CFR493.1236(a)(2): 3075, 2003
6. Clinical laboratory improvement amendments of 1988; final rule. Fed Register. 42CFR493.1289, 2003
7. Bierig JR: Comparing PT results can put a lab's CLIA license on the line. Northfield. CAP Today. 16(2): 84-7, 2002

INDEX

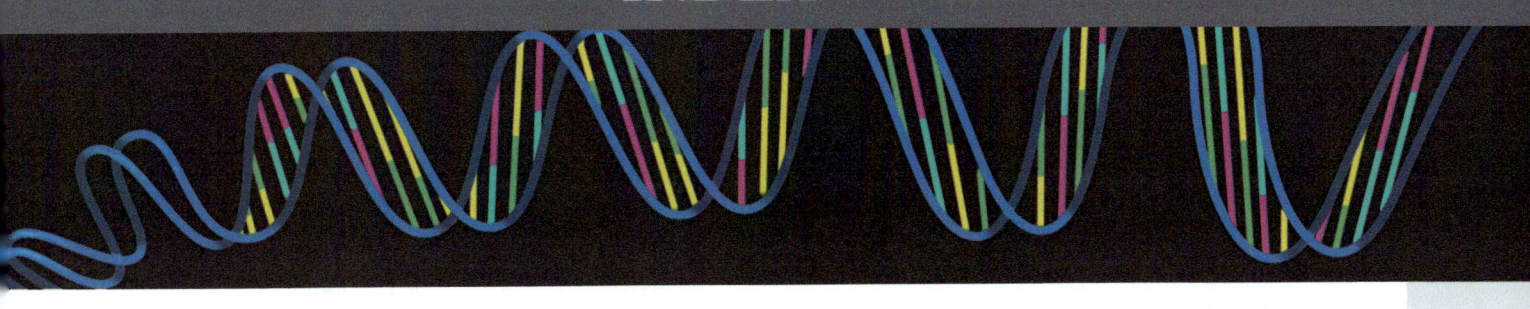

A

Aberrant *MET* signaling, **110–111**
ABL class alterations, **307**
ABL1 fusions, B-lymphoblastic leukemia/lymphoma, *BCR::ABL1*-like (Ph-like ALL), **308**
ABL1 gene, **124**
- chronic myeloid leukemia, *BCR::ABL1*-positive, **137**
- normal function, **42–43**

ABL1 kinase domain, mutations, **44**
ABL2 fusion partners, B-lymphoblastic leukemia/lymphoma, *BCR::ABL1*-like (Ph-like ALL), **308**
ACA. *See* Adrenal cortical adenoma.
ACC. *See* Adrenal cortical carcinoma.
Accreditation, **966–969**
- CAP, **966–968**
    - checklists, **967–968**
    - commissioners, **967**
    - deficiencies, **968**
    - denial or revocation, **968**
    - inspections, **967**
    - probation, **968**
    - programs, **966**
    - standards, **966–967**

Acinar adenocarcinoma, **685**
Acinic cell carcinoma, **509**
- clinicopathologic features, **513**
- differential diagnosis, **512**
- gene expression profiling, **511**
- molecular alterations, **513**
- molecular genetics, **510–511**
- pancreatic ductal adenocarcinoma vs., **616**
- prognosis, **509**
- secretory carcinoma vs., **512**
- in situ hybridization, **510**

Acquired aplastic anemia, pediatric myelodysplastic syndrome and refractory cytopenia of childhood vs., **211–212**
Acquired bone marrow failure disorders, pediatric myelodysplastic syndrome and refractory cytopenia of childhood vs., **212**
Acquired sideroblastic anemias, myelodysplastic syndrome with mutated *SF3B1* vs., **190**
Acral lentiginous melanoma, **789, 790**
Actinic keratosis
- basal cell carcinoma of skin vs., **798**
- cytogenetics, **785**
- differential diagnosis, **786**
- molecular genetics, **785**

Acute basophilic leukemia, **272**
Acute erythroid leukemia, **272**
- myelodysplastic syndrome with *TP53* multihit mutations vs., **205**

Acute leukemia
- blastic plasmacytoid dendritic cell neoplasm vs., **286**
- mixed phenotype, myeloid sarcoma vs., **278**

Acute lymphoblastic leukemia
- acute myeloid leukemia, NOS vs., **273**
- chronic eosinophilic leukemia, NOS vs., **161**

Acute lymphocytic leukemia, blastic plasmacytoid dendritic cell neoplasm vs., **286**
Acute megakaryoblastic leukemia, **272**
- non-Down syndrome-associated, acute myeloid leukemia with t(1;22)/*RBM15::MRTFA* vs., **263**

Acute monocytic leukemia, **272**
- acute promyelocytic leukemia with t(15;17)/*PML::RARA* vs., **251**

Acute myelogenous leukemia. *See* Acute myeloid leukemia.
Acute myeloid leukemia (AML), **232–239**
- with alternative *MECOM* translocations, acute myeloid leukemia with inv(3) or t(3;3)/*GATA2*; *MECOM*, **261**
- with *BCR::ABL1*, **43, 232, 236**
    - chronic myeloid leukemia, *BCR::ABL1*-positive vs., **139**
- biological categories of mutations, **70**
- blastic plasmacytoid dendritic cell neoplasm vs., **286**
- with *CBFB::MYH11* fusion, **236**
- with *CEBPA* mutation, **233, 236**
- chromosomal microarray, **24**
- common genetic mutations and approximate frequencies in, **273**
- conventional, myeloid proliferations associated with Down syndrome vs., **282**
- core-binding factor, **65–66**
- cytogenetics, **234**
- de novo, mutated genes, **71**
- with *DEK::NUP214* fusion, **236**
- diagnostic checklist, **234**
- differential diagnosis, **236**
- extended multigene testing, **70**
- *EZH2* mutation, **100**
- *FLT3*, *NPM1*, and *CEBPA* mutations, **52**
- gene alterations, **234–235**
- gene mutations, **235**
- with inframe basic leucine zipper region (bZIP) *CEBPA* mutation, **232–233, 236**
- with inv(16) or t(16;16)/*CBFB::MYH11*, **244–247**
    - classification, **245**
    - diagnostic checklist, **246**
    - genetic testing, **246**
    - prognosis, **246**

- with inv(3) or t(3;3)/*GATA2; MECOM*, 260–261
    - differential diagnosis, 261
    - molecular genetics, 261
    - prognosis, 261
- juvenile myelomonocytic leukemia vs., 227
- *KIT* mutations, 66
- with *KMT2A* rearrangements, 236
- with maturation, 271, 271–272
- with *MECOM* rearrangements, 236
- with minimal differentiation, 271
- molecular work-up, 135
- with mutated *NPM1*, 232, 236
- with mutated *TP53*, 233, 236
    - acute myeloid leukemia with myelodysplasia-related gene mutations vs., 267
- mutational landscape, 70
- with myelodysplasia-related gene mutations, 232, 233, 236, 264–269
    - acquired genetic alterations, 265
    - acquired molecular genetic alterations induced by exposure to chemotherapy or radiation, 265–266
    - acute myeloid leukemia with t(6;9)/*DEK::NUP214* vs., 259
    - classification, 265
    - cytogenetic abnormalities, 232, 233, 236
    - cytogenetics, 267
    - diagnostic checklist, 267
    - differential diagnosis, 267
    - genetic predisposition, 266
    - genetic testing, 267
    - mutational profile, 267
    - prognosis, 267
    - qualifying cytogenetic abnormalities, 267
- myelodysplastic syndrome with *TP53* multihit mutations vs., 205
- myelodysplastic/myeloproliferative neoplasm, NOS vs., 230
- not otherwise specified (NOS), 270–275
    - acute myeloid leukemia with myelodysplasia-related gene mutations vs., 267
    - acute myeloid leukemia with t(8;21)/*RUNX1::RUNX1T1* vs., 240
    - chromosomal abnormalities, 273
    - differential diagnosis, 273
    - genetic testing, 272–273
    - prognosis, 271
    - recurrent genetic abnormalities, 273
- post cytotoxic exposure, myelodysplastic syndrome, NOS vs., 195
- with recurrent genetic abnormality, 48
    - acute myeloid leukemia with myelodysplasia-related gene mutations vs., 267
    - inv(16)(p13.1q22) or t(16;16)(p13.1;q22), 49
    - myelodysplastic syndrome/acute myeloid leukemia vs., 207
    - t(8;21)(q21.3;q22.12), 48
- *RET* fusion genes, 109
- with *RUNX1::RUNX1T1* fusion, 236
- *SETBP1* mutations, 63
- with t(1;22)(p13.3;q13.1); *RBM15::MRTFA*, myeloid proliferations associated with Down syndrome vs., 282
- with t(1;22)/*RBM15::MRTFA*, 262–263
    - differential diagnosis, 263
    - genetic testing, 263
    - prognosis, 263
- with t(5;17)(q35;q21);*NPM1::RARA*, acute promyelocytic leukemia with t(15;17)/*PML::RARA* vs., 251
- with t(6;9)/*DEK::NUP214*, 258–259
    - differential diagnosis, 259
    - genetic testing, 259
    - prognosis, 259
- with t(8;21)/*RUNX1::RUNX1T1*, 240–243
    - classification, 241
    - cytogenetics, 242
    - differential diagnosis, 240
    - genetic testing, 242
    - prognosis, 241–242
- with t(9;11)/*MLLT3::KMT2A*, 254–257
    - cytogenetics, 256
    - differential diagnosis, 256
    - genetic testing, 256
    - prognosis, 256
- with t(11;17)(q13;q21);*NUMA1::RARA*, acute promyelocytic leukemia with t(15;17)/*PML::RARA* vs., 251
- with t(11;17)(q23;q21); *ZBTB16::RARA*, acute promyelocytic leukemia with t(15;17)/*PML::RARA* vs., 251
- with t(17;17)(q21.2;q21); *STAT5B::RARA*, acute promyelocytic leukemia with t(15;17)/*PML::RARA* vs., 251
- with t(X;17)(p11;q21); *BCOR::RARA*, acute promyelocytic leukemia with t(15;17)/*PML::RARA* vs., 251
- transcripts, reverse transcription PCR, 48–49
- without maturation, 271

Acute myelomonocytic leukemia, 272
- chronic myelomonocytic leukemia vs., 218

Acute promyelocytic leukemia (APL)
- minimal residual disease, 47
- *PML::RARA* fusion, 47, 236
- with t(15;17)/*PML::RARA*, 248–253
    - cytogenetics, 250
    - diagnostic checklist, 251
    - differential diagnosis, 251
    - genetic testing, 250–251
    - prognosis, 249–250
- with variant *RARA* fusions, 251
    - acute promyelocytic leukemia with t(15;17)/*PML::RARA* vs., 251

Acute undifferentiated leukemia of ambiguous lineage, acute myeloid leukemia, NOS vs., 273

ADC. *See* Adenocarcinoma.

Adenocarcinoma
- adenomatoid tumor-like, lung adenocarcinoma, 563
- cervix/vulva/vagina, 738–741
    - differential diagnosis, 740
    - prognosis, 740

INDEX

- colorectal, precancerous lesions, **584–589**
  - chromosomal instability pathway, **585**
  - differential diagnosis, **587**
  - gene mutations, **586–587**
  - genetic testing, **587**
  - mismatch repair (MMR) pathway, **585**
  - prognosis, **586**
  - sporadic polyps, **585**
- diffuse-type, gastric adenocarcinoma vs., **582**
- endometrioid, sex cord-stromal tumors of ovary vs., **778**
- from extrathoracic origin, lung adenocarcinoma vs., **564**
- gastric, **580–583**
  - differential diagnosis, **582**
  - gene mutations, **582**
  - genetic testing, **582**
  - prognosis, **582**
- lung, **560–567**
  - diagnostic checklist, **564**
  - differential diagnosis, **564**
  - mesothelioma vs., **578**
  - molecular genetics, **561–563**
  - prognosis, **561**
- metastatic, cholangiocarcinoma vs., **623**
- NOS
  - adenoid cystic carcinoma vs., **512**
  - HPV-related multiphenotypic sinonasal carcinoma vs., **497**
  - polymorphous carcinoma vs., **521**
- pancreatic ductal, **614–617**
  - differential diagnosis, **616**
  - *KRAS* mutations, **117**
  - molecular genetics, **615–616**
  - prognosis, **615**
- poorly differentiated, small cell neuroendocrine carcinoma vs., **574**
- squamous cell carcinoma, skin vs., **794**

Adenoid cystic carcinoma, **509**
- clinicopathologic features, **513**
- differential diagnosis, **512**
- gene expression profiling, **511**
- HPV-related multiphenotypic sinonasal carcinoma vs., **497**
- lung adenocarcinoma vs., **564**
- microsecretory adenocarcinoma vs., **521**
- molecular alterations, **513**
- molecular genetics, **510–511**
- polymorphous carcinoma vs., **521**
- prognosis, **509**
- secretory carcinoma vs., **513**
- in situ hybridization, **510**

Adenomatoid tumor-like adenocarcinoma, lung adenocarcinoma, **563**

Adenomyoma, atypical polypoid, endometrial intraepithelial neoplasia vs., **743**

Adenosarcoma, low-grade endometrial stromal sarcoma vs., **756**

Adenosquamous carcinoma
- mucoepidermoid carcinoma vs., **512**
- pancreatic ductal adenocarcinoma, **616**

Adrenal cortical adenoma (ACA), **680–683**
- adrenal cortical carcinoma vs., **669**
- diagnostic checklist, **682**
- differential diagnosis, **682**
- genetic testing, **682**

Adrenal cortical carcinoma (ACC), **666–671**
- adrenal cortical adenoma vs., **682**
- differential diagnosis, **669**
- genetic testing, **669**
- pheochromocytoma/paraganglioma vs., **663**
- prognosis, **667**

Adrenocortical adenoma. *See* Adrenal cortical adenoma.
Adrenocortical carcinoma. *See* Adrenal cortical carcinoma.
Adult fibrosarcoma with CD34 expression and NTRK fusions, **897**
Adult granulosa cell tumor (AGCT), **775, 777, 778**
- cytogenetics, **776**
- molecular genetics, **776**

Adult superficial spindle cell sarcoma, **897**
Adult T-cell leukemia/lymphoma (ATLL), **294, 410–415**
- cytogenetics, **411**
- diagnostic checklist, **412**
- differential diagnosis, **412**
- molecular genetics, **411–412**
- peripheral T-cell lymphoma, not otherwise specified vs., **446**
- prognosis, **411**
- T-cell prolymphocytic leukemia vs., **394**

AFH. *See* Angiomatoid fibrous histiocytoma.
Aggressive NK-cell leukemia (ANKL), **402–405**
- blastic plasmacytoid dendritic cell neoplasm vs., **286**
- chronic lymphoproliferative disorder of NK cells vs., **398**
- cytogenetics, **403**
- differential diagnosis, **402**
- extranodal NK-/T-cell lymphoma vs., **408**
- molecular genetics, **403**
- prognosis, **403**

Aggressive systemic mastocytosis, **168**
Agranular CD4(+) NK-cell leukemia. *See* Blastic plasmacytoid dendritic cell neoplasm (BPCDCN).
Aicardi syndrome, choroid plexus tumors, **945**
AIDS patients, EBV-associated smooth muscle tumors, **88**
AKT1 gene, **124**
- meningioma, **949**

Alcohol-related liver disease, **611**
ALK gene, **124**
- functions, **104**
- melanoma, **790**
- rearrangements and mutations, **104–105**
  - testing, **104**

ALK rearrangements
- lung adenocarcinoma, **562**
- papillary thyroid carcinoma, **540**
- primary cutaneous CD30-positive T-cell lymphoproliferative disorders, **439**

ALK(+) anaplastic large cell lymphoma, **300, 446**
- anaplastic large cell lymphoma, ALK-negative vs., **458**

ALK(-) anaplastic large cell lymphoma, **300, 446**
- anaplastic large cell lymphoma, ALK-positive vs., **464**
- peripheral T-cell lymphoma, not otherwise specified vs., **445–446**

ALK(+) large B-cell lymphoma, **104**

INDEX

ALK-positive large B-cell lymphoma, anaplastic large cell lymphoma, ALK-positive vs., **464**
Allele-specific PCR
- *BRAF* mutations, **119**
- *JAK2* mutations, **55**
- *MYD88* L265P mutation, **95**

Allogeneic stem cell transplantation, chronic myeloid leukemia, *BCR::ABL1* positive, **138**
Alterations in chromosomes and DNA, analysis of, common techniques
- amplification methods, **26–29**
- chromosomal microarray, **22–25**
    - aggressive NK-cell leukemia, **403**
    - anaplastic large cell lymphoma, ALK-positive, **464**
    - array-based comparative genomic hybridization, **22–23**
    - Burkitt lymphoma, **388**
    - chromosomal aberrations, **23**
    - Ewing sarcoma, **820**
    - extranodal NK-/T-cell lymphoma, **408**
    - follicular lymphoma, **366**
    - germ cell tumor, ovary, **781**
    - HPV-associated head and neck carcinomas, **496**
    - interdigitating dendritic cell tumor, **485–486**
    - limitations, **23**
    - lung squamous cell carcinoma, **569–570**
    - lymphoplasmacytic lymphoma, **346**
    - melanoma, **789**
    - multiple myeloma (plasma cell myeloma), **357**
    - nodal follicular helper T-cell lymphoma, **451**
    - peripheral T-cell lymphoma, not otherwise specified, **444**
    - primary cutaneous CD30-positive T-cell lymphoproliferative disorders, **440**
    - sex cord-stromal tumors of ovary, **776**
    - single nucleotide polymorphism, **23**
- cytogenetics, **18–21**
- DNA high-resolution melting curve analysis, **30–31**
    - amplicon sizes, **31**
    - fluorescent dyes, **31**
    - pre-HRM specimen preparations, **31**
- DNA methylation analysis, **38–39**
- fluorescence in situ hybridization, **19–20**
    - *BCR::ABL1* fusion, **43**
    - Burkitt lymphoma, **388**
    - diffuse large B-cell lymphoma, **378**
    - *EGFR* amplification, **121**
    - for *ERBB2* (HER2) gene amplifications, **114–115**
    - *KMT2A*-rearranged, **256**
    - lymphoid neoplasms, **296, 297**
    - melanoma, **789**
    - for *MET* amplifications, **112**
    - molecular work-up of myeloid neoplasms, **134**
    - *PML::RARA* fusion, **47**
    - *RET* fusion, **109**
    - *ROS1* fusion, **107**
- high-throughput methods in molecular pathology, **36–37**
- sequencing technologies, **32–35**
    - massively parallel next-generation sequencing, **33–34**

next-generation sequencing, **33, 34**
pyrosequencing, **32–33**
representative examples, **34**
Sanger sequencing, **32**
3rd-generation sequencing, **34**

Alveolar rhabdomyosarcoma, **868, 870, 892**
- differential diagnosis, **872**
- Ewing sarcoma vs., **821**
- genetic findings, **871**
- neuroblastoma vs., **676**

Alveolar soft part sarcoma, **892, 898, 899, 900, 902**
- pheochromocytoma/paraganglioma vs., **663**

AMER1 mutations, Wilms tumor, **645**
AML. *See* Acute myeloid leukemia.
Amplicon sizes, **31**
Amplification methods, **26–29**
Amplification-refractory mutation system, **29**
Ampullary carcinomas, pancreatic ductal adenocarcinoma vs., **616**
Amyloid goiter, medullary thyroid carcinoma vs., **557**
Amyloidosis, lymphoplasmacytic lymphoma, **345**
Analysis of alterations in chromosomes and DNA, common techniques
- amplification methods, **26–29**
- chromosomal microarray, **22–25**
    - aggressive NK-cell leukemia, **403**
    - anaplastic large cell lymphoma, ALK-positive, **464**
    - array-based comparative genomic hybridization, **22–23**
    - Burkitt lymphoma, **388**
    - chromosomal aberrations, **23**
    - Ewing sarcoma, **820**
    - extranodal NK-/T-cell lymphoma, **408**
    - follicular lymphoma, **366**
    - germ cell tumor, ovary, **781**
    - HPV-associated head and neck carcinomas, **496**
    - interdigitating dendritic cell tumor, **485–486**
    - limitations, **23**
    - lung squamous cell carcinoma, **569–570**
    - lymphoplasmacytic lymphoma, **346**
    - melanoma, **789**
    - multiple myeloma (plasma cell myeloma), **357**
    - nodal follicular helper T-cell lymphoma, **451**
    - peripheral T-cell lymphoma, not otherwise specified, **444**
    - primary cutaneous CD30-positive T-cell lymphoproliferative disorders, **440**
    - sex cord-stromal tumors of ovary, **776**
    - single nucleotide polymorphism, **23**
- cytogenetics, **18–21**
- DNA high-resolution melting curve analysis, **30–31**
    - amplicon sizes, **31**
    - fluorescent dyes, **31**
    - pre-HRM specimen preparations, **31**
- DNA methylation analysis, **38–39**
- fluorescence in situ hybridization, **19–20**
    - *BCR::ABL1* fusion, **43**
    - Burkitt lymphoma, **388**
    - diffuse large B-cell lymphoma, **378**
    - *EGFR* amplification, **121**
    - for *ERBB2* (HER2) gene amplifications, **114–115**

INDEX

    KMT2A-rearranged, **256**
    lymphoid neoplasms, **296, 297**
    melanoma, **789**
    for *MET* amplifications, **112**
    molecular work-up of myeloid neoplasms, **134**
    PML::RARA fusion, **47**
    RET fusion, **109**
    ROS1 fusion, **107**
- high-throughput methods in molecular pathology, **36–37**
- sequencing technologies, **32–35**
    massively parallel next-generation sequencing, **33–34**
    next-generation sequencing, **33, 34**
    pyrosequencing, **32–33**
    representative examples, **34**
    Sanger sequencing, **32**
    3rd-generation sequencing, **34**

Analyte-specific reagent (ASR), **929**
Anaplasia, Wilms tumor, **645**
Anaplastic astrocytoma, IDH-mutant. *See* Astrocytoma, IDH-mutant.
Anaplastic ependymoma, ependymal tumors, **933**
Anaplastic gliomas, *IDH1* and *IDH2* mutations, **69**
Anaplastic large cell lymphoma, **294**
- adult T-cell leukemia/lymphoma vs., **412**
- ALK-negative, **446, 456–461**
    cytogenetics, **457**
    differential diagnosis, **458**
    peripheral T-cell lymphoma, not otherwise specified vs., **445–446**
    primary cutaneous CD30-positive T-cell lymphoproliferative disorders, **440**
    prognosis, **457**
- ALK-positive, **104, 446, 462–467**
    cytogenetics, **463**
    differential diagnosis, **464**
    prognosis, **463**
- nodal follicular helper T-cell lymphoma vs., **452**
- testing methods, **297**

Anaplastic thyroid carcinoma, **550–553**
- *ALK* alterations, **105**
- differential diagnosis, **552**
- molecular alterations, **551–552**
- prognosis, **551**

Anemia
- lymphoplasmacytic lymphoma, **345**
- myelodysplastic syndrome, NOS, **193**
- myelodysplastic syndrome with *TP53* multihit mutations vs., **205**

Aneuploidy, **4, 19**
Aneurysmal bone cyst, **895**
- giant cell tumor of bone vs., **835**
- telangiectatic osteosarcoma vs., **814**

Angiofibroma, cellular, **892**
Angioimmunoblastic lymphadenopathy with dysproteinemia. *See* Nodal follicular helper T-cell lymphoma.
Angioimmunoblastic T-cell lymphoma
- *IDH1* and *IDH2* mutations, **69**

  - peripheral T-cell lymphoma, not otherwise specified vs., **445**

Angiomatoid fibrous histiocytoma, **892, 908, 909, 910, 911**
Angiomyxoma, deep (aggressive), **892**
Angiosarcoma, **878, 879, 892**
- atypical vascular lesions vs., **786**
- differential diagnosis, **881**
- epithelioid hemangioendothelioma vs., **881**
- genetic findings, **880**
- hemangioma vs., **881**
- Kaposi sarcoma vs., **881**
- prognosis, **879**

Antibody-based methods
- *IGH* gene rearrangements, **74**
- *TRB* gene rearrangement, **82**

Anti-EGFR monoclonal antibodies, for chemotherapy-refectory metastatic colorectal carcinoma, **121**
Antigen receptor genes, Southern blot analysis, **84–85**
Anti-HGF monoclonal antibodies, **112**
Anti-HGFR antibodies, **112**
APC gene, **124**
- meningioma, **950**

APL. *See* Acute promyelocytic leukemia.
Aplastic anemia
- acquired, pediatric myelodysplastic syndrome and refractory cytopenia of childhood vs., **211–212**
- myelodysplastic syndrome, NOS vs., **195**
- somatic mutations, clonal hematopoiesis and premalignant clonal cytopenia, **183**

ARAF mutations, Langerhans cell histiocytosis, **480**
Arias-Stella reaction, clear cell carcinoma, uterus vs., **752**
ARID1A mutations
- clear cell carcinoma, uterus vs., **752**
- endometrial intraepithelial neoplasia, **743**

Array comparative genomic hybridization, **22–23**
- aberrations detected, **23**
- adult T-cell leukemia/lymphoma, **411**
- enteropathy-associated T-cell lymphoma, **420**
- lymphoid neoplasms, **293**
- melanoma, **789**
- monoclonal gammopathy of undetermined significance, **352**
- myeloid sarcoma, **278**
- splenic marginal zone lymphoma, **327**
- squamous cell carcinoma, skin, **793**
- subcutaneous panniculitis-like T-cell lymphoma, **430**
- T-cell prolymphocytic leukemia, **395**

Asbestos exposure, mesothelioma, **577**
ASPSCR1::TFE3 carcinomas, *TFE3*-rearranged and *TFEB*-altered renal cell carcinomas, **639**
ASR. *See* Analyte-specific reagent.
Astrocytoma
- ependymal tumors vs., **934**
- high-grade, with piloid features
    astrocytoma, IDH-mutant vs., **922**
    pilocytic astrocytoma vs., **926**
- IDH-mutant, **920–923**
    diagnostic checklist, **922**
    differential diagnosis, **922**

v

INDEX

      glioblastoma, IDH wildtype vs., **918**
      molecular genetics, **921**
      oligodendroglioma vs., **929**
      prognosis, **921**
- infiltrating, pilocytic astrocytoma vs., **926**
- pilocytic, **924–927**
      differential diagnosis, **926**
      molecular genetics, **925–926**
      neurofibromatosis 1-associated, **925**
      prognosis, **925**
      sporadic, **925**
- pilomyxoid, pilocytic astrocytoma vs., **926**
- retinoblastoma vs., **952**

Astrocytosis/gliosis, reactive
- astrocytoma, IDH-mutant vs., **921**

ASXL1 mutations
- acute myeloid leukemia, **235**
- atypical chronic myeloid leukemia, **221–222**
- chronic myelomonocytic leukemia, **217**
- mastocytosis, **169**
- myelodysplastic syndrome, NOS, **194**
- myelodysplastic/myeloproliferative neoplasm, NOS, **230**
- myeloproliferative neoplasm, unclassifiable, **163**
- polycythemia vera, **150**

Ataxia telangiectasia, myelodysplastic syndrome, NOS vs., **195**

ATLL. *See* Adult T-cell leukemia/lymphoma.

ATM gene, **124**

ATM mutations
- B-cell prolymphocytic leukemia, **323**
- non-HPV-related head and neck squamous cell carcinoma, **507**
- small lymphocytic lymphoma/chronic lymphocytic leukemia, **319**

Atrophy, preneoplastic conditions, cervix/vulva/vagina vs., **732**

ATRX mutations, astrocytoma, IDH-mutant, **921**

Atypical adenoma, follicular thyroid carcinoma vs., **544**

Atypical adenomatous hyperplasia (AAH), lung adenocarcinoma vs., **564**

Atypical chronic myelogenous leukemia, *BCR::ABL1* negative, chronic myeloid leukemia, *BCR::ABL1*-positive vs., **139**

Atypical chronic myeloid leukemia, **60, 214, 220–223**
- *BCR::ABL1*-negative, chronic myelomonocytic leukemia vs., **218**
- chronic neutrophilic leukemia vs., **146**
- classification, **221**
- cytogenetics, **221**
- differential diagnosis, **222**
- genetic testing, **222**
- molecular genetics, **221–222**
- myelodysplastic/myeloproliferative neoplasm, NOS vs., **230**
- prognosis, **221**
- *SETBP1* mutations, **62–63**

Atypical ductal hyperplasia (ADH) (dysplastic, premalignant), **688–693**
- differential diagnosis, **692**
- molecular genetics, **690**
- as nonobligate precursor, **689**
- prognosis, **689**
- propriety recurrence score, **690–691**

Atypical fibroxanthoma, squamous cell carcinoma, skin vs., **794**

Atypical lipomatous tumor (ALT), **858, 860, 861, 892**
- differential diagnosis, **862**
- prognosis, **859**
- with prominent myxoid stroma, myxoid liposarcoma vs., **862**
- with prominent spindled stromal cells, spindle cell liposarcoma vs., **862**
- sclerosing variant of, dedifferentiated liposarcoma vs., **862**

Atypical lobular endocervical gland hyperplasia, adenocarcinoma, cervix/vulva/vagina vs., **740**

Atypical lymphoid infiltrates
- cytogenetics, **785**
- differential diagnosis, **786**
- molecular genetics, **785**

Atypical (dysplastic) nevi
- cytogenetics, **785**
- differential diagnosis, **786**
- melanoma vs., **790**
- molecular genetics, **785**

Atypical polypoid adenomyoma, endometrial intraepithelial neoplasia vs., **743**

Atypical spindle cell/pleomorphic lipomatous tumor (ASC/PLT), **858, 859, 861**
- differential diagnosis, **862**
- prognosis, **859**

Atypical Spitz nevi/tumors, melanoma vs., **790**

Atypical vascular lesions
- cytogenetics, **785**
- differential diagnosis, **786**
- molecular genetics, **785**

Atypical vascular proliferation, angiosarcoma vs., **881**

AURKA (20q), non-HPV-related head and neck squamous cell carcinoma, **507**

AURKB (17p), non-HPV-related head and neck squamous cell carcinoma, **507**

Autoimmune disorders
- multiple myeloma (plasma cell myeloma) vs., **357**
- subcutaneous panniculitis-like T-cell lymphoma, **429**

Autoimmune lymphoproliferative disorders, pediatric myelodysplastic syndrome and refractory cytopenia of childhood vs., **212**

Autoimmune/collagen vascular diseases, myelodysplastic syndrome, NOS vs., **195**

B

B acute lymphoblastic leukemia, not otherwise specified, B-lymphoblastic leukemia/lymphoma with recurrent genetic abnormalities vs., **304**

B2M (15q), non-HPV-related head and neck squamous cell carcinoma, **506**

BAP1 mutations, melanoma, **790**

INDEX

Basal cell adenoma/adenocarcinoma
- adenoid cystic carcinoma vs., 512
- differential diagnosis, 521
- molecular genetics, 520
- prognosis, 519

Basal cell carcinoma, 796–799
- cytogenetics, 797
- diagnostic checklist, 798
- differential diagnosis, 798
- genetics, 797
- HPV-related multiphenotypic sinonasal carcinoma vs., 497
- molecular genetics, 520, 797
- prognosis, 519, 797
- squamous cell carcinoma, skin vs., 794
- variants, 797–798

Basal-like carcinoma, 720–729
- diagnostic checklist, 725
- differential diagnosis, 724–725
- prognosis, 722–723
- subtypes, 725

Basaloid/small cell variant, squamous cell carcinoma, small cell neuroendocrine carcinoma vs., 574

Basophilic leukemia, acute, 272

Basosquamous basal cell carcinoma, 798

B-cell development, 72–73
- antigen-dependent stages, 73
- antigen-independent stages, 72

B-cell lymphoma
- atypical lymphoid infiltrates vs., 786
- diffuse large, 376–385
    anaplastic thyroid carcinoma vs., 552
    associated with chronic inflammation, 87
    Burkitt lymphoma vs., 390
    cytogenetics, 378
    differential diagnosis, 379
    EBV (+), not otherwise specified, 87
    EZH2 mutation, 99
    fibrin-associated, 87
    molecular genetics, 378
    myeloid sarcoma vs., 278
    not otherwise specified, 87
    prognosis, 377
- mature, molecular changes, 348
- *MYD88* L265P mutation, 94–95
- small lymphocytic lymphoma/chronic lymphocytic leukemia vs., 320

B-cell lymphoproliferative disorders, 299–300

B-cell proliferation, peripheral T-cell lymphoma with, 445

B-cell prolymphocytic leukemia (B-PLL), 322–325
- cytogenetics, 323
- diagnostic checklist, 324
- differential diagnosis, 324
- molecular genetics, 323
- prognosis, 323
- splenic B-cell lymphoma/leukemia, unclassifiable vs., 338

BCOR genetic alterations, sarcoma with, 825
- differential diagnosis, 827
- molecular genetics, 826

BCOR::CCNB3 sarcoma, 825, 826
- differential diagnosis, 827

BCOR-rearranged tumors, 895

BCR gene, normal function, 42

BCR protein, 137

BCR::ABL1 fusion, 42–45
- abnormal oncoprotein, 137
- characteristic types, 139

BCR::ABL1-negative
- atypical chronic myelogenous leukemia, chronic myeloid leukemia, *BCR::ABL1*-positive vs., 139
- myeloproliferative neoplasm
    chronic myeloid leukemia, *BCR::ABL1*-positive vs., 139
    MPL mutations, 57

BCR::ABL1-positive, chronic myeloid leukemia, 136::143
- differential diagnosis, 139
- genetic testing, 138
- prognosis, 138

BCR::ABL1-resistant mutations, 44

BCR::JAK2 fusion, 55

Beckwith-Wiedemann syndrome
- adrenal cortical carcinoma, 667
- Wilms tumor, 644

Benign endometrioid tumors, 769

Benign glandular proliferations, adenocarcinoma, cervix/vulva/vagina vs., 738

Benign histiocytic processes, histiocytic sarcoma vs., 472

Benign monoclonal gammopathy. *See* Monoclonal gammopathy of undetermined significance.

Benign mucinous tumors, 769, 770

Benign serous tumors (BST), 763
- prognosis, 763

Biliary tract cancer, *KRAS* mutations, 117

Bioinformatics, 36, 37

Biologics License Application (BLA), 963

Biphasic synovial sarcoma, desmoplastic small round cell tumor vs., 827

Biphenotypic sinonasal sarcoma (BSS), 531
- cytogenetics, 532
- differential diagnosis, 534
- molecular genetics, 532
- prognosis, 532

BIRC3 mutation, small lymphocytic lymphoma/chronic lymphocytic leukemia, 319

Birt-Hogg-Dubé (BHD) syndrome, chromophobe renal cell carcinoma, 635

Bisulfite conversion dependent, *MGMT* promoter gene methylation assay, 131

Bisulfite conversion methods, 38–39
- measurement, 39

BLA. *See* Biologics License Application.

Bladder and upper tract urothelial carcinoma, EZH2 protein overexpression, 100

Blastema, Wilms tumor, 645

Blastic plasmacytoid dendritic cell neoplasm (BPCDCN), 284–289
- cytogenetics, 285
- differential diagnosis, 286
- molecular genetics, 286
- prognosis, 285

INDEX

Bleeding, lymphoplasmacytic lymphoma, **345**
Bloom syndrome, myelodysplastic syndrome, NOS vs., **195**
Blue cell tumors, small round, Wilms tumor vs., **645**
B-lymphoblastic leukemia/lymphoma, **292, 294**
- *BCR::ABL1* fusion, **43**
- *BCR::ABL1*-like (Ph-like ALL), **306–309**
    - diagnostic checklist, **308**
    - prognosis, **307**
- Burkitt lymphoma vs., **390**
- *KMT2A*-rearranged, acute myeloid leukemia with t(9;11)/*MLLT3::KMT2A* vs., **256**
- recurrent genetic abnormalities, **302–305**
    - classification, **303**
    - diagnostic checklist, **304**
    - differential diagnosis, **304**
    - genetic testing, **304**
    - genetics, **303**
    - prognosis, **303**
- testing methods, **297**
- T-lymphoblastic leukemia/lymphoma vs., **313**
Bone lesions, **895**
Bone marrow failure, myeloproliferative neoplasm, unclassifiable, **163**
Bone marrow failure disorders, acquired, pediatric myelodysplastic syndrome and refractory cytopenia of childhood vs., **212**
Bone marrow failure syndromes
- acute myeloid leukemia, **233**
- myelodysplastic syndrome with *TP53* multihit mutations vs., **205**
Bone marrow fibrosis, myelodysplastic/myeloproliferative neoplasm, NOS, **229**
Bone marrow mastocytosis, **168**
Bone tumors, **895**
- cartilaginous, intermediate and malignant, **838–847**
    - differential diagnosis, **842**
- giant cell tumor, **832–837**
    - cytogenetics, **833–834**
    - differential diagnosis, **835**
    - epigenetics, **834**
    - molecular genetics, **834**
- molecular pathology, **804–809**
    - diagnostic steps, **806**
    - genetic alterations, **807**
    - molecular genetics, **807**
Boveri, Theodor, **18**
BPCDCN. *See* Blastic plasmacytoid dendritic cell neoplasm.
B-PLL. *See* B-cell prolymphocytic leukemia.
BRAF gene, **124**
BRAF mutations, **118–119**
- alterations, **118–119**
- anaplastic thyroid carcinoma, **551**
- B-lymphoblastic leukemia/lymphoma, *BCR::ABL1*-like (Ph-like ALL), **307**
- fusions, **118**
- germline, **119**
- Langerhans cell histiocytosis, **480**
- lung adenocarcinoma, **562**
- melanoma, **789**
- pancreatic intraductal papillary mucinous neoplasm, **621**
- papillary thyroid carcinoma, **539**
- pilocytic astrocytoma, **926**
- poorly differentiated thyroid carcinoma, **547**
- somatic missense, **118**
BRAF proteins, **118**
BRAF V600E mutation
- colorectal adenocarcinoma and precancerous lesions, **586**
- GIST, **592, 593**
- pilocytic astrocytoma, **926**
- Wilms tumor, **645**
BRCA1 mutation
- basal-like carcinoma, **721**
- high-grade serous carcinoma, **765**
BRCA2 mutations, high-grade serous carcinoma, **765**
Breast cancer
- biology and classification, **695**
- *EGFR* amplification, **121**
- EZH2 protein overexpression, **100**
- metaplastic, **710–715**
    - differential diagnosis, **713**
    - gene mutations, **712**
    - prognosis, **711–712**
- *RET* fusion genes, **109**
- triple-negative, **720–729**
    - diagnostic checklist, **725**
    - differential diagnosis, **724–725**
    - immune-enriched subtype, **725**
    - luminal AR, **725**
    - mesenchymal subtype, **725**
    - prognosis, **722–723**
Brenner tumors, **769, 770–771**
Burkitt lymphoma, **87, 294, 299, 386–393**
- cytogenetics, **388**
- diagnostic checklist, **390**
- differential diagnosis, **390**
- diffuse large B-cell lymphoma vs., **379**
- *EZH2* mutation, **99–100**
- molecular changes, **348**
- molecular genetics, **388–389**
- prognosis, **388**
- testing methods, **297**
Burkitt-like lymphoma, chromosomal microarray, **24**
BWS. *See* Beckwith-Wiedemann syndrome.

C

CALR exon 9 frameshift mutations, primary myelofibrosis, **154**
CALR mutations
- atypical chronic myeloid leukemia, **222**
- essential thrombocythemia, **157–158**
- myeloproliferative neoplasm, unclassifiable, **163**
- polycythemia vera, **150**
Calreticulin (*CALR*) gene, **58**
- function, **58–59**

INDEX

- homozygous, knockout mouse, **58**
- mutations, **58–59**

Cancer cytogenetics, **19**

Cancer hotspot next-generation sequencing panels, **124–129**

Cancer testing, *MET* amplifications, **112**

CAP. *See* College of American Pathologists.

Capillary electrophoresis, **78**

Capillary hemangioblastomas, clear cell renal cell carcinoma, **631**

Carcinoma
- basal-like, **720–729**
  - diagnostic checklist, **725**
  - differential diagnosis, **724–725**
  - prognosis, **722–723**
  - subtypes, **725**
- clear cell renal cell, **630–633**
  - differential diagnosis, **632**
  - molecular genetics, **631–632**
  - prognosis, **631**
  - sporadic, **631**
  - *VHL* wildtype, **631**
- hepatocellular, **610–613**
  - adrenal cortical carcinoma vs., **669**
  - cholangiocarcinoma vs., **623**
  - cytogenetics, **612**
  - differential diagnosis, **612**
  - molecular genetics, **612**
  - pheochromocytoma/paraganglioma vs., **663**
  - prognosis, **611**
- neuroendocrine
  - large cell, lung squamous cell carcinoma vs., **570**
  - large cell, small cell neuroendocrine carcinoma vs., **574**
  - olfactory neuroblastoma vs., **534**
  - small cell, **572–575**
  - squamous cell carcinoma, cervix/vulva/vagina vs., **736**
- showing thymus-like differentiation, poorly differentiated thyroid carcinoma vs., **548**
- uterine endometrioid, **744–747**
  - Cancer Genome Atlas molecular subtypes, **745–746**
  - genetic predisposition syndromes, **745**
  - Lynch syndrome-associated, **745**
  - MSI testing, **745**
  - prognosis, **745**
  - sporadic, **745**

Carcinosarcoma, **771**

Cardiac problems, lymphoplasmacytic lymphoma, **345**

Cardiofaciocutaneous syndrome
- *BRAF* mutations, **119**
- *KRAS* mutations, **117**

Carney complex, **543**

Carney triad, pheochromocytoma/paraganglioma, **662**

Carney-Stratakis dyad, pheochromocytoma/paraganglioma, **662, 663**

Cartilaginous tumors, bone, intermediate and malignant, **838–847**
- differential diagnosis, **842**

CASP8 (2q), non-HPV-related head and neck squamous cell carcinoma, **506**

Caspersson, Torbjorn, **18**

β-catenin-activated hepatocellular adenoma, **602–605**
- diagnostic checklist, **604**
- differential diagnosis, **604**
- *HNF1A*-inactivated hepatocellular adenoma vs., **600**
- inflammatory hepatocellular adenoma vs., **608**
- prognosis, **603**

β-catenin-mutated hepatic adenoma. *See* β-catenin-activated hepatocellular adenoma.

CBER. *See* Center for Biologics Evaluation and Research.

CBFB::MYH11, **48–49**

CBL mutations
- atypical chronic myeloid leukemia, **222**
- B-lymphoblastic leukemia/lymphoma, *BCR::ABL1*-like (Ph-like ALL), **307**
- chronic myelomonocytic leukemia, **217**

CCAAT/Enhancer-binding protein alpha (*CEBPA*) gene
- function, **51**
- mutations, **51–52**
  - clinical significance, **52–53**
  - testing, **53**

CCNA1 (13q), non-HPV-related head and neck squamous cell carcinoma, **507**

CCND1 (11q), non-HPV-related head and neck squamous cell carcinoma, **506**

CCNE1 mutations, high-grade serous carcinoma, **765**

CCR4 mutations, adult T-cell leukemia/lymphoma, **412**

CCUS. *See* Clonal cytopenia of undetermined significance.

CD30-positive T-cell lymphoproliferative disorders, primary cutaneous, **438–441**
- molecular alterations, **439–440**
- prognosis, **439**

CD74 (5q), non-HPV-related head and neck squamous cell carcinoma, **507**

CDC. *See* Centers for Disease Control and Prevention.

CDH1 gene, **124**
- non-HPV-related head and neck squamous cell carcinoma, **507**

CDKN2A gene mutation, **124**
- melanoma, **789**
- meningioma, **950**
- non-HPV-related head and neck squamous cell carcinoma, **506**
- pancreatic mucinous cystic neoplasm, **619**
- T-lymphoblastic leukemia/lymphoma, **312**

CDKN2B (9p), non-HPV-related head and neck squamous cell carcinoma, **507**

CEBPA mutations, **50–53**
- acute myeloid leukemia, **234**
- acute myeloid leukemia, NOS, **273**

CEBPB gene, giant cell tumor of bone, **834**

Celiac disease, enteropathy-associated T-cell lymphoma, **417**

Cell adhesion protein expression, **701**

Cellular congenital mesoblastic nephroma, clear cell sarcoma of kidney vs., **649**

Cellular leiomyoma
- leiomyosarcoma vs., **756**
- low-grade endometrial stromal sarcoma vs., **756**

Cellular myofibroma, **897**

INDEX

Cellular schwannoma
- biphenotypic sinonasal sarcoma vs., **534**
- malignant peripheral nerve sheath tumor vs., **888**

Center for Biologics Evaluation and Research (CBER), **961**

Centers for Disease Control and Prevention (CDC), CLIA program, **964**

Centers for Medicare and Medicaid Services (CMS), **958**
- CLIA program, **964**
- LDTs, **965**
- proficiency testing, **968–969**

Central cartilaginous tumors, *IDH1* and *IDH2* mutations, **69**

Central chondrosarcoma, **838, 839, 840**
- differential diagnosis, **842**
- genetic testing, **840**

Centromere, **5**

Certificates, laboratories, **958**

Cervical adenocarcinoma in situ (AIS), preneoplastic conditions, cervix/vulva/vagina, **731**

Cervical intraepithelial neoplasia (CIN)
- EZH2 protein overexpression, **100**
- preneoplastic conditions, cervix/vulva/vagina vs., **731**

Cervical mass, squamous cell carcinoma, cervix/vulva/vagina, **735**

Cervix
- adenocarcinoma, **738–741**
    - differential diagnosis, **740**
    - prognosis, **740**
- preneoplastic conditions, **730–733**
    - differential diagnosis, **732**
    - prognosis, **732**
- squamous cell carcinoma, **734–737**
    - differential diagnosis, **736**
    - prognosis, **735–736**

Checklists, CAP, **967–968**

Chemotherapy, *MET* amplifications, **111–112**

Chemotherapy-refectory metastatic colorectal carcinoma, anti-EGFR monoclonal antibodies for, **121**

Childhood ependymoma, EZH2 protein overexpression, **100**

Childhood-onset mastocytosis, **65**

Chimera, **4**

Chimeric antigen receptor-modified T cell, *TRB* gene rearrangement, **82**

CHIP. *See* Clonal hematopoiesis of indeterminate potential.

Cholangiocarcinoma, **622–623**
- differential diagnosis, **623**
- EZH2 protein overexpression, **101**
- hepatocellular carcinoma vs., **612**
- *IDH1* and *IDH2* mutations, **69**
- molecular genetics, **623**
- prognosis, **623**

Chondroblastoma, **839, 841, 895**
- chondromyxoid fibroma vs., **842**
- clear cell chondrosarcoma vs., **842**
- differential diagnosis, **842**
- genetic testing, **840**
- giant cell tumor of bone vs., **835**

Chondroid lipoma, **892**

Chondromyxoid fibroma, **838, 839, 841–842, 895**
- differential diagnosis, **842**
- genetic testing, **840**

Chondrosarcoma
- central, **838, 839, 840**
    - differential diagnosis, **842**
    - genetic testing, **840**
- clear cell, **838, 839**
    - chondroblastoma vs., **842**
    - differential diagnosis, **842**
- dedifferentiated, **838, 839, 841, 895**
    - conventional central osteosarcoma vs., **814**
    - differential diagnosis of, **842**
    - genetic testing, **840**
- extraskeletal myxoid, **892**
    - epithelioid hemangioendothelioma vs., **881**
- high-grade central, **895**
- low-grade central, **895**
- mesenchymal, **838–839, 840, 841**
    - differential diagnosis, **842**
    - Ewing sarcoma vs., **821**
    - genetic testing, **840**
- periosteal, **838, 839, 841**
    - conventional central osteosarcoma vs., **814**
    - differential diagnosis, **842**
    - grading, **840**
- peripheral, **895**
    - differential diagnosis, **842**
    - secondary, **838, 839**

Chordoma, **895**

Choriocarcinoma
- germ cell tumor, ovary, **782**
- testicular germ cell tumors, **625**

Choroid plexus
- atypical papilloma, choroid plexus tumors, **945**
- carcinoma, choroid plexus tumors, **945**
- normal, choroid plexus tumors vs., **945**
- papilloma, choroid plexus tumors, **945**

Choroid plexus tumors, **944–947**
- differential diagnosis, **945**
- ependymal tumors vs., **934**
- genetic testing, **945**
- grading, **944**

Chromatin, **5**

Chromophobe carcinoma, eosinophilic subtype, oncocytoma vs., **651**

Chromophobe renal cell carcinoma, **634–635**
- clear cell renal cell carcinoma vs., **632**
- differential diagnosis, **635**
- molecular genetics, **635**
- prognosis, **635**

Chromosomal aberrations, **23**

Chromosomal arms, **19**

Chromosomal breakage syndromes, myelodysplastic syndrome, NOS vs., **195**

Chromosomal instability
- choroid plexus tumors, **945**
- pathway, colorectal adenocarcinoma, **585**

Chromosomal microarray, **22–25**
- aggressive NK-cell leukemia, **403**
- anaplastic large cell lymphoma, ALK-positive, **464**

INDEX

- array-based comparative genomic hybridization, 22–23
- Burkitt lymphoma, 388
- chromosomal aberrations, 23
- Ewing sarcoma, 820
- extranodal NK-/T-cell lymphoma, 408
- follicular lymphoma, 366
- germ cell tumor, ovary, 781
- HPV-associated head and neck carcinomas, 496
- interdigitating dendritic cell tumor, 485–486
- limitations, 23
- lung squamous cell carcinoma, 569–570
- lymphoplasmacytic lymphoma, 346
- melanoma, 789
- multiple myeloma (plasma cell myeloma), 357
- nodal follicular helper T-cell lymphoma, 451
- peripheral T-cell lymphoma, not otherwise specified, 444
- primary cutaneous CD30-positive T-cell lymphoproliferative disorders, 440
- sex cord-stromal tumors of ovary, 776
- single nucleotide polymorphism, 23

Chromosomal regions, 19

Chromosome
- categorization and morphology, 5
- human chromosome groups, 6
- numerical chromosome abnormalities, 6
- organization, 4–6
- structure, 4–7

Chromosome analysis (karyotype), molecular work-up of myeloid neoplasms, 134

Chronic eosinophilic leukemia, not otherwise specified, 160–161
- cytogenetics, 161
- differential diagnosis, 161
- genetic testing, 161

Chronic lymphocytic leukemia (CLL), 294, 316–321
- chromosomal microarray, 23–24
- cytogenetics, 318–319
- differential diagnosis, 320
- genetic testing, 319
- mantle cell lymphoma vs., 373
- *MYD88* L265P mutations, 348
- *NOTCH1* mutation, 97
- prognosis, 318
- somatic mutations, 319–320
- splenic B-cell lymphoma/leukemia, unclassifiable vs., 338
- splenic marginal zone lymphoma vs., 329
- testing methods, 297

Chronic lymphoproliferative disorder of NK cells (CLPD-NK), 398–401
- cytogenetics, 399
- differential diagnosis, 398
- gene expression profiling, 399
- molecular genetics, 399
- prognosis, 399

Chronic myelogenous leukemia
- atypical, *BCR::ABL1* negative, chronic myeloid leukemia, *BCR::ABL1*-positive vs., 139
- primary myelofibrosis vs., 154

Chronic myeloid leukemia (CML)
- atypical, 220–223
    - chronic neutrophilic leukemia vs., 146
    - classification, 221
    - cytogenetics, 221
    - differential diagnosis, 222
    - genetic testing, 222
    - molecular genetics, 221–222
    - prognosis, 221
- *BCR::ABL1* fusion, 43
- *BCR::ABL1*-positive, 136–143
    - atypical chronic myeloid leukemia vs., 222
    - chronic myelomonocytic leukemia vs., 218
    - differential diagnosis, 139
    - genetic testing, 138
    - prognosis, 138
- blast phase
    - acute myeloid leukemia with inv(3) or t(3;3)/*GATA2*; *MECOM*, 261
    - acute myeloid leukemia with t(6;9)/*DEK::NUP214* vs., 259
- chronic eosinophilic leukemia, NOS vs., 160
- chronic neutrophilic leukemia vs., 146
- minimal residual disease, 44
- myeloproliferative neoplasm, unclassifiable vs., 164
- polycythemia vera vs., 150
- with thrombocytosis, essential thrombocythemia vs., 158

Chronic myelomonocytic leukemia (CMML), 214, 216–219
- acute myeloid leukemia, NOS vs., 273
- atypical chronic myeloid leukemia vs., 222
- *CSF3R* mutations, 61
- diagnostic checklist, 218
- differential diagnosis, 218
- genetic testing, 218
- molecular genetics, 217
- myelodysplastic syndrome/acute myeloid leukemia vs., 207
- myelodysplastic/myeloproliferative neoplasm, NOS vs., 230
- prognosis, 217
- *SETBP1* mutations, 62
- with *SF3B1* mutation, myelodysplastic syndrome with mutated *SF3B1* vs., 190

Chronic neutrophilic leukemia (CNL), 60, 144–147
- atypical chronic myeloid leukemia vs., 222
- diagnostic checklist, 146
- differential diagnosis, 146
- molecular genetics, 146
- prognosis, 145–146

Chronic NK-cell leukemia, 294

Chronic NK-cell lymphoproliferative disorders, aggressive NK-cell leukemia vs., 402

Chronic pancreatitis, pancreatic ductal adenocarcinoma vs., 616

Chronic viral infections, myelodysplastic/myeloproliferative neoplasm, NOS vs., 230

CIC mutations, oligodendroglioma, 929

INDEX

CIC::DUX4 fusion sarcoma, **824**
- differential diagnosis, **827**

CIC::NUTM1 sarcoma, **897**

CIC-rearranged sarcomas, **824–825, 892**
- differential diagnosis, **827**
- molecular genetics, **826**

Cirrhosis, **611**

Classic hairy cell leukemia, splenic B-cell lymphoma/leukemia, unclassifiable vs., **338**

Classic Hodgkin lymphoma (CHL), **292**
- anaplastic large cell lymphoma, ALK-negative vs., **458**
- anaplastic large cell lymphoma, ALK-positive vs., **464**
- EBV-associated, **88**
- nodal follicular helper T-cell lymphoma vs., **452**
- peripheral T-cell lymphoma, not otherwise specified vs., **446**

Classic leiomyosarcoma, **892**

Classic medulloblastoma, **940**

Claudin-low breast cancer, **723**

Clear cell adenocarcinoma, **739**

Clear cell carcinoma, **519, 769, 770**
- eosinophilic subtype, oncocytoma vs., **651**
- germ cell tumor, ovary vs., **782**
- rhabdoid tumor of kidney vs., **653**
- serous tumors of ovary and fallopian tube vs., **765**
- uterus, **750–753**
    - differential diagnosis, **752**
    - genetic predisposition, **751**
    - genetic testing, **751–752**
    - prognosis, **751**

Clear cell chondrosarcoma, **816, 841, 895**
- chondroblastoma vs., **842**
- differential diagnosis, **842**

Clear cell-containing SG tumors, clear cell carcinoma vs., **521**

Clear cell ependymoma
- ependymal tumors, **933**
- oligodendroglioma vs., **929**

Clear cell papillary renal cell carcinoma
- clear cell renal cell carcinoma vs., **632**
- papillary renal cell carcinoma vs., **637**

Clear cell renal cell carcinoma, **630–633**
- differential diagnosis, **632**
- molecular genetics, **631–632**
- prognosis, **631**
- sporadic, **631**
- *VHL* wildtype, **631**

Clear cell sarcoma, **892**
- kidney, **648–649**
    - differential diagnosis, **649**
    - prognosis, **649**
- malignant peripheral nerve sheath tumor vs., **888**
- of soft tissue, **898, 899, 900–901, 902**
- Wilms tumor vs., **645**

Clear cell sarcoma-like tumor, of GI tract, gastrointestinal stromal tumor vs., **594**

Clear cell tumors, **769, 770**

Clinical Laboratory Improvement Amendments (CLIA), **958, 960**
- regulations, **968–969**

CLL. *See* Chronic lymphocytic leukemia.

Clonal cytopenia of undetermined significance (CCUS)
- clonal hematopoiesis and premalignant clonal cytopenia, **183**
- myelodysplastic syndrome with mutated *SF3B1* vs., **190**

Clonal hematopoiesis and premalignant clonal cytopenia, **182–183**

Clonal hematopoiesis of indeterminate potential (CHIP), clonal hematopoiesis and premalignant clonal cytopenia, **183**

Clonal hematopoietic myeloproliferative neoplasm, chronic eosinophilic leukemia, NOS, **161**

Clonal hematopoietic stem cell disorder, myelodysplastic syndrome with mutated *SF3B1*, **189**

Clonal monocytosis of undetermined significance (CMUS), clonal hematopoiesis and premalignant clonal cytopenia, **183**

Clonality
- criteria, **19**
- testing, **296**
    - *IGH* gene rearrangements, **74**
    - limitations, **297**
    - *TRB* gene rearrangement, **81**
    - *TRG* and *TRD* chain rearrangements, **77–78**

Clone, definition, **19**

Cloud-based software solutions, NGS analysis, **37**

CML. *See* Chronic myeloid leukemia.

CMML. *See* Chronic myelomonocytic leukemia.

CMS. *See* Centers for Medicare and Medicaid Services.

CMUS. *See* Clonal monocytosis of undetermined significance.

CNL. *See* Chronic neutrophilic leukemia.

CNS tumors, EZH2 protein overexpression, **100**

Coagulopathy, lymphoplasmacytic lymphoma, **345**

Coding DNA reference sequence, **14**

Codons, **10**

Cold agglutinin hemolysis, lymphoplasmacytic lymphoma, **345**

Collagen vascular disorders, myelodysplastic/myeloproliferative neoplasm, NOS vs., **230**

College of American Pathologists (CAP)
- accreditation, **966–968**
    - checklists, **967–968**
    - commissioners, **967**
    - deficiencies, **968**
    - denial or revocation, **968**
    - inspections, **967**
    - probation, **968**
    - programs, **966**
    - standards, **966–967**
- proficiency testing, **969**

Colon adenocarcinoma, EZH2 protein overexpression, **101**

Colorectal adenocarcinoma, precancerous lesions, **584–589**
- chromosomal instability pathway, **585**
- differential diagnosis, **587**
- gene mutations, **586–587**
- genetic testing, **587**
- hereditary, **583**
- mismatch repair (MMR) pathway, **585**

- prognosis, **586**
- sporadic polyps, **585**

Colorectal carcinoma
- *BRAF* mutations, **119**
- chromosomal microarray, **24**
- *KRAS* mutations, **117**

Commissioners, CAP, **967**
Composite HE, **880**
Computational hardware, **36**
Congenital amegakaryocytic thrombocytopenia (CAMT), **57**
Congenital dyserythropoietic anemia, myelodysplastic syndrome, NOS vs., **195**
Congenital hematologic disorders, myelodysplastic syndrome, NOS vs., **195**
Congenital mesoblastic nephroma, rhabdoid tumor of kidney vs., **653**
Congenital neutropenia, severe, somatic *CSF3R* mutations in, chronic neutrophilic leukemia vs., **146**
Congenital sideroblastic anemia (CSA), myelodysplastic syndrome with mutated *SF3B1* vs., **190**
Constitutional disorders, *IDH1* and *IDH2* mutations, **69**
Conventional central osteosarcomas, **810–811, 813**
- cytogenetics, **812**
- differential diagnosis, **814**
- gene alterations, **812**

Conventional cytogenetic studies, lymphoid neoplasms, **293**
Conversion, **14, 15**
Copper deficiency
- myelodysplastic syndrome, NOS vs., **195**
- pediatric myelodysplastic syndrome and refractory cytopenia of childhood vs., **212**
- VEXAS syndrome vs., **180**

Copy number variations (CNVs), **22**
- pathogenic, **24**
- resources for interpretation, **24**
- uncertain clinical significance, **24**

Cowden syndrome, uterine endometrioid carcinoma, **745**
Cribriform neuroepithelial tumor, choroid plexus tumors vs., **945**
CRLF2. See Cytokine receptor-like factor 2.
CRTC1::SS18 undifferentiated round cell sarcoma, **897**
Cryoglobulinemia, lymphoplasmacytic lymphoma, **345**
CSA. See Congenital sideroblastic anemia.
CSF1 gene, giant cell tumor of bone, **834**
CSF1R fusion partners, B-lymphoblastic leukemia/lymphoma, *BCR::ABL1*-like (Ph-like ALL), **308**
CSF1R gene, **124**
CSF3R mutations, **60–61**
- atypical chronic myeloid leukemia, **222**
- chronic neutrophilic leukemia, **145**
- germline, chronic neutrophilic leukemia vs., **146**
- myelodysplastic/myeloproliferative neoplasm, NOS, **230**
- in neoplasms, chronic neutrophilic leukemia vs., **146**
- somatic, in severe congenital neutropenia, chronic neutrophilic leukemia vs., **146**

CSF3R protein, **60**
CSNK1A1 gene, myelodysplastic syndrome with del(5q), **201**

C-terminus mutation, *FLT3*, *NPM1*, and *CEBPA* mutations, **51**
CTNNA1 (5q), non-HPV-related head and neck squamous cell carcinoma, **507**
CTNNB1 gene, **124–125**
CTNNB1 mutations
- anaplastic thyroid carcinoma, **551**
- endometrial intraepithelial neoplasia, **743**
- non-HPV-related head and neck squamous cell carcinoma, **507**
- poorly differentiated thyroid carcinoma, **548**
- Wilms tumor, **645**

CTR9 mutations, Wilms tumor, **645**
Cures Act, **960**
Cutaneous anaplastic large cell lymphoma
- anaplastic large cell lymphoma, ALK-negative vs., **458**
- mycosis fungoides/Sézary syndrome vs., **435**

Cutaneous mastocytosis, **168**
CXCL8 (4q), non-HPV-related head and neck squamous cell carcinoma, **507**
CXCR4 mutations, lymphoplasmacytic lymphoma, **346**
Cystadenoma, serous
- pancreatic intraductal papillary mucinous neoplasm vs., **621**
- pancreatic mucinous cystic neoplasm vs., **619**

Cytogenetics, **18–21**
- conventional, *BCR::ABL1* fusion, **43**

Cytokine receptor-like factor 2 (*CRLF2*), B-lymphoblastic leukemia/lymphoma, *BCR::ABL1*-like (Ph-like ALL), **307**
Cytologic dysplasia, reactive disorders with
- myelodysplastic syndrome, NOS vs., **195**
- pediatric myelodysplastic syndrome and refractory cytopenia of childhood vs., **212**

Cytomegalovirus infection
- juvenile myelomonocytic leukemia vs., **227**
- pediatric myelodysplastic syndrome and refractory cytopenia of childhood vs., **212**

Cytopenias
- myelodysplastic syndrome with *TP53* multihit mutations vs., **205**
- myelodysplastic/myeloproliferative neoplasm, NOS vs., **229**
- myeloproliferative neoplasm, unclassifiable, **163**
- reactive (nonneoplastic) causes of, myelodysplastic syndrome, NOS vs., **195**

D

DAPK1 (9q), non-HPV-related head and neck squamous cell carcinoma, **507**
DCC (18q), non-HPV-related head and neck squamous cell carcinoma, **507**
DCSTAMP gene, giant cell tumor of bone, **834**
DDR2 gene mutations, lung adenocarcinoma, **563**
Dedifferentiated chondrosarcoma, **838, 839, 841**
- differential diagnosis, **842**
- genetic testing, **840**

INDEX

Dedifferentiated liposarcomas, **858–859, 860, 861, 892**
- differential diagnosis, **862**
- pleomorphic liposarcoma vs., **862**
- prognosis, **859**

Deep vein thrombosis, monoclonal gammopathy, of undetermined significance, **351**
Deficiencies, CAP, **968**
DEK gene, function, **259**
DEK-NUP214 rearrangement, **259**
del(5q), myelodysplastic syndrome with, **200–203**
- cytogenetics, **201**
- differential diagnosis, **201**
- molecular genetics, **201**
- prognosis, **201**

Deletion, **14, 15, 19**
Deletion/insertion (indel), **14**
Dendritic cell neoplasm
- blastic plasmacytoid, **284–289**
  - cytogenetics, **285**
  - differential diagnosis, **286**
  - molecular genetics, **286**
  - prognosis, **285**
- other than Langerhans cell histiocytosis/Langerhans cell sarcoma, histiocytic sarcoma vs., **472**

Dendritic cell sarcoma
- follicular, **488–491**
  - cytogenetics, **489**
  - differential diagnosis, **490**
  - EBV-associated, **89**
  - inflammatory pseudotumor-like, **89**
  - interdigitating dendritic cell tumor vs., **486**
  - molecular genetics, **489**
  - prognosis, **489**
- inflammatory pseudotumor-like follicular
  - liver, **89**
  - spleen, **89**
- interdigitating
  - follicular dendritic cell sarcoma vs., **490**
  - Langerhans cell histiocytosis vs., **481**

Dendritic cell tumor, interdigitating, **484–488**
- cytogenetics, **485**
- differential diagnosis, **486**
- prognosis, **485**

Dendritic cells, plasmacytoid, nodules of, blastic plasmacytoid dendritic cell neoplasm vs., **286**
Dense histiocyte infiltration, gastric adenocarcinoma vs., **582**
Denys-Drash syndrome, Wilms tumor, **644**
Deoxyribonucleic acid (DNA), **5**
Derivative chromosome, **19**
Dermal-based lymphomas, atypical lymphoid infiltrates vs., **786**
Dermatofibroma, **802–803**
- cytogenetics, **803**
- differential diagnosis, **803**
- genetics, **803**

Dermatofibrosarcoma protuberans, **802–803, 848, 850, 852, 892**
- cytogenetics, **803**
- differential diagnosis, **803, 851**
- genetics, **803**

Desmoid fibromatosis, **848, 849, 852, 892**
- differential diagnosis, **851**
Desmoplastic basal cell carcinoma, **798**
Desmoplastic fibroblastoma, **892**
Desmoplastic melanoma, **789**
- leiomyosarcoma vs., **872**
Desmoplastic small round cell tumor (DSRCT), **824, 892**
- differential diagnosis, **827**
- Ewing sarcoma vs., **821**
- molecular genetics, **826**
- neuroblastoma vs., **676**
Desmoplastic/nodular medulloblastoma, **940**
Developmental disorders, *KRAS* mutations, **117**
Diabetes, metabolic factors, **611**
Diamond-Blackfan anemia, acute myeloid leukemia, **233**
Dideoxynucleotides (ddNTPs), **32**
Differentiated vulvar intraepithelial neoplasia (D-VIN), preneoplastic conditions, cervix/vulva/vagina vs., **731**
Diffuse astrocytoma
- IDH-mutant. *See* Astrocytoma, IDH-mutant.
- *MYB-* or *MYBL1*-altered, astrocytoma, IDH-mutant vs., **922**

Diffuse glioma. *See* Astrocytoma, IDH-mutant.
Diffuse hemispheric glioma, H3G34 mutant
- astrocytoma, IDH-mutant vs., **922**
- glioblastoma, IDH wildtype vs., **918**

Diffuse high-grade glioma, pediatric-type, glioblastoma, IDH wildtype vs., **918**
Diffuse large B-cell lymphoma (DLBCL), **294, 298, 299, 376–385**
- anaplastic thyroid carcinoma vs., **552**
- associated with chronic inflammation, **87**
- Burkitt lymphoma vs., **390**
- cytogenetics, **378**
- differential diagnosis, **379**
- EBV(+)
  - nodal follicular helper T-cell lymphoma vs., **452**
  - not otherwise specified, **87**
- *EZH2* mutation, **99**
- fibrin-associated, **87**
- histiocytic sarcoma vs., **472**
- mantle cell lymphoma vs., **373**
- molecular changes, **348**
- molecular genetics, **378**
- myeloid sarcoma vs., **278**
- not otherwise specified, **87, 377**
- prognosis, **377**

Diffuse low-grade glioma, MAPK pathway-altered, astrocytoma, IDH-mutant vs., **922**
Diffuse malignant mesothelioma, serous tumors of ovary and fallopian tube vs., **765**
Diffuse midline glioma, H3 K27-altered, astrocytoma, IDH-mutant vs., **922**
Diffuse sclerosing variant, papillary thyroid carcinoma, **540**
Digital droplet PCR, *BCR::ABL1* fusion, **44**
Digital ischemia, essential thrombocythemia, **157**
Digital PCR (dPCR), *EGFR* amplification, **121**
Dimeric receptor tyrosine kinase, **110**
Diploid, **4**
Distinctive nested glomoid neoplasm, **897**

INDEX

DLBCL. *See* Diffuse large B-cell lymphoma.
DNA. *See* Deoxyribonucleic acid.
DNA amplification, **31**
DNA digestion, **84**
DNA fingerprinting, Southern blot analysis, **85**
DNA fragments, gel electrophoresis, **85**
DNA high-resolution melting curve analysis, **30–31**
- amplicon sizes, **31**
- *CSF3R* mutations, **61**
- fluorescent dyes, **31**
- *JAK2* mutations, **55**
- *NOTCH1* mutation, **97**
- pre-HRM specimen preparations, **31**
- *SETBP1* mutations, **63**

DNA hybridization, **85**
DNA isolation, **31**
DNA methylation analysis, **38–39**
- astrocytoma, IDH-mutant, **921**
- bisulfite conversion methods, **38–39**
- nonbisulfite-dependent methods, **38**

DNA methyltransferase (DNMT) inhibitors, **39**
DNA microarray technology, lymphoid neoplasms, **293**
DNA polymerase, **8**
- error rates, **8**
- fidelity, **8**

DNA preparation, Southern blot analysis, **84**
DNA repair, **8**
DNA repair gene, **130**
DNA replication, **8–9**
DNA stabilization, in membrane, **85**
DNA strands, dissociation, **8–9**
DNA transcription, **9–10**
DNA translation, **10**
DNMT3A mutations
- acute myeloid leukemia, **234–235**
- acute myeloid leukemia, NOS, **273**
- atypical chronic myeloid leukemia, **222**
- nodal follicular helper T-cell lymphoma, **451**
- T-lymphoblastic leukemia/lymphoma, **312**

Double-hit lymphomas, **299**
Down syndrome
- acute myeloid leukemia, **233**
- myeloid leukemia associated with, acute myeloid leukemia with t(1;22)/*RBM15::MRTFA* vs., **263**
- myeloid proliferations associated with, **280–283**
    cytogenetics, **282**
    diagnostic checklist, **282**
    differential diagnosis, **282**
    prognosis, **281–282**
- pediatric myelodysplastic syndrome and refractory cytopenia of childhood vs., **210**

Driver mutations, **13**
Droplet digital polymerase chain reaction, **29**
Drug reactions, mycosis fungoides/Sézary syndrome vs., **435**
Drugs/medications, myelodysplastic syndrome, NOS vs., **195**
DSRCT. *See* Desmoplastic small round cell tumor.
Dual-probe ISH assay, *ERBB2* (HER2) gene amplifications, **115**

Ductal carcinoma, in situ (DCIS) (dysplastic, premalignant), **688–693**
- differential diagnosis, **692**
- molecular genetics, **690**
- as precursor lesion, **689**
- prognosis, **689**
- propriety recurrence score, **690–691**

Ductal carcinomas, **694–699**
- breast cancer histologic grade and molecular characteristics, **698**
- invasive, molecular subtypes, **698**

Duplex scorpion primers, **28**
Duplication, **14, 15**
DUSP22 rearrangements, primary cutaneous CD30-positive T-cell lymphoproliferative disorders, **439**
Dysembryoplastic neuroepithelial tumor, oligodendroglioma vs., **929**
Dysgerminoma, germ cell tumor, ovary, **781–782**
Dyskeratosis congenita
- acute myeloid leukemia, **233**
- myelodysplastic syndrome, NOS vs., **195**

Dyspareunia, squamous cell carcinoma, cervix/vulva/vagina, **735**
Dysplastic nevi
- cytogenetics, **785**
- differential diagnosis, **786**
- melanoma vs., **790**
- molecular genetics, **785**

E

Early T-cell precursor acute lymphoblastic leukemia, **99, 311**
- gene mutations in, **312**
- prognosis, **311–312**

Ebola virus infection, juvenile myelomonocytic leukemia vs., **227**
EBV-associated human neoplasms, **84–93**
- latent infection, **86–87**
- lytic infection, **86–87**
- structure and genome, **84**
- virion, **84**

EBV(+) diffuse large B-cell lymphoma
- nodal follicular helper T-cell lymphoma vs., **452**

EBV(+) mucocutaneous ulcer, **87**
EBV(+) nodal T-/NK-cell lymphoma, extranodal NK-/T-cell lymphoma vs., **408**
E-cadherin gene (*CDH1*)
- germline mutations, **702**
- mechanism of loss, **701–702**

ECC. *See* Extrahepatic cholangiocarcinoma.
EGFR amplification, **121**
- astrocytoma, IDH-mutant, **921**

EGFR gene, **125**
- alterations, **120–121**
    detection, **121**
- non-HPV-related head and neck squamous cell carcinoma, **506**

INDEX

EGFR mutations, 120–121
- lung adenocarcinoma, 561–562

Elston and Ellis modification of Scarff-Bloom-Richardson histologic grade, 696–697

Embryonal carcinoma, 627
- germ cell tumor, ovary, 782

Embryonal neoplasms, malignant, medulloblastoma, 939

Embryonal rhabdomyosarcoma, 868, 870, 892
- differential diagnosis, 872
- Ewing sarcoma vs., 821
- genetic findings, 871
- malignant peripheral nerve sheath tumor vs., 888

Enchondroma, 895
- central chondrosarcoma vs., 842

Endocervical adenocarcinoma, poorly differentiated, squamous cell carcinoma, cervix/vulva/vagina vs., 736

Endocervical adenocarcinoma in situ
- endometrial intraepithelial neoplasia vs., 743
- preneoplastic conditions, cervix/vulva/vagina, 731

Endocrine tumors, EZH2 protein overexpression, 100

Endometrial adenocarcinoma, adenocarcinoma, cervix/vulva/vagina vs., 740

Endometrial carcinoma
- EZH2 protein overexpression, 100
- prototypical type I, 745
- prototypical type II, 749

Endometrial hyperplasia with atypia, endometrial intraepithelial neoplasia vs., 743

Endometrial intraepithelial neoplasia, 742–743
- differential diagnosis, 743
- molecular genetics, 743
- prognosis, 743

Endometrial polyp, endometrial intraepithelial neoplasia vs., 743

Endometrial stromal nodule, low-grade endometrial stromal sarcoma vs., 756

Endometrioid adenocarcinoma, sex cord-stromal tumors of ovary vs., 778

Endometrioid borderline tumor, 769

Endometrioid carcinoma, 769, 770
- with clear cell changes, not otherwise specified, clear cell carcinoma, uterus vs., 752
- secretory variant, clear cell carcinoma, uterus vs., 752
- with squamous differentiation, clear cell carcinoma, uterus vs., 752
- uterine, 744–747
  - Cancer Genome Atlas molecular subtypes, 745–746
  - genetic predisposition syndromes, 745
  - Lynch syndrome-associated, 745
  - MSI testing, 745, 746
  - prognosis, 745
  - sporadic, 745
- uterine serous carcinoma vs., 749

Endometrioid tumors, 769

Endometriosis, adenocarcinoma, cervix/vulva/vagina vs., 740

Endopredict, 696

Enhancer, 9

Enteropathy-associated NK-/T-cell lymphoma, 446

Enteropathy-associated T-cell lymphoma, 417, 418, 419, 446
- cytogenetics, 420
- diagnostic checklist, 421
- differential diagnosis, 421
- prognosis, 419

Environmental factors, 611

Eosinophilia, myeloid neoplasms with, 135

Eosinophilic cytoplasm, oncocytoma vs., 651

Eosinophilic granuloma. *See* Langerhans cell histiocytosis.

EPD. *See* Extramammary Paget disease.

Ependymal tumors, 932–937
- differential diagnosis, 934
- genetic testing, 934
- prognosis, 933

Ependymoma
- choroid plexus tumors vs., 945
- clear cell, oligodendroglioma vs., 929

Epidermal growth factor receptor (EGFR), 120
- function and structure, 120
- small molecule inhibitors, 121

Epidermotropic T-cell lymphomas, atypical lymphoid infiltrates vs., 786

Epithelial-myoepithelial carcinoma (E-MC)
- differential diagnosis, 521
- HPV-related multiphenotypic sinonasal carcinoma vs., 497
- molecular genetics, 520
- prognosis, 519

Epithelioid hemangioendothelioma, 878, 879, 892
- differential diagnosis, 881
- genetic findings, 880
- prognosis, 879

Epithelioid hemangioma, 892
- angiosarcoma vs., 881
- epithelioid hemangioendothelioma vs., 881

Epithelioid melanoma, malignant peripheral nerve sheath tumor vs., 888

Epithelioid neoplasms, poorly differentiated, diffuse large B-cell lymphoma vs., 379

Epithelioid sarcoma, 892, 898, 899, 900, 902
- rhabdoid tumor of kidney vs., 653
- sclerosing epithelioid fibrosarcoma vs., 851

EPOR fusion partner, B-lymphoblastic leukemia/lymphoma, *BCR::ABL1*-like (Ph-like ALL), 308

EPOR rearrangements, B-lymphoblastic leukemia/lymphoma, *BCR::ABL1*-like (Ph-like ALL), 307

Epstein-Barr virus (EBV)
- associated lymphomas, 87–88
  - in HIV-positive patients, 88
- detection, molecular techniques, 89
- gastric adenocarcinoma, 581
- nonlymphoid neoplasms, 88–89
- pediatric myelodysplastic syndrome and refractory cytopenia of childhood vs., 212

ERBB2 (HER2) amplification
- colorectal adenocarcinoma and precancerous lesions, 586
- lung adenocarcinoma, 562
- serous borderline tumor, 765

INDEX

ERBB2 (HER2) gene, **125**
- amplifications, FISH for, **112, 114–115**
- function, **114**
- overexpression, in cancer, **114**

ERBB2 signaling pathway, activation, gastric adenocarcinoma, **582**

ERBB3 somatic mutation, Langerhans cell histiocytosis, **480**

ERBB4 gene, **125**

Erdheim-Chester disease, Langerhans cell histiocytosis vs., **480–481**

Erythroid leukemia, acute, myelodysplastic syndrome with *TP53* multihit mutations vs., **205**

Erythrophagocytic T-γ lymphoma. *See* Hepatosplenic T-cell lymphoma.

Esophageal squamous cell carcinoma, EZH2 protein overexpression, **101**

Essential thrombocythemia, **156–159**
- *CALR* mutations with, **59**
- cytogenetics, **157**
- differential diagnosis, **158**
- molecular genetics, **157–158**
- myeloproliferative neoplasm, unclassifiable vs., **164**
- polycythemia vera vs., **150**
- primary myelofibrosis vs., **154**
- prognosis, **157**
- sporadic, essential thrombocythemia, **157**

Essential thrombocytosis. *See* Essential thrombocythemia.

Esthesioneuroblastoma, medulloblastoma vs., **940**

ETNK1 mutation, atypical chronic myeloid leukemia, **222**

ETV6::ABL1 fusion, **174**

ETV6::JAK2 fusion, **55**

ETV6::PDGFRB fusion, **176**

Euchromatin, **5**

Ewing family of tumors, olfactory neuroblastoma vs., **534**

Ewing-like sarcomas, Ewing sarcoma vs., **821**

Ewing sarcoma, **818–823, 895**
- atypical, **820–821**
- *CIC*-rearranged sarcomas vs., **827**
- classic, **820**
- cytogenetics, **820**
- differential diagnosis, **821**
- epigenetics, **820**
- genetic predisposition, **819**
- malignant peripheral nerve sheath tumor vs., **888**
- molecular genetics, **820**
- with neural differentiation, **820**
- neuroblastoma vs., **676**
- prognosis, **819**
- round cell sarcoma with *EWSR1*::non-ETS fusions vs., **827**
- sarcoma with *BCOR* genetic alterations vs., **827**
- Wilms tumor vs., **645**

Ewing sarcoma family of tumors
- alveolar rhabdomyosarcoma vs., **872**
- small cell osteosarcoma vs., **814**

EWSR1::non-ETS fusions, round cell sarcoma with, **825–826**
- differential diagnosis, **827**
- molecular genetics, **826**

EWSR1::*SMAD3*-positive fibroblastic tumor, **892**

Exons, **9**

Extrahepatic cholangiocarcinoma (ECC), **622**

Extramammary Paget disease (EPD), preneoplastic conditions, cervix/vulva/vagina, **731, 732**

Extranodal marginal zone lymphoma
- gastrointestinal tract, lymphoplasmacytic lymphoma vs., **347**
- of mucosa-associated lymphoid tissue, **299**

Extranodal NK-/T-cell lymphoma (ENKTL), **406–409**
- aggressive NK-cell leukemia vs., **402**
- cytogenetics, **407**
- differential diagnosis, **408**
- intestinal T-cell lymphoma vs., **421**
- molecular genetics, **408**
- prognosis, **407**

Extraosseous plasmacytoma, medullary thyroid carcinoma vs., **557**

Extrarenal rhabdoid tumor, **898, 899, 901, 902**

Extraskeletal myxoid chondrosarcoma, **898, 899, 901, 902**

EZH2 gene, **125**
- function, **98**
- mutation, **98–101**
    - atypical chronic myeloid leukemia, **222**
    - gain-of-function mutations, **98**
    - loss-of-function mutations, **98**
    - myelodysplastic syndrome, NOS, **194**
    - myeloproliferative neoplasm, unclassifiable, **164**
    - polycythemia vera, **150**
    - somatic, **98**

EZH2 inhibitors, **101**

EZH2 protein, **98**
- overexpression, solid tumors, **100**

F

FAM131B::BRAF fusion gene, pilocytic astrocytoma, **926**

Familial adenomatous polyposis (FAP), **805**
- adrenal cortical carcinoma, **667**
- colorectal adenocarcinoma and precancerous lesions, **585**
- medulloblastoma, **939**

Familial hemophagocytic lymphohistiocytosis, Langerhans cell histiocytosis vs., **481**

Familial neuroblastoma, **674–675**
- *ALK* alterations, **105**

Familial platelet disorder, acute myeloid leukemia, **233**

Familial predisposition syndromes, **233**

Fanconi anemia
- acute myeloid leukemia, **233**
- myelodysplastic syndrome, NOS vs., **195**

FAP. *See* Familial adenomatous polyposis.

FAS mutation, mycosis fungoides/Sézary syndrome, **434**

Fasciitis, nodular, **892**
- inflammatory myofibroblastic tumor vs., **851**

FAT1 (4q), non-HPV-related head and neck squamous cell carcinoma, **506**

INDEX

FBXW7 gene, **125**
- non-HPV-related head and neck squamous cell carcinoma, **507**
- T-lymphoblastic leukemia/lymphoma, **312**
- Wilms tumor, **645**

FDA. *See* Food and Drug Administration.
FDA-approved tests, **929**
FDA-cleared tests, **929**
Federal agencies, regulation of laboratories, **958–959**
Federal laws, IVDs, **960**
Federal Register, **960**
Female genital tract tumors, EZH2 protein overexpression, **100**
FGF1 gene, non-HPV-related head and neck squamous cell carcinoma, **507**
FGFR1 gene, **125**
FGFR1 mutations, **174**
- B-lymphoblastic leukemia/lymphoma, *BCR::ABL1*-like (Ph-like ALL), **307**
- lung adenocarcinoma, **563**
- pilocytic astrocytoma, **926**
- rearrangement, **175**
    detection, **176**
- testing, **175**

FGFR2 gene, **125–126**
- lung adenocarcinoma, **563**

FGFR3 gene, **126**
- lung adenocarcinoma, **563**

FGFR3::TACC3 fusions, glioblastoma, IDH wildtype, **918**
Fibroadenomas, **718**
Fibroblastic tumors, intermediate and malignant, **848–857**
- chromosome and gene alterations, **852**
- differential diagnosis, **851**

Fibroepithelioma of Pinkus, **798**
Fibroma, **775, 777**
- chondromyxoid, **838, 839, 841–842**
    differential diagnosis, **842**
    genetic testing, **840**
- cytogenetics, **776**
- nonossifying, giant cell tumor of bone vs., **835**
- prognosis, **776**
- of tendon sheath, **892**

Fibromatosis
- desmoid, **848, 849, 892**
    differential diagnosis, **851**
- gastrointestinal stromal tumor vs., **594**
- superficial, desmoid fibromatosis vs., **851**

Fibromyxoid sarcoma, low-grade, **849, 850–851**
- differential diagnosis, **851**

Fibrosarcoma, **775, 777**
- adult, dermatofibrosarcoma protuberans vs., **851**
- congenital, embryonal rhabdomyosarcoma vs., **872**
- cytogenetics, **776**
- infantile, **852**
- leiomyosarcoma vs., **872**
- molecular genetics, **777**
- prognosis, **776**

Fibrous dysplasia, **895**
- low-grade central osteosarcoma vs., **814**
- parosteal osteosarcoma vs., **814**
- periosteal osteosarcoma vs., **814**

Fibrous histiocytoma
- dermatofibroma vs., **803**
- dermatofibrosarcoma protuberans vs., **851**

Fibroxanthoma, atypical, squamous cell carcinoma, skin vs., **794**
FIP1L1::PDGFRA fusion, **176**
FISH. *See* Fluorescence in situ hybridization.
5' capping, **9–10**
Flemming, Walther, **18**
Florid vaginal adenosis, adenocarcinoma, cervix/vulva/vagina vs., **740**
FLT3 gene, **126**
- T-lymphoblastic leukemia/lymphoma, **312**

FLT3 ITD mutations
- acute myeloid leukemia, **234**
- acute myeloid leukemia, NOS, **272–273**
- acute myeloid leukemia with inv(16) or t(16;16)/*CBFB::MYH11*, **246**
- acute myeloid leukemia with t(8;21)/*RUNX1::RUNX1T1*, **242**
- myeloid sarcoma, **278**

FLT3 mutations, **50–53, 174**
- acute myeloid leukemia with inv(16) or t(16;16)/*CBFB::MYH11*, **246**
- B-lymphoblastic leukemia/lymphoma, *BCR::ABL1*-like (Ph-like ALL), **307**
- myelodysplastic/myeloproliferative neoplasm, NOS, **230**

FLT3 TKD mutations
- acute myeloid leukemia, **234**
- acute myeloid leukemia with inv(16) or t(16;16)/*CBFB::MYH11*, **246**
- acute myeloid leukemia with t(8;21)/*RUNX1::RUNX1T1*, **242**

FLTS3 mutations
- function, **50**
- mutations, **51**
    clinical significance, **52**
    testing, **53**

Fluorescence in situ hybridization (FISH), **19–20**
- *BCR::ABL1* fusion, **43**
- Burkitt lymphoma, **388**
- diffuse large B-cell lymphoma, **378**
- *EGFR* amplification, **121**
- for *ERBB2* (HER2) gene amplifications, **114–115**
    dual-probe ISH assay, **115**
    methodology, **115**
    pathology review of concurrent H&E, **115**
    predictive cancer testing summary, **115**
    quantitative real-time PCR for evaluation of *ERBB2* gene status, **115**
    single-probe ISH assay, **115**
- karyotype vs., **175**
- *KMT2A*-rearranged, **256**
- lymphoid neoplasms, **293, 296, 297**
- melanoma, **789**
- for *MET* amplifications, **112**
    aberrant *MET* signaling, **110–111, 112**
    MET amplification and chemotherapy, **111–112**
    MET overexpression in tumors, **112**
    predictive cancer testing summary, **112**

INDEX

testing, 112
- molecular work-up of myeloid neoplasms, 134
- *PML::RARA* fusion, 47
- *RET* fusion, 109
- *ROS1* fusion, 107

Fluorescence resonance energy transfer (FRET) probes, 28
Fluorescent dyes, 31
Focal nodular hyperplasia
- β-catenin-activated hepatocellular adenoma vs., 604
- hepatocellular carcinoma vs., 612
- *HNF1A*-inactivated hepatocellular adenoma vs., 600
- inflammatory hepatocellular adenoma vs., 608

Folate deficiency
- myelodysplastic syndrome, NOS vs., 195
- pediatric myelodysplastic syndrome and refractory cytopenia of childhood vs., 212
- VEXAS syndrome vs., 180

Follicular adenoma and carcinoma, papillary thyroid carcinoma vs., 540
Follicular carcinoma, medullary thyroid carcinoma vs., 556
Follicular dendritic cell sarcoma, 488–491
- cytogenetics, 489
- differential diagnosis, 490
- EBV-associated, 89
- inflammatory pseudotumor-like, 89
- interdigitating dendritic cell tumor vs., 486
- molecular genetics, 489
- prognosis, 489

Follicular lesion of uncertain malignant potential, follicular thyroid carcinoma vs., 544
Follicular lymphoma (FL), 294, 298, 299, 362–369
- classification, 363
- cytogenetics, 366
- differential diagnosis, 365
- diffuse, 365
- early and late genetic alterations, 367
- *EZH2* mutation, 99
- genetic abnormalities, 367
- grading, 364–365
- molecular changes, 330, 348
- molecular genetics, 366
- *MYD88* L265P mutations, 348
- nodal follicular helper T-cell lymphoma vs., 452
- pediatric, 365
- pediatric-type, Burkitt lymphoma vs., 390
- prognosis, 364
- reporting pattern, 365
- in situ, 365
- splenic marginal zone lymphoma vs., 329
- testicular, 365
- testing methods, 297
- variants, 365

Follicular neoplasms, basal cell carcinoma of skin vs., 798
Follicular thyroid adenoma, follicular thyroid carcinoma vs., 544
Follicular thyroid carcinoma (FTC), 542–545
- associated inherited syndromes, 543
- cytogenetics, 543
- differential diagnosis, 544
- molecular genetics, 544
- prognosis, 543

Folliculotropic MF, mycosis fungoides/Sézary syndrome, 433
Food, Drug and Cosmetic Act of 1938 (FD&C Act), 960
Food and Drug Administration (FDA), 958–959
- regulations, 960–965
  - IVDs, 960–964
  - LTDs, 964–965
Food and Drug Administration Modernization Act of 1997 (FDAMA), 960, 963
Fractionation by capillary electrophoresis, 74
Fracture callus, conventional central osteosarcoma vs., 814
Fragment sizing analysis, *CALR* mutations, 59
Frameshift, 14
Frasier syndrome, Wilms tumor, 644
FUBP1 mutations, oligodendroglioma, 929

G

G3BP1 gene, myelodysplastic syndrome with del(5q), 201
GAB1::ABL1 spindle cell neoplasm, 897
Gain-of-function mutations, 98
Gallbladder carcinoma, EZH2 protein overexpression, 101
Gammopathy, monoclonal, of undetermined significance, 350–353
- cytogenetics, 352
- multiple myeloma (plasma cell myeloma) vs., 357
- prognosis, 352
Ganglioneuroma, neuroblastoma vs., 676
Gardner fibroma, 852
Gastric adenocarcinoma, 580–583
- differential diagnosis, 582
- gene mutations, 582
- genetic testing, 582
- prognosis, 582
Gastric carcinoma, 89
- EZH2 protein overexpression, 101
Gastric xanthoma, gastric adenocarcinoma vs., 582
Gastroesophageal adenocarcinoma, *EGFR* amplification, 121
Gastrointestinal stromal tumor (GIST), 590–597, 892
- *BRAF* V600E-mutation, 592, 593
- clinical prognostication, 594
- diagnostic checklist, 594
- differential diagnosis, 594
- genetic testing, 593
- *KIT* mutations, 65, 66, 592, 593
- *PDGFRA*-mutated, 592, 593
- prognosis, 591–592
- SDH-deficient, 592, 593
Gastrointestinal tumors, EZH2 protein overexpression, 100–101
GATA1 mutation
- myeloid leukemia of Down syndrome, 281
- normal function, 281
- transient abnormal myelopoiesis, 281
Gaucher disease, Langerhans cell histiocytosis vs., 481
GCTB. *See* Giant cell tumor of bone.

xix

INDEX

Gel electrophoresis, of DNA fragments, **85**
Gene expression profiling
- Burkitt lymphoma, **388–389**
- clear cell carcinoma, uterus, **752**
- diffuse large B-cell lymphoma, **378**
- Ewing sarcoma, **820**
- extranodal NK-/T-cell lymphoma, **408**
- follicular lymphoma, **366**
- germ cell tumor, ovary, **781**
- head and neck mucosal squamous cell carcinoma, non-HPV related, **502**
- hepatosplenic T-cell lymphoma, **425–426**
- lymphoplasmacytic lymphoma, **346**
- mantle cell lymphoma, **372**
- mycosis fungoides/Sézary syndrome, **434**
- nodal follicular helper T-cell lymphoma, **451**
- peripheral T-cell lymphoma, not otherwise specified, **444**
- primary cutaneous CD30-positive T-cell lymphoproliferative disorders, **440**
- small cell neuroendocrine carcinoma, **574**
- squamous cell carcinoma, cervix/vulva/vagina, **736**
- translocation-specific salivary gland tumors, **521**

Gene fusion transcripts, **49**
Gene mutations, **12–15**
Gene sequencing, *CALR* mutations, **59**
Gene-specific hypermethylation, **39**
Genetic predisposition syndrome, uterine endometrioid carcinoma, **745**
Genitourinary tumors, EZH2 protein overexpression, **100**
Genome-wide hypomethylation, **39**
Genomic grade index (GGI), **697**
Genomic instability, leads, **39**
Genomic reference sequence, **14–15**
Genomic sequencing, lymphoid neoplasms, **293**
Genotype vs. phenotype, **13**
Germ cell neoplasia in situ, **626**
Germ cell tumors
- *KIT* mutations, **66**
- metastatic, desmoplastic small round cell tumor vs., **827**
- ovary, **780–783**
    cytogenetics, **781**
    differential diagnosis, **782**
    molecular genetics, **781**
- serous tumors of ovary and fallopian tube vs., **765**
- testicular, **624–629**
    chromosomal microarray, **626**
    cytogenetics, **626**
    epigenetics, **626**
    gene expression profiling, **626**
    microRNAs, **626**
    molecular genetics, **626**
    postpubertal males, **625**
    prepubertal males, **624**
    prognosis, **625**
    spermatocytic tumor, **626**

Germline *CSF3R* mutation, chronic neutrophilic leukemia vs., **146**
Germline *KIT* mutations, mastocytosis, **169**
Germline mutations, **13**
- *BRAF*, **119**
- E-cadherin gene (*CDH1*), **702**
- *FLT3*, *NPM1*, and *CEBPA* mutations, **51**
- *KRAS* gene, **116**

Germline *RET* mutations, **109**
Germline syndromes, osteosarcoma, **811**
Giant cell tumor of bone (GCTB), **832–837, 895**
- cytogenetics, **833–834**
- differential diagnosis, **835**
- epigenetics, **834**
- with malignant transformation, giant cell tumor of bone vs., **835**
- molecular genetics, **834**

Giant cell tumor of soft tissue, **892**
Giant cell-rich osteosarcoma, giant cell tumor of bone vs., **835**
GIST. *See* Gastrointestinal stromal tumor.
GLI1 epithelioid sarcoma, **897**
Glial neoplasms, medulloblastoma vs., **940**
Glioblastoma
- *EGFR* amplification, **121**
- IDH wildtype, **916–919**
    astrocytoma, IDH-mutant vs., **922**
    cytogenetics, **917**
    differential diagnosis, **918**
    molecular genetics, **917–918**
    prognosis, **917**
- *IDH1* and *IDH2* mutations, **69**

Glioblastoma multiforme
- EZH2 protein overexpression, **100**
- *MGMT* promoter methylation, **131**

Glioma
- *BRAF* mutations, **119**
- *IDH1* and *IDH2* mutations, **69**

Glomangiomas, pheochromocytoma/paraganglioma vs., **663**
Glomus tumor, **892**
- gastrointestinal stromal tumor vs., **594**
- pheochromocytoma/paraganglioma vs., **663**

GNA11 gene, **126**
GNA11 mutations, melanoma, **790**
GNAQ gene, **126**
- melanoma, **790**

GNAS gene, **126**
- pancreatic intraductal papillary mucinous neoplasm, **621**

Goblet cell-rich hyperplastic polyp, colorectal adenocarcinoma and precancerous lesions, **585**
Goiter, amyloid, medullary thyroid carcinoma vs., **557**
Gorlin syndrome, medulloblastoma, **939**
Granulocyte colony-stimulating factor (G-CSF)
- acute myeloid leukemia vs., **236**
- *CSF3R* mutations, **60**
- effect, acute myeloid leukemia, NOS vs., **273**
- myelodysplastic/myeloproliferative neoplasm, NOS vs., **230**

Granulomatous disease, Langerhans cell histiocytosis vs., **481**
Granulomatous slack skin, mycosis fungoides/Sézary syndrome, **433**

INDEX

Granulosa cell tumors, **775, 777**
- prognosis, **776**

H

H3F3A gene, giant cell tumor of bone, **834**
Hairy cell leukemia (HCL), **294, 332–335**
- *BRAF* mutations, **119**
- *BRAF* wildtype, **334**
- classic, splenic B-cell lymphoma/leukemia, unclassifiable vs., **338**
- differential diagnosis, **334**
- genetic testing, **334**
- molecular changes, **330, 348**
- molecular findings, **330**
- *MYD88* L265P mutations, **348**
- splenic B-cell lymphoma/leukemia, unclassifiable, **337**
- splenic marginal zone lymphoma vs., **329, 329–330**
- variant
    hairy cell leukemia vs., **334**
    MYD88 L265P mutations, **348**
Hand-Schüller-Christian disease. *See* Langerhans cell histiocytosis.
HAVCR2 germline mutations, subcutaneous panniculitis-like T-cell lymphoma, **429**
HCC. *See* Hepatocellular carcinoma.
HCL. *See* Hairy cell leukemia.
Head and neck mucosal squamous cell carcinoma
- HPV, head and neck mucosal squamous cell carcinoma, non-HPV related vs., **503**
- non-HPV related, **500–505**
    cytogenetics, **502**
    diagnostic checklist, **503**
    differential diagnosis, **503**
    molecular genetics, **502**
    molecular taxonomy, **502–503**
    prognosis, **501**
Head and neck squamous cell carcinoma (HNSCC), *NOTCH1* mutation, **97**
Head and neck tumors, **530–537**
- cytogenetics, **532**
- diagnostic checklist, **534**
- differential diagnosis, **534**
- molecular genetics, **532**
- prognosis, **531–532**
Heavy metal poisoning, myelodysplastic syndrome, NOS vs., **195**
Helicobacter pylori, gastric adenocarcinoma, **581**
Hemangioblastomas, capillary, clear cell renal cell carcinoma, **631**
Hemangioendothelioma, **879**
- composite, **892**
- epithelioid, **878, 879, 892**
    differential diagnosis, **881**
    genetic findings, **880**
    prognosis, **879**
- genetic findings, **880**
- prognosis, **879**
- pseudomyogenic, **892**
Hemangioma
- angiosarcoma vs., **881**
- epithelioid
    angiosarcoma vs., **881**
    epithelioid hemangioendothelioma vs., **881**
Hematologic malignancies, chromosomal microarray, **23–24**
Hematolymphoid neoplasm, VEXAS syndrome vs., **180**
Hematopoiesis, trisomy 21, **281**
Hematopoietic tumors, molecular genetic tests
- *BCR::ABL1* fusion, **42–45**
- calreticulin (*CALR*) gene mutations, **58–59**
- *CSF3R* mutations, **60–61**
    chronic neutrophilic leukemia, **145**
    germline, chronic neutrophilic leukemia vs., **146**
    in neoplasms, chronic neutrophilic leukemia vs., **146**
    somatic, in severe congenital neutropenia, chronic neutrophilic leukemia vs., **146**
- EBV-associated human neoplasms, **84–93**
    latent infection, **86–87**
    lytic infection, **86–87**
    structure and genome, **84**
    virion, **84**
- *EZH2* mutation, **98–101**
    gain-of-function mutations, **98**
    loss-of-function mutations, **98**
    somatic, **98**
- *FLT3*, *NPM1*, and *CEBPA* mutations, **50–53**
- *IDH1* and *IDH2* mutations, **68–69**
    detection, **68**
    somatic, **68**
- immunoglobulin heavy (*IGH*) chain gene
    rearrangements, **72–75**
    B-cell development, **72–73**
    clonality testing, **73–74**
    locus, **73**
    recombination process, **73**
    structure, **72**
- *JAK2* mutations and rearrangements, **54–55**
- *KIT* mutations, **64–67**
    core binding factor acute myeloid leukemia, **65–66**
    gastrointestinal stromal tumor, **65, 66**
    germ cell tumors, **66**
    melanoma, **65, 66**
    systemic mastocytosis, **65, 66**
- *MPL* mutations, **56–57**
    BCR::ABL1-negative myeloproliferative neoplasms, **57**
    molecular approach, **57**
    thrombopoietin receptor, **57**
- *MYD88* mutation, **94–95**
    diagnostic checklist, **95**
- myeloid neoplasms, mutations and gene panel testing, **70–71**
- *NOTCH1* mutation, **96–97**
    diagnostic checklist, **97**
- *PML::RARA* fusion, **46–47**
- reverse transcription PCR for myeloid leukemia transcripts, **48–49**
- *SETBP1* mutations, **62–63**

INDEX

- Southern blot analysis, antigen receptor genes, **84–85**
    - DNA digestion, **84**
    - DNA hybridization, **85**
    - DNA preparation, **84**
    - DNA stabilization, **85**
    - DNA transfer onto nylon or nitrocellulose membrane, **85**
    - gel electrophoresis, **85**
    - interpretation, **85**
    - vs. PCR, in assessment of clonality in lymphoid proliferations, **85**
- T-cell receptor beta (*TRB*) chain gene rearrangements, **80–83**
- T-cell receptor delta (*TRD*) chain, gene arrangements, **76–79**
- T-cell receptor gamma (*TRG*) chain, gene arrangements, **76–79**

Hemophagocytic lymphohistiocytosis
- familial, Langerhans cell histiocytosis vs., **481**
- histiocytic sarcoma vs., **472**

Hemorrhage, essential thrombocythemia, **157**
Hemosiderotic fibrolipomatous tumor (HSFLT), myxoinflammatory fibroblastic sarcoma vs., **851**
Hepatic carcinoma, EZH2 protein overexpression, **101**
Hepatitis B virus (HBV) infection, chronic, hepatocellular carcinoma vs., **611**
Hepatitis C virus (HCV) infection, hepatocellular carcinoma vs., **611**
Hepatitis viruses infection, pediatric myelodysplastic syndrome and refractory cytopenia of childhood vs., **212**

Hepatocellular adenoma
- β-catenin-activated, **602–605**
    - diagnostic checklist, **604**
    - differential diagnosis, **604**
    - *HNF1A*-inactivated hepatocellular adenoma vs., **600**
    - inflammatory hepatocellular adenoma vs., **608**
    - prognosis, **603**
- hepatocellular carcinoma vs., **612**
- *HNF1A*-inactivated, **598–601**
    - β-catenin-activated hepatocellular adenoma vs., **604**
    - diagnostic checklist, **600**
    - differential diagnosis, **600**
    - inflammatory hepatocellular adenoma vs., **608**
    - prognosis, **599**
- inflammatory, **606–609**
    - β-catenin-activated hepatocellular adenoma vs., **604**
    - diagnostic checklist, **608**
    - differential diagnosis, **608**
    - *HNF1A*-inactivated hepatocellular adenoma vs., **600**
    - prognosis, **607**
- unclassifiable
    - β-catenin-activated hepatocellular adenoma vs., **604**
    - *HNF1A*-inactivated hepatocellular adenoma vs., **600**
    - inflammatory hepatocellular adenoma vs., **608**

Hepatocellular carcinoma (HCC), **610–613**
- adrenal cortical carcinoma vs., **669**
- cholangiocarcinoma vs., **623**
- cytogenetics, **612**
- differential diagnosis, **612**
- molecular genetics, **612**
- pheochromocytoma/paraganglioma vs., **663**
- prognosis, **611**

Hepatoid carcinoma, pancreatic ductal adenocarcinoma, **616**
Hepatomegaly, splenic B-cell lymphoma/leukemia, unclassifiable, **337**
Hepatosplenic T-cell lymphoma (HSTCL), **294, 424–427, 446**
- chronic immunosuppression, **425**
- cytogenetics, **425**
- differential diagnosis, **426**
- peripheral T-cell lymphoma, not otherwise specified vs., **446**
- prognosis, **425**

Hepatosplenomegaly, lymphoplasmacytic lymphoma, **345**
HER2 overexpression, **695**
Hereditary diffuse gastric cancer, gastric adenocarcinoma, **581**
Hereditary neutrophilia, **61**
Hereditary retinoblastoma, **805**
- osteosarcoma, **811**

Hereditary thrombocythemia, essential thrombocythemia, **157**
Hereditary tumor syndrome associations, adrenal cortical carcinoma, **667**
Heterochromatin, **5**
Heterozygous interstitial deletion of 5q, myelodysplastic syndrome with del(5q), **201**

HHV6 infection
- juvenile myelomonocytic leukemia vs., **227**

Hibernoma, **892**
- atypical lipomatous tumor vs., **862**

High resolution, **31**
High-grade astrocytoma, with piloid features
- astrocytoma, IDH-mutant vs., **922**
- pilocytic astrocytoma vs., **926**

High-grade B-cell lymphoma
- with 11q aberration, Burkitt lymphoma vs., **378**
- diffuse large B-cell lymphoma vs., **379**
- with *MYC* and *BCL2* rearrangements, **294**
    - Burkitt lymphoma vs., **390**
    - mantle cell lymphoma vs., **373**
- testing methods, **297**

High-grade carcinomas, serous tumors of ovary and fallopian tube vs., **765**
High-grade endometrial stromal sarcoma, **754**
- differential diagnosis, **756**
- genetic tests, **755**

High-grade endometrioid adenocarcinoma, serous tumors of ovary and fallopian tube vs., **765**
High-grade mucoepidermoid carcinoma, salivary duct carcinoma vs., **521**
High-grade myxoid liposarcoma
- differential diagnosis, **862**
- round cell sarcoma with *EWSR1*::non-ETS fusions vs., **827**

High-grade nonendometrioid endometrial carcinoma (NEEC), **749**

INDEX

High-grade pleomorphic sarcoma, conventional central osteosarcoma vs., **814**
High-grade prostatic intraepithelial neoplasia
- molecular genetics, **686**
- prognosis, **685**

High-grade serous carcinoma (HGSC), **763**
- differential diagnosis, **765**
- molecular carcinogenesis, **764**
- prognosis, **763**

High-grade squamous cell carcinoma, olfactory neuroblastoma vs., **534**
High-grade squamous intraepithelial lesion (HSIL), preneoplastic conditions, cervix/vulva/vagina, **731**
High-resolution melting (HRM), **30**
High-resolution melting curve analysis, *EZH2* mutation, **99**
High-throughput methods in molecular pathology, **36–37**
High-throughput test, **28–29**
H(+) ion semiconductor sequencing, **34**
Histiocytic sarcoma, **470–477**
- cytogenetics, **471**
- differential diagnosis, **472**
- diffuse large B-cell lymphoma vs., **379**
- interdigitating dendritic cell tumor vs., **486**
- Langerhans cell histiocytosis vs., **481**
- molecular genetics, **471**
- prognosis, **471**

Histiocytoma
- angiomatoid fibrous, **892**
- fibrous, dermatofibrosarcoma protuberans vs., **851**

Histiocytosis X. *See* Langerhans cell histiocytosis.
Histone deacetylase inhibitors, **39**
Histones, **5**
HIV infection, pediatric myelodysplastic syndrome and refractory cytopenia of childhood vs., **212**
HLA-A (6p), non-HPV-related head and neck squamous cell carcinoma, **507**
HMGAT2::NCOR2 fusion, giant cell-rich bone tumor with, giant cell tumor of bone vs., **835**
HNF1A gene, **126**
HNF1A-inactivated hepatocellular adenoma, **598–601**
- β-catenin-activated hepatocellular adenoma vs., **604**
- diagnostic checklist, **600**
- differential diagnosis, **600**
- inflammatory hepatocellular adenoma vs., **608**
- prognosis, **599**

HNRNPK deletions, mycosis fungoides/Sézary syndrome, **434**
Hodgkin lymphoma
- chronic eosinophilic leukemia, NOS vs., **161**
- classic, **292**
    - anaplastic large cell lymphoma, ALK-negative vs., **458**
    - anaplastic large cell lymphoma, ALK-positive vs., **464**
    - EBV-associated, **88**
    - nodal follicular helper T-cell lymphoma vs., **452**
    - peripheral T-cell lymphoma, not otherwise specified vs., **446**
- myxoinflammatory fibroblastic sarcoma vs., **851**
- nodular lymphocyte-predominant, nodal follicular helper T-cell lymphoma vs., **452**

Hotspot gene panel, targeted, parallel sequencing, **122–123**
- limits, **123**
- technical and interpretive challenges, **123**

Hotspot genes, **122–123**
- mutated, **122–123**
- targeted therapy, **123**

HPV-associated head and neck carcinomas, **494–499**
- chromosomal microarray, **496**
- cytogenetics, **496**
- diagnostic checklist, **497**
- differential diagnosis, **497**
- molecular genetics, **496**
- prognosis, **495–496**

HPV-associated poorly differentiated neuroendocrine carcinomas, **497**
HPV-independent (HPV-I) vulvar squamous cell carcinoma, **735**
HPV-negative head and neck mucosal squamous cell carcinoma (HNMSCC)
- HPV+HNMSCC vs., **497**
- nasopharyngeal EBV-related squamous cell carcinoma vs., **528**

HPV-negative poorly differentiated neuroendocrine carcinoma, HPV-positive poorly differentiated neuroendocrine carcinoma vs., **497**
HPV-positive head and neck mucosal squamous cell carcinoma (HNMSCC), **497**
- HPV-positive poorly differentiated neuroendocrine carcinoma vs., **497**
- infection by HPV types 16 and 18, **495**
- nasopharyngeal EBV-related squamous cell carcinoma vs., **528**

HPV-positive nasopharyngeal carcinoma, **497**
HPV-positive poorly differentiated neuroendocrine carcinoma, **495, 497**
HPV-related multiphenotypic sinonasal carcinoma (HMSC), **495, 497, 531**
HRAS gene, **126**
HRAS mutations
- anaplastic thyroid carcinoma, **551**
- melanoma, **790**
- non-HPV-related head and neck squamous cell carcinoma, **506**
- papillary thyroid carcinoma, **539**
- poorly differentiated thyroid carcinoma, **547**

HRM. *See* High-resolution melting.
HSTCL. *See* Hepatosplenic T-cell lymphoma.
HTLV-I gene, adult T-cell leukemia/lymphoma, **411–412**
HUD. *See* Humanitarian use device.
Human androgen receptor assay (HUMARA), **39**
Human neoplasms, EBV-associated, **84–93**
- latent infection, **86–87**
- lytic infection, **86–87**
- structure and genome, **84**
- virion, **84**

Humanitarian use device (HUD), **963**
Hungerford, David, **18**
Hyalinizing clear cell carcinoma (HCCC)
- differential diagnosis, **521**

xxiii

INDEX

- molecular genetics, **520**
- prognosis, **519**

Hydroa vacciniforme-like lymphoproliferative disorder, **87**

Hypereosinophilia, chronic eosinophilic leukemia, NOS vs., **161**

Hyperplasia
- pseudoepitheliomatous, squamous cell carcinoma, cervix/vulva/vagina vs., **736**
- reactive follicular, follicular lymphoma vs., **365**

I

ICC. *See* Intrahepatic cholangiocarcinoma.
ICUS. *See* Idiopathic cytopenia of undetermined significance.
IDE. *See* Investigational device exemption.
IDH1 gene, **126**
- glioblastoma, IDH wildtype, **917**
- normal function, **68**

IDH1 mutations, **68–69**
- acute myeloid leukemia, **234**
  NOS, **273**
- astrocytoma, IDH-mutant, **921**
- detection, **68**
- myeloproliferative neoplasm, unclassifiable, **163–164**
- oligodendroglioma, **929**
- polycythemia vera, **150**
- somatic, **68**

IDH2 gene, **126–127**
- normal function, **68**

IDH2 mutations, **68–69**
- acute myeloid leukemia, **234**
- astrocytoma, IDH-mutant, **921**
- detection, **68**
- glioblastoma, IDH wildtype, **917**
- mastocytosis, **168**
- myeloproliferative neoplasm, unclassifiable, **163–164**
- nodal follicular helper T-cell lymphoma, **450**
- oligodendroglioma, **929**
- polycythemia vera, **150**
- somatic, **68**

IDH-mutant, astrocytoma, **920–923**
- diagnostic checklist, **922**
- differential diagnosis, **922**
- molecular genetics, **921**
- prognosis, **921**

IDH wildtype, glioblastoma, **916–919**
- cytogenetics, **917**
- differential diagnosis, **918**
- molecular genetics, **917–918**
- prognosis, **917**

Idiopathic cytopenia of undetermined significance (ICUS), clonal hematopoiesis and premalignant clonal cytopenia, **183**

Idiopathic hypereosinophilic syndrome, chronic eosinophilic leukemia, NOS vs., **161**

IGF1R gene, lung adenocarcinoma, **563**
ILNR. *See* Intralobular nephrogenic rests.

Immature teratoma, germ cell tumor, ovary, **782**
Immunoblastic lymphadenopathy. *See* Nodal follicular helper T-cell lymphoma.
Immunocytoma. *See* Lymphoplasmacytic lymphoma.
Immunodeficiency, diffuse large B-cell lymphoma, **377**
Immunodysplastic disease. *See* Nodal follicular helper T-cell lymphoma.
Immunoglobulin heavy (*IGH*) chain gene rearrangements, **72–75**
- B-cell development, **72–73**
- clonality testing, **73–74**
- locus, **73**
- recombination process, **73**
- structure, **72**

In situ hybridization
- acute promyelocytic leukemia with t(15;17)/*PML::RARA*, **250**
- anaplastic large cell lymphoma, ALK-negative, **458**
- anaplastic large cell lymphoma, ALK-positive, **463**
- B-cell prolymphocytic leukemia, **323–324**
- Burkitt lymphoma, **388**
- diffuse large B-cell lymphoma, **379**
- enteropathy-associated T-cell lymphoma, **420**
- Ewing sarcoma, **820**
- extranodal NK-/T-cell lymphoma, **407**
- follicular dendritic cell sarcoma, **489**
- follicular lymphoma, **366**
- hepatosplenic T-cell lymphoma, **425**
- HPV-associated head and neck carcinomas, **496**
- interdigitating dendritic cell tumor, **485**
- lymphoplasmacytic lymphoma, **346**
- mantle cell lymphoma, **372**
- melanoma, **789**
- monoclonal gammopathy of undetermined significance, **352**
- multiple myeloma (plasma cell myeloma), **356–357**
- myeloid sarcoma, **278**
- nodal follicular helper T-cell lymphoma, **450**
- peripheral T-cell lymphoma, not otherwise specified, **444**
- splenic marginal zone lymphoma, **327**
- squamous cell carcinoma, skin, **793**
- subcutaneous panniculitis-like T-cell lymphoma, **429**
- T-cell prolymphocytic leukemia, **395**

In situ squamous cell carcinoma, lung squamous cell carcinoma, **570**
In vitro diagnostic devices, FDA, **929**
In vitro diagnostic products (IVDs), **960**
- 510(k), **962**
- biologics license application, **963**
- class I IVDs without exemption, **963**
- class I/II exemptions, **963**
- classifications, **961**
- de novo request, **962–963**
- FDA guidance, **960–961**
- FDA regulation, **960–964**
- FDA regulatory responsibilities, **961**
- federal laws, **960**
- humanitarian use device, **963**
- investigational device exemption, **962**

INDEX

- premarketing approval process, **961–964**
- presubmission process, **961**
- regulatory controls, **961**

Indolent NK-cell lymphoproliferative disorder of GI tract, **417, 418, 419**

Indolent systemic mastocytosis, **168**

Indolent T-cell lymphoproliferative disorder of GI tract, **417, 418**

Indolent T-lymphoblastic proliferation, T-lymphoblastic leukemia/lymphoma vs., **313**

Infantile fibrosarcoma, **852, 892**

Infantile rhabdomyosarcoma, **892**

Infantile spindle cell sarcoma, with neural features, **897**

Infections
- extranodal NK-/T-cell lymphoma vs., **408**
- myelodysplastic syndrome, NOS, **193**

Infiltrating astrocytoma. See also Astrocytoma, IDH-mutant.
- pilocytic astrocytoma vs., **926**

Infiltrative basal cell carcinoma, **798**

Inflammatory dermatoses
- mycosis fungoides/Sézary syndrome vs., **435**
- squamous cell carcinoma, cervix/vulva/vagina, **735**

Inflammatory hepatocellular adenoma, **606–609**
- β-catenin-activated hepatocellular adenoma vs., **604**
- diagnostic checklist, **608**
- differential diagnosis, **608**
- *HNF1A*-inactivated hepatocellular adenoma vs., **600**
- prognosis, **607**

Inflammatory leiomyosarcoma, **892**

Inflammatory myofibroblastic tumor (IMFT), **848, 849, 852, 892**
- *ALK* alterations, **105**
- with atypia, **756**
- differential diagnosis, **851**
- embryonal rhabdomyosarcoma vs., **872**
- follicular dendritic cell sarcoma vs., **490**
- leiomyosarcoma vs., **756**

Inflammatory pseudotumor-like follicular dendritic cell sarcoma, of liver and spleen, **89**

Infundibulocystic basal cell carcinoma, **798**

Insertion, **14, 15, 19**

Inspections, CAP, **967**

Insular carcinoma. See Poorly differentiated thyroid carcinoma.

Intercalating dyes, **28**

Interdigitating dendritic cell sarcoma
- follicular dendritic cell sarcoma vs., **490**
- Langerhans cell histiocytosis vs., **481**

Interdigitating dendritic cell tumor, **484–488**
- cytogenetics, **485**
- differential diagnosis, **486**
- prognosis, **485**

International Consensus Classification (ICC), **145**

International Prognostic Scoring System-Molecular (IPSSM), myelodysplastic syndrome, **185**

International System for Human Cytogenetic Nomenclature (ISCN) guidelines, **19**

Intestinal T-cell lymphoma, **416–423**
- cytogenetics, **420**
- diagnostic checklist, **421**
- differential diagnosis, **421**
- monomorphic epitheliotropic, **417**
- not otherwise specified, **417, 418, 419**
- prognosis, **420**

Intimal sarcoma, **898, 899, 901, 902**

Intraductal carcinoma
- differential diagnosis, **521**
- molecular genetics, **520**
- prognosis, **519**
- secretory carcinoma vs., **513**

Intraductal papillary mucinous neoplasm
- pancreatic, **620–621**
    - differential diagnosis, **621**
    - prognosis, **621**
- pancreatic mucinous cystic neoplasm vs., **619**

Intrahepatic cholangiocarcinoma (ICC), **622**

Intralobular nephrogenic rests (ILNR), Wilms tumor, **643**

Intrammary nodal metastasis, invasive ductal carcinoma, of no special type with medullary features vs., **707**

Intramuscular myxoma, **892**
- myxofibrosarcoma vs., **851**

Intrathyroid thymic carcinoma, anaplastic thyroid carcinoma vs., **552**

Intronic nucleotides, **14**

Introns, **9**

Invasive carcinoma, ADH and DCIS (dysplastic, premalignant) vs., **692**

Invasive ductal carcinoma
- EZH2 protein overexpression, **100**
- molecular subtypes, **698**
- of no special type with medullary features, **706–709**
    - differential diagnosis, **707**
    - genetic testing, **707**
    - prognosis, **707**

Invasive lobular carcinoma, **701, 703**
- EZH2 protein overexpression, **100**

Invasive melanoma, **789, 790**

Invasive squamous cell carcinoma
- actinic keratosis vs., **786**
- EZH2 protein overexpression, **100**

Inversion (inv), **15, 19**

Investigational device exemption (IDE), **962**

Inv(16) or t(16;16)/*CBFB::MYH11*, acute myeloid leukemia with, **244–247**
- classification, **245**
- diagnostic checklist, **246**
- genetic testing, **246**
- prognosis, **246**

Isocitrate dehydrogenase enzymes, *IDH1* and *IDH2* mutations, **68**

Isolated genitourinary anomalies, Wilms tumor, **644**

IVDs. See In vitro diagnostic products.

INDEX

J

JAK2 exon 12 mutations, **54**
JAK2 fusion partners, B-lymphoblastic leukemia/lymphoma, *BCR::ABL1*-like (Ph-like ALL), **308**
JAK2 gene, **127**
- abnormal function, **54**
- normal function, **54**

JAK2 inhibitors, **55**
JAK2 mutations, **54–55, 174**
- atypical chronic myeloid leukemia, **222**
- essential thrombocythemia, **157**
- myelodysplastic/myeloproliferative neoplasm, NOS, **229**
- myeloid sarcoma, **278**
- myeloproliferative neoplasm, unclassifiable, **163**
- neoplasms with, **55**
- polycythemia vera, **149**
- primary myelofibrosis, **154**

JAK2 rearrangements, **54–55**
- B-lymphoblastic leukemia/lymphoma, *BCR::ABL1*-like (Ph-like ALL), **307**

JAK2 V617F mutation, **54**
- chronic myelomonocytic leukemia, **217**
- essential thrombocythemia, **157**

JAK3 gene, **127**
JMML. *See* Juvenile myelomonocytic leukemia.
Juvenile granulosa cell tumor, **775, 777, 778**
- cytogenetics, **776**
- molecular genetics, **776**

Juvenile myelomonocytic leukemia (JMML), **224–227**
- classification, **225**
- cytogenetics, **226, 227**
- differential diagnosis, **227**
- genetic testing, **227**
- molecular genetics, **226–227**
- prognosis, **226**

Juvenile polyposis
- colorectal adenocarcinoma and precancerous lesions, **586**
- gastric adenocarcinoma, **581**

Juvenile xanthogranuloma, Langerhans cell histiocytosis vs., **481**
Juxtacortical chondroma, peripheral chondrosarcoma vs., **842**

K

Kaposi sarcoma, **878**
- atypical vascular lesions vs., **786**
- differential diagnosis, **881**
- genetic findings, **880–881**

Kaposiform HE, **880**
Karyotype
- description, **19**
- FISH/RT-PCR vs., **175**
- lymphoid neoplasms, **296, 297**
- molecular work-up of myeloid neoplasms, **134**
- *PML::RARA* fusion, **47**

KDR gene, **127**
KEAP1 (19p), non-HPV-related head and neck squamous cell carcinoma, **506**
Keratoacanthoma, squamous cell carcinoma, skin vs., **794**
Keratosis, actinic
- basal cell carcinoma of skin vs., **798**
- cytogenetics, **785**
- differential diagnosis, **786**
- molecular genetics, **785**

KIAA1549::BRAF fusion gene, pilocytic astrocytoma, **925–926**
KIT D816V mutation, mastocytosis, **169**
KIT exon 17 mutations, mastocytosis, **169**
KIT gene, **64, 127**
KIT mutations, **64–67**
- acute myeloid leukemia, **234**
- acute myeloid leukemia with inv(16) or t(16;16)/*CBFB::MYH11*, **246**
- acute myeloid leukemia with t(8;21)/*RUNX1::RUNX1T1*, **242**
- core binding factor acute myeloid leukemia, **65–66**
- gastrointestinal stromal tumor, **65, 66**
- germ cell tumors, **66**
  ovary, **781**
- GIST, **592, 593**
- mastocytosis, **167**
- melanoma, **65, 66, 790**
- myelodysplastic/myeloproliferative neoplasm, NOS, **230**
- systemic mastocytosis, **65, 66**

KMT2A (*MLL*) mutations
- acute myeloid leukemia, NOS, **273**
- non-HPV-related head and neck squamous cell carcinoma, **506**

Kostmann disease, myelodysplastic syndrome, NOS vs., **195**
KRAS gene, **127**
- alterations, **116–117**
- amplifications, **116–117**
- fusion, **117**

KRAS mutations, **116–117**
- acute myeloid leukemia, **234**
- acute myeloid leukemia, NOS, **273**
- acute myeloid leukemia with inv(16) or t(16;16)/*CBFB::MYH11*, **246**
- anaplastic thyroid carcinoma, **551**
- atypical chronic myeloid leukemia, **222**
- B-lymphoblastic leukemia/lymphoma, *BCR::ABL1*-like (Ph-like ALL), **307**
- chronic myelomonocytic leukemia, **217**
- clear cell carcinoma, uterus vs., **752**
- colorectal adenocarcinoma and precancerous lesions, **586**
- endometrial intraepithelial neoplasia, **743**
- low-grade serous carcinoma, **764**
- lung adenocarcinoma, **561**
- mastocytosis, **169**

INDEX

- myelodysplastic/myeloproliferative neoplasm, NOS, 229–230
- pancreatic ductal adenocarcinoma, 615
- pancreatic intraductal papillary mucinous neoplasm, 621
- pancreatic mucinous cystic neoplasm, 619
- papillary thyroid carcinoma, 539
- pilocytic astrocytoma, 926
- poorly differentiated thyroid carcinoma, 547
- serous borderline tumor, 765

KRAS protein, 116

L

Laboratories, regulation, federal agencies, 958–959
Laboratory developed tests (LDTs), 929, 960
- Centers for Medicare and Medicaid Services and FDA regulatory schemes, 965
- CLIA program, 964–965
- CLIA regulations, 964
- FDA regulations, 965
- regulations, 964–965
- regulatory landscape, 965

Laboratory tests, FDA, 929
Lagging strand, 9
Langerhans cell granulomatosis. See Langerhans cell histiocytosis.
Langerhans cell histiocytosis, 478–483
- BRAF mutations, 119
- diagnostic checklist, 481
- differential diagnosis, 480–481
- follicular dendritic cell sarcoma vs., 490
- genetic testing, 480
- histiocytic sarcoma vs., 472
- prognosis, 479

Langerhans cell sarcoma
- histiocytic sarcoma vs., 472
- interdigitating dendritic cell tumor vs., 486
- Langerhans cell histiocytosis vs., 481

Large B-cell lymphoma
- with IRF4 rearrangement, 299
  follicular lymphoma vs., 365–366
- T-cell/histiocyte-rich, nodal follicular helper T-cell lymphoma vs., 452

Large cell neuroendocrine carcinoma
- lung squamous cell carcinoma vs., 570
- small cell neuroendocrine carcinoma vs., 574

Large cell/anaplastic medulloblastoma, 940
Latent membrane protein 1 (LMP1), 527–528
Lauren classification, gastric adenocarcinoma, 582
LDTs. See Laboratory developed tests.
Leading strand, 9
Leiomyoma, gastrointestinal stromal tumor vs., 594
Leiomyosarcoma, 868, 869–870
- biphenotypic sinonasal sarcoma vs., 534
- differential diagnosis, 872
- epigenetics, 871
- genetic findings, 871

- low-grade myofibroblastic sarcoma vs., 851

Lentigo maligna melanoma, 789, 790
LEOPARD syndrome, BRAF mutations, 119
Letterer-Siwe disease. See Langerhans cell histiocytosis.
Leukemia
- acute myeloid. See Acute myeloid leukemia.
- B-cell prolymphocytic, 322–325
  cytogenetics, 323
  diagnostic checklist, 324
  differential diagnosis, 324
  molecular genetics, 323
  prognosis, 323
- Langerhans cell histiocytosis vs., 481
- retinoblastoma vs., 952
- splenic B-cell, unclassifiable, 336–343
  cytogenetics, 337
  differential diagnosis, 338
  prognosis, 337
- T-acute lymphoblastic, 310–315
  antigen receptor gene rearrangements, 312
  differential diagnosis, 313
  gene expression signatures, 312–313
  prognosis, 311–312
  recurrent cytogenetic abnormalities, 312
  somatic gene mutation, 312

Leukemic nonnodal mantle cell lymphoma, splenic B-cell lymphoma/leukemia, unclassifiable vs., 338
Leukemic reticuloendotheliosis. See Hairy cell leukemia.
Leukemogenesis, acute myeloid leukemia, 233
Leukemoid reaction, chronic myeloid leukemia, BCR::ABL1-positive vs., 139
Leukoerythroblastosis, myeloproliferative neoplasm, unclassifiable, 163, 164
Levan, Albert, 18
Levitsky, Grigory Andreevich, 18
Leydig cell tumor, 775, 777
LFS. See Li-Fraumeni syndrome.
Li-Fraumeni syndrome, 805
- adrenal cortical carcinoma, 667
- choroid plexus tumors, 945
- medulloblastoma, 939
- myelodysplastic syndrome with TP53 multihit mutations vs., 205
- osteosarcoma, 811

Light chain deposition disease, lymphoplasmacytic lymphoma, 345
Linux-based software, NGS analysis, 37
Lipoblastoma, 892
- myxoid liposarcoma vs., 862

Lipoma
- atypical lipomatous tumor vs., 862
- conventional, 892
- pleomorphic, 892
  spindle cell liposarcoma vs., 862
- spindle cell, 892
  atypical lipomatous tumor vs., 862
  differential diagnosis, 862
  spindle cell liposarcoma vs., 862

Liposarcoma, 755, 858–867
- dedifferentiated, 858–859, 860, 861, 892
  differential diagnosis, 862

INDEX

      pleomorphic liposarcoma vs., **862**
      prognosis, **859**
- differential diagnosis, **756, 862**
- myxoid, **859, 860, 861, 892**
      differential diagnosis, **862**
      high-grade, **861**
      prognosis, **859**
- myxoid pleomorphic, **861**
      differential diagnosis, **862**
      prognosis, **859**
- pleomorphic, **859, 860, 861, 862**
      dedifferentiated liposarcoma vs., **862**
      differential diagnosis, **862**
      myxoid, **862**
      prognosis, **859**
      spindle cell liposarcoma vs., **862**
- spindle cell, **862**
- well-differentiated, **858, 892**
Liver fatty acid binding protein (L-FABP)-negative hepatic adenoma. *See HNF1A*-inactivated hepatocellular adenoma.
Lobular breast carcinoma, gastric adenocarcinoma vs., **582**
Lobular carcinoma, **700–705**
- classification, **701**
- invasive, classic and variant forms, **701, 703**
- molecular genetics, **702**
- prognosis, **701**
Lobular carcinoma in situ, **702**
- ADH and DCIS (dysplastic, premalignant) vs., **692**
Lobular panniculitis, subcutaneous panniculitis-like T-cell lymphoma vs., **430**
Low-blast-count acute myeloid leukemia, pediatric myelodysplastic syndrome and refractory cytopenia of childhood vs., **212**
Low-frequency gene mutations, **539**
Low-grade adenosquamous carcinoma, **713**
Low-grade astrocytoma. *See* Astrocytoma, IDH-mutant.
Low-grade central osteosarcomas, **810, 811, 812–813**
- differential diagnosis, **814**
Low-grade cribriform cystadenocarcinoma, secretory carcinoma vs., **512**
Low-grade endometrial stromal sarcoma, **754–755**
- differential diagnosis, **756**
- genetic tests, **755**
Low-grade fibromyxoid sarcoma, **849, 850–851, 852, 892**
- differential diagnosis, **851**
Low-grade myxofibrosarcoma, **852**
- myxofibrosarcoma vs., **851**
Low-grade salivary duct carcinoma, secretory carcinoma vs., **512**
Low-grade serous carcinoma (LGSC), **763**
- molecular carcinogenesis, **764**
- prognosis, **763**
Low-grade squamous intraepithelial lesion (LSIL), preneoplastic conditions, cervix/vulva/vagina, **731**
LPL. *See* Lymphoplasmacytic lymphoma.
Lung adenocarcinoma, **560–567**
- diagnostic checklist, **564**
- differential diagnosis, **564**
- mesothelioma vs., **578**
- molecular genetics, **561–563**
- prognosis, **561**
Lung cancer
- chromosomal microarray, **24**
- *EGFR* amplification, **121**
- EZH2 protein overexpression, **101**
- testing algorithms, *MET* amplifications, **112**
Lung carcinosarcoma, *RET* fusion genes, **109**
Lung squamous cell carcinoma, **568–571**
- diagnostic checklist, **570**
- differential diagnosis, **570**
- grading, **570**
- molecular genetics, **569**
- prognosis, **569**
Lupus profundus panniculitis, subcutaneous panniculitis-like T-cell lymphoma vs., **430**
Lymphadenopathy, splenic B-cell lymphoma/leukemia, unclassifiable, **337**
Lymphoblastic leukemia/lymphoma
- Burkitt lymphoma vs., **390**
- myeloid sarcoma vs., **278**
Lymphocytosis, monoclonal B, small lymphocytic lymphoma/chronic lymphocytic leukemia vs., **320**
Lymphoid neoplasms, molecular pathology
- adult T-cell leukemia/lymphoma, **410–415**
- aggressive NK-cell leukemia, **402–405**
- anaplastic large cell lymphoma, ALK-negative, **456–461**
- anaplastic large cell lymphoma, ALK-positive, **462–467**
- B-cell prolymphocytic leukemia, **322–325**
- B-lymphoblastic leukemia/lymphoma, *BCR::ABL1*-like (Ph-like ALL), **306–309**
- B-lymphoblastic leukemia/lymphoma with recurrent genetic abnormalities, **302–305**
- Burkitt lymphoma, **386–393**
- chronic lymphoproliferative disorder of NK cells, **398–401**
- diffuse large B-cell lymphoma, **376–385**
- extranodal NK-/T-cell lymphoma, **406–409**
- follicular lymphoma, **362–369**
- hairy cell leukemia, **332–335**
- hepatosplenic T-cell lymphoma, **424–427**
- intestinal T-cell lymphoma, **416–423**
- lymphoma-associated chromosomal translocations, **298–301**
- lymphoplasmacytic lymphoma, **344–349**
- mantle cell lymphoma, **370–375**
- molecular work-up, **296–297**
- monoclonal gammopathy, of undetermined significance, **350–353**
- multiple myeloma (plasma cell myeloma), **354–361**
- mycosis fungoides/Sézary syndrome, **432–437**
- overview, **292–295**
- peripheral T-cell lymphoma, not otherwise specified, **442–447**
- primary cutaneous CD30-positive T-cell lymphoproliferative disorders, **438–441**
- small lymphocytic lymphoma/chronic lymphocytic leukemia, **316–321**
- splenic B-cell lymphoma/leukemia, unclassifiable, **336–343**

INDEX

- splenic marginal zone lymphoma, **326–331**
- subcutaneous panniculitis-like T-cell lymphoma, **428–431**
- T-cell prolymphocytic leukemia, **394–397**
- T-lymphoblastic leukemia/lymphoma, **310–315**

Lymphoid proliferations, Southern blot vs. PCR, in assessment of clonality, **85**

Lymphoma
- B-cell, *MYD88* L265P mutation, **94–95**
- Burkitt, **386–393**
  - cytogenetics, **388**
  - diagnostic checklist, **390**
  - differential diagnosis, **390**
  - molecular genetics, **388–389**
  - prognosis, **388**
- diffuse large B-cell, **294, 298, 299, 376–385**
  - anaplastic thyroid carcinoma vs., **552**
  - associated with chronic inflammation, **87**
  - Burkitt lymphoma vs., **390**
  - cytogenetics, **378**
  - differential diagnosis, **379**
  - EBV (+), not otherwise specified, **87**
  - *EZH2* mutation, **99**
  - fibrin-associated, **87**
  - histiocytic sarcoma vs., **472**
  - mantle cell lymphoma vs., **373**
  - molecular changes, **348**
  - molecular genetics, **378**
  - myeloid sarcoma vs., **278**
  - not otherwise specified, **87, 377**
  - prognosis, **377**
- EBV-associated, **87–88**
- Ewing sarcoma vs., **821**
- follicular, **294, 298, 299, 362–369**
  - classification, **363**
  - cytogenetics, **366**
  - differential diagnosis, **365**
  - diffuse, **365**
  - early and late genetic alterations, **367**
  - *EZH2* mutation, **99**
  - genetic abnormalities, **367**
  - grading, **364–365**
  - molecular changes, **330, 348**
  - molecular genetics, **366**
  - *MYD88* L265P mutations, **348**
  - nodal follicular helper T-cell lymphoma vs., **452**
  - pediatric, **365**
  - pediatric-type, Burkitt lymphoma vs., **390**
  - prognosis, **364**
  - reporting pattern, **365**
  - in situ, **365**
  - splenic marginal zone lymphoma vs., **329**
  - testicular, **365**
  - testing methods, **297**
  - variants, **365**
- gastric adenocarcinoma vs., **582**
- glioblastoma, IDH wildtype vs., **918**
- invasive ductal carcinoma, of no special type with medullary features vs., **707**
- Langerhans cell histiocytosis vs., **481**
- low-grade, small lymphocytic lymphoma/chronic lymphocytic leukemia vs., **320**
- lymphoplasmacytic, **344–349**
  - differential diagnosis, **347–348**
  - molecular changes, **348**
  - multiple myeloma (plasma cell myeloma) vs., **357**
  - *MYD88* L265P mutations, **348**
  - prognosis, **346**
- mantle cell, **294, 298, 370–375, 372–375**
  - B-cell prolymphocytic leukemia vs., **324**
  - blastoid variant, Burkitt lymphoma vs., **390**
  - cytogenetics, **372**
  - diagnostic checklist, **373**
  - differential diagnosis, **373**
  - follicular lymphoma vs., **365**
  - leukemic nonnodal, splenic B-cell lymphoma/leukemia, unclassifiable vs., **338**
  - molecular changes, **330, 348**
  - molecular genetics, **372**
  - *MYD88* L265P mutations, **348**
  - prognosis, **372**
  - small lymphocytic lymphoma/chronic lymphocytic leukemia vs., **320**
  - splenic marginal zone lymphoma vs., **329**
  - testing methods, **297**
- medulloblastoma vs., **940**
- nasopharyngeal EBV-related squamous cell carcinoma vs., **528**
- olfactory neuroblastoma vs., **534**
- plasmablastic, lymphoplasmacytic lymphoma vs., **348**
- retinoblastoma vs., **952**
- small cell neuroendocrine carcinoma vs., **574**
- splenic B-cell, unclassifiable, **336–343**
  - cytogenetics, **337**
  - differential diagnosis, **338**
  - prognosis, **337**
- testing methods for, **297**
- T-lymphoblastic, **292, 294, 310–315**
  - antigen receptor gene rearrangements, **312**
  - differential diagnosis, **313**
  - *EZH2* mutation, **99**
  - gene expression signatures, **312–313**
  - prognosis, **311–312**
  - recurrent cytogenetic abnormalities, **312**
  - somatic gene mutation, **312**

Lymphoma-associated chromosomal translocations, **298–301**
- *BCL6* rearrangements, **299**
- *DUSP22* rearrangements, **300**
- *IRF4* rearrangements, **299**
- *MYC* rearrangements, **299**
- t(2;5)(P23;Q35); *ALK::NPM1*, **300**
- t(9;14)(P13;Q32); *PAX5::IGH*, **299–300**
- t(11;14)(Q13;Q32); *CCND1::IGH*, **298**
- t(11;18)(Q22;Q21); *BIRC3::MALT1*, **299**
- t(14;18)(Q32;Q21); *IGH::BCL2*, **298–299**
- *TRA* rearrangements, **300**

Lymphomatoid granulomatosis, **87**

Lymphomatoid papulosis, primary cutaneous CD30-positive T-cell lymphoproliferative disorders, **439**

INDEX

Lymphoplasmacytic lymphoma (LPL), **294, 344–349**
- differential diagnosis, **347–348**
- molecular changes, **330, 348**
- multiple myeloma (plasma cell myeloma) vs., **357**
- *MYD88* L265P mutations, **348**
- prognosis, **346**
- splenic marginal zone lymphoma vs., **329**
- testing methods, **297**

Lymphovascular invasion, ADH and DCIS (dysplastic, premalignant) vs., **692**

LYN fusion partner, B-lymphoblastic leukemia/lymphoma, *BCR::ABL1*-like (Ph-like ALL), **308**

Lynch syndrome, **769**
- adrenal cortical carcinoma, **667**
- colorectal adenocarcinoma and precancerous lesions, **585**
- gastric adenocarcinoma, **581**
- uterine endometrioid carcinoma, **745**

M

Malignant melanoma
- diffuse large B-cell lymphoma vs., **379**
- histiocytic sarcoma vs., **472**
- malignant peripheral nerve sheath tumor vs., **888**

Malignant mesothelioma, **578**

Malignant mixed Müllerian tumor (MMMT), undifferentiated uterine sarcoma vs., **756**

Malignant PEComa, leiomyosarcoma vs., **756**

Malignant peripheral nerve sheath tumor (MPNST), **886–891, 892**
- biphenotypic sinonasal sarcoma vs., **534**
- differential diagnosis, **888**
- epithelioid, **887**
- epithelioid variant, **892**
- genetic predisposition, **887**
- genetic testing, **888**
- leiomyosarcoma vs., **872**
- molecular genetics, **887**
- prognosis, **887**
- solitary fibrous tumor vs., **851**
- spindle cell, **888**

MALT lymphoma, splenic marginal zone lymphoma vs., **329**

MammaPrint assay, **696**

Mammary-type myofibroblastoma, **892**

Mantle cell lymphoma (MCL), **294, 298, 370–375**
- B-cell prolymphocytic leukemia vs., **324**
- blastoid variant, Burkitt lymphoma vs., **390**
- cytogenetics, **372**
- diagnostic checklist, **373**
- differential diagnosis, **373**
- follicular lymphoma vs., **365**
- leukemic nonnodal, splenic B-cell lymphoma/leukemia, unclassifiable vs., **338**
- molecular changes, **330, 348**
- molecular genetics, **372**
- *MYD88* L265P mutations, **348**
- prognosis, **372**
- small lymphocytic lymphoma/chronic lymphocytic leukemia vs., **320**
- splenic marginal zone lymphoma vs., **329**
- testing methods, **297**

MAP2K1 mutations, Langerhans cell histiocytosis, **480**

Marginal zone B-cell lymphoma (MALT lymphoma), **294**

Marginal zone hyperplasia, splenic marginal zone lymphoma vs., **329**

Marginal zone lymphoma
- extranodal
    - gastrointestinal tract, lymphoplasmacytic lymphoma vs., **347**
    - molecular changes, **330**
    - splenic marginal zone lymphoma vs., **329**
- molecular changes, **348**
- *MYD88* L265P mutations, **348**
- nodal
    - lymphoplasmacytic lymphoma vs., **347**
    - mantle cell lymphoma vs., **373**
    - splenic marginal zone lymphoma vs., **329**
- small lymphocytic lymphoma/chronic lymphocytic leukemia vs., **320**
- splenic, **326–331**
    - B-cell prolymphocytic leukemia vs., **324**
    - diagnostic checklist, **330**
    - differential diagnosis, **328–330**
    - hairy cell leukemia vs., **334**
    - immunohistochemistry, **330**
    - molecular changes, **330, 348**
    - molecular findings, **330**
    - molecular genetics, **327–328**
    - prognosis, **327**
    - splenic B-cell lymphoma/leukemia, unclassifiable vs., **338**

Marked hepatosplenomegaly, myeloproliferative neoplasm, unclassifiable, **163**

Marker chromosome, **19**

Massively parallel next-generation sequencing, **33–34**

Mast cell activation syndrome, mastocytosis vs., **169**

Mast cell hyperplasia, mastocytosis vs., **169**

Mast cell leukemia, **168**

Mast cell sarcoma, **168**

Mastocytosis, **166–173**
- aggressive systemic, **168**
- bone marrow, **168**
- cutaneous, **168**
- differential diagnosis, **169**
- indolent systemic, **168**
- molecular genetics, **169**
- prognosis, **169**
- smoldering systemic, **168**
- systemic, **168**
    - acute myeloid leukemia with t(8;21)/*RUNX1::RUNX1T1*, **242**
    - with associated hematologic neoplasm, **168**
    - chronic myelomonocytic leukemia vs., **218**
    - diagnostic criteria, **167–168**
    - *KIT* mutations, **65, 66**

Mature B-cell lymphoid neoplasms (B-NHL), **292**

INDEX

Mature B-cell lymphomas, molecular changes, **348**
Mature B-cell neoplasms
- B-cell prolymphocytic leukemia, **322–325**
- Burkitt lymphoma, **386–393**
- diffuse large B-cell lymphoma, **376–385**
- follicular lymphoma, **362–369**
- hairy cell leukemia, **332–335**
- lymphoplasmacytic lymphoma, **344–349**
- mantle cell lymphoma, **370–375**
- monoclonal gammopathy, of undetermined significance, **350–353**
- multiple myeloma (plasma cell myeloma), **354–361**
- small lymphocytic lymphoma/chronic lymphocytic leukemia, **316–321**
- splenic B-cell lymphoma/leukemia, unclassifiable, **336–343**
- splenic marginal zone lymphoma, **326–331**

Mature cystic teratoma, germ cell tumor, ovary, **781, 782**
Mature T- and NK-cell neoplasms
- adult T-cell leukemia/lymphoma, **410–415**
- aggressive NK-cell leukemia, **402–405**
- anaplastic large cell lymphoma, ALK-negative, **456–461**
- anaplastic large cell lymphoma, ALK-positive, **462–467**
- chronic lymphoproliferative disorder of NK cells, **398–401**
- extranodal NK-/T-cell lymphoma, **406–409**
- hepatosplenic T-cell lymphoma, **424–427**
- intestinal T-cell lymphoma, **416–423**
- mycosis fungoides, **432–437**
- peripheral T-cell lymphoma, not otherwise specified, **442–447**
- primary cutaneous CD30-positive T-cell lymphoproliferative disorders, **438–441**
- Sézary syndrome, **432–437**
- subcutaneous panniculitis-like T-cell lymphoma, **428–431**
- T-cell prolymphocytic leukemia, **394–397**

Mature T-cell lymphoid neoplasms (T-NHL), **292**
Mature T-cell lymphoma
- histiocytic sarcoma vs., **472**
- T-lymphoblastic leukemia/lymphoma vs., **313**

Maturing ganglioneuroma, neuroblastoma vs., **676**
MAX gene, pheochromocytoma/paraganglioma, **663**
MDM2 (12q), non-HPV-related head and neck squamous cell carcinoma, **507**
MDS. *See* Myelodysplastic syndrome.
MDS/AML. *See* Myelodysplastic syndrome/acute myeloid leukemia.
MDS/MPN. *See* Myelodysplastic/myeloproliferative neoplasms.
Mechanical artifacts, endometrial intraepithelial neoplasia vs., **743**
MED15::TFE3 carcinomas, *TFE3*-rearranged and *TFEB*-altered renal cell carcinomas, **640**
Mediastinal gray zone lymphoma, diffuse large B-cell lymphoma vs., **379**
Medical Device Amendment of 1976 (MDA76), **960**
Medullary carcinoma
- follicular variant of, follicular thyroid carcinoma vs., **544**
- pancreatic ductal adenocarcinoma, **616**
- papillary thyroid carcinoma vs., **540**

Medullary thyroid carcinoma (MTC), **554–559**
- ATA recommendations for management, **557**
- ATA risk levels, **557**
- differential diagnosis, **556–557**
- distinguishing features between hereditary and sporadic, **557**
- EZH2 protein overexpression, **100**
- genotype-phenotype correlation, **557**
- molecular genetics, **555–556**
- poorly differentiated thyroid carcinoma vs., **548**
- prognosis, **555**
- sporadic, **555**

Medulloblastoma, **938–943**
- differential diagnosis, **940**
- genetic testing, **940**
- prognosis, **939**

Medulloepithelioma, retinoblastoma vs., **952**
Melanoma, **788–791**
- anaplastic thyroid carcinoma vs., **552**
- atypical (dysplastic) nevi vs., **786**
- *BRAF* mutations, **119**
- chromosomal microarray, **24**
- desmoplastic, leiomyosarcoma vs., **872**
- differential diagnosis, **790**
- interdigitating dendritic cell tumor vs., **486**
- invasive, **789, 790**
- *KIT* mutations, **65, 66**
- malignant
    diffuse large B-cell lymphoma vs., **379**
    malignant peripheral nerve sheath tumor vs., **888**
- molecular genetics, **789–790**
- nasopharyngeal EBV-related squamous cell carcinoma vs., **528**
- olfactory neuroblastoma vs., **534**
- prognosis, **789**
- sarcomatoid, malignant peripheral nerve sheath tumor vs., **888**
- in situ and superficial spreading, preneoplastic conditions, cervix/vulva/vagina vs., **732**
- spindle cell
    leiomyosarcoma vs., **872**
    malignant peripheral nerve sheath tumor vs., **888**
- squamous cell carcinoma, cervix/vulva/vagina vs., **736**

Melanoma in situ, **789, 790**
Melanotic Xp11 translocation carcinoma, *TFE3*-rearranged and *TFEB*-altered renal cell carcinomas, **638, 639, 640**
Melting curve analysis, **39**
Meningioma, **948–951**
- cytogenetics, **949**
- differential diagnosis, **950**
- ependymal tumors vs., **934**
- grading, **950**
- molecular genetics, **949–950**
- prognosis, **949**

Merkel cell carcinoma
- basal cell carcinoma of skin vs., **798**
- small cell neuroendocrine carcinoma vs., **574**

Mesenchymal chondrosarcoma, **839, 840, 841, 895**
- differential diagnosis, **842**
- Ewing sarcoma vs., **821**

- genetic testing, 840
Mesenchymal tumor, phosphaturic, 892
Mesoblastic nephroma, cellular congenital, clear cell sarcoma of kidney vs., 649
Mesonephric hyperplasia, adenocarcinoma, cervix/vulva/vagina vs., 740
Mesonephric remnants, preneoplastic conditions, cervix/vulva/vagina vs., 732
Mesonephric-like carcinoma, 771
Mesothelioma, 576–579
 - cytogenetics, 578
 - desmoplastic small round cell tumor vs., 827
 - differential diagnosis, 578
 - malignant, 577
 - molecular genetics, 578
 - molecular testing, 578
 - prognosis, 577
Messenger RNA (mRNA), 5–6, 9, 10
MET (7q), non-HPV-related head and neck squamous cell carcinoma, 506
MET amplifications
 - chemotherapy, 111–112
 - FISH for, 110–113
 - lung adenocarcinoma, 563
 - testing for, 112
MET fusions, glioblastoma, IDH wildtype, 918
MET gene, 127
MET overexpression, in tumors, 111
MET protooncogene, 110
MET signaling, aberrant, 110–111
Metanephric adenoma, Wilms tumor vs., 645
Metaplasia, tubal, preneoplastic conditions, cervix/vulva/vagina vs., 732
Metaplastic breast carcinoma, 710–715
 - differential diagnosis, 713
 - EGFR amplification, 121
 - gene mutations, 712
 - prognosis, 711–712
Metaplastic carcinoma
 - fibromatosis-like, 713
 - with mesenchymal differentiation, 713
Metastases
 - anaplastic thyroid carcinoma vs., 552
 - from uterine endometrial endometrioid carcinoma, surface epithelial tumors of ovary vs., 772
Metastatic adenocarcinoma
 - cholangiocarcinoma vs., 623
 - sinonasal adenocarcinoma vs., 534
Metastatic carcinoma
 - adrenal cortical adenoma vs., 680
 - choroid plexus tumors vs., 945
 - ependymal tumors vs., 934
 - gastric adenocarcinoma vs., 582
 - meningioma vs., 950
 - sclerosing epithelioid fibrosarcoma vs., 851
Metastatic clear cell renal cell carcinoma (RCC), clear cell carcinoma vs., 521
Metastatic colorectal adenocarcinoma, serous tumors of ovary and fallopian tube vs., 765

Metastatic colorectal carcinoma (mCRC), EGFR amplification, 121
Metastatic embryonal tumors, medulloblastoma vs., 940
Metastatic mucinous carcinomas to ovary, surface epithelial tumors of ovary vs., 772
Metastatic neuroendocrine tumors, medullary thyroid carcinoma vs., 557
Metastatic squamous cell carcinoma
 - metaplastic breast carcinoma vs., 713
 - mucoepidermoid carcinoma vs., 512
Metastatic tumors
 - hepatocellular carcinoma vs., 612
 - mesothelioma vs., 578
Metatypical basal cell carcinoma, 798
Methylation assay, MGMT promoter gene, 130–135
Methylation nonspecific primers, 39
Methylation-specific high-resolution melting curve, MGMT promoter gene methylation assay, 131
Methylation-specific PCR, 39
 - MGMT promoter gene methylation assay, 131
Methylation-specific pyrosequencing, MGMT promoter gene methylation assay, 131
O-6-methylguanine-DNA methyltransferase (MGMT) gene, 130
 - expression in tumors, 130
 - promoter gene methylation assay, 130–135
    GBM treatment, 131
    high-grade gliomas, 130–131
    nonmethylated, 131
    status, 131
Mevalonate kinase deficiency, pediatric myelodysplastic syndrome and refractory cytopenia of childhood vs., 212
MGMT (10q), non-HPV-related head and neck squamous cell carcinoma, 507
MGMT promoter methylation, astrocytoma, IDH-mutant, 922
MIBC. See Muscle invasive bladder cancer.
Microcystic stromal cell tumor, 777, 778
 - molecular genetics, 777
Microdeletions, 23, 24
Microglandular hyperplasia, adenocarcinoma, cervix/vulva/vagina vs., 740
Micronodular basal cell carcinoma, 797
Micropapillary carcinoma, lung adenocarcinoma, 564
MicroRNA
 - adult T-cell leukemia/lymphoma, 412
 - extranodal NK-/T-cell lymphoma, 408
 - germ cell tumor, ovary, 781
 - mycosis fungoides/Sézary syndrome, 434–435
Microsatellite instability, colorectal adenocarcinoma and precancerous lesions, 587
Microsecretory adenocarcinoma
 - differential diagnosis, 521
 - molecular genetics, 520
 - prognosis, 519
Microvesicular hyperplastic polyp, colorectal adenocarcinoma and precancerous lesions, 585
MIF (22q), non-HPV-related head and neck squamous cell carcinoma, 507

INDEX

Mild neutrophilic leukocytosis, myeloproliferative neoplasm, unclassifiable, **164**
Minimal residual disease
 - acute promyelocytic leukemia, **47**
 - chronic myeloid leukemia, **44**
MIR30A gene, giant cell tumor of bone, **834**
MIR126 gene, giant cell tumor of bone, **834**
MIR136 gene, giant cell tumor of bone, **834**
miRNA processing genes, mutations, Wilms tumor, **645**
Missense mutation/substitution, **13**
Mitochondrial iron metabolism, primary defects, myelodysplastic syndrome with mutated *SF3B1*, **189**
Mitotically active leiomyoma, leiomyosarcoma vs., **756**
Mixed germ cell tumor, germ cell tumor, ovary, **782**
Mixed phenotype acute leukemia with *BCR::ABL1*, **43**
MLH1 gene, **127**
MLLT1 mutations, Wilms tumor, **645**
Moderately differentiated squamous cell carcinoma, lung squamous cell carcinoma, **570**
Molecular alterations, hepatosplenic T-cell lymphoma, **425**
Molecular beacon probes, **28**
Molecular genetic tests in solid tumors, bone and soft tissue tumors, and CNS tumors
 - *ALK* rearrangements and mutations, **104–105**
 - *BRAF* mutations, **118–119**
 - *EGFR* mutations, **120–121**
 - FISH for *ERBB2* (HER2) gene amplifications, **114–115**
 - FISH for *MET* amplifications, **110–113**
 - *KRAS* mutations, **116–117**
 - *MGMT* promoter gene methylation assay, **130–135**
 - *RET* rearrangements, **108–109**
 - *ROS1* rearrangements, **106–107**
 - targeted hotspot gene panel table, **124–129**
 - targeted hotspot gene panel using massively parallel sequencing, **122–123**
Molecular genetics, multiple myeloma (plasma cell myeloma), **357**
Molecular pathology, high-throughput methods, **36–37**
Molecular pathology of dendritic cell and histiocytic neoplasms
 - follicular dendritic cell sarcoma, **488–491**
 - histiocytic sarcoma, **470–477**
 - interdigitating dendritic cell tumor, **484–488**
 - Langerhans cell histiocytosis, **478–483**
Molecular pathology of lymphoid neoplasms
 - adult T-cell leukemia/lymphoma, **410–415**
 - aggressive NK-cell leukemia, **402–405**
 - anaplastic large cell lymphoma, ALK-negative, **456–461**
 - anaplastic large cell lymphoma, ALK-positive, **462–467**
 - B-cell prolymphocytic leukemia, **322–325**
 - B-lymphoblastic leukemia/lymphoma
    BCR::ABL1-like (Ph-like ALL), **306–309**
    with recurrent genetic abnormalities, **302–305**
 - Burkitt lymphoma, **386–393**
 - chronic lymphoproliferative disorder of NK cells, **398–401**
 - diffuse large B-cell lymphoma, **376–385**
 - extranodal NK-/T-cell lymphoma, **406–409**
 - follicular lymphoma, **362–369**
 - hairy cell leukemia, **332–335**
 - hepatosplenic T-cell lymphoma, **424–427**
 - intestinal T-cell lymphoma, **416–423**
 - lymphoma-associated chromosomal translocations, **298–301**
 - lymphoplasmacytic lymphoma, **344–349**
 - mantle cell lymphoma, **370–375**
 - molecular work-up, **296–297**
 - monoclonal gammopathy, of undetermined significance, **350–353**
 - multiple myeloma (plasma cell myeloma), **354–361**
 - mycosis fungoides/Sézary syndrome, **432–437**
 - nodal follicular helper T-cell lymphoma, **448–455**
 - overview, **292–295**
 - peripheral T-cell lymphoma, not otherwise specified, **442–447**
 - primary cutaneous CD30-positive T-cell lymphoproliferative disorders, **438–441**
 - small lymphocytic lymphoma/chronic lymphocytic leukemia, **316–321**
 - splenic B-cell lymphoma/leukemia, unclassifiable, **336–343**
 - splenic marginal zone lymphoma, **326–331**
 - subcutaneous panniculitis-like T-cell lymphoma, **428–431**
 - T-cell prolymphocytic leukemia, **394–397**
 - T-lymphoblastic leukemia/lymphoma, **310–315**
Molecular pathology of myeloid neoplasms
 - acute myeloid leukemia
    with inv(16) or t(16;16)/*CBFB::MYH11*, **244–247**
    with inv(3) or t(3;3)/*GATA2; MECOM*, **260–261**
    with myelodysplasia-related gene mutations, **264–269**
    not otherwise specified (NOS), **270–275**
    overview, **232–239**
    with t(6;9)/*DEK::NUP214*, **258–259**
    with t(9;11)/*MLLT3::KMT2A*, **254–257**
    with t(1;22)/*RBM15::MRTFA*, **262–263**
    with t(8;21)/*RUNX1::RUNX1T1*, **240–243**
 - acute promyelocytic leukemia with t(15;17)/*PML::RARA*, **248–253**
 - atypical chronic myeloid leukemia, **220–223**
 - blastic plasmacytoid dendritic cell neoplasm, **284–289**
 - chronic eosinophilic leukemia, NOS, **160–161**
 - clonal hematopoiesis and premalignant clonal cytopenia, **182–183**
 - essential thrombocythemia, **156–159**
 - juvenile myelomonocytic leukemia, **224–227**
 - mastocytosis, **166–173**
 - myelodysplastic syndrome
    with del(5q), **200–203**
    mutated *SF3B1*, **188–191**
    NOS, **192–199**
    overview and classification, **184–187**
    with *TP53* multihit mutations, **204–205**
 - myelodysplastic syndrome/acute myeloid leukemia, **206–207**
 - myelodysplastic/myeloproliferative neoplasms, **214–215**
 - myeloid proliferations, associated with Down syndrome, **280–283**

INDEX

- myeloid sarcoma, **276–279**
- myeloid/lymphoid neoplasms with eosinophilia and tyrosine kinase gene fusions, **174–177**
- myeloproliferative neoplasms
    - chronic myeloid leukemia, *BCR::ABL1* positive, **136–143**
    - chronic neutrophilic leukemia, **144–147**
    - polycythemia vera, **148–151**
    - unclassifiable, **162–165**
- primary myelofibrosis, **152–155**
- VEXAS syndrome, **178–181**

Molecular pathology of solid tumors
- adenocarcinoma, cervix/vulva/vagina, **738–741**
- ADH and DCIS (dysplastic, premalignant), **688–693**
- adrenal cortical adenoma, **680–683**
- adrenal cortical carcinoma, **666–671**
- anaplastic thyroid carcinoma, **550–553**
- astrocytoma, IDH-mutant, **920–923**
- basal cell carcinoma, skin, **796–799**
- basal-like and triple-negative breast carcinomas, **720–729**
- bone and soft tissue tumors, **804–809**
- β-catenin-activated hepatocellular adenoma, **602–605**
- cholangiocarcinoma, **622–623**
- choroid plexus tumors, **944–947**
- chromophobe renal cell carcinoma, **634–635**
- clear cell carcinoma, uterus, **750–753**
- clear cell renal cell carcinoma, **630–633**
- clear cell sarcoma of kidney, **648–649**
- colorectal adenocarcinoma, precancerous lesions, **584–589**
- dermatofibroma, **802–803**
- dermatofibrosarcoma protuberans, **802–803**
- ductal carcinomas, **694–699**
- endometrial intraepithelial neoplasia, **742–743**
- ependymal tumors, **932–937**
- Ewing sarcoma, **818–823**
- follicular thyroid carcinoma, **542–545**
- gastric adenocarcinoma, **580–583**
- gastrointestinal stromal tumor, **590–597**
- germ cell tumor, ovary, **780–783**
- giant cell tumor of bone, **832–837**
- glioblastoma, IDH wildtype, **916–919**
- head and neck mucosal squamous cell carcinoma, non-HPV related, **500–505**
- head and neck tumors, **530–537**
- hepatocellular carcinoma, **610–613**
- *HNF1A*-inactivated hepatocellular adenoma, **598–601**
- HPV-associated head and neck carcinomas, **494–499**
- inflammatory hepatocellular adenoma, **606–609**
- intermediate and malignant cartilaginous tumors of bone, **838–847**
- intermediate and malignant myofibroblastic/fibroblastic tumors, **848–857**
- intermediate and malignant vascular tumors, **878–885**
- invasive ductal carcinoma of no special type with medullary features, **706–709**
- liposarcomas, **858–867**
- lobular carcinoma, **700–705**
- lung adenocarcinoma, **560–567**
- malignant peripheral nerve sheath tumor, **886–891**
- medullary thyroid carcinoma, **554–559**
- medulloblastoma, **938–943**
- melanoma, **788–791**
- meningioma, **948–951**
- mesothelioma, **576–579**
- metaplastic breast carcinoma, **710–715**
- muscle sarcomas, **868–877**
- nasopharyngeal EBV-related squamous cell carcinoma, **526–529**
- neuroblastoma, **672–679**
- non-HPV-related head and neck squamous cell carcinoma, **506–507**
- oligodendroglioma, IDH mutant, 1p/19q codeleted, **928–931**
- oncocytoma, **650–651**
- osteosarcomas, **810–817**
- pancreatic ductal adenocarcinoma, **614–617**
- pancreatic intraductal papillary mucinous neoplasm, **620–621**
- pancreatic mucinous cystic neoplasm, **618–619**
- papillary renal cell carcinoma, **636–637**
- papillary thyroid carcinoma, **538–541**
- pheochromocytoma/paraganglioma, **660–665**
- phyllodes tumors, **716–719**
- pilocytic astrocytoma, **924–927**
- poorly differentiated thyroid carcinoma, **546–549**
- premalignant conditions, skin, **784–787**
- preneoplastic conditions, cervix/vulva/vagina, **730–733**
- prostatic adenocarcinoma, acinar type and high-grade prostatic intraepithelial neoplasia, **684–687**
- rare sarcomas of uncertain differentiation with specific molecular alterations, **898–907, 908–915**
- representative genetic findings in bone and soft tissue tumors, **892–897**
- retinoblastoma, **952–955**
- rhabdoid tumor of kidney, **652–653**
- sebaceous tumors, **800–801**
- serous tumors of ovary and fallopian tube, **762–767**
- sex cord-stromal tumors of ovary, **774–779**
- small cell neuroendocrine carcinoma, **572–575**
- small round blue cell sarcomas, **824–831**
- squamous cell carcinoma
    - cervix/vulva/vagina, **734–737**
    - lung, **568–571**
    - skin, **792–795**
- surface epithelial tumors of ovary, **768–773**
- testicular germ cell tumors, **624–629**
- *TFE3*-rearranged and *TFEB*-altered renal cell carcinomas, **638–641**
- translocation-specific salivary gland tumors, **508–517, 518–525**
- urothelial carcinoma, **654–659**
- uterine endometrioid carcinoma, **744–747**
- uterine sarcomas, **754–761**
- uterine serous carcinoma, **748–749**
- Wilms tumor, **642–647**

Molecular work-up of myeloid neoplasms, **134–135**
- global approach to cytogenetic and, **135**
- molecular/genetic techniques commonly used, **134**

INDEX

- purposes of, **134**
Monoclonal B lymphocytosis, small lymphocytic lymphoma/chronic lymphocytic leukemia vs., **312**
Monoclonal gammopathy of undetermined significance, **350–353**
- cytogenetics, **352**
- lymphoplasmacytic lymphoma vs., **348**
- multiple myeloma (plasma cell myeloma) vs., **357**
- prognosis, **352**
Monocytic leukemia, acute, acute promyelocytic leukemia with t(15;17)/*PML::RARA* vs., **251**
Monomorphic epitheliotropic intestinal T-cell lymphoma (MEITL), **417, 418, 419**
Monophasic synovial sarcoma, biphenotypic sinonasal sarcoma vs., **534**
Monosomy, **6**
Monosomy 7, **210**
Morpheaform basal cell carcinoma, **798**
Mosaicism, **4, 6**
MPL gene, **127**
- function, **56–57**
MPL mutations, **56–57**
- atypical chronic myeloid leukemia, **222**
- *BCR::ABL1*-negative myeloproliferative neoplasms, **57**
- essential thrombocythemia, **158**
- molecular approach, **57**
- myeloproliferative neoplasm, unclassifiable, **163**
- polycythemia vera, **150**
- primary myelofibrosis, **154**
- thrombopoietin receptor, **56**
MPNST. *See* Malignant peripheral nerve sheath tumor.
MRTFA (MKL1) gene, function, **263**
Mucinous borderline tumor, **769**
Mucinous carcinoma, **769, 770**
- pancreatic ductal adenocarcinoma, **616**
Mucinous cystic neoplasm, pancreatic, **618–619**
- differential diagnosis, **619**
- prognosis, **619**
Mucinous cystic neoplasm of pancreas. *See* Pancreatic mucinous cystic neoplasm.
Mucoepidermoid carcinoma (MEC), **509**
- clear cell carcinoma vs., **521**
- clinicopathologic features, **513**
- differential diagnosis, **512**
- molecular alterations, **513**
- molecular genetics, **510**
- prognosis, **509**
- in situ hybridization, **510**
Mucosa-associated lymphoid tissue lymphoma, splenic marginal zone lymphoma vs., **329**
Multiple endocrine neoplasia 1 (MEN1), adrenal cortical carcinoma, **667**
Multiple endocrine neoplasia type 2 (MEN2), pheochromocytoma/paraganglioma, **662, 663**
Multiple myeloma (plasma cell myeloma), **294, 354–361**
- asymptomatic, **355**
- chromosomal microarray, **357**
- classification, **355, 358**
- cytogenetics, **356**
- differential diagnosis, **357**
- gene expression profiling, **357**
- genetic abnormalities, **358**
- lymphoplasmacytic lymphoma vs., **348**
- molecular genetics, **357**
- *MYD88* L265P mutations, **348**
- prognosis, **356**
- symptomatic, **355**
Multiplex ligation-dependent probe amplification, **29**
Multiplex polymerase chain reaction, **29**
Muscle invasive bladder cancer (MIBC), **656**
Muscle sarcomas, **868–877**
- differential diagnosis, **872**
- genetic findings, **871–872**
Mutations, types, **13–14**
MUTYH-associated polyposis, colorectal adenocarcinoma and precancerous lesions, **585–586**
MYC mutations
- B-cell prolymphocytic leukemia, **323**
- small lymphocytic lymphoma/chronic lymphocytic leukemia, **320**
MYCN alterations, Wilms tumor, **645**
Mycosis fungoides (MF), **432–437**
- adult T-cell leukemia/lymphoma vs., **412**
- atypical lymphoid infiltrates vs., **786**
- chronic lymphoproliferative disorder of NK cells vs., **398**
- differential diagnosis, **435**
- folliculotropic (pilotropic), **433**
- involving lymph node, peripheral T-cell lymphoma, not otherwise specified vs., **446**
- large cell transformation, primary cutaneous CD30-positive T-cell lymphoproliferative disorders, **439**
- molecular genetics, **434**
- prognosis, **434**
- syringotropic, **435**
MYC-regulated microRNAs, Burkitt lymphoma, **389**
MYD88 gene, **94**
- L265P mutation
    B-cell lymphomas, **94–95**
    testing, **95**
- mutation, **94–95**
    diagnostic checklist, **95**
    lymphoplasmacytic lymphoma, **346**
Myelodysplastic neoplasms
- with low blasts. *See* Myelodysplastic syndrome, not otherwise specified.
- molecular work-up, **135**
Myelodysplastic syndrome (MDS)
- atypical chronic myeloid leukemia vs., **222**
- chromosomal microarray, **24**
- chronic eosinophilic leukemia, NOS vs., **160**
- with del(5q), **184, 200–203**
    cytogenetics, **201**
    differential diagnosis, **201**
    molecular genetics, **201**
    myelodysplastic syndrome with mutated *SF3B1* vs., **190**
    prognosis, **201**
- with excess blasts, **184**
    acute myeloid leukemia, NOS vs., **273**

xxxv

INDEX

acute myeloid leukemia with t(6:9)/*DEK::NUP214* vs., 259
- extended multigene testing, 70–71
- *EZH2* mutation, 100
- with *GATA2*; *MECOM* rearrangement, acute myeloid leukemia with inv(3) or t(3;3)/*GATA2*; *MECOM*, 261
- with isolated del(5q), essential thrombocythemia vs., 158
- molecular work-up, 135
- with mutated *SF3B1* (MDS-*SF3B1*), 184, 188–191
    cytogenetics, 190
    differential diagnosis, 190
    molecular genetics, 190
    prognosis, 190
- with mutated *TP53*, 184
- myelodysplastic/myeloproliferative neoplasm, NOS vs., 230
- not otherwise specified, 192–199
    cytogenetics, 194
    diagnostic checklist, 195
    differential diagnosis, 195
    genetic testing, 195
    molecular genetics, 194
    myelodysplastic syndrome with mutated *SF3B1* vs., 190
    prognosis, 193–194
    with single lineage or multilineage dysplasia, myelodysplastic syndrome with del(5q) vs., 201
    without dysplasia, 184
- overview and classification, 184–187
    International Prognostic Scoring System (Revised), 186
    molecular genetic testing, 185
    mutated genes, 186
    recurring chromosomal abnormalities, 186
    WHO classification, 184–185
- pediatric, 208–213
- post cytotoxic exposure, myelodysplastic syndrome, NOS vs., 195
- *SETBP1* mutations, 62
- subtypes, myelodysplastic syndrome, NOS vs., 195
- with thrombocytosis, essential thrombocythemia vs., 158
- with *TP53* multihit mutations, 204–205
    classification, 205
    diagnostic checklist, 205
    differential diagnosis, 205
    prognosis, 205

Myelodysplastic syndrome/acute myeloid leukemia (MDS/AML), 206–207
- classification, 207
- diagnostic checklist, 207
- differential diagnosis, 207
- genetic testing, 207
- with mutated *TP53*, 184
- with myelodysplasia-related cytogenetic abnormalities, 184
- with myelodysplasia-related gene mutation, 184
- NOS, 184
- prognosis, 207

Myelodysplastic/myeloproliferative neoplasms (MDS/MPN), 214–215
- classification, 214
- diagnostic checklist, 215
- *EZH2* mutation, 100
- myeloproliferative neoplasm, unclassifiable vs., 164
- not otherwise specified (NOS), 228–231
    classification, 229
    cytogenetics, 229
    diagnostic checklist, 230
    differential diagnosis, 230
    genetic testing, 230
    molecular genetics, 229–230
    prognosis, 229
- with ring sideroblasts and thrombocytosis, essential thrombocytosis vs., 158
- with *SF3B1* mutation and thrombocytosis
    myelodysplastic syndrome with mutated *SF3B1* vs., 190
    myelodysplastic/myeloproliferative neoplasm, NOS vs., 230
- unclassifiable, atypical chronic myeloid leukemia vs., 222

Myelofibrosis, primary, 152–155
- with *CALR* mutations, 59
- cytogenetics, 153–154
- differential diagnosis, 154
- essential thrombocythemia vs., 158
- *EZH2* mutation, 100
- genetic testing, 154
- molecular genetics, 154
- polycythemia vera vs., 150
- prognosis, 153

Myeloid leukemia
- acute, 232–239
    with alternative *MECOM* translocations, acute myeloid leukemia with inv(3) or t(3;3)/*GATA2*; *MECOM*, 261
    with *BCR::ABL1*, 43, 232, 236
    biological categories of mutations, 70
    blastic plasmacytoid dendritic cell neoplasm vs., 286
    with *CBFB::MYH11* fusion, 236
    with *CEBPA* mutation, 233, 236
    chromosomal microarray, 24
    common genetic mutations and approximate frequencies in, 273
    conventional, myeloid proliferations associated with Down syndrome vs., 282
    core binding factor, 65–66
    cytogenetics, 234
    de novo, mutated genes, 71
    with *DEK::NUP214* fusion, 236
    diagnostic checklist, 234
    differential diagnosis, 236
    extended multigene testing, 70
    EZH2 mutation, 100
    FLT3, *NPM1*, and *CEBPA* mutations, 52
    gene alterations, 234–235
    gene mutations, 235

xxxvi

INDEX

with inframe basic leucine zipper region (bZIP) *CEBPA* mutation, **232–233**, 236
with inv(16) or t(16;16)/*CBFB::MYH11*, **244–247**
with inv(3) or t(3;3)/*GATA2; MECOM*, **260–261**
juvenile myelomonocytic leukemia vs., 227
KIT mutations, **66**
with *KMT2A* rearrangements, 236
with maturation, **271**, 271–272
with *MECOM* rearrangements, 236
with minimal differentiation, **271**
molecular work-up, **135**
with mutated *NPM1*, 232, 236
with mutated *TP53*, 233, 236
mutational landscape, **70**
with myelodysplasia-related gene mutations, 232, 233, 236, **264–269**
myelodysplastic syndrome with *TP53* multihit mutations vs., **205**
myelodysplastic/myeloproliferative neoplasm, NOS vs., **230**
not otherwise specified (NOS), **270–275**
post cytotoxic exposure, myelodysplastic syndrome, NOS vs., **195**
with recurrent genetic abnormality, **48**
RET fusion genes, **109**
with *RUNX1::RUNX1T1* fusion, **236**
SETBP1 mutations, **63**
with t(1;22)(p13.3;q13.1); *RBM15::MRTFA*, myeloid proliferations associated with Down syndrome vs., **282**
with t(1;22)/*RBM15::MRTFA*, **262–263**
with t(5;17)(q35;q21);*NPM1::RARA*, acute promyelocytic leukemia with t(15;17)/*PML::RARA* vs., **251**
with t(6;9)/*DEK::NUP214*, **258–259**
with t(8;21)/*RUNX1::RUNX1T1*, **240–243**
with t(9;11)/*MLLT3::KMT2A*, **254–257**
with t(11;17)(q13;q21);*NUMA1::RARA*, acute promyelocytic leukemia with t(15;17)/*PML::RARA* vs., **251**
with t(11;17)(q23;q21); *ZBTB16::RARA*, acute promyelocytic leukemia with t(15;17)/*PML::RARA* vs., **251**
with t(17;17)(q21.2;q21); *STAT5B::RARA*, acute promyelocytic leukemia with t(15;17)/*PML::RARA* vs., **251**
with t(X;17)(p11;q21); *BCOR::RARA*, acute promyelocytic leukemia with t(15;17)/*PML::RARA* vs., **251**
transcripts, reverse transcription PCR, **48–49**
without maturation, **271**
- Down syndrome, **281**, 282
  acute myeloid leukemia with t(1;22)/*RBM15::MRTFA* vs., **263**
Myeloid neoplasms, **55**
- blast phase of preexisting, acute myeloid leukemia vs., **236**
- *CALR* mutations, **59**
- with eosinophilia and rearrangements of *PDGFRA*, *PDGFRB*, *FGFR1*, or *PCM1::JAK2*, chronic myelomonocytic leukemia vs., **218**
- with eosinophilia and tyrosine kinase fusion, chronic eosinophilic leukemia, NOS vs., **161**
- *EZH2* mutation, **100**
- *IDH1* and *IDH2* mutations, **69**
- mutations and gene panel testing, **70–71**
- post therapy, pediatric myelodysplastic syndrome and refractory cytopenia of childhood vs., **211**
Myeloid neoplasms, molecular pathology of
- acute myeloid leukemia
    with inv(16) or t(16;16)/*CBFB::MYH11*, **244–247**
    with inv(3) or t(3;3)/*GATA2; MECOM*, **260–261**
    with myelodysplasia-related gene mutations, **264–269**
    not otherwise specified (NOS), **270–275**
    overview, **232–239**
    with t(6;9)/*DEK::NUP214*, **258–259**
    with t(9;11)/*MLLT3::KMT2A*, **254–257**
    with t(1;22)/*RBM15::MRTFA*, **262–263**
    with t(8;21)/*RUNX1::RUNX1T1*, **240–243**
- acute promyelocytic leukemia with t(15;17)/*PML::RARA*, **248–253**
- atypical chronic myeloid leukemia, **220–223**
- blastic plasmacytoid dendritic cell neoplasm, **284–289**
- chronic eosinophilic leukemia, NOS, **160–161**
- clonal hematopoiesis and premalignant clonal cytopenia, **182–183**
- essential thrombocythemia, **156–159**
- juvenile myelomonocytic leukemia, **224–227**
- mastocytosis, **166–173**
- molecular work-up of, **134–135**
    global approach to cytogenetic and, **135**
    molecular/genetic techniques commonly used, **134**
    purposes of, **134**
- myelodysplastic syndrome
    with del(5q), **200–203**
    mutated *SF3B1*, **188–191**
    NOS, **192–199**
    overview and classification, **184–187**
    with *TP53* multihit mutations, **204–205**
- myelodysplastic syndrome/acute myeloid leukemia, **206–207**
- myelodysplastic/myeloproliferative neoplasms, **214–215**
- myeloid proliferations, associated with Down syndrome, **280–283**
- myeloid sarcoma, **276–279**
- myeloid/lymphoid neoplasms with eosinophilia and tyrosine kinase gene fusions, **174–177**
- myeloproliferative neoplasms
    chronic myeloid leukemia, *BCR::ABL1* positive, **136–143**
    chronic neutrophilic leukemia, **144–147**
    polycythemia vera, **148–151**
    unclassifiable, **162–165**
- primary myelofibrosis, **152–155**
- VEXAS syndrome, **178–181**

INDEX

Myeloid proliferations, associated with Down syndrome, 280–283
- cytogenetics, 282
- diagnostic checklist, 282
- differential diagnosis, 282
- prognosis, 281–282

Myeloid sarcoma, 276–279
- acute myeloid leukemia, 236
- acute myeloid leukemia with inv(16) or t(16;16)/*CBFB::MYH11*, 246
- cytogenetics, 277–278
- diagnostic checklist, 278
- differential diagnosis, 278
- diffuse large B-cell lymphoma vs., 379
- genetic testing, 278
- histiocytic sarcoma vs., 472
- molecular genetics, 278
- prognosis, 277

Myeloid/lymphoid neoplasm with eosinophilia and *FGFR1* abnormalities, T-lymphoblastic leukemia/lymphoma vs., 313

Myeloid/lymphoid neoplasms with eosinophilia and tyrosine kinase gene fusions, 174–177
- chronic eosinophilic leukemia, NOS vs., 161
- mastocytosis vs., 169

Myeloma, plasma cell, 354–361
- chromosomal microarray, 357
- classification, 355, 358
- cytogenetics, 356
- differential diagnosis, 357
- gene expression profiling, 357
- genetic abnormalities, 358
- molecular genetics, 357
- prognosis, 356

Myelomonocytic leukemia
- chronic, 216–219
    diagnostic checklist, 218
    differential diagnosis, 218
    genetic testing, 218
    molecular genetics, 217
    myelodysplastic syndrome/acute myeloid leukemia vs., 207
    prognosis, 217
- juvenile, 224–227
    classification, 225
    cytogenetics, 226, 227
    differential diagnosis, 227
    genetic testing, 227
    molecular genetics, 226–227
    prognosis, 226

Myeloproliferative neoplasm-associated mutations, myeloproliferative neoplasm, unclassifiable, 163

Myeloproliferative neoplasms
- in accelerated phase, myelodysplastic syndrome/acute myeloid leukemia vs., 207
- *BCR::ABL1* negative, chronic myeloid leukemia, *BCR::ABL1*-positive vs., 139
- in blast phase, acute myeloid leukemia with myelodysplasia-related gene mutations vs., 267
- *CALR* mutations, 59

- chronic eosinophilic leukemia, NOS, 160–161
- chronic neutrophilic leukemia vs., 146
- essential thrombocythemia, 156–159
- molecular work-up, 135
- myelodysplastic/myeloproliferative neoplasm, NOS vs., 230
- primary myelofibrosis, 152–155
- unclassifiable, 162–165
    cytogenetics, 163
    diagnostic checklist, 164
    differential diagnosis, 164
    genetic testing, 164
    molecular genetics, 163–164

Myoepithelial carcinoma, 908, 909, 911
- differential diagnosis, 521
- molecular genetics, 520
- prognosis, 519
- of soft tissue, 892

Myoepithelioma
- epithelioid hemangioendothelioma vs., 881
- myoepithelial carcinoma vs., 521

Myoepithelioma/myoepithelial carcinoma, pleomorphic adenoma vs., 512

Myofibroblastic sarcoma, low-grade, 848, 849–850
- differential diagnosis, 851
- leiomyosarcoma vs., 872

Myofibroblastic tumor
- inflammatory, 848, 849
    differential diagnosis, 851
    embryonal rhabdomyosarcoma vs., 872
- intermediate and malignant, 848–857
    chromosome and gene alterations, 852
    differential diagnosis, 851

Myopericytoma, 892, 897

Myxofibrosarcoma, 849, 850, 852, 892
- differential diagnosis, 851
- low-grade, myxofibrosarcoma vs., 851

Myxoid chondrosarcoma, extraskeletal, 892, 898, 899, 901, 902
- epithelioid hemangioendothelioma vs., 881

Myxoid leiomyosarcoma, 892

Myxoid liposarcoma, 859, 860, 861
- differential diagnosis, 862
- high-grade, 861
    round cell sarcoma with *EWSR1*::non-ETS fusions vs., 827
- pleomorphic, 892
- prognosis, 859

Myxoid pleomorphic liposarcoma, 861
- differential diagnosis, 862
- prognosis, 859

Myxoinflammatory fibroblastic sarcoma, 849, 850, 892
- differential diagnosis, 851

Myxoma, intramuscular, myxofibrosarcoma vs., 851

Myxopapillary ependymoma, ependymal tumors, 933, 934

INDEX

N

Nanopore-based sequencing, **34**
Nasopharyngeal carcinoma (NPC), **88–89**
Nasopharyngeal EBV-related squamous cell carcinoma, **526–529**
- differential diagnosis, **528**
- genetic factors, **527**
- molecular genetics, **527–528**
- prognosis, **527**

Nasopharyngeal nonkeratinizing differentiated carcinoma, **528**
Nasopharyngeal nonkeratinizing undifferentiated carcinoma, **528**
Nasopharyngeal undifferentiated carcinoma, HPV associated, **497**
Natural killer cells, chronic lymphoproliferative disorder of, **398–401**
- cytogenetics, **399**
- differential diagnosis, **398**
- gene expression profiling, **399**
- molecular genetics, **399**
- prognosis, **399**

Natural killer/T-cell lymphoma (NK-/T-cell lymphoma), **99**
Necrotizing sialometaplasia, mucoepidermoid carcinoma vs., **512**
Neoplasms
- EBV-associated human, **84–93**
    - latent infection, **86–87**
    - lytic infection, **86–87**
    - structure and genome, **84**
    - virion, **84**
- embryonal, malignant, medulloblastoma, **939**
- epithelioid, poorly differentiated, diffuse large B-cell lymphoma vs., **379**
- lymphoid, with eosinophilia and tyrosine kinase fusion, chronic eosinophilic leukemia, NOS vs., **161**
- mature B-cell
    - B-cell prolymphocytic leukemia, **322–325**
    - Burkitt lymphoma, **386–393**
    - diffuse large B-cell lymphoma, **376–385**
    - follicular lymphoma, **362–369**
    - hairy cell leukemia, **332–335**
    - lymphoplasmacytic lymphoma, **344–349**
    - mantle cell lymphoma, **370–375**
    - monoclonal gammopathy, of undetermined significance, **350–353**
    - multiple myeloma (plasma cell myeloma), **354–361**
    - small lymphocytic lymphoma/chronic lymphocytic leukemia, **316–321**
    - splenic B-cell lymphoma/leukemia, unclassifiable, **336–343**
    - splenic marginal zone lymphoma, **326–331**
- mature T- and NK-cell
    - adult T-cell leukemia/lymphoma, **410–415**
    - aggressive NK-cell leukemia, **402–405**
    - anaplastic large cell lymphoma, ALK-negative, **456–461**
    - anaplastic large cell lymphoma, ALK-positive, **462–467**
    - chronic lymphoproliferative disorder of NK cells, **398–401**
    - extranodal NK-/T-cell lymphoma, **406–409**
    - hepatosplenic T-cell lymphoma, **424–427**
    - intestinal T-cell lymphoma, **416–423**
    - mycosis fungoides, **432–437**
    - peripheral T-cell lymphoma, not otherwise specified, **442–447**
    - primary cutaneous CD30-positive T-cell lymphoproliferative disorders, **438–441**
    - Sézary syndrome, **432–437**
    - subcutaneous panniculitis-like T-cell lymphoma, **428–431**
    - T-cell prolymphocytic leukemia, **394–397**
- myeloid, **55**
    - acute myeloid leukemia, not otherwise specified (NOS), **270–275**
    - acute myeloid leukemia, with inv(3) or t(3;3)/*GATA2*; *MECOM*, **260–261**
    - acute myeloid leukemia, with myelodysplasia-related gene mutations, **264–269**
    - acute myeloid leukemia, with t(6;9)/*DEK::NUP214*, **258–259**
    - acute myeloid leukemia, with t(9;11)/*MLLT3::KMT2A*, **254–257**
    - acute myeloid leukemia, with t(1;22)/*RBM15::MRTFA*, **262–263**
    - blastic plasmacytoid dendritic cell neoplasm, **284–289**
    - with eosinophilia and tyrosine kinase fusion, chronic eosinophilic leukemia, NOS vs., **161**
    - *EZH2* mutation, **100**
    - *IDH1* and *IDH2* mutations, **69**
    - mutations and gene panel testing, **70–71**
    - myeloid sarcoma, **276–279**
- myeloproliferative
    - chronic eosinophilic leukemia, NOS, **160–161**
    - chronic myeloid leukemia, *BCR::ABL1* positive, **136–141**
    - chronic neutrophilic leukemia, **144–147**
    - essential thrombocythemia, **156–159**
    - polycythemia vera, **148–151**
    - primary myelofibrosis, **152–155**
    - unclassifiable, **162–165**

Neoplastic conditions, chromosomal microarray, **23–24**
Nephroblastoma. *See* Wilms tumor.
Nephrogenic rests, Wilms tumor, **643**
Nerve sheath tumor, malignant peripheral, **886–891**
- differential diagnosis, **888**
- epithelioid, **887**
- genetic predisposition, **887**
- genetic testing, **888**
- molecular genetics, **887**
- prognosis, **887**
- spindle cell, **888**

Nested polymerase chain reaction, **29**
Neuroblastoma, **672–679**
- differential diagnosis, **676**

INDEX

- familial, **674–675**
    - *ALK* alterations, **105**
- favorable vs. unfavorable histology, **676**
- International Neuroblastoma Pathology Committee classification, **675**
- metastatic, alveolar rhabdomyosarcoma vs., **872**
- olfactory, medulloblastoma vs., **940**
- prognosis, **673–674**
- sporadic, *ALK* alterations, **105**
- staging system, **676**
- Wilms tumor vs., **645**

Neurocytic tumors, medulloblastoma vs., **940**
Neurocytoma, central, oligodendroglioma vs., **929**
Neuroectodermal tumor, primitive
- clear cell sarcoma of kidney vs., **649**
- neuroblastoma vs., **676**
- retinoblastoma vs., **952**

Neuroendocrine carcinoma
- large cell
    - lung squamous cell carcinoma vs., **570**
    - small cell neuroendocrine carcinoma vs., **574**
- olfactory neuroblastoma vs., **534**
- small cell, **572–575**
    - cytogenetics, **573**
    - differential diagnosis, **574**
    - genetic testing, **574**
    - molecular genetics, **574**
    - prognosis, **573**
- squamous cell carcinoma, cervix/vulva/vagina vs., **736**

Neuroendocrine neoplasms, pancreatic ductal adenocarcinoma vs., **616**
Neuroendocrine tumors, pheochromocytoma/paraganglioma vs., **663**
Neuroepithelial tumor
- cribriform, choroid plexus tumors vs., **945**
- dysembryoplastic, oligodendroglioma vs., **929**

Neurofibroma, **892**
- atypical, malignant peripheral nerve sheath tumor vs., **888**

Neurofibromatosis 1 (NF1), **805**
- juvenile myelomonocytic leukemia, **224**
- pheochromocytoma/paraganglioma, **662, 663**
- pilocytic astrocytoma, **925**

Neurofibromatosis 2 (NF2), **805**
- meningioma, **949**

Neurofibromin 1, **925**
Neuropathy, peripheral, monoclonal gammopathy, of undetermined significance, **351**
Neuropathy with ataxia, lymphoplasmacytic lymphoma, **345**
Neutropenia
- myelodysplastic syndrome, NOS, **193**
- myelodysplastic syndrome with *TP53* multihit mutations vs., **205**
- pediatric myelodysplastic syndrome and refractory cytopenia of childhood vs., **209**

Nevoid basal cell carcinoma syndrome, medulloblastoma, **939**
Next-generation sequencing (NGS), **33**
- *ALK* alterations, **105**
- bioinformatics, **36, 37**
- *BRAF* mutations, **119**
- computational hardware, **36**
- data analysis, **36–37**
- diffuse large B-cell lymphoma, **378**
- *EGFR* amplification, **121**
- *EGFR* gene alterations, **121**
- *ERBB2* (HER2) gene amplifications, **115**
- *IGH* gene rearrangements, **74**
- *JAK2* mutations, **55**
- *KRAS* mutations, **117**
- lung squamous cell carcinoma, **569**
- lymphoid neoplasms, **293–294, 296**
- molecular work-up of myeloid neoplasms, **134**
- *MYD88* L265P mutation, **95**
- platforms, **34**
- *PML::RARA* fusion, **47**
- *RET* fusion, **109**
- *ROS1* rearrangements, **107**
- software, **37**
- squamous cell carcinoma, skin, **793**
- targeted hotspot gene panel, **122, 122–123**
- *TRB* gene rearrangement, **82**
- *TRG* and *TRD* chain rearrangements, **78**

NF1. *See* Neurofibromatosis 1.
NF1 mutations
- B-lymphoblastic leukemia/lymphoma, *BCR::ABL1*-like (Ph-like ALL), **307**
- high-grade serous carcinoma, **765**
- pilocytic astrocytoma, **926**

NF2. *See* Neurofibromatosis 2.
NF2 mutations
- ependymal tumors vs., **934**
- meningioma, **949**

NF2-associated ependymomas, ependymal tumors, **933**
NFATC1 gene, giant cell tumor of bone, **834**
NFE2L2 (2q), non-HPV-related head and neck squamous cell carcinoma, **506**
NFKB1 (4q), non-HPV-related head and neck squamous cell carcinoma, **506**
NFKB2 (10q), non-HPV-related head and neck squamous cell carcinoma, **506**
Nijmegen-Breakage syndrome, medulloblastoma, **939**
Nitrocellulose membrane, transfer of DNA to, **85**
NK-cell leukemia, aggressive, **402–405**
- blastic plasmacytoid dendritic cell neoplasm vs., **286**
- chronic lymphoproliferative disorder of NK cells vs., **398**
- cytogenetics, **403**
- differential diagnosis, **402**
- extranodal NK-/T-cell lymphoma vs., **408**
- molecular genetics, **403**
- prognosis, **403**

NK-/T-cell lymphoma, extranodal, **406–409**
- aggressive NK-cell leukemia vs., **402**
- cytogenetics, **407**
- differential diagnosis, **408**
- intestinal T-cell lymphoma vs., **421**
- molecular genetics, **408**
- nasal type, **88**
- prognosis, **407**

NMIBC. *See* Noninvasive bladder cancer.

INDEX

Nodal follicular helper T-cell lymphoma (NTFHL), 448–455
- angioimmunoblastic type, 449, 451
- clinical and laboratory findings, 453
- cytogenetics, 451
- diagnostic checklist, 453
- differential diagnosis, 452
- follicular type, 449, 451
- gene alterations, 450–451
- molecular findings, 453
- NOS, 449, 451
- prognosis, 450

Nodal marginal zone lymphoma
- mantle cell lymphoma vs., 373
- peripheral T-cell lymphoma, not otherwise specified vs., 446

Nodal T follicular helper cell lymphoma
- angioimmunoblastic type, peripheral T-cell lymphoma, not otherwise specified vs., 445
- not otherwise specified, peripheral T-cell lymphoma, not otherwise specified vs., 445

Nodular basal cell carcinoma, 797
Nodular fasciitis, 892
- inflammatory myofibroblastic tumor vs., 851

Nodular lymphocyte-predominant Hodgkin lymphoma, nodal follicular helper T-cell lymphoma vs., 452

Nomenclature, 14–15
Nonbisulfite-dependent methods, 38
Noncanonical *IDH1* mutations, astrocytoma, IDH-mutant, 921
Nonchronic myeloid leukemia myeloproliferative neoplasms, 55
Nonclear cell adenocarcinoma, 739
Nonclonal eosinophilia, chronic eosinophilic leukemia, NOS vs., 161
Nonhematopoietic anaplastic tumors, anaplastic large cell lymphoma, ALK-negative vs., 458
Nonhematopoietic neoplasms, anaplastic large cell lymphoma, ALK-positive vs., 464
Nonhematopoietic tumors, myeloid sarcoma vs., 278
Non-Hodgkin lymphoma, neuroblastoma vs., 676
Non-HPV-associated nasopharyngeal undifferentiated carcinoma, HPV-positive nasopharyngeal carcinoma vs., 497
Non-HPV-related head and neck squamous cell carcinoma, 506–507
Noninvasive bladder cancer (NMIBC), 656
Nonneoplastic disorders, myelodysplastic/myeloproliferative neoplasm, NOS vs., 230
Nonossifying fibroma, giant cell tumor of bone vs., 835
NONO::TFE3 carcinomas, *TFE3*-rearranged and *TFEB*-altered renal cell carcinomas, 640
Nonroutine inspection, CAP, 967
Nonseminomatous germ cell tumors (NSGCTs), malignant, 625
Nonsense mutation/substitution, 13–14
Non-small cell lung cancer
- *ALK* alterations, 104–105
- *BRAF* mutations, 119
- *KRAS* mutations, 117
- *RET* rearrangements, 108, 109
- *ROS1* fusion genes, 107

Noonan syndrome
- *BRAF* mutations, 119
- juvenile myelomonocytic leukemia, 226
- *KRAS* mutations, 117

Noonan syndrome-associated myeloproliferative disorder, 226, 227
NOTCH1 (9p), non-HPV-related head and neck squamous cell carcinoma, 506
NOTCH1 gene, 127–128
- functions, 96
- mutation, 96
  - diagnostic checklist, 97
  - small lymphocytic lymphoma/chronic lymphocytic leukemia, 319–320
  - T-lymphoblastic leukemia/lymphoma, 312

NOTCH1 protein, 96
Novel myxoid mesenchymal tumor, 897
Nowell, Peter, 18
NPM1 gene, 128
NPM1 mutations, 50–53
- acute myeloid leukemia, 234
- acute myeloid leukemia, NOS, 273
- myelodysplastic/myeloproliferative neoplasm, NOS, 229
- myeloid sarcoma, 278

NRAS gene, 128
NRAS mutations
- acute myeloid leukemia, 234
- acute myeloid leukemia, NOS, 273
- acute myeloid leukemia with inv(16) or t(16;16)/*CBFB::MYH11*, 246
- anaplastic thyroid carcinoma, 551
- atypical chronic myeloid leukemia, 222
- B-lymphoblastic leukemia/lymphoma, *BCR::ABL1*-like (Ph-like ALL), 307
- chronic myelomonocytic leukemia, 217
- colorectal adenocarcinoma and precancerous lesions, 586
- mastocytosis, 169
- melanoma, 790
- myelodysplastic syndrome, NOS, 194
- myelodysplastic/myeloproliferative neoplasm, NOS, 229–230
- papillary thyroid carcinoma, 539
- poorly differentiated thyroid carcinoma, 547
- T-lymphoblastic leukemia/lymphoma, 312

N-terminus mutation, *FLT3*, *NPM1*, and *CEBPA* mutations, 51
NTRK mutation, pilocytic astrocytoma, 926
NTRK1 gene fusions
- glioblastoma, IDH wildtype, 918
- lung adenocarcinoma, 563

NTRK1 rearrangements, papillary thyroid carcinoma, 540
NTRK2 fusions, glioblastoma, IDH wildtype, 918
NTRK3 fusions
- B-lymphoblastic leukemia/lymphoma, *BCR::ABL1*-like (Ph-like ALL), 308
- glioblastoma, IDH wildtype, 918

INDEX

NTRK3 mutations, B-lymphoblastic leukemia/lymphoma, *BCR::ABL1*-like (Ph-like ALL), 307
NTRK3 rearrangements, papillary thyroid carcinoma, 540
NTRK-rearranged spindle cell neoplasm, 892, 908, 909, 910, 911
Nucleic acid-based methods
- *IGH* gene rearrangements, 74
- *TRB* gene rearrangement, 82
- *TRG* and *TRD* chain rearrangements, 77–78

Nucleic acid hybridization techniques, EBV detection, 89
Nucleic acids, structure, 4–7
Nucleophosmin (*NPM1*) gene
- function, 50–51
- mutations, 51
   clinical significance, 52
   testing, 53

Nucleotide numbering, 14–15
NUP214 gene, function, 259
NUT (midline) carcinoma (NMC), 531
- cytogenetics, 532
- differential diagnosis, 534
- head and neck mucosal squamous cell carcinoma, non-HPV related vs., 503
- molecular genetics, 532
- prognosis, 531

NUTM1-fusion positive undifferentiated nonmidline tumors, 897
Nutritional deficiencies
- myelodysplastic syndrome, NOS vs., 195
- pediatric myelodysplastic syndrome and refractory cytopenia of childhood vs., 212
- VEXAS syndrome vs., 180

Nylon membrane, transfer of DNA to, 85

O

Obstructive hydrocephalus, ependymal tumors, 933
OFMT. *See* Ossifying fibromyxoid tumor.
Olfactory neuroblastoma (ONB), 531
- cytogenetics, 532
- differential diagnosis, 534
- medulloblastoma vs., 940
- molecular genetics, 532
- prognosis, 532

Oligodendroglioma
- astrocytoma, IDH-mutant vs., 922
- ependymal tumors vs., 934
- IDH mutant, 1p/19q codeleted, 928–931
   differential diagnosis, 929
   molecular genetics, 929
   prognosis, 929
- *IDH1* and *IDH2* mutations, 69
- pilocytic astrocytoma vs., 926
- WHO grade 3, glioblastoma, IDH wildtype vs., 918

Oncocytic tumors, oncocytoma vs., 651
Oncocytoma, 650–651
- diagnostic checklist, 651
- differential diagnosis, 651
- prognosis, 651
- renal, chromophobe renal cell carcinoma vs., 635

Oncocytoma-like epithelioid angiomyolipoma, oncocytoma vs., 650
Oncogenesis, 8, 12
Oncotype DX assay, 695–696
Oral cavity tumors, EZH2 protein overexpression, 101
Ossifying fibromyxoid tumor (OFMT), 892, 908, 909, 910, 911
Osteoblastoma, 895
Osteochondroma, 895
- peripheral chondrosarcoma vs., 842

Osteoclastoma. *See* Giant cell tumor of bone.
Osteoid osteoma, 895
Osteopenia, monoclonal gammopathy, of undetermined significance, 351
Osteoporosis, monoclonal gammopathy, of undetermined significance, 351
Osteosarcomas, 810–817
- clear cell chondrosarcoma vs., 842
- conventional central, 810–811, 813
   cytogenetics, 812
   differential diagnosis, 814
   gene alterations, 812
- dedifferentiated chondrosarcoma vs., 842
- differential diagnosis, 814
- giant cell-rich, giant cell tumor of bone vs., 835
- high grade, 895
- low grade, 895
- low-grade central, 810, 811, 813
   differential diagnosis, 814
- parosteal, 810, 811, 812, 813
   differential diagnosis, 814
- periosteal, 810, 811, 812, 813
   differential diagnosis, 814
- small cell, 810, 811, 813, 814
   differential diagnosis, 814
   Ewing sarcoma vs., 821
- telangiectatic, 810, 811, 812, 813
   differential diagnosis, 814

Ovarian cancer, *EGFR* amplification, 121
Ovarian serous carcinoma, EZH2 protein overexpression, 100
Ovary
- germ cell tumor, 780–783
   cytogenetics, 781
   differential diagnosis, 782
   molecular genetics, 781
- sex cord-stromal tumors of, 774–779
   cytogenetics, 776
   differential diagnosis, 778
   molecular genetics, 776–777
   prognosis, 776

INDEX

P

Paget disease, osteosarcoma, **811**
Pagetoid reticulosis, mycosis fungoides/Sézary syndrome, **433**
Pancreatic adenocarcinoma. *See* Pancreatic ductal adenocarcinoma.
Pancreatic ductal adenocarcinoma (PDA), **614–617**
- differential diagnosis, **616**
- *KRAS* mutations, **117**
- molecular genetics, **615–616**
- prognosis, **615**

Pancreatic infiltrating ductal carcinoma. *See* Pancreatic ductal adenocarcinoma.
Pancreatic intraductal mucinous neoplasm, EZH2 protein overexpression, **101**
Pancreatic intraductal papillary mucinous neoplasm, **620–621**
- differential diagnosis, **621**
- prognosis, **621**

Pancreatic mucinous cystic neoplasm (PMCN), **618–619**
- differential diagnosis, **619**
- pancreatic intraductal papillary mucinous neoplasm vs., **621**
- prognosis, **619**

Pancreatic pseudocyst
- pancreatic intraductal papillary mucinous neoplasm vs., **621**
- pancreatic mucinous cystic neoplasm vs., **619**

Pancreatic tubular adenocarcinoma. *See* Pancreatic ductal adenocarcinoma.
Pancreatitis, chronic, pancreatic ductal adenocarcinoma vs., **616**
Panniculitis
- lobular, subcutaneous panniculitis-like T-cell lymphoma vs., **430**
- lupus profundus, subcutaneous panniculitis-like T-cell lymphoma vs., **430**
- reactive, subcutaneous panniculitis-like T-cell lymphoma vs., **430**
- SLE, subcutaneous panniculitis-like T-cell lymphoma vs., **430**

Papillary carcinoma
- medullary thyroid carcinoma vs., **557**
- solid variant, poorly differentiated thyroid carcinoma vs., **548**
- of thyroid origin, lung adenocarcinoma vs., **564**

Papillary cystitis, urothelial carcinoma vs., **657**
Papillary ependymoma, ependymal tumors, **933**
Papillary hyperplasia, in Graves disease and adenomatous goiter, papillary thyroid carcinoma vs., **540**
Papillary intralymphatic angioendothelioma (PILA)
- genetic findings, **880**
- prognosis, **879**

Papillary renal cell carcinoma (PRCC), **636–637**
- clear cell, papillary renal cell carcinoma vs., **637**
- differential diagnosis, **637**
- prognosis, **637**
- type 1, **637**
- type 2, **637**
- Wilms tumor vs., **645**

Papillary serous carcinoma, clear cell carcinoma, uterus vs., **752**
Papillary thyroid carcinoma (PTC), **538–541**
- *BRAF* mutations, **119**
- cytogenetics, **539**
- differential diagnosis, **540**
- follicular variant of, follicular thyroid carcinoma vs., **544**
- gene fusions, **539–540**
- gene mutations, **539**
- MAPK-related gene alterations, **539**
- prognosis, **539**
- *RET* rearrangements, **108–109**

Papillary tumor, pineal region, choroid plexus tumors vs., **945**
Papilloma, choroid plexus, choroid plexus tumors, **945**
Paracortical hyperplasia, peripheral T-cell lymphoma, not otherwise specified vs., **446**
Paraganglioma (PGL), **660–665**
- differential diagnosis, **663**
- ependymal tumors vs., **934**
- genetic testing, **663**
- medullary thyroid carcinoma vs., **557**
- prognosis, **661**
- tumor distributions, **663**

Parallel sequencing, targeted hotspot gene panel, **122, 122–123**
Parathyroid adenoma and carcinoma, EZH2 protein overexpression, **100**
Parosteal osteosarcomas, **810, 811, 812, 813**
- differential diagnosis, **814**

Paroxysmal nocturnal hemoglobinuria (PNH)
- clonal hematopoiesis and premalignant clonal cytopenia, **183**
- myelodysplastic syndrome, NOS vs., **195**
- pediatric myelodysplastic syndrome and refractory cytopenia of childhood vs., **212**

Parvovirus B19 infection
- juvenile myelomonocytic leukemia vs., **227**
- pediatric myelodysplastic syndrome and refractory cytopenia of childhood vs., **212**

Passenger mutations, **13**
Paternity, Southern blot analysis, **85**
PAX2-inactivating mutations, endometrial intraepithelial neoplasia, **743**
PAX5::JAK2 fusion, **55**
PAX8::PPARG rearrangement
- papillary thyroid carcinoma, **540**

PCM1::JAK2 fusion, **54–55**
PCM1::JAK2 mutations
- detection, **176**
- fusion, **175**
- testing, **175**

PCR. *See* Polymerase chain reaction.
PDA. *See* Pancreatic ductal adenocarcinoma.
PDGFB (22q), non-HPV-related head and neck squamous cell carcinoma, **507**
PDGFRA fusions, glioblastoma, IDH wildtype, **918**

xliii

INDEX

PDGFRA gene, **128**
PDGFRA mutations, **174**
- GIST, **592, 593**
- rearrangement, **174**
    - detection, **176**
    - rare, **176**
- testing, **175**
PDGFRB mutations, **174**
- B-lymphoblastic leukemia/lymphoma, *BCR::ABL1*-like (Ph-like ALL), **308**
- rearrangement, **174–175**
    - detection, **176**
- testing, **175**
PEComa, **756**
Pediatric follicular lymphoma, follicular lymphoma vs., **365**
Pediatric myelodysplastic syndrome (MDS), **208–213**
- classification, **209**
- cytogenetics, **210**
- diagnostic checklist, **212**
- differential diagnosis, **211–212**
- prognosis, **210**
Periampullary carcinomas, pancreatic ductal adenocarcinoma vs., **616**
Perilobular nephrogenic rests (PLNR), Wilms tumor, **643**
Perineurioma, **892**
- myxofibrosarcoma vs., **851**
Periosteal cartilaginous tumors, *IDH1* and *IDH2* mutations, **69**
Periosteal chondrosarcoma, **838, 839, 841**
- differential diagnosis, **842**
- grading, **840**
Periosteal osteosarcomas, **810, 811, 812, 813**
- differential diagnosis, **814**
Peripheral chondrosarcoma
- differential diagnosis, **842**
- secondary, **841**
    - differential diagnosis, **842**
    - grading, **840**
Peripheral nerve sheath tumor, malignant, **886–891**
- differential diagnosis, **888**
- epithelioid, **887**
- genetic predisposition, **887**
- genetic testing, **888**
- leiomyosarcoma vs., **872**
- molecular genetics, **887**
- prognosis, **887**
- solitary fibrous tumor vs., **851**
- spindle cell, **888**
Peripheral neuroblastic tumor. *See* Neuroblastoma.
Peripheral neuropathy, monoclonal gammopathy, of undetermined significance, **351**
Peripheral T-cell lymphoma
- adult T-cell leukemia/lymphoma vs., **412**
- with associated B-cell proliferation, **445**
- with CD30(+) cells, anaplastic large cell lymphoma, ALK-positive vs., **464**
- involving aerodigestive tract, extranodal NK-/T-cell lymphoma vs., **408**
- not otherwise specified, **442–447**
    - anaplastic large cell lymphoma, ALK-negative vs., **458**
    - differential diagnosis, **445–446**
    - intestinal T-cell lymphoma vs., **421**
    - morphologic variants, **445**
    - nodal follicular helper T-cell lymphoma vs., **452, 453**
    - prognosis, **443**
Perivascular epithelioid cell tumor (PEComa), **892, 898, 899, 901, 902**
Peutz-Jeghers syndrome
- adenocarcinoma, cervix/vulva/vagina, **739**
- colorectal adenocarcinoma and precancerous lesions, **586**
- gastric adenocarcinoma, **581**
PGL. *See* Paraganglioma.
PHAT. *See* Pleomorphic hyalinizing angiectatic tumor.
Phenotype, genotype vs., **13**
Pheochromocytoma, **660–665**
- adrenal cortical adenoma vs., **682**
- adrenal cortical carcinoma vs., **669**
- clear cell renal cell carcinoma, **631**
- differential diagnosis, **663**
- genetic testing, **663**
- prognosis, **661**
- tumor distributions, **663**
PHF6 gene mutation, T-lymphoblastic leukemia/lymphoma, **312**
Philadelphia (Ph) chromosome. *See BCR::ABL1* fusion.
Philadelphia-like ALL. *See* B-lymphoblastic leukemia/lymphoma, *BCR::ABL1*-like.
Phosphaturic mesenchymal tumor (PMT), **908, 909, 910, 911**
Phosphodiester bonds, **5**
Phyllodes tumors, **716–719**
- benign, **718**
- borderline, **718**
- classification, **718**
- cytogenetics, **717**
- differential diagnosis, **718**
- malignant, **718**
- molecular genetics, **717**
- prognosis, **717**
- with sarcomatous overgrowth, metaplastic breast carcinoma vs., **713**
PI3K mutations, clear cell carcinoma, uterus, **752**
PI3K-AKT-mTOR pathway alteration, **917**
PI3K-PTEN-AKT pathway, **544**
Piebaldism, *KIT* mutations, **66**
PIK3CA gene, **128**
PIK3CA mutations
- anaplastic thyroid carcinoma, **551–552**
- colorectal adenocarcinoma and precancerous lesions, **586**
- follicular thyroid carcinoma, **544**
- lung adenocarcinoma, **563**
- meningioma, **949–950**
- non-HPV-related head and neck squamous cell carcinoma, **507**
- pancreatic mucinous cystic neoplasm, **619**
Pilocytic astrocytoma, **924–927**
- differential diagnosis, **926**
- molecular genetics, **925–926**
- neurofibromatosis 1-associated, **925**

INDEX

- prognosis, **925**
- sporadic, **925**

Pilomyxoid astrocytoma, pilocytic astrocytoma vs., **926**
Pilotropic MF, mycosis fungoides/Sézary syndrome, **433**
Pineoblastoma, medulloblastoma vs., **940**
Plasma cell myeloma, **298**
- mantle cell lymphoma vs., **373**
- *MYD88* L265P mutations, **348**
- testing methods, **297**

Plasma cell neoplasms, **298**
Plasmablastic lymphoma, **87**
Plasmacytoid dendritic cells, nodules of, blastic plasmacytoid dendritic cell neoplasm vs., **286**
Plasmacytosis, reactive polyclonal, multiple myeloma (plasma cell myeloma) vs., **357**
Pleomorphic adenoma, **509**
- basal cell adenoma/adenocarcinoma vs., **521**
- clinicopathologic features, **513**
- differential diagnosis, **512**
- epithelial-myoepithelial carcinoma vs., **521**
- molecular alterations, **513**
- molecular genetics, **510**
- polymorphous carcinoma vs., **521**
- prognosis, **509**
- in situ hybridization, **510**

Pleomorphic hyalinizing angiectatic tumor (PHAT), **852, 892, 908, 909–910, 911**
- myxoinflammatory fibroblastic sarcoma vs., **851**

Pleomorphic lipoma, **892**
- atypical lipomatous tumor vs., **862**

Pleomorphic liposarcoma, **859, 860, 861, 862, 892**
- dedifferentiated liposarcoma vs., **862**
- differential diagnosis, **862**
- myxoid, **862**
- prognosis, **859**
- spindle cell liposarcoma vs., **862**

Pleomorphic rhabdomyosarcoma, **868, 870–871, 892**
- differential diagnosis, **872**
- genetic findings, **872**

Pleomorphic sarcoma, undifferentiated
- dedifferentiated chondrosarcoma vs., **842**
- high-grade
  - myxofibrosarcoma vs., **851**
  - sclerosing epithelioid fibrosarcoma vs., **851**

PLNR. *See* Perilobular nephrogenic rests.
Ploidy, **4**
PMCN. *See* Pancreatic mucinous cystic neoplasm.
PMF. *See* Primary myelofibrosis.
PML gene, normal function, **46**
PML::RARA fusion, **46–47**
PMT. *See* Phosphaturic mesenchymal tumor.
PNH. *See* Paroxysmal nocturnal hemoglobinuria.
Point mutations, *FLT3*, *NPM1*, and *CEBPA* mutations, **51**
Polyclonal plasmacytosis, reactive, multiple myeloma (plasma cell myeloma) vs., **357**
Polycythemia, secondary, polycythemia vera vs., **150**
Polycythemia vera, **148–151**
- cytogenetics, **150**
- differential diagnosis, **150**
- essential thrombocythemia vs., **158**
- genetic testing, **150**

- myeloproliferative neoplasm, unclassifiable vs., **164**
- primary myelofibrosis vs., **154**
- prognosis, **149**

Polycythemic phase, polycythemia vera, **150**
Polymerase chain reaction (PCR), **26–29**
- acute promyelocytic leukemia with t(15;17)/*PML::RARA*, **250**
- adult T-cell leukemia/lymphoma, **411**
- allele-specific
  - *BRAF* mutations, **119**
  - *JAK2* mutations, **55**
  - *MYD88* L265P mutation, **95**
- anaplastic large cell lymphoma, ALK-negative, **458**
- B-cell prolymphocytic leukemia, **324**
- Burkitt lymphoma, **388**
- chronic lymphoproliferative disorder of NK cells, **399**
- diffuse large B-cell lymphoma, **378**
- digital, *BRAF* mutations, **119**
- droplet digital, **29**
- EBV detection, **89**
- enteropathy-associated T-cell lymphoma, **420**
- extranodal NK-/T-cell lymphoma, **407**
- follicular dendritic cell sarcoma, **489**
- follicular lymphoma, **366**
- hepatosplenic T-cell lymphoma, **425**
- HPV-associated head and neck carcinomas, **496**
- *IGH* gene rearrangements, **74**
- interdigitating dendritic cell tumor, **485**
- *KRAS* mutations, **117**
- lymphoid neoplasms, **293, 297**
- lymphoplasmacytic lymphoma, **346**
- mantle cell lymphoma, **372**
- melanoma, **789**
- *MET* amplifications, **112**
- molecular work-up of myeloid neoplasms, **134**
- multiplex, **29**
- mycosis fungoides/Sézary syndrome, **434**
- nested, **29**
- nodal follicular helper T-cell lymphoma, **450**
- peripheral T-cell lymphoma, not otherwise specified, **444**
- premalignant conditions, skin, **785**
- primary cutaneous CD30-positive T-cell lymphoproliferative disorders, **440**
- quantitative real-time, for *ERBB2* gene status, **115**
- real-time, **28–29**
- restriction site-generating, **29**
- reverse transcription, **28**
- sebaceous carcinoma, **801**
- splenic B-cell lymphoma/leukemia, unclassifiable, **337**
- splenic marginal zone lymphoma, **327**
- squamous cell carcinoma, cervix/vulva/vagina, **736**
- standard, **26–28**
- subcutaneous panniculitis-like T-cell lymphoma, **429**
- T-cell prolymphocytic leukemia, **395**
- *TRB* gene rearrangement, **82**
- *TRG* and *TRD* chain rearrangements, **77**
- variants, **28–29**

Polymorphism, gene mutation vs., **13**
Polymorphous adenocarcinoma (PMC), **509**
- clinicopathologic features, **513**

xlv

INDEX

- differential diagnosis, 512
- molecular alterations, 513
- molecular genetics, 511
- prognosis, 509–510
- in situ hybridization, 510

Polymorphous carcinoma, differential diagnosis, 521

Polymorphous low-grade adenocarcinoma (PLGA), adenoid cystic carcinoma vs., 512

Polyp, endometrial, endometrial intraepithelial neoplasia vs., 743

Polyploidy, 4

Polypoid cystitis, urothelial carcinoma vs., 657

Poorly differentiated adenocarcinoma, small cell neuroendocrine carcinoma vs., 574

Poorly differentiated carcinoma
- anaplastic thyroid carcinoma vs., 552
- squamous cell carcinoma, skin vs., 794

Poorly differentiated chordoma, 895

Poorly differentiated squamous cell carcinoma, lung squamous cell carcinoma, 570

Poorly differentiated thyroid carcinoma (PDTC), 546–549
- differential diagnosis, 548
- molecular alterations, 547–548
- prognosis, 547

Posterior fossa ependymoma, NOS, ependymal tumors, 934

Posterior fossa group A (PFA) ependymoma, ependymal tumors, 933

Posterior fossa group B (PFB) ependymoma, ependymal tumors, 933–934

Postnatal diagnosis, chromosomal microarray, 23

Postpolycythemic myelofibrosis, polycythemia vera, 150

Posttranscription RNA processing, 9–10

Posttranslational modifications, 5, 10
- examples, 6

Posttransplant lymphoproliferative disorder (PTLD), 88

PPARG rearrangement, 544

PRCC. *See* Papillary renal cell carcinoma.

PRCC::TFE3 carcinomas, *TFE3*-rearranged and *TFEB*-altered renal cell carcinomas, 640

Precancerous lesions, colorectal adenocarcinoma, 584–589
- chromosomal instability pathway, 585
- gene mutations, 586–587
- hereditary, 585
- prognosis, 586
- sporadic polyps, 585

Precursor lymphoid neoplasms
- B-lymphoblastic leukemia/lymphoma, *BCR::ABL1*-like (Ph-like ALL), 306–309
- B-lymphoblastic leukemia/lymphoma with recurrent genetic abnormalities, 302–305
- T-lymphoblastic leukemia/lymphoma, 310–315

Precursor T-cell neoplasms. *See* T-lymphoblastic lymphoma.

Precursor T-lymphoblastic leukemia/lymphoma, 97

Premalignant conditions, skin, 784–787
- cytogenetics, 785
- differential diagnosis, 786
- molecular genetics, 785
- prognosis, 785

Premarketing approval process, IVDs, 961–964

Prenatal diagnosis, chromosomal microarray, 23

Preneoplastic conditions, cervix/vulva/vagina, 730–733
- differential diagnosis, 732
- next-generation sequencing, 732
- prognosis, 732

Prepolycythemic phase, polycythemia vera, 150

Prepubertal males, testicular germ cell tumors, 624

Presubmission process, IVDs, 961

Primary cutaneous anaplastic large cell lymphoma, anaplastic large cell lymphoma, ALK-positive vs., 464

Primary cutaneous CD30-positive T-cell lymphoproliferative disorders, 438–441
- molecular alterations, 439–440
- prognosis, 439

Primary cutaneous follicle center lymphoma, follicular lymphoma vs., 365

Primary cutaneous γδ T-cell lymphoma, subcutaneous panniculitis-like T-cell lymphoma vs., 430

Primary cutaneous large cell T-cell lymphoma, CD30(+). *See* Primary cutaneous CD30-positive T-cell lymphoproliferative disorders.

Primary cutaneous small/medium CD4(+) T-cell lymphoma, nodal follicular helper T-cell lymphoma vs., 452

Primary effusion lymphoma (PEL), 88

Primary myelofibrosis (PMF), 152–155
- with *CALR* mutations, 59
- cytogenetics, 153–154
- differential diagnosis, 154
- essential thrombocythemia vs., 158
- *EZH2* mutation, 100
- genetic testing, 154
- molecular genetics, 154
- myeloproliferative neoplasm, unclassifiable vs., 164
- polycythemia vera vs., 150
- prognosis, 153

Primary sarcomas, anaplastic thyroid carcinoma vs., 552

Primary thrombocytosis. *See* Essential thrombocythemia.

Primitive neuroectodermal tumor
- clear cell sarcoma of kidney vs., 649
- neuroblastoma vs., 676
- retinoblastoma vs., 952

Probation, CAP accreditation, 968
- immediate jeopardy, 968
- suspension, 968

Probes, types, 28

Products of conception, chromosomal microarray, 23

Proficiency testing (PT), 966–969
- CAP, 969
- federal regulations, 966

Prolymphocytic leukemia
- B-cell, 322–325
    cytogenetics, 323
    diagnostic checklist, 324
    differential diagnosis, 324
    molecular genetics, 323
    prognosis, 323
- T-cell, 394–397
    cytogenetics, 395

INDEX

differential diagnosis, 394
hepatosplenic T-cell lymphoma vs., 426
molecular genetics, 395
prognosis, 395
Promoter, 9
Promyelocytes, reactive increase in, acute promyelocytic leukemia with t(15;17)/*PML::RARA* vs., 251
Promyelocytic leukemia, acute
- hypergranular (typical), 250
- hypogranular (microgranular), 250
- minimal residual disease, 47
- *PML::RARA* fusion, 47
- with t(15;17)/*PML::RARA*, 248–253
  - cytogenetics, 250
  - diagnostic checklist, 251
  - differential diagnosis, 251
  - genetic testing, 250–251
  - prognosis, 249–250
- with variant *RARA* fusions, 251
Prosigna Breast Cancer Prognostic Gene Signature assay, 696
Prostate adenocarcinoma, EZH2 protein overexpression, 101
Prostate cancer, chromosomal microarray, 24
Prostatic adenocarcinoma, acinar type (PCa), 684–687
- prognosis, 685
Prostatic intraepithelial neoplasia, high-grade, 684–687
- prognosis, 685
Protooncogenes, 12
Pruritus, squamous cell carcinoma, cervix/vulva/vagina, 735
Pseudoangiomatoid carcinoma, angiosarcoma vs., 881
Pseudocarcinomatous hyperplasia, urothelial carcinoma vs., 657
Pseudocyst, pancreatic
- pancreatic intraductal papillary mucinous neoplasm vs., 621
- pancreatic mucinous cystic neoplasm vs., 619
Pseudoendocrine sarcoma, 897
Pseudoepitheliomatous hyperplasia
- squamous cell carcinoma, cervix/vulva/vagina vs., 736
- squamous cell carcinoma, skin vs., 794
Pseudomyogenic hemangioendothelioma, 880, 892
Pseudo-Pelger-Huët abnormality, myelodysplastic/myeloproliferative neoplasm, NOS, 229
PTCH1 alterations, Wilms tumor, 645
PTEN gene, 128
PTEN hamartoma tumor syndromes (PHTS), 543
- colorectal adenocarcinoma and precancerous lesions, 586
PTEN mutations
- anaplastic thyroid carcinoma, 552
- astrocytoma, IDH-mutant, 921
- clear cell carcinoma, uterus vs., 752
- follicular thyroid carcinoma, 544
- high-grade serous carcinoma, 764
- melanoma, 789
- non-HPV-related head and neck squamous cell carcinoma, 506
- T-lymphoblastic leukemia/lymphoma, 312

PTEN-inactivating mutations, endometrial intraepithelial neoplasia, 743
PTGS2 (1q), non-HPV-related head and neck squamous cell carcinoma, 507
PTH1R gene, giant cell tumor of bone, 834
PTK2B rearrangements, B-lymphoblastic leukemia/lymphoma, *BCR::ABL1*-like (Ph-like ALL), 307
PTPN11 gene, 128
PTPN11 mutations, B-lymphoblastic leukemia/lymphoma, *BCR::ABL1*-like (Ph-like ALL), 307
Public Health Service Act of 1944 (PHS Act), 960
Pyrogram, 32
Pyrosequencing, 32–33
- *BRAF* mutations, 119
- *JAK2* mutations, 55
- *KRAS* mutations, 117
- *MYD88* L265P mutation, 95

Q

Quality assurance and regulatory issues
- FDA regulations, 960–965
  - IVDs, 960–964
  - LTDs, 964–965
- federal agencies, and regulation of laboratories, 958–959
- proficiency testing and accreditation, 966–969
Quantitative real-time PCR
- *BCR::ABL1* fusion, 44
- *JAK2* mutations, 55
- *PML::RARA* fusion, 47

R

RAC1 (7p), non-HPV-related head and neck squamous cell carcinoma, 507
Radiation atypia, preneoplastic conditions, cervix/vulva/vagina vs., 732
Radiation exposure, mesothelioma, 577
RARA gene, normal function, 46
RARB (3p), non-HPV-related head and neck squamous cell carcinoma, 507
RAS-associated lymphoproliferative disease, juvenile myelomonocytic leukemia vs., 227
RASSF1 (3p), non-HPV-related head and neck squamous cell carcinoma, 507
RAS-type family mutations, 544
RB1 gene, 128
- non-HPV-related head and neck squamous cell carcinoma, 507
- retinoblastoma, 953
RBM15 gene, function, 263
RBM15::MRTFA (*MKL1*) rearrangement, abnormal function, 263

xlvii

INDEX

Reactive astrocytosis/gliosis, astrocytoma, IDH-mutant vs., 921
Reactive atypia, preneoplastic conditions, cervix/vulva/vagina vs., 732
Reactive condition, myeloproliferative neoplasm, unclassifiable vs., 162
Reactive disorders with cytologic dysplasia, pediatric myelodysplastic syndrome and refractory cytopenia of childhood vs., 212
Reactive (secondary) eosinophilia, chronic eosinophilic leukemia, NOS vs., 161
Reactive follicular hyperplasia, follicular lymphoma vs., 365
Reactive leukocytosis, myeloid proliferations associated with Down syndrome vs., 282
Reactive monocytosis, chronic myelomonocytic leukemia vs., 218
Reactive NK-cell proliferation, chronic lymphoproliferative disorder of NK cells vs., 398
Reactive panniculitis, subcutaneous panniculitis-like T-cell lymphoma vs., 430
Reactive periostitis, parosteal osteosarcoma vs., 814
Reactive polyclonal plasmacytosis, multiple myeloma (plasma cell myeloma) vs., 357
Reactive processes, pilocytic astrocytoma vs., 926
Reactive superficial epithelial changes, clear cell carcinoma, uterus vs., 752
Reactive thrombocytosis, essential thrombocythemia vs., 158
Real-time methylation-specific PCR, 39
- *MGMT* promoter gene methylation assay, 131
Real-time polymerase chain reaction (PCR), 28–29
- mutation-specific, *KRAS* mutations, 117
Refractory cytopenia of childhood (RCC), 208–213
- classification, 209
- cytogenetics, 210
- diagnostic checklist, 212
- differential diagnosis, 211–212
- prognosis, 210
Regressing atypical histiocytosis. *See* Primary cutaneous CD30-positive T-cell lymphoproliferative disorders.
Regulated analytes, 968
Renal cell carcinoma (RCC)
- adrenal cortical adenoma vs., 680
- adrenal cortical carcinoma vs., 669
- chromophobe, 634–635
    differential diagnosis, 635
    molecular genetics, 635
    prognosis, 635
- chromosomal microarray, 24
- clear cell, 630–633
    differential diagnosis, 632
    molecular genetics, 631–632
    prognosis, 631
    sporadic, 631
    VHL wildtype, 631
- EZH2 protein overexpression, 101
- papillary, 636–637
    clear cell, papillary renal cell carcinoma vs., 637
    differential diagnosis, 637

    prognosis, 637
    type 1, 637
    type 2, 637
    Wilms tumor vs., 645
- pheochromocytoma/paraganglioma vs., 663
- succinate dehydrogenase-deficient, oncocytoma vs., 651
- t(6;11), 638, 640
- *TFE3*-rearranged, 638–641
- *TFEB*-altered, 638–641
- Xp11 translocation, 639
Renal medullary carcinoma, nonmedullary, rhabdoid tumor of kidney vs., 653
Renal oncocytoma, chromophobe renal cell carcinoma vs., 635
Repeat expansion, 14
Repeated sequences, `15
Replication fork formation, 9
Respiratory epithelial adenomatoid hamartoma (REAH), sinonasal adenocarcinoma vs., 534
REST mutations, Wilms tumor, 645
Restriction endonuclease digestion, 39
Restriction site-generating polymerase chain reaction, 29
RET::CCDC6 fusion, 539
RET gene
- abnormal function, 108
- fusions, lung adenocarcinoma, 562
- mutations, 109
    germline, 109
    somatic, 109
- normal function, 108
RET rearrangements, 108–109
- targeted therapies, 109
Retiform hemangioendothelioma, 880, 892
Retinoblastoma, 952–955
- differential diagnoses, 952
- hereditary, 805
    osteosarcoma, 811
- molecular genetics, 953
- prognosis, 953
RET::NCOA4 fusion, 540
Reverse transcription polymerase chain reaction (RT-PCR), 28
- karyotype vs., 175
- lymphoid neoplasms, 296
- myeloid leukemia transcripts, 48–49
- *RET* fusion, 109
- *ROS1* fusion, 107
Reversible chain termination sequencing, 34
Revised International Prognostic Scoring System (IPSS-R), 100
- for myelodysplastic syndrome, 185, 186
RFLP analysis, applications of, 85
Rhabdoid predisposition syndrome, choroid plexus tumors, 945
Rhabdoid tumor
- atypical, choroid plexus tumors vs., 945
- atypical teratoid, medulloblastoma vs., 940
- extrarenal, 898, 899, 901, 902

INDEX

- kidney, 652–653
  - clear cell sarcoma of kidney vs., 649
  - diagnostic checklist, 652
  - differential diagnosis, 653
  - prognosis, 653
- soft tissue, 892
- Wilms tumor vs., 645

Rhabdomyosarcoma
- alveolar, 868, 870, 892
  - differential diagnosis, 872
  - genetic findings, 871
  - neuroblastoma vs., 676
- embryonal, 868, 870, 872, 892
  - differential diagnosis, 872
  - genetic findings, 871
  - malignant peripheral nerve sheath tumor vs., 888
- Ewing sarcoma vs., 821
- pleomorphic, 868, 870–871, 892
  - differential diagnosis, 872
  - genetic findings, 872
- sclerosing, 868, 870, 872
  - differential diagnosis, 872
  - genetic findings, 872
  - sclerosing epithelioid fibrosarcoma vs., 851
- spindle cell, 868, 870, 872
  - differential diagnosis, 872
  - genetic findings, 872
  - sclerosing epithelioid fibrosarcoma vs., 851
- uterine sarcomas, 756

RHOA G17V mutation, nodal follicular helper T-cell lymphoma, 450
Ribonucleic acid (RNA), 5
- types, 5–6, 9

Ribosomal RNA (rRNA), 6, 9
Ribosomes, 10
Ribozyme, 6
Ring chromosome, 19
RNA. See Ribonucleic acid.
RNA polymerases, 9
RNA splicing, 9

RNF43 mutations
- pancreatic intraductal papillary mucinous neoplasm, 621
- pancreatic mucinous cystic neoplasm, 619

ROS1 gene
- abnormal function, 106
- non-small cell lung cancer, 107
- other malignancies, 107
- point mutations, 107
- rearrangements, 106–107
- targeted therapy, 107
- testing, 107

ROS1 gene fusions, lung adenocarcinoma, 562
Rosai-Dorfman-Destombes disease, Langerhans cell histiocytosis vs., 481
Rothmund-Thomson syndrome, osteosarcoma, 811

Round cell sarcomas
- with EWSR1::non-ETS fusions, 895
- malignant peripheral nerve sheath tumor vs., 888

Routine inspection, CAP, 967
Rowley, Janet, 18, 42

RPS14 gene, myelodysplastic syndrome with del(5q), 201
RT-PCR. See Reverse transcription polymerase chain reaction.
Rubinstein-Taybi syndrome, medulloblastoma, 939
RUNX1 mutations
- acute myeloid leukemia, 234
- chronic myelomonocytic leukemia, 217
- mastocytosis, 169
- myelodysplastic syndrome, NOS, 194
- myelodysplastic/myeloproliferative neoplasm, NOS, 229
- T-lymphoblastic leukemia/lymphoma, 312

RUNX1::RUNX1T1 fusion, 48, 241

S

Salivary duct carcinoma (SDC)
- differential diagnosis, 521
- molecular genetics, 520
- mucoepidermoid carcinoma vs., 512
- prognosis, 519

Salivary gland carcinoma, lymphoepithelioma-like, 89
Salivary gland intraductal carcinoma, RET fusion genes, 109
Sanger, Frederick, 32
Sanger sequencing, 32
- EGFR gene alterations, 121
- JAK2 mutations, 55
- KRAS mutations, 117
- MYD88 L265P mutation, 95
- NOTCH1 mutation, 97

Sarcoma
- alveolar soft part, 898, 899, 900, 902
- epithelioid, 898, 899, 900, 902
  - sclerosing epithelioid fibrosarcoma vs., 851
- Ewing-like, Ewing sarcoma vs., 821
- follicular dendritic cell, 488–491
  - cytogenetics, 489
  - differential diagnosis, 490
  - molecular genetics, 489
  - prognosis, 489
- intimal, 898, 899, 901, 902
- lung squamous cell carcinoma vs., 570
- mesothelioma vs., 578
- muscle, 868–877
  - differential diagnosis, 872
- small round blue cell, 824–831
  - differential diagnosis, 827
  - mesenchymal chondrosarcoma vs., 842
  - molecular genetics, 826
- synovial, 872, 898, 899–900, 902
- of uncertain differentiation with specific molecular alterations, 898–907, 908–915

Sarcoma-like tumor, clear cell, of GI tract, gastrointestinal stromal tumor vs., 594
Sarcomatoid melanoma, malignant peripheral nerve sheath tumor vs., 888
Satellites, 5
Scar, exuberant, desmoid fibromatosis vs., 851

INDEX

SCC. *See* Squamous cell carcinoma.
Schinzel-Giedion syndrome, **63**
Schwannian stroma-poor neuroblastic tumor. *See* Neuroblastoma.
Schwannoma, **892**
- cellular, malignant peripheral nerve sheath tumor vs., **888**
- ependymal tumors vs., **934**
- gastrointestinal stromal tumor vs., **594**
- meningioma vs., **950**
Schwartz, David, **18**
Sclerosing basal cell carcinoma, **798**
Sclerosing epithelioid fibrosarcoma, **849, 851, 852, 892**
- differential diagnosis, **851**
Sclerosing microcystic adenocarcinoma, microsecretory adenocarcinoma vs., **521**
Sclerosing polycystic adenosis, intraductal carcinoma vs., **521**
Sclerosing rhabdomyosarcoma, **868, 870, 892**
- differential diagnosis, **872**
- genetic findings, **872**
- sclerosing epithelioid fibrosarcoma vs., **851**
Sclerosing stromal tumor, **777**
- cytogenetics, **776**
- molecular genetics, **777**
Scorpion primers, **28**
SDHA gene, pheochromocytoma/paraganglioma, **663**
SDH-deficient GIST, **592, 593**
SDRPL. *See* Splenic diffuse red pulp small B-cell lymphoma.
Sebaceoma, **801**
Sebaceous adenoma (SA), **801**
Sebaceous carcinoma (SC), **801**
- basal cell carcinoma of skin vs., **798**
Sebaceous tumors, **800–801**
- genetics, **801**
- molecular genetics, **801**
- prognosis, **801**
Secondary polycythemia, polycythemia vera vs., **150**
Secretory carcinoma, **509**
- acinic cell carcinoma vs., **512**
- clinicopathologic features, **513**
- differential diagnosis, **512**
- intraductal carcinoma vs., **521**
- microsecretory adenocarcinoma vs., **521**
- molecular alterations, **513**
- molecular genetics, **511**
- prognosis, **510**
- in situ hybridization, **510**
Self-inspection, CAP, **967**
Semiautomated Sanger sequencing, **32**
Seminoma, **625, 627**
Sequence-specific fluorescent labeled probes, **28**
Sequencing
- *CSF3R* mutations, **61**
- *SETBP1* mutations, **63**
Sequencing technologies, **32–35**
- massively parallel next-generation sequencing, **33–34**
- next-generation sequencing, **33, 34**
- pyrosequencing, **32–33**
- representative examples, **34**
- Sanger sequencing, **32**

- 3rd-generation sequencing, **34**
Seromucinous borderline tumor, **771**
Seromucinous tumors, **769**
Serous borderline tumor (SBT), **763**
- molecular carcinogenesis, **764**
- prognosis, **763**
Serous carcinoma, **763, 764**
- actionable genomic alterations, **765**
Serous cystadenoma
- pancreatic intraductal papillary mucinous neoplasm vs., **621**
- pancreatic mucinous cystic neoplasm vs., **619**
Serous tumors of ovary and fallopian tube, **762–767**
- differential diagnosis, **765**
- prognosis, **763**
Serrated polyposis syndrome, colorectal adenocarcinoma and precancerous lesions, **585**
Sertoli cell tumor, **775, 777, 778**
Sertoli-Leydig cell tumor, **775, 777, 778**
- prognosis, **776**
Sessile serrated adenoma, colorectal adenocarcinoma and precancerous lesions, **585**
SET protein, **62**
SETBP1 mutations, **62–63**
- atypical chronic myeloid leukemia, **221**
- chronic myelomonocytic leukemia, **217**
- myelodysplastic/myeloproliferative neoplasm, NOS, **230**
SETBP1 protein, **62**
Severe congenital neutropenia, **61**
- acute myeloid leukemia, **233**
Sex cord-stromal tumors of ovary, **774–779**
- cytogenetics, **776**
- differential diagnosis, **778**
- molecular genetics, **776–777**
- prognosis, **776**
Sex cord tumors
- with annular tubules, **775, 778**
    molecular genetics, **777**
    prognosis, **776**
- NOS, **775, 778**
Sézary syndrome, **432–437**
- chronic lymphoproliferative disorder of NK cells vs., **398**
- differential diagnosis, **435**
- molecular genetics, **434**
- prognosis, **434**
SF3B1 mutations
- chronic myelomonocytic leukemia, **217**
- myelodysplastic syndrome with, **188–191**
    cytogenetics, **190**
    differential diagnosis, **190**
    molecular genetics, **190**
    prognosis, **190**
- small lymphocytic lymphoma/chronic lymphocytic leukemia, **320**
Shaw, Margery Wayne, **18**
Shwachman-Diamond syndrome
- acute myeloid leukemia, **233**
- myelodysplastic syndrome, NOS vs., **195**
Sideroblastic anemia
- acquired, myelodysplastic syndrome with mutated *SF3B1* vs., **190**

INDEX

- congenital, myelodysplastic syndrome with mutated *SF3B1* vs., **190**
- VEXAS syndrome vs., **180**

Signal amplification hybridization, squamous cell carcinoma, cervix/vulva/vagina, **736**

Signet ring stromal tumor, **777**

Silencer, **9**

Single nucleotide polymorphism chromosomal microarray, **23**
- aberrations detected, **23**
- T-cell prolymphocytic leukemia, **395**

Single-molecule real-time (SMRT) sequencing, **34**

Single-probe ISH assay, *ERBB2* (HER2) gene amplifications, **115**

Sinonasal adenocarcinoma (SNAC), **531**
- cytogenetics, **532**
- differential diagnosis, **534**
- molecular genetics, **532**
- prognosis, **531–532**

Sinonasal mucosal melanoma (SMM), **531**
- cytogenetics, **532**
- differential diagnosis, **534**
- molecular genetics, **532**
- prognosis, **532**

Sinonasal sarcoma, biphenotypic, **892**

Sinonasal undifferentiated carcinoma (SNUC), **531**
- cytogenetics, **532**
- differential diagnosis, **534**
- head and neck mucosal squamous cell carcinoma, non-HPV related vs., **503**
- HPV-positive poorly differentiated neuroendocrine carcinoma vs., **497**
- molecular genetics, **532**
- NUT (midline) carcinoma, **534**
- prognosis, **531**

SIX1 mutations, Wilms tumor, **645**

SIX2 mutations, Wilms tumor, **645**

Skin, squamous cell carcinoma, **792–795**
- cytogenetics, **793**
- diagnostic checklist, **794**
- differential diagnosis, **794**
- molecular genetics, **793**
- prognosis, **793**

Skin cancer, EZH2 protein overexpression, **101**

SLE panniculitis, subcutaneous panniculitis-like T-cell lymphoma vs., **430**

SLL. *See* Small lymphocytic lymphoma.

SMAD4 gene, **128–129**

SMAD4 mutations
- pancreatic ductal adenocarcinoma, **615–616**
- pancreatic mucinous cystic neoplasm, **619**

Small B-cell lymphoma, splenic diffuse red pulp
- hairy cell leukemia vs., **334**
- molecular findings, **330**
- splenic B-cell lymphoma/leukemia, unclassifiable, **337**
- splenic marginal zone lymphoma vs., **328–329**

Small B-cell neoplasms, *MYD88* L265P mutations, **348**

Small cell carcinoma
- lung squamous cell carcinoma vs., **570**
- medulloblastoma vs., **940**
- sex cord-stromal tumors of ovary vs., **778**

Small cell neuroendocrine carcinoma, **572–575**
- cytogenetics, **573**
- differential diagnosis, **574**
- genetic testing, **574**
- molecular genetics, **574**
- prognosis, **573**

Small cell osteosarcoma, **810, 811, 813, 814**
- differential diagnosis, **814**
- Ewing sarcoma vs., **821**

Small lymphocytic lymphoma (SLL), **316–321**
- B-cell prolymphocytic leukemia vs., **324**
- cytogenetics, **318–319**
- differential diagnosis, **320**
- genetic testing, **319**
- mantle cell lymphoma vs., **373**
- *MYD88* L265P mutations, **348**
- *NOTCH1* mutation, **97**
- prognosis, **318**
- somatic mutations, **319–320**
- splenic B-cell lymphoma/leukemia, unclassifiable vs., **338**
- splenic marginal zone lymphoma vs., **329**

Small round blue cell sarcomas, **824–831**
- differential diagnosis, **827**
- mesenchymal chondrosarcoma vs., **842**
- molecular genetics, **826**

Small round blue cell tumors, Wilms tumor vs., **645**

Small round cell sarcomas
- high-grade myxoid liposarcoma vs., **862**
- sarcoma with *BCOR* genetic alterations vs., **827**
- small cell osteosarcoma vs., **814**

Small round cell tumor, desmoplastic, **824, 892**
- differential diagnosis, **827**
- Ewing sarcoma vs., **821**
- molecular genetics, **826**
- neuroblastoma vs., **676**

SMARCA4-deficient thoracic sarcoma, **892**

SMARCB1 gene, **129**
- rhabdoid tumor of kidney, **653**

SMARCB1-deficient sinonasal carcinoma (SMARCB1-defSNC), **531**
- cytogenetics, **532**
- differential diagnosis, **534**
- molecular genetics, **532**
- prognosis, **531**

SMARCE1 mutation, meningioma, **950**

SMO gene, **129**
- meningioma, **949**

Smoldering systemic mastocytosis, **168**

Smooth muscle tumor of uncertain malignant potential (STUMP), leiomyosarcoma vs., **756**

Smooth muscle tumors
- EBV-associated, AIDS patients, **88**
- inflamed, inflammatory myofibroblastic tumor vs., **851**

SMZL. *See* Splenic marginal zone lymphoma.

SOCS1 deletions, mycosis fungoides/Sézary syndrome, **434**

Soft tissue angiofibroma, **892**

Soft tissue sarcomas
- clear cell sarcoma of, **898, 899, 900–901, 902**
- genetics, of uncertain differentiation, **902, 911**

INDEX

- primary or metastatic, metaplastic breast carcinoma vs., **713**

Soft tissue tumors
- EZH2 protein overexpression, **101**
- molecular pathology, **804–809**
    - diagnostic steps, **806**
    - genetic alterations, **807**
    - molecular genetics, **807**
- recently described provisional bone, with specific genetic findings, **897**
- representative genetic findings, **892–897**

Solid pseudopapillary neoplasm, pancreatic mucinous cystic neoplasm vs., **619**

Solid tumors, molecular pathology of
- adenocarcinoma, cervix/vulva/vagina, **738–741**
- ADH and DCIS (dysplastic, premalignant), **688–693**
- adrenal cortical adenoma, **680–683**
- adrenal cortical carcinoma, **666–671**
- anaplastic thyroid carcinoma, **550–553**
- astrocytoma, IDH-mutant, **920–923**
- basal cell carcinoma, skin, **796–799**
- basal-like and triple-negative breast carcinomas, **720–729**
- bone and soft tissue tumors, **804–809**
- β-catenin-activated hepatocellular adenoma, **602–605**
- cholangiocarcinoma, **622–623**
- choroid plexus tumors, **944–947**
- chromophobe renal cell carcinoma, **634–635**
- clear cell carcinoma, uterus, **750–753**
- clear cell renal cell carcinoma, **630–633**
- clear cell sarcoma of kidney, **648–649**
- colorectal adenocarcinoma, precancerous lesions, **584–589**
- dermatofibroma, **802–803**
- dermatofibrosarcoma protuberans, **802–803**
- ductal carcinomas, **694–699**
- endometrial intraepithelial neoplasia, **742–743**
- ependymal tumors, **932–937**
- Ewing sarcoma, **818–823**
- follicular thyroid carcinoma, **542–545**
- gastric adenocarcinoma, **580–583**
- gastrointestinal stromal tumor, **590–597**
- germ cell tumor, ovary, **780–783**
- giant cell tumor of bone, **832–837**
- glioblastoma, IDH wildtype, **916–919**
- head and neck mucosal squamous cell carcinoma, non-HPV related, **500–505**
- head and neck tumors, **530–537**
- hepatocellular carcinoma, **610–613**
- *HNF1A*-inactivated hepatocellular adenoma, **598–601**
- HPV-associated head and neck carcinomas, **494–499**
- inflammatory hepatocellular adenoma, **606–609**
- intermediate and malignant cartilaginous tumors of bone, **838–847**
- intermediate and malignant myofibroblastic/fibroblastic tumors, **848–857**
- intermediate and malignant vascular tumors, **878–885**
- invasive ductal carcinoma of no special type with medullary features, **706–709**
- liposarcomas, **858–867**
- lobular carcinoma, **700–705**
- lung adenocarcinoma, **560–567**
- malignant peripheral nerve sheath tumor, **886–891**
- medullary thyroid carcinoma, **554–559**
- medulloblastoma, **938–943**
- melanoma, **788–791**
- meningioma, **948–951**
- mesothelioma, **576–579**
- metaplastic breast carcinoma, **710–715**
- muscle sarcomas, **868–877**
- nasopharyngeal EBV-related squamous cell carcinoma, **526–529**
- neuroblastoma, **672–679**
- non-HPV-related head and neck squamous cell carcinoma, **506–507**
- oligodendroglioma, IDH mutant, 1p/19q codeleted, **928–931**
- oncocytoma, **650–651**
- osteosarcomas, **810–817**
- pancreatic ductal adenocarcinoma, **614–617**
- pancreatic intraductal papillary mucinous neoplasm, **620–621**
- pancreatic mucinous cystic neoplasm, **618–619**
- papillary renal cell carcinoma, **636–637**
- papillary thyroid carcinoma, **538–541**
- pheochromocytoma/paraganglioma, **660–665**
- phyllodes tumors, **716–719**
- pilocytic astrocytoma, **924–927**
- poorly differentiated thyroid carcinoma, **546–549**
- premalignant conditions, skin, **784–787**
- preneoplastic conditions, cervix/vulva/vagina, **730–733**
- prostatic adenocarcinoma, acinar type and high-grade prostatic intraepithelial neoplasia, **684–687**
- rare sarcomas of uncertain differentiation with specific molecular alterations, **898–907, 908–915**
- representative genetic findings in bone and soft tissue tumors, **892–897**
- retinoblastoma, **952–955**
- rhabdoid tumor of kidney, **652–653**
- sebaceous tumors, **800–801**
- serous tumors of ovary and fallopian tube, **762–767**
- sex cord-stromal tumors of ovary, **774–779**
- small cell neuroendocrine carcinoma, **572–575**
- small round blue cell sarcomas, **824–831**
- squamous cell carcinoma
    - cervix/vulva/vagina, **734–737**
    - lung, **568–571**
    - skin, **792–795**
- surface epithelial tumors of ovary, **768–773**
- testicular germ cell tumors, **624–629**
- *TFE3*-rearranged and *TFEB*-altered renal cell carcinomas, **638–641**
- translocation-specific salivary gland tumors, **508–517, 518–525**
- urothelial carcinoma, **654–659**
- uterine endometrioid carcinoma, **744–747**
- uterine sarcomas, **754–761**
- uterine serous carcinoma, **748–749**
- Wilms tumor, **642–647**

INDEX

Solitary fibrous tumor, **848–849, 850, 852, 892**
- differential diagnosis, **851**

Solitary fibrous tumor-hemangiopericytoma spectrum, meningioma vs., **950**

Somatic *CSF3R* mutations, in severe congenital neutropenia, chronic neutrophilic leukemia vs., **146**

Somatic hypermutation, detection, **296–297**

Somatic missense mutations, *BRAF*, **118**

Somatic mutations, **13**
- *KRAS* gene, **116**

Somatic *RET* mutations, **109**

Southern blot analysis, antigen receptor genes, **84–85**
- DNA digestion, **84**
- DNA hybridization, **85**
- DNA preparation, **84**
- DNA stabilization, **85**
- DNA transfer onto nylon or nitrocellulose membrane, **85**
- gel electrophoresis, **85**
- interpretation, **85**
- vs. PCR, in assessment of clonality in lymphoid proliferations, **85**

Southern blot hybridization
- *IGH* gene rearrangements, **74**
- *TRB* gene rearrangement, **81–82**

SPARC (5q), non-HPV-related head and neck squamous cell carcinoma, **507**

Spermatocytic tumor, testicular germ cell tumors, **624, 625, 627**

Spinal ependymoma
- ependymal tumors, **934**
- *MYCN*-amplified, ependymal tumors, **934**

Spindle cell carcinoma, **713**
- metaplastic, phyllodes tumors vs., **718**

Spindle cell lipoma, **892**
- atypical lipomatous tumor vs., **862**
- differential diagnosis, **862**
- spindle cell liposarcoma vs., **862**

Spindle cell liposarcoma, differential diagnosis, **862**

Spindle cell melanoma
- leiomyosarcoma vs., **872**
- malignant peripheral nerve sheath tumor vs., **888**

Spindle cell rhabdomyosarcoma, **868, 870**
- biphenotypic sinonasal sarcoma vs., **534**
- of bone, **895**
- differential diagnosis, **872**
- genetic findings, **872**
- sclerosing epithelioid fibrosarcoma vs., **851**

Spindle cell sarcomas, *BCOR-CCNB3* sarcoma vs., **827**

Spindle cell tumors, **897**

Spindle epithelial tumor, with thymus-like differentiation, anaplastic thyroid carcinoma vs., **552**

Spitz nevi
- atypical, melanoma vs., **790**
- melanoma vs., **790**

Splenic B-cell lymphoma/leukemia
- prominent nucleoli
    molecular findings, **330**
    splenic marginal zone lymphoma vs., **329**
- unclassifiable, **336–343**
    cytogenetics, **337**
    differential diagnosis, **338**
    prognosis, **337**

Splenic B-cell marginal zone lymphoma. *See* Splenic marginal zone lymphoma.

Splenic diffuse red pulp small B-cell lymphoma (SDRPL)
- hairy cell leukemia vs., **334**
- molecular findings, **330**
- splenic B-cell lymphoma/leukemia, unclassifiable, **337**
- splenic marginal zone lymphoma vs., **328–329**

Splenic follicular hyperplasia, splenic marginal zone lymphoma vs., **329**

Splenic lymphoma with circulating villous lymphocytes. *See* Splenic marginal zone lymphoma.

Splenic lymphoma with villous lymphocytes. *See* Splenic B-cell lymphoma/leukemia, unclassifiable.

Splenic marginal zone lymphoma (SMZL), **326–331**
- B-cell prolymphocytic leukemia vs., **324**
- diagnostic checklist, **330**
- differential diagnosis, **328–330**
- hairy cell leukemia vs., **334**
- immunohistochemistry, **330**
- molecular changes, **330**
- molecular findings, **330**
- molecular genetics, **327–328**
- prognosis, **327**
- splenic B-cell lymphoma/leukemia, unclassifiable vs., **338**

Splenomegaly, myelodysplastic/myeloproliferative neoplasm, NOS, **229**

Sporadic aniridia, Wilms tumor, **644**

Sporadic essential thrombocythemia, essential thrombocythemia, **157**

Sporadic medullary thyroid carcinoma, **555**

Sporadic neuroblastoma, *ALK* alterations, **105**

Sporadic polyps, colorectal adenocarcinoma and precancerous lesions, **585**

Sporadic tumors, choroid plexus tumors, **945**

SPTCL. *See* Subcutaneous panniculitis-like T-cell lymphoma.

Squamous cell carcinoma (SCC)
- basal cell carcinoma of skin vs., **798**
- basaloid/small cell variant, small cell neuroendocrine carcinoma vs., **574**
- cervix/vulva/vagina, **734–737**
    cytogenetics, **736**
    differential diagnosis, **736**
    prognosis, **735–736**
- high-grade, olfactory neuroblastoma vs., **534**
- invasive, actinic keratosis vs., **786**
- lung, **568–571**
    diagnostic checklist, **570**
    differential diagnosis, **570**
    grading, **570**
    molecular genetics, **569**
    prognosis, **569**
- metaplastic breast carcinoma, **713**
- metastatic, metaplastic breast carcinoma vs., **713**
- in situ, actinic keratosis vs., **786**

INDEX

- skin, **792–795**
    - cytogenetics, **793**
    - diagnostic checklist, **794**
    - differential diagnosis, **794**
    - molecular genetics, **793**
    - prognosis, **793**
SRC gene, **129**
SRGAP3::RAF1 fusion gene, pilocytic astrocytoma, **926**
SRSF2 mutations
- chronic myelomonocytic leukemia, **217**
- mastocytosis, **169**
- myelodysplastic/myeloproliferative neoplasm, NOS, **230**
- polycythemia vera, **150**
SSBP2::JAK2 fusion, **55**
STAT3 activation, mycosis fungoides/Sézary syndrome, **434**
Steroid cell tumors, **775, 777, 778**
- prognosis, **776**
STK11 gene, **129**
STRN3::JAK2 fusion, **55**
Subcutaneous panniculitis-like T-cell lymphoma (SPTCL), **428–431**
- cytogenetics, **429**
- differential diagnosis, **430**
- extranodal NK-/T-cell lymphoma vs., **408**
- molecular genetics, **429–430**
- prognosis, **429**
Subependymoma, ependymal tumors, **933, 934**
Substitution, **15**
Succinate dehydrogenase-deficient renal cell carcinoma, oncocytoma vs., **651**
Superficial CD34-positive fibroblastic tumor, **892**
Superficial fibromatosis, desmoid fibromatosis vs., **851**
Superficial multicentric basal cell carcinoma, **797**
Superficial spreading melanoma, **789, 790**
Supratentorial ependymoma
- NOS, ependymal tumors, **933**
- *YAP1* fusion positive, ependymal tumors, **933**
- *ZFTA* fusion positive, ependymal tumors, **933**
Surface epithelial tumors of ovary, **768–773**
- differential diagnosis, **772**
- prognosis, **770**
- WHO classification, **769**
Sutton, Walter, **18**
Syndromic association, medullary thyroid carcinoma, **555**
Synovial sarcoma, **892, 898, 899–900, 902**
- biphasic, desmoplastic small round cell tumor vs., **827**
- leiomyosarcoma vs., **872**
- mesothelioma vs., **578**
- monophasic/poorly differentiated, malignant peripheral nerve sheath tumor vs., **888**
- poorly differentiated, Ewing sarcoma vs., **821**
- round cell sarcoma with *EWSR1::*non-ETS fusions vs., **827**
- solitary fibrous tumor vs., **851**
Syringotropic MF, mycosis fungoides/Sézary syndrome, **435**
Systemic infections, multiple myeloma (plasma cell myeloma) vs., **357**

Systemic lupus erythematosus, pediatric myelodysplastic syndrome and refractory cytopenia of childhood vs., **212**
Systemic mastocytosis, **168**
- acute myeloid leukemia with t(8;21)/*RUNX1::RUNX1T1*, **242**
- with associated hematologic neoplasm, **168**
- chronic myelomonocytic leukemia vs., **218**
- diagnostic criteria, **167–168**
- *KIT* mutations, **65, 66**

T

t(3;3)/*GATA2; MECOM*, acute myeloid leukemia with inv(3), **260–261**
- differential diagnosis, **261**
- molecular genetics, **261**
- prognosis, **261**
t(6;9)/*DEK::NUP214*
- acute myeloid leukemia with, **258–259**
    - differential diagnosis, **259**
    - genetic testing, **259**
    - prognosis, **259**
t(6;11) renal cell carcinoma, **638, 640**
t(9;11)/*MLLT3::KMT2A*, acute myeloid leukemia with, **254–257**
- cytogenetics, **256**
- differential diagnosis, **256**
- genetic testing, **256**
- prognosis, **256**
t(9;22)(q34.1;q11.2), **43**
t(15;17)(q24.1;q21.2), **46**
T-acute lymphoblastic leukemia (T-ALL), **310–315**
- antigen receptor gene rearrangements, **312**
- differential diagnosis, **313**
- gene expression signatures, **312–313**
- prognosis, **311–312**
- recurrent cytogenetic abnormalities, **312**
- somatic gene mutation, **312**
T-ALL. *See* T-acute lymphoblastic leukemia.
Tall cell and columnar cell variant, papillary thyroid carcinoma, **540**
TAM. *See* Transient abnormal myelopoiesis (TAM), Down syndrome.
Tanycytic ependymoma, ependymal tumors, **933**
TAP1 (6p), non-HPV-related head and neck squamous cell carcinoma, **507**
TAP2 (6p), non-HPV-related head and neck squamous cell carcinoma, **507**
TAPBP (6p), non-HPV-related head and neck squamous cell carcinoma, **507**
TaqMan probes, **28**
Targetable kinase gene fusions, B-lymphoblastic leukemia/lymphoma, *BCR::ABL1*-like (Ph-like ALL), **308**
Targeted hotspot gene panel table, **124–129**
Targeted sequencing, **34**
- *EZH2* mutation, **99**
T-cell development, **80–81**

INDEX

T-cell differentiation
- antigen-dependent, **80–81**
- antigen-independent, **80**

T-cell large granular lymphocytic (T-LGL) leukemia
- aggressive NK-cell leukemia vs., **402**
- chronic lymphoproliferative disorder of NK cells vs., **398**
- hepatosplenic T-cell lymphoma vs., **426**

T-cell leukemia, **300**
- testing methods for, **297**

T-cell lymphoma, **300**
- adult, **410–415**
    - cytogenetics, **411**
    - diagnostic checklist, **412**
    - differential diagnosis, **412**
    - molecular genetics, **411–412**
    - prognosis, **411**
- angioimmunoblastic
    - *IDH1* and *IDH2* mutations, **69**
    - peripheral T-cell lymphoma, not otherwise specified vs., **445**
- chronic eosinophilic leukemia, NOS vs., **161**
- enteropathy-associated, **416–423, 446**
- epidermotropic, atypical lymphoid infiltrates vs., **786**
- hepatosplenic, **424–427, 446**
    - chronic immunosuppression, **425**
    - cytogenetics, **425**
    - differential diagnosis, **426**
    - peripheral T-cell lymphoma, not otherwise specified vs., **446**
    - prognosis, **425**
- intestinal, **416–423**
    - cytogenetics, **420**
    - diagnostic checklist, **421**
    - differential diagnosis, **421**
    - monomorphic epitheliotropic intestinal T-cell lymphoma, **417**
    - prognosis, **420**
- molecular findings, **446**
- peripheral
    - adult T-cell leukemia/lymphoma vs., **412**
    - with associated B-cell proliferation, **445**
    - involving aerodigestive tract, extranodal NK-/T-cell lymphoma vs., **408**
    - not otherwise specified, **442–447**
- primary cutaneous γδ, subcutaneous panniculitis-like T-cell lymphoma vs., **430**
- subcutaneous panniculitis-like, **428–431**
    - cytogenetics, **429**
    - differential diagnosis, **430**
    - molecular genetics, **429–430**
    - prognosis, **429**

T-cell lymphoproliferative disorders, primary cutaneous CD30-positive, **438–441**
- molecular alterations, **439–440**
- prognosis, **439**

T-cell prolymphocytic leukemia (T-PLL), **394–397**
- cytogenetics, **395**
- differential diagnosis, **394**
- hepatosplenic T-cell lymphoma vs., **426**
- molecular genetics, **395**
- prognosis, **395**

- testing methods, **297**

T-cell receptor (TCR), structure, **76**

T-cell receptor beta (*TRB*) chain gene rearrangements, **80–83**

T-cell receptor delta (*TRD*) chain, gene arrangements, **76–79**

T-cell receptor gamma (*TRG*) chain, gene arrangements, **76–79**

T-cell/histiocyte-rich large B-cell lymphoma
- nodal follicular helper T-cell lymphoma vs., **452**
- peripheral T-cell lymphoma, not otherwise specified vs., **446**

TCR Vβ analysis, by cytometry, **82**

Telangiectatic focal nodular hyperplasia (T-FNH). *See* Inflammatory hepatocellular adenoma.

Telangiectatic hepatic adenoma. *See* Inflammatory hepatocellular adenoma.

Telangiectatic osteosarcomas, **810, 811, 812, 813**
- differential diagnosis, **814**

Telomere, **5**

Tenosynovial giant cell tumor, diffuse or localized, **892**

Teratoid tumor, atypical, choroid plexus tumors vs., **945**

Teratoma, **624**
- germ cell tumor, ovary, **782**
    - immature, **782**
    - mature cystic, **782**
- postpubertal type, **625, 627**
- prepubertal type, **624**

TERT mutations
- clear cell carcinoma, uterus vs., **752**
- follicular thyroid carcinoma, **544**
- melanoma, **790**
- non-HPV-related head and neck squamous cell carcinoma, **507**
- poorly differentiated thyroid carcinoma, **547**

TERT promoter mutations
- meningioma, **950**
- papillary thyroid carcinoma, **539**

Test complexity, FDA, **929**

Testicular germ cell tumors, **624–629**
- chromosomal microarray, **626**
- cytogenetics, **626**
- epigenetics, **626**
- gene expression profiling, **626**
- microRNAs, **626**
- molecular genetics, **626**
- postpubertal males, **625**
- prepubertal males, **624**
- prognosis, **625**
- spermatocytic tumor, **626**

TET2 mutations
- acute myeloid leukemia, **234**
- acute myeloid leukemia, NOS, **273**
- chronic myelomonocytic leukemia, **217**
- mastocytosis, **169**
- myelodysplastic syndrome, NOS, **194**
- myelodysplastic/myeloproliferative neoplasm, NOS, **229**
- myeloproliferative neoplasm, unclassifiable, **163**
- nodal follicular helper T-cell lymphoma, **450**
- polycythemia vera, **150**

INDEX

TFE3-rearranged renal cell carcinoma, **638–641**
TFEB-altered renal cell carcinoma, **638–641**
TGFB1 (19q), non-HPV-related head and neck squamous cell carcinoma, **507**
Thecoma, **775, 777**
- prognosis, **776**

3' rule, **15**
3rd-generation sequencing, **34**
Thrombocythemia, essential
- polycythemia vera vs., **150**
- primary myelofibrosis vs., **154**

Thrombocytopenia
- myelodysplastic syndrome, NOS, **193**
- myelodysplastic syndrome with *TP53* multihit mutations vs., **205**
- pediatric myelodysplastic syndrome and refractory cytopenia of childhood vs., **209**

Thrombocytosis, myeloproliferative neoplasm, unclassifiable, **164**
Thrombopoietin receptor, *MPL* gene function, **56**
Thrombosis, deep vein, monoclonal gammopathy, of undetermined significance, **351**
Thyroid carcinoma
- anaplastic, **550–553**
    - differential diagnosis, **552**
    - molecular alterations, **551–552**
    - prognosis, **551**
- medullary, **554–559**
    - anaplastic thyroid carcinoma vs., **552**
    - ATA recommendations for management, **557**
    - ATA risk levels, **557**
    - differential diagnosis, **556–557**
    - distinguishing features between hereditary and sporadic, **557**
    - genotype-phenotype correlation, **557**
    - molecular genetics, **555–556**
    - poorly differentiated thyroid carcinoma vs., **548**
    - prognosis, **555**
    - sporadic, **555**
- poorly differentiated, **546–549**
    - differential diagnosis, **548**
    - molecular alterations, **547–548**
    - prognosis, **547**
- undifferentiated, poorly differentiated thyroid carcinoma vs., **548**

Tile 21 of Code of Federal Regulations (21 CFR), **960**
TIMP3 (22q), non-HPV-related head and neck squamous cell carcinoma, **507**
TIMP3 promoter hypermethylation, meningioma, **950**
Tjio, Joe Hin, **18**
T-large granular lymphocytic leukemia, **294**
- T-cell prolymphocytic leukemia vs., **394**

T-LBL. *See* T-lymphoblastic lymphoma.
T-lymphoblastic lymphoma (T-LBL), **292, 294, 310–315**
- antigen receptor gene rearrangements, **312**
- differential diagnosis, **313**
- *EZH2* mutation, **99**
- gene expression signatures, **312–313**
- prognosis, **311–312**
- recurrent cytogenetic abnormalities, **312**
- somatic gene mutation, **312**

TNFSF11 gene, giant cell tumor of bone, **834**
TOX mutation, mycosis fungoides/Sézary syndrome, **434**
TP53 gene, **129**
TP53 multihit mutations, myelodysplastic syndrome with, **204–205**
- classification, **205**
- diagnostic checklist, **205**
- differential diagnosis, **205**
- prognosis, **205**

TP53 mutations
- acute myeloid leukemia, **234**
- acute myeloid leukemia, NOS, **273**
- anaplastic thyroid carcinoma, **551**
- astrocytoma, IDH-mutant, **921**
- B-cell prolymphocytic leukemia, **323**
- choroid plexus tumors vs., **945**
- giant cell tumor of bone, **834**
- mycosis fungoides/Sézary syndrome, **434**
- non-HPV-related head and neck squamous cell carcinoma, **506**
- pancreatic ductal adenocarcinoma, **615**
- pancreatic intraductal papillary mucinous neoplasm, **621**
- pancreatic mucinous cystic neoplasm, **619**
- polycythemia vera, **150**
- poorly differentiated thyroid carcinoma, **548**
- small lymphocytic lymphoma/chronic lymphocytic leukemia, **319**
- uterine serous carcinoma, **749**
- Wilms tumor, **645**

TP63 rearrangements, primary cutaneous CD30-positive T-cell lymphoproliferative disorders, **439**
T-prolymphocytic leukemia, **294**
Traditional serrated adenoma, colorectal adenocarcinoma and precancerous lesions, **585**
TRAF7-mutated fibromyxoid spindle cell tumor, **897**
Transcription factors, **9**
Transfer RNA (tRNA), **6, 9, 10**
Transient abnormal myelopoiesis (TAM), Down syndrome, **281, 282**
Transient ischemic attacks, essential thrombocythemia, **157**
Transitional cell carcinoma. *See* Urothelial carcinoma.
Translocation, **14, 15, 19**
Translocation-specific salivary gland tumors, **508–517, 518–525**
- clinicopathologic features, **513**
- diagnostic checklist, **521**
- differential diagnosis, **512, 521**
- molecular alterations, **513**
- molecular genetics, **510–511, 519–520**
- prognosis, **509–510, 519**
- in situ hybridization, **510**

Transposition, **14**
TRB locus, **81**
T regulatory proteins (Tregs), decreased, subcutaneous panniculitis-like T-cell lymphoma, **429**
Trichoblastoma, basal cell carcinoma of skin vs., **798**
Trichoepithelioma, basal cell carcinoma of skin vs., **798**

INDEX

TRIM28 mutations, Wilms tumor, **645**
Triple-negative breast cancer, **720–729**
- diagnostic checklist, **725**
- differential diagnosis, **724–725**
- immune-enriched subtype, **725**
- luminal AR, **725**
- mesenchymal subtype, **725**
- prognosis, **722–723**

Triploidy, **6**
Trisomy, **6**
Trisomy 8
- acute myeloid leukemia with inv(16) or t(16;16)/*CBFB::MYH11*, **246**
- myelodysplastic/myeloproliferative neoplasm, NOS, **229**
- pediatric myelodysplastic syndrome and refractory cytopenia of childhood vs., **210**

Trisomy 21. *See* Down syndrome.
Trophoblastic tumors, **627**
Tubal metaplasia
- adenocarcinoma, cervix/vulva/vagina vs., **740**
- preneoplastic conditions, cervix/vulva/vagina vs., **732**

Tubular adenoma, colorectal adenocarcinoma and precancerous lesions, **585**
Tubulovillous adenoma, colorectal adenocarcinoma and precancerous lesions, **585**
Tumor suppressor genes, **12–13**
Tyrosine kinase gene fusions, molecular work-up, **135**

U

UBA1 germline mutations, VEXAS syndrome, **179**
UBA1 mutation, VEXAS syndrome, **179**
UBA1-acquired mutations, VEXAS syndrome, **179**
Underlying hematopoietic neoplasm, **233**
Undifferentiated carcinoma, **769, 771**
- germ cell tumor, ovary vs., **782**
- high-grade endometrial stromal sarcoma vs., **756**
- pancreatic ductal adenocarcinoma, **616**
- undifferentiated uterine sarcoma vs., **756**

Undifferentiated EBV-related nasopharyngeal carcinoma, head and neck mucosal squamous cell carcinoma, non-HPV related vs., **503**
Undifferentiated pleomorphic sarcoma, **892**
- dedifferentiated liposarcoma vs., **862**
- high-grade
    myxofibrosarcoma vs., **851**
    sclerosing epithelioid fibrosarcoma vs., **851**

Undifferentiated round cell sarcoma of infancy, **897**
Undifferentiated thyroid carcinoma (UTC), poorly differentiated thyroid carcinoma vs., **548**
Undifferentiated uterine sarcoma, **754**
- differential diagnosis, **756**

Uniparental disomy (UPD), **22**
United States Code (U.S.C.), **960**
UPD. *See* Uniparental disomy.
Urothelial carcinoma, **654–659**
- differential diagnosis, **657**
- with local extension, squamous cell carcinoma, cervix/vulva/vagina vs., **736**
- prognosis, **655**

U.S. Department of Health and Human Services, **958, 966**
- CLIA program, **964**

Uterine bleeding, uterine endometrioid carcinoma, **745**
Uterine endometrioid carcinoma, **744–747**
- Cancer Genome Atlas molecular subtypes, **745–746**
- genetic predisposition syndromes, **745**
- Lynch syndrome-associated, **745**
- MSI testing, **745**
- prognosis, **745**
- sporadic, **745**

Uterine leiomyosarcoma, **754**
- differential diagnosis, **756**
- genetic tests, **755**

Uterine sarcomas, **754–761**
- differential diagnosis, **756**
- genetics, **757**

Uterine serous carcinoma (USC), **748–749**
- Cancer Genome Atlas molecular classification, **749**
- differential diagnosis, **749**
- genetic predisposition, **749**
- prognosis, **749**
- recurrent genetic alterations, **749**

Uterine tumor resembling ovarian sex cord tumor (UTROSCT), **756**

V

Vagina
- adenocarcinoma, **738–741**
    differential diagnosis, **740**
    prognosis, **740**
- preneoplastic conditions, **730–733**
    differential diagnosis, **732**
    prognosis, **732**
- squamous cell carcinoma, **734–737**
    differential diagnosis, **736**
    prognosis, **735–736**

Vaginal bleeding, squamous cell carcinoma, cervix/vulva/vagina, **735**
Vaginal intraepithelial neoplasia (VaIN), preneoplastic conditions, cervix/vulva/vagina vs., **731**
Varicella infection, pediatric myelodysplastic syndrome and refractory cytopenia of childhood vs., **212**
Vascular occlusion, essential thrombocythemia, **157**
Vascular tumors, intermediate and malignant, **878–885**
- differential diagnosis, **881**
- genetic findings, **880–881**
- prognosis, **879**

VEGFA (6p), non-HPV-related head and neck squamous cell carcinoma, **507**
VEGFB (11q), non-HPV-related head and neck squamous cell carcinoma, **507**
VEXAS syndrome, **178–181**
- clonal hematopoiesis and premalignant clonal cytopenia, **183**

INDEX

- diagnostic checklist, 180
- differential diagnosis, 180
- myelodysplastic syndrome, NOS vs., 195
- prognosis, 179–180

VHL gene, 129
Viral hepatitis, 611
Viral infection, juvenile myelomonocytic leukemia vs., 227
Vitamin B12 deficiency
- myelodysplastic syndrome, NOS vs., 195
- pediatric myelodysplastic syndrome and refractory cytopenia of childhood vs., 212
- VEXAS syndrome vs., 180

von Hippel-Lindau (VHL) disease, 631
von Hippel-Lindau (VHL) syndrome, pheochromocytoma/paraganglioma, 662, 663
von Waldeyer-Hartz, Wilhelm, 18
Vulva
- adenocarcinoma, 738–741
    - differential diagnosis, 740
    - prognosis, 740
- preneoplastic conditions, 730–733
    - differential diagnosis, 732
    - prognosis, 732
- squamous cell carcinoma, 734–737
    - differential diagnosis, 736
    - prognosis, 735–736

Vulvar dermatoses, adenocarcinoma, cervix/vulva/vagina vs., 740
Vulvar intraepithelial neoplasia (VIN), preneoplastic conditions, cervix/vulva/vagina vs., 731

W

WAGR syndrome, Wilms tumor, 644
Waldenström macroglobulinemia
- molecular changes, 330
- *MYD88* L265P mutations, 348
- splenic marginal zone lymphoma vs., 329

Well-differentiated hepatocellular carcinoma (WDHCC)
- β-catenin-activated hepatocellular adenoma vs., 604
- *HNF1A*-inactivated hepatocellular adenoma vs., 600
- inflammatory hepatocellular adenoma vs., 608

Well-differentiated squamous cell carcinoma, lung squamous cell carcinoma, 570
Werner syndrome, 543
Whipple disease, gastric adenocarcinoma vs., 582
WHO Prognostic Scoring System (WPSS), myelodysplastic syndrome, 185
Whole genome sequencing (WGS), 33
Whole-exome amplification, 29
Whole-exome sequencing (WES), 34
- *CALR* mutations, 59
- *EZH2* mutation, 99

Whole-genome amplification, 29
Wilms tumor, 642–647
- blastema-predominant, clear cell sarcoma of kidney vs., 649
- differential diagnosis, 645
- genetic testing, 645
- metastatic, alveolar rhabdomyosarcoma vs., 872
- neuroblastoma vs., 676
- prognosis, 644

Windows-based software, NGS analysis, 37
Wiskott-Aldrich syndrome, juvenile myelomonocytic leukemia vs., 227
Woringer-Kolopp disease, mycosis fungoides/Sézary syndrome, 433
WPSS. *See* WHO Prognostic Scoring System.
WT1 gene, 129
WT1 mutations
- acute myeloid leukemia, 234
- Wilms tumor, 644

WT2 alterations, Wilms tumor, 644

X

Xanthoma, gastric, gastric adenocarcinoma vs., 582
Xeroderma pigmentosum, myelodysplastic syndrome, NOS vs., 195
Xp11 translocation carcinoma, melanotic, *TFE3*-rearranged and *TFEB*-altered renal cell carcinomas, 638, 639, 640
Xp11 translocation renal cell carcinomas, 639

Y

Yolk sac tumor
- germ cell tumor, ovary, 782
- postpubertal type, 627
- prepubertal type, 624
- sex cord-stromal tumors of ovary vs., 778
- testicular germ cell tumors, 625

Z

ZFTA::RELA-fused ependymoma, ependymal tumors, 933
Zinc deficiency, VEXAS syndrome vs., 180